COMPREHENSIVE
HYPERTENSION

COMPREHENSIVE HYPERTENSION

Gregory Y. H. Lip
M.D., F.R.C.P. (London, Edinburgh, Glasgow), F.E.S.C., F.A.C.C
Professor of Cardiovascular Medicine
Director, Haemostasis, Thrombosis, and Vascular Biology Unit
University Department of Medicine
City Hospital
Birmingham
United Kingdom

John E. Hall, Ph.D.
Arthur C. Guyton Professor and Chair
Department of Physiology and Biophysics
Associate Vice Chancellor for Research
University of Mississippi Medical Center
Jackson, Mississippi
USA

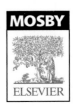

1600 John F. Kennedy Blvd.
Ste 1800
Philadelphia, PA 19103-2899

COMPREHENSIVE HYPERTENSION   ISBN-13: 978-0-323-03961-1

Copyright © 2007 by Mosby, Inc., an affiliate of Elsevier Inc.

Notice

Knowledge and best practice in this field are constantly changing. As new research and experience broaden our knowledge, changes in practice, treatment and drug therapy may become necessary or appropriate. Readers are advised to check the most current information provided (i) on procedures featured or (ii) by the manufacturer of each product to be administered, to verify the recommended dose or formula, the method and duration of administration, and contraindications. It is the responsibility of the practitioner, relying on their own experience and knowledge of the patient, to make diagnoses, to determine dosages and the best treatment for each individual patient, and to take all appropriate safety precautions. To the fullest extent of the law, neither the Publisher nor the Editors assumes any liability for any injury and/or damage to persons or property arising out of or related to any use of the material contained in this book.

Library of Congress Cataloging-in-Publication Data
Comprehensive hypertension / [edited by] Gregory Y.H. Lip, John E. Hall.
    p. cm.
  ISBN 0-323-03961-8
  1. Hypertension. I. Lip, Gregory Y. H. II. Hall, John E. (John Edward), 1946-

RC685.H8C585 2007
616.1'32—dc22   2006048136

Executive Publisher: Natasha Andjelkovic
Senior Developmental Editor: Ann Ruzycka Anderson
Project Manager: Bryan Hayward
Design Direction: Steven Stave

Working together to grow
libraries in developing countries

www.elsevier.com | www.bookaid.org | www.sabre.org

ELSEVIER   BOOK AID International   Sabre Foundation

Printed in China

Last digit is the print number: 9 8 7 6 5 4 3 2 1

CONTENTS

SECTION 4: PHARMACOLOGIC AND NONPHARMACOLOGIC INTERVENTIONS AND TREATMENT GUIDELINES, 947

Section Editors: Daniel W. Jones and Chim C. Lang

CONTRIBUTORS

Vineeta Ahooja, M.D.
Chief Cardiology Fellow
Department of Cardiology
Wayne State University
Detroit, MI
USA

Vamadevan S. Ajay, M.P.H.
Research Fellow
Cardiovascular Health Research
Centre for Chronic Disease Control
New Delhi
India

Laurence Amar, M.D.
Faculté de Médecine René Descartes
Department of Vascular Medicine and
Hypertension
Université René Descartes
Hôpital Européen George Pompidou
Department of Vascular Medicine and
Hypertension
Assistance Publique des Hôpitaux
de Paris
Paris
France

**Lawrence J. Appel, M.D.,
M.P.H.**
Professor of Medicine
Welch Center for Prevention
Epidemiology and Clinical Research
Division of General Internal Medicine
The John Hopkins University School
of Medicine
Baltimore, MD
USA

Michel Azizi, M.D., Ph.D.
Faculté de Médecine René Descartes
Clinical Investigation Center
Université René Descartes
Hôpital Européen George Pompidou
Clinical Investigation Center
Assistance Publique des Hôpitaux
de Paris
Paris
France

George L. Bakris, M.D., F.A.C.P.
Professor and Section Director
Hypertension/Clinical Research Center
Department of Preventive Medicine
Rush Medical College
Rush University Medical Center
Chicago, IL
USA

Lydia A. Bazzano, M.D., Ph.D.
Assistant Professor
Epidemiology and Medicine
Tulane University School of Public
Health and Tropical Medicine
New Orleans, LA
USA

D. Gareth Beevers, M.D., F.R.C.P.
Professor of Medicine
University Department of Medicine
City Hospital
Birmingham
UK

**Lawrence J. Beilin, A.O., M.D.,
F.R.A.C.P.**
Professor
School of Medicine and Pharmacology
University of Western Australia
Perth, Western Australia
Australia

Andrew D. Blann, Ph.D.
Senior Lecturer
University Department of Medicine
University of Birmingham
Consultant Clinical Scientist
University Department of Medicine
City Hospital
Birmingham
UK

Matthew A. Boegehold, Ph.D.
Director
Center for Interdisciplinary Research in
Physiology and Pharmacology
Professor
Department of Physiology and
Pharmacology
West Virginia University
Morgantown, WV
USA

George W. Booz, Ph.D., F.A.H.A.
Assistant Professor
Department of Medicine and Medical
Physiology
The Texas A&M University System
Health Science Center College of
Medicine
Assistant Professor
Division of Pulmonary and Critical
Care Medicine
Scott & White Hospital and Clinic
Research Physiologist (WOC)
The Central Texas Veterans Health
Care System
Division of Molecular Cardiology
The Cardiovascular Research Institute
Temple, TX
USA

**Branko Braam, M.D., Ph.D.,
F.A.S.N.**
Associate Professor
Division of Nephrology and
Immunology, Faculty of Medicine
University of Alberta Hospital
Internist/Nephrologist
Division of Nephrology and
Immunology, Faculty of Medicine
University of Alberta Hospital
Adjunct Assistant Professor of Physiology
Department of Physiology
University of Alberta
Edmonton, Alberta
Canada

Elizabeth L. Brandon, Ph.D.
Postdoctoral Fellow
Physiology and Biophysics
University of Mississippi Medical Center
Jackson, MS
USA

Michael W. Brands, Ph.D.
Professor
Department of Physiology
Medical College of Georgia
Augusta, GA
USA

Mark Britton, M.D., Ph.D.
Physician and Research Scientist
Divisions of General Internal Medicine
and Translational Research and Clinical
Epidemiology
Department of Internal Medicine
Wayne State University
Detroit, MI
USA

Hans R. Brunner, M.D.
Professor Emeritus
Lausanne University
Lausanne
Switzerland
Medizinische Poliklinik
Universitaetsspital
Basel
Switzerland

Beverley Burke, B.Sc.
Clinical Pharmacology
William Harvey Research Institute
Barts and the London School of
Medicine and Dentistry
London
UK

Valerie Burke, M.D., F.R.A.C.P.
School of Medicine and Pharmacology
University of Western Australia
Perth, Western Australia
Australia

Francesco P. Cappuccio, M.D., M.Sc., F.R.C.P., F.F.P.H.
Cephalon Professor
Cardiovascular Medicine and Epidemiology
Consultant Physician
Clinical Sciences Research Institute
Warwick Medical School
Coventry
UK

Robert M. Carey, M.D., M.A.C.P., F.A.H.A.
Harrison Distinguished Professor of Medicine
Department of Medicine
University of Virginia School of Medicine
Charlottesville, VA
USA

Barry L. Carter, Pharm.D., F.A.H.A., F.C.C.P.
Professor
Division of Clinical and Administrative Pharmacy
College of Pharmacy
University of Iowa
Professor
Department of Family Medicine
Roy. J. and Lucille A. Carver College of Medicine
Iowa City, IA
USA

Mark J. Caulfield, F.R.C.P.
Professor
Department of Clinical Pharmacology
William Harvey Research Institute
Barts and the London School of Medicine and Dentistry
London
UK

Yuqing Chen, M.D.
Postdoctoral Researcher
Department of Medicine and Pharmacology
University of California at San Diego
School of Medicine
La Jolla, CA
USA

Jay N. Cohn, M.D., F.A.A.C.
Professor of Medicine
Cardiovascular Division
Director
Rasmussen Center for Cardiovascular Disease Prevention
University of Minnesota Medical Center
Minneapolis, MN
USA

John M. C. Connell, M.D., F.R.C.P., FMed.Sci., F.R.S.E.
Professor of Endocrinology
BHF Glasgow Cardiovascular Research Centre, University of Glasgow
Consultant Endocrinologist
Western Infirmary
Glasgow
Scotland

Anthony Cox, B.Sc., MRPharmS, Clin Dip Pharm
Senior Pharmacovigilance Pharmacist
West Midlands Centre for Adverse Drug Reaction Reporting
Sandwell and West Birmingham Hospitals
NHS Trust
Birmingham
UK

Madhusudan Das, Ph.D.
Visiting Scholar
Department of Medicine and Pharmacology
University of California at San Diego
School of Medicine
La Jolla, CA
USA

Kevin P. Davy, Ph.D.
Associate Professor
Department of Human Nutrition, Foods and Exercise
Director
Human Integrative Physiology Laboratory
Virginia Polytechnic Institute and State University
Blacksburg, VA
USA

Cheryl R. Dennison, R.N., A.N.P., Ph.D.
Assistant Professor
School of Nursing
John Hopkins University
Baltimore, MD
USA

Shant Der Sarkissian, Ph.D.
Post Doctoral Research Associate
Department of Physiology and Functional Genomics
University of Florida
Gainesville, FL
USA

Javier Díez, M.D., Ph.D.
Professor of Vascular Medicine
Department of Medicine
School of Medicine
University of Navarra
Head
Area of Molecular Cardiology
Department of Cardiology and Cardiovascular Surgery
University Clinic of Navarra
Director
Division of Cardiovascular Sciences
Centre for Applied Medical Research
Pamplona
Spain

Peter A. Doris, Ph.D.
Associate Professor of Molecular Medicine
Institute of Molecular Medicine
University of Texas Health Science Center at Houston
Houston, TX
USA

Heather A. Drummond, Ph.D., F.A.H.A.
Assistant Professor
Physiology and Biophysics
University of Mississippi Medical Center
Jackson, MS
USA

Daniel A. Duprez, M.D., Ph.D., F.A.H.A., F.A.C.C., F.E.S.C.
Professor of Medicine
Cardiovascular Division
Medical School
University of Minnesota
Cardiologist
Cardiovascular Division
University Medical Center, Fairview
Director of Research
Rasmussen Center for Cardiovascular Disease Prevention
Cardiovascular Division
Medical School
University of Minnesota
Minneapolis, MN
USA

Fernando Elijovich, M.D., F.A.H.A.
Director
Division of General Internal Medicine
Medical Director
Center for Diagnostic Medicine
Department of Medicine
Scott and White Clinic
Texas A and M University
Temple, TX
USA

Henry L. Elliott, M.D., F.R.C.P.
Senior Lecturer in Medicine and Therapeutics
Division of Cardiovascular and Medical Sciences
University of Glasgow
Consultant Physician
Medicine and Therapeutics
Western Infirmary
Glasgow, Scotland
UK

William J. Elliott, M.D., Ph.D.
Professor of Preventive Medicine, Internal Medicine, and Pharmacology
Department of Preventive Medicine
RUSH Medical College of RUSH University
Attending Physician
Preventive Medicine, Internal Medicine
RUSH University Medical Center
Chicago, IL
USA

David J. Eveson, M.D., M.R.C.P.
Stroke Association Fellow
Cardiovascular Sciences
University Hospitals of Leicester
Leicester
UK

Gregory D. Fink, Ph.D., F.A.H.A.
Professor
Department of Pharmacology and Toxicology
Michigan State University
East Lansing, MI
USA

Nicola Fiotti, M.D.
Assistant Professor in Cardiovascular Diseases
Clinical, Morphological, and Technological Sciences
University of Trieste
Trieste
Italy

John M. Flack, M.D., M.P.H., F.A.H.A.
Professor and Interim Chairman and and Chief
Division of Translational Research and Clinical Epidemiology
Department of Internal Medicine
Wayne State University
Detroit, MI
USA

Joseph T. Flynn, M.D., M.S., F.A.A.P.
Professor of Clinical Pediatrics
Department of Pediatrics
Albert Einstein College of Medicine
Director
Pediatric Hypertension Program
Section of Pediatric Nephrology
Children's Hospital at Montefiore
Bronx, NY
USA

Pierre Foëx, D.M., D.Phil, F.R.C.A., F.Med.Sci.
Professor
Nuffield Department of Anaesthetics
University of Oxford
Honorary Consultant
Nuffield Department of Anaesthetics
The John Radcliffe Hospital
Oxford
UK

Lourdes A. Fortepiani, M.D., Ph.D.
Research Assistant Professor
Department of Physiology
University of Mississippi Medical Center
Jackson, MS
USA

Martin D. Fotherby, M.D., F.R.C.P.
Senior Lecturer
Department of Cardiovascular Sciences
Consultant
Department of Stroke Medicine
University Hospitals of Leicester
Leicester
UK

Fetnat Fouad-Tarazi, M.D.
Division of Cardiology
Department of Medicine
The Cleveland Clinic Foundation
Cleveland, OH
USA

Stanley S. Franklin, M.D., F.A.C.P., F.A.C.C.
Clinical Professor of Medicine
Department of Medicine
Associate Medical Director
UCI Heart Disease Prevention Program
University of California, Irvine
Irvine, CA
USA

Ryan Friese, M.S.
Graduate Student
Department of Bioengineering
University of California, San Diego
La Jolla, CA
USA

John W. Funder, A.O., M.D., Ph.D., F.R.A.C.P.
Professor
Medicine
Monash University
Clayton, Victoria
Professorial Associate
University of Melbourne
Parkville, Victoria
Professor
Institute of Molecular Biosciences
University of Queensland
St. Lucia, Queensland
Senior Fellow
Prince Henry's Institute of Medical Research
Clayton, Victoria
Australia

James J. Galligan, Ph.D., F.A.H.A.
Professor
Department of Pharmacology and Toxicology
Michigan State University
East Lansing, MI
USA

Jeffrey L. Garvin, Ph.D.
Professor
Department of Physiology
Wayne State University
Senior Staff Investigator
Division of Hypertension and Vascular Research
Henry Ford Hospital
Detroit, MI
USA

Christopher L. Gentile, M.S.
Research Associate
Department of Human Nutrition, Foods and Exercise
Virginia Polytechnic Institute and State University
Blacksburg, VA
USA

Jacob George, M.B.Ch.B., M.R.C.P.
Clinical Research Fellow
Department of Medicine and Therapeutics
School of Medicine
University of Dundee
Honorary Senior House Officer
Department of Medicine and Therapeutics
Ninewells Hospital and Medical School
Dundee, Scotland
UK

Lorenzo Ghiadoni, M.D.
Assistant Professor
Department of Internal Medicine
University of Pisa
Pisa
Italy

Carlo Giansante, M.D.
Associate Professor in Internal Medicine
Department of Clinical, Morphological, and Technological Sciences
University of Trieste
Trieste
Italy

Richard E. Gilbert, Ph.D., F.R.A.C.P., F.R.C.P.C.
Professor
Department of Medicine
University of Toronto
Professor
Division of Endocrinology and Metabolism
St. Michael's Hospital
Toronto, Ontario
Canada
Professor
Department of Medicine
University of Melbourne
Melbourne, Victoria
Australia

Sabas I. Gomez, M.D.
Research Fellow
Department of Physiology and Biomedical Engineering
Mayo Clinic
Rochester, MN
USA

Alan H. Gradman, M.D.
Professor
Department of Medicine
Temple University School of Medicine
Chief
Division of Cardiovascular Diseases
Western Pennsylvania Hospital
Pittsburgh, PA
USA

Joey P. Granger, Ph.D.
Department of Physiology and Biophysics
University of Mississippi Medical Center
Jackson, MS
USA

Guido Grassi, M.D.
Full Professor of Medicine
Clinica Medica
Università Milano-Bicocca
Monza
Full Professor of Medicine
Dipartimento di Medicina Clinica
Ospedale San Gerardo
Milan
Italy

**Philip Greenland, M.D.,
F.A.C.P., F.A.C.C., F.A.H.A.**
Harry W. Dingman Professor and
Chairman
Executive Associate Dean for Clinical
and Translational Research
Department of Preventive Medicine
Feinberg School of Medicine
Northwestern University
Chicago, IL
USA

Ehud Grossman, M.D.
Professor of Medicine
Sackler School of Medicine
Tel-Aviv University
Tel-Aviv
Head
Internal Medicine Department and
Hypertension Unit
The Chaim Sheba Medical Center
Tel-Hashomer
Israel

Johannie Gungadoo, B.Sc.
Department of Clinical Pharmacology
William Harvey Research Institute
Barts and the London School of
Medicine and Dentistry
London
UK

John A. Haas, B.S.
Associate in Research
Department of Physiology and
Biomedical Engineering
Mayo Clinic
Rochester, MN
USA

**Peter Y. Hahn, M.D., F.C.C.P.,
D.A.B.S.M.**
Assistant Professor of Medicine
Division of Pulmonary and Critical
Care Medicine
Mayo Clinic College of Medicine
Rochester, MN
USA

John E. Hall, Ph.D.
Arthur C. Guyton Professor and Chair
Department of Physiology and
Biophysics
Associate Vice Chancellor for Research
University of Mississippi Medical Center
Jackson, MS
USA

Bruce A. Hamilton, Ph.D.
Associate Professor
Department of Medicine
Associate Adjunct Professor
Cellular and Molecular Medicine
University of California
San Diego School of Medicine
La Jolla, CA
USA

Joseph R. Haywood, Ph.D.
Professor and Chairperson
Pharmacology and Toxicology
Michigan State University
East Lansing, MI
USA

Jiang He, M.D., D.M.S., Ph.D.
Professor and Chair
Department of Epidemiology
Tulane University School of Public
Health and Tropical Medicine
Clinical Professor of Medicine
Department of Medicine
Tulane University School of Medicine
New Orleans, LA
USA

Marcela Herrera, M.S.
Research Associate
Division of Hypertension and Vascular
Research
Henry Ford Hospital
Detroit, MI
USA

**Martha N. Hill, Ph.D., R.N.
F.A.A.N.**
Dean and Professor of Nursing
Office of the Dean
John Hopkins University
Baltimore, MD
USA

Radu Iliescu, M.D., Ph.D.
Instructor
Department of Physiology and
Biophysics
University of Mississippi Medical Center
Jackson, MS
USA

Chris Isles
Consultant Physician
Renal Unit
Dumfries and Galloway Royal Infirmary
Dumfries
UK

**Joseph L. Izzo, Jr., M.D.,
F.A.C.P., F.A.H.A.**
Professor
Medicine; Pharmacology and Toxicology
SUNY-Buffalo School of Medicine and
Biomedical Sciences
Clinical Director
Medicine
Erie County Medical Center
Buffalo, NY
USA

Rumi Jaumdally
Haemostasis, Thrombosis and Vascular
Biology Unit
University Department of Medicine
City Hospital
Birmingham
UK

Daniel W. Jones, M.D.
Vice Chancellor for Health Affairs
Dean
School of Medicine
University of Mississippi Medical
Center
Jackson, MS
USA

**Patricia M. Kearney,
M.B.B.Ch.B.A.O., M.R.C.P.I.,
M.P.H.**
Honorary Lecturer
Epidemiology and Public Health
University College Cork
Cork
Ireland
Clinical Research Fellow
CTSU
University of Oxford
Oxford
UK

Hein A. Koomans, M.D., Ph.D.
Professor and Chairman
Department of Nephrology and
Hypertension
University Medical Center Utrecht
Internist/Nephrologist
Department of Nephrology and
Hypertension
University Medical Center Utrecht
Utretch
The Netherlands

**Richard A. Krasuski, M.D.,
F.A.C.C.**
Associate Professor
Department of Medicine
Cleveland Clinic Lerner School
of Medicine
Director
Adult Congenital Heart Disease
Services
Cardiovascular Medicine
The Cleveland Clinic
Cleveland, OH
USA

**Henry Krum, Ph.D., F.R.A.C.P.,
F.C.S.A.N.Z.**
Professor
Epidemiology and Preventive Medicine
Monasu University
Alfred Hospital
Clinical Pharmacology
Director
NHMRC CCRE in Therapeutics
Monasu University
Melbourne, Victoria
Australia

Cheryl L. Laffer, M.D., Ph.D., F.A.H.A.
Department of Hypertension, Nephrology
Scott and White Clinic
Texas A and M University
Temple, TX
USA

Chim C. Lang, B.M.Sc., M.D., F.R.C.P.
Professor of Cardiology
Division of Medicine and Therapeutics
Ninewells Hospital and Medical
School
Honorary Consultant Cardiologist
Department of Cardiology
Tayside University Hospitals NHS Trust
Dundee
UK

Nigel J. Langford, M.D., M.R.C.P., M.R.Pharm.S.
Consultant Physician and Clinical
Pharmacologist
West Midlands Centre for Adverse Drug
Reaction Reporting
Sandwell and West Birmingham
Hospitals NHS Trust
Birmingham
UK

Debbie A. Lawlor, Ph.D., M.B., Ch.B.
Consultant Senior Lecturer in
Epidemiology
Department of Social Medicine
University of Bristol
Honorary Consultant in Public Health
North Bristol Acute Trust
Bristol
UK

Dexter L. Lee, Ph.D.
Assistant Professor
Department of Physiology and
Biophysics
Howard University
Washington, D.C.
USA

Bernard I. Lévy, M.D., Ph.D.
Professor
Department of Physiology
University Paris 7
Head
Department of Non-Invasive
Investigations
Hopital Lariboïère
Director
Centre for Cardiovascular Research
Inserm Unit 689
Paris
France

Daniel Link, B.S.
Research Specialist
Internal Medicine
University of Missouri
Columbia, MO
USA

Gregory Y. H. Lip, M.D., F.R.C.P. (London, Edinburgh, Glasgow), F.E.S.C., F.A.C.C.
Professor of Cardiovascular Medicine
Director, Haemostasis, Thrombosis and
Vascular Biology Unit
University Department of Medicine
City Hospital
Birmingham
UK

Graham W. Lipkin, M.D., F.R.C.P.
Honorary Senior Lecturer in Medicine
University of Birmingham
University Hospital Birmingham
Department of Nephrology
Birmingham, West Midlands
UK

Donald M. Lloyd-Jones, M.D., Sc.M., F.A.H.A.
Assistant Professor of Preventive
Medicine and of Medicine (Cardiology)
Feinberg School of Medicine
Northwestern University
Associate Physician
Cardiology
Northwestern Memorial Hospital
Chicago, IL
USA

Thomas E. Lohmeier, Ph.D.
Professor
Physiology and Biophysics
University of Mississippi Medical Center
Jackson, MS
USA

Brona V. Loughrey, B.Sc., M.B., B.Ch., M.R.C.P.
Specialist Registrar
Clinical Biochemistry
Royal Group of Hospitals
Belfast
UK

Thomas M. MacDonald
Professor of Clinical Pharmacology
Division of Medicine and Therapeutics
University of Dundee
Honorary Consultant Physician
Ninewells Hospital and Medical School
Dundee
UK

Robert J. MacFadyen, B.Sc., M.D., F.R.C.P.E., Ph.D.
Consultant Cardiologist and Senior
Lecturer in Medicine
University Department of Medicine and
Department of Cardiology
City Hospital
Birmingham
UK

Sushil K. Mahata, Ph.D.
Professor and VASDHS Principal
Investigator
Hypertension Research Unit
Department of Medicine
University of California, San Diego
School of Medicine
La Jolla, CA
USA

Giuseppe Mancia, M.D.
Full Professor of Medicine and
Chairman
Clinica Medica
Università Milano-Bicocca
Monza, Milan
Italy

Ana Carolina B. Marçano, Ph.D.
Clinical Pharmacology
William Harvey Research Institute
Barts and the London School of
Medicine and Dentistry
London
UK

Jennifer Martin, M.B.Ch.B., M.A., F.R.A.C.P., Ph.D.
Senior Lecturer
Department of Medicine
Melbourne University
Specialist Physician, Clinical
Pharmacologist
Department of Medicine
St. Vincent's Hospital
Melbourne, Victoria
Australia

John C. McGiff, M.D.
Professor and Chair
Department of Pharmacology
New York Medical College
Valhalla, NY
USA

Gordon T. McInnes
Professor of Clinical Pharmacology
Head
Section of Clinical Pharmacology
and Stroke
Medicine Division of Cardiovascular
and Medical Sciences
Gardiner Institute Western Infirmary
Glasgow
UK

Franz H. Messerli, M.D., F.A.C.C., F.A.C.P.
Director, Hypertension Program
Department of Cardiology
St. Lukes-Roosevelt Hospital
Columbia University College
of Physicians and Surgeons
New York, NY
USA

Steven M. Miller, B.Sc.(Hons.), M.B.Ch.B., M.R.C.P., Ph.D.
Clinical Lecturer in Medicine
Faculty of Medicine
University of Glasgow
Glasgow
Scotland

Paul Mitchell, M.B.B.S., M.D., Ph.D., F.R.C.Ophth., F.R.A.N.Z.C.O.
Professor
Department of Ophthalmology
University of Sydney
Sydney, NSW
Director
Ophthalmology
Westmead Hospital
Westmead, NSW
Australia

Jason Moore, Mb.Ch.B., M.R.C.P.
Honorary Lecturer in Medicine
University of Birmingham
Specialist Registrar in Nephrology
Department of Nephrology
University Hospital Birmingham
Birmingham, West Midlands
UK

Trevor A. Mori, Ph.D., C.P. Chem.
School of Medicine and Pharmacology
University of Western Australia
Perth, Western Australia
Australia

Marvin Moser
Clinical Professor of Medicine
Department of Medicine/Cardiology
Yale University School of Medicine
President
High Blood Pressure Foundation, Inc.
New Haven, CT
USA

Maryann N. Mugo, M.D.
Endocrinology Fellow
Department of Internal Medicine
Diabetes and Cardiovascular Disease
Research Center
Division of Endocrinology, Diabetes and
Metabolism
University of Missouri-Columbia
Harry S. Truman Memorial VA Medical
Center
Columbia, MO
USA

Patricia B. Munroe, Ph.D.
Department of Clinical Pharmacology
William Harvey Research Institute
Barts and the London School of
Medicine and Dentistry
London
UK

Nitish Naik, M.D., D.M.
Associate Professor
Department of Cardiology
Doctor
Department of Cardiology
All India Institute of Medical Sciences
New Delhi
India

Samar A. Nasser, P.A.-C., M.P.H.
Physician Assistant
Division of Translational Research and
Clinical Epidemiology
Department of Internal Medicine
Wayne State University
Detroit, MI
USA

Stephen J. Newhouse, M.Sc.
Department of Clinical Pharmacology
William Harvey Research Institute
Barts and the London School of
Medicine and Dentistry
London
UK

Leong L. Ng, M.D.
Pharmacology and Therapeutics Group
Department of Cardiovascular Sciences
Leicester Royal Infirmary
Leicester
UK

Carrie A. Northcott, Ph.D.
Post-Doctoral Fellow
Pharmacology and Toxicology
Michigan State University
East Lansing, MI
USA

Shannon M. O'Connor, B.S.
Research Assistant
Division of Translational Research and
Clinical Epidemiology
Department of Internal Medicine
Wayne State University
Detroit, MI
USA

Daniel T. O'Connor, M.D.
Professor
Department of Medicine and Pharmacology
University of California at San Diego
School of Medicine
La Jolla, CA
USA

Suzanne Oparil, M.D.
Professor of Medicine and Physiology
and Biophysics
Senior Scientist
Center for Aging
Director
Vascular Biology and Hypertension
Program of the Division of
Cardiovascular Disease
Department of Medicine
University of Alabama at Birmingham
Birmingham, AL
USA

Pablo A. Ortiz, Ph.D.
Senior Staff Investigator
Division of Hypertension and Vascular
Research
Henry Ford Hospital
Detroit, MI
USA

Gurusher S. Panjrath, M.D.
Resident
Department of Medicine
Hypertension Program
St. Lukes-Roosevelt Hospital
Columbia University College
of Physicians and Surgeons
New York, NY
USA

Hari Krishnan Parthasarathy, M.B.B.S., M.D., M.R.C.P.
Specialist Registrar
Department of Medicine and Cardiology
Peterborough District Hospital
Peterborough, Cambridgeshire
UK

Ivan J. Perry, M.D., M.Sc., Ph.D., F.R.C.P., F.R.C.P.I., F.F.P.H.M.I., M.F.P.H.
Head of Department
Professor of Public Health
Epidemiology and Public Health
University College Cork
Cork
Ireland

Thomas G. Pickering, M.D., D. Phil.
Professor of Medicine
Director
Behavioral Cardiovascular Health and
Hypertension Program
Division of Cardiology
Columbia Presbyterian Medical Center
New York, NY
USA

Pierre-François Plouin, M.D.
Faculté de Médecine René Descartes
Department of Vascular Medicine and
Hypertension
Université René Descartes
Hôpital Européen Georges Pompidou
Department of Vascular Medicine and
Hypertension
Assistance Publique des Hôpitaux
de Paris
Paris
France

Dorairaj Prabhakaran, M.D., D.M.(Cardiology), M.Sc.
Additional Professor
Department of Cardiology
All India Institute of Medical Sciences
Doctor
Department of Cardiology
All India Institute of Medical Sciences
New Delhi
India

Ian B. Puddey, M.B.B.S., M.D., F.R.A.C.P.
Professor
Faculty of Medicine, Dentistry and
Health Services
University of Western Australia
Nedlands, Western Australia
Australia

John Quilley, Ph.D.
Associate Professor
Department of Pharmacology
New York Medical College
Valhalla, NY
USA

Mohan K. Raizada, Ph.D.
Professor
Department of Physiology and
Functional Genomics
University of Florida
Gainesville, FL
USA

Fangwen Rao, M.D.
Visiting Scholar
Department of Medicine
Center for Medical Genetics
University of California, San Diego
School of Medicine
La Jolla, CA
USA

Jane F. Reckelhoff
Professor
Department of Physiology and
Biophysics
University of Mississippi Medical Center
Jackson, MS
USA

Kolli Srinath Reddy, M.D., D.M.
President
Public Health Foundation of India
Professor
Department of Cardiology
All India Institute of Medical Sciences
Ansari Nagar, New Delhi
India

Damiano Rizzoni, M.D.
Associate Professor of Internal
Medicine
Department of Medical and Surgical
Sciences
University of Brescia
Brescia
Italy

J. Ian S. Robertson, M.D., F.R.C.P., F.R.C.P., M.D.D. (Hons.), M.A., M.B., B.S., F.A.H.A., C.Biol., F.I.Biol., F.R.S.
Formerly Visiting Professor
Prince of Wales Hospital
Chinese University of Hong Kong
Hong Kong
China
Formerly Physician
Medical Research
Council Blood Pressure Unit
Western Infirmary
Glasgow
United Kingdom
Formerly Senior Consultant
Cardiovascular Medicine
Janssen Research Foundation
Belgium

Thompson G. Robinson, M.D., F.R.C.P.
Senior Lecturer
Department of Cardiovascular
Sciences
Consultant
Department of Stroke Medicine
University Hospitals of Leicester
Leicester
UK

J. Carlos Romero, M.D.
Professor
Department of Physiology and
Biomedical Engineering
Mayo Clinic College of Medicine
Rochester, MN
USA

Enrico Agabiti Rosei, M.D.
Full Professor of Internal Medicine
Department of Medical and Surgical
Sciences
University of Brescia
Brescia
Italy

Talma Rosenthal, M.D.
Hypertension Research Unit
Sackler School of Medicine
Tel Aviv University
Tel Aviv
Israel

Dieter Rosskopf, M.D.
Professor
Department of Pharmacology
Research Center for Pharmacology and
Experimental Therapeutics
Ernst-Moritz-Arndt University
Greifswald
Germany

Michael J. Ryan, Ph.D., F.A.H.A.
Assistant Professor
Department of Physiology and Biophysics
University of Mississippi Medical Center
Jackson, MS
USA

Michel E. Safar, M.D.
Professor
Department of Medicine
Université René Descartes
Professor
Diagnosis Center
Hotel-Dieu Hospital
Paris
France

Antonio Salvetti, M.D.
Professor of Internal Medicine
Department of Internal Medicine
University of Pisa
Pisa
Italy

Panteleimon A. Sarafidis, M.D., M.Sc., Ph.D.
Research Fellow
Hypertension/Clinical Research Center
Department of Preventive Medicine
Rush University Medical Center
Chicago, IL
USA

Julio C. Sartori-Valinotti, M.D.
Post-doctoral Fellow
Department of Physiology and
Biophysics
University of Mississippi Medical Center
Jackson, MS
USA

Nicholas J. Schork, Ph.D.
Professor of Family and Preventive
Medicine
Professor of Psychiatry
University of California, San Diego
School of Medicine
La Jolla, CA
USA

John F. Setaro, M.D.
Associate Professor of Medicine
Section of Cardiovascular Medicine
Department of Internal Medicine
Yale University School of Medicine
Attending Physician
Department of Medicine
Yale-New Haven Hospital
New Haven, CT
USA

N. C. Shah, M.B.B.S., M.R.C.P.
School of Medical Practice and
Population Health
Faculty of Health
University of Newcastle
New South Wales
Australia

Julian Shiel, M.D.
Department of Clinical Pharmacology
William Harvey Research Institute
Barts and the London School of
Medicine and Dentistry
London
UK

Ernesto L. Schiffrin, M.D., Ph.D., F.R.C.P.C.
Professor
Department of Medicine
Clinical Research Institute of Montreal
Physician-in-Chief
Department of Medicine
Jewish General Hospital
Montral, Quebec
Canada

Domenic A. Sica, M.D.
Professor and Chairman
Clinical Pharmacology and
Hypertension
Division of Nephrology
Departments of Medicine and
Pharmacology
Virginia Commonwealth University
Health System
Richmond, VA
USA

Alexandre A. da Silva, Ph.D.
Research Assistant Professor
Physiology and Biophysics
University of Mississippi Medical
Center
Jackson, MS
USA

Guillermo B. Silva, M.S.
Research Associate
Division of Hypertension and Vascular
Research
Henry Ford Hospital
Detroit, MI
USA

J. Enrique Silva, M.D., F.A.C.P.
Professor
Department of Medicine
Tufts University Medical School
Chief
Division of Endocrinology and
Metabolism
Department of Medicine
Baystate Medical Center
Springfield, MA
Adjunct Professor
Department of Biology
University of Massachusetts
Amherst, MA
USA

George Davey Smith, D.Sc., F.R.C.P.
Professor
Clinical Epidemiology
Department of Social Medicine
University of Bristol
Honorary Consultant
Public Health Medicine
North Bristol Acute Trust
Bristol
UK

Virend K. Somers, M.D., Ph.D.
Professor
Department of Medicine
Mayo Clinic
Rochester, MN
USA

James R. Sowers, M.D., A.S.C.I., F.A.C.P.
Professor and Director
Diabetes Center
Departments of Medicine and Physiology
University of Arizona Medical Center
Tuscon, AZ
USA

J. David Spence, B.A., M.B.A., M.D., F.R.C.P.C., F.A.H.A.
Professor
Department of Clinical Neurological
Sciences and Medicine
University of Western Ontario
Member, Stroke Service
Department of Clinical Neurological
Sciences
London Health Sciences Centre
Director
Stroke Prevention & Atherosclerosis
Research Centre
Robarts Research Institute
London, Ontario
Canada

Adrian G. Stanley, B.Sc., B.M., M.R.C.P.
Honorary Senior Lecturer (Medical
Education)
Department of Cardiovascular Sciences
University of Leicester
Consultant Physician in Cardiovascular
Medicine
Cardio-Respiratory Directorate
University Hospitals of Leicester
NHS Trust
Leicester
UK

David E. Stec, Ph.D., F.A.H.A.
Assistant Professor
Physiology and Biophysics
University of Mississippi Medical
Center
Jackson, MS
USA

Saverio Stranges, M.D., Ph.D.
Assistant Professor
Department of Social and Preventive
Medicine
School of Public Health and Health
Professions
University at Buffalo
Buffalo, NY
USA

Allan D. Struthers, B.Sc., M.D., F.R.C.P., F.E.S.C.
Professor of Cardiovascular Medicine
and Therapeutics
Division of Medicine and Therapeutics
School of Medicine
University of Dundee
Head of Division and Consultant
Physician
Division of Medicine and Therapeutics
Ninewells Hospital and Medical School
Dundee, Scotland
UK

Craig S. Stump, M.D., Ph.D.
Assistant Professor of Medicine
Internal Medicine—Endocrinology
University of Missouri
Staff Physician
Specialty Care—Endocrinology
Harry S. Truman VA Hospital
Columbia, MO
USA

Fatiha Tabet, B.Sc.
Department of Medicine
Division of Nephrology
Kidney Research Centre
Ottawa Health Research Institute
The Ottawa General Hospital
Department of Hypertension
University of Ottawa
Ottawa, Ontario
Canada

Stefano Taddei, M.D.
Professor
Department of Internal Medicine
University of Pisa
Pisa
Italy

Laurent Taupenot, Ph.D.
Assistant Professor
Department of Medicine
University of California
Biologist
Research Division
VA San Diego Health Care System
San Diego, CA
USA

Muzahir H. Tayebjee, M.B., Ch.B. (Hons), M.R.C.P.
Doctor
Cardiology
Hemel Hempstead General Hospital
Hempstead
United Kingdom
Specialist Registrar in Cardiology
North West Thames Deanery
London
UK

Cleber E. Teixeira, Ph.D.
Pharmacology
State University of Campinas
Campinas, SP
Brazil

Keshari M. Thakali
Department of Pharmacology and
Toxicology
Michigan State University
East Lansing University
East Lansing, MI
USA

Rhian M. Touyz, M.D., Ph.D., F.A.H.A., Fatiha Tabet BSc.
Professor of Medicine
Department of Medicine
Division of Nephrology
Kidney Research Centre
Ottawa Health Research Institute
Doctor
The Ottawa General Hospital
Department of Hypertension
University of Ottawa
Ottawa, Ontario
Canada

Darren Traub, D.O.
Chief Cardiology Fellow
Department of Medicine
Division of Cardiovascular Diseases
Western Pennsylvania Hospital
Pittsburgh, PA
USA

Hung-Fat Tse, M.B.B.S., M.D., M.R.C.P., F.H.K.C.P., F.H.K.A.M., F.R.C.P., F.A.C.C.
Professor of Medicine
Department of Medicine
The University of Hong Kong
Honorary Consultant
Department of Medicine
Queen Mary Hospital
Hong Kong
China

Jason G. Umans, M.D., Ph.D.
Associate Professor
Department of Medicine, Obstetrics,
and Gynecology, and the General
Clinical Research Center
Georgetown University Medical Center
and Penn Medical Lab
Medstar Research Institute
Washington, DC
USA

Puchimada Uthappa, Mb.Ch.B., M.R.C.P.
Honorary Lecturer in Medicine
University of Birmingham
Specialist Registrar in Nephrology
Department of Nephology
University Hospital Birmingham
Birmingham, West Midlands
UK

Anna B. Valina-Toth, B.Sc., M.Sc.
3rd Year M.D./Ph.D. Student
Department of Physiology
Wayne State University
Detroit, MI
USA

George I. Varughese, M.R.C.P., M.R.C.P.
Research Fellow
Haemostasis, Thrombosis and Vascular
Biology Unit
City Hospital
Birmingham
UK

Agostino Virdis, M.D.
Assistant Professor
Department of Internal Medicine
University of Pisa
Pisa
Italy

Stephanie W. Watts, Ph.D., F.A.H.A.
Associate Professor
Department of Pharmacology
and Toxicology
Michigan State University
East Lansing, MI
USA

R. Clinton Webb, Ph.D.
Robert B. Greenblatt Chair
of Endocrinology
Professor and Chairperson of Physiology
Department of Physiology
Medical College of Georgia
Augusta, GA
USA

Gen Wen, M.D., Ph.D.
Project Scientist
Department of Medicine
University of California, San Diego
School of Medicine
La Jolla, CA
USA

Paul K. Whelton, M.D.
Senior Vice President
Health Sciences
Dean
Tulane University School of Medicine
Professor
Departments of Epidemiology and
Medicine
Tulane University School of Medicine
New Orleans, LA
USA

Judith A. Whitworth, A.C., D.Sc., M.D., Ph.D., B.S., F.R.A.C.P.
Professor and Director
The John Curtin School of Medical
Research
The Australian National University
Acton
Australia

Tien Yin Wong, M.B.B.S., M.P.H., Ph.D., F.R.C.S.E., F.R.A.N.Z.C.O.
Professor
Centre for Eye Research Australia
University of Melbourne
Consultant
Ophthalmology
Royal Victorian Eye and Ear Hospital
Melbourne, Victoria
Australia
Consultant
Vitreoretinal Department
Singapore National Eye Centre
Associate Director
Singapore Eye Research Institute
National University of Singapore
Singapore

Ryan M. Woodham, M.D.
Internal Medicine Resident
Department of Internal Medicine
University of Alabama at Birmingham
Birmingham, AL
USA

Kathleen Wyne, M.D., Ph.D., F.A.C.E.
Assistant Professor
Division of Endocrinology and
Metabolism
Department of Internal Medicine
Parkland Memorial Hospital
Zale University Hospital
St. Paul University Hospital
Co-Director
St. Paul Diabetes Management Program
University of Texas Southwestern
Medical Center at Dallas
Dallas, TX
USA

Licy Lorena Yanes, M.D.
Instructor
Department of Physiology and
Biophysics
University of Mississippi Medical
Center
Jackson, MS
USA

Zhekang Ying, Ph.D.
Postdoctoral Fellow
Physiology and Biophysics
University of Mississippi Medical
Center
Jackson, MS
USA

Ian S. Young, B.Sc., M.D., F.R.C.P., F.R.C.P.I., F.R.C.Path.
Professor
Nutrition and Metabolism Group
Centre for Clinical and Population
Sciences
Queen's University
Belfast
UK

Alberto Zanchetti
Emeritus Professor of Medicine
University of Milan
Scientific Director
Istituto Auxologico Italiano
Milan
Italy

Kuixing Zhang, M.D.
Postdoctoral Researcher
Department of Medicine and
Pharmacology
University of California at San Diego
School of Medicine
La Jolla, CA
USA

Lian Zhang
Department of Medicine
University of California, San Diego
School of Medicine
La Jolla, CA
USA

Michael G. Ziegler, M.D.
Professor
Department of Medicine
University of California, San Diego
School of Medicine
La Jolla, CA
USA

PREFACE

Why do we need another textbook of hypertension? Can a single textbook capture the explosion of knowledge in hypertension research and related areas such as vascular biology, genetics, physiology, molecular biology, nephrology, and cardiology? These are reasonable questions, especially when one considers the large number of hypertension textbooks and journals that are already available. Obviously, no single textbook or journal can adequately cover all of these advances. However, there have been few attempts to integrate the basic, clinic, and population science of hypertension research and treatment in a single textbook that can be used by scientists and practicing clinicians. Our goal for *Comprehensive Hypertension* was therefore to assemble the collective knowledge of leading hypertension experts into a comprehensive but readable synopsis of the field.

Comprehensive Hypertension is divided into four major sections: I. Epidemiology; II. Pathophysiology; III. Clinical Approaches; IV. Pharmacologic and Nonpharmacologic Interventions and Treatment Guidelines. Extensive color has been used throughout the book not just for the purpose of making the book attractive, but primarily to better illustrate key points in the figures. Each section is also color coded for quick reference. The section editors and contributors are internationally recognized experts who were selected to provide a comprehensive, but not encyclopedic, perspective of the science of hypertension and its everyday application to treatment of the patient.

The book is intended to be a useful reference for clinicians who provide care for hypertensive patients, for basic and clinical scientists who study the physiology of blood pressure regulation and the pathophysiology of hypertension, and for population scientists concerned with hypertension and related disorders. The book will also be a useful reference for other health care professionals.

In many ways, the field of hypertension research is a great success story. There is a wealth of new information on epidemiology, pathophysiology, and clinical trials. There are also many drugs available that can be used to effectively treat hypertension. However, over one *billion* people worldwide have higher than optimal blood pressure warranting some form of treatment. Hypertension continues to be the number one attributable risk factor for death throughout the world although lowering of blood pressure has been clearly shown to reduce stroke, myocardial infarction, heart failure, and kidney disease. Unfortunately, high blood pressure is often not treated as aggressively as many other conditions that have far less impact on human health. Only a small fraction (usually less than 30 percent) of hypertensive patients are adequately treated, even in countries where major professional and public education efforts have been made to convey the importance of effective treatment. This means that there is still much work to do, not only in understanding the etiology and pathophysiology of hypertension but also in communicating and implementing what we already know to more effective treatment of patients.

We hope that you find our attempts to synthesize this information in a readable but comprehensive textbook is useful, and we invite you to provide feedback on our efforts. We sincerely thank our section editors and contributing authors who have worked hard to make our job as senior editors much easier. We are also grateful to our colleagues at Elsevier, Natasha Andjelkovic (Executive Publisher), Ann Ruzycka Anderson (Senior Developmental Editor), and Bryan Hayward (Production Manager), for facilitating the transition from concept to reality through their editorial and production excellence.

Gregory Y. H. Lip, Birmingham, UK
John E. Hall, Jackson, Mississippi, USA

EPIDEMIOLOGY

*John E. Hall, Gregory Y. H. Lip, and
Paul K. Whelton*

Chapter

1

A Short History of the Study of Hypertension

D. Gareth Beevers and J. Ian S. Robertson

Key Findings

- This introductory chapter covers the history of research into hypertension. Particular attention is given to the measurement of blood pressure, the renin-angiotensin-aldosterone system, and drug trials for the treatment of hypertension.

- We discuss the principal achievements and certain methodological issues, as well as current gaps in our knowledge of the nature of hypertension and its treatment.

- We accept that there are many areas for debate and that some experts may not share our views on various aspects of the history of research into hypertension.

Awareness of the existence of hypertension—raised arterial pressure—as a physiologic or pathophysiologic entity has a long history, stretching back to antiquity. Appreciation of the causes, consequences, and benefits from correcting hypertension became progressively clearer, particularly in the second half of the 20th century, as the topic became the increasing focus of epidemiologic, physiologic, and clinical research. An extensive survey of the concepts and achievements in hypertension research in the 20th century was published in 2004; many of the chapters were written by persons who had participated.[1]

This chapter will briefly outline that history, delineating the pathophysiologic, clinical, and therapeutic relevance of the topic. As far as possible, we propose to economize on references by quoting books and review articles to which the reader is directed for more detailed information.

EARLY HISTORY

Probably the first recorded observations on hypertension were made some 4000 years ago by the Chinese Yellow Emperor, Huang Ti,[2] who noted an association between kidney disease and heart disease, described aphasic apoplexy, and regarded an excessive dietary salt intake as hazardous.

> If too much salt is used in food, the pulse hardens.... When the heart pulse beats vigorously and the strokes are markedly prolonged, the corresponding illness makes the tongue curl up and the patient unable to speak.

A relationship between the quality of the pulse and development of afflictions of the heart and brain was noted by physicians of Thebes in ancient Egypt in the Ebers Papyrus of 1500 BCE, and later in India in the Caraka Samhita of around 150 BCE.[3,4] The early Arabic texts of Masawah, and of the physician Abu Ali al-Hussain ibn Abdulla ibn Sina, usually known as Avicenna (980–1037 CE), also drew attention to abnormalities of the pulse in disease.[5]

CIRCULATION OF THE BLOOD

The significance of many early observations could not, however, be properly appreciated before William Harvey's description in 1628 of the circulation of the blood. In his great work *Exercitatio Anatomica du Motu Cordis et Sanguini in Animabilus*, he correctly set out the concept of blood flowing out from the heart via the arteries, through the periphery, and then returning by way of the veins. Harvey noted that blood went from the heart through the lungs and then back to the heart; however, he was not able to show how blood passed from the arterial to the venous system at the periphery, because no connections were visible to the naked eye. Nevertheless, Harvey rightly supposed that such links existed, but must be too minute to be seen. The Italian Malpighi did observe such capillary vessels, using a microscope, shortly after Harvey's death.[6,7]

EARLY CLINICAL STUDIES: BRIGHT AND MAHOMED

During the 19th century, two physicians working at Guy's Hospital in London made crucial advances toward understanding clinical hypertension.[8,9] In 1836 Richard Bright published an account of a hundred patients with overt renal disease, or proteinuria. Just over half of them had large hearts at *postmortem* examination. He proposed that this cardiac enlargement must be a consequence of an altered quality of the blood or of a raised circulatory pressure. Some 40 years later, Frederick Henry Horatio Akhbar Mahomed, a British physician whose grandfather had migrated from India,[10] worked at the same hospital. Perhaps Mahomed's most important contribution was recognizing in 1874 patients with large-volume pulses who showed no evidence of kidney disease. Mahomed called this condition "chronic Bright's disease without albuminuria," which would now almost certainly be termed essential hypertension. Mahomed went on to note an association between raised arterial pressure and heart attack, stroke, epistaxis, gout, and excessive alcohol consumption, all aspects that remain of considerable epidemiologic interest. Yet another of Mahomed's accomplishments was in improving the sphygmograph, an instrument for the clinical assessment of arterial pressure, as shall shortly be recounted.[7]

BLOOD PRESSURE MEASUREMENT

Crucial to the progress of physiologic and clinical studies on blood pressure was the availability of means for its measurement, and especially its noninvasive measurement. Such methods were developed progressively during the 18th, 19th, and 20th centuries.[7,11]

The first direct measurement of arterial blood pressure was made in 1732 by the Anglican clergyman and distinguished scientist, Stephen Hales, who had a horse tied down to a gate, inserted a brass cannula into its crural artery, and observed that the blood rose up a glass tube to a height of 8 feet 3 inches.[8]

Poiseuille in 1783 adapted from Hales's intra-arterial tube a device that he called a hemodynamometer, comprising a U-shaped tube connected to a shorter tube; the latter could be introduced intra-arterially. The U-tube contained mercury that was separated from the blood by another liquid. By this means Poiseuille could observe arterial pulsation and quantify its pressure.

This approach was elaborated by Hérisson and Gernier, who, instead of inserting a needle or tube into a blood vessel, employed a tightly stretched rubber membrane over the artery. This so-called sphygmograph went on to be refined by Winternitz, Keith, and Ozanam. In 1847, Ludwig had a bird's feather mounted on a float on the mercury surface of the U-tube, and, with the aid of a rotating cylinder carrying smoked paper, was able to record the oscillation of the pulse.

Among several persons who elaborated and modified these procedures was Marey who, in 1860, devised a sphygmograph capable, noninvasively, of transmitting arterial pulsatile variations on to a writing cylinder. The sphygmograph was further improved by Mahomed, who went on to employ the apparatus clinically, and, among other observations, to detect an increase in arterial pressure in patients with scarlet fever and renal damage.

Further crucial advances toward the construction of genuinely robust and reliable devices for the clinical assessment of blood pressure were made by von Bash, Potain, and Mosso.

Then, in two articles published in 1896 and 1897, the Italian Scipione Riva-Rocci described his mercury sphygmomanometer and its method of use. This, with an inflatable cuff for arterial compression was, in essence, the principal apparatus subsequently employed for blood pressure measurement throughout the 20th century, and remains in use to this day. Most impressive are the detailed instructions provided by Riva-Rocci for the maintenance and calibration of the sphygmomanometer, and his emphasis that measurements must be made under favorable resting conditions for the patient. The American neurosurgeon, Harvey Cushing visited Riva-Rocci, and was sufficiently impressed as to order sphygmomanometers to be employed at Johns Hopkins Hospital in Baltimore for the routine measurement of blood pressure in his patients.

Initially only systolic pressure was measurable sphygmomanometrically, taking this as the height of the mercury column at the point of first appearance of the radial pulse distally when the cuff was deflated. Then, in 1905, the Russian army surgeon Nicolai Sergeivich Korotkoff described the results of auscultation over the brachial artery as the cuff on the upper arm was deflated.[8] The pressure at which sounds first were heard has come to be called Korotkoff phase 1, the pressure at sudden muffling of sounds as phase 4, and the point of cessation of sounds as phase 5. Phases 1 and 5 are currently taken as indicating respectively systolic and diastolic arterial pressure, although at one time phase 4 was held by some to denote the diastolic reading.

Such auscultatory blood pressure measurements involved judgment by the observer, and hence could be biased, occasionally compromising epidemiologic studies. Reported values in millimeters of mercury consistently revealed a preference for numbers ending in zero or five. Several devices, including the London School of Hygiene Sphygmomanometer (the Rose Box) and the Hawkesley Random Zero Sphygmomanometer (the Garrow Muddler), were introduced in order to circumvent this problem. With the Rose Box, the observer noted the Korotkoff phases without having a simultaneous view of the mercury column. The Garrow Muddler was designed so that after the blood pressure reading had been obtained, the mercury column settled to a random number between zero and 60 mmHg. This number was then subtracted from the reading obtained by the clinician to obtain the true blood pressure.

The late 20th century saw the introduction of ambulatory blood-pressure monitoring over 24 hours. Such methods are of only minor inconvenience to the subject, who can continue with normal activities, and hence they provide a wealth of physiologic and pathophysiologic information. These approaches also amply confirmed the cautions of Stephen Hales and Riva-Rocci that extraneous stimuli and physical activity could greatly affect the arterial pressure. They also confirmed that a considerable number of patients who had been labeled as hypertensive did in fact have much lower or even normal blood pressures when away from the clinical setting.[7,11]

By the beginning of the 21st century, the mercury sphygmomanometer was becoming progressively superseded by automatic and semiautomatic blood-pressure measuring systems based on oscillometry rather than the auscultatory principles of Korotkoff. These manometers have the advantage that they abolish one source of inaccuracy, namely observer error and bias. There is also increasing concern about the possible toxicity of organic mercury salts.

BLOOD PRESSURE IN POPULATIONS: THE PLATT–PICKERING DEBATE

The ready availability of the mercury sphygmomanometer permitted the survey of blood pressure values across populations, and engendered a crucial and lengthy debate between two prominent English physicians, Robert Platt and George Pickering, in the 1950s and 1960s.[8,12,13]

Platt contended that essential hypertension is an inherited tendency to develop high blood pressure in midlife. In his view this was reflected in a discrete subgroup of subjects wherein hypertension caused serious morbidity. Such patients were, he thought, to be contrasted with another larger population in which the blood pressure rises little if at all with increasing years. Platt hence asserted that

> the frequency distribution of blood pressure in middle age would show a bimodal peak with one peak at a so-called normal level of blood pressure and another peak representing the hypertensive members of the population.

Pickering's very different concept was that essential hypertension represents a quantitative deviation from the norm, a notion requiring that the distribution of blood pressures within populations be continuous, any differences being quantitative rather than qualitative. This idea was not original; Lord Dawson of Penn had stated in 1925 that "hyperpiesia [hypertension] is not a condition with a defined territory; it has no threshold."[14] (Dawson was personal physician to King George V. Not all were impressed by Dawson's skill. A scurrilous jingle ran: "Lord Dawson of Penn has killed so many men; we all have to sing 'God save the King!' ") However, Pickering forcefully developed and promulgated the concept. Blood pressure values in individuals should, according to Pickering, be seen as determined by numerous genetic and environmental influences. Furthermore, adverse cardiovascular events were expected simply to be proportional to the height of the arterial pressure.

The immediate issues were eventually settled in Pickering's favor. Virtually all large population samples have demonstrated a continuous, roughly bell-shaped curve of the distribution of systolic and diastolic blood pressure, the curve being slightly skewed toward the upper end. Hence, it is now accepted that no clear-cut division, other than a quite arbitrary one, can be made between normal blood pressure and "hypertension."

It follows that the distribution of cardiovascular risk, although subject to a range of influences additional to the height of arterial pressure, is also continuous, there being no inferior point of cut-off at which risk ceases. At the highest blood pressure values, there are small numbers of persons at high risk. As lower, but still above-average blood pressures are considered, there is a much larger population in which, overall, the cardiovascular risks, although distinct, are more modest. Further, individuals whose pressures are average for their age are at greater cardiovascular danger than those with values below average. Thus, in general, hypertension is not a disease in the usual sense, but rather an indicator of cardiovascular hazard. These concepts, established only after extensive disputation and no little acrimony, are obviously central to the implementation of antihypertensive drug therapy and preventive medicine.

Geoffrey Rose developed from these ideas a "population strategy" for preventive therapy, whereby he proposed that a modest reduction in blood pressure and hence risk in the population as a whole (including persons whose pressures would be regarded as normal) might greatly reduce the incidence of complications overall. By contrast, directing treatment preferentially toward those with distinctly high pressures would help only a minority.[15] These concepts had wide appeal. However, other researchers questioned the scientific basis of Rose's notions, and were especially concerned that they were being promoted before being tested.[16–18] Remarkably, Tunstall-Pedoe et al.[19] found that between the mid-1980s and mid-1990s, blood pressure fell in 38 different populations, at all levels of readings. This could not, they reasoned, be a consequence of antihypertensive treatment, which would have shown a differential fall only at higher values; these observations remain unexplained.

THE COMPLICATIONS OF HYPERTENSION

The association between raised blood pressure and lesions of the heart, brain, and kidneys had been recognized in the 19th century, notably by Bright and by Mahomed.[8–10] The various complications of hypertension were increasingly clarified in the 20th century, with arterial changes understood as fundamental to those adverse consequences.[20]

Arterial changes

With hypertension, large- and medium-sized arteries (>1 mm in diameter) become thickened, rigid, dilated, and tortuous. Atheroma is prevalent. Smaller arteries evince thickening of the media, intimal expansion, and narrowing of the lumen. It is likely that the upward resetting of the pressure limits in autoregulation of blood flow via various organs that occurs in hypertension results at least in part from such structural changes in small arteries. In the late 20th century, arterial changes were particularly well studied in the brain, where the phenomenon appears to hold true, even though small cerebral arteries are poorly muscled (Figure 1–1).

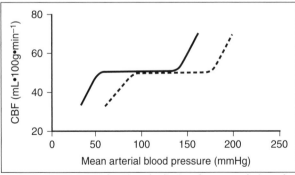

Figure 1–1. Diagram showing the limits of autoregulation of cerebral blood flow (CBF) in a normal person (*continuous line*) and a patient with hypertension (*dotted line*). Cerebral blood flow is held constant over wide limits of systemic arterial pressure. If the systemic blood pressure exceeds the upper limit of autoregulation the brain will be overperfused and become edematous. If the pressure falls below the lower limit of autoregulation, cerebral ischemia, and possible infarction will result. (Redrawn from Kjeldsen SE, Julius S, Hedner T, Hansson L. Stroke is more common than myocardial infarction in hypertension: analysis based on 11 major randomized intervention trials. *Blood Press* 2001;10:190–92.)

Specific to small arteries in the brain are Charcot–Bouchard aneurysms, first described by Charcot and Bouchard in 1868,[21] which were then long neglected and rediscovered by Russell in 1963.[22] These small arteries are typically 0.2 to 1.0 mm in diameter and have attenuated walls; they predispose to intracerebral hemorrhage in hypertension.

The most severe arterial lesions resulting from hypertension occur during the malignant phase, and are the outcome of very high arterial pressure, especially when pressure has risen swiftly. The characteristic lesion of the malignant phase is fibrinoid necrosis or ("plasmatic vasculosis") of small arteries and arterioles, which disrupt as a consequence of the very high blood pressure. An interesting inconsistency emerged in the late 20th century. Malignant-phase hypertension became rare in some countries, such as Australia and Sweden, while remaining common in Britain, notably in Glasgow and Birmingham.[23] This curiosity remains unexplained.

The heart

Patients with very severe hypertension can develop overt hypertensive heart failure without concomitant myocardial damage from coronary artery disease. In such instances, this is often associated with left ventricular diastolic, rather than systolic, dysfunction. While this complication is now becoming infrequent, it remains a problem, particularly in patients of African origin.[24]

Coronary artery atheroma is one of the most common associations of hypertension that has been more thoroughly studied in recent years with greater attention given to mild blood pressure elevation and long-term cardiac functional impairment with left ventricular systolic dysfunction. In the lower ranges of hypertension, coronary arterial disease is usually more prevalent than stroke or cardiac failure. However, in recent trials,[25] strokes have outnumbered heart attacks, possibly because patients at particularly high risk participated in these studies.

The brain

Hypertension is a major cause of intracerebral hemorrhage, which accounts for 20% of all strokes. Many of these catastrophes occur at the site of Charcot–Bouchard microaneurysms of the small arteries deep within the brain.[21,22]

Clinical stroke more often results from cerebral infarction, for which hypertension is again a predisposing factor. Atheromatous plaques can lead to progressive occlusion of arteries or can be a source of emboli that may be composed variously of atheromatous debris and cholesterol crystals, or mixtures of fibrin, leucocytes, and platelets.

A now very rare complication, acute hypertensive encephalopathy, in which headache, confusion, coma, and fits may occur, is almost always superimposed on malignant phase hypertension. Hypertensive encephalopathy is a consequence of the systemic arterial pressure exceeding the upper limit of cerebral autoregulation (Figure 1–1), with resulting overperfusion and cerebral edema. However, in recent years the ready availability of high-resolution computerized tomography and magnetic resonance imaging has revealed brain infarctions in some patients who would have been thought in earlier times to have hypertensive encephalopathy.

The eye

Much interest in hypertension was focused on the eye because the fundus oculi can be inspected directly by means of the ophthalmoscope or retinal camera. The retinal arterial consequences of mild hypertension comprise thickening, irregularity, and tortuosity. Occasionally, emboli may be seen traversing the retinal circulation. Central or segmental retinal arterial or venous occlusions can accompany high blood pressure and may readily be diagnosed ophthalmoscopically.

The onset of the malignant phase can be recognized by the appearance of typically bilateral retinal exudates that may be circumscribed ("hard") or fluffy ("cotton wool spots") and hemorrhages. In the later stages, papilledema and retinal edema may also appear.

The retinal features of hypertension were classified in 1939 by Keith et al.[26] This system was for a time extensively applied, but is today probably obsolete, in part because it embraced the now discredited concept of arterial spasm. Furthermore, examination of these authors' original data demonstrates that their grades III and IV patients had broadly the same adverse prognosis, which is quite different from patients with grades I and II retinopathy. The changes classified as grades I and II are as closely related to the patients' age as to their blood pressure.[27,28]

The kidney

The kidney typically sustains most consequences of the malignant phase, with extensive and progressive fibrinoid necrosis of afferent glomerular arterioles, glomerular infarction, and consequent renal impairment. Hence, in untreated malignant hypertension, provided the course is not terminated abruptly by a catastrophic stroke or cardiac failure, the patient will succumb to renal failure.

The decline of renal function with age is faster with raised arterial pressure, and end-stage renal failure attributable to hypertension became more prevalent in the last decades of the 20th century.[29,30] Although some have questioned whether nonmalignant essential (nonrenal) hypertension is a major cause of renal failure,[31,32] control of blood pressure has been demonstrated in multiple studies to attenuate progression of renal disease (see Chapter 49).

QUANTIFICATION OF RISK—SYSTOLIC AND DIASTOLIC PRESSURE AND COMPOUNDING RISK

It is remarkable that the harmful effects of hypertension were perceived by Bright and Mahomed,[9,10] as well as by Huchard in 1889,[33] before accurate measurements of arterial pressure were achieved. Then, with the introduction of Riva-Rocci's sphygmomanometer, initially only systolic pressure could be assessed. Even after Korotkoff had shown how diastolic might be measured, interest focused on the systolic pressure, and that predilection continued into the 1930s.

The quantitative relationship between arterial pressure and mortality from cardiovascular or renal disease was, from the 1930s onward, consistently shown in data from life insurance companies.[34] That correlation existed for both systolic and diastolic pressures with, for a given pressure level, men being more vulnerable than women.[35]

For a time there was a change of emphasis, and diastolic pressure increasingly came to be regarded as pathogenically the more important, especially in the causation of malignant hypertension. The temporary trend for regarding diastolic pressure as being of greater influence was intriguingly shown in some of Pickering's writings. In the 1968 edition of *High Blood Pressure*, Pickering quoted, and considered at length, insurance company data showing the correlation of risk with both systolic and diastolic pressures.[27] Yet, in discussing the disproportionate elevation of systolic relative to diastolic pressure commonly found in elderly subjects, he stated:

> One might suspect that such patients ... would be more prone to develop cardiovascular accidents ... but I know of no evidence bearing on the question.... [T]his form of hypertension will not be further considered in this book.

Subsequently, prospective epidemiologic studies, most notably the Framingham survey initiated in 1949,[35] clearly underlined once more the pathogenic importance of systolic, as well as of diastolic, pressure. Predominant (often termed "isolated") systolic hypertension clearly denoted hazard. In 2001, a more detailed paper from the Framingham Heart Study reported that after the age of ~40 years, systolic pressure and pulse pressure are more powerful predictions of cardiovascular risk than is diastolic.[36] Almost all long-term population studies now confirm that systolic blood pressure is more predictive than diastolic, although there remains some uncertainty about the prognostic role of diastolic blood pressure in young people who, by virtue of their age, are at low short-term risk.

Surveys such as that from Framingham further emphasized the compounding of cardiovascular and renal dangers of raised blood pressure by additional risk factors. These influences are now seen to include male gender, age, raised serum cholesterol and low density lipoprotein cholesterol, diabetes mellitus and impaired glucose tolerance, cigarette smoking, cold weather, and lower social class. The prevalence of complications is also modified by race/ethnicity and geographical location. More complex or controversial factors include body weight, serum uric acid, circulating levels of renin, angiotensin II and aldosterone, and the consumption of alcohol and salt.[20,37-53]

More recently, Reaven has hypothesized that many of the common cardiovascular risk factors (notably, hypertension, diabetes and impaired glucose tolerance, obesity, and hyperlipidemia), may share a common etiology and outlook mediated by insulin resistance in the so-called "metabolic syndrome." These risk factors cluster and individuals with two or more have a greatly increased risk of cardiovascular disease.[35]

SECONDARY HYPERTENSION

Secondary hypertension is defined as raised blood pressure resulting from a recognizable and often potentially correctable cause, and is thus to be distinguished from the much more prevalent primary ("essential") hypertension. In unselected populations of hypertensive subjects, no more than 1% to 5% of cases are secondary, although a much higher proportion of a given disease may be seen in centers having a particular interest in that condition.[20,54-56]

The principal forms of secondary hypertension are listed in Box 1–1. They are evidently numerous and diverse. These various conditions were identified at irregular intervals throughout the 20th century and additions continue to be made.

Despite their comparative rarity, secondary forms of hypertension have attracted much interest. First, many such syndromes, particularly the rare monogenic forms of hypertension, are readily responsive to correction of the underlying cause. Second, a study of the mechanisms whereby the blood pressure is raised in these disorders facilitates insights into the pathophysiology of essential hypertension; this is a compelling impetus for the study of even very rare forms of secondary hypertension, many of which involve primary excess reabsorption of sodium by the renal tubules.

Box 1–1

Secondary Forms of Hypertension

Renal or renovascular diseases
  Unilateral
  Bilateral
Angiotensinogen-producing tumor
Mineralocorticoid-induced hypertension
  Aldosterone excess: Conn's syndrome and related disorders
  Carcinoma-secreting corticosterone or deoxycorticosterone
  Apparent idiopathic deoxycorticosterone excess
  11β-OHSD deficiency
  17α-hydroxylase deficiency
  11β-hydroxylase deficiency
Pheochromocytoma and related disorders
Intracranial tumor
Guillain–Barré neuropathy
Acromegaly
Cushing's syndrome
Thyroid disease
  Hypothyroidism
  Thyrotoxicosis
Liddle's syndrome
Gordon's syndrome
Endothelin-secreting tumor
Porphyria and hypertension
Hormonal contraceptive use
Drug-induced hypertension: various
Coarctation of the aorta
Pregnancy-induced hypertension

From Robertson JIS, ed. Clinical Aspects of Secondary Hypertension. Vol. 2, *Handbook of Hypertension.* Birkenhäger WH, Reid JL, eds., 1983;2.

Two interesting aspects of secondary hypertension were noted by Pickering in 1955.[27] The first of these was that virtually every such condition can enter the malignant phase, and that such transition was more likely with a rapid rise of blood pressure. The concept can now be broadened, because it is seen to apply not only to the malignant phase but also to all of the vascular complications of hypertension, including cardiac hypertrophy, with the proviso that with aortic coarctation the renal vasculature is protected. Such indiscriminate effects of high blood pressure are modified by concomitant pathophysiology in various syndromes. Thus, considerable evidence has suggested that elevation of angiotensin II can have especially adverse effects on the heart, arteries, and kidney.[37] A further proposal is that aldosterone can induce myocardial extracellular matrix and collagen deposition, although not all studies have supported the notion.[39-43] An excess of circulating catecholamines, as with pheochromocytoma, can cause focal myocardial lesions. In Cushing's syndrome, increased cortisol may promote myocardial hypertrophy independently of blood pressure.

The second of Pickering's 1955 observations[27] was that blood pressure may remain raised in a proportion of cases of secondary hypertension even after the primary cause has been removed or corrected, although the pressure may be more readily controlled with drugs. Such persistent hypertension is probably largely a consequence of hypertension-induced changes, including structural thickening of the walls of resistance arteries, and especially to alterations of the arteries of the kidney. Renal functional impairment has been consistently noted as presaging a less satisfactory fall in blood pressure after correction of the causal abnormality.

PRIMARY ("ESSENTIAL") HYPERTENSION: SEARCH FOR A CAUSE

Appreciation of the remarkable array of disorders that can cause secondary hypertension provided ongoing stimuli and encouragement for investigatingthe pathogenesis of primary, or essential, hypertension. Insights gained therein should obviously facilitate appropriate preventive or therapeutic measures. Geoffrey Rose, however, pointed out that "ever popular terms like idiopathic and essential are actually nonsensical as all diseases must have a cause."[57]

The mind and the sympathetic nervous system

This is an enormous field, which can be only briefly dealt with here. The topic was adumbrated some 2500 years ago by Hippocrates, who clearly perceived a link between mental and physical well-being.[58-60] Almost certainly most laypersons would accept a connection between mental "stress" ("stress" being notoriously difficult to define) and raised blood pressure; by 1931 Hay had embraced the concept medically.[34]

In the mid-19th century, Claude Bernard, Brown-Séquard, and Waller, among others, had shown that the sympathetic nervous system was regulated by centers in the brain, and that stimulation of the sympathetic nerves caused vaso-

constriction. Von Euler in 1946 established that the sympathetic neurotransmitter is noradrenaline (norepinephrine).

Experimental studies in animals by Hess in the 1930s and 1940s demonstrated how emotional and instinctive behavior could be reproduced by exciting discrete groups of neurons. Over the next two decades, Folkow and his colleagues, and subsequently Zanchetti and others, developed these ideas and established that the so-called "defense reaction" would neurogenically induce increases in heart rate and cardiac output; in blood flow through skeletal muscle, heart, and brain at the expense of flow via abdominal organs and skin; and often substantial rises in arterial blood pressure. Folkow went on to link these phenomena with the development of structural changes in resistance arteries, which then reinforced hypertension.

In the 1950s and 1960s, Brod and coworkers showed the pressor effect of forced mental arithmetic. Conversely, Timio and colleagues found that nuns living in seclusion had distinctly lower blood pressure than did control groups of women exposed to the stimuli of urban life but consuming a broadly similar diet.

In the later 20th century, Julius, Esler, and others proceeded to define a syndrome of borderline or mild established essential hypertension in young men and women with sympathetic nervous overactivity, including raised heart rate and cardiac output, with elevated plasma renin. All of these matters are discussed in detail in two recent reviews by Folkow[60] and by Esler.[61]

Adrenal medulla: Adrenaline (epinephrine)

The circulatory effects of intravenous administration of adrenaline (epinephrine) are tachycardia, an increase in systolic blood pressure, and a fall in diastolic blood pressure. These are not features of essential hypertension, leading Pickering to declare in 1955[27]:

> I have never had much doubt that adrenaline is not the agent concerned in producing essential hypertension, since its effects on the circulation are so different from the pattern found in essential hypertension.

However, ideas concerning the sympathetic nervous system mentioned above might link adrenaline with essential hypertension in a more subtle fashion. In 1976 the Glasgow group[62] hypothesized that, because essential hypertension in its early stages can show features of sympathetic nervous system overactivity, the condition may be an exaggeration of the tendency for blood pressure to rise with age. Small increases in pressure resulting from such sympathetic overactivity could cause renal changes, which then maintain the rise in pressure and become the basis of further elevation. According to this group, with more marked hypertension later, the sympathetic element would diminish, but renal vascular resistance would rise.

These concepts were developed further by Brown and MacQuin in 1981,[63] who suggested that a primary abnormality in essential hypertension could be intermittent enhanced release of adrenaline from the adrenal medulla, perhaps as a feature of anxiety and the "defense reaction." Uptake of such episodically excessive circulating adrenaline could then raise blood pressure by facilitating, via presynaptic beta-receptors, noradrenaline release. A substantial body of evidence, reviewed in detail by Nicholls and Richards,[64] has broadly supported these notions.

Adrenal cortex

The review by Nicholls and Richards[61] further concluded that although adrenal cortical hormones might serve to support blood pressure elevation, current evidence is against their having an initiating role in essential hypertension. Certain aspects do, however, merit brief mention here.

Impaired activity of the enzyme 11 beta-hydroxysteroid dehydrogenase-2 (11 β-OHSDH-2) within the kidney limits the normal conversion of cortisol to cortisone, such that intrarenal cortisol gains access to renal mineralocorticoid receptors, and thereby induces mineralocorticoid hypertension. Stewart et al.[65] reported such a case in 1988. This is, of course, overt secondary hypertension. However, the possibility has been raised that milder degrees of such 11 β-OHSDH-2 deficiency within the kidney, or perhaps restricted to vascular smooth muscle, could be responsible for some cases of apparent essential hypertension. Alternatively, a placental deficiency of 11 β-OHSDH could expose the fetus to excessive cortisol, leading to low birth weight and later essential hypertension. These ideas remain to be further explored.

In the early 1960s evidence emerged of a sodium transport inhibitor capable of raising arterial pressure. Later reports indicated the existence of endogenous digitalis-like substances which could inhibit the sodium pump, Na-K-ATPase, and hence stimulate a rise in intracellular sodium and calcium leading to arteriolar constriction. Hamlyn et al.[66] subsequently found evidence that this was possibly a single steroid, ouabain or a closely related isomer, secreted by the adrenal cortex. The validity of these proposals has since, however, been widely questioned, although not refuted.

Aldosterone, the most powerful mineralocorticoid steroid secreted by the adrenal cortex, has interesting and important connotations in essential hypertension. As was indicated in Box 1–1, aldosterone-secreting adenoma (Conn's syndrome) is one among many forms of secondary hypertension, wherein autonomous secretion of an excess of aldosterone by the tumor leads to raised arterial pressure with suppression of the renin–angiotensin system, which is normally a physiologic regulator of aldosterone secretion. Then, in the 1960s and 1970s, it became apparent that a number of hypertensive subjects who did not harbor an adrenocortical adenoma also showed raised aldosterone with low plasma renin levels. This condition was variously termed "idiopathic aldosterone excess," "nontumorous aldosteronism," or "pseudoprimary aldosteronism." In these cases, specific adrenocortical pathology was absent, although nodular changes, or widening, of the zona glomerulosa could sometimes be found, as in essential hypertension. Several groups in the 1970s went on to demonstrate that the aldosterone response to infused angiotensin II became enhanced in essential hypertension. As plasma renin tends to fall with advancing age in essential hypertension, it can readily be seen how such cases might be confused with genuine examples of an aldosterone-secreting tumor.

Indeed, in contrast to patients with aldosterone-secreting adenoma—where plasma angiotensin II and aldosterone are significantly correlated inversely (Figure 1–2A)—in subjects with "idiopathic" aldosterone excess, angiotensin II and aldosterone are positively correlated (Figure 1–2B). Therefore, in the latter aldosterone remains under the physiologic control of the renin–angiotensin system, and these are certainly not instances of "primary" aldosteronism.

Consequently, in 1979 researchers proposed that essential hypertension and so-called nontumorous or "idiopathic" hyperaldosteronism are a continuum of the same condition,[67,68] and this has been repeatedly confirmed in statistical biochemical evaluations.[69,70] Of course, many of these patients, like those with aldosterone-secreting tumors, respond well to potassium-conserving agents such as spironolactone or amiloride.

Despite repeated admonitions, several groups[71–74] continue to describe what is presumably essential hypertension

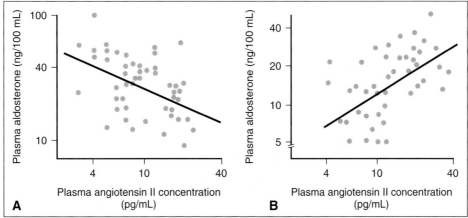

Figure 1–2. Relationship between concurrent basal early morning plasma concentrations of aldosterone and angiotensin II in untreated patients with (**A**) aldosterone-secreting adenoma (r=–0.43, *p*<0.01) and (**B**) idiopathic hyperaldosteronism (r=0.46, *p*<0.01). (Redrawn from Ferris JB, Brown JJ, Fraser R, Lever AF, Robertson JIS in Robertson JIS, ed. *Clinical Aspects of Secondary Hypertension.* Vol. 2, *Handbook of Hypertension.* Amsterdam: Elsevier, 1983:132–161.)

with modestly raised aldosterone, low renin levels, and raised aldosterone/renin ratios but no adrenal tumor, as "primary aldosteronism," and some refer to an "epidemic" of the condition.[75,76] Both tendencies have been roundly attacked by Norman Kaplan.[71]

The kidney and sodium intake

As may be evident from the previous discussion, from the very first glimpses of hypertension in the studies by Bright,[9] the kidney was repeatedly suspected as having a central role in the pathogenesis of hypertension. Others whose work requires mention[77] in this historical account include Franz Volhard, who with Fahr in 1914, provided a detailed description of the renal pathology in Bright's disease; Goldblatt and colleagues, who demonstrated in 1934 that sustained experimental hypertension could be produced by renal artery constriction; and Van Slyke, Homer Smith, and others, who refined the measurement of overall renal function. Then Borst in the Netherlands and Guyton in the United States provided evidence that body salt overload could be involved in raising arterial pressure.

These observations were reinforced by studies of secondary hypertension. Elevated blood pressure in end-stage renal failure was seen to be accompanied by sodium and water retention, and could be alleviated by removal of salt and water at dialysis.[78] With aldosterone-secreting adrenocortical adenoma and consequent aldosterone excess, body sodium content was shown to be increased and the extent of such increase to be closely correlated with hypertension severity. Treatment, either by administration of a potassium-conserving diuretic such as spironolactone or amiloride, or definitively by excision of the tumor, caused blood pressure to fall in proportion to the reduction of body sodium[79] (Figure 1–3).

It can readily be appreciated how these various observations could be linked with proposals made by the Glasgow group,[62] Brown and MacQuin,[63] and Esler and colleagues,[61] that renal lesions caused by sympathetic nervous system overdrive, possibly involving noradrenaline, adrenaline,

and the renin–angiotensin system, could lead to sustained and progressive blood pressure elevation, and hence be involved in the pathogenesis of essential hypertension. In 2002 Johnson et al.[80] elaborated the notion of subtle acquired renal injury as a mechanism of salt sensitivity in hypertension.

Findings pertinent to a different form of secondary hypertension resulting from unilateral renal artery stenosis in which stimulation of the renin–angiotensin system is fundamental to pathogenesis, demonstrated that this form is a syndrome characterized by depletion of body sodium content. Severity of such sodium depletion increases the higher the arterial pressure.[81]

In two large series of patients with untreated essential hypertension during the 1980s, subjects aged less than 40 years had body sodium content that was significantly subnormal, whereas patients aged over 50 had expanded body sodium (Figure 1–4). Independently of age, a significant positive correlation between body sodium content and the level of arterial pressure was reported. In accordance with the findings and concepts mentioned previously, researchers proposed that (1) many young patients with essential hypertension have sodium depletion, perhaps resulting from a natriuretic effect of hypertension caused by a mechanism independent of sodium retention; and (2) in older patients, body sodium content is expanded, possibly as a consequence of hypertension-induced renal changes and/or aldosterone excess.

Meanwhile, various trials had shown modest but distinct declines in blood pressure with dietary sodium restriction. It was emphasized that moderate sodium limitation lasting at least 1 month was most effective; short-term extreme salt deprivation, possibly in part by activating the renin–angiotensin system, could be less impressive. Moreover, the extent of such blood pressure reduction tended to be greater with age; dietary salt restriction was comparatively less effective in young hypertensive subjects. The results of five relevant meta-analyses[84–88] are shown in Table 1–1. The analysis by He and MacGregor[88] is especially relevant, in that only

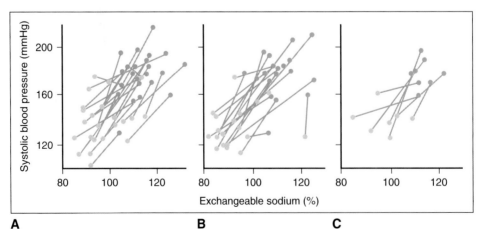

Figure 1–3. Patients with aldosterone-secreting adenoma. Systolic blood pressure related to total exchangeable sodium, expressed as percentage normal in relation to body surface area. **(A)** Before and after surgery. **(B)** Before and during spironolactone. **(C)** Before and during amiloride. (Redrawn from Robertson JIS, Secondary forms of hypertension in Birkenhäger WH, Robertson JIS, Zanchetti A, eds. Hypertension in the twentieth century. *Handbook of Hypertension.* 2004;22: pp. 298–335.)

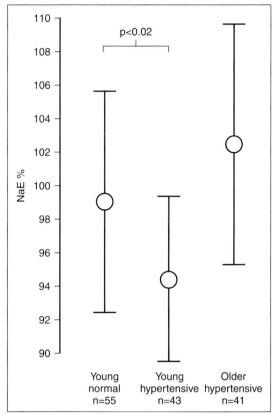

Figure 1–4. Exchangeable sodium (NaE) expressed as percentage normal in terms of body surface area in men. Young hypertensive subjects (aged <35 years) show significantly subnormal body sodium content as compared with young normal subjects. Older hypertensive subjects (aged >50 years) have expanded body sodium. (Data from Johnson RJ, Herrera-Acosta J, Schreiner GF, et al. Subtle acquired renal injury as a mechanism of salt-sensitive hypertension. *N Engl J Med* 2002;346:913–23.)

MEAN REDUCTIONS (MMHG) IN BLOOD PRESSURE (SYSTOLIC/DIASTOLIC) IN FIVE META-ANALYSES OF DIETARY SALT RESTRICTION		
	Overall	
Grobbee and Hofman (81)	3.6/1.98	
	Hypertensive	**Normotensive**
Midgley et al. (82)	3.7/0.9	1.0/0.1
Graudal et al. (84)	3.9/1.9	1.2/0.26
Cutler et al. (83)	4.8/2.5	1.9/1.1
He and MacGregor (85)	4.2/2.4	1.6/0.6

Note: Grobbee and Hofman provided overall figures only; the others analyzed separately those subjects considered initially to be hypertensive or normotensive.

Reprinted by permission from Macmillan Publishers Ltd: from Beevers DG. Salt and cardiovascular disease: not just hypertension. *J Hum Hypertens* 2001;15:749–50.

Table 1–1. Mean Reductions (mmHg) in Blood Pressure (Systolic/Diastolic) in Five Meta-Analyses of Dietary Salt Restriction

studies of moderate salt restriction lasting for at least 1 month were included.

At this juncture, there are no obvious incompatibilities, but recommendations diverge markedly. One group (which includes one of us, DGB)[51] recommends dietary salt restriction regardless of age as a routine part of antihypertensive therapy. Another (which includes JISR)[53] holds that this important issue contains many uncertainties that still require elucidation, and that the appropriateness of salt limitation in young hypertensive subjects is questionable.

Somewhat separate from these arguments is evidence[51,52,88,89] that salt restriction might, *inter alia*, and independently of changes in blood pressure, protect against stroke and left ventricular hypertrophy. Others have conversely worried about the possible cardiovascular hazards of increases in circulating renin, aldosterone, noradrenaline, total cholesterol, and low-density lipoprotein accompanying sodium restriction, and consider that these matters should be subjected to clinical trials.[87] Interestingly, Kaplan and Opie, in a 2006 review entitled "Controversies in hypertension,"[91] evidently discerned no such altercation, and endorsed general dietary salt restriction without reservation.

Urinary sodium and blood pressure

Urinary sodium excretion closely corresponds with the dietary sodium intake. Thus, the epidemiologic assessment of urinary sodium output has attracted much attention because it has been widely assumed that any observed correlation might indicate a causal connection between sodium ingestion and blood pressure. Amid a profusion of studies, two were large and of high methodologic quality.

In 1988 a Scottish report[92] on 7354 men and women aged 40 to 59 years showed only a weak positive correlation between sodium excretion and blood pressure. The authors concluded that sodium had little or no evident independent role in determining blood pressure.

Also in 1988 the Intersalt Cooperative Research Group[93] reported on the relationship in 10,079 men and women aged 20 to 59 years and drawn from 52 centers worldwide. The initial analysis showed a positive association of sodium excretion with median blood pressure, and with the prevalence of (arbitrarily defined) hypertension when all 52 centers were included. However, when four distinctly disparate tribal populations with very low sodium values were excluded, the association disappeared. Meanwhile, in 15 of the individual centers there was a significant positive correlation between sodium excretion and systolic pressure, while a significant negative correlation was reported in two centers. There was also a close relationship between sodium excretion and the increase in blood pressure with age, an effect that persisted even after the four centers with very low salt intake were excluded.

In 1996 a reworking of the "Intersalt" data was published[94] with a more expansive correction for "regression dilution bias." A stronger and significant correlation then emerged between urinary sodium and systolic blood pressure, albeit critics asserted that the reanalysis was inappropriate and invalid.[95]

Whether a genuine correlation might be shown to exist between urinary sodium excretion (and by implication dietary consumption) and blood pressure, it would not, however, permit the conclusion that excessive sodium intake was causal or even contributory. Given the evidence of subnormal body sodium content in young subjects with mild untreated hypertension, their increased sodium consumption could result from an increase in sodium appetite stimulated by that sodium shortfall, probably via angiotensin II.[53]

Genetic aspects

Numerous studies from the 1930s to the present of parent–offspring relationships, natural versus adopted children, and identical and nonidentical twins, have provided evidence of distinct genetic influences on blood pressure in individuals.[96,97] However, one consequence of the controversy between Pickering and Platt,[8,12,13] and the eventual substantiation of Pickering's assertion of the continuous distribution of blood pressure within populations was that blood pressure in individuals was seen as determined by numerous and diverse environmental and genetic influences. Enthusiasm for studies into genetic mechanisms causing raised blood pressure was dampened for several years.

Notwithstanding the smooth continuous but skewed distribution of blood pressures within a given population, there are inevitably a small number of subjects with secondary forms of hypertension concealed within the curve, in whom the causes of any blood pressure elevation are quite distinct. Further, Cusi and Bianchi[97] drew attention to the detailed mathematical analysis performed by McManus[98] on the systolic blood pressures reported in a survey by Bøe et al. in 1957[99] of 67,976 persons over the age of 14 in Bergen, Norway. Pickering had earlier[100] entered an important caveat concerning the systolic readings of Bøe et al. in that they showed marked digit preference—85% ended with 0 and 15% with 5. McManus found that despite the smooth distribution curve apparent on simple inspection of the data, a compound log-normal distribution provided a better and more significant fit than did a single log-normal curve. Although there was only one visible mode, the distribution was shown, in fact, to be compound and "biphasic," as it contained individuals drawn from two separate populations. The appearance of a broadly symmetrical "normal" distribution does not, it was concluded, exclude the existence therein of different discrete distributions due to separate specific genetic (or other) effects. Thus, despite Pickering's earlier concerns, searches for subgroups of essential hypertension with different heritable pathogenetic mechanisms were thereby encouraged.

An increasing resurgence of interest in these aspects occurred, especially during the last three decades of the 20th century. Bianchi and Barlassina,[96] in a major review of the profuse and complex evidence that had accumulated by 2004, concluded that it is unlikely that a single major gene influences essential hypertension. They predicted the imminent identification of a number of gene polymorphisms, each contributing 2% to 10% of genetic variation, depending on the population studied. Further, these authors asserted that gene interactions were likely to be useful targets of future research.

ALCOHOL AND HYPERTENSION

In the 19th century, Mahomed had suggested a link between alcohol excess and hypertension.[10] In a study of French soldiers in 1918, Lian[101] found a clear correlation between alcohol ingestion and the prevalence of hypertension. Such prevalence decreased throughout his classification of "les tres grands buveurs, les grands buveurs, les moyens buveurs, et les sobres."

For a time interest in this relationship declined; Pickering made no mention of the topic in the 1955 and 1968 editions of his book.[27] However, numerous subsequent studies affirmed a likely pressor effect of alcohol ingestion.[102–106] In the 1970s both the Framingham Study and the Copenhagen Heart Study demonstrated a clear relationship between alcohol intake and blood pressure. Even more convincing was the Kaiser Permanente Health Examination Survey of 1977, which confirmed the association in men, women, whites, blacks, and Chinese subjects, independently of educational status and body mass index.[104]

The above results were tempered by repeated observations[44,48] of the apparent protective effect against cardiovascular morbidity of a modest alcoholic intake. That beneficial effect disappeared with high levels of alcohol consumption, which were shown to increase the risk of stroke.[44] The benefit was initially thought to be a property of wine, and especially of red wine, but later studies showed an association with alcohol ingestion regardless of the type of beverage consumed. It has been argued that several meta-analyses of alcohol and cardiovascular disease could have been distorted by the reversion of some subjects to abstinence because of intercurrent illness.[49,50]

BODY WEIGHT

Obesity was recognized by Hippocrates[55,56] as being hazardous to health: "Persons who are naturally of a full habit die suddenly more frequently than those who are slender."

The clinical and epidemiologic measurement of blood pressure in obese persons is particularly subject to error; thus, a suitably large sphygmomanometer cuff must be used on obese persons. Numerous studies[106] have nevertheless confirmed a relationship between body mass index and arterial pressure, and that blood pressure falls with weight reduction. Current estimates from population studies, including the Framingham survey,[35] suggest that excess weight gain may account for as much as 65% to 75% of the risk for essential hypertension.

Hypertension, abdominal obesity, insulin resistance, and dyslipidemia form a cluster that has become known as "the metabolic syndrome." A combination of lifestyle modifications and aggressive antihypertensive drug therapy is recommended for treating patients with this syndrome.[107]

OTHER INFLUENCES

A wide range of other factors may increase blood pressure, including cold weather and high ambient noise levels. Regular exercise, consumption of fresh fruits and vegetables, and the intake of potassium and magnesium can lower blood pressure.[108–110]

RENIN–ANGIOTENSIN SYSTEM

Perhaps the most important contribution to our understanding of the nature of hypertension has been the elucidation of the renin-angiotensin-aldosterone system. Several chapters in this volume are devoted to this system; to avoid repetition, its history is not covered in detail here. Honorable mention must, however, be given to Franz Gross, Jaques Genest, John Laragh, James O. Davis, and, of course, Jerome Conn. In addition, credit for the synthesis of drugs designed to block the system, initially with angiotensin-converting enzyme (ACE) inhibitors and later with angiotensin receptor blockers, must go to Miguel Ondetti, Bernard Rubin, David Cushman, and Pieter Timmermans. This list is, however, intrinsically unfair. Countless others have contributed just as much and many receive recognition elsewhere in this book.

Renin, a protein now recognized as an enzyme, was discovered as a pressor principle in renal extracts by Tigerstedt and Bergman in 1898.[8,37–40,111,112] Elucidation of the complexities of this system comprised a major topic of biochemical, physiologic, and clinical research throughout the 20th century, with numerous and diverse implications for the pathogenesis of hypertension and its treatment.

For three decades after its discovery, renin was largely ignored. Then, in 1934, Goldblatt and colleagues demonstrated that it was possible to produce sustained experimental hypertension by applying constricting clamps to the renal arteries. Surprisingly, although Goldblatt recognized that a humoral substance released from the kidney might be responsible, he did not at first consider renin as a contender. Others did, however, and in 1938 renin was once more extracted from kidneys and partially purified. Delineation of the detailed mode of involvement of renin in the pathogenesis of renovascular hypertension, which was at first thought likely to be simple, turned out to be remarkably intricate.[113]

Kohlstaedt et al. in 1938 and Munoz et al. in 1939 proposed that renin was an enzyme, which was confirmed in 1940 by Page et al. and Braun-Menendez et al. Renin acts on a circulating substrate, angiotensinogen, to form the vasoactive peptide angiotensin II. Details of this complex system as it is currently understood are shown in Figure 1–5. Angiotensinogen was identified chemically by Skeggs et al. in the late 1950s. The amino acid sequences of the bovine and equine octapeptides of angiotensin II were determined, respectively, by Elliott and Peart and by Skeggs et al. in 1956. Angiotensin II was synthesized in the same year.

Practicable assays for circulating renin were introduced in 1963 and 1964, and for angiotensin II in 1971; these were progressively refined in subsequent years. Numerous studies followed that established a wide range of actions attributed to angiotensin II: stimulation of aldosterone and vasopressin secretion, thirst, sodium appetite, a range of direct renal actions, and vagal inhibition (Figure 1–6).

A most important relationship with sodium balance was established in 1963, when it was shown that sodium restriction elevates, and sodium loading depresses, plasma renin.[114] Bing and colleagues pioneered the study of renin in

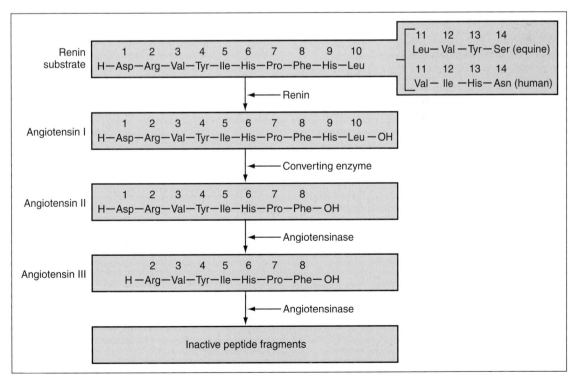

Figure 1–5. Outline of the biochemistry of the renin–angiotensin system. (Redrawn from Nicholls MG, Robertson JIS. The renin system and hypertension. In: Birkenhäger WH, Robertson JIS, Zanchetti A, eds. *Handbook of Hypertension* 2004;22:262–297.)

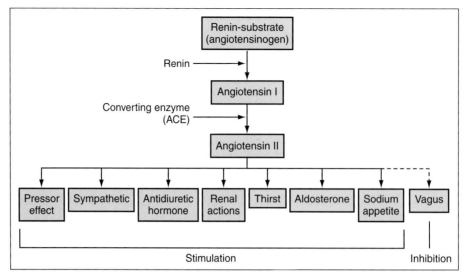

Figure 1–6. The renin–angiotensin system and its principal actions. (Redrawn from Nicholls MG, Robertson JIS. The renin system and hypertension. In: Birkenhäger WH, Robertson JIS, Zanchetti A, eds. *Handbook of Hypertension* 2004;22:262–297.)

extrarenal tissues, with their Danish laboratory reporting the presence of renin in the uterus and salivary glands as early as the 1960s. Renin is now recognized to be present in the brain, heart, blood vessels, adrenal cortex, testis, epididymis, ovary, amniotic fluid, pancreas, and the eye as well.

Two principal receptor subtypes for angiotensin II were identified, namely AT_1 and AT_2. The AT_1 receptor mediates actions of angiotensin II that are indicated in Figure 1–6. Some established, probable, and possible cardiovascular functions of the AT_2 receptor are listed in Table 1–2. Receptor functions comprise an area of intense study in recent years to the present.

By the close of the 20th century, the renin–angiotensin system had been revealed to be widely involved in diverse physiologic processes and clinical disorders. Many of these as they concern humans are listed in Table 1–3.

In the late 20th century, a number of drugs were developed to interrupt the renin–angiotensin system at various sites (Figure 1–5). Thus far, two of the most clinically useful are the ACE inhibitors and the orally active antagonists of the AT_1 receptor. Several effective inhibitors of the enzyme renin were also produced. Initially, none of these possessed adequate oral bioavailability for clinical use, although some recent examples are more promising.[115,116]

One of the least commendable aspects of the study of the renin–angiotensin system has been the reluctance or inability of some researchers to apply proper quantitative standards.[110] Pickering expressed much concern about such deficiencies in 1963,[117] at a time when the first reliable assays for renin were appearing:

> Many workers do not even use a standard ... [but instead employ a] hillbilly method. You cannot compare results from day to day, from one laboratory to another, from country to country.

Even when an international reference preparation of renin was tested and made generally available in 1975,[118] only a few researchers were able and willing to use it. In 1978 one of us (JISR) helped develop a quantitative approach

PHYSIOLOGICAL ROLES OF AT₂ RECEPTOR IN CARDIOVASCULAR SYSTEM	
Action	**Cell or tissue**
Growth inhibition	VSMC Endothelial cell Cardiomyocyte Cardiac fibroblast Embryonic fibroblast
Proapoptosis	VSMC Endothelial cell Cardiomyocyte AT₁ receptor AT₂ receptor (Neuronal cell, R3T3 fibroblast)
Growth promotion	VSMC *in vivo* VSMC in culture Cardiac myocyte
Differentiation	VSMC (neuronal cell)
Decrease in cell matrix	Heart Coronary perivascular cells
Increase in cell matrix	VSMC Cardiac fibroblast Coronary perivascular cells
Decrease in blood pressure	In small arteries
Vasodilatation	Glomerular afferent arteriole
NO production	Kidney Coronary artery and microvessels Aorta
Improvement of cardiac function (LVEDV, LVESV, EF)	Heart
Decrease in chronotrophic effect	Heart

From Nicholls MG, Robertson JIS. The renin system and hypertension. In: Birkenhäger WH, Robertson JIS, Zanchetti A, eds. *Handbook of Hypertension* 2004;22:262–297.

EF, rejection fraction; LVEDV, left ventricular end-diastolic volume; LVESV, left ventricular end-systolic volume; NO, nitric oxide; VSMC, vascular smooth muscle cells.

Table 1–2. Physiological Roles of AT2 Receptor in Cardiovascular System

RENIN SYSTEM IN HEALTH AND DISEASE	
Stimulated	
Certainly or probably involved physiologically, pathophysiologically and/or pathogenically	
Normal pregnancy	Addison's disease and related disorders
Angiotensinogen-secreting tumor	Anorexia nervosa, bulimia nervosa, diuretic abuse, purgative abuse
Renovascular hypertension	Bartter's syndrome and related disorders
Malignant-phase hypertension (some cases)	Vascular and cardiac remodeling
Hemorrhage	Myocardial infarction
Acute circulatory renal failure	Cardiac failure
Multiple organ failure	Chronic renal failure with hypertension
Hepatic cirrhosis	Diabetes insipidus, especially nephrogenic forms
Possibly involved pathophysiologically and/or pathogenically	
Early polycystic kidney disease	Connective tissue diseases
Nephrotic syndrome	Raynaud's phenomenon
Aortic coarctation	Cancerous proliferation
Pheochromocytoma	
Suppressed	
Sodium and fluid excess	Essential hypertension (majority of cases)
Mineralocorticoid hypertension	Primary renin deficiency
Gordon's syndrome	Pregnancy hypertension (i.e., relative to normal pregnancy)
Liddle's syndrome	Syndrome of apparent mineralocorticoid excess

Table 1–3. Renin System in Health and Disease

combining angiotensin II assay with the establishment of relevant dose–response curves.[119] Regrettably, only a few laboratories have since pursued such discipline.

The lack of proper quantification of the renin–angiotensin system continued into the early years of the 21st century, a lamentable deficiency. An analogy may be instructive: consider the difficulties in scientific intercourse if each center were to employ its own peculiar units of blood pressure measurement.

DEVELOPING DRUGS FOR BLOOD PRESSURE REDUCTION

Relationships between hypertension and cardiovascular and renal complications were already becoming clear in the early 20th century, but benefits of reducing blood pressure were by no means apparent. Indeed, it was widely believed that elevated arterial pressure served as a protective response to the narrowing of arterioles, and was necessary in order to maintain perfusion of vital organs. Thus, in 1931 Hay quoted (but did not endorse) the old saw:

> The greatest danger to a man with a high blood pressure lies in its discovery, because then some fool is certain to try and reduce it.[34]

The distinguished American cardiologist, Paul Dudley White, made the following comment:

> Hypertension may be an important compensatory mechanism which should not be tampered with, even were it certain we could control it.[120]

Despite such doubts, attempts at lowering high blood pressure were made, some of them by Hay.[34] In his text-

book on hypertension in 1926, Halls Dally listed a range of procedures[121] directed to that end, almost certainly uniformly futile (Box 1–2).

Effective (but fearsome) antihypertensive measures were subsequently introduced.[26] In 1948, Kempner promulgated his rice and fruit diet, intolerably monotonous if continued for more than a few days, and which probably worked by means of extreme salt restriction. Also in the 1940s and

---

Box 1–2

Selected Antihypertensive Measures Recommended in 1926

Trunecek's solution (sodium chloride, sodium sulphate, sodium bicarbonate, and potassium sulphate)
Total pancreas substance
Calcium salts and atropine (Kylin)
Five grains of blue pill and a saline draught
Thymol oil (oil of thyme)
Benzyl benzoate
Fresh garlic
Dilute hydrochloric acid
Sodium bicarbonate, chloroform, gentia, or rhubarb
Effervescent baths
Douches
Taking the waters at Harrogate, Cheltenham, or Leamington Spa

From Halls Dally JF. *High blood pressure: Its variation and control.* 2nd ed. London: Heinemann, 1926;134–147.

1950s dorsolumbar sympathectomy and extensive bilateral adrenalectomy were performed. These were formidable surgical procedures, with a high incidence of complications and usually unpleasant side effects, although they did reduce blood pressure.[27]

An amusing contemptuous opinion concerning the discomforts of antihypertensive treatment around that time was expressed by S. Weiss of Boston[122]:

> Thus far, what has been done in an effort to reduce the blood pressure? Because of an ill-founded idea that protein was responsible for hypertension and kidney disease, the patient was denied meat and eggs and especially red meat.... His diet was rendered even more unpalatable by withdrawal of salt. Sympathy would doubtless have been extended to this half-starved fellow except that he probably was not able to eat anyway, his teeth having been extracted on the theory that focal infection had something to do with hypertension. Even before this he had sacrificed his tonsils and had his sinuses punctured because of the same theory. In case some food had been consumed, the slight residue was promptly washed out by numerous colonic irrigations.... Of course he was denied alcohol and tobacco as well as coffee and tea.... As a climax to the difficulties of this unfortunate person, he may now fall into the clutches of the neurosurgeon, who is prepared to separate him from his sympathetic nervous system.

Therapeutic expertise did, nevertheless, improve. The earliest effective antihypertensive drugs, the autonomic ganglion–blocking agents, hexamethonium and pempidine, followed logically from surgical sympathectomy, and were introduced in the late 1940s. In subsequent decades, more effective, better-tolerated, and longer-acting, orally effective agents were developed, including, successively, hydralazine, reserpine, thiazide diuretics, guanethidine, methyldopa, beta-blockers, alpha-blockers, clonidine, minoxidil, calcium antagonists, ACE inhibitors, and angiotensin receptor blockers.[123,124]

The more recently introduced drugs provide better blood pressure control. Although the issue is debated, this could be one, but almost certainly not the only, reason for their demonstrable superiority over earlier agents in limiting complications.[23,125–131]

Today, a once-daily dose should produce, 24 hours after ingestion ("trough" drug level) a lowering of systolic pressure by ~10 mmHg and of diastolic pressure by ~8 mmHg. Larger reductions may be achieved with combinations of drugs. These drugs, incidentally, produce somewhat greater changes than have been reported with dietary salt restriction (Table 1–1).

DRUG TREATMENT TRIALS

Hypertension is accompanied by increased cardiovascular morbidity and mortality, but it does not necessarily follow that blood pressure reduction would correct such lesions. Fortunately, however, antihypertensive drugs were developed, and there are now many randomized trials investigating their usefulness.

With the introduction of effective antihypertensive drugs, it was soon determined that they could correct both malignant-phase hypertension (provided that serious renal impairment had not supervened) and overt hypertensive heart failure. Because the course of these conditions, if untreated, was almost invariably fatal, controlled trials were unnecessary, and would, indeed, have been unethical. The early drugs were fairly intolerable; therefore, their use could only be justifiable in patients at very high risk of death.

Demonstration of the ability of antihypertensive drug treatment to prevent complications where the condition had not progressed to the malignant phase or to cardiac failure required controlled trials. In 1964 Hamilton and colleagues[132,133] reported a pioneering study in which initially uncomplicated patients were assigned to antihypertensive drug treatment or simply outpatient review. This trial demonstrated clear benefit from therapy, notably stroke prevention.

Numerous subsequent and larger trials were conducted, and these have been extensively reviewed.[134–137] Strict rules were formulated for the conduct of such studies. These requirements included the allocation of patients at random to control or treatment groups; that the proposed conduct of the trial, especially the method of statistical analysis, be declared at the outset and not subsequently modified; that any additional therapeutic approaches such as dietary or other lifestyle changes should be identical in those allocated to active drug or control; and that the overall system of healthcare must be the same throughout the trial. Whether "open" studies (i.e., non–double-blind investigations) should be accepted without reservation was questioned. Remarkably, these precepts were repeatedly ignored or flouted, such that by the end of the 20th century the situation concerning the benefits of antihypertensive therapy remained depressingly obscure.

The U.S. Veterans Administration (VA) trial of 1967 and 1970[138,139] was designed and initiated as a single study, but was subsequently halted in patients with severe hypertension, with the two resultant patient groups then being analyzed and reported on separately. It is hardly surprising that this behavior engendered much dispute and confusion, with arguments concerning whether it comprised one or two separate trials. As Hampton wrote in 1983,

> The US Veterans' study broke almost every rule of trial design and analysis, and if it were offered to a medical journal today it would probably not be accepted for publication.[134]

Two trials, the Hypertension Detection and Follow-up Program (HDFP)[140,141] and the hypertensive group of those recruited to the Multiple Risk Factor Intervention Trial (MRFIT),[142] were confounded by therapeutic interventions in the treatment group (dietary advice intended to lower body weight, serum cholesterol, and salt intake, plus anti-smoking counseling), which were additional to antihypertensive drugs. Obviously, the effects observed could have been the outcome of the hypertensive drugs, one of the other interventions, or some combination of them.[143,144]

One much-quoted meta-analysis[145] (which, incidentally, accepted several "open" trials for inclusion) discarded the

MRFIT data, explicitly because of potential confounding.[146] Perversely and inexplicably, however, findings from the HDFP were included.

Further, in the HDFP the treatment group was offered a distinctly advantageous overall system of health care. Therefore, it was hardly surprising that mortality from a range of noncardiovascular diseases was lower in the special intervention than in the "control" group. Such benefit can hardly be attributed to the hypertension treatment. As Hampton wrote in 1983,

> The HDFP study ought to be rejected because it was not a proper trial of the treatment of hypertension.... The HDFP seems to show that good care is better than bad care, but it tells us little about hypertension.[134]

Another concern was the inconsistent attitude of trial analysts toward demonstrably unreliable diagnostic criteria for coronary artery disease. In the HDFP, only electrocardiographic data were considered reliable; reports of coronary events elicited by questionnaire or self-reporting were determined to be biased, and thus were initially rejected.[145] It was noted that

> [t]he inclusion of "non-fatal myocardial infarctions" diagnosed by self-reporting or Rose questionnaire has inadvertently but seriously exaggerated the benefits of antihypertensive treatment in HDFP. The large benefits claimed for treatment in young subjects or in women are entirely due to this.[146]

Yet subsequently, and despite clearly recognized flaws, some of the analysts returned, without explanation, to using data that they had themselves earlier condemned as unreliable.[147,148]

Almost certainly the most perceptive and accurate meta-analysis to date was that published by Gueyffier et al. in 1996,[149] which excluded the HDFP, MRFIT, and the part of the VA study dealing with less severe hypertension. The authors found the most impressive treatment benefits in patients aged over 60: 46% reduction in congestive heart failure, 34% in stroke, 23% in cardiovascular mortality (all $p<0.001$); 21% in major coronary events ($p<0.01$); and 10% in all-cause mortality ($p<0.05$). In marked hypertension (entry diastolic pressure at 100 to 130 mmHg), the only complication benefited was congestive cardiac failure, with an 89% reduction in risk ($p<0.001$). In mild-to-moderate hypertension in younger patients, the only

significant benefit was a 49% reduction in stroke ($p<0.001$); the lack of visible benefit concerning coronary events could not be attributed to lower morbidity, because such coronary events were more frequent than stroke in this age group. One of only two trials dealing with recurrent stroke found a significant reduction in the number of deaths with treatment ($p<0.05$).

Sadly, Gueyffier and colleagues soon defected from the standards of that commendably rigorous meta-analysis of 1996. In 1997, Gueyffier, with a different mix of co-authors,[150] addressed the question of differential treatment benefit in men and women. Surprisingly, data from the HDFP, a study that Gueyffier et al. had rejected *in toto* just a year earlier because of its flawed design, were now accepted. Coronary events were computed as elicited by self-reporting, a process already shown to have seriously distorted and exaggerated the apparent benefits of drug treatment in the HDFP ("the large benefits claimed for treatment … in women are entirely due to this"[147]). Thus, the conclusions were guaranteed to be invalid from the outset.

The question of possible differential benefit among several types of antihypertensive agent remains unresolved. As mentioned above, the undoubted protective superiority shown in several studies by more modern drug classes could partly reside in their greater efficacy in lowering blood pressure.[23,124–130] Two trials that addressed this issue[150,151] reached conflicting conclusions. Both trials were, however, seriously confounded by substantial contamination of the treatment groups as initially defined during the course of the studies. The latter ALLHAT study[152] has also been extensively criticized on various other methodologic grounds.[153–155]

It should be apparent from the foregoing that overall the evaluation of antihypertensive treatment trials has been methodologically problematic. At present this deficiency is one of the more embarrassing aspects of research into hypertension. We can, and must, do better.

SUMMARY

This introductory chapter has chronicled progress in our appreciation and understanding of hypertension and its management up to the early 21st century. We hope that the chapter is a useful, if sometimes contentious, perspective on this exciting and therapeutically rewarding subject.

REFERENCES

1. Birkenhäger WH, Robertson JIS, Zanchetti A, eds. *Hypertension in the Twentieth Century: Concepts and Achievements.* Vol. 22, *Handbook of Hypertension.* Amsterdam: Elsevier, 2004.
2. *The Yellow Emperor's Classic of Internal Medicine.* Veith I, trans. Berkeley: University of California Press, 1966.
3. Conrad LI. Arab-Islamic Medicine. In: Bynum WF, Porter R, eds. *Companion Encyclopedia of the History of Medicine.*

Vol. 1. London and New York: Routledge, 1993:676–727.
4. Wujastyk D. Indian medicine. In: Bynum WF, Porter R, eds. *Companion Encyclopedia of the History of Medicine.* Vol. 1. London and New York: Routledge, 1993:755–77.
5. Risse GB. Medical care: the Middle Ages. In: Bynum WF, Porter R, eds. *Companion Encyclopedia of the History of Medicine.* Vol. 1. London and New York: Routledge, 1993:54–7.

6. French R. The Anatomical Tradition. In: Bynum WF, Porter R, eds. *Companion Encyclopedia of the History of Medicine.* Vol. 1. London and New York: Routledge, 1993:81–101.
7. O'Brien E, Fitzgerald D. The history of indirect blood pressure measurement. In: O'Brien E, O'Malley K, eds. *Blood Pressure Measurement.* Vol. 14, *Handbook of Hypertension.* Amsterdam: Elsevier, 1991:1–54.

8. Swales JD, ed. *Classic Papers in Hypertension*. London: Science Press, 1987.

9. Bright R. Tabular view of the morbid appearances in one hundred cases connected with albuminous urine with observations. *Guy's Hosp Rep* 1836;1:380–400.

10. Mahomed FA. The etiology of Bright's disease and the prealbuminuric stage. *Trans Medico-Chirurgical Soc* 1874;57:197–228.

11. Parati G, Mancia G. History of blood pressure measurement from the pre–Riva-Rocci era to the twenty-first century. In: Birkenhäger WH, Robertson JIS, Zanchetti A, eds. *Hypertension in the Twentieth Century: Concepts and Achievements*. Vol. 22, *Handbook of Hypertension*. Amsterdam: Elsevier, 2004:3–32.

12. Robertson JIS. Hypertension: the quantitative versus the qualitative approach. In: Birkenhäger WH, Robertson JIS, Zanchetti A, eds. *Hypertension in the Twentieth Century: Concepts and Achievements*. Vol. 22, *Handbook of Hypertension*. Amsterdam: Elsevier, 2004:125–28.

13. Swales JD. *Platt versus Pickering: An Episode in Recent Medical History*. London: Keynes Press/British Medical Association, 1985.

14. Dawson of Penn: discussion on hyperpiesia. *BMJ* 1925;ii:1161–63.

15. Rose GA. *The Strategy of Preventive Medicine*. Oxford: Oxford University Press, 1992.

16. Skrabanek P. *The Death of Humane Medicine*. London: Social Affairs Unit, 1994.

17. Charlton BG. A critique of Geoffrey Rose's "population strategy" for preventive medicine. *J Royal Soc Med* 1995;88:607–10.

18. Le Fanu J. *The Rise and Fall of Modern Medicine*. London: Little, Brown, 1999:277–80.

19. Tunstall-Pedoe H, Connaghan J, Woodward M, et al. Pattern of declining blood pressure across replicate population surveys of the WHO MONICA project, mid-1980s to mid-1990s, and the role of medication. *BMJ* 2006;332:629–32.

20. Robertson JIS, Ball SG. *Hypertension for the Clinician*. London and Philadelphia: Saunders, 1994.

21. Charcot JM, Bouchard C. Nouvelles recherches sur la pathogénie de l'hémorrhagie cérébrales. *Arch Physiol*;1868:1:110:643,725.

22. Russell RWR. Observations on intracerebral aneurysms. *Brain* 1963;86:425–40.

23. Lip GYH, Beevers M, Beevers DG. The failure of malignant hypertension to decline: a survey of 24 years experience in a multiracial population in England. *J Hypertens* 1994;12:1297–305.

24. Kjeldsen SE, Julius S, Hedner T, Hansson L. Stroke is more common than myocardial infarction in hypertension: analysis based on 11 major randomized intervention trials. *Blood Press* 2001;10:190–92.

25. Graham DI, Lee WR, Cumming AMM, et al. Hypertension and the intracranial and ocular circulations: effect of antihypertensive treatment. In: Robertson

JIS, ed. *Clinical Aspects of Essential Hypertension*. Vol. 1, *Handbook of Hypertension*. Amsterdam: Elsevier, 1983:174–201.

26. Keith NM, Wagener HP, Barker NW. Some different types of essential hypertension: their course and prognosis. *Am J Med Sci* 1939;196:332–43.

27. Pickering GW. *High Blood Pressure*. 2nd ed. London: Churchill, 1968.

28. Dodson PM, Lip GYH, Eames SH, Gibson JM, Bevers DG. Hypertension retinopathy: a review of existing classification systems and a suggestion for a simplified grading system. *J Hum Hypertens* 1996;10:93–98.

29. Schmieder RE, Schädinger H, Messerli FH. Accelerated decline in renal perfusion with aging in essential hypertension. *Hypertension* 1994;23:251–57.

30. Epstein M. Hypertension as a risk factor for progression of chronic renal disease. *Blood Press* 1994;3(Suppl 1):23–28.

31. Kincaid-Smith PS. Renal hypertension. In: Kincaid-Smith PS, Whitworth JA, eds. *Hypertension: Mechanisms and Management*. New York: ADIS Press, 1982:94–101.

32. Beevers DG, Lip GYH. Does non-malignant hypertension cause renal damage? A clinician's view. *J Hum Hypertens* 1996;10:695–9.

33. Zanchetti A. Blood pressure: from systolic to diastolic and back to systolic values as guides to prognosis and treatment. In: Birkenhäger WH, Robertson JIS, Zanchetti A, eds. *Hypertension in the Twentieth Century: Concepts and Achievements*. Vol. 22, *Handbook of Hypertension*. Amsterdam: Elsevier, 2004:143–50.

34. Hay J. The significance of a raised blood pressure. *BMJ* 1931;ii:43–7.

35. Kannel WB. Hypertension as a risk factor: the Framingham contribution. In: Birkenhäger WH, Robertson JIS, Zanchetti A, eds. *Hypertension in the Twentieth Century: Concepts and Achievements*. Vol. 22, *Handbook of Hypertension*. Amsterdam: Elsevier, 2004:129–42.

36. Franklin S, Larson MG, Khan SA, et al. Is pulse pressure useful in predicting risk for coronary heart disease? The Framingham Heart Study. *Circulation* 2001;103:1245–49.

37. Gavras I, Gavras H. Angiotensin II—possible adverse effects on arteries, heart, brain, and kidney: experimental, clinical, and epidemiological evidence. In: Robertson JIS, Nicholls MG, eds. *The Renin–Angiotensin System*. Vol. 1. London and New York: Gower/Mosby, 1993:40.1–40.11.

38. Nicholls MG, Robertson JIS. The renin–angiotensin system in the year 2000. *J Hum Hypertens* 2000;14:649–66.

39. Nicholls MG, Robertson JIS, Inagami T. The renin–angiotensin system in the twenty-first century. *Blood Press* 2001;10:327–43.

40. Robertson JIS. Epidemiology of the renin–angiotensin system in hypertension. In: Bulpitt C, ed. *Handbook of Hypertension* 2000;20:389–427.

41. Matsumura K, Fujii K, Oniki H, et al. Role of aldosterone in left ventricular

hypertrophy in hypertension. *Am J Hypertens* 2006;19:13–18.

42. Stewart AD, Millasseau SC, Dawes M, et al. Aldosterone and left ventricular hypertrophy in Afro-Caribbean subjects with low renin hypertension. *Am J Hypertens* 2006;19:19–24.

43. Milliez P, Girerd X, Plouin P-F, et al. Evidence for an increased rate of cardiovascular events in patients with primary aldosteronism. *J Am Coll Cardiol* 2005;45:1243–48.

44. Gill JS, Zezulka AU, Shipley MJ, et al. Stroke and alcohol consumption. *N Engl J Med* 1986;315:1041–46.

45. Gaziano JM, Buring JE, Breslow JL, et al. Moderate alcohol intake, increased levels of high-density lipoprotein, and its subfractions, and decreased risk of myocardial infarction. *N Engl J Med* 1993;329:1829–34.

46. Palmer AJ, Fletcher AE, Bulpitt CJ, et al. Alcohol intake and cardiovascular mortality in hypertensive patients: report from the Department of Health Hypertension Care Computing Project. *J Hum Hypertens* 1995;12:957–64.

47. Rimm EB, Williams P, Fosher J, et al. Moderate alcohol intake and lower risk of coronary heart disease: meta-analysis of effects on lipids and haemostatic factors. *BMJ* 1999;319:1523–28.

48. Mikamal KJ, Conigrave KM, Mittleman MA, et al. Roles of drinking pattern and type of alcohol consumed in coronary heart disease in man. *N Engl J Med* 2003;348:109–18.

49. Shaper AG, Wannamethee G, Walker M. Alcohol and mortality in British men: explaining the U-shaped curve. *Lancet* 1988;ii:1267–72.

50. Tanne JH. Meta-analysis challenges benefits of moderate drinking. *BMJ* 2006;332:811.

51. Beevers DG. Salt and cardiovascular disease: not just hypertension. *J Hum Hypertens* 2001;15:749–50.

52. Kaplan NM. Evidence in favor of moderate dietary sodium restriction. *Am J Hypertens* 2000;13:8–13.

53. Robertson JIS. Dietary salt and hypertension: a scientific issue or a matter of faith? *J Eval Clin Pract* 2003;9:1–22.

54. Robertson JIS, ed. *Clinical Aspects of Secondary Hypertension*. Vol. 2, *Handbook of Hypertension*. Amsterdam: Elsevier, 1983.

55. Robertson JIS, ed. *Clinical Hypertension*. Vol. 15, *Handbook of Hypertension*. Amsterdam: Elsevier, 1992.

56. Robertson JIS. Secondary forms of hypertension. In: Birkenhäger WH, Robertson JIS, Zanchetti A, eds. *Hypertension in the Twentieth Century: Concepts and Achievements*. Vol. 22, *Handbook of Hypertension*. Amsterdam: Elsevier, 2004:298–335.

57. Rose G. Reflections on changing times. *BMJ* 1990;301:683–87.

58. Hannaway C. Environment and miasmata. In: Bynum WF, Porter R, eds. *Companion Encyclopedia of the History of Medicine*. Vol. 1. London and New York: Routledge, 1993:292–308.

59. Bynum WF. Nosology. In: Bynum WF, Porter R, eds. *Companion Encyclopedia of the History of Medicine*. Vol. 1. London and New York: Routledge, 1993:335–56.

60. Folkow B. Considering "The mind" as a primary cause. In: Birkenhäger WH, Robertson JIS, Zanchetti A, eds. *Hypertension in the Twentieth Century: Concepts and Achievements*. Vol. 22, *Handbook of Hypertension*. Amsterdam: Elsevier, 2004:59–80.

61. Esler M. Looking at the sympathetic nervous system as a primary source. In: Birkenhäger WH, Robertson JIS, Zanchetti A, eds. *Hypertension in the Twentieth Century: Concepts and Achievements*. Vol. 22, *Handbook of Hypertension*. Amsterdam: Elsevier, 2004:81–103.

62. Brown JJ, Lever AF, Robertson JIS, et al. Pathogenesis of essential hypertension. *Lancet* 1976;i:1217–19.

63. Brown MJ, MacQuin I. Is adrenaline the cause of essential hypertension? *Lancet* 1981;ii:1386–89.

64. Nicholls MG, Richards AM. Looking at the adrenals as a primary source. In: Birkenhäger WH, Robertson JIS, Zanchetti A, eds. *Hypertension in the Twentieth Century: Concepts and Achievements*. Vol. 22, *Handbook of Hypertension*. Amsterdam: Elsevier, 2004::104–22.

65. Stewart PM, Corrie JET, Shackleton CHL, et al. Syndrome of apparent mineralocorticoid excess. *J Clin Invest* 1988;82:340–49.

66. Hamlyn JM, Hamilton BP, Manunta P. Endogenous ouabain, sodium balance, and blood pressure: review and a hypothesis. *J Hypertens* 1996;14:151–67.

67. Davies DL, Beevers DG, Brown JJ, et al. Aldosterone and its stimuli in normal and hypertensive man: are essential hypertension and primary hyperaldosteronism without tumour the same condition? *J Endocrinol* 1979;81:79P–91P.

68. Brown JJ, Lever AF, Robertson JIS, et al. Are idiopathic hyperaldosteronism and low-renin hypertension variants of the same condition? *Ann Clin Biochem* 1979;16:380–88.

69. McAreavey D, Murray GD, Lever AF, et al. Similarity of idiopathic aldosteronism and essential hypertension: a statistical comparison. *Hypertension* 1983;5:116–21.

70. Aitchison J, Brown JJ, Ferriss JB, et al. Quadric analysis in the preoperative distinction between patients with and without adrenocortical tumors in hypertension with aldosterone excess and low plasma renin. *Am Hypertens J* 1971;82:660–71.

71. Kaplan NM. Cautions over the current epidemic of primary aldosteronism. *Lancet* 2001;357:953–54.

72. Fraser R, Lever AF, Brown JJ, et al. Cautions over idiopathic aldosteronism. *Lancet* 2001;358:332.

73. Padfield PL. Primary aldosteronism, a common entity? The myth persists. *J Hum Hypertens* 2002;16:159–62.

74. Robertson JIS. Aldosterone excess and essential hypertension. *J Hum Hypertens* 2002;16:527.

75. Stowasser M. Primary aldosteronism: revival of a syndrome. *J Hypertens* 2000;18:363–66.

76. Lim PO, Dow E, Brennan G, et al. High prevalence of primary aldosteronism in the Tayside hypertension clinic population. *J Hum Hypertens* 2000;14:311–15.

77. Birkenhäger WH, De Leeuw PW. Looking at the kidney as a primary source: Experimental and clinical aspects. In: Birkenhäger WH, Robertson JIS, Zanchetti A, eds. *Hypertension in the Twentieth Century: Concepts and Achievements*. Vol. 22, *Handbook of Hypertension*. Amsterdam: Elsevier, 2004:35–58.

78. Brown JJ, Düsterdieck G, Fraser R, et al. Hypertension and chronic renal failure. *Br Med Bull* 1971;27:128–35.

79. Beretta-Piccoli C, Davies DL, Brown JJ, et al. Relation of blood pressure with body and plasma electrolytes in Conn's syndrome. *J Hypertens* 1983;1:197–205.

80. Johnson RJ, Herrera-Acosta J, Schreiner GF, et al. Subtle acquired renal injury as a mechanism of salt-sensitive hypertension. *N Engl J Med* 2002;346:913–23.

81. McAreavey D, Brown JJ, Cumming AMM, et al. Inverse relation of exchangeable sodium and blood pressure in hypertensive patients with renal artery stenosis. *J Hypertens* 1983;1:297–302.

82. Beretta-Piccoli C, Davies DL, Boddy K, et al. Relation of arterial pressure with body sodium, body potassium, and plasma potassium in essential hypertension. *Clin Sci* 1982;63:257–70.

83. Beretta-Piccoli C, Weidmann P, Brown JJ, et al. Body sodium blood volume state in essential hypertension: abnormal relation of exchangeable sodium to age and blood pressure in male patients. *J Cardiovasc Pharmacol* 1984;6(Suppl 1):134–42.

84. Grobbee DE, Hofman A. Does sodium restriction lower blood pressure? *BMJ* 1986;293:27–29.

85. Midgely JP, Matthew AG, Greenwood CMT, et al. Effect of reduced dietary sodium on blood pressure: a meta-analysis of randomized controlled trials. *JAMA* 1996;275:1590–97.

86. Cutler JA, Follman D, Allender PS. Randomized trials of sodium reduction: an overview. *Am J Clin Nutr* 1997;65(Suppl):643–51.

87. Graudal NA, Galløe AM, Garred P. Effects of sodium restriction on blood pressure, renin, aldosterone, catecholamines, cholesterols, and triglyceride: a meta-analysis. *JAMA* 1998;279:1383–91.

88. He FJ, MacGregor GA. Effects of longer-term modest salt reduction on blood pressure: a meta-analysis of randomised controlled trials. Implications for public health. *J Hum Hypertens* 2000;14:846–47.

89. Messerli FH, Schmieder RE, Weir MR. Salt: a perpetrator of hypertensive target organ disease? *Arch Intern Med* 1997;157:2449–52.

90. Antonios TFT, MacGregor GA. Salt—more adverse effects. *Lancet* 1996;348:250–51.

91. Kaplan NM, Opie LH. Controversies in hypertension. *Lancet* 2006;367:168–76.

92. Smith WCS, Crombie IK, Tavendale RT, et al. Urinary electrolyte excretion, alcohol consumption, and blood pressure in the Scottish heart health study. *BMJ* 1988;297:329–30.

93. Intersalt Cooperative Research Group. Intersalt: an international study of electrolyte excretion and blood pressure. Results for 24 hour urinary sodium and potassium excretion. *BMJ* 1988;297:319–28.

94. Elliott P, Stamler J, Nichols R, et al. Intersalt revisited: further analyses of 24 hour urinary sodium excretion and blood pressure within and across populations *BMJ* 1996;312:1249–53.

95. Davey Smith G, Phillips AN. Correction for regression dilution bias in Intersalt was misleading. *BMJ* 1997;315:485–86.

96. Bianchi G, Barlassina C. From familial to genetic hypertension. In: Birkenhäger WH, Robertson JIS, Zanchetti A, eds. *Hypertension in the Twentieth Century: Concepts and Achievements*. Vol. 22, *Handbook of Hypertension*. Amsterdam: Elsevier, 2004:195–215.

97. Cusi D, Bianchi G. Genetic and molecular aspects of hypertension. In: Robertson JIS, ed. *Clinical Hypertension*. Vol. 15, *Handbook of Hypertension*. Amsterdam: Elsevier, 1992:63–94.

98. McManus IC. Bimodality of blood pressure levels. *Stat Med* 1983;2:253–58.

99. Bøe J, Humerfelt S, Wederwang F. Blood pressure in a population: blood pressure readings and height and weight determinations in the adult population of the city of Bergen. *Acta Med Scand* 1957;157(Suppl 321).

100. Pickering GW. The nature of essential hypertension. *Lancet* 1960;ii:1031–32.

101. Lian C. L'alcoholisme cause d'hypertension artérielle. *Bull Acad Med (Paris)* 1915;74:525–28.

102. Beevers DG. Alcohol and hypertension. *Lancet* 1977;ii:114–15.

103. Saunders JB, Beevers DG, Paton A. Alcohol-induced hypertension. *Lancet* 1981;ii:653–56.

104. Klatsky AL. Blood pressure and alcohol consumption. In: Bulpitt CJ, ed. *Epidemiology of Hypertension*. Vol. 20, *Handbook of Hypertension*. Amsterdam: Elsevier, 2000:249–73.

105. Beilin LJ. Alcohol, hypertension, and cardiovascular disease. *J Hypertens* 1995;13:939–42.

106. Beilin LJ. Non-pharmacological management of hypertension: science, consensus, and controversies. In: Birkenhäger WH, Robertson JIS, Zanchetti A, eds. *Hypertension in the Twentieth Century: Concepts and Achievements*. Vol. 22, *Handbook of Hypertension*. Amsterdam: Elsevier, 2004:417–56.

107. Landsberg L. The metabolic syndrome: diabetes, obesity, and hypertension. *Handbook of Hypertension* 2004;22:245–61.

108. He FJ, MacGregor GA. Potassium intake and blood pressure. *Am J Hypertens* 1999;12:849–51.

109. Jee SH, Miller ER, Guallar E, et al. The effect of magnesium supplementation on blood pressure: a meta-analysis of randomized clinical trials. *Am J Hypertens* 2002;15:691–96.

110. Appel LJ, Moore TJ, Obarzanek E, et al. A clinical trial of the effects of dietary patterns on blood pressure. *N Engl J Med* 1997;336:1117–24.

111. Robertson JIS, Nicholls MG, eds. *The Renin-Angiotensin System*. London and New York: Gower/Mosby, 1993.

112. Nicholls MG, Robertson JIS. The renin-angiotensin system and hypertension. In: Birkenhäger WH, Robertson JIS, Zanchetti A, eds. *Hypertension in the Twentieth Century: Concepts and Achievements*. Vol. 22, *Handbook of Hypertension*. Amsterdam: Elsevier, 2004:262–97.

113. Robertson JIS. Renin and the pathophysiology of renovascular hypertension. In: Robertson JIS, Nicholls MG, eds. *The Renin–Angiotensin System*. Vol. 2. London and New York: Gower/Mosby, 1993:55.1–55.34.

114. Brown JJ, Davies DL, Lever AF, et al. Influence of sodium loading and sodium depletion on plasma-renin in man. *Lancet* 1963;ii:278–79.

115. Stanton AV, Barton J, Jensen C, et al. Antihypertensive efficacy of aliskiren (SP100), a new orally-active renin inhibitor. *J Hum Hypertens* 2002;16:899–900.

116. Wood JM, Schnell CR, Cumin F, et al. Aliskiren, a novel, orally effective renin inhibitor, lowers blood pressure in marmosets and spontaneously hypertensive rats. *J Hypertens* 2005;23:417–26.

117. Pickering GW. Concluding remarks. International Symposium on Angiotensin, Sodium, and Hypertension, Quebec, Canada, October 11–14, 1963. *CMAJ* 1964;90:340–41.

118. Bangham DR, Robertson I, Robertson JIS, et al. An international collaborative study of renin assay: establishment of the international reference preparation of human renin. *Clin Sci* 1975;48(Suppl):135–59.

119. Brown JJ, Casals-Stenzel J, Cumming AMM, et al. Angiotensin II, aldosterone, and arterial pressure: a quantitative approach. Arthur C. Corcoran Memorial Lecture by J. Ian S. Robertson. *Hypertension* 1979;1:159–79.

120. White PD. *Heart Disease*. New York: Macmillan, 1931.

121. Halls Dally JF. *High Blood Pressure*. 2nd ed. London: Heinemann, 1926:134–147.

122. Weiss S. (cited in Kannel [35]).

123. Van Zwieten PA, Greenlee WJ, eds. *Antihypertensive Drugs*. Amsterdam: Harwood Academic Publishers, 1997.

124. Van Zwieten PA. Development of antihypertensive drugs: from the bench to the clinic. In: Birkenhäger WH, Robertson JIS, Zanchetti A, eds. *Hypertension in the Twentieth Century: Concepts and Achievements*. Vol. 22, *Handbook of Hypertension*. Amsterdam: Elsevier, 2004:457–86.

125. Heart Outcomes Prevention Evaluation (HOPE) Study Investigators. Effects of an angiotensin-converting-enzyme inhibitor, ramipril, on cardiovascular events in high-risk patients. *N Engl J Med* 2000;342:145–53.

126. Mourad J-J, Safar ME, O'Rourke MF. Who is fooling us? *Lancet* 2002;360:89.

127. Dahlöf B, Devereux RB, Kjeldsen SE, et al. Cardiovascular morbidity and mortality in the losartan intervention for endpoint reduction in hypertension study (LIFE): a randomised trial against atenolol. *Lancet* 2002;359:995–1003.

128. Dahlöf B, Sever PS, Poulter NR, et al. Prevention of cardiovascular events with an antihypertensive regimen of amlodipine adding perindopril as required versus atenolol adding bendrofluazide as required, in the Anglo–Scandinavian cardiac outcomes trial—blood pressure lowering arm (ASCOT-BPLA): a multicentre randomised controlled trial. *Lancet* 2005;366:895–906.

129. Poulter NR, Wedel H, Dahlöf B, et al. Role of blood pressure and other variables in the differential cardiovascular event rates noted in the Anglo–Scandinavian cardiac outcomes trial—blood pressure lowering arm (ASCOT-BPLA). *Lancet* 2005;366:907–13.

130. Staessen JA, Birkenhäger WH. Evidence that new antihypertensives are superior to older drugs. *Lancet* 2005;366:869–71.

131. Kjeldsen SE, Hedner T, Narkiewicz K. Angiotensin receptor blockers and endpoint protection. *Blood Press* 2005;14:195.

132. Hamilton M, Thompson EN, Wisniewski TKM. The role of blood pressure control in preventing complications of hypertension. *Lancet* 1964;i:235–38.

133. Beevers DG. The 40th anniversary of the publication in 1964 of the first trial of the treatment of uncomplicated, severe hypertension by Hamilton, Thompson and Wisniewski. *J Hum Hypertens* 2004;18:831–33.

134. Hampton JR. An appraisal of hypertension trials. *Medicographia* 1983;5(Suppl 1):12–15.

135. Robertson JIS. Hypertension. In: Pitt B, Julian D, Pocock S, eds. *Clinical Trials in Cardiology*. London and Philadelphia: Saunders, 1997:115–60.

136. Robertson JIS. A critique of hypertension treatment trials and of their evaluation. *J Eval Clin Pract* 2001;7:149–64.

137. Robertson JIS. Trials of antihypertensive drug treatment: the strange phenomenon of steadily improving studies yet regressive evaluation. In: Birkenhäger WH, Robertson JIS, Zanchetti A, eds. *Hypertension in the Twentieth Century: Concepts and Achievements*. Vol. 22, *Handbook of Hypertension*. Amsterdam: Elsevier, 2004:487–503.

138. Veterans Administration Cooperative Study Group on Antihypertensive Agents. Effects of treatment on morbidity in hypertension: results in patients with diastolic pressures averaging 115 through 129 mmHg. *JAMA* 1967;202:1028–34.

139. Veterans Administration Cooperative Study Group on Antihypertensive Agents. Effects on morbidity in hypertension. II. Results in patients with diastolic blood pressures averaging 90 through 114 mmHg. *JAMA* 1970;213:1143–52.

140. Hypertension Detection and Follow-up Program Cooperative Group. Five-year findings of the hypertension detection and follow-up program (HDFP). I. Reduction in mortality of persons with high blood pressure, including mild hypertension. *JAMA* 1979;242:2562–71.

141. Hypertension Detection and Follow-up Program Cooperative Group. Five-year findings of the hypertension detection and follow-up program (HDFP). II. Mortality by race, sex, and age. *JAMA* 1979;242:2572–77.

142. Multiple Risk Factor Intervention Trial Group. Multiple risk factor intervention trial: risk factor changes and mortality results. *JAMA* 1982;248:1465–77.

143. Beevers DG. Comments on the hypertension detection and follow-up program (HDFP). *Roy Soc Med Int Congr Symp Series* 1980;26:9–11.

144. Egger M, Davey Smith G. Risks and benefits of treating hypertension: a misleading meta-analysis? *J Hypertens* 1995;13:813–15.

145. Cutler JA, MacMahon SW, Furberg CD. Controlled clinical trials of drug treatment for hypertension: a review. *Hypertension* 1989;13(Suppl 1):36–44.

146. Ramsay LE, Wallis EJ, Yeo WW, et al. The rationale for differing national recommendations for the treatment of hypertension. *Am J Hypertens* 1998;11(Suppl):79–88.

147. Collins R, Peto R, MacMahon S, et al. Blood pressure, stroke, and coronary heart disease. Part 2: short-term reductions of blood pressure: overview of randomised drug trials in their epidemiological context. *Lancet* 1990;335:827–38.

148. MacMahon S. The effects of antihypertensive drug treatment on the incidence of stroke and of coronary heart disease. *Clin Exp Hypertens* 1989;A11:807–23.

149. Gueyffier F, Froment A, Gouton M. New meta-analysis of treatment trials of hypertension: improving the estimate of benefit. *J Hum Hypertens* 1996;10:1–8.

150. Gueyffier F, Boutitie F, Boissel J-P, et al. Effect of antihypertensive drug treatment on cardiovascular outcomes in women and men: meta-analysis of individual patient data from randomized, controlled trials. *Ann Intern Med* 1997;126:761–67.

151. Wing LMH, Reid CM, Ryan P, et al. A comparison of outcomes with angiotensin-converting-enzyme inhibitors and diuretics for hypertension in the elderly. *N Engl J Med* 2003;348:583–92.

152. The ALLHAT officers: The antihypertensive and lipid-lowering treatment to prevent heart attack trial (ALLHAT). *JAMA* 2002;288:2981–97.

153. Meltzer JI. A specialist in clinical hypertension critiques ALLHAT. *Am J Hypertens* 2003;16:416–20.

154. Sjöholm A. ALLHAT: a critical assessment. *Blood Press* 2004;13:75–9.

155. Opie L. Marketing ALLHAT. *Lancet* 2004;363:169–70.

Chapter

2 Blood Pressure in Westernized and Isolated Populations

Lydia A. Bazzano, Jiang He, and Paul K. Whelton

Key Findings

- Cardiovascular disease accounts for 30.9% of global mortality and 10.3% of the global burden of disease.

- Hypertension is estimated to account for 4.4% of the total global burden of disease and contributes to 44% of all ischemic heart disease.

- Gender and race/ethnicity influence age-related changes in blood pressure.

- The distribution of hypertension in Westernized populations is influenced by a number of factors, including age, gender, and racial/ethnic composition of the population under study.

- The lowest prevalence of hypertension for both men and women was in Asia, other than China, and the Pacific Islands.

- Populations who do not demonstrate an age-related rise in blood pressure tend to live in primitive societies isolated from modern lifestyles and have a low salt intake, high level of physical activity, and an absence of obesity. Where there is migration to a more Westernized environment or where "modernization" is occurring *in situ*, blood pressure rises with age and hypertension begins to appear.

Despite recent advances in prevention and treatment, cardiovascular diseases (CVD) remain a major public health problem in both developed and developing countries. Once considered a disease of the industrialized world, it is now apparent that CVD is a public health menace worldwide. Currently CVD accounts for 30.9% of global mortality and 10.3% of the global burden of disease.[1] Worldwide, heart disease and stroke are responsible for nearly 17 million deaths each year, and at present, twice as many deaths from CVD now occur in developing countries compared to developed countries.[2] According to global burden of disease estimates, hypertension is one of the top 10 risk factors for disease worldwide.[2] Hypertension alone is estimated to account for 4.4% of the total global burden of disease and contributes to 44% of all ischemic heart disease.[3]

It has been recognized for some time that a direct positive relationship exists between blood pressure and CVD risk. This relationship has been observed in men and women of all ages, race/ethnic groups, and countries, regardless of other risk factors for CVD; it is strong, graded, and continuous across all levels of blood pressure.[4] Because

hypertension is such a powerful and modifiable risk factor for the development of CVD, understanding the distribution and determinants of blood pressure in populations worldwide is of vital importance. Examining patterns of blood pressure distribution in Westernized or acculturated societies, those in isolated or unacculturated societies, and those in migrants from these societies can shed light on the role of environmental factors in the development of high blood pressures and hypertension.

BLOOD PRESSURE IN WESTERNIZED POPULATIONS

Relationship of blood pressure and age

Many studies in Westernized populations have found remarkably consistent results regarding the relationship of blood pressure to age. Nearly all have demonstrated that mean blood pressure rises with age in Westernized populations, and therefore, so does the incidence and prevalence of hypertension.[5] However, depending on an individual's stage of life, gender, race, initial level of blood pressure and exposure to environmental factors, this general trend may vary a great deal.

Childhood and adolescence

The 1987 report of the Second Task Force on Blood Pressure Control in Children and its 1996 update compiled some of the best available data on the relationship of blood pressure and age in childhood and adolescence.[6,7] Blood pressure measurements recorded on more than 70,000 children aged 1 to 20 who participated in nine cross-sectional surveys, were pooled to create normative blood pressure distribution curves by age. Blood pressure measurements were standardized and were obtained with the child in a seated position using a mercury sphygmomanometer or a Doppler instrument in infants. Among infants and children aged 3 to 12 years, the fourth Korotkoff sound was used to signify diastolic blood pressure, while in adolescents (13 to 18 years), both fourth and fifth Korotkoff sounds were used as markers of diastolic blood pressure. At birth, the average systolic and diastolic pressures were 70 mmHg and 50 mmHg, respectively. There is a rapid and pronounced rise in systolic blood pressure, so that by the end of the first year of life, systolic blood pressure averages 94 mmHg, while diastolic blood pressure rises only 2 mmHg over the same period. Thereafter, there is a tendency for blood pressure to rise with increasing age throughout the remainder of childhood and adolescence. The slope for age-related change in blood pressure is much steeper for systolic (1 to 2 mmHg/year) than for diastolic (0.5 to 1 mmHg/year) blood pressure.

Evidence from the pooled data also reflects the influence of gender on blood pressure. From the age of 4 years onwards, the slope of the age-related change in blood pressure remains fairly constant for boys. For girls the pattern parallels that of boys until adolescence, when the slope for girls becomes considerably flatter than that of boys. Taken as a whole, the evidence suggests little difference in pattern of average blood pressure levels between genders until adolescence. During the teenage years, however, average blood pressure was consistently higher for boys compared to girls. As a consequence, by age 18, boys had average systolic and diastolic blood pressures that were almost 10 and 5 mmHg higher than the corresponding values for girls. There was no evidence for a systematic difference between the average levels of blood pressure in children of different race/ethnicities (white, black, and Mexican American). Data from the Bogalusa Heart Study and the Child and Adolescent Trial for Cardiovascular Health, however, indicate that mean blood pressure level is higher in black compared to white children and lower in Mexican-American compared to black and white children.[8,9]

Adults and the elderly

There is a general tendency for both systolic and diastolic blood pressure to rise during adulthood.[5] The age-related rate of increase is consistently greater for systolic than for diastolic blood pressure. Systolic blood pressure tends to rise until the eighth or ninth decade, whereas diastolic blood pressure tends to remain constant or decline after the fifth decade. As a consequence, pulse pressure increases progressively with aging. This is particularly true during the latter part of life.

The pattern of blood pressure change with age is modified to a certain extent by gender and race/ethnicity. In young adults, systolic and diastolic blood pressures tend to be higher in men than in women; however, the slope of age-related blood pressure increase is steeper for women than for men. As a result, by the seventh decade women tend to have levels of systolic blood pressure that equal or exceed those seen in men. Selective survivorship may explain part of this gender-related difference in blood pressure, as men with high blood pressure earlier on may be less likely to survive and contribute to average blood pressure later in life. Longitudinal analysis of the Framingham cohort and other data sets suggests, however, that selective survivorship only explains a portion of these age-related trends.[10]

Race and ethnicity also influence age-related change in blood pressure. This phenomenon has been well documented in the Third National Health and Nutrition Examination Survey (NHANES III) (Figure 2–1). In men and women, non-Hispanic blacks had the highest and non-Hispanic whites had the lowest average systolic blood pressure, although the differences among the three race/ethnicity groups were small. In women, non-Hispanic whites con-

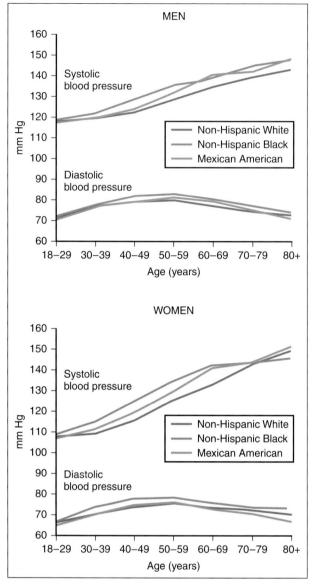

Figure 2–1. Mean systolic and diastolic blood pressures by age and race/ethnicity for men and women. U.S. population 18 years and older.

tinued to have the lowest average systolic blood pressure during the sixth decade. By the seventh decade, however, the three race/ethnicity groups had similar average systolic blood pressure levels. Non-Hispanic black women had a higher average diastolic blood pressure than non-Hispanic white or Mexican-American women. The same was true in men until the end of the fifth decade. Thereafter, diastolic blood pressures were similar in the three race/ethnicity groups.

CLASSIFICATION OF HYPERTENSION

The Sixth Report of the U.S. Joint National Committee for Detection, Evaluation, and Treatment of High Blood Pressure (JNC VI) was published in 1997 and recommended a classification of blood pressure that was adopted by the World Health Organization–International Society of

Hypertension.[11,12] This classification scheme was updated in the Seventh Report (JNC VII), published in 2003 (Table 2–1).[13] These criteria are for individuals who are not on antihypertensive medication and who are not acutely ill. The classification is based on the average of two or more blood pressure readings after an initial screening visit. When systolic blood pressure and diastolic blood pressure fall into different categories, the higher category should be selected to classify the individual's blood pressure.

According to JNC VII criteria, normal blood pressure is defined as a systolic blood pressure less than 120 mmHg and a diastolic blood pressure less than 80 mmHg. Those with a systolic blood pressure between 120 mm and 139 mmHg or diastolic blood pressure between 80 and 89 mmHg are designated as having prehypertension. Hypertension is characterized by a confirmed elevation of systolic (≥140 mmHg) or diastolic (≥90 mmHg) blood pressure. Hypertension is further characterized into two stages according to the patient's level of systolic and diastolic blood pressure. Stage 1 is the milder (systolic 140 to 159 mmHg and/or diastolic 90 to 99 mmHg) and most common form of hypertension. It accounts for approximately 80% of hypertension. Stage 2 hypertension includes those with systolic blood pressure of 160 mmHg or greater and/or diastolic blood pressure of 100 mmHg or greater. Isolated systolic hypertension is defined as systolic blood pressure of 140 mmHg or greater and diastolic blood pressure below 90 mmHg and staged appropriately.

DISTRIBUTION OF HYPERTENSION IN WESTERNIZED POPULATIONS

The distribution of hypertension in Westernized populations is influenced by a number of factors. The incidence and prevalence of hypertension varies by age, gender, and racial/ethnic composition of the population under study. Factors such as environmental exposures, including intake of dietary sodium and potassium, body weight, alcohol consumption, and physical activity, also influence the incidence and prevalence of hypertension; however, those topics are beyond the scope of this chapter.

Age

As discussed previously, there is a large body of data available from Western populations that demonstrates rising mean blood pressure with increasing age. Consequently, the prevalence of hypertension increases with age. In NHANES III, the prevalence of hypertension increased with increasing age (Table 2–2). In the 18- to 24-year-old group, the overall prevalence of hypertension was only 2.6%. The prevalence of hypertension increased to 5.4% in 25- to 34-year-olds and 13.0% in 35- to 44-year-olds. The prevalence rates continued to rise with 27.6% of 45- to 54-year-olds affected and 43.7% of 55- to 64-year-olds. In 65- to 74-year-olds, the overall prevalence was 59.6% and in the 75-and-older age group, it was 70.3%. Several longitudinal cohort studies have also documented that incidence of hypertension increases with age.[14–16]

Gender

Overall the prevalence and incidence of hypertension are slightly higher in men compared to women. In NHANES III, the age-adjusted prevalence of hypertension for all races/ethnicities was 23.5% in men and 23.3% in women. In whites the prevalence was 23.4% in men and 23.1% in women. In blacks the prevalence was slightly higher in women than in men, 28.2% and 27.9%, respectively. The relationship between gender and hypertension is modified by age. In young adults, the prevalence and incidence of hypertension are higher in men than in women. However, by their sixties, women tend to have levels of blood pressure that equal or exceed those seen in men. Consequently, the prevalence of hypertension is higher in women than in men late in life.

CLASSIFICATION OF BLOOD PRESSURE FOR ADULTS AGED 18 AND OLDER ACCORDING TO JNC VII[a]			
Category	Systolic Blood Pressure (mmHg)		Diastolic Blood Pressure (mmHg)
Normal[b]	<120	and	<80
Prehypertension	120–139	and	81–89
Hypertension[c]			
Stage 1	140–159	or	90–99
Stage 2	≥160	or	≥100

[a]Not taking antihypertensive drugs and not acutely ill. When systolic and diastolic pressures fall into different categories, the higher category should be selected to classify the individual's blood pressure status. Isolated systolic hypertension is defined as systolic blood pressure of 140 mmHg or greater and diastolic blood pressure below 90 mmHg and staged appropriately.

[b]Normal blood pressure with respect to cardiovascular disease risk is below 120/80 mmHg. However, unusually low readings should be evaluated for clinical significance.

[c]Based on the average of two or more readings taken at each of two or more visits after an initial screening.

JNC VII, Seventh Report of the U.S. Joint National Committee for Detection, Evaluation, and Treatment of High Blood Pressure.

Source: Chobanian AV, Bakris GL, Black HR, Cushman WC, Green LA, Izzo JL Jr, et al. *Hypertension* 2003;42:1206–52.

Table 2–1. Classification of Blood Pressure for Adults Aged 18 and Older According to JNC VII

PREVALENCE OF HYPERTENSION (%) IN UNITED STATES, 1989–1994								
Age (years)	All Races/Ethnicities[a]			White			Black		
	Total	Men	Women	Total	Men	Women	Total	Men	Women
18–24	2.6	4.6	0.7	2.5	4.6	0.5	2.6	4.1	1.4
25–34	5.4	8.4	2.4	4.9	8.1	1.6	8.2	10.6	6.2
35–44	13.0	16.0	10.2	11.3	14.3	8.5	25.9	29.5	22.9
45–54	27.6	30.0	25.2	25.8	29.1	22.6	46.9	44.3	48.8
55–64	43.7	44.2	43.2	42.1	43.0	41.4	60.0	58.0	63.0
65–74	59.6	55.8	62.7	58.6	54.9	61.7	71.0	65.2	75.6
≥75	70.3	60.5	76.2	69.7	59.0	76.1	75.5	71.3	77.9
Total	23.4	23.5	23.3	23.2	23.4	23.1	28.1	27.9	28.2

[a]Includes race/ethnic groups not shown separately due to small sample sizes.

Source: Wolz M, Cutler J, Roccella EJ, Rohde F, Thone T, Burt V., et al. *Am J Hypertens* 2000;13:103–4 with permission from *The American Journal of Hypertension Ltd.*

Table 2–2. Prevalence of Hypertension (%) in United States, 1989–1994

Race/Ethnicity

In NHANES III the prevalence of hypertension in different racial/ethnic groups was compared. It was found that in the 18- to 49-year-old group, non-Hispanic blacks had prevalence of hypertension of 15% in men and 8% in women, non-Hispanic whites had prevalence of hypertension of 11% in men and 4% in women, and Mexican Americans had the highest prevalence of hypertension in men of 20%, while in women it was only 3%.[17] In the 50- to 69-year-old group, the prevalence was 45% in men and 43% in women among non-Hispanic blacks, 35% and 29% in men and women among non-Hispanic whites, and 37% in both men and in women among Mexican Americans, respectively. Overall the prevalence of hypertension is highest in male and female African Americans. The prevalence of hypertension is higher in white men than Mexican-American men, while the prevalence is higher in Mexican-American women than white women.

Several longitudinal cohort studies have also shown that African Americans have a higher incidence of hypertension than whites.[14,15,18,19] In the Atherosclerosis Risk in Communities Study, the 6-year incidence of hypertension among 45- to 49-year-olds was 13.9% and 12.6% in white men and women, respectively, and 24.9% and 30.3% in African American men and women, respectively.[17] The corresponding incidence of hypertension among participants aged 50 to 64 years was 18.0% and 17.0% in white men and women, respectively, and 28.3% and 29.9% in African-American men and women, respectively. Other longitudinal cohort studies indicated that the incidence of hypertension in African Americans was an average of two times higher than in whites.[14,18,19]

Geographic region

According to a recent study of the global burden of hypertension, 26.4% of the world's adult population in 2000 had hypertension, and 29.2% were predicted to have hypertension by 2025.[20] Regions with the highest estimated prevalence of hypertension had roughly twice the rate of regions with the lowest estimated prevalence. In men, the highest estimated prevalence was in the region of Latin America and the Caribbean, whereas for women, the highest estimated prevalence was in the former socialist economies. The lowest prevalence of hypertension for both men and women was in the region of Asia, other than China, and the Pacific Islands. Rates of hypertension by geographic region and gender are presented in Figure 2–2.

LIFETIME RISK OF HYPERTENSION IN WESTERNIZED POPULATIONS

Although the prevalence of hypertension is a useful indicator of burden of disease in the community, it does not tell us about the risk for developing hypertension in individuals. The individual risk for developing hypertension is best described by incidence or lifetime cumulative incidence statistics. Less information is available about lifetime cumulative incidence of hypertension because it requires follow-up of populations for a prolonged period of time.[14–16,18,19]

The lifetime risk for developing hypertension was estimated among 1298 Framingham Heart Study participants aged 55 to 65 years and free of hypertension at baseline during the 1976–1998 period.[21] For 55-year-old participants, the cumulative risk for developing hypertension was calculated through age 80 while for 65-year-old participants, the risk for developing hypertension was calculated through age 85 years. These follow-up time intervals (25 years for 55-year-olds and 20 years for 65-year-olds) correspond to the current mean residual life expectancies for white individuals at these two ages in the United States. The lifetime risks for developing hypertension were 90% in both 55- and 65-year-old participants (Figure 2–3). The lifetime probability of receiving antihypertensive medication was 60%.[21]

BLOOD PRESSURE IN ISOLATED POPULATIONS

In most Western populations, blood pressure levels rise with advancing age; however, the same is not true in many

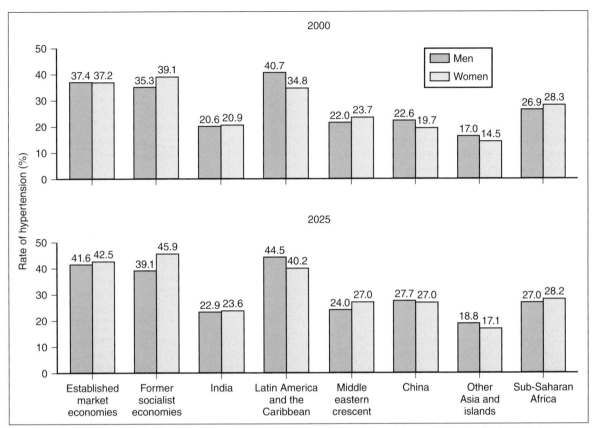

Figure 2–2. Frequency of hypertension in people aged 20 years and older by world region and gender in 2000 (upper) and 2025 (lower). (Redrawn from Kearney PM, Whelton M, Reynolds K, Muntner P, Whelton PK, He J. *Lancet* 2005; 365:217–23 with permission from Elsevier.)

isolated or unacculturated populations. Since 1929, when Donnison[21,22] first described an isolated population in Kenya whose blood pressure did not rise with age, at least 30 similar reports have been published.[23] Other examples of such populations include Melanesians in New Guinea,[24–27] South American Indians,[25,28,29] Pacific Islanders,[8,30–33] Navajo Indians,[34] a rural population in Delhi,[35] Kalahari

Bushmen,[36,37] African Pygmies,[38] and the Yi farmers of southern China.[39] Most of these studies were conducted decades ago and methodology issues exist among them; however, more recent and rigorous studies, such as that among the Yi population,[39] have also shown that blood pressure remains low and does not rise with age in some isolated populations.

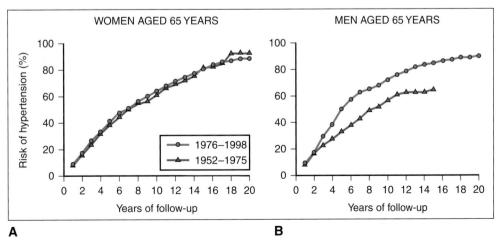

Figure 2–3. Residual lifetime risk of hypertension in women and men aged 65 years of the Framingham Heart Study. (Redrawn from Vasan RS, Beiser A, Seshadri S, Larson MG, Kannel WB, D'Agostino RB, et al. *JAMA* 2002;287:1003–10.)

Africa

Donnison[22] in 1929 was the first to provide evidence suggesting that many Kenyan tribes had low blood pressures that rose little through adulthood.[22] In an area around Lake Victoria in western Kenya, he surveyed the population and medical records of a large hospital located in the region. Among his findings, in surveying approximately 1000 individuals there were no cases of hypertension, and blood pressure levels were low, falling further with advancing age. A more recent study of approximately 2000 male subsistence farmers in Kenya, in an area adjacent to that studied by Donnison[22] decades earlier, confirmed that systolic blood pressure showed no significant rise with age until participants passed 54 years of age and diastolic pressures showed a very small rise with age.[40] In this community, packaged or processed foods were not available, nor were electricity, water supply, or telephone communication, and transportation was primarily on foot within the local community. Most participants were subsistence farmers who engaged in heavy physical labor every day. Mean 24-hour urinary excretion of sodium in this population ranged from 53 to 93 mmol/day, while mean intake of sodium measured by dietary survey was just under 130 mmol/day (3 g/day).[25,40] Of note, both systolic and diastolic blood pressure correlated positively with urinary sodium: potassium ratios in that study, suggesting that cation intake may play an important role in the differences in blood pressure among isolated populations and Westernized populations. A study among the Kung Bushmen living a nomadic, hunter-gatherer lifestyle in Botswana has also shown low blood pressures that increase little with age, and perhaps somewhat decrease with age.[37] In this population, dietary intake of sodium was approximately 86.9 mmol/day (2 g/day), while potassium intake approximated 204.6 mmol/day (8 g/day). Similarly, a study of Bushmen living in the Kalahari Desert, also hunter-gatherers, found an average systolic blood pressure of 100 mmHg, with diastolic pressure approximately 68 mmHg among men, with slightly higher values in women.[36] Again, blood pressure levels in both men and women did not show the age-related increases seen in Westernized populations. Among the Xhosa people of South Africa, blood pressure of those living a traditional lifestyle of subsistence farming in remote villages of the Transkei were low and rose little with advancing age.[41]

South and Central America

Studies examining the blood pressures of isolated populations in South and Central America have included the Cuna Indians, Yanomamo Indians, and Xingu Indians, among other populations.[25,29,42,43] The Yanomamo and Xingu of the tropical rainforests near the equator have very recently been studied as part of an international cooperative study on blood pressures in diverse populations (Figure 2–4).[25] The Yanomamo Indians are perhaps one of the most unacculturated native tribes in South America and possibly in the world. They live in an area of about 200,000 km² located along the border of Brazil and Venezuela. The total population consists of approxi-

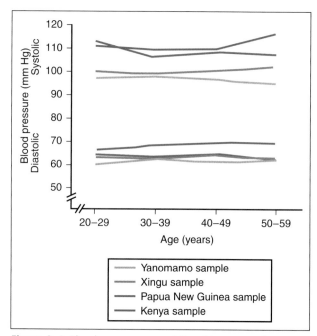

Figure 2–4. Blood pressure-age relationships among four isolated populations studied as part of the International Study of Salt Intake and Blood Pressure. (Redrawn from Carvalho JJ, Baruzzi RG, Howard PF, Poulter N, Alpers MP, Franco LJ, et al. *Hypertension* 1989;14:238–46.)

mately 18,000 individuals, scattered throughout the Amazon rainforest in 200 or so villages composed of 40 to 250 people each. By and large, the Yanomamo are seminomadic, slash-and-burn agriculturalists who live on a diet of locally produced crops and game, supplemented by wild fruits and insects. Dietary staples consist of cooked banana and manioc (cassava). In most villages there is little if any access to salt, refined sugar, alcohol, milk, or other dairy products. Similarly, the Xingu Indians occupy an area of 22,000 km² in the central region of Brazil. Although less isolated than the Yanomamo, the Xingu do not maintain regular contact with non-Indians. The diet of Xingu Indians is principally based on manioc (cassava) and fish. The consumption of meat from game animals is free in some tribes and restricted by taboos in others. The diet also includes, to a lesser extent, corn, sweet potatoes, cara, peanuts, bananas, and wild fruit. Salt and other foods sold in stores are not used regularly. Mean systolic blood pressures among the Yanomamo and Xingu Indians were 101 and 103 mmHg in men and 91 and 96 mmHg in women, respectively. Individuals studied in the Yanomamo villages consumed virtually no salt, while the Xingu Indians had a median intake of about one-third gram of salt daily. Among the Yanomamo Indians, urinary sodium excretion was 0.9 mmol/24 hours, while Xingu Indians had a urinary sodium excretion of 12.5 mmol/24 hours. Those in the sample from Papua New Guinea had a median consumption of 1.5 g of salt daily and the 24-hour urinary excretion of sodium was 37.5 mmol. This contrasts with the median consumption of more than 391.5 mmol/day (9 g/day) and 24-hour urinary sodium excretion of 166 mmol in the rest of this study.[25]

China

Blood pressure has been examined in several isolated populations of China. In 1937, Morse and Beh[44] reported that the blood pressure of aboriginal groups living in mountainous regions of Szechwan, Kweicheo, and Yunnan was low, and rose little with advancing age. Cardiovascular diseases were extremely rare among these populations. More recently, the Yi people from the Szechwan Province have been studied extensively by He et al.[39,45–47]

The Yi people are a minority population in China living in the Liangshan Yi Autonomous Prefecture in southern China, an area covering approximately 70,000 km[2]. The Yi people live in remote mountain districts at 1,500 or more meters above sea level. Their main occupation is agriculture, and they are one of the most primitive societies in China. In the high-mountain regions, isolated from the outside world, the Yi farmers have preserved their own language and lifestyle. Their main crops are potatoes, oats, and buckwheat; they rarely eat meat, except during the Yi New Year in December. Owing to a shortage of water, Yi farmers rarely take a bath and almost never wash their hands, faces, and clothes. Before about 1950, it was extremely difficult for the high-mountain Yi farmers to obtain salt, and although salt is now more readily available, salt consumption has remained quite low. Mountainside Yi farmers have a lifestyle that is in many ways similar to that of the high-mountain Yi farmers, however, they are closer to a highway and have some contact with a more modern lifestyle. Their main staples are rice and corn, but also include potatoes, oats, buckwheat, and beans; they consume more meat and salt than high-mountain Yi farmers. Male Yi farmers, both high-mountain and mountainside residents, smoke home-grown tobacco and consume an average of 30 to 35 g of alcohol daily, corresponding to about three Western alcoholic drinks per day. He et al.[46] studied the blood pressures of 3419 high-mountain Yi farmers and 2936 mountainside Yi farmers, along with 517 Yi migrants who had moved to the county seat, and 1143 Han Chinese who resided in the county seat. They found a mean systolic blood pressure of 101.8 mmHg and 101.2 mmHg among high-mountain men and women, and 100.8 mmHg and 100.1 mmHg among mountainside men and women, respectively. The corresponding mean diastolic blood pressures were 63.0, 63.0, 62.2 and 62.5 mmHg, respectively. In terms of the age–blood pressure relationship, in all groups, blood pressure increased up to the second decade of life. Among men, no further significant increase was seen in systolic blood pressure for high-mountain and mountainside Yi men. Diastolic blood pressure did not increase much with age among high-mountain male farmers, while it increased late in life among the mountainside farmers. Among women, systolic blood pressure remained the same and did not increase with age for high-mountain farmers, but did increase in other groups. Diastolic blood pressure among women increased in all groups but with a very small slope among the high-mountain Yi.

Twenty-four-hour urinary excretions of sodium and potassium were markedly different among Yi mountain groups and Yi migrants to the county seat. For example, high-mountain and mountainside Yi farmers excreted an average of 73.9 and 117.9 mmol of sodium daily, and 58.6 and 48.5 mmol of potassium daily, respectively. Yi migrants excreted a mean of 159.4 mmol of sodium and only 28.3 mmol of potassium daily. Han residents of the county seat excreted 186.0 mmol of sodium and 29.0 mmol of potassium daily, on average, similar to the intakes of Yi migrants.[46]

New Guinea and Pacific Islands

Studies among islanders in isolated populations such as New Guinea and certain Pacific Islands have also demonstrated a lack of age-related blood pressure rise. Sinnett and Whyte[27] studied approximately 1000 members of a New Guinean highland population. The participants were farmers and pig herders with an agriculture-based economy with very little Western influence. They also identified the lack of age-related blood pressure increase and noted that sodium intake was less than 43.5 mmol/day (1 g/day) among the islanders studied. Among the sample of islanders from Papua, New Guinea included in the Intersalt Study, median consumption of sodium was estimated at 65.3 mmol/day (1.5 g/day) and 24-hour excretion of sodium was 37.5 mmol.[25]

Prior et al.[48] examined the populations of the Polynesian Islands of Raratonga and Pukapuka. Among Pukapuka Islanders, an age-related rise in blood pressure was seen only among women and was slight; however, among the Raratonga, blood pressures were higher and increased with age. Dietary surveys and urine analyses revealed a substantially greater mean salt intake among the Raraonga Islanders (mean 24-hour sodium excretion of 50 to 70 mmol in Pukapuka Islanders and 120 to 140 mmol/day in Raratonga Islanders).

Six Solomon Island populations were studied by Page et al.[33] All were rural populations living in villages without access to electricity; however, they varied widely in habitat, way of life, and degree of exposure to Western culture. Among the least acculturated populations, diastolic blood pressure fell with age in males, while among the more acculturated populations, there was no trend with age in males. Systolic pressures in males did not increase with age, whereas in females of the three most acculturated communities, systolic blood pressures did increase with age. In the three most acculturated societies, 24-hour sodium excretions ranged from 50 to 230 mmol, whereas among the least acculturated society, 24-hour urinary sodium excretion was under 20 mmol.

These comparisons of blood pressure in isolated populations suggest that sodium intake plays an important role in determining absolute levels of blood pressure and age–blood pressure relationships. More support for this observation has come from the examination of remote populations in the Intersalt Study.[25] The authors of that study concluded that a certain minimum intake of salt is required to produce a high frequency of hypertension in populations.

MIGRATION STUDIES

Populations that do not demonstrate an age-related rise in blood pressure tend to live in primitive societies isolated from modern lifestyles and have a low salt intake, high level of physical activity, and an absence of obesity. Many studies of those who migrate to a more Westernized environment or who are under modernization *in situ* have shown that blood pressure rises with age and hypertension begins to appear. This change in pattern of blood pressure with aging must be due to an alteration of environmental, rather than genetic influences. Such migrants, therefore, provide a unique population model in which to study the relationship between blood pressure and environmental factors.[39]

In the Tokelau Island Migrant Study, the relationship between blood pressure and migration was studied in a cohort of 654 adult Tokelauans who either remained in their homeland or migrated to New Zealand.[49] Three surveys were conducted between 1968 and 1982. Results showed that both systolic and diastolic blood pressures of migrant men were higher compared with age-matched nonmigrants. In a longitudinal analysis of this cohort, it was noted that blood pressures tended to rise 1 mmHg/year faster among male migrants than among male nonmigrants, and about 0.4 mmHg/year faster among female migrants than among female nonmigrants.[50] Most of this rise in blood pressure could be attributed to weight gain. However, this study did not include a control group of New Zealand local residents.[49,50]

The Yi migrant study is a more recent and significantly larger study of migration from an isolated population to a more Westernized population.[39] In the Yi migrant study, blood pressure was measured in 14,505 persons (8241 Yi farmers, 2575 urban Yi migrants, and 3689 Han urban residents) aged 15 to 89 years. Blood pressure was recorded as the mean of three seated measurements after a 10-minute rest period. At all ages, Yi migrant men had higher mean diastolic pressures than male Yi farmers, and had values similar to Han men. In women, mean systolic and diastolic pressures were lower in Yi farmers in the second half of life, while blood pressures were similar among Yi migrant women and Han women and higher than among Yi farmers. Definite hypertension, defined according to World Health Organization criteria as systolic pressure at least 160 mmHg and/or diastolic pressure at least 95 mmHg and/or use of antihypertensive medication, was extremely rare among Yi farmers (0.66% in men and 0.33% in women). The age-adjusted prevalence of hypertension in male Yi migrants was 4.25%, similar to the 4.91% seen in Han men. For women, age-adjusted prevalence of hypertension was lower among Yi migrants than in Han residents (2.40% and 4.76%, respectively) and much higher than that of Yi farmers. Differences in the prevalence of definite hypertension were especially marked in the oldest age groups. For example, among men aged 65 years and older, the prevalence of definite hypertension was 8.0 times higher in Yi migrants and 13.9 times higher in Han than in Yi farmers.

The contribution of urinary cations to change in blood pressure due to migration was also explored in this study of Yi farmers.[47] Blood pressure and overnight urinary electrolyte levels were measured on 3 consecutive days in 313 Yi farmers, 265 Yi migrants, and 253 urban Han residents, all male. Of the urinary electrolytes, a higher sodium:potassium ratio best explained the higher blood pressure in the migrants. Yi farmers had lower systolic (106.7 mmHg vs. 114.8 mmHg, respectively) and diastolic (66.2 mmHg vs. 71.3 mmHg, respectively) blood pressures than Yi migrants. However, even after adjustment for age, body mass index, alcohol intake, and urinary sodium, potassium, calcium, and magnesium excretion, Yi farmers continued to have lower average blood pressures than Yi migrants. In pooled analyses of all three groups, urinary sodium and calcium were positively related, and urinary potassium and magnesium were inversely related to blood pressure. These results suggest that migration is associated with a higher blood pressure that was partially but not entirely explained by higher levels of adiposity, alcohol, and sodium intake, and lower levels of potassium and magnesium intake.

Poulter et al.[51] examined 325 members of the Luo tribe aged 15 to 34 years who had migrated to Nairobi and 267 controls living in 35 villages on the northern shores of Lake Victoria in western Kenya. They collected medical questionnaires, three 24-hour diet histories, height, weight, pulse, and blood pressure on migrants and controls. In addition, three 12-hour overnight urine samples were collected from all participants and analyzed for sodium, potassium, and creatinine concentrations.

They found that mean systolic blood pressure of migrants was significantly higher than that of controls, and the entire distribution of blood pressure was shifted to higher levels as compared with controls. Mean diastolic blood pressure differences also grew over time. They also concluded that blood pressure differences were not due to selective migration but more likely due to the contribution of dietary and urinary cations. Migrants' mean urinary sodium: potassium ratio was significantly higher than that of controls ($p<0.001$), and weight and pulse rate were also higher among migrants. Their results are highly consistent with that of the Yi migrant study and strongly suggest that urinary sodium:potassium ratio and weight changes are important contributors to increased blood pressure among migrants from a low blood-pressure community, and therefore, may also be an important part of the initiation of essential hypertension.

CONCLUSIONS

High blood pressure is a major risk factor for cardiovascular disease worldwide. In Westernized populations, the pattern of blood pressure is such that most of the population is at increased risk for blood pressure–related cardiovascular diseases. In contrast, the pattern in many isolated populations is such that only a slight fraction if any of the population is at increased risk for blood pressure–related disease. In comparisons of Westernized populations with those isolated populations that demonstrate little or no rise in blood pressure with age, one of the most salient and consistent differences between them is a very low mean sodium intake. Even within isolated populations, those with lower sodium intake and hence lower sodium:potassium excretion ratios in urinary testing, have lower blood pressures and less age-related increase in blood pressure.

Migration studies also lend support the primary role of environmental factors in the development of hypertension. Given that most of the major risk factors for hypertension are modifiable, and strong evidence that hypertension can be prevented altogether, the importance of primary prevention strategies in reducing the global burden of hypertension and cardiovascular diseases cannot be overstated.

REFERENCES

1. Yusuf S, Reddy S, Ourtpuu S, Anand S. Global burden of cardiovascular diseases. Part I: General considerations, the epidemiologic transition, risk factors, and impact of urbanization. *Circulation* 2001;104:2746–53.
2. World Health Organization. The world health report. Shaping the future. Geneva: World Health Organization, 2003.
3. Ezzati M, Hoorn SV, Rodgers A, Lopez AD, Mathers CD, Murray CJ. Estimates of global and regional potential health gains from reducing multiple major risk factors. *Lancet* 2003;362:271–80.
4. Whelton PK, He J, Appel LJ, Cutler JA, Havas S, Kotchen TA, et al. Primary prevention of hypertension: clinical and public health advisory from the national high blood pressure education program. *JAMA* 2002;288:1882–8.
5. Whelton PK Epidemiology of hypertension. *Lancet* 1994;344:101–6.
6. Report of the second task force on blood pressure control in children—1987. Task force on Blood Pressure Control in Children. National Heart, Lung, and Blood Institute, Bethesda, Maryland. *Pediatrics* 1987;79:1–25.
7. National High Blood Pressure Education Program Working Group on Hypertension Control in Children and Adolescents. Update on the 1987 Task Force Report on High Blood Pressure in Children and Adolescents: a working group report from the National High Blood Pressure Education Program. *Pediatrics* 1996; 98:649–58.
8. Berenson GS, Wattigney WA, Webber LS. Epidemiology of hypertension from childhood to young adulthood in black, white, and hispanic population samples. *Public Health Rep* 1996;111(Suppl 2):3–6.
9. Kelder SH, Osganian SK, Feldman HA, Webber LS, Parcel GS, Leupker RV, et al. Tracking of physical and physiological risk variables among ethnic subgroups from third to eighth grade: the child and adolescent trial for cardiovascular health cohort study. *Prev Med* 2002; 34:324–33.
10. Kannel W. B, Gordan T. Evaluation of cardiovascular risk in the elderly: The Framingham Study. *Bull N Y Acad Med* 1978;54:573–91.
11. Joint National Committee on Prevention, Detection, Evaluation, and Treatment of High Blood Pressure. The sixth report of the Joint National Committee on Prevention, Detection, Evaluation, and Treatment of High Blood Pressure. *Arch Intern Med* 1997;157:2413–46.

12. Guidelines subcommittee. 1999 World Health Organization–International Society of Hypertension guidelines for the management of hypertension. *J Hypertens* 1999;17:151–83.
13. Chobanian AV, Bakris GL, Black HR, Cushman WC, Green LA, Izzo JL Jr, et al. Seventh report of the Joint National Committee on Prevention, Detection, Evaluation, and Treatment of High Blood Pressure. *Hypertension* 2003;42:1206–52.
14. Cornoni-Huntley J, LaCroix AZ, Havlik RJ. Race and sex differentials in the impact of hypertension in the United States. The National Health and Nutrition Examination Survey I Epidemiologic Follow-up Study. *Arch Intern Med* 1989;149:780–8.
15. Fuchs FD, Chambless LE, Whelton PK, Nieto FJ, Heiss G. Alcohol consumption and the incidence of hypertension: The atherosclerosis risk in communities study. *Hypertension* 2001;37:1242–50.
16. Vasan RS, Larson MG, Leip EP, Kannel WB, Levy D. Assessment of frequency of progression to hypertension in non-hypertensive participants in the Framingham Heart Study: a cohort study. *Lancet* 2001;358:1682–6.
17. Burt VL, Whelton P, Roccella EJ, Brown C, Cutler JA, Higgins M, et al. Prevalence of hypertension in the U.S. adult population. Results from the third National Health and Nutrition Examination Survey, 1988–1991. *Hypertension* 1995;25:305–13.
18. Apostolides AY, Cutter G, Daugherty SA, Detels R, Kraus J, Wassertheil-Smoller S, et al. Three-year incidence of hypertension in thirteen U.S. Communities. On behalf of the Hypertension Detection and Follow-up Program Cooperative Group. *Prev Med* 1982;11:487–499.
19. Manolio TA, Burke GL, Savage PJ, Sidney S, Gardin JM, Oberman A. Exercise blood pressure response and 5-year risk of elevated blood pressure in a cohort of young adults: the Cardia Study. *Am J Hypertens* 1994;7:234–41.
20. Kearney PM, Whelton M, Reynolds K, Muntner P, Whelton PK, He J. Global burden of hypertension: analysis of worldwide data. *Lancet* 2005; 365:217–23.
21. Vasan RS, Beiser A, Seshadri S, Larson MG, Kannel WB, D'Agostino RB, et al. Residual lifetime risk for developing hypertension in middle-aged women and men: the Framingham Heart Study. *JAMA* 2002;287:1003–10.
22. Donnison CP. Blood pressure in the African native. *Lancet* 1929;i:6–7.

23. Shaper AG. Communities without hypertension. In: Shaper A, Hutt M, Feifar Z, eds. *Cardiovasular Disease in the Tropics*. London: British Medical Association, 1974:77–83.
24. Barnes R. Comparisons of blood pressures and blood cholesterol levels of New Guineans and Australians. *Med J Aust* 1965;192:611–7.
25. Carvalho JJ, Baruzzi RG, Howard PF, Poulter N, Alpers MP, Franco LJ, et al. Blood pressure in four remote populations in the Intersalt Study. *Hypertension* 1989;14:238–46.
26. Maddocks I. Blood pressures in melanesians. *Med J Aust* 1967;1:1123–6.
27. Sinnett PF, Whyte HM. Epidemiological studies in a total highland population, Tukisenta, New Guinea. Cardiovascular disease and relevant clinical, electrocardiographic, radiological and biochemical findings. *J Chronic Dis* 1973;26:265–90.
28. Elliott P, Marmot M. International studies of salt and blood pressure. *Ann Clin Res* 1984;16(Suppl 43):67–71.
29. Oliver WJ, Cohen EL, Neel JV. Blood pressure, sodium intake, and sodium related hormones in the Yanomamo Indians, a "no-salt" culture. *Circulation* 1975;52:146–51.
30. Abbie AA, Schroder J. Blood pressures in Arnhem Land Aborigines. *Med J Aust* 1960;47(2):493–6.
31. Maddocks I. Possible absence of essential hypertension in two complete Pacific Island populations. *Lancet* 1961; 2:396–9.
32. Norman-Taylor W, Rees WH. Blood pressures in three New Hebrides communities. *Br J Prev Soc Med* 1963; 17:141–4.
33. Page LB, Damon A, Moellering RC Jr. Antecedents of cardiovascular disease in six Solomon Islands societies. *Circulation* 1974;49:1132–46.
34. Fulmer HS, Roberts RW. Coronary heart disease among the Navajo Indians. *Ann Intern Med* 1963;59:740–64.
35. Padmavati S, Gupta S. Blood pressure studies in rural and urban groups in Delhi. *Circulation* 1959;19:395–405.
36. Kaminer B, Lutz WP. Blood pressure in bushmen of the Kalahari Desert. *Circulation* 1960;22:289–95.
37. Truswell AS, Kennelly BM, Hansen JD, Lee RB. Blood pressures of Kung Bushmen in northern Botswana. *Am Heart J* 1972;84:5–12.
38. Mann GV, Roels OA, Price DL, Merrill JM. Cardiovascular disease in African Pygmies. A survey of the health status, serum lipids and diet of Pygmies in Congo. *J Chronic Dis* 1962;15:341–71.

39. He J, Klag MJ, Whelton PK, Chen JY, Mo JP, Qian MC, et al. Migration, blood pressure pattern, and hypertension: the Yi migrant study. *Am J Epidemiol* 1991;134:1085–101.

40. Poulter N, Khaw KT, Hopwood BE, Mugambi M, Peart WS, Rose G, et al. Blood pressure and associated factors in a rural Kenyan community. *Hypertension* 1984;6:810–3.

41. Sever PS, Gordon D, Peart WS, Beighton P. Blood-pressure and its correlates in urban and tribal Africa. *Lancet* 1980;2:60–4.

42. Kean BH. The blood pressure of the Cuna Indians. *Am J Trop Med* 1944; 24:341.

43. Lowenstein FW. Blood pressure in relation to age and sex in the tropics and subtropics. A review of the literature and an investigation in two tribes of Brazil Indians. *Lancet* 1961;i:389.

44. Morse WR, Beh YT. Blood pressure amongst aboriginal ethnic groups of Szechwan Province, west China. *Lancet* 1937;i:966–7.

45. He J, Klag MJ, Wu Z, Qian MC, Chen JY, Mo PS, et al. Effect of migration and related environmental changes on serum lipid levels in southwestern Chinese men. *Am J Epidemiol* 1996; 144:839–8.

46. He J, Tell GS, Tang YC, Mo PS, He GQ. Effect of migration on blood pressure: the Yi people study. *Epidemiology* 1991; 2:88–97.

47. Klag MJ, He J, Coresh J, Whelton PK, Chen JY, Mo JP, et al. The contribution of urinary cations to the blood pressure differences associated with migration. *Am J Epidemiol* 1995;142:295–303.

48. Prior IA, Evans JG, Harvey HP, Davidson F, Lindsey M. Sodium intake and blood pressure in two Polynesian populations. *N Engl J Med* 1968; 279:515–20.

49. Beaglehole R, Salmond CE, Hooper A, Huntsman J, Stanhope JM, Cassel JC, et al. Blood pressure and social interaction in Tokelauan migrants in New Zealand. *J Chronic Dis* 1977; 30:803–12.

50. Salmond CE, Joseph JG, Prior IA, Stanley DG, Wessen AF. Longitudinal analysis of the relationship between blood pressure and migration: The Tokelau Island Migrant Study. *Am J Epidemiol* 1985;122:291–301.

51. Poulter NR, Khaw KT, Hopwood BE, Mugambi M, Peart WS, Rose G, et al. The Kenyan Luo migration study: observations on the initiation of a rise in blood pressure. *BMJ* 1990; 300:967–72.

Chapter

3

Regional Differences in Blood Pressure in Developed Countries

Patricia M. Kearney and Ivan J. Perry

Key Findings

- Blood pressure increases with age across regions.

- In younger individuals high blood pressure is more prevalent in men, while in older populations more women than men have high blood pressure.

- The distribution of high blood pressure varies by ethnicity within regions.

- Hypertension is a major public health problem irrespective of age, race/ethnicity, or gender.

- In economically developed countries, the prevalence of hypertension ranges between approximately 20% and 50%, and overall approximately one-third of adults in developed countries are affected.

- The prevalence of hypertension is higher in Europe than in North America or Australia, but overall it is decreasing in most Western countries.

- Population-wide strategies are required for prevention, treatment, and control of hypertension.

- Formal population-level screening programs are required to increase the detection of hypertension.

- Awareness, treatment, and control are required at an individual level.

- Population-level interventions are also required.

Hypertension is an important public health challenge worldwide because of its high prevalence and the concomitant increase in risk of cardiovascular and renal disease.[1,2] It has been identified as the leading global risk factor for mortality and has been ranked third as a cause of disability-adjusted life years.[3] Hypertension is the most important modifiable risk factor for coronary heart disease, stroke, congestive heart failure, chronic renal failure, and peripheral vascular disease.[4–9] Observational epidemiologic studies have demonstrated that elevated blood pressure is related to an increased risk of cardiovascular and renal disease.[6–9] Also, randomized controlled trials have shown that anti-hypertensive drug treatment reduces the morbidity and mortality of cardiovascular and renal disease among patients with hypertension (Table 3–1).[10–12] The treatment of hypertension has improved dramatically over the past 30 years in many countries and this has contributed to the reduction in mortality due to coronary heart disease and stroke that has been observed in some developed countries.[13] However, even in developed countries, most patients with hypertension do not have adequate treatment and control

of their blood pressure.[14,15] Patterns of regional differences in hypertension prevalence may provide insight into the underlying determinants of blood pressure variation and facilitate improvements in hypertension treatment and control.

PREVALENCE OF HYPERTENSION IN DEVELOPED COUNTRIES

It has been estimated that more than one-quarter of the world adult population—totaling nearly 1 billion—had hypertension in 2000 and it is predicted that this proportion will have increased to 29%—1.56 billion—by 2025.[16] In developed countries, the total number of people with hypertension in 2000 was estimated as 333 million, and it is predicted that this number will increase by 24% to 413 million by 2025.[16] In economically developed countries, the prevalence of hypertension ranges between approximately 20% and 50%,[17] and overall approximately one-third of the adult population in developed countries are affected (26.6% of men and 26.1% of women) (Table 3–2).

North America

According to data from the National Health and Nutrition Examination Survey (NHANES) III conducted in 1988–1992, as many as 42.3 million adult residents of the United States have hypertension, defined as having a systolic blood pressure ≥140 mmHg and/or a diastolic blood pressure ≥90 mmHg and/or taking antihypertensive medications. In addition, there are 7.7 million U.S. residents who have been told at least twice by a health professional that they have hypertension. Overall, there are about 50 million adult hypertensives in the United States.[18] The most recent report of the Joint National Committee (JNC) on Prevention, Detection, Evaluation, and Treatment of High Blood Pressure[19] defined a new category, prehypertension (systolic blood pressure of 120 to 139 mmHg or a diastolic blood pressure of 80 to 89 mmHg), which identifies individuals at increased risk of cardiovascular disease. According to data from the NHANES 1999–2000, approximately 60% of American adults (67% of men and 50% of women) had prehypertension or hypertension and 27% had hypertension.[20] A similar prevalence of hypertension was reported in the Canadian Heart Health Survey, a cross-sectional population-based survey that collected data in each of the 10 Canadian provinces between 1986 and 1992.[21] The study reported an overall prevalence of hypertension of 26% in men and 18% in women, which represents 4.1 million Canadian adults.

CHARACTERISTICS OF STUDIES							
Region	Country	Study Year	Age Range	Study Population	Device	Blood Pressure Methods No. of Measures/No. of Visits	Preparation
North America	United States	1988–1994	≥18	National sample of 19,661	Standard mercury	6/2	5-minute rest
	Canada	1986–1992	18–74	National sample of 23,129	Standard mercury	4/2	5-minute rest
Europe	Spain	1990	35–64	National sample of 2,021	Random zero	3/1	—
	England	1998	≥20	National sample of 11,529	Electronic	3/1	5-minute rest
	Germany	1994–1995	25–74	Regional sample of 4,856	Random zero	3/1	30-minute rest
	Greece	1997	18–91	Regional sample of 665	Standard mercury	3/1	5-minute rest
Australia	Australia	1989	25–64	National sample of 19,315	Standard mercury	2/1	—
Japan	Japan	1980	30–74	National sample of 10,346	Standard mercury	1/1	—

Table 3–1. Characteristics of Studies

PREVALENCE OF HYPERTENSION							
Region	Country	Crude Prevalence of Hypertension			Age-Standardized Prevalence of Hypertension		
		Men (%)	Women (%)	Overall (%)	Men (%)	Women (%)	Overall (%)
North America	United States	23.5	23.3	23.4	21.0	19.7	20.3
	Canada	26.0	18.0	22.0	23.5	15.6	21.4
Europe	Spain	46.2	44.3	45.1	41.7	39.0	40.0
	England	43.4	35.0	38.8	34.7	25.7	29.6
	Germany	44.0	32.2	—	38.3	26.4	—
	Greece	30.2	27.1	28.4	18.5	15.9	16.9
Australia	Australia	31.9	20.7	—	30.8	20.1	—
Japan	Japan	50.1	43.3	—	42.7	35.0	38.3

Note: All studies defined hypertension as average BP of ≥140/90 mmHg and/or use of antihypertensive medication.

Table 3–2. Prevalence of Hypertension

Europe

Many studies have estimated the prevalence of hypertension in Western Europe although there are relatively few national studies. The reported prevalence tends to be higher than in equivalent studies in North America.[22] The Spanish National Blood Pressure Study reported a prevalence of hypertension that increased with age and was higher in rural (49.4%) than in urban (43.2%) dwellers.[23] The study estimated that there were 6 million hypertensives aged 35 to 64 years in Spain.[23] The Health Survey for England 1998 was a cross-sectional, household-based nationwide survey of English adults aged 16 years or older.[24] According to the study, 41.5% of men and 33.3% of women had a systolic and/or diastolic blood pressure of ≥140/90 mmHg and/or were receiving antihypertensive therapy.

Australia

The prevalence of hypertension in the Australian general population was estimated as part of the National Heart Foundation's Risk Factor Prevalence Study, which was conducted from 1980 to 1989.[25] The survey was administered to a randomly selected sample as a multicenter cross-sectional survey in 1980, 1983, and 1989. The Australian Institute of Health and Welfare (AIHW) analyzed the data from the National Risk Factor Prevalence Study to obtain estimates of the prevalence of hypertension defined as systolic blood pressure ≥140 mmHg and/or diastolic blood pressure ≥90 mmHg and/or receiving treatment for high blood pressure. According to the AIHW analysis, the prevalence of hypertension in Australian adults aged 25 to 64 years was 31.9% in men and 20.7% in women.[26]

HYPERTENSION AND AGE

There is a large body of data available from Western populations that demonstrates mean blood pressure rises with increasing age.[2,27] While evidence from isolated "acculturated" societies suggests that such an increase in blood pressure is not a biological requirement,[28] in developed countries there is a general tendency for blood pressure to rise progressively with increasing age. As a consequence, there is a concomitant increase in the incidence and prevalence of hypertension with age. The age-related increase in blood pressure, however, varies considerably depending on the individual's stage of life, gender, race/ethnicity, initial level of blood pressure, and exposure to environmental factors.

Childhood and adolescence

Information on the pattern of blood pressure in children and adolescents is provided by the report of the Second Task Force on Blood Pressure Control in Children.[29] This report was based on data from blood pressure measurements on over 70,000 children who participated in nine cross-sectional surveys conducted in the United States and the United Kingdom. At birth, average systolic and diastolic pressures were 70 mmHg and 50 mmHg, respectively. Shortly thereafter, there was a rise in systolic blood pressure, so that by the end of the first year of life it approximated 94 mmHg. Diastolic blood pressure rises by only 2 mmHg over the same time period. For the next 2 to 3 years, systolic and diastolic blood pressures remain stable. Thereafter, there is a tendency for blood pressure to rise with increasing age throughout the remainder of childhood and adolescence. The slope for age-related change in blood pressure is much steeper for systolic (1–2 mmHg/year) than for diastolic (0.5–1 mmHg/year) blood pressure.

The Task Force database provides information on an approximately equal numbers of boys and girls. There is little evidence of a difference in pattern of average blood pressure between the sexes until adolescence. During the teenage years, average blood pressure is consistently higher for boys than for girls. This is particularly true for systolic blood pressure. By age 18, boys have average systolic and diastolic blood pressures that are almost 10 mmHg and 5 mmHg higher, respectively, than the corresponding values for girls. There was no evidence for a systematic difference in average blood pressure between white, black, and Mexican American children in the Task Force database. However, data from the Bogalusa Heart Study and the Child and Adolescent Trial for Cardiovascular Health indicate that mean blood pressure level is higher in black compared to white children and lower in Mexican-American compared to black and white children.[30,31]

Adults and the elderly

There is a general tendency for both systolic and diastolic blood pressure to rise during adult life.[2,27] The age-related rate of rise is consistently higher for systolic than for diastolic blood pressure. Systolic blood pressure tends to rise until the eighth or ninth decade, whereas diastolic blood pressure tends to remain constant or decline after the fifth decade.

As a consequence, pulse pressure increases progressively with aging. This is particularly true during the latter part of life.

The pattern of blood pressure change with age is modified to a certain extent by gender and race/ethnicity. In young adults, systolic and diastolic blood pressures tend to be higher in men than in women. However, the age-related rise in blood pressure with age is steeper for women than for men. As a result, by the seventh decade women tend to have levels of systolic blood pressure that equal or exceed those seen in men. Selective survivorship may explain part of this gender-related difference in blood pressure as men with high blood pressure earlier on may be less likely to survive and contribute to average blood pressure later in life. Longitudinal analysis of the Framingham cohort and other data sets suggests, however, that selective survivorship only explains a portion of these age-related trends.[32]

In NHANES III, the prevalence of hypertension increased with increasing age. In the 18 to 24 age group the overall prevalence of hypertension was only 2.6%. The prevalence of hypertension increased to 5.4% in 25- to 34-year-olds and 13.0% in 35- to 44-year-olds. The prevalence rates continued to rise with 27.6% of 45- to 54-year-olds affected and 43.7% of 55- to 64-year-olds. In 65- to 74-year-olds, the overall prevalence was 59.6% and in over 75-year-olds it was 70.3%. Similar increases in blood pressure with age have been demonstrated in a number of European studies.[23,24,33–35] Across all of these age ranges the prevalence of hypertension is lower in North America than in Europe.[22] However, there was evidence of heterogeneity in mean blood pressure among the European countries at different age groups.[22] In the youngest age groups, Germany, England, and Finland reported the highest prevalence of hypertension, with a lower prevalence of hypertension in Italy and Spain. In the older age groups, Germany and Sweden had the highest levels of hypertension among the European countries while Italy had the lowest mean blood pressure measurements.

HYPERTENSION AND GENDER

Overall the prevalence and incidence of hypertension are slightly higher in men compared to women. In NHANES III, the age-adjusted prevalence of hypertension for all races/ethnicities was 23.5% in men and 23.3% in women. In whites the prevalence was 23.4% in men and 23.1% in women. In blacks the prevalence was slightly higher in women than in men, 28.2% and 27.9%, respectively. The relationship between gender and hypertension is modified by age. In young adults, the prevalence and incidence rates of hypertension are higher in men than in women. For example, in developed countries the overall prevalence of hypertension in young men (20–29 years) is over twice the prevalence in women (14.4% vs. 6.2%, respectively).[16] The prevalence of hypertension remains higher in men than in women up until the sixth decade. However, by their 60s, women tend to have levels of blood pressure that equal or exceed those seen in men. Consequently, the prevalence of hypertension is higher in women than in men at older ages.

HYPERTENSION AND RACE/ETHNICITY

In a worldwide analysis of hypertension prevalence, the effect of race/ethnicity on the prevalence of hypertension differed by gender and by study country, so that overall no clear effect of race/ethnicity on the prevalence of hypertension emerged.[17] In the United States, much interest has focused on the racial/ethnic differences in hypertension, although these differences are only half the size of the differences, for example, between the United States and Europe.[22] In NHANES III, the prevalence of hypertension in different racial/ethnic groups was compared. In both men and women, non-Hispanic blacks had the highest and non-Hispanic whites had the lowest average systolic blood pressure until the end of the fifth decade. In the sixth and later decades, among men, Mexican Americans tended to have the highest average systolic blood pressure, although the differences among the three race/ethnicity groups were small. In women, non-Hispanic blacks continued to have the highest and non-Hispanic whites continued to have the lowest average systolic blood pressure during the sixth decade. By the seventh decade, however, the three race/ethnicity groups had similar average systolic blood pressure levels. Throughout adult life, men had a slightly higher average level of diastolic blood pressure than women did. Non-Hispanic black women had a higher average diastolic blood pressure than non-Hispanic white or Mexican American women. The same was true in men until the end of the fifth decade. Thereafter, diastolic blood pressures were similar in the three race/ethnicity groups. It was found that in the 18 to 49 age group, non-Hispanic blacks had prevalence of hypertension of 15% in men and 8% in women, non-Hispanic whites had prevalence of hypertension of 11% in men and 4% in women, Mexican Americans had the highest prevalence of hypertension in men of 20%, while in women it was only 3%.[18] In the 50 to 69 age group, the prevalence was 45% in men and 43% in women among non-Hispanic blacks; 35% in men and 29% in women among non-Hispanic whites; and 37% in both men and in women among Mexican Americans, respectively. Overall the prevalence of hypertension was highest in male and female African Americans. The prevalence of hypertension was higher in white men than Mexican-American men, while the prevalence was higher in Mexican-American women than white women. Several longitudinal cohort studies have also shown that African Americans have a higher incidence of hypertension than whites.[36–39]

In the Atherosclerosis Risk in Communities Study, the 6-year incidence of hypertension was 13.9% and 12.6% in white men and women, respectively, and 24.9% and 30.3% in African-American men and women, respectively, aged 45 to 49 years.[37] The corresponding incidence of hypertension among participants aged 50 to 64 years was 18.0% and 17.0% in white men and women, and 28.3% and 29.9% in African-American men and women, respectively. Other longitudinal cohort studies indicated that the incidence of hypertension in African Americans was an average of two times higher than in whites.[36,38,39] The effect of race/ethnicity on the prevalence of hypertension was also assessed in the Health Surveys for England. Age-adjusted mean blood pressure levels of older adults were highest among blacks. South Asian men had similar prevalence of hypertension as black men, while South Asian women had similar prevalence of hypertension to white women.

SECULAR TRENDS IN THE PREVALENCE OF HYPERTENSION

Repeated independent cross-sectional surveys in the same populations over time provide information about secular trends in blood pressure and hypertension (Table 3–3). However, attention must be paid to the comparability of the methods of sampling and blood pressure measurement, as well as the definition of hypertension between surveys. Few national data are available to examine the secular trend of hypertension in the general population. Generally speaking, the prevalence of hypertension has declined in most Western populations.[16]

The U.S. National Health and Nutritional Examination Surveys may provide the best data to examine the secular trends of hypertension although there was variation in sample size within each subgroup of the population, in the protocol for blood pressure measurement, and in the potential for measurement error.[40] Overall, hypertension prevalence in the United States has declined progressively since 1971, and the distributions of systolic and diastolic blood pressures have shifted downward during the approximately 30-year period between 1960–1962 and 1988–1991.[40] The decline in the prevalence of hypertension has been consistent across age, gender, and racial/ethnic groups. For example, the age-adjusted prevalence of hypertension defined as blood pressure ≥140/90 mmHg and/or current use of anti-hypertensive medication peaked at 36.3% in 1971–1974 and declined to 20.4% in 1988–1991. Between 1976–1980 and 1988–1991, the prevalence of hypertension among black men aged 50 to 59 years remained relatively stable at 54.7% and 53.3%, respectively. The prevalence for black men aged 60 to 74 increased from 67.0% to 71.2%. In every other age-specific and ethnic group, hypertension prevalence between 1976–1980 and 1988–1991 declined markedly. The proportionate decrease was greatest among 18- to 29-year-olds and least among the 60 to 74 age group. Age-adjusted mean systolic blood pressure decreased from 131 mmHg in 1971–1974 to 119 mmHg in 1988–1991 in the U.S. general population.[40] Mean diastolic pressure decreased from 83 mmHg to 73 mmHg over the same time period. For black men and women, the decline in age-specific systolic blood pressure was greatest between 1971–1974 and 1976–1980; the decline in white men and women was greatest between 1976–1980 and 1988–1991 for most age groups. Age-adjusted diastolic pressure decreased in all subgroups between 1971–1974 and 1988–1991. Age-specific diastolic blood pressure also declined markedly and progressively between 1971–1974 and 1988–1991 for every group. However, while these analyses of data through 1991 have suggested that hypertension is declining, the most recent NHANES survey conducted in 1999–2000 reported a prevalence of hyper-

TRENDS IN PREVALENCE OF HYPERTENSION						
Region	Country	Study	Year	Hypertension Prevalence		
				Men (%)	Women (%)	Overall (%)
North America	United States	NHANES I	1971–1974	40.7	32.1	36.3
		NHANES II	1976–1980	36.8	27.2	31.8
		NHANES III				
		Phase 1	1989–1991	24.9	24.5	25.0
		Phase 2	1991–1994	23.9	26.0	25.0
		NHANES 1999–2000	1999–2000	27.1	30.1	28.7
Europe	Belgium	BIRNH	1980–1985	41.0	30.5	—
		MONICA	1985–1992	26.7	20.0	—
	Finland	FINMONICA	1982	60.7	42.2	—
		FINMONICA	1987	60.5	39.2	—
		FINMONICA	1992	48.3	31.7	—
		FINMONICA	1997	45.9	29.6	—
	England	Health Survey for England	1994	—	—	38.0
		Health Survey for England	1998	41.5	33.3	37.0
	Germany	MONICA Augsburg	1984–1985	37.8	24.6	—
		MONICA Augsburg	1989–1990	37.7	23.5	—
		MONICA Augsburg	1994–1995	39.3	24.8	—
	Greece	Athens	1979–1983	31.0	27.7	—
		Didima	1997	30.2	27.1	28.4
Australia	Australia	Risk Factor Prevalence study	1980	45.6	30.4	—
		Risk Factor Prevalence study	1983	35.1	24.0	—
		Risk Factor Prevalence study	1989	31.9	20.7	—

BIRNH, Belgian Inter-University Research on Nutrition and Health; *FINMONICA*, Finland Monitoring Trends and Determinants in Cardiovascular Disease; *MONICA*, Monitoring Trends and Determinants in Cardiovascular Disease; *NHANES*, National Health and Nutrition Examination Survey.

Table 3–3. Trends in Prevalence of Hypertension

tension of 28.7%, which was an increase of 3.7% from 1988–1991.[41]

The Health Survey for England was conducted in 1998 and updated the findings of a previous survey in 1992.[24] The prevalence of hypertension in those 16 years and older was similar in both surveys, 37% in 1998 and 38% in 1994.[24] The Monitoring Trends and Determinants in Cardiovascular Disease (MONICA) studies were conducted in a number of European countries over the 1980s and 1990s.[42,43] Comparison of the results from the Belgian component of MONICA (1985–1992) with the earlier Belgian Inter-University Research on Nutrition and Health (BIRNH) project (1980–1984) demonstrated a significant decline in the prevalence of hypertension, from 41% and 30.5% to 26.7% and 20% in men and women, respectively.[44] As part of FINMONICA, four independent cross-sectional surveys were conducted in 1982, 1987, 1992, and 1997.[33] The prevalence of hypertension remained stable between 1982 and 1987. There was a significant downward trend in the prevalence of hypertension between 1987 and 1992. During 1992–1997, diastolic blood pressure remained unchanged but the mean systolic blood pressure decreased. In Germany, the MONICA Augsburg Project studied the prevalence of hypertension with three cross-sectional surveys in 1984–1985, 1989–1990, and 1994–1995.[45] In contrast with the

Belgian and Finnish studies, the age-standardized prevalence of hypertension increased slightly from the first to the third survey. In Greece, a 1997 survey[46] reported a prevalence of hypertension that was very similar to a much earlier study in Athens conducted between 1979 and 1983.[47] The prevalence of hypertension in the Australian general population was estimated as part of the National Heart Foundation's Risk Factor Prevalence with surveys administered in 1980, 1983, and 1989.[16] There was a significant reduction in the proportion of the survey participants who were classified as hypertensive during the 1980s.[25]

AWARENESS, TREATMENT, AND CONTROL OF HYPERTENSION

In developed countries, there are relatively high levels of awareness and treatment with approximately one-half to two-thirds of hypertensives aware of their diagnosis and one-third to one-half receiving treatment. Treatment and control of hypertension in the community requires that elevated blood pressure be recognized and that individuals with hypertension receive adequate treatment. The degree of awareness, treatment, and control of hypertension varies considerably among countries (Table 3–4). In addition, hypertension control rates vary by age, gender,

					AWARENESS, TREATMENT, AND CONTROL OF HYPERTENSION			
Region	Country	Study Year	Age Range	Gender	Aware (%)	Hypertensives Treated (%)	Controlled (%)	Treated Hypertensives, Controlled (%)
North America	United States	1988–1992	18–80+	Men	63.0	44.0	19.0	43.0
				Women	76.0	61.0	28.0	46.0
				Total	69.0	53.0	24.0	45.0
	Canada	1986–1992	18–74	Men	53.0	32.0	13.0	40.6
				Women	65.0	49.0	20.0	40.8
				Total	58.0	39.0	16.0	41.0
Europe	Spain	1990	35–64	Men	39.8	27.5	3.7	13.6
				Women	47.7	35.0	5.8	16.5
				Total	44.5	32.0	5.0	15.5
	England	1998	16–75	Men	40.3	25.7	8.0	31.1
				Women	52.2	38.0	10.7	28.2
				Total	46.2	31.8	9.3	29.2
	Germany	1994–1995	25–74	Men	53.8	29.0	9.5	32.8
				Women	67.3	43.4	14.9	34.3
				Total	59.5	35.1	11.8	33.6
	Greece	1997	18–90	Men	50.0	45.2	22.6	50.0
				Women	69.5	61.9	30.5	49.3
				Total	60.8	54.5	27.0	49.5
	Japan	1980	30–74	Men	—	40.5	23.6	55.7
				Women	—	54.5	36.0	65.4

Table 3–4. Awareness, Treatment, and Control of Hypertension

race/ethnicity, socioeconomic status, education, and quality of health care within countries.[48]

Trends in level of awareness, treatment, and control

In the United States, there has been a trend towards greater awareness, treatment, and control of hypertension in the community.[41] During the 12-year interval between NHANES II and III, the proportion of hypertensive patients who were aware of their condition increased from 51% to 73%.[41] Increases in awareness were greater for whites than blacks during this time period. Awareness was higher for women than men among both blacks and whites. For example, 67% of black and white men with hypertension were aware of their diagnosis, while 79% and 82% of black and white women, respectively, were aware of their diagnosis at the time of NHANES III.

The increase in awareness of hypertension between 1976–1980 and 1988–1991 has been accompanied by an increase in the proportion of hypertensives receiving treatment with antihypertensive medications. Overall, the percentage of hypertensives receiving treatment increased from 31% in 1976–1980 to 55% in 1988–1991 in the U.S. population. The large difference in awareness of hypertension between men and women in NHANES III is mirrored by a 19% difference in treatment rates. Less than half of male hypertensives received treatment (46%),

while almost two-thirds of women were on treatment for their high blood pressure (65%). For both genders, the percentage of treatment increased by over 20% between 1976–1980 and 1988–1991, from 21% to 46% in men, and 43% to 65% in women. The percentages of treatment were virtually identical during NHANES III for black and white men at 46% and 47%, and both black and white women at 65%, respectively. The proportion of controlled hypertension increased nearly threefold at the 140/90 mmHg cut-point during the 12 years between NHANES II and III. The control rate of hypertension however remains low at 29%. Control rate is higher in women at 38% than in men at 22%. A greater percentage of whites achieved control than blacks, 31% and 26%, respectively. Control rates among treated hypertensives were higher in women than in men and in blacks than in whites. The overall percentage of treated hypertensives with controlled blood pressure increased from 32% in 1976–1980 to 55% in 1988–1991 in the U.S. general population. NHANES 1999–2000 reported no change in the awareness of hypertension, but a further increase of 6% in hypertension treatment and control.[40]

Increasing levels of awareness, treatment, and control have also been reported in Europe. For example, the Health Survey for England reported increased hypertension awareness, treatment, and control from 46.0%, 31.6%, and 7.1% in 1994 to 52.2%, 38.0%, and 10.7% in 1998, respectively.[24] Among individuals with hypertension, treatment rates were highest among black men and women. Among the treated hypertensives, levels of control did not differ among the three groups of older men but was lower in older South Asian women, compared with white women. In Germany, there was little improvement in the detection rate of hypertension over a 10-year period from 1984–1985 to 1994–1995.[45] Awareness of hypertension remained at approximately 50% in men and 60% in women. The proportion of individuals with hypertension who were receiving drug treatment increased by 7.9% in men and 4.1% in women.[45] Overall, levels of hypertension awareness, treatment, and control in Europe are much lower than in the United States, with levels in Canada lying approximately halfway between these extremes.[15]

PREVENTION

The U.S. National High Blood Pressure Education Program has recommended a combination of population-based and intensive targeted strategies for primary prevention of hypertension.[49] Interventions that have proved effective include weight loss, reduced intake of dietary sodium, moderate alcohol consumption, potassium supplementation, modification of eating habits, and increased physical activity.[49] These lifestyle changes also have positive effects on other cardiovascular risk factors such as obesity and type 2 diabetes. Secondary prevention efforts entail detection, treatment, and control of hypertension.

Although improvements have been made in the detection and treatment of hypertension in developed countries, rates remain far from adequate.[15,17] Interventions to reduce the burden of cardiovascular disease have been successful in some developed regions including Europe, North America, Australia, and New Zealand.[50] These interventions have resulted in substantial reductions in age-adjusted cardiovascular mortality. Personal and nonpersonal health-service interventions have proved cost-effective at both regional and global levels.[51] Although personal health-service strategies have greater potential to reduce the burden of disease, they are less cost-effective than population-wide ones.[51] The availability of analyses of cost-effectiveness allows key decision makers to establish the most appropriate interventions with available resources.

SUMMARY

Hypertension is an important public health problem in developed countries. While the prevalence of hypertension varies among the developed countries, there are some consistent findings. Hypertension prevalence increases with age and tends to be more common in men than in women. There is evidence of a small rural–urban gradient. Over the past decade the prevalence of hypertension has remained stable or decreased in developed countries. The distribution of hypertension within populations is influenced by a number of factors. The prevalence of hypertension varies by age, gender, and racial composition of the population under study. As well as internal factors, the prevalence of hypertension is also affected by environmental exposures, such as intake of dietary sodium and potassium, body weight, alcohol consumption, and physical activity. Any increase in the lifestyle factors of physical inactivity, overweight, high intake of dietary sodium, and low intake of dietary potassium are likely to be accompanied by a concomitant increase in blood pressure.

Awareness of hypertension has improved in the United States and other Western countries over the past decade, but remains inadequate, in particular as only a proportion of those who are aware of their diagnosis are treated, and an even smaller number of those receiving treatment are treated adequately.

An acknowledgment of the global nature of the problem of hypertension is required so that healthcare providers screen for and treat elevated blood pressure. The magnitude of the burden of hypertension, however, requires not only an increase in the awareness, treatment, and control of hypertension, but also concerted efforts targeting the primary prevention of hypertension. The lifetime risk of hypertension for white individuals in the United States has been estimated to be 90% in both 55- and 65-year-old participants.[52] Improvements in the detection, treatment, and control of high blood pressure will not suffice to address a problem that affects a significant proportion of the population. A reduction in average blood pressure could be achieved by lifestyle modification of the general population, which would result in a reduced prevalence of hypertension.

Hypertension is a common public health problem throughout the developed world. It often goes undiagnosed and even when it is identified and treated, few hypertensives achieve adequate control of their blood pressure. The improvements in the awareness, treatment, and control of blood pressure in the United States provide hope that similar advances may be made elsewhere. However, given the high prevalence of hypertension in the community and the difficulties in achieving and maintaining the goals of therapy, lifestyle modification remains an attractive therapeutic option.

REFERENCES

1. He J, Whelton PK. Epidemiology and prevention of hypertension. *Med Clin North Am* 1997;81(5):1077–97.

2. Whelton PK. Epidemiology of hypertension. *Lancet* 1994; 344(8915):101–6.

3. Ezzati M, Lopez AD, Rodgers A, Vander Hoorn S, Murray CJ. Selected major risk factors and global and regional burden of disease. *Lancet* 2002;360(9343):1347–60.

4. Kannel WB. Blood pressure as a cardiovascular risk factor: prevention and treatment. *JAMA* 1996;275(20):1571–6.

5. He J, Whelton PK. Elevated systolic blood pressure and risk of cardiovascular and renal disease: overview of evidence from observational epidemiologic studies and randomized controlled trials. *Am Heart J* 1999;138(3 Pt 2):211–9.

6. MacMahon S, Peto R, Cutler J, et al. Blood pressure, stroke, and coronary heart disease. Part 1: Prolonged differences in blood pressure: prospective observational studies corrected for the regression dilution bias. *Lancet* 1990;335(8692):765–74.

7. Stamler J, Stamler R, Neaton JD. Blood pressure, systolic and diastolic, and cardiovascular risks. US population data. *Arch Intern Med* 1993;153(5): 598–615.

8. Klag MJ, Whelton PK, Randall BL, et al. Blood pressure and end-stage renal disease in men. *N Engl J Med* 1996; 334(1):13–8.

9. He J, Ogden LG, Bazzano LA, Vupputuri S, Loria C, Whelton PK. Risk factors for congestive heart failure in US men and women: NHANES I epidemiologic follow-up study. *Arch Intern Med* 2001;161(7):996–1002.

10. Collins R, Peto R, MacMahon S, et al. Blood pressure, stroke, and coronary heart disease. Part 2: Short-term reductions in blood pressure: overview of randomised drug trials in their epidemiological context. *Lancet* 1990; 335(8693):827–38.

11. Hebert PR, Moser M, Mayer J, Glynn RJ, Hennekens CH. Recent evidence on drug therapy of mild to moderate hypertension and decreased risk of coronary heart disease. *Arch Intern Med* 1993;153(5):578–81.

12. He J, Whelton PK. Selection of initial antihypertensive drug therapy. *Lancet* 2000;356(9246):1942–3.

13. Lenfant C. Reflections on hypertension control rates: a message from the director of the National Heart, Lung, and Blood Institute. *Arch Intern Med* 2002;162(2):131–2.

14. Bhatt DL, Steg PG, Ohman EM, et al. International prevalence, recognition, and treatment of cardiovascular risk factors in outpatients with atherothrombosis. *JAMA* 2006; 295(2):180–9.

15. Wolf-Maier K, Cooper RS, Kramer H, et al. Hypertension treatment and control in five European countries, Canada, and the United States. *Hypertension* 2004;43(1):10–7.

16. Kearney PM, Whelton M, Reynolds K, Muntner P, Whelton PK, He J. Global burden of hypertension:

analysis of worldwide data. *Lancet* 2005;365(9455):217–23.

17. Kearney PM, Whelton M, Reynolds K, Whelton PK, He J. Worldwide prevalence of hypertension: a systematic review. *J Hypertens* 2004;22(1):11–9.

18. Wolz M, Cutler J, Roccella EJ, Rohde F, Thom T, Burt V. Statement from the National High Blood Pressure Education Program: prevalence of hypertension. *Am J Hypertens* 2000;13(1 Pt 1):103–4.

19. Joint National Committee. *The Seventh Report of the Joint National Committee on Prevention, Detection, Evaluation, and Treatment of High Blood Pressure.* Washington, DC: U.S. Department of Health and Human Services, 2004 (NIH publication 04-5230).

20. Wang Y, Wang QJ. The prevalence of prehypertension and hypertension among US adults according to the new Joint National Committee Guidelines. *Arch Intern Med.* 2004;164:2126–2134.

21. Joffres MR, Ghadirian P, Fodor JG, Petrasovits A, Chockalingam A, Hamet P. Awareness, treatment, and control of hypertension in Canada. *Am J Hypertens* 1997;10(10 Pt 1): 1097–102.

22. Wolf-Maier K, Cooper RS, Banegas JR, et al. Hypertension prevalence and blood pressure levels in 6 European countries, Canada, and the United States. *JAMA* 2003;289(18):2363–9.

23. Banegas JR, Rodriguez-Artalejo F, de la Cruz Troca JJ, Guallar-Castillon P, del Rey Calero J. Blood pressure in Spain: distribution, awareness, control, and benefits of a reduction in average pressure. *Hypertension* 1998;32(6):998–1002.

24. Primatesta P, Brookes M, Poulter NR. Improved hypertension management and control: results from the health survey for England 1998. *Hypertension* 2001;38(4):827–32.

25. Bennett SA, Magnus P. Trends in cardiovascular risk factors in Australia. Results from the National Heart Foundation's Risk Factor Prevalence Study, 1980–1989. *Med J Aust* 1994; 161(9):519–27.

26. Australian Institute of Health and Welfare. *National Cardiovascular Disease and Diabetes Database.* Cardiovascular risk factors report. http://www.aihw. gov.au/dataonline/riskfactors/index.cfm Accessed 2 March 2006.

27. Whelton PK, He J, Klag M. Blood pressure in Westernized populations. In Swales JD, ed. *Textbook of Hypertension.* London: Blackwell Scientific, 1994:11–21.

28. He J, Tell GS, Tang YC, Mo PS, He GQ. Effect of migration on blood pressure: the Yi People Study. *Epidemiology* 1991; 2(2):88–97.

29. National Heart, Lung, and Blood Institute. Report of the Second Task Force on Blood Pressure Control in Children—1987. Task Force on Blood Pressure Control in Children. National Heart, Lung, and Blood Institute, Bethesda, Maryland. *Pediatrics* 1987; 79(1):1–25.

30. Berenson GS, Wattigney WA, Webber LS. Epidemiology of hypertension from childhood to young adulthood

in black, white, and Hispanic population samples. *Public Health Rep* 1996;111(Suppl 2):3–6.

31. Kelder SH, Osganian SK, Feldman HA, et al. Tracking of physical and physiological risk variables among ethnic subgroups from third to eighth grade: the Child and Adolescent Trial for Cardiovascular Health cohort study. *Prev Med* 2002;34(3):324–33.

32. Kannel WB, Gordon T. Evaluation of cardiovascular risk in the elderly: the Framingham Study. *Bull N Y Acad Med* 1978;54:573–91.

33. Kastarinen MJ, Salomaa VV, Vartiainen EA, et al. Trends in blood pressure levels and control of hypertension in Finland from 1982 to 1997. *J Hypertens* 1998; 16(9):1379–87.

34. Thamm M. [Blood pressure in Germany—current status and trends]. *Gesundheitswesen* 1999;61:S90–3.

35. Giampaoli S, Palmieri L, Dima F, Pilotto L, Vescio MF, Vanuzzo D. [Socioeconomic aspects and cardiovascular risk factors: experience at the Cardiovascular Epidemiologic Observatory]. *Ital Heart J Suppl* 2001; 2(3):294–302.

36. Cornoni-Huntley J, LaCroix AZ, Havlik RJ. Race and sex differentials in the impact of hypertension in the United States. The National Health and Nutrition Examination Survey I Epidemiologic Follow-up Study. *Arch Intern Med* 1989;149(4):780–8.

37. Fuchs FD, Chambless LE, Whelton PK, Nieto FJ, Heiss G. Alcohol consumption and the incidence of hypertension: the Atherosclerosis Risk in Communities Study. *Hypertension* 2001;37(5):1242–50.

38. Apostolides AY, Cutter G, Daugherty SA, et al. Three-year incidence of hypertension in thirteen U.S. communities. On behalf of the Hypertension Detection and Follow-up Program cooperative group. *Prev Med* 1982;11(5):487–99.

39. Manolio TA, Burke GL, Savage PJ, Sidney S, Gardin JM, Oberman A. Exercise blood pressure response and 5-year risk of elevated blood pressure in a cohort of young adults: the CARDIA study. *Am J Hypertens* 1994;7(3):234–41.

40. Hajjar I, Kotchen TA. Trends in prevalence, awareness, treatment, and control of hypertension in the United States, 1988–2000. *JAMA* 2003; 290 (22):199–206.

41. Burt VL, Cutler JA, Higgins M, et al. Trends in the prevalence, awareness, treatment, and control of hypertension in the adult US population. Data from the health examination surveys, 1960 to 1991. *Hypertension* 1995;26(1):60–9.

42. Geographical variation in the major risk factors of coronary heart disease in men and women aged 35–64 years. The WHO MONICA Project. *World Health Stat Q* 1988;41(3–4):115–40.

43. Wolf HK, Tuomilehto J, Kuulasmaa K, et al. Blood pressure levels in the 41 populations of the WHO MONICA Project. *J Hum Hypertens* 1997;11(11):733–42.

44. De Henauw S, De Bacquer D, Fonteyne W, Stam M, Kornitzer M, De Backer G. Trends in the prevalence, detection, treatment and control of

arterial hypertension in the Belgian adult population. *J Hypertens* 1998; 16(3):277–84.

45. Gasse C, Hense HW, Stieber J, Doring A, Liese AD, Keil U. Assessing hypertension management in the community: trends of prevalence, detection, treatment, and control of hypertension in the MONICA Project, Augsburg 1984–1995. *J Hum Hypertens* 2001;15(1):27–36.

46. Stergiou GS, Thomopoulou GC, Skeva II, Mountokalakis TD. Prevalence, awareness, treatment, and control of hypertension in Greece: the Didima study. *Am J Hypertens* 1999;12:959–65.

47. Moulopoulos SD, Adamopoulos PN, Diamantopoulos EI, Nanas SN, Anthopoulos LN, Iliadi-Alexandrou M. Coronary heart disease risk factors in a random sample of Athenian adults. The Athens Study. *Am J Epidemiol* 1987; 126(5):882–92.

48. He J, Muntner P, Chen J, Roccella EJ, Streiffer RH, Whelton PK. Factors associated with hypertension control in the general population of the United States. *Arch Intern Med* 2002; 162(9):1051–8.

49. Whelton PK, He J, Appel LJ, et al. Primary prevention of hypertension: clinical and public health advisory from The National High Blood Pressure Education Program. *JAMA* 2002; 288(15):1882–8.

50. Thom TJ. International mortality from heart disease: rates and trends. *Int J Epidemiol* 1989;18(Suppl 1):S20–8.

51. Murray CJ, Lauer JA, Hutubessy RC, et al. Effectiveness and costs of interventions to lower systolic blood pressure and cholesterol: a global and regional analysis on reduction of cardiovascular-disease risk. *Lancet* 2003; 361(9359):717–25.

52. Vasan RS, Beiser A, Seshadri S, et al. Residual lifetime risk for developing hypertension in middle-aged women and men: the Framingham Heart Study. *JAMA* 2002;287(8):1003–10.

Regional Differences in Blood Pressure in Developed Countries

Chapter

4

Early-Life Influences on Blood Pressure

Debbie A. Lawlor and George Davey Smith

Key Findings

- Treated and well-controlled hypertensive adults still have a substantial excess mortality and reduced survival compared with normotensive adults. Therefore, identification of the means of preventing hypertension in earlier life is an important objective.

- Blood pressure "tracks" across the life course, such that those at the higher end of the blood pressure distribution in earlier life tend to be at the higher end of the distribution in later life.

- Children of lower socioeconomic status, those whose mothers experienced pregnancy-induced hypertension, whose mothers smoked throughout pregnancy, those with low birth weight, who have high-sodium diets in infancy, and who are obese in childhood or adolescence, tend to have higher blood pressure in adulthood.

- The mechanisms linking these early-life factors to later blood pressure, and the most appropriate means of preventing adult hypertension by intervening in early life, are currently unclear.

- Observational studies with repeat measurements of a range of socioeconomic, behavioral and biological factors assessed over the life course and the use of appropriate statistical methods are required to further understand the temporal relationships between risk factors and the mechanisms that link early-life exposures to future disease.

- There is a need for randomized trials with sufficient resources for long-term follow-up to assess the effects of interventions to reduce maternal smoking, increase breast feeding, reduce salt consumption in infancy, and prevent childhood obesity, on adult blood pressure and associated cardiovascular disease.

Blood pressure in middle-aged and older people is positively and linearly associated with coronary heart disease (CHD) and stroke risk.[1] While treating high blood pressure is beneficial in terms of reducing the occurrence of these outcomes,[2] treated and well-controlled hypertensive adults still have a substantial excess mortality and reduced survival compared with normotensives.[3] Therefore, the identification of the means of preventing hypertension in earlier life is an important objective.

Blood pressure "tracks" across the life course, such that those at the higher end of the blood pressure distribution in earlier life tend to be at the higher end of the distribution in later life.[4] These tracking correlations increase with increasing age in childhood.[5] The strong and increasing tracking correlations from mid-childhood onward suggest that being in the upper end of the blood pressure distribution in middle or older age is largely determined by the middle of one's childhood years and certainly by the time of adolescence.

In this chapter we provide a summary of the current evidence concerning the early-life determinants of adult blood pressure, and discuss how current evidence ought to affect clinical or public health practice, in addition to discussing future research needs in this area. We begin by considering the association between childhood socioeconomic status (SES) and adult blood pressure since childhood SES may be an underlying determinant that acts through several of the other risk factors considered in the chapter. Other risk factors are presented in the chronological order in which they occur in an individual's life course. Of note, many of these exposures act together, rather than in isolation, to have their effect.

EARLY-LIFE SOCIOECONOMIC POSITION

Adverse childhood socioeconomic status (SES) is associated with increased cardiovascular disease (CVD) risk in later life independently of adult SES.[6] There is no strong evidence that childhood SES is associated with higher blood pressure also measured in childhood.[7,8] However, childhood SES does appear to be associated with adult blood pressure, such that those from more adverse childhood SES have higher blood pressure in adulthood, independent of adult SES.[9–11] Consistent with these findings, in the 1946 British birth cohort there was evidence of amplification of the effect of childhood SES on blood pressure, with the difference in blood pressure between manual and nonmanual childhood social class increasing by 1.0 mmHg per 10 years.[11]

There could be several reasons for the increase in the magnitude of the effect of childhood SES on blood pressure over the life course. First, few studies conducted in childhood have adjusted for height, and height may mask any association in childhood, since taller children will tend to be from higher socioeconomic groups,[12,13] but in childhood taller stature is associated with higher blood pressure.[7] Second, there may be latent programming, with a range of adverse environmental exposures in fetal and early postnatal life that are related to socioeconomic disadvantage resulting in abnormal metabolic, structural, and hormonal development that does not manifest itself as elevated blood pressure until later in life. Finally, childhood SES may influence later blood pressure, not through causing permanent damage in childhood or early adulthood, but by setting someone on a trajectory of risk exposures (e.g., poor diet, low levels of physical activity, smoking across the life course), which together result in high blood pressure in later life. In a recent prospective analysis of the Young Finns cohort study, we found that once height was taken into account, childhood SES was strongly associated with blood pressure in childhood (those from the most disadvantaged groups having higher blood pressure).[14] As with other studies we found marked tracking of blood pressure and a strong association between childhood SES and blood pressure in early adulthood. Of note, we found that adjustment for childhood blood pressure resulted in marked attenuation of the association between childhood SES and adult blood pressure, suggesting that adverse childhood SES had a direct effect on blood pressure in childhood, which then tracked into adulthood.[14]

MATERNAL PREGNANCY CHARACTERISTICS

Maternal and pregnancy characteristics have most commonly been related to offspring blood pressure in childhood and adolescence, with very few studies relating these characteristics to adult blood pressure. However, the strong tracking coefficients of blood pressure from late childhood into adulthood (see above) mean that associations with blood pressure in late childhood and adolescence are likely to reflect similar associations into adulthood.

There is also a positive association between pregnancy-induced hypertension or maternal blood pressure measured during pregnancy and offspring blood pressure measured in childhood and adolescence.[15] This may reflect intrauterine effects or the genetic transmission of blood pressure risk from parent to child. The fact that the maternal–offspring blood pressure association is similar to that of the paternal–offspring association suggests that intrauterine effects are unlikely to explain this association.[16]

The small number of studies that have assessed the association between maternal hemoglobin during pregnancy and offspring blood pressure in childhood and adolescence have found inconsistent results, with two studies finding inverse associations,[17,18] one study finding no association,[19] and one study finding a positive association.[20] Maternal smoking during pregnancy has been shown in three studies to be associated with increased offspring blood pressure in childhood and adolescence,[21–23] but two other studies found no such association.[17,20] In the largest study to date (*n*=3864), systolic blood pressure of children whose mothers had smoked throughout pregnancy was on average 0.92 mmHg greater than those whose mothers had never smoked, after adjustment for a range of maternal and infant characteristics, including SES and maternal body mass index (BMI) and gestational hypertension.[23] Blood pressure in children whose mothers

quit smoking early in pregnancy did not differ from those whose mothers had never smoked.

MATERNAL NUTRITION

The "fetal origins hypothesis" suggests that factors which impact on fetal growth have a long-term programming effect on future adult health. In early descriptions of the fetal origins or programming hypothesis, David Barker first suggested that maternal nutrition determined fetal nutrition which in turn impacted upon adult blood pressure and other CVD risk factors through abnormal development, *in utero*, of key systems that determined these CVD risk factors (the so-called Barker hypothesis).

However, it is now acknowledged that maternal nutrition does not equate to fetal nutrition.[24] The fetus of a poorly nourished mother can be well nourished, as nutrients are preferentially directed to the growing fetus. Conversely, a well-nourished mother may have a poorly nourished fetus because of defects in the fetal supply line from the placenta. Much of the direct evidence for an effect of maternal pregnancy diet and fetal nutrition on future blood pressure has come from animal studies, where experimental manipulation during pregnancy is possible.[24–27] One of the great strengths of animal studies is the ability to be able to manipulate maternal nutrition separately from fetal supply line factors and vice versa.[24] In human studies it is impossible to do this. While animal studies have found a direct effect of maternal pregnancy dietary manipulation and reduced fetal supply on blood pressure and other CVD risk factors,[24–27] the generalizability of their findings, as well as the extreme nature of some of the manipulations, such as ligation of umbilical vessels, makes interpreting these results with respect to humans problematic.[24]

The effect of gross maternal pregnancy diet has been assessed in humans using two natural experiments, where pregnant women experienced extreme nutritional deprivation during the World War II.[28–31] These found no effect of starvation during pregnancy on adult blood pressure in their offspring.[28,31] However, this form of extreme starvation does not provide information on variations in maternal diet that occur in contemporary general populations and that might affect future blood pressure in offspring. Further, the offspring of women who actually gave birth to a viable offspring having gone through such extreme nutritional deprivation during pregnancy may be unique in many ways that make these findings difficult to generalize.

In well-characterized rat models, even mild restrictions in maternal protein during pregnancy have been found to be associated with increased blood pressure in offspring.[26,27,32,33] These effects were similar for dietary manipulations at all stages of pregnancy.[32] Results in humans have been mixed. Three historical cohorts found that blood pressure in adulthood was greater among those whose mothers had consumed diets characterized by high levels of animal protein and low levels of carbohydrates in late pregnancy (second half of pregnancy in one study[34] and last trimester in two others[35,36]), but there was no association between maternal diet at other times in pregnancy and offspring blood pressure.[34–36]

In one prospective study there was no association between maternal intake of protein as reported at a mean of 30 weeks gestation and offspring blood pressure in adolescence, although maternal intake of fat was inversely associated with blood pressure in female offspring.[37] In a second prospective study neither maternal intake of protein assessed during the first trimester of pregnancy nor that assessed during the second trimester was associated with offspring blood pressure at a mean age of 6 months,[38] and a third study found no association between the ratio of protein to carbohydrate measured at 32 weeks gestation (nor any other micronutrient) and offspring blood pressure assessed at a mean of 7 years.[39] These inconsistencies may be explained by differences in study design, assessment of dietary intake in pregnancy and age at which blood pressure in the offspring is assessed. Ideally, randomized trials with long-term follow-up should be used to assess the effects of different maternal diets on future blood pressure risk, but such studies are expensive and difficult to conduct.

Observational epidemiologic studies have found that higher intakes of calcium during pregnancy, and by the children themselves in the early postnatal period, is related to lower blood pressure in offspring.[40,41] Further, results from a randomized controlled trial conducted in Argentina found that mean systolic blood pressure at age 7 was lower in those whose mothers had been randomized to 2 g of calcium supplementation per day throughout pregnancy compared to those randomized to placebo, particularly if the child was overweight at age 7.[42] Follow-up was complete for over 85% of both intervention and placebo group, and the mothers remained blind at the 7-year follow-up to which group they had been allocated. Replication of these findings in other populations would be useful.

BIRTH WEIGHT

By January 2005, nearly 100 studies assessing the association of birth weight with blood pressure had been published, and the finding in the majority of these studies of an inverse association has formed a central part of the "fetal origins of chronic disease" or "programming" hypothesis. In nearly all cases, this inverse association was strengthened on adjustment for concurrent body size. Four published systematic reviews of the association have all concluded that an inverse association is apparent, with a magnitude in the region of −1.5 to −2.0 mmHg/kg.[43–46] However, the authors of these reviews and other investigators disagree in their conclusions concerning whether this association is causal, and if causal, whether it is of public health or clinical importance.

The consistency of findings in a range of different populations including children and adults, and populations from high-, middle-, and low-income countries,[45] suggest that the association is unlikely to be fully explained by

confounding factors, since the confounding structures will be different in these different populations. There is also evidence for specificity of the association with birth weight being associated with CVD and its risk factors but not with lung cancer, suggesting that SES and smoking are unlikely to explain the association.[47] Further, in studies where control for potential confounders has been possible, the inverse association between birth weight and blood pressure has been found to be independent of SES, maternal and participant smoking, maternal age, birth order, maternal blood pressure, and alcohol intake.[48–51]

There has been considerable debate about the appropriateness or not of adjusting for contemporary size in studies assessing the association between birth weight and blood pressure in later life.[52,53] In many studies the inverse association between birth weight and later blood pressure is strengthened or only becomes apparent upon adjustment for contemporary weight or BMI. One way to understand this effect of adjustment for contemporary size is to consider a population of adults, all of whom have the same weight or BMI at a particular age. It is differences in the growth trajectories from conception taken by individuals to reach this particular size that predict variations in blood pressure.[16] Trajectories of below average growth *in utero* (representing poor fetal nutrition) and increased growth in childhood (related consumption of high-energy diets) appear to be particularly detrimental.[45,54] However, in humans it is difficult to distinguish between intrauterine and postnatal effects and some have argued that nutrition in infancy is more important than fetal nutrition as a risk factor for high blood pressure and CVD.[55] Alternatively, the possible interaction between intrauterine and postnatal growth may be explained by developmental plasticity—the ability of environmental effects during sensitive developmental periods to affect the mature phenotype.[56,57] The suggestion here is that, through a process of natural selection across generations, the intrauterine environment can "forecast" and prepare a developing human fetus for a postnatal environment of thrift. This preparation will have survival advantages in thrifty environments, but in contemporary Western environments of excessive nutrition the "setting" of metabolic and endocrine pathways for thrift may result in increased risk of hypertension, diabetes, and CVD since the "thrifty"-set metabolic pathways facilitate rapid/accelerated growth in an environment of plenty.[56]

In a recent meta-analysis the magnitude of the effect of birth weight varied by study size, with a weaker association in the larger studies.[46] The authors concluded that publication bias had led to exaggerated conclusions about the effect of birth weight on blood pressure. However, this conclusion fails to recognize that in observational epidemiology, large studies often have lower-quality data. Two very large studies have demonstrated that blood pressure is poorly measured and that the true association of birth weight with blood pressure in these studies is consequently underestimated.[58,59]

A number of investigators have questioned the public health importance of the association, pointing out that even if one accepts an association of the magnitude of −1.5 mmHg/kg, this represents a change in blood pressure of less than 0.2 of a standard deviation for a very substantial (two standard deviations) change in birth weight.[46,60] This weak association has been compared to the much stronger positive association between contemporary weight or BMI and blood pressure.[60] However, while contemporary size will have a direct effect on blood pressure, few investigators imagine that birth weight has a direct effect on blood pressure; rather it acts as a proxy indicator for other exposures, such as fetal nutrition and genetic factors, that may directly affect blood pressure. The associations of birth weight with blood pressure are likely therefore to underestimate the true strength of any association between the real exposure and blood pressure. It is noteworthy that the magnitudes of the associations between birth weight and CHD and stroke (two of the major consequences of high blood pressure) are strong and not dependent on BMI adjustment.[47]

Possible mechanisms for the birth weight–blood pressure association

In terms of how the association between birth weight and adult blood pressure should impact on clinical and public health practice, we need to understand more about the underlying mechanisms. The "fetal origins hypothesis" (also known as the "developmental origins of adult disease and programming" hypothesis) suggests that poor intra-uterine nutrition leads not only to small birth size but also, depending on the timing (or critical period), it "programs" selective changes in body composition, cell size and number, hormonal axes, and metabolism that affect blood pressure and other CVD risk factors.[61] Fetal growth is determined by both maternal and fetal nutrition and it is important to distinguish between the possible effects of maternal nutrition across her life course before pregnancy, maternal nutritional status and diet during pregnancy, and fetal nutrition (i.e., the net supply of metabolic substrate to the fetus) on both fetal growth and future offspring's blood pressure.[24]

In addition to roles for maternal nutrition, diet during pregnancy and the fetal nutrient supply line, it has been suggested that genetic factors might explain the association between birth weight and blood pressure. The same genetic factors may determine both fetal development, and hence birth weight and subsequent risk of insulin resistance and its associated risk factors including elevated blood pressure (the fetal insulin hypothesis).[62,63] While the animal studies discussed above provide proof of principle that fetal programming not explained by genes exists, it is possible that genetic factors and fetal nutritional programming are both relevant to the association of low birth weight with elevated blood pressure in humans.

Examining the association of birth weight with blood pressure within twins has been proposed as a useful research method for distinguishing between fixed maternal factors, pregnancy-related factors, and genetic factors in the association between birth weight and adult disease. A logical progression in these studies is first to treat all of

the twins as individuals and simply assess the association between birth weight and blood pressure in the twin population (*between*-twin study). If an inverse association between birth weight and CVD is found between twins this suggests that twins *per se* do not differ from the general populations in which this association has been demonstrated. A *within*-twin pair analysis is then equivalent to matching on factors that are identical within twin pairs. If there is no association within monozygotic (MZ) pairs between birth weight and blood pressure (i.e., on average the smaller birth-weight MZ twin within any pair has similar blood pressure to the heavier twin), but an inverse association is seen in dizygotic (DZ) twins, then this suggests that factors which are identical between MZ twins (but not DZ twins) explain the association. Since MZ twins are genetically identical, fetal genes would be the most obvious explanation. However, approximately two-thirds of MZ twins share a placenta; therefore the lack of an association specifically within MZ twins may also be consistent with nongenetic placental factors.[64] If there is no association within both MZ and DZ (i.e., when the analysis is undertaken with matching on factors that are identical within either MZ or DZ twin pairs), but there is a between-pairs association, then the association between birth weight and disease would be most simply explained by fixed maternal factors that are identical for both twins in both MZ and DZ pairs. For twins, these factors would include maternal socioeconomic circumstances and environmental exposures in her early life, maternal birth characteristics and growth across her life, maternal age, diet, and smoking and other characteristics during pregnancy. If the within-twin pair associations for both MZ and DZ pairs are similar to the between-twin associations, then this suggests that fetal nutrition (which varies within both twin types) or any other factor that is not identical within twin pairs explains the association.

Studies have examined between- and within-twin pair associations of birth weight and blood pressure, and a recent systematic review and meta-analysis of these studies found a weaker association within-twin pairs than between-twin pairs, suggesting that factors shared by twins (fixed maternal factors from earlier in her life course and at the time of pregnancy) contribute to the association between birth weight and blood pressure in singletons.[65] However, comparisons of paired analyses in MZ and DZ pairs could not provide conclusive evidence for a role for genetic as opposed to shared environmental factors, because of small sample sizes and variations between studies in the methods used for determining zygosity.

Although the within- and between-twin study design looks very elegant, important differences exist between twins and singletons in their growth trajectories, with these differences appearing from very early in gestation, possibly being programmed at conception.[66,67] Thus it is unclear whether one can generalize findings from twin studies to the majority of the population who are single-tons. An extension of the within-twin analysis is a within-family or within-siblings analysis. While the complete control for genetic factors in such a study is not possible, they offer the advantage over twin studies of being more generalizable. In a recent small (N=600 sibling pairs) within-siblings study, the results suggested that the inverse association between birth weight and blood pressure was not explained by fixed maternal factors such as SES, her nutritional status from conception to early adulthood, or maternal genetic factors.[16] Since siblings (as opposed to twins) have experienced different pregnancies and share only 50% of their genes, maternal pregnancy characteristics and genetic factors might explain the association between birth weight and blood pressure. Indeed, in this study adjustment for paternal as well as maternal blood pressure reduced the strength of the association between birth weight and systolic blood pressure of the offspring in childhood, suggesting a potential role for genetic factors. The findings from this small study have now been replicated in a very large (N=103,548 sibling groups) study, providing strong evidence that the birthweight–blood pressure association is not explained by fixed maternal factors (Lawlor DA et al. paper submitted for publication June 2006).

INFANT FEEDING

Two meta-analyses of the association between breast-feeding and blood pressure in later life found very similar pooled estimates despite each including a number of different studies. The pooled estimates suggested an approximate difference in systolic blood pressure of 1 mmHg comparing those who were ever breastfed to those who were exclusively bottle fed.[68,69] Whether this association is causal is difficult to determine since there was evidence of publication bias in both studies and other limitations of the individual studies, including measurement error in determining breastfeeding and confounding.

In one study, published since the most recent of these meta-analyses, parents of children aged 9 and 15 years at examination were asked about exclusive breastfeeding and there was a dose–response association, with greater duration of exclusive breastfeeding being associated with greater reductions in blood pressure.[70] This dose response provides some evidence of causality, but clear evidence for a causal effect requires evidence from randomized controlled trials. The clear benefits of breastfeeding make it impossible to randomize infants to different feeding regimens, but the long-term follow-up of the offspring of women who were randomized to different interventions to promote breastfeeding (if these were effective at increasing breastfeeding) might be one means of determining whether breastfeeding is causally related to blood pressure. The authors of a long-term follow-up of a randomized controlled trial of different feeding regimens in pre-term infants concluded that breast milk had a major beneficial effect on blood pressure and other CVD risk factors in adolescence. However, a recent detailed review of the role of infant feeding on CVD demonstrates that the majority of women randomized to pre-term formula actually also breastfed their children, and concludes that the results really show that individuals in that trial "who were given pre-term formula are more likely to display markers of cardiovascular disease risk."[71]

DIETARY SODIUM INTAKE IN INFANCY AND CHILDHOOD

Among adults, salt intake reduction is associated with small reductions in blood pressure,[72,73] although in childhood urinary sodium levels (a reflection of dietary intake and plasma clearance) do not appear to have a marked effect on blood pressure.[74–78] However, there is evidence that infancy is a sensitive period with respect to the effect of sodium on future blood pressure. In a Dutch study in the early 1980s, infants were randomized to a low or a normal sodium diet for the first 6 months of life. The initial results of that study found that blood pressure in those allocated to the low-sodium diet was 2.1 mmHg lower at the end of the 6-month intervention period, but with further follow-up to 12 months there was no difference between the two groups.[79,80] A 15-year follow-up of the participants found that mean systolic and diastolic blood pressure were markedly lower among the group originally randomized to the low-salt group compared to the high-salt group; mean difference in systolic blood pressure was 3.6 mmHg, and in diastolic blood pressure was 2.2 mmHg.[81] This effect is considerably larger than any reported effects of salt reduction in adults. Interestingly, at the 15-year follow-up there was no difference in mean sodium intake in the two groups, suggesting that the effect was not due to dietary sodium in infancy influencing an individual's taste for salt and later sodium intake. Because of the strong tracking correlations from age 15 onward, this effect of dietary sodium in infancy on blood pressure at age 15 would be likely to have a lasting effect on blood pressure into adulthood. These results should be treated with caution since there was considerable loss to follow-up, with only 35% of the original participants included. Further, their relevance to contemporary populations is unclear since infant formulas contain much less sodium now than they did in the early 1980s when this trial was conducted. To date no other published studies have assessed the effect of random allocation to different dietary sodium levels in infancy and later blood pressure. Since infant formulas in most Western countries now have sodium levels that are equivalent to physiological levels in breast milk, manipulating sodium intake in early infancy in a trial would not be ethical or feasible. However, it is likely that from weaning onward, infant diets will vary considerably in their sodium content, and a randomized controlled trial of the effects of different dietary intake of sodium from weaning age onward in infancy on future blood pressure would be valuable.

CHILDHOOD ADIPOSITY

There is a strong positive relationship between BMI and blood pressure at all stages of the life course.[60] Thus BMI measured in childhood is positively associated with blood pressure in childhood and this association remains throughout life. Since blood pressure tracks from childhood to adulthood, one would therefore expect an association between childhood BMI and adult blood pressure. Several prospective studies have found that BMI or weight measured in childhood is positively associated with blood pressure measured in adulthood.[60] However, this association may not be independent of adult BMI.[82] Increases in BMI during childhood or between childhood and adolescence are also associated with greater blood pressure in adulthood,[83,84] and in a recent Australian study of children, those who changed from being overweight or obese at age 5 to normal weight at age 14 had similar mean blood pressure to those who were normal weight at both ages, whereas those who remained overweight or obese at both ages had higher mean blood pressure.[85]

From a disease prevention perspective, preventing childhood obesity rather than trying to tackle established obesity in adulthood, may be most important since childhood obesity is strongly predictive of adult obesity,[86] and interventions to produce sustained weight loss once obesity is established in either childhood or adulthood are largely ineffective.[87]

CHILDHOOD PHYSICAL ACTIVITY AND FITNESS

Physical activity in childhood could have a direct effect on blood pressure that tracks into adulthood and/or could be strongly correlated with activity levels in adulthood, which in turn are related to adult blood pressure. Increased levels of physical activity and physical fitness are associated with lower blood pressure in childhood.[88–90] In the Harvard Alumni prospective cohort study, participation in vigorous activity while at college in adolescence and early adulthood was associated with a reduced risk of hypertension 16 to 50 years later.[91] However, there was a stronger association between current (adult) activity and blood pressure than between activity levels in earlier life. A systematic review of intervention studies in adults with hypertension concluded that increasing levels of physical activity produced important reductions in blood pressure but only for the duration of regular activity.[92] To our knowledge no intervention studies have examined the long-term effects of increased childhood activity on adult blood pressure.

THE ROLE OF EARLY-LIFE FACTORS IN EXPLAINING POPULATION-LEVEL DIFFERENCES IN MEAN BLOOD PRESSURE

Population variations in mean blood pressure, either between countries or over time, also suggest that early-life factors are important determinants of adult blood pressure. Geographic variations in adult blood pressure, which strongly correlate with variations in CVD rates, have been described for many years.[93] It has been assumed that geographic variations in blood pressure exist only in older adulthood and are not present in childhood.[94] However, there is increasing evidence of geographic variations in blood pressure in childhood, adolescence, and early adulthood that correlate strongly with mean blood pressure in adulthood.[60] Further, downward secular trends in blood pressure, seen in most developed countries, have occurred in all age groups, with important declines in blood pressure levels among children for at least the past 50 years.[95–98] These population findings suggest that the marked declines in blood pressure seen in recent decades are not primarily due to changes in adult risk factors or treatment of those with hypertension since these could not explain the similar declines in children and adolescents. They suggest that early-life factors are important in determining population levels of blood pressure and changes in blood pressure over time.

FUTURE RESEARCH NEEDS AND POLICY IMPLICATIONS

The greatest risk to public health of the associations described in this chapter is likely to be seen in developing countries where the effects of extreme poverty in early life and in earlier generations are increasingly combined with adverse Western diets and lifestyles in adulthood. Despite this risk, very little of the research in this area has been conducted in the developing world.

Work (from developed countries) suggesting that accelerated postnatal growth is detrimental to future high blood pressure and CVD health is a particularly important example of the need to extend this area of research into developing countries. Few would disagree with the suggestion that late weight catch-up in stunted infants or children resulting in the "stunted-(centrally) obese" adult is harmful to cardiovascular health. However, the short-term benefits of catch-up growth for small newborns, particularly in developed countries with continued exposures to infectious diseases and adverse environments, may outweigh any possible long-term detrimental effects.[99] A body of work is underway in this area in developing countries.[100,101]

From a public health policy perspective, understanding the mechanisms and models that underlie the association between early-life risk factors and future blood pressure is important. Individual risk factors will interact with each other and with adult risk factors over the life course to determine future blood pressure. Understanding how different risk factors relate to each other, including temporal relationships, will require development and nurturing by funding agencies and the research community of prospective observational studies with repeat measurements of a range of socioeconomic, behavioral, and biological factors assessed from birth over the life course and across generations. Further, there is a need to develop appropriate statistical methods that model relationships between correlated and temporally related exposures as well as dealing with repeated measurements, hierarchical data, measurement error, and missing values.[102] It is also important to establish randomized trials with sufficient resources for long-term follow-up to assess the effects of (1) interventions to reduce maternal smoking during pregnancy, (2) maternal dietary factors during pregnancy, (3) infant sodium intake, (4) increasing childhood physical activity, and (5) preventing childhood obesity on adult blood pressure and CVD.

SUMMARY

Children from lower-SES households, those whose mothers experience pregnancy-induced hypertension, whose mothers smoke throughout pregnancy, those with low birth weight, who have high-sodium diets in infancy, and who are obese in childhood or adolescence tend to have higher blood pressure in adulthood. However, the mechanisms linking these early-life factors to later blood pressure, and the most appropriate means of preventing adult hypertension by intervening in early life, are currently unclear. Some early-life factors that appear to influence blood pressure—for example, mothers not smoking in pregnancy—have clear benefits irrespective of any possible effect on blood pressure, and should be promoted. However, more research is required to know what early-life interventions will have the greatest public health impact on reducing future hypertension and its associated diseases.

ACKNOWLEDGMENTS

David A. Leon, London School of Hygiene & Tropical Medicine, provided valuable comments on an earlier draft of this chapter.

REFERENCES

1. Lawes CM, Bennett DA, Parag V, et al. Blood pressure indices and cardiovascular disease in the Asia Pacific region: a pooled analysis. *Hypertension* 2003;42:69–75.

2. Blood Pressure Lowering Treatment Trialists' Collaboration. Effects of different blood-pressure-lowering regimens on major cardiovascular events: results of prospectively-designed overviews of randomised trials. *Lancet* 2003;362:1527–35.

3. Andersson OK, Almgren T, Persson B, Samuelsson O, Hedner T, Wilhelmsen L. Survival in treated hypertension: follow up study after two decades. *BMJ* 1998;317:167–71.

4. Nelson MJ, Ragland DR, Syme SL. Longitudinal prediction of adult blood pressure from juvenile blood pressure levels. *Am J Epidemiol* 1992;136:633–45.

5. de Swiet M, Fayers P, Shinebourne EA. Blood pressure in first 10 years of life: the Brompton study. *BMJ* 1992; 304:23–6.

6. Galobardes B, Lynch JW, Davey Smith G. Childhood socioeconomic circumstances and cause-specific mortality in adulthood: systematic review and interpretation. *Epidemiol Rev* 2004;26:7–21.

7. Colhoun HM, Hemingway H, Poulter NR. Socio-economic status and blood pressure: an overview analysis. *J Hum Hypertens* 1998;12:91–110.

8. Batty GD, Leon DA. Socio-economic position and coronary heart disease risk factors in children and young people. Evidence from UK epidemiological studies. *Eur J Public Health* 2002;12:263–72.

9. Blane D, Hart CL, Davey Smith G, Gillis CR, Hole DJ, Hawthorne VM. Association of cardiovascular disease risk factors with socioeconomic position during childhood and during adulthood. *BMJ* 1996;313:1434–8.

10. Wannamethee SG, Whincup PH, Shaper G, Walker M. Influence of fathers' social class on cardiovascular disease in middle-aged men. *Lancet* 1996;348:1259–63.

11. Hardy R, Kuh D, Langenberg C, Wadsworth ME. Birthweight, childhood social class, and change in adult blood pressure in the 1946 British birth cohort. *Lancet* 2003; 362:1178–83.

12. Bobak M, Kriz B, Leon DA, Danova J, Marmot MG. Socioeconomic factors and height of preschool children in the Czech Republic. *Am J Public Health* 1994;84:1167–70.

13. Jansen W, Hazebroek-Kampschreur AA. Differences in height and weight between children living in neighbourhoods of different socioeconomic status. *Acta Paediatr* 1997;86:224–5.

14. Kivimäki M, Lawlor D, Davey Smith G, et al. Early socioeconomic position and blood pressure in childhood and adulthood: The Cardiovascular Risk in Young Finns Study. *Hypertension* 2006;47:39.

15. Taittonen L, Nuutinen M, Turtinen J, Uhari M. Prenatal and postnatal factors in predicting later blood pressure among children: cardiovascular risk in young Finns. *Pediatr Res* 1996;40:627–32.

16. Leon DA, Koupil I, Mann V, et al. Fetal, developmental and parental influences on childhood systolic blood pressure in 600 sib pairs: the Uppsala Family Study. *Circulation* 2005;112:3478–85.

17. Law CM, Barker DJ, Bull AR, Osmond C. Maternal and fetal influences on blood pressure. *Arch Dis Child* 1991; 66:1291–5.

18. Godfrey KM, Forrester T, Barker DJ, et al. Maternal nutritional status in pregnancy and blood pressure in childhood. *Br J Obstet Gynaecol* 1994;101:398–403.

19. Whincup P, Cook D, Papacosta O, Walker M, Perry I. Maternal factors and development of cardiovascular risk: evidence from a study of blood pressure in children. *J Hum Hypertens* 1994;8:337–43.

20. Bergel E, Haelterman E, Belizan J, Villar J, Carroli G. Perinatal factors associated with blood pressure during childhood. *Am J Epidemiol* 2000; 151:594–601.

21. Whincup PH, Cook DG, Shaper AG. Early influences on blood pressure: a study of children aged 5–7 years. *BMJ* 1989;299:587–91.

22. Blake KV, Gurrin LC, Evans SF, et al. Maternal cigarette smoking during pregnancy, low birth weight and subsequent blood pressure in early childhood. *Early Hum Dev* 2000; 57:137–47.

23. Lawlor DA, Najman JM, Sterne J, Williams GM, Ebrahim S, Davey Smith G. Associations of parental, birth, and early life characteristics with systolic blood pressure at 5 years of age: findings from the Mater-University study of pregnancy and its outcomes. *Circulation* 2004; 110:2417–23.

24. Harding JE. The nutritional basis of the fetal origins of adult disease. *Int J Epidemiol* 2001;30:15–23.

25. Benediktsson R, Lindsey RS, Nobel J, Seckl JR, Edwards RW. Glucocorticoid exposure in utero: new model for adult hypertension. *Lancet* 1993; 341:339–41.

26. Jackson AA, Dunn RI, Marchand MC, Langley-Evans SC. Increased systolic blood pressure in rats induced by maternal low protein diet is reversed by dietary supplementation with glycine. *Clin Sci* 2002;103:633–9.

27. Langley-Evans SC, Phillips GJ, Jackson AA. In utero exposure to maternal low protein diets induces hypertension in weaning rats, independently of maternal blood pressure changes. *Clin Nutr* 1994;13:319–24.

28. Roseboom TJ, van der Meulen JH, Ravelli AC, et al. Blood pressure in adults after prenatal exposure to famine. *J Hypertens* 1999;17:325–30.

29. Roseboom TJ, van der Meulen JHP, Osmond C, Barker DJP, Ravelli ACJ, Bleker OP. Plasma lipid profiles in adults after prenatal exposure to the Dutch famine. *Am J Clin Nutr* 2000; 72:1101–6.

30. Ravelli AC, van der Meulen JH, Michels RP, et al. Glucose tolerance in adults after prenatal exposure to famine. *Lancet* 1998;351:173–7.

31. Stanner SA, Bulmer K, Andres C, et al. Does malnutrition in utero determine diabetes and coronary heart disease in adulthood? Results from the Leningrad siege study, a cross sectional study. *BMJ* 1997;315:1342–8.

32. Langley-Evans SC, Welham SJ, Sherman RC, Jackson AA. Weanling rats exposed to maternal low-protein diets during discrete periods of gestation exhibit differing severity of hypertension. *Clin Sci* 1996;91:607–15.

33. Langley-Evans SC, Phillips GJ, Benediktsson R, et al. Protein intake in pregnancy, placental glucocorticoid

metabolism and the programming of hypertension in the rat. *Placenta* 1996;17:169–72.

34. Roseboom TJ, van der Meulen JH, van Montfrans GA, et al. Maternal nutrition during gestation and blood pressure in later life. *J Hypertens* 2001;19:29–34.

35. Campbell DM, Hall MH, Barker DJ, Cross J, Shiell AW, Godfrey KM. Diet in pregnancy and the offspring's blood pressure 40 years later. *Br J Obstet Gynaecol* 1996;103:273–80.

36. Shiell AW, Campbell-Brown M, Haselden S, Robinson S, Godfrey KM, Barker DJ. High-meat, low-carbohydrate diet in pregnancy: relation to adult blood pressure in the offspring. *Hypertension* 2001;38:1282–8.

37. Adair LS, Kuzawa CW, Borja J. Maternal energy stores and diet composition during pregnancy program adolescent blood pressure. *Circulation* 2001;1034–9.

38. Huh SY, Rifas-Shiman SL, Kleinman KP, Rich-Edwards JW, Lipshultz SE, Gillman MW. Maternal protein intake is not associated with infant blood pressure. *Int J Epidemiol* 2005;34:378–4.

39. Leary SD, Ness AR, Emmett PM, Davey Smith G, Headley JE. Maternal diet in pregnancy and offspring blood pressure. *Arch Dis Child* 2005; 90:492–3.

40. McGarvey ST, Zinner SH, Willett WC, Rosner B. Maternal prenatal dietary potassium, calcium, magnesium, and infant blood pressure. *Hypertension* 1991;17:218–24.

41. Gillman MW, Oliveria SA, Moore LL, Ellison RC. Inverse association of dietary calcium with systolic blood pressure in young children. *JAMA* 1992;267:2340–3.

42. Belizan JM, Villar J, Bergel E, et al. Long-term effect of calcium supplementation during pregnancy on the blood pressure of offspring: follow up of a randomised controlled trial. *BMJ* 1997;315:281–5.

43. Law CM, Shiell AW. Is blood pressure inversely related to birth weight? The strength of evidence from a systematic review of the literature. *J Hypertens* 1996;14:935–41.

44. Leon DA, Koupilová I. Birth weight, blood pressure and hypertension: epidemiological studies. In: Barker DJP, ed. *Fetal Origins of Cardiovascular and Lung Disease*. New York: Dekker, 2000:23–48.

45. Huxley RR, Shiell AW, Law CM. The role of size at birth and postnatal catch-up growth in determining systolic blood pressure: a systematic review of the literature. *J Hypertens* 2000;18:815–31.

46. Huxley R, Neil A, Collins R. Unravelling the "fetal origins" hypothesis: is there really an inverse association between birth weight and future blood pressure? *Lancet* 2002;360:59–665.

47. Lawlor DA, Ronalds G, Clark H, Davey Smith G, Leon DA. Birth weight is inversely associated with incident coronary heart disease and stroke among individuals born in the 1950s: findings from the Aberdeen Children of the 1950s prospective cohort study. *Circulation* 2005;112:1414–18.

48. Barker DJ, Bull AR, Osmond C, Simmonds SJ. Fetal and placental size and risk of hypertension in adult life. *BMJ* 1990;301:259–62.

49. Martyn CN, Barker DJ, Jespersen S, et al. Growth in utero, adult blood pressure, and arterial compliance. *British Heart Journal* 1995;73:116–21.

50. Whincup PH, Cook DG, Papacosta O. Do maternal and intrauterine factors influence blood pressure in childhood? *Arch Dis Child* 1992;67:1423–9.

51. Whincup PH, Cook DG, Shaper AG. Early influences on blood pressure: a study of children aged 5–7 years. *BMJ* 1989;299:587–591.

52. Lucas A, Fewtrell MS, Cole TJ. Fetal origins of adult disease-the hypothesis revisited. *BMJ* 1999;319:245–9.

53. Tu YK, West R, Ellison GT, Gilthorpe MS. Why evidence for the fetal origins of adult disease might be a statistical artifact: the "reversal paradox" for the relation between birth weight and blood pressure in later life. *Am J Epidemiol* 2005;161:27–32.

54. Eriksson JG, Forsen T, Tuomilehto J, Osmond C, Barker DJ. Early growth and coronary heart disease in later life: longitudinal study. *BMJ* 2001; 322:949–53.

55. Singhal A, Lucas A. Early origins of cardiovascular disease: is there a unifying hypothesis? *Lancet* 2004; 363:1642–5.

56. Bateson P, Barker D, Clutton-Brock T, et al. Developmental plasticity and human health. *Nature* 2004; 430:419–21.

57. Leon DA. Biological theories, evidence, and epidemiology. *Int J Epidemiol* 2004;33:1167–71.

58. Davies AA, Davey Smith G, Ben-Shlomo Y, Litchfield P. The association between birthweight and blood pressure is statistically robust: findings from a cohort of British Telecom employees working in the United Kingdom. *Pediatr Res* 2003;53 (Suppl 2):9A.

59. Leon DA, Johansson M, Rasmussen F. Gestational age and growth rate of fetal mass are inversely associated with systolic blood pressure in young adults: an epidemiologic study of 165,136 Swedish men aged 18 years. *Am J Epidemiol* 2000;152:597–604.

60. Whincup PH, Cook DG, Geleijnse JM. A life course approach to blood pressure. In: Kuh D, Ben-Shlomo Y, eds. *A Life Course Approach to Chronic Disease Epidemiology*. Oxford: Oxford University Press, 2004:218–39.

61. Barker DJP. *Mothers, Babies and Health in Later Life*. London: Churchill Livingstone, 1998.

62. McKeigue P. Diabetes and insulin action. In: Kuh D, Ben-Shlomo Y, eds. *A Life Course Approach to Chronic Disease Epidemiology*. Oxford: Oxford University Press, 1997:78–100.

63. Hattersley AT, Tooke JE. The fetal insulin hypothesis: an alternative explanation of the association of low birthweight with diabetes and vascular disease. *Lancet* 1999;353:1789–92.

64. Phillips DI. Twin studies in medical research: can they tell us whether diseases are genetically determined? *Lancet* 1993;341:1008–9.

65. McNeill G, Tuya C, Smith WC. The role of genetic and environmental factors in the association between birthweight and blood pressure: evidence from meta-analysis of twin studies. *Int J Epidemiol* 2004; 33:995–1001.

66. Phillips DI, Osmond C. Twins and the fetal origins hypothesis. Many variables differ between twins and singleton infants. *BMJ* 1999;319:517–8.

67. Phillips DI, Davies MJ, Robinson JS. Fetal growth and the fetal origins hypothesis in twins—problems and perspectives. *Twin Res* 2001;4:327–331.

68. Owen CG, Whincup PH, Gilg JA, Cook DG. Effect of breast feeding in infancy on blood pressure in later life: systematic review and meta-analysis. *BMJ* 2003;327:1–7.

69. Martin RM, Gunnell D, Davey Smith G. Breastfeeding in infancy and blood pressure in later life: systematic review and meta-analysis. *Am J Epidemiol* 2005;161:15–26.

70. Lawlor DA, Riddoch C, Page AS, et al. Infant feeding and components of the metabolic syndrome: findings from the European Youth Heart Study. *Arch Dis Child* 2005;90:582–8.

71. Leon DA, Ronalds G. Breast feeding influences on later health—cardiovascular disease. In: Goldberg G, Prentice AM, Prentice A, Simodon K, Fiteau S, eds. *Breast Feeding: Early Life Influences on Later Health*, London, Springer, 2006 (forthcoming).

72. Ebrahim S, Davey Smith G. Lowering blood pressure: a systematic review of sustained effects of non-pharmacological interventions. *J Public Health Med* 1998;20:441–8.

73. Hooper L, Bartlett C, Davey Smith G, Ebrahim S. Systematic review of long term effects of advice to reduce dietary salt in adults. *BMJ* 2002; 325:628.

74. Cooper R, Soltero I, Liu K, Berkson D, Levinson S, Stamler J. The association between urinary sodium excretion and blood pressure in children. *Circulation* 1980;62:97–104.

75. Cooper R, Liu K, Trevisan M, Miller W, Stamler J. Urinary sodium excretion and blood pressure in children: absence of a reproducible association. *Hypertension* 1983;5:135–9.

76. Knuiman JT, Hautvast JG, Zwiauer KF, et al. Blood pressure and excretion of sodium, potassium, calcium and magnesium in 8- and 9-year-old boys from 19 European centres. *Eur J Clin Nutr* 1988;42:847–55.

77. Whincup PH, Cook DG, Papacosta O, Jones SR. Relations between sodium: creatinine and potassium:creatinine ratios and blood pressure in childhood (abstract). *J Hypertens* 1992;10:1434.

78. Geleijnse JM, Grobbee DE, Hofman A. Sodium and potassium intake and blood pressure change in childhood. *BMJ* 1990;300:899–902.

79. Hofman A, Hazebroek A, Valkenburg HA. A randomized trial of sodium intake and blood pressure in newborn infants. *JAMA* 1983;250:370–3.

80. Hoffman A. Sodium intake and blood pressure in newborn: evidence of a causal connection. In: Hoffman A, ed. *Children's Blood Pressure: Report of*

the 88th Ross Conference on Paediatric Research. Columbus, OH: Ross Laboratories, 1989.

81. Geleijnse JM, Hoffman A, Witteman JC, Hazebroek AA, Valkenburg HA, Grobbee DE. Long-term effects of neonatal sodium restriction on blood pressure. *Hypertension* 1997;29:913–7.

82. Holland FJ, Stark O, Ades AE, Peckham CS. Birth weight and body mass index in childhood, adolescence, and adulthood as predictors of blood pressure at age 36. *J Epidemiol Community Health* 1993;47:432–5.

83. Williams S, Poulton R. Birth size, growth, and blood pressure between the ages of 7 and 26 years: failure to support the fetal origins hypothesis. *Am J Epidemiol* 2002;155:849–52.

84. Hardy R, Wadsworth ME, Langenberg C, Kuh D. Birthweight, childhood growth, and blood pressure at 43 years in a British birth cohort. *Int J Epidemiol* 2004;33:121–9.

85. Mamun AA, Lawlor DA, O'Callaghan MJ, Williams GW, Najman JM. The effect of body mass index changes between ages 5 and 14 on blood pressure at age 14: findings from a birth cohort. *Hypertension* 2005;45:1083–7.

86. Parsons TJ, Power C, Logan S, Summerbell CD. Childhood predictors of adult obesity: a systematic review. *Int J Obes* 1999;23:S1–107.

87. Lobstein T, Baur L, Uauy R. Obesity in children and young people: a crisis in public health. *Obes Rev* 2004; 5(Suppl 1):4–85.

88. Andersen LB, Wedderkopp N, Hansen HS, Cooper AR, Froberg K. Biological cardiovascular risk factors cluster in Danish children and adolescents: the European Youth Heart Study. *Prev Med* 2003;37:363–7.

89. Strazzullo P, Cappuccio FP, Trevisan M, et al. Leisure time physical activity and blood pressure in schoolchildren. *Am J Epidemiol* 1988;127:726–33.

90. Kikuchi S, Rona RJ, Chinn S. Physical fitness of 9 year olds in England: related factors. *J Epidemiol Community Health* 1995;49:180–5.

91. Paffenbarger RS Jr, Wing AL, Hyde RT, Jung DL. Physical activity and incidence of hypertension in college alumni. *Am J Epidemiol* 1983;117:245–57.

92. Hagberg JM, Park JJ, Brown MD. The role of exercise training in the treatment of hypertension: an update. *Sports Med* 2000;30:193–206.

93. Marmot MG. Geography of blood pressure and hypertension. *Br Med Bull* 1984;40:380–6.

94. Peart WS. Concepts in hypertension. The Croonian Lecture 1979. *J R Coll Physicians Lond* 1980;14:141–52.

95. Goff DC, Howard G, Russell GB, Labarthe DR. Birth cohort evidence of population influences on blood pressure in the United States, 1887–1994. *Ann Epidemiol* 2001;11:271–9.

96. McCarron P, Davey Smith G, Okasha M. Secular changes in blood pressure in childhood, adolescence and young adulthood: systematic review of trends from 1948 to 1998. *J Hum Hypertens* 2002;16:677–89.

97. McCarron P, Okasha M, McEwen J, Davey Smith G. Changes in blood pressure among students attending Glasgow University between 1948 and 1968: analyses of cross sectional surveys. *BMJ* 2001;322:885–9.

98. Watkins D, McCarron P, Murray L, et al. Trends in blood pressure over 10 years in adolescents: analyses of cross sectional surveys in the Northern Ireland Young Hearts project. *BMJ* 2004;329:139.

99. Victora CG, Barros FC. Commentary: the catch-up dilemma—relevance of Leitch's 'low-high' pig to child growth in developing countries. *Int J Epidemiol* 2001;30:217–20.

100. Yajnik CS. Commentary: fetal origins of cardiovascular risk-nutritional and non-nutritional. *Int J Epidemiol* 2001; 30:57–9.

101. Yajnik CS. The lifecycle effects of nutrition and body size on adult adiposity, diabetes and cardiovascular disease. *Obes Rev* 2002;3:217–24.

102. De Stavola B, Nitsch D, dos Santos Silva I, et al. Statistical issues in life course epidemiology. *Am J Epidemiol* 2006;163:84–96.

Chapter

5

Blood Pressure and the Risks of Cardiovascular Disease and Stroke

Donald M. Lloyd-Jones and Philip Greenland

Key Findings

- Higher levels of blood pressure increase risk for all manifestations of cardiovascular disease (CVD) in a continuous and graded fashion, beginning at levels considered to be well within the "normal" range.

- The vast majority of hypertensive individuals have at least one other risk factor for CVD.

- Hypertension is associated with increased risk even in the absence of other risk factors, but risk increases dramatically when other risk factors are present.

- Elevated systolic blood pressure (SBP) is far more prevalent in the population than elevated diastolic blood pressure (DBP). SBP is at least as strong a risk factor as DBP, and often stronger, in predicting adverse CVD outcomes. SBP is also generally a stronger predictor of CVD events than pulse pressure (SBP minus DBP).

- The relative risks associated with hypertension are higher for heart failure and stroke, indicating a greater etiologic role for hypertension in these manifestations of CVD. Because rates of coronary heart disease (CHD) are substantially higher than rates of stroke and heart failure, hypertension has a greater population impact on CHD.

- Type of first CVD event occurring after hypertension onset varies according to age and sex.

- Younger men tend to experience CHD events first, whereas older men and women at all ages tend to experience stroke.

- Relative risks for CVD are at least as high for older as younger hypertensives, but absolute risks for CVD are substantially higher in older hypertensives, indicating their greater need for blood pressure treatment and control.

- Hypertension is more prevalent, and confers greater risks for CVD, in blacks compared with whites.

Arterial hypertension, or persistent, nonphysiologic elevation of systemic blood pressure, is a major risk factor for all forms of atherosclerotic and atherothrombotic cardiovascular disease (CVD). Moreover, it is now recognized that, beginning at levels well within the so-called "normal" range, higher levels of blood pressure (BP) generally increase risk in a continuous and graded fashion for multiple cardiovascular and noncardiovascular sequelae. Higher levels of BP are associated with increased risk for total mortality, CVD mortality, coronary heart disease (CHD) mortality, myocardial infarction (MI), heart failure (HF), left ventricular hypertrophy (LVH), atrial fibrilla-

tion, stroke, peripheral vascular disease, and renal failure. As discussed below, BP levels exert differential effects on risk for development of each of these endpoints. Individuals with hypertension are at risk for all manifestations of CVD, with concomitant risk factors influencing the manifestation as well. An understanding of the concept of "risk factors" and of epidemiologic measurements of association between a risk factor and disease will serve as an introduction to a detailed examination of BP as a risk factor for CVD and stroke.

The term *risk factor*, referring to an exposure that influences risk for development of disease, was coined in 1961 in a seminal paper from the Framingham Heart Study investigators.[1] Of note, that analysis was among the first to identify substantially elevated risks for CHD among men and women with elevated BP levels. An epidemiologic association between a proposed risk factor and a disease is likely to be causal if it fulfills the following criteria: (1) exposure to the proposed risk factor precedes the onset of disease, (2) there is a strong association (i.e., large relative risk) between exposure and disease incidence, (3) the association between exposure and disease is dose-dependent, (4) exposure is consistently predictive of disease in a variety of populations, (5) the association is independent of other risk factors, and (6) the association is biologically and pathogenically plausible, and is supported by animal experiments as well as clinical investigation.[2] Even more definitive support for an etiologic association between a proposed risk factor and disease can come from clinical intervention trials in which modification of the risk factor (by behavioral or therapeutic interventions) is associated with a decreased incidence of disease. Elevated BP clearly meets all of these criteria, and is accepted as an etiologic risk factor for CVD.

Absolute risk for disease associated with a given exposure is often expressed as the rate of development of new cases of disease per unit of time (or *incidence*) in exposed individuals. This proportion may be compared with the proportion among nonexposed subjects in a variety of ways. The *relative risk* of disease is the ratio of disease incidence among exposed compared with nonexposed individuals. As such, relative risk measures the strength of the association between exposure and disease, but it gives no indication of the absolute risk of disease. The *attributable risk* of a given exposure describes the proportion of the incidence of disease in a population that can be ascribed to the exposure, assuming that a causal relationship exists. The *population attributable risk* (PAR) takes into account the proportion of individuals in the population who are exposed, as well as the relative risk for disease associated with exposure, to allow comparison of the impact of diverse risk factors on the burden of disease in a population. Therefore, attributable risk is a useful concept in determining the public health impact of a given risk factor and in selecting risk factors that should be targeted for prevention programs.[3]

CARDIOVASCULAR DISEASE RISK ACROSS THE SPECTRUM OF BLOOD PRESSURE

Individuals with hypertension, currently defined as untreated systolic BP ≥140 mmHg, or diastolic BP ≥90 mmHg, or receiving therapy for elevated BP, have a two- to three-fold increased risk for all CVD events combined, compared with nonhypertensive individuals. When CVD endpoints are considered individually, *relative* risks with hypertension are greatest for stroke and HF, and somewhat lower for CHD (Figure 5–1, bottom). Nonetheless, because CHD incidence is greater than incidence of stroke and HF, the *absolute* impact of hypertension on CHD is greater than for other manifestations of CVD, as demonstrated by the excess risks shown in Figure 5–1.

Although much of the focus on CVD risk has been on frank hypertension, it is clear that risks for CVD increase at higher BP levels, even within the so-called "normal" range. A recent epidemiologic pooling study of nearly 1 million men and women, which included data on more than 56,000 decedents, revealed that risks for CVD death increase in a continuous fashion at levels starting as low as SBP of 115 mmHg and DBP of 75 mmHg, and possibly lower. For each 20-mmHg increment in SBP or each 10-mmHg increment in DBP, there was approximately a doubling of risk for stroke death and for ischemic heart disease death in both men and women.[4]

Other studies provide confirmation of these findings. Data from more than 347,000 middle-aged men (35 to 57 years old) screened for the Multiple Risk Factor Intervention Trial (MRFIT) provide precise estimates of incremental risks with higher BP levels. As shown in Figure 5–2 (bars), there is a continuous, graded effect of BP on the multivariable-adjusted relative risk for CHD mortality beginning at pressures well below 140 mmHg.[5] Although *relative* risks are clearly highest for men with SBP ≥180 mmHg, these data help make an important point about BP levels in the population at which the majority of CVD events are occurring. In Figure 5–2, the numbers above each bar indicate the number of men in each stratum of SBP at baseline. Although the relative risks were highest for men with SBP ≥180 mmHg, the vast majority of men at baseline had an SBP ≤159 mmHg. Taking into account the number of men in each stratum and the expected rates of CHD death, there is a substantial number of excess CHD deaths occurring at lower BP levels (as shown by the line in Figure 5–2). Thus nearly two-thirds of excess CHD deaths occurred in men with baseline SBP between 130 and 159 mmHg, relatively "mild" levels of elevated BP.

Recent data from the Framingham Heart Study also indicate that the risk associated with BPs in the range of 130 to 139 mmHg systolic or 85 to 89 mmHg diastolic

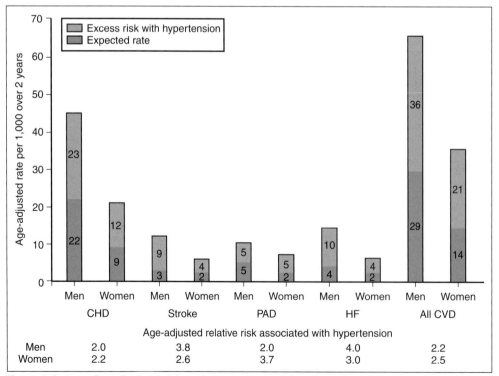

Figure 5–1. Age-adjusted relative risks and excess risks for selected manifestations of cardiovascular disease. Framingham Heart Study, 30-year follow-up. CHD, coronary heart disease; CVD, cardiovascular disease; HF, heart failure; PAD, peripheral arterial disease.

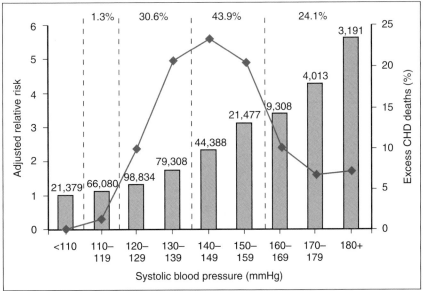

Figure 5–2. Multivariable-adjusted relative risks for coronary heart disease death by systolic blood pressure strata, numbers of men in each stratum, and excess coronary heart disease deaths in each stratum in men aged 35 to 57 years. Multiple Risk Factor Intervention Trial screenees.[5] CHD, coronary heart disease.

are substantial, despite the fact that these levels are not currently classified as hypertension. These "prehypertensive" levels of BP are associated with significantly elevated multivariable-adjusted relative risk for CVD of 2.5 in women and 1.6 in men.[6] In the Physician's Health Study, there was a nearly two-fold increased risk of stroke associated with borderline elevated SBP.[7] Likewise, individuals with SBP between 120 and 139 mmHg or DBP between 80 and 89 mmHg have a high likelihood of progressing to frank hypertension over the next 4 years, especially if they are age 65 or older.[8] For these reasons, JNC 7 (Joint National Committee on Prevention, Detection, Evaluation, and Treatment of High Blood Pressure, Seventh Report) has reclassified the JNC 6 BP categories to place greater emphasis on prevention of hypertension. These previously "normal" and "high-normal" levels (i.e., SBP 120–139 or DBP 80–89) are now classified as "prehypertension."[9]

Although clinical practice guidelines recommend treatment of hypertension in individual patients only when their *current* BP levels cross certain thresholds, there is evidence that *long-term* BP levels confer significant CVD risk over and above current levels. Vasan et al.[10] observed that antecedent time-averaged BP predicted the incidence of CVD events even after adjustment for current BP and other traditional risk factors. Furthermore, antecedent BP (both recent and remote) predicted risk of CVD in both nonhypertensive and hypertensive individuals. Thus, delaying treatment of elevated BP until absolute risk or BP level crosses a threshold may not adequately reduce the risk of CVD events. These findings underscore the importance of preventing hypertension onset and of detecting and controlling elevated BP throughout the life span.[10]

For many CVD endpoints, there is effect modification by gender, with male hypertensives being at higher risk

for CVD events than female hypertensives; HF is a notable exception to this generalization. As discussed below, there is also substantial effect modification by age, with older hypertensives being at similar or higher relative risk but much greater absolute risk than younger ones.[11] Hypertension rarely occurs in isolation, and it confers increased risk for CVD across the spectrum of overall risk factor burden, with increasing importance in the setting of other risk factors.[12] As shown in Figure 5–3, absolute levels of CHD risk increase substantially with increasing risk factor burden, and risk is augmented still further by increases in BP levels from optimal to marked hypertension in both women (Figure 5–3, *A*) and men[13] (Figure 5–3, *B*). Thus BP levels, and the risk they confer, must always be considered in the context of other risk factors and the patient's global risk for CVD.

RISK FACTOR CLUSTERING

Hypertension occurs in isolation very infrequently. A recent assessment of 4962 middle-aged and older individuals from a community-based sample revealed that higher BP stages were associated with a higher mean number of other risk factors and higher rates of clinical CVD and/or target organ damage. Overall, among those with high-normal BP (SBP 130–139 or DBP 85–89 mmHg) or hypertension, only 2.4% had no other CVD risk factors, whereas 59.3% had at least one risk factor, and 38.2% had target organ damage, clinical CVD, or diabetes.[14]

The rising epidemic of obesity within Western societies has led to a greater understanding of the phenomenon of risk factor clustering, and of the pathophysiologic links between hypertension, other risk factors, and risk for CVD. The cluster of risk factors, including central obesity, atherogenic dyslipidemia (with low HDL cholesterol, high

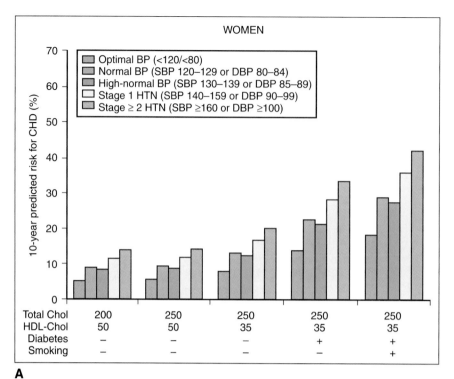

A

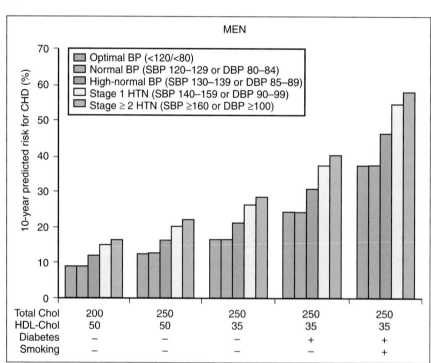

B

Figure 5–3. Predicted 10-year risk for coronary heart disease by level of major risk factors and JNC-VI blood pressure stage in women (**A**) and men (**B**). Calculated from Framingham risk equations published by Wilson et al.[13] BP, blood pressure; Chol, cholesterol; DBP, diastolic blood pressure; HTN, hypertension; SBP, systolic blood pressure.

triglycerides, and small, dense LDL-cholesterol particles), impaired glucose metabolism, vascular inflammation, pro-atherogenic milieu, and elevated BP, has been termed the "metabolic syndrome." Visceral adiposity and insulin resistance appear to play central roles in the development of metabolic syndrome, and elevated BP is a key diagnostic

feature.[15] In some ethnicities, such as blacks, elevated BP is the most common criterion leading to diagnosis of the metabolic syndrome. Hypertension is associated with increased risk for CVD even in the absence of other risk factors, but risk increases dramatically when other risk factors are present, as shown in Figure 5–3.

SYSTOLIC BLOOD PRESSURE, DIASTOLIC BLOOD PRESSURE, PULSE PRESSURE, AND CARDIOVASCULAR DISEASE RISK

Early efforts at understanding risks associated with hypertension, and early clinical intervention trials, focused on DBP, since it was believed that DBP conferred the greater risk for events. Increases in SBP with age were thought to be adaptive, leading to the term "essential" hypertension. Studies of BP patterns with aging in the United States indicate that SBP rises linearly and monotonically with age after about age 30. DBP tends to rise gradually until about age 50, after which it plateaus for approximately 5 to 10 years, and then decreases to the end of the life span.[16,17] These patterns of BP change are largely a function of vascular changes that occur as a result of aging and exposure to environmental and genetic factors that alter vascular function. Specifically, arteriosclerosis, loss of elasticity, and increasing vascular stiffness all contribute to increasing SBP and to decreasing DBP with age. The result of increasing SBP and decreasing DBP in middle-aged and older individuals is a steadily increasing pulse pressure, which is defined as the SBP minus the DBP.

A substantial body of epidemiologic and clinical evidence now indicates that SBP is at least as strong a risk factor as DBP, and often stronger, in prediction of adverse CVD outcomes.[18-20] Kannel et al.[21] were among the first to report on greater risks for CHD associated with SBP than DBP. They concluded that since "the net contribution [to risk] is greater for systolic than for diastolic pressure, the commonly held view concerning the innocuous nature of increased SBP in the elderly requires reevaluation."[21] Although these observations were first published in 1971, it was decades before this concept was widely appreciated and incorporated into clinical practice.

Risk for CVD (including CHD and stroke endpoints, separately or combined) is greater for SBP than DBP whether the two BP components are compared linearly,[20] by quintiles,[19] by deciles (Figure 5–4),[18] or by JNC stage.[18] In addition, SBP predominates when SBP and DBP are considered jointly in multivariable models predicting CVD endpoints.[20] As shown in Figure 5–5, rates of CHD and stroke mortality increase dramatically with increasing SBP at any given level of DBP. However, for any given level of SBP, there is only a modest increase in stroke mortality with increasing DBP, and the trend is nonlinear at higher levels of SBP.[18] In the Cardiovascular Health Study of older Americans, a one-standard-deviation increment in SBP was associated with higher adjusted risk for CHD and stroke than was a one-standard-deviation increment in DBP (or pulse pressure). In models with SBP and DBP together or SBP and pulse pressure together, SBP consistently dominated as the greater risk factor.[20] When men who were screened for inclusion in the Multiple Risk Factor Intervention Trial (MRFIT) were stratified into quintiles of SBP or DBP, risks for each SBP quintile were the same or higher than for the corresponding quintile of DBP.[19] Similar findings were observed when MRFIT screenees were stratified into deciles of SBP and DBP; at every level, SBP was consistently associated with higher

risk for CHD or stroke mortality than the corresponding decile of DBP (Figure 5–4).[18] Finally, when MRFIT screenees were stratified by JNC level of SBP and DBP, SBP level was associated with greater risk for CHD mortality than DBP level at each JNC BP stage.[18]

In fact, when DBP is considered in the context of the SBP level, an *inverse* association between DBP and CHD risk has been observed. Franklin et al.[22] reported that, at any given level of SBP, the relative risks for CHD *decreased* with higher DBP. For example, at an SBP of 150 mmHg, the estimated hazard ratio for CHD was 1.8 at a DBP of 70 mmHg, whereas it was only 1.3 at a DBP of 95 mmHg. The higher the SBP level, the steeper was the decline in CHD risk with increasing DBP. These data provide some evidence for the importance of pulse pressure as a measure of risk, since higher risk was observed in this study when the pulse pressure widened.[22] Pulse pressure will be discussed in greater detail later in this chapter.

Several other lines of evidence contribute to the realization that SBP is a more important predictor of risk in the population, and accounts for a far greater population attributable risk than does DBP. Overall in the U.S. population, elevation of SBP is far more prevalent than elevation of DBP.[23,24] Indeed, isolated systolic hypertension is by far the most common form of hypertension.[24] In addition, SBP correctly classifies JNC stage far better than DBP, and SBP therefore determines need for treatment among high-normal and hypertensive subjects.[23,24] Finally, large clinical trials[25-27] have demonstrated substantial benefit with treatment of isolated systolic hypertension in patients aged ≥60 years. As a result of all of these observations, the Coordinating Committee of the National High Blood Pressure Education Program and the JNC 7 committee recommended that SBP become the major criterion for the diagnosis, staging, and management of hypertension in middle-aged and older patients, who represent the vast majority of hypertensives.[9,28]

In recent years there has been intense interest in pulse pressure as a risk factor for CVD. However, investigators have struggled with how best to "anchor" the pulse pressure. For example, a patient with a BP of 110/60 has the same pulse pressure as a patient with a BP of 170/120 (pulse pressure = 50 mmHg for both), although the latter patient is clearly at higher risk for CVD. Various investigators have anchored the pulse pressure to the DBP, the mean arterial pressure, and the SBP. As discussed above, Franklin et al.[22] observed that higher pulse pressure was associated with greater CHD risk among subjects with the same SBP. Chae et al.[8] found that pulse pressure predicted incident HF in an elderly cohort, even after adjustment for mean arterial pressure, prevalent coronary heart disease, and other HF risk factors. In another study, SBP and pulse pressure conferred similar risk for HF.[29] However, many studies have found that SBP confers greater risk than pulse pressure,[4,20,30] when SBP and pulse pressure are considered separately or as covariates in the same multivariable model. The aforementioned Prospective Studies Collaboration, which pooled data from 61 large epidemiologic studies and nearly 1 million men and women, found that the most informative measure of BP

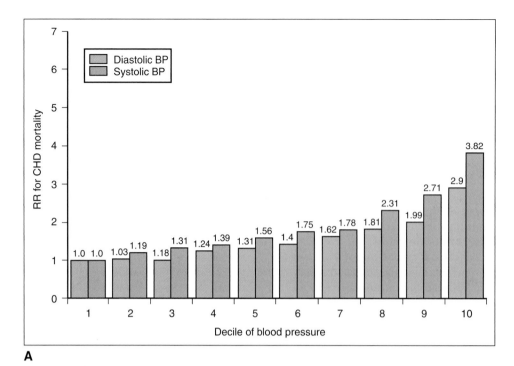

A

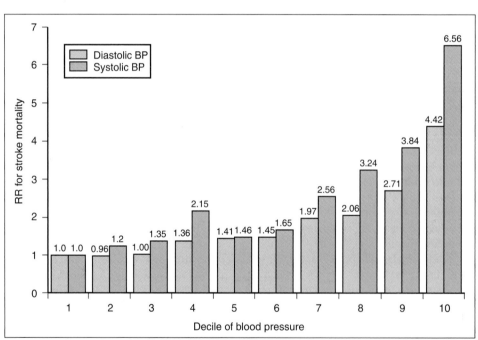

B

Figure 5–4. Relative risks for mortality due to coronary heart disease (**A**) and stroke (**B**), according to decile of systolic and diastolic blood pressure in men aged 35 to 57 years. Multiple Risk Factor Intervention Trial screenees. BP, blood pressure; CHD, coronary heart disease; RR, relative risk. (From Neaton JD, Kuller L, Stamler J, Wentworth DN. Impact of systolic and diastolic blood pressure on cardiovascular mortality. In: Laragh JH, Brenner BM, eds. *Hypertension: Pathophysiology, Diagnosis, and Management.* 2nd ed. New York: Raven Press, 1995:127.)

for prediction of CVD events was the mean of SBP and DBP, which predicted better than SBP or DBP alone, and much better than the pulse pressure.[4] At present, JNC 7 recommends that clinical focus should remain on the SBP in determining need for therapy and achieving goal BP.[9]

BLOOD PRESSURE AND CORONARY HEART DISEASE

Elevated BP is one of the major risk factors contributing to the estimated 1.4 million CHD events that occur in the United States annually.[31] As mentioned above, whereas

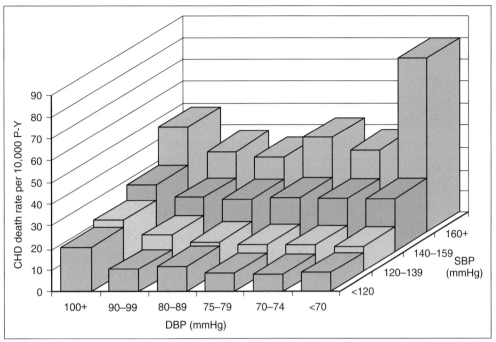

A

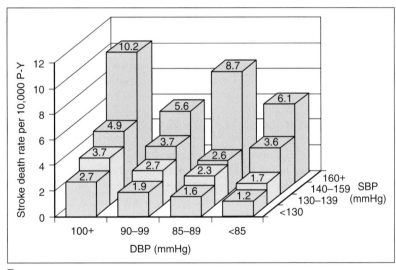

B

Figure 5–5. Death rates (per 10,000 P-Y) from coronary heart disease (**A**) and stroke (**B**) by systolic and diastolic blood pressure levels, considered jointly, in men aged 35 to 57 years. Multiple Risk Factor Intervention Trial screenees. DBP, diastolic blood pressure; P-Y, person-years; SBP, systolic blood pressure. (From Neaton JD, Kuller L, Stamler J, Wentworth DN. Impact of systolic and diastolic blood pressure on cardiovascular mortality. In: Laragh JH, Brenner BM, eds. *Hypertension: Pathophysiology, Diagnosis, and Management.* 2nd ed. New York: Raven Press, 1995:127.)

elevated BP is a major risk factor for CHD, it is a weaker risk factor for CHD, in terms of relative risks, than for stroke or HF. Nonetheless, because hypertension is the most prevalent CHD risk factor, and because the incidence of CHD is greater than the incidence of stroke or HF, the impact of elevated BP is greatest on CHD in the population.

Numerous studies have documented the graded and continuous risk for CHD endpoints associated with higher BP levels. Risk for CHD mortality is not limited to subjects with frank hypertension, however. There is a linear, graded risk for CHD death that extends down even to optimal levels of BP. As shown in Table 5–1, in the Chicago Heart Association Detection Project in Industry, age-adjusted rates for CHD roughly doubled with each 20-mmHg increment in SBP or 10-mmHg in DBP.[32] Similarly, the Prospective Studies Collaboration observed that, beginning at 115 mmHg, the risk for CHD death doubles for

RISKS FOR 25-YEAR CORONARY HEART DISEASE MORTALITY ASSOCIATED WITH SELECTED LEVELS OF BLOOD PRESSURE		
Blood Pressure (mmHg)	Age-Adjusted Rate (per 10,000 person-years)	Multivariable-Adjusted Relative Risk (95% CI)
SBP <120 and DBP<80	5.3	1.39 (0.67–2.86)
SBP 120–129 or DBP 80–84	4.2	1.0 (ref)
SBP 130–139 or DBP 85–89	6.1	1.37 (0.81–2.30)
SBP 140–159 or DBP 90–99	8.2	1.62 (1.00–2.61)
SBP 160–179 or DBP 100–109	15.0	2.51 (1.44–4.37)
SBP ≥180 or DBP ≥110	28.0	3.60 (1.71–7.59)

From Miura K, Daviglus ML, Dyer AR, et al. *Arch Intern Med*. 2001;161:1501.
CI, confidence interval; DBP, diastolic blood pressure; SBP, systolic blood pressure.

Table 5–1. Risks for 25-Year Coronary Heart Disease Mortality Associated with Selected Levels of Blood Pressure

each increase of 20 mmHg in the SBP; similarly, CHD death risk doubles for each increase of 10 mmHg in the DBP beginning at 75 mmHg.[10] Furthermore, the presence of electrocardiographic left ventricular hypertrophy, an important consequence of hypertension, increased risk for CHD over and above elevated BP alone, indicating that duration and severity of hypertension are important determinants of risk, in addition to current BP levels. And, as shown in Figure 5–3, higher BP increases risk incrementally alone and in the presence of other established major CHD risk factors.

BLOOD PRESSURE AND STROKE

Hypertension is the chief factor contributing to the 700,000 strokes that occur each year in the United States. Hypertension is well established as the dominant risk factor for stroke, even when considered in the context of other known risk factors, such as cigarette smoking, atrial fibrillation, MI, and diabetes. Hypertension confers a threefold relative risk for stroke compared with levels <140/<90 mmHg, and approximately 80% of subjects have hypertension prior to the occurrence of a stroke. The attributable risk for stroke associated with hypertension varies between 33% and 53% in different age groups.[33] In adults at age 55 in the Framingham Heart Study, the lifetime risk for stroke was greater than one in six, but it was twice as high among those with hypertension compared with those who had BP of <120/<80 mmHg.[31]

Hypertension works synergistically with other risk factors to increase risk for stroke. For example, the effect of hypertension on risk for stroke is modified substantially by age. Data from 30-year follow-up of the Framingham cohort reveal that there is a linear increase in stroke rates with increasing level of BP, but absolute rates of stroke and transient ischemic attack (TIA) are substantially higher for subjects with hypertension in the age range of 65 to 94 years compared with 35 to 64 years.

As is true for CHD risk prediction, a risk prediction algorithm has been developed to estimate the absolute 10-year risk of an atherothrombotic brain infarct using standard CVD risk factors, plus the presence of atrial fibrillation, heart failure, and coronary disease.[9] In these equations, hypertension represents the predominant risk

factor for stroke, but the risk in people with elevated BP varies over as much as a 10-fold range depending on the degree of exposure to the other risk factors.

Just as with CHD, risk for stroke is not limited to subjects with frank hypertension. There is a linear, graded risk for stroke that extends down even to optimal levels of BP. Beginning at 115 mmHg, the risk for stroke mortality doubles for each increase of 20 mmHg in the SBP; likewise, stroke mortality risk doubles for each increase of 10 mmHg in the DBP beginning at 75 mmHg.[4] Thus at any given age, an individual with SBP of 135 mmHg is at approximately twice the risk, and one with SBP of 155 mmHg at four times the risk, as someone at the same age with an SBP of 115 mmHg.

BLOOD PRESSURE AND HEART FAILURE

With the aging of the population, the concomitant increase in the prevalence of hypertension, and improved survival after MI, HF has become an emerging public health concern. National surveillance data indicate that approximately 4.9 million Americans are living with congestive HF (CHF) currently, with 550,000 incident cases each year. Congestive HF is the leading cause of hospitalization for people aged ≥65 in the United States, with 970,000 hospital discharges in 2002, a major contributor to the estimated annual direct and indirect costs of $28 billion in 2005.[31]

Study of the epidemiology of HF in representative or community-based populations has been problematic, in large part because of the difficulty of devising acceptable clinical and research criteria for the diagnosis of heart failure, which is a syndrome rather than a single clinical entity. However, several criteria[34,35] now exist for diagnosing HF in clinical and epidemiologic research, which has assisted in understanding the risk factors for heart failure.

As with stroke, hypertension is also the dominant risk factor for HF. The overall remaining lifetime risk for HF is one in five for men and women aged ≥40, but at every age there is a stepwise increase in lifetime risk for CHF with increasing BP, with approximately a twofold gradient of risk in those with Stage 2 or treated hypertension compared with those with BP <140/<90 mmHg.[36] From 75%

to 91% of individuals who develop HF have antecedent hypertension.[12,31] In one study, hypertension was associated with hazard ratios for the development of HF of approximately two for men and three for women over the ensuing 18 years.[12] As shown in Figure 5–6, the hazard ratios for HF associated with hypertension (two to three) were far lower than the hazard ratios for HF associated with MI, which were greater than six for both men and women. However, the population prevalence of hypertension was 60%, compared with approximately 6% for MI. Therefore, the PAR of HF, that is, the fraction of HF in this population that was due to hypertension, was 59% in women and 39% in men. The PARs for MI were 13% and 34% for women and men, respectively.[12]

RENAL DISEASE

Hypertension is also a major risk factor for the development of renal disease, and a major cause of the 80,000 deaths from end-stage renal disease that occurred in the United States in 2002.[3] Of the estimated 100,000 cases of incident end-stage renal disease diagnosed in 2002,[31] it was estimated that over 25% were due to hypertension, and more than 40% to diabetes.[37] However, these numbers may substantially underestimate the contribution of BP to the increasing incidence of renal disease, since the data collection form allows only listing of a single diagnostic cause, and hypertension is present in the vast majority of diabetics. Blacks have approximately four times the risk of whites of developing end-stage renal disease, in part due to their significantly higher prevalence of hypertension.[31] In addition to its contribution to end-stage renal disease, elevated BP also occurs in and exacerbates milder forms of chronic kidney disease and worsens proteinuria.

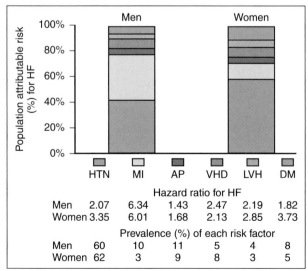

Figure 5–6. Hazard ratios, prevalence, and population-attributable risk percents associated with selected risk factors for heart failure in men and women. Framingham Heart Study.[12] AP, angina pectoris; DM, diabetes mellitus; HF, heart failure; HTN, hypertension; LVH, left ventricular hypertrophy; MI, myocardial infarction; VHD, valvular heart disease.

COMPETING RISKS FOR DIFFERENT CARDIOVASCULAR DISEASE OUTCOMES IN HYPERTENSION

A recent analysis[38] of Framingham Heart Study participants who experienced new-onset hypertension has shed interesting light on the risks for CVD associated with hypertension. Hypertension confers risk for multiple types of CVD events, but there were no previous studies examining which CVD events occur as a first event after hypertension onset in a competing risks framework. Typically, epidemiologic studies follow participants for single outcomes, without considering the joint and competing risks for multiple outcomes. Examining these competing risks in hypertension may be important because the occurrence of one type of CVD event (e.g., stroke) may be associated with greater morbidity and mortality than another type of CVD (e.g., angina), and because the occurrence of one CVD event (e.g., MI) may markedly increase the risk for subsequent CVD events (HF, stroke). Focusing efforts on preventing the first event after hypertension onset could therefore have important implications on longevity and quality of life, and different strategies may be needed to prevent diverse outcomes.

In this study, 645 men and 702 women (mean age: 55±12 years in men, 59±12 years in women) who were free of CVD and had new-onset hypertension after 1977 were included. At all ages following the onset of hypertension, CVD was more likely to occur as a first event than non-CVD death. The 12-year competing cumulative incidence of any CVD endpoint as a first event in men was 24.7%, compared with 9.8% for noncardiovascular death (hazards ratio [HR]=2.53, 95% confidence interval [CI]=1.83–3.50); in women, the competing incidences were 16.0% versus 10.1%, respectively (HR=1.58, 95% CI=1.13–2.20). The contrast between risk for CVD and non-CVD death was most striking in men with hypertension onset at age <60 years; in this group, the 12-year risk of CVD was 19.9% compared with 3.5% for non-CVD death (HR=5.67, 95% CI=3.07–10.46). For both men and women, there was a dramatic rise in stroke and HF as first hard CVD events with hypertension onset at age ≥60 years, compared with <60 years. As shown in Figure 5–7, types of first hard CVD events differed by gender and age at hypertension onset: in men younger than 60, hard CHD events were the most common first events, whereas in older men and in women at all ages stroke was the most common first event.[38]

These results may have important implications for primary prevention strategies. For example, in women and older men with new-onset hypertension, hypertensive-related CVD events (stroke, HF) predominate as first events. Thus clinicians and patients may want to focus their major efforts on achieving BP control, specifically aiming to lower the risk of stroke and HF in these subgroups, especially given the impressive reductions in stroke and HF documented in antihypertensive therapy trials. In younger men with new-onset hypertension, prevention might be tailored toward antihypertensive therapy plus use of lipid-lowering medications and aspirin, for which

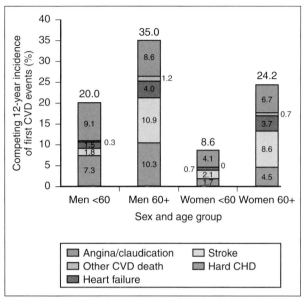

Figure 5–7. Competing 12-year incidence for different types of first cardiovascular disease events by age and sex among new-onset hypertensive men and women in the Framingham Heart Study.[38] CHD coronary heart disease; CVD, cardiovascular disease.

there are impressive data on preventing major nonfatal and fatal CHD events. Recent clinical trials support the approach of using these ancillary treatments to prevent CHD in hypertensive patients.[39,40]

BLOOD PRESSURE IN THE ELDERLY AND MINORITY GROUPS

The elderly are among the fastest growing segments of the U.S. population,[41] and they also have the greatest prevalence of hypertension.[31,42] Hypertension occurs in the absence of other CVD risk factors only rarely in older persons,[14] and it is often accompanied by a clustering of other risk factors. The prevalence of three or more coexisting risk factors is four times higher among hypertensive than among normotensive older individuals.[43]

As discussed above, older hypertensive patients appear to be at risk for a somewhat different spectrum of first CVD events than younger patients. Among new-onset hypertensives aged <60, the most common first major CVD event after 12 years of follow-up was an MI or hospitalization for unstable angina. Conversely, in those with hypertension onset at age ≥60 years, the most common first major CVD event was a stroke, particularly among older women.[38] Whereas the risk for CHD increases steadily with increasing age, the risks for HF and atrial fibrillation increase more dramatically among older compared with younger hypertensives.[35,44]

In a recent analysis of BP risks for CVD among adults across the age spectrum, relative risks for CVD associated with increasing BP stage did not decline with advancing age, and absolute risks increased markedly (Figure 5–8). Among participants aged ≥80 years, major cardiovascular

events occurred in 9.5% of the normal BP (referent) group, 19.8% of the prehypertension group (HR=1.9, 95% CI=0.9–3.9), 20.3% of the Stage 1 hypertension group (HR=1.8, 95% CI=0.8–3.7) and 24.7% of the Stage 2/treated hypertension group (HR=2.4, 95% CI=1.2–4.6).[11]

Hypertension has a greater impact in some race/ethnic groups than in others. Hypertension is more prevalent in blacks than in whites.[42] In addition, there is evidence to suggest that hypertension may confer differential risks for CVD, depending on race/ethnicity. For example, in a multivariable analysis from the Atherosclerosis Risk in Communities study, hypertension was a particularly strong risk factor for CHD among black women, with hazard ratios as follows: black women, 4.8 (95% CI=2.5–9.0), white women, 2.1 (CI=1.6–2.9), black men, 2.0 (CI=1.3–3.0), and white men, 1.6 (CI=1.3–1.9).[45] Further studies of the impact of BP on CVD across ethnic groups are needed.

SUMMARY AND PERSPECTIVES

In summary, elevated BP levels increase the risk for all manifestations of CVD, as well as total mortality and renal disease, in a continuous and graded fashion, beginning at levels at least as low as 115/75 mmHg. Increases in SBP with aging are the major cause of hypertension diagnosis in the population, and increases in SBP confer substantial risk for CVD events, regardless of age. Hypertension rarely occurs in isolation; rather, it is usually accompanied by other CVD risk factors that jointly and synergistically increase hypertension-related risks for CVD. Hypertension increases relative risks for stroke and heart failure most dramatically, but because CHD is more common, hypertension has its greatest impact in increasing the population risk for CHD. With the aging of the population and the worldwide obesity epidemic, the burden of hypertension and of its sequelae is likely to increase substantially. Greater efforts are therefore needed to prevent the development of hypertension, to control BP levels after the onset of hypertension, and to control associated risk factors in order to optimize CVD prevention across the population.

Future research should continue to define the risks associated with elevated BP, especially in minority groups and women. Epidemiologic data can continue to help us understand population trends in BP and suggest strategies for primordial prevention (prevention of risk factor development), and primary and secondary prevention of CVD once elevated BP is present. A better understanding is needed of the changes in arterial stiffness that are observed with aging, in order to determine whether there are lifestyle or other interventions that can prevent the age-related increases in SBP and pulse pressure. In addition, research into the links between elevated BP and other CVD risk factors may yield novel insights and new targets for therapy. Research into defining successful means for weight reduction and weight maintenance may provide the greatest public health benefit with regard to BP levels.

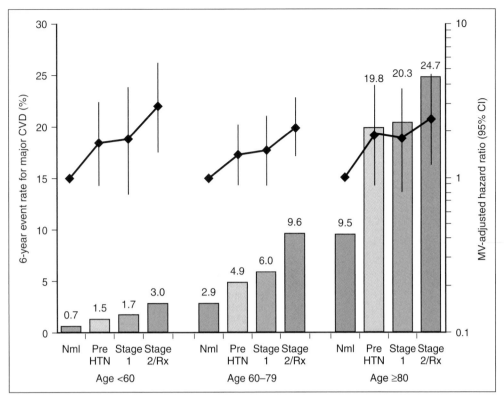

Figure 5–8. Six-year event rates (shown by the columns and on the left axis) and multivariable-adjusted relative risks with 95% confidence intervals (shown by the diamonds and lines and on the right axis) for major cardiovascular disease events by age group and blood pressure stage. Framingham Heart Study.[11] CVD, cardiovascular disease; HTN, hypertension; Nml, normal; MV, multivariable. Blood pressure is stratified as follows: normal (untreated systolic <120 and diastolic <80 mm Hg); prehypertension (untreated systolic 120–139 or diastolic 80–89 mm Hg); Stage 1 hypertension (untreated systolic 140–159 or diastolic 90–99 mm Hg); and Stage 2 (untreated systolic ≥160 or diastolic ≥100 mm Hg) or treated hypertension.

REFERENCES

1. Kannel WB, Dawber TR, Kagan A, et al. Factors of risk in the development of coronary heart disease—six-year follow-up experience. *Ann Intern Med* 1961; 55:33.

2. Hill AB. The environment and disease: association or causation? *Proc R Soc Med* 1965;58:295.

3. Hennekens CH, Buring JE. *Epidemiology in Medicine.* Boston: Little, Brown and Co., 1987.

4. Prospective Studies Collaboration. Age-specific relevance of usual blood pressure to vascular mortality: a meta-analysis of individual data for one million adults in 61 prospective studies. *Lancet* 2002;360:1903.

5. Stamler J, Stamler R, Neaton JD. Blood pressure, systolic and diastolic, and cardiovascular risks. US population data. *Arch Intern Med* 1993;153:598.

6. Vasan RS, Larson MG, Leip EP, et al. Assessment of frequency of progression to hypertension in non-hypertensive participants in the Framingham Heart Study: a cohort study. *Lancet* 2001; 358:1682.

7. O'Donnell CJ, Ridker PM, Glynn RJ, et al. Hypertension and borderline isolated systolic hypertension increase

risks of cardiovascular disease and mortality in male physicians. *Circulation* 1997;95:1132.

8. Chae CU, Pfeffer MA, Glynn RJ, et al. Increased pulse pressure and risk of heart failure in the elderly. *JAMA* 1999; 281:634.

9. Chobanian AV, Bakris GL, Black HR, et al. Seventh report of the Joint National Committee on Prevention, Detection, Evaluation, and Treatment of High Blood Pressure. *Hypertension* 2003;42:1206.

10. Vasan RS, Massaro JM, Wilson PWF, et al. Antecedent blood pressure and risk of cardiovascular disease: the Framingham Heart Study. *Circulation* 2002;105:48.

11. Lloyd-Jones DM, Evans JC, Levy D. Hypertension in adults across the age spectrum: current outcomes and control in the community. *JAMA* 2005; 294:466.

12. Levy D, Larson MG, Vasan RS, et al. The progression from hypertension to congestive heart failure. *JAMA* 1996; 275:1557.

13. Wilson PW, D'Agostino RB, Levy D, et al. Prediction of coronary heart disease using risk factor categories. *Circulation* 1998;97:1837.

14. Lloyd-Jones DM, Evans JC, Larson MG, et al. Cross-classification of JNC VI blood pressure stages and risk groups in the Framingham Heart Study. *Arch Intern Med* 1999;159:2206.

15. Reaven GM. Banting lecture 1988. Role of insulin resistance in human disease. *Diabetes Care* 1988;37:1595.

16. Burt VL, Whelton P, Roccella EJ, et al. Prevalence of hypertension in the US adult population: results from the Third National Health and Nutrition Examination Survey, 1988–1991. *Hypertension* 1995;25:305.

17. Franklin SS, Gustin W, Wong ND, et al. Hemodynamic patterns of age-related changes in blood pressure. The Framingham Heart Study. *Circulation* 1997;96:308.

18. Neaton JD, Kuller L, Stamler J, Wentworth DN. Impact of systolic and diastolic blood pressure on cardiovascular mortality. In: Laragh JH, Brenner BM, eds. *Hypertension: Pathophysiology, Diagnosis, and Management.* 2nd ed. New York: Raven Press, 1995:127.

19. Neaton JD, Wentworth DN. Serum cholesterol, blood pressure, cigarette smoking, and death from coronary

heart disease: overall findings and differences by age for 316,099 white men. *Arch Intern Med* 1992;152:56.

20. Psaty BM, Furberg CD, Kuller LH, et al. Association between blood pressure level and the risk of myocardial infarction, stroke, and total mortality. *Arch Intern Med* 2001;161:1183.

21. Kannel WB, Gordon T, Schwartz MJ. Systolic versus diastolic blood pressure and risk of coronary heart disease; the Framingham Study. *Am J Cardiol* 1971;27:335.

22. Franklin SS, Khan SA, Wong ND, et al. Is pulse pressure useful in predicting risk for coronary heart disease? The Framingham Heart Study. *Circulation* 1999;100:354.

23. Lloyd-Jones DM, Evans JC, Larson MG, et al. Differential impact of systolic and diastolic blood pressure level on JNC-VI staging. *Hypertension* 1999;34:381.

24. Franklin SS, Jacobs MJ, Wong ND, et al. Predominance of isolated systolic hypertension among middle-aged and elderly US hypertensives. *Hypertension* 2001;37:869.

25. SHEP Cooperative Research Group. Prevention of stroke by antihypertensive drug treatment in older persons with isolated systolic hypertension. Final results of the Systolic Hypertension in the Elderly Program (SHEP). *JAMA* 1991; 265:3255.

26. Liu L, Wang JG, Gong L, et al. Comparison of active treatment and placebo in older Chinese patients with isolated systolic hypertension. Systolic Hypertension in China (Syst-China) Collaborative Group. *J Hypertens* 1998; 16(12 Pt 1):1823.

27. Staessen JA, Fagard R, Thijs L, et al. Randomised double-blind comparison of placebo and active treatment for older patients with isolated systolic hypertension. The Systolic Hypertension in Europe (Syst-Eur) Trial Investigators. *Lancet* 1997;350:757.

28. Izzo JL, Levy D, Black HR. Importance of systolic blood pressure in older Americans. *Hypertension* 2000;35:1021.

29. Haider AW, Larson MG, Franklin SS, Levy D. Systolic blood pressure, diastolic blood pressure, and pulse pressure as predictors of risk for congestive heart failure in the Framingham Heart Study. *Ann Intern Med* 2003;138:10.

30. Miura K, Dyer AR, Greenland P, et al. Pulse pressure compared with other blood pressure indexes in the prediction of 25-year cardiovascular and all-cause mortality rates: the Chicago Heart Association Detection Project in Industry Study. *Hypertension* 2001; 38:232.

31. American Heart Association. *Heart disease and stroke statistics—2005 update.* Dallas, TX: American Heart Association, 2004.

32. Miura K, Daviglus ML, Dyer AR, et al. Relationship of blood pressure to 25-year mortality due to coronary heart disease, cardiovascular diseases, and all causes in young adult men: the Chicago Heart Association Detection Project in Industry. *Arch Intern Med* 2001;161:1501.

33. Wolf PA, Abbott RD, Kannel WB. Atrial fibrillation as an independent risk factor for stroke: the Framingham Study. *Stroke* 1991;22:8:983.

34. Schellenbaum GD, Rea TD, Heckbert SR, et al. Survival associated with two sets of diagnostic criteria for congestive heart failure. *Am J Epidemiol* 2004; 160:628.

35. Ho KK, Pinsky JL, Kannel WB, Levy D. The epidemiology of heart failure: the Framingham Study. *J Am Coll Cardiol* 1993;22:6A.

36. Lloyd-Jones DM, Larson MG, Leip EP, et al. Lifetime risk for developing congestive heart failure: the Framingham Heart Study. *Circulation* 2002;106:3068.

37. U.S. Renal Data System. *USRDS 2003 Annual Data Report.* Bethesda, MD: National Institute of Diabetes and Digestive and Kidney Diseases, National Institutes of Health (NIH), U.S. Department of Health and Human Services, 2003.

38. Lloyd-Jones DM, Leip EP, Larson MG, et al. Novel approach to examining first cardiovascular events after hypertension onset. *Hypertension* 2005;45:39.

39. Hansson L, Zanchetti A, Carruthers SG, et al. Effects of intensive blood-pressure lowering and low-dose aspirin in patients with hypertension: principal results of the Hypertension Optimal Treatment (HOT) randomised trial. *Lancet* 1998;351:1755.

40. Sever PS, Dahlof B, Poulter NR, et al. Prevention of coronary and stroke events with atorvastatin in hypertensive patients who have average or lower-than-average cholesterol concentrations, in the Anglo-Scandinavian Cardiac Outcomes Trial—Lipid Lowering Arm (ASCOT-LLA): a multicentre randomised controlled trial. *Lancet* 2003;361:1149.

41. Meyer J. *Age: 2000. Census 2000 Brief.* Washington, DC: U.S. Department of Commerce, Economics and Statistics Administration, U.S. Census Bureau, 2001.

42. Fields LE, Burt VL, Cutler JA, et al. The burden of adult hypertension in the United States 1999 to 2000. A rising tide. *Hypertension* 2004;44:398.

43. Kannel WB, Wilson PW, Silbershatz H, D'Agostino RB. Epidemiology of risk factor clustering in elevated blood pressure. In: Gotto AM, L'Enfant C, Paoletti R, eds. *Multiple Risk Factors in Cardiovascular Disease.* New York: Kluwer Academic Publishers, 1998:325.

44. Benjamin EJ, Levy D, Vaziri SM, et al. Independent risk factors for atrial fibrillation in a population- based cohort. The Framingham Heart Study. *JAMA* 1994;271:840.

45. Jones DW, Chambless LE, Folsom AR, et al. Risk factors for coronary heart disease in African Americans: the Atherosclerosis Risk in Communities Study, 1987–1997. *Arch Intern Med* 2002;162:2565.

Chapter

6 Lifestyle and Blood Pressure

Lydia A. L. Bazzano and Jiang He

Key Findings

- Among environmental risk factors, diet and nutrition play key roles, as well as physical inactivity, alcohol consumption, obesity, and stress, which clearly have an effect on blood pressure and the development of hypertension.

- Reduced dietary sodium intake lowers blood pressure in both normotensive and hypertensive individuals, reduces the incidence of hypertension, and may reduce the cardiovascular disease in overweight individuals.

- Potassium supplementation lowers blood pressure in both hypertensive and normotensive persons, although this may differ by level of dietary sodium intake.

- There is an inverse association between dietary protein intake and blood pressure. Increasing fiber intake has beneficial effects on blood pressure in both normotensive and hypertensive subjects, while supplementation of the diet with omega-3 polyunsaturated fatty acids reduces blood pressure.

- There is an inverse relationship between physical activity and blood pressure.

- A positive and independent association between alcohol consumption and elevated blood pressure is noted. Overweight and obesity also play an important role in the development of hypertension.

- Psychological and emotional stress may also contribute to the development of hypertension.

Hypertension is an important public health challenge worldwide. Its high prevalence and subsequent increased risk for developing cardiovascular diseases including heart attack, stroke, and chronic kidney disease have placed it as the leading risk factor for all-cause mortality, and a major cause of life-years adjusted disability.[1] A recent study on the global burden of hypertension found that 26.4% of the adult population in 2000 had hypertension and 29.2% were projected to have hypertension by the year 2025. This translates to approximately 972 million persons, with 333 million in economically developed countries and 639 million in economically developing countries who had hypertension in 2000. In 2025, 1.56 billion adults are expected to have hypertension.[2]

Hypertension is a complex disorder that is influenced by genetic and environmental factors as well as their interaction. Genetic factors may determine individuals' susceptibility to environmental risk factors and risk of developing hypertension. However, the environmental factors must be present to trigger the pathogenesis of the disease in most persons with hypertension. Among environmental risk factors, diet and nutrition play key roles, with intakes of sodium, potassium, fats, fiber, and protein clearly having an effect on blood pressure and the development of hypertension. Physical inactivity, alcohol consumption, obesity, and stress also play important roles in the development of hypertension.

DIET AND BLOOD PRESSURE

Sodium intake

Clinical trials have demonstrated that reduced dietary sodium intake lowers blood pressure in both normotensive and hypertensive individuals, reduces the incidence of hypertension, and may reduce the cardiovascular disease in overweight individuals.[3-6] Evidence from the Trials of Hypertension Prevention, Phase II (TOHP II), showed that overweight participants with high normal blood pressures could reduce their blood pressures with sodium restriction and avoid the development of hypertension. In this trial, 2382 men and women (aged 30 to 54) with a diastolic blood pressure 83 to 89 and systolic blood pressure less than 140 who were 110% to 165% of ideal body weight were randomized to usual care, salt restriction, weight reduction, or both.[4] Sodium restriction was associated with a 50- and 40-mEq decline in sodium intake at 6 and 36 months, respectively. Compared to usual care, systolic and diastolic blood pressure fell at 6 months by 2.9 and 1.6 mmHg with salt restriction. At 48 months, the relative risk of developing hypertension was 16% to 22% lower with lifestyle intervention than among those assigned to usual care.

The randomized controlled Trial of Nonpharmacologic Interventions in the Elderly (TONE) included a total of 975 men and women aged 60 to 80 years with systolic blood pressure less than 145 mmHg and diastolic blood pressure less than 85 mmHg while receiving treatment with a single antihypertensive medication. Of these participants, 585 obese participants were randomized to reduced sodium intake, weight loss, both, or usual care, and 390 nonobese participants were randomized to either reduced sodium intake or usual care groups. After 3 months of intervention, withdrawal of the single antihypertensive agent was attempted. As shown in Figure 6–1, participants who were assigned to reduce their sodium intake were significantly less likely to be diagnosed with high blood

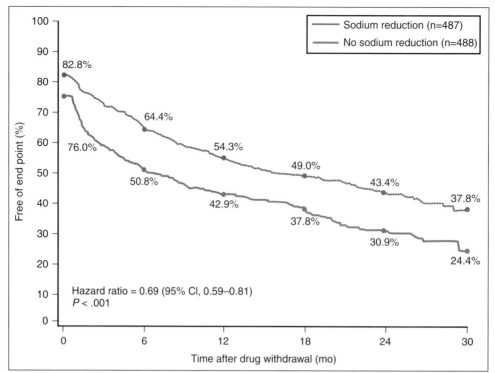

Figure 6–1. Percentages of the 487 participants who were, and the 488 who were not, assigned to the reduced sodium intake intervention who remained free of cardiovascular events and high blood pressure and did not have an antihypertensive agent prescribed during follow-up. (Adapted from Whelton PK, et al. *JAMA* 1998;279:839–46.)

pressure at a follow-up visit, be treated with an anti-hypertensive agent again, or have a cardiovascular event during the follow-up period as compared to those not assigned to reduce sodium intake (relative hazard ratio, 0.69; 95% confidence interval [CI]=0.59 to 0.81, $p<0.001$). Compared to the usual care group, the obese participants who were assigned to reduce sodium intake had a relative hazard of 0.60 (95% CI=0.45–0.80, $p<0.001$) for the combined endpoint.[5]

The Dietary Approaches to Stop Hypertension (DASH)-Sodium trial tested the blood pressure effects of three levels of sodium reduction in two diet groups.[6] The three sodium levels were 143 mmol/d, reflecting typical U.S. consumption; 106 mmol/d, reflecting the upper limit of current U.S. recommendations; and 65 mmol/d, targeted at further reduction of blood pressure. In the control diet, which was designed to reflect a typical American diet, reducing sodium intake from the higher to the intermediate level significantly reduced systolic blood pressure by 2.1 mmHg, and reducing sodium intake from the intermediate to the lower level further decreased systolic blood pressure by 4.6 mmHg. In the DASH diet group, corresponding reductions in systolic blood pressure were 1.3 and 1.7 mmHg, respectively. The combination of DASH diet with lower sodium level reduced systolic blood pressure by 7.1 mmHg in nonhypertensive persons, and 11.5 mmHg in hypertensive persons.[6]

At least three meta-analyses of randomized controlled trials have also shown that sodium reduction decreases blood pressure and prevents hypertension.[7–9] In all of these studies, sodium reduction was associated with a significant reduction in systolic blood pressure among normotensive persons. Cutler et al.[9] estimated that an average reduction of 77 mmol/day in dietary sodium intake resulted in a reduction of 2.8 mmHg in systolic blood pressure and 1.5 mmHg in diastolic blood pressure (Table 6–1).

While controversy remains as to whether reducing salt intake reduces the morbidity and mortality of cardiovascular diseases, some prospective cohort studies have suggested that a high sodium intake is associated with increased risk of cardiovascular disease. For example, in the National Health and Nutrition Examination Survey I Epidemiologic Follow-up Study (NHEFS), a 100-mmol higher level of sodium intake among obese persons was associated with a 32% increase in stroke incidence, 89% increase in stroke mortality, 44% increase in coronary heart disease mortality, 61% increase in cardiovascular disease mortality and a 39% increase in mortality from all causes.[3]

Potassium intake

Observational epidemiologic studies have identified an inverse association between dietary intake of potassium and blood pressure level within and across populations.[10] The large-scale high-quality data from the International Study of Salt and Blood Pressure (INTERSALT), including more than 10,000 participants from 52 population samples in 32 countries worldwide, provide the most precise and accurate observational estimates of the effect of potassium on blood pressure.[11,12] After adjustment for age, sex, body

SUMMARY OF REDUCTIONS IN BLOOD PRESSURE (MMHG) IN RESPONSE TO VARIOUS INTERVENTIONS BASED ON EVIDENCE FROM RECENT META-ANALYSES			
Intervention	Meta-Analysis	Change in Blood Pressure (95% Confidence Interval)	
		Systolic	Diastolic
Sodium reduction	Cutler et al., 1997[9]	–2.8 (–2.4 to –1.7)	–1.5 (–1.9 to –1.1)
Potassium supplementation	Whelton et al., 1997[15]	–3.1 (–4.3 to –1.9)	–1.9 (–3.4 to –0.5)
Fish oil supplementation	Geleijnse et al., 2002[68]	–2.1 (–3.2 to –1.0)	–1.6 (–2.2 to –1.0)
Physical activity	Whelton et al., 2002[82]	–3.8 (–4.9 to –2.7)	–2.6 (–3.4 to -1.8)
Alcohol reduction	Xin et al., 2001[91]	–3.3 (–4.1 to –2.5)	–2.0 (–2.6 to –1.5)
Weight loss	Neter et al., 2003[93]	–4.4 (–5.9 to –2.9)	–3.6 (–4.9 to –2.3)

Table 6–1. Summary of Reductions in Blood Pressure (mmHg) in Response to Various Interventions Based on Evidence from Recent Meta-Analyses

mass index, alcohol consumption and urinary sodium excretion and correction for regression dilution bias, a 50-mmol per day increase in urinary potassium excretion was associated with a 3.36 mmHg lower systolic blood pressure and 1.87 mmHg lower diastolic blood pressure.

Diets low in potassium have also been implicated in the higher prevalence of hypertension in African Americans.[13,14] Grim et al.[13] studied blood pressure and electrolyte intake in a random sample of the African American and white populations of Evans County, Georgia. The prevalence of hypertension was higher in African Americans compared to their counterparts who were white. Sodium intake, assessed by collecting duplicate diets and 24-hour urine specimens, was similar in African Americans and whites. Potassium intake, on the other hand, was significantly lower in African Americans than in whites: 24 versus 40 mmol per day for men and 27 versus 36 mmol per day in women, respectively. Likewise in the Veterans Administration Cooperative Study on Antihypertensive Agents, 24-hour urinary excretion of sodium was similar in African American and white untreated hypertensives, but African Americans excreted 62% less potassium than their counterparts who were white, or 45 versus 73 mmol per day.[14]

Randomized controlled trials document that potassium supplementation lowers blood pressure in both hypertensive and normotensive persons.[15] In a meta-analysis of 33 randomized controlled trials, potassium supplementation (median, 75 mmol/day) lowered systolic blood pressure by 3.1 mmHg (95% CI=–4.3 to –1.9) and diastolic blood pressure by 1.9 (95% CI=–3.9 to –0.5) (Figure 6–2) (Table 6–1). Conversely, a low dietary potassium intake has been associated with elevated blood pressure levels in randomized trials.[16,17]

The effects of potassium supplementation may differ by level of dietary sodium intake. When diets concurrently include high sodium levels, the effects of an increase in potassium intake are enhanced,[15] and may be blunted in those with a low baseline level of sodium intake. In their meta-analysis of randomized trials of potassium supplementation, Whelton et al.[15] found a dose-response relationship between change in 24 hour urinary potassium and effect size in trials in which the participants were consuming a diet high in sodium ($p<0.001$).

Increased dietary potassium intake has also been associated with lower risk of stroke or cardiovascular diseases. Khaw and Barrett-Connor[18] examined the relationship between potassium intake and stroke mortality among 859 male and female retirees in Southern California and identified a strong inverse association (relative risk [RR]=0.60, 95% CI=0.44–0.82).[18] Likewise, Ascherio et al.[19] identified an inverse association among the partici-

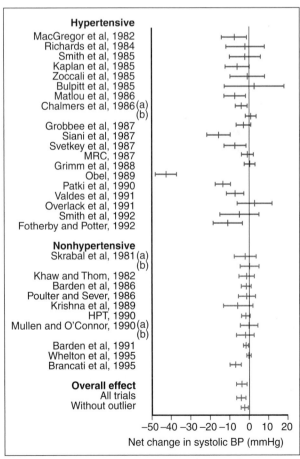

Figure 6–2. Average net change in systolic BP and corresponding 95% confidence interval after treatment with oral potassium supplementation in 32 randomized controlled trials. BP, blood pressure; MRC, Medical Research Council; HPT, Hypertension Prevention Trial. (Adapted from Whelton PK, et al. *JAMA* 1997;277:1624–32.)

pants in the Health Professionals' Follow-up Study. In the first National Health and Nutrition Examination Survey Epidemiologic Follow-up Study, Bazzano et al.[20] examined the relationship between dietary potassium intake and the risk of stroke in a representative sample of 9805 U.S. men and women. Over an average of 19 years of follow-up, participants consuming a low-potassium diet at baseline (<34.6 mmol potassium/24 hours) experienced a 28% higher hazard of stroke (RR=1.28, 95% CI=1.11–1.47, p<0.001) than other participants, after adjustment for established cardiovascular disease risk factors.

Fruits, vegetables and legumes are major sources of potassium in the diet. One cup of orange juice contains approximately 473 mg of potassium, one cup of cooked peas contains approximately 384 mg of potassium, and one medium-sized baked potato contains 926 mg of potassium.[21] Dairy products, meats, and nuts are also important dietary sources of potassium. Suggested goal intakes for individuals in the United States are approximately 4.5 to 4.7 g per day or 115 to 120 mmol per day.

Dietary fat intake

A diet high in fat often includes energy in excess of that expended and so results in weight gain, which in turn can lead to increased blood pressure. When the relationship between total dietary fat intake and blood pressure has been investigated, after accounting for adiposity or change in body weight, conflicting results have been found. Total dietary fat intake has not been associated with blood pressure in cross-sectional epidemiologic studies[22–25]; however, intake of dietary saturated fats was associated with hypertension in two Finnish studies[22,23] and oleic acid was inversely correlated with blood pressure in two small clinical studies.[26,27] Many other studies found no such association.[25,26,28,29] Prospective studies have shown conflicting results. In the Nurses' Health Study, dietary fatty acids showed no association with the 4-year incidence of hypertension,[30] while analyses of the Multiple Risk Factor Intervention Trial (MRFIT) data showed positive associations between blood pressure and saturated fats and an inverse association with polyunsaturated fats.[31] With a few exceptions,[32–34] trials testing the effects of substituting carbohydrates or unsaturated fats for animal fat have not demonstrated significantly lower blood pressures.[35–38] However, most of these trials were small and did not have the power to detect changes in blood pressure less than 3 to 5 mmHg.

Fat moderation has been one of the aspects of more complex interventions to prevent hypertension. For example, in the DASH study of dietary patterns, 459 adults with systolic blood pressures of less than 160 mmHg and diastolic blood pressures of 80 to 95 mmHg were fed a control diet that was low in fruits, vegetables, and dairy products, with a fat content typical of the average diet in the United States for 3 weeks, and then were randomly assigned to receive the control diet, a diet rich in fruits and vegetables, or a "combination" diet rich in fruits, vegetables, and low-fat dairy products and with reduced saturated (6% vs. 16% of energy) and total fat (27% vs. 37% of energy) for the next 8 weeks.[39] At baseline, the mean (± standard deviation) systolic and diastolic blood pressures were 131.3±10.8 mmHg and 84.7±4.7 mmHg, respectively. The combination diet reduced systolic and diastolic blood pressure by 5.5 and 3.0 mmHg more, respectively, than the control diet (p<0.001 for each); and the fruits-and-vegetables diet reduced systolic blood pressure by 2.8 mmHg more (p<0.001) and diastolic blood pressure by 1.1 mmHg more than the control diet (p=0.07). Among the 133 subjects with hypertension, the combination diet reduced systolic and diastolic blood pressure by 11.4 and 5.5 mmHg more, respectively, than the control diet (p<0.001 for each); among the 326 subjects without hypertension, the corresponding reductions were 3.5 mmHg (p<0.001) and 2.1 mmHg (p=0.003).[39] While the possible effects of consuming a diet reduced in total and saturated fat on blood pressure cannot be distinguished from other components of the "combination" diet in this trial, it is likely from previous trials that those effects were small.

If present, the potential effects of polyunsaturated fatty acids (specifically, the n-6 variety) on blood pressure may be related to the modulation of prostaglandin synthesis. The deprivation of linoleic acid during a salt-loading study resulted in a significantly elevated blood pressure in the rat.[40] At the same time, total prostaglandin metabolites were reduced significantly. Cox et al.[41] found that urinary excretion of prostaglandin E_2 was dependent on dietary intake of linoleic acid. Tobian et al.[42] found that feeding high levels of linoleic acid to salt-sensitive Dahl rats on a high-salt diet reduced blood pressure and increased PGE_2 levels in the renal papilla, thereby facilitating the transport of sodium and increasing capacity for sodium excretion.[43,44]

Dietary protein intake

Extensive evidence from observational studies supports an inverse association between dietary protein intake and blood pressure independent of body fat and body weight. These data have been reviewed several times over the past decade,[45–49] and at least two meta-analyses of these data have been published.[45,49] Recently two large observational studies have reported results on the relationship between dietary protein intake and blood pressure.[31,50] The INTERSALT study analyzed data from 24-hour urinary samples of more than 10,000 participants for markers of protein intake. Inverse associations were significant (p<0.001) for two of three markers of protein intake and blood pressure with adjustment for 24-hour excretions of sodium, potassium, calcium, and magnesium; body mass index; and alcohol intake.[50] The International Study of Macronutrients and Blood Pressure (INTERMAP) analyzed data from 4680 men and women aged 40 to 59 from 17 population samples in China, Japan, the United Kingdom, and the United States. To assess diet, blood pressure, and other variables, participants were seen at four visits, four 24-hour dietary recalls were done, and two timed 24-hour urine specimens collected. A significant inverse relationship between vegetable protein and blood pressure was identified independent of body weight, but not animal or total protein and blood pressure.

Inverse associations were also found in analyses of the MRFIT cohort.[31]

In the most recent review of this literature, 26 cross-sectional analyses were identified from 18 different studies, with 16 of these identifying an inverse relationship between protein or a marker of its intake and blood pressure or hypertension.[48] In the same review, five longitudinal studies were identified, which have reported on dietary protein intake and blood pressure or incidence of hypertension. Of those, three reports found no association, two found an inverse association, and one found an inverse association between vegetable protein and both systolic and diastolic blood pressure, and a direct association between animal protein and change in systolic blood pressure.[51]

Trials of protein supplementation or substitution of protein for carbohydrate or fat in the diet have produced inconsistent results. Early studies investigated responses to low- and high-protein diets with added beef or soy protein and addition of one egg per day to the diet.[52–54] These studies did not find a significant association between intervention diets and blood pressure during the study period. More recently, trials of soybean protein supplementation have demonstrated lower blood pressures in the intervention group participants.[47,55,56] He et al.[57] collected data from 302 participants, aged 35 to 64 years, with an initial untreated systolic blood pressure of 130 to 159 mmHg, diastolic blood pressure of 80 to 99 mmHg, or both. Study participants were randomized to receive 40 g of isolated soybean protein supplement per day or a complex carbohydrate control for 12 weeks, and blood pressures were obtained at baseline, and at 6 and 12 weeks. Body weight was maintained in both groups without significant change. Compared to the control group, the net changes in systolic and diastolic blood pressure were −4.31 mmHg (95% CI=−2.11−−6.51 mmHg, $p<0.001$) and −2.76 mmHg (95% CI=−1.35−−4.16 mmHg, $p<0.001$), respectively after 12 weeks (Figure 6–3). In addition, increased protein intake has been a feature of more complex interventions such as the combination (fruit, vegetable, and low-fat dairy) diet in the DASH trial. In that combination diet, 17.9% of energy was derived from protein versus 13.8% of energy in the control diet.[39]

The mechanism by which dietary protein influences blood pressure is largely unknown. However, dietary protein intake could influence blood pressure through the actions of its many constituent amino acids. For instance, both tyrosine and tryptophan lower blood pressure when injected intraperitoneally in animal models.[58,59] Arginine is a metabolic precursor of nitric oxide, and the amino acid cysteine influences nitric oxide metabolism,[50] while tyrosine and phenylalanine affect the synthesis of catecholamines in the central nervous system.[60]

Dietary fiber intake

Observational and experimental studies have demonstrated that increasing fiber intake has beneficial effects on blood pressure in both normotensive and hypertensive subjects.[46,61] Clinical trials have shown wide variation in blood pressure responses to dietary fiber supplemen-

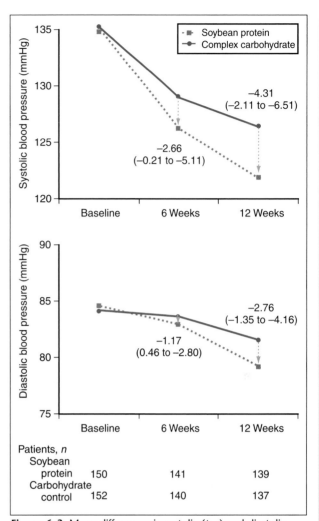

Figure 6–3. Mean differences in systolic (*top*) and diastolic (*bottom*) blood pressures and 95% confidence intervals among trial participants randomized to receive soybean protein supplementation or complex carbohydrate. (Adapted from He J, et al. *Ann Intern Med* 2005;143:1–9.)

tation.[46] For example, a recent randomized, placebo-controlled trial of fiber supplementation involved 110 trial participants aged 30 to 65 years who had untreated, but higher-than-optimal blood pressure or stage 1 hypertension who were randomly assigned to receive 8 g/day of water-soluble fiber from oat bran or a control intervention. An average of the nine measurements was used to determine mean blood pressure at the baseline and termination visits. The net changes in systolic blood pressure were −1.8 mmHg (95% CI=−4.3 to 0.8) following 12 weeks, −2.2 mmHg (95% CI=−5.3 to 1.0) following 6 weeks, and −2.0 mmHg (95% CI=−4.4 to 0.3) for an average of the 6- and 12-week visits. The corresponding net changes in diastolic blood pressure were −1.2 mmHg (95% CI=−3.0 to 0.5) following 12 weeks, −0.8 mmHg (95% CI=−3.1 to 1.4) following 6 weeks, and −1.0 mmHg (95% CI=−2.6 to 0.5) for an average of the 6- and 12-week visits.[61]

Given the many clinical trials of dietary fiber and blood pressure which may have lacked power to detect small but meaningful blood pressure effects, a meta-analysis of randomized placebo-controlled trials of the effects of fiber supplementation on blood pressure was conducted by Whelton et al.[62] They identified 25 randomized controlled trials, and abstracted data on study design, sample size, participant and intervention characteristics, duration of follow-up, and change in mean blood pressure. Fiber supplementation (average dose of 10.7 g/d) was associated with a significant –1.65 mmHg (95% CI=–2.70 to –0.61) change in diastolic and a non-significant –1.15 mmHg (95% CI=–2.68 to 0.39) change in systolic blood pressure. A significant reduction in both systolic and diastolic blood pressure was observed in trials conducted among participants with hypertension: –5.95 mmHg (95% CI=–9.50—2.40) and –4.20 mmHg (95% CI= –6.55—1.85), respectively. Similarly, trials with a duration of intervention at least 8 weeks long also showed significant reductions in both systolic and diastolic blood pressures, –3.12 mmHg (95% CI=–5.68—0.56) and –2.57 mmHg (95% CI=–4.01—1.14), respectively.[62] Fiber supplementation was also a part of the DASH study interventions. Both the fruit and vegetable and the combination diets included 31 g of fiber daily versus the control diet which included 9 g of fiber daily.[39]

Moreover, dietary fiber intake may also favorably influence other cardiovascular risk factors resulting in lower risk of coronary heart disease. For example, in the large NHEFS cohort, a higher intake of dietary fiber appeared to be associated with a reduced risk of coronary heart disease.[20] Beneficial effects of fiber were related to water-soluble types of fiber more so than insoluble fiber in that study.

The potential effect of dietary fiber intake on blood pressure may have several mechanisms, given that dietary fiber has multifaceted effects on both digestion and absorption of nutrients. Soluble fiber increases insulin sensitivity in both diabetics and normal subjects.[62–64] Insulin resistance and its concomitant compensatory hyperinsulinemia have been suggested to play a role in the etiology and pathogenesis of hypertension,[65] although this concept has been controversial. A diet supplemented with fiber may also form a component of weight-loss strategies, and reducing body weight is another mechanism by which a dietary fiber may aid in the prevention of hypertension.[66,67]

Fish and fish oil

Several lines of evidence suggest that supplementation of the diet with omega-3 polyunsaturated fatty acids, commonly referred to as fish oils, reduces blood pressure by altering prostaglandin synthesis. However, many of the clinical trials of fish oil supplementation have been of insufficient size to detect relevant blood pressure changes. At least three meta-analyses of clinical trials of fish oil supplementation and blood pressure have been conducted.[68–70] All three of these found significant antihypertensive effects of fish oil. The most recent, conducted in 2002, analyzed 36 trials of fish oil supplementation and found that intake of fish oil (median dose 3.7 g/day) reduced systolic blood pressure by 2.1 mmHg (95% CI=–1.0—3.2, p<0.01) and diastolic blood pressure by 1.6 mmHg (95% CI=–1.0—2.2, p<0.01). Restricting their

analysis to double-blind trials demonstrated blood pressure reductions of 1.7 mmHg (95% CI=–0.3—3.1) systolic and 1.5 mmHg (95% CI=–0.6—2.3) diastolic.[68] These estimates correspond well with those of the meta-analysis conducted by Appel et al.[69] Weighted pooled estimates of 11 clinical trials of fish oil supplementation and blood pressure in normotensive individuals yielded systolic blood pressure reductions of 1.0 mmHg (95% CI= –2.0–0.0) and diastolic reductions of 0.5 mmHg (95% CI=–1.2–0.2). In six trials of hypertensives, weighted pooled estimates of systolic and diastolic blood pressure changes were –5.5 mmHg (95% CI=–8.1—2.9) and –3.5 mmHg (95% CI=–5.0—2.1), respectively.[69]

Dietary pattern

People manipulate their diets by choosing foods rather than nutrients. Consequently, studies of food intake and blood pressure have become as important as those of nutrient intake. Epidemiologic studies have suggested that a dietary pattern that includes abundant fruits, vegetables, and low-fat diary products may lower blood pressure.

Several observational studies of fruit and vegetable intake have shown an association with lower blood pressures.[71–74] For example, in a cross-sectional study conducted among 4393 Spanish men and women, blood pressure was inversely associated with fruit and vegetable consumption as measured by food frequency questionnaire.[71] Among 1710 men enrolled in the Chicago Western Electric cohort and followed for 7 years, average systolic blood pressure/diastolic blood pressure increase was 1.9/0.3 mmHg per year. The systolic blood pressure of men who consumed 14 to 42 cups of vegetables a month (0.5 to 1.5 cups/day) versus less than 14 cups a month (<0.5 cups/day) was estimated to rise 2.8 mmHg less in 7 years (p<0.01). The systolic blood pressure of men who consumed 14 to 42 cups of fruit a month versus less than 14 cups a month was estimated to increase 2.2 mmHg less in 7 years (p<0.05).[72] A study in children of the Framingham Children's study suggests similar effects of consuming a diet high in fruits and vegetables.[73] Fruits and vegetables are major sources of potassium and fiber in the diet of most peoples worldwide.

Low-fat dairy products may also play a role in the prevention of hypertension and the lowering of blood pressure. Most diary products provide significant amounts of calcium and protein, both of which likely contribute to blood pressure lowering effects. Several meta-analyses of the association between calcium intake and blood pressure have substantiated a small blood pressure–lowering effect of calcium supplementation.[75–78]

The DASH clinical trial demonstrated that manipulation of dietary pattern with increased consumption of fruits, vegetables, and low-fat dairy products while maintaining constant energy consumption, lowers blood pressure and may prevent the onset of hypertension.[39] The combination diet significantly lowered blood pressure in all major subgroups including men, women, African Americans, non-African Americans, hypertensives, and normotensives. The effect of the DASH combination diet in hypertensive individuals is similar in magnitude to drug monotherapy for hypertension, and from a public health perspective, wide adoption of the DASH dietary pattern may shift the population blood pressure distribution downward, thereby reducing the risk of blood pressure–related cardiovascular diseases.

PHYSICAL ACTIVITY AND BLOOD PRESSURE

Observational epidemiologic studies have demonstrated a consistent inverse relationship between physical activity and blood pressure independent of body weight and adiposity. In a Japanese cohort of 6017 men aged 35 to 60 years, a walk of 21 minutes or more compared with 10 minutes or less was associated with a 29% lower risk of hypertension (p for trend=0.02).[79] In the Atherosclerosis Risk in Communities Study cohort, white men who performed the most leisure activity (primarily walking and cycling) had 34% lower odds of developing hypertension over 6 years compared with those who were least active (odds ratio=0.66, 95% CI=0.47–0.94, p for trend=0.01).[80] In that study, leisure physical activity was not associated with the incidence of hypertension in white women or African Americans.

Evidence from randomized controlled trials also supports the role of physical activity in lowering blood pressure. At least two meta-analyses of randomized trials of aerobic exercise effects on blood pressure have been conducted to date.[81,82] Kelley conducted a meta-analysis among women aged 18 years and older, including 10 randomized trials with 732 participants. Overall, a significant reduction in systolic, by –2 mmHg (95% CI=–3 to –1 mmHg) and diastolic, by –1 mmHg (95% CI=–2 to –1 mmHg), blood pressure was observed in these women.[81] In the meta-analysis by Whelton et al.,[82] 54 randomized controlled trials with 2419 men and women participants were included in the analysis (Figure 6–4) (Table 6–1). Pooled estimates showed that aerobic exercise was associated with a significant reduction in mean systolic and diastolic blood pressure: –3.84 mmHg (95% CI=–4.97–−2.72) and –2.58 mmHg (95% CI=–3.35–−1.81), respectively.[82]

Some of the mechanisms by which physical activity reduces blood pressure may be independent of body weight. For instance, aerobic exercise improves insulin sensitivity and lowers insulin levels, which have been implicated in the pathogenesis of hypertension.[83] Physical activity may also lower blood pressure by causing weight loss.[84] Therefore, promoting physical activity could have substantial public health benefits as a means to reduce blood pressure.

ALCOHOL CONSUMPTION AND BLOOD PRESSURE

Moderation of alcohol intake is an important part of efforts to prevent hypertension and decrease blood pressure. Observational epidemiologic studies have demonstrated a positive and independent association between alcohol consumption and elevated blood pressure.[85–87] Several clinical trials of the effects of alcohol

reduction on blood pressure have been conducted.[88–91] However, most of these studies have had small sample sizes and have reported inconsistent findings. One trial of 641 U.S. military veterans also failed to show a decrease in blood pressure with alcohol reduction.[90] In that study, veterans with an average intake of three or more drinks per day and with diastolic blood pressures between 0 and 99 mmHg were randomly assigned to either a cognitive-behavioral alcohol reduction program or observation for 15 to 24 months. The intervention group reduced alcohol intake by an average of 1.3 drinks per day compared with the control group; however, this net reduction was less than the anticipated minimum of two drinks per day. The intervention group had a 1.2/0.7 mmHg greater reduction in blood pressure than the control group (p=0.17 for systolic and p=0.18 for diastolic) for the 6-month primary endpoint. One explanation for the lack of significant reduction in blood pressure in this study is the relatively small change in alcohol intake of these veterans.

Because of the large number of studies with small sample sizes, and the importance of even small reductions in blood pressure, meta-analysis of these randomized controlled trials has been conducted by Xin et al.[91] Fifteen randomized controlled trials with a total of 2234 participants were included. Overall, alcohol reduction was associated with a significant reduction in mean systolic and diastolic blood pressures of –3.31 (95% CI=–4.10–−2.52) and –2.04 mmHg (–2.58–−1.49), respectively (Figure 6–5) (Table 6–1). A dose–response relationship was seen between the mean percentage of alcohol reduction and mean blood pressure reduction in this study.

BODY WEIGHT AND BLOOD PRESSURE

Overweight and obesity play important roles in the development of hypertension. Several studies support the role of weight loss in the prevention and treatment of hypertension. The TONE trial was designed to determine whether weight loss or dietary sodium reduction would produce satisfactory blood pressure control after withdrawal of antihypertensive drug therapy, using a factorial design.[5] The average reduction in weight for obese participants assigned to weight loss was approximately 3.5 to 4.5 kg, versus an average of 0.9-kg reduction for those no assigned to the weight-loss arm. At the trial endpoint, 39% of those randomized to weight loss remained off antihypertensive medication with a blood pressure of less than 150/90 mmHg and without a blood pressure–related complication, compared with 26% of those not assigned to weight loss 30 months after the attempted withdrawal of antihypertensive drug therapy.

He et al.[92] examined the relationship between long-term weight loss and hypertension by studying 181 men and women who participated in the TOHP, phase I (TOHP I). At baseline in 1987–1988, participants were aged 30 to 54 years and had diastolic blood pressure of 80 to 89 mmHg and systolic blood pressure of less than 160 mmHg. They were randomly assigned to one of two 18-month lifestyle modification interventions (aimed at either weight loss or dietary sodium reduction) or to a

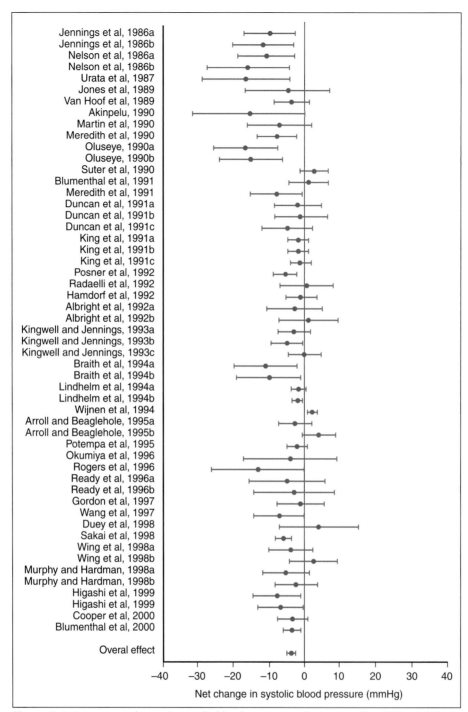

Figure 6–4. Average net change in systolic blood pressure and corresponding 95% confidence intervals related to aerobic exercise intervention in 53 randomized controlled trials. (Adapted from Whelton SP, et al. *Ann Intern Med* 2002;136:493–503.)

usual care group. Post-trial follow-up was conducted in 1994 and 1995. Blood pressure was measured by blinded observers with a random-zero sphygmomanometer, and incident hypertension was defined as a systolic blood pressure of at least 160 mmHg or a diastolic blood pressure of at least 90 mmHg, or treatment with an antihypertensive medication. After 7 years of follow-up, the incidence of hypertension was 18.9% in the weight-loss group and 40.5% in its control group. In logistic regression analysis adjusted for baseline age, gender, race,

physical activity, alcohol consumption, education, body weight, systolic blood pressure, and urinary sodium excretion, the odds of hypertension was reduced by 77% (odds ratio 0.23, 95% CI=0.07–0.76, *p*=0.02) in the weight-loss group compared with their control groups. Similar significant reductions in blood pressure and hypertension were found in the TOHP, phase II.[84]

Evidence from a meta-analysis of randomized controlled trials of the influence of weight reduction on blood pressure also supports weight loss as an important inter-

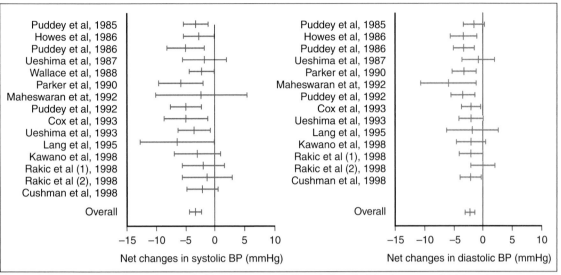

Figure 6–5. Average net change in systolic blood pressure (*left*) and diastolic blood pressure (*right*) and corresponding 95% confidence intervals related to alcohol reduction intervention in 15 randomized controlled trials. (Adapted from Xin X, et al. *Hypertension* 2001;38:1112–7.)

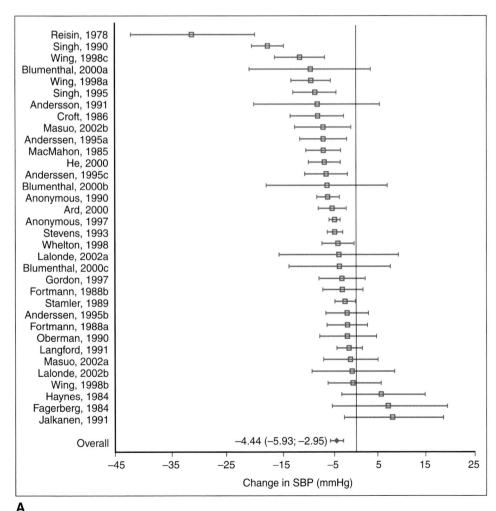

A

Figure 6–6. Blood pressure effects in randomized controlled trials of weight reduction. *Open squares* represent average net changes in systolic blood pressure and diastolic blood pressure in individual trials (or trial strata), with 95% confidence intervals. (Adapted from Neter, et al. *Hypertension* 2003:42:878–84.)

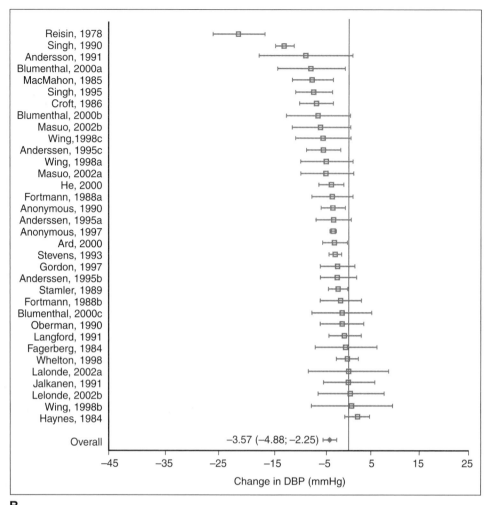

B

Figure 6–6.—cont'd

vention for the prevention and treatment of hypertension.[93] Twenty-five randomized controlled trials published between 1966 and 2002 with a total of 4874 participants were included. Authors found that a net weight reduction of 5.1 kg (95% CI=–6.03—4.25) by means of energy restriction increased physical activity or both reduced systolic blood pressure by 4.4 mmHg (95% CI=–5.93—2.95) and diastolic blood pressure by –3.57 mmHg (95% CI=–4.88—2.25) (Figure 6–6) (Table 6–1).

STRESS AND BLOOD PRESSURE

Psychological and emotional stress may also contribute to the development of hypertension and incremental increases in blood pressure via the body's sympathetic nervous system.[94] Trials of relaxation techniques ranging from transcendental meditation to biofeedback have shown small but potentially important improvements in blood pressure with use of these noninvasive methods.[95–97] Unfortunately, several of these trials have methodologic weaknesses that may have affected their results.[97]

In one well-conducted randomized trial, Schneider et al.[98] tested the short-term efficacy of two stress-reduction

techniques in the treatment of mild hypertension in older African Americans. A total of 127 individuals aged 55 to 85 years with prehypertension or stage I hypertension were randomized to a 3-month transcendental meditation (TM) or progressive muscle relaxation (PMR) or educational control (EC) program, which included information on lifestyle factors, and were followed in a primary care, inner-city health center. Of these, 16 did not complete follow-up blood pressure measurements. Both active intervention groups showed significant reductions in systolic and diastolic blood pressures compared with the EC group. Compared with the EC group, the TM group showed a reduction of 10.7 mmHg in systolic (p=0.0002) and 6.4 mmHg diastolic (p=0.00005) blood pressure. Compared with the EC group, the PMR group showed adjusted reductions of 4.7 mmHg in systolic (p=0.054) and 3.3 mmHg in diastolic (p=0.02) blood pressures. The reductions in the TM group were significantly greater than in the progressive muscle relaxation group for both systolic blood pressure (p=0.02) and diastolic blood pressure (p=0.03).[98] The findings of this study and others suggest that psychosocial interventions in hypertensive and prehypertensive individuals warrant more investigation.

SUMMARY

In 2000, nearly 927 million people worldwide were affected by high blood pressure. The need for lifestyle interventions in the prevention and treatment of hypertension is increasingly a priority. Since the majority of cardiovascular events occur in individuals with high normal or mildly elevated blood pressure, public health strategies to shift population blood pressure to a lower level is of utmost importance in order to reduce the burden of cardiovascular disease. Even small reductions in blood pressure, if applied to an entire population, could have an enormous beneficial effect on cardiovascular events. The effects of changes in dietary patterns, including reduced consumption of sodium, increased intake of potassium, and certain foods, and increasing physical activity, moderation of alcohol intake and weight loss have been documented in well conducted randomized clinical trials.[99] On the other hand, the effects of dietary fat, fiber, protein, fish oil, and psychosocial stress need to be further examined. Evidence suggests that even small changes in blood pressure due to lifestyle change of the population would result in significantly lower rates of hypertension and cardiovascular diseases worldwide.

REFERENCES

1. Ezzati M, Lopez AD, Rodgers A, Vander Hoorn S, Murray CJ. Selected major risk factors and global and regional burden of disease. *Lancet* 2002;360:1347–60.

2. Kearney PM, Whelton M, Reynolds K, Muntner P, Whelton PK, He J. Global burden of hypertension: analysis of worldwide data. *Lancet* 2005; 365:217–23.

3. He J, Ogden LG, Vupputuri S, Bazzano LA, Loria C, Whelton PK. Dietary sodium intake and subsequent risk of cardiovascular disease in overweight adults. *JAMA* 1999;282:2027–34.

4. Trials of Hypertension Prevention Collaborative Research Group. Effects of weight loss and sodium reduction intervention on blood pressure and hypertension incidence in overweight people with high-normal blood pressure. The trials of hypertension prevention, Phase II. *Arch Intern Med* 1997;157:657–67.

5. Whelton PK, Appel LJ, Espeland MA, Applegate WB, Ettinger WH Jr, Kostis JB, et al. Sodium reduction and weight loss in the treatment of hypertension in older persons: a randomized controlled trial of nonpharmacologic interventions in the elderly (TONE). Tone Collaborative Research Group. *JAMA* 1998;279:839–46.

6. Sacks FM, Svetkey LP, Vollmer WM, Appel LJ, Bray GA, Harsha D, et al. Effects on blood pressure of reduced dietary sodium and the dietary approaches to stop hypertension (DASH) diet. DASH-Sodium Collaborative Research Group. *N Engl J Med* 2001;344:3–10.

7. Midgley JP, Matthew AG, Greenwood CM, Logan AG. Effect of reduced dietary sodium on blood pressure: a meta-analysis of randomized controlled trials. *JAMA* 1996;275:1590–7.

8. Graudal NA, Galloe AM, Garred P. Effects of sodium restriction on blood pressure, renin, aldosterone, catecholamines, cholesterols, and triglyceride: a meta-analysis. *JAMA* 1998;279:1383–91.

9. Cutler JA, Follmann D, Allender PS. Randomized trials of sodium reduction: an overview. *Am J Clin Nutr* 1997; 65(Suppl. 2):643S–51S.

10. He J, Whelton PK. Potassium, blood pressure, and cardiovascular disease: an epidemiologic perspective. *Cardiol Rev* 1997;5:255–60.

11. INTERSALT Cooperative Research Group. INTERSALT: an international study of electrolyte excretion and blood pressure. Results for 24 hour urinary sodium and potassium excretion. *BMJ* 1988;297:319–28.

12. Dyer AR, Elliott P, Shipley M, Stamler R, Stamler J. Body mass index and associations of sodium and potassium with blood pressure in intersalt. *Hypertension* 1994;23:729–36.

13. Grim CE, Luft FC, Miller JZ, Meneely GR, Battarbee HD, Hames CG, et al. Racial differences in blood pressure in Evans County, Georgia: Relationship to sodium and potassium intake and plasma renin activity. *J Chronic Dis* 1980;33:87–94.

14. Veterans Administration Cooperative Study Group on Antihypertensive Agents. Urinary and serum electrolytes in untreated black and white hypertensives. *J Chronic Dis* 1987; 40:839–47.

15. Whelton PK, He J, Cutler JA, Brancati FL, Appel LJ, Follmann D, et al. Effects of oral potassium on blood pressure. Meta-analysis of randomized controlled clinical trials. *JAMA* 1997;277:1624–32.

16. Krishna GG, Kapoor SC. Potassium depletion exacerbates essential hypertension. *Ann Intern Med* 1991; 115:77–83.

17. Krishna GG, Miller E, Kapoor S. Increased blood pressure during potassium depletion in normotensive men. *N Engl J Med* 1989;320:1177–82.

18. Khaw KT, Barrett-Connor E. Dietary potassium and stroke-associated mortality. A 12-year prospective population study. *N Engl J Med* 1987; 316:235–40.

19. Ascherio A, Rimm EB, Giovannucci EL, Colditz GA, Rosner B, Willett WC, et al. A prospective study of nutritional factors and hypertension among US men. *Circulation* 1992;86:1475–84.

20. Bazzano LA, He J, Ogden LG, Loria CM, Whelton PK. Dietary fiber intake and reduced risk of coronary heart disease in US men and women: the National Health and Nutrition Examination Survey I Epidemiologic Follow-up Study. *Arch Intern Med* 2003;163:1897–904.

21. U.S. Department of Agriculture, Agricultural Research Service. USDA National Nutrient Database for Standard Reference. Release 18. Washington, DC: U.S. Department of Agriculture, 2005.

22. Salonen JT, Salonen R, Ihanainen M, Parviainen M, Seppanen R, Kantola M, et al. Blood pressure, dietary fats, and antioxidants. *Am J Clin Nutr* 1988; 48:1226–32.

23. Salonen JT, Tuomilehto J, Tanskanen A. Relation of blood pressure to reported intake of salt, saturated fats, and alcohol in healthy middle-aged population. *J Epidemiol Community Health* 1983;37:32–7.

24. Reed D, McGee D, Yano K, Hankin J. Diet, blood pressure, and multicollinearity. *Hypertension* 1985;7:405–10.

25. Gruchow HW, Sobocinski KA, Barboriak JJ. Alcohol, nutrient intake, and hypertension in US adults. *JAMA* 1985; 253:1567–70.

26. Rubba P, Mancini M, Fidanza F, Gautiero G, Salo M, Nikkari T, et al. Adipose tissue fatty acids and blood pressure in middle-aged men from southern Italy. *Int J Epidemiol* 1987; 16:528–31.

27. Williams PT, Fortmann SP, Terry RB, Garay SC, Vranizan KM, Ellsworth N, et al. Associations of dietary fat, regional adiposity, and blood pressure in men. *JAMA* 1987;257:3251–6.

28. Elliott P, Fehily AM, Sweetnam PM, Yarnell JW. Diet, alcohol, body mass, and social factors in relation to blood pressure: the Caerphilly heart study. *J Epidemiol Community Health* 1987; 41:37–43.

29. Joffres MR, Reed DM, Yano K. Relationship of magnesium intake and other dietary factors to blood pressure: the Honolulu Heart Study. *Am J Clin Nutr* 1987;45:469–75.

30. Witteman JC, Willett WC, Stampfer MJ, Colditz GA, Sacks FM, et al. A prospective study of nutritional factors and hypertension among us women. *Circulation* 1989;80:1320–7.

31. Stamler J, Caggiula A, Grandits GA, Kjelsberg M, Cutler JA. Relationship to blood pressure of combinations of dietary macronutrients. Findings of the Multiple Risk Factor Intervention Trial (MRFIT). *Circulation* 1996;94:2417–23.

32. Iacono JM, Puska P, Dougherty RM, Pietinen P, Vartiainen E, Leino U, et al. Effect of dietary fat on blood pressure in a rural finnish population. *Am J Clin Nutr* 1983;38:860–9.

33. Puska P, Iacono JM, Nissinen A, Korhonen HJ, Vartianinen E, Pietinen P, et al. Controlled, randomised trial of the effect of dietary fat on blood pressure. *Lancet* 1983;1:1–5.

34. Puska P, Iacono JM, Nissinen A, Vartiainen E, Dougherty R, Pietinen P, et al. Dietary fat and blood pressure: an intervention study on the effects of a low-fat diet with two levels of polyunsaturated fat. *Prev Med* 1985; 14:573–84.

35. Sacks FM, Rouse IL, Stampfer MJ, Bishop LM, Lenherr CF, Walther RJ. Effect of dietary fats and carbohydrate on blood pressure of mildly hypertensive patients. *Hypertension* 1987;10:452–60.

36. Mutanen M, Kleemola P, Valsta LM, Mensink RP, Rasanen L. Lack of effect on blood pressure by polyunsaturated and monounsaturated fat diets. *Eur J Clin Nutr* 1992;46:1–6.

37. Aro A, Pietinen P, Valsta LM, Salminen I, Turpeinen AM, Virtanen M, et al. Lack of effect on blood pressure by low fat diets with different fatty acid compositions. *J Hum Hypertens* 1998; 12:383–9.

38. Morris MC, Sacks FM. Dietary fats and blood pressure. In: Swales J, ed. *Textbook of Hypertension*. Oxford: Blackwell, 1994:605–18.

39. Appel LJ, Moore TJ, Obarzanek E, Vollmer WM, Svetkey LP, Sacks FM, et al. A clinical trial of the effects of dietary patterns on blood pressure. DASH Collaborative Research Group. *N Engl J Med* 1997;336:1117–24.

40. Rosenthal J, Simone PG, Silbergleit A. Effects of prostaglandin deficiency on natriuresis, diuresis, and blood pressure. *Prostaglandins* 1974;5:435–40.

41. Cox JW, Rutecki GW, Francisco LL, Ferris TF. Studies of the effects of essential fatty acid deficiency in the rat. *Circ Res* 1982;51:694–702.

42. Tobian L, Ganguli M, Johnson MA, Iwai J. Influence of renal prostaglandins and dietary linoleate on hypertension in Dahl S rats. *Hypertension* 1982;4:149–53.

43. Stokes JB. Effect of prostaglandin e2 on chloride transport across the rabbit thick ascending limb of Henle. Selective inhibitions of the medullary portion. *J Clin Invest* 1979;64:495–502.

44. Stokes JB, Kokko JP. Inhibition of sodium transport by prostaglandin e2 across the isolated, perfused rabbit collecting tubule. *J Clin Invest* 1977; 59:1099–104.

45. Obarzanek E, Velletri PA, Cutler JA. Dietary protein and blood pressure. *JAMA* 1996;275:1598–603.

46. He J, Whelton PK. Effect of dietary fiber and protein intake on blood pressure: a review of epidemiologic evidence. *Clin Exp Hypertens* 1999;21:785–96.

47. Burke V, Hodgson JM, Beilin LJ, Giangiulioi N, Rogers P, Puddey IB. Dietary protein and soluble fiber reduce ambulatory blood pressure in treated hypertensives. *Hypertension* 2001; 38:821–6.

48. Elliott P. Protein intake and blood pressure in cardiovascular disease. *Proc Nutr Soc* 2003;62:495–504.

49. Liu L, Ikeda K, Sullivan DH, Ling W, Yamori Y. Epidemiological evidence of the association between dietary protein intake and blood pressure: a meta-analysis of published data. *Hypertens Res* 2002;25:689–95.

50. Stamler J, Elliott P, Kesteloot H, Nichols R, Claeys G, Dyer AR, et al. Inverse relation of dietary protein markers with blood pressure. Findings for 10,020 men and women in the intersalt study. INTERSALT Cooperative Research Group. International Study of Salt and Blood Pressure. *Circulation* 1996;94:1629–34.

51. Stamler J, Liu K, Ruth K. J, Pryer J, Greenland P. Eight-year blood pressure change in middle-aged men: relationship to multiple nutrients. *Hypertension* 2002;39:1000–6.

52. Sacks FM, Kass EH. Low blood pressure in vegetarians: effects of specific foods and nutrients. *Am J Clin Nutr* 1988; 48:795–800.

53. Sacks FM, Marais GE, Handysides G, Salazar J, Miller L, Foster JM, et al. Lack of an effect of dietary saturated fat and cholesterol on blood pressure in normotensives. *Hypertension* 1984; 6:193–8.

54. Sacks FM, Wood PG, Kass EH. Stability of blood pressure in vegetarians receiving dietary protein supplements. *Hypertension* 1984;6:199–201.

55. Teede HJ, Dalais FS, Kotsopoulos D, Liang YL, Davis S, McGrath BP. Dietary soy has both beneficial and potentially adverse cardiovascular effects: a placebo-controlled study in men and postmenopausal women. *J Clin Endocrinol Metab* 2001;86:3053–60.

56. He J, Wu XG, Gu DF, Duan XF, Whelton PK. Soybean protein supplementation and blood pressure: a randomized, controlled clinical trial. *Circulation* 1998; 101:711 (abstract).

57. He J, Gu D, Wu X, Chen J, Duan X, Chen J, et al. Effect of soybean protein on blood pressure: a randomized, controlled trial. *Ann Intern Med* 2005; 143:1–9.

58. Sved AF, Fernstrom JD, Wurtman RJ. Tyrosine administration reduces blood pressure and enhances brain norepinephrine release in spontaneously hypertensive rats. *Proc Natl Acad Sci U S A* 1979;76:3511–4.

59. Sved AF, Van Itallie CM, Fernstrom JD. Studies on the antihypertensive action of l-tryptophan. *J Pharmacol Exp Ther* 1982;221:329–33.

60. Acworth IN, During MJ, Wurtman RJ. Tyrosine: effects on catecholamine release. *Brain Res Bull* 1988;21:473–7.

61. He J, Streiffer RH, Muntner P, Krousel-Wood MA, Whelton PK. Effect of dietary fiber intake on blood pressure: a randomized, double-blind, placebo-controlled trial. *J Hypertens* 2004; 22:73–80.

62. Whelton SP, Hyre AD, Pedersen B, Yi Y, Whelton PK, He J. Effect of dietary fiber intake on blood pressure: a meta-analysis of randomized, controlled clinical trials. *J Hypertens* 2005; 23:475–81.

63. Anderson JW, Zeigler JA, Deakins DA, Floore TL, Dillon DW, Wood CL, et al. Metabolic effects of high-carbohydrate, high-fiber diets for insulin-dependent diabetic individuals. *Am J Clin Nutr* 1991;54:936–43.

64. Fukagawa NK, Anderson JW, Hageman G, Young VR, Minaker KL. High-carbohydrate, high-fiber diets increase peripheral insulin sensitivity in healthy young and old adults. *Am J Clin Nutr* 1990;52:524–8.

65. Ferrannini E, Buzzigoli G, Bonadonna R, Giorico MA, Oleggini M, Graziadei L, et al. Insulin resistance in essential hypertension. *N Engl J Med* 1987; 317:350–7.

66. Rossner S, von Zweigbergk D, Ohlin A, Ryttig K. Weight reduction with dietary fibre supplements. Results of two double-blind randomized studies. *Acta Med Scand* 1987;222:83–8.

67. Ryttig KR, Tellnes G, Haegh L, Boe E, Fagerthun H. A dietary fibre supplement and weight maintenance after weight reduction: a randomized, double-blind, placebo-controlled long-term trial. *Int J Obes* 1989;13:165–71.

68. Geleijnse JM, Giltay EJ, Grobbee DE, Donders AR, Kok FJ. Blood pressure response to fish oil supplementation: metaregression analysis of randomized trials. *J Hypertens* 2002;20:1493–9.

69. Appel LJ, Miller ER 3rd, Seidler AJ, Whelton PK. Does supplementation of diet with 'fish oil' reduce blood pressure? A meta-analysis of controlled clinical trials. *Arch Intern Med* 1993; 153:1429–38.

70. Morris MC, Sacks F, Rosner B. Does fish oil lower blood pressure? A meta-analysis of controlled trials. *Circulation* 1993; 88:523–33.

71. Alonso A, de la Fuente C, Martin-Arnau AM, de Irala J, Martinez JA, Martinez-Gonzalez MA. Fruit and vegetable consumption is inversely associated with blood pressure in a Mediterranean population with a high vegetable-fat intake: The Seguimiento Universidad de Navarra (SUN) study. *Br J Nutr* 2004; 92:311–9.

72. Miura K, Greenland P, Stamler J, Liu K, Daviglus ML, Nakagawa H. Relation of vegetable, fruit, and meat intake to 7-year blood pressure change in middle-aged men: the Chicago Western Electric study. *Am J Epidemiol* 2004; 159:572–80.

73. Moore LL, Singer MR, Bradlee ML, Djousse L, Proctor MH, Cupples LA, et al. Intake of fruits, vegetables, and dairy products in early childhood and subsequent blood pressure change. *Epidemiology* 2005;16:4–11.

74. Beitz R, Mensink GB, Fischer B. Blood pressure and vitamin c and fruit and vegetable intake. *Ann Nutr Metab* 2003;47:214–20.

75. Greenland S. Re: "Comments on a meta-analysis of the relation between dietary calcium intake and blood pressure." *Am J Epidemiol* 1999; 149:786–7.

76. Birkett NJ. Comments on a meta-analysis of the relation between dietary calcium intake and blood pressure. *Am J Epidemiol* 1998;148:223–8; discussion 232–3.

77. Bucher HC, Cook RJ, Guyatt GH, Lang JD, Cook DJ, Hatala R, et al. Effects of dietary calcium supplementation on blood pressure. A meta-analysis of randomized controlled trials. *JAMA* 1996;275:1016–22.

78. Allender PS, Cutler JA, Follmann D, Cappuccio FP, Pryer J, Elliott P. Dietary calcium and blood pressure: a meta-analysis of randomized clinical trials. *Ann Intern Med* 1996;124:825–31.

79. Hayashi T, Tsumura K, Suematsu C, Okada K, Fujii S, Endo G. Walking to work and the risk for hypertension in men: the Osaka Health Survey. *Ann Intern Med* 1999;131:21–6.

80. Pereira MA, Folsom AR, McGovern PG, Carpenter M, Arnett DK, Liao D, et al. Physical activity and incident hypertension in black and white adults: the Atherosclerosis Risk in Communities Study. *Prev Med* 1999;28:304–12.

81. Kelley GA. Aerobic exercise and resting blood pressure among women: a meta-analysis. *Prev Med* 1999;28:264–75.

82. Whelton SP, Chin A, Xin X, He J. Effect of aerobic exercise on blood pressure: a meta-analysis of randomized, controlled trials. *Ann Intern Med* 2002; 136:493–503.

83. Brown MD, Moore GE, Korytkowski MT, McCole SD, Hagberg JM. Improvement of insulin sensitivity by short-term exercise training in hypertensive African American women. *Hypertension* 1997; 30:1549–53.

84. Stevens VJ, Obarzanek E, Cook NR, Lee IM, Appel LJ, Smith West D, et al. Long-term weight loss and changes in blood pressure: results of the trials of hypertension prevention, Phase II. *Ann Intern Med* 2001;134:1–11.

85. Yoshita K, Miura K, Morikawa Y, Ishizaki M, Kido T, Naruse Y, et al. Relationship of alcohol consumption to 7-year blood pressure change in Japanese men. *J Hypertens* 2005; 23:1485–90.

86. Russell M, Cooper ML, Frone MR, Peirce RS. A longitudinal study of stress, alcohol, and blood pressure in community-based samples of blacks and non-blacks. *Alcohol Res Health* 1999;23:299–306.

87. Okubo Y, Miyamoto T, Suwazono Y, Kobayashi E, Nogawa K. Alcohol consumption and blood pressure in Japanese men. *Alcohol* 2001;23:149–56.

88. Kawano Y, Abe H, Takishita S, Omae T. Effects of alcohol restriction on 24-hour ambulatory blood pressure in Japanese men with hypertension. *Am J Med* 1998;105:307–11.

89. Rakic V, Puddey IB, Burke V, Dimmitt SB, Beilin LJ. Influence of pattern of alcohol intake on blood pressure in regular drinkers: a controlled trial. *J Hypertens* 1998;16:165–74.

90. Cushman WC, Cutler JA, Hanna E, Bingham SF, Follmann D, Harford T, et al. Prevention and Treatment of Hypertension Study (PATHS): effects of an alcohol treatment program on blood pressure. *Arch Intern Med* 1998; 158:1197–207.

91. Xin X, He J, Frontini MG, Ogden LG, Motsamai OI, Whelton PK. Effects of alcohol reduction on blood pressure: a meta-analysis of randomized controlled trials. *Hypertension* 2001; 38:1112–7.

92. He J, Whelton PK, Appel LJ, Charleston J, Klag MJ. Long-term effects of weight loss and dietary sodium reduction on incidence of hypertension. *Hypertension* 2000;35:544–9.

93. Neter JE, Stam BE, Kok FJ, Grobbee DE, Geleijnse JM. Influence of weight reduction on blood pressure: a meta-analysis of randomized controlled trials. *Hypertension* 2003;42:878–84.

94. Markovitz JH, Matthews KA, Kannel WB, Cobb JL, D'Agostino RB. Psychological predictors of hypertension in the framingham study. Is there tension in hypertension? *JAMA* 1993;270: 2439–43.

95. Eisenberg DM, Delbanco TL, Berkey CS, Kaptchuk TJ, Kupelnick B, Kuhl J, et al. Cognitive behavioral techniques for hypertension: are they effective? *Ann Intern Med* 1993;118:964–72.

96. Nakao M, Yano E, Nomura S, Kuboki T. Blood pressure-lowering effects of biofeedback treatment in hypertension: a meta-analysis of randomized controlled trials. *Hypertens Res* 2003;26:37–46.

97. Canter PH, Ernst E. Insufficient evidence to conclude whether or not transcendental meditation decreases blood pressure: results of a systematic review of randomized clinical trials. *J Hypertens* 2004;22:2049–54.

98. Schneider RH, Staggers F, Alxander CN, Sheppard W, Rainforth M, Kondwani K, et al. A randomised controlled trial of stress reduction for hypertension in older African Americans. *Hypertension* 1995;26:820–7.

99. Whelton PK, He J, Appel LJ, Cutler JA, Havas S, Kotchen TA, et al. Primary prevention of hypertension: clinical and public health advisory from the National High Blood Pressure Education Program. *JAMA* 2002;288:1882–8.

Chapter

7

Dietary Fats and Blood Pressure

Trevor A. Mori, Valerie Burke, and Lawrence J. Beilin

Key Findings

- Population studies provide support for a protective effect of omega-3 (ω3) fatty acids against atherosclerotic heart disease and sudden death. Evidence suggests that ω3 fatty acids also provide protection against stroke, particularly ischemic stroke.

- Omega-3 fatty acids have multiple effects leading to improvements in blood pressure, cardiac function, arterial compliance, vascular function, and lipid metabolism, as well as reduced cytokine formation, and antiplatelet and anti-inflammatory effects.

- In humans, the two principal ω3 fatty acids, eicosapentaenoic acid (EPA) and docosahexaenoic acid (DHA), have differential effects on blood pressure, vascular reactivity, heart rate, and serum lipids.

- In population studies, lower blood pressure is associated with higher polyunsaturated fat intake and higher blood pressure with higher saturated fat intake, but population studies cannot define effects of specific nutrients and may be confounded by lifestyle factors.

- There have been no consistent effects of omega-6, monounsaturated, or saturated fats on blood pressure, but some studies suggest that monounsaturated fat may lower blood pressure, particularly in hypertension and diabetes.

- Complex dietary changes such as those eaten by many vegetarians are associated with lower blood pressures and less obesity and reduce blood pressure in randomized controlled trials. Such diets are characterized by increased fruit and vegetables and nuts, relatively high levels of low-fat dairy products, and hence poly- and monounsaturates and lower levels of saturated fats than in a typical Western diet.

- The Dietary Approaches to Stop Hypertension trials showed that the blood pressure–lowering effect of increased fruit and vegetables could be retained in the presence of lean meat, poultry, and fish, and enhanced by reduction in saturated fats and increased polyunsaturates or monounsaturates from low-fat dairy products.

- These complex dietary patterns probably lower blood pressure through effects of multiple nutrients and micronutrients, including effects of dietary fiber, potassium, magnesium, antioxidants, and effects of fats on endothelial and vascular function.

This chapter reviews evidence for effects of different types and quantities of dietary fats on blood pressure. As more recent evidence is available concerning specific effects of omega-3 (ω3) polyunsaturates, they are considered in more detail in relation to their overall effects on cardiovascular disease. The focus is primarily on human studies, although animal data are considered where they are concordant with clinical data and throw additional light on mechanisms.

OMEGA-3 POLYUNSATURATED FATTY ACIDS

There is considerable evidence from clinical, experimental, and epidemiologic studies that the ω3 fatty acids, derived from fish and fish oils, are protective against atherosclerotic heart disease and sudden coronary death.[1–2] Omega-3 fatty acids have multiple biological effects leading to improvements in blood pressure[3–6] and cardiac function,[7] arterial compliance,[8,9] endothelial function and vascular reactivity,[10,11] lipid metabolism,[12,13] reduced neutrophil/ monocyte cytokine formation,[14] and antiplatelet[15] and anti-inflammatory effects.[16] Recent evidence has demonstrated that in humans, eicosapentaenoic acid (EPA) (20:5 ω3) and docosahexaenoic acid (DHA) (22:6 ω3), the two main ω3 fatty acids, have differential effects on lipids,[17–19] blood pressure,[20] heart rate,[20] and vascular reactivity.[10]

Observational studies

Bang and Dyerberg[21] first showed a low incidence of coronary deaths in Greenland Eskimos consuming a high-fat diet rich in ω3 fatty acids derived from seal and whale blubber, compared with Danes who ate a typical Western diet.[21] These observations recognized that EPA[22] and DHA[23] accounted for prolonged bleeding time, decreased platelet adhesiveness, and low plasma triglycerides in these individuals.

Numerous prospective population studies have confirmed a relationship between increased fish consumption and lower rates of coronary mortality and/or sudden death. The Zutphen study showed that men eating as little as one fish meal a week had more than a 50% lower coronary death rate than those who never or rarely ate fish.[24] A follow-up study by the same authors demonstrated that a small consumption of fish protected against coronary heart disease mortality in an elderly population.[25] Similarly, the Cardiovascular Health Study reported an inverse association between fish consumption and fatal ischemic heart disease in an elderly population (>65 years).[26,27] Interestingly, the association held for tuna, broiled or baked fish, but not fried fish or fish sandwiches.[27] In the same cohort, consumption of fish such as tuna, broiled or baked fish, but not fried fish, was also associated with a reduced incidence of congestive heart failure.[28] An inverse association between fish consumption and coronary heart disease mortality was also shown in a study from Sweden[29] and in two studies from Finland in patients with established coronary artery disease.[30,31]

Data from the Multiple Risk Factor Intervention Trial (MRFIT) showed that when men comprising the control group were divided into quintiles according to their mean ω3 fatty acid intake, there were significant inverse correlations between ingestion of fish oils and coronary heart disease, all cardiovascular diseases, and all-cause mortality, with the highest quintile having a 40% to 50% lower mortality rate.[32] The Chicago Western Electric study in middle-aged men showed that those who ate >35 g of fish daily had a 38% reduced risk of death from coronary heart disease at the 30-year follow-up, with a dose-dependent effect of increasing fish consumption.[33] In addition, the U.S. Physicians' Health Study reported that consumption of more than one fish meal per week conferred a 52% risk-adjusted reduction in sudden cardiac death compared with men that consumed fish less than monthly.[34] The study, however, did not show a significant association between fish consumption and overall cardiovascular endpoints.[35] In a follow-up of the same cohort, prospective, nested, case–control analysis among men followed for up to 17 years, showed that baseline blood levels of ω3 fatty acids were inversely related to the risk of sudden death.[36] Men in the third and fourth quartile had an adjusted relative risk of 0.28 and 0.19, respectively, relative to those in the lowest quartile.

Hu et al.[37] have shown in the Nurses' Health Study that higher consumption of fish and ω3 fatty acids was also associated with a lower risk of coronary heart disease in women. Women consuming two to four fish meals per week had an adjusted relative risk of 0.69 compared with those who ate less than one fish meal per month. In a subanalysis of diabetic women from the same cohort, two to four fish meals per week was associated with an adjusted relative risk of 0.64 for coronary heart disease and 0.67 for total mortality compared with those who ate less than one fish meal per month.[38]

In a case–control study of patients with primary cardiac arrest, Siscovick et al.[39] reported that eating the equivalent of one fatty fish meal per week in the month prior to the event was equivalent to a 50% reduction in risk of a primary event. Burchfiel et al.[40] showed in the Honolulu Heart Program that consumption of fish at least twice a week was associated with a 65% risk reduction in Japanese-American men who were heavy smokers.

Recent findings have shown that fish consumption was also associated with a reduction in the incidence of atrial fibrillation in an elderly population[41] and in patients undergoing coronary bypass surgery.[42]

Not all studies have shown associations between fish consumption and cardiovascular events,[43] possibly due to the uncertainty of estimation of usual dietary fish consumption, failure to distinguish fatty- from low-fat fish, and the complex correlation between diet and other lifestyle factors. In a systematic review, Marckmann et

al.[44] suggested that the discrepancy between studies may also relate to differences in the study populations, with only high-risk individuals benefiting from increasing their fish consumption. The authors proposed that a 40- to 60-g/day fish intake would confer a 50% reduction in death from coronary heart disease in high-risk populations. These findings have been supported in similar meta-analyses.[45–47]

The strongest evidence for a protective effect of ω3 fatty acids is from two randomized controlled trials in patients who had previous heart attacks. In the Diet and Reinfarction Trial, men who had recovered from a myocardial infarction were randomized to either a "usual care" group or they were advised to increase their ω3 fatty acid intake by eating two to three servings of fatty fish weekly.[48] Those men who increased dietary fish consumption and/or took fish oil supplements had a 29% reduction over 2 years in sudden cardiac death. The GISSI Prevenzione study[49] involved patients who had survived a myocardial infarction within the previous 3 months. These patients were randomized in a factorial, open-label, controlled design to either fish oil (1 g daily), vitamin E (300 mg daily), both interventions, or no treatment. After 3.5 years, fish oil supplementation was associated with a 30% reduction in cardiac mortality, a 20% reduction in total mortality and a 45% decrease in sudden death, whereas vitamin E had no significant effect. The combination of fish oil with vitamin E did not increase the benefit compared with fish oil alone. In a subsequent report, the authors demonstrated that a significant reduction in sudden death was apparent 4 months after commencing the program.[50]

There is less evidence for benefits of fish on blood pressure from population studies, although this may be in part due to methodologic issues. However, a cross-sectional comparison of Bantu fisherfolk with non–fish-eating Bantu farmers showed that the former had a much lower increase in blood pressure with ageing.[51] Paradoxically, the high incidence of hypertension in Japan occurs despite high fish intake, although this may be due to very high salt consumption.

An inverse association between increasing intakes of ω3 fatty acids and risk of stroke has been shown in the Nurses' Health Study,[52] in men participating in the Health Professional Follow-up Study,[53] and in the Cardiovascular Health Study.[54] In all reports, the effect was observed for ischemic but not hemorrhagic stroke.

Clinical trials

Randomized controlled trials of fish oils or dietary fish consumption provide unequivocal evidence for a blood pressure–lowering effect of ω3 fatty acids. Meta-analyses have shown such an effect in hypertensives.[3–5] In a meta-analysis of 31 placebo-controlled trials of effects of fish oils on blood pressure, Morris et al.[4] found an overall reduction of –3.0/–1.5 mmHg with a significant dose–response effect estimated at –0.66/–0.35 mmHg/g ω3 fatty acid. The hypotensive effect was strongest in hypertensive (treated and untreated) subjects (–3.4/–2.0 mmHg). Appel et al.[3] estimated that blood pressure fell 1.0/0.5 mmHg in normotensives (11 trials) and 5.5/3.5 mmHg in untreated hypertensives (6 trials) with an average intake of more than 3 g/day of ω3 fatty acids. More recently, Geleijnse et al.,[5] in a meta-analysis of 36 trials, showed that ω3 fatty acids reduced blood pressure by –2.1/–1.6 mmHg. Blood pressure–lowering effects tended to be greater in older (>45 years) (–3.5/–2.4) and hypertensive (>140/90 mmHg) (–4.0/–2.5) individuals.

The study by Bonaa et al.[55] is most conclusive in terms of clinical trials. This population-based study involved untreated mildly hypertensive subjects randomized to 6 g/day of 85% EPA and DHA or 6 g/day corn oil for 10 weeks. Relative to the corn oil group, the group treated with fish oil had a –6.4/–2.8 mmHg decrease in blood pressure. In addition, blood pressure reductions were inversely related to baseline plasma phospholipid ω3 fatty acids. Other placebo-controlled studies have demonstrated significant benefits of dietary ω3 fatty acids on blood pressure in hypertensives.[56–60] Prisco et al.[61] showed that 24-hour ambulatory blood pressure was reduced by 5 to 6 mmHg after taking 3.44 g/day of ω3 fatty acids for 2 months, in mild essential hypertensive, normolipidemic men. Toft et al.[62] also confirmed that in essential hypertensives blood pressures fell by 3.8/2.0 mmHg more than controls after 16 weeks of 4 g/day of fish oil containing 85% EPA plus DHA.

The blood pressure–lowering effects of ω3 fatty acids are potentiated by sodium restriction[63] and concomitant usage of antihypertensive drugs. In this regard, fish oils amplified the hypotensive action of the β-adrenergic receptor blocker propranolol in mild-to-moderate hypertensives,[64] but there was no additional benefit in hypertensives on ACE inhibition.[65] However, fish oils may be a useful adjunct to antihypertensive therapy with β-blockers or diuretics.[66] Others have shown that ω3 fatty acids reduced blood pressure by 3.1/1.8 mmHg in treated hypertensives who were taking β-blockers alone, diuretics alone, or a combination of the two.[66]

Vandongen et al.[67] compared the effects of 12 weeks of fish meals or fish oil supplements providing 2.2 to 6.3 g/day (mean intake 3.65 g/day) of ω3 fatty acids in the setting of a high- or low-fat diet in 120 men with high-normal blood pressure. Although individual subgroups showed no significant falls in blood pressure, in all the groups combined there was a significant inverse correlation between the falls in systolic and diastolic blood pressure and heart rate, and increases in ω3 and decreases in ω6 fatty acids in platelet phospholipids.

Studies from our Unit examined whether dietary ω3 fatty acids in the form of dietary fish had independent and additive effects to weight control on blood pressure.[68] In a factorial design study, 63 overweight, treated hypertensives were randomized to weight loss alone by calorie restriction, a daily fish meal (approximately 3.65 g/day ω3 fatty acids), the two combined, or a control diet, for 4 months. The final 4 weeks involved weight stabilization for the weight control groups whose weight fell an average 5.6 kg. Twenty-four–hour ambulatory blood pressures showed significant independent and additive effects of dietary fish and weight loss. Relative to controls, daytime

blood pressures fell by 6.0/3.0 mmHg in the fish group, 5.5/2.2 in the weight loss group, and 13.0/9.3 with the combination (Figure 7–1). Fish consumption was also associated with significant reductions in heart rate by three to four beats per minute, suggesting an autonomic/cardiac component to the blood pressure reduction.

The antihypertensive effect of eicosapentaenoic acid versus docosahexaenoic acid

There is evidence that DHA and EPA have differential effects on lipid metabolism[17–19,69] and platelet aggregation.[70] Blood pressure control is also differentially affected by EPA and DHA. In humans, Mori et al.[20] showed that DHA, but not EPA, significantly reduced 24-hour (–5.8/–3.3 mmHg) and daytime (awake) (–3.5/–2.0 mmHg) blood pressure, relative to the placebo in overweight, mildly hypercholesterolemic subjects (Figure 7–2). Patients were given 4 g daily of highly purified EPA, DHA, or olive oil (placebo) capsules, while continuing their usual diets for 6 weeks. These effects were

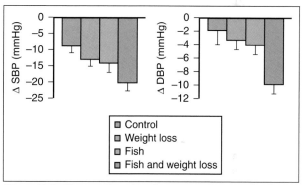

Figure 7–1. Changes from baseline to post-intervention in 24-hour ambulatory SBPs and DBPs during awake hours in the control, weight loss, fish, and combined weight loss and fish groups. Data are shown as mean plus standard error of the mean. DBP, diastolic blood pressure; SBP, systolic blood pressure.

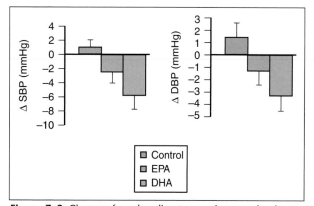

Figure 7–2. Changes from baseline to post-intervention in 24-hour ambulatory systolic and diastolic blood pressures in the control (olive oil), EPA, and DHA groups. Data are shown as mean plus standard error of the mean. DHA, docosahexaenoic acid; EPA, eicosapentaenoic acid.

accompanied by significant improvements in endothelial and smooth muscle function in the forearm microcirculation with DHA but not EPA, as well as reduced vasoconstrictor responses.[10] The study also showed that DHA, but not EPA, significantly reduced 24-hour, awake and asleep heart rate by 3.5, 3.7, and 2.8 bpm, respectively.[20] In contrast, Woodman et al.[18] showed that neither EPA nor DHA given as 4-g doses daily for 6 weeks, decreased blood pressure in treated hypertensive, type 2 diabetic patients. Possible explanations for the lack of an anti-hypertensive effect may have been related to concomitant use of other pharmacologic agents, presence of glycemia, and increased blood pressure variability in these diabetic patients.

Mechanisms for antihypertensive effects of omega-3 fatty acids
Vascular function and the role of nitric oxide

Benefits on blood pressure following dietary ω3 fatty acids are likely to be due to changes in vascular, cardiac, and/or autonomic function. Fish oil supplementation in hypertensive rats increased endothelial relaxation in aortic rings exposed to acetylcholine[71] and decreased pressor reactivity of perfused mesenteric resistance vessels.[72] Yin et al.[71] showed that increased endothelial relaxant effects were due at least in part to suppression of thromboxane A_2 (TXA_2) or cyclic endoperoxides, with the additional effect of enhanced endothelial nitric oxide (NO) synthesis. Studies in humans have shown that fish oils reduced forearm vascular reactivity to angiotensin II and noradrenaline.[73–75] The blunting effect of fish oils on noradrenaline and angiotensin II responses in human forearm resistance arteries were antagonized by oral administration of indomethacin, suggesting that ω3 fatty acids, at least in part, modify cyclooxygenase-derived prostanoids.[76] Indomethacin *per se*, at the dose given, did not affect responses to the two agonists.

Fish oils had a minimal effect on acetylcholine-induced vasodilation or reactive hyperemia in forearms of healthy subjects.[76] However, ω3 fatty acids restored impaired responses to endothelium-dependent vasodilators in patients with coronary artery disease,[77,78] as well as in animal models, including the SHR,[71] the glucocorticoid-induced hypertensive rat,[79] and the hypercholesterolemic and atherosclerotic pig,[80] all characterized by endothelial damage. Vasodilatory responses to acetylcholine in hypercholesterolemic subjects were also enhanced by dietary fish oil in the absence of changes in total cholesterol.[81]

Individuals with type 2 diabetes who received ω3 fatty acids supplements have improved forearm vasodilator responses to acetylcholine, but not to glyceryl trinitrate, suggesting that fish oils may protect against vasospasm and thrombosis by enhancing NO release and suppressing thromboxane.[82] Additional evidence that ω3 fatty acids affect production or release of NO, was from studies demonstrating enhanced responses to endothelium-dependent vasodilators such as bradykinin, serotonin, ADP, and thrombin, in rings of coronary arteries taken from pigs fed cod-liver oil.[83] In addition, EPA potentiated

in vitro NO release evoked by IL-1β in vascular smooth muscle cells[84] and in endothelial cells in response to ADP and bradykinin.[85]

Omega-3 fatty acids may also improve endothelial function in systemic large arteries in humans. Goodfellow et al.[86] showed a significant improvement in flow-mediated dilatation of the brachial artery following 4 months with 4 g daily of ω3 fatty acids, in subjects with hyperlipidemia. The improvement was confined to endothelial-dependent responses.

Studies in rats have shown differential effects of EPA and DHA on vascular function.[87,88] Engler et al.[88] reported that in aortic rings EPA and DHA induced endothelium-dependent and independent vasodilation, respectively. McLennan et al.[87] demonstrated that DHA was also more effective than EPA at inhibiting thromboxane-like vasoconstrictor responses in the aortas from spontaneously hypertensive rats (SHR). They suggested that DHA prevented thromboxane-induced contraction and perhaps restored the vasoconstrictor/vasodilator balance following impairment of the normal NO-related processes. Whether DHA inhibits thromboxane synthetase or thromboxane A_2/prostaglandin H_2 receptor function remains uncertain.

Indirect evidence for a beneficial effect of DHA but not EPA on endothelial function in humans was obtained by measuring serum and urinary nitrate output.[89] However, these results are only suggestive of increased NO production in endothelial cells, since nitrates are also derived from other sources. Mori et al.[10] reported that DHA, but not EPA, improved vasodilator responses to endogenous and exogenous NO donors and attenuated vasoconstrictor response to noradrenaline in the forearm microcirculation of overweight subjects with hyperlipidemia. The mechanisms were predominantly endothelium independent, based on enhanced vasodilatory responses following co-infusion of acetylcholine with L-NMMA and infusion of nitroprusside, both of which are endothelium independent. However, the data do not preclude an endothelial component in the dilatory responses associated with DHA. These findings were associated with a reduction in blood pressure in these patients following supplementation with DHA, but not EPA.[20] Yin et al.[71] previously showed an endothelial-independent vasodilatory effect of ω3 fatty acids in perfused mesenteric resistance vessels from SHR.

The favorable effects of DHA on vasoreactivity[10] may be attributable to direct and indirect effects of DHA on the arterial wall. DHA incorporation into endothelial membranes could increase membrane fluidity, calcium influx, and endogenous synthesis and release of NO. Additional mechanisms may include direct effects of DHA on receptor-stimulated NO release, enhanced release of vasodilator prostanoids, and/or endothelial-derived hyperpolarizing factor, consistent with experimental evidence.[79] Enhanced vasodilator response to sodium nitroprusside may be due increased biotransformation to NO or increased reactivity of smooth muscle cells to vasorelaxation as a result of decreased calcium influx.[90] Increased release of cyclooxygenase-derived vasodilatory metabolites may have accounted for the decreased vasoconstrictor response to noradrenaline following DHA.[10] Vasodilator effects of DHA could also be related to increased basal production of NO in smooth muscle cells as a consequence of decreased release of platelet-derived growth factor (PDGF),[91] since induction of NOS in vascular smooth muscle cells is inhibited by PDGF.[92]

Vascular compliance

Blood pressure is strongly influenced by arterial compliance, which in turn is influenced by endothelial function. In this regard, McVeigh et al.[8] showed that compliance in the large arteries and more peripheral vasculature, as measured by pulse-contour analysis, improved significantly after 6 weeks of fish oil compared with olive oil, in type 2 diabetic individuals. There were no changes in mean arterial blood pressure, cardiac output, stroke volume, or systemic vascular resistance. In patients with dyslipidemia, EPA and DHA supplementation improved arterial compliance by 35% and 27%, respectively.[9] There was no significant difference in the effect between EPA and DHA.

Vasodilator and vasoconstrictor prostanoids

The antihypertensive effect of ω3 fatty acids may also relate to modulation of vasodilator and vasoconstrictor prostanoids. Omega-3 fatty acids suppress production of thromboxane B_2 (TXB_2), a metabolite of the vasoconstrictor and potent aggregator TXA_2.[93] Diets rich in ω3 fatty acids decreased TXA_2 with concomitant increased TXA_3, the analogous but significantly less biologically active EPA-derived metabolite, in patients with atherosclerosis.[94] An increase in prostaglandin I_3 (prostacyclin, PGI_3), derived from EPA and equipotent in the vasodilatory and antiaggregatory activities to the arachidonic acid-derived prostaglandin I_2 (PGI_2), without a fall in PGI_2, was reported following ω3 fatty acids.[94,95] It was suggested that a significant increase in total prostacyclin (PGI_2 and PGI_3) formation, together with reduced total thromboxane (TXA_2 and TXA_3), may explain altered endothelial and vascular responses following dietary ω3 fatty acids.

Plasma noradrenaline and adenosine triphosphate levels

Hashimoto et al.[96] showed that rats fed DHA intragastrically had reduced plasma noradrenaline levels and increased adenyl purines such as adenosine triphosphate (ATP), released both spontaneously and in response to noradrenaline from segments of caudal artery. Furthermore, plasma adenyl purines were significantly inversely associated with blood pressure. This finding is noteworthy, in view of the fact that ATP causes vasodilation by stimulating the release of NO from endothelial cells, by a direct action on vascular smooth muscle cells and by hyperpolarizing smooth muscle cells. The authors suggested that DHA-accelerated ATP release from vascular endothelial cells, in conjunction with reduced plasma noradrenaline, may have been responsible for the fall in blood pressure associated with ω3 fatty acids.[96]

Membrane function/membrane fluidity

Incorporation of ω3 fatty acids into plasma and cellular membranes likely alters the physicochemical structure of the membrane leading to changes in fluidity, flexibility, permeability, and function of the membrane and membrane-bound proteins. It is plausible this may affect enzyme activity, receptor affinity, and transport capacity of the cell, including synthesis and/or release of NO. Hashimoto et al.[97] showed that DHA had a greater effect than EPA in increasing membrane fluidity of endothelial cells cultured from rat thoracic aortas, a finding that may have significance in view of the greater effect of DHA compared to EPA on maintaining vascular function and reducing blood pressure in humans.[10,20]

Cardiac function

A reduction in heart rate in animals[98,99] and humans[18,20,67,68,100,101] following dietary ω3 fatty acids suggests a significant cardiac component associated with the antihypertensive effects. This is possibly mediated by effects on autonomic nerve function or β-adrenoreceptor activity. In a recent meta-analysis of 30 studies, ω3 fatty acids were shown to reduce heart rate overall by –1.6 bpm, with greater reductions in trials with baseline heart rate >69 bpm (–2.5 bpm) and in trials of >12 weeks duration (–2.5 bpm).[102]

Data from human studies also strongly suggest that ω3 fatty acids increase heart rate variability in patients at high risk of sudden cardiac death and in healthy individuals,[103,104] supporting an antiarrhythmic effect of ω3 fatty acids.

In humans, Mori et al.[20] reported that heart rate was reduced by DHA, but not EPA. The authors showed that in overweight, mildly hyperlipidemic, but otherwise healthy men given 4 g daily of EPA, DHA, or olive oil for 6 weeks, 24-hour, awake, and asleep heart rate fell –3.5, –3.7, and –2.8 bpm, respectively, following DHA. Interestingly, EPA resulted in a small, but nonsignificant rise in heart rate. In a follow-up trial of similar design in type 2 diabetic individuals, the same authors confirmed that DHA, but not EPA, significantly reduced clinic standing and supine heart rates (–5.8 and –3.9 bpm, respectively) compared with the placebo.[18] Differential effects of EPA and DHA on heart rate were supported by the findings of Grimsgaard et al.[100]

Omega-3 fatty acids are incorporated into myocardial cells altering electrophysiologic function in a manner that reduces the vulnerability to ventricular fibrillation.[7] The antiarrhythmic effects of ω3 fatty acids are most likely related to their ability to inhibit the fast, voltage-dependent sodium current and the L-type calcium currents.[7] Evidence of potassium channel modulation has also been provided.[7] Moreover, the free fatty acids and not phospholipid-bound fatty acids conferred the inhibitory effect.[7] McLennan et al.[87] also showed that DHA, but not EPA, prevented ischemia-induced cardiac arrhythmias in hooded Wistar rats fed purified oils, confirming differential effects demonstrated in humans.[18,20,100]

SATURATED, MONOUNSATURATED, AND OMEGA-6 POLYUNSATURATED FATTY ACIDS

Possible mechanisms

There are plausible mechanisms that link the type or amount of dietary fats and blood pressure. These include effects on prostaglandin synthesis,[105] endothelial function,[106] vascular reactivity,[107,108] changes in lipid composition of cell membranes, resulting in modification of transport processes,[109] and insulin resistance, which is increased by saturated fatty acids.[110] Antioxidants present in dietary fats, such as polyphenols in olive oil,[111] could also influence blood pressure.

While some studies suggest that saturated, monounsaturated, or ω6 fatty acids affect blood pressure, evidence is inconsistent and, overall, reviewers consider that these dietary fats do not have a modifying role.[112,113] Because interest has moved from a focus on individual nutrients to the benefits of a prudent diet, as used in the Dietary Approaches to Stop Hypertension (DASH) trials,[114] there have been few relevant clinical trials since these reviews.

Observational studies

In cross-sectional studies, lower blood pressure has been associated with polyunsaturated fat or polyunsaturated/saturated (P/S) fat ratio, and higher blood pressure with saturated fats.[115–117] However, other studies have reported contradictory findings[118,119]; more recently, the large National Health and Nutritional Examination Survey III in the United States found that higher intake of monounsaturated and polyunsaturated fats was associated with higher blood pressure.[120] In a study of 1000 Australian schoolchildren at ages 9 and 12, no relation was found between dietary fat type or quantity and blood pressure.[121,122]

Cross-sectional studies that have examined fatty acids in adipose tissue, red cells, or plasma also show no consistent effect of saturated or ω6 PUFA or P/S ratio on blood pressure.[117,123,124]

In large prospective studies, no association between the incidence of hypertension and intake of saturated, polyunsaturated, or monounsaturated fats has been found.[118,119,125]

Population studies cannot recognize effects of specific nutrients, while dietary patterns may be confounded by other lifestyle factors such as obesity and physical activity. Smoking and alcohol consumption, both of which are associated with higher intake of fat and lower consumption of fruits and vegetables,[126,127] can affect interpretation. Inaccuracies in recording food intake also influence results.[128] While measurement of tissue fatty acids avoids errors in dietary data, levels are affected by metabolic processes and by lifestyle, particularly alcohol consumption[129] and smoking.[130]

Clinical studies

Many early studies that investigated associations between dietary fats and blood pressure had design flaws. These included uncontrolled interventions, multiple changes in nutrients, failure to allow for familiarization in measurement of blood pressure, and failure to control for lifestyle factors.[112,131]

Saturated and omega-6 fatty acids

Randomized controlled trials in normotensive individuals have shown no consistent effects on blood pressure with dietary modifications to change the intake of saturated fat, polyunsaturated fat, or the P/S ratio.[132–134] Changes in the P/S ratio achieved by using supplements combined with a standard low-fat diet, rather than changes in foods, also showed no effect on blood pressure.[135] Linoleic acid supplements have produced no change[136] or reduction in blood pressure.[137]

Studies in hypertensives have also shown no consistent effects of saturated fat, ω6 polyunsaturated fat, or P/S ratio on blood pressure. This applies to both the use of modified diets[138] and dietary supplements.[139,140]

Monounsaturated fatty acids

In most studies, no effect of monounsaturated fatty acids on blood pressure in normotensives has been seen, using either dietary change[141,142] or fatty acid supplements.[143] However, in a randomized controlled trial in normotensive young men, systolic and diastolic blood pressure fell relative to controls during 4-week periods of a diet rich in monounsaturated fat.[144] The authors suggested that effects may be mediated by improvements in glucose homeostasis.

In a small study of hypertensive women that compared oleic acid-rich safflower oil and olive oil as sources of monounsaturated fats,[145] systolic and diastolic blood pressures were lower with the olive oil diet. In patients treated with antihypertensive drugs, a diet rich in monounsaturated fat from extra-virgin olive oil was associated with lower blood pressure and a greater reduction in the dose of drugs needed to control hypertension than a similar diet based on sunflower oil.[111] The authors suggested that the improvements were related to antioxidant polyphenols present in the olive oil rather than to differences in fatty acid composition of the two diets.

Although diets high in monounsaturated fats have been reported to improve glycemic control, lipid profile, and blood pressure in type 2 diabetes, their use is controversial.[146] In a controlled trial in type 2 diabetics, replacement of 20% of energy from carbohydrates with 20% of energy from monounsaturated fat, providing a total of 50% energy from fat, was associated with lower blood pressure.[147] This observation does not distinguish between the effects of lower carbohydrates and higher monounsaturated fats. However, blood pressure in diabetics also fell with a diet containing 30% energy from fat, of which 10% was monounsaturated, relative to an isoenergetic diet in which polyunsaturates replaced the monounsaturates.[148]

In studies that report lower blood pressure associated with olive oil as a source of monounsaturated fat, it is not clear whether any effects relate to the type of fat, dietary patterns, or to other components of olive oil, such as antioxidants. Responses may differ in patients with type 2 diabetes mellitus.

Trans fatty acids

Trans fatty acids, formed in the process of hardening polyunsaturated fats in the manufacture of margarines and shortening, contribute 2% to 4% of energy in a typical diet in the United States.[149] These fatty acids have properties intermediate between cis unsaturated and saturated fatty acids and can increase blood cholesterol.[150]

Trans fatty acids have not been shown to affect blood pressure. In normotensive men and women, blood pressure did not differ significantly between diets containing 8% to 10% of energy as oleic acid, trans fatty acids, or saturated fatty acids.[151,152] Substitution of 20% of energy from fat with soybean oil, semiliquid margarine, soft margarine, partially hydrogenated soybean oil, solid margarine, or butter showed no effect on blood pressure in a small crossover trial that may have included treated hypertensives.[153]

The way in which fats are cooked is another relatively unexplored issue, with one study reporting an association between the risk of hypertension and the intake of excess polar compounds in cooking oil and the use of sunflower oil.[154]

In summary, except for ω3 fatty acids, there is no consistent evidence for specific effects of the type or amount of dietary fat on blood pressure in humans, independent of other dietary components and lifestyle factors. Complex dietary changes, which include modification of dietary fats, patterned on lacto-ovo-vegetarian diets[155,156] and those as used in the DASH trials,[114] offer an effective and palatable approach to prevention and treatment of hypertension.

DIETARY FATS AS PART OF COMPLEX DIETARY CHANGES

Whereas there is clear-cut evidence concerning blood pressure–lowering effects of ω3 fatty acids of marine origin, data on effects on blood pressure of saturated, monounsaturated, or shorter chain polyunsaturated fats or on the ratio of polyunsaturated to saturated fats are more difficult to interpret. As outlined above cross-sectional and prospective population data show inconsistent associations between these fats and blood pressure levels or the prevalence of hypertension. In a study of dietary and lifestyle factors on the prevalence of hypertension across five Westernized countries, only fish fatty acids contributed to the attributable risk.[157] On the other hand, the Chicago Western Electric study of 8-year blood pressure changes in middle-aged men showed an independent association between the Keys dietary lipid score and systolic blood pressure, while vegetable protein, vitamin C and beta carotene, were inversely related.[158] With recent attention on the health benefits of a "Mediterranean"-type diet, it is interesting that in a large study from Greece adherence to such a diet was inversely associated with blood pressure, with intake of olive oil, fruit, and vegetables all having statistically significant effects.[159]

However, reports on populations in which differences in dietary fats are part of more complex dietary changes have been more consistent in terms of associations with blood pressure. Since the early twentieth century, there have been reports showing that strict lacto-ovo-vegetarians or vegans had lower blood pressures and less hypertension than meat eaters.[160–163] By comparing Seventh Day Adventist vegetarians with another religious group, meat-eating Mormons, Rouse et al.[164] were able to show that these effects were most likely due to diet rather than other lifestyle factors. As vegetarian populations tended to eat less saturated fats and more polyunsaturates, this led to suggestions that a high P/S ratio diet might predispose to lower blood pressures.[165] However, diets of vegetarians and vegans are characterized by a wide variety of nutrients and whole-food differences compared with regular meat eaters as well as lower BMI and several other lifestyle differences that could influence blood pressure. Although differences in BMI are attributed by some to the blood pressure differences between vegetarians and meat eaters,[166] this is not the entire explanation.[164] Factor analysis of dietary patterns related to blood pressure differences between Seventh Day Adventist vegetarians and Mormon meat eaters in Western Australia suggested that combinations of changes in polyunsaturated, fiber, and vitamin C might be responsible.[167]

Several more recent cross-sectional population studies suggest that combinations of nutrients including fruit, vegetables, and low-fat dairy products contribute to lower blood pressures.[168,169] A recently published but "historical" prospective analysis on 1710 men in the Chicago Western Electric Study from 1958 to 1966 also supported the concept that diets high in fruit and vegetables and lower in meats other than fish reduced the risk of developing hypertension.[170]

Randomized controlled trials of dietary interventions have thrown more light on the issue and can be divided into two broad categories. The first refers to trials that have restricted dietary changes to fats alone, without substantially altering intake of other nutrients or micronutrients. Such trials are difficult to conduct without altering total caloric intake, which can itself affect blood pressure. Studies of this nature have already been described in this review, and have generally been negative with regard to effects of saturated and ω6 polyunsaturates on blood pressure. The secondary category of dietary trials also attempts to increase the ratio of polyunsaturated to saturated fats, but in the process affects intake of all major food groups, usually increasing consumption of fruit, nuts, vegetables, and fish, while reducing consumption of high-fat dairy products, meat, and poultry. This results not only in changes in dietary fats, but also in the type and amount of protein and carbohydrates, and in a range of micronutrients including antioxidant vitamins and other antioxidants, fiber, and fiber types. Furthermore, such diets are usually characterized by an increase in lower glycemic index foods, in minerals such as potassium and magnesium, and sometimes a reduction in sodium intake.

There is good evidence from randomized controlled trials that such complex dietary changes reduce blood pressure and some evidence that dietary fat patterns contribute to these changes. Randomized controlled trials of lacto-ovo-vegetarian diets and in regular meat eaters showed falls in blood pressure in both normotensives[155] and untreated hypertensives.[156] These trials involved an increase in P/S ratio from around 0.3 to 1.0, along with other nutrient changes. Iacono et al.[171] and Puska et al.[172] conducted dietary trials increasing P/S ratio in hypercholesterolemic subjects and consistently showed falls in blood pressure. They concluded that changes in the amount and type of fat were responsible; however, their interventions also involved complex dietary changes characterized by an increased consumption of fruit, vegetables, and low-fat dairy products at the expense of high-fat dairy and meat products. Following a series of studies that focused on individual nutrient changes in fats, fiber, or protein type, it was concluded that lower blood pressures induced by vegetarian diets were probably due to a combination of complex dietary changes rather than any specific dietary component.[173] A small study of the effects of a "prudent" diet in normotensives[174] also showed that it was not necessary to exclude meat from dietary patterns similar to those eaten by vegetarians to achieve blood pressure reduction.

It was on the basis of these various strands of evidence pointing to effects of complex dietary patterns and with the clear-cut blood pressure lowering effects of vegetarian diets, the DASH trial[114] was designed to determine whether diets more acceptable to the general population would lower blood pressure in subjects with high normal blood pressure or mild hypertension. This landmark trial included three arms, a control group who continued the normal Western diet, a group who substantially increased fruit and vegetable consumption, and a third group who ate the "DASH combination diet," which also decreased saturated fat intake and increased consumption of low-fat dairy products.[114] There was a progressively greater blood pressure reduction across the three groups with a significantly greater effect of the combination diet. Although the DASH trial provides the best evidence for a role of dietary fats on blood pressure as part of a more complex dietary change, it is not as conclusive as the authors suggested, as the group who changed their fat intake also altered their intake of meat products and increased fish intake and consumption of low-fat dairy products containing other nutrients and minerals. Moreover, although there were no significant weight changes during the 8-week study, there was a reduction in estimated calorie intake with the complex DASH diet that might have contributed to blood pressure reduction.

Subsequent studies on effects of DASH-type diets on blood pressure, such as the DASH salt study,[175] have all included the whole dietary package and are thereby unable to throw further light on the contribution of fats *per se* to changes in blood pressure.[176] Moreover, in the PREMIER study, the DASH combination-diet regimen achieved no additional blood pressure reduction over and above standard measures for weight control, increased physical activity and modest sodium and alcohol restriction.[176] The original DASH study was a "proof of principle" trial in which the meals were all provided at communal canteens where the volunteers were strictly supervised. Interestingly, the "acceptability" of and adherence to the full recommendations of the DASH diet as regards increased fruit and vegetable consumption in noninstitutionalized individuals were not borne out in the more relaxed environment of the PREMIER study nor in an Australian study in which sodium restriction but not the DASH package lowered blood pressure.[177]

Further evidence of the contribution of monounsaturated fats comes from a study in which the complete carbohydrate-rich DASH diet was compared with two arms, one of which was enriched with protein and the other with predominantly unsaturated fats at the expense of carbohydrates in a 6-week cross-over design.[178] Compared with the carbohydrate-rich diet, the unsaturated fat diet further decreased blood pressure by 1.3 mmHg overall and by 2.9 mmHg in hypertensives. Unfortunately, there was no standard Western diet control group.

CONCLUSIONS

There is sound evidence for blood pressure lowering–effects of ω3 fatty acids of marine origin taken in either the form of fish oil supplements or regular intake of fish to provide 3 to 4 g of ω3 fatty acids daily. Lesser amounts of ω3 fatty acids have an antiarrhythmic effect in subjects at a high risk of heart disease. Clinical trials suggest that omega-3 fatty acids reduce the risk of coronary heart deaths in patients with prior heart disease, while population studies suggest that higher fish consumption protects against ischemic heart disease and ischemic stroke in the general population. Omega-6 polyunsaturates and monounsaturates when substituted for saturated fatty acids may have some blood pressure–lowering effect if they are part of complex dietary changes that include substantial increases in consumption of fruit, nuts, and vegetables and low-fat dairy products. These effects can be enhanced by moderation of salt intake.

From the clinical and public health viewpoint of optimum diets for preventing and managing hypertension, it is probably not critical whether increases in P/S ratio effectively lower blood pressure, as the improvements in lipid profile resulting from these changes in dietary fats are sufficient justification as measures to reduce long-term cardiovascular risk. More important from the blood pressure viewpoint is the type and amount of ω3 fatty acids and the effects of various types of fats on cardiac rhythm stability, atherosclerosis, thrombosis, endothelial function, satiety, total caloric intake, and palatability. For example, high saturated fat consumption as part of high-calorie diets also contributes to increasing rates of obesity and will have an importance influence on blood pressure through this mechanism.

REFERENCES

1. Schmidt EB, Arnesen H, de Caterina R, et al. Marine n-3 polyunsaturated fatty acids and coronary heart disease. Part I. Background, epidemiology, animal data, effects on risk factors and safety. *Thromb Res* 2005;115:163–70.
2. Schmidt EB, Arnesen H, Christensen JH, et al. Marine n-3 polyunsaturated fatty acids and coronary heart disease. Part II. Clinical trials and recommendations. *Thromb Res* 2005; 115:257–262.
3. Appel LJ, Miller ER. III, Seidler AJ, Whelton PK. Does supplementation of diet with 'fish oil' reduce blood pressure? *Arch Intern Med* 1993; 153:1429–38.
4. Morris MC, Sacks F, Rosner B. Does fish oil lower blood pressure? A meta-analysis of controlled trials. *Circulation* 1993;88:523–33.
5. Geleijnse JM, Giltay EJ, Grobbee DE, et al. Blood pressure response to fish oil supplementation: meta-regression analysis of randomized trials. *J Hypertens* 2002;20:1493–9.
6. Beilin LJ, Mori TA. Dietary ω3 fatty acids. In: PK Whelton, J He, GT Louis, eds. *Lifestyle Modification for the Prevention and Treatment of Hypertension.* New York: Marcel Dekker, Inc., 2003:275–300.
7. Leaf A, Kang JX, Xiao YF, Billman GE. Clinical prevention of sudden cardiac death by n-3 polyunsaturated fatty acids and mechanism of prevention of arrhythmias by n-3 fish oils. *Circulation* 2003;107:2646–52.
8. McVeigh GE, Brennan GM, Cohn JN, et al. Fish oil improves arterial compliance in non-insulin-dependent diabetes mellitus. *Arterioscler Thromb* 1994;14:1425–9.
9. Nestel P, Shige H, Pomeroy S, et al. The n-3 fatty acids eicosapentaenoic acid and docosahexaenoic acid increase systemic arterial compliance in humans. *Am J Clin Nutr* 2002; 76:326–30.
10. Mori TA, Watts GF, Burke V, et al. Differential effects of eicosapentaenoic acid and docosahexaenoic acid on forearm vascular reactivity of the microcirculation in hyperlipidaemic, overweight men. *Circulation* 2000; 102:1264–9.
11. Chin JP. Marine oils and cardiovascular reactivity. *Prostaglandins Leuk Essent Fatty Acids* 1994; 50:211–22.
12. Harris WS. n-3 Fatty acids and lipoproteins: comparison of results from human and animal studies. *Lipids* 1996;31:243–52.
13. Harris WS. n-3 Fatty acids and serum lipoproteins: human studies. *Am J Clin Nutr* 1997;65(Suppl 5):1645S–54S.
14. Calder PC. Polyunsaturated fatty acids, inflammation, and immunity. *Lipids* 2001,36:1007–24.
15. Knapp HR. Dietary fatty acids in human thrombosis and hemostasis. *Am J Clin Nutr* 1997;65:1687S–98S.
16. Mori TA, Beilin LJ. ωFatty acids and inflammation. *Curr Atheroscler Rep* 2004;6:461–7.
17. Mori TA, Bao DQ, Burke V, et al. Purified eicosapentaenoic acid and docosahexaenoic acid have differential effects of on serum lipids and lipoproteins, LDL—particle size, glucose and insulin, in mildly hyperlipidaemic men. *Am J Clin Nutr* 2000;71:1085–94.
18. Woodman RJ, Mori TA, Burke V, et al. Effects of purified eicosapentaenoic acid and docosahexaenoic acid on glycaemic control, blood pressure and serum lipids in treated-hypertensive type 2 diabetic patients. *Am J Clin Nutr* 2002;76:1007–15.
19. Grimsgaard S, Bonaa KH, Hansen JB, Nordoy A. Highly purified eicosapentaenoic acid and docosahexaenoic acid in humans have similar triacylglycerol-lowering effects but divergent effects on serum fatty acids. *Am J Clin Nutr* 1997;66:649–59.
20. Mori TA, Bao DQ, Burke V, et al. Docosahexaenoic acid but not eicosapentaenoic acid lowers ambulatory blood pressure and heart rate in humans. *Hypertension* 1999; 34:253–60.
21. Bang HO, Dyerberg J, Nielsen AB. Plasma lipid and lipoprotein pattern in Greenlandic west-coast Eskimos. *Lancet* 1971;1:1143–5.
22. Dyerberg J, Bang HO, Stoffersen E, et al. Eicosapentaenoic acid and prevention of thrombosis and atherosclerosis? *Lancet* 1978;2:117–9.
23. Sanders TA, Vickers M, Haines AP. Effect on blood lipids and haemostasis of a supplement of cod-liver oil, rich in eicosapentaenoic and docosahexaenoic acids, in healthy young men. *Clin Sci* 1981;61:317–24.
24. Kromhout D, Bosschieter EB, de Lezenne Coulander C. The inverse relation between fish consumption and 20-year mortality from coronary heart disease. *N Engl J Med* 1985; 312:1205–9.
25. Kromhout D, Feskens EJ, Bowles CH. The protective effect of a small amount of fish on coronary heart disease mortality in an elderly population. *Int J Epidemiol* 1995;24:340–5.
26. Lemaitre RN, King IB, Mozaffarian D, et al. n-3 Polyunsaturated fatty acids, fatal ischemic heart disease, and nonfatal myocardial infarction in older adults: the Cardiovascular Health Study. *Am J Clin Nutr* 2003;77:319–25.
27. Mozaffarian D, Lemaitre RN, Kuller LH, et al. Cardiac benefits of fish consumption may depend on the type of fish meal consumed: the Cardiovascular Health Study. *Circulation* 2003;107:1372–7.
28. Mozaffarian D, Bryson CL, Lemaitre RN, et al. Fish intake and risk of incident heart failure. *J Am Coll Cardiol* 2005; 45:2015–21.
29. Norell SE, Ahlbom A, Feychting M, Pedersen NL. Fish consumption and mortality from coronary heart disease. *BMJ* 1986;293:26.
30. Erkkila AT, Lehto S, Pyorala K, Uusitupa MI. n-3 Fatty acids and 5-y risks of death and cardiovascular disease events in patients with coronary artery disease. *Am J Clin Nutr* 2003;78:65–71.
31. Erkkila AT, Lichtenstein AH, Mozaffarian D. Herrington DM. Fish intake is associated with a reduced progression of coronary artery atherosclerosis in postmenopausal women with coronary artery disease. *Am J Clin Nutr* 2004;80:626–32.
32. Dolecek TA. Epidemiological evidence of relationships between dietary polyunsaturated fatty acids and mortality in the multiple risk factor intervention trial. *Proc Soc Exp Biol Med* 1992;200:177–82.
33. Daviglus ML, Stamler J, Orencia AJ, et al. Fish consumption and the 30-year risk of fatal myocardial infarction. *N Engl J Med* 1997; 336:1046–53.
34. Albert CM, Hennekens CH, O'Donnell CJ, et al. Fish consumption and risk of sudden cardiac death. *JAMA* 1998; 279:23–8.
35. Morris MC, Manson JE, Rosner B, et al. Fish consumption and cardiovascular disease in the physicians' health study: a prospective study. *Am J Epidemiol* 1995;142:166–75.
36. Albert CM, Campos H, Stampfer MJ, et al. Blood levels of long-chain n-3 fatty acids and the risk of sudden death. *N Engl J Med* 2002;346:1113–8.
37. Hu FB, Bronner L, Willett WC, et al. Fish and omega-3 fatty acid intake and risk of coronary heart disease in women. *JAMA* 2002;287:1815–21.
38. Hu FB, Cho E, Rexrode KM, et al. Fish and long-chain omega-3 fatty acid intake and risk of coronary heart disease and total mortality in diabetic women. *Circulation* 2003;107:1852–7.
39. Siscovick DS, Raghunathan TE, King I, et al. Dietary intake and cell membrane levels of long-chain n-3 polyunsaturated fatty acids and the risk of primary cardiac arrest. *JAMA* 1995;274:1363–7.
40. Burchfiel CM, Reed DM, Strong JP, et al. Predictors of myocardial lesions in men with minimal coronary atherosclerosis at autopsy. The Honolulu Heart Program. *Ann Epidemiol* 1996;6(2):137–46.
41. Mozaffarian D, Psaty BM, Rimm EB, et al. Fish intake and risk of incident atrial fibrillation. *Circulation* 2004; 110:368–73.
42. Calo L, Bianconi L, Colivicchi F, et al. N-3 Fatty acids for the prevention of atrial fibrillation after coronary artery bypass surgery: a randomized, controlled trial. *J Am Coll Cardiol* 2005;45:1723–8.
43. Ascherio A, Rimm EB, Stampfer MJ, et al. Dietary intake of marine n-3 fatty acids, fish intake, and the risk of coronary disease among men. *N Engl J Med* 1995;332:977–82.
44. Marckmann P, Gronbaek M. Fish consumption and coronary heart disease mortality. A systematic review of prospective cohort studies. *Eur J Clin Nutr* 1999;53(8):585–90.
45. Bucher HC, Hengstler P, Schindler C, Meier G. n-3 Polyunsaturated fatty acids in coronary heart disease: a meta-analysis of randomized controlled trials. *Am J Med* 2002; 112:298–304.
46. He K, Song Y, Daviglus ML, et al. Greenland P. Accumulated evidence on fish consumption and coronary

heart disease mortality: a meta-analysis of cohort studies. *Circulation* 2004;109:2705–11.

47. Whelton SP, He J, Whelton PK, Muntner P. Meta-analysis of observational studies on fish intake and coronary heart disease. *Am J Cardiol* 2004;93:1119–23.

48. Burr ML, Fehily AM, Gilbert JF, et al. Effects of changes in fat, fish, and fibre intakes on death and myocardial reinfarction: diet and reinfarction trial (DART). *Lancet* 1989;2:757–61.

49. GISSI-Prevenzione Investigators. Dietary supplementation with n-3 polyunsaturated fatty acids and vitamin E after myocardial infarction: results of the GISSI-Prevenzione trial. Gruppo Italiano per lo Studio della Sopravvivenza nell'Infarto miocardico. *Lancet* 1999;354:447–55.

50. Marchioli R, Barzi F, Bomba E, et al. GISSI-Prevenzione Investigators. Early protection against sudden death by n-3 polyunsaturated fatty acids after myocardial infarction: time-course analysis of the results of the Gruppo Italiano per lo Studio della Sopravvivenza nell'Infarto Miocardico (GISSI)-Prevenzione. *Circulation* 2002; 105:1897–903.

51. Pauletto P, Puato M, Caroli MG, et al. Blood pressure and atherogenic lipoprotein profiles of fish-diet and vegetarian villagers in Tanzania: the Lugalawa study. *Lancet* 1996; 348:784–8.

52. Iso H, Rexrode KM, Stampfer MJ, et al. Intake of fish and omega-3 fatty acids and risk of stroke in women. *JAMA* 2001;285:304–312.

53. He K, Rimm EB, Merchant A, et al. Fish consumption and risk of stroke in men. *JAMA* 2002;288(24):3130–6.

54. Mozaffarian D, Longstreth WT, Lemaitre RN, et al. Fish consumption and stroke risk in elderly individuals—the Cardiovascular Health Study. *Arch Int Med* 2005;165(2):200–6.

55. Bonaa KH, Bjerve, KS, Straume B, et al. Effect of eicosapentaenoic acid and docosahexaenoic acid on blood pressure in hypertension. A population-based intervention trial from the Tromso study. N Engl J Med 1990;322:795–801.

56. Knapp HR, FitzGerald GA. The antihypertensive effects of fish oil. A controlled study of polyunsaturated fatty acid supplements in essential hypertension. *N Engl J Med* 1989; 320:1037–43.

57. Radack K, Deck C, Huster G. The effects of low doses of n-3 fatty acid supplementation on blood pressure in hypertensive subjects. A randomized controlled trial. *Arch Intern Med* 1991;151:1173–80.

58. Norris PG, Jones CJ, Weston MJ. Effect of dietary supplementation with fish oil on systolic blood pressure in mild essential hypertension. *BMJ* 1986; 293:104–5.

59. Singer P, Berger I, Luck K, et al. Long-term effect of mackerel diet on blood pressure, serum lipids and thromboxane formation in patients with mild essential hypertension. *Atherosclerosis* 1986;62:259–65.

60. Levinson PD, Iosiphidis AH, Saritelli AL, et al. Effects of n-3 fatty acids in essential hypertension. *Am J Hypertens* 1990;3:754–60.

61. Prisco D, Paniccia R, Bandinelli B, et al. Effect of medium-term supplementation with a moderate dose of n-3 polyunsaturated fatty acids on blood pressure in mild hypertensive patients. *Thromb Res* 1998;91:105–12.

62. Toft I, Bonna KH, Ingebretsen OC, et al. Effects of n-3 polyunsaturated fatty acids on glucose homeostasis and blood pressure in essential hypertension. A randomized, controlled trial. *Ann Intern Med* 1995;123:911–8.

63. Cobiac L, Nestel PJ, Wing LM, Howe PRC. A low sodium diet supplemented with fish oil lowers blood pressure in the elderly. *J Hypertens* 1992;10:87–92.

64. Singer P, Melzer S, Goschel M, Augustin S. Fish oil amplifies the effect of propranolol in mild essential hypertension. *Hypertension* 1990; 16:682–91.

65. Howe PR, Lungershausen YK, Cobiac L, et al. Effect of sodium restriction and fish oil supplementation on BP and thrombotic risk factors in patients treated with ACE inhibitors. *J Hum Hypertens* 1994;8:43–9.

66. Lungershausen YK, Abbey M, Nestel PJ, Howe PR. Reduction of blood pressure and plasma triglycerides by omega-3 fatty acids in treated hypertensives. *J Hypertens* 1994; 12:1041–5.

67. Vandongen R, Mori TA, Burke V, et al. Effects on blood pressure of ω3 fats in subjects at increased risk of cardiovascular disease. *Hypertension* 1993;22:371–9.

68. Bao DQ, Mori TA, Burke V, et al. Effects of dietary fish and weight reduction on ambulatory blood pressure in overweight hypertensives. *Hypertension* 1998;32:710–7.

69. Rambjor GS, Walen AI, Windsor SL, Harris WS. Eicosapentaenoic acid is primarily responsible for hypotriglyceridemic effect of fish oil in humans. *Lipids* 1996;31:S45–9.

70. Woodman RJ, Mori TA, Burke V, et al. Effects of purified eicosapentaenoic acid and docosahexaenoic acid on platelet, fibrinolytic and vascular function in type 2 diabetic patients. *Atherosclerosis* 2003;166:85–93.

71. Yin K, Chu ZM, Beilin LJ. Blood pressure and vascular reactivity changes in spontaneously hypertensive rats fed fish oil. *Br J Pharmacol* 1991;102:991–7.

72. Chu ZM, Yin K, Beilin LJ. Fish oil feeding selectively attenuates contractile responses to noradrenaline and electrical stimulation in the perfused mesenteric resistance vessels of spontaneously hypertensive rats. *Clin Exp Pharmacol Physiol* 1992; 19:177–81.

73. Lorenz R, Spengler U, Fischer S, et al. Platelet function, thromboxane formation and blood pressure control during supplementation of the western diet with cod liver oil. *Circulation* 1983;67:504–11.

74. Yoshimura T, Matsui K, Ito M, et al. Effects of highly purified eicosapentaenoic acid on plasma beta thromboglobulin level and vascular reactivity to angiotensin II. *Artery* 1987;14:295–303.

75. Chin JPF, Gust AP, Nestel PJ, Dart AM. Fish oils dose-dependently inhibit vasoconstriction of forearm resistance vessels in humans. *Hypertension* 1993; 21:22–8.

76. Chin JPF, Gust AP, Dart AM. Indomethacin inhibits the effects of dietary supplementation with fish oils on vasoconstriction of human forearm resistance vessels in vivo. *J Hypertens* 1993;11:1229–34.

77. Vekshtein VI, Yeung AC, Vita JA. et al. Fish oil improves endothelium-dependent relaxation in patients with coronary artery disease. *Circulation* 1989;80(Suppl II):II-434.

78. Fleischhauer FJ, Yan W-D, Fischell TA. Fish oil improves endothelium-dependent coronary vasodilation in heart transplant recipients. *J Am Coll Cardiol* 1993;21:982–9.

79. Yin K, Chu ZM, Beilin LJ. Study of mechanisms of glucocorticoid hypertension in rats: Endothelial related changes and their amelioration by dietary fish oils. *Br J Pharmacol* 1992;106:435–42.

80. Shimokawa H, Vanhoutte PM. Dietary cod-liver oil improves endothelium-dependent response in hypercholesterolaemic and atherosclerotic porcine arteries. *Circulation* 1988;78:1421–30.

81. Chin JPF, Dart AM. Therapeutic restoration of endothelial function in hypercholesterolaemic subjects: effect of fish oils. *Clin Exp Pharmacol Physiol* 1994;21:749–55.

82. McVeigh GE, Brennan GM, Johnston GD, et al. Dietary fish oil augments nitric oxide production or release in patients with type 2 (non-insulin dependent) diabetes mellitus. *Diabetologia* 1993;36:33–8.

83. Shimokawa H, Lam JYT, Chesebro JH, et al. Effects of dietary supplementation with cod-liver oil on endothelium-dependent response in porcine coronary arteries. *Circulation* 1987; 76:898–905.

84. Schini VB, Durante W, Catovsky S, Vanhoutte PM. Eicosapentaenoic acid potentiates the production of nitric oxide evoked by interleukin-1β in cultured vascular smooth muscle cells. *J Vasc Res* 1993;30:209–17.

85. Boulanger C, Schini VB, Hendrickson H, Vanhoutte PM. Chronic exposure of cultured endothelial cells to eicosapentaenoic acid potentiates the release of endothelium-derived relaxing factor(s). *Br J Pharmacol* 1990;99:176–80.

86. Goodfellow J, Bellamy MF, Ramsey MW, et al. Dietary supplementation with marine omega-3 fatty acids improve systemic large artery endothelial function in subjects with hypercholesterolemia. *J Am Coll Cardiol* 2000;35(2):265–70.

87. McLennan P, Howe P, Abeywardena M, et al. The cardiovascular protective role of docosahexaenoic acid. *Eur J Pharmacol* 1996;300:83–9.

88. Engler MB, Engler MM, Ursell PC. Vasorelaxant properties of n-3 polyunsaturated fatty acids in aortas from spontaneously hypertensive and normotensive rats. *J Cardiovasc Risk* 1994;1:75–80.

89. Harris WS, Rambjor GS, Windsor SL, Diederich D. n-3 Fatty acids and urinary excretion of nitric oxide metabolites in humans. *Am J Clin Nutr* 1997;65:459–64.

90. Chin JP, Dart AM. How do fish oils affect vascular function? *Clin Exp Pharmacol Physiol* 1995;22:71–81.

91. Fox PL, DiCorleto PE. Fish oils inhibit endothelial cell production of platelet-derived growth factor-like protein. *Science* 1988;241:453–546.

92. Schini VB, Durante W, Elizondo E, et al. The induction of nitric oxide synthase activity is inhibited by TGF-α_1, PDGF$_{AB}$ and PDGF$_{BB}$ in vascular smooth muscle cells. *Eur J Pharmacol* 1992;216:379–83.

93. Fischer S, Weber PC. Thromboxane A_3 (TXA$_3$) is formed in human platelets after dietary eicosapentaenoic acid (C20:5 ω3). *Biochem Biophys Res Commun* 1983;116(3):1091–9.

94. Knapp HR, Reilly IA, Alessandrini P, FitzGerald GA. In vivo indexes of platelet and vascular function during fish-oil administration in patients with atherosclerosis. *N Engl J Med* 1986; 314(15):937–42.

95. Fischer S, Weber PC. Prostaglandin I$_3$ is formed in vivo in man after dietary eicosapentaenoic acid. *Nature* 1984; 307(5947):165–8.

96. Hashimoto M, Shinozuka K, Gamoh S, et al. The hypotensive effect of docosahexaenoic acid is associated with the enhanced release of ATP from the caudal artery of aged rats. *J Nutr* 1999;129:70–6.

97. Hashimoto M, Hossain S, Yamasaki H, et al. Effects of eicosapentaenoic acid and docosahexaenoic acid on plasma membrane fluidity of aortic endothelial cells. *Lipids* 1999; 34:1297–304.

98. Billman GE, Hallaq H, Leaf A. Prevention of ischemia-induced ventricular fibrillation by omega 3 fatty acids. *Proc Natl Acad Sci USA* 1994;91(10):4427–30.

99. McLennan PL, Barnden LR, Bridle TM, et al. Dietary fat modulation of left ventricular ejection fraction in the marmoset due to enhanced filling. *Cardiovasc Res* 1992;26:871–7.

100. Grimsgaard S, Bonaa KH, Hansen JB, Myhre ESP. Effects of highly purified eicosapentaenoic acid and docosahexaenoic acid on hemodynamics in humans. *Am J Clin Nutr* 1998;68:52–9.

101. Dallongeville J, Yarnell J, Ducimetiere P, et al. Fish consumption is associated with lower heart rates. *Circulation* 2003;108(7):820–5.

102. Mozaffarian D, Geelen A, Brouwer IA, et al. Effect of fish oil on heart rate in humans - A meta-analysis of randomized controlled trials. *Circulation* 2005;112(13):1945–52.

103. Christensen JH, Schmidt EB. n-3 Fatty acids and the risk of sudden cardiac death. *Lipids* 2001;36(Suppl):S115–8.

104. Christensen JH. n-3 Fatty acids and the risk of sudden cardiac death. Emphasis on heart rate variability. *Danish Med Bull* 2003;50(4):347–67.

105. Codde JP, Beilin LJ. Prostaglandins and experimental hypertension: a review with special emphasis on the effect of dietary lipids. *J Hypertens* 1986; 4:675–86.

106. Fuentes F, Lopez-Miranda F, Sanchez E, et al. Mediterranean and low-fat diets improve endothelial function in hypercholesterolaemic men. *Ann Intern Med* 2001;134:1115–9.

107. Straznicky NE, Louis WJ, McGrade P, Howes LG. The effects of dietary lipid modification on blood pressure, cardiovascular reactivity and sympathetic activity in man. *J Hypertens* 1993;11:427–37.

108. Goode GK, Heagerty AM. In vitro responses of human peripheral small arteries hypercholesterolemia and effects of therapy. *Circulation* 1995; 91:2898–903.

109. Muriana FJG, Ruizgutierrez V, Guerrero A, Montilla C, et al. Olive oil normalizes the altered distribution of membrane cholesterol and Na+-Li+ countertransport activity in erythrocytes of hypertensive patients. *J Nutr Biochem* 1997;8:205–10.

110. Storlein LH, Baur LA, Kritekos AD, et al. Dietary fats and insulin action. *Diabetologia* 1996;39:621–31.

111. Ferrara LA, Raimondi AS, Episcopo L, et al. Olive oil and reduced need for antihypertensive medications. *Arch Intern Med* 2000;160:837–42.

112. Sacks FM. Dietary fats and blood pressure: a critical review of the evidence. *Nutr Rev* 1989;47:291–300.

113. Morris MC. Dietary fats and blood pressure. *J Cardiovasc Risk* 1994; 1:21–30.

114. Appel LJ, Moore TJ, Obarzanek E, et al. A clinical trial of the effects of dietary patterns on blood pressure. DASH Collaborative Research Group. *N Engl J Med* 1997;336(16):1117–24.

115. Salonen JT, Salonen R, Ihanainen M, et al. Blood pressure, dietary fats and antioxidants. *Am J Clin Nutr* 1988; 48:1226–32.

116. Stamler J, Cagguila A, Kjelsberg M, Cutler JA. Relationship to blood pressure of combinations of dietary macronutrients. Findings of the Multiple Risk Factor Intervention Trial. *Circulation* 1996;94:2417–23.

117. Oster P, Arab L, Schellenberg B, et al. Linoleic acid and blood pressure. *Prog Food Nutr Sci* 1980;4:39–40.

118. Witteman J, Willett WC, Stampfer MJ, et al. A prospective study of nutritional factors and hypertension among US women. *Circulation* 1989;80:1320–7.

119. Ascherio A, Rimm EB, Giovannucci EL, et al. A prospective study of nutritional factors and hypertension among US men. *Circulation* 1992;86:1475–84.

120. Hajjar I, Kotchen T. Regional variations of blood pressure in the United States are associated with regional variations in dietary intakes: The NHANES-III data. *J Nutr* 2003;133:211–4.

121. Jenner DA, English DR, Vandongen R, et al. Diet and blood pressure in 9-year old Australian children. *Am J Clin Nutr* 1988;47: 1052–9.

122. Jenner DA, Vandongern R, Beilin LJ. Relationships between blood pressure and measures of dietary energy intake, physical fitness and physical activity in Australian children aged 11–12. *J Epidemiol Commun Health* 1992; 46:108–13.

123. Grimsgaard S, Bonaa KH, Jacobsen BK, et al. Plasma saturated and linoleic fatty acids are independently associated with blood pressure. *Hypertension* 1999;34:478–83.

124. Riemersma RA, Wood DA, Bulter S, et al. Linoleic acid content in adipose tissue and coronary heart disease. *BMJ* 1986;292:1423–7.

125. Ascherio A, Hennekens C, Willett WC, et al. Prospective study of nutritional factors, blood pressure, and hypertension among US women. *Hypertension* 1996;27(5):1065–72.

126. McPhillips JB, Eaton CB, Gans KM, et al. Dietary differences in smokers and non-smokers from two southeastern New England communities. *J Am Diet Assoc* 1994; 94:287–92.

127. Herbeth B, Didelot-Barthelemy L, Lemoine A, Le Devehat C. Dietary behaviour of French men according to alcohol drinking pattern. *J Stud Alcohol* 1988;49:268–72.

128. Willett W. *Nutritional Epidemiology*. New York: Oxford University Press, 1998.

129. Romon M, Nuttens M-Cc, Theret N, et al. Comparison between fat intake assessed by a 3-day food record and phospholipid fatty acid composition of red blood cells: results from the Monitoring of Cardiovascular Diseases—Lille Study. *Metabolism* 1995;44:1139–45.

130. Oliver MF. Cigarette smoking, polyunsaturated fats, linoleic acid and coronary heart disease. *Lancet* 1989; ii:1241–2.

131. Rouse IL, Beilin LJ. Nutrition, blood pressure and hypertension. *Med J Aust* 1983;(Suppl):S19–23.

132. National Heart Diet Study Research Group. The National Diet Heart Study final report. *Circulation* 1968; 37(Suppl 3):I1–428.

133. Brussaard JH, van Raaij JMA, stasse-Wolthuis M, et al. Blood pressure and diet in normotensive volunteers: absence of an effect of dietary fibre, protein or fat. *Am J Clin Nutr* 1981; 34:2023–9.

134. Uusitupa MI, Sarkkinen ES, Torpstrom J, et al. Long term effects of four fat-modified diets on blood pressure. *J Hum Hypertens* 1994;8:209–18.

135. Margetts BM, Beilin LJ, Armstrong BK, et al. Blood pressure and dietary polyunsaturated and saturated fats: a controlled trial. *Clin Sci* 1985; 69:165–75.

136. Bing RF, Heagerty AM, Swales JD. Dietary changes in membrane lipids and leucocyte calcium. *J Cardiovasc Pharmacol* 1988;12(Suppl 3):S110–3.

137. Heagerty AM, Ollerenshaw JD, Robertson DI, et al. Influence of dietary linoleic acid on leucocyte sodium transport and blood pressure. *BMJ* 1986;293:295–7.

138. Sciarrone SC, Rouse I, Rogers P, Beilin LJ. A factorial study of fat and fibre changes and sodium restriction in blood pressure in human hypertensive subjects. *Clin Exp Pharmacol Physiol* 1990;17:197–201.

139. Sacks FM, Rouse IL, Stampfer MJ, et al. Effect of dietary fats and carbohydrate on blood pressure of mildly hypertensive patients. *Hypertension* 1987;10:452–60.

140. Deferne JL, Leeds AR. The antihypertensive effect of dietary supplementation with a 6-desaturated

essential fatty acid concentrate as compared with sunflower seed oil. *J Hum Hypretens* 1992;6:113–9.

141. Aro A, Pietinen P, Valsta LM, et al. Lack of effect on blood pressure by low fat diets with different fatty acid compositions. *J Hum Hypertens* 1998; 12:383–9.

142. Mutanen M, Kleemola P, Valsta LM, et al. Lack of effect on blood pressure by polyunsaturated and monounsaturated fat diets. *Eur J Clin Nutr* 1992;46:1–6.

143. Sacks FM, Stamfer MJ, Munoz A, et al. Effect of linoleic and oleic acids on blood pressure, blood viscosity and erythrocyte cation transport. *J Am Coll Nutr* 1987;6:179–85.

144. Espino-Montoro A, Lopez-Miranda J, Castro P, et al. Monounsaturated fatty acid enriched diets lower plasma insulin levels and blood pressure in healthy young men. *Nutr Metab Cardiovasc Dis* 1996;6:147–54.

145. Ruitz-Gutierrez V, Muriana FJG, Guerrero A, et al. Plasma lipids, erythrocyte membrane lipids and blood pressure of hypertensive women after ingestion of dietary oleic acid from two different sources. *J Hypertens* 1996;14:1483–90.

146. Ros E. Dietary cis-monounsaturated fatty acids and metabolic control in type 2 diabetes. *Am J Clin Nutr* 2003; 78(Suppl):617S–25S.

147. Rasmussen OW, Thomsen C, Hansen KW, et al. Effects on blood pressure, glucose, and lipid levels of a high-monounsaturated fat diet compared with a high-carbohydrate diet in NIDDM subjects. *Diabetes Care* 1993; 16:1565–71.

148. Thomsen C, Rasmussen OW, Hansen KW, et al. Comparison of the effects on the diurnal blood pressure, glucose, and lipid levels of a diet rich in monounsaturated fatty acids with a diet rich in polyunsaturated fatty acids in type 2 diabetic subjects. *Diabetes Med* 1995;12:600–6.

149. Expert Panel on Trans Fatty Acids and Coronary Heart Disease. Trans fatty acids and coronary heart disease risk. Report of the Expert Panel on Trans Fatty Acids and Coronary Heart Disease. *Am J Clin Nutr* 1995; 62:655S–708S.

150. ASCN/AIN Task Force on Trans Fatty Acids. Position paper on trans fatty acids. *Am J Clin Nutr* 1996;63:663–70.

151. Mensink RP, de Louw MHJ, Katan MB. Effects of dietary trans fatty acids on blood pressure in normotensive subjects. *Eur J Clin Nutr* 1991; 45:375–82.

152. Zock PL, Blijlevens RAMT, de Vries JHM, Katan MB. Effects of stearic acid and trans fatty acids versus linoleic acid on blood pressure in normotensive women and men. *Eur J Clin Nutr* 1993; 47:437–44.

153. Lichtenstein AH, Erkkila AT, Lamarche B, Schwab US, Jalbert SM, Ausman LM. Influence of hydrogenated fat and butter on CVD risk factors: remnant-like particles, glucose and insulin, blood pressure and C-reactive protein. *Atherosclerosis* 2003;171:97–107.

154. Soriguer F, Rojo-Martinez G, Dobarganes MC, et al. Hypertension is related to the degradation of dietary frying oils. *Am J Clin Nutr* 2003; 78:1092–7.

155. Rouse IL, Beilin LJ, Armstrong BK, Vandongen R. Blood-pressure-lowering effect of a vegetarian diet: controlled trial in normotensive subjects. *Lancet* 1983;1:5–10.

156. Margetts BM, Beilin LJ, Vandongen R, Armstrong BK. Vegetarian diet in mild hypertension: a randomised controlled trial. *BMJ* 1986;293:1468–71.

157. Geleijnse JM, Kok FJ, Grobbee DE. Impact of dietary and lifestyle factors on the prevalence of hypertension in Western populations. *Eur J Public Health* 2004;14:235–9.

158. Stamler J, Liu K, Ruth KJ, et al. Eight-year blood pressure change in middle-aged men: relationship to multiple nutrients. *Hypertension* 2002; 39:1000–6.

159. Psaltopoulou T, Naska A, Orfanos P, et al. Olive oil, the Mediterranean diet, and arterial blood pressure: the Greek European Prospective Investigation into Cancer and Nutrition (EPIC) study. *Am J Clin Nutr* 2004;80:1012–8.

160. Saile F. Influence of vegetarian food on blood pressure. *Med Klin* 1930; 26:929–31.

161. Groen JJ, Tijong KB, Koster et al. The influence of nutrition and ways of life on blood cholesterol and the prevalence of hypertension and coronary heart disease among Benedictine and Trappist monks. *Am J Clin Nutr* 1962;10:456–70.

162. Sacks F, Rosner B, Kass EH. Blood pressure in vegetarians. *Am J Epidemiol* 1977;100:390–8.

163. Burke V, Beilin LJ. Vegetarian diets and high blood pressure—an update. *Nutr Metab Cardiovasc Dis* 1994; 4:103–12.

164. Rouse IL, Armstrong BK, Beilin LJ. The relationship of blood pressure to diet and lifestyle in two religious populations. *J Hypertens* 1983; 1:65–71.

165. Rouse IL, Beilin LJ. Vegetarian diet and blood pressure. *J Hypertens* 1984;2(3): 231–40.

166. Appleby PN, Davey GK, Key TJ. Hypertension and blood pressure among meat eaters, fish eaters, vegetarians and vegans in EPIC-Oxford. *Public Health Nutr* 2002; 5:645–54.

167. Rouse IL, Beilin LJ, Mahoney DP, et al. Nutrient intake, blood pressure, serum and urinary prostaglandins and serum thromboxane B2 in a controlled trial with a lacto-ovo-vegetarian diet. *J Hypertens* 1986;4:241–50.

168. He J, Klag MJ, Whelton PK, et al. Dietary macronutrients and blood pressure in southwestern China. *J Hypertens* 1995;13:1267–74.

169. Falkner B, Sherif K, Michel S, Kushner H. Dietary nutrients and blood pressure in urban minority adolescents at risk for hypertension. *Arch Pediatr Adolesc Med* 2000; 9:918–22.

170. Miura K, Greenland P, Stamler J, et al. Relation of vegetable, fruit, and meat intake to 7-year blood pressure change in middle-aged men. *Am J Epidemiol* 2004;159: 572–80.

171. Iacono J, Marshall M, Dougherty R, et al. Reduction in blood pressure associated with high polyunsaturated fat diets that reduce blood cholesterol in man. *Prev Med* 1975;4:426–43.

172. Puska P, Iacono J, Nissinen A, et al. Controlled, randomised trial of the effect of dietary fat on blood pressure. *Lancet* 1983;I:1–5.

173. Rouse IL, Beilin LJ. Vegetarian and other complex diets, fibre intake and blood pressure. In: Laragh JH, Brenner BM, eds. *Hypertension: Pathophysiology, Diagnosis and Management.* New York: Raven Press, 1989:241–55.

174. Kestin M, Rouse I, Correll R, Nestel P. Cardiovascular disease risk factors in free-living men: comparison of two prudent diets, one based on lactoovovegetarianism and the other allowing lean meat. *Am J Clin Nutr* 1989;50:280–7.

175. Obarzanek E, Proschan MA, Vollmer WM, et al. Individual blood pressure responses to changes in salt intake: results from the DASH-Sodium trial. *Hypertension* 2003;42:459–67.

176. Appel LJ, Champagne CM, Harsha DW, et al. Effects of comprehensive lifestyle modification on blood pressure control: main results of the PREMIER clinical trial. *JAMA* 2003; 289:2083–93.

177. Nowson CA, Worsley A, Margerison C, et al. Godfrey SJ. Blood pressure response to dietary modifications in free-living individuals. *J Nutr* 2004; 13:2322–9.

178. Appel LJ, Sacks FM, Carey VJ, et al. Effects of protein, monosaturated fat, and carbohydrate intake on blood pressure and seum lipids. Results of the OmniHeart randomized trial. *JAMA* 2005;294:2455–64.

Chapter

8 Effects of Dietary Patterns

Lawrence J. Appel

Key Findings

- Of the environmental factors that influence blood pressure (i.e., diet, sedentary lifestyle, toxins, and psychosocial factors), dietary factors have a major, and likely predominant, role in determining blood pressure.

- Dietary modifications that lower blood pressure are a reduced sodium intake, increased potassium intake, weight loss (among those who are overweight or obese), and moderation of alcohol consumption (among those who drink).

- Certain dietary patterns (vegetarian, Dietary Approaches to Stop Hypertension [DASH]-style, and Mediterranean diets) are also associated with reduced blood pressure.

- Evidence from clinical trials has often documented subadditive effects among established risk factors, that is, the combined effect of two or more blood pressure–reducing components is less than the sum of blood pressure reductions from each component alone.

Elevated blood pressure results from environmental factors, genetic factors, and interactions among these factors. Of the environmental factors that influence blood pressure (i.e., diet, sedentary lifestyle, toxins, and psychosocial factors), dietary factors have a major, and likely predominant, role in blood pressure homeostasis. A substantial body of evidence strongly supports the concept that multiple aspects of diet affect blood pressure. Dietary modifications that lower blood pressure are reduced sodium intake, increased potassium intake, weight loss (among those who are overweight or obese), and moderation of alcohol consumption (among those who drink).[1] A very high intake of n-3 polyunsaturated fatty acids from pill supplements (commonly termed "fish oil") also lowers blood pressure but at doses that are commonly associated with side effects.

Certain dietary patterns (vegetarian, Dietary Approaches to Stop Hypertension [DASH]-style, and Mediterranean diets) are also associated with reduced blood pressure. The blood pressure lowering effects of these dietary patterns reflects the cumulative effects of their constituent nutrients that include the well-established factors that affect blood pressure (e.g., potassium) and perhaps other factors (e.g., fiber, meat) whose effect on blood pressure is uncertain. To a limited extent, available research has explored whether the blood pressure effects of individual nutrients are additive, synergistic, or subadditive. Evidence from clinical trials has often documented subadditive effects among estab-

lished risk factors, that is, the combined effect of two or more blood pressure-reducing components is less than the sum of blood pressure reductions from each component alone.[2–4] Nonetheless, the cumulative effects, even if subadditive, can be substantial and have major public health benefits.

The primary objective of this chapter is to review the effects of selected dietary patterns (vegetarian, DASH-style, and Mediterranean diets) on blood pressure. In addition to lowering blood pressure, these dietary patterns have also been associated with a reduced risk of cardiovascular disease, particularly coronary heart disease. In this chapter, I also review the effects of dietary carbohydrate and protein on blood pressure. See Chapter 7 for a review of the effects of fat on blood pressure.

VEGETARIAN DIETS

Vegetarian diets have long been associated with reduced blood pressure.[5] In non-Western societies that consume a largely plant-based diet, hypertension is rare, while migration from these often rural societies to more urban societies is associated with a rise in blood pressure and increased prevalence of hypertension.[6,7] In industrialized countries, where hypertension is commonplace, individuals who consume a vegetarian diet have substantially lower blood pressure than nonvegetarians. Some of the lowest blood pressures observed in industrialized countries have been documented in strict vegetarians living in Massachusetts. Vegetarians also experience a lower, age-related rise in blood pressure[8,9] (Figure 8–1). Importantly, observational studies from Europe and the United States have consistently documented that vegetarian diets are associated with a reduced risk of coronary heart disease.[10]

Aspects of a vegetarian lifestyle that might affect blood pressure include nondietary factors (e.g., physical activity), well-established dietary risk factors for elevated blood pressure (e.g., sodium, potassium, weight, alcohol), and other aspects of a vegetarian diet (e.g., high fiber, no meat). As discussed in the next section, observational studies have to a very limited extent controlled for the well-established determinants of blood pressure.

Weight certainly accounts for part of the blood pressure–lowering effect of a vegetarian lifestyle. On average, vegetarians weigh considerably less than nonvegetarians. However, in analyses that adjust for or stratify by weight, an effect of vegetarian diets on blood pressure often persists.[8,11] Fewer studies have determined whether reduced sodium

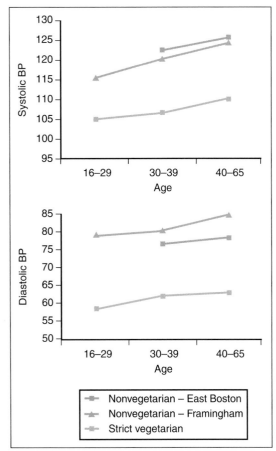

Figure 8–1. Blood pressure by age in a strict vegetarian population in Boston and in nonvegetarian populations in East Boston and Framingham, Massachusetts. (Adapted from Sacks FM, Kass EH. *Am J Clin Nutr* 1988;48(Suppl 3):795–800.)

and/or increased potassium are responsible for the blood pressure–lowering effects of vegetarian diets. Although data are limited, vegetarians tend to consume more potassium than nonvegetarians. The high intake of potassium, a nutrient that lowers blood pressure,[12] likely results from consumption of fruits and vegetables. Available evidence indicates that the salt intake of vegetarians is similar to and potentially exceeds that of nonvegetarians; such findings suggest that the blood pressure–lowering effects of a vegetarian diet can be further improved by reducing salt intake. In a matched-pairs analysis of vegetarians and non-vegetarians, Armstrong et al.[13] documented that vegetarians had higher urinary potassium excretion (62.9 mmol/day) than the nonvegetarians (54.8 mmol/day), while the urinary excretion of sodium was nonsignificantly higher in the vegetarians (mean of 169.7 vs. 61.2 mmol/day). Such data are consistent with evidence that an increased intake of fruits and vegetables[14,15] lowers blood pressure. It is doubtful that physical activity accounts for the lower blood pressure of vegetarians. Armstrong et al.[8] noted that vegetarians and nonvegetarians had similar levels of self-reported, leisure-time physical activity and had similar occupations.

Two trials, one in nonhypertensives[16] and another in hypertensives,[17] have documented that adoption of a vegetarian diet can reduce blood pressure. Other trials have explored the relationship between animal products and specific nutrients (e.g., saturated fat) on blood pressure.[9] In a trial of nonhypertensive individuals,[16] consumption of a vegetarian diet, similar in nutrient composition to a ovolactovegetarian diet, led to significant reductions in systolic blood pressure (5–6 mmHg) and diastolic blood pressure (2–3 mmHg), compared to a nonvegetarian diet. In the trial of hypertensives,[17] an ovolactovegetarian diet compared to a nonvegetarian diet reduced systolic blood pressure by 5 mmHg but not diastolic blood pressure; sodium and potassium intakes appeared similar in the vegetarian and nonvegetarian diets. Still, neither trial tightly controlled these aspects of the diets. In a series of small trials, exchanging meat and eggs for vegetable products and reducing saturated fat had no significant impact on blood pressure.[9,18]

In summary, both observational studies and clinical trials indicate that adoption of a vegetarian diet can lower blood pressure. It is likely that the effects on blood pressure result from several factors. While vegetarians tend to weigh less than nonvegetarians and tend to consume more potassium, other aspects of vegetarian diet, yet to be elucidated, also contribute to the blood pressure–lowering effects of these diets.

MEDITERRANEAN-STYLE DIETS

In view of the heterogeneous cultures and agricultural patterns of the Mediterranean region, the "Mediterranean" diet is a not a single diet. Rather, this term applies to dietary patterns that emphasize fruits, vegetables, bread, cereals, potatoes, beans, nuts, and seeds; that include olive oil, dairy products, fish, poultry, wine, and eggs; and that are reduced in red meat.[19] As such, these diets tend to be low in saturated fat and high in monounsaturated fat, fiber, and folic acid.[20] Although detailed information on the nutrient composition of Mediterranean diets is sparse, such diets are presumably rich in other nutrients, such as potassium. Despite the difficulties of characterizing a Mediterranean-style diet, interest in such diets is considerable because of their apparent health benefits, particularly a reduced risk of coronary heart disease. Recent observational studies have documented that the reduced risk of coronary heart disease from a Mediterranean-style diet extends to the general population,[21] those with prior coronary heart disease,[22] and older-aged adults.[23]

In addition to reducing the risk of coronary heart disease, Mediterranean-style diets appear to reduce blood pressure. Early evidence came from the landmark Seven Countries Study. Specifically, in parts of Greece where traditional diets are eaten, the prevalence of hypertension was half that of Western Europe and the United States.[24] Subsequently, a cross-sectional study of 1154 Greek women and 1128 Greek men free of cardiovascular disease documented that consumption of a Mediterranean-style diet was associated with a 26% reduced prevalence of hypertension, even after controlling for potential confounders.[25]

In a recent observational study, the Greek European Investigation into Cancer and Nutrition (EPIC) study, greater adherence to a Mediterranean diet was associated with lower blood pressure.[26] In this study, higher blood pressure was associated with a lower intake of olive oil, fruit, and vegetables, and a higher intake of meat, meat products, and cereals. The authors speculate that the high salt intake of cereals accounted for the direct association of cereal intake with blood pressure.

Few trials have tested the effects of Mediterranean-style diets on blood pressure. In one small-scale study that enrolled nonhypertensive adults residing in southern Italy, replacement of their usual diet with a diet increased in saturated fats and reduced in monounsaturated fat and carbohydrate led to an increase in blood pressure.[27] A modified Mediterranean-style diet with increased α-linolenic acid had no effect on blood pressure in the Lyon Diet Heart Study.[28,29]

THE DASH-STYLE DIETARY PATTERNS

In the early 1990s, when the DASH research effort was initiated, the well-established, dietary determinants of blood pressure were weight, salt, and alcohol. However, several lines of evidence suggested that other dietary factors likely influence blood pressure. As discussed previously, vegetarian diets were associated with lower blood pressure in both observational studies and clinical trials. In other observational studies, an increased intake of potassium, calcium, magnesium, fiber, and protein were each associated with lower blood pressure. Still, in clinical trials in which these nutrients were tested separately, reductions in blood pressure were typically small and/or inconsistent.

In this setting, the original DASH trial tested whether modification of whole dietary patterns might affect blood pressure.[30] The DASH trial tested two hypotheses: (1) that increased intake of fruits and vegetables lowers blood pressure, and (2) that an overall healthy dietary pattern (initially known as the "combination" diet, now called the "DASH" diet) lowers blood pressure. The DASH trial was the first of a series of three large, controlled feeding studies testing the effects of dietary patterns on blood pressure. Subsequently, the DASH-Sodium trial[4] tested the main and interactive effects of sodium reduction and dietary patterns, while the OmniHeart trial[31] determined whether partial substitution of carbohydrate with protein or monounsaturated fat could further lower blood pressure.

In contrast to previous diet–blood pressure trials, which often were supplement trials or behavioral intervention studies, the DASH trial was a feeding study, in which participants received all of their food for 11 weeks. After a 3-week run-in on a control diet that is typical of what many Americans eat, participants were randomized to eat for 8 weeks one of the following three diets: (1) continuation of the control diet, (2) a "fruits and vegetables" diet, or (3) the DASH diet. The DASH diet emphasized fruits, vegetables, and low-fat dairy products; included whole grains, poultry, fish and nuts; and was reduced in fats, red meat, sweets, and sugar-containing beverages (Table 8–1). This diet was rich in potassium, magnesium,

calcium, and fiber, and was reduced in total fat, saturated fat, and cholesterol; it was also somewhat increased in protein, because previous observational studies had noted an inverse association of protein intake with blood pressure.[32,33] The control diet had a nutrient composition that was typical of that consumed by many Americans at the time the trial was designed. Its potassium, magnesium, and calcium levels were comparatively low, while its macronutrient profile and fiber content corresponded to average U.S. consumption. The fruits and vegetables diet was rich in potassium, magnesium, and fiber, but otherwise similar to the control diet, that is, the macronutrient profile of the fruits and vegetables diet and the control diet were similar.

All three diets contained similar amounts of sodium (approximately 3000 mg/day). Energy intake was adjusted to maintain body weight. Permissible alcohol intake during the trial was no more than two drinks per day. In this fashion, the study directly controlled the major, established dietary determinants of blood pressure (salt, weight, and alcohol).

DASH participants were 459 adults with prehypertension or stage 1 hypertension, that is, a systolic blood pressure of less than 160 mmHg and diastolic blood pressure of 80 to 95 mmHg (not on medication). The mean age was 45 years, average blood pressure was 131/85 mmHg, and 29% had stage 1 hypertension (systolic blood pressure 140–159 mmHg and/or diastolic blood pressure 90–95 mmHg). By design, African Americans comprised 60% of the population.

Among all participants, the DASH diet significantly lowered mean systolic blood pressure by 5.5 mmHg and mean diastolic blood pressure by 3.0 mmHg. The fruits and vegetables diet also significantly reduced blood pressure but to a lesser extent, about 50% of the effect of the DASH diet. Such findings are consistent with other studies, which indicate that increased fruit and vegetable intake can lower blood pressure.[14,15] The effect of the DASH diet was relatively rapid; the full effect was apparent at 2 weeks and was sustained until the end of feeding 6 weeks later (see Figure 8–2). In subgroup analyses, the DASH diet significantly lowered blood pressure in all major subgroups (blacks, nonblacks, men, women, hypertensives, and nonhypertensives). However, the effects of the DASH diet in black participants (6.9/3.7 mmHg) were significantly greater than corresponding effects in nonblack participants (3.3/2.4 mmHg). The effects in hypertensive individuals (11.6/5.3 mmHg) were particularly striking and were significantly greater than the effects in nonhypertensive (3.5/2.2 mmHg) individuals.[34]

Results from the DASH trial have led some individuals to question the importance of established dietary risk factors for elevated blood pressure. To this end, the subsequent DASH-Sodium trial provided convincing empirical support for recommendations to simultaneously implement sodium reduction with the DASH diet. The DASH-Sodium trial tested the effects of sodium reduction and the DASH diet, alone and combined, on blood pressure. While sodium reduction alone and the DASH diet alone each lowered blood pressure, the combination of sodium reduction with the DASH diet led to the largest blood

NUTRIENT TARGETS AND AVERAGE DAILY SERVINGS OF FOOD GROUPS BY DIET IN DASH TRIAL[a]			
	Control Diet	Fruits and Vegetables Diet	DASH Diet
Nutrients			
Fat (% kcal)	37	37	27
Saturated fat	16	16	6
Monounsaturated fat	13	13	13
Polyunsaturated fat	8	8	8
Carbohydrates (% kcal)	48	48	55
Protein (% kcal)	15	15	18
Cholesterol (mg/day)	300	300	150
Fiber (g/day)	9	31	31
Potassium (mg/day)	1700	4700	4700
Magnesium (mg/day)	165	500	500
Calcium (mg/day)	450	450	1240
Sodium (mg/day)	3000	3000	3000
Servings of Food Groups (servings/day)			
Fruits and juices	1.6	5.2	5.2
Vegetables	2.0	3.3	4.4
Grains	8.2	6.9	7.5
Low-fat dairy	0.1	0.0	2.0
Regular-fat dairy	0.4	0.3	0.7
Nuts, seeds, and legumes	0.0	0.6	0.7
Beef, pork, and ham	1.5	1.8	0.5
Poultry	0.8	0.4	0.6
Fish	0.2	0.3	0.5
Fat, oils, and salad dressing	5.8	5.3	2.5
Snacks and sweets	4.1	1.4	0.7

Adapted from Appel LJ, Moore TJ, Obarzanek E, Vollmer WM, Svetkey LP, Sacks FM, et al. *N Engl J Med* 1997;336(16):1117–24. Copyright 1997 Massachusetts Medical Society.

DASH, Dietary Approaches to Stop Hypertension.

[a]For 2100-kcal energy level.

Table 8–1. Nutrient Targets and Average Daily Servings of Food Groups by Diet in DASH Trial[a]

pressure reductions.[4] Overall, adoption of the DASH diet should supplement, rather than supplant, established lifestyle changes to reduce blood pressure.

The DASH diet, as well as the diets studied in OmniHeart trial (discussed later), are safe and broadly applicable to the general population. However, because of their relatively high potassium, phosphorus, and protein content, these diets are not recommended in persons with stage 3 or 4 chronic kidney disease, that is, an estimated glomerular filtration rate of less than 60 mL/min/1.73 m²².[35]

Speculation about the effective (and ineffective) components of the DASH diet has been considerable. The diet that emphasized fruits and vegetables resulted in blood pressure reductions that were approximately half of the total effect of the DASH diet. Fruits and vegetables are rich in potassium, magnesium, fiber, and many other nutrients. Of these nutrients, potassium is best established as a means to lower blood pressure, particularly in persons with low intake, in persons with hypertension, and in blacks.[36]

Aside from testing fruits and vegetables, the DASH trial was not designed to identify the specific nutrients and foods responsible for the observed reductions in blood pressure. Compared to the fruits and vegetables diet, the combination diet had more vegetables, low-fat dairy products, fish, calcium, protein, and complex carbohydrate, and was lower in saturated fat, monounsaturated fat, total fat, cholesterol, and red meat. Hence, inferences about the effects of specific nutrients and foods are largely speculative, and rely more on the interpretation of data from other studies than on results of the DASH trial itself.

While the blood pressure reductions from the DASH diet are impressive, it is plausible that this carbohydrate-rich dietary pattern can be improved by replacing some carbohydrate with either protein or monounsaturated fat. With this objective, the OmniHeart trial compared the effects of three healthy dietary patterns—a diet rich in carbohydrate (similar to the DASH diet), a second rich in protein (about half from plant sources), and a third diet

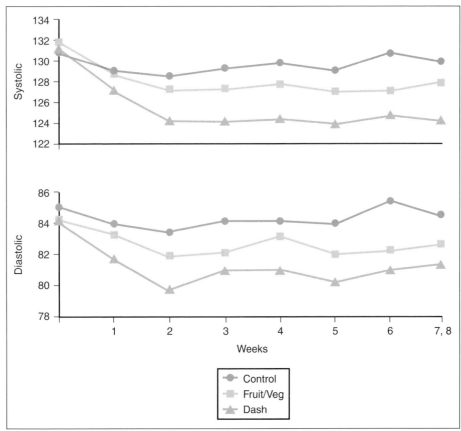

Figure 8–2. Blood pressure by week during the Dietary Approaches to Stop Hypertension feeding study in three diets (control diet, "fruits and vegetables diet," and "DASH diet"). (Adapted from Appel LJ, Moore TJ, Obarzanek E, Vollmer WM, Svetkey LP, Sacks FM, et al. *N Engl J Med* 1997;336(16):1117–24. Copyright 1997 Massachusetts Medical Society.)

rich in unsaturated fat (predominantly monounsaturated fat)[31] (Table 8–2). All three diets were reduced in saturated fat, cholesterol, and sodium, and rich in fruit, vegetables, fiber, potassium, and other minerals at recommended levels. As displayed in Figure 8–3, *A* and *B*, each diet lowered systolic blood pressure. Furthermore, substituting some of the carbohydrate (approximately 10% of total kilocalories) with either protein (about half from plant sources) or with unsaturated fat (mostly monounsaturated fat) further lowered blood pressure.

Results from the DASH, DASH-Sodium, and OmniHeart trials have important clinical and public health implications. The effect of DASH-style diets in hypertensives is similar in magnitude to drug monotherapy for hypertension. Hence, these dietary patterns should be an effective initial treatment for hypertension before prescription of drug therapy. Although none of the trials enrolled medication-treated hypertensives, DASH-style diets, similar to other effective lifestyle changes, should also be an effective adjuvant therapy.

From a public health perspective, DASH-style diets may be an effective means to prevent hypertension. In addition, adoption of a DASH-style diet could shift the population blood pressure distribution downward, thereby reducing the risk of blood pressure–related cardiovascular disease. It has been estimated that a population-wide reduction in blood pressure of the magnitude observed in

the DASH trial could reduce stroke incidence by 27% and coronary heart disease by 15%. In addition to reducing blood pressure, the DASH-style diets are nutrient-rich and meet each of the major nutrient recommendations established by the Institute of Medicine.[37,38]

DASH-Sodium and OmniHeart were controlled feeding studies. To determine the feasibility and effects of the DASH diet in the context of established lifestyle recommendations, the PREMIER trial tested the effects of two multifactorial interventions in comparison to an advice-only control group. One lifestyle intervention attempted to reduce weight, lower sodium intake, and increase physical activity. One of the interventions also included the DASH diet. Those assigned to the latter group increased their intake of fruits, vegetables, and dairy products but, in the contrast to the DASH feeding studies, did not achieve the nutrient and food group targets of the DASH diet. Still, the best blood pressure control was consistently observed in the group that also received the DASH diet.[39,40]

CARBOHYDRATE

A complex body of evidence suggests that both type and amount of carbohydrate affect blood pressure.[41] Worldwide, there are many societies that eat carbohydrate-rich, low-fat diets that have low blood pressure levels compared to Western populations.[42] Still, data from observational

NUTRIENT TARGETS AND AVERAGE DAILY SERVINGS OF FOODS BY DIET AT 2100 KCAL IN OMNIHEART TRIAL			
	CARB[b]	PROT	UNSAT
Nutrient Targets (% kcal)[a]			
Fat	27	27	*37*
Saturated fat	6	6	6
Monounsaturated fat	13	13	*21*
Polyunsaturated fat	8	8	*10*
Carbohydrate[c]	*58*	48	48
Protein[d]	15	*25*	15
Meat	5.5	9	5.5
Dairy	4	4	4
Plant	5.5	12	5.5
Food Groups (servings/day)			
Fruits and juices	6.6	3.8	4.8
Vegetables	4.4	5.4	6.3
Grains	5.3	5	4.2
Low-fat dairy products	1.4	2.3	1.6
High-fat dairy products	0.7	0.2	0.3
Legumes, nuts, seeds, and other vegetable protein	1.3	3	1.2
Beef, pork, and ham	0.9	1.1	1
Poultry	1.6	2.6	1.8
Fish	1.1	1.3	1
Egg product substitute	0.2	1.1	0.1
Desserts and sweets	4.6	2.5	1.7
Fats and oils	6	3.5	12

Adapted from Appel LJ, Sacks FM, Carey VJ, Obarzanek E, Swain JF, Miller ER 3rd, et al. *JAMA* 2005;294(19):2455–64.

[a]By design, the following nutrient targets were similar in each diet: cholesterol <150 mg/day, fiber ≥30 mg/day, sodium 2300 mg (100 mmol)/day, potassium 4700 mg (120 mmol)/day, magnesium 500 mg/day, and calcium 1200 mg/day.

[b]Nutrient targets in the DASH diet were identical to those in the CARB diet, except that in DASH, the proportion of kilocalories from protein was 18% and from carbohydrate was 55%. Bolded italic text highlights major differences between diets.

[c]The glycemic index of the three diets was moderate and similar (68 in CARB, 71 in PROT, and 75 in UNSAT).

[d]The average daily intake of soy protein was 0.5 g in CARB, 7.3 g in PROT, and 0.5 g in UNSAT.

CARB, similar to the DASH diet; *DASH*, Dietary Approaches to Stop Hypertension; *PROT*, rich in protein, about half from plant sources; *UNSAT*, rich in monounsaturated fat.

Table 8–2. Nutrient Targets and Average Daily Servings of Foods by Diet at 2100 kcal in OmniHeart Trial

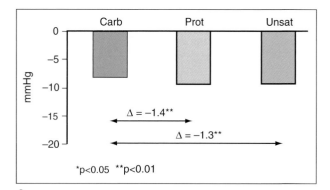

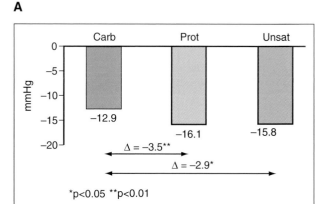

Figure 8–3. Effects of three healthy dietary patterns tested in the OmniHeart feeding study on systolic blood pressure in all participants (**A**) and in hypertensive participants (**B**). *CARB*, similar to the DASH diet; *PROT*, rich in protein, about half from plant sources; *UNSAT*, rich in monounsaturated fat. (Adapted from Appel LJ, Brands MW, Daniels SR, Karanja N, Elmer PJ, Sacks FM, et al. *Hypertension* 2006;47(2):296–308.)

studies that specifically examined the effect of carbohydrate intake on blood pressure have been inconsistent (direct in one study,[32] no association in another,[43] and inverse association in another[44]). In early trials, typically small, increasing carbohydrates by reducing total fat generally did not reduce blood pressure.[45] In contrast, the recently completed OmniHeart feeding study documented that in the setting of a healthy diet similar to the DASH diet, partial substitution of carbohydrate with either protein (about half from plant sources) or monounsaturated fat

lowers blood pressure; importantly, the type of carbohydrate in each diet, as indicated by the total dietary glycemic index, was moderate and virtually identical in each diet.[31]

Some trials have tested the effects of acute sugar consumption on blood pressure. In several[46,47] but not all studies,[48] consumption of sugars increased blood pressure. Consistent with these studies are results from a weight-loss trial in which a low glycemic index–diet reduced blood pressure to a greater extent than a standard high glycemic index.[49] Potential mechanisms for a direct effect on blood pressure include interactions with salt intake, promotion of salt retention,[46,50] and increased catecholamine production or release with stimulation of the sympathetic nervous system.[51–54] Overall, additional research is warranted prior to making specific recommendations about the amount and type of carbohydrates as a means to lower blood pressure.

PROTEIN

A paradigm shift has occurred regarding the effects of dietary protein intake on blood pressure. The prevailing belief regarding protein's effect on blood pressure has been that there is either no association[55] or a direct association.[8,42,56] As highlighted below, the best available evidence is that increased protein intake, particularly from plant sources, can lower blood pressure.

As reviewed by Obarzanek et al.[57] and subsequently by He and Whelton,[58] an extensive, and generally consistent, body of evidence from observational studies has documented significant inverse associations between protein intake and blood pressure. Observational studies also suggest that an increased protein intake, especially protein from plant sources, might prevent cardiovascular disease.[59,60] Among the earliest findings were observations from the 1970s and 1980s in Asian countries, especially Japan and China, in which there was an inverse association between protein intake and rates of hypertension and stroke.[61,62] Subsequently a large number of observational studies reproduced this relationship. Recently two major observational studies, the International Study on Macronutrients and Blood Pressure (INTERMAP) and the Chicago Western Electric Study, documented significant inverse relationships between protein intake and blood pressure.[44,63] In these studies, protein from plant sources was associated with lower blood pressure, while protein from animal sources had no effect.

Some trials have also examined the effects of increased protein intake on blood pressure. Most of these trials tested soy-based interventions on blood pressure. In some but not all of these trials, soy supplementation replacing carbohydrates reduced blood pressure.[64,65] One of the most persuasive studies is a recent large trial conducted in China which documented that increased protein intake from soy supplements, replacing carbohydrates, lowered blood pressure.[66] In the recently completed OmniHeart study, partial substitution of carbohydrates with protein (about half from plant sources) lowered blood pressure.[31]

Several mechanisms by which protein might lower blood pressure have been proposed. One potential set of mechanisms focuses on the biological effects of constituent amino acids. Synthesis of catecholamines in the central nervous system is affected by the intake of tyrosine and phenylalanine.[67] Tyrosine[68] and tryptophan[69] lower blood pressure when injected intraperitoneally into animals. Histidine (a precursor for the synthesis of histamine) contributes to regulation of sympathetic nervous system[70] and dilation of peripheral vessels.[71] Arginine is the metabolic precursor of nitric oxide, a powerful vasodilator

EFFECTS OF DIETARY FACTORS AND DIETARY PATTERNS ON BLOOD PRESSURE: SUMMARY OF THE EVIDENCE		
	Hypothesized Effect	Evidence
Weight	Direct	++
Sodium chloride (salt)	Direct	++
Potassium	Inverse	++
Magnesium	Inverse	+/−
Calcium	Inverse	+/−
Alcohol	Direct	++
Vitamin C	Inverse	+/−
Fat		
Saturated fatty acids	Direct	+/−
Omega-3 polyunsaturated fatty acids	Inverse	++
Omega-6 polyunsaturated fatty acids	Inverse	+/−
Monounsaturated fatty acids	Inverse	+
Trans fatty acids	Uncertain	+/−
Protein		
Total protein	Uncertain	+
Vegetable protein	Inverse	+
Animal protein	Uncertain	+/−
Carbohydrate	Direct	+
Fiber	Inverse	+
Cholesterol	Direct	+/−
Dietary patterns		
Vegetarian diets	inverse	++
DASH-type dietary patterns	inverse	++
Mediterranean diets	inverse	+

Adapted from Appel LJ, Brands MW, Daniels SR, Karanja N, Elmer PJ, Sacks FM, et al. *Hypertension* 2006;47(2):296–308.

Key to evidence: +/− = limited or equivocal evidence; + = suggestive evidence, typically from observational studies and some clinical trials; ++ = persuasive evidence, typically from clinical trials.

DASH, Dietary Approaches to Stop Hypertension.

Table 8–3. Effects of Dietary Factors and Dietary Patterns on Blood Pressure: Summary of the Evidence

that acts on the endothelium.[72] According to Moncada and Higgs,[72] increased ingestion of arginine may reverse vascular reactivity changes and reduce intimal thickness in atherosclerosis, reduce the excessive proliferation of smooth muscle cells in hypertension, and lower blood pressure. Taurine may reduce blood pressure by natriuretic and diuretic effects in the kidney or inhibitory effects on the renin angiotensin system.[73] Alternatively or concomitantly, biologically active peptides (e.g., peptides with angiotensin-converting enzyme inhibitor activity) may lower blood pressure.[74]

In aggregate, data from clinical trials, in conjunction with evidence from animal studies and observational studies, support the hypothesis that substitution of carbohydrates with increased intake of protein, particularly from plants, can lower blood pressure. However, it remains uncertain whether the effects result from increased protein or reduced carbohydrate.

SUMMARY

A substantial body of evidence strongly supports the concept that multiple dietary factors affect blood pressure

(Table 8–3). Dietary modifications that effectively lower blood pressure are weight loss, reduced salt intake, increased potassium intake, and moderation of alcohol consumption (among those who drink). Available evidence is sufficiently strong to conclude that certain dietary patterns—specifically, DASH-style diets, vegetarian diets, and perhaps Mediterranean-style diets—also lower blood pressure. Substitution of carbohydrate with protein from plant sources or monounsaturated fat also reduces blood pressure. Other dietary factors may affect blood pressure, but the effects are small and/or the evidence is uncertain.

DASH-style diets, vegetarian diets, and Mediterranean-style diets, while distinctive, share several common features. Each is rich in fruits, vegetables, and other plant products such as nuts and seeds, and each is reduced in saturated fat and meats. Each diet has several variants, thereby enhancing their generalizability and appeal. Efforts to enhance the adoption of these dietary patterns are warranted in view of their beneficial effects on blood pressure and cardiovascular disease.

REFERENCES

1. Appel LJ, Brands MW, Daniels SR, Karanja N, Elmer PJ, Sacks FM, et al. Dietary approaches to prevent and treat hypertension: a scientific statement from the American Heart Association. *Hypertension* 2006;47(2):296–308.
2. Chalmers J, Morgan T, Doyle A, Dickson B, Hopper J, Mathews J, et al. Australian National Health and Medical Research Council dietary salt study in mild hypertension. *J Hypertens Suppl* 1986;4(6):S629–37.
3. Trials of Hypertension Prevention Collaborative Research Group. Effects of weight loss and sodium reduction intervention on blood pressure and hypertension incidence in overweight people with high-normal blood pressure. The Trials of Hypertension Prevention, Phase II. *Arch Intern Med* 1997;157(6):657–67.
4. Sacks FM, Svetkey LP, Vollmer WM, Appel LJ, Bray GA, Harsha D, et al. Effects on blood pressure of reduced dietary sodium and the Dietary Approaches to Stop Hypertension (DASH) diet. DASH-Sodium Collaborative Research Group. *N Engl J Med* 2001;344(1):3–10.
5. Berkow SE, Barnard ND. Blood pressure regulation and vegetarian diets. *Nutr Rev* 2005;63(1):1–8.
6. Poulter NR, Khaw K, Hopwood BE, Mugambi M, Peart WS, Sever PS. Determinants of blood pressure changes due to urbanization: a longitudinal study. *J Hypertens Suppl* 1985;3(3):S375–7.
7. He J, Klag MJ, Whelton PK, Chen JY, Mo JP, Qian MC, et al. Migration, blood pressure pattern, and hypertension: the Yi Migrant Study. *Am J Epidemiol* 1991;134(10):1085–101.

8. Armstrong B, van Merwyk AJ, Coates H. Blood pressure in Seventh-Day Adventist vegetarians. *Am J Epidemiol* 1977;105(5):444–9.
9. Sacks FM, Kass EH. Low blood pressure in vegetarians: effects of specific foods and nutrients. *Am J Clin Nutr* 1988;48(Suppl 3):795–800.
10. Key TJ, Fraser GE, Thorogood M, Appleby PN, Beral V, Reeves G, et al. Mortality in vegetarians and nonvegetarians: detailed findings from a collaborative analysis of 5 prospective studies. *Am J Clin Nutr* 1999;70(Suppl 3):516S–24S.
11. Melby CL, Goldflies DG, Hyner GC, Lyle RM. Relation between vegetarian/nonvegetarian diets and blood pressure in black and white adults. *Am J Public Health* 1989;79(9):1283–8.
12. Whelton PK, He J, Cutler JA, Brancati FL, Appel LJ, Follmann D, et al. Effects of oral potassium on blood pressure. Meta-analysis of randomized controlled clinical trials. *JAMA* 1997;277(20):1624–32.
13. Armstrong B, Clarke H, Martin C, Ward W, Norman N, Masarei J. Urinary sodium and blood pressure in vegetarians. *Am J Clin Nutr* 1979;32(12):2472–6.
14. John JH, Ziebland S, Yudkin P, Roe LS, Neil HA, Oxford Fruit and Vegetable Study Group. Effects of fruit and vegetable consumption on plasma antioxidant concentrations and blood pressure: a randomised controlled trial. *Lancet* 2002;359(9322):1969–74.
15. Alonso A, de la Fuente C, Martin-Arnau AM, de Irala J, Martinez JA, Martinez-Gonzalez MA. Fruit and vegetable consumption is inversely associated with blood pressure in a Mediterranean

population with a high vegetable-fat intake: the Seguimiento Universidad de Navarra (SUN) Study. *Br J Nutr* 2004;92(2):311–9.
16. Rouse IL, Beilin LJ, Armstrong BK, Vandongen R. Blood-pressure-lowering effect of a vegetarian diet: controlled trial in normotensive subjects. *Lancet* 1983;1(8314–5):5–10.
17. Margetts BM, Beilin LJ, Vandongen R, Armstrong BK. Vegetarian diet in mild hypertension: a randomised controlled trial. *BMJ (Clin Res Ed)* 1986;293(6560):1468–71.
18. Sacks FM, Marais GE, Handysides G, Salazar J, Miller L, Foster JM, et al. Lack of an effect of dietary saturated fat and cholesterol on blood pressure in normotensives. *Hypertension* 1984;6(2 Pt 1):193–8.
19. Kris-Etherton P, Eckel RH, Howard BV, St Jeor S, Bazzarre TL. AHA Science Advisory: Lyon Diet Heart Study. Benefits of a Mediterranean-style, National Cholesterol Education Program/American Heart Association Step I Dietary Pattern on Cardiovascular Disease. *Circulation* 2001;103(13):1823–5.
20. Kok FJ, Kromhout D. Atherosclerosis—epidemiological studies on the health effects of a Mediterranean diet. *Eur J Nutr* 2004;43(Suppl 1):I/2–5.
21. Trichopoulou A, Costacou T, Bamia C, Trichopoulos D. Adherence to a Mediterranean diet and survival in a Greek population. *N Engl J Med* 2003;348(26):2599–608.
22. Trichopoulou A, Bamia C, Trichopoulos D. Mediterranean diet and survival among patients with coronary heart disease in Greece. *Arch Intern Med* 2005;165(8):929–35.

23. Knoops KT, de Groot LC, Kromhout D, Perrin AE, Moreiras-Varela O, Menotti A, et al. Mediterranean diet, lifestyle factors, and 10-year mortality in elderly European men and women: the HALE project. *JAMA* 2004;292(12):1433–9.

24. Keys A. *Seven Countries: A Multivariate Analysis of Death and Coronary Heart Disease.* Cambridge, MA: Harvard University Press, 1980.

25. Panagiotakos DB, Pitsavos CH, Chrysohoou C, Skoumas J, Papadimitriou L, Stefanadis C, et al. Status and management of hypertension in Greece: role of the adoption of a Mediterranean diet: the Attica study. *J Hypertens* 2003;21(8):1483–9.

26. Psaltopoulou T, Naska A, Orfanos P, Trichopoulos D, Mountokalakis T, Trichopoulou A. Olive oil, the Mediterranean diet, and arterial blood pressure: the Greek European Prospective Investigation into Cancer and Nutrition (EPIC) study. *Am J Clin Nutr* 2004;80(4): 1012–8.

27. Struzzullo P, Ferro-Luzzi A, Siani A, et al. Changing the Mediterranean diet: effect on blood pressure. *J Hypertens* 1986;4:407–12.

28. de Lorgeril M, Renaud S, Mamelle N, Salen P, Martin JL, Monjaud I, et al. Mediterranean alpha-linolenic acid-rich diet in secondary prevention of coronary heart disease. *Lancet* 1994;343(8911): 1454–9 (see comments) (published erratum appears in *Lancet* 1995; 345(8951):738).

29. de Lorgeril M, Salen P, Martin JL, Monjaud I, Delaye J, Mamelle N. Mediterranean diet, traditional risk factors, and the rate of cardiovascular complications after myocardial infarction: final report of the Lyon Diet Heart Study. *Circulation* 1999;99(6):779–85.

30. Appel LJ, Moore TJ, Obarzanek E, Vollmer WM, Svetkey LP, Sacks FM, et al. A clinical trial of the effects of dietary patterns on blood pressure. DASH Collaborative Research Group. *N Engl J Med* 1997;336(16):1117–24.

31. Appel LJ, Sacks FM, Carey VJ, Obarzanek E, Swain JF, Miller ER 3rd, et al. Effects of protein, monounsaturated fat, and carbohydrate intake on blood pressure and serum lipids: results of the OmniHeart randomized trial. *JAMA* 2005; 294(19):2455–64.

32. Stamler J, Caggiula A, Grandits GA, Kjelsberg M, Cutler JA. Relationship to blood pressure of combinations of dietary macronutrients. Findings of the Multiple Risk Factor Intervention Trial (MRFIT). *Circulation* 1996;94(10): 2417–23.

33. Stamler J, Elliott P, Kesteloot H, Nichols R, Claeys G, Dyer AR, et al. Inverse relation of dietary protein markers with blood pressure. Findings for 10,020 men and women in the INTERSALT Study. INTERSALT Cooperative Research Group. International Study of Salt and Blood Pressure. *Circulation* 1996;94(7): 1629–34.

34. Svetkey LP, Simons-Morton D, Vollmer WM, Appel LJ, Conlin PR, Ryan DH, et al. Effects of dietary patterns on blood pressure: subgroup analysis of the Dietary Approaches to Stop Hypertension (DASH) randomized clinical trial. *Arch Intern Med* 1999; 159(3):285–93.

35. National Kidney Foundation. K/DOQI Clinical Practice Guidelines on Hypertension and Antihypertensive Agents in Chronic Kidney Disease. *Am J Kidney Dis* 2004;43(Suppl. 1):S1–290.

36. Brancati FL, Appel LJ, Seidler AJ, Whelton PK. Effect of potassium supplementation on blood pressure in African Americans on a low-potassium diet. A randomized, double-blind, placebo-controlled trial. *Arch Intern Med* 1996;156(1):61–7.

37. Institute of Medicine. *Dietary Reference Intakes for Energy, Carbohydrate, Fiber, Fat, Fatty Acids, Cholesterol, Protein, and Amino Acids.* Washington, DC: National Academy Press, 2002.

38. Institute of Medicine. *Dietary Reference Intakes: Water, Potassium, Sodium Chloride, and Sulfate.* Washington, DC: National Academy Press, 2004.

39. Appel LJ, Champagne CM, Harsha DW, Cooper LS, Obarzanek E, Elmer PJ, et al. Effects of comprehensive lifestyle modification on blood pressure control: main results of the PREMIER clinical trial. *JAMA* 2003;289(16):2083–93.

40. Elmer PJ, Obarzanek E, Vollmer WM, Simons-Morton D, Stevens VJ, Rohm Young D, et al. Effects of comprehensive lifestyle modification on diet, weight, physical fitness, and blood pressure control: 18-month results of PREMIER, a randomized trial. *Ann Intern Med* 2006;144:485–95.

41. Hodges RE, Rebello T. Carbohydrates and blood pressure. *Ann Intern Med* 1983;98(5 Pt 2):838–41.

42. Sacks FM, Rosner B, Kass EH. Blood pressure in vegetarians. *Am J Epidemiol* 1974;100(5):390–8.

43. Reed D, McGee D, Yano K, Hankin J. Diet, blood pressure, and multicollinearity. *Hypertension* 1985;7(3 Pt 1):405–10.

44. Stamler J, Liu K, Ruth KJ, Pryer J, Greenland P. Eight-year blood pressure change in middle-aged men: relationship to multiple nutrients. *Hypertension* 1999;39(5):1000–6.

45. Morris MC. Dietary fats and blood pressure. *J Cardiovasc Risk* 1994;1(1): 21–30.

46. Rebello T, Hodges RE, Smith JL. Short-term effects of various sugars on antinatriuresis and blood pressure changes in normotensive young men. *Am J Clin Nutr* 1983;38(1):84–94.

47. Israel KD, Michaelis OE 4th, Reiser S, Keeney M. Serum uric acid, inorganic phosphorus, and glutamic-oxalacetic transaminase and blood pressure in carbohydrate-sensitive adults consuming three different levels of sucrose. *Ann Nutr Metab* 1983;27(5):425–35.

48. Visvanathan R, Chen R, Horowitz M, Chapman I. Blood pressure responses in healthy older people to 50 g carbohydrate drinks with differing glycaemic effects. *Br J Nutr* 2004; 92(2):335–40.

49. Pereira MA, Swain J, Goldfine AB, Rifai N, Ludwig DS. Effects of a low-glycemic load diet on resting energy expenditure and heart disease risk factors during weight loss. *JAMA* 2004; 292(20):2482–90.

50. Preuss HG. Interplay between sugar and salt on blood pressure in spontaneously hypertensive rats. *Nephron* 1994;68(3): 385–7.

51. Bunag RD, Tomita T, Sasaki S. Chronic sucrose ingestion induces mild hypertension and tachycardia in rats. *Hypertension* 1983;5(2):218–25.

52. Fournier RD, Chiueh CC, Kopin IJ, Knapka JJ, DiPette D, Preuss HG. Refined carbohydrate increases blood pressure and catecholamine excretion in SHR and WKY. *Am J Physiol* 1986; 250(4 Pt 1):E381–5.

53. Gradin K, Nissbrand H, Ehrenstom F, Henning M, Persson B. Adrenergic mechanisms during hypertension induced by sucrose and/or salt in the spontaneously hypertensive rat. *Naunyn Schmiedebergs Arch Pharmacol* 1988;337(1):47–52.

54. Young JB, Landsberg L. Stimulation of the sympathetic nervous system during sucrose feeding. *Nature* 1977;269(5629):615–7.

55. Meyer TW, Anderson S, Brenner BM. Dietary protein intake and progressive glomerular sclerosis: the role of capillary hypertension and hyperperfusion in the progression of renal disease. *Ann Intern Med* 1983;98(5 Pt 2):832–8.

56. McCarron DA, Henry HJ, Morris CD. Human nutrition and blood pressure regulation: an integrated approach. *Hypertension* 1982;4(5 Pt 2):III2–13.

57. Obarzanek E, Velletri PA, Cutler JA. Dietary protein and blood pressure. *JAMA* 1996;275(20):1598–603.

58. He J, Whelton PK. Effect of dietary fiber and protein intake on blood pressure: a review of epidemiologic evidence. *Clin Exp Hypertens* 1999;21(5–6):785–96.

59. Hu FB, Stampfer MJ, Manson JE, Rimm E, Colditz GA, Speizer FE, et al. Dietary protein and risk of ischemic heart disease in women. *Am J Clin Nutr* 1999;70(2):221–7 (see comments).

60. Kelemen LE, Kushi LH, Jacobs DR Jr, Cerhan JR. Associations of dietary protein with disease and mortality in a prospective study of postmenopausal women. *Am J Epidemiol* 2005;161(3): 239–49.

61. Liu LS. Hypertension studies in China. *Clin Exp Hypertens* 1989;11(5–6):859–68.

62. Yamori Y, Horie R, Nara Y, Kihara M, Ikeda K, Mano M, et al. Dietary prevention of hypertension in animal models and its applicability to human. *Ann Clin Res* 1984;16 Suppl 43:28–31.

63. Elliott P, Stamler J, Appel L, Dennis B, Dyer AR, Kesteloot H, et al. Relationship of dietary protein to blood pressure: the INTERMAP Study. *Arch Intern Med* 2006;166:79–87.

64. Teede HJ, Dalais FS, Kotsopoulos D, Liang YL, Davis S, McGrath BP. Dietary soy has both beneficial and potentially adverse cardiovascular effects: a placebo-controlled study in men and postmenopausal women. *J Clin Endocrinol Metab* 2001;86(7): 3053–60.

65. Burke V, Hodgson JM, Beilin LJ, Giangiulioi N, Rogers P, Puddey IB. Dietary protein and soluble fiber reduce ambulatory blood pressure in treated hypertensives. *Hypertension* 2001;38(4): 821–6.

66. He J, Gu D, Wu X, Chen J, Duan X, Chen J, et al. Effect of soybean protein on blood pressure: a randomized, controlled trial. *Ann Intern Med* 2005; 143(1):1–9.

67. Anderson GH. Proteins and amino acids: effects on the sympathetic nervous system and blood pressure regulation. *Can J Physiol Pharmacol* 1986;64(6):863–70.

68. Sved AF, Fernstrom JD, Wurtman RJ. Tyrosine administration reduces blood pressure and enhances brain norepinephrine release in spontaneously hypertensive rats. *Proc Natl Acad Sci U S A* 1979;76(7):3511–4.

69. Sved AF, Van Itallie CM, Fernstrom JD. Studies on the antihypertensive action of L-tryptophan. *J Pharmacol Exp Ther* 1982;221(2):329–33.

70. Akins VF, Bealer SL. Central nervous system histamine regulates peripheral sympathetic activity. *Am J Physiol* 1991;260(1 Pt 2):H218–24.

71. Bender DA. Histidine. In: Bender DA, et al., eds. *Amino Acid Metabolism.* 2nd ed. Chichester: John Wiley, 1985: 188–200.

72. Moncada S, Higgs A. The L-arginine–nitric oxide pathway. *N Engl J Med* 1993;329:2003–12.

73. Martin DS. Dietary protein and hypertension: where do we stand? *Nutrition* 2003;19(4):385–6.

74. FitzGerald RJ, Murray BA, Walsh DJ. Hypotensive peptides from milk proteins. *J Nutr* 2004;134(4):980S–8S.

PATHOGENESIS

*Joey P. Granger and
Leong L. Ng*

Chapter
9
Renovascular Hypertension: Pathophysiology and Evaluation of Renal Function

Sabas I. Gomez, John A. Haas, and J. Carlos Romero

Definition

Renovascular hypertension (RVH) is the elevation of blood pressure (BP) that follows the incomplete occlusion of one or both renal arteries.

In humans, the partial occlusion of one renal artery is produced by fibromuscular dysplasia or atherosclerosis.

In animals, RVH is induced by constricting the renal artery with a clamp or with a stent that induces intimal arterial hyperplasia.

Key Findings

- Experimental reduction of renal perfusion pressure (RPP) leads to an initial increase in plasma renin activity (PRA) that correlates with both the degree of the stenosis and the increase in blood pressure. In a later phase, plasma renin activity is "normalized" at the same time that there is a progressive elevation of oxidative stress, which from that point on correlates with the increase of BP.

- The increase in BP tends to restore renal blood flow (RBF) in the stenotic kidney and it increases RPP in the contralateral kidney, producing a compensatory natriuresis. This equilibrium could persist for years when the stenosis is mild.

- In cases with severe stenosis, the increase in BP needed to restore RBF is so large that it is followed by cardiac insufficiency and volume depletion (through natriuresis in the contralateral kidney), which lead to renal failure.

- Unilateral constriction of a renal artery produces a decrease in renal volume on the stenotic side, while it increases the volume of the contralateral kidney. In the stenotic kidney, the degree of the stenosis correlates with a fall in RBF, glomerular filtration rate (GFR), tubular sodium load, and sodium excretion. In the contralateral kidney, there is a marked opposite directional change in all of these parameters.

- This sequence of events is reproduced by the intravenous infusion of small subpressor doses of angiotensin II (Ang II), which stimulates the production of oxidative stress and chronically increases BP in the same fashion as that seen in RVH.

- Slow pressor responses are greatly facilitated by sodium overload. Sodium depletion abolishes slow pressor responses along with the "side effects" of angiotensin such as cardiac hypertrophy, inflammation, or stimulation of oxidative stress.

- All changes in renal hemodynamics and renal tubular function can be estimated with three-dimensional computerized tomography that has high temporal resolution.

Clinical Implications

- Accurate determinations of changes in renal hemodynamic and tubular function in both the stenotic and contralateral kidneys plus the level of oxygen consumption with BOLD-MRI will allow the clinician to evaluate renal function more accurately as well as better determine the efficacy of revascularization on medical treatment.

In 1937, Goldblatt et al.[1,2] demonstrated that in the dog, constriction of one renal artery (two-kidney, one-clip Goldblatt hypertension, or 2KD-1CGH) without disturbing the contralateral kidney is followed by a significant increase in mean arterial pressure (MAP). However, the mechanisms responsible for hypertension in this model are still debatable.[3–5] These problems, along with the lack of knowledge about the specific changes induced in the stenotic kidney by arterial constriction, as well as in the contralateral kidney by the development of hyperplasia, has made it difficult to assess renal function, and thereby to predict the clinical outcomes of surgical interventions or medical treatments that are directed to correct the stenosis[6–8] or to reduce hypertension by medical treatment.

This chapter examines new developments in the pathogenesis of renovascular hypertension that have been obtained by the application of novel x-ray and magnetic resonance imaging (MRI) techniques.

EFFECTS OF RENAL ARTERIAL CONSTRICTION ON RENAL HEMODYNAMICS AND SODIUM EXCRETION

In the stenotic kidney, the acute decrease of renal perfusion pressure (RPP) below the range of autoregulation (<75 mmHg), is accompanied by a proportional and transient decrease in renal blood flow (RBF) and glomerular filtration rate (GFR),[9,10] and by a very prominent fall in tubular fluid dynamics (TFD) and urinary sodium excretion.[11,12] These changes are followed by a significant increase in the renal content of renin[13] and plasma renin activity (PRA).[3,10,14,15] These elevations of PRA are most likely responsible for the immediate increase in sodium retention and in MAP (about 20 to 40 mmHg, depending on the severity of the stenosis), which reaches a plateau and stabilizes within the following 2 weeks.[10,15] In fact, during the acute phase of hypertension, PRA correlates with the increase in MAP,[10,16] while the administration of angiotensin II (Ang II) converting enzyme or Ang II receptor antagonists produces a rapid (<1 hour) normalization of MAP.[17–19] This increase of MAP does not affect RBF or GFR in the contralateral kidney because of a vasoconstrictor response due to renal autoregulation.[11,12] Pressure natriuresis in the contralateral kidney is significantly increased; however, it is blunted by the antinatriuretic effect of high levels of circulating Ang II.[4,20] Under these conditions, a rather unstable equilibrium is reached where the hypertension and antinatriuresis due to activation of the renin-angiotensin system (RAS) improves perfusion of the stenotic kidney without imposing a significant functional load on the contralateral kidney.[10] This marks the transition to stable chronic phase (Figure 9–1, A), which equilibrium can be broken by changes in the degree of stenosis and/or in fluid volumes. For example, in well-controlled studies, Ferrario et al.[21] and Leenen and de Jong[22] showed that in animals with mild renal stenosis, RBF was restored with moderate elevations of systemic blood pressure (BP), while the animals with severe renal artery stenosis required very high levels of BP. This increase of BP overwhelms the antinatriuretic effects of Ang II, producing a marked increase in sodium excretion in the contralateral kidney. This response could lead to volume depletion and a significant fall in MAP, which stimulates more release of renin inducing an even more pronounced vasoconstriction. All of these changes could easily precipitate renal failure (Figure 9–1, B). Wilson et al.[23] were the first to characterize this vicious circle in rabbits, which was later on studied in more detail by Möhring et al.[24] in rats, while Barraclough[25] showed that this outcome could occur in humans. This response,

similar to that occurring in the chronic phase of 2KD-1CGH, represents a compromise between the level of increase in BP (which is needed to restore the function in the stenotic kidney) and the ability of the contralateral kidney to maintain fluid volume in spite of pressure-induced natriuresis.[5,10,26] Such equilibrium is an important feature because the tendency toward volume depletion will render hypertension almost entirely dependent on the levels of plasma renin. In these circumstances, high BP can be normalized by blocking Ang II.

On the contrary, excessive sodium retention or an amount of sodium retention inappropriate to the existing levels of Ang II will render hypertension very dependent on volume or oxidative stress and endothelin,[27] while blockade of the RAS will have a smaller effect[17,19] on both oxidative stress and endothelin, and on MAP. This assumption is well illustrated by a study we conducted to assess the role of Ang II and sodium intake in rabbits having severe and moderate 2KD-1CGH.[28] In these animals, severe hypertension (BP increased from control levels of 80±3 mmHg to 117±3 mmHg) occurred with high levels of plasma renin activity (21.6 ng/mL/h). This was accompanied by high levels of plasma creatinine and ECFV depletion (as measured with inulin). Correction of volume depletion with a high-sodium diet for 10 days decreased PRA, while BP fell from 117±3 to 98±2.5 mmHg and also improved plasma creatinine. The same effect was obtained after intravenous administration of 1000 ng/kg/min of saralasin (a peptide analog that blocks Ang II). In contrast, moderate 2KD-1CGH, which elicited a BP level of 97±2 mmHg, was not altered by a high-sodium diet, volume expansion, or angiotensin antagonist (Figure 9–2). In this study, there was no attempt to define the effects of volume depletion. However, in pilot studies, volume depletion with diuretics failed to increase BP in moderately hypertensive rabbits, in spite of a very signifi-

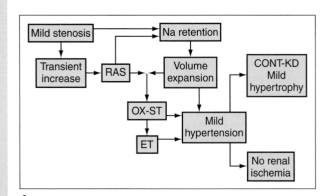

A

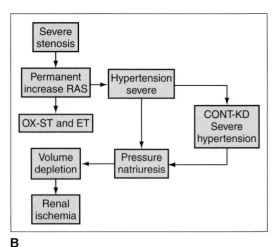

B

Figure 9–1. Effects of mild (**A**) and severe (**B**) stenosis during the development of unilateral renovascular hypertension. In mild stenosis, the increase in systemic blood pressure is sufficient to restore renal circulation in the stenotic kidney, but is not enough to provoke in the contralateral kidney pressure natriuresis, thus reaching an equilibrium. This is in contrast with the effect of severe stenosis (**B**), which needs a very significant elevation of blood pressure to restore the perfusion of the stenotic kidney. This induces pressure natriuresis, which is followed by volume depletion that aggravates renal ischemia; the most likely outcome of this latter decompensation is renal insufficiency. CONT-KD, contralateral kidney; ET, endothelin; OX-ST, oxidative stress; RAS, renal artery stenosis.

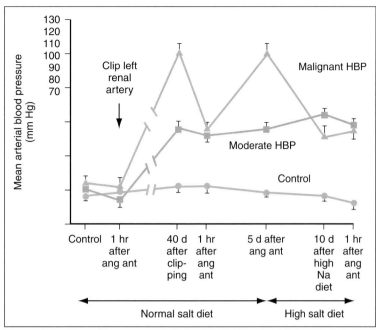

Figure 9–2. Effect of intravenous infusion of angiotensin II[1,8] (ang ant) on normotensive rabbits and after the development of renovascular hypertension during normal and high salt intake. Vertical bars represent mean plus standard error.

cant increase in PRA. These may be due to the fact that the increase in PRA, produced by diuretics, is secondary to volume depletion, whereas in the development of severe RVH, the increase in PRA occurs first and volume depletion is secondary to hypertension (pressure natriuresis). Discussion about the possibility of activating a secondary hypertensive mechanism has relied upon the assumption that the level of Ang II is inappropriate with the existing fluid volumes or vice versa.[27] However, the significance of circulating levels of Ang II remains ill defined. Nishiyama et al.[29] and van Kats et al.[30] have shown that the infusion of minute amounts of Ang II is rapidly accumulated in the kidney yielding cortical and medullary levels that were 20 and 19 times higher, respectively, than the concentration in plasma.[29] These results raise a question on the extent to which the inverse correlation that exists between circulating plasma Ang II and extracellular fluid volumes may be less significant than the relationship between the intrarenal concentration of Ang II (in renal interstitium) versus renal interstitial pressure. As pointed out in an extensive review on this subject, the interstitial pressure of the kidney is highly positively correlated with changes in extracellular fluid volumes.[27]

Finally, it should be emphasized that high levels of circulating Ang II do not necessarily stimulate oxidative stress, as occurs in severe sodium restriction. In order for Ang II to stimulate oxidative stress, the levels should be inappropriately high with respect to fluid volumes. Under these conditions, there is a reduction of nitric oxide (NO) and a production of significant levels of peroxynitrites and isoprostanes (ISOP).[27] These changes appear to favor an increase in the synthesis of endothelin which could be stimulated by Ang II or by some components of oxidative stress.[31,32] In this manner, the decrease in the concen-

tration of the vasodilator NO with a concomitant elevation of ISOP and endothelin will significantly enhance the vasoconstrictor effect of Ang II, which explains the slow pressor response, or they may sustain hypertension *per se* without a prominent participation of Ang II.[27]

There are some additional aspects with respect to the equilibrium among Ang II, sodium balance, oxidative stress, and endothelin that deserve comment. In the majority of cases, the functional equilibrium between the stenotic kidney and the contralateral kidney is achieved and can last for years, during which the effects of high BP on the contralateral kidney are characterized by development of progressive arterial hyperplasia, glomerular obsolescence, renal hyperplasia, and nephrosclerosis.[33] Meanwhile, the stenotic kidney undergoes vascular and tubular atrophy and mitotic hyperplastic transformation with different degrees of inflammation.[26,34] All these anatomic alterations in both kidneys are assumed to be accompanied by specific changes in tissue perfusion index (TPI=milliliters of blood per gram of tissue), RBF distribution, and TFF in superficial and deep nephrons. In the past, these changes have only been partially assessed by micropuncture studies in superficial nephrons.[26,35,36] We intend in this overview to examine the results of recent studies performed with the use of novel noninvasive computerized tomography with high temporal resolution. This technique has allowed evaluation of the specific hemodynamic and tubular functional changes that coexist with defined renal anatomic alterations in each kidney. Renal ischemia is measured indirectly by estimating with MRI the renal levels of deoxyhemoglobin (dHb), and allows a significant advance in diagnosis of the stenosis, and more accurate predictability of successful stenosis repair or revascularization.

ROLE OF RENIN-ANGIOTENSIN SYSTEM

Earlier studies reported that the inhibition of Ang II formation with converting enzyme inhibitor (CEI) produced a significant decrease of MAP only when administered in the early phase of 2KD-1CGH (within the first 2 weeks).[4,17–19] However, no immediate effects on BP (1 to 2 hours) were noticed when these maneuvers were performed in the chronic phase (more than 4 weeks) of hypertension.[19,26] These results were interpreted as indicating that the early phase of 2KD-1CGH was "renin dependent," while another mechanism was responsible for the maintenance of hypertension in the chronic phase.[26] At that time, some investigators thought that in the chronic phase of hypertension, the increase in total peripheral resistance was due to arteriolar hyperplasia. However, this assumption was not supported by experimental evidence showing that chronic hypertension was completely reversed by removing the renal arterial constriction or by removal of the clipped kidney.[23,37] Furthermore, Miller et al.[38] showed that the chronic phase of 2KD-1CGH was blunted if the formation of Ang II was inhibited prior to the constriction of the renal artery with CEI. These observations in animals have correlative observations in humans.[39–41] In general, the Sixth Report of the Joint National Committee on Prevention, Detection, Evaluation, and Treatment of High Blood Pressure (JNC 6) explicitly recognizes the potential for BP reduction to slow the progression of renal disease in essential hypertension. Nonetheless, the major stumbling block in RVH (as opposed to essential hypertension) is that the reduction of systemic pressure can aggravate the underperfusion of the stenotic kidney,[42] particularly when the therapy is supplemented by diuretics.[42,43] However, reduction of BP is very beneficial in the contralateral kidney.[43–45] In one of these studies, the administration of Ang II converting enzyme produced a shrinking of the stenotic kidney with fibrosis and marked atrophy (called medical nephrectomy) while the structure and function of the contralateral kidney were preserved.[46] The damage in the stenotic kidney was not attributed to the effect of BP reductions because it was not seen during administration of minoxidil; however, the beneficial effects of BP reduction in the contralateral kidney were more evident with CEI than with minoxidil.[46] The lack of information about oxidative stress and endothelin and the relative effects on these processes produced by CEI or minoxidil make interpretation of the results difficult. In general, all other studies show that there is great variability of antihypertensive treatments to restore BP or renal function.[42]

THE SO-CALLED SLOW PRESSOR RESPONSES TO ANGIOTENSIN II

The reasons for the variable efficacy of CEI and Ang II antagonist to lower BP during the chronic phase of Goldblatt hypertension are consistent with the fact that the levels of PRA are within the range found in normotensive animals.[10,15,19,47,48] The occasional hypotensive response to CEI has been explained by assuming that the

blockade of ACE (which is also a kininase II) produces simultaneously an accumulation of (unmetabolized) bradykinin. However, experimental data have failed to support this assumption.[49]

Another possibility to explain how normal levels of Ang II maintain high levels of BP in 2KD-1CGH is that Ang II activates an independent vasoconstrictor mechanism that initially potentiates its pressor effect and that later on may act, to a certain extent, independent of Ang II. In fact, it has been shown that the intravenous infusion of a small (subpressor) concentration of Ang II, one not sufficient to acutely produce any significant increase in BP, induces very sustained hypertension when given for several days.[20,50] This response should be distinguished from the "fast pressor responses," which are characterized by a rapid elevation of BP (reaching a maximal response in 1 to 2 minutes) that follows the infusion of large doses (60 to 800 ng/mL/kg) of Ang II.[51] In contrast, the "slow or indirect pressor effect" developed progressively and may reach a maximum following 7 to 10 days of intravenous infusion.[4,20,52,53] In a study conducted by Brown et al.,[53] it was shown that the infusion of 10 ng/kg/min of Ang II to normotensive rats increases BP by 40 mmHg, reaching a plateau on the 7th day of infusion. These levels of BP could only be reached in normotensive rats by the rapid infusions of 270 ng/kg/min of Ang II, in which case the circulating levels of Ang II measured 1 minute after was approximately 2220 pg/mL of Ang II. In contrast, the rats with a chronic infusion of Ang II, having a similar level of hypertension, exhibited circulating levels of Ang II (230 pg/mL) that were slightly elevated with respect to those recorded in normotensive untreated rats (150 pg/mL). Blockade of Ang II with Ang II receptor antagonist produced, in the group chronically infused with Ang II, a reversal of hypertension in the following 7 hours. These studies have been confirmed and extended by Hu et al.[54] who showed that slow responses can be induced not only by Ang II (3 ng/kg/min), but also by very minute amounts (0.3 ng/kg/min) of recombinant renin.[54] Under these conditions, the levels of circulating Ang II (6±2 ng/mL) do not differ from those measured during the control period (5±2 ng/mL)[54] (Figure 9–3). Because of the time required for the development of the slow responses, it is tempting to postulate that this phenomenon occurs after the initial phase (1 week) in the development of RVH, and that the chronic phase is better characterized by the increase in oxidative stress and endothelin.

SODIUM BALANCE

Brunner et al.[55] have shown that the physiologic levels of PRA correlate inversely with the amount of sodium intake in normotensive or hypertensive patients. This relationship indicates that for any given level of sodium intake, the existing levels of Ang II and NO are within the range needed to maintain sodium balance and normal arterial pressure. Reciprocally, one can also say that any plasma level of PRA that is within the normal range can induce hypertension if it is inappropriately high with respect to fluid volume. These characteristics have been eloquently

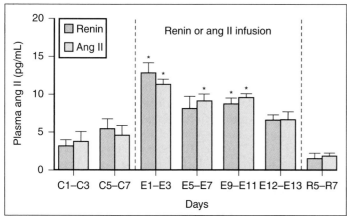

Figure 9–3. Plasma angiotensin II (vertical axis) level during renin (orange bars) or angiotensin (green bars) infusions of 3 ng of angiotensin per minute. *$p<0.05$ versus control period. C, control days; E, experimental days; R, recovery days.

exposed by the studies of DeClue et al.,[56] who showed that if circulating levels of Ang II are clamped by a continuous infusion of Ang II at the rate of 5 ng/kg/min, then the level of BP is determined by the amount of sodium intake (Figure 9–4). Moreover, under similar conditions where circulating levels of Ang II have been clamped (5 ng/kg/min), and the intake of sodium chloride has been set at 500 mEq/day, administration of a diuretic (furosemide) tends to normalize BP by reducing fluid volumes (to levels that are presumably appropriate to the concentration of Ang II). Krieger and Cowley[57] lend support to the previous finding by showing that Ang II–induced hypertension can be prevented if volume expansion is prevented by controlling sodium intake.

The concept of excessive levels of Ang II with respect to the level of sodium intake was first introduced by Hollenberg et al.,[58] showing that some hypertensive individuals are incapable of lowering the level of renin activity during volume and expansion. They call this group "nonmodulators," and the alteration was corrected by the administration of CEIs because it brought the levels of Ang II to a level appropriate to the existing fluid volume. There is also evidence that the chronic phase of moderate RVH exhibits many of the characteristics of the slow pressor responses to Ang II. For example, during the first month of the development of hypertension, there is a significant correlation between the elevation of systemic plasma renin activity and the absolute increase in MAP from control levels. As mentioned previously, during this phase renin plays a predominant role in sustaining hypertension. In contrast, after 2 months of the development of hypertension, the levels of plasma renin activity are nearly normal and exhibit a very poor correlation with BP. In contrast, the circulating level of isoprostane, which as mentioned previously is a marker of oxidative stress, exhibits a poor correlation during the first month of the development of hypertension. However, after 2 months the level of circulating isoprostane is proportional and correlates with increases in BP. Interestingly, all the studies mentioned thus far indicate that the elements which participate in chronic phase of renovascular hypertension

may not be different than those participating in essential hypertension. In both forms of hypertension, the kidney plays an important role[59]—it evolves with normal levels of plasma renin or angiotensin, there is a secondary activation of oxidative stress, and both are characterized by an isolated increase in total peripheral resistance. These similarities have been emphasized by Hall.[60]

OXIDATIVE STRESS

Two of the major components of oxidative stress are superoxide and hydrogen peroxide (H_2O_2). Superoxide and H_2O_2 can be generated in many vascular cells, and are derived from NADPH oxidase, cyclooxygenase, lipoxygenase, heme oxygenases, peroxidases, and hemoproteins such as heme and hematin.[27] The mechanism(s) by which Ang II causes production of superoxide has not been entirely elucidated. However, Mollnau et al.[61] found that chronic (7 days) Ang II infusion increased expression of nox 1, gp91(phox), and p22(phox) subunits of NADPH oxidase via a protein kinase C mechanism.[27] This Ang II–mediated increase in the production of superoxide then sets into motion a series of events that play important roles in hypertension.

Under normal conditions (Figure 9–5, left), the superoxide that is produced in the cell combines with superoxide dismutase (SOD), which converts it to H_2O_2. H_2O_2 is further metabolized to H_2O by the action of catalase and glutathione peroxidase, but under pathologic conditions (Figure 9–5, right) when an oxidative environment is present in cells, H_2O_2 can be a source of hydroxyl radicals.[27] Also, under oxidative conditions, tetrahydrobiopterin (BH_4), a cofactor required for the NO synthase (NOS) activity, can

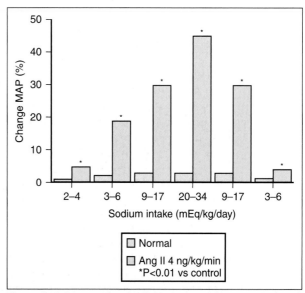

Figure 9–4. Percent changes in mean arterial pressure induced by progressive elevation of sodium intake (horizontal axis) in normal dogs and dogs receiving a continuous intravenous infusion of angiotensin. Ang II, antiotension II; MAP, mean arterial pressure.

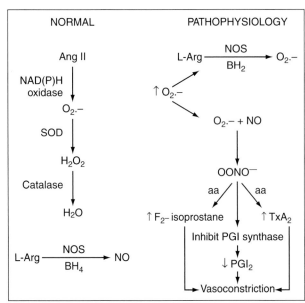

NORMAL   PATHOPHYSIOLOGY

Figure 9–5. Normal physiology (*left*). Angiotensin II (Ang II) has been shown to upregulate synthesis of NAD(P)H oxidase subunits to produce superoxide (O_2^-). Under normal conditions, superoxide will be converted by superoxide dismutase (SOD) to hydrogen peroxide (H_2O_2). Hydrogen peroxide is converted to water via the actions of catalase. In the presence of tetrahydrobiopterin (BH_4), nitric oxide synthase (NOS) produces nitric oxide (NO) from L-arginine (L-Arg). Pathophysiology (*right*). Under oxidative conditions, BH_4 is converted to dihydrobiopterin (BH_2), and NOS produces superoxide (O_2^-). A combination of O_2^- and NO is peroxynitrite (ONOO$^-$). Peroxynitrite produces vasoconstriction by converting arachidonic acid (aa) to F_2^- isoprostanes and by increasing thromboxane A_2 (TxA_2). Peroxynitrite also causes vasoconstriction by inhibiting prostacyclin (PGI_2) synthase and thereby decreasing vasodilator prostacyclin (PGI_2).

be oxidized to dihydrobiopterin (BH_2). In this case, NOS will produce superoxide rather than NO,[62–64] making this another mechanism by which ROS can be produced and NO concentrations can be reduced.

RECENT ADVANCES IN THREE-DIMENSIONAL COMPUTERIZED TOMOGRAPHY WITH TEMPORAL RESOLUTION IN MEASURING CHANGES IN INTRARENAL DISTRIBUTION OF BLOOD FLOW AND TUBULAR DYNAMICS

Romero and Lerman[65] surveyed the major advances made in the exploration of renal function since the development of static and dynamic computerized tomography (CT). One of the most important steps toward the estimation of organ blood flow was made by a team of investigators at the Mayo Clinic who developed the first three-dimensional (3D) computerized tomography scanner with high temporal resolution.[66] This instrument was successfully used to measure changes in intrarenal distribution of blood flow, and the accuracy of these determinations was better than with any other method, including inert gases, thermodynamics, microspheres, and so on.[67,68]

The theoretical basis to study renal function from image reconstruction was published in 1986.[69] Furthermore, 3D tomography with temporal resolution is an excellent methodology to study changes in total RBF, medullary and cortical blood flow, and renal volume.[70] Jaschke et al.[71] were the first to indicate the convenience of electron-beam CT to study the distribution of blood flow. Electron-beam CT measures functional changes in both kidneys during the development of RVH. Excellent correlations were found between RBF measured with electromagnetic flow probes and electron-beam CT and between GFR measured with inulin and electron-beam CT (Figure 9–6).

Electron-beam CT scanning during the renal passage of contrast media, which behaves like inulin (filtered in the glomeruli and not reabsorbed by the renal tubules), yields a profile of density changes in proximal tubules, descending and ascending segments of the loop of Henle, distal nephrons, and collecting ducts, which reflects tubular reabsorption in these segments (Figure 9–7). This concept was confirmed by measuring changes in contrast medium concentration along the renal tubules induced by furosemide.[72] This diuretic reduces sodium chloride reabsorption in the thick ascending loop of Henle. Consequently, electron-beam CT estimations showed a decrease in tubular fluid transit time and a concomitant enhancement of tubular fluid concentration from the proximal to the loop of Henle, while both transit times in distal tubules and collecting ducts were shortened along with a fall in tubular fluid concentrations.

CHANGES IN RENAL HEMODYNAMICS IN STENOTIC AND CONTRALATERAL KIDNEYS IN RENOVASCULAR HYPERTENSIVE PIGS

Results of studies conducted before and after the development of hypertension due to unilateral renal arterial constriction in swine are illustrated in Figure 9–8. It can be seen that during the control period when the MAP in the aorta was 105±3 mmHg, the right and the left kidney exhibited a volume of 75±3 and 78±3 cm³, respectively. Under these conditions the blood flow to each of these kidneys was 323±5 mL/min and 340±6 mL/min, respectively. Tissue perfusion, the amount of blood perfusing each gram of tissue, was 4.31±0.3 for the right kidney and 4.37±.4 mL/cm³ for the left kidney. After 1 month of renal arterial constriction, when MAP was 145±5 mmHg, there was a significant reduction in volume in the stenotic kidney to 68±3 cm³, whereas the contralateral kidney volume increased by 66% to 125±5 cm³. These changes were accompanied by an 18% reduction in blood flow to 276±7 mL/min in the stenotic kidney, whereas in the contralateral kidney renal blood flow was increased by 78% to 576 mL/min. It should be noted that in spite of this opposite directional change in both kidneys, the amount of kidney blood flow per gram of tissue remained relatively constant. Flow per gram of kidney weight decreased only by 0.06% (to 4.07±0.3 mL/cm³) in the stenotic kidney, while the same flow increase by only 0.07% in the contralateral kidney to 4.61 cm³. These

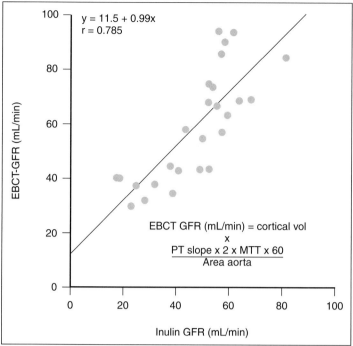

$$y = 11.5 + 0.99x$$
$$r = 0.785$$

$$\text{EBCT GFR (mL/min)} = \frac{\text{cortical vol}}{\text{PT slope} \times 2 \times \text{MTT} \times 60} \times \text{Area aorta}$$

Figure 9–6. Correlation between measurement of glomerular filtration rate performed with inulin (horizontal axis) or with electron beam computerized tomography (vertical axis). GFR, glomerular filtration rate; EBCT, electron beam computerized tomography.

results could be interpreted as indicating that renal parenchyma adjusts itself to the amount of blood that is received. Furthermore, histologic analysis also suggests that in the stenotic kidney, the reduction of renal parenchyma is mainly due to a replacement of interstitial fibrosis along with degenerative changes in renal tubules. Renal fibrosis is also present in the contralateral kidney, but the increase in volume is mainly accounted for by an increase in renal tubular volume and vascular hypertrophy.

Highly relevant to hemodynamic changes in the stenotic and contralateral kidney described above is the fact that in the stenotic kidney RBF, GFR, and distal delivery of tubular fluid correlated with the severity of the stenosis. This strongly suggests that the major determinant of the decrements in hemodynamic and renal tubular parameters as well as tissue damage was dependent on the fall of renal perfusion pressure distal to the clip. In the contralateral kidney, the increments in blood flow, GFR, and distal delivery of tubules as well as tissue volume did not correlate well with an increase in perfusion pressure, perhaps due to the tendency of the kidney to autoregulate blood flow when renal perfusion pressure is increased.

RENAL OXYGEN CONSUMPTION, TUBULAR REABSORPTION, AND RENAL ISCHEMIA

Renal oxygen consumption has been conventionally divided into (1) a small, but constant, basal oxygen uptake, and (2) a variable functional oxygen uptake. More precisely, the basal oxygen consumption is the oxygen uptake that occurs in the nonfiltering kidney without tubular reabsorption. The functional oxygen consumption is the total oxygen uptake needed to reabsorb sodium. The existence of these two components, basal and functional oxygen consumption, was demonstrated by Lassen et al.[73] in 1961. These investigators decreased renal perfusion pressure from 100 mmHg to 50 mmHg. Under these conditions, the glomerular capillary hydrostatic pressure decreased from 60 to 30 mmHg, below the glomerular capillary colloidal osmotic pressure. In the absence of GFR, oxygen consumption, which is determined by the very basal metabolic needs of the renal tissue, was calculated to be 1 μmol/g/min of O_2.[73] This consumption is comparable to that observed in other epithelial secretory tissue, such as the submaxillary gland, parotid gland, and pancreas in resting conditions.[73] Interestingly, as renal perfusion pressure was increased above 50 mmHg, renal oxygen consumption increased proportionally, exhibiting a high correlation with both glomerular filtration rate (tubular sodium load) and sodium reabsorption (Figure 9–9). Under these conditions, the renal oxygen consumption increased to 6 μmol/g/min. These observations led to the notion that suprabasal oxygen consumption is determined by the amount of sodium being reabsorbed in the renal tubules.

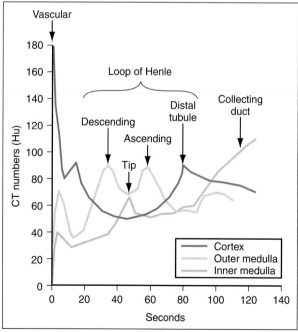

Figure 9–7. Changes in x-ray density (CT numbers) in the cortex, outer medulla, and inner medulla during the passage of x-ray contrast media that behaves like inulin. The time at which the peaks of density were detected in the renal cortex (proximal and distal tubules) in the outer medulla (descending and ascending loop of Henle) and in the inner medulla (tip of the loop of Henle and collecting duct) are represented in the horizontal axis. CT, computerized tomography.

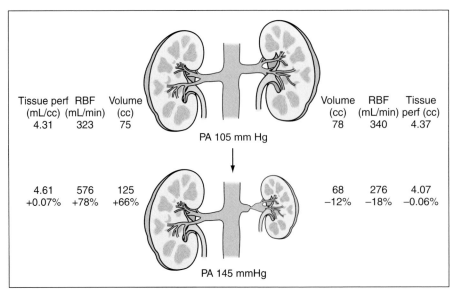

Figure 9–8. Changes in tissue perfusion, renal blood flow, renal volume, and arterial pressure induced by stenosis of renal artery. PA, arterial pressure; RBF, renal blood flow; Tissue perf, tissue perfusion; Vol, renal volume.

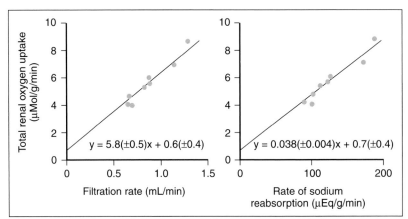

Figure 9–9. Correlations between total renal oxygen uptake with the values of glomerular filtration rate (*left*) and the rate of sodium tubular reabsorption (*right*).

Such observations raised the question of whether all renal tubular segments have the same energy requirement and thus equivalent oxygen consumption. In this regard, early studies indicated that energy requirement is a major characteristic of distal tubules because mannitol infusions, which inhibit proximal sodium reabsorption, do not alter oxygen consumption.[74] In contrast, saline infusions, which tend to decrease significantly proximal sodium reabsorption and at the same stimulate distal tubular reabsorption, significantly increase oxygen consumption.[74–76] Furthermore, these observations agree with the finding that the enzymes responsible for gluconeogenesis, such as glucose 6-phosphatase, fructose-1, 6-diphosphatase, and phosphoenolpyruvate carboxykinase, are limited to the proximal tubules.[77] Gluconeogenesis is an energy-requiring process that by its very nature does not proceed in the same cell in which glycolysis provides energy. Oxidative metabolism, chiefly of fat, is therefore the major source of energy in

the proximal tubular cells of a cortex.[75] On the other hand, the enzymes that participate in glycolysis—hexokinase, phosphofructokinase, and pyruvate kinase—predominate in distal segments of the nephron, such as medullary ascending limb, cortical thick limb, distal convoluted tubules, and the entire collecting duct.[77]

In agreement with all these observations, it was also found that the concentration of Na-K-ATPase is five to eight times higher in the distal than in the proximal tubules.[78] This enzyme is mainly responsible for metabolic active transport of sodium from the tubular lumen to the renal interstitium. Na-K-ATPase is inhibited by ouabain, ethacrynic acid, and furosemide. In a study performed in anesthetized dogs where mannitol was given first to inhibit proximal tubular sodium reabsorption (mannitol diuresis), ouabain reduced sodium potassium ATPase activity in the kidney by 75%. Under these conditions, sodium reabsorption was decreased by 40% and renal oxygen consumption by 45%. Contrasting with these findings was the observation that the administration of acetazolamide, an inhibitor of carbonic anhydrase (which accounts for most of the sodium reabsorption in the proximal tubules), reduced total Na reabsorption to a level further down than that induced by ouabain without decreasing oxygen consumption.[79]

It should be emphasized here that for years it was assumed that the kidney was supplied with more than enough oxygen to perform its work because, under conditions where the renal artery contains 8.8 μmol/mL of oxygen, the vein shows a concentration of 7.3 μmol/mL. Thus the renal artery–venous difference of O_2 concentration is very small, averaging 1.4 μmol/mL.[77] However, when one considers that the kidney blood supply is 20% of total cardiac output per minute, it becomes apparent that the whole organ has a high oxygen consumption.[77] This is particularly true for the outer medulla where oxygen consumption represents 79% of the total supply. For comparative purposes, it should be stated that the outer medulla consumes 79% of its oxygen supply, while the heart consumes 65%[77] (Table 9–1).

When considering the blood and oxygen supplied to the cortex and the medulla, there are additional characteristics that are determined by the special anatomic arrangement of the intrarenal vasculature. For example, small intrarenal arteries run in parallel to small intrarenal veins. This allows the rapid transfer of oxygen from the artery to the vein, decreasing hemoglobin saturation before blood reaches the peripheral vasculature. This transfer of oxygen is particularly prominent in the renal medulla where oxygen passes from the descending to the ascending vasa recta. This accounts for the small arterial venous differences of oxygen in the kidney and also for the observation that oxygen concentration in the vein is higher than in peripheral capillaries. This characteristic places the outer medulla in a relatively vulnerable situation because of the high oxygen consumption associated with a relatively low oxygen supply. Oxygen delivered to the outer medulla is 7.6 mL/min/100 g of tissue, where oxygen consumption is 6 mL/min/100g of tissue (Table 9–1). This explains the selective injury produced in thick ascending limb segments under conditions of renal ischemia produced by controlled hemorrhage, or after prolonged renal vasoconstriction, because it is induced by blockade of prostaglandin synthesis in dogs submitted to sodium depletion and simultaneously the administration of contrast x-ray medium.[80,81]

In agreement with all these data are preliminary studies indicating that, in the stenotic kidney, the decrease of renal blood flow, GFR, and tubular sodium load is proportional to the degree of renal stenosis. In these studies, the amount of fluid reaching the distal tubules, as well as tubular concentration of solutes, falls in proportion to the decrease in RBF and GFR. Consequently, in these kidneys, there is a proportional decrease in oxygen consumption. Under these conditions, the amount of oxygen consumption, which is inhibited by the administration of furosemide (an inhibitor of the Na-2Cl-K co-transporter), is also proportionally decreased. From all of these observations, we have hypothesized that the fall in the so-called furosemide-induced suppression of oxygen consumption (FISOC) can be used as an index of distal tubular sodium reabsorption, and will correlate with the ability of the kidney to recover after recirculation is reestablished by surgical interventions or by percutaneous transluminal renal artery angioplasty (PTRAA).

In the contralateral kidney, the opposite is likely to be observed. A significant increase of O_2 consumption can be predicted on the basis of a 66% increase in total renal volume (renal hypertrophy), a 78% elevation of RBF, and 60% increase in GFR observed in previous studies. These changes are also attended by proportional elevations of distal tubular fluid flow and Na reabsorption. FISOC should be increased. However, these changes in the contralateral kidney, which reflect a compensatory reaction to minimize the decreased function of the stenotic kidney, create vulnerability to decrements in RPP. Since the ability of the contralateral kidney to autoregulate is significantly decreased, the minimum perfusion pressure needed to maintain RBF, GFR, and Na excretion in the contralateral kidney is not known. Hence, a fall in MAP that follows the PTRAA could precipitate renal insufficiency, if recirculation of the stenotic kidney is not sufficient to restore renal function and compromises renal circulation and everyday function in the contralateral kidney.

RATIO OF OXYGEN CONSUMPTION TO OXYGEN DELIVERY IN OUTER MEDULLA OF KIDNEY AND OTHER ORGANS				
Region or Organ	O_2 Delivery	Rate of Blood Flow (mL/min/100 g)	O_2 Consumption	O_2 Consumption/O_2 Delivery (%)
Hepatoportal	11.6	58	2.20	18
Kidney	84.0	420	6.80	8
Outer medulla	7.6	190	6.00	79
Brain	10.8	54	3.70	34
Skin	2.6	13	0.38	15
Skeletal muscle	0.5	2.7	0.18	34
Heart	16.8	84	11.0	65
Reprinted by permission from Macmillan Publishers Ltd: from Epstein FH. *Kidney Int* 1997;51:381–5.				

Table 9–1. Ratio of Oxygen Consumption to Oxygen Delivery in Outer Medulla of Kidney and Other Organs

SUMMARY

Renovascular hypertension is a form of secondary hypertension, that is, an underlying disease is leading to the cause of elevated BP. The renal vascular (renovascular) alteration is a narrowing of the artery(s) to one or both kidneys. This reduction of blood flow leads to the affected kidney or kidneys to mistakenly respond as if the BP is low. The primary mechanistic response to this stimulus is to secrete hormones that increase peripheral vascular resistance by inducing vasoconstriction and, secondarily, to signal the body to retain salt and water, which causes an increase in BP. The ensuing cascade of events involves many pathogenic mechanisms, including the renin-angiotensin system and oxidative stress, and varies depending on the presence of a functioning contralateral kidney. We have developed 3D imaging techniques of the kidney that allow for quantification and assessment of kidney function, thus making early detection and evaluation of the disease possible.

REFERENCES

1. Goldblatt H, Lynch J, Hanzal RF, Summerville WW. Studies on experimental hypertension. I. The production of persistent elevation of systolic blood pressure by means of renal ischemia. *J Exp Med* 1934;59:347–78.
2. Goldblatt H. Studies on experimental hypertension. III. The production of persistent hypertension in monkeys (Macaque) by renal ischemia. *J Exp Med* 1937;65:671–75.
3. Brown JJ, Davies DL, Morton JJ, et al. Mechanism of renal hypertension. *Lancet* 1976;1:1219–21.
4. Caravaggi AM, Bianchi G, Brown JJ, et al. Blood pressure and plasma angiotensin II concentration after renal artery constriction and angiotensin infusion in the dog. (5-Isoleucine) angiotensin II and its breakdown fragments in dog blood. *Circ Res* 1976;38:315–21.
5. Romero JC, Feldstein AE, Rodriguez-Porcel MG, Cases-Amenos A. New insights into the pathophysiology of renovascular hypertension. *Mayo Clin Proc* 1997;72:251–60.
6. Wilcox CS. Ischemic nephropathy: noninvasive testing. *Semin Nephrol* 1996;16:43–52.
7. Novick AC. Options for therapy of ischemic nephropathy: role of angioplasty and surgery. *Semin Nephrol* 1996;16:53–60.
8. Textor SC. Revascularization in atherosclerotic renal artery disease. *Kidney Int* 1998;53:799–811.
9. London GM, Safar ME. Renal hemodynamics in patients with sustained essential hypertension and in patients with unilateral stenosis of the renal artery. *Am J Hypertens* 1989;2:244–52.
10. Bianchi G, Baldoli E, Lucca R, Barbin P. Pathogenesis of arterial hypertension after the constriction of the renal artery leaving the opposite kidney intact both in the anaesthetized and in the conscious dog. *Clin Sci* 1972; 42:651–64.
11. Selkurt EE, Hall PW, Spencer MP. Influence of graded arterial pressure decrement on renal clearance of creatinine, p-amino-hippurate and sodium. *Am J Physiol* 1949;159:369–78.
12. Shipley RE, Study RS. Changes in renal blood flow, extraction of inulin, glomerular filtration rate, tissue pressure and urine flow with acute alterations of renal artery blood pressure. *Am J Physiol* 1951;167:676–88.
13. Regoli D, Hess R, Brunner HB, et al. Interrelationship of renin content in kidneys and blood pressure in renal hypertensive rats. *Arch Int Pharmacodyn Ther* 1962;140:416–26.
14. Swales JD, Thurston H, Queiroz FP, et al. Dual mechanism for experimental hypertension. *Lancet* 1971;2:1181–4.
15. Romero JC, Lazar JD, Hoobler SW. Effects of renal artery constriction and subsequent contralateral nephrectomy on the blood pressure, plasma renin activity, and plasma renin substrate concentration in rabbits. *Lab Invest* 1970;22:581–7.
16. Lerman LO, Schwartz RS, Grande JP, et al. Noninvasive evaluation of a novel swine model of renal artery stenosis. *J Am Soc Nephrol* 1999;10:1455–65.
17. Romero JC, Mak SW, Hoobler SW. Effect of blockade of angiotensin–1 converting enzyme on the blood pressure of renal hypertensive rabbits. *Cardiovasc Res* 1974;8:681–7.
18. Masaki Z, Ferrario CM, Bumpus FM, et al. The course of arterial pressure and the effect of Sar1-Thr8-angiotensin II in a new model of two-kidney hypertension in conscious dogs. *Clin Sci Mol Med* 1977;52:163–70.
19. Gavras H, Brunner HB, Vaughan ED, Laragh JH. Angiotensin-sodium interaction in blood pressure maintenance of renal hypertensive and normotensive rats. *Science* 1973;180:1369–71.
20. Lever AF. The fast and the slowly developing pressor effect of angiotensin II. In: Robertson JIS, Nicholls MG, eds. *The Renin Angiotensin System.* London: Gower Medical Publishing, 1993:28.1–9.
21. Ferrario CM, Blumle C, Nadzam GR, McCubbin JW. An externally adjustable renal artery clamp. *J Appl Physiol* 1971; 31:635–7.
22. Leenen FHH, de Jong W. Plasma renin and sodium balance during the development of moderate and severe renal hypertension in rats. *Circ Res* 1975;36:179–86.
23. Wilson C, Byrom FB. The vicious circle in chronic Bright's disease: experimental evidence from the hypertensive rat. *Q J Med* 1941;10:65–94.
24. Mohring J, Mohring B, Naumann HJ, et al. Salt and water balance and renin activity in renal hypertension of rats. *Am J Physiol* 1975;228:1847–55.
25. Barraclough MA. Sodium and water depletion with acute malignant hypertension. *Am J Med* 1966; 40:265–72.
26. Martinez-Maldonado M. Pathophysiology of renovascular hypertension. *Hypertension* 1991;17:707–19.
27. Reckelhoff JF, Romero JC. Role of oxidative stress in angiotensin-induced hypertension. *Am J Physiol Regul Integr Comp Physiol* 2003;284:R893–912.
28. Romero JC, Holmes DR, Strong CG. The effect of high sodium intake and angiotensin antagonist in rabbits with severe and moderate hypertension induced by constriction of one renal artery. *Hypertension* 1977;40: I-17–I-23.
29. Nishiyama A, Seth DM, Navar LG. Renal interstitial fluid concentrations of angiotensins I and II in anesthetized rats. *Hypertension* 2002;39:129–34.
30. van Kats JP, de Lannoy LM, Jan Danser AH, et al. Angiotensin II type 1 (AT1) receptor-mediated accumulation of angiotensin II in tissues and its intracellular half-life in vivo. *Hypertension* 1997;30:42–9.
31. Haas JA, Krier JD, Bolterman RJ, et al. Low-dose angiotensin II increases free isoprostane levels in plasma. *Hypertension* 1999;34:983–6.
32. Reckelhoff JF, Zhang H, Srivastava K, et al. Subpressor doses of angiotensin II increase plasma F(2)-isoprostanes in rats. *Hypertension* 2000;35:476–9.
33. Heptinstall RH. Hypertension II: secondary forms. In: Heptinstall RH, ed. *Pathology of the Kidney.* Vol. 2. 4th ed. Boston: Little, Brown, and Co, 1992:1029–95.
34. Cantin M, Solymoss B, Benchimol S, et al. Metaplastic and mitotic activity of the ischemic (endocrine) kidney in experimental renal hypertension. *Am J Pathol* 1979;96:545–65.
35. Ploth DW, Schnermann J, Dahlheim H, et al. Autoregulation and tubuloglomerular feedback in normotensive and hypertensive rats. *Kidney Int* 1977;12:253–67.
36. Bonvalet JP, Berjal G, de Rouffignac D. Single glomular filtration rate of superficial and juxta-medullary nephrons in the rat during different types of arterial hypertension. *Pflugers Arch* 1973;340:133–44.
37. Wilson C, Ledingham JM, Floyer MA. Experimental renal and renoprival hypertension. In: Rouller C, Mueller AF, eds. *The Kidney: Morphology, Biochemistry, Physiology.* New York: Academic Press, 1971:155.
38. Miller ED Jr, Samuels AI, Haber E, Barger AC. Inhibition of angiotensin conversion and prevention of renal

hypertension. *Am J Physiol* 1975; 228:448–53.

39. Svetkey LP, Himmelstein SI, Dunnick NR, et al. Prospective analysis of strategies for diagnosing renovascular hypertension. *Hypertension* 1989; 14:247–57.

40. Staessen J, Bulpitt C, Fagard R, et al. Long-term converting-enzyme inhibition as a guide to surgical curability of hypertension associated with renovascular disease. *Am J Cardiol* 1983;51:1317–22.

41. Hricik DE. Angiotensin-converting enzyme inhibition in renovascular hypertension: the narrowing gap between functional renal failure and progressive renal atrophy. *J Lab Clin Med* 1990;115:8–9.

42. Textor SC, Wilcox CS. Renal artery stenosis: a common, treatable cause of renal failure? *Annu Rev Med* 2001; 52:421–42.

43. van de Ven PJ, Beutler JJ, Kaatee R, et al. Angiotensin converting enzyme inhibitor-induced renal dysfunction in atherosclerotic renovascular disease. *Kidney Int* 1998;53:986–93.

44. Wilcox CS, Smith TB, Frederickson ED. The captopril GFR renogram in renovascular hypertension. *Clin Nucl Med* 1988;14:107.

45. Menard J, Michel JB, Plouin PF. A cautious view of the value of angiotensin-converting enzyme inhibition in renovascular disease. In: Robertson JIS, Nicholls MG, eds. *The Renin-Angiotensin System*. London: Gower Medical, 1993:89.1–9.

46. Jackson B, Franze L, Sumithran E, Johnston CI. Pharmacologic nephrectomy with chronic angiotensin converting enzyme inhibitor treatment in renovascular hypertension in the rat. *J Lab Clin Med* 1990;115:21–7.

47. Brunner HR, Kirshman JD, Sealey JE, Laragh JH. Hypertension of renal origin: evidence for two different mechanisms. *Science* 1971;174:1344–6.

48. Watkins BE, Davis JO, Hanson RC, et al. Incidence and pathophysiological changes in chronic two-kidney hypertension in the dog. *Am J Physiol* 1976;231:954–60.

49. Carretero OA, Scicli G. The kallikrein-kinin system as a regulator of cardiovascular and renal function. In: Laragh JH, Brenner BM, eds. *Hypertension: Pathophysiology, Diagnosis, and Management*. 2nd ed. New York: Raven Press, 1995:983–99.

50. McCubbin JW, DeMoura RS, Page IH, Olmsted F. Arterial hypertension elicited by subpressor amounts of angiotensin. *Science* 1965;149:1394–5.

51. Page IH, Helmer OM. A crystalline pressor substance (angiotonin) resulting from the action between renin and renin activation. *J Exp Med* 1940; 71:29–42.

52. Simon G, Abraham G, Cserep G. Pressor and subpressor angiotensin II

administration. Two experimental models of hypertension. *Am J Hypertens* 1995;8:645–50.

53. Brown JJ, Casals-Stenzel J, Cumming AM, et al. Angiotensin II, aldosterone and arterial pressure: a quantitative approach. Arthur C. Corcoran Memorial Lecture. *Hypertension* 1979;1:159–79.

54. Hu L, Catanzaro DF, Pitarresi TM, et al. Identical hemodynamic and hormonal responses to 14-day infusions of renin or angiotensin II in conscious rats. *J Hypertens* 1998;16:1285–98.

55. Brunner HR, Laragh JH, Baer L, et al. Essential hypertension: renin and aldosterone, heart attack and stroke. *N Engl J Med* 1972;286:441–9.

56. DeClue JW, Guyton AC, Cowley AW Jr, et al. Subpressor angiotensin infusion, renal sodium handling, and salt-induced hypertension in the dog. *Circ Res* 1978; 43:503–12.

57. Krieger JE, Cowley AW Jr Prevention of salt angiotensin II hypertension by servo control of body water. *Am J Physiol* 1990;258:H994–1003.

58. Hollenberg NK, Chenitz WR, Adams DF, Williams GH. Reciprocal influence of salt intake on adrenal glomerulosa and renal vascular responses to angiotensin II in normal man. *J Clin Invest* 1974; 54:34–42.

59. Rettig R, Folberth C, Stauss H, et al. Role of the kidney in primary hypertension: a renal transplantation study in rats. *Am J Physiol* 1990; 258:F606–11.

60. Hall JE. Renal function in one-kidney, one-clip hypertension and low renin essential hypertension. *Am J Hypertens* 1991;4:523S–33S.

61. Mollnau H, Wendt M, Szocs K, et al. Effects of angiotensin II infusion on the expression and function of NAD(P)H oxidase and components of nitric oxide/cGMP signaling. *Circ Res* 2002; 90:E58–65.

62. Stroes E, Hijmering M, van Zandvoort M, et al. Origin of superoxide production by endothelial nitric oxide synthase. *FEBS Lett* 1998;438:161–4.

63. Vasquez-Vivar J, Hogg N, Martasek P, et al. Tetrahydrobiopterin-dependent inhibition of superoxide generation from neuronal nitric oxide synthase. *J Biol Chem* 1999;274:26736–42.

64. Xia Y, Tsai AL, Berka V, Zweier JL. Superoxide generation from endothelial nitric-oxide synthase. A Ca2+/calmodulin-dependent and tetrahydrobiopterin regulatory process. *J Biol Chem* 1998; 273:25804–8.

65. Romero JC, Lerman LO. Novel noninvasive techniques for studying renal function in man. *Semin Nephrol* 2000;20:456–62.

66. Ritman EL, Kinsey JH, Robb RA, et al. Three-dimensional imaging of heart, lungs, and circulation. *Science* 1980; 210:273–80.

67. Knox FG, Ritman EL, Romero JC. Intrarenal distribution of blood flow:

evolution of a new approach to measurement. *Kidney Int* 1984; 25:473–9.

68. Iwasaki T, Ritman EL, Fiksen-Olsen MJ, et al. Renal cortical perfusion—preliminary experience with the dynamic spatial reconstructor (DSR). *Ann Biomed Eng* 1985;13:259–71.

69. Bentley MD, Fiksen-Olsen MJ, Knox FG, et al. The use of the dynamic spatial reconstructor to study renal function (International Symposium on Primary Hypertension). In: Kaufman W, ed. *Primary Hypertension*. Berlin and Heidelberg: Springer Verlag, 1986: 126–41.

70. Lerman LO, Bentley MD, Bell MR, et al. Quantitation of the in vivo kidney volume with cine computed tomography. *Invest Radiol* 1990; 25:1206–11.

71. Jaschke W, Lipton MJ, Boyd DP, et al. Attenuation changes of the normal and ischemic canine kidney. Dynamic CT scanning after intravenous contrast medium bolus. *Acta Radiol Diagn (Stockh)* 1985;26:321–30.

72. Lerman LO, Rodriguez-Porcel M, Sheedy PF 2nd, Romero JC. Renal tubular dynamics in the intact canine kidney. *Kidney Int* 1996;50:1358–62.

73. Lassen NA, Munck O, Thaysen JH. Oxygen consumption and sodium reabsorption in the kidney. *Acta Physiol Scand* 1961;51:371–84.

74. Kiil F, Aukland K, Refsum HE. Renal sodium transport and oxygen consumption. *Am J Physiol* 1961; 201:511–6.

75. Dirks JH, Cirksena WJ, Berliner RW. The effects of saline infusion on sodium reabsorption by the proximal tubule of the dog. *J Clin Invest* 1965;44:1160–70.

76. Rector FC Jr, Vangiesen G, Kiil F, Seldin DW. Influence of expansion of extracellular volume on tubular reabsorption of sodium independent of changes in glomerular filtration rate and aldosterone activity. *J Clin Invest* 1964;43:341–8.

77. Epstein FH. Oxygen and renal metabolism. *Kidney Int* 1997;51:381–5.

78. Schmidt U, Guder WG. Sites of enzyme activity along the nephron. *Kidney Int* 1976;9:233–42.

79. Mathisen O, Raeder M, Sejersted OM, Kiil F. Effect of acetazolamide on glomerular balance and renal metabolic rate. *Scand J Clin Lab Invest* 1976; 36:617–25.

80. Agmon Y, Peleg H, Greenfeld Z, et al. Nitric oxide and prostanoids protect the renal outer medulla from radiocontrast toxicity in the rat. *J Clin Invest* 1994;94:1069–75.

81. Jones DP. Renal metabolism during normoxia, hypoxia, and ischemic injury. *Annu Rev Physiol* 1986;48:33–50.

Chapter

10 Left Ventricular Physiology and Pathophysiology in Hypertension

George W. Booz

Key Findings

- The left ventricle in hypertension undergoes remodeling that eventually proves detrimental to heart function.

- Specific events include cardiac muscle hypertrophy, interstitial fibrosis, and increased mass with or without increased wall thickness.

- A common feature of the left ventricular (LV) remodeling is impaired relaxation (diastolic dysfunction), often accompanied by impaired contractility.

- Increased LV mass is an important risk factor for cardiovascular disease, including ventricular arrhythmias and heart failure.

Clinical Implications

- Atrial fibrillation and stroke, secondary to left arterial enlargement, may occur with LV hypertrophy.

- Compromised oxygen delivery makes the hypertrophied myocardium susceptible to ischemic damage, and patients with LV hypertrophy are more likely to exhibit renal damage.

In hypertension, the left ventricle undergoes hypertrophy as a compensatory mechanism to reduce wall stress and maintain pump function in the face of the increased afterload. The introduction of echocardiography as a diagnostic tool, however, has established that the increased left ventricular (LV) mass observed in hypertension cannot be construed simply as a compensatory process, but represents an important, independent predictor of morbidity and mortality.[1,2] In fact, LV hypertrophy, which is generally defined based on LV mass normalized to body size (LV mass index), represents a stronger risk factor than blood pressure for adverse cardiovascular events. At which point increased LV mass ceases to be compensatory and becomes deleterious in hypertension is not known, but the concept of inappropriate LV mass or excess mass beyond that predicted based on gender, body height, and hemodynamic burden has been introduced to better address this issue.[3–7] Inappropriate LV mass not only predicts cardiovascular risk independent of other risk factors, such as age and blood pressure (as does conventionally defined LV mass), but also in the presence or absence of echocardiographic LV hypertrophy. The idea of inappropriate LV mass also underscores a major difference between the appropriate (physiologic) LV hypertrophy produced by exercise and that observed with

hypertension. Additionally, unlike what occurs with exercise, hypertension induces changes in both the contractile and supportive compartments of the heart that are maladaptive and eventually prove detrimental to normal pump function.[8]

ANATOMY AND BIOCHEMISTRY

An increase in cardiac workload brought on by conditions that cause volume or pressure overload results in an increase in LV mass as a primary adaptive mechanism. Pure pressure overload is thought to induce a concentric pattern of left ventricle hypertrophy due to the replication of sarcomeres in parallel.[9,10] In this form of hypertrophy, the increase in LV mass is accompanied by a thickening of the septal and posterior walls (the ratio of LV wall thickness to cavity diameter increases), as a compensatory mechanism to maintain normal wall stress. With volume overload, in contrast, individual muscle fibers elongate due to the addition of sarcomeres in series. Consequently, LV mass increases, but relative wall thickness remains normal, resulting in LV dilation and an eccentric pattern of hypertrophy. Echocardiography reveals, however, that the overall geometric response of the heart to arterial hypertension can follow any one of four patterns (Figure 10–1), with approximately half of all patients exhibiting a normal LV geometry (Table 10–1).[11–13] These different patterns of adaptation are not simply attributable to differences in severity or duration of hypertension, but are thought to reflect the variable impact of preload on the left ventricle due to changes in blood volume and/or venous compliance, as well as LV dilation due to the growing inadequacy of (concentric) hypertrophy to compensate for increased afterload. Additionally, genetic factors and an association of obesity with eccentric hypertrophy influence the geometric pattern. A normal LV mass with increased relative wall thickness (concentric remodeling) is proposed to be a consequence of volume underload from pressure natriuresis "canceling out" the effect of pressure overload, which does not occur with concentric hypertrophy.[12,13] At the other extreme, concomitant pressure and volume overload is thought to result in a pattern of eccentric hypertrophy. Indices of systemic hemodynamics and cardiac performance in hypertensive patients are consistent with this interpretation (Table 10–1). Additionally, stroke volume is positively related to the LV minor/major hemiaxis ratio at end-diastole. At the lower extreme, with the most elliptic cavities, are patients

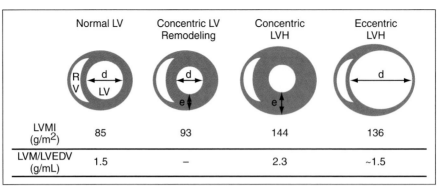

Figure 10–1. Left ventricular geometric patterns in hypertensive patients. Echocardiography shows that the left ventricle can adapt any one of four geometric patterns in response to hypertension, reflecting the relative contributions of pressure and volume overloads. LVMI, left ventricular mass index; RWT, relative wall thickness; RW, right ventricle; LV, left ventricle; LVH, left ventricular hypertrophy; d, left ventricular chamber diameter; e, left ventricular wall thickness. (Values are from Ganau A, Devereux RB, Roman MJ, de Simone G, Pickering TG, Saba PS, et al. *J Am Coll Cardiol* 1992;19:1550–8.)

HEMODYNAMICS AND CARDIAC PERFORMANCE ASSOCIATED WITH VARIOUS LEFT VENTRICLE GEOMETRIC PATTERNS IN HYPERTENSION				
	Normal Left Ventricle	**Concentric Remodeling**	**Concentric Hypertrophy**	**Eccentric Hypertrophy**
Prevalence	52%	13%	8%	27%
Left ventricular mass	—	—	↑	↑
Relative wall thickness	—	↑	↑	—
Blood pressure	↑	↑	↑↑↑	↑↑
Stroke index	—	↓	—	↑
Cardiac index	—	↓	—	↑
Total peripheral resistance	↑	↑↑↑	↑↑	—

Reprinted from Patterns of left ventricular hypertrophy and geometric remodeling in essential hypertension. Ganau A, et al. *J Am Coll Cardiol* 1992;19:1550–8. Copyright 1992 with permission from The American College of Cardiology Foundation.

Table 10–1. Hemodynamics and Cardiac Performance Associated with Various Left Ventricle Geometric Patterns in Hypertension

with concentric remodeling. At the upper end, with the most spherical cavities, are patients with eccentric hypertrophy.

LV hypertrophy associated with arterial hypertension represents primarily an increase in the size of individual muscle fibers, accompanied by interstitial and perivascular fibrosis due to an accumulation of fibrillar collagen.[10,14] These changes result from both mechanical forces acting on the heart, as well as pressure-overload activation of the sympathetic and renin angiotensin system (Figure 10–2).[14,15] Additionally, both pressure and volume overload induce expression of a number of growth and fibrotic factors by cardiac fibroblasts and myocytes, including angiotensin II, IL-6 family cytokines, endothelin-1, insulin-like growth factor I, and TGF-β.[16,17] Hypertrophy at the level of the cardiac myocyte represents an increase in protein content, but is distinguishable from physiologic hypertrophy because of an accompanying gene expression profile that is presumably maladaptive. Specifically, expression of genes associated with embryonic development (e.g., those for β-myosin heavy chain, skeletal α-actin, as well as atrial and brain natriuretic peptides) is increased, and expression of some adult cardiac muscle genes, (e.g., α-myosin heavy-chain and sarcoplasmic reticulum Ca^{2+}-ATPase) is decreased.[18] The hypertrophied heart charac-

teristically exhibits decreased β-adrenergic responsiveness. In part, this is due to increased myocardial levels of β-ARK1, a kinase responsible for homologous desensitization of β-adrenergic receptors. Alterations in metabolism occur as well in the hypertrophied myocardium. These include reduced fatty acid oxidation, increased glucose uptake, and glycolysis, and less coupling of glycolysis to the tricarboxylic acid cycle.[19,20] The myocardial fibrosis seen in hypertension results from increased collagen type I and III synthesis by fibroblasts, but there are also changes in the ratio and cross linking of the collagen types.[14,21] Changes in the activity of enzymes that degrade collagen, matrix metalloproteinases (MMPs), occur in a temporal fashion: initially activity is increased, followed by a chronic phase of normal activity, which gives way to increased activity and collagen degradation that contributes to chamber dilation.[22,23] During the compensatory phase of LV hypertrophy, the increase in extracellular collagen contributes to myocardial stiffness, abnormalities of cardiac function, and the increased frequency of ventricular arrhythmias commonly observed in hypertensive patients.[21] Additionally, by constraining vasodilation of intramyocardial coronary arteries, perivascular fibrosis has a part in the decreased coronary reserve frequently seen in hypertension.[24]

GENETICS

Early observations that the magnitude of LV hypertrophy varies considerably among individuals with the same levels of blood pressure, and may even be absent, suggested that genetics plays a role in hypertension-related LV hypertrophy. Support for this has been provided by analyses of epidemiologic studies that attempted to parse the impact of independent determinants of LV hypertrophy, such as age, gender, blood pressure, and body mass index (BMI), from a contribution of heredity. One of the first such analyses, of the largely Caucasian population–based Framingham Heart Study, suggested indeed that heredity has a greater impact on LV mass than systolic blood pressure.[24] Combined large-population studies have provided estimates for heritability of LV mass that fall within a range of 0.2 to 0.8.[25–30] This broad range likely reflects not only a contribution of shared genes and familial environment, but also ethnic differences among genes responsible for LV hypertrophy and remodeling.

An increased risk of concentric remodeling and concentric, but not eccentric, LV hypertrophy was found among siblings of affected subjects in echocardiographic substudies of the population-based MONICA Augsburg surveys.[31] After adjusting for age, blood pressure, and BMI, the risk elevation related to a familial disposition of LV hypertrophy was 1.4 to 1.7. Several analyses involving juvenile twins reached the conclusion that inherited factors strongly influence interindividual variability of LV mass.[32–34] Additionally, after adjusting for other confounders, black identical twins exhibited a higher intraclass correlation coefficient for LV mass than black fraternal twins. A similar finding was reached in a recent population-based study of healthy adult twins, suggesting that LV phenotype has a significant genetic determination that may be independent of age or environment.[30]

The issue of ethnic or racial differences in LV mass among hypertensive adults is one of particular relevance for black hypertensive Americans, who experience substantially higher rates of stroke, coronary heart disease, and heart failure than white Americans.[35,36] A higher prevalence of increased LV mass was observed in young black adults compared with their white counterparts in a cohort of the prospective Coronary Artery Disease Risk Development in Young Adults (CARDIA) Study[37] and in a longitudinal study of children.[38] In an analysis of the Hypertension Genetic Epidemiology Network (HyperGEN) Study, substantial differences were noted in prevalence and magnitude of cardiac structure changes between blacks and whites undergoing treatment for hypertension.[36] Blacks had increased LV mass and relative wall thickness in multivariable models that adjusted for important confounders.

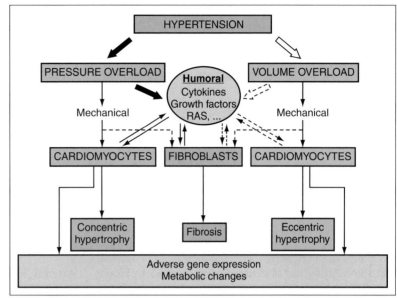

Figure 10–2. Hypertension-induced remodeling of the left ventricle reflects the dual contribution of mechanical and humoral stimuli resulting from both pressure overload (predominately) and volume overload. A greater contribution of humoral stimuli (endocrine, paracrine, and autocrine) occurs with pressure overload. These stimuli act on both fibroblasts to increase perivascular and interstitial fibrosis, and on cardiomyocytes to induce pathologic hypertrophy, which entails adverse changes in gene expression and metabolism. Both cardiomyocytes and fibroblasts produce cytokines and growth factors, which can amplify left ventricular remodeling in an autocrine/paracrine manner.

Adjusted LV internal dimension was smaller in blacks than whites, consistent with the predominant pattern of concentric LV hypertrophy in hypertension.

Which genes influence susceptibility of the left ventricle to hypertrophy in hypertension is not known to any great degree. The focus to date has been on genes of hormonal systems, such as the renin-angiotensin-aldosterone system, activated in hypertension and implicated in LV hypertrophy. Likely due to a number of factors, including small sample size, absence of Hardy-Weinberg equilibrium, genotyping errors, and differences in population background, many of these studies have produced contradictory results. A prime example is studies involving an insertion/deletion (I/D) polymorphism of a 287-bp Alu element in intron 16 of the ACE gene. This polymorphism seemed a good candidate to influence LV hypertrophy, since the DD genotype is linked to enhanced ACE activity. In this case, meta-analysis of contradictory case–control studies showed LV hypertrophy overall was not associated with the D allele; however, in untreated patients, the DD genotype exhibited a higher risk of cardiac hypertrophy compared to the II genotype, suggesting that the D allele may worsen LV hypertrophy if hypertension is not controlled.[39] Carriers of the Glu27 allele of the β_2 adrenergic receptor,[40] and noncarriers of the 192 base pair allele of a cytosine-adenosine repeat in the IGF-I promoter[41] were reported to be at higher risk for developing cardiac hypertrophy. A +9/−9 exon 1 polymorphism of the B_2 bradykinin receptor[42] and single nucleotide polymorphisms (SNPs) in the angiotensinogen, apolipoprotein B, angiotensin II type 1 receptor (AT_1), and α_2-adrenoreceptor genes, have all been shown to impact on the magnitude of regression of LV hypertrophy during antihypertensive treatment.[43,44] The G1675A polymorphism associated with reduced expression of the angiotensin-II type 2 receptor (AT_2),[45] and the –344C/T promoter polymorphism of the aldosterone synthase gene, associated with increased plasma aldosterone levels, have also been linked to LV hypertrophy.[46]

PHYSIOLOGY AND PATHOPHYSIOLOGY

Increased systolic blood pressure associated with increased peripheral resistance and arterial stiffening is an important determinant of LV hypertrophy. Blood pressure, however, is also affected by cardiac performance, and mathematical modeling based on clinical data suggests that the heart makes a substantial contribution to increased blood pressure in hypertension. One such analysis showed that the contribution of cardiac pump function to blood pressure in hypertensive patients is a function of the remodeling process, with estimates of 21%, 65%, and 108% for concentric remodeling, concentric hypertrophy, and eccentric hypertrophy, respectively.[47] For hypertensive patients with a normal geometry of the left ventricle, the estimated contribution was 55%.

A number of associations between target organ damage and LV remodeling have been described in hypertension. Patients with LV hypertrophy are more likely to exhibit kidney damage, carotid plaguing, or increased carotid intima-media thickness.[48] The risk of target organ damage can be further stratified by LV geometric pattern, the risk being highest with concentric and intermediate with eccentric hypertrophy.[2,49–51] Cardiac hypertrophy *per se* does not explain this relationship, as concentric remodeling of the left ventricle, that is, increased wall thickness with normal LV mass, represents an independent predictor of increased cardiovascular risk in hypertensive patients as well.[13] The higher levels of blood pressure and neurohormonal activation seen with concentric hypertrophy (predominant pressure overload) likely explain the greater risk of target organ damage, since each of these parameters impacts on cardiac, vascular, and renal remodeling. LV concentric hypertrophy is associated with especially high arterial pressure, and patients with this pattern of remodeling have the most advanced retinopathy on funduscopic examination, and the most severe abnormalities in arterial structure and function, including greater arterial hypertrophy, arterial stiffness, and increased total peripheral resistance.[52,53] In mild to moderate hypertension, abnormalities in carotid arterial structures are most severe with concentric remodeling or hypertrophy. Perhaps not surprisingly, concentric geometry is more likely to be associated with cerebrovascular events. Concentric LV hypertrophy is also associated with the greatest renal dysfunction, and is likely to potentiate the decline in glomerular filtration rate with aging.[54] On the other hand, while lower systemic arterial stiffness is associated with eccentric hypertrophy, so also is aortic root dilation, and those individuals may be at higher risk of an adverse event.[55]

Left arterial (LA) enlargement, symptomatic of hypertensive heart disease, commonly occurs in hypertensive patients with LV hypertrophy, and represents a risk factor for arterial fibrillation and stroke.[56] Left arterial enlargement occurs in response to stiffening of the ventricle and increased LV end-diastolic pressure, but may also be secondary to changes in systolic LV function. When observed in patients with normal systolic function by echocardiography, LA enlargement is generally interpreted as an early sign of reduced diastolic LV function. In middle-aged and older hypertensive patients with LV hypertrophy, LA enlargement was found to be especially prevalent among patients who were obese, older, female, or had eccentric LV geometry.[57] The degree of LV hypertrophy did not impact on the occurrence of LA enlargement, nor did the presence of atrial fibrillation or mitral regurgitation.

PATHOPHYSIOLOGY

Arterial hypertension is commonly accompanied by impaired LV systolic performance as assessed by mid-wall fractional shortening using echocardiography.[58] Measuring midwall shortening kinetics identifies patients with systolic dysfunction despite normal LV chamber performance and has independent prognostic value. Among asymptomatic normotensive or hypertensive adults, lower midwall shortening is associated with less favorable indices of arterial structure and function, and hemodynamics.[58] Depressed myocardial contractility has been observed in young patients (~33 years old) with borderline to mild hypertension, exhibiting concentric LV remodeling, and thus represents an early consequence of increased blood pressure independent of an increase in LV mass.[59] In older individuals (~66 years old) with Stage I to II hypertension, LV systolic performance was shown to worsen as LV mass and relative wall thickness increased either separately or together, when assessed as either endocardial or midwall shortening.[60] The prevalence of depressed endocardial fractional shortening was highest among individuals with eccentric hypertrophy, while impaired midwall shortening predominated among those with concentric remodeling or hypertrophy. However, in a large population with untreated hypertension, LV hypertrophy was found to be a determinant of impaired midwall systolic function independent of concomitant changes in chamber geometry.[61]

A moderate impairment in diastolic function as evidenced by a slight increase in atrial filling peak velocity has been noted to accompany LV geometric remodeling in the early stages of hypertension.[62] Others have noted that a relatively modest prolongation of isovolumic relaxation time (IVRT) may occur in hypertension before any systolic dysfunction, even when contractility is monitored at the level of the midwall.[63] The less severely abnormal relaxation is independent of geometry or load and could be due to metabolic abnormalities. Overall, when measured as midwall shortening, the progression in the impairment of systolic function parallels those in diastolic function,[64] likely because factors thought to contribute to abnormal diastolic filling, such as impaired calcium handling, increased interstitial fibrosis, and subendocardial ischemia, might also impact on systolic function. In otherwise healthy, unmedicated patients with moderate hypertension and normal conventional measures of systolic function, subnormal midwall shortening was highly correlated with abnormal diastolic function, identified by late (A) LV inflow velocity greater than early (E) velocity and longer IVRT.[65] The latter parameter differs among individuals grouped according to LV geometry, primarily due to a positive correlation with LV mass. A subsequent report showed that depressed LV midwall performance and impaired diastolic filling (prolonged IVRT and abnormal E/A ratio) were interrelated independent of covariates, yet also related to LV mass independently of one another.[66]

Among moderate hypertensive patients with LV hypertrophy, *inappropriate* LV mass was independently associated with higher prevalence of systolic and diastolic abnormalities.[4,5] The percentage of patients with systolic myocardial dysfunction was 43% and 79% for those with eccentric and concentric LV hypertrophy, respectively. Notably, the prevalence of prolonged IRVT was high (65% to 77%) among all patients with LV hypertrophy, regardless of classification as appropriate or inappropriate. This finding is consistent with diastolic dysfunction preceding abnormal systolic function in hypertension. Among patients with mild hypertension and LV hypertrophy, inappropriate LV mass was associated with concentric LV geometry and reduced midwall systolic mechanics.[67] Among patients with moderate to severe hypertension, inappropriately high LV mass was associated with lower systolic function (ejection fraction, midwall shortening, and circumferential end-systolic stress) and diastolic function (prolonged IVRT and lower mitral E/A ratio), independent of LV hypertrophy, concentric geometry, and other covariates.[4]

In hypertensive patients without LV hypertrophy, myocardial oxygen consumption per unit weight is increased. LV hypertrophy is accompanied by a normalization of oxygen consumption, but the ratio between cardiac work and oxygen utilization or myocardial efficiency is reduced. Possible explanations include a greater oxygen demand of a more active interstitial compartment in LV hypertrophy, as well as alterations in substrate utilization and mechanics of hypertrophied muscle fibers. However, not all studies have observed reduced myocardial efficiency with left ventricular hypertrophy, possibly because of differences in the geometric pattern of LV hypertrophy in the populations. Myocardial efficiency was found to be more reduced in hypertrophied hearts that exhibited a concentric compared to eccentric pattern.[68] Myocardial perfusion reserve and hyperemic myocardial blood flow are also reduced in the hypertrophied left ventricle; however, in this case, an impact of LV geometric pattern has not been consistently observed.[68,69] Impaired myocardial blood flow is thought to be due for the most part to reduced intramyocardial coronary density because of increased interstitial fibrosis. Compromised oxygen delivery makes the hypertrophied myocardium more susceptible to ischemic damage, particularly during exercise.

While studies have shown that the reversal of LV hypertrophy with antihypertensive treatment is associated with a reduced risk for subsequent cardiovascular disease,

few have addressed the prognostic impact of geometric structure during treatment. Perhaps not unexpectedly, the persistence of concentric hypertrophy during hypertensive treatment is associated with lower systolic performance, as well as greater cardiovascular morbidity and mortality.[70] However, the incidence of cardiovascular events is greater in patients presenting as well with LV concentric remodeling during treatment, that is, normal LV mass but increased wall thickness. The close association between concentric geometry (both concentric hypertrophy and remodeling) and cardiovascular events is likely explained by a number of factors, including more severe abnormalities in diastolic filling, lower myocardial contractility, and a higher risk of arrhythmias, as well as more pronounced vascular remodeling.

CLINICAL IMPLICATIONS AND PERSPECTIVES

Echocardiographic determination of LV hypertrophy in patients with hypertension is a strong independent predictor of cardiovascular morbidity and mortality, with those exhibiting concentric LV hypertrophy having the greatest risk.[2,49–51] This geometric pattern of hypertrophy is associated with especially high arterial pressure and dramatic alterations in arterial structure, which affects the coronary arteries as well and may lead to myocardial infarction. Partly as a consequence of postinfarction remodeling, the left ventricle begins to adapt an eccentric geometry. Thus in arterial hypertension, the common clinical course for LV remodeling is thought to be concentric LV remodeling, concentric LV hypertrophy, followed by eccentric LV hypertrophy due to postinfarction remodeling (as well as growing wall stress, and fluid retention). Consistent with this scenario, cardiovascular disease, including coronary artery disease, is more common among patients with eccentric LV geometry than those with more concentric LV geometry.[71]

Most patients with LV hypertrophy are asymptomatic, but angina, dyspnea, syncope, and sudden death do occur. Both the electrocardiogram and echocardiogram are commonly used to diagnose LV hypertrophy. The former is useful as an initial screen to detect LA or LV hypertrophy, arterial fibrillation, ventricular arrhythmias, and myocardial ischemia. An echocardiogram provides information on chamber dimensions and wall thickness of the left atrium and left ventricle, wall motion abnormalities, and LV performance (ejection fraction). Echocardiographic determination of the concentric phenotype during treatment may also prove to have utility for assessing treatment effectiveness.

While hypertrophy is generally considered to be a compensatory response of the left ventricle to arterial hypertension, the hypertrophied LV hypertrophy eventually undergoes decompensation and transition to a dilated cardiomyopathy and heart failure (Figure 10–3). At that stage, the heart is unable to pump sufficient blood to meet the metabolic demands of organs and tissues, and as LV end-diastolic and LA pressures increase, pulmonary venous congestion and pulmonary congestion ensue.

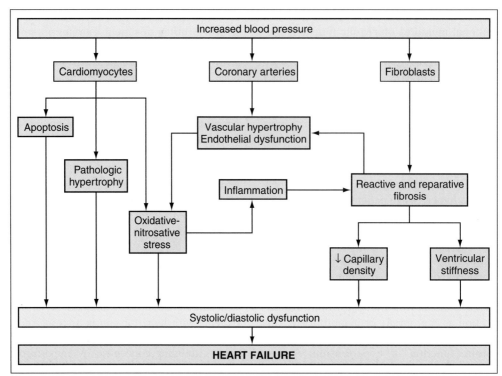

Figure 10–3. Systolic and/or diastolic dysfunction in hypertension results from the impact of increased blood pressure on cardiomyocytes, coronary arteries, and cardiac fibroblasts. Reduced oxygen delivery to cardiomyocytes due to impaired vessel function and decreased capillary density may result from increased fibrosis, which also contributes to increased ventricular stiffness. Compromised oxygen delivery, along with endothelial dysfunction and the altered expression and cellular localization of nitric oxide synthase isoforms by cardiomyocytes, may result in oxidative-nitrosative stress. In turn, oxidative-nitrosative stress may impair cardiomyocyte contractility and relaxation, contribute to cardiomyocyte apoptosis, and create an inflammatory state that further stimulates reactive fibrosis. Pathologic hypertrophy of cardiomyocytes has also been proposed to be associated with activation of G-protein coupled signaling events linked to apoptosis.

Heart failure is a leading cause of death in the developed world, and while life expectancy has been increased through drug development, a diagnosis of heart failure generally proves fatal.[72] Concentric or eccentric hypertrophy both may progress to heart failure. Although there is evidence that cardiac myocyte cell death is one contributing factor, the specific mechanisms responsible for transition of hypertrophy into heart failure are still unknown. Oxidative-nitrosative stress and/or NO-redox disequilibrium are likely contributing factors as well.[73,74] In approximately half of the cases, heart failure is associated with reduced contractility (systolic heart failure). Heart failure resulting from hypertension may also be associated with normal LV function, that is, ejection fraction (diastolic heart failure). Compared to patients with systolic heart failure, patients with heart failure and preserved ejection fraction are generally older, female, and have a history of hypertension.[72,75] The etiology of heart failure with preserved ejection fraction, the contribution of systolic-ventricular and arterial stiffening, and its optimal treatment are questions currently being investigated.[72,75,76]

SUMMARY

Hypertension exerts profound effects on LV geometry and structure that involve contractile and noncontractile compartments, which can prove detrimental to normal pump function of the heart. The LV geometric remodeling often seen in hypertension represents an important independent predictor of morbidity and mortality, with a concentric pattern of hypertrophy presenting the highest risk. A common feature of LV remodeling in hypertension is impaired relaxation (diastolic dysfunction) due to interstitial fibrosis, abnormal Ca^{2+} homeostasis, modifications of myofilament Ca^{2+} sensitivity, and possible increased stiffness within the sarcomere. The degree of diastolic dysfunction progresses with the severity of hypertension, and is often accompanied by impaired contractility. Aging also has a greater negative impact on diastolic function than systolic function, which may explain the high incidence of diastolic heart failure with preserved systolic function in the elderly. Increased myocardial fibrosis is thought to contribute to the effect of aging on diastolic function. The effect of aging on other components of diastolic function needs to be explored, as well as the impact of gender on aging-associated LV remodeling, given the greater incidence of diastolic heart failure with preserved systolic function among women. In light of recent evidence in rats, linking reactive fibrosis and diastolic dysfunction associated with hypertension to macrophage accumulation,[77] a future avenue to explore is the role of inflammation in diastolic dysfunction and the impact that aging has on the inflammatory process. The question of whether oxidative-nitrosative stress in the myocardium as a putative causative factor in precipitating the inflammatory response could serve as a therapeutic target to ameliorate myocardial fibrosis and diastolic dysfunction in hypertensive hearts will need to be answered.[78]

In hypertension, the left ventricle commonly undergoes hypertrophy to compensate for the increased afterload, but if hypertension is poorly controlled or untreated, the left ventricle decompensates and heart failure follows. The events responsible for the transition of hypertrophy to heart failure are not well understood, although a loss of cardiac muscle seems to be involved. The role that increased extracellular matrix degradation plays, due to enhanced activity of MMPs, has not been well explored. Finally, regression of LV hypertrophy is associated with a lower overall risk of cardiovascular disease. Weight loss, exercise, salt restriction, and lowering blood pressure with most antihypertensive agents produce regression. Another strategy might be to exploit intrinsic regulators of cardiac hypertrophy that have been identified in the past few years, including the antihypertrophic NO-cGMP system. Given the report that persistence of concentric hypertrophy during hypertensive treatment is associated with greater cardiovascular morbidity and mortality, developing strategies that aggressively target the concentric phenotype warrants special attention.

REFERENCES

1. Levy D, Garrison RJ, Savage DD, Kannel WB, Castelli WP. Prognostic implications of echocardiographically determined left ventricular mass in the Framingham Heart Study. N Engl J Med 1990; 322:1561–6.
2. Koren MJ, Devereux RB, Casale PN, Savage DD, Laragh JH. Relation of left ventricular mass and geometry to morbidity and mortality in uncomplicated essential hypertension. Ann Intern Med 1991;114:345–52.
3. de Simone G, Palmieri V, Koren MJ, Mensah GA, Roman MJ, Devereux RB. Prognostic implications of the compensatory nature of left ventricular mass in arterial hypertension. J Hypertens 2001;19:119–25.
4. Palmieri V, Wachtell K, Gerdts E, Bella JN, Papademetriou V, Tuxen C, et al. Left ventricular function and hemodynamic features of inappropriate left ventricular hypertrophy in patients with systemic hypertension: the LIFE study. Am Heart J 2001;141:784–91.
5. Palmieri V, Wachtell K, Bella JN, Gerdts E, Papademetriou V, Nieminen MS, et al. Usefulness of the assessment of the appropriateness of left ventricular mass to detect left ventricular systolic and diastolic abnormalities in absence of echocardiographic left ventricular hypertrophy: the LIFE study. J Hum Hypertens 2004;18:423–30.
6. de Simone G, Verdecchia P, Pede S, Gorini M, Maggioni AP. Prognosis of inappropriate left ventricular mass in hypertension: the MAVI study. Hypertension 2002;40:470–6.
7. de Simone G, Kitzman DW, Palmieri V, Liu JE, Oberman A, Hopkins PN, Bella JN, Rao DC, Arnett DK, Devereux RB. Association of inappropriate left ventricular mass with systolic and diastolic dysfunction: the HyperGEN study. Am J Hypertens 2004;17:828–33.
8. Selvetella G, Hirsch E, Notte A, Tarone G, Lembo G. Adaptive and maladaptive hypertrophic pathways: points of convergence and divergence. Cardiovasc Res 2004;63:373–80.
9. Devereux RB, Roman MJ. Left ventricular hypertrophy in hypertension: stimuli, patterns, and consequences. Hypertens Res 1999;22:1–9.

10. Hunter JJ, Chien KR. Signaling pathways for cardiac hypertrophy and failure. N Engl J Med 1999;341(17):1276–83.
11. Reichek N. Patterns of left ventricular response in essential hypertension. J Am Coll Cardiol 1992;19:1559–60.
12. Ganau A, Devereux RB, Roman MJ, de Simone G, Pickering TG, Saba PS, et al. Patterns of left ventricular hypertrophy and geometric remodeling in essential hypertension. J Am Coll Cardiol 1992;19:1550–8.
13. Verdecchia P, Schillaci G, Borgioni C, Ciucci A, Battistelli M, Bartoccini C, et al. Adverse prognostic significance of concentric remodeling of the left ventricle in hypertensive patients with normal left ventricular mass. J Am Coll Cardiol 1995;25:871–8.
14. Gonzalez A, Lopez B, Diez J. Fibrosis in hypertensive heart disease: role of the renin-angiotensin-aldosterone system. Med Clin North Am 2004;88:83–97.
15. Dzau VJ. The role of mechanical and humoral factors in growth regulation of vascular smooth muscle and cardiac myocytes. Curr Opin Nephrol Hypertens 1993;2:27–32.
16. Hefti MA, Harder BA, Eppenberger HM, Schaub MC. Signaling pathways in cardiac myocyte hypertrophy. J Mol Cell Cardiol 1997;29:2873–92.
17. Schluter KD, Piper HM. Regulation of growth in the adult cardiomyocytes. FASEB J 1999;(Suppl 13):S17–22.
18. Chien KR, Zhu H, Knowlton KU, Miller-Hance W, van-Bilsen M, O'Brien TX, et al. Transcriptional regulation during cardiac growth and development. Annu Rev Physiol 1993;55:77–95.
19. Lehman JJ, Kelly DP. Gene regulatory mechanisms governing energy metabolism during cardiac hypertrophic growth. Heart Fail Rev 2002;7:175–85.
20. Leong HS, Brownsey RW, Kulpa JE, Allard MF. Glycolysis and pyruvate oxidation in cardiac hypertrophy—why so unbalanced? Comp Biochem Physiol A Mol Integr Physiol 2003;135:499–513.
21. Lopez B, Gonzalez A, Varo N, Laviades C, Querejeta R, Diez J. Biochemical assessment of myocardial fibrosis in hypertensive heart disease. Hypertension 2001;38:1222–6.

22. Janicki JS, Brower GL, Gardner JD, Chancey AL, Stewart JA Jr. The dynamic interaction between matrix metalloproteinase activity and adverse myocardial remodeling. Heart Fail Rev 2004;9:33–42.
23. Hein S, Arnon E, Kostin S, Schonburg M, Elsasser A, Polyakova V, et al. Progression from compensated hypertrophy to failure in the pressure-overloaded human heart: structural deterioration and compensatory mechanisms. Circulation 2003; 107:984–91.
24. Post WS, Larson MG, Myers RH, Galderisi M, Levy D. Heritability of left ventricular mass: the Framingham Heart Study. Hypertension 1997;30:1025–8.
25. Schunkert H, Erdmann J. Well kept secrets of the genome. Eur Heart J 2003;24:501–3.
26. Bleumink GS, Schut AF, Sturkenboom MC, Deckers JW, van Duijn CM, Stricker BH. Genetic polymorphisms and heart failure. Genet Med 2004; 6(6):465–74.
27. Kuznetsova T, Staessen JA, Olszanecka A, Ryabikov A, Stolarz K, Malyutina S, et al. Maternal and paternal influences on left ventricular mass of offspring. Hypertension 2003;41:69–74.
28. Bella JN, MacCluer JW, Roman MJ, Almasy L, North KE, Best LG, et al. Heritability of left ventricular dimensions and mass in American Indians: the Strong Heart Study. J Hypertens 2004; 22:281–6.
29. Arnett DK, Hong Y, Bella JN, Oberman A, Kitzman DW, Hopkins PN, et al. Sibling correlation of left ventricular mass and geometry in hypertensive African Americans and whites: the HyperGEN study. Hypertension Genetic Epidemiology Network. Am J Hypertens 2001;14:1226–30.
30. Swan L, Birnie DH, Padmanabhan S, Inglis G, Connell JM, Hillis WS. The genetic determination of left ventricular mass in healthy adults. Eur Heart J 2003;24:577–82.
31. Schunkert H, Brockel U, Hengstenberg C, Luchner A, Muscholl MW, Kurzidim K, et al. Familial predisposition of left ventricular hypertrophy. J Am Coll Cardiol 1999;33:1685–91.

32. Adams TD, Yanowitz FG, Fisher AG, Ridges JD, Nelson AG, Hagan AD, et al. Heritability of cardiac size: an echocardiographic and electrocardiographic study of monozygotic and dizygotic twins. *Circulation* 1985;71:39–44.

33. Harshfield GA, Grim CE, Hwang C, Savage DD, Anderson SJ. Genetic and environmental influences on echocardiographically determined left ventricular mass in black twins. *Am J Hypertens* 1990;3:538–43.

34. Verhaaren HA, Schieken RM, Mosteller M, Hewitt JK, Eaves LJ, Nance WE. Bivariate genetic analysis of left ventricular mass and weight in pubertal twins (the Medical College of Virginia twin study). *Am J Cardiol* 1991; 68:661–8.

35. Chobanian AV, Bakris GL, Black HR, Cushman WC, Green LA, Izzo JL Jr, et al. Seventh report of the Joint National Committee on Prevention, Detection, Evaluation, and Treatment of High Blood Pressure. *Hypertension* 2003; 42:1206–52.

36. Kizer JR, Arnett DK, Bella JN, Paranicas M, Rao DC, Province MA, et al. Differences in left ventricular structure between black and white hypertensive adults: the Hypertension Genetic Epidemiology Network study. *Hypertension* 2004;43:1182–8.

37. Lorber R, Gidding SS, Daviglus ML, Colangelo LA, Liu K, Gardin JM. Influence of systolic blood pressure and body mass index on left ventricular structure in healthy African-American and white young adults: the CARDIA study. *J Am Coll Cardiol* 2003;41:955–60.

38. Dekkers C, Treiber FA, Kapuku G, Van Den Oord EJ, Snieder H. Growth of left ventricular mass in African American and European American youth. *Hypertension* 2002;39:943–51.

39. Kuznetsova T, Staessen JA, Wang JG, Gasowski J, Nikitin Y, Ryabikov A, et al. Antihypertensive treatment modulates the association between the D/I ACE gene polymorphism and left ventricular hypertrophy: a meta-analysis. *J Hum Hypertens* 2000;14:447–54.

40. Iaccarino G, Lanni F, Cipolletta E, Trimarco V, Izzo R, Iovino GL, et al. The Glu27 allele of the β2 adrenergic receptor increases the risk of cardiac hypertrophy in hypertension. *J Hypertens* 2004;22:2117–22.

41. Bleumink GS, Schut AF, Sturkenboom MC, Janssen JA, Witteman JC, van Duijn CM, et al. A promoter polymorphism of the insulin-like growth factor-I gene is associated with left ventricular hypertrophy. *Heart* 2005;91:239–40.

42. Hallberg P, Lind L, Michaelsson K, Karlsson J, Kurland L, Kahan T, et al. B2 bradykinin receptor (B2BKR) polymorphism and change in left ventricular mass in response to antihypertensive treatment: results from the Swedish Irbesartan Left Ventricular Hypertrophy Investigation versus Atenolol (SILVHIA) trial. *J Hypertens* 2003;21:621–4.

43. Liljedahl U, Kahan T, Malmqvist K, Melhus H, Syvanen AC, Lind L, et al. Single nucleotide polymorphisms predict the change in left ventricular mass in response to antihypertensive treatment. *J Hypertens* 2004;22:2321–8.

44. Kurland L, Melhus H, Karlsson J, Kahan T, Malmqvist K, Ohman P, et al. Polymorphisms in the angiotensinogen and angiotensin II type 1 receptor gene are related to change in left ventricular mass during antihypertensive treatment: results from the Swedish Irbesartan Left Ventricular Hypertrophy Investigation versus Atenolol (SILVHIA) trial. *J Hypertens* 2002;20:657–63.

45. Kuznetsova T, Staessen JA, Thijs L, Kunath C, Olszanecka A, Ryabikov A, et al. Left ventricular mass in relation to genetic variation in angiotensin II receptors, renin system genes, and sodium excretion. *Circulation* 2004; 110:2644–50.

46. Stella P, Bigatti G, Tizzoni L, Barlassina C, Lanzani C, Bianchi G, et al. Association between aldosterone synthase (CYP11B2) polymorphism and left ventricular mass in human essential hypertension. *J Am Coll Cardiol* 2004; 43:265–70.

47. Segers P, Stergiopulos N, Westerhof N. Quantification of the contribution of cardiac and arterial remodeling to hypertension. *Hypertension* 2000; 36:760–5.

48. Cushman WC. The burden of uncontrolled hypertension: morbidity and mortality associated with disease progression. *J Clin Hypertens (Greenwich)* 2003;5(Suppl 2):14–22.

49. Bella JN, Roman MJ, Pini R, Schwartz JE, Pickering TG, Devereux RB. Assessment of arterial compliance by carotid midwall strain-stress relation in hypertension. *Hypertension* 1999;33:793–9.

50. Roman MJ, Pickering TG, Schwartz JE, Pini R, Devereux RB. Relation of arterial structure and function to left ventricular geometric patterns in hypertensive adults. *J Am Coll Cardiol* 1996;28:751–6.

51. Shigematsu Y, Hamada M, Mukai M, Matsuoka H, Sumimoto T, Hiwada K. Clinical evidence for an association between left ventricular geometric adaptation and extracardiac target organ damage in essential hypertension. *J Hypertens* 1995;13:155–60.

52. Blake J, Devereux RB, Herrold EM, Jason M, Fisher J, Borer JS, et al. Relation of concentric left ventricular hypertrophy and extracardiac target organ damage to supranormal left ventricular performance in established essential hypertension. *Am J Cardiol* 1988;62:246–52.

53. Ghali JK, Liao Y, Cooper RS. Influence of left ventricular geometric patterns on prognosis in patients with or without coronary artery disease. *J Am Coll Cardiol* 1998;31:1635–40.

54. Fesler P, Du Cailar G, Ribstein J, Mimran A. Left ventricular remodeling and renal function in never-treated essential hypertension. *J Am Soc Nephrol* 2003;14:881–7.

55. Bella JN, Wachtell K, Boman K, Palmieri V, Papademetriou V, Gerdts E, et al. Relation of left ventricular geometry and function to aortic root dilatation in patients with systemic hypertension and left ventricular hypertrophy (the LIFE study). *Am J Cardiol* 2002;89:337–41.

56. Jennings GL. The left atrium in hypertension: next to the chamber of power. *J Hypertens* 2004;22:1473–4.

57. Gerdts E, Oikarinen L, Palmieri V, Otterstad JE, Wachtell K, Boman K, et al. Correlates of left atrial size in hypertensive patients with left ventricular hypertrophy: the Losartan Intervention for Endpoint Reduction in Hypertension (LIFE) study. *Hypertension* 2002;39:739–43.

58. Devereux RB, de Simone G, Pickering TG, Schwartz JE, Roman MJ. Relation of left ventricular midwall function to cardiovascular risk factors and arterial structure and function. *Hypertension* 1998;31:929–36.

59. Palatini P, Visentin P, Mormino P, Pietra M, Piccolo D, Cozzutti E, et al. Left ventricular performance in the early stages of systemic hypertension. HARVEST Study Group. Hypertension and Ambulatory Recording Venetia Study. *Am J Cardiol* 1998;81:418–23.

60. Wachtell K, Rokkedal J, Bella JN, Aalto T, Dahlof B, Smith G, et al. Effect of electrocardiographic left ventricular hypertrophy on left ventricular systolic function in systemic hypertension (the LIFE study). Losartan Intervention for Endpoint. *Am J Cardiol* 2001;87:54–60.

61. Schillaci G, Vaudo G, Pasqualini L, Reboldi G, Porcellati C, Verdecchia P. Left ventricular mass and systolic dysfunction in essential hypertension. *J Hum Hypertens* 2002;16:117–22.

62. Palatini P, Visentin P, Mormino P, Mos L, Canali C, Dorigatti F, et al. Structural abnormalities and not diastolic dysfunction are the earliest left ventricular changes in hypertension. HARVEST Study Group. *Am J Hypertens* 1998;11:147–54.

63. de Simone G, Greco R, Mureddu G, Romano C, Guida R, Celentano A, et al. Relation of left ventricular diastolic properties to systolic function in arterial hypertension. *Circulation* 2000;101: 152–7.

64. Schussheim AE, Diamond JA, Jhang JS, Phillips RA. Midwall fractional shortening is an independent predictor of left ventricular diastolic dysfunction in asymptomatic patients with systemic hypertension. *Am J Cardiol* 1998;82: 1056–9.

65. Wachtell K, Smith G, Gerdts E, Dahlof B, Nieminen MS, Papademetriou V, et al. Left ventricular filling patterns in patients with systemic hypertension and left ventricular hypertrophy (the LIFE study). Losartan Intervention for Endpoint. *Am J Cardiol* 2000;85: 466–72.

66. Wachtell K, Papademetriou V, Smith G, Gerdts E, Dahlof B, Engblom E, et al. Relation of impaired left ventricular filling to systolic midwall mechanics in hypertensive patients with normal left ventricular systolic chamber function: the Losartan Intervention for Endpoint Reduction in Hypertension (LIFE) study. *Am Heart J* 2004;148:538–44.

67. Palmieri V, de Simone G, Roman MJ, Schwartz JE, Pickering TG, Devereux RB. Ambulatory blood pressure and metabolic abnormalities in hypertensive subjects with inappropriately high left ventricular mass. *Hypertension* 1999;34:1032–40.

68. Akinboboye OO, Chou RL, Bergmann SR. Myocardial blood flow and efficiency in concentric and eccentric left ventricular hypertrophy. *Am J Hypertens* 2004;17: 433–8.

69. Schafer S, Kelm M, Mingers S, Strauer BE. Left ventricular remodeling impairs

coronary flow reserve in hypertensive patients. *J Hypertens* 2002;20:1431–7.

70. Muiesan ML, Salvetti M, Monteduro C, Bonzi B, Paini A, Viola S, et al. Left ventricular concentric geometry during treatment adversely affects cardiovascular prognosis in hypertensive patients. *Hypertension* 2004;43:731–8.

71. Zabalgoitia M, Berning J, Koren MJ, Stoylen A, Nieminen MS, Dahlof B, et al. Impact of coronary artery disease on left ventricular systolic function and geometry in hypertensive patients with left ventricular hypertrophy (the LIFE study). *Am J Cardiol* 2001;88:646–50.

72. Hunt SA, Baker DW, Chin MH, Cinquegrani MP, Feldman AM, Francis GS, et al. ACC/AHA guidelines for the evaluation and management of chronic heart failure in the adult: executive summary. A report of the American College of Cardiology/American Heart Association Task Force on Practice Guidelines (Committee to Revise the 1995 Guidelines for the Evaluation and Management of Heart Failure) developed in collaboration with the International Society for Heart and Lung Transplantation, endorsed by the Heart Failure Society of America. *Circulation* 2001;104:2996–3007.

73. Giordano FJ. Oxygen, oxidative stress, hypoxia, and heart failure. *J Clin Invest* 2005;115:500–8.

74. Hare JM, Stamler JS. NO/redox disequilibrium in the failing heart and cardiovascular system. *J Clin Invest* 2005;115:509–17.

75. Hogg K, Swedberg K, McMurray J. Heart failure with preserved left ventricular systolic function; epidemiology, clinical characteristics, and prognosis. *J Am Coll Cardiol* 2004; 43:317–27.

76. Kass DA, Bronzwaer JG, Paulus WJ. What mechanisms underlie diastolic dysfunction in heart failure? *Circ Res* 2004;94:1533–42.

77. Kuwahara F, Kai H, Tokuda K, Takeya M, Takeshita A, Egashira K, et al. Hypertensive myocardial fibrosis and diastolic dysfunction: another model of inflammation? *Hypertension* 2004;43: 739–45.

78. Weber KT. From inflammation to fibrosis: a stiff stretch of highway. *Hypertension* 2004;43:716–9.

Chapter

11 Hemodynamics of Hypertension

Joseph L. Izzo, Jr.

Key Findings

- In hypertension at any age, increased or inappropriately high sympathetic nervous system (SNS) activity causes or exacerbates a fundamental hemodynamic imbalance that includes both inappropriately high cardiac output and inappropriately high systemic vascular resistance (SVR).

- Hypertensive individuals appear to make a transition from a high-output, low-resistance state to a low-output, high-resistance state as they age. It is not clear that such a transition occurs in most individuals with hypertension or if this transition is part of the usual aging process.

- Arterial pressure and cardiac output must vary to meet different physiologic, thermoregulatory, and metabolic demands and hemodynamic responses to physiologic and metabolic stimuli vary within and across individuals. Under stimulated conditions, either flow or resistance may change based on the nature of the stimulus and the underlying disease state.

- The generation of systolic pressure is far more complex in its physiology than the generation of diastolic blood pressure (BP) and systolic BP contains information about both nonpulsatile and pulsatile flow.

- An in-depth analysis of a systolic pulse contour yields the concept of "ventricular–vascular interactions" during systole. During early systole, the interaction of the left ventricle and the aorta generate a forward pressure wave and an initial systolic peak pressure (usually called P1). In late systole, the interaction of the forward pressure wave and flow discontinuities in the peripheral arterial tree generate reflected pressure waves that often augment P1 (forming P2). The observed systolic pulse contour is the sum of these "ventricular–vascular interactions."

- Increased pulse pressure (PP) (generally P1) is sometimes due to an isolated increase in stroke volume (severe anemia, hyperdynamic hypertension, aortic insufficiency, thyrotoxicosis, vitamin deficiency, or arteriovenous shunting, renal failure) but the etiology of wide PP or isolated systolic hypertension is predominantly due to increased central arterial stiffness.

- Stiffening of the aorta and carotid arteries has another important homeostatic consequence: increased blood pressure variability. With collagen deposition and calcification, baroreflex mechanoreceptors are restrained in their ability to stretch, thus reducing the effect of an important negative feedback loop controlling SNS outflow.

- At all points along the arterial tree, forward- and backward-traveling waves summate to create the unique morphology of the pressure wave at a particular point. Central and peripheral pressure waveforms differ because of the relative timing differences of the incident and reflected waves at the two sites.

- As pressure waves travel downstream, the forward pressure wave is amplified due to increased impedance in arteries of decreasing caliber, causing PP amplification. The wall composition also changes with arterial size; in the thoracic aorta, there is a predominance of elastin over collagen, but in the peripheral conduit arteries, there is more collagen than elastin. Importantly, not all segments of the arterial tree become stiffer with aging or disease.

- Cardiac and vascular target organ damage is a predictable interrelated consequence of the systolic hypertension with direct implications for cardiovascular symptoms and pathology. Increased central systolic BP increases cardiac afterload and leads to left ventricular hypertrophy. Increased central arterial stiffness and cardiac afterload cause decreased exercise tolerance, diastolic dysfunction, and eventually, heart failure. Ischemic heart disease is exacerbated as well due to reduced diastolic pressure and reduced coronary filling, especially in response to systemic vasodilation.

By its very name, *hypertension* is essentially a hemodynamic syndrome. This statement does not contradict the observations that hypertension is associated with a diverse series of metabolic, functional, and structural abnormalities. Rather, it stipulates that hypertension is not a lesser byproduct of a broader "metabolic syndrome." While central obesity appears to contribute in parallel to metabolic abnormalities (e.g., insulin resistance) and increased systolic and diastolic blood pressure, the syndrome of hypertension in the population over age 50 is also directly related to increased stiffness of the aorta and central arteries, with accompanying increases in systolic blood pressure, decreases in diastolic blood pressure, and widening of pulse pressure. There is little to suggest that "essential" hypertension has a primary genetic basis; rather it is best characterized as an acquired, age-related syndrome that occurs primarily in highly industrialized societies. Remarkably, the pathogenesis of systolic hypertension is still poorly understood, probably owing in large measure to its complexity. Current research has begun to focus on arterial wall pathophysiology, but other mechanisms, especially inappropriately high activity of the sympathetic nervous system (SNS), appear to play a causal or permissive role in all forms of hypertension. The syndrome of hypertension is thus a highly heterogeneous condition best described by its intrinsic hemodynamic abnormalities.

BASIC HEMODYNAMICS

Ohm's Law and circulation

The classical approach to the hemodynamics of hypertension applies the same principles that govern an electrical circuit (Ohm's Law). In this steady-state model:

Mean arterial pressure (voltage) = Cardiac output (current) × Systemic vascular resistance (impedance)

In extending this simplified model to the investigation of human hemodynamics, mean arterial pressure (MAP) has been historically determined from peripheral sphygmomanometry using the following formula:

MAP = diastolic blood pressure + 1/3 pulse pressure

This approximation of mean pressure holds for heart rates above 55 to 60; if bradycardia is present, MAP is somewhat overestimated. A more accurate approximation of MAP can also be obtained by oscillometric blood pressure (BP) methods that identify MAP as the pressure at which the maximum oscillatory amplitude of the pulse occurs. Systemic resistance is mathematically more closely related to diastolic pressure or MAP than to systolic pressure.

Pressure-volume homeostasis

There is a certain degree of BP homeostasis that can be explained as counter-regulation of cardiac output and systemic vascular resistance (SVR); if one increases, the other tends to fall. Yet the primary physiologic mechanisms that defend arterial pressure itself (SNS, renin-angiotensin system, renal salt-water handling) do not correspond directly to any flow-resistance model. BP regulation is better explained by the concept of pressure–volume homeostasis. Foremost in BP counter-regulation is the SNS, which responds instantaneously and chronically to both pressure and volume signals.[1,2] Circulatory SNS homeostasis involves two major inhibitory baroreflexes that control SNS outflow: the aorto-carotid baroreflex that responds to changes in arterial pressure or "afterload," and the cardiopulmonary baroreflex that responds to changes in cardiac filling or "preload." Under usual physiologic circumstances, both of these reflexes work in tandem to prevent hypoperfusion and hypotension. If there is a sudden fall in arterial pressure, aorto-carotid mechanoreceptors are "unloaded" and afferent signals are sent to the brainstem instantly to stimulate SNS outflow to the heart and vasculature.[3] If blood volume and cardiac preload are suddenly reduced, cardiac mechanoreceptors are unloaded and SNS activation proceeds via the same brainstem centers affected by aorto-carotid baroreflex unloading.[3–5] Conversely, salt loading or extracellular volume expansion suppresses SNS activity. During upright postural adaptation, the degree of SNS stimulation correlates strongly with the degree of reduction in cardiac stroke volume caused by gravitational blood pooling.[6] In contrast, acute increases in central blood volume lead to withdrawal of SNS activity, with ensuing renal vasodilation, enhanced natriuresis, and dilation of systemic arteries and veins, independent of aorto-carotid baroreflex function.[7] Thus the cardiopulmonary baroreflex system can override a normal aorto-carotid system, especially during postural adaptation or other conditions that affect central blood volume.[6–10]

SNS overactivity in hypertension

In hypertension at any age, there is increased or inappropriately high SNS activity,[11–15] which causes or exacerbates a fundamental hemodynamic imbalance that includes *both* inappropriately high cardiac output and inappropriately high SVR. High cardiac sympathetic drive has been demonstrated via pharmacologic blockade of beta-receptors,[16,17] and by radiotracer methods that reveal high cardiac norepinephrine turnover.[18] High peripheral vascular sympathetic tone and increased alpha-adrenergic receptor dependency[19] occur in association with altered fatty acid metabolism in vascular smooth muscle cells, creating a potential link to obesity-related hypertension.[20] Increased plasma catecholamines[11,12,15] have been repeatedly demonstrated in hypertensive individuals, both young and old. The etiology of the high SNS activity in hypertension is undoubtedly complex, but SNS overactivity is associated with obesity,[21] aging,[11,12] and higher BP in general.[11,12,15] In chronic hypertension, baroreflexes cannot fully compensate for inappropriate SNS activity and cannot restore elevated BP back to normotensive levels due to the phenomena of resetting and blunting. Aorto-carotid baroreflexes quickly *reset* at any pressure level so that acute increases or decreases in BP affect SNS activity equally in normotensive people and those with early hypertension. The only change is in the set-point of the response. With chronic hypertension, however, aorto-carotid baroreflexes also become *blunted*, in that an acute increase in blood pressure causes less SNS suppression.[22] Abnormal cardiopulmonary baroreflex activity in hypertension[23] also contributes to abnormal pressure–volume homeostasis. For example, the high muscle SNS nerve traffic in hypertensives cannot be suppressed to a normal degree during salt loading.[13]

Pressure-flow imbalances in aging and hypertension

Steady-state hemodynamic studies have yielded a view that hypertension is caused by an isolated increase in SVR. Yet in most people with diastolic or systolic hypertension, it can be argued that cardiac output is also inappropriately high.[19,24–28] Arterial pressure is more tightly regulated than cardiac output but neither is a highly regulated physiologic variable and wide intra-individual variations in BP and blood flow are necessary to meet diverse physiologic demands. In the population at large, cardiac output at rest varies by at least threefold,[6,24] creating a very broad overlap between normal and hypertensive individuals in cardiac output or SVR. With or without hypertension, aging has a marked effect on systemic hemodynamics. Early in life, heart rate and cardiac output are relatively high, while later in life, heart rate and cardiac output decrease.[11,12,15] In cross-sectional studies, SVR increases at least until middle age,[12] while pulse pressure continues to increase with advancing age[29] due to continuous increases in central arterial stiffness.

Thus the BP configuration in later years is usually isolated systolic hypertension.[30,31]

There are certain recurring hemodynamic patterns that have been described in the population. At one extreme is "hyperdynamic," or high-output hypertension,[32,33] which occurs in younger individuals with early or "borderline" hypertension, and is associated with normal or low SVR.[15] At the other extreme, older individuals, especially those with long-standing high blood pressure, typically manifest high SVR and normal-to-low cardiac output.[11,12] Hypertensive individuals thus appear to make a transition from a high-output, low-resistance state to a low-output, high-resistance state as they age.[34] Yet it is not clear that such a transition occurs in most individuals with hypertension or if this transition is part of the usual aging process. One prospective 20-year follow-up study documents within-individual transitions from high cardiac output to high SVR but the study group only included those with hyperdynamic hypertension,[35] not the larger group who manifest isolated systolic hypertension as the only sign of the condition. In the Framingham study, systolic hypertension usually precedes diastolic hypertension.[36] Thus the best available information suggests that the vast majority of older hypertensives never manifest either diastolic hypertension or a hyperdynamic phase of the disorder, despite the fact that inappropriately high cardiac output at any age exacerbates hypertension.[37] It is also likely that the apparent age-related transition from high flow to high resistance is due to the peculiar form of selection bias intrinsic to cross-sectional studies.

In longstanding hypertension, structural cardiac and vascular maladaptations further sustain the high blood pressure. The degree of left ventricular hypertrophy (LVH) is closely related to the individual's chronic systolic blood pressure.[38] Some studies suggest that LVH may be at least partially a result of chronically high SNS activity.[39] Over time, arteriolar smooth-muscle hypertrophy[40,41] also appears to sustain the inappropriately high SVR. Fortunately, these chronic structural changes are at least partially reversible because adequate long-term treatment of hypertension favorably affects both LVH[42] and vascular smooth-muscle hypertrophy[41] and reduces overall cardiovascular risk.[42]

Hemodynamic stress response patterns

Arterial pressure and cardiac output must vary to meet various physiologic, thermoregulatory, and metabolic demands, and hemodynamic responses to physiologic and metabolic stimuli vary within and across individuals. Under stimulated conditions, either flow or resistance may change based on the nature of the stimulus and the underlying disease state. During physiologic extremes such as bicycle exercise, the cardiac output of conditioned individuals can increase by over four-fold.[24] Even during relatively mild stresses such as the assumption of the upright posture, gravitational pooling and diminished venous return cause a decrease in upright cardiac output by about 20% compared to the supine posture.[6,43] Mental and physical stress can be used as laboratory probes to partially differentiate hypertensives from normotensives; hypertensives tend to respond to mental or physical stress with a combined pattern of increased cardiac output and peripheral vasoconstriction, whereas normotensives tend to respond with increased cardiac output alone.[26,44] Psychosocial-physiologic differences in stress responses can also be demonstrated; the presence of a personality profile characterized by suppressed anger or hostility defines a subpopulation of individuals that responds with vasoconstriction after mental stress rather than increased cardiac output.[45] A variety of subacute or chronic environmental adaptations also affect resting cardiac output and SVR. In the northern latitudes, for example, resting supine cardiac output is about 15% lower in the winter than the summer in normal and borderline hypertensive individuals.[43]

There is an important conservation mechanism that further modifies flow-resistance relationships and permits selective flow redistribution. Flow distribution across organ beds is made possible by selective vasoconstriction, which allows diverse physiologic adaptations with the least possible increase in cardiac work. Under usual resting or lightly stimulated conditions, about 40% of cardiac output goes to skeletal muscle, while about 20% to 25% each goes to the brain and kidneys. In response to various physiologic stimuli, both total cardiac output and the fractional flow sent to each major organ bed can vary widely. Modulation in organ perfusion is dependent on a variety of systemic and local vasoregulatory mechanisms, including regional SNS activity and the influences of circulating hormones such as vasopressin.[46]

Limitations of steady-state hemodynamic model

As can be gleaned from the foregoing discussion, there are major limitations to the use of steady-state hemodynamic formulas to describe chronic hypertension. In the past, it was assumed that the syndrome of hypertension could be described adequately by the concept of increased SVR (i.e., diastolic hypertension) with normal cardiac output but this is a gross oversimplification of the problem. The simplified steady-state model is still useful as a teaching aid but it does not fully explain critical features of pulsatile flow or hypertensive target organ damage. First, the components of Ohm's Law do not correspond to the physiologic control mechanisms: there are no constant flow or resistance sensors in the body, and circulatory systems are pulsatile, not constant-flow systems. Second, the physiologic variation in SVR is extremely wide within and between individuals, with extremely broad overlap between normal and hypertensive individuals.[11,24,47,48] Third, it is now clear that the consequences of hypertension are much more closely related to systolic blood pressure, which is only partially dependent on systemic resistance.[49,50] Finally, hemodynamic profiling has not proved to be a useful guide to therapy in chronic hypertension; antihypertensive drugs, which exert complex actions on the neuroendocrine and hemodynamic mechanisms, often lead to parallel reductions in cardiac output and systemic resistance.

There are also practical problems that plague the measurement of flow and resistance in humans. Invasive studies are neither practical nor definitive, and the wide physiologic variability of flow and resistance in everyday life makes threshold values essentially meaningless. Noninvasive studies of systemic hemodynamics are also technically difficult to reproduce. Doppler flow studies are difficult because of the peculiar geometry of the aortic root. The integral of a peripheral pulse contour could be used to estimate stroke volume were it not for the presence of reflected waves and other peripheral pulse transmission phenomena. Echocardiographic (ECG) determination is subject to substantial variations in results because of differences in ventricular geometry, and is relatively costly. Nuclear studies are expensive, cumbersome, and time consuming, and cannot detect acute hemodynamic changes. Impedance cardiography using ECG-gated variation in thoracic impedance can be used to derive stroke volume. While within-subject changes are relatively reliable using this technique, interindividual comparisons require a population-based algorithm that can be influenced by variable thoracic-abdominal anatomic configurations and altered conductivity within the thorax.

PULSATILE HEMODYNAMICS

The National Heart, Lung, and Blood Institute has redefined the approach to hypertension by focusing on systolic rather than diastolic pressure as the principal clinical endpoint for diagnosis and monitoring of hypertension, ending the twentieth-century view that hypertension is simply an elevation of diastolic BP.[49] The Joint National Committee in its seventh report has reiterated this position[51] and professional organizations worldwide have subsequently concurred. Systolic pressure is very highly correlated with pulse pressure (PP = systolic – diastolic pressure), and both are independent cardiovascular disease risk predictors.[52] Systolic pressure is preferred over PP as a clinical management variable, however, because it is almost identical to PP in its predictive value in epidemiologic studies. Systolic BP has been the principal dependent variable in successful clinical trials,[53] is easier to understand, and is more accurately determined.[49] Detection methods have also changed; oscillometric methods are becoming more widely used. They are reasonably reliable for the detection of mean and systolic pressures but depend on proprietary algorithms that differ among manufacturers,[54] and are intrinsically not as accurate in estimating diastolic BP or PP.[55]

Pulse as biological signal

The generation of systolic pressure is far more complex in its physiology than the generation of diastolic BP and systolic BP contains information about both nonpulsatile and pulsatile flow. Teleologically, it can be argued that systolic pressure and PP are more physiologically relevant to short-term and long-term BP control because normal cardiovascular homeostasis requires cyclical stretch to generate feedback signals. It is attractive to speculate that the cardiac stretch and peripheral pulse volume are the primary biological signals sensed by cardiac and arterial smooth-muscle mechanoreceptors. Cellular stretch, further modified by other deformation signals in some cells (e.g., endothelium) alter cell function via changes in ion transport, cell metabolism, and production of autacoids and vasoactive substances, all of which can affect local and regional blood flow.[56] At the same time, afferent fibers from specialized mechanoreceptors communicate with the central nervous system to regulate systemic flow. This integrated model provides the necessary information for systemic and regional cardiovascular homeostasis.

Ventricular–vascular interactions and pulse contours

An in-depth analysis of a systolic pulse contour yields the concept of "ventricular–vascular interactions" during systole (Figure 11–1). During early systole, the interaction of the left ventricle and the aorta generate a forward pressure wave and an initial systolic peak pressure (usually called P1). In late systole, the interaction of the forward pressure wave and flow discontinuities in the peripheral arterial tree generate reflected pressure waves that often augment P1 (forming P2). The observed systolic pulse contour is the sum of these "ventricular–vascular interactions" (Figure 11–2). Hypertension can be subdivided into its hemodynamic components using these concepts (Figure 11–2). In this model, increased systemic resistance causes increases in both systolic BP and diastolic BP, whereas increased systolic BP can result from increased cardiac stroke volume or increased aortic impedance (due to decreased aortic diameter or increased aortic stiffness). Increased aortic stiffness also leads to a decrease in diastolic BP through alteration in capacitance and reduced diastolic "runoff" (Figure 11–3).

Systolic hypertension: Aortic abnormalities

Large arteries serve two major interrelated functions: transfer of blood to peripheral organs (the conduit or

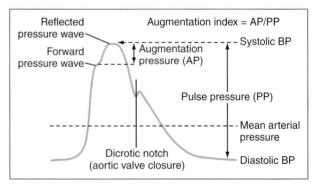

Figure 11–1. Anatomy of a central pulse wave. Several different physical forces determine the morphology of a pulse contour, which is the result of a series of ventricular–vascular interactions. Early systolic interactions of the ventricle and the aorta determine the height of the forward pressure wave (P1). Later in systole, a primary reflected wave returns to the aortic root where it summates with the decaying forward wave (P2), augmenting central systolic pressure, especially in older individuals with hypertension.

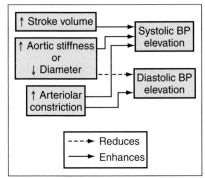

Figure 11–2. Pathogenesis of systolic and diastolic hypertension. Diastolic BP elevation occurs principally as a result of systemic vasoconstriction. Systolic BP elevation is the result of increased diastolic BP as well as increased cardiac stroke volume, increased aortic stiffness, or decreased aortic diameter. Central pulse pressure is also affected by the timing and magnitude of reflected pressure waves, whereas peripheral pulse pressure is predominantly determined by the forward pressure wave (see text). BP, blood pressure.

transmission function) and partial damping of cardiac pulsation (the compliance or capacitance function). Circulatory pulsation is reflected clinically by the amplitude of the PP, which is determined by the underlying series of ventricular–vascular interactions. Increased PP (generally P1) is sometimes due to an isolated increase in stroke volume (severe anemia, hyperdynamic hypertension, aortic insufficiency, thyrotoxicosis, vitamin deficiency, or arteriovenous shunting, renal failure[57]), but the etiology of wide PP or isolated systolic hypertension (ISH) is predominantly due to increased central arterial stiffness.[49] Whether or not the diastolic (or mean) pressure is elevated depends on the concomitant degree of elevation of systemic resistance (Figure 11–1). In normal young people, the elastic recoil function of the proximal aorta serves to dampen the impact of pulsatile flow (i.e., it narrows the PP) by retaining a fraction of each cardiac stroke volume in the central arteries during systole and then delivering this retained volume to the distal circulation during diastole (Figure 11–3).[58] Because the normal aorta functions as a capacitance chamber (Windkessel model) and a passive third pumping chamber, pulsatile flow is damped and PP is relatively narrow. When central arteries are intrinsically smaller, or if they stiffen with aging and hypertension, the capacitance and damping functions of the aorta are diminished and more of each individual stroke volume is forced through the resistance arterioles during systole. The amplitude of the forward pressure wave (and PP) increases, and the systolic peak itself becomes sharper,[59] independent of any changes in cardiac output or systemic resistance. With aging, because of the reduction in the elastic recoil function of the aorta, the fraction of each stroke volume retained in the aorta during systole is decreased. Consequently, there is a

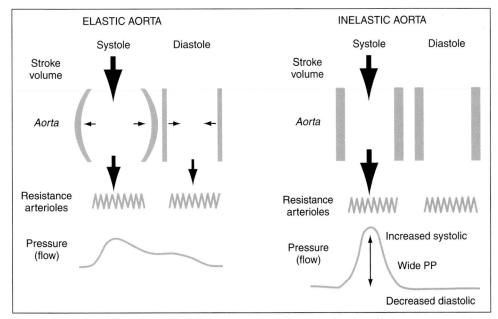

Figure 11–3. Capacitance function of the aorta and pathogenesis of wide pulse pressure. In individuals with elastic central arteries (usually younger people, *left panel*), the aorta is distended by each cardiac stroke volume. The result is a diminution of systolic flow, with the retained remnant of each stroke volume delivered by aortic elastic recoil to the periphery during diastole. This phenomenon represents normal capacitance or damping of cardiac pulsation. As vessels stiffen (usually older people, *right panel*), the fraction of stroke volume delivered during systole increases and the pressure and flow during diastole decrease. The hallmark of central arterial stiffness (reduced capacitance and damping) is thus a widened PP. PP, pulse pressure. (Adapted from Izzo JL Jr, *J Am Geriatr Soc* 1982;30:352–9: Blackwell Scientific.)

corresponding reduction in diastolic flow and BP and a net widening of PP. Degenerative stiffening of the aorta and central arteries is sometimes called *arteriosclerosis* to differentiate it from *atherosclerosis,* the occlusive result of endovascular inflammatory disease, lipid oxidation, and plaque formation. At a cellular level, arteriosclerosis is the result of age and hypertension-related adaptations in the tunica media, including the breakdown of the elastin network, increased collagen deposition, and vascular smooth-muscle hypertrophy.[60–63]

It has been taught that an age-related increase in aortic diameter is a major contributing factor to increased impedance and wide PP.[64] This line of reasoning, however, runs counter to the basic principles of arterial biomechanics and to the observed trends in large observational studies. The input impedance of an artery is *directly* proportional to the root of its "effective stiffness" (wall elasticity-thickness product) and *inversely* proportional to the root of the fifth power of its diameter. With aging and hypertension, wall thickness and intrinsic wall stiffness do increase but these changes are accompanied by age-related increases in aortic diameter.[65] It seems most plausible that the age-related increase in diameter serve to counteract (rather than cause) the age-related increases in effective arterial stiffness and the wide PP. In smaller individuals, including women, isolated systolic hypertension begins with a smaller aortic diameter and normal aortic wall properties. Mitchell et al.[66] have reported an inverse relationship between aortic diameter and systolic BP in middle-aged individuals with systolic hypertension (with or without diastolic hypertension). An inverse relationship between aortic size and systolic blood pressure (or PP) was also observed in recent studies, such as the Framingham Heart study and the LIFE study.[31,65,67,68]

The idea that wide PP hypertension is not simply "burned-out" diastolic hypertension is also supported by the Framingham and NHANES databases to the effect that the onset of hypertension in middle-aged individuals begins with elevated systolic pressure (and normal diastolic pressure).[31,69] The most rational interpretation of current data is that individuals with smaller aortas have an intrinsic tendency toward wide PP as a result of increased aortic impedance. Age-related dilatation of the aorta also occurs but does not fully compensate for the increased systolic BP load. Aging and hypertension-related increases in aortic wall thickness and changes in intrinsic wall composition are maladaptive compensations for increased aortic diameter (and load) that exacerbates the wide PP.

Stiffening of the aorta and carotid arteries has another important homeostatic consequence: increased blood pressure variability. With collagen deposition and calcification, baroreflex mechanoreceptors are restrained in their ability to stretch, thus reducing the effect of an important negative feedback loop controlling SNS outflow.[22] In response to an increase in cardiac output, the absence of the aortocarotid baroreflex allows maintenance of a higher heart rate and vascular resistance than would normally occur, thus leading to a prolonged increase in systolic pressure after stimulation. Conversely, vasodilation after exercise or a large meal is met with a lessened counter-regulatory SNS-mediated vasoconstriction, and pressure remains low for a longer period of time.[70–72]

Pulse wave reflection and augmentation

Late systolic ventricular–vascular interactions involve the impact of reflected pressure waves, which arise at points of "impedance mismatch" (where the flow and pressure waves are not perfectly matched). Common reflection sites are branch points, constrictions, areas of turbulence, or areas of change in wall stiffness. Reflected waves can be characterized by two basic properties: timing and amplitude. Timing is a function of pulse wave velocity (PWV), which is directly dependent on arterial stiffness and the distance to the reflecting site and inversely dependent on arterial diameter. The amplitude of the reflected wave is dependent on the reflection coefficient generated in the distal circulation and is usually characterized as the augmentation pressure (increment over the incident wave caused by the reflected wave) or augmentation index (AI), the fraction of total PP attributable to the reflected wave) (Figure 11–2), usually corrected for height[73] or gender[74] and heart rate.[75]

At all points along the arterial tree, forward- and backward-traveling waves summate to create the unique morphology of the pressure wave at a particular point. Central and peripheral pressure waveforms differ because of the relative timing differences of the incident and reflected waves at the two sites. Since these pattern differences are somewhat predictable, the central waveform theoretically can be recreated from the corresponding peripheral waveform using a generalized transfer function. Yet there remains considerable debate about the reliability of this approach.[55,74,76–82] Overall, even if the nuances of the central waveform are lost in the application of a fixed transfer function, central systolic pressure can be reasonably estimated from the radial pressure waveform.[55,78] In contrast, central PP cannot be as easily estimated because of intrinsic inaccuracies in the measurement of peripheral diastolic pressure.[55]

There is a popular misconception that AI is primarily a measure of arterial stiffness. Instead, the principal determinant of AI is the reflection coefficient, which is strongly influenced by peripheral vasomotor tone. AI correlates strongly with DBP, MAP, and SVR.[83,84] The peripheral circulatory contribution to AI has been demonstrated by the instantaneous increases in AI that occur during acute infusion of vasoconstrictors such as norepinephrine,[85,86] angiotensin II,[86,87] or endothelin.[88] Conversely, nitrovasodilators immediately diminish AI.[89–92] In experiments in which AI and PWV have been measured simultaneously, acute changes in AI are far greater than the corresponding changes in PWV. There is a small effect of age or arterial stiffness on AI, but overall AI is only weakly related to arterial stiffness.

Pulse pressure amplification and microcirculation

As pressure waves travel downstream, the forward pressure wave is amplified due to increased impedance in arteries of decreasing caliber, causing *pulse pressure amplification*.[93] Wall composition also changes with arterial size; in the thoracic aorta, there is a predominance of elastin over collagen, but in the peripheral conduit arteries, there is more collagen than elastin. Importantly, not all segments of the arterial tree become stiffer with aging or disease. In hypertensives[94] and diabetics,[95] the brachial arteries demonstrate normal or increased age-related compliance, at least in part due to their relatively larger diameters compared to normal individuals. It seems likely that this enhanced compliance serves as an important offload mechanism that transfers the capacitance function a little further downstream.

In normal young people, brachial systolic pressure is often 10 to 20 mm Hg higher than aortic root systolic pressure, but with very wide interindividual variation. It has been said that there is a diminution of pulse pressure amplification (PPA) with aging,[62] but this statement is based on the comparison of peak pressures at the radial artery, which is almost exclusively related to the amplitude of the forward wave (P1) compared to the sum P1 and the reflected wave at the aortic root.[62] Newer studies are beginning to compare central and peripheral P1 values to learn more about the properties of large arteries independent of wave reflection.[96] The practical importance of variability in PPA is that brachial cuff blood pressures do not provide uniformly accurate information about central or distal systolic pressure or PP. Thus, in order to obtain more relevant information about a given patient, it will be necessary to use measures other than a standard blood pressure cuff applied to the arm.

Hypertensive target-organ damage

Thus, it can be seen that cardiac and vascular target organ damage are predictable interrelated consequences of the systolic hypertension with direct implications for cardiovascular symptoms and pathology. Increased central systolic BP increases cardiac afterload and leads to left ventricular hypertrophy.[97] Increased central arterial stiffness and cardiac afterload (Figure 11–4) cause decreased exercise tolerance,[98,99] diastolic dysfunction, and eventually, heart failure.[98,100–102] Ischemic heart disease is exacerbated as well due to reduced diastolic pressure and reduced coronary filling,[103] especially in response to systemic vasodilation.[104,105]

It is highly likely that PP markedly affects normal microcirculatory function and structure and that wide PP contributes to organ dysfunction. For example, glomerular filtration rate (GFR) is PP-dependent,[106] and therefore PP must affect salt and water excretion. Renal pulsation itself is probably critical to the maintenance of normal excretory function because kidneys with reduced pulsatility (e.g., a rejecting or ischemic renal allograft or the Page model of perinephritic scarring) have reduced GFR[107,108] with hypertension. In individuals with "prehypertensive" blood pressures, higher PP is associated with higher cardiac output and reduced capillary density.[109] This phenomenon of "microcirculatory rarefaction" has been reported in individuals with insulin resistance[110,111] and salt-sensitive hypertension,[112] and is histologically similar to focal renal

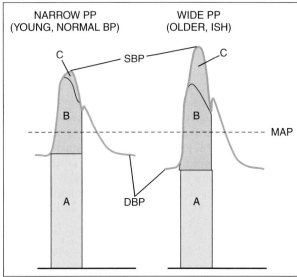

Figure 11–4. Central pulse contours and cardiac workload in aging and hypertension. Cardiac workload (the integral of the central pulse contour during systole) can be decomposed into relative contributions of diastolic pressure (**A**), the early systolic interaction of ventricular emptying with aortic impedance (**B**), and the late systolic interaction of ventricular emptying with the distal circulation and reflected waves (**C**). With advancing age, central PP (systolic – diastolic) widens. In this example, MAP and early systolic load (**B**) remain constant, diastolic pressure load (**A**) decreases, and late-systolic load (**C**) markedly increases. The net result for the older individual is central ISH and increased cardiac load due to the need for left ventricle to sustain contraction until late systole to counteract the effects of increased wave reflection. This pattern leads to concentric left ventricular hypertrophy and is associated with peripheral target-organ damage. ISH, isolated systolic hypertension; MAP, mean arterial pressure; PP, pulse pressure.

glomerulosclerosis, the hallmark lesion of progressive renal failure. To complete the cycle, PP has been found to correlate with the degree of albuminuria,[113] and central arterial stiffness correlates inversely with GFR.[114–117] Systolic hypertension or wide PP is the principal etiologic finding in ischemic stroke[52] and the PWV is directly related to the severity of carotid plaques.[118] It is also likely that the cerebral microcirculation in hypertension is affected similarly to the kidneys, because systolic hypertension and wide PP are associated with leukoariosis, lacunar infarcts, and dementia,[119] which appear to be close correlates of glomerular capillary hypertension, focal glomerulosclerosis, and chronic kidney disease, respectively.

Vascular smooth muscle hypertrophy is also likely to be a primary response to increased PP. In hypertension, there is increased arteriolar wall thickness relative to the luminal diameter of resistance arterioles,[41,120] a phenomenon that serves to sustain systemic resistance (and therefore systolic BP) at an inappropriate level. Additional stiffening of the aorta further elevates systolic pressure BP, thus creating a "vicious cycle," where increased PP leads to further increases in PP. Fortunately, there is some reversibility of this structural abnormality because arteriolar hypertrophy is partially reversible with vasodilator drugs such as angiotensin-converting enzyme inhibitors. In contrast, beta-blocker drugs, which do not tend to reduce PP, do not reduce the increased arteriolar wall-to-lumen ratio found in essential hypertension.[41]

SUMMARY

Hypertension is a hemodynamic syndrome first described as an anomaly of increased resistance to steady-state flow. Although this "classical" approach retains some utility as a teaching model and for classifying pharmacologic responses, a pulsatile model is necessary to explain important features of the pathogenesis and natural history of hypertension. Age-related changes in pulsatile hemo-dynamics, exacerbated by the presence of hypertension, form the basis for a series of interdependent functional and structural changes that also have metabolic implications. The pathogenesis of hypertension and its consequences are not linearly related but rather form a "vicious cycle" that, in effect, leads to premature cardiovascular aging. Central arterial stiffness and wave reflections modify the systolic pulse contour and lead to specific patterns of target organ damage that extend simultaneously from the heart to microcirculations. These continuously evolving interactive pathophysiologic changes in hypertension are thus both causes and effects of this ubiquitous hemodynamic syndrome.

REFERENCES

1. Chapleau MW, Hajduczok G, Abboud FM. Pulsatile activation of baroreceptors causes central facilitation of baroreflex. *Am J Physiol* 1989;256:H1735–41.
2. Hajduczok G, Chapleau MW, Ferlic RJ, Mao HZ, Abboud FM. Gadolinium inhibits mechanoelectrical transduction in rabbit carotid baroreceptors. Implication of stretch-activated channels. *J Clin Invest* 1994;94:2392–2396.
3. Izzo JL Jr, Taylor AA. The sympathetic nervous system and baroreflexes in hypertension and hypotension. *Curr Hypertens Rep* 1999;1:254–63.
4. Luft FC, Rankin LI, Henry DP, Bloch R, Grim CE, Weyman AE, et al. Plasma and urinary norepinephrine at extremes of sodium intake in normal man. *Hypertension* 1979;1:261–266.
5. Romoff MS, Kreusch G, Campese VM, Wang MS, Friedler RM, Weidmann P, et al. Effect of sodium intake on plasma catecholamines in normal subjects. *J Clin Endocrinol Metab* 1979;48:26–31.
6. Izzo JL Jr, Sander E, Larrabee PS. Effect of postural stimulation on systemic hemodynamics and sympathetic nervous activity in systemic hypertension. *Am J Cardiol* 1990;65:339–342.
7. Guo GB, Thames MD. Abnormal baroreflex control in renal hypertension is due to abnormal baroreceptors. *Am J Physiol* 1983;245:420–8.
8. Thames MD, Johnson LN. Impaired cardiopulmonary baroreflex control of renal nerves in renal hypertension. *Circ Res* 1985;57:741–7.
9. Simon AC, Safar ME, Weiss YA, London GM, Milliez PL. Baroreflex sensitivity and cardiopulmonary blood volume in normotensive and hypertensive patients. *Br Heart J* 1977;39:799–805.
10. Tidgren B, Hjemdahl P, Theodorsson E, Nussberger J. Renal responses to lower body negative pressure in humans. *Am J Physiol* 1990;259:F573–9.
11. Messerli FH, Frohlich ED, Suarez DH, Reisin E, Dreslinski GR, Dunn FG, Cole FE. Borderline hypertension: relationship between age, hemodynamics and circulating catecholamines. *Circulation* 1981;64:760–4.
12. Izzo JL Jr, Smith RJ, Larrabee PS, Kallay MC. Plasma norepinephrine and age as determinants of systemic hemodynamics in men with established essential hypertension. *Hypertension* 1987;9:415–9.
13. Anderson EA, Sinkey CA, Lawton WJ, Mark AL. Elevated sympathetic nerve activity in borderline hypertensive humans. Evidence from direct intraneural recordings. *Hypertension* 1989;14:177–83.
14. Esler M, Lambert G, Jennings G. Increased regional sympathetic nervous activity in human hypertension: causes and consequences. *J Hypertens* 1990; (Suppl 8):S53–7.
15. Julius S, Krause L, Schork NJ, Mejia AD, Jones KA, van de Ven C, et al. Hyperkinetic borderline hypertension in Tecumseh, Michigan. *J Hypertens* 1991;9:77–84.
16. Hansson L, Zweifler AJ, Julius S, Hunyor SN. Hemodynamic effects of acute and prolonged beta-adrenergic blockade in essential hypertension. *Acta Med Scand* 1974;196:27–34.
17. Grossman E, Rosenthal T, Peleg E, Holmes C, Goldstein DS. Oral yohimbine increases blood pressure and sympathetic nervous outflow in hypertensive patients. *J Cardiovasc Pharmacol* 1993;;22:22–6.
18. Esler MD, Jennings GL, Johns J, Burke F, Little PJ, Leonard P. Estimation of 'total' renal, cardiac and splanchnic sympathetic nervous tone in essential hypertension from measurements of noradrenaline release. *J Hypertens Suppl* 1984;2:S123–5.
19. Egan B, Panis R, Hinderliter A, Schork N, Julius S. Mechanism of increased alpha adrenergic vasoconstriction in human essential hypertension. *J Clin Invest* 1987; 80:812–7.
20. Stepniakowski KT, Lu G, Miller GD, Egan BM. Fatty acids, not insulin, modulate alpha1-adrenergic reactivity in dorsal hand veins. *Hypertension* 1997;30:1150–5.
21. Ward KD, Sparrow D, Landsberg L, Young JB, Vokonas PS, Weiss ST. Influence of insulin, sympathetic nervous system activity, and obesity on blood pressure: the Normative Aging Study. *J Hypertens* 1996; 14:301–8.
22. Goldstein DS. Arterial baroreflex sensitivity, plasma catecholamines, and pressor responsiveness in essential hypertension. *Circulation* 1983; 68(2):234–40.
23. Julius S, Cottier C, Egan B, Ibsen H, Kiowski W. Cardiopulmonary mechanoreceptors and renin release in humans. *Fed Proc* 1983;42:2703–8.
24. Julius S, Conway J. Hemodynamic studies in patients with borderline blood pressure elevation. *Circulation* 1968;38:282–8.
25. Esler MD, Julius S, Randall OS, Ellis CN, Kashima T. Relation of renin status to neurogenic vascular resistance in borderline hypertension. *Am J Cardiol* 1975;36:708–15.
26. Wilson MF, Sung BH, Pincomb GA, Lovallo WR. Exaggerated pressure response to exercise in men at risk for systemic hypertension. *Am J Cardiol* 1990;66:731–6.
27. Egan B, Schmouder R. The importance of hemodynamic considerations in essential hypertension. *Am Heart J* 1988;116(2 part 2):594–9.
28. Izzo JL Jr. Sympathoadrenal activity, catecholamines, and the pathogenesis of vasculopathic hypertensive target-organ damage. *Am J Hypertens* 1989; 2:305S–12S.
29. Burt VL, Whelton P, Roccella EJ, Brown C, Cutler JA, Higgins M, et al. Prevalence of hypertension in the US adult population: results from the Third National Health and Nutrition Examination Survey, 1988–1991. *Hypertension* 1995;25:305–13.
30. Franklin SS, Gustin WT, Wong ND. Hemodynamic patterns of age-related changes in blood pressure. *Circulation* 1997;96:308–15.
31. Franklin SS, Jacobs MJ, Wong ND, L'Italien GJ, Lapuerta P. Predominance of isolated systolic hypertension among middle-aged and elderly US hypertensives: analysis based on National Health and Nutrition Examination Survey (NHANES) III. *Hypertension* 2001;37:869–74.

32. Frohlich ED, Dustan HP, Page IH. Hyperdynamic beta-adrenergic circulatory state. *Arch Intern Med* 1966;117:614–9.

33. Messerli FH, De Carvalho JG, Christie B, Frohlich ED. Systemic and regional hemodynamics in low, normal and high cardiac output borderline hypertension. *Circulation* 1978; 58:441–8.

34. Julius S. Transition from high cardiac output to elevated vascular resistance in hypertension. *Am Heart J* 1988; 116(2 part 2):600–6.

35. Lund-Johansen P. Twenty-year follow-up of hemodynamics in essential hypertension during rest and exercise. *Hypertension* 1991;18(Suppl 3): III-54–61.

36. Franklin SS, Pio JR, Wong ND, Larson MG, Leip EP, Vasan RS, et al. Predictors of new-onset diastolic and systolic hypertension: the Framingham Heart Study. *Circulation* 2005;111:1121–7.

37. Korner PI, Jennings GL, Esler MD. Pathogenesis of human primary hypertension: a new approach to the identification of causal factors and to therapy. *J Hypertens Suppl* 1986; 4:149–53.

38. Verdecchia P, Angeli F, Gattobigio R, Guerrieri M, Benemio G, Porcellati C. Does the reduction in systolic blood pressure alone explain the regression of left ventricular hypertrophy? *J Hum Hypertens* 2004;18:S23–8.

39. Schlaich MP, Kaye DM, Lambert E, Sommerville M, Socratous F, Esler MD. Relation between cardiac sympathetic activity and hypertensive left ventricular hypertrophy. *Circulation* 2003;108:560–5.

40. Egan B, Julius S. Vascular hypertrophy in borderline hypertension: relationship to blood pressure and sympathetic drive. *Clin Exp Hypertens A* 1985; A7(2–3):243–55.

41. Schiffrin EL, Deng LY, Larochelle P. Progressive improvement in the structure of resistance arteries of hypertensive patients after 2 years of treatment with an angiotensin I–converting enzyme inhibitor. Comparison with effects of a beta-blocker. *Am J Hypertens* 1995; 8:229–36.

42. Verdecchia P, Angeli F, Borgioni C, Gattobigio R, de Simone G, Devereux RB, et al. Changes in cardiovascular risk by reduction of left ventricular mass in hypertension: a meta-analysis. *Am J Hypertens* 2003;16:895–9.

43. Izzo JL Jr, Larrabee PS, Sander E, Lillis LM. Hemodynamics of seasonal adaptation. *Am.J Hypertens* 1990; 3:405–7.

44. Sung BH, Wilson MF, Izzo JL Jr, Ramirez L, Dandona P. Moderately obese, insulin-resistant women exhibit abnormal vascular reactivity to stress. *Hypertension* 1997;30:848–53.

45. Schneider RH, Egan BM, Johnson EH, Drobny H, Julius S. Anger and anxiety in borderline hypertension. *Psychosomatic Med* 1986;48:242–8.

46. Hirsch AT, Dzau VJ, Majzoub JA, Creager MA. Vasopressin-mediated forearm vasodilation in normal humans. Evidence for a vascular vasopressin V2 receptor. *J Clin Invest* 1989;84:418–26.

47. Safar ME, Weiss YA, Levenson JA, London GM, Milliez PL. Hemodynamic study of 85 patients with borderline hypertension. *Am J Cardiol* 1973; 31:315–9.

48. Messerli FH, Christie B, DeCarvalho JG, Aristimuno GG, Suarez DH, Dreslinski GR, et al. Obesity and essential hypertension. Hemodynamics, intravascular volume, sodium excretion, and plasma renin activity. *Arch Int Med* 1981;141:81–5.

49. Izzo JL Jr, Levy D, Black HR. Clinical Advisory Statement: Importance of systolic blood pressure in older Americans. *Hypertension* 2000; 35:1021–4.

50. Izzo JL Jr. Arterial stiffness and the systolic hypertension syndrome. *Curr Opin Cardiol* 2004;19:341–52.

51. Chobanian AV, Bakris GL, Black HR, Cushman WC, Green LA, Izzo JL Jr, et al. The seventh report of the Joint National Committee on Prevention, Detection, Evaluation, and Treatment of High Blood Pressure: JNC 7 Express. *JAMA* 2003;289:2560–72.

52. Domanski MJ, Davis BR, Pfeffer MA, Kastantin M, Mitchell GF. Isolated systolic hypertension: prognostic information provided by pulse pressure. *Hypertension* 1999; 34:375–80.

53. Black H, Kuller L, O'Rourke M, et al. The first report of the Systolic and Pulse Pressure (SYPP) Working Group. *J Hypertens* 1999;17(Suppl 5):S1–12.

54. Sims AJ, Reay CA, Bousfield DR, Menes JA, Murray A. Low-cost oscillometric non-invasive blood pressure monitors: device repeatability and device differences. *Physiol Measurement* 2005;26:441–5.

55. Smulyan H, Siddiqui DS, Carlson RJ, London GM, Safar ME. Clinical utility of aortic pulses and pressures calculated from applanated radial-artery pulses. *Hypertension* 2003; 42:150–5.

56. Rubanyi GM, Freay AD, Kauser K, Johns A, Harder DR. Mechanoreception by the endothelium: mediators and mechanisms of pressure- and flow-induced vascular responses. *Blood Vessels* 1990;27:246–57.

57. Tozawa M, Iseki K, Iseki C, Takishita S. Pulse pressure and risk of total mortality and cardiovascular events in patients on chronic hemodialysis. *Kidney Int* 2002;61:717–26.

58. Izzo JL Jr. Hypertension in the elderly: a pathophysiologic approach to therapy. *J Am Geriatr Soc* 1982; 30:352–9.

59. Chadwick RS, Goldstein DS, Keiser HR. Pulse-wave model of brachial arterial pressure modulation in aging and hypertension. *Am J Physiol* 1986; 251:H1–11.

60. Avolio A, Fa-Quan D, Wei-Qiang L, Yao-Fei L, Zhen-Dong H, Lian-Fen X, et al. Effects of aging on arterial distensibility in populations with high and low prevalence of hypertension: comparison between urban and rural communities in China. *Circulation* 1987;71:202–10.

61. Avolio A. Genetic and environmental factors in the function and structure of the arterial wall. *Hypertension* 1995; 26:23–37.

62. O'Rourke MF, Kelly RP. Wave reflection in the systemic circulation and its implications in ventricular function. *J Hypertens* 1993;11:327–37.

63. Avolio A, Jones D, Tafazzoli-Shadpour M. Quantification of alterations in structure and function of elastin in the arterial media. *Hypertension* 1998; 32:170–5.

64. Isnard RN, Pannier BM, Laurent S, London GM, Diebold B, Safar ME. Pulsatile diameter and elastic modulus of the aortic arch in essential hypertension: a noninvasive study. *J Am Coll Cardiol* 1989;13:399–405.

65. Vasan RS, Larson MG, Levy D. Determinants of echocardiographic aortic root size. The Framingham Heart Study. *Circulation* 1995; 91:734–40.

66. Mitchell GF, Lacourciere Y, Ouellet JP, Izzo JL Jr, Neutel J, Kerwin LJ, et al. Determinants of elevated pulse pressure in middle-aged and older subjects with uncomplicated systolic hypertension: the role of proximal aortic diameter and the aortic pressure-flow relationship. *Circulation* 2003;108:1592–8.

67. Vasan RS, Larson MG, Benjamin EJ, Levy D. Echocardiographic reference values for aortic root size: the Framingham Heart Study. *J Am Soc Echocardiogr* 1995;8:793–800.

68. Bella JN, Wachtell K, Boman K, Palmieri V, Papademetriou V, Gerdts E, et al. Relation of left ventricular geometry and function to aortic root dilatation in patients with systemic hypertension and left ventricular hypertrophy (the LIFE study). *Am J Cardiol* 2002;89:337–41.

69. Haider AW, Larson MG, Franklin SS, Levy D. Systolic blood pressure, diastolic blood pressure, and pulse pressure as predictors of risk for congestive heart failure in the Framingham Heart Study. *Ann Int Med* 2003;138:10–6.

70. Tonkin AL, Wing LM, Morris MJ, Kapoor V. Afferent baroreflex dysfunction and age-related orthostatic hypotension. *Clin Sci* 1991;81:531–8.

71. Floras JS, Sinkey CA, Aylward PE, Seals DR, Thoren PN, Mark AL. Postexercise hypotension and sympathoinhibition in borderline hypertensive men. *Hypertension* 1989;14:28–35.

72. Jansen RW, Kelly-Gagnon MM, Lipsitz LA. Intraindividual reproducibility of postprandial and orthostatic blood pressure changes in older nursing-home patients: relationship with chronic use of cardiovascular medications. *J Am Geriatr Soc* 1996; 44:383–9 [erratum], *J Am Geriatr Soc* 1996;44(6):722].

73. McGrath BP, Liang YL, Kotsopoulos D, Cameron JD. Impact of physical and physiological factors on arterial function. *Clin Exp Pharmacol Physiol* 2001;28:1104–7.

74. Hope SA, Tay DB, Meredith IT, Cameron JD. Comparison of generalized and gender-specific transfer functions for the derivation of aortic waveforms. *Am J Physiol Heart Circ Physiol* 2002;283:H1150–6.

75. Gatzka CD, Cameron JD, Dart AM, Berry KL, Kingwell BA, Dewar EM, et

al. Correction of carotid augmentation index for heart rate in elderly essential hypertensives. ANBP2 Investigators. Australian Comparative Outcome Trial of Angiotensin-Converting Enzyme Inhibitor- and Diuretic-Based Treatment of Hypertension in the Elderly. *Am J Hypertens* 2001; 14:573–7.

76. Kelly R, Hayward C, Ganis J, Daley J, Avolio A, O'Rourke MF. Noninvasive registration of the arterial pressure pulse waveform using high-fidelity applanation tonometry. *J Vasc Med Biol* 1989;1:142–149.

77. Karamanoglu M, O'Rourke MF, Avolio AP, Kelly RP. An analysis of the relationship between central aortic and peripheral upper limb pressure waves in man. *Eur Heart J* 1993; 14:160–167.

78. Chen CH, Nevo E, Fetics B, Pak PH, Yin FC, Maughan WL, et al. Estimation of central aortic pressure waveform by mathematical transformation of radial tonometry pressure. Validation of generalized transfer function. *Circulation* 1997;95:1827–36.

79. Segers P, Carlier S, Pasquet A, Rabben SI, Hellevik LR, Remme E, et al. Individualizing the aorto-radial pressure transfer function: feasibility of a model-based approach. *Am J Physiol Heart Circ Physiol* 2000;279:H542–9.

80. Hope SA, Meredith IT, Cameron JD. Reliability of transfer functions in determining central pulse pressure and augmentation index. *J Am Coll Cardiol* 2002;40:1196 (author reply 1196–7).

81. Hope SA, Meredith IT, Cameron JD. Is there any advantage to using an arterial transfer function? *Hypertension* 2003;42:e6–7 (author reply e6–7).

82. Hoeks AP, Meinders JM, Dammers R. Applicability and benefit of arterial transfer functions. *J Hypertens* 2003; 21:1241–3.

83. Izzo JL Jr, Manning TS, Shykoff BE. Office blood pressures, arterial compliance characteristics, and estimated cardiac load. *Hypertension* 1999;38:1467–70.

84. Nurnberger J, Dammer S, Opazo Saez A, Philipp T, Schafers RF. Diastolic blood pressure is an important determinant of augmentation index and pulse wave velocity in young, healthy males. *J Hum Hypertens* 2003;17:153–8.

85. Wilkinson IB, Franklin SS, Hall IR, Tyrrell S, Cockcroft JR. Pressure amplification explains why pulse pressure is unrelated to risk in young subjects. *Hypertension* 2001;38:1461–6.

86. Wilkinson IB, MacCallum H, Hupperetz PC, van Thoor CJ, Cockcroft JR, Webb DJ. Changes in the derived central pressure waveform and pulse pressure in response to angiotensin II and noradrenaline in man. *J Physiol* 2001;530:541–50.

87. Rehman A, Rahman AR, Rasool AH. Effect of angiotensin II on pulse wave velocity in humans is mediated through angiotensin II type 1 (AT(1)) receptors. *J Hum Hypertens* 2002; 16:261–6.

88. Vuurmans TJ, Boer P, Koomans HA. Effects of endothelin-1 and

endothelin-1 receptor blockade on cardiac output, aortic pressure, and pulse wave velocity in humans. *Hypertension* 2003;41:1253–8.

89. Westling H, Jansson L, Jonson B, Nilsen R. Vasoactive drugs and elastic properties of human arteries in vivo, with special reference to the action of nitroglycerine. *Eur Heart J* 1984; 5:609–16.

90. Nichols WW, O'Rourke MF, Avolio AP, Yaginuma T, Pepine CJ, Conti CR. Ventricular/vascular interaction in patients with mild systemic hypertension and normal peripheral resistance. *Circulation* 1986; 74:455–62.

91. Yaginuma T, Avolio A, O'Rourke M, Nichols W, Morgan JJ, Roy P, et al. Effect of glyceryl trinitrate on peripheral arteries alters left ventricular hydraulic load in man. *Cardiovasc Res* 1986; 20:153–60.

92. Stokes GS, Barin ES, Gilfillan KL. Effects of isosorbide mononitrate and AII inhibition on pulse wave reflection in hypertension. *Hypertension* 2003; 41:297–301.

93. O'Rourke MF, Yaginuma T. Wave reflections and the arterial pulse. *Arch Intern Med* 1984;144:366–71.

94. van der Heijden-Spek JJ, Staessen JA, Fagard RH, Hoeks AP, Boudier HA, Van Bortel LM. Effect of age on brachial artery wall properties differs from the aorta and is gender dependent: a population study. *Hypertension* 2000;35:637–42.

95. Kimoto E, Shoji T, Shinohara K, Inaba M, Okuno Y, Miki T, Koyama H, Emoto M, Nishizawa Y. Preferential stiffening of central over peripheral arteries in type 2 diabetes. *Diabetes* 2003;52:448–52.

96. Laurent P, Albaladejo P, Blacher J, Rudnichi A, Smulyan H, Safar ME. Heart rate and pulse pressure amplification in hypertensive subjects. *Am J Hypertens* 2003;16:363–70.

97. Izzo JL Jr, Gradman AH. Mechanisms and management of hypertensive heart disease: from left ventricular hypertrophy to heart failure. *Med Clin North Am* 2004;88:1257–71.

98. Hundley WG, Kitzman DW, Morgan TM, Hamilton CA, Darty SN, Stewart KP, et al. Cardiac cycle-dependent changes in aortic area and distensibility are reduced in older patients with isolated diastolic heart failure and correlate with exercise intolerance. *J Am Coll Cardiol* 2001;38:796–802.

99. Bonapace S, Rossi A, Cicoira M, Franceschini L, Golia G, Zanolla L, Marino P, Zardini P. Aortic distensibility independently affects exercise tolerance in patients with dilated cardiomyopathy. *Circulation* 2003; 107:1603–8.

100. Palmieri V, Bella JN, Roman MJ, Gerdts E, Papademetriou V, Wachtell K, et al. Pulse pressure/stroke index and left ventricular geometry and function: the LIFE Study. *J Hypertens* 2003;21:781–7.

101. Gates PE, Tanaka H, Graves J, Seals DR. Left ventricular structure and diastolic function with human ageing. Relation to habitual exercise and arterial stiffness. *Eur Heart J* 2003; 24:2213–20.

102. Matsumoto Y, Hamada M, Hiwada K. Aortic distensibility is closely related to the progression of left ventricular hypertrophy in patients receiving hemodialysis. *Angiology* 2000; 51:933–41.

103. Kingwell BA, Waddell TK, Medley TL, Cameron JD, Dart AM. Large artery stiffness predicts ischemic threshold in patients with coronary artery disease. *J Am Coll Cardiol* 2002;40:773–9.

104. Ohtsuka S, Kakihana M, Watanabe H, Sugishita Y. Chronically decreased aortic distensibility causes deterioration of coronary perfusion during increased left ventricular contraction. *J Am Coll Cardiol* 1994; 24:1406–14.

105. Vinereanu D, Nicolaides E, Boden L, Payne N, Jones CJ, Fraser AG. Conduit arterial stiffness is associated with impaired left ventricular subendocardial function. *Heart (British Cardiac Society)* 2003;89:449–50.

106. Smith A, Karalliedde J, De Angelis L, Goldsmith D, Viberti G. Aortic pulse wave velocity and albuminuria in patients with type 2 diabetes. *J Am Soc Nephrol* 2005;16:1069–75.

107. Takata M, Denton KM, Anderson WP. Renal and systemic vascular conductances in renal wrap hypertension in rabbits. *J Hypertens* 1988;6:719–22.

108. Denton KM, Anderson WP, Korner PI. Renal blood flow and glomerular filtration rate in renal wrap hypertension in rabbits. *J Hypertens* 1983;1:351–5.

109. Sullivan JM, Prewitt RL, Josephs JA. Attenuation of the microcirculation in young patients with high-output borderline hypertension. *Hypertension* 1983;5:844–851.

110. Isaksson H, Cederholm T, Jansson E, Nygren A, Ostergren J. Therapy-resistant hypertension associated with central obesity, insulin resistance, and large muscle fibre area. *Blood Pressure* 1993;2:46–52.

111. Julius S, Gudbrandsson T, Jamerson K, Andersson O. The interconnection between sympathetics, microcirculation, and insulin resistance in hypertension. *Blood Pressure* 1992;1:9–19.

112. Johnson RJ, Gordon KL, Suga S, Duijvestijn AM, Griffin K, Bidani A. Renal injury and salt-sensitive hypertension after exposure to catecholamines. *Hypertension* 1999; 34:151–9.

113. Cirillo M, Stellato D, Laurenzi M, Panarelli W, Zanchetti A, De Santo NG. Pulse pressure and isolated systolic hypertension: association with microalbuminuria. The GUBBIO Study Collaborative Research. *Kidney Int* 2000;58:1211–8.

114. London GM, Guerin AP, Marchais SJ, Pannier B, Safar ME, Day M, Metivier F. Cardiac and arterial interactions in end-stage renal disease. *Kidney Int* 1996;50:600–8.

115. London GM, Guerin AP, Pannier B, Marchais SJ, Benetos A, Safar ME. Arterial wave reflections and increased systolic and pulse pressure in chronic uremia: study using noninvasive carotid pulse waveform registration. *Hypertension* 1992;20:10–19.

116. Blacher J, Demuth K, Guerin AP, Safar ME, Moatti N, London GM. Influence of biochemical alterations on arterial stiffness in patients with end-stage renal disease. *Arterioscler Throm Vasc Biol* 1998;18:535–41.

117. Groothoff JW, Gruppen MP, Offringa M, de Groot E, Stok W, Bos WJ, et al. Increased arterial stiffness in young adults with end-stage renal disease since childhood. *J Am Soc Nephrol* 2002;13:2953–61.

118. Zureik M, Bureau JM, Temmar M, Adamopoulos C, Courbon D, Bean K, et al. Echogenic carotid plaques are associated with aortic arterial stiffness in subjects with subclinical carotid atherosclerosis. *Hypertension* 2003; 41:519–27.

119. Mangiarua EI, Lee RM. Morphometric study of cerebral arteries from spontaneously hypertensive and stroke-prone spontaneously hypertensive rats. *J Hypertens* 1992; 10:1183–90.

120. Folkow B. "Structural factor" in primary and secondary hypertension. *Hypertension* 1990;16(1):89–101.

Chapter 12

The Arterial System in Human Hypertension

Daniel A. Duprez and Jay N. Cohn

Key Findings

- Structural and functional properties of the arterial wall are altered in hypertension even at the early stages of the disease.

- Arterial stiffness is the most important cause of increasing systolic and pulse pressure, and of increasing pulse pressure with aging.

- Morbidity and mortality associated with hypertension are primarily related to arterial damage and may affect one or several organs.

Clinical Implications

- Considering the potential implications of arterial assessment in the prevention of cardiovascular disease, evaluation of the arterial effects of antihypertensive treatment is recommended.

The principal function of the arterial system is to deliver an adequate supply of blood to tissues and organs. In performing this primary conduit function, the arteries transform the pulsatile flow generated by ventricular contraction into a continuous flow of blood in the periphery. This latter cushioning function is dependent on the mechanical properties of the arterial walls.

Blood pressure (BP) is a powerful cardiovascular (CV) risk factor that acts on the arterial wall and is responsible in part for various CV events, such as cerebrovascular accidents and ischemic heart disease.[1] In clinical practice, two specific and arbitrary points of the BP curve, peak systolic BP (SBP) and end-diastolic BP (DBP), are used to define the CV risk factor. Because the goal of drug treatment of hypertension is to prevent CV complications, it appears likely that the totality of the BP curve, not simply two specific and arbitrary points, should be considered to act mechanically on the arterial wall and therefore should be used to propose an adequate definition of high BP (Figure 12–1).

PHYSIOLOGIC ROLE OF ARTERIES

Traditionally the BP curve has been considered to contain a steady component, mean BP, and a pulsatile component, the pulse pressure. Hemodynamic research has shifted away from a steady-flow approach toward a pulsatile flow approach because the former is less predictive in relation to cardiovascular morbidity and mortality.[2,3] The growing importance of pulsatile pressure indices paralleled the notion that not only increases in systemic vascular resistance but also increases in arterial stiffness are important in the pathophysiology of hypertension.[4]

A current approach consists of considering the BP curve as the summation of a steady component, mean arterial blood pressure (MAP), and a pulsatile component, pulse pressure (PP). MAP, the product of cardiac output multiplied by total peripheral resistance, is the pressure for the steady flow of blood and oxygen to peripheral tissues and organs. The pulsatile component, PP, is the consequence of intermittent ventricular ejection from the heart. PP is influenced by several cardiac and vascular factors, but it is the role of large conduit arteries, mainly the aorta, to minimize pulsatility. In addition to the pattern of left ventricular ejection, the determinants of PP (and SBP) are the cushioning capacity of arteries and the timing and intensity of wave reflections. The former is influenced by arterial stiffness, usually expressed in the quantitative terms of compliance and distensibility. The latter result from the summation of a forward wave coming from the heart and propagating at a given speed (pulse wave velocity, or PWV) toward the origin of resistance vessels and a backward wave returning toward the heart from particular sites characterized by specific reflection indices.[5,6] Information about the interaction between the left ventricle and the physical properties of the arterial circulation can be derived by the descriptive and quantitative analysis of the arterial pressure pulse waveform.[7,8]

Ejection of blood into the aorta generates a pressure wave that is propagated to other arteries throughout the body. As in elastic conduits, this forward-traveling pressure wave may be reflected at all points of structural and/or functional discontinuity of the arterial tree. From these different points of discontinuity, mainly located in the distal arteries at the branching origins of arterioles, a reflected wave is generated that travels backward toward the ascending aorta. Thus incident and reflected pressure waves are in constant interaction along the arterial circuit and are summed up into the actual pressure wave. The final amplitude and shape of the measured aortic BP wave are determined by the phase relationship (timing) between the two component waves. The timing of incident and reflected pressure waves depends on pulse wave velocity, the traveling distance of pressure waves, and the duration of ventricular ejection. In young subjects, under physiological conditions, the backward pressure wave returns from the distal arterial compartment during diastole,

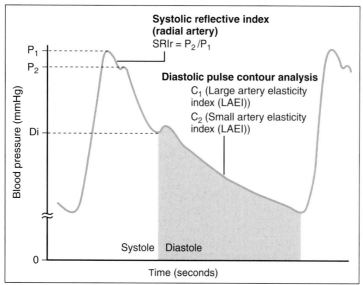

Figure 12–1. In clinical practice two specific and arbitrary points of the blood pressure curve, peak SBP and end DBP, are used to define normotension and hypertension. Several parameters are derived from the blood pressure curve to provide information about the arterial system. This figure illustrates some examples: SRI is derived from the ratio of the second over the first peak of the systolic part of the radial artery wave form (P_2/P_1). C_1 (large artery elasticity index) and C_2 (small artery elasticity index) are derived from diastolic pulse contour analysis of the radial artery waveform. Augmentation pressure is the difference between the second and the first peak of the systolic part of the radial artery waveform ($P_2 - P_1$). The augmentation index is the ratio $P_2 - DBP/P_1 - DBP$. DBP, diastolic blood pressure; SBP, systolic blood pressure; SRI, systolic reflective index. (From Duprez DA, Kaiser DR, Whitwam W, et al. *Am J Hypertens* 2004;17:647–653 with permission from *The American Journal of Hypertension Ltd.*)

making PP higher in peripheral than in central arteries. This physiological phenomenon, called PP amplification, is influenced by pulse wave velocity. With heightened PWV, the reflecting sites of the distal compartment appear "closer" to the ascending aorta, and the reflected waves occur earlier, being more closely in phase with incident waves in this region. Such an earlier return of wave reflections means that the reflected wave affects the central arteries during systole and not during diastole. This disturbed signal results in an augmentation of aortic and ventricular pressures during systole and reduces aortic pressure during diastole. Hence, altered mechanical properties of the aortic wall influence the level of aortic SBP (which is increased) and DBP (which is decreased) as a consequence of early wave reflections. Finally, all these findings taken together indicate that a disturbed pressure signal arising from the distal arteries through disturbed wave reflections may alter the heart-vessel coupling and lead to increased CV risk. Evidence for this pathophysiologic mechanism arises from studies of pulsatile arterial hemodynamics, as highlighted recently by the role of pulse wave velocity and wave reflections as independent factors in CV risk in hypertension and various CV diseases.[9–11]

Wave reflections alter the ventricular-vascular coupling not only through increased arterial stiffness and changed timing, but also through modifications in their amplitude. Such possibilities depend on the reflectance properties of the arterial tree, which arise from the distal part of the arterial tree. They are influenced by the geometry, number, structure, and function of smaller muscular arteries and arterioles. Thus acute and active arterial and arteriolar constriction results in earlier aortic wave reflections at the aortic level and hence increased PP. It appears that elastic arteries buffer the pulsations, muscular arteries actively alter propagation velocity, and arterioles serve as major reflection sites. Each of these alterations (or their combination) enables cross-talk between the proximal and distal compartments of the arterial tree, which leads to the predominant or selective increases of SBP and PP observed in aged and/or hypertensive populations at high CV risk.[12,13] In the presence of decreased ventricular ejection, these frequency-dependent factors disturb the heart-vessel coupling, increase the load of the heart, and favor cardiac hypertrophy, coronary ischemia, and ultimately CV death.[14]

The interest in the arterial cushioning function of pulsatile flow has given us a myriad of indices generated by various noninvasive measurement techniques, which only indirectly measure the desired arterial stiffness characteristics. Given their complexity in describing the structure and function of these indirect approaches, simplified mathematical models have been developed.[15,16] However, it is important to recognize that different parts of the arterial system have different functions. The proximal large arteries buffer the pulsations; the more distal or muscular arteries alter propagation velocities and vascular impedance, and serve as major reflection sites. Each of these alterations or their combination enables a cross-talk between the proximal and distal compartments of the arterial tree.

PHYSIOLOGIC EFFECTS OF VASCULAR WALL ALTERATIONS

All arteries exhibit compliance characteristics that can be defined as the increase in caliber for a given rise in pressure (dV/dP, where dV is the change in artery volume over a linear length and dP is the rise in pressure during the cardiac cycle). Only the smaller arteries and arterioles provide major resistance to flow, which is exquisitely sensitive to changes in the caliber of these microvessels. The role of compliance in the conduit arteries is a critical determinant of their storage capacity during systole. Much of the stroke volume delivered by the ventricle is accommodated in the pressure-dependent increase in arterial caliber, and this volume is released during diastole to help maintain diastolic pressure. When compliance of these conduit arteries is reduced, the result is less storage of stroke volume and/or a greater increase in systolic pressure to distend the noncompliant arterial bed. Increased workload on the left ventricle and a decrease in aortic diastolic pressure are the hemodynamic accompaniments of reduced large artery compliance, which will lead to an increase in systolic blood pressure as it is observed in systolic hypertension and in diabetes.[17,18]

Compliance of the more distal arterial system at sites of tapering and at branch points serves to cushion the arterial pulse wave during its transmission through the arterial bed. The less the cushioning effect the greater the magnitude and frequency of oscillations or reflections that appear to have their origin at these sites in the vascular bed. The pressure response to these oscillations results from a complex interaction of the storage volume of these cushioning vessels, compliance of the more proximal arterial system, and pulse wave velocity that influences the rate at which these reflections are transmitted back to the root of the aorta. Compliance of the arterioles also will influence pulsatile vascular resistance. To the extent that pulsatile pressure is transmitted to the arterioles, the caliber of these vessels, and thus the resistance, will vary throughout the cardiac cycle, depending on the compliance of these vessels. Another possible effect of compliance alteration is its influence on shear force at the arterial wall. Such alterations in shear force may contribute to endothelial damage and to the atherosclerotic process in the conduit arteries.[18,20]

Arterial stiffness is determined by its visco-elastic properties, which are in turn dependent on the structure (or composition) and function of the vessel wall.[21] Alterations in the extracellular matrix of the media and adventitia have long been implicated in the pathogenesis of age- and blood pressure-related increase in arterial stiffness. There is now good evidence that acute and low-grade chronic inflammation is associated with stiffening of the large arteries[22] (Figure 12–2). This is likely to promote atheroma formation and increase cardiovascular risk. The exact mechanisms responsible for arterial stiffening remain to be elucidated but are likely to reflect both functional and structural changes in the vessel wall. It is possible that inflammation may be involved in the initiation as well as development of hypertension, with the exertion of proinflammatory actions through several mediators,

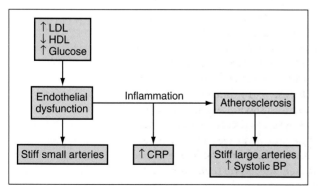

Figure 12–2. Role of vascular inflammation on large and small arteries stiffness in the pathogenesis of arterial hypertension. BP, blood pressure; CRP, C-reactive protein. (From Duprez DA, Somasundaram PE, Sigurdsson G, et al. *J Hum Hypertens* 2005;19:515–9.)

including adhesion molecules, chemokines, growth factors, heat shock proteins, endothelin-1, and angiotensin.[23,24] Indeed, even a persistent low-grade inflammatory state could result in a high but within "normal range" concentrations of inflammatory cytokines. Moreover, low-grade inflammation has been associated with endothelial damage and dysfunction and consequently will lead to impaired vasodilation and hypertension.

CONTROL OF ARTERIAL TONE

An increase in arterial tone has traditionally been viewed as the hallmark for elevated blood pressure. Although some have suggested that an increase in cardiac output with normal vascular resistance is the initial hemodynamic abnormality in patients with hypertension,[25] the chronic hypertensive state usually is associated with an increase in total systemic vascular resistance. This increase in resistance is generally attributed to an increase in vascular tone.[26] The mechanism for this increase is, however, cryptic. The role of the sympathetic nervous system, the renin-angiotensin system, electrolyte changes, alterations in release of endothelial relaxing factor, increased release of endothelial constricting factors, and other factors that mediate tissue blood flow autoregulation have all been implicated in the process.[1] Neural and hormonal influences that alter tone of the arteriole, and thus the calculated systemic vascular resistance, also play a role in the larger conduit arteries. An increase in smooth muscle tone in the muscular arteries that represent most of the conduit vessels will alter the pressure-to-volume relationship in these vessels and result in a decrease in arterial compliance or elasticity.[27]

The problem of identifying an abnormality in arterial tone related to some neural or hormonal effect is compounded by the fact that during daily life, arterial tone and blood pressure changes are continuously induced by alterations in neurohormonal activity. During exercise, emotional or temperature stress, and even during periods of standing, these systems may be activated and an alteration in regional or systemic vascular tone may result. Therefore, the dilemma in identifying individuals with elevated blood pressure from the normal fluctuations of blood pressure in normotensive individuals is intensified. Attempts to define the hypertensive state by the degree of blood pressure elevation or the sustained nature of this elevation during 24-hour monitoring often serves as the only distinguishing feature between the normotensive individual with fluctuations in arterial tone and the hypertensive who is thought to be at risk for cardiovascular events.

CONTROL OF ARTERIAL STRUCTURE

Although hypertension was traditionally viewed as a disease of increased arterial tone, the vascular structural abnormality in hypertensive disease has become the focus of more recent investigation. Those same neural and hormonal influences that alter arterial tone appear also to induce changes in arterial structure. Thus the blood pressure increase and the hormones that produce arterial constriction both tend to stimulate arterial growth, whereas blood pressure reduction and hormones that induce vasodilation tend to induce growth regression. Growth of both vascular smooth muscle cells and connective tissue may be induced by hemodynamic and hormonal influences.

Vascular remodeling (Figure 12–3) is considered an adaptive response to elevation of arterial pressure to normalize the wall tension. In essential hypertension, large artery remodeling is characterized by an increase in media thickness–lumen diameter ratio and cross-sectional area. This augmentation of media mass, or hypertrophic remodeling, is explained by changes in size or number of vascular smooth muscle cells and matrix collagen deposition.[28] In resistance arteries (diameter ≤300 μm), essential hypertension is associated with a reduced lumen and increased media thickness–lumen ratio but without cross-sectional area increase, producing a type of remodeling designated as inward eutrophic remodeling.[29] To explain this different response between large and small arteries, it is suggested that small arteries are not submitted to an augmented wall stress because they are initially constricted.[30] This remodeling of the vascular structure is dependent not only on blood pressure but also on blood flow and hormonal environment, in which the renin-angiotensin-aldosterone system plays a crucial role.

Arterial injury is considered as the starting point for what is called arterial remodeling.[31] Once the endothelium has been injured, an immunologic cascade sets in. Cell surface molecules that mediate interaction of leucocytes and endothelium such as vascular and intercellular cell adhesion molecule 1 (VCAM-1 and ICAM-1) get upregulated.[32] Inflammatory cells are therefore directed to the site of injury by chemoattractant factors such as monocyte chemoattracting protein 1 (MCP-1). Secretion of chemokines and cytokines by endothelial and lymphoid cells upholds the process of inflammation. Macrophage-colony stimulating factor (M-CSF) effects an upregulation of the scavenger receptors on the activated macrophages and by this stimulates the uptake of oxidized lipoproteins and the formation of foam cells. Growth factors like platelet-derived growth factor (PDGF) expressed by endothelial cells induce a migration of smooth muscle cells into the intima of the atheromatous lesion, which is subjected to intracellular matrix degradation mainly evoked by metalloproteinases (MMPs).[33] The growth of an atherosclerotic plaque is compensated by caliber expansion of the whole vessel, while keeping the lumen size steady, the so-called positive remodeling. As soon as the plaque exceeds a certain dimension, the lumen gets affected, leading to arterial stenosis, the so-called negative remodeling. Minor decreases in the lumen of small arteries and arterioles will significantly increase resistance. Accordingly, these segments of the arterial tree are known as resistance arteries, and they may play an important role in the development of hypertension and may also contribute to its complications.[34] The vascular changes in resistance arteries that result in decreased lumen size in hypertension may be structural, mechanical, or functional. Extracellular matrix remodeling is very important in the process of vascular remodeling. With chronic vasoconstriction, the small arteries may become embedded in the remodeled extracellular matrix and may not return to their vasodilated state.[35]

The arterial structural changes that accompany hypertension may serve as a distinguishing feature between the normotensive individual with fluctuating blood pressure and vascular resistance and the truly hypertensive individual at risk for vascular events. Furthermore, this abnormality of structure may exist even in the absence of an elevated blood pressure and thus may identify individuals in the normotensive range who are at risk for cardiovascular events. Preliminary studies have suggested that a reduction in small artery compliance can be detected in subjects with a parental history of hypertension even before their pressure is significantly elevated.[36] No other simple technique, except the crude measurement of so-called risk factors, is able to identify this at-risk population.

SEQUENTIAL CHANGES IN HYPERTENSION

Abnormalities of the arterial vasculature that precede cardiovascular morbid events are likely to occur in a temporal sequence (Figure 12–4). The initial abnormalities appear to be functional, in large part related to endothelial dysfunction associated with decreased bioavailability of NO.[37] A decrease in constitutive release of NO, which maintains low small artery tone, may be the initial abnormality, but it is soon accompanied by a decrease in stimulated release of endothelial vasodilators, as manifested by a reduction in flow-mediated dilation of conduit arteries.[38,39] These functional abnormalities of the vasculature should precede and are mechanistic precursors of the structural alterations that are responsible for thickening of the conduit artery wall,[40] increases in pulse

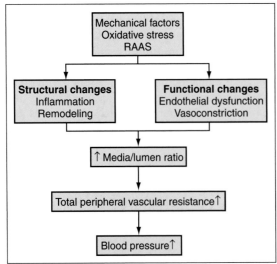

Figure 12–3. The effect of structural and functional changes of the arterial system in the pathogenesis of arterial hypertension. RAAS, renin-angiotensin-aldosterone system.

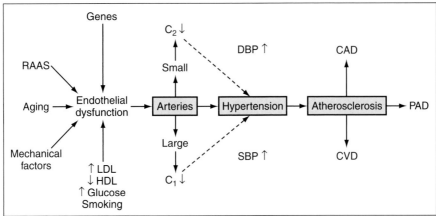

Figure 12–4. Temporal sequence of arterial changes in arterial hypertension. The functional defect starts predominantly in the small arteries as endothelial dysfunction. Structural dysfunction occurs later and affects large and small arteries leading to the reduction of small (C_1) and large arterial elasticity (C_1). This will lead to increase of diastolic and systolic blood pressure. Further damage of the arterial system in arterial hypertension leads then to atherothrombotic complications, such as acute myocardial infarction, stroke, and PAD. CAD, coronary artery disease; CVD, cardiovascular disease; DBP, diastolic blood pressure; PAD, peripheral arterial disease; SBP, systolic blood pressure; RAAS, renin-angiotensin-aldosterone system.

pressure,[41] and atherosclerotic plaque development.[42] These structural changes may also result in additional functional abnormalities. But cross-sectional studies suggest that this sequence of vascular manifestations of vascular disease is not always detectable.

Functional and structural changes in the artery wall precede and accompany atherosclerosis and its obstructive and thrombotic events. These changes should alter the volume increment that occurs in the arterial bed during the systolic pressure increase with each cardiac cycle. A variety of techniques developed in recent years provide quantitation of these pathophysiologic changes in the arterial wall (Figure 12–5). Because aging produces changes similar to those observed in atherosclerosis, all methods for evaluation must be corrected for age and, perhaps, gender.[43] Thus to serve as a useful surrogate for disease progression, the method must provide insight into disease presence independent of age. Furthermore, if arterial wall compliance, elasticity, or stiffness is to serve as a valuable surrogate for efficacy of therapy, it should be tracked with disease progression and regression.

An understanding of the sequential changes that occur in the arterial system is crucial in order to appreciate the temporal influence on the occurrence of cardiovascular disease and its response to treatment. Diagnostic procedures are currently designed to assess the extent and severity of vascular disease after the development of symptoms or when morbid events occur. The diagnostic challenge must be to detect abnormal structure and function in the vascular system before the development of symptoms or signs of cardiovascular disease.[13] By providing a direct assessment of abnormal structure or tone in the arterial vasculature, alterations in arterial compliance may improve risk stratification and identify individuals with early vascular damage who are predisposed to future vascular events.[44]

EFFECTS OF AGING

Available evidence suggests that the incidence of systolic hypertension is increasing in individuals over 50 years of age. The reasons for this evolution are quite simple[45] (Figure 12–6). First, prolongation of the duration of life is responsible for an increased number of older individuals with increased systolic blood pressure (SBP). Second, the goal for treatment of systolic-diastolic hypertension in middle-aged subjects has been based on the reduction of diastolic blood pressure (DBP). Because it is much easier

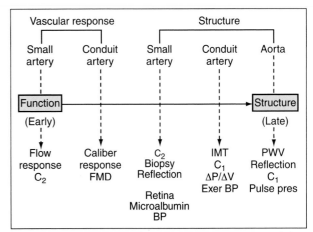

Figure 12–5. Methods to study the sequential changes of the arterial system in arterial hypertension. ΔP/ΔV, pressure/volume relationship of a single artery; C_1, large artery elasticity index; C_2, small artery elasticity index; exer BP, blood pressure rise in response to a standardized exercise test; flow response, response to acetylcholine; FMD, flow-mediated vasodilation; IMT, intima-medial thickness of carotid artery; reflection, augmentation index; retina, retinal vasculature; pulse pres, auscultatory pulse pressure; PWV, pulse wave velocity.

to control DBP (<90 mmHg) than SBP (<140 mmHg), and because, with age, DBP tends spontaneously to be reduced and SBP to be enhanced, this situation contributes *per se* to increase the incidence of systolic hypertension in the elderly. All these findings are important to consider, as the pathophysiologic mechanisms of systolic hypertension involve not only altered vascular resistance, the classical hallmark of high blood pressure (BP), but also changes of stiffness and wave reflections, which refer to conduit arteries, mainly the aorta and its principal branches.

Adaptations in the arterial vasculature play a critical role in influencing cardiovascular hemodynamics with advancing age.[46] The generalized structural and functional changes in the arterial circulation contribute to alterations in regional blood flow, progression of atherogenesis, and the microvascular abnormalities that occur during senescence.[47] In large arteries, aging results in progressive deposition of calcium salts, fraying and fragmentation of elastin, and an increase in the number and cross-linking of collagen fibers that alter the compliance characteristics of the vessel wall.[48] A rigid aorta is less able to buffer the pulsatile output from the heart; it contributes to an increase in systolic blood pressure and left ventricular afterload and a decrease in diastolic blood pressure and impaired coronary perfusion. Recent evidence suggests that an increase in pulse pressure is accompanied by progressive vessel wall damage and atherogenesis, and is associated with an increase in cardiac morbidity and mortality rates.[49]

While it is generally accepted that the structural and functional changes associated with aging impair compliance of the arterial circulation, these studies have been confined to the large conduit arteries and have emphasized that changes in pulsatile arterial function do not progress in a uniform or consistent manner in all arteries.[50] Prior studies that used pulse wave velocity to estimate the stiffness of arterial segments have indicated that the aorta stiffens progressively at an accelerated rate compared with other arterial segments. Echo-tracking technology has revealed that age-related changes in pulsatile function are nonhomogeneous within localized arterial segments of elastic and muscular arteries and that the compliance characteristics of the radial artery may paradoxically increase with age.[51] In contrast to the marked heterogeneity in the physical characteristics of localized arterial segments with aging, consistent and predictable changes occur in the arterial pulse contour regardless of the site of measurement. These changes reflect alterations in total arterial compliance and can be quantified with the pulse contour analysis technique, which provides an assessment not only of the physiologic behavior of the large conduit arteries that serve a capacitance function, but also of the smaller arteries that represent the predominant site of reflected waves or oscillations in the arterial bed.[43]

THERAPEUTIC RESPONSE IN HYPERTENSION

The goal of therapeutic interventions to lower blood pressure is the reduction of the risk of cardiovascular events. Because these events are directly related to structural abnormalities in arterial circulation, it is intuitive that an effective therapy should slow or reverse these abnormal structural changes. Efforts have also been made to identify a favorable effect of drug therapy on arterial compliance measurements. These have been studied by both pulse contour analysis and by ultrasound estimates of arterial wall thickness and distensibility. Preliminary studies have shown favorable effects of a number of drug interventions on these arterial characteristics.[52] Of course, any antihypertensive agent would be expected to reduce arterial stiffness because BP reduction *per se* unloads the stiff components of the arterial wall such as collagen. However, it seems likely that pharmacologic treatment can improve arterial stiffness beyond BP reduction.[53]

Pharmacologic trials often focus on large proximal elastic arteries (such as the aorta and the common carotid artery) because they represent the largest contribution to

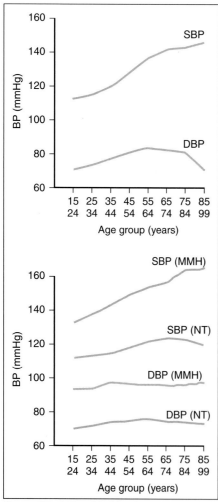

Figure 12–6. Trend in blood pressure with age in the overall population from the Argentine Blood Pressure Study. BP, blood pressure; DBP, diastolic blood pressure; MMH, mild to moderate hypertension; NT, normotension; SBP, systolic blood pressure. (From Galarza CR, Alfie J, Waisman GD, et al. *Hypertension* 1997;30:809–16.)

systemic compliance and therefore have the most impact on left ventricular load. Although muscular arteries, like the brachial, radial, and femoral arteries, contribute only modestly to total compliance, they are of interest to determine the contribution of smooth muscle relaxation to the increase in arterial compliance. Improving compliance of distal muscular arteries reduces the contribution of wave reflections to left ventricular afterload, but also is a marker for improved endothelial function that should favorably affect the long-term structural abnormalities in the large and small arteries. Reducing mechanical stress, either steady or pulsatile, at the site of proximal elastic or distal muscular arteries, is also a desirable goal of drug treatment.

In most pharmacologic studies, the elastic properties of large arteries have been assessed noninvasively. Direct techniques include measurements of carotid-femoral pulse wave velocity (PWV), an index of aortic stiffness, and or measurements of cross-sectional distensibility and compliance (carotid, femoral, and radial arteries). Indirect techniques are frequently based on models of local (brachial) or systemic circulations.[54] Small artery behavior is best assessed by pulse contour analysis. Late systolic pressure augmentation of a reflected wave can be detected in radial artery waveform recordings. More reliably, the diastolic decay of the radial pulse wave can be subjected to computer analysis that utilizes a modified Windkessel model to calculate both large and small artery compliance that quantitates the functional and structural status of both vascular segments.[7,10,12,16,44]

Whether classes of antihypertensive agents vary in their efficacy to affect arterial structure and thus influence arterial compliance via a pressure-independent mechanism is controversial and remains to be evaluated in large-scale trials or in meta-analysis of smaller studies. Most published studies have included small groups of patients (<20 patients/group), and are thus underpowered to conclude a lack of efficacy of one drug versus another. Moreover, several studies are short-term studies in which the effect of antihypertensive on the arterial system was studied during a period of 4 weeks or less. Long-term studies are much more important to know the effect of the antihypertensive agent on the vascular tree beyond blood pressure lowering.[55,56]

Despite these limitations, it is thus far generally accepted that angiotensin-converting enzyme inhibitors, angiotensin-II receptor blockers, aldosterone antagonists, calcium antagonists (especially dihydropyridines), and nitrates share a similar ability to decrease arterial stiffness in hypertensive patients in long-term studies. The effect on large artery stiffness is dependent to a considerable extent on reducing blood pressure, whereas the effect on small artery stiffness is predominantly influenced by improved endothelial function. It is also well accepted that the nonselective β blocker propranolol and the selective β$_1$ blocker atenolol are less efficacious during long-term treatment than β blockers with vasodilating properties.[57] Nonspecific vasodilators have only a moderate effect to decrease arterial stiffness, while diuretics have nearly no effect or a minor effect in reducing arterial stiffness.

Table 12–1 summarizes the effects of antihypertensive drugs on arterial stiffness.

The early *in vivo* diagnosis and follow-up of subclinical progression of arteriosclerosis is important for the evaluation of efficient preventive and therapeutic interventions. The carotid artery intima media thickness (IMT) is a reliable surrogate marker of arteriosclerosis and could be easily investigated with high resolution B-mode sonography. Due to its good reproducibility, the IMT measurement is optimal for tracking the progression or regression of atherosclerotic disease. The increase of IMT is influenced by numerous vascular risk factors (age, smoking, hypertension, dyslipidemia) and positively associated with the incidence of vascular events in the arterial vasculature (stroke, myocardial infarct). Studies of antihypertensive medication have confirmed that lowering blood pressure significantly reduces the progression of IMT. It is likely but not documented that reduced progression of IMT is accompanied by a decrease of future vascular events.[58,59]

The hope for the future is that a practical noninvasive screening technique will be used to assess the function and structure of the arterial wall in subjects with hypertension or even subjects at risk to develop hypertension. The effect of antihypertensive therapy on the functional and structural vessel wall abnormality can then be monitored during therapeutic intervention. Thus a drug regimen that did not favorably affect the arterial structure or function in a given patient could be replaced by another drug regimen that might be more effective. The correction of the arterial wall abnormality could then serve as a guide to therapeutic efficacy rather than the absolute level of blood pressure, which now serves as the surrogate marker. How the blood pressure changes and the arterial wall changes might relate needs to be intensively studied. Furthermore, it would be necessary to confirm that a favorable effect on the arterial wall is associated with a reduction of morbid events. It is therefore now important to assess the efficacy of any new antihypertensive strategy with regard to not only its ability to reduce blood pressure, but also its impact on structural and functional alterations in large and small arteries.[60]

EFFECT OF ANTIHYPERTENSIVE DRUGS ON ARTERIAL STIFFNESS	
Antihypertensive Agent	**Arterial Stiffness**
Diuretics	=
Beta blockers	= or ↑
Beta blockers with vasodilating properties	↓
Calcium antagonists	↓
ACE inhibitors	↓↓
Angiotensin II receptor blockers	↓↓
Aldosterone receptor blockers	↓↓
Nitrate	↓
Nonspecific vasodilator	↓

Table 12–1. Effect of Antihypertensive Drugs on Arterial Stiffness

CONCLUSIONS

Recognition that the artery wall is an important target of the disease we aim to treat has stressed the need for monitoring techniques to identify effective treatments in trials and to track individual patients for the natural history of their disease and the efficacy of interventions. Although data using existing technologies are still limited in scope and follow-up, pulse wave analysis is particularly attractive because of its simplicity and apparent sensitivity. Pulse wave velocity also is relatively simple, but its confinement to the aorta and large conduit arteries limits its application to identifying structural changes in the large arteries. Reproducibility and freedom from extraneous

influences are critical to the application of methods for monitoring. Blood pressure measurement itself is neither reliably reproducible nor free from extraneous influences. Nonetheless, BP has served in population studies as a guide to cardiovascular risk. Its use in individuals, however, usually is buttressed by repeated measurements, either in the office or at home, by exclusion of outlying measurements, and by awareness of environmental conditions at the time of measurement. Assessment of the mechanical properties of the small and large arteries has the potential to be far more sensitive and specific for detecting CV disease and the response to drug therapy than the BP alone.[44]

REFERENCES

1. Cohn JN. Arteries, myocardium, blood pressure and cardiovascular risk towards a revised definition of hypertension. *J Hypertens* 1998;16:2117–24.
2. Glasser SP, Arnett DK, McVeigh GM, et al. Vascular compliance and cardiovascular disease: a risk factor or a marker? *Am J Hypertens* 1997;10:1175–89.
3. Madhaven S, Ooi WL, Cohen H, Alderman MH. Relation of pulse pressure and blood pressure reduction to the incidence of myocardial infarction. *Hypertension* 1994;23:395–401.
4. McVeigh GE, Burns DE, Finkelstein SM, et al. Reduced vascular compliance as a marker for essential hypertension. *Am J Hypertens* 1991;4:245–51.
5. Duprez DA, Kaiser DR, Whitwam W, et al. Determinants of radial artery pulse wave analysis in asymptomatic individuals. *Am J Hypertens* 2004;17:647–53.
6. O'Rourke MF, Staessen JA, Vlachopoulos C, et al. Clinical applications of arterial stiffness; definitions and reference values. *Am J Hypertens* 2002;15:426–44.
7. Finkelstein SM, Cohn JN. First- and third-order models for determining arterial compliance. *J Hypertens* 1992;10(Suppl):S11–4.
8. McVeigh GE. Pulse waveform analysis and arterial wall properties. *Hypertension* 2003;41:1010–1.
9. Laurent S, Boutouyrie P, Asmar R, et al. Aortic stiffness is an independent predictor of all-cause mortality in hypertensive patients. *Hypertension* 2001;37:1236–41.
10. Grey E, Bratteli C, Glasser SP, et al. Reduced small artery but not large artery elasticity is an independent risk marker for cardiovascular events. *Am J Hypertens* 2003;16:265–9.
11. Weber T, Auer J, O'Rourke MF, et al. Arterial stiffness, wave reflections, and the risk of coronary artery disease. *Circulation* 2004;109:184–9.
12. Cohn JN, Quyyumi AA, Hollenberg NK, Jamerson KA. Surrogate markers for cardiovascular disease: functional markers. *Circulation* 2004;109(Suppl 1):IV31–46.
13. Cohn JN, Hoke L, Whitwam W, et al. Screening for early detection of cardiovascular disease in asymptomatic individuals. *Am Heart J* 2003;146(4):679–85.
14. Duprez DA, De Buyzere ML, Rietzschel ER, et al. Inverse relationship between aldosterone and large artery compliance in chronically treated heart failure patients. *Eur Heart J* 1998;19:1371–6.
15. Davies JI, Struthers AD. Pulse wave analysis and pulse wave velocity: a critical review of their strengths and weaknesses. *J Hypertens* 2003;21:463–72.
16. McVeigh GE. Pulse waveform analysis and arterial wall properties. *Hypertension* 2003;41:1010–1.
17. Beltran A, McVeigh G, Morgan D, et al. Arterial compliance abnormalities in isolated systolic hypertension. *Am J Hypertens* 2001;14:1007–11.
18. McVeigh GE. Arterial compliance in hypertension and diabetes mellitus. *Am J Nephrol* 1996;16:217–22.
19. Duprez DA, De Buyzere MM, De Bruyne L, et al. Small and large artery elasticity indices in peripheral arterial occlusive disease (PAOD). *Vasc Med* 2001;6:211–4.
20. Duprez DA, De Buyzere ML, De Backer TL, et al. Relationship between arterial elasticity indices and carotid artery intima-media thickness. *Am J Hypertens* 2000;13:1226–32.
21. Barenbrock M, Spieker C, Kerber S, et al. Different effects of hypertension, atherosclerosis and hyperlipidaemia on arterial distensibility. *J Hypertens* 1995;13(12 Pt 2):1712–27.
22. Duprez DA, Somasundaram PE, Sigurdsson G, et al. Relationship between C-reactive protein and arterial stiffness in an asymptomatic population. *J Hum Hypertens* 2005;19:515–9.
23. McEniery CM, Wilkinson IB. Large artery stiffness and inflammation. *J Hum Hypertens* 2005;19:507–9.
24. Boos CJ, Lip GYH. Elevated high-sensitive C-reactive protein, large arterial stiffness and atherosclerosis: a relationship between inflammation and hypertension? *J Hum Hypertens* 2005;19:511–3.
25. Messerli FH, Frohlich ED, Suarez DH, et al. Borderline hypertension: relationship between age, hemodynamics and circulating catecholamines. *Circulation* 1981;64:760–4.
26. Clement DL, Duprez D. Circulatory changes in muscle and skin arteries in primary hypertension. *Hypertension* 1984;6(6 Pt 2):III122–27.
27. Duprez DA, De Buyzere ML, Verloove HH, et al. Influence of the arterial blood pressure and nonhemodynamic factors on regional arterial wall properties in moderate essential hypertension. *J Hum Hypertens* 1996;10:251–6.
28. Lehoux S, Tedgui A. Signal transduction of mechanical stresses in the vascular wall. *Hypertension* 1998;32:338–45.
29. Mulvany MJ, Baumbach GL, Aalkjaer C, et al. Vascular remodeling. *Hypertension* 1996;28:505–6.
30. Martinez-Lemus LA, Hill MA, Bolz SS, et al. Acute mechanoadaptation of vascular smooth muscle cells in response to continuous arteriolar vasoconstriction: implications for functional remodeling. *FASEB J* 2004; 18:708–10.
31. Intengan HD, Schiffrin EL. Vascular remodeling in hypertension: roles of apoptosis, inflammation, and fibrosis. *Hypertension* 2001;38(3 Pt 2):581–7.
32. Davies MJ, Gordon JL, Gearing AJ, et al. The expression of the adhesion molecules ICAM-1, VCAM-1, PECAM, and E-selectin in human atherosclerosis. *J Pathol* 1993;171:223–10.
33. Newby AC. Dual role of matrix metalloproteinases (matrixins) in intimal thickening and atherosclerotic plaque rupture. *Physiol Rev* 2005;85:1–31.
34. Rizzoni D, Porteri E, Boari G, et al. Prognostic significance of small artery structure in hypertension. *Circulation* 2003;108:2230–5.
35. Intengan HD, Schiffrin EL. Structure and mechanical properties of resistance arteries in hypertension role of adhesion molecules and extracellular matrix determinants. *Hypertension* 2000;36:312–8.
36. Weber MA, Smith DH, Neutel JM, Graettinger WF. Arterial properties of early hypertension. *J Hum Hypertens* 1991;5:417–23.
37. McVeigh GE, Allen PB, Morgan DR, et al. Nitric oxide modulation of blood vessel tone identified by arterial

waveform analysis. *Clin Sci (Lond)* 2001;100:387–93.

38. Clarkson P, Celermajer DS, Powe AJ, et al. Endothelium-dependent dilatation is impaired in young healthy subjects with a family history of premature coronary disease. *Circulation* 1997; 96:3378–83.

39. Anderson TJ, Uehata A, Gerhard MD, et al. Close relation of endothelial function in the human coronary and peripheral circulation. *J Am Coll Cardiol* 1995;26:1235–41.

40. Barenbrock M, Hausberg M, Kosch M, et al. Flow-mediated vasodilation and distensibility in relation to intima-media thickness of large arteries in mild essential hypertension. *Am J Hypertens* 1999;12:973–9.

41. Lee KW, Blann AD, Lip GY. High pulse pressure and nondipping circadian blood pressure in patients with coronary artery disease: relationship to thrombogenesis and endothelial damage/dysfunction. *Am J Hypertens* 2005;18:104–15.

42. Ross R. The pathogenesis of atherosclerosis: a perspective for the 1990s. *Nature* 1993;362:801–9.

43. McVeigh GE, Bratteli CW, Morgan DJ, et al. Age-related abnormalities in arterial compliance identified by pressure pulse contour analysis. *Hypertension* 1999;33:1392–8.

44. Cohn JN, Duprez DA, Grandits GA. Arterial elasticity as part of a comprehensive assessment of cardiovascular risk and drug treatment. *Hypertension* 2005;46:217–20.

45. Galarza CR, Alfie J, Waisman GD, et al. Diastolic pressure underestimates age-related hemodynamic impairment. *Hypertension* 1997;30:809–16.

46. Lund-Johansen P. Twenty-year follow-up of hemodynamics in essential hypertension during rest and exercise. *Hypertension* 1991;18(Suppl 5):III54–61.

47. Pepe S, Lakatta EG. Aging hearts and vessels: masters of adaptation and survival. *Cardiovasc Res* 2005;66:190–3.

48. Robert L. Aging of the vascular wall and atherogenesis: role of the elastin-laminin receptor. *Atherosclerosis* 1996; 123:169–79.

49. London GM. Role of arterial wall properties in the pathogenesis of systolic hypertension. *Am J Hypertens* 2005;18(1 Pt 2):19S–22S.

50. Khder Y, Bray Des Boscs L, et al. Endothelial, viscoelastic and sympathetic factors contributing to the arterial wall changes during aging. *Cardiol Elderly* 1996;4:161–5.

51. Van Merode T, Brands PJ, Hoeks APG, Reneman RS. Different effects of aging on elastic and muscular arterial bifurcations in men. *J Vasc Res* 1996; 33:47–52.

52. Asmar R. Effect of antihypertensive agents on arterial stiffness as evaluated by pulse wave velocity: clinical implications. *Am J Cardiovasc Drugs* 2001;1:387–97.

53. Weber T, Auer J, Eisserer G, et al. Arterial stiffness and cardiovascular drugs. *Curr Pharm Design* 2003; 9:1049–63.

54. O'Rourke MF, Staessen JA, Vlachopoulos C, et al. Clinical applications of arterial stiffness; definitions and reference values. *Am J Hypertens* 2002;15:426–44.

55. White WB, Duprez D, St. Hillaire R, et al. Effects of the selective aldosterone blocker eplerenone versus the calcium antagonist amlodipine in systolic hypertension. *Hypertension* 2003; 41:1021–6.

56. Ting CT, Chen CH, Chang MS, Yin FCP. Short- and long-term effects of antihypertensive drugs on arterial reflections, compliance and impedance. *Hypertension* 1995;26:524–30.

57. McEniery CM, Schmitt M, Qasem A, et al. Nebivolol increases arterial distensibility in vivo. *Hypertension* 2004; 44:305–10.

58. Zanchetti A, Bond MG, Hennig M, et al. Calcium antagonist lacidipine slows down progression of asymptomatic carotid atherosclerosis: principal results of the European Lacidipine Study on Atherosclerosis (ELSA), a randomized, double-blind, long-term trial. *Circulation* 2002; 106:2422–7.

59. Terpstra WF, May JF, Smit AJ, et al. Effects of amlodipine and lisinopril on intima-media thickness in previously untreated, elderly hypertensive patients (the ELVERA trial). *J Hypertens* 2004; 22:1309–16.

60. Duprez DA, Florea N, Killpatrick B, et al. Valsartan increases small arterial elasticity in asymptomatic individuals. *Am J Hypertension* 2005;18(5Pt2):224A.

Chapter

13 Resistance Vessels in Hypertension

Michel E. Safar and Bernard I. Lévy

Key Findings

- The blood pressure curve involves two different components: a steady component corresponding to mean arterial pressure and to continuous flow within small resistance arteries, and a pulsatile component corresponding to pulsatile pressure and flow within large arteries.

- The two hemodynamic components are in constant interaction not only through neurohumoral pathways but also through the transit of wave reflections.

- Survival in subjects with hypertension requires adaptive mechanisms, including the structure and function of resistance vessels, that affect the entire cardiovascular system.

- A clear knowledge of the continuous cross-talk observed between the different components of the vascular tree is needed to understand cardiovascular risk.

The aorta takes origin from the left ventricle and almost immediately curves, in a three-dimensional way, giving off branches to the heart, head, and upper and lower limbs (macrocirculation). Beyond the early branches, the total cross-sectional area of the arterial tree begins to expand dramatically. Whereas the total cross-section increases, the average diameter is reduced, reflecting the increased number of bifurcations toward arterioles (microcirculation).[1,2] Along the arterial and arteriolar tree, the forces governing flow are dependent on the pressure generated by the heart. This quantity, which is the difference between the actual pressure and its hydrostatic component, is commonly referred to as "blood pressure" (BP).[1] It is the gradient of pressure, which drives the flow. The distribution of this pressure gradient through the circulation, which is largely dissipated in forcing the blood through the microcirculation, is the origin of vascular resistance. The behavior of vascular resistance in the presence of high BP is the subject of this chapter, taking into account, that within the arterial tree, the heart is an intermittent, but not a steady, pump. Increased vascular resistance is considered a hallmark of hypertension.

HEMODYNAMICS, HISTOPATHOLOGY, AND BIOCHEMISTRY

BP profile along the arterial tree

At the end of ventricular ejection, the pressure in the aorta falls much more slowly than in the left ventricle because the large central arteries, and particularly the aorta, are elastic and thus act as a reservoir during systole, storing some of the ejected blood, which is then forced out into the peripheral vessels during diastole (Windkessel effect). Then the pressure pulse generated by ventricular contraction travels along the aorta as a *wave* (Figure 13–1, *A*). It is possible to calculate its velocity (pulse wave velocity [PWV]) from the delay between two waves located at two different sites, if the distance between measuring sites is known (Figure 13–2). Furthermore, when simultaneous BP measurements are made at different points all along the aorta, it appears that the pressure wave changes shape as it travels down the aorta. Whereas the systolic blood pressure (SBP) actually increases with distance from the heart, the *mean* level of the arterial pressure (MAP) falls slightly (about 4 mmHg) during the same course along the length of the aorta (Figure 13–1, *A*). Thus the amplitude of the pressure oscillation between systole and diastole (the pulse pressure [PP]) nearly doubles (Figure 13–1). The process of PP amplification continues in the branches of the aorta out to the level of about the third generation of branches. Thereafter both PP and MAP decrease rapidly to the levels found in the microcirculation where a quasi steady flow is observed. Thus whereas the macrocirculation is characterized by pulsatile flow as well as by the propagation of a pressure wave, PWV and PP amplification, the microcirculation is influenced by steady flow, and hence follows Poiseuille's law. Under this condition, the pressure gradient becomes proportional to the velocity and viscosity of blood, to the length of the arteriolar tree, and mostly is inversely proportional to the fourth power of vascular diameter.

Several animal studies have examined the hydrostatic pressure profile along the macro and microcirculation, that is, between the heart and capillaries.[1–3] The general consensus is that the BP decrease occurs predominantly in precapillary vessels ranging from 10 to 300 μm. Conversely, a very high vascular resistance (which represents the mechanical forces that are opposed to blood flow) builds up abruptly from larger to smaller arteries, over a transitional short length of the path between arteries and veins, thus causing a dramatic decrease in MAP. At the same time, the PP amplitude decreases, resulting in almost completely steady flow through resistance vessels. A further contribution to opposition to flow derives also from the reflection of arterial pulsations that cannot enter the high resistance vessels and are summated with pressure waves approaching the area of high resistance[1,2] (Figure 13–1, *B* and *C*). This area of reflection, which is directly related to the number

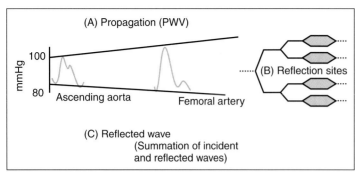

Figure 13–1. Pressure wave along the arterial tree. **A,** Forward pressure wave is propagated from the heart toward the microvascular network at a given pulse wave velocity; pulse pressure is higher in peripheral than in central arteries due to a higher SBP and a slightly lower DBP. **B,** Pressure wave is reflected and the principal reflection sites are located in the microvascular network. **C,** Backward pressure wave returns toward the heart at the same PWV as the pressure wave. The arterial BP curve is in fact the summation of the incident and reflected pressure waves at each point of the arterial (aortic) tree. BP, blood pressure; DBP, diastolic blood pressure; PWV, pulse wave velocity; SBP, systolic blood pressure.

and geometric properties of arteriolar bifurcations,[1] will be analyzed in detail at the end of this chapter.

Histomorphometric characteristics of the arterial wall

The basic architecture of arterial and arteriolar vessels is usually described in terms of cross-sectional arrangement of vascular smooth muscle (VSM) cells and extracellular matrix (ECM). The former predominates in arterioles (microcirculation) and the latter in large arteries (macro-circulation).[4] Large arteries are mainly constituted, within the media, of lamellae of elastic material with intervening layers of VSM cells, collagen fibers, and ground substance. In the proximal aorta, elastin is the dominant component, while in the distal aorta the collagen to elastin ratio is reversed, and in peripheral arteries, collagen predominates. Thereafter, VSM cells become the quasi-exclusive material of the vascular wall. This description is consistent with the chemical properties and gene expression of elastin, collagen, and VSM cells along the aorta and its branches.[5]

The protein product of the elastin gene is synthesized by VSM cells and secreted as a monomer, tropoelastin.[2–4] After post-translational modification, tropoelastin is cross-linked and organized into elastin polymers that form concentric rings of elastic fenestrated lamellae around the arterial lumen. Elastin-deficient mice die from an occlusive fibrocellular pathology caused by subendothelial proliferation and accumulation of VSM cells in early neonatal life.[6] Thus elastin is a crucial signaling molecule that directly controls VSM cell biology and stabilizes arterial structure and resting vessel diameter. On the other hand, vascular collagen is determined at a very young developmental stage, and thereafter remains quite stable due to a very low turnover. Nevertheless, the proportion of collagen types I and III has a differential mechanical impact on stiffness of the vessel wall.[7] Furthermore, neurohumoral factors, particularly those related to angiotensin II and aldosterone, modulate collagen accumulation.[8] Finally,

collagen is also subjected to important chemical modifications, such as breakdown, cross-linking or glycation, resulting in marked changes in stiffness along the vessel wall.[3]

ECM is responsible for the passive mechanical properties of the arteries, in particular of the aorta and its main branches.[1,2] In a cylindrical vessel, when the transmural pressure rises, a curvilinear pressure-diameter curve ensues, mainly due to the recruitment of elastin at low pressure and of collagen fibers at high pressure.[1,2] Nevertheless, several other molecules, through their role in cell–cell and cell–matrix attachments, may contribute to the three-dimensional repartition of mechanical forces within the arterial wall.[3] As an example, in rat proximal elastic arteries, the main VSM cell type consists of desmin-negative cells with high levels of connexins C_x43. In small- to medium-sized muscular arteries, the main VSM cell type is desmin-positive with low levels of C_x43.[9] Interestingly, in mice lacking desmin, isobaric carotid stiffness is increased.[10]

VSM cells do not represent a homogenous population. For the same genomic background, there are different mixtures of phenotypes, involving not only contractile and secretory properties but also proliferative and apoptotic behavior.[3,11] The distribution of each of these phenotypes is mainly influenced by age, location within the vascular tree, and presence of underlying pathologic factors. Contractile properties, which are mainly expressed in arterioles, are responsible for the active mechanical properties of small and large vessels.[1–3] Changes in VSM tone may occur either directly or through signals arising from endothelial cells. Endothelium is a source of substances, particularly nitric oxide (NO), and of signal transduction mechanisms[12] that necessarily influence the biophysical properties of vessels.[1–3] Many of these signals are influenced by blood flow through the mechanism of endothelium-dependent dilatation, which is not restricted to vessels of particular size (muscular or musculoelastic). In contrast, the role of mediators arising from endothelium predominates in muscular distal arteries.[12,13] The wall–lumen ratio of such vessels is influenced by the local differential effects of NO and other vasodilating (bradykinin, prostaglandins) or vasoconstrictive (norepinephrine, angiotensin, endothelin) agents. Whether such arteriolar changes may modify the pattern of wave reflections issued from distal VSM cells is the subject of recent research.[3]

VASCULAR DEVELOPMENT AND GENETICS

The pulsatile component of BP represents a direct continuation of the heart beat and originates at the proximal part of the thoracic aorta. This is necessarily the module of hemodynamic forces that predominates during the early phase of vascular development, and must be rapidly brought under control at birth for cardiovascular (CV) survival. In contrast to PP, the optimal MAP may be achieved only from the distal part of the arterial tree, where the microvascular network develops and Poiseuille's law is applicable.

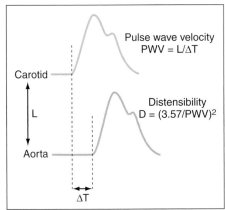

Figure 13–2. PWV measurement between the common carotid artery and the origin of common femoral artery (end of the aorta): the time delay (ΔT) between the noninvasive BP recordings is measured using a foot-to-foot method; the PWV is obtained from the distance (L) between the two recordings and ΔT. BP, blood pressure; PWV, pulse wave velocity.

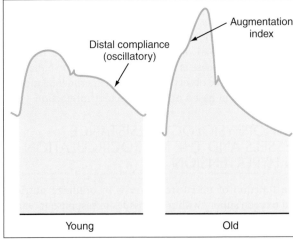

Figure 13–3. Aortic BP in younger and older subjects for the same MAP (i.e., the same cross-sectional area under the curve). The shapes of the aortic blood BP curves differ markedly in younger and older subjects. The latter has a higher SBP and lower DBP due to increased arterial stiffness and early wave reflections. These early wave reflections cause a supplementary increase of SBP during systole, called the augmentation index, and mainly observed in older subjects. Another index of wave reflection may be calculated in diastole (called here, distal or oscillatory compliance). BP, blood pressure; DBP, diastolic blood pressure; MAP, mean arterial pressure; SBP, systolic blood pressure.

Accordingly, the steady phenomenon of MAP occurs at a later phase of CV development.

As shown from the previous hemodynamic descriptions, the BP curve results from the interaction between two different components: a steady one, corresponding to MAP, and a pulsatile one corresponding to PP (Figure 13–3). Studies of rats and knockout mice indicate that the genetics of each of these two components may be analyzed separately.[10,14] Genome-wide linkage analysis has shown the importance of identifying genetic factors in subjects with high PP independently of MAP.[15] Thus for genetic studies, an evaluation of the totality of the BP curve, mainly of the aortic curve, is necessary for an adequate description of the main phenotypes of hypertension. From this viewpoint, an important finding in subjects with hypertension results from studies of the ACE I/D gene polymorphism. (Other genetic findings are developed in other chapters of this book.) Staessen et al.[16] were the first to show that the DD genotype was significantly associated with hypertension, but mostly with isolated systolic hypertension in the elderly. In this population, the DD genotype is associated not only with increased PP but also with increased arterial stiffness and accelerated increase of PP with age.[16,17] Furthermore, more recent research suggests that the combination of two or three specific gene polymorphisms (ACE, aldosterone synthase and alpha-adducin gene polymorphisms) affect SBP, PP, and vessel wall properties more profoundly than a single genotype.[16]

Whatever the gene polymorphisms may be, blood vessel development is primarily issued from the *in situ* differentiation of endothelial cells from the mesoderm and their coalescence into primary vessels.[13,18] Subsequent remodeling of the primary vascular plexus into a more mature vascular system occurs through a process known as angiogenesis. This involves sprouting, splitting, and remodeling of

capillaries, which leads to reorganization of the primary vessels into large and small vessels, and hence dominantly contributes to the progressive increase of vascular resistance, and thereby MAP. Hormonal factors such as angiotensin II participate in this process.[13,18] Nevertheless, a major point is that vessels adapt to flow in order to optimize the shear stress to which they are subjected. Flow not only shapes the global patterning of the arterial tree, but also regulates the activation of several biochemical markers such as ephrin B2 and neuropilin.[18]

For the understanding of resistance vessels development, it is worth noting that Poiseuille's law recognizes arteriolar length and the fourth power of vascular radius as the most important geometric factors determining the resistance of microvascular network. Thus the resistance of a tree-like branched network can be described by relatively simple extensions of Poiseuille's classic equation.[18] Nevertheless, the number of blood vessels coupled in parallel is also an important factor to consider. Computer simulations have shown that elimination of a number of small arterioles from a vascular bed (rarefaction) causes an increase in total resistance.[19] In the particular case of arcade-like networks, the situation is quite difficult to define, as they contain arteriolar branches that are coupled both in series and in parallel. In these networks, resistance is determined by the combined contribution of the length and diameter of individual arterioles, their branching angles, the location of their branching points, and the number of branches.[18] Thus in order to identify vascular resistance, it is important to define not only the absolute number of blood vessels, but also the nature of the changes in the network. Interestingly, this network may serve as sites of wave reflections (see above). A model developed by Green[19] has demonstrated that removal of arteriolar segments causes an increase in resistance, and that the extent of the increase is sufficient to explain the enhanced vascular resistance observed in several experimental models of hypertension based on microvascular rarefaction.

PATHOPHYSIOLOGY: RESISTANCE VESSELS AND THE MICROCIRCULATION IN HYPERTENSION

The function of microcirculation is to optimize nutrient and oxygen supply within the tissues in response to variations of demand, and to minimize large fluctuations of hydrostatic pressure in the capillaries causing disturbances in capillary exchange.[13,18] In hypertension, the main question is to determine under which conditions a large drop in hydrostatic pressure may be achieved from the larger to the smaller arteries without any deleterious effect on tissue blood flow causing organ damage.[18]

Location and main characteristics of peripheral vascular resistances in chronic hypertension

As mentioned previously, the pressure drop along the vascular bed occurs predominantly in precapillary vessels ranging from 10 to 300 μm in diameter.[1–3,18] Studies of skeletal muscle in spontaneously hypertensive rats (SHR) have concluded that pressure is elevated approximately proportionally throughout the precapillary vasculature.[1–3,18] DeLano et al.[20] found that if the measured pressures are normalized by the systemic MAP, pressures are virtually identical in normotensive rats and SHR at all the locations studied. These results suggest that because the major pressure drop occurs in the smallest arteries and arterioles, these vessels represent the principal site of the increased vascular resistance in hypertension. The most striking evidence results from the marked increase of resistance that occurs when the vasculature is maximally relaxed.[21] From Poiseuille's law, it appears that altered minimum vascular resistance could be the result of a diminution of the lumen diameter of individual vessels, of vessels being longer, or of their rarefaction (a decreased number of vessels connected in parallel).[13,18] Thus it seems likely that, in hypertension, the structure and function of microcirculation may be altered in different ways, and does not involve necessarily a vessel diameter narrowing. A first possibility is that the mechanisms regulating vasomotor tone may be abnormal, leading to enhanced vasoconstriction, reduced vasodilating responses, and/or altered autoregulation.[13,18] Another possibility is the presence of anatomic alterations of the structure of individual precapillary resistance vessels, such as increases in their wall-to-lumen ratios[20,21] or reduction of the density (rarefaction) of arterioles or capillaries within a given vascular bed.[13,18] It seems likely that the relative contribution of these factors may differ in various vascular beds and may vary according to hypertension models.

Hypertensive changes in vasomotor tone and autoregulation

The most obvious mechanism increasing resistance to blood flow in arterioles is vasoconstriction. Only small changes in lumen size are required to make large adjustments in flow and pressure. Vasomotor tone in resistance arteries is controlled by local or metabolic regulation and by the sympathetic nervous system.[13,18] In addition, paracrine substances, mostly released by the endothelial cells, play a key role in the control of local vasomotor tone. Endothelin and prostaglandin H2/thromboxane A^2 are important vasoactive candidates to consider in the mechanisms of hypertension.[13,18]

The tone of the microcirculation and, consequently, the levels of tissue perfusion are tightly coupled to the status of tissue oxygen consumption. When oxygen requirements are increased, blood inflow increases accordingly.[2] The ability of a vascular bed to constrict and dilate in order to maintain flow during changes of perfusion pressure, independently of any systemic neurohumoral regulation, is termed "autoregulation." In coronary circulation, autoregulation is most effective between pressures of 60 and 160 mmHg.[22] Importantly, chronic hypertension shifts the range of pressures over which autoregulation occurs in the myocardium, so that flow will begin to decline at greater pressure. A similar hemodynamic mechanism has been observed within renal and cerebral circulations.[1–3,20] The nature of the signaling molecules that participate in the local autoregulation process remains poorly understood. In experimental hypertension, vasoconstriction seems to be particularly enhanced at the initial stages when arterial pressure increases rapidly, producing a rapid increase in myogenic tone.[23] On the other hand, a loss of vasodilating properties, particularly of endothelial origin, has been also reported in other animal models.[13,18,24]

Structural factors of increased vascular resistance: Increased wall–lumen ratio and/or microcirculation rarefaction

Hypertrophy of the vascular wall, resulting in decreased lumen size, and medial hypertrophy, resulting in heightened vasodilated vascular resistance, are concepts that received considerable attention in models of secondary hypertension.[18,21,24] Increases in the media–lumen ratio of small arteries have been widely documented in several forms of experimental secondary hypertension.[18,21] These changes are consistent with the view that vessels maintain constant wall stress in the face of changing pressure. Resistance arteries at the beginning of the resistance section of the vascular bed (±300 μm) exhibit only weak myogenic responses and remodel with a combination of lumen reduction and wall hypertrophy. Small resistance arteries (50 to 10 μm), where most hemodynamic resistance is located, are protected against increased circumferential wall stress and do not hypertrophy during chronic hypertension. Thus it is not clear whether arterioles undergo increases in wall–lumen ratio in primary hypertension. SHR arterioles have not been reported to show consistently either reduced luminal diameter or wall thickening (reviewed by Struijker-Boudier et al.[25]). In hypertensive humans, reduced arteriolar lumen diameters are difficult to demonstrate,[21,25] since only *in vitro* determinations are available and three-dimensional measurements cannot be easily done. Thus in hypertensive humans, the expression "altered structure of the arterial wall," is often somewhat ambiguous. A narrowed lumen with resulting increased media–lumen ratio can occur without any change in the amount of material in the vessel wall.[21] Conversely, an increased media–lumen ratio may not cause a narrowed lumen, and an increased amount of wall material (demonstrated by an increase of the wall cross-sectional area) is not necessarily accompanied by a smaller lumen or elevated media–lumen ratio.[13,18] Finally, in hypertensive humans, the structural changes and impaired vasodilator capacity resulting from the increased wall–lumen ratio contribute to CV complications.[18,21,26] Nevertheless, these changes are not always directly related to BP level. They cannot represent the exclusive mechanism responsible for high MAP in subjects with essential hypertension.

Independently of changes in wall–lumen ratio, Hutchins et al.[27] first described up to 50% rarefaction of the microvasculature in the cremaster muscles of SHR, and Prewitt et al.[28] subsequently found rarefaction of capillaries and arterioles in SHR gracilis muscle. There is now much evidence that the development of hypertension is accompanied by a diminished density of arterioles and capillaries in skeletal muscle in both animal models and human hypertension.[29–31] Rarefaction[13,18] can be either functional, resulting from vasoconstriction strong enough to close the vascular lumen and prevent the perfusion of a capillary bed, or structural, in which case the vessels are absent or their density is decreased in perfused tissues. Because functional rarefaction of the capillary beds in skeletal muscles of normotensive animals has been described in the past,[13,18] only arteriolar and capillary structural rarefaction may greatly contribute to the basic mechanisms of hypertension. Previously, we discussed to what extent the structural rarefaction of the microvascular network may contribute to the increase in vascular resistance and MAP. It is possible that this process may result from the net effect of combined growth and apoptosis.[3,11,18,25] Furthermore, the rarefaction process may predominate in specialized organs or tissues, such as the kidney.[13,18] Numerous experimental studies and significant statistical associations between reduced nephron numbers and high BP strongly suggest the latter possibility.[3]

CLINICAL IMPLICATIONS AND PERSPECTIVES: CROSS-TALK BETWEEN HEART AND RESISTANCE VESSELS

Studies in hypertension have constantly shown consistent links between cardiac function and resistance vessels, as well as the role of small vessels in end-organ damage. These links are traditionally described as exclusively due to specific neurohumoral or cellular mechanisms. However, sophisticated mechanical factors may also participate in this cross-talk.[2,3]

Ejection of blood into the aorta generates a BP wave that is propagated to other arteries throughout the body. As in elastic conduits, this forward traveling pressure wave is reflected at all points of structural and/or functional discontinuity of the arterial tree, that is, mainly at the origin of resistance arteries (Figure 13–1, *B*). Thus a reflected wave is generated that travels backward toward the ascending aorta (Figure 13–1, *C*). Incident and reflected pressure waves are in constant interaction along the arterial circuit and are summed up into the actual pressure wave. The final amplitude and shape of the measured aortic BP wave are determined by the phase relationship (timing) between the two components of these waves. In younger subjects, under physiologic conditions with elastic arteries, the backward pressure wave returns from the distal arterioles during diastole, making PP higher in peripheral than in central arteries and boosting coronary perfusion.[2,3] In older subjects with rigid arteries and hence heightened PWV, the reflecting sites corresponding to arteriolar branching appear "closer" to the ascending aorta and the reflected waves occur earlier (Figure 13–3), being more closely in phase with incident waves in this region. Such an earlier return of wave reflections results in an augmentation of aortic and ventricular pressures during systole and reduces aortic pressure during diastole, favoring myocardial ischemia (Figure 13–3). Hence, altered mechanical properties of the aortic wall influence the level of aortic SBP (which is increased) and DBP (which is decreased). Finally, a disturbed pressure signal arising from arterioles modifies wave reflections, worsens the heart–vessel coupling and favors CV complications. Evidence for this pathophysiologic process has been highlighted by the role of PWV and wave reflections as independent CV risk factors in subjects with hypertension and other CV diseases.[32–35]

Importantly, wave reflections alter the ventricular–vascular coupling not only through increased arterial stiffness and change in timing but also through modifications in their amplitude. This process depends on reflectance properties of the vascular bed, which mainly arise from microvascular network. Every change in the local properties of an artery may be the site of partial reflection of the pressure wave, in the same way that any discontinuity in a stretched string is a source of reflection. These reflections are influenced by the geometry, number, structure, and function of smaller muscular arteries and arterioles, and finally microvascular rarefaction. Taylor[36] previously reported that an increase of the arterial cross-sectional area at peripheral bifurcations causes a delay of wave reflections with subsequent selective decreases of SBP and PP through changes in the peripheral reflection pattern. In subjects with hypertension, an opposite pattern has been described, resulting from hypertrophy and/or remodeling of arteriolar vessels.[3] Furthermore, age influences greatly all these modifications and tends to increase SBP and PP more rapidly in the central than in the distal arteries, causing a reduction of SBP and PP amplification. This reduction also constitutes an independent predictor of CV mortality in hypertensive subjects.[37]

SUMMARY

In summary, the present description has shown that, within the vascular tree, elastic arteries buffer the pulsations, muscular arteries actively alter propagation velocity, and arterioles serve not only as resistance vessels but also as major reflection sites. Within the CV system, all these alterations (or their combination) enable a continuous cross-talk between the heart and the microvascular network.[2,3] Disturbance of these frequency-dependent alterations favors a predominant increase of SBP and PP, as observed in aged and/or hypertensive populations with high CV risk. This process contributes to increasing the heart's load and favors cardiac hypertrophy and coronary ischemia, finally causing CV death. The consequences of these findings on the clinical aspects of systolic or systolic–diastolic hypertension and on the strategy for CV diseases remain to be taken into consideration in the future.

ACKNOWLEDGMENTS

This study was performed with the help of INSERM and GPH-CV (Groupe de Pharmacologie et d'Hémodynamique Cardiovasculaire), Paris. We thank Anne Safar, MD, for helpful and stimulating discussions.

REFERENCES

1. Caro CG, Pedley TJ, Schroter RC, Seed WA. *The Mechanics of the Circulation*. New York and Toronto: Oxford University Press, 1978.
2. Nichols WW, O'Rourke M. *McDonald's Blood Flow in Arteries. Theoretical, Experimental and Clinical Principles*. 4th ed. Sydney, Auckland: Arnold E. London, 1998.
3. Safar ME, Levy BI, Struijker-Boudier H. Current perspectives on arterial stiffness and pulse pressure in hypertension and cardiovascular diseases. *Circulation* 2003;107(22):2864–9.
4. Glagov S. Hemodynamic risk factors: mechanical stress, mural architecture, medial nutrition and vulnerability of arteries to atherosclerosis. In: Wissler RW and Geer JC, eds. *The Pathogenesis of Atherosclerosis*. Baltimore: Williams & Wilkins, 1972:164–99.
5. Davidson JM, Hill KE, Mason ML, Giro G. Longitudinal gradients of collagen and elastin gene expression in the porcine aorta. *J Biol Chem* 1985;260:1901–8.
6. Li DY, Brooke B, Davis EC, et al. Elastin is an essential determinant of arterial morphogenesis. *Nature* 1998;393:276–80.
7. Fleischmayer R, Perlish JS, Burgeson RE, Shaikh-Bahai F. Type I and type III collagen interactions during fibrillogenesis. *Ann N Y Acad Sci* 1990;580:161–75.
8. Safar ME, Thuilliez C, Richard V, Benetos A. Pressure-independent contribution of sodium to large artery structure and function in hypertension. *Cardiovasc Res* 2000;46:269–76.
9. Ko YS, Coppen SR, Dupont E, et al. Regional differentiation of desmin, connexin43, and connexin45 expression patterns in rat aortic smooth muscle. *Arterioscler Thromb Vasc Biol* 2001;21:355–64.
10. Lacolley P, Challande P, Boumaza S, et al. Mechanical properties and structure of carotid arteries in mice lacking desmin. *Cardiovasc Res* 2001;51:178–87.
11. Hamet P. Proliferation and apoptosis of vascular smooth muscle in hypertension. *Curr Opin Nephrol Hypertens* 1995;4:1–7.
12. Davies PF. Flow-mediated endothelial mechanotransduction. *Physiol Rev* 1995;75:519–60.

13. Levy BI, Ambrosio G, Pries AR, Struijker-Boudier HAJ. Microcirculation in hypertension. A new target for treatment? *Circulation* 2001;104:735–40.
14. Lacolley P, Labat C, Pujol A, et al. Increased carotid wall elastic modulus and fibronectin in aldosterone-salt treated rats—effects of eplerenone. *Circulation* 2002;106:2848–53.
15. Destefano AL, Larson MG, Mitchell GF, et al. Genome-wide scan for pulse pressure in the National Heart, Lung and Blood Institute's Framingham Heart Study. *Hypertension* 2004;44(2):152–5.
16. Staessen JA, Wang JG, Brand E, et al. Effects of three candidate genes on prevalence and incidence of hypertension in a Caucasian population. *J Hypertens* 2001;19:1349–58.
17. Safar ME, Lajemi M, Rudnichi A, et al. Angiotensin-converting enzyme D/I gene polymorphism and age-related changes in pulse pressure in subjects with hypertension. *Arterioscler Thromb Vasc Biol* 2004;24:782–6.
18. Struijker Boudier HA, Ambrosio G. *Microcirculation and Cardiovascular Disease*. London: Lippincott Williams & Wilkins, 2000.
19. Green JF. *Mechanical Concepts in Cardiovascular and Pulmonary Physiology*. Philadelphia: Lea & Fiberger, 1977.
20. Delano FA, Schmid-Schonbein GW, Skalak TC, Zweifach BW. Penetration of the systemic blood pressure into the microvasculature of rat skeletal muscle. *Microvasc Res* 1991;41:92–110.
21. Folkow B. Physiological aspects of primary hypertension. *Physiol Rev* 1982;62:347–504.
22. Hoffman JIE. A critical view of coronary reserve. *Circulation* 1987;75(Suppl I):6–11.
23. Meininger GA, Lubrano VM, Granger HJ. Hemodynamic and microvascular responses in the hindquarters during the development of renal hypertension in rats. Evidence for the involvement of an autoregulatory component. *Circ Res* 1984;55:609–22.
24. Mulvany MJ, Aalkjaer C. Structure and function of small arteries. *Physiol Rev* 1990;70:921–61.
25. Struijker-Boudier HA, Le Noble JLML, Messing MWJ, et al. The microcirculation and hypertension. *J Hypertens* 1992;10 (suppl 7):S147–56.

26. Schiffrin EL, Deng LY. Structure and function of resistance arteries of hypertensive patients treated with a β-blocker or a calcium channel antagonist. *J Hypertens* 1996;14:1247–55.
27. Hutchins PM, Bond RF, Green HD. Participation of oxygen in the local control of skeletal muscle microvasculature. *Circ Res* 1974;40(4):85–93.
28. Prewitt RL, Chen II, Dowell R. Development of microvascular rarefaction in the spontaneously hypertensive rat. *Am J Physiol* 1982;243(2):H243–51.
29. Greene AS, Tonellato PJ, Lui J, et al. Microvascular rarefaction and tissue vascular resistance in hypertension. *Am J Physiol* 1989;256:H126–31.
30. Antonios TF, Singer DRJ, Markandu ND. Rarefaction of skin capillaries in borderline essential hypertension suggests an early structural abnormality. *Hypertension* 1999;34:655–8.
31. Sullivan JM, Prewitt RL, Joseph JA. Attenuation of the microcirculation in young patients with high-output borderline hypertension. *Hypertension* 1983;5:844–51.
32. Blacher J, Guerin A, Pannier B, et al. Impact of aortic stiffness on survival in end-stage renal failure. *Circulation* 1999;99:2434–9.
33. Laurent S, Boutouyrie P, Asmar R, et al. Aortic stiffness is an independent predictor of all-cause mortality in hypertensive patients. *Hypertension* 2001;37:1236–41.
34. London GM, Blacher J, Pannier B, et al. Arterial wave reflections and survival in end-stage renal failure. *Hypertension* 2001;38:434–438.
35. Meaume S, Benetos A, Henry OF, et al. Aortic pulse wave velocity predicts cardiovascular mortality in subjects >70 years of age. *Arterioscler Thromb Vasc Biol* 2001;21:2046–50.
36. Taylor MG. Wave travel in arteries and the design of the cardiovascular system. In: Attinger EO, ed. *Pulsatile Blood Flow*. New York: McGraw-Hill, 1964:343–7.
37. Safar ME, Blacher J, Pannier B, et al. Central pulse pressure and mortality in end-stage renal disease. *Hypertension* 2002;39:735–8.

Chapter

14

The Endothelium in Hypertension: Assessment and Clinical Aspects of Micro- and Macrovascular Function

Andrew D. Blann

Definition

- Endothelial function refers to the ability of the endothelium to adequately perform its physiological roles, such as in the regulation of blood pressure and in hemostasis.

Key Findings

- Endothelial function can be objectively quantified.
- Endothelial function is involved in the pathogenesis of cardiovascular disease. Diverse pathological processes that damage the endothelium therefore precipitate its dysfunction.

Clinical Implications

- Hypertension and thrombosis, and therefore increased risk of adverse cardiovascular events such as myocardial infarction, stroke and heart failure, result from endothelial dysfunction.

The endothelium is important in several physiological and pathological processes, with direct involvement in regulation of local blood flow (via vessel tone), regulation of vessel permeability, regulation of the clotting cascade (via expression of anticoagulant and procoagulant factors), and regulation of leukocyte and fluid movements into the media and therefore the tissues.[1,2] Thus, if the maintenance of endothelial function is important in minimizing or slowing the development and progression of heart disease and atherosclerosis it follows that the converse is also true (i.e., that loss of vascular integrity is associated with an increased risk of developing, for example, left ventricular hypertrophy and atherothrombotic disease). Indeed, Virchow introduced the concept that loss of endothelial integrity is a part of the pathogenesis of thrombosis over 150 years ago.

In the present day, this concept is supported by the fact that endothelial function is impaired in all of the classical (e.g., diabetes mellitus, hypertension, smoking, hypercholesterolemia) and several emerging cardiovascular risk factors (Table 14–1). Given the role of the endothelium in regulating the coagulation cascade, the link between endothelial dysfunction and disease development may be an alteration in the balance of procoagulant and anticoagu-

lant factors, resulting in abnormal coagulability and the consequences of inappropriate thrombogenesis such as myocardial infarction, congestive heart failure, and stroke.[3–5]

ASSESSING ENDOTHELIAL FUNCTION AND DYSFUNCTION

Before describing endothelium damage/dysfunction, we first briefly revisit vascular physiology. The vascular endothelium comprises a vast number of flattened orthogonal cells that line the entire vascular tree. Broadly speaking, the endothelium impacts onto cardiovascular disease in (at least) two independent but potentially overlapping areas: thrombosis/hemostasis and the regulation of blood pressure. In the former, the endothelium expresses/secretes/releases both procoagulants (e.g., von Willebrand factor, tissue factor, factor V) and anticoagulants (e.g., thrombomodulin, heparin, prostacyclin). Vascular tone and blood pressure are regulated by the balance between vasodilators (e.g., nitric oxide, NO) and vasoconstrictors (e.g., endothelin). It is clear, therefore, that disruption of vascular physiology can have a fundamental influence on both thrombosis and hypertension.[6,7]

Thus, given the central role of the endothelium in preventing the development and progression of atherothrombotic disease it is clearly desirable to be able to assess the endothelium in terms of its structural and functional integrity. Plasma proteins have long been used as assessors in these terms. Some of these assessor molecules can be relatively easily measured in the laboratory, although not all (e.g., tissue factor) are specific for the endothelium and others (e.g., NO) are virtually impossible to measure simply and directly. Of those that have potential as markers of endothelial function, increased levels of plasma von Willebrand factor (vWf) have long been taken to imply an insult to the endothelium[8] and are present in all risk factors for atherosclerosis as well as in frank vascular disease. Increased levels also predict adverse cardiovascular outcome. Increased levels of other plasma markers (tissue plasminogen activator, soluble E selectin, and soluble thrombomodulin) have also been described as reflecting endothelial perturbation.[2,9]

Recently, a more physiological view of the assessment of large vessel endothelial function has been developed [i.e., flow-mediated dilatation (FMD)].[10,11] This uses a cuff to occlude the brachial artery, followed by assessment of blood flow distal to the occlusion (using high-frequency ultrasound) following reversal of the occlusion. The release of the cuff causes endothelial-dependent vasodilatation, which is thought to be mediated via shear stress causing release of NO from endothelial cells. The change in diameter of the brachial artery is therefore a measure of the endothelium-dependent vasodilatation. The endothelium-independent response can be assessed by the use of sublingual nitrate medications that act directly on the smooth muscle cells.

Laser Doppler with iontophoresis is a relatively novel method of assessing *microvascular* endothelial function in an area of skin. Iontophoresis uses a small electric current to deliver vasoactive substances such as acetylcholine or sodium nitroprusside through the skin. Acetylcholine stimulates the endothelial cells to produce NO, and therefore measures the endothelial-dependent response. Sodium nitroprusside is a NO donor that directly stimulates the smooth muscle of the skin arterioles and thus bypasses the endothelial cell.[12,13]

Probably the strongest evidence of *severe* damage to the vasculature by a factor or factors known or unknown is the appearance of circulating endothelial cells (CECs) in the plasma.[14–16] These cells can be identified in the blood using immunomagnetic separation and by flow cytometry, and represent either damaged endothelial cells that have broken off the vessel wall and are thus circulating, or progenitor cells migrating from the bone marrow to repair a site of endothelial damage. The debate regarding their purpose or significance continues, but in either case CECs appear to be markers of severe endothelial damage. Clinically, they are associated with the presence of, and prognosis following, myocardial infarction—with elevated numbers of CECs at 48 hours post myocardial infarction predicting major adverse cardiac events at 30 days and 1 year.[15,16] Thus,

technically CECs are not so much a direct marker of endothelial function as a marker of the degree of damage done to this tissue, and as such are a tool of vascular biologists. These aspects are summarized in Box 14–1.

ENDOTHELIAL FUNCTION IN HYPERTENSION AND CARDIOVASCULAR DISEASE

Endothelial dysfunction/damage is present in all classical cardiovascular risk factors and in clear disease (Table 14–1, which also highlights some possible mechanisms). Evidence of this has been provided from changes in vascular function defined by altered release of specific molecules (e.g., vWf, tissue plasminogen activator) into the blood, and altered reactivity of large vessels (e.g., the brachial artery) to changes in blood flow (i.e., FMD)(Box 14–1). Indeed, the literature is dominated by these two methods. As endothelial damage is associated with increased plasma vWf, and as endothelial dysfunction is associated with impaired (i.e., reduced) FMD, in theory the two ought to correlate inversely if they are themselves related. This has been demonstrated in a study largely of patients with hypertension but often with other risk factors[17] (Figure 14–1). Thus, patients with the highest vWf also generally have the most adverse (i.e., lowest) FMD. Similarly, those with good FMD have low vWf. However, this study is unusual in that almost all workers chose one of these two approaches.

As yet, microvascular function—as assessed, for example, by laser Doppler iontophoresis—is a relatively new technique that has made relatively little impact on cardiovascular pathophysiology.[12,13] However, relevant studies

---

Box 14–1

Assessment of Endothelial Function and Integrity

- Changes (almost always an increase) in specific plasma proteins such as von Willebrand factor, soluble E selectin, and soluble thrombomodulin.
- Changes (generally an impairment) in response to altered blood flow in large vessels such as the brachial artery (i.e., flow-mediated dilatation, FMD). This may be due to impaired release of nitric oxide by a damaged endothelium.
- Changes (generally an impairment) in response to pharmacological stimulation (e.g., microelectrically driven transdermal acetylcholine) in small blood vessels such as those of the forearm (i.e., laser-Doppler iontophoresis).
- Increased numbers of circulating endothelial cells in the plasma are likely to reflect direct damage to the mural endothelium.

MAJOR PATHOLOGICAL MECHANISMS LEADING TO VASCULAR DYSFUNCTION	
Risk Factor	**Possible Mechanism Primary**
Hypercholesterolemia	Cytotoxic oxidized LDL
Smoking	Carbon monoxide, hypoxia
Diabetes	Hyperglycemia
Hypertension[a]	Hydrostatic pressure
Hyperhomocysteinemia	Unclear: homocysteine itself (?)
Inflammation	Excessive cytokine stimulation
Secondary	
Obesity	Unclear/compound
Physical inactivity	Unclear/poor overall cardiovascular health
Renal disease	Uremia
Liver disease	Hyperbilirubinemia
Insufficient antioxidants	Poor diet deficient in vitamins, etc.

a. Hypertension may be a primary or secondary pathological process because it can be a cause or consequence of endothelial dysfunction (see text for discussion). Although male sex and increasing age are often cited as risk factors for atherosclerosis, these can hardly be described as major pathological mechanisms and are certainly not treatable.

Table 14–1. Major Pathological Mechanisms Leading to Vascular Dysfunction

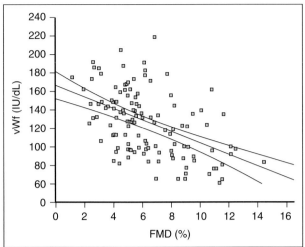

Figure 14–1. Correlation between von Willebrand factor and FMD. The correlation line between FMD and von Willebrand factor is shown, with 95% confidence intervals [FMD = flow-mediated dilatation; vWf = von Willebrand factor]. Correlation between FMD and vWf: r=-0.517, p<0.001. (Redrawn from Felmeden DC, Blann AD, Spencer CGC, et al. A comparison of flow mediated dilatation and von Willebrand factor as markers of endothelial cell function in health and in hypertension: Relationship to cardiovascular risk and the effects of treatment. *Blood Coag Fibrinolysis* 2003;14:425–31, with permission.)

are emerging. For example, advanced age is associated with endothelial dysfunction, and reduced arterial elasticity parallels changes in impaired endothelium-dependent vasodilation. It appears that reduced arterial elasticity may be used as a noninvasive measure for the determination of endothelial function.[18] Farkas et al.[19] used similar technology to demonstrate impaired microvascular responses in essential hypertension compared to normotensives, although notably the plasma marker vWf was no different. Weight reduction and exercise are effective in improving body mass index in the obese, but also in improving macrovascular function (brachial artery FMD).[20] However, this program did not improve microvascular reactivity as evaluated by laser-Doppler perfusion imaging after iontophoresis with acetylcholine, or as evaluated by levels of plasma marker vWf. One hesitates to jump to the conclusion that large-vessel reactivity is more sensitive than small-vessel reactivity or plasma markers, as these may reflect different aspects of endothelial pathophysiology.

The most recent marker of vascular damage, CECs, has also (as yet) made little impact in hypertension. The potential mechanisms of endothelial cell detachment from the vessels are multiple and not exclusive. Different experimental models have documented that denudation of the vessels can be triggered by mechanical injury, defective adhesive properties of the endothelial cells, protease- or cytokine-mediated detachment, or the activation of an apoptotic program. Therefore, if increased numbers of CECs do indeed reflect a damaged endothelium such levels should correlate with other assessment methods (e.g., plasma markers and with FMD). Indeed, Rajagopalan et al.[21] found an inverse correlation between CECs and FMD. Kas-Deelen et al.[22] found that CECs strongly (*p*<0.001) correlated

with vWf but not with soluble E selectin, whereas Makin et al.[23] also correlated CECs with vWf and plasma tissue factor. Because vWf is essentially the gold standard plasma marker for endothelial damage,[8,9] this is strong evidence that CECs also reflect severe vascular disturbance. Moving to hypertension, correlations between pulmonary artery blood pressure and CEC number have been reported.[24,25] This relationship may be due to the high blood pressure damaging and thus converting mural endothelial cells into CECs. Notably, it is established that the plasma marker of endothelial damage (vWf) is raised in hypertension.[26–28]

If endothelial damage/dysfunction is present, can it be reversed by intervention? Many antihypertensive drugs are known to prevent or reduce progression of arterio-occlusive disease, and many also reduce major cardiovascular endpoints, but often the mechanisms behind this cardiovascular protection remain elusive.

ANTIHYPERTENSIVE THERAPY AND THE ENDOTHELIUM

Evidence of endothelial perturbation in hypertension include increased release of vWf[17,26–28] and impaired FMD.[17,29] Furthermore, both of these markers predict adverse cardiovascular outcome,[30–32] and (as mentioned) they have an inverse relationship[17] (Figure 14–1). Clinically, there is of course considerable evidence that successful treatment of hypertension by virtually all classes of drugs lowers cardiovascular risk,[33–39] and it is attractive to presume that this benefit is the direct consequence of lower blood pressure—although other mechanisms cannot be ruled out. Thus, these large epidemiological studies are generally unable to answer more complex questions of the mechanism of this benefit at the level of the molecule and/or cell.

With regard to studies on antihypertensive therapy and the endothelium, most are relatively small and of short duration. In addition, adequate blood pressure control with monotherapy is difficult, and in many instances two or more drugs are needed. Many existing studies cannot dissect out the effects of individual drugs or the associated nonpharmacological methods (e.g., salt restriction, weight loss, and so on), which is part of modern holistic hypertension management.

Calcium channel blockers (CCBs)

In general, although CCBs tend to improve endothelial function[40–47] the mechanism of this is debatable. One route may be by improving blood pressure: another effect could be due to direct action on the endothelial cells (for example, in acting on cell membrane calcium channels to reduce the influx of calcium into cells).[48,49] By decreasing calcium flux into smooth muscle cells, CCBs enhance the vasodilatation produced by NO.[50] It has been suggested that these drugs may restore NO availability through an antioxidant mechanism, and that they may enhance NO action through inhibition of superoxide-induced NO decomposition in the vessel wall.[51–53]

Alternatively, CCBs may also act by reducing the production of endothelins.[54] The potentiation by ET-1 of vasoconstriction produced by other agonists such as noradrenaline and serotonin is also inhibited by CCBs.[55] Nifedipine has been shown to improve endothelial function in patients with hypercholesterolemia independently of the effect on blood pressure.[56] CCBs may not all be the same. For example, Ding et al.[57] reported that nifedipine and diltiazem (but not verapamil) up-regulated endothelial nitric oxide synthase (NOS) expression, implying that the dihydropyridine and benzothiazepine classes (but not the phenylalkylamine class of drugs) are better for improving the endothelial function.

ACE inhibitors (ACEIs)

Large clinical trials such as the HOPE and PROGRESS studies[33,34] (using ramipril and perindopril) have suggested that ACEIs have a role over and above their antihypertensive effect in reducing vascular complications. They may improve blood pressure and endothelial function via different mechanisms beyond inhibiting the renin-angiotensin system alone. One such mechanism is to reduce the inactivation of bradykinin, causing an augmentation of NO release.[58] Another is stabilizing the beta 2-receptor, reducing oxidative stress and tissue ET-1 levels,[59] and preventing the formation of angiotensin II (which can cause endothelial dysfunction by inhibiting NOS activity). Another mechanism induces oxidative stress and increases the levels of NO.[60–62] Numerous other trials of ACEIs have been shown to improve endothelial function.[63–70] For example, the TREND study (Trial on Reversing Endothelial Dysfunction)[68] looked at endothelial function in normotensive patients with coronary artery disease and found that quinapril significantly improved coronary artery diameter in response to acetylcholine after 6 months of treatment.

Angiotensin II receptor blockers (ARBs)

ARBs are a relatively new class of drugs, and although losartan has been shown to be more effective than atenolol in reducing vascular endpoints[71] data on their role in improving endothelial function is limited. In studies comparing losartan[72] or irbesartan[73] with beta blockers, the ARBs have been shown to have a beneficial effect on endothelial function and to be superior to the beta blockers in this effect (although one study found them equally effective).[74] However, a small study by Li Saw Hee et al.[67] did not show any changes in plasma endothelial marker vWf after 8 weeks of therapy with losartan.

Alpha and beta blockers

The available data do not appear to support the hypothesis that endothelial function is tremendously improved by these agents. In experimental animal models, carvedilol (but not propanolol) appears to protect against endothelial damage,[75] but studies in human hypertensives on the effects of beta blockers on endothelial function have given varying results. Seljeflot et al.[76] showed that treatment with atenolol and doxazosin causes a decrease in levels of vWf, but these tended to correlate with the blood pressure reduction and could be just a reflection of the lowered blood pressure. Indirect measurements of endothelial function, such as with gluteal skin biopsy or forearm blood flow, do not show any improvement when using atenolol.[72,73] One study using nevibolol[77] did show an improvement in the forearm blood flow after treatment. Thus, beta blockers may improve endothelial function solely by their blood-pressure-lowering properties and whether or not they have any additional influence(s) on the endothelium remains uncertain. The same may be true with alpha blockers, and for both classes the improvement with treatment appears to correlate with the amount of blood pressure reduction.

CONCLUSIONS AND PERSPECTIVES

Numerous large international trials have clearly shown that the successful treatment of hypertension brings cardiovascular benefit. However, although eminent opinion states that the endothelium is important in this risk factor linking the two may not be straightforward and debate continues.[50,78–83] Endothelial dysfunction has been identified in patients with virtually every known cardiovascular risk factor, and its presence predicts future adverse events. It is clear that most workers favor vWf as a plasma marker of damage to the endothelium,[26–28,76] although others have used endothelin-1 and soluble E selectin.[28,84,85]

Treatment of hypertension generally results in an improvement in endothelial function that accompanies the reduced cardiovascular risk. Although there are considerable data on the genetics of hypertension,[86–88] unlike the risk of left ventricular hypertrophy (and on ACE polymorphisms, for example) there are as yet no well-recognized genetic polymorphisms influencing the endothelium that are likely to impact clinical medicine directly. These topics are dealt with extensively in other chapters of this book.

Current clinical resources do not allow for routine measurement of endothelial function in individual patients, except in research settings. In addition, markers of endothelial function have been used to predict increased cardiovascular risk in populations but not in individuals. To be useful in predicting an individual's specific cardiovascular risk, a test must have an acceptable positive and negative predictive value, and this is emphatically not the case for the current measures of endothelial function available. In addition, many of these tests are time consuming and operator dependent, which reduces the likelihood of them becoming useful clinical tests. However, in a research setting these tests are often extremely useful parameters that provide information on the effectiveness of a drug or an intervention in reducing cardiovascular risk in a population.

REFERENCES

1. Cines DB, Pollak ES, Buck CA, et al. Endothelial cells in physiology and in the pathophysiology of vascular disorders. *Blood* 1998;91:3527–61.
2. Blann AD. Endothelial cell activation, injury, damage and dysfunction: Separate entities or mutual terms? *Blood Coagul Fibrinolysis* 2000; 11:623–30.
3. Drexler H, Hayoz D, Munzel T, et al. Endothelial function in congestive heart failure. *Am Heart J* 1993;126:761–64.
4. Burnett JC Jr. Coronary endothelial dysfunction in the hypertensive patient: From myocardial ischemia to heart failure. *J Hum Hypertens* 1997;11:45–9.
5. Vallet B, Wiel E. Endothelial cell dysfunction and coagulation. *Crit Care Med* 2001;29:S36–41.
6. Blann AD. How a damaged blood vessel wall contributes to thrombosis and hypertension. *Pathophysiol Haemost Thromb* 2004;33:445–48.
7. Pearson JD. Normal endothelial cell function. *Lupus* 2000;9:183–88.
8. Boneu B, Abbal M, Plante J, Bierme R. Factor-VIII complex and endothelial damage. *Lancet* 1975;i:1430.
9. Blann AD, Taberner DA. A reliable marker of endothelial cell dysfunction: Does it exist? *Br J Haematol* 1995;90:244–48.
10. Celermajer DS, Sorensen KE, Gooch VM, et al. Non-invasive detection of endothelial dysfunction in children and adults at risk of atherosclerosis. *Lancet* 1992;340:1111–15.
11. Li J, Zhao SP, Li XP, et al. Non-invasive detection of endothelial dysfunction in patients with essential hypertension. *Int J Cardiol* 1997;61:165–69.
12. Morris SJ, Shore AC. Skin blood flow responses to the iontophoresis of acetylcholine and sodium nitroprusside in man: Possible mechanisms. *J Physiol* 1996;496:531–42.
13. Belcaro G, Labropoulos N, Laurora G, et al. Laser Doppler skin perfusion pressure in normal and vascular subjects with rest pain: An universal measurement? *J Cardiovasc Surg* 1994;35:7–9.
14. Blann AD, Woywodt A, Bertolini F, et al. Circulating endothelial cells: Biomarker of vascular disease. *Thromb Haemostas* 2005;93:228–35.
15. Mutin M, Canavy I, Blann A, et al. Direct evidence of endothelial injury in acute myocardial infarction and unstable angina by demonstration of circulating endothelial cells. *Blood* 1999;93:2951–58.
16. Lee KW, Lip GYH, Tayebjee M, et al. Circulating endothelial cells, von Willebrand factor, interleukin-6 and prognosis in patients with acute coronary syndromes. *Blood* 2005;105:526–32.
17. Felmeden DC, Blann AD, Spencer CGC, et al. A comparison of flow mediated dilatation and von Willebrand factor as markers of endothelial cell function in health and in hypertension: Relationship to cardiovascular risk and the effects of treatment. *Blood Coag Fibrinolysis* 2003;14:425–31.
18. Tao J, Jin YF, Yang Z, et al. Reduced arterial elasticity is associated with endothelial dysfunction in persons of advancing age: Comparative study of noninvasive pulse wave analysis and laser Doppler blood flow measurement. *Am J Hypertens* 2004;17:654–59.
19. Farkas K, Kolossvary E, Jarai Z, et al. Non-invasive assessment of microvascular endothelial function by laser Doppler flowmetry in patients with essential hypertension. *Atherosclerosis* 2004; 173:97–102.
20. Hamdy O, Ledbury S, Mullooly C, et al. Lifestyle modification improves endothelial function in obese subjects with the insulin resistance syndrome. *Diabetes Care* 2003;26:2119–25.
21. Rajagopalan S, Somers EC, Brook RD, et al. Endothelial cell apoptosis in systemic lupus erythematosus: A common pathway for abnormal vascular function and thrombosis propensity. *Blood* 2004;103:3677–83.
22. Kas-Deelen AM, Harmsen MC, De Maar EF, et al. Acute rejection before cytomegalovirus infection enhances von Willebrand factor and soluble VCAM-1 in blood. *Kidney Int* 2000; 58:2533–42.
23. Makin A, Chung NAY, Silverman SH, et al. Assessment of endothelial damage in atherosclerotic vascular disease by quantification of circulating endothelial cells. *Eur Heart J* 2004;25:371–76.
24. Bull TM, Golpon H, Hebbel RP, et al. Circulating endothelial cells in pulmonary hypertension. *Thromb Haemostas* 2003; 90:698–703.
25. Del Papa N, Colombo G, Fracchiolla N, et al. Circulating endothelial cells as a marker of ongoing vascular disease in systemic sclerosis. *Arthritis Rheum* 2004; 50:1296–1304.
26. Blann AD, Naqvi T, Waite M, McCollum CN. von Willebrand factor and endothelial cell damage in essential hypertension. *J Hum Hypertens* 1993; 7:107–11.
27. Preston RA, Ledford M, Materson BJ, et al. Effects of severe, uncontrolled hypertension on endothelial activation: Soluble vascular cell adhesion molecule-1, soluble intercellular adhesion molecule-1 and von Willebrand factor. *J Hypertens* 2002;20:871–77.
28. Hlubocka Z, Umnerova V, Heller S, et al. Circulating intercellular cell adhesion molecule-1, endothelin-1 and von Willebrand factor-markers of endothelial dysfunction in uncomplicated essential hypertension: The effect of treatment with ACE inhibitors. *J Hum Hypertens* 2002;16:557–62.
29. Panza JA, Quyyumi AA, Brush JE Jr, Epstein SE. Abnormal endothelium-dependent vascular relaxation in patients with essential hypertension. *N Eng J Med* 1990;323:22–7.
30. Blann AD, Waite MA. von Willebrand factor and soluble E-selectin in hypertension: Influence of treatment and value in predicting the progression of atherosclerosis. *Coronary Artery Dis* 1996;7:143–47.
31. Lip GY, Blann AD, Edmunds E, Beevers DG. Baseline abnormalities of endothelial function and thrombogenesis in relation to prognosis in essential hypertension. *Blood Coagul Fibrinolysis* 2002;13:35–41.
32. Perticone F, Ceravolo R, Pujia A, et al. Prognostic significance of endothelial dysfunction in hypertensive patients. *Circulation* 2001;104:191–96.
33. Yusuf S, Sleight P, Pogue J, et al. Effects of an angiotensin-converting-enzyme inhibitor, ramipril, on cardiovascular events in high-risk patients. The Heart Outcomes Prevention Evaluation Study Investigators. *N Eng J Med* 2000; 342:145–53.
34. PROGRESS Collaborative Group. Randomised trial of a perindopril-based blood-pressure-lowering regimen among 6,105 individuals with previous stroke or transient ischaemic attack. *Lancet* 2001;358:1033–41.
35. Dickstein K, Kjekshus J; OPTIMAAL Steering Committee of the OPTIMAAL Study Group. Effects of losartan and captopril on mortality and morbidity in high-risk patients after acute myocardial infarction: The OPTIMAAL randomised trial. Optimal Trial in Myocardial Infarction with Angiotensin II Antagonist Losartan. *Lancet* 2002;360:752–60.
36. Dahlof B, Devereux RB, Kjeldsen SE, et al.; LIFE Study Group. Cardiovascular morbidity and mortality in the losartan intervention for endpoint reduction in hypertension study (LIFE): A randomised trial against atenolol. *Lancet* 2002;359:995–1003.
37. Pitt B, Zannad F, Remme WJ, et al. The effect of spironolactone on morbidity and mortality in patients with severe heart failure. Randomized Aldactone Evaluation Study Investigators. *N Eng J Med* 1999;341:709–17.
38. Pitt B, Remme W, Zannad F, et al.; The Eplerenone Post-Acute Myocardial Infarction Heart Failure Efficacy and Survival Study Investigators. Eplerenone, a selective aldosterone blocker, in patients with left ventricular dysfunction after myocardial infarction. *N Eng J Med* 2003;348:1309–21.
39. Julius S, Kjeldsen SE, Weber M, et al.; VALUE Trial Group. Outcomes in hypertensive patients at high cardiovascular risk treated with regimens based on valsartan or amlodipine: The VALUE randomised trial. *Lancet* 2004; 363:2022–31.
40. Taddei S, Virdis A, Ghiadoni L, et al. Lacidipine restores endothelium-dependent vasodilation in essential hypertensive patients. *Hypertension* 1997;30:1606–12.
41. Taddei S, Virdis A, Ghiadoni L, et al. Restoration of nitric oxide availability after calcium antagonist treatment in essential hypertension. *Hypertension* 2001;37:943–48.
42. The ENCORE Group. Effect of nifedipine and cerivastatin on coronary endothelial function in patients with coronary artery disease: The ENCORE I Study (Evaluation of nifedipine and cerivastatin on recovery of coronary endothelial function). *Circulation* 2003;107:422–28.
43. On YK, Kim CH, Sohn DW, et al. Improvement of endothelial function by amlodipine and vitamin C in essential hypertension. *Korean J Intern Med* 2002; 17:131–37.
44. Schiffrin EL, Pu Q, Park JB. Effect of amlodipine compared to atenolol on

small arteries of previously untreated essential hypertensive patients. *Am J Hypertens* 2002;15:105–10.

45. Taddei S, Virdis A, Ghiadoni L, et al. Effect of calcium antagonist or beta blockade treatment on nitric oxide-dependent vasodilation and oxidative stress in essential hypertensive patients. *J Hypertens* 2001;19:1379–86.

46. Millgard J, Hagg A, Sarabi M, Lind L. Captopril, but not nifedipine, improves endothelium-dependent vasodilation in hypertensive patients. *J Hum Hypertens* 1998;12:511–16.

47. Luscher TF, Yang Z. Calcium antagonists and ACE inhibitors: Effect on endothelium and vascular smooth muscle. *Drugs* 1993;46(Suppl 2):121–32.

48. Erne P, Bolli P, Burgisser E, Buhler FR. Correlation of platelet calcium with blood pressure: Effect of antihypertensive therapy. *New Eng J Med* 1984; 310:1084–88.

49. Yang ZH, von Segesser L, Bauer E, et al. Different activation of the endothelial L-arginine and cyclooxygenase pathway in the human internal mammary artery and saphenous vein. *Circ Res* 1991;68:52–60.

50. Taddei S, Virdis A, Ghiadoni L, Salvetti A. Endothelial dysfunction in hypertension: Fact or fancy?. *J Cardiovasc Pharmacol* 1998;32(Suppl 3):S41–47.

51. Lupo E, Locher R, Weisser B, Vetter W. In vitro antioxidant activity of calcium antagonists against LDL oxidation compared with alpha-tocopherol. *Biochem Biophys Res Comm* 1994;203:1803–08.

52. Mak IT, Boehme P, Weglicki WB. Antioxidant effects of calcium channel blockers against free radical injury in endothelial cells: Correlation of protection with preservation of glutathione levels. *Circ Res* 1992;70:1099–1103.

53. Yang J, Fukuo K, Morimoto S, et al. Pranidipine enhances the action of nitric oxide released from endothelial cells. *Hypertension* 2000;35:82–5.

54. Haug C, Voisard R, Baur R, et al. Effect of diltiazem and verapamil on endothelin release by cultured human coronary smooth-muscle cells and endothelial cells. *J Cardiovasc Pharmacol* 1998;31(Suppl 1):S388–91.

55. Yang ZH, Richard V, von Segesser L, et al. Threshold concentrations of endothelin-1 potentiate contractions to norepinephrine and serotonin in human arteries: A new mechanism of vasospasm? *Circulation* 1990;82:188–95.

56. Verhaar MC, Honing ML, van Dam T, et al. Nifedipine improves endothelial function in hypercholesterolemia, independently of an effect on blood pressure or plasma lipids. *Cardiovasc Res* 1999;42:752–60.

57. Ding Y, Vaziri ND. Nifedipine and diltiazem but not verapamil up-regulate endothelial nitric-oxide synthase expression. *J Pharmacol Exp Therapeut* 2000;292:606–09.

58. Kohno M, Yokokawa K, Minami M, et al. Plasma levels of nitric oxide and related vasoactive factors following long-term treatment with angiotensin-converting enzyme inhibitor in patients with essential hypertension. *Metab Clin Experimental* 1999;48:1256–59.

59. Ruschitzka F, Noll G, Luscher TF. Angiotensin converting enzyme inhibitors and vascular protection in hypertension. *J Cardiovasc Pharmacol* 1999;34:S1–12.

60. Munzel T, Keaney JF Jr. Are ACE inhibitors a "magic bullet" against oxidative stress? *Circulation* 2001;104:1571–74.

61. Zhuo JL, Mendelsohn FA, Ohishi M. Perindopril alters vascular angiotensin-converting enzyme, AT(1) receptor, and nitric oxide synthase expression in patients with coronary heart disease. *Hypertension* 2002;39:634–38.

62. Jain S, Rajeshwari J, Khullar M, Kumari S. Enalapril acts through release of nitric oxide in patients with essential hypertension. *Renal Fail* 2001;23:651–57.

63. Koh KK, Bui MN, Hathaway L, et al. Mechanism by which quinapril improves vascular function in coronary artery disease. *Am J Cardiol* 1999;83:327–31.

64. Higashi Y, Sasaki S, Nakagawa K, et al. Effect of the angiotensin-converting enzyme inhibitor imidapril on reactive hyperemia in patients with essential hypertension: Relationship between treatment periods and resistance artery endothelial function. *J Am Coll Cardiol* 2001;37:863–70.

65. Taddei S, Virdis A, Ghiadoni L, et al. Antihypertensive drugs and reversing of endothelial dysfunction in hypertension. *Curr Hypertens Rep* 2000;2:64–70.

66. Nielsen FS, Rossing P, Gall MA, et al. Lisinopril improves endothelial dysfunction in hypertensive NIDDM subjects with diabetic nephropathy. *Scand J Clin Lab Investig* 1997;57:427–34.

67. Li-Saw-Hee FL, Beevers DG, Lip GY. Effect of antihypertensive therapy using enalapril or losartan on haemostatic markers in essential hypertension: A pilot prospective randomised double-blind parallel group trial. *Int J Cardiol* 2001;78:241–46.

68. Mancini GB, Henry GC, Macaya C, et al. Angiotensin-converting enzyme inhibition with quinapril improves endothelial vasomotor dysfunction in patients with coronary artery disease. The TREND (Trial on Reversing Endothelial Dysfunction) Study. *Circulation* 1996;94:258–65.

69. Fox KM; European Trial on Reduction of Cardiac Events with Perindopril in Stable Coronary Artery Disease Investigators. Efficacy of perindopril in reduction of cardiovascular events among patients with stable coronary artery disease: The EUROPA study. *Lancet* 2003;362:782–88.

70. Hirooka Y, Imaizumi T, Masaki H, et al. Captopril improves impaired endothelium-dependent vasodilation in hypertensive patients. *Hypertension* 1992;20:175–80.

71. Dahlof B, Devereux RB, Kjeldsen SE, et al. Cardiovascular morbidity and mortality in the losartan intervention for endpoint reduction in hypertension study (LIFE): A randomised trial against atenolol. *Lancet* 2002;359:995–1003.

72. Schiffrin EL, Park JB, Intengan HD, Touyz RM. Correction of arterial structure and endothelial dysfunction in human essential hypertension by the angiotensin receptor antagonist losartan. *Circulation* 2000;101:1653–59.

73. Makris TK, Stavroulakis GA, Krespi PG, et al. Fibrinolytic/hemostatic variables in arterial hypertension: Response to treatment with irbesartan or atenolol. *Am J Hypertens* 2000;13:783–88.

74. von zur Muhlen B, Kahan T, Hagg A, et al. Treatment with irbesartan or atenolol improves endothelial function in essential hypertension. *J Hypertens* 2001;19:1813–18.

75. Christopher TA, Lopez BL, Yue TL, et al. Carvedilol, a new beta-adrenoreceptor blocker, vasodilator and free-radical scavenger, exerts an anti-shock and endothelial protective effect in rat splanchnic ischemia and reperfusion. *J Pharmacol Exp Therapet* 1995; 273:64–71.

76. Seljeflot I, Arnesen H, Andersen P, et al. Effects of doxazosin and atenolol on circulating endothelin-1 and von Willebrand factor in hypertensive middle-aged men. *J Cardiovasc Pharmacol* 1999;34:584–88.

77. Tzemos N, Lim PO, MacDonald TM. Nebivolol reverses endothelial dysfunction in essential hypertension: A randomized, double-blind, crossover study. *Circulation* 2001;104:511–14.

78. Rizzoni D, Porteri E, Castellano M, et al. Endothelial dysfunction in hypertension is independent from the etiology and from vascular structure. *Hypertension* 1998;31:335–41.

79. Puddu P, Puddu GM, Zaca F, Muscari A. Endothelial dysfunction in hypertension. *Acta Cardiol* 2000;55:221–32.

80. Taddei S, Virdis A, Ghiadoni L, et al. Endothelial dysfunction in hypertension. *J Nephrol* 2000;13:205–10.

81. Kaplan NM. The endothelium as prognostic factor and therapeutic target: What criteria should we apply? *J Cardiovasc Pharmacol* 1998;32(Suppl 3):S78–80.

82. Nadar S, Blann AD, Lip GYH. Endothelial dysfunction: Methods of assessment and application to hypertension. *Current Pharmacol Design* 2004;10:3591–606.

83. Nadar S, Blann AD, Lip GYH. Antihypertensive therapy and endothelial function. *Current Pharmacol Design* 2004;10:3607–14.

84. Blann AD, Tse W, Maxwell SJR, Waite MA. Increased levels of the soluble adhesion molecule E-selectin in essential hypertension. *J Hypertension* 1994;12:925–28.

85. DeSouza CA, Dengel DR, Macko RF, et al. Elevated levels of circulating cell adhesion molecules in uncomplicated essential hypertension. *Am J Hypertens* 1997;10:1335–41.

86. Dominiczak AF, Brain N, Charchar F, et al. Genetics of hypertension: Lessons learnt from mendelian and polygenic syndromes. *Clin Exp Hypertens* 2004;26:611–20.

87. Tanira MO, Al Balushi KA. Genetic variations related to hypertension: A review. *J Hum Hypertens* 2005;19:7–19.

88. Luft FC. Geneticism of essential hypertension. *Hypertension* 2004;43:1155–91.

Chapter

15

Vascular Remodeling and Rarefaction in Hypertension

Matthew A. Boegehold

Definitions

In established hypertension, structural changes within the resistance vasculature involve vascular wall remodeling to produce smaller passive diameters and/or the regression and loss of small arterioles from the network ("structural rarefaction").

A structural reduction in passive vessel diameters can occur through inward vascular wall growth ("hypertrophic inward remodeling") or rearrangement of existing wall elements without wall growth ("eutrophic inward remodeling").

Key Findings

- Vascular wall remodeling can be triggered by a pressure-dependent increase in circumferential wall stress and/or the local actions of various growth factors. Ongoing investigations are continuing to provide important details on the intracellular signaling pathways through which this remodeling occurs.

- The structural rarefaction of arterioles can be triggered by a prolonged cessation of luminal flow that accompanies intense vasoconstriction, or by a reduction in the local concentrations of angiotensin II and/or other endogenous trophic factors.

- In addition to contributing to increased total peripheral resistance (and therefore elevated arterial pressure), the functional consequences of vascular wall remodeling include a reduced capacity for maximal dilation and altered responsiveness to vasoactive stimuli, whereas those for arteriolar and capillary rarefaction include increased heterogeneity in local blood flow and alterations in transcapillary exchange—including a reduced efficiency for tissue oxygen delivery.

Clinical Implications

- Because structural changes in the resistance vasculature may contribute importantly to some types of end-organ damage in hypertensive individuals, antihypertensive therapy is becoming increasingly more focused on reversing these changes.

When fully established, most forms of primary and secondary hypertension are characterized by a normal cardiac output and elevated total peripheral resistance (TPR). Because the chronic elevation in arterial pressure is usually attributable to increased TPR, a long-standing goal of hypertension research has been to define the mechanisms that underlie the development and maintenance of this increased resistance. From a physiologic standpoint, it is equally important to understand the effect of a sustained increase

in vascular resistance on local blood flow and its regulation in various organs, and the effect of any attendant flow abnormalities on organ function and the progression of end-organ damage. This information is critical for the development of more effective clinical strategies to treat hypertension and its consequences. Some of this information has been obtained from studies on human subjects, but because detailed investigation of the resistance vasculature and its function often requires invasive procedures more of this information has been obtained from various animal models of hypertension. The rat is the most common species used for this purpose. Investigators have developed a variety of rat models that exhibit hypertension of genetic origin—such as the spontaneously hypertensive rat (SHR)—or hypertension that has been experimentally induced, such as the two-kidney one-clip rat. Although there may be some differences between humans and other mammals in the regulatory mechanisms that influence blood pressure and blood flow, there are also many similarities that justify the use of these animal models.[1]

As discussed in earlier chapters, the primary resistance vessels in most organs and tissues include the arterioles as well as the small feed arteries located immediately upstream from the microcirculation. These feed arteries, which typically range between 100 and 350 μm in luminal diameter, are often referred to as "resistance arteries." The actual distribution of total vascular resistance between the resistance arteries and the true arterioles can vary depending on the vascular bed. Although *in vivo* microvascular pressure measurements generally indicate that the arterioles control most of the resistance, there are some organs (such as the brain) in which as much as 50% of total vascular resistance is attributable to the resistance arteries.[2]

Structural changes have been found throughout the resistance vasculature of hypertensive individuals, and these changes can contribute importantly to the maintenance of increased TPR. In early studies, these structural changes were inferred from findings that hemodynamic resistance in the absence of vascular tone ("passive resistance") is elevated in hypertensive patients and animals.[3] From direct observations of the vasculature, we now know that these changes include (1) alterations in vessel wall structure that lead to reduced luminal diameters and increased responsiveness to vasoconstrictors and (2) a loss of arterioles and capillaries from microvascular networks, which can also have profound effects on the exchange of water and solutes between the vascular compartment and surrounding tissues. Recent studies have provided detailed information on the cellular and molecular mechanisms that underlie these structural changes, and continuing efforts to further clarify these pathways represent an important focus of current hypertension research.

There is also mounting evidence to indicate that changes in vascular wall structure and network architecture not only contribute to the development and maintenance of high blood pressure but may play a major role in the development of some types of end-organ damage that occur in hypertensive individuals. Because end-organ damage is the ultimate cause of the morbidity and mortality associated with hypertension, the prevention or reversal of these structural changes has become an important goal in the therapeutic management of hypertension.

ANATOMY AND BIOCHEMISTRY

Direct observations of the vasculature in different forms of hypertension have revealed that the increased vascular resistance of most organs is ultimately due to a reduction in the inner diameter of resistance vessels and/or a reduction in the number of these vessels being perfused in parallel. This latter phenomenon is commonly referred to as "microvascular rarefaction." These abnormalities are often localized to specific regions of the resistance vessel network, although the relative importance of reduced diameters versus rarefaction to the overall resistance increase can vary from one organ to another, and can also change within any particular organ as hypertension develops.[1]

Reduced inner diameters through vessel wall remodeling

In hypertension, the inner diameter of resistance vessels may be functionally reduced through sustained vasoconstriction[4,5] and/or structurally reduced through anatomic remodeling of the vessel wall.[6] Because the resistance of each vessel is inversely related to the fourth power of its radius, a relatively small decrease in radius can produce a large increase in resistance to flow. Studies in which different stages of hypertension have been compared indicate that functional and structural reductions in diameter are not always independent of each other, but are often linked in a temporal sense. In early (developing) hypertension, inner diameters are reduced primarily through an active increase in resting vascular tone. The mechanisms by which tone could be increased in relation to microvascular rarefaction are discussed later in this chapter, and are described in more detail elsewhere in this book. This sustained constriction often leads to vascular wall remodeling, so that structurally reduced diameters predominate in the established stage of hypertension.[1]

Traditionally, the ratio of a vessel's wall thickness to its lumen diameter (the "wall-to-lumen ratio") has been used to quantify the changes in vessel wall structure associated with hypertension. However, because this ratio can also change acutely with vascular tone it is not by itself an exclusive index of structural changes. Instead, changes in vessel wall structure and mass are more accurately determined by measuring a vessel's inner and outer circum-

ference after vascular tone has been abolished, and then calculating the cross-sectional area of the passive wall.

Vessel wall remodeling that would lead to reduced inner diameters can occur through one of two general processes. The first involves inward growth of the wall due to smooth muscle hypertrophy or hyperplasia. Hypertrophy refers to an increase in cell size associated with increased protein synthesis, whereas hyperplasia refers to an increase in cell number associated with DNA synthesis. For resistance vessels, this wall growth most often occurs exclusively by smooth muscle hypertrophy, and is therefore referred to as "hypertrophic inward remodeling." The second process involves the rearrangement of existing wall elements around a smaller lumen with no net wall growth, referred to as "eutrophic inward remodeling."[7] Inward remodeling, whether hypertrophic or eutrophic, leads to increased flow resistance at maximum vasodilation.[8] More importantly, and particularly in the case of hypertrophic inward remodeling, any prevailing level of vascular tone will produce a smaller inner diameter due to the encroachment of wall elements into the lumen[9] (Figure 15–1).

As hypertension develops, the larger conduit arteries can also undergo a form of remodeling that is characterized by an increase in wall mass—typically involving a combination of smooth muscle hypertrophy and hyperplasia, with increased extracellular matrix deposition. However, in contrast to the changes that take place in the resistance vessels this wall growth in larger arteries is typically directed outward so that lumen diameter is not reduced ("hypertrophic outward remodeling").[10]

The hypertrophic inward remodeling of resistance vessels can be triggered by numerous stimuli. One major stimulus appears to be blood pressure itself, or more specifically the increase in circumferential vascular wall stress that accompanies a chronic elevation of pressure. Experimentally, protection of a vascular bed from increased pressure during the onset of hypertension has often been found to prevent structural changes from developing in the resistance vasculature.[10] Figure 15–2 illustrates the known elements of the signaling pathway through which a pressure-dependent increase in circumferential wall stress can stimulate inward growth of the resistance vessel wall. This may be expressed as an equation:

$$\text{Circumferential wall stress} = P_t\, r/W$$

where P_t = transmural pressure (the difference between luminal pressure and pressure outside the vessel, which can also be thought of as vascular distending pressure), r = vessel radius, and W = wall thickness.

This mechanical wall stress is transmitted to the vascular smooth muscle cells via elements of the extracellular matrix, which connect to the cell membrane at focal adhesion sites. A number of different molecules at these adhesion sites could act as primary mechanosensors that would transmit this stress across the cell membrane and into the cell interior. There is strong evidence that the family of membrane-spanning glycoproteins known as integrins often serve this role, triggering a complex intracellular phosphorylation cascade upon activation.[10,11] Early

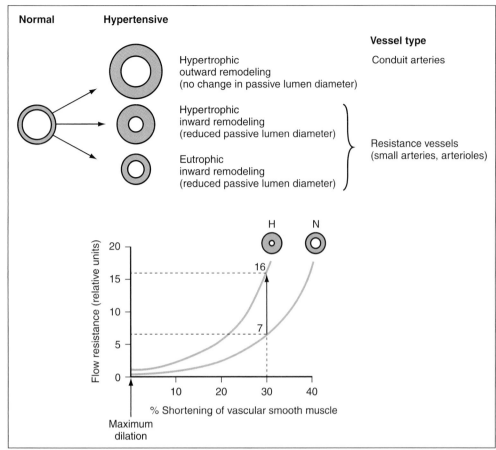

Figure 15–1. Types of vascular remodeling associated with hypertension, and the effect of hypertrophic inward remodeling on vascular resistance at different levels of vascular tone. Because a vessel's resistance is inversely related to the fourth power of its radius, a relatively small difference in luminal diameters between the normotensive and hypertensive conditions can translate into a large difference in flow resistance. H, vessel from hypertensive individual; N, vessel from normotensive individual.

in this cascade, focal adhesion kinase (FAK)—which is directly associated with the integrin β-subunit— undergoes both autophosphorylation and additional phosphorylation through interaction with phosphorylated tyrosine kinases such as c-Src. This leads to binding of a complex containing growth factor receptor-bound protein 2 (Grb2) and the guanine nucleotide exchange factor son-of-sevenless (Sos), and then to activation of the small GTP-binding protein Ras. Ras activation triggers activation of the mitogen-activated protein (MAP) kinase cascade and phosphorylation of extracellular signal-regulated kinase (ERK 1/2). Once phosphorylated, ERK 1/2 can translocate to the cell nucleus, where it phosphorylates various transcription factors to alter the expression of proto-oncogenes such as c-fos and c-jun.

Angiotensin II (Ang II) and other endogenous growth factors can also play a central role in the hypertrophic remodeling of resistance vessels.[6,10] Figure 15–3 illustrates the elements of the signaling pathways through which these factors may promote inward wall growth. The activation of smooth muscle membrane receptors for epidermal growth factor (EGF), platelet-derived growth factor (PDGF), or insulin-like growth factor 1 (IGF-1) triggers activation of Ras and the MAP kinase cascade, leading to increased

ERK 1/2 phosphorylation, with upstream events that include an increase in the activity of c-Src and other tyrosine kinases.[12] Angiotensin II (acting via the g-protein-coupled AT_1 receptor) also activates these pathways, either directly or through an NAD(P)H oxidase-dependent increase in reactive oxygen species (ROS).[13] Various ROS, most notably superoxide anion and hydrogen peroxide, can serve as important signaling molecules in this process by triggering the phosphorylation and activation of C-src and FAK.[14] Interestingly, Ang II can also induce the transactivation of growth factor receptors, either through ROS generation or other pathways.[12]

Eutrophic inward remodeling is also a complex process, but is currently less well understood than hypertrophic inward remodeling. Eutrophic remodeling is known to involve numerous events, including the rearrangement of vascular smooth muscle cells, changes in extracellular matrix deposition, and changes in cell-cell or cell-matrix interactions.[6] In contrast to the hypertrophic inward remodeling triggered by elevated wall stress or growth factors, eutrophic inward remodeling apparently does not depend on activation of tyrosine kinases or the MAP kinase cascade.[15] This form of remodeling can be triggered by a chronic increase in vascular tone, which is apparently

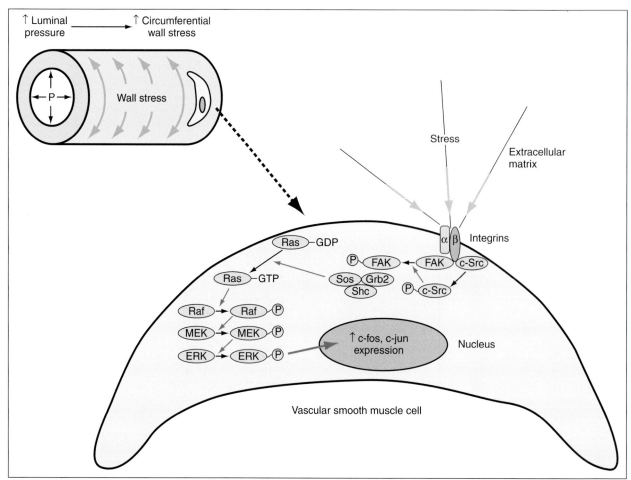

Figure 15–2. Known elements of the signaling pathway through which a pressure-related increase in circumferential wall stress leads to hypertrophy of vascular smooth muscle cells. FAK, focal adhesion kinase; cSrc, cSrc kinase; Grb2, growth factor receptor-bound protein 2; Sos, the guanine nucleotide exchange factor son-of-sevenless, Shc is an adaptor protein, Ras is a GTP-binding protein, Raf is a tyrosine kinase; MEK, mitogen-activated protein kinase/extracellular signal-regulated kinase kinase; ERK, extracellular signal-regulated kinase.

linked to subsequent rearrangement of the extracellular matrix through the activity of β-integrins.[15] Recent findings also suggest that this matrix rearrangement depends on the activity of tissue-type transglutaminases, which are constitutively expressed multifunctional enzymes associated with β-integrins and which can catalyze the formation of stabilizing crosslinks between rearranged matrix proteins.[16]

Eutrophic remodeling could also occur through apoptosis (programmed cell death) in the outer regions of the vessel wall, which would reduce external vessel diameter, coupled with increased cellular growth toward the lumen, which would reduce internal vessel diameter. However, the exact role of apoptosis in vascular remodeling remains unclear, and this type of eutrophic remodeling may only occur in certain forms of hypertension.[6]

Reduced number of perfused vessels (rarefaction)

In the hypertensive state, vascular rarefaction may be defined as either a reversible closure of vessels due to intense vasoconstriction ("functional rarefaction") or a frank loss of vessels from the network ("structural rarefaction"). Either scenario will lead to increased vascular resistance

due to the reduction in the number of parallel pathways available for flow conduction at that level of the resistance vessel network (Figure 15–4). Although vessel wall remodeling can occur in both the resistance arteries and true arterioles of hypertensive individuals, rarefaction is generally limited to distal segments of the arteriolar network and to the capillary beds. Arteriolar and capillary rarefaction has been widely documented in many animal models of hypertension,[1] and in the skin, skeletal muscle, conjunctiva, and intestine of hypertensive humans.[17]

In a manner somewhat analogous to eutrophic resistance vessel remodeling, there is often a clearly defined progression from constriction-induced functional rarefaction in developing hypertension to structural rarefaction in established hypertension, and this progression offers some insight into the mechanisms that underlie this transition.[1,18] In early hypertension, an intense constriction of some arterioles can lead to cessation of their perfusion. A sustained lack of perfusion will in turn lead to atrophy and degeneration of endothelial as well as vascular smooth muscle cells (Figure 15–5), resulting in the actual loss of vessels from the network.[19] Because the initial functional rarefaction is a manifestation of intense sustained

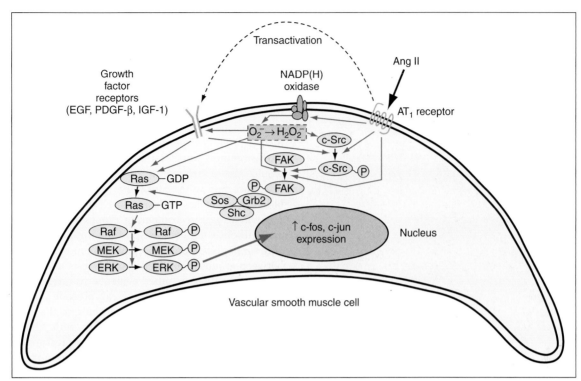

Figure 15–3. Known elements of the signaling pathways through which angiotensin II (Ang II) and other growth receptors lead to hypertrophy of vascular smooth muscle cells. EGF, epidermal growth factor; PDGF-β, the β isoform of platelet-derived growth factor; IGF-1, insulin-like growth factor 1. Other abbreviations same as in Fig. 15–2.

vasoconstriction, any mechanism that promotes increased vascular tone in the hypertensive state could theoretically lead to functional rarefaction. These mechanisms include (1) a reduced availability of endothelial nitric oxide or an increased production of endothelium-derived vasoconstrictors such as endothelin, prostaglandin H_2, or thromboxane A_2,[20] (2) an increased responsiveness of vascular smooth muscle to oxygen,[5] neurally released norepinephrine,[2] or pressure-dependent (myogenic) stimuli,[21] and (3) a chronic increase in the activity of the sympathetic nervous system.[22]

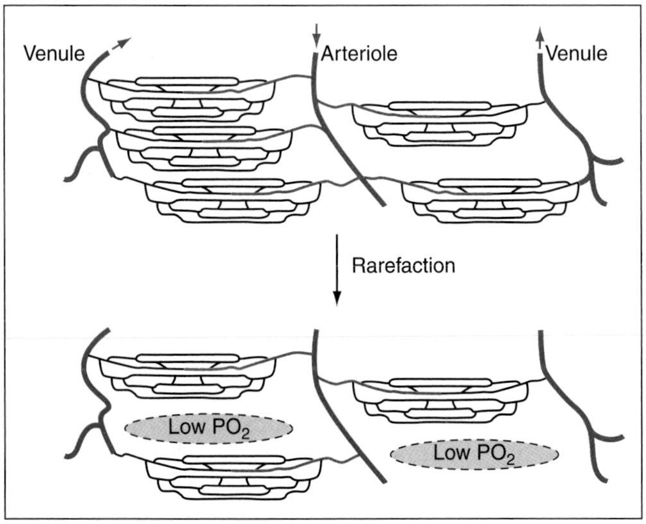

There have been some reports of structural arteriolar rarefaction in hypertensive individuals without any evidence of a preceding functional rarefaction.[23] This raises the possibility that the presence of fewer vessels in the arteriolar network could reflect a decreased capacity for angiogenesis, such that normal network development does not occur in growing individuals who are susceptible to hypertension.[24] However, the experimental evidence that directly addresses this hypothesis is modest and at times conflicting,[25] and further studies are necessary to critically evaluate this possibility. Structural rarefaction could also occur independently of constriction if the actions of one or more endogenous trophic factors become suppressed, leading to a regression of previously existing vessels. In addition to its well-recognized roles in the control of renal function and systemic hemodynamics, Ang II (acting via the AT_1 receptor) is an important trophic factor necessary to normal angiogenesis and vascular wall growth and to the maintenance of normal vascular wall and network structure.[26] In forms of hypertension characterized by suppression of the renin-angiotensin system, microvascular rarefaction has been linked to a decrease in circulating Ang II levels—presumably through the withdrawal of these trophic actions.[26]

Figure 15–4. Rarefaction of terminal arterioles and capillaries can contribute to increased vascular resistance (through a reduction in the number of parallel pathways for flow conduction), and can reduce transcapillary solute and water exchange (through a reduction in total capillary surface area and an increase in mean diffusion distance).

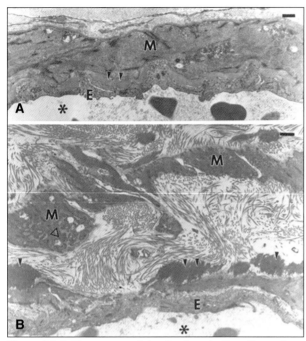

Figure 15–5. The process of structural rarefaction. Shown here are electron micrographs of normal (A) and dissociating (B) arterioles in rat skeletal muscle during reduced renal mass hypertension. In B, smooth muscle (M) cells of the dissociating arteriole have become separated from the endothelium (E). Also evident is the partial or complete loss of the basement membrane and increased presence of collagen in the region underlying the smooth muscle. Arrowheads indicate elastin, and asterisks identify the vessel lumen. Rough endoplasmic reticulum is evident in the vicinity of the open triangle in the M cell to the left. Bar = 1 μm. (Reproduced from Hansen-Smith FM, Morris LW, Greene AS, Lombard JH. Rapid microvessel rarefaction with elevated salt intake and reduced renal mass hypertension in rats. *Circ Res* 1996; 79:324–30, with permission).

GENETICS

Blood pressure is a continuous normally distributed variable that is polygenic (determined by the behavior of many interacting genes) and strongly influenced by environmental variables. Assessing the genetic underpinnings of one particular aspect of hypertension, such as structural changes within the resistance vasculature, is therefore a complex and difficult task. In considering whether there may be a genetically based predisposition among some individuals to develop vascular remodeling or rarefaction with hypertension, it is important to first understand whether these structural changes are actually a cause or consequence of hypertension. A demonstration of remodeling or rarefaction in young individuals who have hypertensive parents, and may therefore be predisposed to hypertension, could yield important information in this regard. However, the current data on this point are somewhat contradictory. For the most part, resistance vessel remodeling and arteriolar rarefaction have been observed in individuals who are already hypertensive,[17] and it has been well documented that vascular wall remodeling and rarefaction can readily occur in response to sustained

increases in pressure (as discussed previously) or blood flow (through changes in luminal shear stress).[10,27] Therefore, alterations in resistance vessel structure or network architecture associated with hypertension are often considered a secondary response to the hypertensive condition. This, in turn, has given rise to the concept that remodeling and rarefaction represent a form of "structural autoregulation" to maintain normal tissue blood flows over a prolonged period in the face of increased organ perfusion pressures.[23] In this event, such vascular changes would not contribute to the initial rise in peripheral resistance but rather contribute to its maintenance once blood pressure has been increased. Consistent with this view, investigators comparing groups of offspring with and without a family predisposition for hypertension, but with similar blood pressures, have not reported a difference between groups in minimal vascular resistance.[17]

However, there is other evidence to suggest that the initiation of structural changes can precede the increase in arterial pressure, and thus contribute to the genesis of hypertension. For example, patients with "borderline hypertension" (in which elevated blood pressure is intermittent and relatively modest) have been found to exhibit the same degree of structural capillary rarefaction as those with established hypertension.[28] In addition, some investigators have reported that there is capillary rarefaction in association with a familial predisposition to essential hypertension.[29]

Thus, in some individuals there may be a genetic predisposition to the development of such structural changes, although the extent to which these early changes would contribute to any subsequent rise in total peripheral resistance is not known. Because remodeling of resistance vessels appears to have a causal role in hypertension-related end-organ damage (see material following), findings of a genetic susceptibility to cardiac and renal damage in hypertensive individuals may also reflect the heritability of structural changes.[30]

PHYSIOLOGY AND PATHOPHYSIOLOGY

In many forms of hypertension, TPR is elevated in direct proportion to arterial pressure. Cardiac output tends to be normal, and there is often little or no change in its fractional distribution among different organs—indicating a fairly uniform increase in vascular resistance throughout the peripheral circulation.[31,32] Under these conditions, tissue blood flows are preserved at or near normal values in hypertensive individuals.[32] The elevated arterial pressure is transmitted well into the microvasculature, but the increased resistance of small arteries and arterioles effectively dissipates this pressure increase such that pressure in the smallest arterioles is often normal in hypertensive individuals[2] (Figure 15–6). Therefore, in addition to preventing tissue overperfusion increased precapillary resistance in the hypertensive state can effectively shield most capillary networks from abnormally high hydrostatic pressures, which in turn would prevent excessive transcapillary water filtration and tissue edema. The exact contribution of structural versus functional changes to the overall increase in

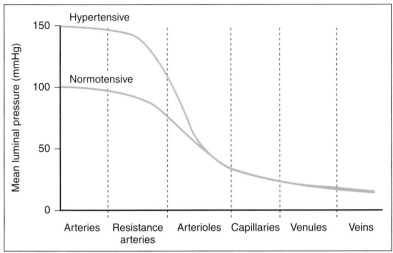

Figure 15–6. Shift in peripheral vascular pressure profile associated with hypertension. In the hypertensive individual, the increased slope of the pressure drop across the resistance arteries and arterioles reflects an increased resistance to flow, due in part to vascular remodeling and rarefaction.

precapillary resistance can vary from organ to organ in hypertensive individuals, and (as implied previously) can change with the stage of hypertension.

If structural remodeling of the resistance vasculature leads to reduced luminal diameters at any given level of vascular tone, the hemodynamic resistance of these vessels will clearly be increased. The extent to which this remodeling increases the overall vascular resistance of an organ or tissue will depend not only on the magnitude of the diameter reductions but on the fraction of total resistance that normally resides in the remodeled vessels. The fractional distribution of hemodynamic resistance within any vascular bed can be experimentally determined from localized pressure measurements, which provide information on the network's pressure profile (such as that shown in Figure 15–6) and thereby allowing the investigator to calculate the dissipation of pressure across each of the series-coupled segments (e.g., feed arteries, proximal arterioles, distal arterioles, capillaries, and so on). To date, this detailed information has only been obtained in animal models of hypertension, where it has revealed a considerable degree of variability in the hemodynamic importance of structural changes. For example, a structural reduction in arteriolar diameters has been estimated to account for most of the increased resistance to blood flow in the cremaster muscle of rats with two-kidney one-clip hypertension,[33] whereas similar changes contribute little to increased hindquarter vascular resistance in the SHR.[34]

Rarefaction is more localized within the resistance network than is remodeling, occurring only among the smallest arterioles.[23] However, because these vessels are responsible for a considerable fraction of total network resistance in many vascular beds the impact of rarefaction on whole-organ resistance can also be substantial. Experimental and theoretical studies indicate that in some forms of hypertension the fraction of the total increase in network vascular resistance due to arteriolar rarefaction can approach that due to active increases in microvascular tone.[18,35]

Whether occurring through eutrophic or hypertrophic remodeling, a structural reduction in resistance vessel diameters can also provide a mechanical advantage for resistance vessels by reducing circumferential wall stress. In this event, less smooth muscle force generation would be required to maintain resting vascular diameter at any level of transmural pressure.[4,36] Consequently, a remodeled arteriole can maintain its active diameter and participate in flow regulation at higher luminal pressures than can a normal arteriole[36,37]—an adaptation that is clearly advantageous in the hypertensive state. This adaptation is evident in some vascular beds during autoregulation, which is defined here as the tendency of an organ to maintain constant blood flow despite changes in perfusion pressure.

As shown in Figure 15–7, the range of pressures over which vascular resistance can be adjusted to preserve normal blood flow (i.e., an organ's "autoregulatory range") can be shifted upward in hypertensive individuals.

The mechanical advantage associated with resistance vessel remodeling can be reinforced if there is also an increased contribution of passive wall elements to total wall tension. This would further reduce the level of active force required to offset elevated luminal pressure.[4] However, that portion of total wall tension attributable to passive (as opposed to active) tension is largely determined by passive wall distensibility, and studies conducted in hypertensive animals indicate that this characteristic does not uniformly change with hypertension in all vascular beds. For example, passive arteriolar wall distensibility is decreased in the intestine of the SHR[4] but is increased in the cerebral cortex of the stroke-prone SHR—possibly due to a dispro-

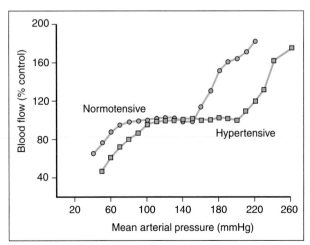

Figure 15–7. Shift in the cerebral circulation autoregulatory curve associated with spontaneous hypertension in rats. (Adapted from Harper SL Bohlen HG. Microvascular adaptation in the cerebral cortex of adult spontaneously hypertensive rats. *Hypertension* 1984;6:408–19).

portionate increase in more distensible wall elements (i.e., smooth muscle and elastin).[38] Furthermore, the passive distensibility of mesenteric, coronary, and cremaster muscle resistance vessels from SHR are not different from those of their normotensive counterparts.[21,39,40]

In many tissues, local blood flow regulation is the result of a complex interplay among metabolic, myogenic, and endothelium-dependent mechanisms. In hypertension, each of these mechanisms can be altered by molecular and/or biochemical changes within the endothelium or smooth muscle of resistance vessels.[20,41] However, structural changes may also be important in this regard. The magnitude of resistance vessel constriction in response to any stimulus is determined in part by the length/tension relationship of its vascular smooth muscle such that a maximal response will occur only when resting smooth muscle length is within some optimal range. If this resting length is changed by vessel wall remodeling, this could produce a nonspecific change in vascular responsiveness to constrictor stimuli. Furthermore, remodeling not only reduces a vessel's capacity for maximal dilation but can be accompanied by a reduced responsiveness to vasodilators at submaximal concentrations.[42] To the extent there are changes in responsiveness to vasoconstrictor and/or vasodilator stimuli, and to the extent rarefaction can limit the network's capacity for homogenous flow distribution, structural changes in the resistance vasculature could have profound effects on local blood flow regulation. Mathematical modeling suggests that the ability of a tissue to regulate its own oxygen delivery can become compromised in hypertensive individuals due to the heterogeneous distribution of blood flow that accompanies microvascular rarefaction, leaving the PO_2 in some tissue regions highly sensitive to changes in tissue metabolism.[43]

The loss of small arterioles, and by extension the capillaries that arise from them, also has important consequences for solute and water exchange between the vascular compartment and surrounding tissue. For example, rarefaction of only the most distal arterioles, which could have a relatively modest effect on total network resistance and blood flow, could dramatically reduce the efficiency of tissue oxygen delivery by increasing the heterogeneity of flow among those capillaries that remain perfused.[35] Separate from, but possibly potentiated by, this flow heterogeneity an overall reduction in the number of perfused capillaries and small arterioles will lead to decreased oxygen delivery due to (1) a reduction in the total capillary surface area available for exchange and (2) an increase in the mean diffusion distance between any respiring cell and the nearest perfused vessel (Figure 15–4). This reduction in oxygen delivery has been confirmed with direct measurements of tissue PO_2 in tissues that exhibit arteriolar and capillary rarefaction in the hypertensive state.[43,44]

CLINICAL IMPLICATIONS AND PERSPECTIVES

Resistance vessels from untreated hypertensive patients often exhibit structurally reduced diameters due to eutrophic remodeling, and in some cases also exhibit hypertrophic

remodeling.[12,17] In addition to the contribution they make to increased total peripheral resistance, these changes in resistance vessel structure can also play an important role in the development of some types of end-organ damage associated with hypertension. Resistance artery remodeling is clearly evident in patients with mild (early) hypertension before the onset of any clinically relevant end-organ damage.[45] Other studies have demonstrated that hypertension-associated stroke linked to small vessel infarction is due in part to structural changes in the cerebral microvasculature,[29] and that small artery remodeling contributes to the mechanisms of hypertension-associated renal failure.[46] The prognostic value of these structural changes has also been recognized. The degree to which subcutaneous small arteries are remodeled has been found to be a strong predictor of fatal and nonfatal cardiac, cerebral, and renal events in hypertensive patients— independent of other known cardiovascular risk factors.[47]

The functional and structural rarefaction of arterioles and capillaries is also well documented in untreated hypertensive patients.[17,28,48,49] The contribution of rarefaction to end-organ damage is less clear, although disruption of normal tissue oxygen and nutrient delivery could clearly lead to compromised organ function.

In light of the importance of resistance vessel remodeling in contributing to end-organ damage, and the possible problems in tissue solute-water transport posed by rarefaction, the normalization of microvascular structure and hemodynamics should be an important goal of antihypertensive therapy. Although such therapy has often been directed toward reversing the abnormal constriction of resistance vessels, recent therapeutic efforts have been increasingly directed toward reducing or reversing the changes in vascular structure associated with hypertension and toward reducing or reversing microvascular rarefaction. In fact, some antihypertensive agents have been found to exert their effects through both an acute change in vascular function (vasodilation) and chronic improvements in vessel and network structure.

Depending on the therapeutic strategy employed and the duration of treatment, antihypertensive therapy may partially or completely reverse the structural remodeling of resistance vessels in hypertensive humans.[17] However, there are clear differences among the major classes of antihypertensive agents with respect to their impact on resistance vessel structure, and these differences are not related to the magnitude of blood pressure reduction. For example, there is little evidence that either diuretics or beta-blockers can reverse vascular remodeling or rarefaction,[29,50] whereas calcium antagonists are effective in reducing both arteriolar remodeling and capillary rarefaction—at least in animal models of hypertension.[51] Angiotensin-converting enzyme (ACE) inhibitors are also effective in reversing the remodeling of resistance vessels in both animal models and hypertensive patients, although there are conflicting results on the ability of these agents to reverse rarefaction.[29,50] In some cases, antagonists of Ang II (AT_1) receptors can also reverse microvascular remodeling and rarefaction. Certain combinations of antihypertensive agents are also effective in reversing these structural changes, and in some cases these combinations can be more effective than either agent given alone.[29]

Additional studies are required to more clearly determine the extent to which resistance vessel remodeling and rarefaction can be primary (i.e., causal) events in the development of hypertension, and to more completely understand the intracellular signaling pathways that trigger and sustain these structural changes. This is particularly true in the case of eutrophic remodeling, where the possible involvement of cellular apoptosis is intriguing yet poorly understood. Another unresolved issue of obvious importance for hypertension research is the elucidation of those mechanisms responsible for the onset and progression of hypertension-related organ damage, including the exact role of vascular remodeling in these processes. Finally, although not specifically discussed in relation to structural changes studies to evaluate the contributions of inflammation and reactive oxygen species to this target-organ damage also appear to hold much promise in helping to understand these pathologic changes.[14,41] This information is of obvious value in developing more effective therapeutic strategies for the prevention and treatment of hypertension and its consequences.

SUMMARY

In hypertensive individuals, increased vascular resistance can be due in part to structural changes in the diameter of individual resistance vessels (through vascular wall remodeling) or structural changes in the architecture of resistance vessel networks (through rarefaction). The relative influences of remodeling versus rarefaction on vascular resistance, as well as the fraction of the overall resistance increase attributable to structural versus functional changes in general, can vary from organ to organ within a hypertensive individual and depends on the form of hypertension and its developmental stage.

The hypertrophic inward remodeling of resistance vessels can be triggered by numerous stimuli, including pressure-dependent increases in vascular wall stress and the actions of different vascular growth factors. In contrast, the eutrophic inward remodeling of these vessels can be triggered by sustained vasoconstriction. Investigators are continuing to make important progress in defining the intracellular signaling pathways through which these and other stimuli lead to inward vascular remodeling. The structural rarefaction of arterioles and capillaries can occur in response to a constriction-dependent cessation of vessel perfusion, leading to degradation of vascular wall elements or to a decrease in the availability of one or more endogenous vascular growth or trophic factors.

It is unclear whether some of these structural changes within the resistance vasculature can precede the onset of hypertension (and therefore contribute to its development) or whether they represent a secondary adaptation to the hypertensive state (and therefore contribute to the maintenance of increased TPR and arterial pressure). Nevertheless, it is becoming apparent that in addition to their effects on TPR these changes may also have important effects on the regulation of tissue blood flow and transcapillary exchange.

Because resistance vessel remodeling may also play a role in the development of hypertension-related end-organ damage, the reversal of changes in vascular structure is becoming an important focus of antihypertensive therapy. However, additional studies are needed to clearly determine which classes of hypertensive agents (alone or in combination) are most effective in achieving this goal.

REFERENCES

1. Prewitt RL, Hashimoto H, Stacy DL. Microvascular alterations in hypertension. In: McDonagh P (ed.). *Microvascular Perfusion and Transport in Health and Disease.* Basel: Karger, 1987:31–59.
2. Bohlen HG. The microcirculation in hypertension. *J Hypertension* 1989;7(Suppl 4):S117–24.
3. Mulvany MJ. Contractile properties of resistance vessels related to cellular. In: Lee RMKW (ed.). *Blood Vessel Changes in Hypertension: Structure and Function, Volume I.* Boca Raton, FL: CRC Press, 1989:1–24.
4. Bohlen HG, Lash JM. Active and passive arteriolar regulation in spontaneously hypertensive rats. *Hypertension* 1994;23:757–64.
5. Lombard JH, Hinojosa-Laborde C, Cowley AW Jr. Hemodynamics and microcirculatory alterations in reduced renal mass hypertension. *Hypertension* 1989;13:128–38.
6. Intengan HD, Schiffrin EL. Structure and mechanical properties of resistance arteries in hypertension: Role of adhesion molecules and extracellular matrix determinants. *Hypertension* 2000;36:312–18.

7. Heagerty AM, Aalkjaer C, Bund SJ, et al. Small artery structure in hypertension: Dual processes of remodeling and growth. *Hypertension* 1993;21:391–97.
8. Sexton WL, Korthuis RJ, Laughlin MH. Vascular flow capacity of hindlimb skeletal muscles in spontaneously hypertensive rats. *J Appl Physiol* 1990;69:1073–79.
9. Folkow B, Hallbeck M, Lundgren Y, Weiss L. Background of increased flow resistance and vascular reactivity in spontaneously hypertensive rats. *Acta Physiol Scand* 1970;80:93–106.
10. Prewitt RL, Rice DC, Dobrian AD. Adaptation of resistance arteries to increases in pressure. *Microcirculation* 2002;9:295–304.
11. Lehoux S, Tedgui A. Signal transduction of mechanical stresses in the vascular wall. *Hypertension* 1998;32:338–45.
12. Schiffrin EL, Touyz RM. From bedside to bench to bedside: Role of renin-angiotensin-aldosterone system in remodeling of resistance arteries in hypertension. *Am J Physiol* 2004;287:H435–46.
13. Hughes AD. AT$_1$-signaling in vascular smooth muscle. *JRAAS* 2000;1:125–30.

14. Griendling KK, Sorescu D, Lassegue B, Ushio-Fukai M. Modulation of protein kinase activity and gene expression by reactive oxygen species and their role in vascular physiology and pathophysiology. *Art Thromb Vasc Biol* 2000;20:2175–83.
15. Bakker ENTP, Buus CL, VanBavel E, Mulvany MJ. Activation of resistance arteries with endothelin-1: From vasoconstriction to functional adaptation and remodeling. *J Vasc Res* 2004;41:174–82.
16. Bakker ENTP, Buus CL, Spaan JAE, et al. Small artery remodeling depends on tissue-type transglutaminase. *Circ Res* 2005;96:119–26.
17. Shore AC, Tooke JE. Microvascular function in human essential hypertension. *J Hypertension* 1994;12:717–28.
18. Hernandez I, Greens AS. Hemodynamic and microcirculatory changes during development of renal hypertension. *Am J Physiol* 1995;268:H33–38.
19. Hansen-Smith FM, Morris LW, Greene AS, Lombard JH. Rapid microvessel rarefaction with elevated salt intake and reduced renal mass hypertension in rats. *Circ Res* 1996;79:324–30.

SECTION
2

PATHOGENESIS

20. Koller A. Signaling pathways of mechanotransduction in arteriolar endothelium and smooth muscle cells in hypertension. *Microcirculation* 2002;9:277–94.
21. Falcone JC, Granger HJ, Meininger GA. Enhanced myogenic activation in skeletal muscle arterioles from spontaneously hypertensive rats. *Am J Physiol* 1993; 265:H1847–55.
22. Hart MN, Heistad DD, Brody MJ. Effect of chronic hypertension and sympathetic denervation on wall/lumen ratio of cerebral vessels. *Hypertension* 1980;2:419–23.
23. Prewitt RL, Hashimoto H, Stacy DL. Structural and functional rarefaction of microvessels in hypertension. In: Lee RMKW (ed.). *Blood Vessel Changes in Hypertension: Structure and Function, Volume II.* Boca Raton, FL: CRC Press, 1989:71–89.
24. LeNoble FAC, Stassen FRM, Hacking WJG, Struijker-Boudier HAJ. Angiogenesis and hypertension. *J Hypertension* 1988; 16:1563–72.
25. Sane DC, Anton L, Brosnihan KB. Angiogenic growth factors and hypertension. *Angiogenesis* 2004; 7:193–201.
26. Greene AS. Life and death in the microcirculation: A role for angiotensin II. *Microcirculation* 1998;5:101–07.
27. Skalak TC, Price RJ. The role of mechanical stresses in microvascular remodeling. *Microcirculation* 1996; 3:143–65.
28. Antonios TFT, Singer DRJ, Markandu ND, et al. Rarefaction of skin capillaries in borderline essential hypertension suggests an early structural abnormality. *Hypertension* 1999;34:655–58.
29. Levy BI, Ambrosio G, Pries AR, Struijker-Boudier HAJ. Microcirculation in hypertension: A new target for treatment? *Circulation* 2001;104:735–40.
30. Arnett DK. Heritability of hypertension and target organ damage. In: Izzo JL Jr, Black HR (eds.). *Hypertension Primer, Third Edition: The Essentials of High Blood Pressure.* Dallas: American Heart Association, 2003:227–29.
31. Boegehold MA, Huffman LJ, Hedge GA. Peripheral vascular resistance and regional blood flows in hypertensive Dahl rats. *Am J Physiol* 1991;261:R934–38.
32. Coleman TG, Hall JE. Systemic hemodynamics and regional blood flow regulation. In: Izzo JL Jr, Black HR (eds.). *Hypertension Primer, Third Edition: The Essentials of High Blood Pressure.* Dallas: American Heart Association, 2003:111–14.
33. Ono Z, Prewitt RL, Stacy DL. Arteriolar changes in developing and chronic stages of two-kidney, one clip hypertension. *Hypertension* 1989;14:36–43.
34. Prewitt RL, Reilly CK, Wang DH. Pressure-flow curves reflect arteriolar responses in perfused rat hindquarters. *Hypertension* 1994;23:223–28.
35. Greene AS, Tonellato PJ, Lui J, et al. Microvascular rarefaction and tissue vascular resistance in hypertension. *Am J Physiol* 1989;256:H126–31.
36. Baumbach GL, Heistad DD. Cerebral circulation in chronic arterial hypertension. *Hypertension* 1988;12:89–95.
37. Harper SL, Bohlen HG. Microvascular adaptation in the cerebral cortex of adult spontaneously hypertensive rats. *Hypertension* 1984;6:408–19.
38. Baumbach GL, Walmsley JG, Hart MN. Composition and mechanics of cerebral arterioles in hypertensive rats. *Am J Pathol* 1988;133:464–71.
39. Garcia SR, Izzard AS, Heagerty AM, Bund SJ. Myogenic tone in coronary arteries from spontaneously hypertensive rats. *J Vasc Res* 1997;34:109–16.
40. Izzard AS, Bund SJ, Heagerty AM. Myogenic tone in mesenteric arteries from spontaneously hypertensive rats. *Am J Physiol* 1996;270:H1–6.
41. Boegehold MA. Microvascular structure and function in salt-sensitive hypertension. *Microcirculation* 2002;9:225–41.
42. Frisbee JC, Lombard JH. Chronic elevations in salt intake and reduced renal mass hypertension compromise mechanisms of arteriolar dilation. *Microvasc Res* 1998;56:218–27.
43. Greene AS, Tonellato PJ, Zhang Z, et al. Effect of microvascular rarefaction on tissue oxygen delivery in hypertension. *Am J Physiol* 1992;256:H126–31.
44. Lombard JH, Frisbee JC, Greene AS, et al. Microvascular flow and tissue PO_2 in skeletal muscle of chronic reduced renal mass hypertensive rats. *Am J Physiol* 2000;279:H2295–2302.
45. Park JB, Schiffrin EL. Small artery remodeling is the most prevalent (earliest?) form of target organ damage in mild essential hypertension. *J Hypertens* 2001;19:921–30.
46. Klahr S, Morrissey J. Progression of chronic renal disease. *Am J Kidney Dis* 2003;41:S3–7.
47. Rizzoni D, Porteri E, Boari GEM, et al. Prognostic significance of small-artery structure in hypertension. *Circulation* 2003;108:2230–35.
48. Hernandez N, Torres SH, Finol HJ, Vera O. Capillary changes in skeletal muscle of patients with essential hypertension. *The Anatomical Record* 1999;256:425–32.
49. Serne EH, Gans ROB, Maaten JC, et al. Impaired skin capillary recruitment in essential hypertension is caused by both functional and structural capillary rarefaction. *Hypertension* 2001;38:238–42.
50. Thybo NK, Stephens N, Cooper A, et al. Effect of antihypertensive treatment on small arteries of patients with previously untreated essential hypertension. *Hypertension* 1995;25:474–81.
51. Kobayashi N, Kobayashi K, Hara K, et al. Benidipine stimulates nitric oxide synthase and improves coronary circulation in hypertensive rats. *Am J Hypertens* 1999;12:483–91.

166

Chapter

16

The RhoA/Rho-Kinase Signaling Pathway in Vascular Smooth Muscle Contraction: Biochemistry, Physiology, and Pharmacology

Cleber E. Teixeira and R. Clinton Webb

Key Findings

- Contraction of the vascular smooth muscle is initiated, and to a lesser extent maintained, by a rise in the concentration of free Ca^{2+} in the cell cytoplasm. As a result, several signaling pathways trigger a Ca^{2+}/calmodulin interaction to stimulate phosphorylation of the myosin light chain (MLC).

- It is well established that the Ca^{2+} signal is not the sole factor that regulates vascular smooth muscle contraction, because alterations of the Ca^{2+} sensitivity in the contractile apparatus are also known to play an important role. Ca^{2+} sensitivity of smooth muscle reflects the ratio of activities of MLC kinase and MLC phosphatase, which determines the level of MLC phosphorylation.

- Ca^{2+} sensitization of the contractile proteins is widely attributed to the monomeric G protein RhoA and mediated by its effector, Rho-kinase, to inhibit the dephosphorylation of MLC in the presence of basal (Ca^{2+} dependent or independent) or increased MLC kinase activity, thereby maintaining force generation.

- In animal and human studies, the Ca^{2+} sensitization mediated by the Rho-kinase signaling pathway has been shown to be substantially involved in the pathogenesis of hypertension, vasospasm, atherosclerosis, pulmonary hypertension, stroke, and heart failure.

- Because changes mediated by the abnormal activation of the RhoA/Rho-kinase signaling are implicated in the pathogenesis of several cardiovascular diseases, intervention with this pathway may potentially have therapeutic consequences.

INTRODUCTION

Sheets or layers of smooth muscle cells constitute the walls of various organs and tubes in the body, including the blood vessels, stomach, intestines, bladder, airways, uterus, and the penile and clitoral cavernosal sinuses. In its differentiated state, the primary function of smooth muscle is mechanical, to generate force. This force may be utilized to perform many functions, including maintenance and regulation of circulation, gastrointestinal motility, expulsion of the fetus, regulation of light admitted to the retina, regulation of intraocular pressure in the eye, and the behavior of the urogenital tract. When made to contract, the smooth muscle cells shorten and propel the luminal content of the organ, or the cell shortening varies the diameter of a tube to regulate the flow of its content. Smooth muscle cells lack the striated banding pattern found in cardiac and skeletal muscle, and they receive neural innervation from the autonomic nervous system. In addition, the contractile state of smooth muscle is controlled by hormones, autocrine/paracrine agents, and other local chemical signals. Smooth muscle cells also develop tonic and phasic contractions in response to changes in load or length. Regardless of the stimulus, smooth muscle cells use cross-bridge cycling between actin and myosin to develop force, and Ca^{2+} ions serve to initiate the underlying molecular signaling that leads to contraction.

The vascular smooth muscle cell is a highly specialized cell whose principal function is contraction. It expresses a variety of contractile proteins, ion channels, and signaling molecules that regulate the contractile process. Upon contraction, vascular smooth muscle cells shorten, thereby decreasing the diameter of a blood vessel in order to regulate the blood flow and pressure. In this chapter, we focus primarily on the contractile phenotype of vascular smooth muscle cells and describe the molecular signaling pathways involved in the regulation of contraction, particularly the role of the RhoA/Rho-kinase signaling in contractile processes and the pathophysiological implications of this pathway.

THE CONTRACTILE MECHANISM OF THE VASCULAR SMOOTH MUSCLE

In the intact body, the process of smooth muscle cell contraction is regulated principally by pharmacomechanical (ligand-mediated activation of cell surface receptors) and electromechanical (stretch, intraluminal pressure) activation of the contractile proteins myosin and actin.[1] A change in membrane potential, brought on by the firing of action potentials or by activation of stretch-dependent ion channels in the plasma membrane, can also trigger contraction. For contraction to occur, myosin light-chain kinase (MLC kinase) must phosphorylate the 20-kDa light chain of myosin, enabling the molecular interaction of myosin with actin. Energy released from ATP by myosin ATPase activity results in the cycling of the myosin cross-bridges with actin for contraction.[2,3] Counteracting the pulling forces exerted by external tension, cells can generate contractile force. Actin-myosin fibers contract following myosin light-chain phosphorylation, and by insertion of these fibers into focal contacts associated with the plasma membrane tension develops within a cell, accompanied by inward cell contraction.

The extent of cell contraction depends on the external tension pulling outward. Eventually, a state of equilibrium between internal contractile force and external tension is achieved. There are two types of contractility: isotonic contraction (in which there is shortening of actin-myosin filaments and therefore cell contraction) and isometric contraction, in which filament shortening does not occur but tension increases. Thus, contractile activity in smooth muscle is determined primarily by the phosphorylation state of the light chain of myosin, a highly regulated process. In some smooth muscle cells, the phosphorylation of the light chain of myosin is maintained at a low level in the absence of external stimuli (i.e., no receptor or mechanical activation).[4] This activity results in what is known as vascular tone, which can be defined as the degree of constriction of a blood vessel relative to its maximal diameter in the dilated state.

Under basal conditions, most resistance and capacitance vessels exhibit some degree of smooth muscle contraction that determines the diameter or tone of the vessel. Vascular tone is also partially determined by a multitude of vasoconstrictor factors such as norepinephrine, angiotensin II, vasopressin, and 5-hydroxytryptamine—as well as by vasodilator factors such as nitric oxide, bradykinin, and prostacyclin. These factors can be divided into extrinsic factors (which originate outside the blood vessel) and intrinsic factors, which originate in the vessel itself. Extrinsic factors primarily serve the function of regulating arterial pressure by altering systemic vascular resistance, whereas intrinsic mechanisms are concerned with regulation of local blood flow within an organ.[5]

Ca^{2+}-dependent contraction

The state of contraction of smooth muscle is known to depend on cytosolic Ca^{2+} levels. A rise in the concentration of cytoplasmic Ca^{2+} is the trigger for vascular contraction.[6] However, contraction in smooth muscle, unlike striated muscle, is regulated to a large extent by a mechanism independent of membrane potential—in which agonists induce contraction without membrane depolarization. Contraction of smooth muscle is initiated by a Ca^{2+}-mediated change in the thick (myosin) filaments, whereas in striated muscle Ca^{2+}-mediated contraction is initiated by changes in the thin (actin) filaments. In response to specific stimuli in smooth muscle (for instance, the α-adrenoceptor agonist norepinephrine released from the sympathetic nerve endings within the arterial wall), the intracellular concentration of Ca^{2+} rapidly increases and then declines to a level that is elevated above basal in the continued presence of the agonist.[7] This initial increase in cytosolic Ca^{2+} arises from Ca^{2+} released from intracellular stores (sarcoplasmic reticulum) and the latter as of entry from the extracellular space via receptor-operated Ca^{2+} channels.[8]

The biochemical signals that trigger Ca^{2+} release involve activation of phospholipase C (PLC) by heterotrimeric G-proteins upon binding of agonists to the seven transmembrane receptors on the smooth muscle cell membrane.[9] PLC is specific for the membrane lipid phosphatidylinositol 4,5-biphosphate (PIP$_2$) to catalize the formation of two potent second messengers, inositol 1,4,5-triphosphate (IP$_3$) and diacylglycerol (DAG). The binding of IP$_3$ to specific receptors on the sarcoplasmic reticulum results in the release of Ca^{2+} into the cytosol. The primary target protein of this initial rise in intracellular Ca^{2+} is believed to be calmodulin (CaM). A Ca^{2+}-CaM complex allows a subsequent interaction with MLC kinase, resulting in a conformational change of the CaM-MLC kinase and thus exposing the catalytic site. This sequence of events leads to the activation of MLC kinase and the phosphorylation of Ser19 of the 20-kDa regulatory light chain of myosin (MLC$_{20}$). It is widely accepted that the degree of MLC$_{20}$ phosphorylation is the essential factor that determines the extent to which the vascular smooth muscle contracts: MLC$_{20}$ phosphorylation promotes contraction whereas MLC$_{20}$ dephosphorylation, following a reduction in intracellular Ca^{2+}, results in relaxation.

The second messenger (DAG) activates protein kinase C (PKC), which phosphorylates specific target proteins. There are several PKC isozymes in smooth muscle cells, such as PKCα and β (DAG and Ca^{2+} dependent) or PKCε (DAG dependent), and each has a tissue-specific role. In many cases PKC has contraction-promoting effects such as phosphorylation of many kinases, as well as various ion channels and ion transporters. Phorbol esters constitute a group of synthetic compounds known to activate PKC, mimic the action of DAG, and cause contraction of smooth muscle.[10,11] Finally, L-type Ca^{2+} channels (voltage-operated Ca^{2+} channels) in the membrane also open in response to membrane depolarization induced by stretch of the smooth muscle cell, which has been proposed to play an important role in myogenic reactivity and tone.[5,12]

Ca^{2+} sensitization mechanism

Using fluorescence Ca^{2+} indicators to measure intracellular Ca^{2+}, it has been revealed that the Ca^{2+} concentration does not necessarily parallel the degree of smooth muscle contraction.[13] Subsequent studies in permeabilized vascular smooth muscle showed that GTPγS and G-protein-coupled receptor agonists could increase contractile force without increasing intracellular Ca^{2+}.[14,15] The extent of MLC$_{20}$ phosphorylation or force of contraction induced by agonist stimulation is higher than that predicted by the actual Ca^{2+} concentration in the cell, the so-called Ca^{2+} sensitization. Thus, an additional mechanism of regulation that can modify the levels of MLC$_{20}$ phosphorylation and degree of contraction independently of Ca^{2+} concentration has been proposed. Most importantly, it is understood that the increased MLC$_{20}$ phosphorylation via a GTP-binding protein is due to the inhibition of MLC phosphatase rather than to activation of MLC kinase.[16,17] The small GTPase RhoA (a member of the Rho subfamily of the Ras superfamily of monomeric GTPases) and its effector Rho-associated kinase (Rho-kinase) are responsible for the Ca^{2+} sensitization induced by agonist stimulation and are thought to act by inhibiting MLCP activity.[18]

SIGNAL TRANSDUCTION REGULATING CA²⁺ SENSITIVITY

Until recently, the molecular mechanism by which RhoA regulates smooth muscle contraction was largely unknown. However, the signaling pathway that involves the downstream effector of RhoA (Rho-kinase) has been shown to play a crucial role in the Ca²⁺ sensitization of smooth muscle contraction.[19,20] Further, analyses using inhibitory probes specific for Rho-kinase have revealed that Rho-kinase-mediated Ca²⁺ sensitization is involved in a variety of cardiovascular diseases, suggesting that Rho-kinase could be a therapeutic target.[21]

Small Rho GTPases

Rho family GTPases function to control a multitude of cellular processes, including actin cytoskeletal rearrangements, cell movement, and smooth muscle contraction.[22,23] These proteins act as binary molecular switches that are turned on and off (i.e., cycle between an inactive GDP-bound and an active GTP-bound state) in response to a variety of stimuli. To become activated, RhoA must be targeted via its geranylgeranylated C-terminus to the membrane. In the GTP-bound active state, RhoA is conformationally primed to engage downstream effectors such as Rho-kinase in order to transduce signals that influence diverse biological responses. When the bound GTP is hydrolyzed to GDP, RhoA returns to the inactive basal state.[22]

Regulation of RhoA activity

Three classes of regulatory proteins are involved in balancing RhoA between the GTP-bound active and GDP-bound inactive states: (1) GTPase-activating proteins (GAPs), which act by negative regulation through increases in the intrinsic GTPase activity of RhoA to accelerate the return of the protein to the inactive state, (2) guanine nucleotide dissociation inhibitors (GDIs), which sequester the GDP-bound form of RhoA and regulate the intracellular localization of the protein by preventing binding to the membrane, and (3) Rho-specific guanine nucleotide exchange factors (GEFs), which stimulate the GTP-GDP exchange reaction (Figure 16–1).

RhoGDIs

Three isoforms of RhoGDI have been identified to date: the ubiquitously expressed RhoGDI$_\alpha$ (GDI1), the hematopoietic cell-selective RhoGDI$_\beta$ (GDI2), and RhoGDI$_\gamma$, which is restricted to lung, brain, and testis.[24,25] RhoGDI acts as an endogenous inhibitor for RhoA through two mechanisms: stabilizing RhoA in its inactive GDP-bound form, and translocating RhoA-GDP to the cytosol after extracting it from the membrane. Although RhoGDI is able to interact with both the GTP- and GDP-bound Rho, the binding of GDP to Rho increases the affinity for RhoGDI more than ten times.[26] Overexpression or exogenous administration of high concentrations of RhoGDI in tissues inhibits Rho-mediated biological activity.[27,28] In a cell-free system derived from rat kidney, RhoA is extracted from the brush border membrane after addition of a gluthatione S-trans-

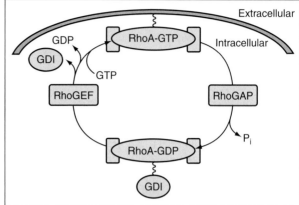

Figure 16–1. Regulation of RhoA activity. Rho GTPases function as molecular switches that control cell function by cycling between two interconvertible forms: a GDP-bound "inactive" form and a GTP-bound "active" form. In resting cells, the cytosolic inactive form of RhoA is complexed with RhoGDI (guanine nucleotide dissociation inhibitor). The rate-limiting step of the GDP/GTP exchange (which is the dissociation of GDP) is promoted by the association of a GEF (guanine nucleotide exchange factor), the activity of which may be regulated by an upstream signal such as the activation of heterotrimeric G-proteins. The GTP-bound form of RhoA is converted into the GDP-bound form due to its intrinsic GTPase activity, which is stimulated by a GAP (GTPase-activating protein).

ferase (GST)-GDI fusion protein.[29] The ability of RhoGDI to extract RhoA from the plasma membrane is not solely dependent on the exchange of nucleotide on RhoA. Phosphorylation of RhoA on Ser188 by cyclic AMP-dependent protein kinase (PKA) has been shown to increase the RhoA interaction with RhoGDI, even at the GTP-bound state.[30] Forskolin, an adenylyl cyclase activator, markedly reduces the amount of active RhoA in renal CD8 cells according to RhoA-GTP pull-down assay and Western blot analysis. Phosphorylation of RhoA and decreased membrane fraction of GDI by forskolin treatment lead to increased RhoGDI-RhoA complexes in the cytosol.[31] Transfection of human microvascular endothelial cells with adenovirus encoding the PKA inhibitor gene blocks the inhibitory effect of forskolin on RhoA.[32] These studies suggest that phosphorylation of RhoA is an alternative mechanism to inhibit RhoA activity, independently of its nucleotide-bound state.

RhoGEFs

RhoGEFs receive upstream signals that trigger the various signal transduction cascades that involve small GTP-binding proteins, and for that reason they are regarded as the main regulators of RhoA activity.[33,34] A group of RhoGEFs characterized by a unique motif resembling a "regulator of G-protein signaling" (RGS) domain at the N-terminal have been identified and these were shown to bind to the activated α-subunit of heterotrimeric G-proteins.[35] Currently, this group of RhoGEF proteins comprises three members: p115RhoGEF, PDZ-RhoGEF, and leukemia-associated RhoGEF (LARG). The RGS domain of these GEFs also functions as a GAP, accelerating G$_\alpha$-intrinsic GTPase activity.[36,37] Binding of G_α subunits to these proteins stimulates GEF activity toward RhoA, and as a consequence RhoGEFs operate as nodes connecting signal transduction cascades modulated by large and small GTPases.[33,35] It has been reported that $G_{\alpha12}$ and $G_{\alpha13}$ (the members of the G_{12} family) can physically associate with p115RhoGEF, PDZ-RhoGEF, and LARG.[38-40] Mutation of $G_{\alpha13}$ on residues Glu229, Lys204, or Arg232 attenuates the activation of p115RhoGEF and LARG—as well as the subsequent RhoA activation.[41,42] In addition, $G_{\alpha q}/G_{\alpha11}$ was also reported to activate RhoGEFs and thus lead to the activation of RhoA.[43,44]

These RhoGEFs, like other GEFs, contain a Dbl homology (DH) domain and a pleckstrin homology (PH) domain linked in tandem. Crystallographic studies provided the physical evidence that RhoGEFs directly interact with RhoA via both DH and PH domains.[45] The DH domain is thought to be responsible for catalyzing the nucleotide exchange reaction, whereas the PH domain may stabilize the binding of DH domain to RhoA and direct the subcellular localization of RhoA to the membrane, allowing RhoA to interact with actin.[46,47] In some cases, the PH domain can also modulate the nucleotide exchange activity of the DH domain.[48] Indeed, it has been demonstrated that the DH/PH domains of LARG catalyze nucleotide exchange more efficiently than the DH domain alone.[49] In their inactive state, the RGS domain and the DH domain have reciprocal inhibitory effects. When G_α is activated, the RGS domain of RhoGEF binds to G_α and exposes the DH domain (which is able to interact with RhoA and initiate nucleotide exchange).[35] It has also been demonstrated that p115RhoGEF mediates thrombin-induced cytoskeletal rearrangement, and a direct phosphorylation of p115RhoGEF by PKCα is observed within 1 minute of thrombin stimulation.[50] Inhibition of PKCα results in attenuation of thrombin-induced RhoA activation, suggesting that G_{12} and PKCα pathways may run in parallel to modulate RhoGEF activity.

RhoGAPs

The RhoGAP family is defined by the presence of a conserved RhoGAP domain in the primary sequences that consists of about 150 amino acids and shares at least 20% sequence identity with other family members. The RhoGAP domain is distinct from the GAP modules responsible for turning off other classes of GTPases (e.g., Ras, Ran, or ARF), and it is sufficient for the binding to GTP-bound Rho proteins and accelerating their GTPase activity.[51] RhoGAPs inhibit RhoA through enhancing the intrinsic rate of GTP hydrolysis, and thus active RhoA is converted into inactive RhoA-GDP. The basic mechanism of GTPase stimulation relies on the stabilization of the highly mobile switch regions and the transition state of the GTP-hydrolysis reaction by supplying a catalytic arginine to the active site.[52-55] This mechanism is predicted based on crystallographic studies demonstrating that Arg85 on RhoGAP engages the GTPase active site and stabilizes the transition state of the GTP hydrolysis.[56] Therefore, GAPs position the catalytically crucial Gln63 in an appropriate conformation toward a nucleophilic water molecule, which

hydrolyses GTP and neutralizes developing negative charges on the leaving group during the phosphoryl-transfer reaction. Replacement of this so-called "arginine finger" by an Ala greatly diminishes the catalytic capacity of the respective GAPs, which are still able to bind the GTPase with high affinity.[57-59] Several GAPs have been identified to selectively interact with Rho, such as Graf, p122RhoGAP, and p190RhoGAP.[60-62]

Measurement of RhoA activity

Activation of the RhoA protein is associated with the exchange of GDP for GTP and the translocation of the active GTP-bound RhoA from the cytosol to the membrane.[63,64] RhoA activation can therefore be assessed by both measurement of the amount of cellular GTP-RhoA and detection of the RhoA protein in membrane fractions by Western blot analysis. These approaches are commonly used for the assessment of RhoA activity.[63,65-67] The method used for measuring the amount of GTP-RhoA is based on the specific binding of GTP-RhoA (but not GDP-RhoA) to the RB domain of RhoA effectors.[68] The RB domain of rhotekin[68] and mDia[69] are used in this pull-down assay to precipitate active GTP-RhoA from protein extracts from cells or tissues. Activation of RhoA based on increased GTP binding has been more difficult to demonstrate, but a few groups have reported increased binding of radio-labeled guanine nucleotides to RhoA following receptor stimulation. Formylmethionylleucylphenylalanine (fMLP) increased both [^{32}P]GTP- and [^{32}P]GDP-bound RhoA in leukocytes.[70,71] [^{35}S]GTPγS binding to RhoA was increased in response to fMLP in leukocytes and in response to thrombin in rat aortic smooth muscle cells.[71,72] α_2-Adrenergic receptor stimulation increased [^{32}P]GTP binding to RhoA and decreased [^{32}P]GDP-RhoA binding in preadipocytes.[73] Expression of various constitutively activated G_α subunits of heterotrimeric G proteins in COS-7 cells has also been shown to increase RhoA-[^{32}P]GTP binding.[74]

Rho-associated kinase and MLC phosphorylation

The identification and functional analysis of RhoA effectors shed light on the signaling pathway linking RhoA to the regulation of the MLC phosphatase activity (i.e., the MLC_{20} phosphorylation level). As described previously, although RhoA may mediate Ca^{2+} sensitization an intact plasma membrane is required for this event because RhoA does not inhibit MLC phosphatase directly.[75] Following the demonstration that the membrane translocation of RhoA is temporally associated with Ca^{2+} sensitization,[65] and given that the active RhoA-GTP complex is presumably membrane bound whereas MLC phosphatase is cytosolic, a "diffusible cofactor" would be necessary to establish the signal transduction pathway. Rho-kinase was then identified as the downstream effector of RhoA mediating Ca^{2+} sensitization. Indeed, Rho-kinase is one of the best characterized RhoA effectors and exists in two isoforms: ROKα (also called ROCK2) and ROKβ (also known as p160ROCK or ROCK1).[76] In addition to Rho-kinase, several other proteins have been identified as effectors of Rho, including protein kinase N (PKN), rhophilin, rhotekin, citron, p140mDia, and citron kinase.[77,78] However, the roles of those effectors of Rho other than Rho-kinase remain to be examined.

Rho-kinases are serine/threonine protein kinases that contain an N-terminal catalytic kinase domain, a coiled-coil domain in the middle portion, and a putative C-terminal PH domain split by an insertion of a cystein-rich region.[76] The Rho-binding (RB) domain of Rho-kinase is localized in the C-terminal portion of the coiled-coil domain, and Rho-kinase activity is enhanced by binding GTP-RhoA.[76,79,80] The expression of Rho-kinase is accelerated by inflammatory stimuli (such as angiotensin II and IL-1β) through PKC/NF-κB pathway,[81] with a negative modulation by physiological concentrations of estrogen and a positive modulation by clinical concentrations of nicotine.[82] Remnant lipoproteins also upregulate Rho-kinase in human coronary vascular smooth muscle cells.[83] Indeed, mRNA expression of Rho-kinase is enhanced at the inflammatory and arteriosclerotic arterial lesions in animals[84,85] and humans,[86] causing hypercontraction of the artery.

The targets of Rho-kinase have been identified, and include the myosin-binding subunit (MBS) of myosin phosphatase, ERM (ezrin, radixin, moesin) family, adducin, intermediate filament (vimentin), Na^+-H^+ exchanger, and LIM-kinase1.[87] Among these, one of the main substrates of Rho-kinase is MLCP, which is physiologically responsible for the dephosphorylation of the MLC_{20} of myosin II. This phosphatase comprises three subunits: a 37-kDa phosphatase catalytic subunit, a 110- to 130-kDa myosin binding subunit (MBS)—also called myosin phosphatase target subunit (MYPT1)—and a 20-kDa subunit with unknown function.[88,89] MBS is ubiquitously expressed with a relatively higher concentration in smooth muscle cells. With the PP1c-binding domain on the N-terminal region and the myosin binding domain on the C-terminal region, MBS targets MLC phosphatase to the myosin filaments and increases the catalytic activity of PP1c.[90] Phosphorylation of MBS at Thr696 is believed to decrease PP1c catalytic activity, which inhibits MLC phosphatase and maintains the MLC_{20} phosphorylation level. Activated Rho-kinase phosphorylates the MBS to inhibit MLC phosphatase activity.[91] Therefore, Rho-kinase and MBS are believed to regulate the level of MLC_{20} phosphorylation cooperatively, and this regulatory mechanism plays important roles in a variety of cellular functions, particularly in smooth muscle contraction. Indeed, agonists such as prostaglandin $F_{2\alpha}$, lysophosphatidic acid, and angiotensin II have been shown to increase phosphorylation of MBS at Thr696 and to enhance Ca^{2+} sensitivity through activation of Rho-kinase.[91–93] In chicken amnion smooth muscle and rat tail artery, Rho-kinase inhibits MLC phosphatase through phosphorylation of MBS at Thr850 and thus reduces the binding of MLC phosphatase to MLC.[94–96]

TOOLS AND METHODS TO PROBE THE RHOA/RHO-KINASE PATHWAY

The C3 exoenzyme isolated from *Clostridium botulinum* is the most commonly used toxin for the examination of the functional role of RhoA because it specifically inhibits RhoA through ADP-ribosylation at Asn41 and has little effect on other proteins of the Rho family. The inhibition of RhoA by C3 exoenzyme is thought to block the dissociation of RhoA and RhoGDI complex and prevent the activation of RhoA by RhoGEF, in that the RhoA activators GTPγS and PIP_2 are unable to release RhoA from RhoGDI in the presence of C3.[97] ADP-ribosylation of RhoA does not appear to interfere with its nucleotide binding, RhoGTPase activity, or interaction with downstream effectors such as Rho-kinase.[63,97,98] On the other hand, cytotoxic necrotizing factors (CNF)-1 and -2 (first isolated from *Eschirichia coli*) have been shown to turn RhoA into a constitutively active form by deamidating Gln63 to Glu, which blocks the RhoGAP-increased GTP hydrolysis.[99,100] CNF-1 and -2 also affect other RhoGTPases, such as Rac and CDC42.[101] Recently, CNF_Y identified in *Yersinia pseudo-tuberculosis* strains has been demonstrated to selectively activate RhoA without activation of Rac or CDC42.[102] The kinase activity-deficient form of Rho-kinase or the C-terminal fragments that lack the kinase activity should theoretically serve as the dominant-negative form of Rho-kinase in cells.[19] Thus, the C-terminal fragment of Rho-kinase that contains the RB domain—deficient in Rho-binding activity after point mutations and the PH domain [RB/PH(TT)]—serves as the dominant-negative form that specifically inhibits Rho-kinase.[19,85]

Several compounds have been developed and reported to specifically inhibit Rho-kinase activity in an ATP competitive manner. As a result, the availability of specific Rho-kinase inhibitors has enabled the evaluation of the physiological roles of Rho-kinase in vascular smooth muscle. The pyridine derivative Y-27632 ((R)-(+)-*trans*-N-(4-pyridyl)-4-(1-aminoethyl)-cyclohexanecarboxamide), a highly selective inhibitor of Rho-kinase, has proved to be a useful pharmacological tool to examine the role of Rho-kinase in various cellular functions.[103] It competes for the ATP binding site on Rho-kinase, thus preventing the Rho-kinase-mediated phosphorylation of MLC phosphatase and resulting in relaxation of smooth muscle. Y-27632 is transported into cells by a carrier-facilitated diffusion mechanism to inhibit Rho-kinase activity. Therefore, the extracellular concentration of Y-27632 is similar to the intracellular concentration. The K_i value of Y-27632 for Rho-kinase is approximately 200-fold lower than that for other protein kinases involved in smooth muscle contractility, such as PKC, PKA, and MLC kinase.[103,104] Although Y-27632 is relatively less selective for the Ca^{2+}-dependent PKC isoforms, it is a potent inhibitor of the Ca^{2+}-independent PKCδ and PKCε isoforms, which have been shown to mediate Ca^{2+} sensitization.[104,105] Y-27632 has minimal effects on intracellular Ca^{2+} at the low micromolar range, whereas it significantly inhibits the rise of cytosolic Ca^{2+} levels at higher concentrations.[106–109]

Another family of compounds derived from isoquinolinesulfonamide shows selectivity for Rho-kinase. The compound HA-1077, or fasudil hydrochloride ((5-isoquinolinesulfonyl)homopiperazine)— with a K_i value of 0.3 μM—also competes for the ATP binding site on Rho-kinase. However, HA-1077 is also a potent inhibitor of PKA and PKC—with K_i values of approximately 1 μM and 9.3 μM, respectively.[110] It has been recently demonstrated that hydroxyfasudil, a major active metabolite of fasudil after oral administration, has a more specific inhibitory effect on Rho-kinase.[111,112] The K_i value of hydroxyfasudil is 0.17 μM for Rho-kinase, 18 μM for PKC, and 140 μM for MLC kinase.[111] The compound H-1152 ((S)-(+)-2-methyl-1-[(4-methyl-5-isoquinolinyl)sulfonyl] homopiperazine) is similar in structure to fasudil, with the exception of two extra methyl groups, which significantly enhance its inhibitory effect and selectivity for Rho-kinase. Its K_i value for Rho-kinase is approximately 1.6 nM, which makes this compound 400 times more potent to inhibit Rho-kinase among other kinases, such as PKA, PKC, and MLC kinase.[113]

The biological activities of RhoA and Rho-kinase can also be manipulated by overexpression of constitutively active and dominant-negative mutants of RhoA or Rho-kinase as well as the RhoGTPase regulators. The dominant-negative RhoA (T19NRhoA) is generated by substitution of Asp for Thr at position 19, which leads to increased affinity for RhoGEF and decreased GTP binding—competing with exogenous RhoA for RhoGEF.[114] The substitution of Leu for Glu at position 63 results in a constitutively active RhoA (V14RhoA). Rho-kinase dominant-negative and active mutants are also used to investigate RhoA/Rho-kinase-mediated Ca^{2+} sensitization.[115,116] Recently, small-interference RNA (siRNA) has emerged as a new powerful tool to selectively silence the expression of the target gene. This post-transcriptional gene silencing by these 21 to 25 nucleotides leads to degradation of target mRNAs. Anti-RhoA siRNA has been reported to successfully knock down RhoA expression in cells.[117,118]

RHO-KINASE AND VASCULAR SMOOTH MUSCLE CONTRACTION

Agonists (norepinephrine, endothelin, thromboxane, and so on) that bind to G-protein-coupled receptors produce contraction by increasing both the cytosolic Ca^{2+} concentration and the Ca^{2+} sensitivity of the contractile apparatus (Figure 16–2).[119] The increased sensitivity toward Ca^{2+} results from inhibition of MLC phosphatase activity, leading to increased MLC_{20} phosphorylation and tension at a constant Ca^{2+} concentration. This Ca^{2+}-sensitizing effect is ascribed to the activation of RhoA that stimulates Rho-kinase, which in turn phosphorylates the regulatory subunit of MLC phosphatase and inhibits its activity.[19,20,119] Y-27632 has been widely used to inhibit Rho-kinase and was originally developed as a relaxant of vascular smooth muscle. This compound completely inhibits agonist-induced contraction of both intact and permeabilized strips of vascular smooth muscle.[104] In addition, the Rho-kinase inhibitor fasudil antagonizes contractions of rabbit aortic smooth muscle in response to prostaglandin $F_{2\alpha}$ ($PGF_{2\alpha}$), which has been shown to comprise a Ca^{2+}-sensitizing mechanism characterized by the inhibition of MLC_{20} dephosphorylation through Rho-kinase-induced MBS phosphorylation.[93]

Smooth muscle cells, especially in the smaller arteries and arterioles, are intrinsically active—and this myogenic responsiveness plays a key role in blood flow control and regulation of peripheral resistance. Although an increase in intracellular Ca^{2+} is necessary for the initiation of myogenic responsiveness, a major component of myogenic activation results from an increase in Ca^{2+} sensitivity—as demonstrated by the ability of Y-27632 to suppress myogenic tone without significant changes in the intracellular Ca^{2+} levels.[120] In addition, it has been shown that ROKα is expressed in mesenteric and celiac arteries, contributing to the control of perfusion pressure.[121,122] These studies underlie the physiological importance of the RhoA/Rho-kinase signaling pathway in the maintenance of microvascular constriction and ultimately in the control of vascular resistance.

With regard to the involvement of Rho-kinase in the regulation of Ca^{2+} sensitivity in human arteries, Y-27632 has been demonstrated to strongly relax agonist-induced but not KCl-induced contraction.[123] In addition, the relaxation produced by Y-27632 was not dependent on a decrease in cytosolic Ca^{2+}, suggesting that a Rho-kinase-associated pathway is involved in agonist-induced Ca^{2+} sensitization of human small omental arteries.[123] Several additional reports demonstrate that the RhoA/Rho-kinase signaling plays a key role in agonist-induced contraction of other types of smooth muscle, including cerebral arteries, coronary artery, and pulmonary vasculature.[124-126] Recently, the increase in intracellular Ca^{2+} concentrations induced by either membrane depolarization or receptor stimulation has been shown to activate the RhoA/Rho-kinase pathway in vascular smooth muscle and thus contribute to the regulation of Ca^{2+} sensitivity.[106-109] However, the upstream signaling pathways that regulate the mechanism of Ca^{2+}-mediated activation of RhoA and the identification of the GEF involved, if any, still remain largely unidentified.

As illustrated previously, several studies have helped to clarify the biochemical basis for the regulation of MLC_{20} phosphorylation and dephosphorylation, which coordinate the degree of contraction in the vascular smooth muscle. The involvement of the RhoA/Rho-kinase signaling pathway in the regulation of the Ca^{2+} sensitivity, and to a certain extent of Ca^{2+} handling, is at present evident. However, the intracellular signal transduction that connects the contractile stimulation to such molecular networks regulating the Ca^{2+} sensitivity has yet to be revealed. Hence, even though several reports have discussed the involvement of the RhoA/Rho-kinase pathway in the regulation of the vascular tone and Ca^{2+} sensitivity it remains to be elucidated as to how this pathway is activated by the contractile stimuli that cause Ca^{2+} sensitization.

REGULATION OF THE RHOA/RHO-KINASE PATHWAY BY NO

Relaxation of vascular smooth muscle results from a decrease in cytosolic Ca^{2+} concentration and/or reduced Ca^{2+} sensitivity of the contractile apparatus. Physiologically released

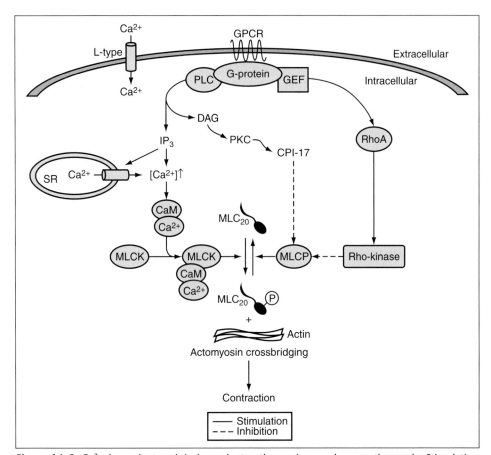

Figure 16–2. Ca^{2+}-dependent and -independent pathways in vascular smooth muscle. Stimulation of G-protein-coupled receptors (GPCR) leads to stimulation of phospholipase C (PLC), which catalyzes the formation of inositol 1,4,5-triphosphate (IP_3) and diacylglycerol (DAG). IP_3 activates receptors located on the sarcoplasmic reticulum (SR), causing Ca^{2+} release and subsequent increases in intracellular Ca^{2+} concentration. Following binding to calmodulin (CaM), the Ca^{2+}/CaM complex stimulates the myosin light-chain kinase (MLCK), which phosphorylates the myosin light chain (MLC20) and results in smooth muscle contraction. Opening of L-type Ca^{2+} channels due to membrane depolarization also causes intracellular Ca^{2+} to increase and elicit contraction. After activation by DAG, protein kinase C (PKC) phosphorylates the PKC-potentiated inhibitor protein of 17 kDa (CPI-17), which decreases myosin phosphatase (MLCP) activity through phosphorylation. Activation of GPCR also stimulates RhoA activity, secondary to the stimulation of a Rho guanine nucleotide exchange factors (GEFs). The activated RhoA stimulates Rho-kinase, which in turn phosphorylates the myosin binding subunit of MLCP—leading to increased MLC20 phosphorylation in a Ca^{2+}-independent manner. This process is hence referred to as Ca^{2+} sensitization.

endothelium-derived nitric oxide (NO) elevates cGMP, the second messenger responsible for relaxation of vascular smooth muscle and subsequently enlargement of the vessel lumen.[127] Cyclic GMP-induced relaxation involves activation of the cGMP-dependent protein kinase (cGK). The potent vasodilator action of the NO/cGMP pathway has been ascribed to a decrease in cytosolic Ca^{2+} through activation of multiple mechanisms, which might involve reduced IP_3 synthesis, inhibition of Ca^{2+} release from IP_3-sensitive stores, or phosphorylation of Ca^{2+} and K^+ channels.[128] In addition, the NO/cGMP signaling pathway has been demonstrated to phosphorylate recombinant RhoA via cGK at Ser188,[66] which results in inhibition of RhoA-induced stress fiber formation. In addition, the NO donor sodium nitroprusside and constitutively active cGK

were shown to inhibit the phenylephrine-induced translocation of RhoA from the cytosolic to the membrane fraction in rat aorta, indicating that the NO/cGMP pathway mediates inactivation of RhoA.[66] Indeed, endogenous NO-induced vasorelaxation has also been demonstrated to be mediated in part by inhibition of RhoA/Rho-kinase signaling in rat aorta and celiac artery.[122,129] Another study demonstrated that NOS inhibition in intact rats enhances α_2-adrenoreceptor-stimulated RhoA/Rho-kinase in isolated aortic segments. Acute and chronic NOS inhibition augmented sensitivity to Y-27632-induced relaxation in α_2-adrenoreceptor-constricted aorta, supporting the concept that the inhibitory effect of NO on RhoA/Rho-kinase signaling is less active in chronic NOS-inhibited hypertensive aorta.[130]

RHOA/RHO-KINASE SIGNALING IN CARDIOVASCULAR DISEASES

The contractile state of vascular smooth muscle controls the vessel lumen size, and an abnormal increase in vascular smooth muscle tone is involved in the pathogenesis of vascular diseases. Consequently, a better understanding of the molecular mechanism regulating vascular tone is crucial to establish new strategies for the prevention and management of vascular diseases, such as hypertension and atherosclerosis. Increased vascular resistance is centrally involved in the pathogenesis of hypertension, but the molecular mechanisms leading to increased resistance are not well defined. Alteration of RhoA/Rho-kinase-mediated regulation of vascular tone has attracted considerable attention because it emerges as a potential cause of increased vascular resistance. For that purpose, pathological as well as physiological roles of Rho-kinase have been evaluated using the aforementioned Rho-kinase inhibitors.[21]

Hypertension

In spontaneously hypertensive rats (SHRs), agonist-induced Ca^{2+} sensitization was found to be enhanced, and both expression and activity of Rho-kinase are elevated even before the development of hypertension.[131] Administration of Y-27632 preferentially reduced systemic blood pressure in various rat models of systemic hypertension irrespective of the mechanisms of hypertension.[104] On the other hand, comparable doses of Y-27632 did not significantly affect blood pressure in normotensive animals, suggesting that the RhoA/Rho-kinase pathway is substantially involved in the pathogenesis of hypertension. Application of Rho-kinase inhibitors or dominant-negative Rho-kinase into the nucleus tractus solitarii causes sustained decrease in heart rate and blood pressure in SHRs but not in normotensive Wistar-Kyoto (WKY) rats, suggesting that Rho-kinase may also be involved in the regulation of central mechanisms of hypertension.[93]

The precise mechanisms for the activation of the RhoA-Rho-kinase signaling pathway in vascular smooth muscle in hypertensive models have not been fully determined. In this regard, molecular and functional studies have addressed the contribution of the RhoA-Rho-kinase signaling pathway in vascular smooth muscle cells as well as in ring segments obtained from hypertensive animals. The finding that Y-27632-induced dilation of the basilar artery *in vivo* is enhanced during chronic hypertension provided evidence that basal Rho-kinase activity may be enhanced in the cerebral circulation in this disease.[132] Interestingly, angiotensin II has been recently shown to elicit constriction of isolated basilar arteries via Rho-kinase signaling, an effect that may be enhanced during chronic hypertension.[133] Conversely, no apparent role for RhoA or Rho-kinase has been demonstrated in altered carotid artery contractility observed during chronic angiotensin-II-induced hypertension,[134] reflecting signaling differences between vascular beds. RhoA activation is usually detected in the aortae of various hypertensive rat models—namely, stroke-prone spontaneously hypertensive rats (SHRSP), L-NAME-treated rats, renal hypertensive rats, and DOCA-salt rats—where

it is not in normotensive controls.[135,136] The increased levels of active RhoA could be ascribed to either a shift in the balance of GDP-RhoA/GTP-RhoA or to increased expression of RhoA in the hypertensive state. For example, both the activation of RhoA and the resultant phosphorylation of MBS at Thr696 by Rho-kinase were enhanced when compared to WKY in aortic smooth muscle cells isolated from SHRSP,[136] suggesting an increased activity of this pathway in this hypertensive model.

Although some reports have shown increased expression and activation of RhoA and the upregulation of Rho-kinase RNA, others have detected no significant differences in the expression of the molecular components of this pathway.[135,136] It is likely that alterations in the RhoA-Rho-kinase pathway could be consequential to a causative upstream event in the hypertensive state. In this scenario, the demonstration of increased mRNA expression of the three RGS-containing RhoGEFs (PDZ-RhoGEF, LARG, and p115RhoGEF) in the aortas from 12-week-old SHRSP (REFS), in a stage where mean systolic blood pressure was higher (187 ± 5 mmHg) when compared to normotensive WKY rats (126 ± 2 mmHg), suggests that the activation of RhoA is a consequence rather than a cause of hypertension.[137]

Intra-arterial administration of fasudil induced marked vasodilator responses of the forearm circulation (along with a decrease in vascular resistance) in hypertensive patients compared with normotensive control subjects, whereas those in response to sodium nitroprusside were similar between the two groups.[138] This suggests that Rho-kinase is also implicated in the increased peripheral vascular resistance observed in human hypertension. It remains to be elucidated whether long-term inhibition of Rho-kinase also alleviates hypertensive vascular disease or cardiac hypertrophy in humans.

Coronary vasospasm

Coronary vasospasm plays an important role in a wide variety of ischemic heart diseases, not only in variant angina but in other forms of angina pectoris, myocardial infarction, and sudden death.[139] Experimental studies using a porcine model of coronary vasospasm have demonstrated evidence for an involvement of Rho-kinase in this disorder, whereby both arterial spasm and the associated increase in MBS phosphorylation are sensitive to Y-27632.[84] Furthermore, increased Rho-kinase mRNA expression is localized to the spastic site of the artery. Gene transfer of dominant-negative Rho-kinase has also been found to abolish coronary vasospasm, as well as to decrease the phosphorylation levels of ERM proteins (which are known downstream targets of Rho-kinase).[115] In addition, direct PKC activation has been shown to induce coronary spasm, which was attenuated by hydroxyfasudil and associated with increased levels of membrane-bound RhoA.[140] This was the first study to suggest an interaction between PKC and RhoA/Rho-kinase in coronary artery spasm, with RhoA/Rho-kinase presumably located downstream of PKC in the signaling pathway. Thus, Rho-kinase may represent a more specific and therefore preferable target for the treatment of coronary vasospasm.

In other studies, long-term treatment with a nonhypotensive dose of fasudil significantly suppressed coronary vascular lesion formation in SHRs,[141] strongly indicating that Rho-kinase is also involved in the pathogenesis of hypertensive vascular disease (which is distinct from that of systemic hypertension). The therapeutic effects of fasudil were also studied in a rat model with long-term infusion of angiotensin II, which is also characterized by hypertension and coronary vascular lesions. Similarly, fasudil significantly suppressed the coronary vascular lesion formation and improved the endothelial vasodilator function along with a decrease in the endothelial production of superoxide anions.[112]

In patients with vasospastic angina pectoris, intracoronary fasudil markedly inhibited acetylcholine-induced coronary spasm as well as the related myocardial ischemia, suggesting that Rho-kinase is largely involved in the pathogenesis of coronary spasm in humans.[142] In addition, fasudil is effective in treating patients with microvascular angina, indicating an involvement of Rho-kinase-mediated hyperreactivity of coronary microvessels.[143] Clinical trials on the antianginal effects of fasudil in patients with stable effort angina have demonstrated that the long-term oral treatment with the Rho-kinase inhibitor is effective in ameliorating exercise tolerance in patients with adequate safety profiles.[144] Furthermore, fasudil is useful for the treatment of intractable coronary spasm resistant to maximal vasodilator therapy with calcium channel blockers and nitrates after coronary artery bypass surgery.[145]

Cerebral vasospasm

Cerebral vasospasm is a potentially fatal complication that can occur when major cerebral arteries are exposed to clotted blood following subarachnoid hemorrhage (SAH). The involvement of Rho-kinase in cerebral vasospasm was first demonstrated in a canine model of SAH where spasm and associated enhanced phosphorylation of both MLC and MBS in the basilar artery were inhibited by Y-27632.[146] Increased expression of both RhoA and Rho-kinase mRNA have also been detected in rat basilar artery following SAH,[147] which may account for the apparent enhanced activity of this pathway during SAH. More recently, increased phosphorylation of MLC phosphatase was reported in basilar arteries of rabbits after SAH—and increased vasoconstriction to serotonin was found to be markedly reduced by fasudil[148]—suggesting that augmented Rho-kinase activity contributes to the exaggerated cerebral artery contractility following SAH.

Oxyhemoglobin is a central candidate as a mediator of cerebral vasospasm after SAH, in that it is a constrictor released during clot lysis. Y-27632, fasudil, and the PKC inhibitor Ro-32-0432 have been reported to relax rabbit basilar arteries precontracted with oxyhemoglobin. In addition, oxyhemoglobin also induces the translocation of RhoA (as well as PKCα and PKCε) in cultured cerebrovascular smooth muscle cells and intact basilar arteries.[149] Taken together, these observations support the notion that oxyhemoglobin may elicit cerebral artery spasm through the activation of both the RhoA/Rho-kinase and the PKC signaling pathways.[150]

Atherosclerosis

Atherosclerosis is characterized by vascular abnormalities including endothelial dysfunction, poor availability of NO, and inflammation. The first evidence for a link between RhoA/Rho-kinase signaling and regulation of NO production was the observation that RhoA can negatively regulate endothelial NO synthase (eNOS) mRNA expression in cultured human endothelial cells.[151] More recent studies have demonstrated that Rho-kinase may contribute to the regulation of the expression of plasminogen activator inhibitor-1 (PAI-1), whose increased production is thought to contribute to the development of atherosclerosis. For example, Y-27632 and dominant-negative Rho-kinase have both been shown to prevent angiotensin-II-induced increases in PAI-1 mRNA expression.[152,153] In addition, chronic administration of Y-27632 decreases atherosclerotic plaque size and inflammatory cell accumulation within atherosclerotic plaques in mice,[154] providing the first direct link between Rho-kinase and atherosclerotic lesion formation.

A recent report showed that thrombin stimulation of endothelial cells can lead to increased arginase activity, which in turn competes with eNOS for the substrate L-arginine and limiting NO production. Inhibition of RhoA or Rho-kinase has been reported to prevent the thrombin-evoked increases in arginase activity, whereas constitutively active RhoA or Rho-kinase could enhance enzyme activity.[155] Higher RhoA expression and arginase activity were also found in atherosclerotic aortae of apoE-deficient mice, thus introducing the concept that by increasing arginase activity the RhoA/Rho-kinase signaling pathway may suppress NO production and lead to endothelial dysfunction and atherosclerosis. Another mechanism linking RhoA/Rho-kinase to vascular NO production is the inhibition of endothelial Rho-kinase that increases phosphatidylinositol 3-kinase (PI3K) activity and phosphorylated Akt, resulting in enhanced NO production.[156,157] These findings raise the possibility that Rho-kinase may tonically inhibit PI3K activity in the endothelium and the consequent NO production.

Both *in vivo* gene transfer of dominant-negative Rho-kinase[158] and long-term treatment with a Rho-kinase inhibitor[159,160] have also been shown to suppress balloon-injury-induced neointimal formation in animals *in vivo*. Long-term treatment with MCP-1 and oxidized low-density lipoproteins (ox-LDL) causes vascular lesions characterized by neointimal formation and constrictive remodeling in porcine coronary arteries *in vivo*. Long-term oral treatment with fasudil significantly suppressed this vascular lesion formation, caused at least in part by the inhibition of macrophage migration *in vivo*.[161]

Pulmonary hypertension

Primary pulmonary arterial hypertension is a fatal disease characterized by endothelial dysfunction, vascular smooth muscle cell hypercontraction and proliferation, and inflammatory cell migration, in which Rho-kinase may also be substantially involved. Long-term treatment with fasudil suppresses the development of monocrotaline-induced pulmonary hypertension in rats when started simultaneously with (and even induces a marked regression when started after) establishment of pulmonary hypertension.[162] Inhalation of fasudil may also be effective in reducing pulmonary vascular resistance in animal models of pulmonary hypertension with various etiologies.[163] Because prostacyclin lacks inhibitory effects on Rho-kinase, a combination therapy with prostacyclin and a Rho-kinase inhibitor may provide a useful therapeutic strategy for this fatal disorder.[164] Intravenous infusion of fasudil significantly reduces pulmonary vascular resistance in patients with pulmonary hypertension, indicating an involvement of Rho-kinase pathway in the pathogenesis of pulmonary hypertension in humans.[165]

Stroke

In a rat model of stroke (lacunar infarction) caused by pharmacological damage of endothelial cells and subsequent thrombotic occlusion, intraperitoneal administration of fasudil shortly after the endothelial damage reduces cerebral infarct size and resultant neurological deficit.[166] In a rat model of microembolization stroke, intravenous administration of hydroxyfasudil prevents neutrophil accumulation, reduces cerebral infarct size, and improves neurological functions,[167] suggesting the efficacy of fasudil/hydroxyfasudil for the treatment of ischemic brain damage. A clinical trial with an intravenous form of fasudil in the acute phase of stroke demonstrates that the Rho-kinase inhibitor exerts beneficial effects on ischemic neuronal damage without serious adverse effects.[168]

Heart failure

In a dog model of tachypacing-induced heart failure, the Ca^{2+}-sensitizing mechanism of conduit artery (femoral artery) is augmented, resulting in the enhanced vasoconstrictor response to norepinephrine. Treatment with Y-27632 attenuates this response without a significant change in intracellular Ca^{2+} concentrations in the vascular smooth muscle cells, suggesting an involvement of the RhoA/Rho-kinase pathway in the increased vasoconstrictor response in heart failure.[169] In patients with heart failure, intra-arterial infusion of fasudil causes a preferential increase in forearm blood flow compared with control subjects, suggesting an involvement of the Rho-kinase pathway in the increased peripheral vascular resistance in heart failure in humans.[170]

RHO-KINASE INHIBITORS FOR THE TREATMENT OF CARDIOVASCULAR DISEASE

Small molecule inhibitors are extremely useful for dissecting complex cellular events that require that coordination and regulation of many proteins. By inhibiting a specific component of a biochemical network, one can deduce its function in the process. Following G-protein-coupled receptors, protein kinases have become the second most important class of targets for drug discovery over the last 20 years. Although only four kinase inhibitors have reached the market to date (Fasudil for Rho-kinase,

Rapamycin for TOR, Gleevec for BCR-Abl, and Iressa for EGFR), many more are already in clinical development.

Fasudil was approved in 1995 for the treatment of cerebral vasospasm, a painful and potentially deadly result of subarachnoid hemorrhage. This drug has significant vasodilatory activity[171] and is currently undergoing clinical trials for the treatment of angina pectoris.[144] Fasudil has a heptameric homopiperazine ring at the position of the methyl-piperazine ring of H7, and further derivitization of fasudil led to H-1152—with two additional methyl groups, one at the isoquinoline ring and the other at the homopiperazine ring. H-1152 has a better inhibitory profile than fasudil and Y-27632, with an IC_{50} value for Rho-kinase in the low nanomolar range and a reportedly enhanced selectivity (Figure 16–3).[113]

The common feature of all protein kinases is the ATP binding at highly conserved binding interactions at the ATP binding site. The prevalence of cardiovascular diseases associated with Rho-kinase dysregulation underscores the need for therapeutic Rho-kinase inhibitors, with the caveat that they must be highly selective for their dysregulated targets to avoid inhibition of other ubiquitous kinases—in that most protein kinase inhibitors are ATP competitive and as such should be tested rigorously for cross-reactivity with other kinases. The effects of fasudil are attributed to

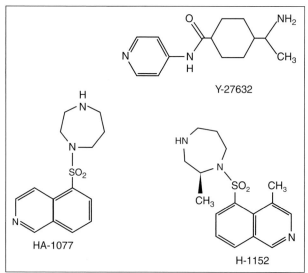

Figure 16–3. Structures of Rho-kinase inhibitors.
Several inhibitors with a relatively high degree of specificity toward Rho-kinase have been developed over the past few years. The most widely used is Y-27632, which inhibits agonist-induced contraction of vascular smooth muscle and shows efficacy in normalizing high blood pressure in different rat models of hypertension. This is therefore a potential therapeutic drug. This drug was originally reported to inhibit the two isoforms of Rho-kinase, and to exert its antihypertensive effect by preventing Rho-kinase from inhibiting myosin phosphatase. Such an effect causes a decrease in MLC20 phosphorylation and vascular smooth muscle relaxation, and hence dilation of blood vessels. The compound HA-1077, also known as fasudil hydrochloride, shows efficacy for the treatment of cerebral vasospasm and causes vasodilation of the forearm circulation in hypertensive patients. H-1152 is a parent molecule of the latter compound and is a novel inhibitor showing higher selectivity and potency in inhibiting Rho-kinase.

inhibition of Rho-kinase,[79] although its *in vitro* activity is not strictly limited to Rho-kinase because other protein kinases (such as PKA, PRK2, MSK1, and S6K1) are also inhibited by fasudil, although to a lesser extent.[172] Likewise, Y-27632 and the close molecule Y-32885 inhibit PRK2 and Rho-kinase at similar concentrations.[172]

Recently, a large number of structurally unrelated scaffolds of Rho-kinase inhibitors have been designed using pharmacophore information obtained from the results of high-throughput screening and structural information from a homology model of Rho-kinase. Consequently, potent platforms for developing Rho-kinase inhibitors (such as pyridine, 1H-indazole, isoquinoline, and phthalimide) were identified using a docking simulation based on the ligand-binding pocket of Rho-kinase. Thus, potent and selective Rho-kinase inhibitors were obtained with little cross-reactivity against other kinases, such as MAP kinase, PKA, PKC, and some receptor tyrosine kinases.[173]

The development of cell-permeant Rho-kinase inhibitors has great advantages for the study of signaling transduction, in that they can be rapidly used to assess the physiological roles of Rho-kinase in cells and tissues. Inhibition of the endogenous enzyme avoids the need for overexpression of dominant-negative and constitutively active Rho-kinase, which can cause the specificity of signaling to lead to erroneous conclusions. Although fasudil is the only clinically available Rho-kinase inhibitor at present with minimal adverse effects so far, careful development of more selective and potent Rho-kinase inhibitors is needed because clinical studies suggest that Rho-kinase inhibition may be useful for the treatment of a wide spectrum of cardiovascular diseases—including angina pectoris, hypertension, and heart failure. Therefore, the availability of potent and selective Rho-kinase inhibitors is extremely useful in helping to delineate their pharmacological profile, safety, and therapeutic potential in the treatment of cardiovascular disorders.

PERSPECTIVES

Much has been learned in the past several years about the involvement of the RhoA/Rho-kinase pathway in a variety of cardiovascular diseases, although many aspects of signaling upstream and downstream of this pathway remain unclear. In various animal models, Rho-kinase inhibitors can be used to treat these diseases. These findings make the RhoA/Rho-kinase-mediated signaling pathway a promising new target for therapeutic interventions in diseases as common as hypertension. The near future will probably bring an increasing number of clinical trials to evaluate new strategies aiming at the inhibition of RhoA/Rho-kinase pathway with Rho-kinase inhibitors or gene-therapeutic approaches. It remains unclear whether the disorders associated with the RhoA/Rho-kinase pathway observed in animal models are indeed applicable to human patients. Studies aiming to elucidate the role of Rho-kinase in the pathogenesis of cardiovascular diseases have already been started, and more studies are needed to confirm the potential therapeutic importance and clinical usefulness of Rho-kinase inhibitors. Nevertheless, Rho-kinase is widely expressed in the organism and although the clinical trials with fasudil demonstrated its efficacy and safety profile in humans this should be interpreted with cautious optimism. RhoGEFs receive the upstream signals that trigger the various signal transduction cascades that involve small GTP-binding proteins. Therefore, the ability to block them specifically could be useful as a therapeutic intervention for the treatment of hypertension. The suitability of this family of RGS-containing RhoGEFs as therapeutic targets represents a daunting task, basically due to the limited knowledge about their role in physiologic and pathophysiologic processes in the cardiovascular system. Further, the mechanisms of regulation and the cellular contexts within which they act still need to be elucidated. How each RhoGEF interacts with RhoA in a tightly regulated manner poses the major challenge of this field. The revelation of the nature of this interaction may then provide the basic framework for developing novel therapeutic strategies for treating hypertension.

ACKNOWLEDGMENTS

This study was supported by grants from the National Institutes of Health (HL-71138, HL-74167). Cleber E. Teixeira is funded by a postdoctoral fellowship (No. 0425437B) from the American Heart Association (Southeast Affiliate).

REFERENCES

1. Somlyo AV, Somlyo AP. Intracellular signaling in vascular smooth muscle. *Adv Exp Med Biol* 1993;346:31–8.

2. Kamm KE, Stull JT. The function of myosin and myosin light chain kinase phosphorylation in smooth muscle. *Annu Rev Pharmacol Toxicol* 1985;25:593–620.

3. Hai CM, Murphy RA. Ca²⁺, crossbridge phosphorylation, and contraction. *Annu Rev Physiol* 1989;51:285–98.

4. Barany M, Barany K. Protein phosphorylation during contraction and relaxation. In: Barany M (ed.). *Biochemistry of Smooth Muscle Contraction.* San Diego, CA: Academic Press, 1996;321–39.

5. Davis MJ, Hill MA. Signaling mechanisms underlying the vascular myogenic response. *Physiol Rev* 1999;79:387–423.

6. Himpens B, Missiaen L, Casteels R. Ca²⁺ homeostasis in vascular smooth muscle. *J Vasc Res* 1995;32:207–19.

7. Kasai Y, Yamazawa T, Sakurai T, Taketani Y, Iino M. Endothelium-dependent frequency modulation of Ca²⁺ signaling in individual vascular smooth muscle cells of the rat. *J Physiol* 1997;504:349–57.

8. Wier WG, Morgan KG. α₁-Adrenergic signaling mechanisms in contraction of resistance arteries. *Rev Physiol Biochem Pharmacol* 2003;150:91–139.

9. Somlyo AP, Somlyo AV. Signal transduction by G-proteins, rho-kinase and protein phosphatase to smooth muscle and non-muscle myosin II. *J Physiol* 2000;522:177–85.

10. Way KJ, Chou E, King GL. Identification of PKC-isoform-specific biological actions using pharmacological approaches. *Trends Pharmacol Sci* 2000;21:181–87.

11. Brose N, Rosenmund C. Move over protein kinase C, you've got company: Alternative cellular effectors of diacylglycerol and phorbol esters. *J Cell Sci* 2002;115:4399–411.

12. Moosmang S, Schulla V, Welling A, Feil R, Feil S, Wegener JW, et al. Dominant

role of smooth muscle L-type calcium channel Cav1.2 for blood pressure regulation. *EMBO J* 2003;22:6027–34.

13. Bradley AB, Morgan KG. Alterations in cytoplasmic calcium sensitivity during porcine coronary artery contractions as detected by aequorin. *J Physiol* 1987;385:437–48.

14. Nishimura J, Kolber M, van Breemen C. Norepinephrine and GTPγS increase myofilament Ca^{2+} sensitivity in α-toxin permeabilized arterial smooth muscle. *Biochem Biophys Res Commun* 1988;157:677–83.

15. Fujiwara T, Itoh T, Kubota Y, Kuriyama H. Effects of guanosine nucleotides on skinned smooth muscle tissue of the rabbit mesenteric artery. *J Physiol* 1989;408:535–47.

16. Kitazawa T, Gaylinn BD, Denney GH, Somlyo AP. G-protein-mediated Ca^{2+} sensitization of smooth muscle contraction through myosin light chain phosphorylation. *J Biol Chem* 1991;266:1708–15.

17. Kitazawa T, Masuo M, Somlyo AP. G protein-mediated inhibition of myosin light-chain phosphatase in vascular smooth muscle. *Proc Natl Acad Sci USA* 1991;88:9307–10.

18. Noda M, Yasuda-Fukazawa C, Moriishi K, Kato T, Okuda T, Kurokawa K, et al. GTPγS-induced enhancement of phosphorylation of 20 kDa myosin light chain in vascular smooth muscle cells: Inhibition of phosphatase activity. *FEBS Lett* 1995;367:246–50.

19. Fukata Y, Amano M, Kaibuchi K. Rho-Rho-kinase pathway in smooth muscle contraction and cytoskeletal reorganization of non-muscle cells. *Trends Pharmacol Sci* 2001;22:32–9.

20. Somlyo AP, Somlyo AV. Ca^{2+} sensitivity of smooth muscle and nonmuscle myosin II modulated by G proteins, kinases, and myosin phosphatase. *Physiol Rev* 2003;83:1325–58.

21. Wettschureck N, Offermanns S. Rho/Rho-kinase mediated signaling in physiology and pathophysiology. *J Mol Med* 2002;80:629–38.

22. Etienne-Manneville S, Hall A. Rho GTPases in cell biology. *Nature* 2002;420:629–35.

23. Sorokina EM, Chernoff J. Rho-GTPases: New members, new pathways. *J Cell Biochem* 2005;94:225–31.

24. Olofsson B. Rho guanine dissociation inhibitors: Pivotal molecules in cellular signalling. *Cell Signal* 1999;11:545–54.

25. DerMardirossian C, Bokoch GM. GDIs: Central regulatory molecules in Rho GTPase activation. *Trends Cell Biol* 2005;15:356–63.

26. Sasaki T, Kato M, Takai Y. Consequences of weak interaction of rho GDI with the GTP-bound forms of rho p21 and rac p21. *J Biol Chem* 1993;268:23959–63.

27. Gong MC, Gorenne I, Read P, Jia T, Nakamoto RK, Somlyo AV, et al. Regulation by GDI of RhoA/Rho-kinase-induced Ca^{2+} sensitization of smooth muscle myosin II. *Am J Physiol Cell Physiol* 2001;281:C257–69.

28. Wei L, Imanaka-Yoshida K, Wang L, Zhan S, Schneider MD, DeMayo FJ, et al. Inhibition of Rho family GTPases by Rho GDP dissociation inhibitor disrupts cardiac morphogenesis and inhibits cardiomyocyte proliferation. *Development* 2002;129:1705–14.

29. Bilodeau D, Lamy S, Desrosiers RR, Gingras D, Beliveau R. Regulation of Rho protein binding to membranes by rhoGDI: Inhibition of releasing activity by physiological ionic conditions. *Biochem Cell Biol* 1999;77:59–69.

30. Lang P, Gesbert F, Delespine-Carmagnat M, Stancou R, Pouchelet M, Bertoglio J. Protein kinase A phosphorylation of RhoA mediates the morphological and functional effects of cyclic AMP in cytotoxic lymphocytes. *EMBO J* 1996;15:510–19.

31. Tamma G, Klussmann E, Procino G, Svelto M, Rosenthal W, Valenti G. cAMP-induced AQP2 translocation is associated with RhoA inhibition through RhoA phosphorylation and interaction with RhoGDI. *J Cell Sci* 2003;116:1519–25.

32. Qiao J, Huang F, Lum H. PKA inhibits RhoA activation: A protection mechanism against endothelial barrier dysfunction. *Am J Physiol Lung Cell Mol Physiol* 2003;284:L972–80.

33. Schmidt A, Hall A. Guanine nucleotide exchange factors for Rho GTPases: Turning on the switch. *Genes Dev* 2002;16:1587–609.

34. Rossman KL, Sondek J. Larger than Dbl: New structural insights into RhoA activation. *Trends Biochem Sci* 2005;30:163–65.

35. Fukuhara S, Chikumi H, Gutkind JS. RGS-containing RhoGEFs: The missing link between transforming G proteins and Rho? *Oncogene* 2001;20:1661–68.

36. Hollinger S, Hepler JR. Cellular regulation of RGS proteins: Modulators and integrators of G protein signaling. *Pharmacol Rev* 2002;54:527–59.

37. Kurose H. $G_{\alpha12}$ and $G_{\alpha13}$ as key regulatory mediator in signal transduction. *Life Sci* 2003;74:155–61.

38. Hart MJ, Jiang X, Kozasa T, Roscoe W, Singer WD, Gilman AG, et al. Direct stimulation of the guanine nucleotide exchange activity of p115 RhoGEF by $G_{\alpha13}$. *Science* 1998;280:2112–14.

39. Fukuhara S, Murga C, Zohar M, Igishi T, Gutkind JS. A novel PDZ domain containing guanine nucleotide exchange factor links heterotrimeric G proteins to Rho. *J Biol Chem* 1999;274:5868–79.

40. Suzuki N, Nakamura S, Mano H, Kozasa T. $G_{\alpha12}$ activates Rho GTPase through tyrosine-phosphorylated leukemia-associated RhoGEF. *Proc Natl Acad Sci USA* 2003;100:733–38.

41. Nakamura S, Kreutz B, Tanabe S, Suzuki N, Kozasa T. Critical role of lysine 204 in switch I region of $G_{\alpha13}$ for regulation of p115RhoGEF and leukemia-associated RhoGEF. *Mol Pharmacol* 2004;66:1029–34.

42. Grabocka E, Wedegaertner PB. Functional consequences of $G_{\alpha13}$ mutations that disrupt interaction with p115RhoGEF. *Oncogene* 2005;24:2155–65.

43. Booden MA, Siderovski DP, Der CJ. Leukemia-associated Rho guanine nucleotide exchange factor promotes $G_{\alpha q}$-coupled activation of RhoA. *Mol Cell Biol* 2002;22:4053–61.

44. Chikumi H, Vazquez-Prado J, Servitja JM, Miyazaki H, Gutkind JS. Potent activation of RhoA by $G_{\alpha q}$ and G_q-coupled receptors. *J Biol Chem* 2002;277:27130–34.

45. Derewenda U, Oleksy A, Stevenson AS, Korczynska J, Dauter Z, Somlyo AP, et al. The crystal structure of RhoA in complex with the DH/PH fragment of PDZRhoGEF, an activator of the Ca^{2+} sensitization pathway in smooth muscle. *Structure* 2004;12:1955–65.

46. Cerione RA, Zheng Y. The Dbl family of oncogenes. *Curr Opin Cell Biol* 1996;8:216–22.

47. Zheng Y. Dbl family guanine nucleotide exchange factors. *Trends Biochem Sci* 2001;26:724–32.

48. Blomberg N, Baraldi E, Nilges M, Saraste M. The PH superfold: A structural scaffold for multiple functions. *Trends Biochem Sci* 1999;24:441–45.

49. Kristelly R, Gao G, Tesmer JJ. Structural determinants of RhoA binding and nucleotide exchange in leukemia-associated Rho guanine-nucleotide exchange factor. *J Biol Chem* 2004;279:47352–62.

50. Holinstat M, Mehta D, Kozasa T, Minshall RD, Malik AB. Protein kinase Cα-induced p115RhoGEF phosphorylation signals endothelial cytoskeletal rearrangement. *J Biol Chem* 2003;278:28793–98.

51. Moon SY, Zheng Y. Rho GTPase-activating proteins in cell regulation. *Trends Cell Biol* 2003;13:13–22.

52. Gamblin SJ, Smerdon SJ. GTPase-activating proteins and their complexes. *Curr Opin Struct Biol* 1998;8:195–201.

53. Scheffzek K, Ahmadian MR, Wiesmuller L, Kabsch W, Stege P, Schmitz F, et al. Structural analysis of the GAP-related domain from neurofibromin and its implications. *EMBO J* 1998;17:4313–27.

54. Kosloff M, Selinger Z. Substrate assisted catalysis: Application to G proteins. *Trends Biochem Sci* 2001;26:161–66.

55. Vetter IR, Wittinghofer A. The guanine nucleotide-binding switch in three dimensions. *Science* 2001;294:1299–304.

56. Rittinger K, Walker PA, Eccleston JF, Nurmahomed K, Owen D, Laue E, et al. Crystal structure of a small G protein in complex with the GTPase-activating protein rhoGAP. *Nature* 1997;388:693–97.

57. Ahmadian MR, Stege P, Scheffzek K, Wittinghofer A. Confirmation of the arginine-finger hypothesis for the GAP-stimulated GTP-hydrolysis reaction of Ras. *Nat Struct Biol* 1997;4:686–89.

58. Leonard DA, Lin R, Cerione RA, Manor D. Biochemical studies of the mechanism of action of the Cdc42-GTPase-activating protein. *J Biol Chem* 1998;273:16210–15.

59. Graham DL, Eccleston JF, Lowe PN. The conserved arginine in rho-GTPase-activating protein is essential for efficient catalysis but not for complex formation with Rho.GDP and aluminum fluoride. *Biochemistry* 1999;38:985–91.

60. Homma Y, Emori Y. A dual functional signal mediator showing RhoGAP and phospholipase C-delta stimulating activities. *EMBO J* 1995;14:286–91.

61. Taylor JM, Macklem MM, Parsons JT. Cytoskeletal changes induced by GRAF, the GTPase regulator associated with focal adhesion kinase, are mediated by Rho. *J Cell Sci* 1999;112:231–42.

62. Haskell MD, Nickles AL, Agati JM, Su L, Dukes BD, Parsons SJ. Phosphorylation of p190 on Tyr1105 by c-Src is necessary but not sufficient for EGF-induced actin disassembly in C3H10T1/2 fibroblasts. *J Cell Sci* 2001;114:1699–708.

63. Fujihara H, Walker LA, Gong MC, Lemichez E, Boquet P, Somlyo AV, at al. Inhibition of RhoA translocation and calcium sensitization by in vivo ADP-ribosylation with the chimeric toxin DC3B. *Mol Biol Cell* 1997;8:2437–47.

64. Laufs U, Marra D, Node K, Liao JK. 3-Hydroxy-3-methylglutaryl-CoA reductase inhibitors attenuate vascular smooth muscle proliferation by preventing rho GTPase-induced down-regulation of p27(Kip1). *J Biol Chem* 1999;274:21926–31.

65. Gong MC, Fujihara H, Somlyo AV, Somlyo AP. Translocation of rhoA associated with Ca^{2+} sensitization of smooth muscle. *J Biol Chem* 1997;272:10704–09.

66. Sauzeau V, Le Jeune H, Cario-Toumaniantz C, Smolenski A, Lohmann SM, Bertoglio J, et al. Cyclic GMP-dependent protein kinase signaling pathway inhibits RhoA-induced Ca^{2+} sensitization of contraction in vascular smooth muscle. *J Biol Chem* 2000;275:21722–29.

67. Sauzeau V, Le Jeune H, Cario-Toumaniantz C, Vaillant N, Gadeau AP, Desgranges C, et al. P_{2Y1}, P_{2Y2}, P_{2Y4}, and P_{2Y6} receptors are coupled to Rho and Rho kinase activation in vascular myocytes. *Am J Physiol Heart Circ Physiol* 2000;278:H1751–61.

68. Ren XD, Kiosses WB, Schwartz MA. Regulation of the small GTP-binding protein Rho by cell adhesion and the cytoskeleton. *EMBO J* 1999;18:578–85.

69. Kimura K, Tsuji T, Takada Y, Miki T, Narumiya S. Accumulation of GTP-bound RhoA during cytokinesis and a critical role of ECT2 in this accumulation. *J Biol Chem* 2000;275:17233–36.

70. Laudanna C, Campbell JJ, Butcher EC. Role of Rho in chemoattractant-activated leukocyte adhesion through integrins. *Science* 1996;271:981–83.

71. Laudanna C, Campbell JJ, Butcher EC. Elevation of intracellular cAMP inhibits RhoA activation and integrin-dependent leukocyte adhesion induced by chemoattractants. *J Biol Chem* 1997;272:24141–44.

72. Seasholtz TM, Majumdar M, Kaplan DD, Brown JH. Rho and Rho kinase mediate thrombin-stimulated vascular smooth muscle cell DNA synthesis and migration. *Circ Res* 1999;84:1186–93.

73. Betuing S, Daviaud D, Pages C, Bonnard E, Valet P, Lafontan M, et al. $G_{\beta\gamma}$-independent coupling of α_2-adrenergic receptor to p21(rhoA) in preadipocytes. *J Biol Chem* 1998;273:15804–10.

74. Gohla A, Harhammer R, Schultz G. The G-protein G_{13} but not G_{12} mediates signaling from lysophosphatidic acid receptor via epidermal growth factor receptor to Rho. *J Biol Chem* 1998;273:4653–59.

75. Gong MC, Iizuka K, Nixon G, Browne JP, Hall A, Eccleston JF, et al. Role of guanine nucleotide-binding proteins — ras-family or trimeric proteins or

both — in Ca^{2+} sensitization of smooth muscle. *Proc Natl Acad Sci USA* 1996;93:1340–45.

76. Amano M, Fukata Y, Kaibuchi K. Regulation and functions of Rho-associated kinase. *Exp Cell Res* 2000;261:44–51.

77. Hall A. Rho GTPases and the actin cytoskeleton. *Science* 1998;279:509–14.

78. Kaibuchi K, Kuroda S, Amano M. Regulation of the cytoskeleton and cell adhesion by the Rho family GTPases in mammalian cells. *Annu Rev Biochem* 1999;68:45986.

79. Matsui T, Amano M, Yamamoto T, Chihara K, Nakafuku M, Ito M, et al. Rho-associated kinase, a novel serine/threonine kinase, as a putative target for small GTP binding protein Rho. *EMBO J* 1996;15:2208–16.

80. Chen XQ, Tan I, Ng CH, Hall C, Lim L, Leung T. Characterization of RhoA-binding kinase ROKα implication of the pleckstrin homology domain in ROKα function using region-specific antibodies. *J Biol Chem* 2002;277:12680–88.

81. Hiroki J, Shimokawa H, Higashi M, Morikawa K, Kandabashi T, Kawamura N, et al. Inflammatory stimuli upregulate Rho-kinase in human coronary vascular smooth muscle cells. *J Mol Cell Cardiol* 2004;37:537–46.

82. Hiroki J, Shimokawa H, Mukai Y, Ichiki T, Takeshita A. Divergent effects of estrogen and nicotine on Rho-kinase expression in human coronary vascular smooth muscle cells. *Biochem Biophys Res Commun* 2005;326:154–59.

83. Oi K, Shimokawa H, Hiroki J, Uwatoku T, Abe K, Matsumoto Y, et al. Remnant lipoproteins from patients with sudden cardiac death enhance coronary vasospastic activity through upregulation of Rho-kinase. *Arterioscler Thromb Vasc Biol* 2004;24:918–22.

84. Kandabashi T, Shimokawa H, Miyata K, Kunihiro I, Kawano Y, Fukata Y, et al. Inhibition of myosin phosphatase by upregulated rho-kinase plays a key role for coronary artery spasm in a porcine model with interleukin-1β. *Circulation* 2000;101:1319–23.

85. Shimokawa H. Rho-kinase as a novel therapeutic target in treatment of cardiovascular diseases. *J Cardiovasc Pharmacol* 2002;39:319–27.

86. Kandabashi T, Shimokawa H, Mukai Y, Matoba T, Kunihiro I, Morikawa K, et al. Involvement of rho-kinase in agonists-induced contractions of arteriosclerotic human arteries. *Arterioscler Thromb Vasc Biol* 2002;22:243–48.

87. Shimokawa H, Takeshita A. Rho-kinase is an important therapeutic target in cardiovascular medicine. *Arterioscler Thromb Vasc Biol* 2005;25:1767–75.

88. Hartshorne DJ, Ito M, Erdodi F. Myosin light chain phosphatase: Subunit composition, interactions and regulation. *J Muscle Res Cell Motil* 1998;19:325–41.

89. Ito M, Nakano T, Erdodi F, Hartshorne DJ. Myosin phosphatase: structure, regulation and function. *Mol Cell Biochem* 2004;259:197–209.

90. Tanaka J, Ito M, Feng J, Ichikawa K, Hamaguchi T, Nakamura M, et al. Interaction of myosin phosphatase target subunit 1 with the catalytic subunit of type 1 protein phosphatase. *Biochemistry* 1998;37:16697–703.

91. Kimura K, Ito M, Amano M, Chihara K, Fukata Y, Nakafuku M, et al. Regulation of myosin phosphatase by Rho and Rho-associated kinase (Rho-kinase). *Science* 1996;273:245–48.

92. Feng J, Ito M, Ichikawa K, Isaka N, Nishikawa M, Hartshorne DJ, et al. Inhibitory phosphorylation site for Rho-associated kinase on smooth muscle myosin phosphatase. *J Biol Chem* 1999;274:37385–90.

93. Ito K, Shimomura E, Iwanaga T, Shiraishi M, Shindo K, Nakamura J, et al. Essential role of rho kinase in the Ca^{2+} sensitization of prostaglandin $F_{2\alpha}$-induced contraction of rabbit aortae. *J Physiol* 2003;546:823–36.

94. Velasco G, Armstrong C, Morrice N, Frame S, Cohen P. Phosphorylation of the regulatory subunit of smooth muscle protein phosphatase 1M at Thr850 induces its dissociation from myosin. *FEBS Lett* 2002;527:101–04.

95. Stevenson AS, Matthew JD, Eto M, Luo S, Somlyo AP, Somlyo AV. Uncoupling of GPCR and RhoA-induced Ca^{2+}-sensitization of chicken amnion smooth muscle lacking CPI-17. *FEBS Lett* 2004;578:73–9.

96. Wilson DP, Susnjar M, Kiss E, Sutherland C, Walsh MP. Thromboxane A_2-induced contraction of rat caudal arterial smooth muscle involves activation of Ca^{2+} entry and Ca^{2+} sensitization: Rho-associated kinase-mediated phosphorylation of MYPT1 at Thr-855, but not Thr-697. *Biochem J* 2005;389:763–74.

97. Genth H, Gerhard R, Maeda A, Amano M, Kaibuchi K, Aktories K, et al. Entrapment of Rho ADP-ribosylated by Clostridium botulinum C3 exoenzyme in the Rho-guanine nucleotide dissociation inhibitor-1 complex. *J Biol Chem* 2003;278:28523–27.

98. Sehr P, Joseph G, Genth H, Just I, Pick E, Aktories K. Glucosylation and ADP ribosylation of rho proteins: Effects on nucleotide binding, GTPase activity, and effector coupling. *Biochemistry* 1998;37:5296–304.

99. Boquet P. Bacterial toxins inhibiting or activating small GTP-binding proteins. *Ann NY Acad Sci* 1999;886:83–90.

100. Aktories K, Schmidt G, Just I. Rho GTPases as targets of bacterial protein toxins. *Biol Chem* 2000;381:421–26.

101. Aktories K, Schmidt G. A new turn in Rho GTPase activation by Escherichia coli cytotoxic necrotizing factors. *Trends Microbiol* 2003;11:152–55.

102. Hoffmann C, Pop M, Leemhuis J, Schirmer J, Aktories K, Schmidt G. The Yersinia pseudotuberculosis cytotoxic necrotizing factor (CNFY) selectively activates RhoA. *J Biol Chem* 2004;279:16026–32.

103. Ishizaki T, Uehata M, Tamechika I, Keel J, Nonomura K, Maekawa M, et al. Pharmacological properties of Y-27632, a specific inhibitor of rho-associated kinases. *Mol Pharmacol* 2000;57:976–83.

104. Uehata M, Ishizaki T, Satoh H, Ono T, Kawahara T, Morishita T, et al. Calcium sensitization of smooth muscle mediated by a Rho-associated protein kinase in hypertension. *Nature* 1997;389:990–94.

105. Eto M, Kitazawa T, Yazawa M, Mukai H, Ono Y, Brautigan DL. Histamine-

induced vasoconstriction involves phosphorylation of a specific inhibitor protein for myosin phosphatase by protein kinase C α and δ isoforms. *J Biol Chem* 2001;276:29072–78.

106. Ito S, Kume H, Honjo H, Katoh H, Kodama I, Yamaki K, et al. Possible involvement of Rho kinase in Ca^{2+} sensitization and mobilization by MCh in tracheal smooth muscle. *Am J Physiol Lung Cell Mol Physiol* 2001;280:L1218–24.

107. Mita M, Yanagihara H, Hishinuma S, Saito M, Walsh MP. Membrane depolarization-induced contraction of rat caudal arterial smooth muscle involves Rho-associated kinase. *Biochem J* 2002;364:431–40.

108. Ghisdal P, Vandenberg G, Morel N. Rho-dependent kinase is involved in agonist-activated calcium entry in rat arteries. *J Physiol* 2003;551:855–67.

109. Sakamoto K, Hori M, Izumi M, Oka T, Kohama K, Ozaki H, et al. Inhibition of high K+-induced contraction by the ROCKs inhibitor Y-27632 in vascular smooth muscle: Possible involvement of ROCKs in a signal transduction pathway. *J Pharmacol Sci* 2003;92:56–69.

110. Nagumo H, Sasaki Y, Ono Y, Okamoto H, Seto M, Takuwa Y. Rho kinase inhibitor HA-1077 prevents Rho-mediated myosin phosphatase inhibition in smooth muscle cells. *Am J Physiol Cell Physiol* 2000;278:C57–65.

111. Shimokawa H, Seto M, Katsumata N, Amano M, Kozai T, Yamawaki T, et al. Rho-kinase-mediated pathway induces enhanced myosin light chain phosphorylations in a swine model of coronary artery spasm. *Cardiovasc Res* 1999;43:1029–39.

112. Higashi M, Shimokawa H, Hattori T, Hiroki J, Mukai Y, Morikawa K, et al. Long-term inhibition of Rho-kinase suppresses angiotensin II-induced cardiovascular hypertrophy in rats in vivo: Effect on endothelial NAD(P)H oxidase system. *Circ Res* 2003;93:767–75.

113. Sasaki Y, Suzuki M, Hidaka H. The novel and specific Rho-kinase inhibitor (S)-(+)-2-methyl-1-[(4-methyl-5-isoquinoline)sulfonyl]-homopiperazine as a probing molecule for Rho-kinase-involved pathway. *Pharmacol Ther* 2002;93:225–32.

114. Feig LA. Tools of the trade: Use of dominant-inhibitory mutants of Ras-family GTPases. *Nat Cell Biol* 1999;1:E25–27.

115. Morishige K, Shimokawa H, Eto Y, Kandabashi T, Miyata K, Matsumoto Y, et al. Adenovirus-mediated transfer of dominant-negative rho-kinase induces a regression of coronary arteriosclerosis in pigs in vivo. *Arterioscler Thromb Vasc Biol* 2001;21:548–54.

116. Pawlak G, Helfman DM. Post-transcriptional down-regulation of ROCKI/Rho-kinase through an MEK-dependent pathway leads to cytoskeleton disruption in Ras-transformed fibroblasts. *Mol Biol Cell* 2002;13:336–47.

117. Deroanne C, Vouret-Craviari V, Wang B, Pouyssegur J. EphrinA1 inactivates integrin-mediated vascular smooth muscle cell spreading via the Rac/PAK pathway. *J Cell Sci* 2003;116:1367–76.

118. Pille JY, Denoyelle C, Varet J, Bertrand JR, Soria J, Opolon P, et al. Anti-RhoA and anti-RhoC siRNAs inhibit the proliferation and invasiveness of MDA-MB-231 breast cancer cells in vitro and in vivo. *Mol Ther* 2005;11:267–74.

119. Somlyo AP, Somlyo AV. From pharmacomechanical coupling to G-proteins and myosin phosphatase. *Acta Physiol Scand* 1998;164:437–48.

120. VanBavel E, van der Meulen ET, Spaan JA. Role of Rho-associated protein kinase in tone and calcium sensitivity of cannulated rat mesenteric small arteries. *Exp Physiol* 2001;86:585–92.

121. Buyukafsar K, Arikan O, Ark M, Secilmis A, Un I, Singirik E. Rho-kinase expression and its contribution to the control of perfusion pressure in the isolated rat mesenteric vascular bed. *Eur J Pharmacol* 2004;485:263–68.

122. Teixeira CE, Jin L, Ying Z, Palmer T, Priviero FB, Webb RC. Expression and functional role of the RhoA/Rho-kinase pathway in rat coeliac artery. *Clin Exp Pharmacol Physiol* 2005;32:817–24.

123. Martinez MC, Randriamboavonjy V, Ohlmann P, Komas N, Duarte J, Schneider F, et al. Involvement of protein kinase C, tyrosine kinases, and Rho kinase in Ca^{2+} handling of human small arteries. *Am J Physiol Heart Circ Physiol* 2000;279:H1228–2138.

124. Janssen LJ, Lu-Chao H, Netherton S. Excitation-contraction coupling in pulmonary vascular smooth muscle involves tyrosine kinase and Rho kinase. *Am J Physiol Lung Cell Mol Physiol* 2001;280:L666–74.

125. Nobe K, Paul RJ. Distinct pathways of Ca^{2+} sensitization in porcine coronary artery: Effects of Rho-related kinase and protein kinase C inhibition on force and intracellular Ca^{2+}. *Circ Res* 2001;88:1283–90.

126. Miao L, Dai Y, Zhang J. Mechanism of RhoA/Rho kinase activation in endothelin-1- induced contraction in rabbit basilar artery. *Am J Physiol Heart Circ Physiol* 2002;283:H983–89.

127. Llorens S, Jordan J, Nava E. The nitric oxide pathway in the cardiovascular system. *J Physiol Biochem* 2002;58:179–88.

128. Lucas KA, Pitari GM, Kazerounian S, Ruiz-Stewart I, Park J, Schulz S, et al. Guanylyl cyclases and signaling by cyclic GMP. *Pharmacol Rev* 2000;52:375–414.

129. Chitaley K, Webb RC. Nitric oxide induces dilation of rat aorta via inhibition of rho-kinase signaling. *Hypertension* 2002;39:438–42.

130. Carter RW, Begaye M, Kanagy NL. Acute and chronic NOS inhibition enhances α_2-adrenoreceptor-stimulated RhoA and Rho kinase in rat aorta. *Am J Physiol Heart Circ Physiol* 2002;283:H1361–69.

131. Mukai Y, Shimokawa H, Matoba T, Kandabashi T, Satoh S, Hiroki J, et al. Involvement of Rho-kinase in hypertensive vascular disease: A novel therapeutic target in hypertension. *FASEB J* 2001;15:1062–64.

132. Chrissobolis S, Sobey CG. Evidence that Rho-kinase activity contributes to cerebral vascular tone in vivo and is enhanced during chronic hypertension: Comparison with protein kinase C. *Circ Res* 2001;88:774–79.

133. Faraci FM, Lamping KG, Modrick ML, Ryan MJ, Sigmund CD, Didion SP. Cerebral vascular effects of angiotensin II: New insights from genetic models. *J Cereb Blood Flow Metab* 2005;(in press).

134. Ryan MJ, Didion SP, Mathur S, Faraci FM, Sigmund CD. Angiotensin II-induced vascular dysfunction is mediated by the AT1A receptor in mice. *Hypertension* 2004;43:1074–79.

135. Seko T, Ito M, Kureishi Y, Okamoto R, Moriki N, Onishi K, et al. Activation of RhoA and inhibition of myosin phosphatase as important components in hypertension in vascular smooth muscle. *Circ Res* 2003;92:411–18.

136. Moriki N, Ito M, Seko T, Kureishi Y, Okamoto R, Nakakuki T, et al. RhoA activation in vascular smooth muscle cells from stroke-prone spontaneously hypertensive rats. *Hypertens Res* 2004;27:263–70.

137. Ying Z, Jin L, Dorrance AM, Webb RC. Increased expression of mRNA for regulator of G protein signaling domain-containing Rho guanine nucleotide exchange factors in aorta from stroke-prone spontaneously hypertensive rats. *Am J Hypertens* 2004;17:981–85.

138. Masumoto A, Hirooka Y, Shimokawa H, Hironaga K, Setoguchi S, Takeshita A. Possible involvement of Rho-kinase in the pathogenesis of hypertension in humans. *Hypertension* 2001;38:1307–10.

139. Shimokawa H. Cellular and molecular mechanisms of coronary artery spasm: Lessons from animal models. *Jpn Circ J* 2000;64:1–12.

140. Kandabashi T, Shimokawa H, Miyata K, Kunihiro I, Eto Y, Morishige K, et al. Evidence for protein kinase C-mediated activation of Rho-kinase in a porcine model of coronary artery spasm. *Arterioscler Thromb Vasc Biol* 2003;23:2209–14.

141. Shimokawa H, Morishige K, Miyata K, Kandabashi T, Eto Y, Ikegaki I, et al. Long-term inhibition of Rho-kinase induces a regression of arteriosclerotic coronary lesions in a porcine model in vivo. *Cardiovasc Res* 2001;51:169–77.

142. Masumoto A, Mohri M, Shimokawa H, Urakami L, Usui M, Takeshita A. Suppression of coronary artery spasm by the Rho-kinase inhibitor fasudil in patients with vasospastic angina. *Circulation* 2002;105:1545–47.

143. Mohri M, Shimokawa H, Hirakawa Y, Masumoto A, Takeshita A. Rho-kinase inhibition with intracoronary fasudil prevents myocardial ischemia in patients with coronary microvascular spasm. *J Am Coll Cardiol* 2003;41:15–9.

144. Shimokawa H, Hiramori K, Iinuma H, Hosoda S, Kishida H, Osada H, et al. Anti-anginal effect of fasudil, a Rho-kinase inhibitor, in patients with stable effort angina: A multicenter study. *J Cardiovasc Pharmacol* 2002;40:751–61.

145. Inokuchi K, Ito A, Fukumoto Y, Matoba T, Shiose A, Nishida T, et al. Usefulness of fasudil, a Rho-kinase inhibitor, to treat intractable severe coronary spasm after coronary artery bypass surgery. *J Cardiovasc Pharmacol* 2004;44:275–77.

146. Sato M, Tani E, Fujikawa H, Kaibuchi K. Involvement of Rho-kinase-mediated phosphorylation of myosin light chain in enhancement of cerebral vasospasm. *Circ Res* 2000;87:195–200.

147. Miyagi Y, Carpenter RC, Meguro T, Parent AD, Zhang JH. Upregulation of rho A and rho kinase messenger RNAs in the basilar artery of a rat model of subarachnoid hemorrhage. *J Neurosurg* 2000;93:471–76.

148. Watanabe Y, Faraci FM, Heistad DD. Activation of Rho-associated kinase during augmented contraction of the basilar artery to serotonin after subarachnoid hemorrhage. *Am J Physiol Heart Circ Physiol* 2005;288:H2653–58.

149. Wickman G, Lan C, Vollrath B. Functional roles of the rho/rho kinase pathway and protein kinase C in the regulation of cerebrovascular constriction mediated by hemoglobin: Relevance to subarachnoid hemorrhage and vasospasm. *Circ Res* 2003;92:809–16.

150. Lan C, Das D, Wloskowicz A, Vollrath B. Endothelin-1 modulates hemoglobin-mediated signaling in cerebrovascular smooth muscle via RhoA/Rho kinase and protein kinase C. *Am J Physiol Heart Circ Physiol* 2004;286:H165–73.

151. Laufs U, Liao JK. Post-transcriptional regulation of endothelial nitric oxide synthase mRNA stability by Rho GTPase. *J Biol Chem* 1998;273:24266–71.

152. Takeda K, Ichiki T, Tokunou T, Iino N, Fujii S, Kitabatake A, et al. Critical role of Rho-kinase and MEK/ERK pathways for angiotensin II-induced plasminogen activator inhibitor type-1 gene expression. *Arterioscler Thromb Vasc Biol* 2001;21:868–73.

153. Kobayashi N, Nakano S, Mita S, Kobayashi T, Honda T, Tsubokou Y, et al. Involvement of Rho-kinase pathway for angiotensin II-induced plasminogen activator inhibitor-1 gene expression and cardiovascular remodeling in hypertensive rats. *J Pharmacol Exp Ther* 2002;301:459–66.

154. Mallat Z, Gojova A, Sauzeau V, Brun V, Silvestre JS, Esposito B, et al. Rho-associated protein kinase contributes to early atherosclerotic lesion formation in mice. *Circ Res* 2003;93:884–88.

155. Ming XF, Barandier C, Viswambharan H, Kwak BR, Mach F, Mazzolai L, et al. Thrombin stimulates human endothelial arginase enzymatic activity via RhoA/ROCK pathway: Implications for atherosclerotic endothelial dysfunction. *Circulation* 2004;110:3708–14.

156. Wolfrum S, Dendorfer A, Rikitake Y, Stalker TJ, Gong Y, Scalia R, et al. Inhibition of Rho-kinase leads to rapid activation of phosphatidylinositol 3-kinase/protein kinase Akt and cardiovascular protection. *Arterioscler Thromb Vasc Biol* 2004;24:1842–47.

157. Budzyn K, Marley PD, Sobey CG. Opposing roles of endothelial and smooth muscle phosphatidylinositol 3-kinase in vasoconstriction: Effects of rho-kinase and hypertension. *J Pharmacol Exp Ther* 2005;313:1248–53.

158. Eto Y, Shimokawa H, Hiroki J, Morishige K, Kandabashi T, Matsumoto Y, et al. Gene transfer of dominant negative Rho kinase suppresses neointimal formation after balloon injury in pigs. *Am J Physiol Heart Circ Physiol* 2000;278:H1744–50.

159. Sawada N, Itoh H, Ueyama K, Yamashita J, Doi K, Chun TH, et al. Inhibition of rho-associated kinase results in suppression of neointimal formation of balloon-injured arteries. *Circulation* 2000;101:2030–33.

160. Shibata R, Kai H, Seki Y, Kato S, Morimatsu M, Kaibuchi K, et al. Role of Rho-associated kinase in neointima formation after vascular injury. *Circulation* 2001;103:284–89.

161. Miyata K, Shimokawa H, Kandabashi T, Higo T, Morishige K, Eto Y, et al. Rho-kinase is involved in macrophage-mediated formation of coronary vascular lesions in pigs in vivo. *Arterioscler Thromb Vasc Biol* 2000;20:2351–58.

162. Abe K, Shimokawa H, Morikawa K, Uwatoku T, Oi K, Matsumoto Y, et al. Long-term treatment with a Rho-kinase inhibitor improves monocrotaline-induced fatal pulmonary hypertension in rats. *Circ Res* 2004;94:385–93.

163. Nagaoka T, Fagan KA, Gebb SA, Morris KG, Suzuki T, Shimokawa H, et al. Inhaled Rho kinase inhibitors are potent and selective vasodilators in rat pulmonary hypertension. *Am J Respir Crit Care Med* 2005;171:494–99.

164. Abe K, Morikawa K, Hizume T, Uwatoku T, Oi K, Seto M, et al. Prostacyclin does not inhibit rho-kinase: An implication for the treatment of pulmonary hypertension. *J Cardiovasc Pharmacol* 2005;45:120–24.

165. Fukumoto Y, Matoba T, Ito A, Tanaka H, Kishi T, Hayashidani S, et al. Acute vasodilator effects of a Rho-kinase inhibitor, fasudil, in patients with severe pulmonary hypertension. *Heart* 2005;91:391–92.

166. Toshima Y, Satoh S, Ikegaki I, Asano T. A new model of cerebral microthrombosis in rats and the neuroprotective effect of a Rho-kinase inhibitor. *Stroke* 2000;31:2245–50.

167. Satoh S, Utsunomiya T, Tsurui K, Kobayashi T, Ikegaki I, Sasaki Y, Asano T. Pharmacological profile of hydroxy fasudil as a selective rho kinase inhibitor on ischemic brain damage. *Life Sci* 2001;69:1441–53.

168. Shibuya M, Hirai S, Seto M, Satoh S, Ohtomo E. Effects of fasudil in acute ischemic stroke: Results of a prospective placebo-controlled double-blind trial. *J Neurol Sci* 2005;238:31–9.

169. Hisaoka T, Yano M, Ohkusa T, Suetsugu M, Ono K, Kohno M, et al. Enhancement of Rho/Rho-kinase system in regulation of vascular smooth muscle contraction in tachycardia-induced heart failure. *Cardiovasc Res* 2001;49:319–29.

170. Kishi T, Hirooka Y, Masumoto A, Ito K, Kimura Y, Inokuchi K, et al. Rho-kinase inhibitor improves increased vascular resistance and impaired vasodilation of the forearm in patients with heart failure. *Circulation* 2005;111:2741–47.

171. Ono-Saito N, Niki I, Hidaka H. H-series protein kinase inhibitors and potential clinical applications. *Pharmacol Ther* 1999;82:123–31.

172. Davies SP, Reddy H, Caivano M, Cohen P. Specificity and mechanism of action of some commonly used protein kinase inhibitors. *Biochem J* 2000;351:95–105.

173. Breitenlechner C, Gassel M, Hidaka H, Kinzel V, Huber R, Engh RA, Bossemeyer D. Protein kinase A in complex with Rho-kinase inhibitors Y-27632, Fasudil, and H-1152P: Structural basis of selectivity. *Structure* 2003;11:1595–607.

Chapter

17

Matrix Metalloproteinases and the Extracellular Matrix

Muzahir H. Tayebjee and Gregory Y. H. Lip

Key Findings

- The extracellular matrix (ECM) has structural and functional roles.

- In hypertension, changes in the cardiac and vascular ECM are manifested, for example, as left ventricular hypertrophy.

- Matrix metalloproteinases (MMPs) and their inhibitors, tissue inhibitors of matrix metalloproteinases (TIMPs), have key roles in modulating the structure and function of ECM.

- In hypertension, the assessment of circulating MMP and TIMP may be useful noninvasive markers of tissue structure and function and provide prognostic information.

The extracellular matrix (ECM) is the connecting tissue that surrounds the cellular elements of solid organs. Like tissue cement, it forms a substrate to hold cells together. The ECM is also a dynamic structure that is integral to organ function. Apart from providing structural support, the ECM is fundamental to cell-cell signaling.

The ECM is composed of structural proteins (collagen and elastin), specialized proteins (e.g., fibrillin and fibronectin), and proteoglycans. Within this complex network are signal receptor proteins and enzymes that control the turnover of this highly complex system. The ECM, although ubiquitous, has variable composition in different organs. Various factors can affect the structure of ECM, including stretch and pressure, inflammation, perfusion or ischemia, and prevailing growth factors. In disease states, the changes in ECM can be important in organ repair but also detrimental. For example, a growing body of evidence suggests that the composition of cardiac ECM changes as hypertension progresses.

Matrix metalloproteinases (MMPs) and their endogenous inhibitors, tissue inhibitors of metalloproteinases (TIMPs), are ubiquitous to ECM and are thought to play a major role in ECM remodeling. Indeed, there is growing evidence that these compounds are involved in tissue turnover in normal physiology as well as in pathology (e.g., as seen in the cardiac fibrosis associated with hypertensive left ventricular hypertrophy).

The study of MMPs and TIMPs is important because they could have potential diagnostic and therapeutic value. This might allow identification of groups of patients where matrix turnover is damaging the heart or vascular response to injury. Furthermore, understanding the mechanisms of these responses might allow the development of novel pharmacological agents alone or in combination with other treatment to prevent deterioration in heart and vascular function—seen, for example, in end-stage heart failure.

ANATOMY/BIOCHEMISTRY

There are more than 20 identified MMPs important in the ECM, and they have been classified according to their substrate specificity [i.e., collagenases, gelatinases, stromelysins, matrilysin, macropage elastase, and membrane-type MMP (MT-MMP)]. Each enzyme has also been given a numerical classification. For example, interstitial collagenase is MMP-1. This numerical classification scheme is used in this text.[1]

Each MMP is made up of a propeptide active site and a zinc-binding domain. To activate the enzyme, the propeptide must be cleaved to allow water to bind to zinc (Figure 17–1). Apart from MMP-7, all other MMPs contain a carboxyterminal hemopexin (PEX) domain. Calcium occupies a "hole" within this site. It is this site that determines the enzyme interactions. For example, this site is important for the interaction of TIMP-1 with MMP-9. Various other domains also exist. For example, fibronectin repeats in MMP-2 and MMP-9, which bind gelatin.[2] Nevertheless, it should be noted that the enzymes responsible for forming ECM precursors are located intracellularly, and post-translational modification occurs within the ECM (e.g., cleavage of the amino terminal of procollagen by procollagen N proteinase).

The composition of ECM at any given time is dependent on the balance between the rate of formation and breakdown. The regulation of ECM components is controlled at the transcriptional level and is mediated by growth factors such as human growth hormone and platelet-derived growth factor. The main control systems of current interest are in the regulation of the key structural MMPs.

The MMP activity associated with ECM turnover can be effected at the transcriptional level, where local cytokine production (TNFα or decorin) can regulate synthesis of both MMP and TIMP. The peptide is produced as an inactive proenzyme, and constant background expression occurs at a low level over and above which many of the MMP series are induced during pathological processes. Metalloproteinases are generally not stored in large quantities, and need to be actively transcribed for activity. However, neutrophils during the inflammatory response are unique

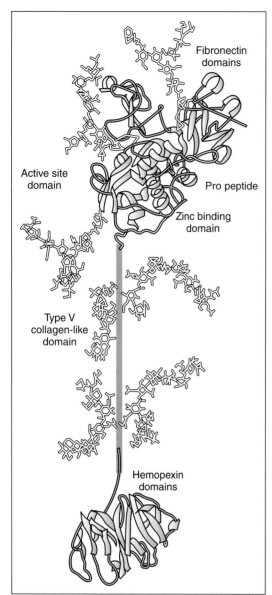

Figure 17–1. The 3D structure of MMP-1. (From Van den Steen PE, Opdenakker G, Wormald MR, et al. Matrix remodelling enzymes, the protease cascade and glycosylation. *Biochimica et Biophysica Acta* 2001;1528:61–73, with permission.)

Labels in figure: Fibronectin domains; Active site domain; Pro peptide; Zinc binding domain; Type V collagen-like domain; Hemopexin domains

collagen synthesis is stimulated by angiotensin II (in high concentrations) and aldosterone when added to the culture medium. This increased synthesis could be inhibited by adding specific aldosterone and angiotensin II receptor antagonists. Angiotensin II has been found to stimulate collagen synthesis and regulate collagen degradation by increasing the concentration of TIMP-1 and hence attenuating endothelial cell interstitial MMP-1 activity. The balance between MMP-1 and TIMP-1 is thought to be important in the pathology of hypertensive heart and vascular disease.[4]

Growth factors and cytokines have also been closely implicated in the regulation of MMP/TIMP function and synthesis. Tumor necrosis factor alpha (TNFα), a pro-inflammatory and immunoregulatory cytokine, regulates (and in turn can be regulated by) TIMPs and MMPs. The exact nature of the control system is yet to be determined, but TIMPs prevent post-translational activation of TNFα. Moreover, anti-TNF α therapy seems to be associated with a reduction in serum MMP-1 and MMP-3. Similarly, platelet-derived growth factor (PDGF) and interleukin-1 (IL-1) both stimulate MMP synthesis. Conversely, transforming growth factor beta (TGF β), heparin, corticosteroids, TIMP-1 (inducible by cytokines), TIMP-2 (mainly constitutive), and TIMP-3 inhibit MMP synthesis and activity. Metalloproteinases may also play a role in regulating cytokine activity. For example, MMP-9 can activate IL-1β, and MMP-3 is able to degrade activated IL-1β.[5]

Given the important role of the tissue-blood interface in the process of vascular function and clotting, it is of considerable importance that components of the clotting cascade affect the post-translational activity of MMPs. Indeed, plasmin is a potent activator of most MMPs, and can cleave precursor MMP propeptides to the active molecules. Human urokinase-type plasminogen activator (uPA) and uPA receptors are expressed by monocytes and macrophages and can activate MMPs. Because macrophages accumulate at "sites of inflammation," this localized presentation of MMP activators results in localized proteolytic activity (e.g., at leading edges of cells). MMP-3 can cleave plasmin, which can activate even more MMP-3 and thus result in positive feedback mechanisms that amplify enzyme activity in a manner similar to that of the clotting cascade (as well as interacting with it). Furthermore, thrombin has been shown to result in the activation of active MMP-2. This can occur either directly by increasing the catalysis of pro-MMP-2 or indirectly by increasing the expression of MT-1 MMP, and by speeding the intracellular transit of this enzyme to the cell surface (where MT1-MMP proceeds to activate transcribed MMP-2).[3]

Using human umbilical vein endothelial cells and abdominal aorta endothelial cell tissue culture, it has been suggested that oxidized low-density lipoprotein can induce the expression of MMP-1 and reduce the synthesis of TIMP-1, therefore favoring collagen degradation. This is a key interaction because it may be one of the mechanisms leading to plaque progression and instability. Raised serum ox-LDL has been associated with increased circulating

in that they do manufacture, store, and quickly release MMPs. Control over MMP activity can also be exerted at the post-translational (zymogens and inhibitory enzyme) level. In molecular terms, the enzyme activity can be modulated by a cysteine switch mechanism whereby the MMP is folded by the binding of cysteine via a disulphide bond to the zinc molecule in the active site, which prevents access to the enzyme active site. *In vitro* treatments such as proteolysis, heat, or alkylation allow a change in its conformation to facilitate analysis of the total fraction of enzymatic activity.[3]

There is a substantial body of evidence that ECM turnover is regulated by the renin-angiotensin-aldosterone system, which in turn regulates MMPs and TIMPs. Tissue culture experiments using rat fibroblasts have shown that

MMP-9 levels in patients with increased generalized cardiovascular risk factors and appears to play a supporting role for MMPs as a means by which lipoproteins interact in atherosclerotic plaque pathology.[6]

Finally, these enzymes also have effects on the cell cycle. MMP-7 can cleave the Fas ligand to produce soluble FasL, which is able to induce apoptosis. Moreover, using rat smooth muscle tissue culture techniques and transfecting cells with TIMP-1, -2, and -3 it was found that TIMP-1 did not affect cell proliferation but TIMP-2 over-expression caused a dose-dependent reduction in proliferation, and overexpression of TIMP-3 actually increased apoptosis.[7]

GENETICS

This is a relatively new area in MMP and TIMP biology. There is little clinically relevant information about this topic, which is covered in the next section.

PHYSIOLOGY AND PATHOPHYSIOLOGY

Hypertension has a major impact on the circulation, and hence on many organ systems. For example, the development of LVH and diastolic and systolic heart failure, myocardial infarction, and stroke occur along with increasing atherosclerosis and renal failure because of the effect of raised blood pressure on the microcirculation. Most of these changes relate to altered structure of the ECM, and because of this it is likely that MMPs and TIMPs are involved in this process.

To date, the majority of studies have focused on changes in collagen turnover (the predominant cardiovascular ECM protein) and cardiac structure that can occur in hypertension and on how MMPs and TIMPs may have a role in this process. In particular, there is increased deposition of collagen, a change in the ratio of collagen subtype, and differential cross linking. The synthesis and breakdown of collagen leads to the production of end peptides; for example, carboxy-terminal propeptide of procollagen type I (PCIP) (a marker of collagen type I synthesis). These fragments are released into tissue and the systemic circulation and can be measured by radio-immunoassay. Circulating peptides are reliable surrogates of ECM turnover and have an established role in clinical medicine. In animal experimental models of hypertension, these markers can be used to assess ECM turnover in tissue extracts. Indeed, the serum PCIP is increased in spontaneously hypertensive rats, mirroring quantitative increases in type I collagen in the myocardium when compared with normotensive Wistar-Kyoto rats.[8] These results therefore demonstrate altered collagen turnover hypertension and possibly contribute to an increase in myocardial stiffness. Cell culture studies of myocardial fibroblasts from genetically hypertensive rats have also indicated that these fibroblasts play an important role in fibrosis by producing increased amounts of types I and III collagen.[9]

What role could MMPs and TIMPs play in abnormal ECM turnover in hypertension? In hypertensive salt-sensitive rats, TIMP-2, TIMP-4, and MMP-2 expression is increased in the myocardium—particularly at the time when LVH progresses to left ventricular dilatation and failure.[10] The activity of MMP-2 appears to be increased during the development of LVH before heart failure develops in untreated hypertensive rats, although other MMPs may have roles as well. Furthermore, it is thought that MMP-2 may also be involved in facilitating muscle growth by digesting surrounding ECM (in that the tensile strength of cardiac muscle is reduced by incubating myocytes with excess MMP-2) and that this effect is reversed by anti-MMP-2 antibody and TIMP.[11] Although there is controversy as to the timescale of MMP-2 activation, it is clear is that MMP-2 is important in the progression of LVH to ventricular dilatation and the emergence of heart failure—an effect it probably mediates by reducing matrix binding. Although MMP-2 has been highlighted, it is more than likely that other MMPs and TIMPs are involved in this process.

Animal studies have postulated a role for MMPs and TIMPs in abnormal ECM turnover. However, it is generally accepted that results obtained from experimental animal models cannot be extrapolated directly to humans. Indeed, the etiology of human hypertension is multifactorial and takes time to develop. Animal studies, on the other hand, often rely on surgical, severe dietetic, or genetic manipulation to cause hypertension. Furthermore, obtaining tissue samples from humans is difficult (and often impossible) for ethical reasons. Therefore, much of the evidence about the importance of MMPs and TIMPs in humans has come from plasma and serum analysis together with noninvasive tissue assessment. Fortuitously, there are similarities between results obtained in animal experiments and humans, allowing inferences on pathophysiology to be made. Because these are more relevant clinically, they are focused on here.

Work from our laboratory and others have demonstrated an increase in circulating MMP-9 and TIMP-1 in hypertension but a reduction in MMP-1 compared with healthy human controls. These changes were associated with an increase in levels of plasma PCIP and carboxy-terminal telopeptide of type I collagen (CITP) (marker of collagen degradation), which constitutes indirect evidence that MMPs and TIMPs could be implicated in abnormal ECM turnover in hypertension. A crucial question is what abnormal ECM turnover occurs in hypertension? Hypertension is a systemic disease and affects many major organs (in particular, the arterial tree and the heart), and circulating MMPs and TIMPs could therefore originate from many places in the body. The clinical value of measuring circulating MMPs and TIMPs relies on knowledge of their origin, but as discussed previously human tissue studies are difficult and other indirect methods are required in locating the source.[4]

Recently, there have been several studies using echocardiography as a noninvasive assessment of cardiac structure and function to demonstrate a link between abnormalities in ECM and MMPs and TIMPs in hypertension. Echocardiography can give an estimate of left ventricular mass, and Doppler imaging allows the study of blood flow patterns within the heart. Tissue Doppler imaging in particular has played an important role in characterizing diastolic dysfunction. This modality offers better assessment of left ventricular relaxation during diastole as compared to transmitral flow assessment because e' (which represents early left ventricular relaxation) decreases progressively as disease advances but E (passive ventricular filling as measured by standard Doppler assessment) decreases and then pseudonormalizes and becomes higher than normal as disease advances.

Tissue inhibitor of metalloproteinase-1, which is raised in patients with hypertension, is associated with several abnormal echocardiographic parameters. Circulating TIMP-1 correlates positively with left ventricular mass (E/e') and negatively with e' (Figure 17–2). Furthermore, a strong link was seen between a TIMP-1 value of >500 ng/mL and reversal of the Doppler E/A ratio of transmitral flow. These findings, although not directly from cardiac tissue, are interesting because they do suggest a role for TIMP-1. Collagen type 1 is a principal determinant cardiac ECM and is therefore a major determinant of left ventricular compliance. Collagen type I is composed of thick strands, imparting strength and rigidity to the ECM. However, excess type I collagen will result in loss of ventricular compliance and elasticity. Hence, passive left ventricular filling in diastole is reduced, as the ventricle is less compliant. Tissue inhibitor of metalloproteinase-

1 is thought to increase tissue concentrations of collagen type I by inhibiting MMPs. Therefore, TIMP-1 may be a key mediator of left ventricular diastolic dysfunction through definition of the ventricular matrix composition and may have a role in the development of symptomatic diastolic heart failure.[12,13]

Of note, there is an interesting link between MMP-1 and TIMP-1. In patients with untreated hypertension, serum CITP and MMP-1 decrease and levels of TIMP-1 rise. In the presence of LVH, MMP-1 and CITP levels are lower and predictably TIMP-1 levels are higher. Following a year's treatment with angiotensin-converting enzyme therapy, levels of CITP and MMP-1 increased but levels of TIMP-1 decreased. Collagen type 1 is a major substrate for MMP-1, and is degraded by MMP-1. Therefore, it is not surprising that there is an inverse relationship between TIMP-1 and MMP-1, and modulation of either may have potential clinical benefit[4] (Figure 17–3).

Left ventricular hypertrophy is not an ideal prognostic marker in hypertension. Although echocardiography is a simple technique, it requires time and expertise to perform. The resting ECG is not sensitive enough. Because there is a relationship between TIMP-1 and left ventricular structure it is plausible that measurement of circulating TIMP-1 could be used to track LVH over a period of time, and may provide prognostically useful information. Although appealing, carefully conducted

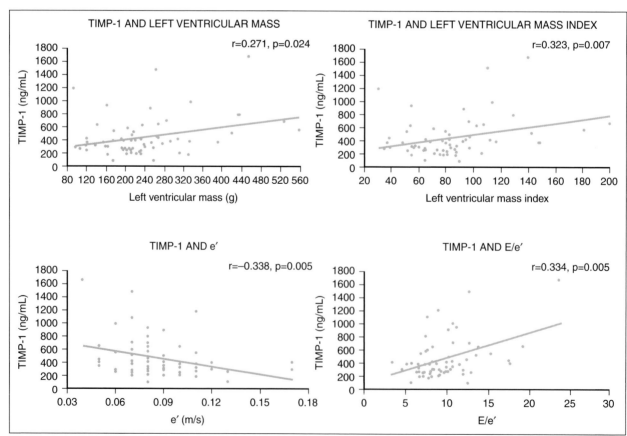

Figure 17–2. The relationship between echocardiographic parameters of left ventricular mass and diastolic function and TIMP-1. (Adapted from Tayebjee MH, Nadar SK, MacFadyen RJ, Lip GY. Tissue inhibitor of metalloproteinase-1 and matrix metalloproteinase-9 levels in patients with hypertension: Relationship to tissue Doppler indices of diastolic relaxation. *Am J Hypertens* 2004;17:770–74 with permission from *The American Journal of Hypertension Ltd.*)

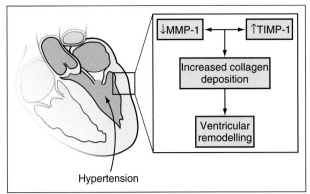

Figure 17–3. In hypertension, a change in tissue concentrations of MMP-1 and TIMP-1 would alter cardiac matrix turnover and affect ventricular mechanics. These changes may be central to abnormal ventricular remodeling and diastolic dysfunction. (MMP-1, matrix metalloproteinase-1; TIMP-1, tissue inhibitor of metalloproteinase-1).

prospective studies are necessary before bringing this into practice. Further, to date no studies have demonstrated a prognostic role for TIMP-1.

Matrix metalloproteinase-9 (MMP-9), on the other hand, has shown some promise as a prognostic marker. Raised circulating levels have been observed in hypertension, coronary artery disease (both stable and unstable), diabetes, and peripheral vascular disease. It is a gelatinase, and is unique in that it can be released rapidly from neutrophils by exocytosis. For this reason it has been implicated in the pathophysiology of plaque rupture in unstable coronary artery disease. This effect is in part mediated by weakening of plaque ECM following release by plaque inflammatory cells. In a large study of patients with stable coronary artery disease, higher circulating levels of MMP-9 were associated with a poorer outcome from cardiovascular events. Moreover, certain alleles of MMP-9 are associated with a poorer prognosis. In patients with hypertension, there is a modest correlation with MMP-9 and Framingham cardiovascular risk scores. Interestingly, treatment of hypertension reduces MMP-9.[3]

From a matrix turnover point of view, what is the role of MMP-9? As discussed previously, increasing arterial stiffness is well recognized and is associated with alterations in the ECM that are principally associated with increased deposition of type I collagen at the expense of the other constituents. For these changes in the ECM composition to occur, there must be a shift in the turnover of ECM. Collagen type I is not a major substrate for MMP-9, and hence raised tissue activity and concentrations may reflect the breakdown of components other than collagen type I in order to facilitate collagen changes mediated by other MMPs. Circulating concentrations of MMP-1 (involved principally in the breakdown of collagen type I) appear to be seen in lower levels in patients with hypertension, and this will favor the maintenance of a stiffer and more fibrous myocardial and/or arterial ECM. Therefore, increased MMP-9 in cardiac and vascular tissue may be "making more space" for the deposition of collagen type I.[14]

Patients with long-standing hypertension sometimes develop hypertensive dilated cardiomyopathy. However, little is known about the changes in MMP and TIMP activity in humans in the context of transition from normal to impaired left ventricular function. There is evidence from studies of myocardial infarction and dilated cardiomyopathy that metalloproteinase activity changes as the ventricle remodels and dilates. Myocardial MMP-9 has shown to be upregulated (and MMP-1 downregulated[15]), and there is an increase in the MMP-9–to–TIMP-1 and MMP-9–to–TIMP-2 ratio.[16,17] MMP-2 and MMP-3 both rise during the development of nonischemic dilated cardiomyopathy and could represent a similar pattern to that seen during hypertensive heart failure. The precise roles of MMPs and TIMPs are unknown, but they almost certainly have a pivotal role in changing the structure and function of cardiac ECM. Indeed, assessment of these MMPs and TIMPs in patients may help in identifying individuals at risk, and therefore it has been speculated that these markers may be of prognostic value.

CLINICAL IMPLICATIONS AND PERSPECTIVES

There is growing evidence now of the fact that MMPs and TIMPs could potentially be used to track the changes in the structure of ECM and may therefore have clinical use. Diastolic dysfunction has been studied more extensively, and results indicate that TIMP-1 may be a useful predictor of this. Nevertheless, the precise role of TIMP-1 in clinical practice has yet to be defined by large-scale studies. One of the potential drawbacks is the large variance in TIMP-1 even in normal individuals. In addition, although assessment of circulating TIMP-1 is easy it must be borne in mind that the total concentration will be a result of "tissue leak" from many organs and is hence not cardiac or vascular specific. Future studies could examine whether there are cardiac-specific isoforms that would increase the specificity of the analysis.

Assessment of matrix metalloproteinase, on the other hand, could have a role in predicting cardiovascular prognosis in patients with hypertension. This could help in better risk stratification. However, because of variance and specificity this analysis will depend on larger-scale studies to determine clinical value. In clinical practice there is a tendency to measure concentration rather than activity, the former being easier. Unfortunately, there is not always a direct link between the two and enzyme activity could be low in the context of high concentration because of inactive enzyme. This point is crucial, especially in the case of MMP-9, where its role in plaque turnover (for example) is a consequence of its activity. More work is needed to decide on whether concentration can be used as a surrogate of activity.

It is being recognized that it may be more useful to study the MMP/TIMP ratio or examine MMP-TIMP complexes rather than the assessment of a single MMP. We have recently demonstrated in gestation hypertension that in normal pregnancy the MMP/TIMP ratio is higher and that with the development of hypertension this ratio falls. In normal pregnancy, the rise in the MMP/TIMP ratio favors activated metalloproteinase activity, and among other actions suggests favoring ECM breakdown. Theoretically, this will obviously be important in the invasion of the uterine wall by the cytotrophoblast. The significant fall in this ratio during gestational hypertension does suggest a milieu that acts against myometrial invasion. The subsequent compromise to placental perfusion can result in relative or absolute fetal hypoxia and disordered placental function. It is important to recognize that this does not provide any information on enzyme

activity. Nevertheless, this model does suggest that MMPs and TIMPs could be useful assessments of matrix structure—especially because the tissue being studied is relatively large (i.e., placenta versus heart).[18]

What about the use of MMP and TIMP modulators clinically? Unfortunately, specific compounds that inhibit MMPs have not really proved beneficial. This may be due to the fact that systemic therapy is not organ or tissue targeted; that is, whereas enzyme inhibition will be beneficial in one area the effects of this would be detrimental in another. Indeed, there is evidence that MMP and TIMP levels vary in different cells. However, indirect manipulation of MMP and TIMP activities has been shown to be beneficial. Use of antihypertensive therapy, drugs that affect the renin-angiotenisn-aldosterone system, and statins have reversed altered MMP and TIMP levels when assessed in tissue and in blood.[4,14]

SUMMARY

Clearly changes in the cardiac and vascular ECM occur in hypertension, the former resulting in left ventricular hypertrophy, diastolic dysfunction, and in some cases hypertensive dilated cardiomyopathy. Arterial stiffness and atherosclerosis are potential consequences of the latter (Figure 17–4). Matrix metalloproteinases and their inhibitors have key roles in mediating these changes. Their main role clinically could be in the noninvasive assessment of tissue structure and prognosis rather than therapy. However, because of the large numbers of MMPs and TIMPs and roles that are not yet clearly defined much more work is needed before they can be considered useful clinical markers.

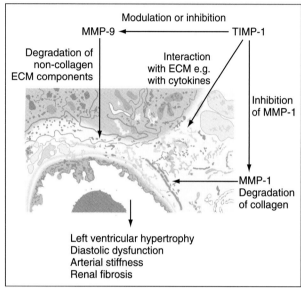

Figure 17–4. Speculative interaction among MMP-1, MMP-9, and TIMP-1 in hypertension.

REFERENCES

1. McCawley L, Matrisian L. Matrix metalloproteinases:they're not just for matrix anymore! *Curr Opin Cell Biol* 2001;13:534–40.

2. Van den Steen PE, Opdenakker G, Wormald MR, et al. Matrix remodelling enzymes, the protease cascade and glycosylation. *Biochimica et Biophysica Acta* 2001;1528:61–73.

3. Tayebjee MH, Lip GY, MacFadyen RJ. Matrix metalloproteinases in coronary artery disease: Clinical and therapeutic implications and pathological significance. *Curr Med Chem* 2005; 12:917–25.

4. Tayebjee MH, MacFadyen RJ, Lip GYH. Extracellular matrix biology: A new frontier in linking the pathology and therapy of hypertension? *J Hypertens* 2003;21:2211–18.

5. Sternlicht MD, Werb Z. How matrix metalloproteinases regulate cell behaviour. *Annu Rev Cell Dev Biol* 2001;17:463–516.

6. Kalela A, Koivu TA, Hoyhtya M, et al. Association of serum MMP-9 with autoantibodies against oxidized LDL. *Atherosclerosis* 2002;160:161–65.

7. Baker A, Zaltsman A, George S, Newby A. Divergent effects of tissue inhibitor of metalloproteinase-1, -2, or -3 overexpression on rat vascular smooth muscle cell invasion, proliferation, and death in vitro: TIMP-3 promotes apoptosis. *J Clin Invest* 1998;101: 1478–87.

8. Díez J, Panizo A,Gil M, et al. Serum markers of collagen type I metabolism in spontaneously hypertensive rats relation to myocardial fibrosis. *Circulation* 1996;93:1026–32.

9. Philips N. Bashey RI. Jimenez SA. Collagen and fibronectin expression in cardiac fibroblasts from hypertensive rats. *Cardiovasc Res* 1994;28:1342–47.

10. Iwanaga Y, Aoyama T, Kihara Y, et al. Excessive activation of matrix metalloproteinases coincides with left ventricular remodeling during transition from hypertrophy to heart failure in hypertensive rats. *J Am Coll Cardiol* 2002;39:1384–91.

11. Mujumdar V, Smiley L, Tyagi S. Activation of matrix metalloproteinase dilates and decreases cardiac tensile strength. *Int J Cardiol* 2001;79:277–86.

12. Lindsay M, Maxwell P, Dunn F. TIMP-1 a marker of left ventricular diastolic dysfunction and fibrosis in hypertension. *Hypertension* 2002;40:136–41.

13. Tayebjee MH, Nadar SK, MacFadyen RJ, Lip GY. Tissue inhibitor of metalloproteinase-1 and matrix metalloproteinase-9 levels in patients with hypertension: Relationship to tissue Doppler indices of diastolic relaxation. *Am J Hypertens* 2004; 17:770–74.

14. Tayebjee MH, Nadar S, Blann AD, et al. Matrix metalloproteinase-9 and tissue inhibitor of metalloproteinase-1 in hypertension and their relationship to cardiovascular risk and treatment: A substudy of the Anglo-Scandinavian Cardiac Outcomes Trial (ASCOT). *Am J Hypertens* 2004;17:764–69.

15. Spinale FG, Coker ML, Heung LJ, et al. A matrix metalloproteinase induction/ activation system exists in the human left ventricular myocardium and is upregulated in heart failure. *Circulation* 2000;102:1944–49.

16. Reinhardt D, Sigusch H, Hensse J, et al. Cardiac remodelling in end stage

heart failure: Upregulation of matrix
metalloproteinase (MMP) irrespective
of the underlying disease, and evidence
for a direct inhibitory effect of ACE
inhibitors on MMP. *Heart* 2002;88:
525–30.

17. Wilson EM, Gunasinghe HR, Coker ML,
et al. Plasma matrix metalloproteinase
and inhibitor profiles in patients with
heart failure. *J Card Fail* 2002;8:390–98.
18. Tayebjee MH, Karalis I, Nadar S,
Beevers DG, MacFadyen RJ, Lip GY.

Circulating matrix metalloproteinase-9
(MMP-9) and tissue inhibitors of
metalloproteinases -1 and -2 (TIMP-1
&2) levels in gestational hypertension.
Am J Hypertens 2005;18:325–29.

Chapter

18

Cell Membranes (Blood Cell and Platelet Membranes in Human Essential Hypertension)

Dieter Rosskopf

Key Findings

- Enhanced activities of Na^+/Li^+ countertransport and Na^+/H^+ exchange in blood cells is a frequent finding in hypertension.

- The physiological roles and the molecular identity of Na^+/Li^+ countertransport remain to be resolved.

- Studies with cell lines from hypertensive individuals indicate that the enhanced activity of Na^+/H^+ exchange is genetically fixed.

- The Na^+/H^+ exchanger isoform 1 (NHE1), the sole mediator of this transport in blood cells, has been excluded as a candidate gene in hypertension.

- An altered regulation of NHE1 is the most likely cause of the observed abnormality.

- Polymorphisms in signaling proteins (e.g., in the G protein β3 subunit) may contribute to the genetically fixed enhancement of NHE1 activity.

INTRODUCTION

Blood cells have been intensively studied in hypertension research for several reasons. First, blood cells are easily accessible and can be obtained noninvasively in contrast to other (more obvious) target tissues in hypertension research. Given the huge number of cells, purification of blood cells and of blood cell membranes is simple. Packed erythrocytes or red cell ghosts (i.e., erythrocyte membrane particles devoid of hemoglobin) can be obtained in large volumes, which was essential for early biochemical and cell physiologic studies. Second, platelets were addressed as model "cells" for vascular smooth muscle and endothelial cells because they share similar receptor systems and signal transduction pathways. In addition, platelets are involved in the pathogenesis of thromboembolic and atherosclerotic processes frequently associated with hypertension (a topic separately addressed in the following chapter).

Third, as molecular biology and genetics emerged, lymphocytes were the prime source of blood DNA. Furthermore, lymphocytes (together with macrophages) are the only blood cells that can be kept alive for several days in cell culture. Immortalization of human B lymphocytes with Epstein-Barr virus (EBV) is (other than outgrowth of fibroblasts from skin specimens) the only method for the routine establishment of human cell lines for limitless supply of biological material from a given human individual. Fourth, in recent years macrophages have been intensively studied for their involvement in atherosclerosis [with special emphasis on inflammation (together with granulocytes and lymphocytes), lipid metabolism, and as models for angiogenesis]. Fifth, abnormalities observed in blood cells are in part considered "intermediate phenotypes" in hypertension. Following this concept, intermediate phenotypes are genetically determined, do not contribute directly to the pathogenesis of hypertension, and may be useful in classifying different types of hypertension and in identifying causative (genetic) factors.

The "model function" (or better "surrogate function") of blood cells, however, involves inherent problems. First, it has been postulated that abnormalities identified in blood cells are representative of similar alterations in key mechanisms of blood pressure regulation (including renal ion handling or cell signaling in resistance vessels). Modern transcriptome or proteome analyses, however, indicate a limited overlap in the expression of such systems between different cell types.

Second, taking blood cells *ex vivo* from hypertensive donors in search of intermediate phenotypes inherently presents the problem that these cells have "experienced" a hypertensive circulation and a hypertensive neurohumoral milieu. Therefore, it is often impossible to distinguish between primary and secondary effects (i.e., between causative factors and epiphenomena of a hypertensive circulation). One possible solution to this dilemma is the mentioned immortalization of human B lymphocytes with EBV and their subsequent characterization after long-term culture. Alterations observed under such conditions have a high probability of indicating a primary defect.

Third, red blood cells lack a nucleus and platelets are subcellular components shed from megakaryocytes (thus preventing the application of advanced techniques from molecular biology and genetics). It is impossible to review here all findings on blood cells in hypertension given the limited space of this chapter and the conjecture that many known biological systems expressed in blood cells have been investigated for a role in hypertension. Many of these systems are extensively covered in other chapters of this book, where their key relevance is obvious. Here we focus on those systems for which guiding contributions originated from the investigation of blood cells.

With the emergence half a century ago of evidence that altered renal sodium processing may contribute to the pathogenesis of hypertension, cellular cation homeostasis became an important research area.[1] Intracellular Na^+ concentration was reported to be increased in red and white blood cells in hypertension, although this notion was later challenged. Likewise, there exist many reports of altered blood cell Na^+ transport mechanisms (including passive Na^+ fluxes, Na^+/K^+ ATPase activity, and $Na^+/K^+/Cl^-$ transport activity).[2] (See also Figure 18–1.) With the advent of prophylactic lithium therapy in mood disorders, a Na^+/Li^+ countertransport (SLC) activity was discovered in red blood cells that set the intracellular Li^+ concentration below the serum concentration.[3] More than a quarter of a century ago, Canessa and co-workers reported in a seminal publication an enhanced SLC activity in hypertension, a finding that set in motion many clinical, epidemiologic, and genetic studies. There are currently more than a thousand reports on this subject.[4,5,6]

Today, enhanced SLC activity is the best-characterized intermediate phenotype in hypertension. Because Li^+ is virtually absent from body fluids, SLC activity was considered an artificial transport mode. Hence, it was logical that the discovery of Na^+/H^+ transport mechanisms gave rise to the notion that Na^+/Li^+ countertransport is only a peculiar transport mode under highly artificial conditions. Thus, many groups moved to the analysis of cellular Na^+/H^+ transport activity, which was subsequently found to be enhanced in hypertension.[7–10] Despite many efforts, it remains still open whether blood cell Na^+/Li^+ and Na^+/H^+ exchange is mediated by an identical protein. Searches for genetic polymorphisms in the gene for the Na^+/H^+ exchanger isoform expressed in blood cells remained unsuccessful, and genome-wide linkage analysis excluded this gene as a candidate gene in hypertension.[11] Likewise, the variation in SLC activity could not be attributed to genetic markers in the NHE1 gene.[12] Na^+/H^+ exchanger activity is modulated by many different intracellular signaling systems.

Taking into consideration that Ca^{2+} concentrations are elevated in platelets from hypertensive subjects, the interplay between Na^+/H^+ exchange activity and cellular signaling was intensively studied and led to the identification of a polymorphism in a heterotrimeric G protein supposed to be linked to enhanced Na^+/H^+ exchange activity (a notion that still awaits formal proof).[13] Following this route, we will focus here on abnormalities in Na^+/H^+ exchange and Na^+/Li^+ countertransport, and we will address basic functions and abnormalities of G protein signaling in hypertension.

ANATOMY, BIOCHEMISTRY, AND PHYSIOLOGY

Fundamental information on the generation, function, and fate of blood cells and the key organs involved can be found in many excellent textbooks of hematology and physiology.

Cation transport mechanisms in blood cells: Na^+/Li^+ countertransport

With concepts of abnormal renal Na^+ handling[1] and based on the at that time unproven assumption that relevant ion carriers could exist in blood cells and display similar abnormalities as in the kidney, a multitude of studies have utilized the ready availability and suitability of erythrocytes for transport studies in hypertension.[2,10] Transport physiologists have characterized several Na^+ transport systems in blood cells and most of them could meanwhile be attributed to distinct transporter proteins/genes on a molecular level (Figure 18–1). These Na^+ transport systems include the amiloride-sensitive Na^+/H^+ exchanger, the ouabain-sensitive Na^+ pump, sodium-dependent and -independent Cl^-/HCO_3^- exchangers (inhibited by DIDS, a stilbene sulphonate), and a furosemide-sensitive $Na^+-K^+-2Cl^-$ cotransporter.

Under physiological conditions, the Na^+ pump (also called the Na^+/K^+ ATPase) transports Na^+ out of cells and thus constitutes the driving force behind the other transport systems (which cause an influx of Na^+). Measurements of the maximum Na^+ transport rates for these transporter modes indicate that Na^+/H^+ exchange exhibits the highest Na^+ transport capacity, followed by the Na^+-dependent Cl^-/HCO_3^- exchange (most likely a coupled transport process), and finally by the $Na^+-K^+-2Cl^-$ cotransporter differing by almost one order of magnitude each. Furthermore, using radioactive Na^+ isotopes transport modes as Na^+-coupled Na^+ transport have been described (today best attributed to concerted actions of the previously cited transporters and the sodium pump). Of note, all of these transporters accept lithium ions for sodium ions, a fact that mirrors similar electrochemical properties of Na^+ and Li^+.

An Na^+/Li^+ exchange activity was identified in red cells with the introduction of lithium therapy.[3] For measure-

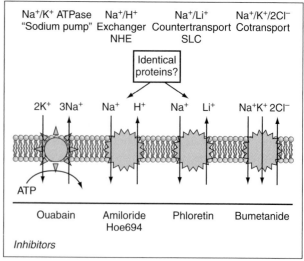

Figure 18–1. Major cation transporters in blood cells. Shown is the physiological transport mode and indicated are typical inhibitors.

ment of SLC, red cells are loaded with lithium (according to the standard procedure in the seminal report by Canessa et al.) to 13 mmol/L, and aliquots are allowed to leak into ouabain-containing medium in the presence or absence of 150 mmol/l Na^+.[4] Here, Na^+ influx is coupled in a 1:1 stoichiometry to Li^+ efflux. In comparison with the other Na^+ transporters mentioned previously, maximum Na^+ influx rates mediated by SLC are one order of magnitude lower than Na^+ influx by Na^+/H^+ exchange and are in the range of $Na^+/K^+/2Cl^-$ cotransport. SLC activity is inhibited by phloretin. Exposure to N-ethylmaleimide, an alkylating agent, results in altered SLC kinetics which was taken as an early hint for the involvement of a transport protein. Initially, SLC was thought to be confined to red blood cells.[5,6] Subsequent studies, however, demonstrated SLC activity in fibroblasts and lymphoblasts[14,15] among others.

The physiological role of SLC is a puzzling question because plasma is normally lacking Li^+. One concept proposes that SLC catalyzes an equimolar Na^+/Na^+ exchange that is physiologically silent and of low activity compared with other Na^+ transport modes. Such a concept, however, is again not a satisfying answer to its physiological role. This led to concepts that Na^+/Li^+ exchange is a special transport mode of Na^+/H^+ exchangers.

Na^+/H^+ exchange

Na^+/H^+ exchange (NHE) as a transport mode was first described in 1976. Its first isoform (NHE1) was cloned[16] in 1989, followed by the identification and cloning of at least five more NHE isoforms.[17] NHE1, the ubiquitously expressed "housekeeping" isoform, is of key importance for intracellular pH (pH_i) regulation and cellular volume control. NHE2, NHE3, and NHE4 are predominantly expressed in polarized epithelia, and NHE5 is confined to the brain. In concerted actions together with carbonic anhydrase enzyme and Cl^-/HCO_3^- exchange mechanisms, the epithelial isoforms mediate vectorial Na^+ transport thereby driving water fluxes and bicarbonate transport. Newly identified isoforms (NHE6 through NHE9) have been localized to intracellular structures, and their precise functions remain elusive. A novel nomenclature for the respective genes refers to SLC9A1-9 for NHE isoforms 1 through 9.[18-20]

Here, we will focus on NHE1, the isoform expressed in blood cells. In addition to its "housekeeping" functions in pH_i and volume regulation, NHE1 activity has been implicated in cell cycle regulation, proliferation, migration, adhesion, and resistance to apoptosis. The transporter is an integral plasma membrane protein and mediates under physiological conditions the exchange of intracellular H^+ for extracellular Na^+, with the Na^+ gradient established by the Na^+/K^+ pump as the driving force. Intracellular acidification activates the exchanger, which acts to reestablish the pH_i to a certain set point. Kinetically, this is an allosteric regulation by intracellular H^+ mediated by a proposed H^+ sensor in the molecule which is further modified by additional regulatory modifications of the transport protein.

Subtle fluctuations in steady-state pH_i affect the action of many biomolecules and may even be used for regulatory purposes. Therefore, the fine control of pH_i is of fundamental importance in sustaining a suitable milieu for stable enzymatic activity, protein interactions, and ultimately cell function and survival. To this end, cells express several pH_i-regulating mechanisms, including Na^+/H^+ exchange and Na^+-dependent and -independent Cl^-/HCO_3^- exchangers. Under hypoxic conditions (e.g., during myocardial or cerebral ischemia) an uncontrolled acidification by excess metabolic acid production occurs, causing gross damage to the cell. Here, pH_i-regulating processes (including NHE1) guard against uncontrolled acidification by maintaining intracytoplasmic acid/base balance.[21]

Cellular volume control is of similar vital importance, and adaptations are obviously necessary during cell growth and division. Protons (in contrast to Na^+ ions) are not osmotically active. Thus, an exchange of intracellular H^+ for extracellular Na^+ is accompanied by a net influx of water and NHE1 activation, an important mechanism in fighting volume shrinkage and in inducing volume increase. The fine control of such processes, however, requires the concerted action of several ion-transporting systems other than NHE1.[20] Potent inhibitors of NHE1 are pyrazone derivatives (amiloride, dimethylamiloride, ethylisopropylamiloride) and benzoylguanidine derivatives (cariporide, HOE694, eniporide).[21] Available evidence suggests that these compounds affect the interaction of NHE1 with Na^+. Kinetic properties, molecular and cellular regulations, and susceptibilities to inhibitors differ considerably among various NHE isoforms.

On a molecular level, NHE1, the prototypic Na^+/H^+ exchanger, consists of 12 conserved membrane-spanning domains at the N-terminus of the protein, followed by a long intracellular C-terminus. This intracellular domain comprises numerous predicted phosphorylation sites for different kinases and binding sites for other ancillary factors. It thus appears to serve as the major regulatory domain of NHE1 (Figure 18–2A). The extended loop between transmembrane domains 9 and 10 is supposed to form part of the ion conduction pathway. There is some limited evidence suggesting a higher order of NHE1 molecules *in vivo* (for instance, as homodimers or tetramer complexes).

Na^+/H^+ exchangers are subject to an intensive and complex regulation in addition to their kinetic control by Na^+ and H^+ ions. Many hormones, neurotransmitters, and growth factors activate NHE1, thereby causing an intracellular alkalinization and volume increases that frequently precede cell proliferation. Hence, NHE1 has also been considered a "growth factor activatable" Na^+/H^+ exchanger. Such stimuli (e.g., serum, growth factors, thrombin, angiotensin II, a-adrenoceptor agonists, and many more) are transmitted by membrane receptors of the G protein-coupled receptor family or by the family of receptor tyrosine kinases. This activation converges on the common mitogen-activated protein kinase (MAP kinase) pathway and involves a mitogen-activated extracellular-signal-related kinase (MEK-ERK)-p90[rsk].

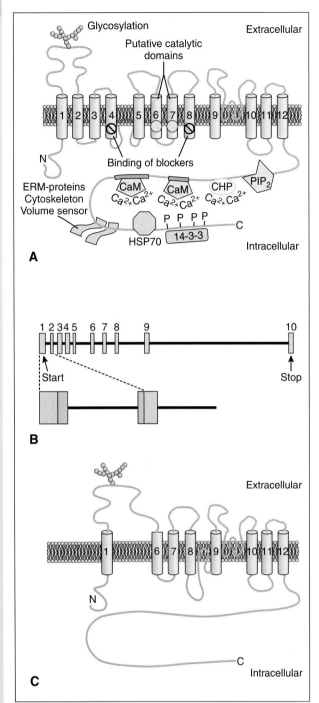

Figure 18–2. (A) Topological model of the Na⁺/H⁺ exchanger isoform 1. The transporter consists of 12 transmembrane domains and a long cytoplasmic domain, which is involved in regulation of the transport activity. Indicated are the putative binding sites for interacting proteins: CaM (Ca/Calmodulin), HSP70 (heat shock protein), PIP2 (phosphatidylinositol-4,5-bisphosphate), ERM (esrin-radixin-moesin protein binding), and CHP (calcineurin-homolog protein). **(B)** Gene structure and alternative splicing leading to the putative variant DNHE1. Parts from exons 1 and 2 that are alternatively spliced are indicated in red. **(C)** Putative structure of DNHE1, a variant of NHE1 assumed to mediate Na⁺/Li⁺ exchange.

This latter kinase phosphorylates a conserved serine of NHE1, which in turn can bind multifunctional scaffolding proteins of the 14-3-3 class that can mediate a further assembly of additional signaling molecules. NHE1 is also a substrate for the p160 Rho-associated kinase (p160ROCK), which transduces signals from integrin receptors involved in cell adhesion and spreading. The platelet-derived growth factor receptor can activate NHE1 by a second pathway in addition to the MAP kinase pathway, which involves an Nck-interacting kinase (NIK). The mechanism whereby phosphorylation of the intracellular NHE1 C-terminus translates into increased cation transport remains unexplained. Available evidence suggests that NHE1 forms a multiprotein complex, and it has been proposed that carbonic anhydrase binds to modified sites on NHE1. The local production of H⁺ could in turn stimulate NHE1 by the common kinetic mechanisms.

In addition to 14-3-3 proteins and carbonic anhydrase, Ca²⁺/calmodulin is an important binding partner that increases NHE1 transport activity and appears to integrate signals from stimuli that lead to an increase in cellular Ca²⁺ concentrations. The Ca²⁺-binding phosphoproteins CHP1 and CHP2 (calcineurin B homologous protein) and tescalcin also bind to NHE1. Association with these proteins is also accompanied by an increase in steady-state pH$_i$. Furthermore, binding of the phosphoinositide phosphatidylinositol 4,5 bisphosphate (PIP$_2$) has been demonstrated to be critical for optimal NHE1 activity, which would connect the exchanger to a complex regulation by systems affecting the phosphoinositide content.[19-23]

Finally, NHE1 can interact with members of the ERM family of actin-binding proteins (which include ezrin, radixin, and moesin). Here, NHE1 serves as a membrane anchor for cytoskeleton proteins and can act as a scaffold protein to generate multiprotein complexes in signal transduction. In accord with the distribution of such interacting proteins, NHE1 molecules are not evenly distributed on the plasma membrane but accumulate in certain microdomains. The interaction with ERM proteins is important for the reorganization of the actin cytoskeleton and in turn for the control of cell morphology, adhesion, and migration. Interestingly, this function appears to be at least in part independent of the cation transporting function. Taken together, we have to envisage NHE1 not only as an important ion transporter that fundamentally affects cellular homeostasis but as a highly complex integrator for a vast array of different extracellular signals (Figure 18–3 summarizes some of these pathways).

Given this complex regulation and the ubiquitous expression of NHE1, it is difficult to predict its physiological role *in vivo*, a question that has now been addressed with several mouse models. In one spontaneous mutant mouse model, a nonsense mutation (Lys442) in NHE1 occurs that causes a highly reduced transport activity. These mice are termed SWE (slow-wave epilepsy) mice,

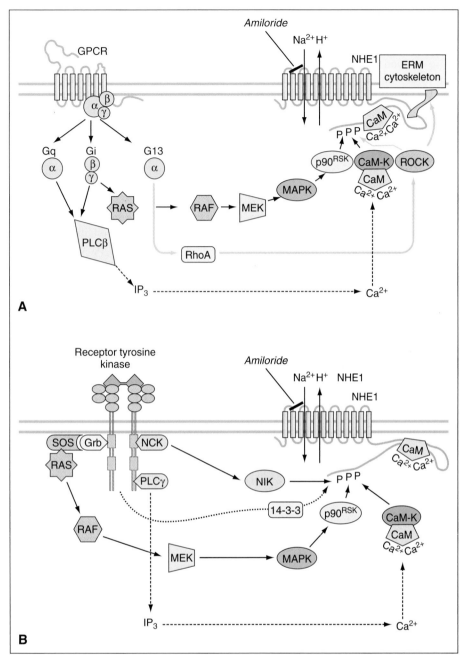

Figure 18–3. Examples for the complex regulation of NHE1 by signal transduction events. (**A**) Activation by G protein-coupled receptor. (**B**) Receptor tyrosine kinases (e.g., platelet-derived growth factor receptor). Pathways have been explained in the main body of the text.

referring to one characteristic of a more complex phenotype in homozygous animals that includes growth retardation, seizures (grand mal and petit mal), locomotor ataxia, and high mortality before weaning.[24] In a targeted NHE1 knockout animal model a similar phenotype has been observed.[25] In addition, these mice had a reduced parotid gland secretion, were resistant to experimental cardiac ischemia/reperfusion injuries, and exhibited a decreased renal HCO_3^- absorption and a distinctly altered gene expression in the brain.

Heterotrimeric G proteins

We will learn in the "Pathophysiology" section of this chapter that increased activity of NHE1 is a frequent observation in primary hypertension. Genetic studies argued against a genetic defect in NHE1 that causes hypertension, a notion that sparked an intensive search for abnormalities in the complex regulation of NHE1 in hypertension. One approach was to investigate G protein-coupled signal transduction in hypertension, which resulted in the identification of a functional polymorphism in a G protein β subunit. Here, we present some essential information on the functions of heterotrimeric G proteins.[26–30] Their name relates to two main characteristics: their ability to bind guanine nucleotides and their composition of three different subunits termed Gα, Gβ, and Gγ. Gβ and Gγ form a stable dimer and act as a functional monomer.

The Gα subunit carries the enzymatic activity of the complex in that it mediates the hydrolytic conversion of GTP into GDP. The crucial function of heterotrimeric G proteins is to relay the activation from an agonist-bound receptor to various intracellular effector systems. The family of G protein-coupled receptors (GPCR) counts more than one thousand members (the largest family of membrane receptors in our genome). All GPCR consist of seven membrane-spanning domains, which led to the synonyms *heptahelical receptors* and *serpentine receptors*. Typical members of this class of receptors are all adrenergic receptors, angiotensin II receptors, thrombin receptors, and many more.

The inactive heterotrimeric G protein consists of a Gα subunit and a Gβγ dimer. The Gα subunit has bound GDP. Upon interaction with an activated GPCR, the Gα subunit changes its conformation and releases GDP (Figure 18–4). The GDP is replaced by GTP and in its GTP-bound state the Gα subunit takes an activated conformation with low affinity for the Gβγ dimer. Subsequently, GTP-bound Gα subunits interact with their respective effector systems (e.g., adenylyl cyclases) and modulate their activity. Like-

wise, free Gβγ dimers are also effective regulators of many effector systems. The GTPase activity of the Gα subunit mediates a hydrolytic cleavage of GTP into GDP, which terminates its active conformation. Upon association of the GDP-bound Gα with a Gβγ dimer, the "GTPase cycle" is closed and the heterotrimeric G protein is ready for another round of activation.

At present, more than 20 Gα, 5 Gβ, and 12 Gγ genes have been identified in the human genome. Together, they give rise to (theoretically) more than a thousand different heterotrimers, which may explain the observed receptor and effector specificity in G protein-mediated cell signaling. Currently, G proteins are further subdivided according to their Gα subunit. $G\alpha_S$, the "stimulatory G protein," was identified based on its ability to activate adenylyl cyclases. Likewise, $G\alpha_i$ (the "inhibitory G protein") diminishes the activity of adenylyl cyclase isoforms. There are actually several isoforms in the $G\alpha_i$ family ($G\alpha_{i1}$, $G\alpha_{i2}$, $G\alpha_{i3}$, $G\alpha_o$), with sometimes distinct functions. In addition to inhibiting adenylyl cyclase activity, activation of $G\alpha_i$ has been linked to many more cellular effects, including activation of potassium channels, activation of kinase pathways, and initiation of cell proliferation. Most likely, these latter functions are attributable to the release of Gβγ subunits.

Another subfamily of Gα proteins, the $G\alpha_q$ family, with the members $G\alpha_q$, $G\alpha_{11}$, $G\alpha_{14}$, and $G\alpha_{15}$ is predominantly involved in the activation of phospholipase Cβ isoforms, which results in the generation of inositol trisphosphate and ultimately in an increase of intracellular Ca^{2+}. $G\alpha_{12}$ and $G\alpha_{13}$ mediate the activation of small G proteins of the rho family, which are implicated in the regulation of cell shape and motility. Free Gβγ dimers are also important and versatile regulators of many effector systems, including adenylyl cyclases, phospholipase Cβ isoforms, PI3 kinases, potassium and calcium channel isoforms, and several kinase systems associated with cell proliferation. In principle, Gβγ dimers are released upon activation of any Gα subunit. $G\alpha_i$ proteins, however, are the most frequently expressed Gα class of G proteins on a molar level, which makes them a main source of free Gβγ subunits.

Historically, G proteins have also been classified according to their susceptibility to modification by bacterial toxins. Hence, $G\alpha_S$ proteins are activated by treatment with cholera toxin whereas members of the $G\alpha_i$ family are inhibited upon exposure to pertussis toxin. Therefore, $G\alpha_i$ proteins are frequently referred to as "pertussis toxin-sensitive" or "PTX-sensitive" G proteins.

The crucial advantage of this highly complex system of different G proteins and effector systems is its ability to integrate and fine-tune many different signals into a cellular response. For instance, adenylyl cyclase activity (and thus the generation of cAMP) is stimulated by the $G\alpha_S$ pathway, is inhibited by $G\alpha_i$ proteins, and can further be modulated by released Gβγ subunits and Ca^{2+} transients elicited by activation of $G\alpha_q$. Within the last decade, additional regulators of this system have been identified that deserve mention. RGS proteins are "regulators of G protein signaling" and serve to accelerate the GTPase activity of Gα subunits and thus to terminate G protein-mediated signals.[31]

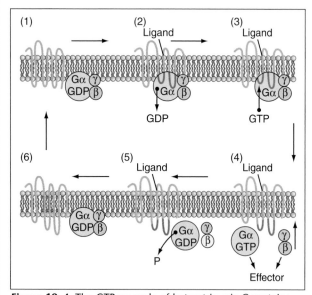

Figure 18–4. The GTPase cycle of heterotrimeric G proteins. Binding of a ligand to a heptahelical receptor induces a conformational change that is transduced to interacting Gα proteins[2] (GDP-bound, inactive). An ensuing conformational change of the Gα subunits induces a GDP/GTP exchange[3] and the dissociation of the now activated Gα subunit (GTP-bound) from the Gβγ dimer and the receptor. Gβγ subunit and activated Gα subunit modulate effector systems.[4] The endogenous GTPase activity of the Gα subunit hydrolyzes GTP to GDP and leading to a reassociation and potentially another round of the GTPase cycle.[5,6]

Similarly, G protein receptor kinases (GRKs) inhibit once-activated GPCRs, thus counteracting unbalanced cell activation.[32] In the context of hypertension research, GRK4 has attained some interest because genetic polymorphisms of this gene have been associated with hypertension.[33] GRK4 expression is confined to the kidneys, where it regulates dopamine receptor 1 activity. One polymorphism causes an amino acid exchange of the gene, which becomes constitutively active resulting in a sustained down-regulation of dopamine receptor signaling.[33]

PATHOPHYSIOLOGY

Na⁺/Li⁺ countertransport

Following the seminal report by Canessa et al. of an enhanced SLC activity in primary hypertension, more than hundred independent reports confirmed this result.[4–6] Subsequent studies showed that enhanced SLC activity is also associated with type I diabetes, especially in the context of hypertension (i.e., insulin resistance, hyperlipidemia, gravidity with and without hypertension, and renal and cardiac hypertrophy). Increased SLC activity has also been demonstrated in rapid progressive IgA nephropathy and in diabetic patients with proliferative retinopathy.[4–6] Enhanced SLC activity is one of the strongest predictors for diabetic nephropathy. Within the context of hypertension, SLC activity has been associated with phenotypes of non-modulating hypertension and an enhanced total body exchangeable Na⁺.

An increase in SLC activity has not only been confined to red blood cells from hypertensive individuals but has been detected *ex vivo* in skin fibroblasts[15] and lymphoblasts from hypertensive patients,[14] which may be taken as a clue for a generalized membrane abnormality that prevails in cell culture indicating a genetic determination. It is important to note that these findings always refer to the mean Na⁺/Li⁺ exchange activity in hypertension and that there is a considerable overlap between values of normotensive and hypertensive subjects. SLC activity is modulated by different factors. Addition of insulin in physiological concentrations to erythrocytes from fasted individuals results in increased maximal SLC transport rates. Alcohol intake or use of steroids also affects SLC activity.

Despite intensive efforts, the mechanisms that contribute to altered SLC kinetics are currently not understood. Several hypotheses have been proposed, including concepts of genetic variants in the (so far, unidentified) transporter gene or of circulating factors in hypertension that activate SLC with insulin. According to another model, enhanced SLC activity mirrors (more or less nonspecifically) an altered lipid composition of the plasma membrane that results in an enhanced "membrane viscosity."[34] Experimental modification of the lipid composition has been accompanied by changes in SLC activity and studies in normo- and hyperlipidemic individuals or upon treatment with lipid-lowering agents have demonstrated modulatory effects on SLC activity. Despite considerable efforts, a consistent model demonstrating

how changes in the lipid composition cause altered SLC activity is still missing.

Based on the observation that exposure of red cells to N-ethylmaleimide result in a modulation of SLC activity, speculations have been put forward that thiol modifications (e.g., by oxidation) of transporters or associated proteins contribute to the observed kinetic abnormalities.[35] Taken together, the exact mechanisms that cause altered SLC activity remain to be unraveled. A major hindrance in these attempts is the unresolved question of which protein mediates SLC such that the direct investigative modification of the systems by methods of modern molecular biology is prevented. Hence, it is generally understood that SLC does not constitute a physiologically relevant ion exchange that directly causes hypertension, but rather represents a sensitive indicator for aspects of a membrane abnormality that may cause (or is itself caused by) the underlying pathology (i.e., primary hypertension). In this scenario, enhanced SLC activity remains a valuable marker for a predisposition to essential hypertension and for the rate of progression of several renal diseases and diabetic complications.

Na⁺/H⁺ exchange

Based on the still unproven hypothesis that SLC is a specialized transport mode of Na⁺/H⁺ exchange,[7] many groups have tested this assumption in different cell types from hypertensive humans and in animal models of hypertension. A considerable body of evidence on this topic has been accumulated that correlates an increased Na⁺/H⁺ exchange activity with hypertension, although with some controversy.[9,36,37] Increased activity of Na⁺/H⁺ exchange was first described in human platelets, followed by similar reports in erythrocytes and lymphocytes.[7,8]

In these cell types, Na⁺/H⁺ exchange activity is almost exclusively mediated by the NHE1 isoform, which was subsequently considered a target gene for hypertension research. In addition, enhanced Na⁺/H⁺ exchange activity was also observed in various tissues from spontaneously hypertensive rats, including vascular smooth muscle cells.[36,37] Furthermore, an enhanced NHE1 activity was also observed in patients with diabetic nephropathy, analogous with findings with SLC.[38] Another similarity with SLC is the substantial overlap in NHE1 activities between normotensive and hypertensive individuals, which precludes its use for diagnostic purposes.

Several hypotheses were put forward about how an increase in Na⁺/H⁺ exchange activity could translate in a rise in blood pressure. First, it was claimed that an enhanced Na⁺/H⁺ exhange upon expression of an analogous activity in the kidney could cause an increased Na⁺ reabsorption. Current evidence, however, suggests that NHE3 is crucial for this function. Other concepts attributed increased NHE1 activity (e.g., in vascular smooth muscle cells) to elevated intracellular Na⁺ levels that could inhibit Na⁺/Ca²⁺ exchange and ultimately result in increased Ca²⁺ concentrations (which were again frequently but not unequivocally observed in blood platelets).[39] Alternatively, it has been suggested that high NHE1 activity leads to an increased proliferation, and ultimately by media hyperplasia of blood vessels to hypertension. None of these concepts has been proven so far.

The cloning of NHE1 allowed extending this research to a molecular level.[17] Most authors agree that in humans and in SHR animals enhanced NHE1 activity is not accompanied by an enhanced expression of NHE1 transcripts or NHE1 protein.[40-43] This is in striking contrast to the finding that unselective overexpression of NHE1 in transgenic mice causes a salt-sensitive form of hypertension.[44] On the one hand, this underscores that NHE1 may actually contribute to blood pressure regulation. On the other hand, it demonstrates that animal models are sometimes of limited relevance for human hypertension.

As explained in the introduction to this chapter, research on blood cells in hypertension bears the inherent challenge of discriminating between cause and effect, i.e., between potential primary factors and epiphenomena of the disease. One way of circumventing this problem is the use of cell lines from individuals with a certain hypertension-associated cellular phenotype. If such a phenotype is sustained in many generations of cell culture, it is plausibile to conclude that a genetic basis for this observation exists.

Two principal models allow for the generation of individual human cell lines: (1) the immortalization of B lymphoblasts with the EBV and (2) the outgrowth of skin fibroblasts from tiny biopsies. Using EBV-transformed lymphoblasts from patients with hypertension[40,43] and from patients with diabetes[45] and diabetic nephropathy,[46] a sustained increase in NHE1 activity could be demonstrated that prevailed in cell culture. Later, some findings were repeated with human skin fibroblasts.[47] Again, the enhancement of NHE1 activity was not related to an increased NHE1 transcript or protein expression. Together, these observations strengthened the notion that NHE1 is a prime candidate gene of human hypertension. Extensive sequencing efforts and linkage analyses, however, ruled out this possibility.[11]

NHE1 is subject to a complex and multifaceted regulation integrating many different outside and inside signals of mammalian cells. Current concepts suggest that the increased NHE1 activity is a genetically determined marker for alterations in the upstream regulation of NHE1. This notion is further strengthened by experimental evidence showing an increased phosphorylation of the NHE1 proteins in hypertension with increased NHE1 activity in humans and rats.[48,49] In diabetic nephropathy, however, increased NHE1 activity was not accompanied by an altered phosphorylation of the protein.[50] Furthermore, increased phosphorylation was not the only factor involved in the increased NHE1 activity in hypertension.

Because NHE1 is a substrate for several kinases, one strategy for unraveling an "initial" abnormality is to systematically follow these signaling pathways from the NHE1 protein upstream. Hence, an increased activity of the MAP kinase cascade has been reported in cells with enhanced NHE1 activity.[51] Again, it is not clear whether this is the prime cause of enhanced NHE1 activity. Thus,

it remains open whether we will ever find such an "initial" abnormality. The chances are that there exist different factors contributing to an enhanced sensitivity of cells from hypertensive subjects. In such a scenario, an enhanced NHE1 activity could be a common integrator of various factors with a strong genetic basis.

G proteins and hypertension

Tightly linked to concepts of an enhanced reactivity of cells from some hypertensive patients, as mirrored by an enhanced NHE1 activity, we systematically began to investigate signal transduction upstream of NHE1 using the generated EBV lymphoblasts and skin fibroblasts.[52,53] A crucial observation was that Ca^{2+} signals, elicited by typical GPCRs, are also increased in cells lines from hypertensive individuals. Treatment with pertussis toxin abolished these differences, indicating the involvement of $G\alpha_i$ type G proteins.[52] A systematic sequencing strategy resulted in the discovery of a genetic polymorphism in *GNB3* (C825T), the gene for the Gβ3 subunit associated with hypertension.[13]

Mechanistically, this polymorphism is associated with the occurrence of two alternative splice variants termed Gβ3s and Gβ3s2.[13,54] Gβ subunits together with Gγ subunits in a stable dimer are potent regulators of many effector systems.[27] Protein crystallization studies have resolved the structure of the Gβγ dimer. The Gβ protein consists of seven regular protein motifs called WD domains. These seven domains, which are highly conserved in all eukaryotes, form a propeller protein that exhibits a very compact and stable structure. This highly coordinated stable structure allows Gβ proteins to assemble and coordinate other proteins which is how Gβγ dimers regulate effector systems.[55] The splicing to Gβ3s or Gβ3s2 causes the loss of the equivalent of one WD domain upon translation of such transcripts (Figure 18–5).[54]

Expression of these variants is associated with an increased signal transduction, as indicated by enhanced Ca^{2+} signals, accelerated proliferation, or increased

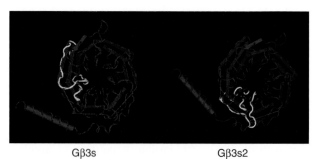

Gβ3s   Gβ3s2

Figure 18–5. Models of Gβ3s and Gβ3s2. Based on the protein crystallization data obtained from the highly homologous protein Gβ1, the structure of the Gβ3 protein is depicted (without Gα and Gγ). The picture shows the typical propeller structure consisting of seven WD domains ("propeller blades") and an N-terminal helical extension. The yellow ribbons indicate the structural elements that are missing in Gβ3s and Gβ3s2, caused by alternative splicing. In both cases the equivalent of one WD domain is missing, leading to a proposed structure of six WD domains.

stimulated GTPγS binding (a measure of G protein activation).[56] It is difficult to explain how the loss of one WD domain translates into the gain-of-function of the system. One theory suggests that Gβγ dimers containing Gβ3s or Gβ3s2 are less suited to stabilize a Gα subunit in its GDP-bound form as a heterotrimer. This could result in an increased sensitivity of such a heterotrimer toward activation by a receptor.[56] Although these concepts contain some plausibility, conclusive proof is missing.

Overexpression of Gβ3s or Gβ3s2 in different cell types and model systems mimics some of these issues, whereas other features are missing (e.g., the activation of certain effector systems by Gβ3s or Gβ3s2).[54,57] Overexpressing G protein components into cell lines is a routine method of analyzing this system but bears some problems because it grossly disturbs a finely controlled balance of endogenous G-protein-signaling components. Presently, we have to conclude that despite considerable efforts the molecular nature by which a polymorphism in *GNB3* translates into a complex phenotype is as yet unresolved which contrasts with the considerable amount of data from genetic association studies.

Given that the 825T allele of the mentioned *GNB3* C825T polymorphism sensitizes signal transduction in all cell types where Gβ3 is expressed, it is relatively easy to speculate that an enhanced signal transduction may affect vessel reactivity, the activity of the vegetative nerve system, or the signaling by vasoactive agonists (including angiotensin II and endothelins). This could ultimately result in hypertension. Again, a final proof of these concepts is missing. The discovery of the *GNB3* C825T polymorphism is a sequel of studies on NHE1 exchange activity. A convincing association, however, of the *GNB3* 825T allele with enhanced NHE1 activity (or SLC activity) in large human samples has not been demonstrated. A small sample could not describe a linkage between cation transport activities and *GNB3* polymorphisms.[58] Other relevant results from association studies pertaining to Gβ3 are summarized in the section following.

GENETICS

SLC activity has been shown to be heritable to a high extent, but the genetic mechanisms have been difficult to identify so far. Several studies suggest that 50 to 80% of the population variation in SLC activity is attributable to genetic effects, with additional evidence for segregation at a single locus.[59] Increased SLC activity is already detectable in children and adolescents.[60] Similar associations between SLC activity and the phenotypic characteristics described have been demonstrated in many ethnic groups, including whites, Asians, and blacks.[61] In blacks, however, absolute SLC activity is lower than in the other ethnic groups.

An important yet unresolved question is whether Na+/Li+ countertransport is an artificial transport mode of the ubiquitous NHE1, a debate starting shortly after the discovery of SLC. NHE1 and SLC differ in their susceptibility to inhibitors. Whereas NHE1 is potently blocked by amiloride derivatives, these compounds do not affect

SLC activity which is inhibited by phloretin, a compound that, conversely, does not affect NHE1.

The cloning strategy for NHE1 involved the application of a suicide selection process that relied on the acceptance of Li+ for Na+.[17] Expression of the NHE1 cDNA in Xenopus oocytes conferred both Na+/H+ exchange and Na+/Li+ exchange activity.[62] At first glance, this might represent a convincing argument for the molecular identities of NHE1 and SLC. The observation, however, that SLC became amiloride sensitive in Xenopus oocytes was difficult to understand and could be interpreted as the susceptibility to inhibition changes in oocytes or the fact that NHE1 is able to mediate SLC but only in the amphibian system.[62]

Two more recent reports addressed this issue again. In 2001, Kammerer et al. reported an analysis of the variances in SLC activity in 634 non-inbred baboons comprising 11 pedigrees, a primate model for primary hypertension.[63] The heritability attributable to SLC activity in this model was almost 60%. In a multipoint genome-wide screen they found evidence for a possible quantitative trait locus (QTL) on baboon chromosome 5, which is homologous to human chromosome 4. This locus, which comprises a wide-stretched region of chromosome 5, was calculated to contribute two-thirds of the observed total genetic variability of SLC activity. This finding contrasts with the localization of the human NHE1 gene (SLC9A1) on chromosome 1. On the other hand, it is not imperative that genetic abnormalities that affect transport activity reside in the transporter gene itself. Polymorphisms in regulating pathways or interacting proteins can also cause genetically fixed transport abnormalities. Hence, these results underscore again the heritability of SLC but do not answer the question of identity.

In 2003, Zerbini et al. argued that SLC is mediated by a splice variant of NHE1 referred to as DNHE1.[64] Here, alternative splicing occurs with non-canonical splice sites in exon 1 and exon 2 (Figure 18–2B and C). By immunoblotting they demonstrated the existence of an immunoreactive protein with the predicted size of DNHE1 together with NHE1 in membranes from red cells and reticulocytes in similar amounts. Upon expression of the respective cDNA in fibroblasts lacking NHE1, an amiloride-insensitive but phloretin-sensitive SLC activity was measured. By semiquantitative RT-PCR, an enhanced transcript expression of NHE1 plus DHNE1 was observed in mRNA prepared from whole blood of individuals with high SLC activity compared to subjects with low SLC activity. For a final answer, these results require independent reproduction. Notably, alternative splicing at non-canonical sites is a rare event and the predicted topology of DNHE1 raises some concern.

As mentioned in the "Pathophysiology" section of this chapter, the NHE1 has been considered an important candidate gene for hypertension research (which would also be true for a finally identified SLC gene). Intensive searches for polymorphisms in *NHE1*, however, did not result in the identification of functional or otherwise useful polymorphisms. Conversely, genetic linkage analyses provide good evidence that there is no relevant association between the locus for NHE1 and hypertension.[11,12]

Searching for genetic polymorphisms in genes of proteins involved in NHE1 regulation led to the discovery of a C825T polymorphism in the gene *GNB3* encoding the Gβ3 subunit of heterotrimeric G proteins. In association studies, the T allele of *GNB3* has been associated with the risk for hypertension. Interestingly, a common polymorphism in *GNAS* (the gene for Gα$_S$) has also been associated with essential hypertension.[65]

Pertaining to the *GNB3* C825T polymorphism, several reports reproduced the original finding whereas other groups could not.[66–69] A major problem is the fact that there is a considerable variance in genotype distribution within different ethnicities.[70] Whereas the C allele is the predominant allele in Caucasians, in blacks the T allele prevails. Asians have intermediate frequencies. Hence, there is a high risk for disparate population admixture in case-control studies. The *GNB3* gene comprises a comparably short stretch of 6 kB DNA on chromosome 12. This explains why in Caucasians two haplotypes explain more than 95% of the observed variability.[71,72] In other words, genotyping at the C825T locus provides information for six additional tightly linked polymorphisms. In Asians and in blacks, the situation is more complicated. Because we do not know which of the identified polymorphisms are ultimately necessary for alternative splicing to Gβ3s or Gβ3s2 different ethnic-dependent haplotype structures could be one solution to some discrepancies observed.

Numerous association studies dealing with the *GNB3* C825T polymorphism have provided additional information on the phenotype of hypertension linked to this polymorphism, although the results remained controversial.[73] There is no obvious association between *GNB3* polymorphisms and the severity of hypertension.[73] Several studies, however, suggest a higher risk for left ventricular hypertrophy[74] and stroke[75] in carriers of the *GNB3* 825T allele. The 825T allele was further linked to lower renin levels in hypertension.[67] Normotensive carriers with this allele were shown to exhibit reduced peripheral resistance and increased renal plasma flow.

The 825T allele was also linked to obesity and speculations were raised whether this gene contributes to the pathogenesis of a metabolic syndrome.[70] Of note, birth weight was also influenced by this polymorphism, an interesting finding as to the ongoing debate on birth weight and cardiovascular risk.[76] Of special interest is the observation that carriers of the 825T allele are subject to a better response to treatment with thiazide diuretics, a finding that was further modulated by effects of gender and ethnicity.[77] Altogether, the T allele of the *GNB3* C825T polymorphism is associated with a complex phenotype. Some results in this field are promising. Nevertheless, many questions regarding the mechanisms remain unanswered.

CLINICAL IMPLICATIONS AND PERSPECTIVES

At present, increased SLC activity is a well-described intermediate phenotype in hypertension and related diseases. The enhanced activity precedes the development of primary hypertension and diabetic nephropathy. The measurement of SLC activity is comparably easy and its reproducibility in different laboratories is high. Furthermore, SLC activity remains rather constant within one individual over time. Nevertheless, enthusiasm for measuring SLC has diminished for three main reasons. First, there is considerable overlap in SLC activity between normotensive and hypertensive patients or between diabetic patients with and without nephropathy. Refined kinetic analyses that determine V_{max} and K_M values for external Na$^+$ may lead to a better prediction, but they increase costs considerably. Second, knowledge about SLC activity does not change the therapeutic regimes for hypertension or diabetic nephropathy. Third, we have not yet understood the reasons for the kinetic abnormalities on a molecular level and the final pieces of this puzzle are still missing, which include the questions of its molecular identity and which genotypes are linked to SLC activity. There is first direct evidence that a splice variant of NHE1 mediates SLC. However, available evidence excludes the NHE1 gene as a candidate gene for hypertension. Together, this may explain why SLC activity determination has not become a routine method in clinical medicine.

The NHE1 gene has been excluded as contributing to hypertension pathogenesis. Other attempts, however, have studied the role of NHE1 in cardiovascular diseases especially in the context to reperfusion injury and an increased Na$^+$ load upon intracellular acidosis. Therapeutic drugs have been developed to inhibit these mechanisms, unfortunately without a significant benefit. These attempts have left several novel compounds for inhibition of NHE1. We are beginning to learn that NHE1 is not only an ion carrier but an integrator of many signals and an anchor protein for the regulation of the cytoskeleton. In the area of translational medicine, such NHE1-blocking compounds could in the end be useful for treating disease states not identified so far.

More than 200 studies have investigated the *GNB3* C825T polymorphism and described a complex phenotype that extends from cardiovascular medicine into other fields, including psychiatry and psychology, which is compatible with the diverse functions of G proteins expressed in all human cells. Although promising, the predictive value of this polymorphism (e.g., for individualized medicine, in diagnosis, or for pre-identification of responders) is limited. Observed effects with this polymorphism result from statistical comparisons between groups and are relevant for basic science purposes but have limited value for individual subjects or individualized medicine.

For scientific purposes, especially with case-control studies, it is of utmost importance to exclude confounding effects by different ethnic admixtures in case-control studies because *GNB3* C825T genotype frequencies vary extremely among the major ethnicities. Nevertheless, one can imagine that the *GNB3* C825T polymorphism together with other polymorphisms will be addressed in innovative diagnostic tools (e.g., in the field of pharmacogenetics with "SNP chip" or similar approaches).

SUMMARY

Enhanced activity of SLC, first identified in human red cells, is a well-characterized intermediate phenotype in hypertension and diabetic nephropathy. Its physiological role, however, remains elusive. Some speculate that SLC is an artificial transport mode Na$^+$/H$^+$ exchanger, especially of the Na$^+$/H$^+$ exchanger isoform NHE1. Different susceptibilities toward inhibitors argue against this notion. A recent report claims that SLC is mediated by a cryptic splice variant of NHE1, termed DNHE1, and not by the mature NHE1 protein.

Increased activity of Na$^+$/H$^+$ exchange is also a well-characterized characteristic of blood cells from hypertensive subjects. In both cases, however, there is a broad overlap between values from normotensive and hypertensive subjects (which diminishes the value for individualized diagnostic and, ultimately, for therapeutic decisions). The increased activity observed in blood cells is attributable to the activity of NHE1. Fundamental functions of NHE1 are protection from intracellular acidification and cell volume control. The activity of this transporter is subject to a complex regulation by phosphorylation and by interactions with ancillary proteins. Current understanding suggests that NHE1 is a multiprotein complex with tight connections to the cytoskeleton and other pH-regulating mechanisms.

In cell lines from hypertensive individuals (immortalization of B lymphocytes with the EBV or generation of human skin fibroblasts), the enhanced activity is retained under cell culture conditions implying genetic mechanisms. Studies with cells taken *ex vivo* and experiments with immortalized cells indicate that alterations in the expression of NHE1 transcripts or protein do not contribute to the observed abnormality. Refined analyses present evidence that the phosphorylation of NHE1 is enhanced in hypertension. The NHE1 is a highly regulated transporter and available evidence suggests that upstream signaling systems may contribute to the activation of this exchanger in hypertension.

G proteins relay signals from many receptors to intracellular effectors. They consist of three different subunits termed Gα, Gβ, and Gγ. Experiments with immortalized cells from hypertensive individuals indicated that the sensitivity of this system is increased in hypertension, that this propensity to enhanced signal transduction remains stable under cell culture conditions, and that such an enhanced signal transduction could cause the activation of NHE1. Systematic sequencing of many genes from components of this system led to the discovery of a polymorphism (C825T) in the gene of the G protein subunit Gβ3 (*GNB3*).

Several association studies have reproduced these findings. Controversial reports, however, also exist. The distribution of the *GNB3* alleles varies significantly between different ethnicities, a potentially important confounder. Although the contribution of this polymorphism to the genesis of hypertension is limited, promising results indicate that this polymorphism could be used for prediction of an antihypertensive therapy (pharmacogenetic use) as shown for diuretics.

REFERENCES

1. Tobian L, Binion JT. Tissue cations and water in essential hypertension. *Circulation* 1952;5:754–58.

2. Garay R. Typology of Na$^+$ transport abnormalities in erythrocytes from essential hypertensive patients: A first step towards the diagnosis and specific treatment of different forms of primary hypertension. *Cardiovasc Drug Ther* 1990;4:373–78.

3. Duhm J, Eisenried F, Becker BF, Greil W. Studies on the lithium transport across the red cell membrane. I. Li$^+$ uphill transport by the Na$^+$-dependent Li$^+$ counter-transport system of human erythrocytes. *Pflügers Arch* 1976; 364:147–55.

4. Canessa M, Adragna N, Solomon HS, et al. Increased sodium-lithium countertransport in red cells of patients with essential hypertension. *N Engl J Med* 1980;302:772–76.

5. West IC, Rutherford PA, Thomas TH. Sodium-lithium countertransport: Physiology and function. *J Hypertens* 1998;16:3–13.

6. Zerbini G, Gabellino D, Ruggiere D, Maestroni A. Increased sodium-lithium countertransport activity: A cellular dysfunction common to essential hypertension and diabetic nephropathy. *J Am Soc Nephrol* 2004;15:S81–84.

7. Livne A, Balfe JW, Veitch R, et al. Increased platelet Na$^+$/H$^+$ exchange rates in essential hypertension: Application of a novel test. *Lancet* 1987;i:533–36.

8. Canessa M, Morgan K, Goldszer R, et al. Kinetic abnormalities of the red blood cell sodium-proton exchange in hypertensive patients. *Hypertension* 1991;17:340–48.

9. Ng LL. Sodium proton exchanger (NHE) isoforms: Potential relevance to hypertension and its complications. *Nephrol Dial Transplant* 1998;13:2994–96.

10. Orlov SN, Adragna NC, Adarichev VA, Hamet P. Genetic and biochemical determinants of abnormal monovalent ion transport in primary hypertension. *Am J Physiol* 1999;276:C511–36.

11. Lifton RP, Hunt SC, Williams RR, et al. Exclusion of the Na$^+$-H$^+$ antiporter as a candidate gene in human essential hypertension. *Hypertension* 1991;17:8–14.

12. Dudley CR, Giuffra LA, Raine AE, Reeders ST. Assessing the role of APNH, a gene encoding for a human amiloride-sensitive Na$^+$/H$^+$ antiporter, on the interindividual variation in red cell Na$^+$/Li$^+$ countertransport. *J Am Soc Nephrol* 1991;2:937–43.

13. Siffert W, Rosskopf D, Siffert G, et al. Association of a human G-protein β3 subunit variant with hypertension. *Nat Genet* 1998;18:45–48.

14. Völzke H, Gruska S, Vogelgesang D, et al. Intracellular calcium and sodium-lithium countertransport in type 2 diabetic patients with and without albuminuria. *Endocr J* 2006 (e-published ahead of press).

15. Zerbini G, Podesta F, Meregalli G, et al. Fibroblast Na -Li countertransport rate is elevated in essential hypertension. *J Hypertens* 2001;19:1263–69.

16. Murer H., Hopfer U, Kinne R. Sodium/proton antiport in brush-border-membrane vesicles isolated from rat small intestine and kidney. *Biochem J* 1976;154:597–604.

17. Sardet C, Franchi A, Pouysségur J. Molecular cloning, primary structure and expression of the human growth factor-activatable Na$^+$/H$^+$ antiporter. *Cell* 1989;56:271–80.

18. Bobulescu IA, Di Sole F, Moe OW. Na$^+$/H$^+$ exchangers: Physiology and link to hypertension and organ ischemia. *Curr Opin Nephrol Hypertens* 2005; 14:485–94.

19. Fliegel L. The Na$^+$/H$^+$ exchanger isoform 1. *Int J Biochem Cell Biol* 2005;37:33–37.

20. Orlowski J, Grinstein S. Diversity of the mammalian sodium/proton exchanger SLC9 gene family. *Pflügers Arch* 2004; 447:549–65.

21. Linz WJ, Busch AE. NHE-1 inhibition: From protection during acute ischaemia/reperfusion to prevention/reversal of myocardial remodelling. *Naunyn Schmiedebergs Arch Pharmacol* 2003;368:239–46.

22. Hayashi H, Szaszi K, Grinstein S. Multiple modes of regulation of Na⁺/H⁺ exchangers. *Ann NY Acad Sci* 2002; 976:248–58.

23. Putney LK, Denker SP, Barber DL. The changing face of the Na⁺/H⁺ exchanger, NHE1: Structure, regulation, and cellular actions. *Annu Rev Pharmacol Toxicol* 2002;42:527–52.

24. Cox GA, Lutz CM, Yang CL, et al. Sodium/hydrogen exchanger gene defect in slow-wave epilepsy mutant mice. *Cell* 1997;91:139–48.

25. Cox GA, Lutz CM, Yang CL, et al. Targeted disruption of the murine Nhe1 locus induces ataxia, growth retardation, and seizures. *Am J Physiol Cell Physiol* 1999;276:C788–95.

26. Koelle MR. Heterotrimeric G protein signaling: Getting inside the cell. *Cell* 2006;126:25–27.

27. Wettschureck N, Offermanns S. Mammalian G proteins and their cell type specific functions. *Physiol Rev* 2005;85:1159–1204.

28. Cabrera-Vera TM, Vanhauwe J, Thomas TO, et al. Insights into G protein structure, function, and regulation. *Endocr Rev* 2003;24:765–81.

29. Morris AJ, Malbon CC. Physiological regulation of G protein-linked signaling. *Physiol Rev* 1999;79:1373–1430.

30. Gudermann T, Schöneberg T, Schultz G. Functional and structural complexity of signal transduction via G-protein-coupled receptors. *Annu Rev Neurosci* 1999; 20:399–427.

31. Willars GB. Mammalian RGS proteins: Multifunctional regulators of cellular signalling. *Semin Cell Dev Biol* 2006; 17:363–76.

32. Penela P, Murga C, Ribas C, et al. Mechanisms of regulation of G protein-coupled receptor kinases (GRKs) and cardiovascular disease. *Cardiovasc Res* 2006;69:46–56.

33. Felder RA, Sanada H, Xu J, et al. G protein-coupled receptor kinase 4 gene variants in human essential hypertension. *Proc Natl Acad Sci USA* 1999;99:3872–77.

34. Chi Y, Mota de Freitas D, Sikora M, Bansal VK. Correlations of Na⁺-Li⁺ exchange activity with Na⁺ and Li⁺ binding and phospholipid composition in erythrocyte membranes of white hypertensive and normotensive individuals: A nuclear magnetic resonance investigation. *Hypertension* 1996;27:456–64.

35. Mead P, Wilkinson R, Thomas TH. Thiol protein defect in sodium-lithium countertransport in subset of essential hypertension. *Hypertension* 1999; 34:1275–80.

36. Siffert W, Düsing R. Na⁺/H⁺ exchange in hypertension and in diabetes mellitus: Facts and hypotheses. *Basic Res Cardiol* 1996;91:179–90.

37. Rosskopf D, Düsing R, Siffert W. Membrane sodium-proton exchange and primary hypertension. *Hypertension* 1993;21:607–17.

38. Ng LL, Davies JE. Abnormalities in Na⁺/H⁺ antiporter activity in diabetic nephropathy. *J Am Soc Nephrol* 1992; 3:S50–55.

39. Aviv A. The links between cellular Ca²⁺ and Na⁺/H⁺ exchange in the pathophysiology of essential hypertension. *Am J Hypertens* 1996;9:703–07.

40. Ng LL, Sweeney FP, Siczkowski M, et al. Na⁺-H⁺ antiporter phenotype, abundance, and phosphorylation of immortalized lymphoblasts from humans with hypertension. *Hypertension* 1995;25:971–77.

41. Siczkowski M, Davies JE, Ng LL. Sodium-hydrogen antiporter protein in normotensive Wistar-Kyoto rats and spontaneously hypertensive rats. *J Hypertens* 1994;12:775–81.

42. Kelly MP, Quinn PA, Davies JE, Ng LL. Activity and expression of Na⁺-H⁺ exchanger isoforms 1 and 3 in kidney proximal tubules of hypertensive rats. *Circ Res* 1997;80:853–60.

43. Rosskopf D, Frömter E, Siffert W. Hypertensive sodium-proton exchanger phenotype persists in immortalized lymphoblasts from essential hypertensive patients: A cell culture model for human hypertension. *J Clin Invest* 1993;92: 2553–59.

44. Kuro-o M, Hanaoka K, Hiroi Y, et al. Salt-sensitive hypertension in transgenic mice overexpressing Na⁺-proton exchanger. *Circ Res* 1995;76:148–53.

45. Ng LL, Davies JE, Siczkowski M, et al. Abnormal Na⁺/H⁺ antiporter phenotype and turnover of immortalized lymphoblasts from type 1 diabetic patients with nephropathy. *J Clin Invest* 1994;93:2750–57.

46. Davies JE, Siczkowski M, Sweeney FP, et al. Glucose-induced changes in turnover of Na⁺/H⁺ exchanger of immortalized lymphoblasts from type I diabetic patients with nephropathy. *Diabetes* 1995;44:382–88.

47. Siczkowski M, Davies JE, Sweeney FP, et al. Na⁺/H⁺ exchanger isoform-1 abundance in skin fibroblasts of type I diabetic patients with nephropathy. *Metabolism* 1995;44:791–95.

48. Siczkowski M, Davies JE, Ng LL. Na⁺-H⁺ exchanger isoform 1 phosphorylation in normal Wistar-Kyoto and spontaneously hypertensive rats. *Circ Res* 1995;76: 825–31.

49. Ng LL, Sweeney FP, Siczkowski M, et al. Na⁺-H⁺ antiporter phenotype, abundance, and phosphorylation of immortalized lymphoblasts from humans with hypertension. *Hypertension* 1995;25:971–77.

50. Sweeney FP, Siczkowski M, Davies JE, et al. Phosphorylation and activity of Na⁺/H⁺ exchanger isoform 1 of immortalized lymphoblasts in diabetic nephropathy. *Diabetes* 1995;44:1180–85.

51. Sweeney FP, Quinn PA, Ng LL. Enhanced mitogen-activated protein kinase activity and phosphorylation of the Na⁺/H⁺ exchanger isoform-1 of human lymphoblasts in hypertension. *Metabolism* 1997;46:297–302.

52. Siffert W, Rosskopf D, Moritz A, et al. Enhanced G protein activation in immortalized lymphoblasts from patients with essential hypertension. *J Clin Invest* 1995;96:759–66.

53. Pietruck F, Moritz A, Montemurro M, et al. Selectively enhanced cellular signaling by Gi proteins in essential hypertension: Gα₁₂, Gα₁₃, Gα₁, and Gβ₂ are not mutated. *Circ Res* 1996;79: 974–83.

54. Rosskopf D, Manthey I, Habich C, et al. Identification and characterization of Gβ3s2, a novel splice variant of the G-protein β3 subunit. *Biochem J* 2001; 371:223–32.

55. Sprang SR. G protein mechanisms: Insights from structural analysis. *Annu Rev Biochem* 1997;66:639–78.

56. Rosskopf D, Koch K, Habich C, et al. Interaction of Gβ3s, a splice variant of the G-protein Gβ3, with Gγ- and Gα-proteins. *Cell Signal* 2003;15:479–88.

57. Ruiz-Velasco V, Ikeda SR. A splice variant of the G protein beta 3-subunit implicated in disease states does not modulate ion channels. *Physiol Genomics* 2003;13:85–95.

58. Poch E, Gonzalez-Nunez D, Compte M, De la Sierra A. G-protein β3-subunit gene variant, blood pressure and erythrocyte sodium/lithium countertransport in essential hypertension. *Br J Biomed Sci* 2002; 59:101–04.

59. Hasstedt SJ, Wu LL, Ash KO, et al. Hypertension and sodium-lithium countertransport in Utah pedigrees: Evidence for major-locus inheritance. *Am J Hum Genet* 1988;43:14–22.

60. Weder AB. Cation transport markers as predictors of hypertension. *Am J Hypertens* 1991;4:633S–37S.

61. Ragone E, Strazzullo P, Siani A, et al. Ethnic differences in red blood cell sodium/lithium countertransport and metabolic correlates of hypertension: An international collaborate study. *Am J Hypertens* 1998;11:935–41.

62. Busch S, Burckhardt BC, Siffert W. Expression of the human sodium/ proton exchanger NHE-1 in Xenopus laevis oocytes enhances sodium/proton exchange activity and establishes sodium/lithium countertransport. *Pflügers Arch* 1995;429:859–69.

63. Kammerer CM, Cox LA, Mahaney MC, et al. Sodium-lithium countertransport activity is linked to chromosome 5 in baboons. *Hypertension* 2001;37:398–402.

64. Zerbini G, Maestroni A, Breviario D, et al. Alternative splicing of NHE-1 mediates Na-Li countertransport and associates with activity rate. *Diabetes* 2003;52:1511–18.

65. Jia H, Hingorani AD, Sharma P, et al. Association of the G(s)alpha gene with essential hypertension and response to beta-blockade. *Hypertension* 1999; 34:8–14.

66. Schunkert H, Hense HW, Doring A, et al. Association between a polymorphism in the G protein β3 subunit gene and lower renin and elevated diastolic blood pressure levels. *Hypertension* 1998; 32:510–13.

67. Benjafield AV, Jeyasingam CL, Nyholt DR, et al. G-protein β3 subunit gene (GNB3) variant in causation of essential hypertension. *Hypertension* 1998; 32:1094–97.

68. Brand E, Herrmann SM, Nicaud V, Ruidavets JB, Evans A, Arveiler D, et al. The 825C/T polymorphism of the G-protein subunit beta3 is not related to hypertension. *Hypertension* 1999; 33:1175–78.

69. Dong Y, Zhu H, Sagnella GA, et al. Association between the C825T polymorphism of the G protein β3-subunit gene and hypertension in blacks. *Hypertension* 1999;34:1193–96.

70. Siffert W, Forster P, Jöckel KH, et al. Worldwide ethnic distribution of the G protein β3 subunit 825T allele and its association with obesity in Caucasian, Chinese, and Black African individuals. *J Am Soc Nephrol* 1999;10:1921–30.

71. Rosskopf D, Busch S, Manthey I, Siffert W. G protein β 3 gene: Structure, promoter, and additional polymorphisms. *Hypertension* 2000; 36:33–41.

72. Rosskopf D, Manthey I, Siffert W. Identification and ethnic distribution of major haplotypes in the gene GNB3 encoding the G-protein β3 subunit. *Pharmacogenetics* 2002;12:209–20.

73. Siffert W. G protein polymorphisms in hypertension, atherosclerosis, and diabetes. *Annu Rev Med* 2005;56:17–28.

74. Poch E, Gonzalez D, Gomez-Angelats E, et al. G-Protein β(3) subunit gene variant and left ventricular hypertrophy in essential hypertension. *Hypertension* 2000;35:214–18.

75. Morrison AC, Doris PA, Folsom AR., et al. G-protein β3 subunit and α-adducin polymorphisms and risk

of subclinical and clinical stroke. *Stroke* 2001;32:822–28.

76. Hocher B, Slowinski T, Stolze T, et al. Association of maternal G protein β3 subunit 825T allele with low birthweight. *Lancet* 2000;355:1241–42.

77. Turner ST, Schwartz GL, Chapman AB, Boerwinkle E. C825T polymorphism of the G Protein β3-subunit and antihypertensive response to a thiazide diuretic. *Hypertension* 2001;37:739–43.

Chapter

19 Arterial and Venous Function in Hypertension

Keshari M. Thakali, James J. Galligan, Gregory D. Fink, and Stephanie W. Watts

Key Findings

- Arteries carry blood away from the heart to tissues at a relatively high pressure. By contrast, veins carry blood back to the heart at considerably lower pressures.

- Arteries and veins are structurally and compositionally different, with arteries providing elastic resistance to flow and veins providing blood storage capacity.

- Arteries and veins are innervated by both the sympathetic and sensory nervous systems.

- Differences in vessel innervation, mechanics, receptor handling, endothelial cell function, and vascular smooth muscle cell growth exist between arteries and veins.

- Venous adaptations in response to high blood pressure have not been adequately studied as they have been in arteries, and hypertension-induced changes in contractility and remodeling are likely to occur differently in arteries and veins.

- An index of venomotor tone is increased in hypertension, suggesting that venous function contributes to this disease.

Hypertension has long been associated with arterial changes that increase total peripheral resistance in hypertension (see Chapters 16 and 30). Although there is no question of the relevance of arterial function to hypertension, the role of the venous system in hypertension is far from clear. The venous system, the "other half" of the vascular component of the cardiovascular system, has not been heavily studied because it is a low-pressure system that does not determine total peripheral resistance and has thus been viewed as largely unimportant in acute or chronic changes in blood pressure. However, a growing body of literature suggests that the ability of the venous system to redistribute functional blood volume can significantly alter blood pressure in a manner relevant to hypertension. The goal of this chapter is to present basic facts about arterial and venous vessels, highlighting differences where they are known. These facts are integrated into a picture of a current viewpoint as to how these differences may influence the physiology and pathophysiology of hypertension. In this chapter, we do not discuss the pulmonary and portal circulations, nor pulmonary and portal hypertension, and invite the reader to consult recent excellent reviews on these subjects.[1-4] It should be noted that many of the comments that follow are general and necessarily broad sweeping. Vessel function and responsiveness—be it arterial or venous—can be tissue and species dependent, and thus care should be taken in applying statements made here to all arteries and all veins.

ANATOMY/BIOCHEMISTRY

A safe rule of thumb to remember with respect to vessel function is that structure determines function. Arteries carry blood away from the heart at a relatively high pressure, whereas veins carry blood back to the heart at a relatively low pressure. This movement of blood, dependent on the pumping action of the heart, is critical for providing necessary oxygen and nutrients to all tissues—allowing for exchange of nutrients and waste products, and then for returning the blood to the heart for reoxygenation and removal of gaseous waste. Because the duties of arteries and veins are different, one can appreciate that their structure would be different.

The arterial and venous circulations are connected through capillaries, the site at which gas and solutes are exchanged. The development of the artery/capillary/venous system is coordinated. In development, arterial endothelial cells provide the ligand Ephrin B2, which can interact with the venous EphB4 tyrosine kinase receptor.[5] Interactions between the Eph receptors and Eph ligands have emerged as a dominant theme in cell movement and tissue boundary development.[6] The expression of Ephrin B2 in arterial and EphB4 in venous endothelial cells, respectively, is faithfully carried on into adulthood—and thus is described as a stable difference between arterial and venous vascular smooth muscle cells.[5] Thus, the ephrin system (at least in the developing and adult mouse) is one that demarks arterial and venous tissue.

Structure

Fig. 19–1 depicts a cross section of a rendered artery and vein. Both artery and vein are composed of the following similar layers.

- The innermost layer (or tunica intima), which contains functioning endothelial cells, and in the case of the artery an elastic lamina.

- The tunica media, which is largely composed of smooth muscle, elastin, and collagen.

- The tunica adventitia, which is collagenous but sometimes composed of smooth muscle cells. The vasa vasorum (small blood vessels that integrate into the adventitia) provide nutrients to the blood vessel itself.

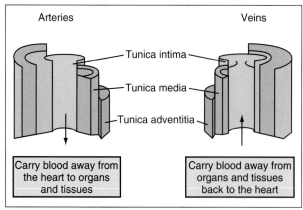

Figure 19–1. Structure of arteries and veins. Blood vessels are comprised of three layers: the innermost tunica intimia, the tunica media, and the tunica adventitia.

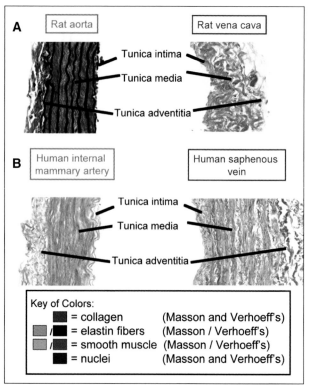

Figure 19–2. Histologic sections of Verhoeff-Masson-trichrome-stained rat thoracic aorta and vena cava (**A**) and Masson-trichrome-stained human internal mammary artery and saphenous vein (**B**). Verhoeff-Masson trichrome stain key: blue = collagen, pinkish purple = smooth muscle, black = elastin fibers, and dark purple = nuclei. Masson trichrome stain key: blue = collagen, pinkish purple = smooth muscle, red = elastin fibers, and dark purple = nuclei.

Several differences exist between the structure of an artery and a vein. The layers of the blood vessel are more clearly delineated in an artery compared to a vein, and this is particularly illustrated when viewing the thoracic vena cava versus the thoracic aorta from the same rat (Figure 19–2, A). This is less apparent when comparing arteries and veins from humans (Figure 19–2, B). The media of an artery is typically thicker than that of a vein, and the elastic component of a vein is small when compared to that of an artery. Similarly, larger veins possess venous valves that in conjunction with contraction of the vessel assist in moving blood toward the heart. Collectively, these differences enable the arterial side to handle the high pressures produced by cardiac contraction and the necessity of bringing the blood to tissues, whereas the venous side acts in capacitive circulation—allowing blood to pool and serve as a low-pressure reservoir for blood. The ability of veins to accommodate a large percentage of total circulating blood volume (~70%) is an important fact for understanding how venous function could influence blood pressure.

Innervation

The sympathetic and sensory nervous systems innervate both arteries and veins.[7,8] There have been few reports of nitroxidergic (nitric oxide, NO) autonomic nerves innervating blood vessels.[9] Interestingly, whereas most systemic blood vessels have been described as being largely independent of parasympathetic innervation studies in the human greater saphenous vein demonstrate the presence of acetylcholinesterase-containing nerve fibers in the adventitial medial border.[10] Axons of sympathetic and sensory neurons travel from ganglia paravascularly, ultimately arborizing in the adventitia and penetrating the vessels. Figure 19–3, A depicts fluorescence of norepinephrine in an artery versus a vein (sympathetic innervation), as well as staining of the sensory neuropeptide calcitonin gene-related peptide (Figure 19–3, B; CGRP, a marker for sensory nerves). Both vessel types are innervated by the sympathetic nervous system. However, it is apparent that the venous system is less densely innervated than the arterial system and that the sympathetic fibers that innervate veins are limited to

primarily venous adventitia, whereas sympathetic fibers on arteries typically penetrate the media.[11]

Nonetheless, there is an important difference in how the sympathetic nervous system stimulates the artery and vein, thereby causing them to contract. Veins respond to a lower frequency of stimulation compared to arteries. If one performs a frequency response curve for a vein versus an artery, the response of the vein will be shifted leftward compared to the artery. An example of this is the mesenteric vascular bed in which veins respond to nerve stimulation at a frequency of 1 to 2 Hz, whereas arteries respond at a higher frequency (10 to 20 Hz).[7,12] Thus, at any nonmaximal level of stimulation veins will respond with a greater contraction compared to arteries. Another difference between arterial and venous innervation is the fact that these two blood vessel types receive their innervation from separate sympathetic postganglionic neurons[13] and perivenous sympathetic nerves release more norepinephrine when compared to norepinephrine release from periarterial sympathetic nerves.[14] Finally, veins (of the mesentery) lack the ATP-dependent rapid excitatory junction potentials observed in arteries.[12]

Function

An exhaustive list of functional differences between arteries and veins is beyond the scope of this chapter. Here, we

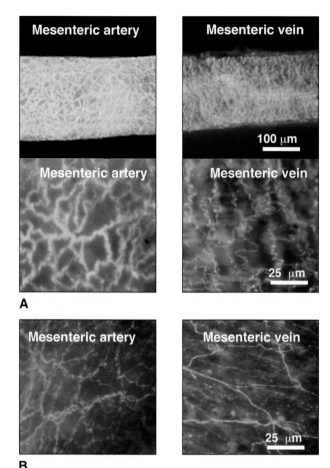

A

B

Figure 19–3. Comparison of sympathetic (**A**) and sensory (**B**) innervation of rat mesenteric arteries and veins. Sympathetic innervation of arteries and veins was compared using glyoxylic acid fluorescence staining of catecholamines. Calcitonin-gene-related peptide (CGRP) immunoreactivity was used to compare sensory innervation of arteries and veins.

focus on those aspects of vessel function that are likely relevant to changes in vessel activity in hypertension.

Contractility

Change in the tone of an artery will result in alterations of total peripheral resistance, whereas similar changes in the vein results in changes in compliance/capacitance. Ours and other laboratories have observed numerous differences in arterial versus venous contractile responsiveness, and these differences range from the basic to agonist specific.

Because of smaller muscular content, a vein is not able to contract with the same magnitude of force as does an artery and is thus not handled in the same way experimentally. For example, if a comparably sized rat thoracic vena cava and rat thoracic aorta ring were mounted in isolated tissue baths for measurement of isometric contraction, the passive tension applied to the vein to bring smooth muscle cells to their optimum length is less (aorta, 4 g; vena cava, 1 g) and the maximum contraction to a receptor-independent agonist (e.g., KCl) is also less (e.g., 100-mM KCl aorta, 1.5 to 2.5 g; vena cava, 0.5 g). When one views the speed of contraction of an isolated vein compared to an artery, veins respond more quickly than

do arteries. This is evidenced by experimental measures such as time to half-maximal contraction (Figure 19–4). One can argue that this might be influenced by the receptor agonist used to elicit the concentration response curve. However, this same difference in speed of contraction is seen when the largely receptor-independent agonist potassium chloride (KCl) is used. Thus, the speed of mechanical contraction is different. We have begun to understand these differences by studying the forms of myosin heavy chains (MHCs) expressed in an artery and vein that contribute to the rate of actin/myosin association.

Similarly, differences in endothelial cell function exist. Our laboratory has not been able to obtain maximum relaxation to an agonist that stimulates production of vasorelaxant substances from the endothelial cell of the vein. A similar disparity was observed in the left circumflex artery versus middle cardiac vein of the pig,[15] and in comparison of acetylcholine-induced relaxation in the human saphenous vein and internal mammary artery.[16] A direct measure of NO in endothelial cells suggests that venous endothelial cells produce lower basal levels of NO compared to arterial endothelial cells, yet veins express a greater density of NOS proteins compared to arteries.[17] A comparison of other endothelial-cell-derived substances has not been performed.

Differences in general sensitivity to adrenergic stimuli have been observed. For example, isolated veins (large and small) do not respond with a robust contraction to agonists of adrenergic receptors when compared to arteries, yet both arteries and veins are innervated by the sympathetic nervous system. Perez-Rivera has demonstrated that mesenteric veins (mouse) do not desensitize to adrenergic stimuli to the same degree observed in mesenteric

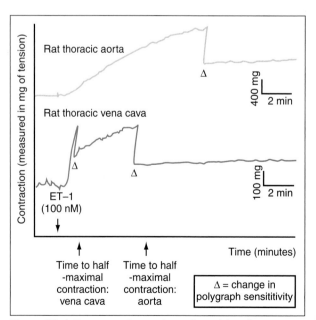

Figure 19–4. Representative tracings of arterial and venous contraction (measured in milligrams of tension) to the vasoconstrictor endothelin-1 (ET-1) demonstrate that veins contract faster than arteries. The time to half-maximal contraction to ET-1 (100 nM) is significantly shorter in rat thoracic vena cava compared to thoracic aorta.

arteries from the same bed[18] and may have a complement of adrenergic receptors not present in arteries. Similarly, venous and arterial adrenergic vasoconstriction differs in response to hypoxia and metabolic inhibition in that veins appear to be relatively insensitive to hypoxia inhibition whereas arterial tone is potently antagonized by the same signals.[19] Intuitively, this makes sense because the veins necessarily operate under low-oxygen conditions.

One of the most interesting differences observed between arteries and veins is their intrinsically different response to endothelin-1 (ET-1). ET-1 is a vasoactive peptide produced within the endothelial cells of both veins and arteries. ET-1 exerts its physiological effects through combination with plasma membrane receptors, the ET_A and ET_B receptor. When the responses of multiple arteries and veins from different species are compared, three striking differences can be culled. First, veins are more sensitive to the contractile effect of ET-1 (threshold for initiating response is lower) and ET-1 is more potent (EC_{50} value or effective concentration necessary to cause a half-maximal contraction is lower).[20] Second, veins respond to agonist of the ET_B receptor such as sarafotoxin 6C (S6c) or IRL-1620 with contraction, whereas arteries generally do not contract to these same agonists (Fig. 19–5). Third, arteries desensitize completely to ET-1, whereas veins maintain at least a partial response to ET-1 in the same conditions that would cause an artery to desensitize.[21] These findings suggest that veins may be more responsive or continue to respond to ET-1 in conditions of chronic ET-1 exposure.

Growth

The previous section listed differences in arterial versus venous contractile responses. Differences are also observed in the parameter of growth (or mitogenesis). Specifically, isolated smooth muscle cells from a vein and artery behave differently in response to stretch. In cells placed in a Flexercell (an apparatus that provides cyclical and constant stretch to cells plated on flexible substrate), venous smooth muscle cells responded to cyclical stretch with mitogenesis/growth and arterial smooth muscle cells did not.[22]

There has been the suggestion that in venous-to-arterial grafts it is the venous smooth muscle cell and *not* the surrounding arterial smooth muscle cells that are responsible for the arterialization of the vein. In other words, it is the vein that provides the cells that allow it to change to resemble an artery (thicker media). This is supported by the findings that smooth muscle cells from human saphenous vein have a higher growth rate than those from a human internal mammary artery.[23] Comparable findings were observed in rabbit saphenous vein and internal mammary artery.[24] An interesting difference between the arterial and venous smooth muscle cells in the rabbit was that arterial smooth muscle cells produced greater levels of the inhibitory proteoglycan decorin.[24] The lack of sufficient decorin production may be one reason for the greater synthetic rates of venous smooth muscle cells.

The endothelial cell of the vein seems particularly capable of producing signals that stimulate cellular growth.[25] Previously, we suggested that venous endothelial cells may produce less NO compared to arterial endothelial cells—another means by which growth may be promoted. Moreover, endothelial cells from veins do not respond with proliferation to minimally oxidized LDL as do arterial endothelial cells.[26]

Reactive oxygen species (ROS)

Both NO and superoxide have been measured in arteries and veins. These reactive substances have been associated with altered contractility and remodeling of blood vessels. Guzik et al.[16] demonstrated lower steady-state levels of both NO and reactive oxygen species (superoxide, peroxynitrite) in the human saphenous vein when compared to the human internal mammary artery, but the vessels were similar when parameters of NO bioavailability and superoxide/peroxynitrite production were compared. This suggests that although the overall systems of vasoactive ROS production may be lower in a vein than in an artery there does not appear to be differences in the balance between superoxide production and NO availability. This group has also shown that the source of superoxide in a

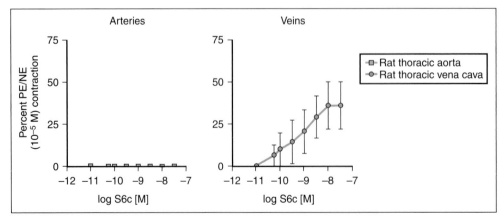

Figure 19–5. Differences in arterial and venous ET_B receptor function. Veins from sham normotensive and DOCA-salt hypertensive rats contract to sarafotoxin 6c (S6c), an ET_B receptor-specific agonist, whereas arteries for sham normotensive and DOCA-salt hypertensive rats do not contract to this agonist. Data are represented as mean ± SEM. NE, norepinephrine; PE, phenylephrine.

human vein and artery differs, with the NAD(P)H oxidase system being a proportionately greater source in veins and xanthine oxidase the predominant producer in arteries. In addition, the subunit composition of the NAD(P)H oxidase enzyme differed in arteries versus veins. Veins expressed more nox 2, whereas arteries expressed quantitatively greater more nox 4. These measures in human vessels were preceded by measures in rats in which venules and arterioles of both Dahl salt-sensitive (Dahl-S) and salt-resistant (Dahl-R) were stained for tetranitroblue tetra-zolium dye as a measure of superoxide content.[27]

Superoxide is converted to hydrogen peroxide (H_2O_2) by the catalytic action of superoxide dismutases, and hydrogen peroxide has received significant attention as a long-lived signaling molecule compared to superoxide. Veins responded to exogenous H_2O_2 with greater contraction than did arteries.[28] The work described here suggests intrinsic differences in the ROS produced by an artery and a vein and how arteries and veins utilize ROS in signaling. We invite readers to consult Chapter 30 for further details on reactive oxygen species.

GENETICS

There is little relevant information about differences in molecular genetics that control function of a normal artery versus a normal vein, although venous function is highly hereditable in humans.[29] Even less information is available in regard to how this control may change in hypertension. Adams et al. compared expression of 4048 genes in macaque aorta and vena cava and observed that mRNA expression of 68 out of 4048 genes were elevated in aorta compared to vena cava, with the largest difference in mRNA occurring in a regulator of G-protein signaling (RGS) 5. A similar pattern of increased RGS5 expression was also observed in rat arteries compared to veins.[30] RGS proteins are GTPase activating proteins and function to inhibit GPCR signaling. RGS5 overexpression inhibits endothelin-1-induced increases in intracellular calcium.[31] On a purely speculative note, increased arterial RGS5 expression may explain differences in venous and arterial reactivity to vasoactive hormones and peptides, although this has yet to be shown experimentally.

One recent study investigated the impact of NOSIII gene polymorphism (T-786C, G894T) on endothelium-dependent and -independent venodilation in the human, but findings were negative in that vasodilation to bradykinin and sodium nitroprusside did not differ between wild-type humans and those with a single nucleotide polymorphism.[32] Thus, differences in the gene expression between arteries and veins is an area ripe for investigation.

PHYSIOLOGY AND PATHOPHYSIOLOGY: FOCUS ON HYPERTENSION

A large body of work exists to support changes in arterial structure, function, and biochemistry in hypertension, and Chapter 12 in this book reviews this work. In general, arteries demonstrate changes in both their contractile ability and their structure.

Structurally, arteries undergo a process of remodeling in hypertension, an adaptive response of the artery to preserve its structural integrity against higher-than-normal pressures. The vascular smooth muscle cells in the media can become larger in size (hypertrophy), undergo mitogenesis (hyperplasia), and rearrange themselves such that the lumen of the blood vessel is smaller. This remodeling is accompanied by altered patterns of collagen secretion and activation of matrix metalloproteases and growth factors. Figure 19–6 shows Masson Trichrome staining of small mesenteric arteries and veins from sham normotensive and deoxycorticosterone acetate (DOCA)-salt hypertensive rats in which smooth muscle is stained pinkish-purple, collagen is stained blue, and nuclei are stained dark purple. The mesenteric artery wall from the DOCA-salt hypertensive rat is thicker when compared to the mesenteric artery from the sham normotensive rat. Other modifications can occur, but the end result is a stronger artery with a functional reduction in the lumen diameter. Because the resistance to blood flow is inversely related to the fourth power of the radius of the diameter, the changes in wall thickness and lumen diameter that occur in hypertension contribute to the disease. Functionally, arteries from hypertensive subjects show the following *in vitro* characteristics: (1) a general increase in sensitivity to contractile agonists such as serotonin, (2) a general decrease in sensitivity to relaxant agonist such as isoproterenol or acetylcholine, and (3) generation of spontaneous tone and oscillatory contractions.

Changes in venous reactivity have not been comparably studied, and venous structure under the condition of hypertension is not well investigated. For example, Aalkjaer et al. observed increased wall thickness and decreased lumen diameter in small mesenteric arteries from spontaneously hypertensive rats compared to their normotensive WKY counterparts, but did not observe any difference in wall thickness or lumen diameter from corresponding small mesenteric veins.[33] Figure 19–6 demonstrates that there are few obvious changes in structure in mesenteric veins from DOCA-salt hypertensive rats compared to sham normotensive rats, in that wall thickness is not different. It is unclear whether venous lumen diameter is consistently decreased in hypertension. Contractile experiments using isolated veins suggest that unlike an artery a vein does not dramatically change its response to agonists such as ET-1 and NE.[14,20] Similarly, there appears to be little change in neurogenic responses of splanchnic veins in hypertension (DOCA-salt based) yet a potentiated neurogenic response in arteries from the same rats.[14] Thus, in hypertension veins do not appear to possess the same altered structural characteristics as do arteries, and venous function seems uncompromised. A question therefore arises as to whether veins play a role in the development and maintenance of high blood pressure.

VENOCONSTRICTION AS A CAUSE AND/ OR CONTRIBUTOR TO HYPERTENSION

Ultimately, the differences in arterial and venous structure and function enable these two blood vessel types to

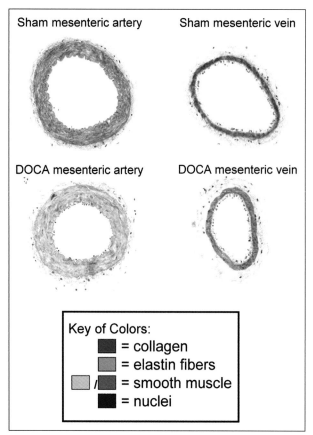

Figure 19–6. Masson trichrome staining of small mesenteric arteries and veins from sham normotensive and DOCA-salt hypertensive rats. Masson trichrome stain key: blue = collagen, pinkish purple = smooth muscle, red = elastin fibers, and dark purple = nuclei.

serve a different but complementary physiologic purpose in the body and specifically for determination of blood pressure. One model that encapsulates the complementary function of the venous and arterial system is the Coleman-Guyton model (Figure 19–7). One can immediately envision how changes in arterial function change total peripheral resistance (TPR) and thus blood pressure, whereas changes in venous function can alter venous return and modify cardiac output (CO). There is ample evidence to support the important role of arterial function in both maintenance of normal and elevated blood pressure. Drug treatment of human hypertension relies heavily upon reducing arterial function through blockade of adrenergic receptors, L-type voltage gated calcium channels, or formation of the vaso-constrictor angiotensin II. The reader is directed to Section IV in this book, which highlights these treatments. The present chapter briefly presents what is understood as to the physiologic and pathophysiologic roles of the venous system in determination of blood pressure.

The spontaneously hypertensive rat (SHR) shows an elevation of CO early in hypertension,[34] and this is validated in the young human with mild or borderline essential hypertension who has an elevated CO in the absence of an elevated TPR in early stages of blood pressure elevation.[35] These data suggest that changes in venous function may be an initiating factor in these cases of hypertension. A measure of venous function *in vivo* is mean circulatory filling pressure (MCFP). This is the average resting pressure throughout the circulation when the pumping action of the heart is stopped. It is determined by both blood volume and venomotor tone. Our group has recently measured MCFP in DOCA-salt animals immediately following implantation of DOCA. If

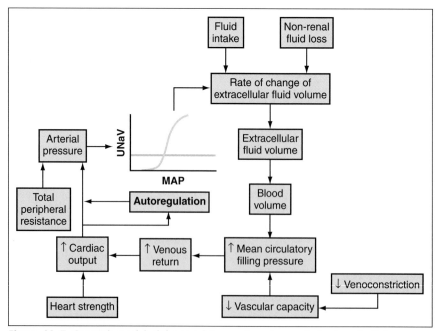

Figure 19–7. Guyton's model of the circulatory system demonstrates how both increases in arterial and venous tone can elevate blood pressure.

the hypothesis that MCFP (and thus venous functioning) is important to the initiation of blood pressure elevation, MCFP should rise before a rise in blood pressure or blood volume. This is, in fact, what we observed.[36] These important data suggest that venous function contributes to the rise in blood pressure. Others have observed an increase in MCFP in the adult SHR compared to WKY.[37] The question then becomes what causes venoconstriction. The finding by Martin et al. that pharmacologic ganglionic blockade resulted in a larger fall in MCFP in SHR compared to WKY suggests that the sympathetic nervous system may play a role in elevation of MCFP in the SHR. Similar observations have been made in the DOCA-salt model. This idea is supported by studies in which sympathetic input to small mesenteric resistance veins on the SHR and reduced-renal mass hypertensive rats was enhanced compared to normotensive controls.[38] If tone is elevated similarly in sympathetic neurons that innervate arteries and veins, changes in tone in veins may be greater than in arteries.

Venous changes observed in experimental settings of normal and high blood pressure are also observed, to some degree, in the human. In 1969, Walsh demonstrated that venous distensibility (and thus compliance) was reduced in essential hypertension.[39] Safar and London[40, 41] measured a decreased capacitance of the venous system in human hypertension, suggesting that venous contractility or structure had been altered. These were followed by studies suggesting that central (or trunk) blood volume (but not total blood volume) was increased in hypertension.[42]

Genetic polymorphisms may play an important role in the decreased venous capacitance observed in human essential hypertension. A polymorphism (C825T) in the G-protein β3 (*GNB3*) subunit has been associated with hypertension.[43] The 825T allele of *GNB3* is characterized by enhanced G-protein signaling, and carriers of the 825T allele exhibit increased responsiveness to vasoactive hormones and peptides.[44, 45] Mitchell et al. observed that carriers of the C825T polymorphism of *GNB3* responded with enhanced venoconstriction to ET-1 and adrenergic agonists.[46] Whether enhanced venoconstriction in response to vasoactive peptides or increased sympathetic activity is causally linked to essential hypertension in carriers of the 825T allele of *GNB3* has yet to be established.

CLINICAL IMPLICATIONS AND PERSPECTIVES

The important message from this collective work is that venous function should be viewed as a parameter that can be modified for potential therapeutic treatment of hypertension. At the very least, venous changes and participation in blood pressure determination should be considered in evaluating physiologic models of hypertension.

SUMMARY

This chapter summarized both *in vitro* and *in vivo* experimental findings that underscore important basic differences in arterial versus venous structure, function, and signaling (Figure 19–8). These two different sides of the circulation respond to hypertension in different manners, such that the manipulation of the venous side presents an interesting and unique means of altering elevated blood pressure.

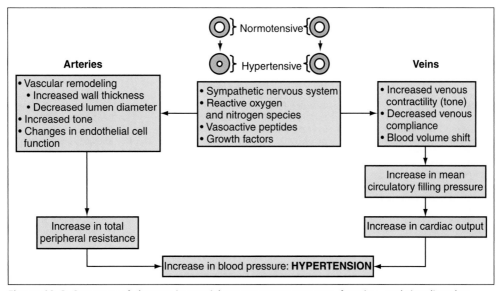

Figure 19–8. Summary of changes in arterial versus venous structure, function, and signaling that occur during the development and maintenance of hypertension.

REFERENCES

1. Farber HW, Loscalzo J. Pulmonary arterial hypertension. *N Engl J Med* 2004;351:1655–65.

2. McLaughlin VV, Rich S. Pulmonary hypertension. *Curr Probl Cardiol* 2004;29:575–634.

3. Mela M, Mancuso A, Burroughs A. Drug treatment for portal hypertension. *Ann Hepatol* 2002;1:102.

4. Knechtle SJ. Portal hypertension: from Eck's fistula to TIPS. *Ann Surg* 2003;238:S49–55.

5. Shin D, Garcia-Cardena G, Hayashi S, et al. Expression of ephrinB2 identifies a stable genetic difference between arterial and venous vascular smooth muscle as well as endothelial cells, and marks subsets of microvessels at sites of adult neovascularization. *Dev Biol* 2001;230:139–50.

6. Boyd AW, Lackmann M. Signals from Eph and Ephrin proteins: A developmental tool kit. *Science's STKE* 11 December 2001.

7. Kreulen DL. Properties of the venous and arterial innervation in the mesentery. *J Smooth Muscle Res* 2003;39:269–79.

8. Manzini S, Perretti F, Tramontana M, et al. Neurochemical evidence of calcitonin gene related peptide-like immunoreactivity (CGRP-LI) release from capsaicin sensitive nerves in rat mesenteric arteries and veins. *Gen Pharmacol* 1991;22:275–78.

9. Toda N, Okamura T. The pharmacology of nitric oxide in the peripheral nervous system of blood vessels. *Pharmacol Rev* 2003;55:271–324.

10. Amenta F, Cavallotti C, Dotta F, et al. The autonomic innervation of the human greater saphenous vein. *Acta Histochem* 1983;72:111–16.

11. Brandao F. A comparative study of the role played by some inactivation pathways in the disposition of the transmitter in the rabbit aorta and the saphenous vein of the dog. *Blood Vessels* 1976;13:309–18.

12. Hottenstein OD, Kreulen DL. Comparison of the frequency dependence of venous and arterial responses to sympathetic nerve stimulation in guinea pigs. *J Physiol* 1987;384:153–67.

13. Browning KN, Zheng ZL, Kreulen DL, Travagli RA. Two populations of sympathetic neurons project selectively to mesenteric artery or vein. *Am J Physiol* 1999;276:H1263–72.

14. Luo M, Hess MC, Fink GD, et al. Differential alterations in sympathetic neurotransmission in mesenteric arteries and veins in DOCA-salt hypertensive rats. *Auton Neurosci* 2003;104:47–57.

15. Zhang RZ, Yang Q, Yim APC, et al. Different role of nitric oxide and endothelium-derived hyperpolarizing factor in endothelium-dependent hyperpolarization and relaxation in porcine coronary arterial and venous system. *J Cardiovasc Pharmacol* 2004;43:839–50.

16. Guzik TJ, West NEJ, Pillai R, et al. Nitric oxide modulates superoxide release and peroxynitrite formation in human blood vessels. *Hypertension* 2002;39:1088–94.

17. de Sousa MG, Yugar-Toledo JC, Rubira M, et al. Ascorbic acid improves impaired venous and arterial endothelium dependent dilation in smokers. *Acta Pharmacological Sinica* 2005;26:447–52.

18. Perez-Rivera AA, Fink GD, Galligan JJ. Increased reactivity of murine mesenteric veins to adrenergic agonists: Functional evidence supporting increased α_1-adrenoceptor reserve in veins compared with arteries. *J Pharmacol Exp Ther* 2004;308:350–57.

19. Leech CJ, Faber JE. Differential sensitivity of venular and arteriolar α-adrenergic receptor constriction to inhibition by hypoxia. *Circ Res* 1996;78:1064–74.

20. Watts SW, Fink GD, Northcott CA, Galligan JJ. Endothelin-1-induced venous contraction is maintained in DOCA-salt hypertension: Studies with receptor agonists. *Br J Pharmacol* 2002;137:69–79.

21. Thakali K, Fink GD, Watts SW. Arteries and veins desensitize differently to endothelin. *J Cardiovasc Pharmacol* 2004;43:387–93.

22. Dethlefsen SM, Shepro D, D'Amore PA. Comparison of the effects of mechanical stimulation on venous and arterial smooth muscle cells in vitro. *J Vasc Res* 1996;33:405–13.

23. Yang Z, Oemar BS, Carrel T, et al. Different proliferative properties of smooth muscle cells of human arterial and venous bypass vessels. *Circulation* 1998;97:181–87.

24. Wong AP, Nili N, Strauss BH. In vitro differences between venous and arterial-derived smooth muscle cells: Potential modulatory role of decorin. *Cardiovasc Res* 2005;65:702–10.

25. Waybill PN, Chinchilli VM, Ballermann BJ. Smooth muscle cell proliferation in response to co-culture with venous and arterial endothelial cells. *J Vasc Interv Radiol* 1997;8:375–81.

26. Ulrich-Merzenich G, Metzner C, Bhonde RR, et al. Simultaneous isolation of endothelial and smooth muscle cells from human umbilical artery or vein and their growth response to low-density lipoproteins. *In vitro Cell Dev Biol* 2002;38:265–72.

27. Swei A, Lacy F, DeLano FA, Schmid-Schonbein GW. Oxidative stress in the Dahl hypertensive rat. *Hypertension* 1997;30:1628–33.

28. Thakali K, Demel SL, Fink GD, Watts SW. Endothelin-1 (ET-1)-induced contraction in veins is independent of hydrogen peroxide (H_2O_2). *Am J Physiol Heart Circ Physiol* 2005;289(3):H1115–22.

29. Brinsuk M, Tank J, Luft FC, et al. Heritability of venous function in humans. *Arterioscler Thromb Vasc Biol* 2004;24:207–11.

30. Adams LD, Geary RL, McManus B, Schwartz SM. A comparison of aorta and vena cava medial message expression by cDNA array analysis identifies a set of 68 consistently differentially expressed genes, all in aortic media. *Circ Res* 2000;87:623–31.

31. Zhou J, Moroi K, Nishiyama M, et al. Characterization of RGS5 in regulation of G protein-coupled receptor signaling. *Life Sci* 2001;68:1457–69.

32. Fricker R, Hesse C, Weiss J, et al. Endothelial venodilator response in carriers of genetic polymorphisms involved in NO synthesis and degradation. *Br J Clin Pharmacol* 2004;58:169–77.

33. Aalkjaer C, Mulvany MJ. Morphological and mechanical properties of small mesenteric arteries and veins in spontaneously hypertensive rats. *Acta Physiol Scand* 1979;107:309–12.

34. Smith TL, Hutchins PM. Central hemodynamics in the developmental stage of spontaneous hypertension in the unanesthetized rat. *Hypertension* 1979;1:508–17.

35. Lund-Johansen P. Hemodynamics of essential hypertension. In: Swales JD (ed.). *Textbook of Hypertension.* Oxford: Blackwell Scientific Publications, 1994:61.

36. Fink GD, Watts SW, Galligan JJ. Venoconstriction in the development of DOCA-salt hypertension. [Abstract]. *Hypertension* 2002;40:418.

37. Martin DS, Rodrigo MC, Appelt CW. Venous tone in the developmental stages of spontaneous hypertension. *Hypertension* 1998;31:139–44.

38. Willems WJ, Harder DR, Contney SJ, et al. Sympathetic supraspinal control of venous membrane potential in spontaneous hypertension in vivo. *Am J Physiol* 1982;243(3):C1016.

39. Walsh JA, Hyman C, Maronde RF. Venous distensibility in essential hypertension. *Cardiovasc Res* 1969;3:338–49.

40. Safar ME, London DM. Venous system in essential hypertension. *Clin Sci* 1985;69:497–504.

41. Safar ME, London GM. Arterial and venous compliance in sustained essential hypertension. *Hypertension* 1987;10:133–39.

42. Julius S. Interaction between renin and the autonomic nervous system in hypertension. *Am Heart J* 1988;116:611–16.

43. Benjafield AV, Jeyasingam CL, Nyholt DR, et al. G-protein beta3 subunit gene (GNB3) variant in causation of essential hypertension. *Hypertension* 1998;32:1094–97.

44. Wenzel RR, Siffert W, Bruck H, et al. Enhanced vasoconstriction to endothelin-1, angiotensin II and noradrenaline in carriers of the GNB3 825T allele in the skin microcirculation. *Pharmacogenetics* 2002;12:489–95.

45. Mitchell A, Buhrmann S, Seifert A, et al. Venous response to nitroglycerin is enhanced in young, healthy carriers of the 825T allele of the G protein beta3 subunit gene (GNB3). *Clin Pharmacol Ther* 2003;74:499–504.

46. Mitchell A, Luckebergfeld B, Buhrmann S, et al. Effects of systemic endothelin A receptor antagonism in various vascular beds in men: In vivo interactions of the major blood pressure-regulating systems and associations with the GNB3 C825T polymorphism. *Clin Pharmacol Ther* 2004;76:396.

Chapter

20 Sodium Pumps

Peter A. Doris

Definition

The sodium pump is a membrane ion transport complex that plays a central role in renal sodium reabsorption.

Key Findings

- Renal transport of ions by the sodium pump is subject to regulation.
- Disturbances in pump function may be linked to hypertension through alterations in the pump itself, as reported in the Dahl salt-sensitive rat.
- Abnormal regulation may also alter function: defective dopaminergic regulation of the pump occurs in the spontaneously hypertensive rat, whereas defective interactions with cytoskeletal components participating in pump regulation create hypertension in the Milan hypertensive rat.

Clinical Implications

- Abnormalities in pump activity in rat models suggest that human hypertension may also be influenced by polymorphisms in pump structural or regulatory genes.

Few aspects of cell biology are more fundamental than the fact that cells are separated from their surrounding environment by a membrane. This cell membrane encloses the soluble cell proteins and is largely impermeable to them. These proteins (at normal cellular pH) are predominantly negatively charged and are neutralized by potassium ions, which are much more abundant in the intracellular fluid (~150 mmol/L) compared to the extracellular fluid (~4 mmol/L). The cell membrane is permeable to potassium ions, allowing these ions to enter to neutralize proteins. However, the proteins generate an osmotic effect that tends to draw water into the cells across the relatively water-permeable membrane. Swelling of cells is prevented by opposing the osmotic pressure generated by intracellular proteins with a high concentration of sodium ions outside the cell (~140 mmol/L), while maintaining a low intracellular sodium content (~15 mmol/L).

A central question in cell physiology for several decades in the middle of the last century concerned the mechanism producing this distribution of ions, essential to protect the cell from bursting as a result of osmotic swelling. Among the alternative explanations considered, the possibility that the cell membrane was impermeable to sodium was favored—in part because it exempted the cell from the high-energy cost implicit in any biological process to redistribute ions. However, the fact that there is some sodium inside the cell suggested that this explanation might be false. The alternative explanation proposed that the transmembrane gradient of sodium is sustained by an energy-dependent secretory process to remove sodium from inside the cell. This explanation was proven to be correct and ignited a search to find and characterize the protein responsible for this activity. The work of Jens Skou, Robert Post, and others led to the identification of a membrane ATPase that could transport sodium ions asymmetrically from inside the cell in exchange for potassium ions outside the cell and showed that this enzymatic activity could be inhibited by plant-derived steroids and steroid glycosides related to digitalis.[1,2] By this means, the activity and eventually the identity of the sodium pump became known. With these fundamental observations achieved, the path was opened to develop ever more detailed understanding of the sodium/potassium-ATPase that is the sodium pump. This understanding now extends beyond the key role played by the pump in solving the osmotic problem of the cell and includes understanding of its role in creating the membrane potential in excitable cells, coupling the transport of other substances into and out of cells, and (of greatest significance to this chapter) its role in achieving directional transepithelial ion transport.

Among the ion transporting epithelia, the renal epithelium (comprised of about 1 million nephrons per kidney) is remarkable for the enormous quantity of fluid and electrolytes that pass across it. The adult kidneys filter about 150 L of fluid from the blood each day. The majority of this fluid (>99%) and the solutes it contains (principally sodium and chloride) are reabsorbed, leaving only a fraction of the filtered material to be excreted. The sodium pump provides the main driving force of renal reabsorption. Extensive evidence now shows that blood pressure links to renal sodium reabsorption via the pressure-natriuresis mechanism.[3,4] Elevation of blood pressure in the vessels perfusing the kidneys results in reduced reabsorption of fluid and electrolytes by the nephrons and consequently increased sodium excretion. This relationship appears to be altered in hypertension so that a higher level of blood pressure is required to maintain sufficient sodium excretion. In this manner, the persistently elevated blood pressure of hypertension can be regarded as an adaptive response directed toward maintenance of sodium homeostasis.[4] Given the key role played by the sodium pump in this process, there has been great interest in the possibility that abnormality of sodium/potassium-ATPase function or its regulation can be a causative factor in the pathogenesis of hypertension. This chapter examines the structure/function relationships of the sodium pump, its distribution and regulation, and evidence implicating the sodium pump in the pathogenesis of hypertension.

BIOCHEMISTRY

The P-type ATPase family includes four known mammalian isoforms of the alpha subunit of sodium/potassium-ATPase, as well as the sarcoplasmic reticulum and plasma membrane calcium-ATPases and the gastric and non-gastric H+/K+-ATPases (Table 20–1). In the kidney, only the alpha 1 isoform of the Na+/K+-ATPase is expressed. The 100-kD alpha subunits of Na+/K+-ATPase, as well as the H+/K+-ATPases, are associated with a glycoprotein beta subunit that is required via co-translational assembly for maturation, stability, targeting, and functional activity of the protein.[5,6] Several isoforms of this beta subunit are encoded in the genome, but only the beta 1 subunit is expressed in the kidney.[7] The kidney alpha-beta heterodimers have an additional subunit that is a member of the FXYD family of proteins, named for an invariant amino acid motif present in family members.[8] Many of the seven members of the FXYD family have been shown to be associated with the sodium pump, but in the kidney only FXYD2 (gamma subunit) and FXYD4 (CHIF, corticosteroid hormone-inducible factor) are expressed and appear to modulate some aspects of pump function.

The sodium pump is an integral membrane protein in which the alpha subunit possesses 10 transmembrane spanning domains, whereas the beta subunit and any associated FXYD proteins each have a single transmembrane domain[9] (Figure 20–1). The family feature uniting the P-type ATPases arises from the existence of a transient phosphorylated intermediate during the pump cycle. This intermediate is formed as the gamma phosphate of ATP is transferred to the aspartate residue in a motif (DKTGT) that is common to the P-type ATPase. Although the high-resolution structure of the sodium/potassium-ATPase has not been obtained directly it has been inferred by homology mapping to the closely related sarcoplasmic reticulum Ca-ATPase (SERCA), whose crystals have been analyzed at 2.6A resolution.[10] This provides an important opportunity to begin to connect the extensive biochemical and physiologic understanding of the pump to its three-dimensional structure.

PHYSIOLOGY

To effect unidirectional transport across the renal epithelium, the sodium pump is distributed to the basolateral border of the nephron and occurs throughout its length. However, highest abundance occurs in the proximal tubules, the medullary thick ascending limb, and the distal tubule and adjacent connecting tubule.[11] The bulk of salt and water reabsorption occurs in the proximal tubule and is reflected in the high abundance of sodium pump in this region. Distal regions of the nephron are responsible for adjusting the final reabsorption of sodium, with aldosterone providing a dominant role in regulation at this site by controlling access of sodium ions to intracellular sites where sodium can be engaged by the pump and reabsorbed.[12] Distal tubule adjustments provide fine control of sodium excretion, whereas proximal tubule reabsorption contributes to the bulk recovery of filtered plasma fluid and electrolyte. Sodium reabsorption driven by the sodium pump in the ascending limb and distal convolution occurs in a region

THE P-TYPE ATPASES		
Group	Gene	Function
Ib	ATP7A	Cu++-transporting ATPase, alpha polypetide
	ATP7B	Cu++-transporting ATPase, beta polypetide
IIa	ATP2A1	Sarcoplasmic reticulum Ca++-ATPase (SERCA1)
	ATP2A2	Sarcoplasmic reticulum Ca++-ATPase (SERCA2)
	ATP2A3	Sarcoplasmic reticulum Ca++-ATPase (SERCA3)
IIb	ATP2B1	Plasma membrane type reticulum Ca++-ATPase (PMCA1)
	ATP2B2	Plasma membrane type reticulum Ca++-ATPase (PMCA2)
	ATP2B3	Plasma membrane type reticulum Ca++-ATPase (PMCA3)
	ATP2B4	Plasma membrane type reticulum Ca++-ATPase (PMCA4)
IIc	ATP1A1	Na+, K+-ATPase, alpha 1 subunit
	ATP1A	Na+, K+-ATPase, alpha 2 subunit
	ATP1A3	Na+, K+-ATPase, alpha 3 subunit
	ATP1A4	Na+, K+-ATPase, alpha 4 subunit
	ATP4A	Gastric H+-K+-ATPase, alpha subunit

The P-type ATPases are a large and ubiquitous family of proteins with a characteristic pattern of conserved amino acid residues, including the DKTGTLT motif providing the aspartate residue (D) that is transiently phosphorylated by ATP during the pump cycle. This transmembrane protein generally has 10 membrane-inserted helices with large and conserved domains in the cytoplasmic loops linking M2 and M3 and M4 and M5. This table provides the members of the major groups represented in mammals. Many groups contain members that are present only in lower organisms.

Table 20–1. The P-Type ATPases

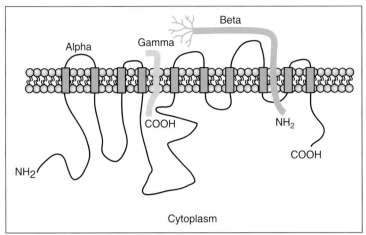

Figure 20–1. The structure of the sodium pump complex in kidney incorporating catalytic (alpha), structural (beta), and modulatory (gamma) subunits. The catalytic alpha subunit contains 10 membrane-inserted helices. The intracytoplasmic N-terminus is an important site of regulatory phosphorylation leading to engagement with the clathrin-coated pit mechanism of endocytosis. The second (large) intracytoplasmic loop contains the ATP catalytic site that is transiently phosphorylated during the ion transport cycle. The beta subunit is glycosylated at its extracytoplasmic surface.

of the nephron that is highly water impermeable, thereby allowing dilution of the tubular content as a result of pump-mediated fluid reabsorption. At the same time, osmolarity of the adjacent interstitial fluid is increased, providing a key mechanism allowing the establishment of a medullary concentration gradient by which renal concentration can occur. Thus, sodium pump function is adapted to perform specialized physiologic roles in different nephron regions. Although its action does not differ, its role is modified by virtue of the other properties of those regions and of the effect of upstream handling of renal filtrate that determines what is delivered.

REGULATION

The subcellular localization of the sodium pump has been the subject of much recent investigation that has revealed that the pump can be found in both plasma membrane and endosomal membranes.[13] In this regard, the pump is not unlike G-protein-coupled membrane receptors that can undergo internalization from the plasma membrane after binding ligand.[14] Just as G-protein-coupled receptors can be in locations providing or preventing access to ligand, so too the sodium pump appears to exist in pools distributed between the basolateral membrane from which pump-mediated transepithelial sodium reabsorption can occur and intracellular endosomal membrane compartments from which site net transepithelial reabsorption cannot be driven.

Although the sodium pump is synthesized de novo in the endoplasmic reticulum as a membrane-resident protein and is transported through the Golgi to the cell surface, its presence in the plasma membrane appears to require stabilizing interactions with the actin cytoskeleton.[15] These interactions with actin involve ankyrin, fodrin, and adducin. Furthermore, the interaction between plasma-membrane-inserted sodium pump and the actin cytoskeleton is a dynamic one in which movement out of the cell membrane by interaction with AP2 protein and clathrin via clathrin-coated pits can result in withdrawal of the sodium pump into endosomal membranes.[16–18] Although this pump movement has been studied most extensively in the proximal tubule, it appears to represent a pump recycling mechanism by which the level of transepithelial ion transport can be modulated by altering the distribution of the pump between internal and external cell membranes. Interactions with AP2 and clathrin appear to be initiated by post-translational modification of the sodium pump on the alpha subunit, and considerable effort has been made to determine the kinases involved and the amino acid targets subject to phosphorylation.

The sodium pump also incorporates an extracellular receptor. The existence and identity of an endogenous ligand for this receptor continues to be a persistent controversy in sodium pump biology.[19,20] The receptor clearly is able to bind cardiotonic steroid drugs, such as the plant-derived cardiac steroid glycosides of the digitalis family, as well as structurally similar non-glycoside steroids produced as skin venoms by some amphibians. That these drugs and venoms evince an ion transport inhibitory action in response to liganding of the receptor is clear. This ion transport inhibition by cardiotonic steroids appears to be the biological basis of their therapeutic action[21] that has been, and continues to be, exploited as an effective remedy for heart failure in Western medicine for hundreds of years and in traditional Chinese medicine for several millennia. The functional significance of endogenous ligand binding to the receptor site has remained obscured by several critical gaps in knowledge and understanding. For example, difficulties in identification of the chemical structure of the endogenous ligand continue to pose a real obstacle to the acceptance of the concept that this receptor site functions as an evolutionarily conserved tool of homeostasis.[22] Another problem is that the universal distribution of the sodium pump suggests a lack of specificity of response to sodium pump ligands. An endogenous ligand could potentially affect essentially all cells in the body, and lack of specificity is a reasonable concern. In some species, the binding affinity of the receptor site incorporated in the alpha 1 subunit shows a high ligand off-rate.[23] This results in rapid ligand dissociation kinetics and thus proves problematic for a concept that invokes a role of the endogenous ligand as an inhibitor of the ion transport action of the pump wherein the biological consequence of ion transport inhibition presumably requires a shift in transmembrane ion gradients that are more readily achieved by ligands that have low receptor off-rates and so provide a persistent inhibition of ion transport. Indeed, some recent evidence suggests that the endogenous ligand is not a glycoside but rather a cardiotonic steroid similar or identical to a major cardiotonic steroid produced by amphibians.[24] Aglycone cardiotonic steroids lack the stabilizing influence on receptor binding that is provided by the sugar residues incorporated in glycosides.[25]

Recent information has come to light suggesting that existing concepts of the actions of cardiotonic steroids on the sodium pump are incomplete and pointing to a role of the ligand-sodium pump complex that lies outside ion transport. This new evidence suggests that ligand binding of the cardiotonic steroid site of the alpha subunit creates a signal transduction complex that results in activation of mitogen-activated kinase pathways leading to a number of potential biological outcomes, notably cell growth and proliferation.[26–30] Additional evidence suggests interaction between the ouabain-liganded sodium pump and the inositol trisphosphate receptors that contribute to signaling via the induction of calcium oscillations.[31] A substantial body of evidence from several sources has now accumulated in support of this signal transduction property,[32,33] and a model encompassing some of the notable features is presented in Figure 20–2. This raises anew the question of the existence

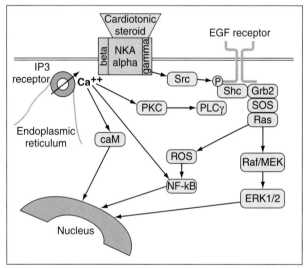

Figure 20–2. The signal transduction pathways proposed for cardiotonic steroid signaling through Na/K-ATPase. Na/K-ATPase may interact directly with the IP3 receptor in ER and initiate calcium oscillations, perhaps via a calcium-induced calcium release mechanism. Na/K-ATPase may also transactivate EGF receptor through Src, leading to association of Shc with phosphorylated EGFR, recruitment of Grb2, SOS, and conversion of Ras to its GTP-bound form. Ras-GTP signaling may activate mitochondrial reactive oxygen species generation (ROS) and operate through Raf1 (MAP3K) to initiate ERK1/2 signaling via MAP2K (MEK1). Interestingly, ERK1/2 activation by EGFR appears to result from internalized EGFR present in endosome and can be blocked when internalization is blocked. Thus, early endosomes may act as a signal coordination complex in which CS redirect Na/K-ATPase to the early endosomes and receptor tyrosine kinase acts on endosomal EGFR to initiate ERK1/2 signaling. Both ROS and calcium oscillations may act to suppress I-κB inhibition of NF-κB. These and signals resulting from activation of calmodulin (CaM) may all contribute to activation of transcriptional programs increasing cell growth and division. The role of Na:Ca exchange to elevate intracellular calcium that may be important in the inotropic action of cardiac glycosides in the heart is not included in this diagram because there is little evidence of this mechanism in kidney.

and functional role of endogenous cardiotonic steroids and offers some solutions to dilemmas that impede elucidation and acceptance of endogenous cardiotonic steroids. For example, the problem of organ or cell type specificity of endogenous cardiotonic steroid binding to the sodium pump might be accommodated by the coupling of the pump to second-messenger signaling functions only in selective tissues or cell types. The problem of cardiac glycoside-resistant isoforms is also resolved because signal transduction mechanisms do not require the persistent binding and sustained inhibition of ion transport to mediate their effects. Receptor-ligand interactions in signaling processes are generally highly transient and utilize rapid receptor on- and off-rates. Indeed, the rat isoform of the sodium pump that has a rapid ligand binding on- and off-rate and is thus highly resistant (IC50 = 10^{-5}M to 10^{-6}M) to the ion transport inhibition of cardiotonic steroids is fully sensitive to the signal transduction activation resulting from ligand-sodium pump interaction with ERK activation and growth responses detectible at 10^{-9}M and below.[32]

The continuing evolution of insight into sodium pump biology suggests that there remains much unexplored scope to increase understanding of the role of the pump in the genesis of hypertension. However, much existing evidence has been developed already, particularly as the result of genetic investigations in animal models of hypertension in which the diversity and complexity of the disease phenotype is more restricted than in human populations.

GENETICS

The role of heritable factors in the genesis of essential hypertension demonstrates an extreme range when considered from the perspective of individual patients. Very rarely, mutations in a single gene can create hypertension.[34] Such mutations (because of the resulting hypertensive end-organ injury) can be seriously maladaptive, and barring the sustained intervention of modern therapies (and probably even in spite of them) are rapidly selected against in nature. The presence in the population of Mendelian forms of hypertension reflects both a small number of new mutations arising in pedigrees that were previously unaffected as well as a limited degree of transmission of these mutations from founders to their progeny. Many of the single gene mutations that produce hypertension do so by directly or indirectly affecting mechanisms of renal sodium reabsorption that are ultimately driven by the action of the sodium pump.[35]

In most hypertensive patients, genetic factors play a significant but smaller role. This role is strongly modified by environmental variables and aging processes. Heritability represents the degree of similarity in a trait that can be attributed to the sharing of alleles that occurs among related individuals. Twin studies were the first to demonstrate that blood pressure is a heritable trait,[36,37] and broader family studies confirm the heritability of blood pressure levels.[38,39] Overall, blood pressure has a heritability of about 30 to 40%. However, and in contrast with single-gene Mendelian forms of hypertension, this heritability shows no simple pattern of transmission within families. This fact suggests that the inheritance of blood pressure levels and hypertension susceptibility may be polygenic and that susceptibility alleles of multiple genes may interact within individuals as well as between the individual and their environment (diet, lifestyle, exercise, stress, and so on) to create the heritability of blood pressure. Although remarkable progress has been made to uncover gene mutations contributing to rare Mendelian forms of hypertension, efforts to identify genes and the variation they contain that contribute to common polygenic hypertension are confronted by substantial obstacles arising not only in the effect of environmental variation but from within the genetic architecture of disease susceptibility.[40–42] These arise from the possibility that the allelic variation contributing to hypertension is greater in society as a whole than within affected families. Thus, the causal alleles segregating in two different families might partially overlap, or may be completely independent. This allows an unknown degree of genetic heterogeneity. Given the fact that blood pressure is subject to regulation via an extremely broad range of physiologic systems (endocrine, vascular, autonomic, renal), the potential for variation in a very large number of genes to contribute to population patterns of hypertension occurrence cannot be discounted. Each additional gene involved in hypertension in the population reduces the power of population gene mapping studies to localize that gene to a particular region of a particular chromosome, the first step necessary on the path to identifying the gene. The task is made more difficult by the likelihood that some hypertension gene variants are capable of epistatic interaction.[43,44] This interaction means that the effect of the gene variant on the phenotype is affected by other gene variation in a multiplicative, rather than simple additive, way. This can increase the difficulty of gene identification because the effect of the causative allele in a given individual is strongly affected by variation at other sites within the genome.

Given the complexity of the heritability of hypertension in humans it is not surprising that animal models of the disease that provide a homogenous genetic mechanism and allow greater opportunities to extend genetic evidence directly to altered function have been a useful means of understanding the mechanism of polygenic hypertension. Several rat models of hypertension have been inbred to genetic homogeneity. Inbreeding results in identical copies of each gene at every locus on every diploid chromosome, which thus further simplifies the genetic background in which hypertension alleles function. These models have taken advantage of natural allelic variation affecting blood pressure and hypertension susceptibility. By selecting from outbred rat populations those individuals with higher blood pressures (at baseline or under salt loading) and selectively breeding these individuals to concentrate hypertension alleles within individual animals, numerous inbred models of hypertension have been developed—including the SHR (and various substrains),[45] the Dahl salt-sensitive rat,[46] the Milan hypertensive rat,[47] the Sabra rat,[48] and the New Zealand hypertensive rat.[49] In the first three of the strains mentioned, evidence suggests that sodium pump function is directly or indirectly altered as part of the genetic mecha-

nism leading to hypertension. This is perhaps not completely surprising because of the key role of the sodium pump in renal transepithelial sodium reabsorption. It also stresses the importance of a full understanding of sodium pump biology as an important aid to uncovering the genetic and pathogenetic basis of hypertension in humans.

The Dahl salt-sensitive rat (SS) possesses a nonsynonymous mutation in the alpha 1 subunit of the sodium pump.[50] This polymorphism results in the substitution of leucine for glutamine at amino acid position 276 (Q276L), which alters the hydrophobicity of a region of the pump that is involved in the formation of the transmembrane pore. There has been considerable controversy over the existence of this sequence variation, and before exploring the evidence that this variant is responsible for a pump-mediated role in the genesis of hypertension the main facts of the controversy should first be considered.

The initial report identified the polymorphism and indicated that it alters the hydropathy profile of a region of the protein believed to be involved in coordination of ion binding, resulting in a reduction in potassium ion transport and a putative role in hypertension.[50] This report appeared almost concurrently with a co-segregation study performed by another group that addressed whether a restriction fragment polymorphism located in or nearby the alpha 1 subunit was associated with blood pressure levels in Dahl SS measured by tail cuff. These authors concluded that it was not, or rather that it did not act with sufficiently large effect to be detected by the rather imprecise tail cuff blood pressure measurements used.[51] Similarly, only pulse pressure showed a significant positive association with inheritance of SS alleles of the sodium pump when blood pressures were determined in directly cannulated anesthetized animals.[52] Another study using more precise telemetry measurements did report linkage between the alpha 1 subunit in Dahl SS and inheritance of blood pressure.[53] The sodium pump polymorphism reported in Dahl SS rats could not be confirmed by another group using restriction digestion at the mutant site of PCR-amplified genomic DNA and was also undetected by resequencing the gene.[54] The polymorphism reported creates an interesting stem-loop structure that might contribute to sequencing errors or to amplification-induced mutation. The absence of the reported nonsynonymous polymorphism was also confirmed by another group using restriction digestion of PCR-amplified DNA as well as mini-sequencing reactions.[55]

Because of this contradictory data, the initial report of sodium pump polymorphism has been extended and confirmed by its originators very thoroughly using a range of techniques directed to DNA and RNA sequence coding the alpha 1 subunit gene as well as to the pump protein itself.[56,57] Furthermore, the generation of a transgenic rat in which the Dahl salt-resistant (SR) rat gene was reconstructed (including the proximal 5′ regulatory sequence and some 3′ untranslated sequence) and expressed in the Dahl SS rat resulted in phenotypic shifts in blood pressure, renal injury, and extended life span—all consonant with a role of the Dahl SS sodium pump in hypertension.[53] Although this transgenic model is not as complete a genetic test as would be achieved by a knock-out/knock-in strategy, it is still supportive of the role of the Dahl SS allele in the generation of hypertension. Furthermore, a recent report indicates that amino acid sequencing of the alpha subunit from Dahl SS confirms the expected amino acid change, that decreased potassium and increased sodium affinity of the partially purified pump protein is observed in Dahl SS kidney, and that susceptibility to proteolytic cleavage differs in a manner consonant with altered hydrophobicity of the pump predicted from the amino acid substitution.[56]

This contradictory evidence may find a rational explanation, although one that accounts for all of the discrepant results that have been recorded among investigations of Dahl SS is not yet forthcoming. Before reaching a conclusion about the role of the sodium pump in Dahl SS hypertension, it is important to recognize that all gene variation exists in haplotypes that distinguish one allele from another by sequence variation at one or more sites within the gene and adjacent chromosomal sequence. It has become clear from investigation of this model that even excluding the Dahl Q276L polymorphism at least two haplotypes of the alpha 1 subunit exist and differ between Dahl SS and Dahl SR rats. This is apparent because detailed sequence analysis performed during the course of investigating the Dahl SS rat has revealed additional intronic polymorphisms[52,55] in this gene. At least one of these polymorphisms is also present in some other inbred laboratory rat strains.[55] It is worthwhile to consider where and how such gene haplotypes arise. Haplotypes represent adjacent sequence variation on the same haploid chromosome. Most often this is single-nucleotide polymorphism, although deletions, insertions, and sequence repeats are not uncommon. By virtue of its close proximity in the same genomic locus, the resulting sequence variation tends to be inherited as a unit and is separated from adjacent sequence variation by recombination only very rarely. A new haplotype can be created by a novel mutation or by a recombination event occurring at the locus of the haplotype that creates a new combination of existing sequence variation on the same chromosome. By genetic drift or natural selection, the newly created haplotype may become more frequent in a wild population.

Genes (such as the alpha 1 subunit gene) that are multi-exon genes covering tens of thousands of bases may contain extensive natural variation in wild animals that has been carried forward in laboratory strains—allowing the possibility that two distinct haplotypes of the alpha 1 subunit gene might become fixed when generating any contrasting inbred strains. At present, five single-nucleotide polymorphisms in the rat alpha 1 subunit gene are recorded in the public NCBI database (dbSNP). These five SNPs permit the existence of up to 25 different haplotypes of the rat alpha 1 subunit. Because much of the gene sequence outside the specific polymorphisms that have been the subject of investigation in Dahl SS and other hypertensive rat strains has gone uninvestigated or incompletely investigated, it is not yet possible to determine whether all functional sequence variation responsible for an effect of the alpha 1 subunit on sodium pump function has been uncovered.

In addition to the well-validated but controversial studies of sodium pump gene variation in the genesis of hypertension in Dahl SS rats, it is notable that disease gene mapping studies have placed hypertension susceptibility in the same locus as the alpha subunit of the sodium pump in another distinct model of the disease, SHR (and SHR-SP).[58–60]

In SHR, extensive physiologic evidence indicates an abnormality in the regulation of proximal tubule sodium reabsorption that precedes the development of hypertension. Nephron micropuncture studies in young SHR have demonstrated increased proximal sodium reabsorption.[61,62] This has been extended to conscious animals in studies using fractional reabsorption of lithium, an indicator of proximal sodium reabsorption that provides further support of altered renal sodium handling in SHR.[63] In older SHR animals, changes in proximal sodium reabsorption are lost.[61] However, sustaining proximal sodium reabsorption in mature hypertensive animals required a much higher renal perfusion pressure, indicating that the pressure/natriuresis relationship is shifted to allow the acquisition of sodium balance by sustaining a higher level of blood pressure. Similar abnormalities of proximal tubular sodium reabsorption have been observed using lithium clearance in the Dahl SS model of hypertension.[64] Because the sodium pump drives proximal sodium reabsorption, it must have primary or secondary involvement in the abnormal sodium reabsorption.

As indicated previously, regulation of sodium pump activity is achieved in part by phosphorylation events that are the output of signal transduction systems.[65,66] Dopamine clearly plays an important role in regulation of proximal tubule sodium reabsorption and appears to do so through regulation of the activity of both proximal tubule luminal sodium entry pathways and the active transport of sodium by the pump in proximal tubule basolateral membranes.[65,67] Felder and Jose have developed an extensive series of studies demonstrating that dopamine-mediated inhibition of proximal tubule sodium reabsorption, which occurs via the cAMP-coupled D1 receptor, is deficient in SHR in spite of increased local renal dopamine production.[68] This is accompanied by a redistribution of dopamine receptors from the cell surface that is similar to the ligand-induced G-protein-coupled receptor desensitization/internalization phenomenon.[69] This work has led to vigorous investigation of sequence variation in the dopamine receptor as well as its regulatory kinase (GRK4). Unfortunately, none of these gene targets has resulted in evidence for gene variation in the induction of hypertension in SHR. The issue of whether dopamine signaling deficits are secondary to changes in ion transport mechanisms that are autonomously able to increase sodium reabsorption that then drives secondarily increased dopamine-mediated inhibitory responses (and consequently leads to receptor desensitization) has not been finally answered. What is clear at present is that among the genes involved in dopamine signaling of increased proximal tubule sodium reabsorption and elevated blood pressure in SHR the alpha 1 subunit of the pump is notable in being located in a chromosomal region that has consistently been shown to associate with the inheritance of elevated blood pressure.

Positional mapping evidence that the chromosomal locus containing the alpha 1 subunit is involved in the genesis of hypertension has been further strengthened by the generation of a congenic SHR substrain in which substitution of this locus with the corresponding one from WKY results in a significant reduction in blood pressure.[58] Abnormalities in the sodium pump in young SHR include the pump's altered subcellular distribution with a greater proportion of the available pump protein present in the basolateral membrane (Figure 20–3) and a smaller portion in endosomal compartments.[70] This shift is apparent during the period when proximal tubule sodium reabsorption is increased prior to the onset of hypertension. When hypertension is mature, this altered distribution is restored to normal. Here again, however, it is unclear whether the altered subcellular targeting of the pump protein is a primary genetic phenomenon or secondary to dysregulation in some other pathway.

Whether genetic alterations in the sodium pump are responsible *per se* for elevation of blood pressure in SHR and Dahl SS rats is not yet completely clear. In the case of SHR, the field might be moved forward by determining whether the dopamine signaling deficits and sodium pump subcellular localization alterations are repaired in the congenic model in which the SHR alpha 1 sodium pump locus is replaced by that of WKY. Such insight could begin to sort out whether dopamine signaling defects and altered subcellular localization are attributable to sequence variation in a locus containing the renal alpha subunit or whether they arise from another region of the genome.

By selective breeding from out-bred Wistar rats, Bianchi and colleagues created another rat model of hypertension: the Milan hypertensive strain (MHS).[47] This model unequivocally indicates the capacity of mechanisms altering renal sodium pump function to generate increased blood pressure.

Early investigations pointed to a renal abnormality in MHS with increased proximal tubule sodium reabsorption as a key element.[71] Alterations of ion handling were also observed in other cell types, including erythrocytes.[72] Ultimately, the alpha subunit of adducin (one of several cytoskeletal proteins believed to influence actin cytoskeleton dynamics) was found to be polymorphic in MHS.[73] Reciprocal congenic strains isolating the two adducin variant alleles in normotensive and hypertensive rats confirms the effect of variation at this locus on blood pressure.[74] This adducin polymorphism expressed in cultured renal proximal tubule cells impairs dopamine-mediated endocytosis of the sodium pump and blocks the interaction between the sodium pump and adaptin subunits necessary to mediate the cytoskeletal interactions that effect internalization of the pump.[74] Consequently, there is increased stability of pump protein inserted in the basolateral membrane, inhibition of the normal recycling of pump protein from the basolateral membrane to intracellular membrane sites, and an increase in both sodium pump activity and sodium reabsorption.

This work in MHS stimulated an investigation of the existence of polymorphisms in the alpha, beta, and gamma subunits of adducin in humans. The identification of such variation has led to a number of studies that have not yet generated a completely clear consensus of the likely role of naturally occurring common variation in these genes in the pathogenesis of hypertension in humans. Indeed, the challenges that must be confronted by such studies are rather great. First, a decision must be made to study a categorical (hypertension versus normotension) or a quantitative trait (blood pressure level). Second, it must be recognized that there is likely genotypic heterogeneity in hypertension in humans and that the portion of phenotypic variation, if any, affected by adducin polymorphism may make identification difficult unless populations are large and the susceptibility allele is reasonably frequent and able to modify the trait substantially. Furthermore, the hypertension phenotype is heterogeneous, and various classifiers may be used to distinguish subtypes that meaningfully relate to the underlying genetic mechanism. Depending on the unknown extent of genetic heterogeneity and the size of the study population, it may be necessary to select a subgroup of hypertensives (e.g., salt sensitive) to demonstrate the effect of adducin polymorphism. This may explain the dissonant findings that have emerged in human genetic studies of adducin. Several studies examining linkage and association of variation in or around adducin genes report positive findings, whereas others do not. A recently published meta-analysis of these many studies summarizes the evidence for adducin involvement in salt-sensitive hypertension and reaches an understandably cautious conclusion.[75] This cautious conclusion in humans contrasts with that in rats and may be related to the fact that clear and consistent functional consequences of MHS adducin polymorphism on membrane ion transport are apparent in MHS. Similar evidence at the *in vitro* cellular level of functional consequence of human adducin variation is limited and is derived principally from studies of erythrocytes,[76,77] with evidence of altered renal ion transport limited to indirect studies.[78]

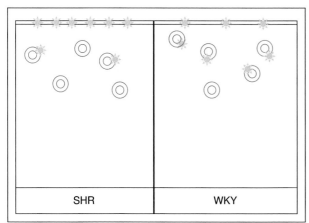

Figure 20–3. Altered subcellular distribution of Na/K-ATPase in basolateral membrane of renal proximal tubules in SHR. Sodium pumps (star) are distributed between endosomes (double circle) and the basolateral membrane (upper border). In young SHR, the abundance of sodium pump protein in the basolateral membrane is almost twice that in WKY, whereas pump abundance in the late endosomes is reduced in SHR compared to WKY. This mistargeting may contribute to the excess sodium reabsorption observed during the development of hypertension in this model.

PHARMACOLOGY

The observations of a key abnormality in sodium-pump-mediated renal sodium reabsorption in MHS has led to a pharmacological approach to alter sodium pump function as a means of treating hypertension and related disorders. Part of the rationale of this approach appears to reside in the finding of increased immuno- and bioassay measurement of levels of endogenous cardiotonic steroid in MHS[79] and the potential role of this material in elevation of blood pressure. This stimulated the identification of a cardiac glycoside, PST2238, which has reduced cardiac activity and is able to correct the abnormal sodium pump function and blood pressure in MHS.[80,81] It is interesting that PST2238 appears to be able to regulate sodium pump function in hypertension, whereas the dopamine inhibition of the pump is suppressed. These effects appear to develop over relatively long time courses. Dopamine regulation of sodium pump activity leading to transepithelial ion transport is inhibited in MHS, and this appears related to its inability to initiate sodium pump internalization from the basolateral membrane to internal endosomes.[82] Ouabain has recently also been shown to be able to cause internalization of the sodium pump in renal epithelial cells. If PST2238 acts as a ouabain agonist with respect to internalization, this might explain the inhibitory effect on pump function activated by adducin polymorphism. However, exposure to ouabain appears to mimic the adducin polymorphism in producing increased pump activity, and PST2238 also antagonizes this effect. Other antagonistic effects of PST2238 on ouabain-induced pump function have recently been reported.[83] Clearly, considerable fundamental pharmacological investigation is required to understand the mechanism of PST2238 action. However, present evidence in this nascent field suggests that abnormal pump function contributing to hypertension may be corrected by specific pharmacotherapies targeting the cardiotonic steroid binding site of the pump.

SUMMARY

Sodium pump activity drives renal sodium reabsorption and provides a potential mechanism by which altered regulation can contribute to hypertension. Altered regulation of the pump can be primary or secondary. In animal models, evidence consonant with a primary role of the pump attributable to allelic variation in the pump has been obtained in animal models. In the Dahl SS rat, this evidence is centered on polymorphism in the renal catalytic subunit of the pump but has been disputed. In SHR and New Zealand hypertensive rat models, positional mapping approaches point to an important hypertension locus in the region of the renal catalytic subunit gene, and in SHR there is a shift in subcellular targeting of the pump in the renal proximal tubule during the development. SHR also shows altered regulation of proximal tubule pump activity by dopaminergic signaling. Further work is required to determine whether alterations in pump function in these models are due to primary genetic variation in the gene encoding the renal catalytic unit of the pump, although this is consistent with available data. In human essential hypertension, many obstacles impede the identification of genes and their pathogenetic process in contributing to hypertension susceptibility, although in some hypertensive subgroups interesting parallels have been observed between rat models and human hypertension—including altered proximal tubule sodium handling and abnormal regulation of the renal sodium pump by dopamine signal transduction mechanisms.

REFERENCES

1. Post RL. Seeds of sodium, potassium ATPase. *Annu Rev Physiol* 1989;51:1–15.
2. Skou JC. Nobel Lecture: The identification of the sodium pump. *Biosci Rep* 1998;18:155–69.
3. McDonough AA, Leong PK, Yang LE. Mechanisms of pressure natriuresis: How blood pressure regulates renal sodium transport. *Ann N Y Acad Sci* 2003;986:669–77.
4. Guyton AC. Blood pressure control—special role of the kidneys and body fluids. *Science* 1991;252:1813–16.
5. Caplan MJ, Forbush B III, Palade GE, Jamieson JD. Biosynthesis of the Na,K-ATPase in Madin-Darby canine kidney cells: Activation and cell surface delivery. *J Biol Chem* 1990;265:3528–34.
6. Geering K. The functional role of the beta-subunit in the maturation and intracellular transport of Na,K-ATPase. *FEBS Lett* 1991;285:189–93.
7. Hayward AL, Hinojos CA, Nurowska B, et al. Altered sodium pump alpha and gamma subunit gene expression in nephron segments from hypertensive rats. *J Hypertens* 1999;17:1081–87.
8. Sweadner KJ, Rael E. The FXYD gene family of small ion transport regulators or channels: cDNA sequence, protein signature sequence, and expression. *Genomics* 2000;68:41–56.
9. Horisberger JD. Recent insights into the structure and mechanism of the sodium pump. *Physiology* (Bethesda) 2004;19:377–87.
10. Toyoshima C, Inesi G. Structural basis of ion pumping by Ca2+-ATPase of the sarcoplasmic reticulum. *Annu Rev Biochem* 2004;73:269–92.
11. Cheval L, Doucet A. Measurement of Na-K-ATPase-mediated rubidium influx in single segments of rat nephron. *Am J Physiol* 1990;259:F111–21.
12. Booth RE, Johnson JP, Stockand JD. Aldosterone. *Adv Physiol Educ* 2002;26:8–20.
13. Chibalin AV, Katz AI, Berggren PO, Bertorello AM. Receptor-mediated inhibition of renal Na(+)-K(+)-ATPase is associated with endocytosis of its alpha- and beta-subunits. *Am J Physiol* 1997;273:C1458–65.
14. Ferguson SS, Downey WE III, Colapietro AM, et al. Role of beta-arrestin in mediating agonist-promoted G protein-coupled receptor internalization. *Science* 1996;271:363–66.
15. Marrs JA, Napolitano EW, Murphy-Erdosh C, et al. Distinguishing roles of the membrane-cytoskeleton and cadherin mediated cell-cell adhesion in generating different Na+,K(+)-ATPase distributions in polarized epithelia. *J Cell Biol* 1993;123:149–64.
16. Done SC, Leibiger IB, Efendiev R, et al. Tyrosine 537 within the Na+,K+-ATPase alpha-subunit is essential for AP-2 binding and clathrin-dependent endocytosis. *J Biol Chem* 2002;277:17108–11.
17. Ogimoto G, Yudowski GA, Barker CJ, et al. G protein-coupled receptors regulate Na+,K+-ATPase activity and endocytosis by modulating the recruitment of adaptor protein 2 and clathrin. *Proc Natl Acad Sci USA* 2000;97:3242–47.
18. Yudowski GA, Efendiev R, Pedemonte CH, et al. Phosphoinositide-3 kinase binds to a proline-rich motif in the Na+,K+-ATPase alpha subunit and regulates its trafficking. *Proc Natl Acad Sci USA* 2000;97:6556–61.
19. Hansen O. No evidence for a role in signal-transduction of Na+/K+-ATPase interaction with putative endogenous ouabain. *Eur J Biochem* 2003;270:1916–19.

20. Schoner W, Bauer N, Muller-Ehmsen J, et al. Ouabain as a mammalian hormone. *Ann NY Acad Sci* 2003;986:678–84.

21. Reuter H, Henderson SA, Han T, et al. The Na+-Ca2+ exchanger is essential for the action of cardiac glycosides. *Circ Res* 2002;90:305–08.

22. Doris PA, Bagrov AY. Endogenous sodium pump inhibitors and blood pressure regulation: An update on recent progress. *Proc Soc Exp Biol Med* 1998;218:156–67.

23. Allen JC, Schwartz A. A possible biochemical explanation for the insensitivity of the rat to cardiac glycosides. *J Pharmacol Exp Ther* 1969;168:42–6.

24. Bagrov AY, Fedorova OV, Dmitrieva RI, et al. Characterization of a urinary bufodienolide Na+,K+-ATPase inhibitor in patients after acute myocardial infarction. *Hypertension* 1998;31:1097–103.

25. Wallick ET, Dowd F, Allen JC, Schwartz A. The nature of the transport adenosine triphosphatase-digitalis complex. VII. Characteristics of ouabagenin-Na+,K+-adenosine triphosphatase interaction. *J Pharmacol Exp Ther* 1974;189:434–44.

26. Abramowitz J, Dai C, Hirschi KK, et al. Ouabain- and marinobufagenin-induced proliferation of human umbilical vein smooth muscle cells and a rat vascular smooth muscle cell line, A7r5. *Circulation* 2003;108:3048–53.

27. Aydemir-Koksoy A, Abramowitz J, Allen JC. Ouabain-induced signaling and vascular smooth muscle cell proliferation. *J Biol Chem* 2001;276:46605–11.

28. Haas M, Askari A, Xie Z. Involvement of Src and epidermal growth factor receptor in the signal-transducing function of Na+/K+-ATPase. *J Biol Chem* 2000;275:27832–37.

29. Kometiani P, Li J, Gnudi L, Kahn BB, et al. Multiple signal transduction pathways link Na+/K+-ATPase to growth-related genes in cardiac myocytes: The roles of Ras and mitogen-activated protein kinases. *J Biol Chem* 1998;273:15249–56.

30. Xie Z, Askari A. Na(+)/K(+)-ATPase as a signal transducer. *Eur J Biochem* 2002;269:2434–39.

31. Miyakawa-Naito A, Uhlen P, Lal M, et al. Cell signaling microdomain with Na,K-ATPase and inositol 1,4,5-trisphosphate receptor generates calcium oscillations. *J Biol Chem* 2003;278:50355–61.

32. Dmitrieva RI, Doris PA. Ouabain is a potent promoter of growth and activator of ERK1/2 in ouabain-resistant rat renal epithelial cells. *J Biol Chem* 2003;278:28160–66.

33. Liu J, Periyasamy SM, Gunning W, et al. Effects of cardiac glycosides on sodium pump expression and function in LLC-PK1 and MDCK cells. *Kidney Int* 2002;62:2118–25.

34. Lifton RP. Molecular genetics of human blood pressure variation. *Science* 1996;272:676-80.

35. Lifton RP, Gharavi AG, Geller DS. Molecular mechanisms of human hypertension. *Cell* 2001;104:545–56.

36. Luft FC. Twins in cardiovascular genetic research. *Hypertension* 2001;37:350–56.

37. Ward R. Familial aggregation and genetic epidemiology of blood pressure. In: Laragh JH, Brenner BM (eds.). *Hypertension: Pathophysiology, Diagnosis and Management, Second Edition.* New York: Raven Press, 1995.

38. Fava C, Burri P, Almgren P, et al. Heritability of ambulatory and office blood pressure phenotypes in Swedish families. *J Hypertens* 2004;22:1717–21.

39. Kotchen TA, Kotchen JM, Grim CE, et al. Genetic determinants of hypertension: identification of candidate phenotypes. *Hypertension* 2000;36:7–13.

40. Doris PA. Hypertension genetics, single nucleotide polymorphisms, and the common disease: Common variant hypothesis. *Hypertension* 2002;39:323–31.

41. Harrap SB. Where are all the blood-pressure genes? *Lancet* 2003;361:2149–51.

42. Luft FC. Geneticism of essential hypertension. *Hypertension* 2004;43:1155–59.

43. Moore JH. A global view of epistasis. *Nat Genet* 2005;37:13–14.

44. Moore JH. The ubiquitous nature of epistasis in determining susceptibility to common human diseases. *Hum Hered* 2003;56:73–82.

45. Okamoto K, Aoki K. Development of a strain of spontaneously hypertensive rats. *Jpn Circ J* 1963;27:282–93.

46. Rapp JP, Dene H. Development and characteristics of inbred strains of Dahl salt-sensitive and salt-resistant rats. *Hypertension* 1985;7:340–49.

47. Bianchi G, Baer PG, Fox U, et al. Changes in renin, water balance, and sodium balance during development of high blood pressure in genetically hypertensive rats. *Circ Res* 1975;36:153–61.

48. Ben-Ishay D, Kobrin I, Saliternick-Vardi R, et al. The Sabra hypertension prone (H) and hypertension resistant (N) rat strain. *Paroi Arterielle* 1980;6:157–59.

49. Simpson FO, Phelan EL, Clark DW, et al. Studies on the New Zealand strain of genetically hypertensive rats. *Clin Sci Mol Med Suppl* 1973;45(Suppl 1):15s–21.

50. Herrera VL, Ruiz-Opazo N. Alteration of alpha 1 Na+,K(+)-ATPase 86Rb+ influx by a single amino acid substitution. *Science* 1990;249:1023–26.

51. Rapp JP, Dene H. Failure of alleles at the Na+, K(+)-ATPase alpha 1 locus to cosegregate with blood pressure in Dahl rats. *J Hypertens* 1990;8:457–62.

52. Zicha J, Negrin CD, Dobesova Z, et al. Altered Na+-K+ pump activity and plasma lipids in salt-hypertensive Dahl rats: relationship to Atp1a1 gene. *Physiol Genomics* 2001;6:99–104.

53. Herrera VL, Xie HX, Lopez LV, et al. The alpha1 Na,K-ATPase gene is a susceptibility hypertension gene in the Dahl salt-sensitiveHSD rat. *J Clin Invest* 1998;102:1102–11.

54. Simonet L, St Lezin E, Kurtz TW. Sequence analysis of the alpha 1 Na+,K(+)-ATPase gene in the Dahl salt-sensitive rat. *Hypertension* 1991;18:689–93.

55. Barnard R, Kelly G, Manzetti SO, Harris EL. Neither the New Zealand genetically hypertensive strain nor Dahl salt-sensitive strain has an A1079T transversion in the alpha1 isoform of the Na(+),K(+)-ATPase gene. *Hypertension* 2001;38:786–92.

56. Kaneko Y, Cloix JF, Herrera VL, Ruiz-Opazo N. Corroboration of Dahl S Q276L alpha1Na,K-ATPase protein sequence: impact on affinities for ligands and on E1 conformation. *J Hypertens* 2005;23:745–52.

57. Ruiz-Opazo N, Barany F, Hirayama K, Herrera VL. Confirmation of mutant alpha 1 Na,K-ATPase gene and transcript in Dahl salt-sensitive/JR rats. *Hypertension* 1994;24:260–70.

58. Jeffs B, Negrin CD, Graham D, et al. Applicability of a "speed" congenic strategy to dissect blood pressure quantitative trait loci on rat chromosome 2. *Hypertension* 2000;35:179–87.

59. Kloting I, Kovacs P, van den Brandt J. Quantitative trait loci for body weight, blood pressure, blood glucose, and serum lipids: Linkage analysis with wild rats (Rattus norvegicus). *Biochem Biophys Res Commun* 2001;284:1126–33.

60. Samani NJ, Gauguier D, Vincent M, et al. Analysis of quantitative trait loci for blood pressure on rat chromosomes 2 and 13: Age-related differences in effect. *Hypertension* 1996;28:1118–22.

61. Arendshorst WJ, Beierwaltes WH. Renal and nephron hemodynamics in spontaneously hypertensive rats. *Am J Physiol* 1979;236:F246–51.

62. Kato S, Miyamoto M, Kato M, et al. Renal sodium metabolism in spontaneously hypertensive rats: Renal micropuncture study of the rate of 22Na recovery by the microinjection method. *J Hypertens* 1986;4(Suppl 3):S255–56.

63. Biollaz J, Waeber B, Diezi J, et al. Lithium infusion to study sodium handling in unanesthetized hypertensive rats. *Hypertension* 1986;8:117–21.

64. Roos JC, Kirchner KA, Abernethy JD, Langford HG. Differential effect of salt loading on sodium and lithium excretion in Dahl salt-resistant and -sensitive rats. *Hypertension* 1984;6:420–44.

65. Chibalin AV, Ogimoto G, Pedemonte CH, et al. Dopamine-induced endocytosis of Na+,K+-ATPase is initiated by phosphorylation of Ser-18 in the rat alpha subunit and is responsible for the decreased activity in epithelial cells. *J Biol Chem* 1999;274:1920–27.

66. Chibalin AV, Pedemonte CH, Katz AI, et al. Phosphorylation of the catalyic alpha-subunit constitutes a triggering signal for Na+,K+-ATPase endocytosis. *J Biol Chem* 1998;273:8814–19.

67. Chen C, Lokhandwala MF. Inhibition of Na+,K(+)-ATPase in rat renal proximal tubules by dopamine involved DA-1 receptor activation. *Naunyn Schmiedebergs Arch Pharmacol* 1993;347:289–95.

68. Zeng C, Sanada H, Watanabe H, et al. Functional genomics of the dopaminergic system in hypertension. *Physiol Genomics* 2004;19:233–46.

69. Jose PA, Eisner GM, Drago J, et al. Dopamine receptor signaling defects in spontaneous hypertension. *Am J Hypertens* 1996;9:400–05.

70. Hinojos CA, Doris PA. Altered subcellular distribution of Na+,K+-ATPase in proximal tubules in young spontaneously hypertensive rats. *Hypertension* 2004;44:95–100.

71. Bianchi G, Ferrari P, Cusi D, et al. Genetic aspects of ion transport systems in hypertension. *J Hypertens Suppl* 1990;8:S213–18.

72. Bianchi G, Ferrari P, Cusi D, et al. Cell membrane abnormalities and genetic hypertension. *J Clin Hypertens* 1986;2:114–19.

73. Salardi S, Modica R, Ferrandi M, et al. Characterization of erythrocyte adducin from the Milan hypertensive strain of rats. *J Hypertens Suppl* 1988;6:S196–98.

74. Tripodi G, Florio M, Ferrandi M, et al. Effect of Add1 gene transfer on blood pressure in reciprocal congenic strains of Milan rats. *Biochem Biophys Res Commun* 2004;324:562–68.

75. Beeks E, Kessels AG, Kroon AA, et al. Genetic predisposition to salt-sensitivity: A systematic review. *J Hypertens* 2004;22:1243–49.

76. Glorioso N, Filigheddu F, Cusi D, et al. Alpha-Adducin 460Trp allele is associated with erythrocyte Na transport rate in North Sardinian primary hypertensives. *Hypertension* 2002;39:357–62.

77. Grant FD, Romero JR, Jeunemaitre X, et al. Low-renin hypertension, altered sodium homeostasis, and an alpha-adducin polymorphism. *Hypertension* 2002;39:191–96.

78. Manunta P, Burnier M, D'Amico M, et al. Adducin polymorphism affects renal proximal tubule reabsorption in hypertension. *Hypertension* 1999;33:694–97.

79. Ferrandi M, Manunta P, Balzan S, et al. Ouabain-like factor quantification in mammalian tissues and plasma: Comparison of two independent assays. *Hypertension* 1997;30:886–96.

80. Ferrandi M, Barassi P, Minotti E, et al. PST 2238: A new antihypertensive compound that modulates renal Na-K pump function without diuretic activity in Milan hypertensive rats. *J Cardiovasc Pharmacol* 2002;40:881–89.

81. Ferrari P, Ferrandi M, Torielli L, et al. Antihypertensive compounds that modulate the Na-K pump. *Ann NY Acad Sci* 2003;986:694–701.

82. Efendiev R, Krmar RT, Ogimoto G, et al. Hypertension-linked mutation in the adducin alpha-subunit leads to higher AP2-mu2 phosphorylation and impaired Na+,K+-ATPase trafficking in response to GPCR signals and intracellular sodium. *Circ Res* 2004;95:1100–08.

83. Ferrandi M, Molinari I, Barassi P, et al. Organ hypertrophic signaling within caveolae membrane subdomains triggered by ouabain and antagonized by PST 2238. *J Biol Chem* 2004;279:33306–14.

Chapter 21

Platelet and Coagulation Abnormalities

George I. Varughese and Gregory Y. H. Lip

Key Findings

- Hypertension is associated with the flow of blood under high pressures, yet the complications of hypertension, such as myocardial infarction or stroke are paradoxically thrombotic rather than hemorrhagic.

- Increasing evidence suggests that hypertension fulfills the prerequisites of the Virchow triad for thrombogenesis, leading to a prothrombotic or hypercoagulable state.

- Hypertension leads to changes in platelets, endothelium, and coagulation and fibrinolytic pathways that help to promote the induction and the maintenance of this prothrombotic state.

- Study of the prothrombotic state in hypertension is of paramount importance, as understanding the pathophysiologic processes underlying it can help prevent many of the thrombosis-related complications associated with hypertension.

Clinical Implications

- The prothrombotic state in hypertension can to a certain extent be reversed by the treatment of hypertension, although different antihypertensive agents may have variable effects in reversing these changes.

- Some of the effects are related to blood pressure normalization, but drugs such as those acting on the renin-angiotensin-aldosterone system appear to have an effect over and above this.

- Antiplatelet agents have been shown to confer a degree of benefit to high-risk hypertensive patients, as long as their blood pressure is well controlled.

Hypertension is a well-recognized risk factor for coronary artery disease, atherosclerosis, and cerebrovascular disease. In hypertension, the arterial walls are exposed to the flow of blood under high pressures; nonetheless the common complications of hypertension (such as myocardial infarction or stroke) are ironically thrombotic rather than hemorrhagic—the so-called "thrombotic paradox of hypertension."[1] Hypertension fulfills the basic rudiments of the Virchow's triad—that is, abnormalities in the vessel wall, bloodstream, and blood constituents—described more than 150 years ago, thus enhancing thrombogenesis.[2] In the 21st century, we recognize "abnormalities of the vessel wall" to comprise endothelial damage or dysfunction, while "abnormalities in the blood constituents" include abnormalities in hemostatic and fibrinoloytic factors, as well as platelet activation, and "flow abnormalities" as abnormal shear stress and impaired flow reserve. While Virchow originally referred to venous thrombosis, the basic concepts of the triad can be applied to arterial thrombosis in hypertension. These have also had considerable clinical importance due to the prospect for reversing some of the underlying pathologic mechanisms by effective treatments.

PLATELET ABNORMALITIES AND CHANGES IN HYPERTENSION

Platelets in patients who have hypertension differ from those of normotensive subjects in their size, shape, volume, and life span, and they also demonstrate an increased tendency to aggregate.[3-5] Abnormal platelet aggregation as well as increased plasma markers of platelet activation are present in the setting of hypertension.[6-9] Biochemical indices released from platelets in those with hypertension such as beta-thromboglobulin[10,11] and soluble P-selectin[12,13] also show evidence of increased platelet activation, as reflected by abnormalities in their levels.[14-16] In addition, there is evidence of raised intraplatelet calcium levels[17-19] in the setting of hypertension.

The increased shear stress contributes to platelet activation in hypertension, leading to an increased release of platelet microparticles.[20] Platelet microparticles are a relatively novel discovery[21] and high levels of platelet microparticles are seen in patients with severe hypertension compared to normotensive individuals.[22] These microparticles may add to a prothrombotic state by promoting thrombin generation and platelet adhesion to the vessel wall. Indeed, they contain glycoproteins IIb and IIIa, as well as P-selectin and thrombospondin, leading to binding to the subendothelial matrix causing even greater platelet activation and binding, thus causing a vicious cycle of a greater propensity to thrombosis.

Neuroendocrine factors, such as alterations in angiotensin II and catecholamine levels can also affect the platelets in patients with hypertension, which are more sensitive to increased levels of catecholamines[23] that in turn are potential stimulators for platelet activation and aggregation (Box 21–1). Other subtle factors, such as the increased expression of adrenoceptors[24] and increased viscosity of the blood in hypertensive patients, enhance platelet activation.[25]

Finally, many commonly coexistent conditions with hypertension, such as diabetes,[26] atrial fibrillation, and congestive heart failure, are also well recognized to activate platelets.[27,28]

ABNORMALITIES OF ENDOTHELIUM IN HYPERTENSION AND IMPLICATIONS IN PLATELETS

The endothelium, which forms the margin between the blood and the vessel wall, is also exposed to increased pressure forces in patients with high blood pressure. This can cause a variety of insults to the endothelium resulting in endothelial damage and dysfunction, which eventually leads to platelet aggregation (Box 21–2). The endothelium plays a crucial role in cardiovascular pathophysiology, being the preliminary target for initiating the prothrombotic disease process.[29,30] The integrity of the endothelium is important in order to prevent atherothrombotic disease,[31] as it has many pro- and anti-coagulant properties.[32] Hence endothelial perturbation in hypertension can culminate in even more definitive vascular damage and atherosclerosis.

Nitric oxide (NO), which is mainly derived from the endothelium, plays a significant part in controlling vascular tone and it has been proposed that a reduction in endogenous NO is associated with impaired vasodilatation and a rise in peripheral vascular resistance in hypertension. Studies have shown that resting NO activity is reduced in people with high blood pressure.[33] This fact is further substantiated by reports suggesting that the excretion of the metabolic end product of NO is decreased in the urine

of patients with high blood pressure in comparison to the normotensive population.[34]

Endothelium-dependent vasodilatation in response to acetylcholine (which is NO mediated) has been noted to be impaired both in the forearm circulation[35-38] and coronary vascular bed[39] in patients with hypertension.

The role of superoxide anion (O_2^-) and its involvement in oxidative stress has also been related to various cardiovascular diseases as well as hypertension.[40] The availability of superoxide anion (O_2^-) influences the synthesis of NO, and hence can alter endothelial function.[41] Consequently, a decrease in NO leads to impaired vasodilatation and a subsequent increase in peripheral vascular resistance, contributing further to hypertension,[42,43] again setting up a vicious cycle (Figure 21–1, *A*).

Vascular endothelial growth factor (VEGF) is recognized to act on the endothelium (Figure 21–1, *B*) to induce differentiation and proliferation and therefore angiogenesis due to paracrine or autocrine effects.[44] VEGF may also induce a procoagulant state in the endothelium.[45-47] Platelets carry VEGF,[48] and once thrombus formation occurs, a dysfunctional endothelium will have impaired antiplatelet activity.[31] VEGF is higher in the setting of hypertension[49,50] could also have other implications, such as the development of collaterals. Paradoxically, the high levels

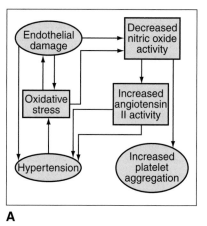

A

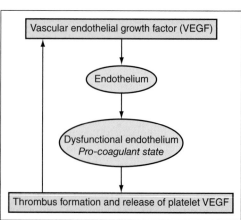

B

Figure 21–1. A, Hypertension, endothelial damage, and platelet dysfunction. **B,** Effects of vascular endothelial growth factor on the endothelium and platelets.

of VEGF seen in hypertension may also be the result of release from platelets when they form thrombi.[51]

ABNORMALITIES OF FIBRINOLYSIS AND COAGULATION IN HYPERTENSION

The whole process of thrombogenesis is due to a fine equilibrium between the coagulation and fibrinolytic pathways, and many of the blood constituents associated with hypertension and its complications are components of these pathways.

For example, the fibrinolytic system is crucial in averting intravascular thrombosis (Figure 21–2), and the final outcome of the fibrinolytic activity depends on the equilibrium between plasminogen activators, such as tissue-type plasminogen activator (t-PA) and plasminogen activator inhibitors (PAI). These components are synthesized in the endothelial and smooth muscle cells of the vascular wall.

The progression of events in fibrinolysis involves the activation of plasminogen to plasmin. Plasmin then helps in the lysis of fibrin and also enhances the activation of certain anti-inflammatory cytokines, such as transforming growth factor-beta (TGF-β). The latter also inhibits the migration and proliferation of smooth muscle cells. This inhibition is important, as it is a vital phase in the formation of atherosclerotic lesions.

The abnormalities in coagulation and fibrinolytic pathways associated with hypertension may lead to an increased risk of thrombotic events due to the enhanced coagulability and impaired fibrinolysis.[52–56] Certainly there is an obvious association between rising blood pressure and impaired fibrinolysis in hypertensive patients without established cardiovascular disease, or known risk factors for cardiovascular disease, even after correcting other variables like age, gender, and body mass index.[57] Similarly, high fibrin D-dimer levels (a degradation product of fibrin) have been reported in patients with hypertension,[58] and are an index of ongoing intravascular fibrin formation and thrombogenesis. Such fibrin degradation products may be of prognostic value in determining arterial thrombotic events.[59]Hypertension can lead to atrial fibrillation, which in itself can cause a prothrombotic state.[60–63] The duration of atrial fibrillation is not relevant, and even in patients with new onset nonrheumatic atrial fibrillation (nonsustained and <48 hours duration), there are increased concentrations of soluble thrombomodulin and von Willebrand factor (vWf) (as indices of endothelial damage or dysfunction) and fibrin D-dimer (an index of thrombogenesis); the latter persist up to 30 days after cardioversion.[60] Hemostatic markers for platelet activity, such as platelet factor-4 and beta-thromboglobulin (TG), have also been shown to be raised in patients with nonvalvular atrial fibrillation.[61] The raised plasma levels of vWf in this condition are even predictive of vascular events and stroke.[62]

Congestive heart failure (CHF) carries a poor prognosis with a high mortality rate, frequent hospitalizations, and an increased risk of thrombotic complications, such as stroke. Cytokines may contribute to the progression and prothrombotic state of CHF, including the proinflammatory interleukin-6 (IL-6). The procoagulant properties of these cytokines may be mediated via tissue factor (TF), a potent clotting activator. Indeed, IL-6 and TF are predictors of poor prognosis in chronic CHF.[64] Abnormal levels of soluble P-selectin, vWF, and hemorheological indices may also contribute to a hypercoagulable state in CHF,[65] especially in female patients and in those with the more severe New York Heart Association class.[66] Treatment with angiotensin-converting enzyme inhibitors improves the prothrombotic state in these patients.

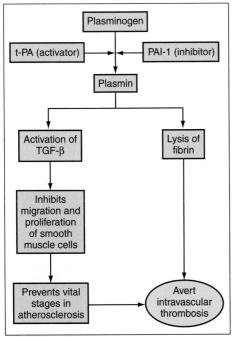

Figure 21–2. Role of the fibrinolytic system in averting thrombosis.

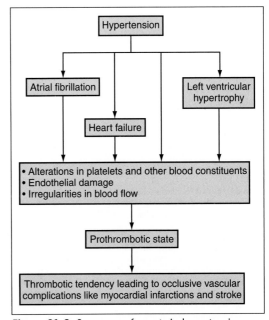

Figure 21–3. Sequence of events in hypertensive cardiovascular disease leading to the prothrombotic state.

Patients with left ventricular (LV) hypertrophy are at high risk for complications associated with hypertension.[58] Unsurprisingly, hypertensive patients with LV hypertrophy (defined as a LV mass index >134 g/m^2 in men or >110 g/m^2 in women) had higher plasma fibrinogen compared with those without LV hypertrophy. The high plasma fibrinogen levels were related to blood pressures, LV mass index (and LV hypertrophy), and left atrial size.[58]

A flow diagram illustrating an overview of the mechanisms in the pathogenesis of the prothrombotic state in patients with hypertension and hypertensive cardiovascular diseases is shown in Figure 21–3.

CONCLUSIONS

Abnormalities in hemorheologic factors and abnormal thrombogenesis and endothelial damage/dysfunction may act synergistically to increase the risk of thrombogenesis and atherosclerosis in hypertensive patients. Thus hypertension leads to abnormalities in platelets, coagulation, and fibrinolysis that eventually lead to a prothrombotic state, causing deaths related to cardiovascular disease and stroke.[67] Many of these abnormalities can be related to hypertensive target organ damage, and effectively reversed by antihypertensive treatment.[68]

REFERENCES

1. Lip GYH. Hypertension, platelets, and the endothelium: the "thrombotic paradox" of hypertension (or "Birmingham paradox") revisited. *Hypertension* 2003;41:199–200.
2. Virchow R. Phlogose und thrombose in gerasystem. In: Virchow R, ed. *Gesammelte Abhandlungen zur Wissenchaftichen Medicin.* Frankfurt: Von Meidinger Sohn, 1856:458–636.
3. Gleerup G, Winther K. Decreased fibrinolytic activity and increased platelet function in hypertension. Possible influence of calcium antagonism. *Am J Hypertens* 1991;4(2 Pt 2):168S–71S.
4. Stott DJ, Saniabadi AR, Inglis GC, et al. Serotonin and platelet aggregation in patients with essential hypertension compared with a normotensive control group. *Drugs* 1988;36(Suppl 1):78–82.
5. Tofler GH, Brezinski D, Schafer AI, et al. Concurrent morning increase in platelet aggregability and the risk of myocardial infarction and sudden cardiac death. *N Engl J Med* 1987;316(24):1514–8.
6. Felmeden DC, Spencer CG, Chung NA, et al. Relation of thrombogenesis in systemic hypertension to angiogenesis and endothelial damage/dysfunction (a substudy of the Anglo-Scandinavian Cardiac Outcomes Trial [ASCOT]). *Am J Cardiol* 2003;92(4):400–5.
7. Minuz P, Patrignani P, Gaino S, et al. Determinants of platelet activation in human essential hypertension. *Hypertension* 2004;43(1):64–70.
8. Preston RA, Jy W, Jimenez JJ, et al. Effects of severe hypertension on endothelial and platelet microparticles. *Hypertension* 2003;41(2):211–7.
9. Taddei S, Virdis A, Ghiadoni L, et al. Endothelial dysfunction in hypertension. *J Cardiovasc Pharmacol* 2001;38(Suppl 2):S11–4.
10. Blann AD, Lip GYH, Islim IF, Beevers DG. Evidence of platelet activation in hypertension. *J Hum Hypertens* 1997;11:607–9.
11. Kjeldsen SE, Gjesdal K, Eide I, et al. Increased beta-thromboglobulin in essential hypertension: interactions between arterial plasma adrenaline, platelet function and blood lipids. *Acta Med Scand* 1983;213(5):369–73.
12. Goto S, Tamura N, Eto K, et al. Functional significance of adenosine 5′-diphosphate receptor (P2Y(12)) in platelet activation initiated by binding of von Willebrand factor to platelet GP

Ib alpha induced by conditions of high shear rate. *Circulation* 2002;105:2531–6.
13. Spencer CG, Gurney D, Blann AD, et al. Von Willebrand factor, soluble P-selectin, and target organ damage in hypertension: a substudy of the Anglo-Scandinavian Cardiac Outcomes Trial (ASCOT). *Hypertension* 2002;40:61–6.
14. Gupta S, Gupta VK, Dhamija RK, Kela AK. Platelet aggregation patterns in normotensive and hypertensive subjects. *Indian J Physiol Pharmacol* 2002;46(3):379–82.
15. Fornitz GG. Platelet function and fibrinolytic activity in borderline and mild hypertension. The influence of age, exercise, smoking and antihypertensive therapy. *Dan Med Bull* 2002;49(3):210–26.
16. Lemne C, Vesterqvist O, Egberg N, et al. Platelet activation and prostacyclin release in essential hypertension. *Prostaglandins* 1992;44(3):219–35.
17. Quan Sang KH, Devynck MA. Increased platelet cytosolic free calcium concentration in essential hypertension. *J Hypertens* 1986;4:567–74.
18. Erne P, Burgisser E, Bolli P, et al. Free calcium concentration in platelets closely relates to blood pressure in normal and essentially hypertensive subjects. *Hypertension* 1984;6(2 Pt 2):I166–9.
19. Le Quan Sang KH, Benlian P, Kanawati C, et al. Platelet cytosolic free calcium concentration in primary hypertension. *J Hypertens* Suppl 1985;3(Suppl 3):S33–6.
20. Nomura S, Imamura A, Okuno M, et al. Platelet-derived microparticles in patients with arteriosclerosis obliterans: enhancement of high shear-induced microparticle generation by cytokines. *Thromb Res* 2000;98:257–68.
21. Nomura S. Function and clinical significance of platelet-derived microparticles. *Int J Hematol* 2001;74(4):397–404.
22. Preston RA, Jy W, Jimenez JJ, et al. Effects of severe hypertension on endothelial and platelet microparticles. *Hypertension* 2003;41:211–7.
23. Vlachakis ND, Aledort L. Platelet aggregation in relationship to plasma catecholamines in patients with hypertension. *Atherosclerosis* 1979;32(4):451–60.
24. Varani K, Gessi S, Caiazza A, et al. Platelet alpha2-adrenoceptor alterations in patients with essential hypertension. *Br J Clin Pharmacol* 1999;47(2):167–72.

25. Letcher RL, Chien S, Pickering TG, et al. Direct relationship between blood pressure and blood viscosity in normal and hypertensive subjects. Role of fibrinogen and concentration. *Am J Med* 1981;70:1195–202.
26. Hippisley-Cox J, Pringle M. Prevalence, care, and outcomes for patients with diet-controlled diabetes in general practice: cross sectional survey. *Lancet* 2004;364(9432):423–8.
27. Kamath S, Blann AD, Lip GY. Platelets and atrial fibrillation. *Eur Heart J* 2001;22(24):2233–42.
28. Vinik AI, Erbas T, Park TS, et al. Platelet dysfunction in type 2 diabetes. *Diabetes Care* 2001;24(8):1476–85.
29. Ross R. Atherosclerosis is an inflammatory disease. *Am Heart J* 1999;138(5 Pt 2):S419–20.
30. Mutin M, Canavy I, Blann A, et al. Direct evidence of endothelial injury in acute myocardial infarction and unstable angina by demonstration of circulating endothelial cells. *Blood* 1999;93(9):2951–8.
31. Blann AD. Endothelial cell activation, injury, damage and dysfunction: separate entities or mutual terms? *Blood Coagul Fibrinolysis* 2000;11(7):623–30.
32. Cines DB, Pollak ES, Buck CA, et al. Endothelial cells in physiology and in the pathophysiology of vascular disorders. *Blood* 1998;91(10):3527–61.
33. Forte P, Copland M, Smith LM, et al. Basal nitric oxide synthesis in essential hypertension. *Lancet* 1997;349(9055):837–42.
34. Palmer RM, Ashton DS, Moncada S. Vascular endothelial cells synthesize nitric oxide from L-arginine. *Nature* 1988;333(6174):664–6.
35. Panza JA, Casino PR, Kilcoyne CM, Quyyumi AA. Role of endothelium-derived nitric oxide in the abnormal endothelium-dependent vascular relaxation of patients with essential hypertension. *Circulation* 1993;87(5):1468–74.
36. Panza JA, Quyyumi AA, Brush JE Jr, Epstein SE. Abnormal endothelium-dependent vascular relaxation in patients with essential hypertension. *N Engl J Med* 1990;323(1):22–7.
37. Hirooka Y, Imaizumi T, Harada S, et al. Endothelium-dependent forearm vasodilation to acetylcholine but not to substance P is impaired in patients with heart failure. *J Cardiovasc Pharmacol* 1992;20(Suppl 12):S221–5.

38. Linder L, Kiowski W, Buhler FR, Luscher TF. Indirect evidence for release of endothelium-derived relaxing factor in human forearm circulation in vivo. Blunted response in essential hypertension. *Circulation* 1990;81(6):1762–7.

39. Egashira K, Suzuki S, Hirooka Y, et al. Impaired endothelium-dependent vasodilation of large epicardial and resistance coronary arteries in patients with essential hypertension. Different responses to acetylcholine and substance P. *Hypertension* 1995;25(2):201–6.

40. Hamilton CA, Brosnan MJ, McIntyre M, et al. Superoxide excess in hypertension and ageing: a common cause of endothelial dysfunction. *Hypertension* 2001, 37:529–34.

41. Moncada S, Higgs A. The L-arginine-nitric oxide pathway. *New Eng J Med* 1993;329:2002–12.

42. Chowdhary S, Townend JN. Nitric oxide and hypertension: not just an endothelium derived relaxing factor! *J Hum Hypertens* 2001;15:219–27.

43. Vallance P, Collier J. Biology and clinical relevance of nitric oxide. *BMJ* 1994;309(6952):453–7.

44. Dvorak HF, Brown LF, Detmar M, Dvorak AM. Vascular permeability factor/vascular endothelial growth factor, microvascular hyperpermeability, and angiogenesis. *Am J Pathol* 1995;146(5):1029–39.

45. Mechtcheriakova D, Wlachos A, Holzmuller H, et al. Vascular endothelial cell growth factor-induced tissue factor expression in endothelial cells is mediated by EGR-1. *Blood* 1999;93(11):3811–23.

46. Camera M, Giesen PL, Fallon J, et al. Cooperation between VEGF and TNF-alpha is necessary for exposure of active tissue factor on the surface of human endothelial cells. *Arterioscler Thromb Vasc Biol* 1999;19(3):531–7.

47. Huang YQ, Li JJ, Hu L, et al. Thrombin induces increased expression and secretion of VEGF from human FS4 fibroblasts, DU145 prostate cells and CHRF megakaryocytes. *Thromb Haemost* 2001;86(4):1094–8.

48. Banks RE, Forbes MA, Kinsey SE, et al. Release of the angiogenic cytokine vascular endothelial growth factor (VEGF) from platelets: significance for VEGF measurements and cancer biology. *Br J Cancer* 1998;77(6):956–64.

49. Blann AD, Belgore FM, McCollum CN, et al. Vascular endothelial growth factor and its receptor, Flt-1, in the plasma of patients with coronary or peripheral atherosclerosis, or type II diabetes. *Clin Sci (Lond)* 2002;102(2):187–94.

50. Belgore FM, Blann AD, Li-Saw-Hee FL, et al. Plasma levels of vascular endothelial growth factor and its soluble receptor (SFlt-1) in essential hypertension. *Am J Cardiol* 2001;87(6):805–7, A9.

51. Banks RE, Forbes MA, Kinsey SE, et al. Release of the angiogenic cytokine vascular endothelial growth factor (VEGF) from platelets: significance for VEGF measurements and cancer biology. *Br J Cancer* 1998;77(6):956–64.

52. Tomiyama H, Kimura Y, Mitsuhashi H, et al. Relationship between endothelial function and fibrinolysis in early hypertension. *Hypertension* 1998;31 (1 Pt 2):321–7.

53. Makris TK, Stavroulakis GA, Krespi PG, et al. Fibrinolytic/hemostatic variables in arterial hypertension: response to treatment with irbesartan or atenolol. *Am J Hypertens* 2000;13:783–8.

54. Aigbe A, Famodu AA. Haemorheological and fibrinolytic activity in hypertensive Nigerians. *Clin Hemorheol Microcirc* 1999;21:415–20.

55. Eliasson M, Jansson J, Nilsson P, Asplund K. Enhanced levels of t-PA Ag in essential hypertension. A popular based study in Sweden. *J Hypertens* 1997;15:349–56.

56. Wall U, Jem C, Bergbrant A, Jem S. Enhanced levels of tPA-Ag in borderline hypertension. *Hypertension* 1995;26:796–800.

57. Poli KA, Tofler GH, Larson MG, et al. Association of blood pressure with fibrinolytic potential in the Framingham offspring population. *Circulation* 2000;101:264–9.

58. Lip GY, Blann AD, Jones AF, et al. Relationship of endothelium, thrombogenesis, and hemorheology in systemic hypertension to ethnicity and left ventricular hypertrophy. *Am J Cardiol* 1997;80:1566–71.

59. Fowkes FG, Lowe GD, Housley E, et al. Cross linked fibrin degradation products, progression of peripheral arterial disease, and risk of coronary heart disease. *Lancet* 1993;342:84–6.

60. Marin F, Roldan V, Climent VE, et al. Plasma von Willebrand factor, soluble thrombomodulin, and fibrin D-dimer concentrations in acute onset non-rheumatic atrial fibrillation. *Heart* 2004;90(10):1162–6.

61. Inoue H, Nozawa T, Okumura K, et al. Prothrombotic activity is increased in patients with nonvalvular atrial fibrillation and risk factors for embolism. *Chest* 2004;126(3):687–92.

62. Conway DS, Pearce LA, Chin BS. Prognostic value of plasma von Willebrand factor and soluble P-selectin as indices of endothelial damage and platelet activation in 994 patients with nonvalvular atrial fibrillation. *Circulation* 2003;107(25):3141–5.

63. Chung NA, Belgore F, Li-Saw-Hee FL, et al. Is the hypercoagulable state in atrial fibrillation mediated by vascular endothelial growth factor? *Stroke* 2002;33(9):2187–91.

64. Chin BS, Blann AD, Gibbs CR, et al. Prognostic value of interleukin-6, plasma viscosity, fibrinogen, von Willebrand factor, tissue factor and vascular endothelial growth factor levels in congestive heart failure. *Eur J Clin Invest* 2003;33(11):941–8.

65. Lip GY, Pearce LA, Chin BS, et al. Effects of congestive heart failure on plasma von Willebrand factor and soluble P-selectin concentrations in patients with non-valvar atrial fibrillation. *Heart* 2005;91(6):759–63.

66. Gibbs CR, Blann AD, Watson RD, Lip GY. Abnormalities of hemorheological, endothelial, and platelet function in patients with chronic heart failure in sinus rhythm: effects of angiotensin-converting enzyme inhibitor and beta-blocker therapy. *Circulation* 2001;103(13):1746–51.

67. He FJ, MacGregor GA. Cost of poor blood pressure control in the UK: 62,000 unnecessary deaths per year. *J Hum Hypertens* 2003;17(7):455–7.

68. Nadar S, Lip GY. The prothrombotic state in hypertension and the effects of antihypertensive treatment. *Curr Pharm Des* 2003;9(21):1715–32.

Chapter

22 Role of Cytokines and Inflammation in Hypertension

Michael J. Ryan

Key Findings

- Numerous studies suggest an association between increased serum cytokines and essential hypertension, although a causal relationship has yet to be definitively determined.

- Cytokines have pleiotropic effects to mediate immune responses. The physiologic actions of cytokines are dependent on intracellular pathways activated by cell surface receptors.

- Inflammatory cytokines may regulate neurohumoral pathways like the renin-angiotensin or endothelin system, and alter vascular, heart, and renal function to promote hypertension.

- Cytokines are thought to play an integral role in the progression of certain forms of hypertension including preeclampsia, pulmonary hypertension, and autoimmune and metabolic disorders.

- Single nucleotide polymorphisms that occur in cytokine gene sequences may be genetically associated with hypertension.

- Inflammation and cytokines may become important therapeutic targets as more is understood about their role in the progression of hypertension.

Inflammation is a complex physiologic response to tissue injury that is mediated by numerous cell types and peptides called cytokines. A typical inflammatory response involves increased blood flow and vascular permeability along with recruitment of macrophages and monocytes to an injured area. Recently, the notion that inflammation may be important in the development of cardiovascular disease has been bolstered by evidence that atherosclerosis, once thought to be a lipid storage disease, requires cytokines, adhesion molecules, and immune cells (reviewed in Libby, Ridker, and Maseri[1]). Cytokines have also been suggested to play an important role in the progression of heart disease, stroke, aneurysm, renal disease, and hypertension.

Historically, investigators attempting to understand the pathogenesis of hypertension have focused on renal, vascular, cardiac, neurohumoral, genetic, and environmental factors. However, like atherosclerosis, investigators have observed a relationship between inflammatory cytokines and blood pressure suggesting that hypertension may be a chronic inflammatory condition. As a result, attention has turned toward understanding the role that these inflammatory cytokines play in the development of hypertension. While growing evidence suggests an association between hypertension and several markers of inflammation, the mechanisms by which chronic increases in pro-inflammatory cytokines promote hypertension are just now being examined. Thus this is an important and emerging area of research interest. The focus of this chapter will be to examine what is currently known about the relationship between inflammatory cytokines and hypertension. Particular attention will be given to this relationship in humans and animal models of hypertension, as well as neurohumoral and organ systems that are affected by cytokines.

CYTOKINES

Cytokines comprise a group of proteins that are secreted by cells of the innate and adaptive immune system, but can be produced and released by virtually any cell type. The physiologic actions of these proteins are the result of a balance between pro-inflammatory and anti-inflammatory cytokines that are released when the immune system is challenged with either a foreign microbe or some other antigen.

There are three main classes of cytokines based on their functional properties. These include cytokines involved in the innate immune response, the adaptive immune response, and those that promote leukocyte maturation. The biological actions of cytokines are diverse, but most often promote increased cell adhesion molecule expression (endothelial activation), increased production and release of cytokines from endothelial and immune cells, recruitment of lymphocytes and monocytes, and generation of reactive oxygen species important for the oxidative burst to destroy foreign antigens. During severe inflammatory reactions, similar to what is observed during sepsis, cytokines mediate increased body temperature (fever), reduced food intake, and impaired vascular smooth muscle and heart contractility. The latter actions promote reduced blood pressure and shock. Indeed, a great deal is understood about the effect of large increases in inflammatory cytokines on vascular function and blood pressure. In contrast, despite recent evidence suggesting that hypertension may be a mild chronic inflammatory condition, there has been relatively little attention paid to the effects of chronic moderate increases in cytokines and how they regulate blood pressure.

At the cell level, cytokines bind to plasma membrane receptors of which there are several types mediating multiple and complex signaling pathways. These pathways have been extensively reviewed by others.[2–6] Tumor necrosis factor alpha (TNF-α) and interleukin-1 (IL-1) have similar pro-inflammatory signaling pathways. The intracellular domain of the receptor activates MAP-kinase signaling pathways (p38MAPK, JNK) and leads to phosphorylation of Jun and an increase in the AP1 transcription factor. Activation of these receptors also leads to inhibition of IκB (by phosphorylating it), thus allowing NFκB to regulate gene expression. This is considered the inflammatory signaling pathway. Alternatively, these cytokines can activate an apoptotic pathway, although it is not yet clear how activation of this pathway is chosen over the inflammatory path. Other cytokines, including interleukins 4, 6, 10, and 12, and interferon gamma (IFNγ) typically activate the JAK/STAT signaling cascade. After receptor binding, STAT proteins are recruited to the cytoplasmic domain of the receptor containing a Janus kinase (JAK). JAK phosphorylates the inactive STAT proteins, allowing them to form a homodimer and translocate to the nucleus where they can regulate gene transcription. Activation of these pathways has been implicated in the regulation of blood pressure, and therefore may be important clinical targets for the treatment of hypertension.

CYTOKINES AND ESSENTIAL HYPERTENSION

Evidence that chronic inflammation may be important in the progression of hypertension stems from data showing that cytokines are increased in the serum of individuals with essential hypertension. While there are numerous cytokines, this chapter will focus primarily on TNF-α, interleukin-6 (IL-6), and C-reactive protein (CRP), which have been implicated in the development of hypertension.

Tumor necrosis factor alpha

TNF-α is the principal cytokine that mediates inflammatory responses, and typically acts in a paracrine or autocrine fashion. When produced in high amounts, TNF-α can be detected in the circulation. It is primarily produced by phagocytes, T cells, natural killer cells, and mast cells, but can also be released from other cell types including endothelial cells. Newly generated TNF-α is formed as a 27-kD membrane-bound protein that is cleaved by metalloproteinases to form a 17-kD protein. These form a homotrimer that can bind to cell surface receptors (TNFR1 and TNFR2) located on virtually every cell type in the body. Binding to its receptor leads to downstream activation of NFκB to regulate the expression of numerous genes and also promotes cleavage of the receptors to generate soluble TNF-α receptors (sTNFR1, sTNFR2). These have been used as a serum marker for increased TNF activity and inflammation.

In humans there is growing evidence that TNF-α is elevated in individuals with essential hypertension. For example, TNF-α appears to be an independent risk factor for predicting hypertension in adults, even after adjusting for body mass index, age, and family history of previous cardiovascular disease.[7] The relationship between TNF-α and blood pressure is also evident in apparently healthy individuals.[8] The authors of these studies suggested that hypertension may be promoting inflammation; however, whether cytokines are a causal factor in the progression of hypertension has not been determined. There is some evidence to suggest that TNF-α could promote hypertension through activating the potent vasoconstrictor endothelin-1 (ET-1).[9]

Further understanding of how TNF-α can promote hypertension will most certainly be aided through studies of experimentally induced hypertension in animal models. Similar to humans, a relationship between blood pressure and serum levels of TNF-α has been reported in rats with hypertension induced by DOCA salt, nitric oxide synthase inhibition, or the two-kidney-one-clip model.[10] These animals, in addition to hypertension, have increased blood pressure variability and decreased baroreceptor sensitivity, which suggests a role for cytokines in mediating central regulation of blood pressure.

There is also evidence at the cellular level consistent with a role for TNF-α in promoting hypertension. For example, treatment of human umbilical vein endothelial cells (HUVEC) with either TNF-α or lipopolysaccharide (LPS, endotoxin) induces endothelial expression of cell-adhesion molecules, a response that is inhibited by a p38 MAP-kinase antagonist. Importantly, pharmacologic inhibition of p38 MAP kinase in stroke-prone spontaneously hypertensive rats prevented hypertension and improved renal function in this model.[11,12] These data implicate TNF-α signaling pathways as potentially important for the progression of hypertension.

Interleukin-6

IL-6 is one of the few inflammatory cytokines that acts in an endocrine fashion. Its primary function is to recruit neutrophils to inflamed tissue and stimulate antibody release from B lymphocytes. IL-6 also promotes the release of acute-phase reactants such as CRP from the liver, which will be discussed in greater detail below. In humans, several lines of evidence suggest that IL-6 is associated with, and often predictive of, the development of hypertension. Numerous studies report that elevated serum IL-6 levels are observed in individuals with hypertension independent of other cardiovascular risk factors.[7,10,13] Like TNF-α, these studies largely promote the notion that inflammation is caused by hypertension; however, plasma levels of IL-6 can be used to predict the development of hypertension. As an example, enhanced IL-6 response to stress in normotensive individuals predicted the development of hypertension at a 3-year follow-up visit.[14]

Recently, the role for IL-6 in the progression of hypertension has become clearer through experimentation in animal models. It has been recently shown that angiotensin-mediated hypertension (Figure 22–1) and psychosocial stress–induced hypertension (placing a male mouse into a cage formerly occupied by another male mouse) are attenuated in IL-6 knockout mice.[15,16] These data and those from human studies support an important pathophysiologic role for IL-6 in the development of hypertension. The cellular mechanisms by which IL-6 can promote hypertension have not yet been clearly defined,

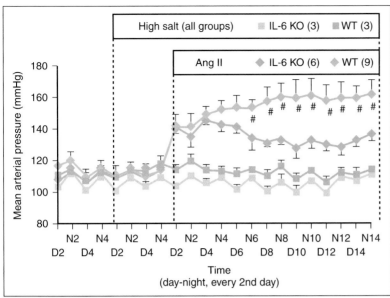

Figure 22–1. Infusion of angiotensin II causes an increase in blood pressure that is significantly attenuated in interleukin-6 knockout mice. Experiments were performed in wild-type and knockout mice placed on a high salt diet and measurements of blood pressure were made using radiotelemetry. (Redrawn from Lee DL, Sturgis LC, Labazi H, Osborne Jr JB, Fleming C, Pollock JS, et al. *Am J Physiol Heart Circ Physiol* 2005;209:H935–40. Used with permission.)

although like TNF-α, there is evidence that IL-6 can promote oxidative stress. In addition, IL-6 is a potent stimulator of acute-phase reactants from the liver, which may also play a role in the progression of hypertension.

C-Reactive protein

Acute-phase reactants are liver-derived plasma proteins that increase in response to infection. C-reactive protein (CRP) belongs to this class of circulating peptides and is a widely used clinical marker for inflammation. It is important for opsonization (making an antigen susceptible to the actions of phagocytes) and also activates the complement cascade. Several studies have reported elevated CRP in hypertensive patients and that it predicts the development of hypertension in otherwise healthy individuals.[17–20] The degree to which CRP levels associate with hypertension varies among ethnic populations. For example, among hypertensive individuals, the highest levels of CRP are observed in Chinese, followed by African Americans and Caucasians.[21] Similar correlations between CRP and hypertension were also reported in Korean and Colombian populations.[22,23] No relationship was observed among participants of Hispanic descent.[21] Although some studies suggest that there are no gender differences in serum CRP levels as they relate to hypertension,[21] there is evidence that hormone replacement therapy in postmenopausal women is associated with increased serum CRP in apparently healthy women.[24] This may be an important area for further investigation given the current debate on safety, particularly with regard to cardiovascular outcomes, in women who are prescribed hormone therapy.

To date, animal studies examining the role of CRP in the development of hypertension have not been performed.

However, two recent studies have begun to address the potential cellular mechanism for how CRP might promote hypertension. In isolated human aortic endothelial cells (HAEC), CRP has been shown to attenuate the production of the potent vasodilators prostacyclin and nitric oxide. CRP can also attenuate expression of the thrombolytic enzyme tissue plasminogen activator (tpA), which is an important anticoagulant.[25] In a separate study, investigators showed a potential mechanism for CRP-mediated endothelial dysfunction. They demonstrated that CRP activated HAECs in culture leading to increased monocyte adhesion. Endothelial activation was promoted by impairing endothelial nitric oxide synthase (eNOS) activity caused by reduced phosphorylation at ser1179.[26] Thus the ability of CRP to cause endothelial dysfunction may be an important contributing mechanism to the subsequent development of hypertension.

Other cytokines

In addition to those already discussed, numerous other cytokines have been implicated in the development of hypertension in humans and/or animal models, including IL-1β, monocyte chemoattractant protein 1 (MCP-1), interleukin 2 (IL-2), *regulated on activation normal T expressed and secreted* (RANTES), and transforming growth factor β (TGF-β).[27–29] TGF-β is considered to be an anti-inflammatory cytokine that inhibits the proliferation of lymphocytes and leukocytes. However, evidence suggests that TGF-β directly correlates with mean arterial pressure, systolic pressure, and diastolic pressure in patients with end-stage renal disease.[30] TGF-β can promote hypertension through activation of the RAS or endothelin systems[30,31]; however, profibrotic actions of TGF-β have also been implicated in target organ damage that contributes to hypertension. This is supported by evidence that TGF-β is significantly associated with renal injury and hypertension independently of blood pressure.[29] Therefore, a large number of studies on the role of TGF-β in promoting hypertension have focused on tissue injury.

Although much of the evidence discussed above indicates a prohypertensive relationship between cytokines and blood pressure, there is evidence for antihypertensive actions of cytokines. For example, subcutaneous injection of IFN-γ once a week for 10 weeks lowered blood pressure and reduced glomerular sclerosis in Dahl salt-sensitive (DahlSS) rats on a high-salt diet.[32] Similarly, subcutaneous infusion of interleukin-2 (IL-2) prevented the development of hypertension when administered to young spontaneously hypertensive rats (SHR) and normalized blood pressure in SHRs with established hypertension.[33] Therefore, the effects of cytokines on blood pressure are likely the result of a balance between pro- and anti-inflammatory actions of these immune response mediators.

NEUROHUMORAL AND ORGAN SYSTEMS AFFECTED BY CYTOKINES

The mechanisms by which inflammatory cytokines contribute to the development of hypertension have become an important area of research. While cellular and molecular mechanisms for cytokine actions continue to be uncovered, there is considerable evidence for the effect of cytokines on organ systems that are vital for the regulation of blood pressure. This section will focus on neurohumoral, vascular, renal, central, and cardiac effects of pro-inflammatory cytokines.

Renin-angiotensin system

The renin-angiotensin system (RAS) is the most powerful endocrine system in the body, and is critical for regulating renal function, body fluid homeostasis, and vascular tone. The well-known biochemical cascade for the generation of angiotensin II (Ang II) begins with renin release from juxtaglomerular cells of the kidney and culminates in the generation of Ang II by angiotensin converting enzyme (ACE). The effects of Ang II to increase blood pressure can be attributed to altered renal function, increased peripheral vascular resistance, and increased sympathetic nerve activity. In addition to its renal, vascular, and central effects, there is now evidence supporting a pro-inflammatory mechanism for Ang II in the progression of hypertension.

In humans, several studies demonstrate that blockade of RAS, either with angiotensin receptor blockers (ARB) or ACE inhibitors, lowers serum amounts of cytokines including TNF-α, IL-6, CRP, and MCP-1.[34-36] The expression of TGF-β is also modified by blockade of RAS. For example, treatment of individuals with newly diagnosed, but never treated, essential hypertension had increased serum levels of TGF-β that were markedly reduced following treatment with the ARB losartan.[37] In peripheral blood monocytes isolated from individuals with essential hypertension, *in vitro* stimulation with Ang II caused an increased production of IL-1β that was prevented by preincubation with an ARB.[38] Thus Ang II can have direct effects on the physiologic function of cells from the immune system.

The pro-inflammatory actions of Ang II have been reported in animal models of hypertension as well. Increased aortic expression IL-1β, TNF-α, IL-6, and their downstream signaling mediator NFκB, are attenuated after treatment with ARBs in the SHR model of hypertension. Triple therapy, however, did not alter cytokine expression in this study, demonstrating that RAS was critical for the increased inflammatory markers.[39] In transgenic rats overexpressing human renin and in the two-kidney-one-clip model of hypertension, serum levels of MCP-1 and renal macrophage infiltration were significantly reduced, along with blood pressure, after treatment with the ARB valsartan.[40] Finally, the effect of RAS to promote inflammation was demonstrated in numerous studies using a rat transgenic for human renin and human angiotensinogen. This model has hypertension, cardiac hypertrophy, and renal damage. In addition, TNF-α, adhesion molecule, and monocyte attachment have been reported in renal vessels and kidney homogenates from these animals. Treatment of these rats

with ARB or ACE inhibitors lowers blood pressure and attenuates the expression of these inflammatory markers.[41-43] Therefore, data from human and animal studies support a pro-inflammatory role for RAS in the progression of hypertension and suggest another important therapeutic benefit for administering ARBs and ACE inhibitors to lower blood pressure.

Currently available data regarding the regulation of RAS by cytokines are conflicting. Experiments using an *in vitro* model of juxtaglomerular cells suggest that TNF-α and IL-1β inhibit renin gene transcription.[44-46] To the contrary, TNF-α and IL-1β have been shown to increase renin release in rat renal cortical slices[47] and a bolus infusion of IL-1β in Wistar rats increases blood pressure (measured by tail cuff) and plasma renin activity.[48] Using similar amounts of TNF-α in HepG2 cells (liver carcinoma) it has been shown that TNF-α stimulates transcription of the angiotensinogen gene.[49] While differences in the models and methodologies used may account for the disparities, these experiments were all performed with an acute exposure to inflammatory cytokines. The effect of chronically elevated cytokines on components of RAS in whole animals remains to be elucidated.

Endothelin

Another endocrine peptide that has been implicated in the development of hypertension is ET-1. ET-1 is a 21–amino acid peptide generated from cleavage of the precursor pre-proendoethlin and is widely recognized as the most potent vasoconstrictor. Like Ang II, it has vascular, renal, and central effects (Reviewed in Miyauchi and Masaki[50], and Simonson[51]) to mediate blood pressure. Although it has not been extensively examined in humans, presently available data suggest a relationship among ET-1, inflammation, and hypertension.[9,28]

Several studies using animal models of hypertension have examined this relationship. For example, stroke-prone SHR rats fed a high-salt diet have increased renal expression of pre-proendothelin and TGF-β, the latter of which is attenuated by pharmacologic blockade of the ETa receptor.[52] Evidence also indicates that inflammatory cytokines promote the generation and release of ET-1, suggesting a feed-forward mechanism to promote inflammation. For example, incubation of vascular smooth muscle cells (VSMC) with TNF-α causes NFκB and STAT1 translocation to the nucleus and increased expression of ET-1.[53] Inhibitors of NFκB and STAT1 abrogated the ET-1–stimulating actions of TNF-α.

Vascular

The vascular wall is an important target for the physiologic actions of both Ang II and ET-1. Activation of vascular endothelial cells is critical to the inflammatory response as it facilitates the attachment of monocytes and can lead to impaired endothelial function. Endothelial dysfunction can be promoted through numerous mechanisms, including reductions in the generation and availability of nitric oxide or in the generation of reactive oxygen species. Impaired vascular function promotes end organ damage and leads to increased peripheral vascular resistance that each contribute to the development of hypertension.

In humans with hypertension, considerable data support a role for inflammatory cytokines to alter vascular function. Levels of TNF-α, IL-6, and CRP have been shown to independently associate with increased arterial stiffness, velocity, and thickness in humans with essential hypertension.[54–57] Individuals with high levels of circulating CRP were more likely to develop peripheral artery disease and hypertension, making CRP a potential predictor of future peripheral vascular disease in apparently healthy men.[58] The effects of CRP to alter vessel function are supported by data showing that elevated levels of CRP are associated with impaired forearm blood flow in patients with coronary artery disease. Interestingly, individuals that also had elevated serum interleukin 10 (IL-10), an anti-inflammatory cytokine, did not have impaired flow responses. The mechanism by which IL-10 protected the endothelium was through reduced oxidative stress.[59] This study demonstrates the important balance that exists between pro- and anti-inflammatory cytokines.

The effects of inflammatory cytokines on vascular function have often been studied in animals given LPS, which causes a large increase in the generation of TNF-α. LPS impairs endothelial-dependent relaxation through generation of reactive oxygen species. There is also evidence for a large increase in iNOS during these acute reactions. High levels of nitric oxide can be toxic to cell function. While these studies suggest a role for cytokines in modulating endothelial function, the infusion of LPS leads to a reduction in blood pressure similar to what occurs during sepsis. Therefore, these large increases in cytokines do not reflect levels observed during hypertension. The effect of chronic moderately elevated inflammatory cytokines on endothelial function is not yet clear. Circulating and attached monocytes with increased expression of cell adhesion molecules have been reported in SHR but not Wistar Kyoto (WKY) or Sprague Dawley (SD) rats. In addition, vascular tissue isolated from SHRs has higher expression and releases greater amounts of TNF-α and IL-1β compared to controls,[60] suggesting that vessels during hypertension may be sensitized to generate cytokines and contribute to impaired function. Other studies have shown that infusion or incubation with IL-6 or TNF-α (at levels observed during hypertension) can cause impaired endothelial-dependent relaxation in peripheral conduit vessels.[61–64] While these data are important, studies using conduit vessels have greater significance for understanding the progression of atherosclerosis and less for the development of hypertension. Therefore, it will be critical to examine the effect of inflammatory cytokines on smaller resistance vessels from the kidneys, which are important for long-term blood pressure regulation.

Renal

The importance of the kidneys in the long-term regulation of blood pressure is well known, and there is evidence to suggest that inflammation may play an important role in altering renal function. For example, high levels of CRP are associated with increased blood pressure, and those with renal damage (measured by microalbuminuria) had the highest serum CRP levels.[65] However, while serum CRP levels correlate with blood pressure and cardiovascular risk, it does not always associate with renal function.[66] Thus the association between serum CRP and renal function in humans is not clear. Studies on the relationship between other inflammatory cytokines and renal function in humans is limited with the exception of TGF-β levels that correlate with not only hypertension but also with proteinuria and renal fibrosis.[37]

Recent evidence demonstrates a potentially critical role for TGF-β in the regulation of kidney function and blood pressure in animal models. For example, treatment of DahlSS rats with a neutralizing antibody to TGF-β lowered blood pressure, reduced fibrosis, proteinuria, and sclerosis in rats on a high-salt diet.[67] The effect of TGF-β on renal microvessel autoregulation was assessed *ex vivo* using the juxtamedullary nephron technique. In this study, the authors demonstrated that TGF-β, but not other growth factors, completely abolished the autoregulatory response of rat renal afferent arterioles. The mechanism by which this occurred was dependent on the generation of reactive oxygen species, since autoregulatory responses were restored after treatment with tempol.[68] Therefore, similar to other cytokines, reactive oxygen species may be an important mechanism contributing to the effects of TGF-β on blood pressure.

Evidence suggests that other cytokines may also modulate renal function. Inhibition of p38 MAP kinase, a key downstream signaling mechanism mediating the cellular actions of cytokines, has been shown to reduce renal damage and attenuate TNF-α and IL-1β expression in kidneys from DahlSS rats.[69] The RAS transgenic rat model of hypertension described above has increased renal expression of TNF-α and renal vascular expression of cell adhesion molecules that is attenuated by treatment with the corticosteroids, Etanercept (TNF-α antagonist), MMF (inhibitor of T/B cell proliferation), or blockade of RAS.[42,43] TNF-α expression has also been shown to be increased in the medullary thick ascending limb in rats with Ang II–mediated hypertension.[70] Taken together, studies in humans and animal models support a role for inflammatory cytokines in modulating renal function.

Central nervous system

The central nervous system is recognized as a short-term regulator of blood pressure, but also has important long-term effects in arterial pressure through altered renal sympathetic nerve activity. It has long been recognized that inflammatory cytokines have central effects to increase activity of the hypothalamic pituitary axis. HPA activation increases the release of adrenocorticotropin hormone (ACTH) leading to increased corticosteroid production. Corticosteroids have general immunosuppressive actions; however, chronic increases can promote hypertension by augmenting sodium and water retention in the kidneys.

The actions of specific inflammatory cytokines on central nervous system–mediated changes in blood pressure and renal function were recently examined in a study by Zhang et al.[71] The authors examined, in anesthetized rats, the effect of acute forebrain TNF-α infusion on sympathetic nerve activity, blood pressure, and heart rate. Infusion of TNF-α increased arterial pressure, heart rate, and renal sympathetic nerve activity through the actions of prostaglandins in the paraventricular nucleus. Others have demonstrated that intracisternal or intravenous infusion of IL-1β increases blood pressure in a prostaglandin-dependent manner in rats.[72] The circumventricular organ, area postremus, and choroid plexus are likely sites of cytokine action since these regions do not have a blood–brain barrier. While these studies indicate a prohypertensive action of cytokines in the brain and central nervous system, there are studies that suggest a role for cytokines to suppress sympathetic activity. Ye et al.[73] showed that infusion of IL-1β into the lateral ventricle of rats causes a decrease in blood pressure that is reversed by using a neutralizing antibody to IL-1β. They further demonstrated that IL-1β has a tonic inhibitory effect on sympathetic nerve activity.[74] These data indicate that the effect of cytokines on central control of blood pressure may be subject to regional actions within the brain.

Another cytokine that acts in the brain to regulate blood pressure is leptin. Leptin is typically associated with metabolism and is recognized as a satiety factor in rodents; however, it promotes immune responses and increases renal sympathetic nerve activity and blood pressure through centrally mediated mechanisms. The leptin receptor is similar in structure to the IL-6 receptor. Predominantly produced by adipocytes, leptin is increased during obesity and metabolic syndrome, of which one of the major phenotypes is hypertension. The role of inflammatory cytokines during hypertension and metabolic syndrome will be discussed later in this chapter.

Cardiac

Heart function may also be affected by inflammatory cytokines under pathologic conditions. Individuals with heart failure have a deteriorating condition where the failing heart cannot supply enough blood and oxygen to meet metabolic demand. This leads to activation of RAS and increased sodium and water retention, which exacerbates hypertension and heart failure. Recent evidence supports a role for cytokines in the progression to heart failure. Data from the Framingham Heart Study show that the incidence of heart failure was increased with increased inflammatory markers IL-6, TNF-α, and CRP. IL-6 was the best predictor of heart failure in this study.[75] Other studies showed that as heart failure progresses, levels of CRP, IL-1β, and TNF-α, along with soluble receptors for TNF-α, increase.[76,77] Additionally, individuals with rheumatoid arthritis (a chronic inflammatory disease) have an increased risk for developing heart failure and patients treated with anti-TNF-α therapy were less likely to have heart failure.[78]

Similar to humans, evidence from animal models suggests a role for inflammation in heart failure. For example, cardiac muscle from SHR has increased number of mast cells that express high levels of TNF-α, IL-6, NFκB, and TGF-β.[79] In addition, treatment of DahlSS rats with ARB or ACE inhibitors reduces cardiac macrophage infiltration, IL-6, and TGF-β expression.[80]

SPECIAL EXAMPLES OF INFLAMMATION AND HYPERTENSION

Preeclampsia

Preeclampsia is defined by hypertension and proteinuria during the third trimester of pregnancy that resolves upon delivery of the placenta. One cause of preeclampsia is thought to be due to reduced uterine perfusion pressure to the fetus. Women with preeclampsia have increased cardiovascular risk later in life as do infants born to preeclamptic mothers. Growing evidence points to a role for inflammatory cytokines as a causative factor in the development of preeclampsia. Several studies in humans suggest that serum cytokines including IL-2, TNF-α, IL-6, and CRP are elevated in women with preeclampsia and can even be predictive for the development of preeclampsia when measured early in the pregnancy.[81–83] Interestingly, in a 20-year follow-up after a preeclamptic pregnancy, women have an increased ratio of pro-inflammatory to anti-inflammatory cytokines.[84]

Our understanding of the pathophysiology of preeclampsia has been aided by the development of animal models. Alexander et al.[85] demonstrated a potential role for cytokines in preeclampsia when infusion of TNF-α caused hypertension in pregnant but not virgin rats. The Granger laboratory has recently developed a reduced uterine perfusion pressure (RUPP) model of preeclampsia in the rat by restricting blood flow in the uterine arteries. These animals develop hypertension, general endothelial dysfunction, and proteinuria similar to what is observed in humans. LaMarca et al.[86,87] demonstrated that these rats, like humans, have elevated levels of TNF-α (Figure 22–2), and that hypertension mediated by TNF-α infusion in pregnant rats can be ameliorated with blockade of the endothelin system. Increased levels of TNF-α or IL-6 can cause endothelial dysfunction in pregnant rats, suggesting that inflammatory cytokines are also important for the impaired vessel function during preeclampsia.[61,62,64] Infusion of IL-6 either during early or late pregnancy in the rat leads to hypertension in the offspring by age 5 weeks, which supports a role for cytokines in not only causing preeclampsia but also for increasing cardiovascular risk in offspring.[88]

Metabolic syndrome

Metabolic syndrome is a disorder that can be characterized by insulin resistance, obesity, hyperglycemia, and hypertension. Oftentimes this leads to the development of type II diabetes. Although this disorder is an amalgamation of numerous phenotypes, several studies have reported increased serum cytokines in individuals with metabolic syndrome as a potential underlying mechanism. TNF-α, IL-6, CRP, TGF-β, and leptin are all directly correlated with increased body mass index,[89] and CRP and IL-6 have been shown to associate with fasted insulin levels in addition to blood pressure.[90] Studies suggest that increased cytokines can raise the likelihood of developing metabolic syndrome.[91] Elevated cytokines can also promote diabetes through negatively regulating insulin receptor signaling.

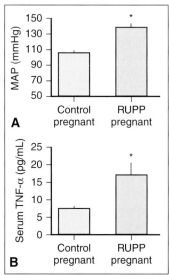

Figure 22–2. MAP and serum concentration of TNF-α are significantly increased in RUPP rat model of preeclampsia at day 19 of gestation. MAP, mean arterial pressure; RUPP, reduced uterine perfusion pressure. (Adapted from Babbette B, LaMarca D, Bennett WA, Alexander BT, Cockrell K, Granger JP. *Hypertension* 2005;46(4):1022–5.)

The mechanisms by which inflammatory cytokines might promote metabolic syndrome are not yet clear.

Pulmonary hypertension

Pulmonary hypertension results from altered vascular function (constriction and thickening) that leads to increased pressure in the arteries supplying the lungs. Inflammatory cytokines have been implicated in vascular dysfunction that is prevalent during pulmonary hypertension. Serum levels of IL-1β and IL-6 are reportedly increased,[27] and lung biopsies from individuals with primary pulmonary hypertension showed increased expression of RANTES.[92] RANTES attracts T lymphocytes and monocytes, which are the most abundant infiltrates in pulmonary hypertension. Like other cytokines, RANTES activates ET-1,[93] which plays an important role in the pathogenesis of pulmonary hypertension.[94]

A role for cytokines has also been demonstrated in experimental models of pulmonary hypertension. For example, transgenic mice overexpressing TNF-α develop pulmonary hypertension,[95] while TNF-α receptor knockout mice do not develop pulmonary hypertension in response to bleomycin, an anticancer therapy that induces pulmonary fibrosis and hypertension in rodents.[96] Bleomycin-induced pulmonary hypertension in mice is mediated by TNF-α and downstream mediators NFκB and AP1.[96] IL-6 infusion has been shown to cause pulmonary hypertension in rats that is preventable by neutralizing IL-6 antibodies.[97] ET-1 may also play an important role in IL-6–mediated pulmonary hypertension based on data from cell culture studies

showing that pulmonary artery smooth muscle cells have an augmented production of pre-proendothelin and ET-1 in response to TNF-α or IFN-γ.[98] These data are consistent with a role for the endothelin system in cytokine-mediated hypertension, and is similar to what has been reported in preeclampsia.

Chronic inflammatory disease

Individuals with chronic inflammatory diseases (systemic lupus erythematosus [SLE], rheumatoid arthritis, scleroderma, sarcoidosis, etc.) are at great risk for the development of cardiovascular disease in general and hypertension in particular. For example, studies have shown that more than 50% of patients with SLE, the prototypical autoimmune disorder, have hypertension that is not necessarily dependent on renal damage typically associated with SLE.[99–101] Individuals with SLE have been shown to have increased circulating and tissue levels of inflammatory cytokines. An association with CRP was observed in patients with SLE and hypertension and cardiovascular risk,[102] and serum from patients with SLE increases IL-6 release from isolated endothelial cells.[103] Despite this high level of cardiovascular risk and hypertension, there have been surprisingly few studies aimed at investigating the role that inflammatory cytokines play in the progression of hypertension during chronic inflammatory disorders such as SLE.

GENETIC VARIATION OF CYTOKINES

From individual to individual there is variation in the DNA sequences that determine genetic makeup. Throughout the human genome, thousands of single nucleotide substitutions have been identified and are referred to as single nucleotide polymorphisms (SNP). These SNPs may have significant effects on whether a DNA sequence is appropriately transcribed and translated or have no affect at all. SNPs can be used as genetic markers to identify relationships with certain diseases. For example, consider a base pair change from G to C at position X in a gene that is vital for blood pressure regulation. If the mutation occurs at a high frequency in a population of hypertensive patients, that SNP is considered to be associated with hypertension. While a genetic association suggests a relationship between genotype and phenotype, it does not provide information on functional changes that occur as a result of the polymorphism. Furthermore, investigators often come to different conclusions about genetic associations because numerous factors, including population size and makeup, can influence the results. Many studies have been performed in humans by examining common SNPs that associate with hypertension, including SNPs identified in inflammatory cytokines.

Tumor necrosis factor alpha

In humans, there is evidence that the TNF-α gene locus associates with obesity-related hypertension.[104] Within the TNF-α gene, two common SNPs have been identified in the promoter region (G-238A and G-308A). There is evidence supporting an association of these SNPs with hypertension in Japanese and Argentine populations[105,106];

however, this association was not evident in Chinese subjects.[107,108] These disparate results can likely be attributed to different populations studied. Whether mutations in TNF-α are important for the development of hypertension remains to be elucidated.

Interleukin-6

Several SNPs for IL-6 have been identified in humans including a G-174C and G-636C in the promoter region, and an intronic C1691G. The G-636C allele is associated with hypertension in Japanese women, while the C1691G allele is associated with hypertension in men.[109] A separate study of Japanese women found no association between several IL-6 polymorphisms and blood pressure. The G-174C allele in the IL-6 promoter has been shown to be significantly associated with hypertension. However it is interesting to note that in one study, individuals with the GC or CC genotype were at greatest risk for having increased diastolic pressure and left ventricular hypertrophy[110] while other investigators found the GG genotype to have the strongest association with hypertension.[111]

C-Reactive protein

Although numerous studies demonstrate an association between serum levels of CRP and blood pressure, the evidence supporting genetic associations between CRP SNPs and hypertension is weak. The G1059C polymorphism for CRP was previously reported to be a marker for cardiovascular risk.[112] However, while the frequency of this SNP has been associated with blood pressure, the association was not significant when adjusted for other cardiovascular risk factors.[113]

Other cytokines

Polymorphisms in other cytokines have been examined with respect to hypertension, but have failed to reveal a genetic association (TGF-β, T10C; IFN-γ, T874A; and IL-1β; taq dimorphism +3892) with the exception of an arginine allele in codon 25 of TGF-β that is increased in hypertensive patients.[114]

IMPLICATIONS FOR THERAPY

Although the mechanisms by which inflammatory cytokines contribute to the progression of hypertension continue to be elucidated, it is clear that they play an important role. Therefore, treatments that mitigate inflammation will likely have great benefit for patients with hypertension. Blockade of the RAS with ARBs or ACE inhibitors is one of the most common pharmacologic treatments for hypertension. These drugs have a myriad of cardiovascular benefits to which anti-inflammation can be added. Many patients use HMG CoA reductase inhibitors, or statins, to safely regulate cholesterol and reduce cardiovascular risk. Importantly, statins have been shown to be anti-inflammatory.[115,116] While they may not have significant blood pressure–lowering capabilities acutely, the long-term benefit of statin therapy on hypertension could be significant.

The thiazolidinedione (TZD) drug family was developed over the past 15 years, and is currently used to improve insulin sensitivity in otherwise resistant patients. TZDs are potent activators of the nuclear transcription factor, peroxisome proliferator activated receptor gamma (PPARγ). Evidence suggests in human and animal models that they reduce blood pressure and attenuate the expression of pro-inflammatory cytokines. There is currently a great deal of research regarding the potential cardiovascular benefits of these drugs.

Corticosteroids are commonly used as general immunosuppressive therapy for patients with chronic inflammatory disease. Unfortunately, chronic corticosteroid use can lead to increased blood pressure as a result of its mineralocorticoid actions to increase sodium and water retention by the kidneys. This precludes corticosteroids from being an effective anti-inflammatory treatment of hypertension. To the contrary, there are anti-inflammatory therapies commonly recommended for humans to reduce cardiovascular risk. Many physicians prescribe a low-dose, nonsteroidal, anti-inflammatory regimen (i.e., aspirin) for individuals with increased cardiovascular risk. Aspirin is also commonly used to treat symptoms of chronic inflammatory diseases. Cyclosporine is a general immunosuppressive drug that prevents lymphocytes from producing inflammatory cytokines. It is used in humans who have undergone organ transplants or in those with chronic inflammatory disease. Evidence in rodents suggests that the inhibition of cytokines by cyclosporine can reduce blood pressure.[117] As more is learned about the role that inflammatory cytokines play in the progression of cardiovascular disease, anti-inflammatory drugs may become more common for the treatment of hypertension.

CONCLUSIONS

The role that inflammation and cytokines play in the progression of hypertension is an emerging area of research interest that will continue to garner attention. There is strong supporting evidence to show that increased cytokines are associated with numerous forms of hypertension. These inflammatory mediators can regulate, and be regulated by, neurohumoral pathways that have long been implicated in the development of hypertension. The effect of cytokines on the development of hypertension is not limited to these endocrine systems, but rather can be vital to altering function in multiple organ systems, including the brain, kidneys, heart, and vasculature. Moreover, there is evidence to support genetic associations between variant SNPs in cytokines and hypertension. Despite growing evidence supporting a role for cytokines in the progression of cardiovascular disease, there are few studies that demonstrate a direct role for cytokines in the progression of hypertension. Therefore, providing definitive evidence and mechanisms for the role of cytokines in hypertension will be important for the development of future therapies.

REFERENCES

1. Libby P, Ridker PM, Maseri A. Inflammation and atherosclerosis. *Circulation* 2002;105(9):1135–43.

2. Miyajima A, Kitamura T, Harada N, Yokota T, Arai K. Cytokine receptors and signal transduction. *Annu Rev Immunol* 1992;10:295–331.

3. Dong C, Davis RJ, Flavell RA. MAP kinases in the immune response. *Annu Rev Immunol* 2002;20:55–72.

4. Leonard WJ. Role of Jak kinases and STATs in cytokine signal transduction. *Int J Hematol* 2001;73(3):271–7.

5. Sweeney SE, Firestein GS. Signal transduction in rheumatoid arthritis. *Curr Opin Rheumatol* 2004;16(3):231–7.

6. Wajant H, Pfizenmaier K, Scheurich P. Tumor necrosis factor signaling. *Cell Death Differ* 2003;10(1):45–65.

7. Stumpf C, John S, Jukic J, Yilmaz A, Raaz D, Schmieder RE, et al. Enhanced levels of platelet P-selectin and circulating cytokines in young patients with mild arterial hypertension. *J Hypertens* 2005;23(5):995–1000.

8. Bautista LE, Vera LM, Arenas IA, Gamarra G. Independent association between inflammatory markers (C-reactive protein, interleukin-6, and TNF-alpha) and essential hypertension. *J Hum Hypertens* 2005;19(2):149–54.

9. Cottone S, Vadala A, Vella MC, Mule G, Contorno A, Cerasola G. Comparison of tumour necrosis factor and endothelin-1 between essential and renal hypertensive patients. *J Hum Hypertens* 1998;12(6):351–4.

10. Wang DS, Xie HH, Shen FM, Cai GJ, Su DF. Blood pressure variability, cardiac baroreflex sensitivity and organ damage in experimentally hypertensive rats. *Clin Exp Pharmacol Physiol* 2005;32(7):545–52.

11. Lenhard SC, Nerurkar SS, Schaeffer TR, Mirabile RC, Boyce RW, Adams DF, et al. p38 MAPK inhibitors ameliorate target organ damage in hypertension. Part 2. Improved renal function as assessed by dynamic contrast-enhanced magnetic resonance imaging. *J Pharmacol Exp Ther* 2003;307(3):939–46.

12. Ju H, Behm DJ, Nerurkar S, Eybye ME, Haimbach RE, Olzinski AR, et al. p38 MAPK inhibitors ameliorate target organ damage in hypertension. Part 1. p38 MAPK-dependent endothelial dysfunction and hypertension. *J Pharmacol Exp Ther* 2003;307(3):932–8.

13. Chae CU, Lee RT, Rifai N, Ridker PM. Blood pressure and inflammation in apparently healthy men. *Hypertension* 2001;38(3):399–403.

14. Brydon L, Steptoe A. Stress-induced increases in interleukin-6 and fibrinogen predict ambulatory blood pressure at 3-year follow-up. *J Hypertens* 2005;23(5):1001–7.

15. Lee DL, Sturgis LC, Labazi H, Osborne Jr JB, Fleming C, Pollock JS, et al. Angiotensin II hypertension is attenuated in interleukin-6 knockout mice. *Am J PhysiolHeart Circ Physiol* 2005;209:H935–40.

16. Lee DL, Leite R, Fleming C, Pollock JS, Webb RC, Brands MW. Hypertensive response to acute stress is attenuated in interleukin-6 knockout mice. *Hypertension* 2004;44(3):259–63.

17. King DE, Egan BM, Mainous AG, III, Geesey ME. Elevation of C-reactive protein in people with prehypertension. *J Clin Hypertens (Greenwich)* 2004;6(10):562–8.

18. Schillaci G, Pirro M, Gemelli F, Pasqualini L, Vaudo G, Marchesi S, et al. Increased C-reactive protein concentrations in never-treated hypertension: the role of systolic and pulse pressures. *J Hypertens* 2003;21(10):1841–6.

19. Patel JV, Lim HS, Nadar S, Tayebjee M, Hughes EA, Lip GY. Abnormal soluble CD40 ligand and C-reactive protein concentrations in hypertension: relationship to indices of angiogenesis. *J Hypertens* 2006;24(1):117–21.

20. Niskanen L, Laaksonen DE, Nyyssonen K, Punnonen K, Valkonen VP, Fuentes R, et al. Inflammation, abdominal obesity, and smoking as predictors of hypertension. *Hypertension* 2004;44(6):859–65.

21. Lakoski SG, Cushman M, Palmas W, Blumenthal R, D'Agostino RB, Jr., Herrington DM. The relationship between blood pressure and C-reactive protein in the Multi-Ethnic Study of Atherosclerosis (MESA). *J Am Coll Cardiol* 2005;46(10):1869–74.

22. Bautista LE, Lopez-Jaramillo P, Vera LM, Casas JP, Otero AP, Guaracao AI. Is C-reactive protein an independent risk factor for essential hypertension? *J Hypertens* 2001;19(5):857–61.

23. Sung KC, Suh JY, Kim BS, Kang JH, Kim H, Lee MH, et al. High sensitivity C-reactive protein as an independent risk factor for essential hypertension. *Am J Hypertens* 2003;16(6):429–33.

24. Ridker PM, Hennekens CH, Rifai N, Buring JE, Manson JE. Hormone replacement therapy and increased plasma concentration of C-reactive protein. *Circulation* 1999;100(7):713–6.

25. Singh U, Devaraj S, Jialal I. C-reactive protein decreases tissue plasminogen activator activity in human aortic endothelial cells: evidence that C-reactive protein is a procoagulant. *Arterioscler Thromb Vasc Biol* 2005;25(10):2216–21.

26. Mineo C, Gormley AK, Yuhanna IS, Osborne-Lawrence S, Gibson LL, Hahner L, et al. FcgammaRIIB mediates C-reactive protein inhibition of endothelial NO synthase. *Circ Res* 2005;97(11):1124–31.

27. Humbert M, Monti G, Brenot F, Sitbon O, Portier A, Grangeot-Keros L, et al. Increased interleukin-1 and interleukin-6 serum concentrations in severe primary pulmonary hypertension. *Am J Respir Crit Care Med* 1995;151(5):1628–31.

28. Parissis JT, Korovesis S, Giazitzoglou E, Kalivas P, Katritsis D. Plasma profiles of peripheral monocyte-related inflammatory markers in patients with arterial hypertension. Correlations with plasma endothelin-1. *Int J Cardiol* 2002;83(1):13–21.

29. Derhaschnig U, Shehata M, Herkner H, Bur A, Woisetschlager C, Laggner AN, et al. Increased levels of transforming growth factor-beta1 in essential hypertension. *Am J Hypertens* 2002;15(3):207–11.

30. Li B, Khanna A, Sharma V, Singh T, Suthanthiran M, August P. TGF-beta1 DNA polymorphisms, protein levels, and blood pressure. *Hypertension* 1999;33(1 Pt 2):271–5.

31. Kurihara H, Yoshizumi M, Sugiyama T, Takaku F, Yanagisawa M, Masaki T, et al. Transforming growth factor-beta stimulates the expression of endothelin mRNA by vascular endothelial cells. *Biochem Biophys Res Commun* 1989;159(3):1435–40.

32. Ishimitsu T, Uehara Y, Numabe A, Tsukada H, Ogawa Y, Iwai J, et al. Interferon gamma attenuates hypertensive renal injury in salt-sensitive Dahl rats. *Hypertension* 1992;19(6 Pt 2):804–8.

33. Tuttle RS, Boppana DP. Antihypertensive effect of interleukin-2. *Hypertension* 1990;15(1):89–94.

34. Vazquez-Oliva G, Fernandez-Real JM, Zamora A, Vilaseca M, Badimon L. Lowering of blood pressure leads to decreased circulating interleukin-6 in hypertensive subjects. *J Hum Hypertens* 2005;19(6):457–62.

35. Fliser D, Buchholz K, Haller H. Antiinflammatory effects of angiotensin II subtype 1 receptor blockade in hypertensive patients with microinflammation. *Circulation* 2004;110(9):1103–7.

36. Manabe S, Okura T, Watanabe S, Fukuoka T, Higaki J. Effects of angiotensin II receptor blockade with valsartan on pro-inflammatory cytokines in patients with essential hypertension. *J Cardiovasc Pharmacol* 2005;46(6):735–9.

37. Laviades C, Varo N, Diez J. Transforming growth factor beta in hypertensives with cardiorenal damage. *Hypertension* 2000;36(4):517–22.

38. Dorffel Y, Latsch C, Stuhlmuller B, Schreiber S, Scholze S, Burmester GR, et al. Preactivated peripheral blood monocytes in patients with essential hypertension. *Hypertension* 1999;34(1):113–7.

39. Sanz-Rosa D, Oubina MP, Cediel E, de Las HN, Vegazo O, Jimenez J, et al. Effect of AT1 receptor antagonism on vascular and circulating inflammatory mediators in SHR: role of NF-kappaB/IkappaB system. *Am J PhysiolAm J Physiol Heart Circ Physiol* 2005;288(1):H111–5.

40. Hilgers KF, Hartner A, Porst M, Mai M, Wittmann M, Hugo C, et al. Monocyte chemoattractant protein-1 and macrophage infiltration in hypertensive kidney injury. *Kidney Int* 2000;58(6):2408–19.

41. Muller DN, Dechend R, Mervaala EM, Park JK, Schmidt F, Fiebeler A, et al. NF-kappaB inhibition ameliorates angiotensin II-induced inflammatory damage in rats. *Hypertension* 2000;35(1 Pt 2):193–201.

42. Mervaala EM, Muller DN, Park JK, Schmidt F, Lohn M, Breu V, et al. Monocyte infiltration and adhesion molecules in a rat model of high human renin hypertension. *Hypertension* 1999;33(1 Pt 2):389–95.

43. Muller DN, Shagdarsuren E, Park JK, Dechend R, Mervaala E, Hampich F, et al. Immunosuppressive treatment protects against angiotensin II-induced renal damage. *Am J Pathol* 2002;161(5):1679–93.

44. Pan L, Wang Y, Jones CA, Glenn ST, Baumann H, Gross KW. Enhancer-dependent inhibition of mouse renin transcription by inflammatory cytokines. *Am J PhysiolAm J Physiol Renal Physiol* 2005;288(1):F117–24.

45. Petrovic N, Kane CM, Sigmund CD, Gross KW. Downregulation of renin gene expression by interleukin-1. *Hypertension* 1997;30(2 Pt 1):230–5.

46. Todorov V, Muller M, Schweda F, Kurtz A. Tumor necrosis factor-alpha inhibits renin gene expression. *Am J Physiol Regul Integr Comp Physiol* 2002;283(5):R1046–51.

47. Chen LS, Cuddy MP, LaVallette LA. Regulation of human renin gene promoter activity: a new negative regulatory region determines the responsiveness to TNF alpha. *Kidney Int* 1998;54(6):2045–55.

48. Andreis PG, Neri G, Meneghelli V, Mazzocchi G, Nussdorfer GG. Effects of interleukin-1 beta on the renin-angiotensin-aldosterone system in rats. *Res Exp Med (Berl)* 1992;192(1):1–6.

49. Brasier AR, Li J, Wimbish KA. Tumor necrosis factor activates angiotensinogen gene expression by the Rel A transactivator. *Hypertension* 1996;27(4):1009–17.

50. Miyauchi T, Masaki T. Pathophysiology of endothelin in the cardiovascular system. *Annu Rev Physiol* 1999;61:391–415.

51. Simonson MS. Endothelins: multifunctional renal peptides. *Physiol Rev* 1993;73(2):375–411.

52. Tostes RC, Touyz RM, He G, Ammarguellat F, Schiffrin EL. Endothelin A receptor blockade decreases expression of growth factors and collagen and improves matrix metalloproteinase-2 activity in kidneys from stroke-prone spontaneously hypertensive rats. *J Cardiovasc Pharmacol* 2002;39(6):892–900.

53. Woods M, Wood EG, Bardswell SC, Bishop-Bailey D, Barker S, Wort SJ, et al. Role for nuclear factor-kappaB and signal transducer and activator of transcription 1/interferon regulatory factor-1 in cytokine-induced endothelin-1 release in human vascular smooth muscle cells. *Mol Pharmacol* 2003;64(4):923–31.

54. Manabe S, Okura T, Watanabe S, Higaki J. Association between carotid haemodynamics and inflammation in patients with essential hypertension. *J Hum Hypertens* 2005;19(10):787–91.

55. Yasmin, McEniery CM, Wallace S, Mackenzie IS, Cockcroft JR, Wilkinson IB. C-reactive protein is associated with arterial stiffness in apparently healthy individuals. *Arterioscler Thromb Vasc Biol* 2004;24(5):969–74.

56. Kullo IJ, Seward JB, Bailey KR, Bielak LF, Grossardt BR, Sheedy PF, et al. C-reactive protein is related to arterial wave reflection and stiffness in asymptomatic subjects from the community. *Am J Hypertens* 2005;18(8):1123–9.

57. Mahmud A, Feely J. Arterial stiffness is related to systemic inflammation in essential hypertension. *Hypertension* 2005;46(5):1118–22.

58. Ridker PM, Cushman M, Stampfer MJ, Tracy RP, Hennekens CH. Plasma concentration of C-reactive protein and risk of developing peripheral vascular disease. *Circulation* 1998 10;97(5):425–8.

59. Fichtlscherer S, Breuer S, Heeschen C, Dimmeler S, Zeiher AM. Interleukin-10 serum levels and systemic endothelial vasoreactivity in patients with coronary artery disease. *J Am Coll Cardiol* 2004 7;44(1):44–9.

60. Liu Y, Liu T, McCarron RM, Spatz M, Feuerstein G, Hallenbeck JM, et al. Evidence for activation of endothelium and monocytes in hypertensive rats. *Am J Physiol* 1996;270(6 Pt 2):H2125–31.

61. Orshal JM, Khalil RA. Reduced endothelial NO-cGMP-mediated vascular relaxation and hypertension in IL-6-infused pregnant rats. *Hypertension* 2004;43(2):434–44.

62. Orshal JM, Khalil RA. Interleukin-6 impairs endothelium-dependent NO-cGMP-mediated relaxation and enhances contraction in systemic vessels of pregnant rats. *Am J Physiol Regul Integr Comp Physiol* 2004;286(6):R1013–23.

63. Davis JR, Giardina JB, Green GM, Alexander BT, Granger JP, Khalil RA. Reduced endothelial NO-cGMP vascular relaxation pathway during TNF-alpha-induced hypertension in pregnant rats. *Am J Physiol Regul Integr Comp Physiol* 2002;282(2):R390–9.

64. Giardina JB, Green GM, Cockrell KL, Granger JP, Khalil RA. TNF-alpha enhances contraction and inhibits endothelial NO-cGMP relaxation in systemic vessels of pregnant rats. *Am J Physiol Regul Integr Comp Physiol* 2002;283(1):R130–43.

65. Tsioufis C, Dimitriadis K, Chatzis D, Vasiliadou C, Tousoulis D, Papademetriou V, et al. Relation of microalbuminuria to adiponectin and augmented C-reactive protein levels in men with essential hypertension. *Am J Cardiol* 2005;96(7):946–51.

66. Menon V, Wang X, Greene T, Beck GJ, Kusek JW, Marcovina SM, et al. Relationship between C-reactive protein, albumin, and cardiovascular disease in patients with chronic kidney disease. *Am J Kidney Dis* 2003;42(1):44–52.

67. Dahly AJ, Hoagland KM, Flasch AK, Jha S, Ledbetter SR, Roman RJ. Antihypertensive effects of chronic anti-TGF-beta antibody therapy in Dahl S rats. *Am J Physiol Regul Integr Comp Physiol* 2002;283(3):R757–67.

68. Sharma K, Cook A, Smith M, Valancius C, Inscho EW. TGF-beta impairs renal autoregulation via generation of ROS. *Am J Physiol Renal Physiol* 2005;288(5):F1069–77.

69. Tojo A, Onozato ML, Kobayashi N, Goto A, Matsuoka H, Fujita T. Antioxidative effect of p38 mitogen-activated protein kinase inhibitor in the kidney of hypertensive rat. *J Hypertens* 2005;23(1):165–74.

70. Ferreri NR, Zhao Y, Takizawa H, McGiff JC. Tumor necrosis factor-alpha-angiotensin interactions and regulation of blood pressure. *J Hypertens* 1997;15(12 Pt 1):1481–4.

71. Zhang ZH, Wei SG, Francis J, Felder RB. Cardiovascular and renal sympathetic activation by blood-borne TNF-alpha in rat: the role of central prostaglandins. *Am J Physiol Regul Integr Comp Physiol* 2003;284(4):R916–27.

72. Takahashi H, Nishimura M, Sakamoto M, Ikegaki I, Nakanishi T, Yoshimura M. Effects of interleukin-1 beta on blood pressure, sympathetic nerve activity, and pituitary endocrine functions in anesthetized rats. *Am J Hypertens* 1992;5(4 Pt 1):224–9.

73. Ye S, Mozayeni P, Gamburd M, Zhong H, Campese VM. Interleukin-1beta and neurogenic control of blood pressure in normal rats and rats with chronic renal failure. *Am J Physiol Heart Circ Physiol* 2000;279(6):H2786–96.

74. Campese VM, Ye S, Zhong H. Downregulation of neuronal nitric oxide synthase and interleukin-1beta mediates angiotensin II-dependent stimulation of sympathetic nerve activity. *Hypertension* 2002;39(2 Pt 2):519–24.

75. Vasan RS, Sullivan LM, Roubenoff R, Dinarello CA, Harris T, Benjamin EJ, et al. Inflammatory markers and risk of heart failure in elderly subjects without prior myocardial infarction: the Framingham Heart Study. *Circulation* 2003;107(11):1486–91.

76. Tsioufis C, Stougiannos P, Kakkavas A, Toutouza M, Mariolis A, Vlasseros I, et al. Relation of left ventricular concentric remodeling to levels of C-reactive protein and serum amyloid A in patients with essential hypertension. *Am J Cardiol* 2005;96(2):252–6.

77. Testa M, Yeh M, Lee P, Fanelli R, Loperfido F, Berman JW, et al. Circulating levels of cytokines and their endogenous modulators in patients with mild to severe congestive heart failure due to coronary artery disease or hypertension. *J Am Coll Cardiol* 1996;28(4):964–71.

78. Wolfe F, Michaud K. Heart failure in rheumatoid arthritis: rates, predictors, and the effect of anti-tumor necrosis factor therapy. *Am J Med* 2004;116(5):305–11.

79. Shiota N, Rysa J, Kovanen PT, Ruskoaho H, Kokkonen JO, Lindstedt KA. A role for cardiac mast cells in the pathogenesis of hypertensive heart disease. *J Hypertens* 2003;21(10):1935–44.

80. Yoshida J, Yamamoto K, Mano T, Sakata Y, Nishikawa N, Nishio M, et al. AT1 receptor blocker added to ACE inhibitor provides benefits at advanced stage of hypertensive diastolic heart failure. *Hypertension* 2004;43(3):686–91.

81. Qiu C, Luthy DA, Zhang C, Walsh SW, Leisenring WM, Williams MA. A prospective study of maternal serum C-reactive protein concentrations and risk of preeclampsia. *Am J Hypertens* 2004;17(2):154–60.

82. Conrad KP, Miles TM, Benyo DF. Circulating levels of immunoreactive cytokines in women with preeclampsia. *Am J Reprod Immunol* 1998;40(2):102–11.

83. Dong M, He J, Wang Z, Xie X, Wang H. Placental imbalance of Th1- and Th2-type cytokines in preeclampsia. *Acta Obstet Gynecol Scand* 2005;84(8):788–93.

84. Freeman DJ, McManus F, Brown EA, Cherry L, Norrie J, Ramsay JE, et al. Short- and long-term changes in plasma inflammatory markers associated with preeclampsia. *Hypertension* 2004;44(5):708–14.

85. Alexander BT, Cockrell KL, Massey MB, Bennett WA, Granger JP. Tumor necrosis factor-alpha-induced hypertension in pregnant rats results in decreased renal neuronal nitric oxide synthase expression. *Am J Hypertens* 2002;15(2 Pt 1):170–5.

86. LaMarca BB, Bennett WA, Alexander BT, Cockrell K, Granger JP. Hypertension produced by reductions in uterine perfusion in the pregnant rat: role of tumor necrosis factor-alpha. *Hypertension* 2005;46(4):1022–5.

87. LaMarca BB, Cockrell K, Sullivan E, Bennett W, Granger JP. Role of endothelin in mediating tumor necrosis factor-induced hypertension in pregnant rats. *Hypertension* 2005;46(1):82–6.

88. Samuelsson AM, Ohrn I, Dahlgren J, Eriksson E, Angelin B, Folkow B, et al. Prenatal exposure to IL-6 results in hypertension and increased hypothalamic-pituitary-adrenal axis activity in adult rats. *Endocrinology* 2004;145:4897–4911.

89. Bullo M, Garcia-Lorda P, Megias I, Salas-Salvado J. Systemic inflammation, adipose tissue tumor necrosis factor, and leptin expression. *Obes Res* 2003;11(4):525–31.

90. Fernandez-Real JM, Vayreda M, Richart C, Gutierrez C, Broch M, Vendrell J, et al. Circulating interleukin 6 levels, blood pressure, and insulin sensitivity in apparently healthy men and women. *J Clin Endocrinol Metab* 2001;86(3):1154–9.

91. Pedrinelli R, Dell'Omo G, Di B, V, Pellegrini G, Pucci L, Del PS, et al. Low-grade inflammation and microalbuminuria in hypertension. *Arterioscler Thromb Vasc Biol* 2004;24(12):2414–9.

92. Dorfmuller P, Zarka V, Durand-Gasselin I, Monti G, Balabanian K, Garcia G, et al. Chemokine RANTES in severe pulmonary arterial hypertension. *Am J Respir Crit Care Med* 2002;165(4):534–9.

93. Molet S, Furukawa K, Maghazechi A, Hamid Q, Giaid A. Chemokine- and cytokine-induced expression of endothelin 1 and endothelin-converting enzyme 1 in endothelial cells. *J Allergy Clin Immunol* 2000;105(2 Pt 1):333–8.

94. Reents S. Predisposing factors for severe, uncontrolled hypertension in an inner-city minority population. *N Engl J Med* 1993 21;328(3):214.

95. Fujita M, Mason RJ, Cool C, Shannon JM, Hara N, Fagan KA. Pulmonary hypertension in TNF-alpha-overexpressing mice is associated with decreased VEGF gene expression. *J Appl Physiol* 2002;93(6):2162–70.

96. Ortiz LA, Champion HC, Lasky JA, Gambelli F, Gozal E, Hoyle GW, et al. Enalapril protects mice from pulmonary hypertension by inhibiting TNF-mediated activation of NF-kappaB and AP-1. *Am J Physiol Lung Cell Mol Physiol* 2002;282(6):L1209–21.

97. Miyata M, Sakuma F, Yoshimura A, Ishikawa H, Nishimaki T, Kasukawa R. Pulmonary hypertension in rats. 2. Role of interleukin-6. *Int Arch Allergy Immunol* 1995;108(3):287–91.

98. Wort SJ, Woods M, Warner TD, Evans TW, Mitchell JA. Cyclooxygenase-2 acts as an endogenous brake on endothelin-1 release by human pulmonary artery smooth muscle cells: implications for pulmonary hypertension. *Mol Pharmacol* 2002;62(5):1147–53.

99. Budman DR, Steinberg AD. Hypertension and renal disease in systemic lupus erythematosus. *Arch Intern Med* 1976;136(9):1003–7.

100. Selzer F, Sutton-Tyrrell K, Fitzgerald S, Tracy R, Kuller L, Manzi S. Vascular stiffness in women with systemic lupus erythematosus. *Hypertension* 2001;37(4):1075–82.

101. Swaak AJ, van den Brink HG, Smeenk RJ, Manger K, Kalden JR, Tosi S, et al. Systemic lupus erythematosus: clinical features in patients with a disease duration of over 10 years, first evaluation. *Rheumatology (Oxford)* 1999;38(10):953–8.

102. Barnes EV, Narain S, Naranjo A, Shuster J, Segal MS, Sobel ES, et al. High sensitivity C-reactive protein in systemic lupus erythematosus: relation to disease activity, clinical presentation and implications for cardiovascular risk. *Lupus* 2005;14(8):576–82.

103. Yoshio T, Masuyama JI, Kohda N, Hirata D, Sato H, Iwamoto M, et al. Association of interleukin 6 release from endothelial cells and pulmonary hypertension in SLE. *J Rheumatol* 1997;24(3):489–95.

104. Pausova Z, Deslauriers B, Gaudet D, Tremblay J, Kotchen TA, Larochelle P, et al. Role of tumor necrosis factor-alpha gene locus in obesity and obesity-associated hypertension in French Canadians. *Hypertension* 2000;36(1):14–9.

105. Sookoian S, Garcia SI, Gianotti TF, Dieuzeide G, Gonzalez CD, Pirola CJ. The G-308A promoter variant of the tumor necrosis factor-alpha gene is associated with hypertension in adolescents harboring the metabolic syndrome. *Am J Hypertens* 2005;18(10):1271–5.

106. Izawa H, Yamada Y, Okada T, Tanaka M, Hirayama H, Yokota M. Prediction of genetic risk for hypertension. *Hypertension* 2003;41(5):1035–40.

107. Sheu WH, Lee WJ, Lin LY, Chang RL, Chen YT. Tumor necrosis factor alpha-238 and -308 polymorphisms do not associate with insulin resistance in hypertensive subjects. *Metabolism* 2001;50(12):1447–51.

108. Lee SC, Pu YB, Thomas GN, Lee ZS, Tomlinson B, Cockram CS, et al. Tumor necrosis factor alpha gene G-308A polymorphism in the metabolic syndrome. *Metabolism* 2000;49(8):1021–4.

109. Tanaka C, Mannami T, Kamide K, Takiuchi S, Kokubo Y, Katsuya T, et al. Single nucleotide polymorphisms in the interleukin-6 gene associated with blood pressure and atherosclerosis in a Japanese general population. *Hypertens Res* 2005;28(1):35–41.

110. Losito A, Kalidas K, Santoni S, Jeffery S. Association of interleukin-6-174G/C promoter polymorphism with hypertension and left ventricular hypertrophy in dialysis patients. *Kidney Int* 2003;64(2):616–22.

111. Jeng JR, Wang JH, Liu WS, Chen SP, Chen MY, Wu MH, et al. Association of interleukin-6 gene G-174C polymorphism and plasma plasminogen activator inhibitor-1 level in Chinese patients with and without hypertension. *Am J Hypertens* 2005;18(4 Pt 1):517–22.

112. Suk HJ, Ridker PM, Cook NR, Zee RY. Relation of polymorphism within the C-reactive protein gene and plasma CRP levels. *Atherosclerosis* 2005;178(1):139–45.

113. Davey SG, Lawlor DA, Harbord R, Timpson N, Rumley A, Lowe GD, et al. Association of C-reactive protein with blood pressure and hypertension: life course confounding and Mendelian randomization tests of causality. *Arterioscler Thromb Vasc Biol* 2005;25(5):1051–6.

114. Frossard PM, Gupta A, Pravica V, Perrey C, Hutchinson IV, Lukic ML. A study of five human cytokine genes in human essential hypertension. *Mol Immunol* 2002;38(12–13):969–76.

115. Marz W, Winkler K, Nauck M, Bohm BO, Winkelmann BR. Effects of statins on C-reactive protein and interleukin-6 (the Ludwigshafen Risk and Cardiovascular Health study). *Am J Cardiol* 2003;92(3):305–8.

116. Tsiara S, Elisaf M, Mikhailidis DP. Early vascular benefits of statin therapy. *Curr Med Res Opin* 2003;19(6):540–56.

117. Mervaala E, Muller DN, Park JK, Dechend R, Schmidt F, Fiebeler A, et al. Cyclosporin A protects against angiotensin II–induced end-organ damage in double transgenic rats harboring human renin and angiotensinogen genes. *Hypertension* 2000;35(1 Pt 2):360–6.

Chapter

23 Role of the Kidney in Hypertension

Joey P. Granger and John E. Hall

Key Findings

- Experimental and theoretical evidence strongly support a central role for the kidneys in the long-term regulation of body fluid volume and arterial pressure.

- A pivotal part of the renal-body fluid feedback control system for long-term blood pressure regulation is the renal-pressure natriuresis mechanism whereby increases in renal perfusion pressure lead to significant increases in sodium and water excretion.

- Renal-pressure natriuresis is abnormal in all types of experimental and clinical hypertension.

- Hypertension is an important compensatory mechanism that allows maintenance of sodium balance when renal-pressure natriuresis is impaired.

- Impaired renal-pressure natriuresis and chronic hypertension can be caused by factors that either reduce glomerular filtration rate and/or increase tubular reabsorption.

- A shift of renal-pressure natriuresis can occur as a result of intrarenal abnormalities such as enhanced formation of angiotensin II, reactive oxygen species, and endothelin (via ET_A receptor activation) or decreased synthesis of nitric oxide or natriuretic prostanoids. In other instances, the altered kidney function is caused by extrarenal disturbances, such as increased sympathetic nervous system activity or excessive formation of antinatriuretic hormones such as aldosterone.

Although severe kidney disease has been recognized for more than 100 years to be closely associated with hypertension, the importance of more subtle renal dysfunction in the pathogenesis of essential hypertension has not been as well appreciated, partly because there are no obvious renal defects in most hypertensive patients. Many of the measurements that are commonly used to evaluate kidney function, such as glomerular filtration rate (GFR), renal blood flow, serum creatinine, and sodium excretion are often within the normal range, at least in the early stages of primary (essential) hypertension. On the other hand, increased total peripheral vascular resistance is an obvious abnormality found in most patients with hypertension, leading many to focus mainly on the mechanisms of peripheral vasoconstriction as a cause of hypertension.

An interesting fact to consider is that almost all forms of experimental hypertension are caused by obvious insults to the kidneys that alter renal hemodynamics or tubular reabsorption. For example, constriction of the renal arteries (e.g., Goldblatt hypertension), compression of the kidneys (e.g., perinephritic hypertension), or administration of sodium-retaining hormones (e.g., mineralocorticoids or angiotensin II [Ang II]) are all associated with either initial reductions in renal blood flow and GFR or increases in tubular reabsorption prior to development of hypertension. As blood pressure rises, the initial renal changes are obscured by compensations that restore kidney function toward normal. The rise in blood pressure then initiates a cascade of cardiovascular changes, including increased peripheral vascular resistance that may be more striking than the initial disturbance of kidney function. For this reason the importance of renal dysfunction in causing hypertension has often been underestimated.

Although specific abnormalities of kidney function are difficult to identify in most patients with primary hypertension, there is one aspect of kidney function, the renal-pressure natriuresis mechanism, that is abnormal in all types of experimental and clinical hypertension.[1-3] Renal-pressure natriuresis refers to the effects of increased arterial pressure to raise sodium excretion and is usually accompanied by "pressure diuresis" (increased water excretion). In hypertension, a normal rate of sodium excretion (equal to sodium intake) is maintained despite elevated blood pressure, which would normally cause natriuresis and diuresis.[1-3] This indicates that pressure natriuresis and diuresis are reset in hypertensive subjects. Although the causes of this resetting have been examined in many forms of experimental hypertension and secondary forms of human hypertension, the mechanisms that cause abnormal pressure natriuresis in patients with primary hypertension are not completely understood. Before discussing factors that contribute to abnormal pressure natriuresis in hypertension, we will briefly discuss the basic feedback systems that link renal excretion of sodium and water with altered blood pressure regulation in hypertension.

RENAL–BODY FLUID FEEDBACK SYSTEM FOR LONG-TERM BLOOD PRESSURE REGULATION

Arterial pressure is the product of cardiac output and total peripheral vascular resistance, and moment-to-moment regulation of blood pressure is closely linked to factors that alter either cardiac function or peripheral vascular resistance. However, long-term blood pressure regulation is more complex because it is closely intertwined with control of body fluid volume, which is determined by the balance between fluid intake and renal excretion. Even transient imbalances between fluid intake and excretion can alter extracellular fluid volume and cardiac output, and eventually peripheral vascular resistance, through autoregulatory mechanisms that are activated secondary to changes in blood pressure.[1,4]

Under steady-state conditions, there must be a precise balance between the intake and output of fluid and electrolytes. Otherwise, continued expansion or contraction of body fluid volumes would eventually lead to complete circulatory collapse. In fact, it is much more critical to maintain water and electrolyte balances than to maintain a normal level of blood pressure and, as discussed later, chronic hypertension provides a means of restoring fluid balance when intrarenal and neurohumoral mechanisms are unable to maintain a normal rate of fluid excretion, equal to intake, after a disturbance that impairs kidney function.

Pressure natriuresis, a key component of renal–body fluid feedback

The effect of increased blood pressure to cause natriuresis and diuresis can be shown in acute studies, and is even more impressive with chronic increases in blood pressure.[1,3] If kidney function is not impaired, increased arterial pressure raises sodium excretion, and as long as excretion exceeds intake, extracellular fluid volume continues to decrease, reducing venous return and cardiac output until blood pressure returns to normal and fluid intake and output are re-established (Figure 23–1). Conversely, when blood pressure falls below normal, the kidneys retain sodium and water until arterial pressure is restored to the normal set-point. In this way, pressure natriuresis acts as a key component of a feedback system that normally stabilizes blood pressure and body fluid volumes.

An important feature of renal pressure natriuresis is that various hormonal and neural control systems can amplify or blunt the basic effect of blood pressure on sodium and water excretion.[2,3] For example, during chronic increases in sodium intake, only small changes in blood pressure are needed to maintain sodium balance in many people. One of the reasons for this insensitivity of blood pressure to salt intake is that secretion of antinatriuretic hormones

(e.g., Ang II and aldosterone) is reduced and secretion of natriuretic hormones (e.g., atrial natriuretic peptide) is increased; the hormonal changes then enhance the effectiveness of pressure natriuresis and allow sodium balance to be maintained with minimal increases in blood pressure. Excessive activation of these antinatriuretic systems or deficiency of natriuretic hormones, however, can reduce the effectiveness of pressure natriuresis, thereby necessitating greater increases in blood pressure to maintain sodium balance (as discussed later in this chapter).

Another important characteristic of renal-pressure natriuresis is that it is part of an integral control system with infinite feedback gain.[1] This means that it continues to operate until blood pressure is restored to the original set-point, which is determined by the various intrarenal and neurohumoral mechanisms that control the kidney's ability to excrete sodium and water. Therefore, as long as renal-pressure natriuresis is unaltered, disturbances that tend to raise blood pressure, such as increased cardiac pumping ability or increased peripheral vascular resistance, will not cause chronic hypertension. For sodium balance to be maintained in the face of increased arterial pressure, there must be a concomitant shift of pressure natriuresis to higher blood pressures.

Renal-pressure natriuresis impairment in all forms of experimental and human hypertension

In all forms of hypertension that have been studied, there is a shift of renal-pressure natriuresis that sustains the hypertension.[1–4] The shift of pressure natriuresis can be caused by *intrarenal* disturbances that increase tubular reabsorption or reduce renal blood flow and GFR in some cases. In other instances, the altered kidney function is caused by *extrarenal* disturbances, such as increased sympathetic nervous system (SNS) activity or excessive formation of antinatriuretic hormones, which reduce the kidney's ability to excrete sodium and water, shift pressure natriuresis, and eventually raise arterial pressure.

As discussed later, some renal abnormalities (e.g., increased preglomerular resistance caused by renal artery stenosis) cause a parallel shift of pressure natriuresis toward higher blood pressures without reducing the slope, and are therefore associated with hypertension that is relatively salt-insensitive; thus, the degree of hypertension is not greatly exacerbated by high sodium intake. Other abnormalities of kidney function (e.g., excessive sodium reabsorption in distal parts of the nephron) reduce the slope of pressure natriuresis and cause salt-sensitive hypertension.[2,3] Effective treatment of hypertension therefore requires correction of abnormal pressure natriuresis, either by directly increasing renal excretory capability or indirectly by reducing extrarenal antinatriuretic and antidiuretic influences on the kidneys.

MECHANISMS OF IMPAIRED RENAL-PRESSURE NATRIURESIS IN HYPERTENSION

Impaired renal-pressure natriuresis and chronic hypertension can be caused by factors that either reduce GFR or

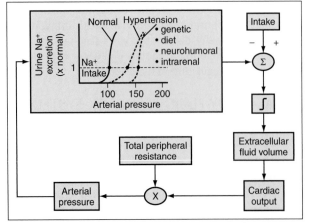

Figure 23–1. Basic renal–body fluid feedback mechanism for long-term regulation of blood pressure and body fluid volumes.

increase tubular reabsorption. Since tubular reabsorption and GFR are both approximately 100-fold greater than urinary excretion of sodium and water, relatively small changes in either of these variables can potentially have large effects on urinary excretion. Under steady-state conditions, a chronic reduction in GFR must be perfectly compensated for by mechanisms that decrease tubular reabsorption if renal excretion is to be returned toward normal and sodium and fluid balance are maintained. Likewise, a sustained increase in tubular reabsorption must be compensated for by increased GFR. Otherwise, fluid retention would continue, eventually causing circulatory collapse.

If intrinsic renal mechanisms or neurohumoral adjustments are capable of returning renal excretion to normal in the face of insults to the kidneys, hypertension may not develop—even with major disturbances—such as loss of functional kidney mass. However, the fact that hypertension occurs so frequently indicates that intrinsic renal mechanisms and neurohumoral controls may not be powerful enough to completely prevent alterations in renal excretion when there are major abnormalities of glomerular filtration or tubular reabsorption. In these instances, increased arterial pressure helps to maintain perfect glomerulotubular balance and normal rates of sodium and water excretion, equal to intake, despite abnormal kidney function. The general types of renal abnormalities that can cause chronic hypertension include (1) increased preglomerular resistance, (2) decreased glomerular capillary filtration coefficient, (3) reduced numbers of functional nephrons, and (4) increased tubular reabsorption (Figure 23–2 and Table 23–1).

Hypertension caused by generalized increases in preglomerular resistance

Examples of a generalized increase in preglomerular resistance are those caused by suprarenal aortic coarctation or

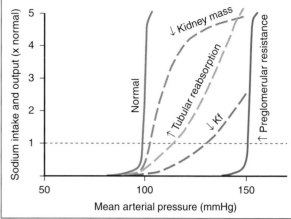

Figure 23–2. Steady-state relationships between arterial pressure and urinary sodium excretion and sodium intake for subjects with normal kidneys and four general types of renal dysfunction that cause hypertension: decreased kidney mass, increased reabsorption in distal and collecting tubules, reductions in glomerular capillary filtration coefficient (K_F), and increased preglomerular resistance. Note that increased preglomerular resistance causes *salt-insensitive* hypertension, whereas the other renal abnormalities cause *salt-sensitive* hypertension.

constriction of one of the renal arteries and removal of the contralateral kidney (e.g., one-kidney, one-clip Goldblatt hypertension). Immediately after constriction of the renal artery or aortic coarctation, renal blood flow is reduced to the kidneys and there is a rapid rise in plasma renin activity and transient sodium retention. Within a few days, sodium excretion returns to normal and sodium balance is reestablished. If sodium intake is normal and adequate volume is available, plasma renin activity also returns to normal in

CAUSES AND CHARACTERISTICS OF SALT-SENSITIVE AND SALT-INSENSITIVE HYPERTENSION						
Causes	Blood Pressure	Pressure Natriuresis	Renal Blood Flow	Glomerular Filtration Rate	Plasma Renin Activity	Glomerulosclerosis[a]
Salt-Sensitive Hypertension						
1. Decreased kidney mass	↑, ⟷	Decreased slope	↓	↓	↓	Yes
2. Decreased glomerular capillary filtration coefficient (K_f)	↑	Decreased slope	↑	↓, ⟷	↑, ⟷	Yes
3. Increased distal and collecting tubule reabsorption	↑	Decreased slope	↑	↑	↓	Yes
Salt-Insensitive Hypertension						
1. Increased preglomerular resistance	↑	Parallel Shift	↓, ⟷	↓, ⟷	↑, ⟷	No
2. Increased reabsorption in proximal tubules and loops of Henle	↑	Parallel Shift	↑	↑	↑, ⟷	Yes
[a]Glomerulosclerosis is predicted to occur secondary to hypertensive stimuli that cause chronic increases in glomerular hydrostatic pressure and/or hyperfiltration of surviving nephrons.						

Table 23–1. Causes and Characteristics of Salt-Sensitive and Salt-Insensitive Hypertension

the established phase of hypertension. At this point, most indices of renal function are nearly normal, including pressure distal to the stenosis if the constriction is not too severe. The rate at which renal function returns to normal and the time course for development of hypertension depend on the severity of the stenosis, sodium intake, and rate of Ang II formation.[1,5]

How do these experimental models of increased preglomerular resistance relate to human hypertension, other than the obvious conditions of aortic coarctation or renal artery stenosis? When Harry Goldblatt[6] first produced hypertension in dogs by constricting the main renal artery, his goal was to produce an experimental model that mimicked the pathologic changes found in human essential hypertension. As a pathologist, Goldblatt noted that many hypertensive patients at autopsy had nephrosclerosis, and he hypothesized that essential hypertension might be caused by diffuse renal arteriolar sclerosis, particularly in preglomerular vessels. Presumably, functional or pathologic increases in preglomerular resistance at other sites besides the main renal arteries, such as the interlobular arteries or afferent arterioles, could also increase arterial pressure through the same mechanisms activated by clipping the renal artery. For example, widespread structural increases in afferent arteriolar resistance (e.g., nephrosclerosis) or functional increases in resistance caused by excessive activation of the sympathetic nervous system or high levels of catecholamines (e.g., pheochromocytoma) would also cause hypertension through the same mechanisms as constriction of the main renal artery.

An observation that led many investigators to question whether Goldblatt hypertension is relevant to human essential hypertension was the finding that many hypertensive patients have no obvious indication of renal ischemia. Renal blood flow and GFR are nearly normal and plasma renin activity may be normal (or even slightly reduced) in many hypertensive patients. However, as previously discussed there is little indication of renal ischemia, even in experimental Goldblatt hypertension after compensatory increases in blood pressure have occurred.

It is interesting to note that some patients with primary hypertension have the same characteristics seen in the one-kidney, one-clip Goldblatt model of hypertension, including nearly normal levels of GFR and plasma renin activity, a parallel shift of pressure natriuresis to higher blood pressures, and a relatively salt-insensitive form of hypertension.[1,2,5] Indeed, studies in hypertensive patients have shown that drug therapy which decreases preglomerular resistance, such as calcium channel blockers, causes a parallel shift of pressure natriuresis toward lower blood pressures.[7] Thus, primary hypertension in some patients may be caused by functional or pathologic increases in preglomerular resistance. This is almost certainly the case in patients who have severe arthrosclerotic lesions in the renal blood vessels.

Hypertension caused by nonhomogeneous, patchy increases in preglomerular resistance

In the two-kidney, one-clip Goldblatt model of hypertension, there is a nonhomogeneous increase in preglomerular

resistance with ischemia occurring in nephrons of the clipped kidney, while nephrons in the contralateral untouched kidney have increased single nephron blood flow and GFR. The underperfused clipped kidney secretes large amounts of renin, whereas the untouched kidney secretes very little renin.[1,3]

An important distinction between a generalized increase in preglomerular resistance and patchy, nonhomogeneous increases in preglomerular resistance is the evolution of renal injury associated with hypertension. When there is a generalized increase in preglomerular resistance, caused by renal artery stenosis of a single kidney, the glomeruli are protected from the damaging effects of increased blood pressure. In the two-kidney, one-clip model, however, the glomeruli of the untouched kidney are subjected to the full effects of increased blood pressure. With prolonged hypertension, pathological changes in the untouched kidney add to the impairment of overall renal excretory capability. At this stage, removal of the clipped kidney only partially restores arterial pressure to normal. However, removal of the contralateral untouched kidney and unclipping the stenotic kidney normalizes blood pressure. Thus, in this model chronic exposure to high blood pressure in the untouched kidney apparently causes structural changes as well as functional changes that in turn contribute to the progression of hypertension.

The relevance of experimental models of nonhomogeneous increases in preglomerular resistance to human hypertension is obvious in cases of stenosis in only one renal artery with the contralateral kidney being unaffected. Eventually, the contralateral kidney becomes injured, leading to further amplification of hypertension and loss of kidney function if the hypertension is untreated. In some patients with essential hypertension, there may also be patchy nephrosclerosis within each kidney providing a clinical counterpart to the two-kidney Goldblatt model of hypertension. In these instances, the ischemic nephrons secrete large amounts of renin and the nonischemic nephrons vasodilate and initially have increased single nephron GFR.[8] However, the combined effects of hypertension and hyperfiltration eventually damage the nephrons that were initially nonischemic, leading to progressive nephron loss.

Hypertension caused by decreased glomerular capillary filtration coefficient

Reducing the glomerular capillary filtration coefficient (K_f) initially lowers GFR and sodium excretion. Renal vasodilation of afferent arterioles and increased renin release occur via macula densa feedback due to reduced NaCl delivery to the macula densa. The initial sodium retention and increased Ang II formation lead to increased arterial pressure, which helps to restore GFR and renin release toward normal. After these compensations, the main persistent abnormalities of kidney function are reduced filtration fraction, increased glomerular hydrostatic pressure, and increased renal blood flow.

Unfortunately, these compensatory increases in arterial pressure and glomerular hydrostatic pressure, which are needed to offset a fall in K_f and to restore sodium excretion to normal, may also lead to additional renal dysfunction over a period of years by causing further glomerular injury; this further reduces K_f and requires additional increases in blood pressure to maintain normal water and electrolyte balances. Such a sequence may initiate progressive kidney damage.

The clinical counterparts of this sequence may be found in hypertension caused by glomerulonephritis or by other conditions that cause thickening and damage to the glomerular capillary membranes, such as chronic diabetes mellitus.[9]

Effects of reduced numbers of functional nephrons

A factor that contributes to salt sensitivity of blood pressure and decreased plasma renin activity in some hypertensive patients is a loss of functional nephrons. Complete loss of nephrons (such as surgical reduction of kidney mass) in the absence of other abnormalities usually does not lead to significant hypertension.[1,3] In contrast, loss of functional nephrons due to ischemia or infarction of renal tissue usually causes marked hypertension that is initially due to increased renin secretion in the early stages and then is eventually mediated by additional abnormalities, such as immunological renal injury, in the established phase of the hypertension.[10]

Considering our previous discussion, one might predict that reductions in the number of functional nephrons should impair renal excretory capability and cause hypertension regardless of whether the loss was associated with renal ischemia. Yet, experimental studies have shown that surgical removal of large amounts of the kidney, to the point that uremia occurs, rarely causes severe hypertension as long as sodium intake is normal.[1,11] The reason that loss of entire nephrons *per se*, without ischemia in the remaining nephrons, does not cause usually cause marked hypertension is that overall glomerular filtration and tubular reabsorption capability are simultaneously reduced so that balance between filtration and reabsorption can be maintained without major adaptive changes in blood pressure. However, reducing the number of functional nephrons makes the kidneys very susceptible to additional insults that impair their function or to additional challenges of sodium homeostasis. Thus, hypertension associated with excess mineralocorticoids is much more severe after reducing kidney mass. Likewise, the kidney's ability to increase sodium excretion in response to the additional challenge of high sodium intake is accompanied by much larger increases in blood pressure when kidney mass is reduced.[1,3,11]

With the loss of entire nephrons, each surviving nephron must excrete greater amounts of sodium and water to maintain balance. This is achieved by increasing GFR and decreasing reabsorption in the remaining nephrons, resulting in increased sodium chloride delivery to the macula densa and suppression of renin release. This, in turn, impairs the kidney's ability to further decrease renin release during high sodium intake. Therefore, after loss of kidney mass blood pressure become very salt sensitive.

Although the functional effects of nephron loss may not cause hypertension in the absence of high salt intake or other insults to the kidney, compensatory changes that take place after nephron loss may eventually damage the surviving nephrons.[9] For example, renal vasodilation and increased single-nephron GFR may, over long periods of time, lead to glomerulosclerosis and reductions in K_f. These pathologic changes, in addition to the loss of functional nephrons, may eventually shift pressure natriuresis sufficiently to cause severe hypertension.

What is the relevance of experimental models produced by surgically removing kidney mass to human hypertension? With normal aging there is gradual loss of functional nephrons after age 40 and this loss of nephrons is accelerated by renal diseases, such as glomerulonephritis, diabetes mellitus, or long-standing hypertension. Thus, even though hypertension may not begin with loss of nephrons, chronic elevations in glomerular pressure and other metabolic abnormalities that are often associated with hypertension may eventually cause injury to the glomeruli and progressive nephron loss that amplifies the hypertension and makes blood pressure more salt sensitive.

Loss of functional nephrons by partial renal infarction

The experimental model of surgical reduction of kidney mass should not be confused with the model of infarction hypertension produced by tying off branches of the renal artery, the so-called "5–6 ablation" model. This model is usually produced by removing one kidney and obstructing two of the three branches of the renal artery of the remaining kidney. In the infarction model, hypertension develops even without a high sodium intake due to ischemia of the surviving nephrons, activation of the renin-angiotensin system, and immune-mediated injury of the kidney.[9,10] In reality, the 5–6 renal ablation hypertension is a model of severe patchy renal ischemia with characteristics similar to that described for the one-kidney, one-clip Goldblatt model or nonhomogeneous patchy glomerulosclerosis.

Hypertension caused by increased tubular reabsorption

Hypertension can also be caused by factors that raise tubular reabsorption, such as excessive formation of mineralocorticoids or Ang II. The severity of hypertension depends on the degree to which tubular reabsorption is stimulated and on other factors such as the functional kidney mass and sodium intake. When kidney function is otherwise normal, mineralocorticoids may have only moderate hypertensive effects.[1,3] However, with loss of functional nephrons, the hypertensive potency of mineralocorticoids is greatly enhanced.

Increased distal and collecting tubule reabsorption causes salt-sensitive hypertension

One feature of hypertension caused by increased distal or collecting tubular reabsorption is that it is usually salt sensitive, with increased sodium intake exacerbating the hypertension. Increased reabsorption at sites beyond the macula densa, such as the distal tubules and collecting tubules, causes a salt-sensitive form of hypertension because it also elicits chronic increases in sodium chloride delivery to the macula densa that, in turn, suppresses renin secretion.[1-4] The increased distal tubule sodium chloride delivery occurs as a compensation for increased distal and collecting tubular reabsorption in order to maintain sodium balance. The reduction of renin secretion to very low levels, characteristic of disorders associated with increased distal or collecting tubular reabsorption, prevents further suppression of Ang II formation during high sodium intake, and therefore makes blood pressure salt sensitive.

In addition, blood pressure caused by increased tubular reabsorption is often associated with a tendency toward extracellular volume expansion. However, when increased tubular reabsorption is associated with marked peripheral vasoconstriction, such as occurs with very high levels of Ang II, the degree of volume expansion depends on the relative effects of the vasoconstrictor on the peripheral blood vessels and the renal blood vessels.[1,12] With severe peripheral vasoconstriction and decreased vascular capacitance, relatively small amounts of volume retention can lead to marked hypertension.

Increased proximal reabsorption causes salt-insensitive hypertension

If increased tubular reabsorption occurs in the proximal tubules or loop of Henle, prior to the macula densa, a salt-insensitive form of hypertension usually results. Increased tubular reabsorption prior to the macula densa tends to increase renin secretion and elicits a compensatory renal vasodilation that raises GFR and renal plasma flow. However, as hypertension develops, the macula densa sodium chloride delivery and renin secretion return to nearly normal, and the renin-angiotensin system (RAS) is fully capable of responding to additional challenges such as increased sodium intake. Therefore, high sodium intake is accompanied by appropriate suppression of renin release and Ang II formation, which permits sodium balance to be maintained with only small increases in blood pressure.[3,12] Nevertheless, the pressure natriuresis mechanisms are shifted to higher blood pressures parallel to the normal curve, and the severity of the hypertension depends on the degree to which reabsorption is increased in the proximal tubules and loops of Henle.

SALT-SENSITIVE AND SALT-INSENSITIVE HYPERTENSION

Salt sensitivity of blood pressure is a quantitative phenotype, rather than following the bi-modal categorization of "salt sensitive" or "salt insensitive," and there is considerable heterogeneity of blood pressure responses to changes in sodium intake in normotensive as well as in hypertensive subjects.[13,14]

Although various methods have been used to assess salt sensitivity, most protocols involve relatively short-term changes in sodium intake, typically over a few days. Weinberger et al.[13] defined salt sensitivity as a 10-mmHg or greater change in mean blood pressure from the level measured after a 4-hour infusion of 2 liters of normal saline compared to the level measured the morning after 1 day of a low (10 mmol) sodium diet and administration of three doses of furosemide. With this definition, 51% of hyper-

tensive and 26% of normotensive subjects were found to be salt sensitive.[13] However, there has been little effort to determine the repeatability of salt sensitivity in the same persons over long periods of time (years), and it is not known whether short-term blood pressure responses reliably predict the long-term effects of changes in salt intake.

What are the factors that contribute to salt sensitivity of blood pressure? From clinical observations it is clear that there are many demographic and pathophysiologic conditions associated with salt sensitivity.[3,12] Older individuals are usually more salt sensitive than young people, and African–Americans are often more salt sensitive than Caucasians. It should be recognized, however, that there are many exceptions to these generalizations and considerable heterogeneity exists in the blood pressure responses to changes in salt intake even in these populations.

Genetic factors independent of race have been linked to salt sensitivity of blood pressure. For example, genetic abnormalities that increase distal and collecting tubule sodium reabsorption or that cause excess secretion of sodium-retaining hormones (e.g., mineralocorticoids) cause salt-sensitivity of blood pressure.[14,15] Also, diabetes mellitus, renal diseases that cause loss of nephron function, and abnormalities of the RAS are all associated with increased salt sensitivity of blood pressure.[12-14] All of these examples appear to share two common pathways to the salt sensitivity of blood pressure: (1) loss of functional nephrons, or (2) reduced responsiveness of the RAS.

Loss of functional nephrons as a major cause of salt-sensitive blood pressure

As discussed previously, the effect of nephron loss to enhance salt sensitivity has been well established from experimental and clinical studies. Figure 23–3 shows the effect of surgically reducing kidney mass on salt sensitivity in dogs. As long as sodium intake was normal, surgical reduction of kidney mass by 25%, or even as much as 70%, did not markedly alter blood pressure.[11] However, after loss of kidney mass, blood pressure became exquisitely sensitive to changes in sodium intake, and with high sodium intake blood pressure rose by approximately 40 mmHg.

How is this experimental study conducted in dogs relevant to human hypertension? Even in normal healthy people, there appears to be about a 10% decrease in the number of functional nephrons per decade of life after age 40.[16,17] By age 70 the average healthy individual would be predicted to have at least a 30% decrease in the number of functional nephrons. When there is underlying renal disease, hypertension, or diabetes, the loss of nephrons with aging is greatly exacerbated. Other less common causes of nephron loss include primary renal diseases such as glomerulonephritis, acquired renal disease caused by analgesic abuse, uncontrolled diabetes mellitus, and developmental causes due to poor maternal nutrition or placental ischemia.

Reduced responsiveness of the RAS as a major cause of salt-sensitive blood pressure

The RAS is the most powerful hormonal system in the body for controlling sodium excretion and therefore plays

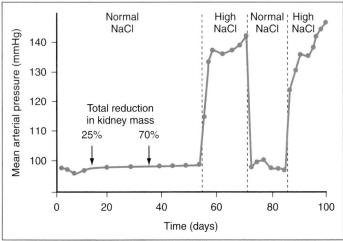

Figure 23–3. The effect of reducing kidney mass on salt sensitivity in dogs. Note that as long as sodium chloride intake was normal, surgical reduction of kidney mass by 25% or even 70% did not markedly alter arterial pressure. However, after loss of kidney mass, blood pressure became exquisitely sensitive to high sodium chloride intake. (Data from Langston JB, Guyton AC, Douglas BH, Dorsett PE. *Circulation Res* 1963;12:508–12.)

a major role in determining salt sensitivity of blood pressure.[18] With high sodium intake, suppression of the RAS permits normal excretion of sodium and water without substantial increases in blood pressure. Conversely, activation of the RAS is a primary mechanism for preventing a reduction in blood pressure during low sodium intake.

Figure 23–4 shows the importance of changes in Ang II formation in maintaining blood pressure relatively constant during variations in salt intake from 5 mmol/day up to 80, 240, and 500 mmol/day for 8 days at each level.

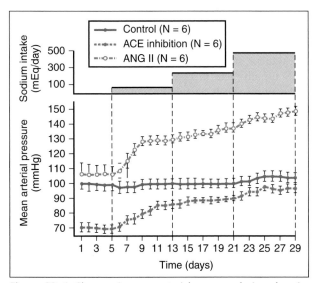

Figure 23–4. Changes in mean arterial pressure during chronic changes in sodium intake from a low level of 5 mmol/day to 80, 240, and 500 mmol/day in normal control dogs, after ACE inhibition, or when Ang II was infused at a constant low dose (5 ng/kg/min) to prevent Ang II from being suppressed when sodium intake was raised. (Data from Hall JE, Guyton AC, Smith MJ Jr, Coleman TG. *Am J Physiol* 1980;239:F271–80.)

In normal dogs, with a functional RAS, there were only small increases in blood pressure associated with this 100-fold range of sodium intakes.[19] However, when Ang II was infused at a low level that had initially little effect on blood pressure but which prevented Ang II from being suppressed as sodium intake was raised, blood pressure became very salt sensitive. After blockade of Ang II formation, blood pressure also became salt sensitive, although pressure was maintained at a much lower level, especially when sodium intake was low.[19] Thus, one of the major functions of the RAS is to permit wide variations in intake and excretion of sodium without large fluctuations in blood pressure that would otherwise be needed to maintain sodium balance.

What clinical conditions can lead to reduced responsiveness of the RAS? Focal nephrosclerosis or patchy preglomerular vasoconstriction, as occurs with renal infarcts, leads to increased renin secretion in ischemic nephrons and suppressed renin secretion in overperfused nephrons.[8] In ischemic as well as overperfused nephrons, the ability to adequately suppress renin secretion during high salt intake is impaired.

Another cause of reduced responsiveness of the RAS is increased distal and collecting tubular sodium reabsorption, as occurs with mineralocorticoid excess or mutations that increase distal and collecting tubule reabsorption (e.g., Liddle's syndrome). In these conditions, excess sodium retention causes almost complete suppression of renin secretion, and therefore an inability to further decrease renin release during high sodium intake. As a result, blood pressure becomes very salt sensitive. It is interesting that every known form of monogenetic hypertension discovered in humans thus far is mediated by a common pathway—excess renal tubular sodium chloride reabsorption that, in turn, impairs renal-pressure natriuresis and causes salt-sensitive hypertension.[15]

As discussed previously, not all renal abnormalities cause salt-sensitive hypertension. Some, such as generalized diffuse increases in preglomerular resistance, cause a parallel shift of pressure natriuresis and hypertension, but do not cause salt sensitivity of blood pressure. Salt sensitivity is not increased in this form of hypertension because the RAS system is fully capable of appropriate suppression during high sodium intake, and sodium balance is maintained with minimal increases in blood pressure.

Salt-sensitive subjects may have greater target-organ injury

What is the clinical significance of salt sensitivity besides the obvious fact that it provides insight into the pathogenesis of hypertension and it indicates which patients may benefit most from reduction of salt intake? Perhaps less obvious is that salt sensitivity may also predict which patients are at greatest risk for hypertensive target-organ injury. Salt-sensitive forms of hypertension caused by increased distal tubular reabsorption, nephron loss, or inability to suppress Ang II formation are usually associated with glomerular hyperfiltration and increased glomerular hydrostatic pressure that is further amplified by the hypertension[3,12] (Table 23–1). Together the hypertension and renal hyperfiltration promote glomerular injury and may eventually cause loss of nephron function. Clinical studies support this concept and have demonstrated that salt-sensitive subjects typically have an increase in glomerular hydrostatic pressure and albumin excretion when given a salt load, whereas salt-resistant subjects have lower glomerular hydrostatic pressure and less urinary albumin excretion.[20]

There is also evidence that salt-sensitive subjects may die earlier than subjects who are salt resistant. In a study by Weinberger et al.[21] in which subjects were followed for more than 20 years, normotensive subjects with increased salt sensitivity died almost a the same rate as hypertensive subjects and much faster than salt-resistant subjects who were normotensive. Whether this increased risk was related to hemodynamic or blood pressure effects of salt or to other effects is still unclear. It is also not known whether long-term high salt intake, lasting over many years, may cause a person who is initially "salt insensitive" to become "salt sensitive" due to gradual renal injury.

THE RENIN-ANGIOTENSIN SYSTEM

The RAS is perhaps the most powerful hormone system for regulating body fluid volumes and arterial pressure, as evidenced by the effectiveness of various RAS blockers in reducing blood pressure in normotensive and hypertensive subjects. Although the RAS has many components, its most important effects on blood pressure regulation are exerted by Ang II, which participates in both short-term and long-term control of arterial pressure. Ang II is a powerful vasoconstrictor and helps maintain blood pressure in conditions associated with acute volume depletion (e.g., hemorrhage), sodium depletion, or circulatory depression (e.g., heart failure). The long-term effects of Ang II on blood pressure, however, are closely intertwined with volume homeostasis through direct and indirect effects on the kidneys.

When the RAS is fully functional, the chronic renal-pressure natriuresis curve is steep, and sodium balance can be maintained over a wide range of intakes with minimal changes in blood pressure (Figure 23–5). One reason for the effectiveness of the normal pressure natriuresis mechanism is that Ang II levels are suppressed during high sodium intake and increased when sodium intake is restricted, thereby adjusting renal sodium excretion appropriately without the need to invoke large changes in blood pressure to maintain sodium balance.

Blockade of the RAS, with Ang II–receptor blockers (ARBs) or angiotensin-converting enzyme (ACE) inhibitors increases renal excretory capability so that sodium balance can be maintained at reduced blood pressures.[19] However, blockade of the RAS also reduces the slope of pressure natriuresis and makes blood pressure salt sensitive.[19] Inappropriately high levels of Ang II reduce renal excretory capability and impair pressure natriuresis, thereby reducing the slope and necessitating increased blood pressure to maintain sodium balance.

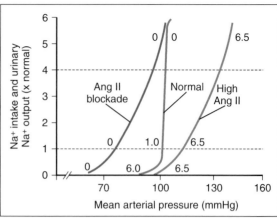

Figure 23–5. Steady-state relationships between arterial pressure and sodium intake and excretion under normal conditions with a fully functional renin-angiotensin system, after blockade of Ang II formation with an ACE inhibitor, and after Ang II infusion at a low dose to prevent Ang II levels from being supressed when sodium intake was increased. The numbers along the curves are estimated Ang II levels expressed as times normal. (Modified from data in Hall JE, Guyton AC, Smith MJ Jr, Coleman TG. *Am J Physiol* 1980;239:F271–80.)

Mechanisms for the potent antinatriuretic effects of Ang II include renal hemodynamic effects as well as direct and indirect effects to increase tubular reabsorption.[18] In most physiologic conditions, such as reduced sodium intake or renal ischemia, increased Ang II causes renal vasoconstriction but does not reduce GFR.[18] Instead, Ang II increases renal sodium reabsorption through multiple hemodynamic and tubular effects.

Ang II–mediated efferent arteriolar constriction attenuates GFR reductions in underperfused kidneys

Physiological activation of the RAS usually occurs as compensation for conditions that cause underperfusion of the kidneys, such as sodium depletion or hemorrhage. The RAS usually acts in concert with other autoregulatory mechanisms, such as tubuloglomerular feedback (TGF) and myogenic activity, to maintain a relatively constant GFR when kidney perfusion is threatened.[18,22] In these cases, administration of ARBs or ACE inhibitors may further reduce GFR, even though renal blood flow is preserved. The impairment of GFR after RAS blockade is due, in part, to inhibition of the constrictor effects of Ang II on efferent arterioles, as well as reduced arterial pressure.[18]

The effects of Ang II appear to be most important when renal perfusion pressure is reduced to low levels, near the limits of autoregulation, or when other disturbances such as sodium depletion are superimposed on low perfusion pressure. Clinically, the importance of the constrictor effects of Ang II on efferent arterioles becomes especially important in patients with renal artery stenosis and/or sodium depletion who may have substantial decreases in GFR when treated with RAS blockers.[23,24]

The relatively weak constrictor action of Ang II on preglomerular vessels is related, in part, to selective protection of these vessels by autacoid mechanisms such as prostaglandins or nitric oxide (NO). After blockade of prostaglandin synthesis or inhibition of EDNO, Ang II infusion caused marked constriction of preglomerular as well as postglomerular vessels (see Hall[18] and Hall et al.[25] for review). When the ability of the kidneys to produce these autacoids is impaired by treatment with nonsteroidal anti-inflammatory drugs or by chronic vascular disease (e.g., atherosclerosis), increased levels of Ang II may reduce GFR by constricting afferent and efferent arterioles.

Increased Ang II exacerbates glomerular injury in overperfused kidneys

Although blockade of the vasoconstrictor effects of Ang II on the efferent arterioles may cause a further decline in GFR in underperfused nephrons, RAS blockade may be beneficial when nephrons are hyperfiltering and Ang II is not appropriately suppressed. For example, in diabetes mellitus and in certain forms of hypertension associated with glomerulosclerosis and nephron loss, Ang II blockade, by decreasing efferent arteriolar resistance and arterial pressure, lowers glomerular hydrostatic pressure and attenuates glomerular hyperfiltration.[25–27] Clinical and experimental studies indicate that RAS blockers are more effective than other antihypertensive agents in preventing glomerular injury, even with similar reductions in blood pressure[28,29]; this appears to be due partly to a greater reduction in glomerular hydrostatic pressure caused by vasodilation of efferent arterioles after blockade of the RAS.

Do nonhemodynamic effects of Ang II cause renal injury?

Ang II has also been suggested to cause glomerular injury through direct actions that promote vascular smooth muscle, increased collagen formation, and production of extracellular matrix by mesangial cells, in addition to its hemodynamic effects.[30,31] Much of the evidence supporting this hypothesis comes from *in vitro* studies, often using supraphysiologic concentrations of Ang II. Although *in vivo* studies have demonstrated greater renoprotective effects of RAS blockers compared to other antihypertensive drugs, decreases in glomerular hydrostatic pressure due to efferent arteriolar vasodilation may have contributed to these beneficial effects. Moreover, in studies where arterial pressure was measured very accurately using 24-hour telemetry, the renoprotective effects of RAS blockade appear to be due largely to hemodynamic effects including the reductions in arterial pressure.[32]

The concept that Ang II directly mediates renal injury independent of blood pressure is difficult to reconcile with the finding that physiologic activation of the RAS is not associated with vascular, glomerular, or tubulointerstitial injury as long as the kidney is not overperfused or exposed to high blood pressure. For example, sodium depletion does not cause renal injury despite marked increases in renal Ang II levels. Also, the clipped kidney of the two-kidney, one-clip Goldblatt model of hypertension is exposed to high Ang II levels, but is protected from increased arterial pressure by the clip on the renal artery and has no visible injury as long as the stenosis is not too severe.

However, the nonclipped kidney, exposed to lower Ang II concentrations but higher blood pressures, has marked focal segmental glomerular sclerosis as well as tubulointerstitial changes characteristic of hypertension.[33] These observations suggest that the hemodynamic effects of Ang II are necessary for many of the glomerular, tubular, interstitial proliferative, and other phenotypic changes that occur in Ang II–dependent hypertension.

Ang II–mediated changes in peritubular capillary dynamics promote increased tubular reabsorption

Ang II–mediated constriction of efferent arterioles stabilizes GFR, but also reduces renal blood flow and peritubular capillary hydrostatic pressure, and increases peritubular colloid osmotic pressure as a result of increased filtration fraction.[18] These changes, in turn, reduce the hydrostatic pressure of renal interstitial fluid and raise interstitial fluid colloid osmotic pressure, thereby increasing the driving force for fluid reabsorption across tubular epithelial cells and reducing back-leak of sodium from the intercellular spaces into the tubules.

The effects of Ang II on renal hemodynamics and interstitial fluid dynamics may also alter reabsorption in more distal parts of the tubule. For example, reductions in renal medullary blood flow due to efferent arteriolar constriction or to direct effects of Ang II on the vasa recta may enhance reabsorption in the loop of Henle and collecting ducts.[18,34] Thus, there are several pathways by which subtle changes in renal hemodynamics, without major changes in GFR, may mediate the effects of Ang II to enhance renal sodium reabsorption.

Ang II directly stimulates proximal tubular sodium reabsorption

The proximal tubule was the first site at which Ang II was shown to directly stimulate sodium and fluid transport in the nephron. This effect occurs at very low Ang II concentrations (10^{-13} to 10^{-10} M) and is mediated by actions on the luminal and basolateral membranes[35] (Figure 23–6). Ang II stimulates the sodium-hydrogen antiporter on the luminal membrane and increases sodium-potassium-ATPase activity as well as sodium-bicarbonate co-transport on the basolateral membrane. These effects appear to be due in part to inhibition of an adenyl cyclase and increased phospholipase C activity. These combined actions of Ang II greatly enhance proximal tubular sodium reabsorption by increasing sodium entry into the epithelial cells, sodium extrusion into the interstitial fluid, and uptake of sodium and fluid into the peritubular capillaries.[36]

Ang II increases sodium reabsorption in loop of Henle, macula densa, and distal nephron segments

In vivo microperfusion studies have shown that Ang II, in physiologic concentrations, increases bicarbonate reabsorption in the loop of Henle and stimulates sodium-potassium-2-chloride transport in the medullary thick ascending loop of Henle (TALH).[37,38] Ang II stimulates multiple ion transporters in the distal parts of the nephron, which include

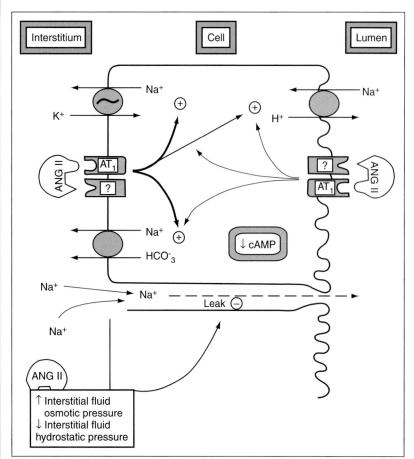

Figure 23–6. Ang II increases proximal tubular reabsorption by binding to receptors on the luminal and basolateral membranes and stimulating Na^+/H^+ antiporter, Na^+/HCO_3^- co-transport, and Na^+/K^+ ATPase activity. ANG II also increases reabsorption by increasing interstitial fluid colloid osmotic pressure and decreasing interstitial fluid hydrostatic pressure.

hydrogen-ATPase activity as well as epithelial sodium channel activity in the cortical collecting ducts.[34,39]

Ang II may also stimulate ion transport in the macula densa epithelial cells, a nephron site that may be particularly important in determining the final urine excretion of sodium. The macula densa is a crucial component of TGF, which operates to maintain a relatively constant delivery of sodium chloride to the distal tubules by feedback regulation of afferent and efferent arteriolar resistances and therefore GFR. Ang II amplifies TGF feedback sensitivity, probably by stimulating macula densa sodium chloride transport.[25,40] In this way, enhanced feedback sensitivity permits a decrease in distal sodium chloride delivery without compensatory increases in GFR via TGF. Decreased distal tubular sodium chloride delivery, caused by the multiple proximal tubule and vascular actions of Ang II, combines with other actions of Ang II on the distal nephron sites to reduce sodium excretion and exert powerful antinatriuretic effects. For this reason, Ang II is one of the most powerful sodium-retaining hormones in the body, and therefore exerts important effects on renal pressure natriuresis and long-term blood pressure regulation. Conversely, blockade of Ang II provides a means of enhancing renal excretory capability, thereby allowing sodium balance to be maintained at greatly reduced arterial blood pressures.

ALDOSTERONE

Aldosterone is also a powerful sodium-retaining hormone, and consequently has important effects on pressure natriuresis and long-term regulation blood pressure. The primary sites of actions of aldosterone on sodium reabsorption are in distal tubules, cortical collecting tubules, and collecting ducts where aldosterone stimulates sodium reabsorption and potassium secretion. These effects are due mainly to binding of aldosterone to intracellular mineralocorticoid receptors (MR) and activation of transcription by target genes.[41] These, in turn, stimulate synthesis or activation of the sodium-potassium ATPase pump on the basolateral epithelial membrane and activation of amiloride-sensitive sodium channels on the luminal side of the epithelial membrane. These effects are termed "genomic" because they are mediated by activation of gene transcription and require 60 to 90 minutes to occur after administration of aldosterone.

Aldosterone is also thought to exert more rapid *nongenomic* effects on the kidney and cardiovascular system.[42] Aldosterone increases the sodium current in the principal cells of the cortical collecting tubule through activation of the amiloride-sensitive channel and stimulates the sodium-hydrogen exchanger in a few minutes after application (see Funder[42] and Wehling et al.[43] for reviews). In vascular smooth muscle cells, aldosterone stimulates sodium influx by activating the sodium-hydrogen exchanger in less than 4 minutes. Acute aldosterone administration may rapidly reduce forearm blood flow in humans,[44] although some investigators have found either no change or an increase in blood flow.[45] The putative membrane receptor and the cell-signaling mechanisms responsible for these rapid nongenomic actions of aldosterone have not been identified, especially with physiologic levels of aldosterone. Thus, the importance of the nongenomic effects of aldosterone on long-term regulation of renal-pressure natriuresis and blood pressure are still unclear.

The overall effects of aldosterone on renal pressure natriuresis are similar to those observed for Ang II. With low sodium intake, increased aldosterone helps prevent sodium loss and reductions in blood pressure. Conversely, during high sodium intake, suppression of aldosterone helps to prevent excessive sodium retention and attenuates an increase in blood pressure.

Excess aldosterone secretion reduces the slope of pressure natriuresis so that blood pressure becomes very salt sensitive. Thus, increasing plasma aldosterone 6- to 10-fold cause marked hypertension when sodium intake is normal or elevated, but there is very little effect on blood pressure when sodium intake is low.[1,46]

In recent years, interest has turned once again to the role of aldosterone and activation of MR in human hypertension. Some investigators have suggested that hyperaldosteronism or excess activation of MR may be more common than previously believed, especially in patients with resistant hypertension. For example, the prevalence of primary aldosteronism has been reported to be almost 20% among patients referred to specialty clinics for resistant hypertension. Many of these resistant patients are overweight or obese.[47]

Regardless of the prevalence of primary aldosteronism, there is emerging evidence that antagonism of MR may provide an important therapeutic tool for preventing target organ injury and reducing blood pressure in hypertension.[47–49] We have previously shown, for example, antagonism of MR attenuated sodium retention, hypertension, and glomerular hypofiltration in obese dogs fed a high-fat diet.[50] This finding was somewhat surprising in view of the fact that plasma aldosterone concentration was only slightly elevated in obesity.[51] However, even mild increases of plasma aldosterone may contribute to increased blood pressure when accompanied by marked sodium retention and volume expansion since aldosterone greatly enhances salt sensitivity of blood pressure.

Another possible explanation for the effectiveness of MR antagonisms in obese, insulin-resistant patients is that there may be enhanced sensitivity to the effects of aldosterone due to increased abundance of epithelial sodium channels (ENaC), which would amplify the effects of MR activation on sodium reabsorption and blood pressure. It is also possible that the marked effects of MR blockade to reduce blood pressure in obesity are mediated partly by glucocorticoid activation of the MR. Normally the MR is "protected" from activation by glucocorticoids due to the effects of 11β-hydroxysteroid dehydrogenase 2 (11β-HSD2) which converts active cortisol into inactive cortisone (see Chapter 68). Reductions in 11β-HSD2 in the renal tubules would therefore lead to increased MR activation by cortisol, causing sodium retention, hypokalemia, and hypertension. Although studies in some experimental models of hypertension, such as the Dahl salt-sensitive rat, have shown reduced expression of 11β-HSD2 in the kidney, there have been few studies that have assessed the potential role of this mechanism in human obesity hypertension.

THE SYMPATHETIC NERVOUS SYSTEM

The SNS is an important short-term and long-term controller of arterial pressure. Sympathetic vasoconstrictor fibers are distributed to almost all regions of the vasculature as well as to the heart, and activation of the SNS can raise blood pressure in a few seconds by causing vasoconstriction, increased cardiac pumping capability, and increased heart rate. Conversely, sudden inhibition of SNS activity can decrease arterial pressure to as low as half normal within less than a minute. Therefore, changes in SNS activity caused by various reflex mechanisms, central nervous system

(CNS) ischemia, or activation of higher centers in the brain provide powerful and rapid, moment-to-moment regulation of arterial pressure.

The SNS plays an important role in long-term regulation of arterial pressure and in the pathogenesis of hypertension by activation of the renal sympathetic nerves.[52] There is extensive innervation of the renal blood vessels, the juxtaglomerular apparatus, and the renal tubules and excessive activation of these nerves causes sodium retention, increased renin secretion, and impaired renal-pressure natriuresis.[52] Except for extreme circumstances, such as severe hemorrhage or other conditions associated with marked circulatory depression, activation of the renal sympathetic nerves is usually not great enough to cause marked reductions in renal blood flow or GFR. However, even mild increases of renal sympathetic activity stimulate renin secretion and sodium reabsorption in multiple segments of the nephron, including the proximal tubule, the loop of Henle, and more distal segments.[52] Thus, the renal nerves provide a mechanism by which the various reflex mechanisms and higher CNS centers can contribute to long-term regulation of arterial pressure.

The preganglionic neurons that synapse with the renal sympathetic postganglionic fibers are located in the lower thoracic and upper lumbar segments of the spinal cord and receive multiple inputs from various regions of the brain, including the brain stem, forebrain, and cerebral cortex. These complex neural pathways provide multiple pathways by which neural reflexes and higher CNS centers can influence renal SNS activity and chronic regulation of arterial pressure.[53,54]

Evidence for a role of the renal nerves in hypertension comes from multiple studies showing that renal denervation reduces blood pressure in various models of experimental hypertension.[52] For example, complete renal denervation attenuates the development of hypertension in spontaneously hypertensive rats[52] as well as in obese hypertensive dogs.[55] Renal denervation may also delay or attenuate increased blood pressure in several forms of experimental hypertension, although some studies have not found an important role for the renal nerves in various forms of secondary hypertension. In Ang II hypertension, for example, *decreased* renal sympathetic activity appears to attenuate the rise in blood pressure.[56]

Human primary hypertension, especially when associated with obesity, is often associated with increased renal sympathetic activity.[57] Although the mechanisms that cause activation of renal sympathetic nerves in primary hypertension or in most experimental models are still unclear, we will briefly discuss three that have attracted considerable interest.

Resetting of baroreceptor reflexes in hypertension

The importance of the arterial baroreceptors in buffering moment-to-moment changes in blood pressure is clearly evident in baroreceptor-denervated animals in which there is extreme variability of blood pressure caused by normal daily activities.[58] Although blood pressure increases to very high levels or falls to low levels throughout the day after baroreceptor denervation, the average 24-hour mean arterial pressure is not markedly altered.

Although the arterial baroreceptors provide a powerful means for moment-to-moment regulation of arterial pressure, their role in long-term blood pressure regulation has been controversial. One reason that the baroreceptors have often been considered to be relatively unimportant in chronic regulation of blood pressure is that they tend to reset within a few days to the level of blood pressure to which they are exposed.[58] Therefore, in most forms of chronic hypertension, the arterial baroreflexes are reset to higher blood pressures. To the extent that resetting of baroceptors occurs, this would attenuate their potency as a long-term controller of blood pressure.

Some experimental studies, however, suggest that the baroreceptors may not completely reset and therefore contribute to long-term blood pressure regulation (see Chapter 24). Thus, with prolonged increases in arterial pressure, the baroreflexes may contribute to *reductions* in renal sympathetic activity and promote sodium and water excretion. This, in turn, may attenuate the rise in arterial blood pressure.[56] Although impairment of baroreflexes contributes to increased lability of blood pressure, there is little evidence that baroreceptor dysfunction plays a major role in *causing* chronic hypertension.

Although impaired baroreflexes may not cause chronic hypertension directly by altering SNS activity, increased blood pressure lability, accompanied by periodic large increases in blood pressure, may cause gradual renal injury and eventually lead to chronic hypertension. Studies in experimental animals have shown that baroreceptor-denervated animals have significant structural changes in the kidneys, including glomerular injury.[59]

Does chronic stress cause hypertension by SNS activation?

Acute physiologic stresses, including pain, exercise, exposure to cold, and mental stress, can all lead to increased SNS activity and transient hypertension. It is also widely believed, however, that chronic stress may lead to long-term increases in blood pressure. Support for this concept comes largely from a few epidemiological studies showing that populations or groups, such as air traffic controllers and lower socioeconomic groups, who are believed to lead more stressful lives also have increased prevalence of hypertension.[60] (See Chapter 42 for further discussion of psychosocial stress and hypertension.) Currently, however, there is limited evidence for a direct cause-and-effect relationship between psychosocial stress and chronic hypertension. Further experimental studies are needed to determine (1) if intermittent psychosocial stresses can indeed lead to chronic SNS activation hypertension, and (2) the mechanisms that link psychosocial stresses to chronic hypertension.

Obesity as major cause of SNS activation in primary hypertension

Population studies indicate that excess weight gain is one of the best predictors for development of human primary hypertension (see Chapter 38). Risk estimates from the Framingham Heart Study, for example, suggest that approximately 78% of hypertension in men and 65% in women can be attributed to excess weight gain.[61]

The mechanisms responsible for obesity hypertension appear to be closely linked to increased renal SNS activity. Obese persons have elevated SNS activity in various tissues, including the kidneys and skeletal muscle, as assessed by microneurography, tissue catecholamine spillover, or other methods.[51] Studies in experimental animals and humans indicate that combined α- and β-adrenergic blockade markedly attenuates the hypertension associated with obesity.[51,57,62] Moreover, the renal sympathetic efferent nerves mediate much of the chronic effects of SNS activation on blood pressure in obesity since bilateral renal denervation greatly attenuates the sodium retention and hypertension in obese dogs.[55] Thus, obesity increases renal sodium reabsorption, impairs pressure natriuresis, and causes hypertension in part by increasing renal SNS activity.

The mechanisms that increase renal SNS activity in obesity have not been fully elucidated, although several potential mediators have been suggested including hyperinsulinemia, increased Ang II, activation of chemoreceptor-mediated reflexes associated with sleep apnea, and hyperleptinemia. One of the most promising of these mechanisms is hyperleptinemia.[63]

Leptin is released by adipocytes in proportion to the degree of adiposity and acts on various regions of the hypothalamus to regulate body weight by decreasing appetite and increasing energy expenditure due to increased SNS activity (Figure 23–7). Studies in rodents indicate that increases in plasma leptin to levels comparable found in severe obesity can also raise arterial pressure via SNS activation.[64] Support for the possibility that leptin may be an important link among obesity, renal SNS activation, and hypertension is the finding that rodents with leptin deficiency or mutations of the leptin receptor have little or no increase in blood pressure despite severe obesity when compared to their lean controls.[63,65] Also, obese children with leptin gene mutations have early-onset morbid

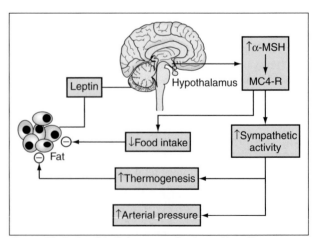

Figure 23–7. Possible links among leptin and its effects on the hypothalamus, sympathetic activation, and hypertension. Leptin may mediate much of its effects on appetite and sympathetic activity by stimulating other neurochemical pathways, including α-melanocyte–stimulating hormone, which activates melanocortin 4-receptors (MC4-R).

obesity, but no indication of the SNS activation that would usually accompany obesity.[66] These observations suggest that hyperleptinemia may be an important factor in linking obesity with renal SNS activation and hypertension in humans as well as in rodents (see Chapter 38).

The stimulatory effect of leptin on SNS activity is mediated by interaction with other hypothalamic factors, especially the proopiomelanocortin pathway. In a recent study, antagonism of the melanocortin 3/4 receptors (MC3/4R) completely abolished the acute effects of leptin on renal SNS activity as well as the chronic effects on blood pressure.[67] Likewise, the chronic hypertensive effects of leptin were completely abolished in MC3/4R knock-out (KO) mice.[68] These observations indicate that a functional MC-4R is important in linking obesity and hyperleptinemia with increased SNS activity and hypertension.

Thus, obesity is a key factor in causing primary hypertension in many patients via activation of renal sympathetic activity. The leptin-hypothalamic-melanocortin system appears to link excess adiposity with increased SNS activity in rodents and may be important in humans, although further studies are needed to determine the quantitative importance of this pathway.

THE ENDOTHELIN SYSTEM

In 1988, Yanagisawa et al.[69] characterized an endothelial-derived vasoconstrictor, a 21 amino acid peptide subsequently called endothelin. Endothelin-1 (ET-1) is derived from a 203 amino acid peptide precursor, preproendothelin, which is cleaved after translation to form proendothelin.[70–74] In the presence of a converting enzyme located within the endothelial cells, proendothelin or big endothelin is cleaved to produce the 21 amino acid peptide, endothelin. ET-1 receptor–binding sites have been identified throughout the body with the greatest numbers of receptors in the kidneys and lungs.[70–74]

While the biochemical and molecular nature of endothelin has been well characterized, the physiologic importance of endothelin in the regulation of renal and cardiovascular function has yet to be fully elucidated.[70–74] ET-1 can either elicit a prohypertensive, antinatriuretic effect by activating ET_A receptors in the kidneys or an antihypertensive, natriuretic effect via renal ET_B receptor activation.[75] Thus, the ability of ET-1 to influence blood pressure regulation and renal-pressure natriuresis is highly dependent on where ET-1 is produced and which ET receptor type is activated (Figure 23–8).

Endothelin-1 reduces pressure natriuresis and increases blood pressure via endothelin Type A receptor activation

ET_A receptors are primarily located on vascular smooth muscle cells. These receptors are thought to be involved in mediating ET-1 vasoconstriction and cellular proliferation in various disease states.[70–74] Although ET_A receptors may play a role in certain forms of hypertension, these receptors do not appear to have a major influence on cardiovascular and renal function under normal physiologic conditions.

ET-1, via ET_A receptor activation, exerts a variety of actions within the kidney that, if sustained chronically, could contribute to the development of hypertension and progressive renal injury.[70–74] ET-1 decreases GFR and renal plasma flow through vascular smooth muscle and mesangial cell contraction. Long-term effects of ET-1 on the kidney include mesangial cell proliferation and extracellular matrix deposition as well as vascular smooth muscle hypertrophy in renal resistance vessels.[70–74] Previous studies have indicated that expression of ET-1 is greatly enhanced in animal models of severe hypertension with renal vascular hypertrophy and in models of progressive renal injury.[76–81] In addition, treatment with endothelin receptor antagonists attenuated the hypertension and small-artery morphologic changes and improved kidney function in these models.[77,81]

Several lines of evidence suggest that ET-1 may play an important role in salt-sensitive forms of hypertension. Dahl salt-sensitive (DS) rats placed on a high sodium diet are characterized by an attenuated pressure natriuresis, development of hypertension, and extensive renal lesions in the form of glomerulosclerosis, renal arteriolar and tubular injury, and progressive renal failure in late phases of the disease. There is growing evidence to support the hypothesis that ET-1, acting via an ET_A receptor, may play a role in mediating some of the renal injury of DS hypertension. Studies have demonstrated that prepro-ET-1 mRNA and vascular responsiveness to ET-1 are increased in the renal cortex of DS rats compared with Dahl salt-resistant (DR) rats.[76,77] In addition, a positive correlation between ET-1 generation in the renal cortex and the extent of glomerulosclerosis has been reported in DS hypertensive rats.[70–74] Also supporting a role of ET-1 in DS hypertension is a study indicating that acute infusion of a nonselective ET_A-ET_B receptor antagonist directly into the renal interstitium improved renal hemodynamic and excretory functions in DS rats but not in DR rats.[76] Moreover, chronic blockade of ET_A receptors attenuates the hypertension and proteinuria, and ameliorates the glomerular and tubular damage associated with high salt intake in DS rats.[77] An important unanswered question is whether the beneficial effect of the ET_A blockade in reducing renal injury is mediated through reducing blood pressure or through direct renal mechanisms.

Recent studies have also suggested an important interaction between ET-1 and the RAS. Renal ET-1 synthesis is enhanced in various animal models of chronic Ang II–induced hypertension.[78–82] In addition, the renal and hypertensive effects of Ang II are markedly attenuated or completely abolished by ET_A receptor antagonists.[78–82] The quantitative importance of ET-1 in mediating the chronic hypertensive actions of Ang II may depend on the level of dietary sodium intake.

ET-1 is also involved in the pathophysiology of hypertension in the pregnancy disorder pre-eclampsia. Pre-eclampsia is associated with hypertension, proteinuria, and endothelial dysfunction.[83–85] Because endothelial damage is a known stimulus for ET-1 synthesis, increases in the production of ET-1 and activation of ET_A receptors may participate in the pathophysiology of hypertension during

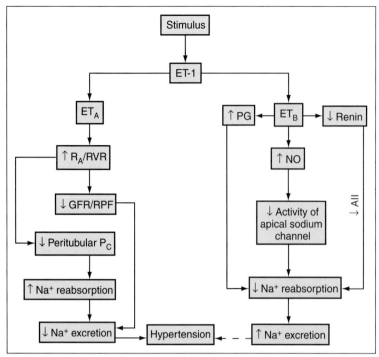

Figure 23–8. Summary of the pro- and anti-hypertensive actions of endothelin-1 (ET-1). The ability of ET-1 to influence blood pressure regulation and renal pressure-natriuresis is highly dependent on where ET-1 is produced and which renal ET receptor type is activated. ET-1 can elicit a prohypertensive antinatriuretic effect by activating ET_A receptors in the kidneys. Activation of renal ET_A receptors increases renal vascular resistance (RVR), which decreases renal plasma flow (RPF) and glomerular filtration rate (GFR), and enhances sodium reabsorption by decreasing peritubular capillary hydrostatic pressure (Pc). The net effect of renal ET_A receptor activation would be increases in sodium retention and blood pressure. Conversely, ET-1 can elicit an antihypertensive natriuretic effect via ET_B receptor activation. Activation of the renal ET_B receptor leads to enhanced synthesis of nitric oxide (NO) and prostaglandin E2 (PG) and suppression of the renin-angiotensin system. The net effect of renal ET_B receptor activation would be decreases in sodium retention and blood pressure.

One potential mechanism for enhanced ET-1 production is via transcriptional regulation of the ET-1 gene by tumor necrosis factor alpha (TNF-α). TNF-α is elevated in pre-eclamptic women and has been implicated in the disease processes. Chronic infusion of TNF-α in pregnant rats, at a rate to mimic plasma levels (two- to three-fold increase) observed in women with pre-eclampsia significantly increases blood pressure.[89] The increase in arterial pressure produced by a two- to three-fold elevation in plasma levels of TNF-α in pregnant rats is associated with significant increases in local production of endothelin in the kidney, placenta, and vasculature.[90] Moreover, the increase in mean arterial pressure in response to TNF-α is completely abolished in pregnant rats treated with an ET_A receptor antagonist.[90] Collectively, these findings suggest that endothelin, via ET_A receptor activation, plays an important role in mediating TNF-α–induced hypertension in pregnant rats.

Endothelin-1 enhances sodium excretion and minimizes salt-induced increases in blood pressure via ET_B receptor activation

While much attention has been given to the role of ET-1 in the pathophysiology of cardiovascular and renal disease acting via an ET_A receptor, recent studies indicate an important physiologic role for ET-1 in the regulation of sodium balance and arterial pressure via ET_B receptor activation.[91–97] The most compelling evidence that the endothelin system may play a significant role in the regulation of sodium balance and arterial pressure are the reports that transgenic animals deficient in ET_B receptors develop severe salt-sensitive hypertension.[95] Additional evidence comes from studies indicating that pharmacologic antagonism of ET_B receptors produces significant hypertension in rats.[96,98]

Although *systemic* ET_B receptor blockade produces significant hypertension that is salt sensitive, the physiologic mechanisms involved in mediating the hypertension are still unknown. Since ET_B receptors are located on multiple cell types through the body, including endothelial cells and renal epithelial cells, both intrarenal and extrarenal mechanisms may mediate the hypertension produced by chronic disruption of ET_B receptor. However, several recent studies suggest that the renal endothelin system plays a major role in controlling blood pressure under high sodium intake conditions. To examine the role of endothelial cell ET_B receptors in salt-sensitive hypertension, Bagnall et al.[99] generated an endothelial cell-specific ET_B receptor KO mice using a Cre-*loxP* approach. They reported that ablation of ET_B receptors exclusively from endothelial cells produces endothelial dysfunction in the absence of hypertension. In contrast to models of total ET_B receptor ablation, the

pre-eclampsia. Alexander et al.[86] examined the role of ET-1 in mediating the hypertension in a placental ischemic model of pre-eclampsia.[87] Using an RNase protection assay, they found that renal expression of preproendothelin was significantly elevated in both the medulla and the cortex of the pregnant rats with chronic reductions in uterine perfusion pressure compared with control pregnant rats. Moreover, they reported that chronic administration of the selective ET_A receptor antagonist markedly attenuated the increase in mean arterial pressure in pregnant rats with chronic reductions in uterine perfusion pressure. In sharp contrast to the response in reduced uterine perfusion pressure rats, ET_A receptor blockade had no significant effect on blood pressure in the normal pregnant animal. These findings suggest that ET-1 plays a major role in mediating the hypertension produced by chronic reductions in uterine perfusion pressure in pregnant rats.

Sera from pregnant rats exposed to chronic reductions in uterine perfusion increases endothelin production by cultured endothelial cells.[88] The exact mechanism linking enhanced renal production of ET-1 to placental ischemia in pregnant rats or in women with pre-eclampsia is unknown.

blood pressure response to a high-salt diet was unchanged in endothelial cell–specific ET_B receptor KOs compared to control mice. These important findings suggest that nonendothelial cell ET_B receptors are important for regulation of blood pressure.

The renal medulla and hypertension: Role of endothelin-1 and ET_B receptors

There is growing evidence that ET-1, acting through the renal medullary ET_B receptors, is involved in the regulation of sodium balance and blood pressure under normal physiologic conditions.[75,100-103] The kidney is an important site of ET-1 production, and ET_B receptors are expressed at important renal sites of ET-1 synthesis, particularly in the renal medulla.[75] Some of the first studies using synthetic ET-1 demonstrated that nonpressor doses of ET-1 produced significant natriuresis and diuresis.[72] It is now known that ET_B receptors are located in various parts of the nephron, including the proximal tubule, medullary thick ascending limb, collecting tubule, and the inner medullary collecting duct.[72,102,103] The highest concentration of ET_B receptors appears to be on the inner medullary collecting duct in the renal medulla.[75,92-94] Activation of ET_B receptors has been reported to inhibit sodium and water reabsorption along various parts of the nephron.[72] Taken together, these data indicate that ET-1, via ET_B receptors, may influence the renal handling of sodium and water. The exact mechanism whereby ET_B receptor activation inhibits sodium reabsorption is unclear but could involve other autacoid factors such as nitric oxide, PGE2, and/or 20 HETE (Figure 23–9).

For the renal ET-1 system to be an important control system for the regulation of sodium balance, the production of renal ET-1 should change in response to variations in sodium intake. Moreover, blockade of ET_B receptors

should result in a salt-sensitive form of hypertension. Although there are ample data showing that ET-1 can influence sodium reabsorption, there is a paucity of data in the literature examining the relationship between sodium intake and renal production of ET-1. A study by Pollock and Pollock,[98] however, has shown a positive correlation between sodium intake and renal excretion of ET-1. Convincing evidence for a role of renal ET-1 in controlling sodium excretion and arterial pressure during chronic changes in sodium intake has come from several other studies. Gariepy et al.[97] demonstrated that rats deficient in ET_B receptor expression display salt-sensitive hypertension. Likewise, Pollock and Pollock[98] reported that chronic pharmacological blockade of the ET_B receptor in rats resulted in hypertension that was sensitive to dietary sodium intake. Moreover, Ohuchi et al.[101] reported elevation in blood pressure by genetic and pharmacologic disruption of the ET_B receptor in mice.

In a recent report by Ge et al.,[100] selective disruption of the ET_B receptor in the collecting duct cells of mice was found to produce significant hypertension that was salt sensitive (Figure 23–9). Collecting duct ET_B KO mice on a normal sodium diet were hypertensive.[100] Collecting duct ET_B KO mice on a high-sodium diet had worsened hypertension, reduced urinary sodium excretion, and weight gain.[100] These findings provide strong evidence that the collecting-duct ET_B receptor is an important physiologic regulator of renal sodium excretion and blood pressure.

Role of endothelin in human hypertension

Although ET-1 clearly plays a significant role in the pathogenesis of some forms of experimental hypertension, especially salt-sensitive models, its role in human primary hypertension is unclear. Bosentan, a combined ET_A/ET_B receptor antagonist, significantly lowered blood pressure in a large double-blind clinical trial, indicating that the endothelin system plays a role in maintaining blood pressure in human hypertension.[104] However, the magnitude of the blood pressure reduction by bosentan was almost the same as that observed in normotensive humans. While this observation suggests that endothelin probably does not play a major role in contributing to increases in blood pressure in most patients with essential hypertension, blockade of the antihypertensive ET_B receptor may have masked an important role of endothelin in essential hypertension via ET_A receptor activation. Therefore, the importance of ET-1 in human essential hypertension deserves further investigation.

NITRIC OXIDE

The vascular endothelium releases a short-acting substance caled nitric oxide (NO) that induces local relaxation. Intravenous infusion of competitive inhibitors of the enzyme responsible for NO production (nitric oxide synthase) induced rapid increases in blood pressure in various species of animals.[105] These effects were rapidly reversed with intravenous infusion of L-arginine, the substrate for NO synthase. These studies suggested that tonic release of nitric oxide by vascular endothelium may be important for

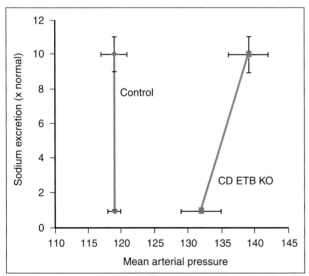

Figure 23–9. Collecting duct-specific knockout of the endothelin B receptor (CD ETB KO) causes a hypertensive shift in the pressure natriuresis relationship. (Data from Ge Y, Bagnall A, Stricklett P, Strait K, Webb D, Kotelevtsev Y, et al. *Am J Physiol Renal Physiol* 2006 [Epub before print].)

regulation of vascular function. To investigate this concept further, the long-term effects of nitric oxide synthase inhibitors were examined in various animal models and were found to cause sustained hypertension associated with reductions in renal hemodynamics and pressure natriuresis.[105] The magnitude of the increase in blood pressure was also dependent on the dietary sodium intake.[105] These findings have led to the concept that NO is not only important in the long-term regulation of sodium balance and blood pressure, but also to the notion that abnormalities in NO production result in altered pressure natriuresis and a salt-sensitive form of hypertension.

Nitric oxide enhances pressure natriuresis via hemodynamic and tubular mechanisms

The renal effector mechanisms whereby reductions in NO synthesis alter pressure natriuresis can be divided into hemodynamic and tubular components, each of which may be modulated by processes that are intrinsic and extrinsic to the kidney (Figure 23–10). For example, reductions in NO synthesis could lead to a decrease in renal sodium excretory function by directly increasing basal renal vascular resistance or by enhancing the renal vascular responsiveness to vasoconstrictors such as Ang II or norepinephrine.[105–114] Reductions in NO synthesis also reduce sodium excretory function either through direct effects on tubular transport or through changes in intrarenal physical factors such as renal interstitial hydrostatic pressure or medullary blood flow.[106–108] Inhibition of NO synthesis reduces renal interstitial fluid hydrostatic pressure (RIHP) and urinary sodium excretion.[109] Furthermore, normalization of the blunted pressure natriuretic response in Dahl S rats pro-

duced during stimulation of NO production results from improvement in the kidney's ability to generate RIHP in response to changes in renal perfusion pressure.[109] Thus, changes in RIHP appear to be an important component of the effect of NO on sodium reabsorption *in vivo*.

Most investigators attribute the alterations in RIHP to changes in flow and pressure in the medullary circulation.[107] Consistent with this hypothesis are observations that the acute infusion of an NO synthase inhibitor directly into the renal medulla significantly reduces papillary blood flow, RIHP, and urinary sodium and water excretion without affecting the GFR or systemic pressure.[107–109] Chronic medullary interstitial infusion of NO synthase inhibitors in conscious rats results in sustained reductions in medullary blood flow, sustained sodium and water retention, and hypertension, which are all reversed when the infusion is discontinued.[107] These findings demonstrate that reductions in medullary blood flow may be another important mechanism whereby inhibition of NO in the kidney leads to a hypertensive shift in pressure natriuresis.

Inhibition of NO synthesis may have direct effects on renal tubule transport. NO has direct effects on sodium uptake in cultured cortical collecting duct cells by altering apical sodium channels.[106] Sodium transport in the cortical collecting duct *in vivo* is mediated through changes in cyclic GMP. Micropuncture studies have shown NO synthase inhibitors decrease proximal tubule reabsorption in anesthetized rats.[106] This effect has been attributed to antagonism of Ang II–mediated sodium transport. An effect of NO on proximal reabsorption has also been inferred from changes in lithium clearance induced during inhibition of NO production. Thus, NO can affect sodium reabsorption via direct effects on tubular transport or indirectly via alteration in medullary blood flow or renal interstitial hydrostatic pressure.

Nitric oxide interacts with the renin-angiotensin system

Another mechanism whereby NO synthesis inhibition may reduce pressure natriuresis is via activation of the RAS.[105] Inhibition of NO production enhances renin release from rat cortical kidney slices. Inhibitors of NO synthesis also increase plasma renin activity *in vivo*, an effect that is dependent on the macula densa mechanism.[111]

Several lines of evidence suggest that impaired NO production may play an important role in the regulation of sodium balance and in pathogenesis of salt-sensitive hypertension.[108,110] An increase in renal NO production or release as evidenced by increased urinary excretion of NO metabolites or the NO second messenger, cyclic GMP, has been

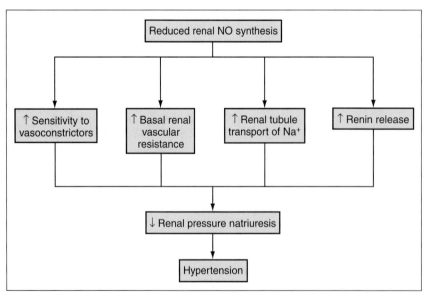

Figure 23–10. The renal effector mechanisms whereby reductions in NO synthesis decrease pressure natriuresis and increase blood pressure. A reduction in nitric oxide (NO) synthesis leads to a decrease in renal sodium excretory function by directly increasing basal renal vascular resistance, enhancing renal vascular responsiveness to vasoconstrictors such as ANGII or norepinephrine, or activating the renin-angiotensin system. Reductions in NO synthesis also reduce sodium excretory function through direct effects on tubular transport or through changes in intrarenal physical factors such as renal interstitial hydrostatic pressure or medullary blood flow.

reported to be essential for the maintenance of normotension during a dietary salt challenge. Prevention of this increase in renal NO production resulted in salt-sensitive hypertension.[110]

There is also ample experimental evidence demonstrating that NO synthesis is impaired in some vascular beds in human essential hypertension. The extent to which these observations reflect effects of the hypertensive process or reflect important mechanisms for the pathogenesis of the hypertensive condition remains unclear.

ATRIAL NATRIURETIC PEPTIDE

Atrial natriuretic peptide (ANP) is a 28 amino-acid peptide synthesized and released from atrial cardiocytes in response to stress. Once ANP is released from the atria, it enhances sodium excretion through extrarenal and intrarenal mechanisms.[115,116] ANP increases GFR while having no effect on renal blood flow. However, increased GFR is not a prerequisite for ANP to enhance sodium excretion. ANP may alter tubular sodium reabsorption either directly by inhibiting the active tubular transport of sodium or indirectly via alterations in medullary blood flow, physical factors, and intrarenal hormones.[115]

ANP inhibits renin and aldosterone synthesis

Atrial natriuretic peptide also has important actions at several sites of the RAS cascade.[115] Intrarenal or intravenous infusion of ANP reduces the renin secretion rate by a macula densa mechanism, since ANP failed to reduce renin secretion in nonfiltering kidneys. The reduction in renin secretion decreases intrarenal levels of Ang II, which could contribute to ANP-induced natriuresis. When intrarenal levels of Ang II were prevented from decreasing, the natriuretic effects of ANP were blunted.[115,116]

ANP also decreases aldosterone release from the adrenal zona glomerulosa cells.[115,116] Two mechanisms for ANP-induced suppression of aldosterone release have been suggested: (1) direct action on adrenal glomerulosa cells, and (2) reduced circulating levels of Ang II due to suppressed renin secretion under *in vivo* conditions.[115] Although the suppression of aldosterone release would not play a role in mediating the acute natriuretic responses to ANP, decreases in circulating levels of aldosterone could contribute to the long-term actions of ANP on sodium balance and arterial pressure regulation.

ANP plays role in short-term and long-term volume regulation

Plasma levels of ANP are elevated in numerous physiologic conditions associated with enhanced sodium excretion.[115,116] Acute saline of blood volume expansion consistently elevates circulating levels of ANP. Some, but not all, investigators have reported that chronic increases in dietary sodium intake raise circulating levels of ANP. Several studies have reported that infusions of exogenous ANP at rates that result in physiologically relevant plasma concentrations, comparable to those observed during volume expansion, have significant renal and cardiovascular effects.[115–117]

Infusion of ANP at a rate that causes a twofold increase in plasma ANP elicits significant natriuresis, especially in the presence of other natriuretic stimuli, such as high renal perfusion pressure.[115–117] Long-term physiologic elevations in plasma ANP also shift the renal-pressure natriuresis relationship and reduce arterial pressure.[117]

Blockade of ANP system produces salt-sensitive hypertension

The development of genetic mouse models that exhibit chronic alterations in expression of the genes for ANP or its receptors (NPR-A, NPR-C) have also provided compelling evidence for a role of ANP in chronic regulation of renal pressure natriuresis and blood pressure.[118] Transgenic mice overexpressing ANP gene are hypotensive relative to the nontransgenic litter mates, whereas mice harboring functional disruptions of the ANP or NPR-A genes are hypertensive. The ANP gene "knock-out" mice develop a salt-sensitive form of hypertension in association with failure to adequately suppress the RAS. These findings suggest that genetic deficiencies in ANP or natriuretic receptor activity could play a role in the pathogenesis of salt-sensitive hypertension.

RENAL EICOSANOIDS

Renal eicosanoids are thought to be important mediators of vascular function, sodium and water homeostasis, and renin release.[119] Cyclooxygenase metabolizes arachidonic acid into prostaglandin (PG) G_2 and subsequently to PGH_2, which is then further metabolized by tissue-specific isomerases to PGs and thromboxane.

Although the kidney produces many types of PGs with multiple functions, the major renal prostaglandin that controls sodium excretion is probably PGE_2.[115] However, production of other arachidonate acid metabolites, such as prostacyclin, thromboxane, and 20-HETE, may also influence renal-pressure natriuresis and blood pressure regulation. The largest production of PGE_2 occurs in the medulla with decreasing synthesis in the cortex. PGE_2 is synthesized and rapidly inactivated and, once synthesized, is released and not stored. Once released, PGE_2 influences sodium transport by several intrarenal mechanisms.

Despite numerous reports that PGs may contribute to the natriuresis of acute physiologic perturbations, the importance of endogenous renal PGs in the long-term regulation of sodium balance remains unclear.[115] Increases in dietary sodium intake have little or no effect on urinary PG excretion. In addition, nonspecific cyclooxygenase inhibitors do not affect the sodium excretory or blood pressure responses to chronic alterations in dietary sodium intake. Thus, it appears that endogenous renal PGs may not play a major role in regulating sodium excretion during chronic changes in sodium intake.[115]

While long-term administration of PG synthesis inhibitors has very little effect on volume and/or arterial pressure regulation under normal physiologic conditions, renal PGs may be important in pathophysiologic states associated with enhanced activity or the RAS.[115] *In vitro* and *in vivo* studies indicate that renal PGs protect the preglomerular vessels from excessive Ang II–induced vasoconstriction.[115] In the absence of this protective mechanism in pathophysiologic states, the renal vasculature could be exposed to the potent vasoconstrictor actions of Ang II. This could lead to significant impairment of renal hemodynamics, reduced excretory function, and hypertension.

Inhibitors of COX-2 enzyme increase blood pressure and reduce renal-pressure natriuresis

There are at least two distinct cyclooxygenases, COX-1 and COX-2.[53] COX-1 is called the *constitutive* enzyme because of its wide tissue distribution, while COX-2 has been termed as *inducible* because of its more restricted basal expression and its upregulation by inflammatory and/or proliferative stimuli.[119] Based on the concept that COX-1 performs cellular housekeeping functions for normal physiologic activity, and COX-2 acts at inflammatory sites, it was initially hypothesized that the renal effects of nonsteroidal anti-inflammatory drugs might be linked to COX-1 inhibition.[119] However, increasing experimental and clinical evidence has indicated that COX-2 metabolites may play a role in the regulation of renal function under various physiologic and pathophysiologic conditions.[119] COX-2 inhibition has been shown to decrease urine sodium excretion and induce mild to moderate increases in arterial pressure. Moreover, blockade of COX-2 activity can have deleterious effects on renal blood flow and GFR. In addition to physiologic regulation of COX-2 expression in the kidney, increased renal cortical COX-2 expression is seen in experimental models associated with altered renal hemodynamics and progressive renal injury. Long-term treatment with selective COX-2 inhibitors ameliorates functional and structural renal damage in these conditions.[119]

Eicosanoids produced by cytochrome P450 monooxygenase metabolism of arachidonic acid alter renal-pressure natriuresis

In addition to renal PGs generated via the COX pathway, other eicosanoids that inhibit tubular sodium transport are produced by cytochrome P450 (CYP) monooxygenase metabolism of arachidonic acid.[120] CYP enzymes metabolize arachidonic acid primarily to 20-hydroxyeicosatetraenoic acid (20-HETE) and epoxyeicosatrienoic acids (EETs). 20-HETE is a potent constrictor of renal arterioles that may have an important role in autoregulation of renal blood flow and tubuloglomerular feedback (Figure 23–11).[120] 20-HETE and EETs also inhibit sodium reabsorption in the proximal tubule and TALH (Figure 23–11). Compelling evidence suggests that the renal production of CYP metabolites of arachidonic acid is altered in genetic and experimental models of hypertension, and that this system

contributes to the resetting of pressure natriuresis and the development of hypertension. In the spontaneously hypertensive rat (SHR), the renal production of 20-HETE is increased, and inhibitors of the formation of 20-HETE decrease arterial pressure.[120] Blockade of 20-HETE synthesis also reduces blood pressure or improves renal function in deoxycorticosterone acetate (DOCA) salt, Ang II-infused, and Lyon hypertensive rats.[120] In contrast, 20-HETE formation is reduced in the thick ascending limb of Dahl S rats and this contributes to elevated sodium reabsorption.[120] Enhanced 20-HETE synthesis improves pressure natriuresis and lowers blood pressure in Dahl S rats, whereas inhibitors of 20-HETE production promote the development of hypertension in Lewis rats.[120]

Studies in humans also suggest that CYP metabolites may play a role in sodium homeostasis. Urinary 20-HETE excretion is regulated by salt intake and is differentially regulated in salt-sensitive versus salt-resistant subjects.[121,122] Moreover, there appears to be a strong negative relationship between the excretion of 20-HETE and body mass index, suggesting that some factor related to obesity may be responsible for decreased synthesis or excretion of this eicosanoid in hypertension.[121,122] These observations support the possibility that impaired renal production of 20-HETE could contribute to attenuated renal-pressure natriuresis in human hypertension, especially when associated with obesity. However, further mechanistic studies are needed to test the importance of 20-HETE in human hypertension.

OXIDATIVE STRESS

Oxidative stress occurs when the total oxidant production exceeds the antioxidant capacity. Recent studies suggest that reactive oxygen species (ROS) may play a role in the initiation and progression of cardiovascular dysfunction

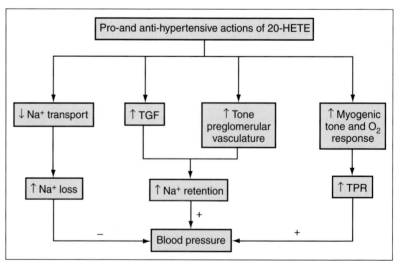

Figure 23–11. Summary of the pro- and anti-hypertensive actions of 20-HETE. 20-HETE produced in the renal tubules inhibits sodium transport and lowers blood pressure. In the renal vasculature and glomerulus, 20-HETE is a constrictor that lowers glomerular filtration rate, promotes sodium retention, and increases arterial pressure. In the peripheral circulation, 20-HETE increases vascular tone and increases blood pressure. TGF, tubuloglomerular feedback; TPR, total peripheral resistance. (Redrawn from Roman RJ. *Physiol Rev* 2002;82:131–85. Used with permission.)

associated with diseases such as hyperlipidemia, diabetes mellitus, and hypertension.[123–127] In many forms of hypertension, the increased ROS are derived from NAD(P)H oxidases, which could serve as a triggering mechanism for uncoupling endothelial NOS by oxidants.[123]

ROS produced by migrating inflammatory cells and/or vascular cells have distinct functional effects on each cell type.[123] These effects include endothelial dysfunction, renal tubule sodium transport, cell growth, migration, inflammatory gene expression, and matrix regulation. ROS, by affecting renal hemodynamics and renal tubule cell function (Figure 23–12), can alter renal pressure natriuresis and blood pressure regulation.[123–127]

Growing experimental evidence supports a role for ROS in various animal models of sodium-sensitive hypertension.[125–129] The Dahl salt-sensitive (S) rat has increased vascular and renal superoxide production and increased levels of H_2O_2. The renal protein expression of superoxide dismutase is decreased in the kidney of Dahl S rats, and long-term administration of Tempol, a superoxide dismutase mimetic, significantly decreases arterial pressure and renal damage. Another salt-sensitive model, the stroke-prone spontaneously hypertensive rat (SHRSP), has elevated levels of superoxide and decreased total plasma antioxidant capacity. Superoxide production is also increased in the deoxycorticosterone acetate (DOCA)-salt hypertensive rat. Treatment of the DOCA-salt rats with apocynin, an NADPH oxidase inhibitor, decreases aortic superoxide production and arterial pressure.

The importance of oxidative stress in human hypertension is unclear. An imbalance between total oxidant production and the antioxidant capacity in human hypertension has been reported to occur in some but not all studies.[123] The equivocal findings in human studies are most likely due to the difficulty of assessing oxidative stress in humans. Moreover, most recent human studies have found that vitamin E and C supplementation has little or no effect on blood pressure.[123]

INFLAMMATORY CYTOKINES

Epidemiologic and experimental studies have revealed an association between biochemical markers of systemic inflammation and cardiovascular disease such as atherosclerosis, heart failure, and hypertension.[130–134] While significant progress has been made in our understanding of the role of inflammatory cytokines in pathogenesis of atherosclerotic disease, the quantitative importance of cytokines in the pathogenesis and progression of hypertension has yet to be fully elucidated.

Important blood-pressure regulatory systems such as the RAS and SNS interact with the proinflammatory cytokines such as interleukin-6 (IL-6) and tumor necrosis factor-alpha (TNF-α). The SNS stimulates the release of proinflammatory cytokines and sympathetic nerves may also serve as a source of cytokines.[135] There is also experimental evidence that proinflammatory cytokines may activate the SNS.[135] Ang II enhances the synthesis of TNF-α and IL-6, and stimulates chemokine monocyte chemoattractant protein-1 (MCP-1) and nuclear factor-kappa B.[136] Ang II also increases the production of ROS, including hydrogen peroxide, that participate in the process of inflammation.[137,138]

Proinflammatory cytokines also affect vascular function and endothelium-derived factors involved in cardiovascular regulation. TNF-α and IL-6 have both been shown to induce structural as well as functional alterations in endothelial cells.[131,139,140] These cytokines enhance the formation of a number of endothelial cell substances such as endothelin, reduce acetylcholine-induced vasodilatation, and destabilize the mRNA of endothelial NO synthase.[131,140] Thus, endothelial dysfunction associated with many forms of hypertension may, in part, be mediated by proinflammatory cytokines.

Also supporting a potential role for cytokines in the regulation of arterial pressure are findings that plasma levels of proinflammatory cytokines correlate with increased blood pressure in certain forms of human hypertension and experimental animal models of hypertension.[131,139] Moreover, several recent studies have demonstrated that chronic increases in plasma levels of cytokines, comparable to concentrations observed in hypertension associated with pre-eclampsia, result in significant and sustained increases in arterial pressure. For example, Alexander et al.[141] and Lamarca et al.[89] reported that a twofold elevation in the plasma levels of TNF-α significantly increased arterial pressure and renal vascular resistance in pregnant rats, and Orshal et al.[142]

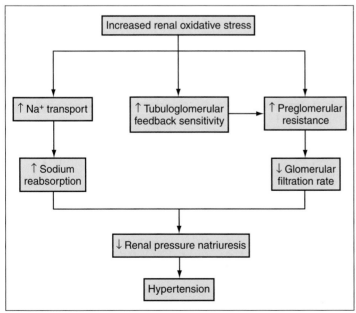

Figure 23–12. Renal effector mechanisms whereby reactive oxygen species decrease pressure natriuresis and increase blood pressure. An increase in renal oxidative stress decreases renal pressure natriuresis by increasing basal renal vascular resistance or enhancing tubuloglomerular feedback, both of which would decrease the glomerular filtration rate. Renal oxidative stress also reduces sodium excretion by direct effects on renal tubular transport.

reported similar findings infusing IL-6 for 5 days in pregnant rats. While these studies demonstrate that increasing plasma levels of cytokines comparable to concentrations observed in certain forms of hypertension can lead to significant elevations in blood pressure, the quantitative role of endogenous cytokines in mediating in increases in arterial pressure in various forms of hypertension associated with enhanced formation of proinflammatory cytokines remains unclear.

A recent study by Lee et al.[143] tested the role of endogenous IL-6 in mediating the hypertension caused by Ang II in male C57BL6 and IL-6 KO (IL-6 KO) mice. The major finding from this study was that the hypertension caused by chronic Ang II excess depends significantly on the presence of IL-6. Mice with the knock-out of IL-6 had significantly lower mean arterial pressure than wild-type mice during 2 weeks of Ang II infusion. While these findings clearly demonstrate a quantitatively significant role for IL-6 in mediating the chronic hypertensive response to angiotensin II in mice, the importance of inflammatory cytokines in the pathogenesis and progression of the various forms of human hypertension is unclear and is currently an important area of investigation.

SUMMARY

Experimental evidence collected over the last several decades has clearly demonstrated a central role of renal-pressure natriuresis in long-term blood pressure regulation and its impairment in all forms of hypertension, including human essential hypertension. Although the exact causes of impaired renal-pressure natriuresis in hypertension are still unclear, it is likely that multiple extrarenal neurohumoral and intrarenal defects contribute to abnormal pressure natriuresis and increased blood pressure in various forms of human hypertension. Intrarenal defects may include abnormalities such as enhanced formation of angiotensin II, reactive oxygen species, and endothelin (via ET_A receptor activation) or decreased synthesis of NO or natriuretic prostanoids. In other instances, extrarenal disturbances, such as increased SNS activity or excessive formation of antinatriuretic hormones such as aldosterone may lead to a reduction in renal-pressure natriuresis. With longstanding hypertension, structural damage in the kidney may further shift pressure natriuresis and exacerbate hypertension.

Because of the central role for the kidneys in the long-term regulation of arterial pressure and its importance in the pathophysiology of hypertension, a better understanding of the various factors that contribute to impaired renal-pressure natriuresis is warranted. Identification of factors that influence renal-pressure natriuresis will continue to lead to novel therapies for treating hypertension, one of the major risk factors of cardiovascular diseases.

REFERENCES

1. Guyton AC. Arterial pressure and hypertension. In: *Circulatory Physiology II*. Philadelphia: W.B. Saunders, 1980.
2. Hall JE, Mizelle HL, Hildebrandt DA, Brands MW. Abnormal pressure natriuresis: a cause or a consequence of hypertension? *Hypertension* 1990;15:547–59.
3. Hall JE, Guyton AC, Brands MW. Pressure-volume regulation in hypertension. *Kidney Int* 1996;49(Suppl 55):S35–41.
4. Guyton AC. Abnormal renal function and autoregulation in essential hypertension. *Hypertension* 1991;18(Suppl 5):III49–53.
5. Hall JE. Renal function in one-kidney, one-clip hypertension and low renin essential hypertension. *Am J Hypertens* 1991;4:523S–33S.
6. Goldblatt H, Lynch J, Hanzal RF, Summerville WW. Studies on experimental hypertension. I. The production of persistent elevation of systolic blood pressure by means of renal ischemia. *J Exp Med* 1934;59:347–80.
7. Kimura G, Brenner BM. The renal basis for salt sensitivity in hypertension. In: Laragh JH, Brenner BM, eds. *Hypertension: Pathophysiology, Diagnosis, and Management*. New York: Raven Press, 1995:1569–88.
8. Laragh JH. Nephron heterogeneity: clue to the pathogenesis of essential hypertension and effectiveness of angiotensin-converting enzyme inhibitor treatment. *Am J Med* 1989;87:2S–14S.
9. Brenner BM. Nephron adaptation to renal injury or ablation. *Am J Physiol* 1985;249:F324-37.
10. Norman RA Jr, Galloway PG, Dzielak DJ, Huang M. Mechanisms of partial renal infarct hypertension. *J Hypertens* 1988;6:397–403.
11. Langston JB, Guyton AC, Douglas BH, Dorsett PE. Effect of changes in salt intake on arterial pressure and renal function in partially nephrectomized dogs. *Circulation Res* 1963;12:508–12.
12. Hall JE, Brands MW, Shek EW. Central role of the kidney and abnormal fluid volume control in hypertension. *J Hum Hypertens* 1996;10:633–39.
13. Weinberger MH. Salt sensitivity of blood pressure in humans. *Hypertension* 1996;27:481–90.
14. Johnson RJ, Rodriguez-Iturbe B, Nakagawa T, et al. Subtle renal injury is likely a common mechanism for salt-sensitive essential hypertension. *Hypertension* 2005;45:326–30.
15. Lifton RP. Molecular genetics of human blood pressure variation. *Science* 1996;272:676–80.
16. Dunhill MS, Halley W. Some observations on the quantitative anatomy of the kidney. *J Pathol* 1973;110:113–61.
17. Hall JE, Coleman TG, Guyton AC. The renin-angiotensin system: normal physiology and changes in older hypertensives. *J Am Geriatric Soc* 1989;37:801–13.
18. Hall JE. Control of sodium excretion by angiotensin II: intrarenal mechanisms and blood pressure regulation. *Am J Physiol* 1986;250:R960–72.
19. Hall JE, Guyton AC, Smith MJ Jr, Coleman TG. Blood pressure and renal function during chronic changes in sodium intake: role of angiotensin. *Am J Physiol* 1980;239:F271–80.
20. Campese VM. Salt sensitivity in hypertension. Renal and cardiovascular implications. *Hypertension* 1994;23:531–50.
21. Weinberger MH, Fineberg NS, Fineberg SE, Weinberger M. Salt sensitivity, pulse pressure, and death in normal and hypertensive humans. *Hypertension* 2001;37: 429–32.
22. Schnermann J, Briggs J. Function of the juxtaglomerular apparatus: local control of glomerular dynamics. In: Seldin DW, Giebisch G, eds. *The Kidney: Physiology and Pathophysiology*, 2nd ed. New York: Raven Press, 1992:1249–90.
23. Hricik DE. Captopril-induced renal insufficiency and the role of sodium balance. *Ann Intern Med* 1985;103:222–23.
24. Textor SC, Tarazi RC, Novick AC, et al. Regulation of renal haemodynamics and glomerular filtration in patients with renovascular hypertension during converting enzyme inhibition with captopril. *Am J Med* 1984;76:29–37.

25. Hall JE, Guyton AC, Brands MW. Control of sodium excretion and arterial pressure by intrarenal mechanisms and the renin-angiotensin system. In: Laragh JH, Brenner BM, eds. *Hypertension: Pathophysiology, Diagnosis and Management*, 2nd ed. New York: Raven Press, 1995:1451–75.

26. Anderson S, Rennke HG, Brenner BM. Therapeutic advantage of converting enzyme inhibitors in arresting progressive renal disease associated with systemic hypertension in the rat. *J Clin Inv* 1986;77:1993–2000.

27. Parving HH, Hommel E, Smidt UM. Protection of kidney function and decrease in albuminuria by captopril in insulin dependent diabetics with nephropathy, *BMJ* 1988;297:1086–91.

28. Lewis EM, Hunsicker LG, Bain RP, Rohde ED. The effect of angiotensin-converting enzyme inhibition on diabetic nephropathy. *N Engl J Med* 1993;329:1456–62.

29. Brenner BM, Cooper ME, de Zeeuw D, et al. Effects of losartan on renal and cardiovascular outcomes in patients with type 2 diabetes and nephropathy. *N Engl J Med* 2001;345:861–69.

30. Matsuaka M, Hymes J, Ichikawa I. Angiotensin in progressive renal diseases: theory and practice. *J Am Soc Nephrol* 1996;7:2025–43.

31. Ketteler M, Noble NA, Border WA. Transforming growth factor-B and angiotensin: the missing link from glomerular hyperfiltration to glomerulosclerosis? *Ann Rev Physiol* 1995;57:279–95.

32. Griffin KA, Abu-Amarah I, Picken M, Bidani AK. Renoprotection by ACE inhibition or aldosterone blockade is blood pressure-dependent. *Hypertension* 2003;41:201–206.

33. Eng E, Veniants M, Floege J, et al. Renal proliferative and phenotypic changes in rats with two-kidney, one-clip Goldblatt hypertension. *Am J Hypertens* 1994;7:177–85.

34. Hall JE, Granger JP. Regulation of fluid and electrolyte balance in hypertension: role of hormones and peptides. In: Battegay EJ, Lip GHY, Bakris GL, eds. *Hypertension: Principles and Practice*. Boca Raton, FL: Taylor & Francis, 2005:121–42.

35. Harris PJ, Young JA. Dose-dependent stimulation and inhibition of proximal tubular sodium reabsorption by angiotensin II in the rat kidney. *Pflugers Arch* 1977;367:295–97.

36. Navar LG, Harrison-Bernard LM, Nishiyama A, Kobori H. Regulation of intrarenal angiotensin II in hypertension. *Hypertension* 2002;39:316–22.

37. Capasso G, Unwin R, Ciani F, et al. Bicarbonate transport along the loop of Henle. II. Effects of acid-base, dietary and neurohumoral determinants. *J Clin Invest* 1994; 94:830–38.

38. Amlal H, LeGoff C, Vernimmen C, et al. ANG II controls Na$^+$-K$^+$(NH$_4^+$)-2Cl$^-$ cotransport via 20-HETE and PKC in medullary thick ascending limb. *Am J Physiol* 1998;274:C1047–56.

39. Peti-Peterdi J, Warnock DG, Bell PD. Angiotensin II directly stimulates ENaC activity in the cortical collecting duct via AT(1) receptors. *J Am Soc Nephrol* 2002;13:1131–35.

40. Schnermann J, Levine DZ. Paracrine factors in tubuloglomerular feedback: adenosine, ATP, and nitric oxide. *Annu Rev Physiol* 2003;65:501–29.

41. Fuller PJ, Young MJ. Mechanisms of mineralocorticoid action. *Hypertension* 2005;46:1227–35.

42. Funder JW. The nongenomic actions of aldosterone. *Endocr Rev* 2005;26:313–21.

43. Wehling M, Kasmayr J, Theisen K. Rapid effects of mineralocorticoids on sodium-proton exchanger: genomic or nongenomic pathway? *Am J Physiol* 1991;260:E719–26.

44. Romagni P, Rossi F, Guerrini L, et al. Aldosterone induces contraction of the resistance arteries in man. *Atherosclerosis* 2003;166:345–49.

45. Gunaruwan P, Schmitt M, Taylor J, et al. Lack of rapid aldosterone effects on forearm resistance vasculature in health. *J Renin Angiotensin Aldosterone Syst* 2002;3:123–25.

46. Hall JE, Granger JP, Smith MJ Jr, Premen AJ. Role of renal hemodynamics and arterial pressure in aldosterone "escape." *Hypertension* 1984;6(Suppl I):I183–92.

47. Calhoun DA, Nishizaka MK, Zaman MA, et al. Hyperaldosteronism among black and white subjects with resistant hypertension. *Hypertension* 2002;40:892–96.

48. Krum H, Nolly H, Workman D, et al. Efficacy of eplerenone added to renin-angiotensin blockade in hypertensive patients. *Hypertension* 2002;40:117–23.

49. Rocha R, Stier CT Jr. Pathophysiological effects of aldosterone in cardiovascular tissues. *Trends Endocrinol Metab* 2001;12:308–14.

50. de Paula RB, da Silva AA, Hall JE. Aldosterone antagonism attenuates obesity-induced hypertension and glomerular hyperfiltration. *Hypertension* 2004;43:41–47.

51. Hall JE. The kidney, hypertension, and obesity. *Hypertension* 2003;41:625–33.

52. DiBona GF. Neural control of the kidney: past, present, and future. *Hypertension* 2003;4:621–24.

53. Guyenet PG. The sympathetic control of blood pressure. *Nat Rev* 2006;7:335–46.

54. Dampney RAL, Horiuchi J, Killinger S, et al. Long-term regulation of arterial blood pressure by hypothalamic nuclei: some critical questions. *Clin Exper Pharmacol Physiol* 2005;32:419–25.

55. Kassab S, Kato T, Wilkins FC, et al. Renal denervation attenuates the sodium retention and hypertension associated with obesity. *Hypertension* 1995;25:893–97.

56. Lohmeier TE, Hildebrandt DA, Warren S, et al. Recent insights into the interactions between the baroreflex and the kidneys in hypertension. *Am J Physiol Regul Integr Comp Physiol* 2005;288:R828–36.

57. Esler M. The sympathetic system and hypertension. *Am J Hypertens* 2000;13:99S–105S.

58. Cowley AW Jr. Long-term control of arterial blood pressure. *Physiol Rev* 1992;72:231–300.

59. Orfila C, Damase-Michel C, Lepert JC, et al. Renal morphological changes after sinoaortic denervation in dogs. *Hypertension* 1993;21:758–66.

60. Kaplan NM. *Kaplan's Clinical Hypertension*, 8th ed. Philadelphia: Lippincott Williams & Wilkins, 2002.

61. Garrison RJ, Kannel WB, Stokes J, et al. Incidence and precursors of hypertension in young adults: the Framingham Offspring Study. *Prev Med* 1987;16:234–51.

62. Wofford MR, Anderson DC, Brown CA, et al. Antihypertensive effect of alpha and beta adrenergic blockade in obese and lean hypertensive subjects. *Am J Hypertens* 2001;14:164–68.

63. Hall JE, Hildebrandt DA, Kuo JJ. Obesity hypertension: role of leptin and sympathetic nervous system. *Am J Hypertens* 2001;14:103s–15s.

64. Shek EW, Brands MW, Hall JE. Chronic leptin infusion increases arterial pressure. *Hypertension* 1998;31:409–14.

65. Mark AL, Shaffer RA, Correia ML, et al. Contrasting blood pressure effects of obesity in leptin-deficient ob/ob mice and agouti yellow mice. *J Hypertens* 1999;17:1949–53.

66. Ozata M, Ozdemir IC, Licinio J. Human leptin deficiency caused by a missense mutation: multiple endocrine defects, decreased sympathetic tone, and immune system dysfunction indicate new targets for leptin action, greater central than peripheral resistance to the effects of leptin, and spontaneous correction of leptin-mediated defects. *J Clin Endocrinol Metab* 1999;10:3686–95.

67. daSilva AA, Kuo JJ, Hall JE. Role of hypothalamic melanocortin 3/4 receptors in mediating the chronic cardiovascular, renal, and metabolic actions of leptin. *Hypertension* 2004;43:1312–17.

68. Tallam LS, da Silva AA, Hall JE. Melanocortin-4 receptor mediates chronic cardiovascular and metabolic actions of leptin. *Hypertension* 2006;48:58–64.

69. Yanagisawa M, Kurihara H, Kimura S, et al. A novel potent vasoconstrictor peptide produced by vascular endothelial cells. *Nature* 1988;332:411–15.

70. Kohan D. Endothelins in the normal and diseased kidney. *Am J Kidney Dis* 1997;29:2–26.

71. Schiffrin EL. Endothelin: potential role in hypertension and vascular hypertrophy. *Hypertension* 1995;25:1135–43.

72. Simonson MS, Dunn MJ. Endothelin peptides and the kidney. *Annu Rev Physiol* 1993;55:249–65.

73. Schiffrin EL. Vascular endothelin in hypertension. *Vascul Pharmacol* 2005;43:19–29.

74. Granger JP. Endothelin. *Am J Physiol Regul Integr Comp Physiol* 2003;285:R298–301.

75. Kohan DE. The renal medullary endothelin system in control of sodium and water excretion and systemic blood pressure. *Curr Opin Nephrol Hypertens* 2006;15:34–40.

76. Kassab S, Novak J, Miller T, et al. Role of endothelin in mediating the attenuated renal hemodynamics in Dahl salt-sensitive hypertension. *Hypertension* 1997;30:682–86.

77. Kassab S, Miller M, Novak J, et al. Endothelin-A receptor antagonism attenuates the hypertension and renal injury in Dahl salt-sensitive rats. *Hypertension* 1998;31:397–402.

78. Alexander BT, Cockrell KL, Rinewalt AN, et al. Enhanced renal expression of preproendothelin mRNA during chronic angiotensin II hypertension. *Am J Physiol Regul Integr Comp Physiol* 2001;280:R1388–392.

79. Ballew JR, Fink GD. Role of ET-1$_A$ receptors in experimental ANG II-induced hypertension in rats. *Am J Physiol Regul Integr Comp Physiol* 2001;281:R150–54.

80. d'Uscio LV, Moreau P, Shaw S, et al. Effects of chronic ET-1$_A$-receptor blockade in angiotensin II–induced hypertension. *Hypertension* 1997;29:435–41.

81. Perez del Villar C, Garcia Alonso CJ, Feldstein CA, et al. Role of endothelin in the pathogenesis of hypertension. *May Clin Proc* 2005;80:84–96.

82. Sasser JM, Pollock JS, Pollock DM. Renal endothelin in chronic angiotensin II hypertension. *Am J Physiol Regul Integr Comp Physiol* 2002;283:R243–48.

83. Granger JP, Alexander BT, Llinas MT, et al. Pathophysiology of hypertension during preeclampsia: linking placental ischemia with endothelial dysfunction. *Hypertension* 2001;38:718–22.

84. Khalil RA, Granger JP. Vascular mechanisms of increased arterial pressure in preeclampsia: lessons from animal models. *Am J Physiol Regul Integr Comp Physiol* 2002;283:R29–45.

85. Wilkins FC Jr, Alberola A, Mizelle HL, et al. Systemic hemodynamics and renal function during long-term pathophysiological increases in circulating endothelin. *Am J Physiol Regul Integr Comp Physiol* 1995;268:R375–81.

86. Alexander BT, Rinewalt AN, Cockrell KL, et al. Endothelin-A receptor blockade attenuates the hypertension in response to chronic reductions in uterine perfusion pressure. *Hypertension* 2001;37:485–89.

87. Granger JP, LaMarca BBD, Cockrell K, et al. Reduced uterine perfusion pressure (RUPP) model for studying cardiovascular-renal dysfunction in response to placental ischemia. *Methods Mol Med* 2006;122:383–92.

88. Roberts L, LaMarca B, Fournier L, et al. Enhanced endothelin synthesis by endothelial cells exposed to sera from pregnant rats with decreased uterine perfusion. *Hypertension* 2006;47:615–18.

89. LaMarca BB, Bennett WA, Alexander BT, et al. Hypertension produced by reductions in uterine perfusion in the pregnant rat. Role of tumor necrosis factor-α. *Hypertension* 2005;46:1022–25.

90. LaMarca BB, Cockrell K, Sullivan E, et al. Role of endothelin in mediating tumor necrosis factor-induced hypertension in pregnant rats. *Hypertension* 2005;46:82–86.

91. Dean R, Zhuo J, Alcorn D, et al. Cellular localization of endothelin receptor subtypes in the rat kidney following in vitro labeling. *Clin Exp Pharmacol Physiol* 1996;23:524–31.

92. Jones CR, Hiley CR, Pelton JT, Miller RC. Autoradiographic localization of endothelin binding sites in kidney. *Eur J Pharmacol* 1989;163:379–82.

93. Karet FE, Kuc RE, Davenport AP. Novel ligands BQ123 and BQ3020 characterize endothelin receptor subtypes ET-1A and ET-1B in human kidney. *Kidney Int* 1993;44:36–42.

94. Nambi P, Pullen M, Wu HL, et al. Identification of endothelin receptor subtypes in human renal cortex and medulla using subtype-selective ligands. *Endocrinology* 1992;131:1081–86.

95. Gariepy CE, Cass DT, Yanagisawa M. Null mutation of endothelin-B receptor gene in spotting lethal rats causes aganglionic megacolon and white coat color. *Proc Natl Acad Sci U S A* 1996;93:867–72.

96. Strachan FE, Spratt JC, Wilkinson IB, et al. Systemic blockade of the endothelin-B receptor increases peripheral vascular resistance in healthy men. *Hypertension* 1999;33:581–85.

97. Gariepy CE, Ohuchi T, Williams SC, et al. Salt-sensitive hypertension in endothelin-B receptor-deficient rats. *J Clin Invest* 2000;105:925–33.

98. Pollock DM, Pollock JS. Evidence for endothelin involvement in the response to high salt. *Am J Physiol Renal Physiol* 2001;281:F144–50.

99. Bagnall AJ, Kelland NF, Gulliver-Sloan F, et al. Deletion of endothelial cell endothelin B receptors does not affect blood pressure or sensitivity to salt. *Hypertension* 2006;48:286–93.

100. Ge Y, Bagnall A, Stricklett P, Strait K, Webb D, Kotelevtsev Y, et al. Collecting duct-specific knockout of the endothelin B receptor causes hypertension and sodium retention. *Am J Physiol Renal Physiol* 2006 [Epub before print].

101. Ohuchi T, Kuwaki T, Ling G, et al. Elevation of blood pressure by genetic and pharmacological disruption of the ETB receptor in mice. *Am J Physiol Regul Integr Comp Physiol* 1999;276:R1071–77.

102. Kohzuki M, Johnston CI, Chai SY, et al. Localization and endothelin receptors in the rat kidney. *Eur J Pharmacol* 1989;160:193–94.

103. Michel H, Backer A, Meyer-Lehnert H, et al. Rat renal, aortic and pulmonary endothelin-1 receptors: effects of changes in sodium and water intake. *Clin Sci (Colch)* 1993;85:593–97.

104. Krum H, Viskoper RJ, Lacourciere Y, Budde M, Charlon V. The effect of an endothelin-receptor antagonist, bosentan, on blood pressure inpatients with essential hypertension. Bosentan Hypertension Investigators. *N Engl J Med* 1998;338:784–90.

105. Schnackenberg CG, Kirchner K, Patel A, Granger JP. Nitric oxide, the kidney, and hypertension. *Clin Exp Pharmacol Physiol* 1997;24:600–606.

106. Ortiz PA, Garvin JL. Role of nitric oxide in the regulation of nephron transport. *Am J Physiol Renal Physiol* 2002;282:F777–84.

107. Cowley AW Jr, Mori T, Mattson D, Zou AP. Role of renal NO production in the regulation of medullary blood flow. *Am J Physiol Regul Integr Comp Physiol* 2003;284:R1355–69.

108. Granger JP, Alexander BT. Abnormal pressure natriuresis in hypertension: role of nitric oxide. *Acta Physiologica Scandinavia* 2000;168:161–68.

109. Nakamura T, Alberola A, Granger JP. Role of renal interstitial pressure as a mediator of sodium retention during blockade of endothelium derived nitric oxide hypertension. *Hypertension* 1993;21:956–960.

110. Sanders PW. Sodium intake, endothelial cell signaling, and progression of kidney disease. *Hypertension* 2004;43:142–46.

111. Schnackenberg C, Tabor B, Strong M, Granger JP. Intrarenal NO blockade enhances renin secretion rate by a macula densa mechanism. *Am J Physiol* 1997;272:R879–86.

112. Schnackenberg C, Wilkins C, Granger JP. Role of nitric oxide in modulating the vasoconstrictor actions of angiotensin II in preglomerular and postglomerular vessels in dogs. *Hypertension* 1995;26:1024–29.

113. Granger JP, Alberola A, Salazer F, Nakamura T. Control of renal hemodynamics during intrarenal systemic EDNO synthesis blockade. *J Cardiovasc Pharmacol* 1992;20:S160–62.

114. Granger JP, Novak J, Schnackenberg C, Williams S, Reinhart G. Role of renal nerves in mediating the hypertensive effects of nitric oxide synthesis inhibition. *Hypertension* 1996;27:613–18.

115. Knox FG, Granger JP. Control of sodium excretion: an integrative approach. In: Windhager E, ed. *Handbook of Renal Physiology*. New York: Oxford University Press, 1992:927–67.

116. Vesely DL. Atrial natriuretic peptides in pathophysiological diseases. *Cardiovasc Res* 2001;51:647–58.

117. Granger JP, Opgenorth TJ, Salazar J, Romero JC, Burnett JC Jr. Long-term hypotensive and renal effects of chronic infusions of atrial natriuretic peptide in conscious dogs. *Hypertension* 1986;8:II112–16.

118. Melo LG, Steinhelper ME, Pang SC, Tse Y, Ackermann U. ANP in regulation of arterial pressure and fluid-electrolyte balance: lessons from genetic mouse models. *Physiol Genomics* 2000;3:45–58.

119. Cheng HF, Harris RC. Cyclooxygenases, the kidney, and hypertension. *Hypertension* 2004;43:525–30.

120. Roman RJ. P-450 metabolites of arachidonic acid in the control of cardiovascular function. *Physiol Rev* 2002;82:131–85.

121. Laffer CL, Laniado-Schwartzman M, Wang MH, Nasjletti A, Elijovich F. Differential regulation of natriuresis by 20-hydroxyeicosatetraenoic acid in human salt-sensitive versus salt-resistant hypertension. *Circulation* 2003;107:574–78.

122. Laffer CL, Laniado-Schwartzman M, Wang MH, Nasjletti A, Elijovich F. 20-HETE and furosemide-induced natriuresis in salt-sensitive essential hypertension. *Hypertension* 2003;41:703–08.

123. Taniyama Y, Griendling KK. Reactive oxygen species in the vasculature: molecular and cellular mechanisms. *Hypertension* 2003;42:1075–81.

124. Wilcox CS. Reactive oxygen species: roles in blood pressure and kidney function. *Curr Hypertens Rep* 2002;4:160–66.

125. Manning RD Jr, Meng S, Tian N. Renal and vascular oxidative stress and salt-sensitivity of arterial pressure. *Acta Physiol Scand* 2003;179:243–50.

126. Reckelhoff JF, Romero JC. Role of oxidative stress in angiotensin-induced hypertension. *Am J Physiol Regul Integr Comp Physiol* 2003;284:R893–912.

127. Romero JC, Reckelhoff JF. State-of-the-art lecture. Role of angiotensin and oxidative stress in essential hypertension. *Hypertension* 1999;34:943–49.

128. Sedeek M, Alexander BT, Abram SR, Granger JP. Role of oxidative stress in endothelin-induced hypertension in rats. *Hypertension* 2003;42:806–10.

129. Garvin JL, Ortiz PA. The role of reactive oxygen species in the regulation of tubular function. *Acta Physiol Scand* 2003;179:225–32.

130. Chae CU, Lee RT, Rifai N, Ridker PM. Blood pressure and inflammation in apparently healthy men. *Hypertension* 2001;38:399–403.

131. Conrad KP, Benyo DF. Placental cytokines and the pathogenesis of preeclampsia. *Am J Reprod Immunol* 1997;37:240–49.

132. Donners MM, Daemen MJ, Cleutjens KB, Heeneman S. Inflammation and restenosis: implications for therapy. *Ann Med* 2003;35:523–31.

133. Sattar N, McCarey DW, Capell H, and McInnes IB. Explaining how "high-grade" systemic inflammation accelerates vascular risk in rheumatoid arthritis. *Circulation* 2003;108:2957–63.

134. Siwik DA, Colucci WS. Regulation of matrix metalloproteinases by cytokines and reactive oxygen/nitrogen species in the myocardium. *Heart Fail Rev* 2004;9:43–51.

135. Zhang ZH, Wei SG, Francis J, Felder RB. Cardiovascular and renal sympathetic activation by blood-borne TNF in rat: the role of central prostaglandins. *Am J Physiol Regul Integr Comp Physiol* 2003;284:R916–27.

136. Han Y, Runge MS, Braiser AR. Angiotensin II induces interleukin-6 transcription in vascular smooth muscle cells through pleiotropic activation of nuclear factor-kappa B transcription factors. *Circ Res* 1999;84:695–703.

137. Ruiz-Ortega M, Ruperez M, Lorenzo O, Esteban V, Blanco J, Mezzano S, Egido J. Angiotensin II regulates the synthesis of proinflammatory cytokines and chemokines in the kidney. *Kidney Int* 2002;82:12–22.

138. Sanz-Rosa D, Oubina MP, Cediel E, De Las Heras N, Vegazo O, Jimenez J, et al. Effect of AT1 receptor antagonism on vascular and circulating inflammatory mediators in SHR: Role of NFκB/IκB system. *Am J Physiol Heart Circ Physiol* 2005;288:H111–15.

139. Granger JP, Alexander BT, Llinas MT, Bennett WA, Khalil RA. Pathophysiology of preeclampsia: linking placental ischemia/hypoxia with microvascular dysfunction. *Microcirculation* 2002;9:147–60.

140. Giardina JB, Green GM, Cockrell KL, Granger JP, Khalil RA. TNF enhances contraction and inhibits endothelial NO-cGMP relaxation in systemic vessels of pregnant rats. *Am J Physiol Regul Integr Comp* 2002;283:R130–43.

141. Alexander BT, Massey MB, Cockrell KL, Bennett WA, Granger JP. Elevations in plasma TNF in pregnant rats decreases renal nNOS and iNOS and results in hypertension. *Am J Hypertens* 2002;15:170–75.

142. Orshal JM, Khalil RA. Reduced endothelial NO-cGMP-mediated vascular relaxation and hypertension in IL-6-infused pregnant rats. *Hypertension* 2004;43:434–444.

143. Lee DL, Sturgis LC, Labazi H, Osborne Jr JB, Fleming C, Pollock JS, et al. Angiotensin II hypertension is attenuated in interleukin-6 knockout mice. *Am J Physiol Heart Circ Physiol* 2006;290:H935–40.

Chapter

24

The Baroreflex in the Pathogenesis of Hypertension

Thomas E. Lohmeier and Heather A. Drummond

Key Findings

- Experimental studies have clearly demonstrated incomplete baroreflex resetting of sympathetic activity during chronic alterations in arterial pressure.

- Baroreflex suppression of renal sympathetic nerve activity is sustained in experimental hypertension, a response expected to attenuate the rise in arterial pressure.

- Chronic electrical activation of the carotid baroreflex has sustained effects to suppress sympathetic activity and to lower arterial pressure, especially when hypertension is associated with increased sympathetic activity, such as in obesity.

- Acute determinations of baroreflex function in human subjects indicate that baroreflex suppression of sympathetic outflow is impaired in obesity hypertension, but whether this contributes to chronic sympathetic activation is unclear at present.

There is now considerable evidence that the sympathetic nervous system plays a key role in the pathogenesis of primary hypertension, but the determinants of sympathetic activation are unresolved.[1–8] In contrast to primary hypertension, some forms of secondary hypertension appear to be associated with suppression of the sympathetic nervous system.[9–11] Because the arterial baroreflex is a powerful buffering mechanism that counteracts short-term fluctuations in arterial pressure by mediating reciprocal changes in sympathetic and parasympathetic activity, there has been considerable interest in the possibility that this reflex might also play a role in long-term control of arterial pressure. This is highlighted by reports that primary hypertension is often associated with baroreflex dysfunction.[3,5] However, the possibilities that sustained activation of the baroreflex account for the apparent sympathoinhibition present in secondary hypertension, and that impaired baroreflex function leads to increased sympathetic activity in hypertension, are merely conjecture at the present time. This uncertainty is due, in part, to the paucity of techniques available to assess the long-term effects of the baroreflex on sympathetic activity and organ function.

Until the last several years, there has been little direct evidence that either supports or refutes the possibility that baroreflexes play a role in pathogenesis of hypertension. Nonetheless, as recently reviewed,[12] two key observations, made decades ago, are often mentioned to discount the potential role of baroreflexes in long-term control of arterial pressure: (1) baroreceptors reset, and (2) baroreceptor deafferentation (sinoaortic denervation) (SAD) produces little or no sustained increase in arterial pressure.

Regarding the baroreceptor resetting argument, it is well established that baroreceptors reset in the direction of change in arterial pressure, which diminishes the initial alteration in sympathetic activity induced by the baroreflex in response to a disturbance in arterial pressure.[13,14] Consequently, resetting of the baroreceptors decreases the ability of the baroreflex to serve as a long-term compensatory mechanism for the control of arterial pressure. However, because of technical limitations inherent in long-term recordings of nerve activity, the degree of baroreflex resetting associated with chronic changes in arterial pressure has not been determined with any certainty. Most direct information relating to sympathetic baroreflex resetting has come from *acute* studies in anesthetized animals subjected to various experimental preparations designed to mimic blood pressure–baroreceptor interactions under more physiologic conditions. Electrophysiologic techniques used in anesthetized animals to record baroreceptor afferent nerve activity in chronic hypertension also support the concept of baroreceptor resetting. However, these studies too are incapable of determining the precise degree of chronic baroreceptor resetting that occurs under normal daily activity. Therefore, although considerable resetting of the baroreflex occurs both acutely and chronically, the time course and extent of chronic resetting is unclear. Consequently, the uncertainty regarding the *long-term* baroreflex relationships between arterial pressure and sympathetic activity in response to interventions that result in sustained alterations in arterial pressure prohibit any definitive conclusions regarding the ability of the baroreflex to chronically alter sympathetic activity and regulate arterial pressure.

The other argument frequently made to discount an important role of the baroreflex in the pathogenesis of hypertension is that the rise in arterial pressure following SAD is largely transient, and that little or no hypertension occurs chronically.[14–16] The presumption then is that if complete loss of the sympathoinhibitory effects of baroreceptor input fails to chronically increase central sympathetic output, then it is unlikely that natural alterations in baroreceptor activity could have long-term effects on sympathetic activity and arterial pressure. However, because of technical limitations precluding chronic measurement of nerve activity, time-dependent changes in sympathetic activity following SAD have not been directly established. Instead, they are often assumed based on changes in arterial pressure or circulating levels of norepinephrine (NE). Both represent imprecise indices of alteration in sympathetic activity. Therefore, one cannot discount the possibility that SAD produces sustained increases in sympathetic activity, but no hypertension, because non-neural compensatory mechanisms are activated to reduce arterial pressure. An additional concern with using SAD as a model for understanding baroreflex function is that central reorganization of baroreflex circuitry occurs after baroreceptor deafferentation, which appears to diminish the efferent sympathetic response to loss of baroreceptor input.[17] Furthermore, as discussed later in this chapter, recent studies by Thrasher[16,18] in chronically instrumented dogs clearly illustrate a dichotomy between complete loss of baroreceptor input by deafferentation and the more physiologic response to sustained reductions in barorecep-tor activity when arterial pressure is chronically reduced.

In light of the uncertainties regarding the sustained effects of baroreflexes on sympathetic activity, what new information is needed to better understand the role of baroreflexes in long-term control of arterial pressure? Because the kidneys play a critical role in long-term regu-lation of arterial pressure by virtue of their ability to regulate body fluid volumes,[19,20] it is critical to determine whether baroreflexes have sustained effects on renal excre-tory function.[12] As illustrated in Figure 24–1, and discussed later, one way that the baroreflex could alter the function of the renal body–fluid feedback mechanism for long-term control of arterial pressure is by producing chronic changes in renal sympathetic nerve activity (RSNA). This chapter will emphasize recent studies that support the hypothesis that baroreflex suppression of RSNA is

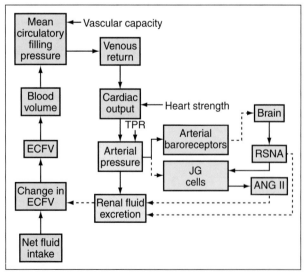

Figure 24–1. Interaction of arterial baroreceptors (*green shading*) with the renal body fluid feedback mechanism (*blocks with blue and beige shading*), including pressure natriuresis (*blocks with beige shading*). Dashed lines indicate inhibition. Ang II, angiotensin II; ECFV, extracellular fluid volume; JG, juxtaglomerular; RSNA, renal sympathetic nerve activity; TPR, total peripheral resistance.

sustained in hypertension, which leads to increased renal excretory function, a response that favors a reduction in arterial pressure.

ANATOMY/BIOCHEMISTRY

Afferent limb of baroreflex

Arterial baroreceptors are located in the aortic arch and carotid sinuses, and are formed by small nerve endings present in the adventitia of these vessels (Figure 24–2, A).[21,22] In most species, baroreceptor nerve endings are located near the adventitial-medial border. Baroreceptors are mechanosensors that are activated by pressure-induced vessel wall stretch or strain.[21] Mechanosensitive ion channels are believed to be a critical component of such mechanosensors.[23,24] As illustrated in Figure 24–2, *B*, activation of these channels increases permeability to sodium and calcium, leading to a generator potential in the mechanoreception zone.[23,24] In turn, the current from the mechanoreception zone flows into the spike initiation zone, which activates voltage-gated Na+ channels result-ing in axonal discharge. Thus the process of mechano-transduction is the initiating step in baroreception that results in an electric signal (neural discharge).[23,24]

The mechanosensing property of baroreceptors is likely due to the coupling of mechanosensitive ion channels with cytoskeletal membrane and extracellular proteins.

Terminals of myelinated and unmyelinated barorecep-tors intertwine within the adventitia, making it difficult to study baroreceptor pressure encoding.[22–24] Because of experimental limitations, understanding the molecular identity and mechanisms of baroreceptor mechanotrans-duction has required investigators to apply information from other organisms and sensory systems to unravel the mystery of baroreceptor mechanotransduction. Specifically, research on mechanosensory transduction in the nematode *Caenorhabditis elegans* has advanced our understanding of mechanotransduction.[25–28] Genetic screens in the nematode revealed a number of genes required for the nematodes' ability to respond to touch. It is now known that these genes are related to a group of mammalian genes in the degenerin/epithelial Na+ channel (DEG/ENaC) family, which includes members of the acid-sensing ion channel (ASIC) family.[27,28] Several studies suggest that ENaC and/or ASIC proteins may form the pore of mechano-sensitive ion channel complexes in baroreceptor neurons.[27–29] The role of other mechanosensitive ion channels from other gene families is unknown.[27]

The presence of two distinct types of baroreceptors is well known.[21] Generally speaking, baroreceptors are classi-fied based on their discharge properties and degree of myelination.[30] One group is formed by neurons with large myelinated afferent fibers. These baroreceptors have lower activation thresholds and fire more rapidly upon stimu-lation. These are often referred to as type I baroreceptors. The other group is formed by neurons with unmyelinated or small poorly myelinated afferent fibers. These baro-receptors tend to have higher activation thresholds and discharge at lower frequencies. They are referred to as

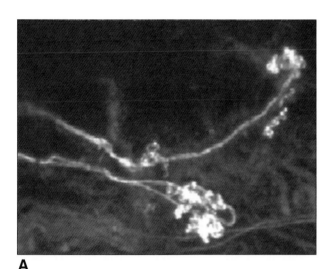

A

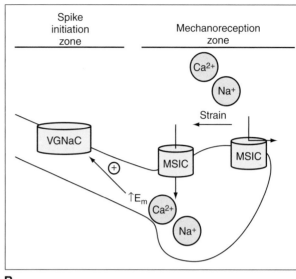

B

Figure 24–2. Baroreceptor sensory nerve ending and mechanoelectrical coupling. **A,** A fluorescently labeled nerve ending in the aortic arch. **B,** Schematic representation of proposed mechanoelectrical coupling in baroreceptor nerve endings. Mechanosensitive ion channels activated by strain increase Na^+ and/or Ca^{2+} entry, which activates voltage gated Na^+ channels, resulting in the generation of an action potential. MSIC, mechanosensitive ion channels; VGNaC, voltage-gated Na^+ channels.

type II baroreceptors. These two receptor types may have a differential role in the regulation of arterial pressure.[31] For example, type II baroreceptors show less resetting than type I baroreceptors and, therefore, may be more important in long-term control of arterial pressure.[32] How differences in mechanotransduction might account for the specific discharge properties of baroreceptor subtypes is poorly understood.

Baroreceptor afferents from the carotid sinus travel in the carotid sinus nerve (Hering's nerve) before joining the glossopharyngeal nerve. The afferent fibers from aortic baroreceptors pass centrally via the vagus nerves. Baroreceptor afferents in both the glossopharyngeal and vagus nerves terminate in the nucleus of the tractus solitarius (NTS) in the medulla of the brain.

Central baroreflex circuitry

An article by Pilowsky and Goodchild[33] updates recent advances in understanding the central baroreflex pathways and neurotransmitters mediating the sympathetic baroreflex, and interested readers are referred to this excellent review. A simplified diagram of the medullary circuitry comprising the sympathetic baroreflex and its integration into the chronic feedback control of arterial pressure is provided in Figure 24–3. Since the renal body–fluid feedback mechanism plays a central role in the long-term control of arterial pressure, this schema for the chronic regulation of arterial pressure is based upon alterations in RSNA linking baroreflex induced changes in central sympathetic output to renal excretory function. Renal sympathetic outflow consists of neuronal discharges from sympathetic preganglionic motor neurons in the intermediolateral cell column of the spinal cord. These motor neurons are controlled, in part, by bulbospinal sympathoexcitatory neurons located in the rostral ventrolateral medulla (RVLM), a nucleus whose activity is modu-

lated by the baroreflex. Specifically, acute recording studies have demonstrated that baroreflex inhibition of the RVLM is achieved by a circuit which activates neurons in the NTS, the site of termination of baroreceptor inputs. In turn, NTS neurons activate inhibitory neurons in the caudal ventrolateral medulla (CVLM) that project to the RVLM. Consequently, if baroreflex resetting is incomplete in chronic hypertension, then activation of neurons in the NTS and CVLM and attendant suppression of sympatho-excitatory RVLM neurons should be sustained responses to hypertension. This would favor sustained suppression of RSNA. Studies discussed later in this chapter support this hypothesis.

Efferent limb of baroreflex

The postganglionic fibers to the kidneys innervate the vasculature, tubules, and renin containing juxtaglomeru-

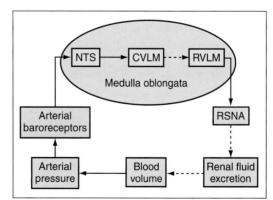

Figure 24–3. Arterial baroreceptors, the medullary neurons comprising the baroreflex, and the link to the renal body–fluid feedback mechanism via the renal nerves. CVLM, caudal ventrolateral medulla; NTS, nucleus of the tractus solitarius; RVLM, rostral ventrolateral medulla.

lar cells.[34,35] Increases in RSNA decrease sodium excretion by promoting sodium reabsorption, decreasing renal blood flow and glomerular filtration rate, and increasing renin release.[34,35] The NE released from adrenergic nerve terminals exerts direct vasoconstrictor and tubular effects that decrease sodium excretion by activation of postjunctional α_1-adrenoceptors receptors. Additionally, because increases in RSNA stimulate renin secretion, the generation of ANG II contributes indirectly to the antinatriuretic effects of noradrenergic stimulation (Figure 24–1). ANG II increases sodium reabsorption and reduces blood flow by acting on ANG II-type AT_1 receptors located on the tubules and vasculature.

Stimulation of renin secretion by the renal nerves is achieved by activation of both α_1-and β_1-adrenoceptors.[34,35] Noradrenergic stimulation of α_1-adrenoceptors may increase renin secretion in two ways: (1) by reducing the stretch of the afferent arteriole and the associated juxtaglomerular cells (the intrarenal baroreceptor) through constriction of the upstream vasculature, and (2) by decreasing the delivery of sodium chloride to the macula densa through promotion of sodium reabsorption in the proximal tubule and loop of Henle. Noradrenergic stimulation of renin secretion is also achieved by activating β_1-adrenergic receptors located on the juxtaglomerular cells themselves.

Numerous acute studies have been conducted to elucidate the complex interactions between the renal sympathetic nerves and the renin-angiotensin system in the control of renal function.[34,35] However, while much progress has been made in understanding the acute interactions between these pathways in the control of renal function, a precise definition of the long-term quantitative interrelationships is still needed. An understanding of the direct versus the indirect effects of the renal nerves on renal function is complicated by the time dependency of these interactions, which prohibit extrapolation of the findings from acute studies to chronic conditions such as hypertension. There are few chronic studies that have attempted to determine the relative importance of the direct and indirect pathways in promoting sodium retention. The evidence we have suggests that the indirect pathway has an increasingly important role in promoting sodium retention, as angiotensin II (Ang II) is generated during more prolonged periods of adrenergic stimulation.[35-37]

PHYSIOLOGY

Long-term regulation of arterial pressure is closely linked to volume homeostasis through the renal body–fluid feedback mechanism (Figure 24–1).[19,20] Increases in body fluid volume and arterial pressure cause the kidneys to increase salt and water excretion. In turn, the pressure natriuresis and diuresis reduces body fluid volume until arterial pressure returns to control levels. Conversely, when arterial pressure falls too low, the kidneys retain fluid, and body fluid volume increases, returning arterial pressure toward normal.

In response to disturbances in body fluid volume and arterial pressure, there are changes in several extrarenal and intrarenal factors. These contribute to long-term regulation of arterial pressure by affecting the sensitivity of the pressure natriuresis mechanism.[20] One especially important feedback mechanism for long-term blood pressure control is the renin-angiotensin-aldosterone system. Under normal conditions, elevations in body fluid volume suppress this potent sodium-retaining system. Suppression of the renin-angiotensin-aldosterone system increases the sensitivity of pressure natriuresis and minimizes increments in body fluid volume and arterial pressure. Just the opposite changes occur for regulation of arterial pressure when body fluid volume is reduced. In contrast to the well-established role of the renin-angiotensin-aldosterone system, it is unclear whether, and to what extent, the arterial baroreflex also contributes to long-term feedback control of arterial pressure.

The baroreflex plays an important role in short-term regulation of arterial pressure by mediating changes in peripheral resistance, vascular capacity (a determinant of mean circulatory filling pressure and, thus, venous return), and cardiac function (Figure 24–1). However, due to the renal body–fluid feedback mechanism for long-term control of arterial pressure, these autonomic responses, even if sustained chronically, would not be expected to produce long-term changes in arterial pressure, unless they were associated with a simultaneous effect on pressure natriuresis.[12,19,20] In the absence of a change in renal excretory function, any sympathetically mediated alterations in arterial pressure would result in similar directional changes in the renal excretion of sodium, which would return body fluid volume and arterial pressure toward control. Consequently, if the baroreflex were to play a role in the chronic regulation of arterial pressure during disturbances in body fluid volume and arterial pressure, then the baroreflex must in some way have a sustained effect to alter renal excretory function. Because chronic changes in renal adrenergic activity alter renal excretory function,[12,36,38] one way in which the baroreflex could alter pressure natriuresis and produce long-term changes in arterial pressure is by chronically influencing RSNA (Figure 24–1).

Chronic unloading of baroreceptors results in neurogenic hypertension

To examine the role of baroreflexes in mediating sustained alterations in sympathetic activity, Thrasher determined arterial pressures responses for up to 5 weeks of carotid baroreceptor unloading in chronically instrumented dogs.[16,18] In these studies, baroreceptors in the aortic arch and one carotid sinus were denervated, leaving one carotid sinus with intact innervation. After several days of control measurements, baroreceptor unloading was achieved by ligation of the common carotid artery proximal to the innervated sinus. In response to unloading of carotid baroreceptors, there was sustained hypertension for the duration of the study (5 weeks). The initial days of baroreceptor unloading were associated with sodium retention and increased renin secretion, responses consistent with increased RSNA. In the chronic phase of the hypertension, however, increments in plasma renin activity were not statistically significant, presumably due to the effects of increased arterial pressure to counteract neurally mediated renin secretion. These studies are consistent with the hypothesis that increased RSNA and attendant activation of the renin-angiotensin system are sustained baroreflex responses to reduced arterial pressure. However, confirmation of this hypothesis must await the demonstration that renal denervation markedly attenuates or completely abolishes baroreflex-mediated hypertension.

Thrasher[16] also compared chronic arterial pressure responses in dogs with SAD to dogs subjected to baroreceptor unloading. In contrast to the sustained hypertension produced by chronic unloading of baroreceptors, increases in arterial pressure following SAD were transient, persisting ~2 weeks. Thus the dichotomy between the arterial pressure responses to SAD and baroreceptor unloading questions the relevance of the former traditional approach for elucidating chronic baroreflex-mediated sympathetic responses. The sustained hypertension following chronic baroreceptor unloading suggests that complete central resetting does not occur in response to a more physiologic stimulus—reduced pulse synchronous input from baroreceptors—and indicates that resetting of the baroreflex is incomplete when arterial pressure is chronically reduced. These studies support the concept that the baroreflex can have long-term effects on sympathetic activity and arterial pressure.

Role of baroreflexes in chronic regulation of arterial pressure during increased sodium intake

Increased salt intake is a frequent challenge to the regulation of body fluid volume and arterial pressure. During chronic increases in salt intake, it is widely recognized that suppression of the renin-angiotensin-aldosterone system minimizes volume expansion and increments in arterial pressure by increasing renal excretory function. In contrast, the role of the nervous system in defending against chronic perturbations in body fluid volume and arterial pressure is unclear. To determine whether baroreflex-induced suppression of sympathetic activity contributes to the chronic regulation of arterial pressure during sustained increases in sodium intake, arterial pressure responses to increased salt intake have been assessed in rats with and without intact arterial baroreflexes.[39–41] The results of these studies are consistent in that they demonstrate little or no change in arterial pressure in response to chronic increases in salt intake when baroreflexes are intact but significant increases in arterial pressure following SAD. While these studies indicate that sustained activation of the baroreflex contributes to arterial pressure regulation during chronic increases in salt intake, they do not address the efferent mechanisms that mediate this neural response. Neural mechanisms do promote sodium excretion by inhibiting RSNA during acute increments in body fluid volume and renal denervation impairs the natriuretic response to an acute salt load.[34,35] Therefore, if baroreflex-mediated inhibition of RSNA were a sustained response to chronic increases in salt intake, the resultant increase in renal excretory func-

tion would be expected to minimize volume retention and concomitant increments in arterial pressure.

The issue of whether reflex-induced renal sympathoinhibition is a long-term response for defending volume homeostasis is unsettled because of technical difficulties in long-term monitoring of changes in RSNA and the attendant sodium excretory responses. Therefore, the effects of the baroreflex on renal excretory function during chronic increases in salt intake have been deduced from sodium balance determinations in rats with and without intact baroreflexes.[40,41] Unfortunately, the results from this approach have been inconsistent. In one study, DiBona and Sawin[41] found that the reported salt-sensitive hypertension in rats with SAD was associated with greater retention of sodium than in control rats subjected to a high-salt intake, suggesting that baroreflex activation normally minimizes volume expansion by chronically enhancing renal excretory function, presumably by inhibiting RSNA. In contrast to these findings, an earlier study by Osborn and Hornfeldt[40] found no significant difference in sodium balance between baroreceptor-intact and baroreceptor-denervated rats fed a high-salt diet, despite an increase in mean arterial pressure (MAP) present only in rats with SAD. However, it should be emphasized that one confounding issue in interpreting sodium balance studies in the face of changes in neural activity is that alterations in the sympathetic nervous system simultaneously modulate vascular capacity and renal excretory function, responses that have opposing effects on blood volume. Specifically, baroreflex-induced renal sympathoinhibition would promote sodium excretion and decrease blood volume, whereas baroreflex-induced decreases in sympathetic constriction of the vasculature would favor sodium retention and increase blood volume. For this reason, in the absence of knowledge about the volume-holding capacity of the circulatory system (which can not be directly measured), changes in sodium balance provide limited insight into the impact of neurally induced alterations in body fluid volume on arterial pressure. Long-term changes in arterial pressure are not necessarily related to alterations in blood volume *per se*, but are instead related to the ratio of blood volume to the volume holding capacity of the circulation (the mean circulatory filling pressure, which can be measured).[19] Thus the long-term influence of alterations in reflex function on renal excretory function and the attendant changes in arterial pressure cannot be deduced with certainty from measurements of sodium balance alone. This point is clearly evident from the response to direct electrical activation of the carotid baroreflex. As illustrated below, chronic electrical activation of the carotid baroreflex produces a sustained reduction in arterial pressure, but this response is associated with the retention and not the loss of sodium.[42,43]

To determine whether the renal nerves contribute to sodium homeostasis during chronic increments in salt intake, Lohmeier et al.[44] conducted studies in dogs with unilateral renal denervation and surgical division of the urinary bladder into hemibladders to allow separate 24-hour urine collection from denervated and intact kidneys. This is a powerful model for exposing a functional role of the renal nerves because both kidneys are exposed to the same perfusion pressure and hormonal influences. Consequently, any differences in sodium excretion between the kidneys can be attributed to the effects of the renal nerves on renal excretory function. In this study, sodium excretion rates in the two kidneys were approximately equal during the control period. However, when sodium intake was chronically increased eight-fold, the innervated kidney excreted significantly more sodium than the contralateral denervated kidney. Taken in the context of the rat SAD studies and experiments in dogs with both NE and Ang II hypertension, these results are consistent with the hypothesis that baroreflex-mediated renal sympathoinhibition is a sustained response that promotes sodium excretion during increments in salt intake, thus contributing to the chronic regulation of body fluid volume and arterial pressure.

Renal nerves chronically promote sodium excretion in secondary hypertension
Norepinephrine-induced hypertension

Activation of the sympathetic nervous system, including sympathetic outflow to the kidneys, is commonly associated with primary hypertension.[1–8] In contrast, results from microneurographic studies in human subjects suggest that the sympathetic nervous system is suppressed in secondary hypertension.[9–11] However, whether this sympathoinhibition includes the neural outflow to the kidneys has not been established.

We reasoned that the split-bladder preparation, in combination with unilateral renal denervation, might provide a novel and effective approach for determining whether inhibition of RSNA and attendant increments in renal excretory function are long-term compensatory responses following the induction of secondary hypertension. However, an initial concern was whether the denervated kidney in the split-bladder preparation might be supersensitive to circulating NE.[34] If so, this could confound interpretation of the renal responses to NE. Therefore, we first elected to investigate renal excretory responses during the induction of hypertension induced by chronic infusion of NE.[45] Figure 24–4 illustrates changes in the relative 24-hour excretion rates of sodium from denervated (DEN) and innervated (INN) kidneys in dogs after 4 to 5 days of progressively higher rates of NE infusion. In this study, infusion of NE at rates producing increments in plasma levels of NE as high as ~3000 pg/mL or ~30 times normal had no influence on the relative excretion rates of sodium between the innervated and denervated kidneys (DEN/INN). This indicated that denervated kidneys were not supersensitive to either physiologic or pathophysiologic increases in plasma NE concentration. However, at the highest tested infusion rate of NE which produced pharmacologic levels of NE (~70 times normal) and hypertension, there was a persistently higher rate of sodium excretion from innervated compared to denervated kidneys, as reflected by the decrease in the DEN/INN. This last finding is consistent with the possibility that denervated kidneys are supersensitive to pharmacologic levels of circulating NE. Alternately, the higher rate of sodium

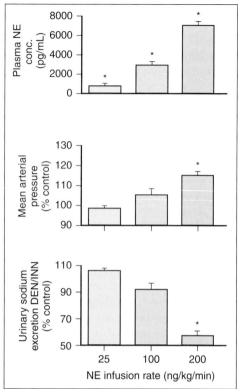

Figure 24–4. Chronic effects of NE infusion on plasma NE conc., mean arterial pressure, and the relative 24-hour excretion rates of sodium from DEN and INN kidneys. *$p<0.05$ versus control before NE infusion. conc., concentration; DEN, denervated kidneys; INN, innervated kidneys; NE, norepinephrine.

excretion from innervated versus denervated kidneys at rates of NE infusion causing hypertension, also suggest another possibility—that sustained sympathoinhibition and attendant loss of sodium might be a long-term compensatory response to the hypertension. If so, similar changes in the relative excretion rates of sodium between innervated and denervated kidneys might also be expected in other forms of secondary hypertension. Further, if renal sympathoinhibition and attendant increments in sodium excretion are mediated by the baroreflex, then SAD should abolish this response.

Angiotensin II–induced hypertension

In view of the well-established sympathoexcitatory effects of Ang II and studies in rats suggesting that the sympathetic nervous system contributes to Ang II hypertension,[46] we reasoned that the Ang II infusion model of hypertension would provide a particularly challenging test of the baroreflex suppression hypothesis. That is, if Ang II–mediated increases in RSNA contribute to hypertension and are more pronounced than the actions of the baroreflex in suppressing renal sympathetic outflow, then there should be *less* sodium excreted from innervated than denervated kidneys during Ang II infusion. In fact, just the opposite response occurred.[47] During a 5-day infusion of Ang II, which produced a three- to five-fold increase in plasma levels of the peptide, MAP increased 30-35 mmHg in the absence of a change in heart rate (Figure 24–5). Additionally, during Ang II infusion, total sodium excretion (from both kidneys) decreased for 1 to 2 days before sodium balance was subsequently achieved at the elevated MAP (Figure 24-6). Moreover, as in NE-mediated hypertension, the hypertension induced by Ang II infusion in dogs with an intact baroreflex was associated with a relative *increase* in sodium excretion from innervated versus denervated kidneys, as reflected by the *fall* in the DEN/INN. This differential effect on sodium excretion occurred in the absence of differences in either glomerular filtration rate or renal plasma flow between kidneys, indicating the predominant influence of the renal nerves was mediated via actions on tubular function. In a subsequent investigation of longer duration, the sustained decrease in the DEN/INN for sodium excretion was found to persist for 10 days of Ang II infusion,[48] supporting the longevity of this response. These studies are consistent with earlier findings in chronically instrumented dogs indicating decreased renal NE spillover (an indirect index of RSNA) during long-term infusion of Ang II.[49] More recently, Barrett et al.[50] have confirmed this regional sympathetic response to Ang II hypertension by making direct recordings of RSNA in chronically instrumented rabbits. Using elegant technology to directly record RSNA, 24 h/day, these investigators demonstrated distinct suppression of RSNA throughout the duration of a 7-day period of hypertension induced by Ang II infusion. Thus taken together, the above studies in chronically instrumented animals provide no support for the hypothesis that increased RSNA impairs sodium excretion and con-

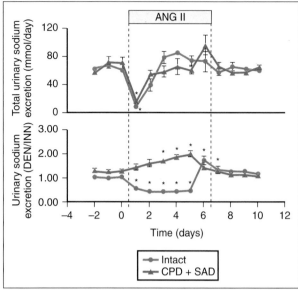

Figure 24–6. Daily rates of sodium excretion from both DEN and INN kidneys during chronic infusion of Ang II before (intact baroreceptor afferents) and after CPD+SAD. *$p<0.05$ versus control. Ang II, angiotensin II; CPD, cardiopulmonary denervation; DEN, denervated kidneys; INN, innervated kidneys; SAD, sinoaortic denervation.

tributes to Ang II hypertension. Rather, these studies indicate that suppression of RSNA is a chronic compensatory response, which may actually attenuate the antinatriuretic and hypertensive effects of Ang II.

Recent studies in both the dog and rabbit strongly support the hypothesis that the arterial baroreflex produces sustained inhibition of RSNA during Ang II hypertension. After determining the hemodynamic and renal excretory responses to chronic Ang II infusion in the intact state, dogs with split bladders and unilateral renal denervation were subjected to deafferentation of cardiopulmonary and sinoaortic baroreceptors (CPD+SAD). This was followed by repeating the 5-day infusion of Ang II (Figures 24–5 and 24–6).[47] In contrast to the baroreflex intact state, in which there was no change in heart rate during Ang II hypertension, there was sustained tachycardia throughout the 5 days of Ang II infusion following CPD+SAD. Because the denervation procedure abolished the vagal innervation of the heart, the increase in heart rate during Ang II infusion indicates prolonged activation of cardiac sympathetic outflow. Regarding the kidneys, following CPD+SAD the DEN/INN for sodium excretion actually *increased* during Ang II infusion, a response diametrically opposite to that observed when the reflexes were intact. Thus in the absence of the baroreflexes, increased circulating levels of Ang II decreased renal excretory function more in innervated kidneys than denervated ones, presumably by increasing RSNA. That the functional differences in sodium excretion between innervated and denervated kidneys are truly related to differences in RSNA is strongly supported by direct 24-hour recordings of RSNA in rabbits chronically infused with Ang II.[51] In this study, the suppression of RSNA that was previously reported in rabbits with Ang II hypertension was totally abolished following SAD. Thus

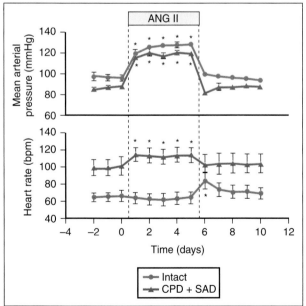

Figure 24–5. Effects of chronic infusion of Ang II on mean arterial pressure and heart rate in dogs before (intact baroreceptor afferents) and after cardiopulmonary and sinoaortic denervation (CPD+SAD). *$p<0.05$ versus control. Dogs also had split bladders and unilateral renal denervation. Ang II, angiotensin II; bpm, beats per minute; CPD, cardiopulmonary denervation; SAD, sinoaortic denervation.

these studies clearly indicate that arterial baroreflexes have sustained effects in Ang II hypertension to inhibit RSNA and promote renal excretory function, suggesting a potential compensatory role in attenuating hypertension. However, despite the ability of baroreflex activation to increase renal excretory function in both dogs and rabbits with Ang II hypertension, it should be noted that baroreceptor deafferentation did not influence the degree of hypertension in these studies, confirming an earlier report by Cowley and DeClue.[52] This may indicate that baroreflex inhibition of RSNA has a relatively weak capacity to shift pressure natriuresis to a lower arterial pressure level in the presence of high circulating levels of the potent sodium-retaining hormones Ang II and aldosterone. This contention receives direct support from the MAP responses to chronic electrical activation of the carotid baroreflex in dogs with Ang II hypertension,[43] as discussed below. The unimpressive effects of baroreflex activation on MAP in Ang II hypertension, however, do not discount the possibility that the baroreflex may have an important compensatory role in attenuating the severity of other more prevalent forms of hypertension.[53]

Sustained activation of neurons in central baroreflex pathway in both primary and secondary hypertension

To further test the hypothesis that the baroreflex is chronically activated in hypertension, we used Fos-like (Fos-Li) protein immunochemistry to determine sites of neuronal activation in the baroreflex pathway. This methodology is based on the principle that stimulation of neurons results in the activation of immediate early genes, including c-*fos*, which in turn lead to the expression of transcriptional regulatory proteins, including Fos and Fos-related proteins. Fos and Fos-related proteins can be measured by immunohistochemistry and, therefore, quantification of Fos-Li staining can serve as a convenient marker for neuronal activation.[54] Advantages of this methodology include the fact that: (1) it can be used to map a large number of activated neurons rather than just the activity of individual neurons, and (2) it can be used in animals that remain conscious during the induction of hypertension circumventing the confounding influence of anesthesia and surgical stress on neuronal activation.

Angiotensin II–induced hypertension

To complement the results discussed above from the Ang II model of hypertension, Ang II was infused both acutely (2 hours) and chronically (5 days) into two groups of dogs, and Fos-Li staining in these dogs was compared to that of a third control group administered saline alone.[55] Responses to chronic Ang II infusion are illustrated in Figure 24–7. MAP increased ~20 and 35 mmHg after acute and chronic Ang II infusion, respectively, and was unchanged in controls. During acute Ang II infusion, there were significant increases in Fos-Li staining in the NTS and CVLM, but no increase in staining in RVLM neurons. As baroreflex suppression of sympathoexcitatory neurons in the RVLM is mediated by activation of NTS and CVLM neurons (Figure 24–3), these acute responses were

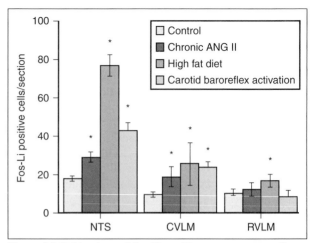

Figure 24–7. Numbers of Fos-Li–positive neurons per section in various regions of the medulla in control dogs and in dogs chronically infused with Ang II, fed a high-fat diet, and subjected to prolonged electrical activation of the carotid baroreflex. Ang II, angiotensin II; CVLM, caudal ventrolateral medulla; NTS, nucleus of the tractus solitarius; RVLM, rostral ventrolateral medulla. *$p<0.05$ versus control.

expected and they confirmed the findings of others in both the rat and rabbit.[56,57] Moreover, a novel finding in this study was that this same pattern of central activation was observed during *chronic* infusion of Ang II. Therefore, this study further supports the hypothesis that the baroreflex is chronically activated in this model of secondary hypertension.

Obesity-induced hypertension

Given the dogma that baroreflexes reset and are an unimportant, long-term determinant of sympathetic activity and arterial pressure, and the mounting experimental evidence that the sympathetic nervous system is activated in primary hypertension, the contention that baroreflex inhibition of sympathetic activity is a sustained response in most forms of clinical hypertension meets with considerable skepticism. While the results from the Ang II model of hypertension clearly indicated that sustained activation of the baroreflex is present for as long as 10 days of hypertension (the duration of the studies), critical support for prolonged baroreflex activation in long-standing hypertension was still needed. This was provided from a study in dogs with chronic obesity hypertension.[58] In this study, dogs were fed either a regular diet or an identical diet with the addition of 0.5 to 0.9 kg of cooked beef fat to induce obesity hypertension, the most prevalent form of primary hypertension in human subjects. After 6 weeks on the high-fat diet, MAP was elevated ~15 mmHg in association with an increase in body weight of ~50%. There were no changes in either body weight or MAP in the control group. Results of Fos-Li immunoreactivity in medullary neurons are illustrated in Figure 24–7. The number of Fos-Li–positive cells in the NTS and the CVLM were three to five times greater in obese than in control dogs, results qualitatively similar to those observed during chronic Ang II hypertension (Figure 24–7). This suggests that neurons subserving the baroreflex were chronically activated in this clinically relevant model of primary hypertension. However, a notable difference between the models of hypertension was the increased staining of RVLM neurons in obese dogs. As spinally projecting neurons in the RVLM provide tonic excitatory input drive to sympathetic preganglionic neurons that control sympathetic output to the peripheral circulation, the increased Fos-Li staining in RVLM neurons is consistent with reports of increased sympathetic activity in obesity hypertension.[1,2,4–6,59] Taken together, these results suggest that sympathoexcitatory inputs into the RVLM predominate over the inhibitory effects of the baroreflex in obesity hypertension. Nonetheless, these results suggest sustained activation of the baroreflex in primary as well as secondary hypertension. As baroreflex inhibition of sympathetic nerve activity is progressively impaired during the evolution of obesity hypertension,[5,6] baroreflex dysfunction may make an increasingly important contribution to sympathetic activation in the later stages of this form of hypertension.

Chronic electrical activation of carotid baroreflex

To determine the time dependency and underlying mechanisms of the blood pressure–lowering effects of the baroreflex, independent of temporal alterations in mechanotransduction at the level of the baroreceptors, we revitalized an earlier approach for the nonpharmacologic treatment of hypertension—chronic electrical activation of the carotid baroreflex.[42,43,53,60] While experimental and clinical studies initiated in the mid-1960s established that that the severity of hypertension could be attenuated by electrical activation of the carotid baroreflex, the results of these studies were sketchy, nonquantitative, and fraught with technical complications.[60] Using state-of-the-art technology, studies have been conducted in dogs that have provided quantitative insight into the temporal and

mechanistic responses to prolonged electrical activation of the baroreflex. These studies were achieved by chronically implanting electrodes around both carotid arteries and using an externally adjustable pulse generator to electrically activate the carotid baroreflex.

Responses in normotensive dogs

Because of the dogma that baroreflexes are unable to produce sustained alterations in sympathetic activity and arterial pressure, the first study using this new technology was designed to critically evaluate the cardiovascular, neurohormonal, and renal excretory responses to prolonged baroreflex activation (PBA) in normotensive dogs.[42] To achieve this goal, chronically instrumented dogs maintained on a fixed diet to facilitate water and electrolyte balance determinations were subjected to 7 days of PBA after control measurements. Immediately following baroreflex activation, MAP decreased ~25 mmHg in association with a modest reduction in heart rate. These acute responses reflect the reciprocal effects of baroreflex activation to suppress the sympathetic and stimulate the parasympathetic nervous systems. Moreover, both the hypotension (Figure 24–8) and the bradycardia were sustained throughout the entire 7 days of PBA with no evidence for temporal diminution of these responses. Sustained reductions in MAP were associated with a ~35% decrease in plasma NE concentration, a response consistent with suppression of the sympathetic nervous system. Taken together, these data indicate that PBA can lead to substantial reductions in MAP by suppressing the sympathetic nervous system. Further, because baroreceptor afferent activity is constant during PBA, these sustained responses may indicate that central mechanisms do not normally make an important contribution to baroreflex resetting.

An additional observation was that PBA leads to chronic activation of neurons contributing to the baroreflex pathway (Figure 24–7). While not unexpected, this finding lends credence to the results from the Fos-Li studies discussed previously, indicating sustained activation of the baroreflex in experimental models of both primary and secondary hypertension.

Before daily sodium balance was achieved at a reduced arterial pressure, a moderate amount of sodium was retained during the first 24 hours of PBA (Figure 24–9). Maintenance of sodium balance at a reduced arterial pressure indicates PBA produces sustained increases in renal excretory function, presumably by chronically suppressing RSNA.[12] However, despite the renal actions of PBA favoring the excretion of sodium, there was net sodium retention, not sodium loss, during chronic baroreflex-mediated suppression of

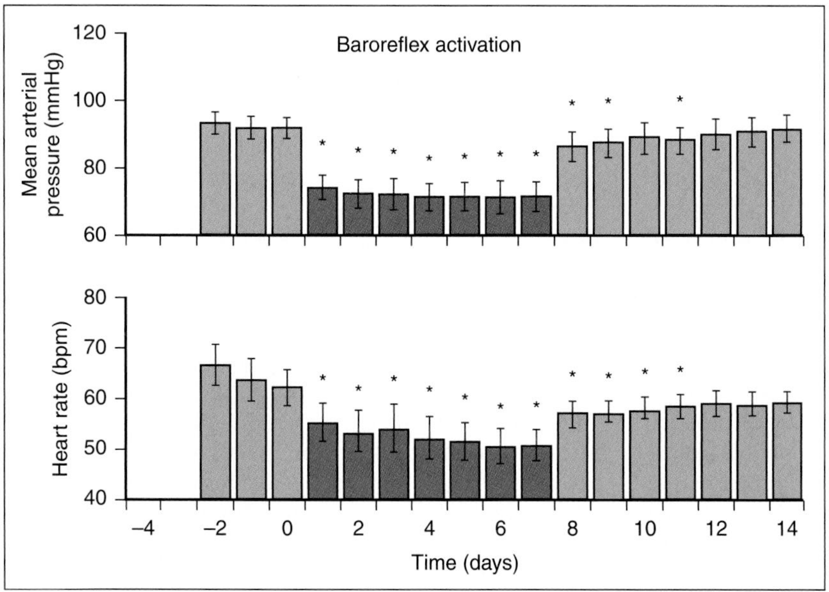

Figure 24–8. Effects of prolonged bilateral electrical activation of the carotid baroreflex on mean arterial pressure and heart rate. *$p<0.05$ versus control.

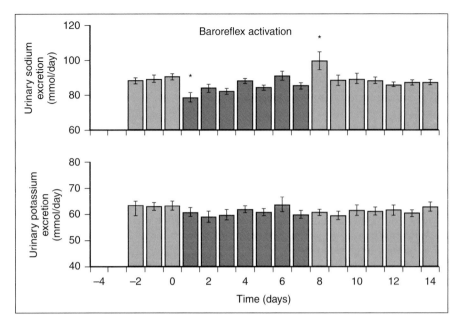

Figure 24–9. Effects of prolonged bilateral electrical activation of the carotid baroreflex on daily rates of sodium and potassium excretion. *$p<0.05$ versus control.

the sympathetic nervous system. Net sodium retention during the first 24 hours of PBA reflects the ability of sympathoinhibition to increase vascular capacity and decrease arterial pressure.[12,19] As discussed earlier, sodium balance determinations do not necessarily reflect the true impact of changes in neural activity on renal excretory function. It should be emphasized once again that if baroreflex activation had not simultaneously increased renal excretory capacity, the initial fall in MAP during PBA would not have been sustained, despite a persistent decrease in vasoconstriction induced by sympathetic inhibition.[12,19]

A possible mechanism for mediating the long-term blood pressure–lowering effects of the baroreflex is suppression of RSNA. This may be the critical response that links decreased central output to increased renal excretory function, but this remains to be evaluated experimentally. In this regard, a particularly important finding in the study illustrated in Figures 24–8 and 24–9 was that plasma renin activity and plasma aldosterone concentration did not increase concomitantly with the fall in arterial pressure induced by PBA. Quantitative studies in chronically instrumented dogs have demonstrated that reductions in renal perfusion pressure greater than ~15 mmHg normally result in substantial increases in renin secretion.[61–63] Therefore, the failure of plasma renin activity to increase despite reductions in MAP of 20 to 25 mmHg would indicate that PBA exerts sustained inhibitory effects on renin secretion. Because alterations in renal adrenergic activity produce directionally similar changes in renin secretion, reflex suppression of RSNA may be the primary mechanism that accounts for the sustained inhibitory effects on renin secretion during PBA.[62] Furthermore, because the renin-angiotensin-aldosterone system has powerful long-term effects on renal excretory function and arterial pressure, baroreflex-mediated suppression of renin secretion may

contribute importantly to the chronic blood pressure-lowering effects of the baroreflex. That is, in the absence of the renal sympathoinhibitory effects on renin secretion, pressure-dependent activation of the renin-angiotensin-aldosterone system may greatly diminish the blood pressure–lowering effects of PBA. Thus suppression of both the direct and indirect (via renin release) actions of the renal nerves on sodium reabsorption likely contributes to the chronic effects of the baroreflex to reduce arterial pressure (Figure 24–1).

Responses in angiotensin II hypertension

To evaluate quantitatively the impact of increased activity of the renin-angiotensin-aldosterone system on the long-term blood pressure–lowering response to PBA, the baroreflex was chronically activated after induction of hypertension by infusion of Ang II.[43] MAP responses to PBA under control conditions and after the induction of Ang II hypertension in the same dogs are illustrated in Figure 24–10. Under control conditions, MAP (93±1mmHg) decreased ~20 mmHg in association with a ~55% decrease in plasma NE concentration during PBA, but there were no significant changes in plasma renin activity. These responses under control conditions were comparable to those reported in our earlier study (Figures 24–8 and 24–9). During chronic infusion of Ang II, there was a threefold elevation in plasma aldosterone concentration and MAP increased 30 to 35 mmHg (to 129±3 mmHg). Additionally, plasma NE concentration decreased ~25%. Most importantly, during the next 7 days of baroreflex activation/Ang II infusion, reductions in MAP (Figure 24–10) and plasma NE concentration were markedly diminished compared to responses in the control state. In fact, during PBA, plasma NE concentration failed to decrease significantly from its already depressed values during Ang II infusion. This presumably reflects prior

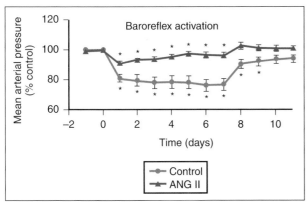

Figure 24–10. Effects of prolonged bilateral electrical activation of the carotid baroreflex on mean arterial pressure in the normotensive control state and then after the induction of Ang II hypertension. *p<0.05 versus control. Ang II, angiotensin II.

activation of the baroreflex. The final reduction in arterial pressure was less than 25% of the control response. While the natural engagement of the baroreflex during Ang II hypertension undoubtedly contributed to the reduced sympathetic response to PBA, it is unlikely that this was a major factor in the diminished MAP response to PBA. If endogenous activation of the baroreflex produced appreciable sympathoinhibitory reductions of MAP in Ang II hypertension, then one would expect SAD to exacerbate Ang II hypertension. As mentioned above, it does not.[51,52] Therefore, despite baroreflex suppression of RSNA in Ang II hypertension, it would appear that neurally induced increments in renal excretory function are markedly depressed by high circulating levels of the potent sodium-retaining hormones Ang II and aldosterone. Presumably, it is for this reason that PBA has reduced blood pressure-lowering effects in Ang II hypertension. Whether this is the primary reason that accounts for the diminished blood pressure response, this study emphasizes the potential importance of renin inhibition in permitting a robust fall in arterial pressure during PBA.

Responses in obesity hypertension

Excess weight gain and obesity are believed to play a major role in causing increased arterial pressure in the majority of patients with primary hypertension.[1,2,59] Although the mechanisms that account for obesity-induced hypertension are not clearly understood, there is considerable evidence from experimental and clinical studies that activation of the sympathetic nervous system, including sympathetic outflow to the kidneys, plays a causal role in promoting increased arterial pressure.[1,2,5–7,59] Additionally, because increased RSNA increases renin release, the renin-angiotensin system may also contribute to obesity hypertension.[59] Consequently, if the baroreflex has the capacity to chronically inhibit RSNA, this form of hypertension may be especially sensitive to PBA.

The influence of PBA on arterial pressure was studied in dogs with obesity-induced hypertension.[53] After 4 weeks of a high-fat diet, body weight and MAP were increased by ~50% and 15%, respectively, in association with an

approximate twofold elevation in plasma NE concentration, consistent with sympathetic activation. Although plasma renin activity increased substantially during the initial weeks of the high-fat diet, values returned to control levels as the hypertension progressed. This temporal normalization of plasma renin activity during the evolution of obesity hypertension may reflect the opposing effects of increased arterial pressure and sympathetic activity on renin secretion. Most importantly, the sympathetic and arterial pressure responses to PBA during week 5 of obesity hypertension were dramatic. Throughout the entire 7 days of PBA, plasma NE concentration and MAP were reduced to or below control levels. Furthermore, despite the fall in MAP, plasma renin activity did not increase during PBA. These findings emphasize the potential importance of the baroreflex in opposing the activation of the sympathetic nervous system and the hypertension often associated with obesity. Once again, these findings are also consistent with the hypothesis that reflex suppression of renin secretion contributes importantly to the long-term antihypertensive effects of PBA.

CLINICAL IMPLICATIONS AND PERSPECTIVES

While novel approaches in animals provide strong evidence linking increased renal excretory function to sustained baroreflex activation in chronic hypertension, it should be emphasized that experimental observations have been made over weeks to months, rather than months to years. Thus the duration of experimental studies may be inadequate to truly reflect baroreflex function in clinical hypertension. Further, the techniques used in experimental studies have been invasive and, in most instances, not feasible for human investigation. Therefore, because of experimental limitations, there is little direct evidence from human studies to indicate that sustained baroreflex activation is a relevant long-term compensatory mechanism in human hypertension. A major impediment in advancing this concept is that physiologic and pathophysiologic alterations in sympathetic activity are regionally heterogeneous (Table 24–1), and assessment of sympathetic outflow to the kidneys is not readily achieved in human subjects, particularly in regards to baroreflex function. Consequently, support for this concept and, therefore, its clinical importance, are largely based on a surrogate for RSNA-sympathetic outflow to skeletal muscle, which is measured by microneurography. Another caveat in the interpretation of the clinical studies is that direct assessment of baroreflex modulation of sympathetic activity in human hypertension by traditional techniques is based solely on *acute* changes in nerve traffic in response to either spontaneous or induced changes in arterial pressure. It is not clear from these *acute* studies whether diminished arterial baroreflex buffering of sympathetic nerve traffic translates into *long-term* alterations in sympathetic outflow.

Efferent postganglionic nerve traffic in subcutaneous nerves distributed to skeletal muscle (and skin) vasculature can be measured directly by microneurography, and

REGIONAL SYMPATHETIC ACTIVITY IN PATHOPHYSIOLOGIC CONDITIONS					
Regions	Early CHF	Advanced CHF	Nonobese HT	Obesity	Obesity HT
Cardiac	↑	↑↑	↑	↓	⇌
Renal	⇌	↑	↑	↑	↑
Muscular	⇌	↑	↑	↑	↑↑
Plasma	⇌	↑	⇌↑	⇌↑	⇌↑

CHF, chronic heart failure; HT, hypertension.

Data from Grassi G, Cattaneo B, Seravalle G, et al. *Hypertension* 1998;31:68–72; Grassi G, Seravalle G, Dell'Oro R, et al. *Hypertension* 2000;36:538–42; Grassi G, Seravalle G, Quarti-Trevano F, et al. *Hypertension* 2003;42:873–7; Rumantir M, Vaz M, Jennings G, et al. *J Hypertens* 1999;17:1125–33; and Rundqvist B, Elam M, Bergmann-Sverrisdottir Y, et al. *Circulation* 1997;95:169–75.

Table 24–1. Regional Sympathetic Activity in Pathophysiologic Conditions

this technique has been used extensively to determine changes in sympathetic activity and baroreflex function in various pathophysiologic states, including hypertension and heart failure (Table 24–1). In contrast, regional sympathetic activation to internal organs, including the heart and kidneys, cannot be measured directly and must be inferred from measurement of organ-specific NE spillover (Table 24–1). While the NE spillover technique does permit estimation of sympathetic activity to internal organs, it cannot be used to assess dynamic changes in sympathetic activity, which are measured by microneurography to assess sympathetic baroreflex function. Consequently, baroreflex control of RSNA must be surmised from measurements of sympathetic outflow to skeletal muscle. Simultaneous measurements of efferent postganglionic muscle sympathetic nerve activity and renal NE spillover do indicate a correlation between the two in resting, healthy normotensive men.[64] Further, while it is not uncommon for there to be a disparity between sympathetic outflow to skeletal muscle and to internal organs, including the heart, this disparity does not appear to apply to the renal circulation (Table 24–1).[3,5–7,65] As illustrated in Table 24–1, there appears to be a concordance between sympathetic outflow to skeletal muscle and the kidneys in a number of pathophysiologic states, but this may not always hold.

Microneurographic studies in patients with secondary hypertension

Activation of the sympathetic nervous system is not commonly present in secondary hypertension.[3,9–11] In fact, microneurographic studies in patients with secondary hypertension are consistent with the hypothesis that the baroreflex responds to hypertension by chronically suppressing RSNA, thus increasing sodium excretion in a compensatory fashion. In patients with adrenal pheochromocytoma, measurements of sympathetic nerve activity to skeletal muscle indicate that the hypertension induced by high circulating levels of catecholamines is associated with decreased central sympathetic outflow.[10] This finding is also consistent with the sustained increase in neurally-induced sodium excretion that occurs in dogs with hypertension induced by chronic infusion of NE, and suggests that the sympathoinhibition in patients with pheochromocytoma may include the sympathetic outflow to the

kidneys, as well as to skeletal muscle. Additionally, sympathetic outflow to skeletal muscle is suppressed in patients with primary aldosteronism,[9] another form of secondary hypertension. In contrast to patients with pheochromocytoma and primary aldosteronism, microneurographic studies in patients with renovascular hypertension are inconsistent and have indicated increased, normal, or decreased sympathetic activity.[3,9,11,66,67] As renovascular hypertension may be associated with activation of the renin-angiotensin system, the basis for these inconsistent findings may lie in the opposing effects of circulating levels of Ang II and baroreflex inhibition on sympathetic activity. Recall that RSNA is suppressed in experimental hypertension induced by infusion of Ang II as long as the inhibitory effects of the baroreflex are operative. However, following deafferentation of the baroreceptors, the sympathoexcitatory effects of high plasma levels of Ang II appear to manifest, resulting in either normal or increased RSNA.[47,51] Indeed, in renovascular hypertension, there is a direct relationship between increments in sympathetic activity and circulating levels of Ang II.[66] The various sympathetic responses recorded in renovascular hypertension may thus reflect the net temporal opposing effects of Ang II and the baroreflex.

Microneurographic and regional norepinephrine spillover studies in patients with primary hypertension

Microneurographic recordings of efferent postganglionic sympathetic nerve traffic to skeletal muscle vasculature and measurements of whole-body and region-specific NE spillover have provided strong evidence for increased sympathetic activity in primary hypertension.[1–8] As sympathetic activation occurs both in the initial and sustained phases of primary hypertension, and includes the renal circulation, these responses are consistent with the notion that increased RSNA plays a causal role in impairing pressure natriuresis and in promoting increased arterial pressure throughout the entire evolution of the hypertensive process. However, while net sympathetic outflow is increased in primary hypertension, this does not necessarily exclude a sustained inhibitory influence of the baroreflex on sympathetic activity. Rather, this may indicate that central excitatory inputs predominate over the inhibitory effects of the baroreflex on sympathetic activity.

If this notion is correct, then baroreflex dysfunction may provide an additional stimulus to increased central sympathetic outflow.

The mechanisms that account for activation of the sympathetic nervous system in primary hypertension have not been determined with certainty. Numerous hypotheses have emerged over the years, including attributing the sympathoexcitation to increased plasma levels of Ang II and leptin. One of most long-standing hypotheses is that impaired baroreflex restraint of sympathetic nerve traffic leads to increases in sympathetic activity in primary hypertension. Initial support for this hypothesis was based on studies demonstrating impaired baroreflex control of heart rate in patients with hypertension. However, subsequent microneurographic studies demonstrated that while there is impaired baroreflex modulation of vagal tone, baroreflex control of sympathetic activity is not abnormal in lean hypertensive patients.[3,5] Thus if one were to extrapolate these acute baroreflex responses to long-term modulation of sympathetic outflow to the kidneys, it would appear that an impaired ability of the baroreflex to inhibit sympathetic activity cannot account for the increased RSNA and arterial pressure in nonobese subjects with primary hypertension. Still, this reasoning may not apply to patients with primary hypertension associated with obesity.

Many patients with primary hypertension are overweight. As in lean patients with primary hypertension, activation of the sympathetic nervous system, including sympathetic outflow to the kidneys, is a characteristic feature of obesity hypertension.[1,2,5–7,59] Further, as in lean patients with hypertension, the mechanisms that account for sympathetic activation in obesity remain uncertain. Much interest has been directed to the possibility that leptin released from adipose tissue acts centrally to stimulate sympathetic activity. The results from microneurographic studies in patients with obesity hypertension present an additional possibility. These studies have demonstrated that patients with obesity hypertension, in contrast to lean hypertensive subjects, have impaired baroreflex control of sympathetic activity.[5,6] Therefore, it is conceivable that impaired baroreflex restraint of sympathetic outflow might result in the activation of the sympathetic nervous system and contribute to the hypertension commonly present in obesity. However, in the context of this chapter, it should be emphasized that this explanation is dependent upon the following unsubstantiated physiologic responses. First, the baroreflex must produce sustained inhibition of sympathetic activity in obesity hypertension. This possibility receives support from the observations indicating there is sustained activation of the baroreflex in dogs with chronic obesity hypertension.[58] Second, impaired baroreflex restraint of sympathetic activity must include sympathetic outflow to the kidneys, as well as to skeletal muscle. Finally, deficiencies in baroreflex function must include *long-term*, as well as *acute*, alterations in renal sympathetic outflow. It is not likely that these critical issues will be resolved with the current methodology available for human investigation. Nonetheless, because PBA has potent sympathoinhibitory and antihypertensive effects in experimental obesity-induced hypertension,[53] the possibility that baroreflex dysfunction may contribute importantly to the pathogenesis of obesity hypertension should not be dismissed and merits further investigation.

Baroreflex and antihypertensive therapy

Sympathetic responses to chronic antihypertensive therapy, as assessed by microneurography, are inconsistent and probably influenced by differences in drug class, pharmacokinetics, and pharmacodynamics, as well as experimental protocols. Nonetheless, observations in several studies are consistent with the hypothesis that baroreflex resetting is incomplete during antihypertensive therapy. Although reflex activation of the sympathetic nervous system is neither a surprising nor an uncommon response to acute drug-induced reductions in arterial pressure, some studies employing microneurography have reported sustained increases in sympathetic activity in hypertensive subjects during chronic antihypertensive therapy.[21,27,68] While these clinical studies may be interpreted to support the notion of incomplete baroreflex resetting, it is problematic to attribute increases in sympathetic activity during either dietary sodium restriction or diuretic administration to baroreceptor unloading and not to the sympathoexcitatory effects associated with concomitant activation of the renin-angiotensin system. However, increases in sympathetic outflow to muscle have been reported even when reductions in arterial pressure have been achieved with either a diuretic-Ang II blocker combination or an Ang II receptor blocker alone,[68,70] antihypertensive drugs that attenuate the actions of Ang II.

If baroreflex unloading does lead to sustained sympathetic activation, as recent experimental studies suggest, this obviously would be an undesirable response because reflex tachycardia and sympathoexcitation have untoward effects on the heart and oppose the blood pressure–lowering effects of antihypertensive therapy. Sympathetic antagonism with either drugs that act centrally or device-based therapy for baroreflex activation are logical choices to reduce the sympathetic activation commonly associated with primary hypertension. The marked sympathoinhibitory and antihypertensive responses to PBA in obesity-induced hypertension provide a strong rationale for sympathetic antagonism in the treatment of primary hypertension, and highlight the potential importance of the baroreflex in the pathogenesis of hypertension.

SUMMARY

Because SAD does not lead to sustained hypertension, and resetting is a common feature of the baroreflex, the prevailing dogma for the latter part of the 20th century was that baroreflexes do not chronically influence sympathetic activity and arterial pressure. More recently, the interpretation of these studies has been challenged as novel experimental approaches in chronically instrumented animals have provided solid evidence that baroreflex resetting is incomplete during chronic alterations in arterial pressure. Recent experimental studies have also shown that baroreflex suppression of sympathetic activity, including sympathetic outflow to the kidneys, is a sustained response in chronic hypertension. Because baroreflex suppression of RSNA persistently increases the renal excretion of sodium, contrary to established dogma, these studies indicate that the baroreflex may play a compensatory role in attenuating the severity of hypertension. While the above observations in hypertensive animals have been made over a time course of weeks to over a month, a caveat in the interpretation of these studies is that their duration may be too short to provide an accurate indication of baroreflex function in clinical hypertension persisting for many years. Thus future studies must include hypertensive protocols lasting for at least several months. Unfortunately, current technology is inadequate for elucidating the long-term functional effects of the baroreflex in human subjects.

Although further experimental validation is needed, the renal nerves may be the critical link between baroreflex-induced alterations in central sympathetic outflow and renal excretory responses that lead to long-term changes in arterial pressure. Consequently, difficulties inherent in monitoring RSNA in human subjects pose a major obstacle to determining the role of the baroreflex in the pathogenesis of clinical hypertension. Despite this imposing limitation, studies using microneurography to directly measure postganglionic sympathetic nerve activity in skeletal muscle as a surrogate for RSNA have provided some intriguing results. First, microneurographic studies suggest that sympathetic activity may be suppressed in patients with secondary hypertension. This observation, while not providing direct evidence, supports the possibility advanced by animal experiments that activation of the baroreflex may account for sustained renal sympathoinhibition in hypertension, a response expected to attenuate the increase in arterial pressure. Another potentially relevant observation from microneurographic studies is that the evolution of obesity hypertension is associated with progressive baroreflex dysfunction. If this impairment in the ability of the baroreflex to evoke *acute* changes in muscle sympathetic nerve activity also reflects *long-term* alterations in sympathetic outflow to the kidneys, then impaired baroreflex restraint of nerve traffic may contribute to the increased renal sympathoexcitation and increased arterial pressure in this most prevalent form of primary hypertension. This possibility merits serious consideration because PBA has potent sympathoinhibitory and antihypertensive effects in experimental obesity hypertension.

Technology allowing chronic activation of the carotid baroreflex by electrical stimulation has provided new insight into the role of the baroreflex in long-term control of arterial pressure. A unique aspect of this technology is that it permits a critical, quantitative assessment of the mechanisms that mediate the long-term blood pressure–lowering effects of the baroreflex. Initial studies using this approach have demonstrated impressive sustained reductions in arterial pressure in both normotensive and hypertensive dogs. If fact, baroreflex-induced reductions in arterial pressure have been so dramatic that human clinical trials have already been initiated to evaluate the clinical application of this technology in the treatment of resistant hypertension.[60] In addition to providing a better understanding of long-term baroreflex control of arterial pressure in humans, these clinical trials may pave the way for a novel, nonpharmacologic approach for the treatment of hypertension.

REFERENCES

1. Esler M. The sympathetic system and hypertension. *Am J Hypertens* 2000;13:99S–105S.
2. Esler M, Rumantir M, Wiesner G, et al. Sympathetic nervous system and insulin resistance: from obesity to diabetes. *Am J Hypertens* 2001;14:304S–9S.
3. Grassi G, Cattaneo B, Seravalle G, et al. Baroreflex control of sympathetic nerve activity in essential and secondary hypertension. *Hypertension* 1998;31: 68–72.
4. Grassi G. Counteracting the sympathetic nervous system in essential hypertension. *Curr Opin Nephrol Hypertens* 2004;13: 513–9.
5. Grassi G, Seravalle G, Dell'Oro R, et al. Adrenergic and reflex abnormalities in obesity-related hypertension. *Hypertension* 2000;36:538–42.
6. Grassi G, Seravalle G, Quarti-Trevano F, et al. Effects of hypertension and obesity on the sympathetic activation of heart failure patients. *Hypertension* 2003;42: 873–7.
7. Rumantir M, Vaz M, Jennings G, et al. Neural mechanisms in human obesity-related hypertension. *J Hypertens* 1999; 17:1125–33.

8. Smith P, Graham L, Mackintosh A, et al. Relationship between central sympathetic activity and stages of human hypertension. Am *J Hypertens* 2004;17:217–22.
9. Miyajima E, Yamada Y, Yoshida Y, et al. Muscle sympathetic nerve activity and renovascular hypertension and primary aldosteronism. *Hypertension* 1991; 17:1057–62.
10. Grassi G, Seravalle G, Turri C, Mancia G. Sympathetic nerve traffic responses to surgical removal of pheochromocytoma. *Hypertension* 1999;34:461–5.
11. Grassi G, Esler M. The sympathetic nervous system in renovascular hypertension: lead actor or 'bit' player? *J Hypertens* 2002;20:1071–3.
12. Lohmeier T, Hildebrandt D, Warren S, et al. Recent insights into the interactions between the baroreflex and the kidneys in hypertension. *Am J Physiol Regul Integr Comp Physiol* 2005;288:R828–36.
13. Chapleau M, Hajduczok G, Abboud F. Resetting of the arterial baroreflex: peripheral and central mechanism. In: Zucker I and Gilmore J, eds.

Reflex Control of the Circulation. Boca Raton, FL: CRC Press, 1991:165–94.
14. Cowley A Jr. Long-term control of arterial blood pressure. *Physiol Rev* 1992;72:231–300.
15. Cowley A, Liard J, Guyton A. Role of the baroreceptor reflex in daily control of arterial blood pressure and other variables in dogs. *Circ Res* 1973;32:564–76.
16. Thrasher T. Effects of chronic baroreceptor unloading on blood pressure in the dog. *Am J Physiol Regul Integr Comp Physiol* 2005;288:R863–71.
17. Ito S, Sved A. Influences of GABA in the nucleus of the solitary tract on blood pressure in baroreceptor-denervated rats. *Am J Physiol Regul Integr Comp Physiol* 1997;273:R1657–62.
18. Thrasher T. Unloading arterial baroreceptors causes neurogenic hypertension. *Am J Physiol Regul Integr Comp Physiol* 2002;282:R1044–53.
19. Guyton A. *Arterial Pressure and Hypertension.* Philadelphia: W.B. Saunders, 1980.
20. Hall J, Brands M. The renin-angiotensin-aldosterone systems: renal mechanisms and circulatory homeostasis. In: Seldin

D and Giebisch G, eds. *The Kidney: Physiology and Pathophysiology*, 2nd ed. New York: Raven Press, 1992:1455–504.

21. Downing S. Baroreceptor regulation of the heart. In: Berne R, ed. *The Cardiovascular System: Handbook of Physiology*. Baltimore: Waverly Press, 1979:621–52.

22. Krauhs J. Structure of rat aortic baroreceptors and their relationship to connective tissue. *J Neurocytol* 1979;8:401–14.

23. Chapleau M, Cunningham J, Sullivan M, et al. Structural versus functional modulation of the arterial baroreflex. *Hypertension* 1995;26:341–7.

24. Chapleau M, Hajduczok G, Sharma R, et al. Mechanisms of baroreceptor activation. *Clin Exp Hypertens* 1995; 17:1–13.

25. Garcia-Anoveros J, Corey D. The molecules of mechanosensation. *Annu Rev Neurosci* 1997;20:567–94.

26. Gillespie P, Walker R. Molecular basis of mechanosensory transduction. *Nature* 2001;413:194–202.

27. Welsh M, Price M, Xie J. Biochemical basis of touch perception: mechanosensory function of degenerin/ epithelial Na+ channels. *J Biol Chem* 2002;277:2369–72.

28. Bianchi L, Driscoll M. Protons at the gate: DEG/ENaC ion channels help us feel and remember. *Neuron* 2002; 34:337–40.

29. Drummond H, Welsh M, Abboud F. ENaC subunits are molecular components of the arterial baroreceptor complex. *Ann N Y Acad Sci* 2001;940:42–7.

30. Seagard J, van Brederode J, Dean C, et al. Firing characteristics of single-fiber carotid sinus baroreceptors. *Circ Res* 1990;66:1499–1509.

31. Seagard J, Hopp F, Drummond H, Van Wynsberghe A. Selective contribution of two types of carotid sinus baroreceptors to the control of blood pressure. *Circ Res* 1993;72: 1011–22.

32. Seagard J, Gallenberg L, Hopp F, Dean C. Acute resetting in two functionally different types of carotid baroreceptors. *Circ Res* 1992;70: 559–65.

33. Pilowsky P, Goodchild A. Baroreceptor reflex pathways and neurotransmitters: 10 years on. *J Hypertens* 2002;20: 1675–88.

34. DiBona G, Kopp U. Neural control of renal function. *Physiol Rev* 1997;77: 75–197.

35. Van Vliet B, Hall J, Lohmeier T, Mizelle H. In: Bennett T and Gardiner S, eds. *Renal Circulation: Nervous Control of Blood Vessels*. London: Harwood Academic Publishers, 1996:371–433.

36. Reinhart G, Lohmeier T, Hord C. Hypertension induced by chronic renal adrenergic stimulation is angiotensin dependent. *Hypertension* 1995;25: 940–9.

37. Le Fevre M, Guild S, Ramchandra R, et al. Role of angiotensin II in the neural control of renal function. *Hypertension* 2003;41:583–91.

38. Jacob F, Ariza P, Osborn J. Renal denervation lowers arterial pressure independent of dietary sodium intake in normal rats. *Am J Physiol Heart Circ Physiol* 2003;284:H2302–10.

39. Howe P, Rogers P, Minson J. Influence of dietary sodium on blood pressure in baroreceptor-denervated rats. *J Hypertens* 1985;3:457–60.

40. Osborn J, Hornfeldt B. Arterial baroreceptor denervation impairs long-term regulation of arterial pressure during dietary salt loading. *Am J Physiol Heart Circ Physiol* 1998;275:H1558–66.

41. DiBona G, Sawin L. Effect of arterial baroreceptor denervation on sodium balance. *Hypertension* 2002;40:547–51.

42. Lohmeier T, Irwin E, Rossing M, et al. Prolonged activation of the baroreflex produces sustained hypotension. *Hypertension* 2004;43:306–11.

43. Lohmeier T, Dwyer T, Hildebrandt D, et al. Influence of prolonged baroreflex activation on arterial pressure in angiotensin hypertension. *Hypertension* 2005;46:1194–1200.

44. Lohmeier T, Hildebrandt D, Hood W. Renal nerves promote sodium excretion during long-term increases in salt intake. *Hypertension* 1999;33:487–92.

45. Lohmeier T, Reinhart G, Mizelle H, et al. Renal denervation supersensitivity revisited. *Am J Physiol Regul Integr Comp Physiol* 1998;275:R1239–46.

46. Fink G. Long-term sympatho-excitory effect of angiotensin II: a mechanism of spontaneous and renovascular hypertension. *Clin Exp Pharmacol Physiol* 1997;24:91–5.

47. Lohmeier T, Lohmeier J, Haque A, Hildebrandt D. Baroreflexes prevent neurally induced sodium retention in angiotensin hypertension. *Am J Physiol Regul Integr Comp Physiol* 2000;279: R1437–48.

48. Lohmeier T, Lohmeier J, Reckelhoff J, Hildebrandt D. Sustained influence of the renal nerves to attenuate sodium retention in angiotensin hypertension. *Am J Physiol Regul Integr Comp Physiol* 2001;281:R434–43.

49. Carroll R, Lohmeier T, Brown A. Chronic angiotensin II infusion decreases renal norepinephrine overflow in conscious dogs. *Hypertension* 1984;6:675–81.

50. Barrett C, Ramchandra R, Guild S, et al. What sets the long-term level of renal sympathetic nerve activity: a role for angiotensin II and baroreflexes? *Circ Res* 2003;92:1330–6.

51. Barrett C, Guild S, Ramchandra R, Malpas S. Baroreceptor denervation prevents sympathoinhibition during angiotensin II–induced hypertension. *Hypertension* 2005;46:1–5.

52. Cowley A Jr, DeClue J. Quantification of baroreceptor influences on arterial pressure changes seen in primary angiotensin-induced hypertension in dogs. *Circ Res* 1976;39:779–87.

53. Lohmeier T, Dwyer T, Irwin E, et al. Prolonged activation of the baroreflex abolishes obesity-induced hypertension. *Hypertension* 2005;46:816.

54. Dampney R, Li Y, Hirooka Y, et al. Use of c-fos functional mapping to identify the central baroreceptor reflex pathway: advantages and limitations. *Clin Exp Hypertens* 1995;17:197–208.

55. Lohmeier T, Lohmeier J, Warren S, et al. Sustained activation of the central baroreceptor pathway in angiotensin hypertension. *Hypertension* 2002;39: 550–6.

56. Li Q, Sullivan M, Dale W, et al. Fos-like immunoreactivity in the medulla after acute and chronic angiotensin II infusion. *J Pharmacol Exp Ther* 1998;284:1165–73.

57. Potts P, Hirooka Y, Dampney R. Activation of brain neurons by circulating angiotensin II: direct effects and baroreceptor-mediated secondary effects. *Neuroscience* 1999;90:581–94.

58. Lohmeier T, Warren S, Cunningham J. Sustained activation of the central baroreceptor pathway in obesity hypertension. *Hypertension* 2003;43: 96–102.

59. Hall J, Hildebrandt D, Kuo J. Obesity hypertension: role of leptin and sympathetic nervous system. *Am J Hypertens* 2001;14:103S–15S.

60. Lohmeier T, Barrett A, Irwin E. Prolonged activation of the baroreflex: a viable approach for the treatment of hypertension? *Curr Sci* 2005;7:193–8.

61. Kirchheim H, Finke R, Hackenthal E, et al. Baroreflex sympathetic activation increases activation threshold pressure for the pressure-dependent renin release in conscious dogs. *Pfleugers Arch* 1985; 405:127–35.

62. Peters T, Kaczmarczyk G. Plasma renin activity during hypotensive responses to electrical stimulation of carotid sinus nerves in conscious dogs. *Clin Exp Pharm Physiol* 1994;21:1–8.

63. Yang H, Lohmeier T, Kivlighn S, et al. Sustained increases in plasma epinephrine concentration do not modulate renin secretion. *Am J Physiol Endocrinol Metab* 1989;257:E57–64.

64. Wallin B, Thompson J, Jennings G, Esler M. Renal noradrenaline spillover correlates with muscle sympathetic activity in humans. *J Physiology* 1996; 491:881–7.

65. Rundqvist B, Elam M, Bergmann-Sverrisdottir Y, et al. Increased cardiac adrenergic drive precedes generalized sympathetic activation in human heart failure. *Circulation* 1997;95:169–75.

66. Johansson M, Elam M, Rundqvist B, et al. Increased sympathetic nerve activity in renovascular hypertension. *Circulation* 1999;99:2537–42.

67. Morlin C, Fagius J, Hagg A, et al. Continuous recording of muscle nerve sympathetic activity during percutaneous transluminal angioplasty in renovascular hypertension in man. *J Hypertens* 1990; 8:239–44.

68. Fu Q, Zhang R, Witkowski S, et al. Persistent sympathetic activation during chronic antihypertensive therapy: a potential mechanism for long term morbidity? *Hypertension* 2005;45: 513–21.

69. Grassi G, Dell'Oro R, Seravalle G, et al. Short- and long-term neuroadrenergic effects of moderate dietary sodium restriction in essential hypertension. *Circulation* 2002;106:1957–61.

70. Heusser K, Vitkovsky J, Raasch W, et al. Elevation of sympathetic activity by eprosartan in young male subjects. *Am J Hypertens* 2003;16:658–64.

Chapter

25 Central Nervous System Control of Blood Pressure

Carrie A. Northcott and Joseph R. Haywood

Definitions

■ The central nervous system (CNS) consists of a network of interconnected neurons located in the brain and spinal cord that receives, interprets, and responds to various stimuli through humoral and neurochemical signals controlling physiologic functions.

Key Findings

■ The CNS plays a significant role in blood pressure maintenance by maintaining a balance that occurs between output systems which include the sympathetic and parasympathetic divisions of the autonomic nervous system, pituitary hormones, and the renin-angiotensin system.

Clinical Implications

■ Central mechanisms controlling blood pressure are complex, and the full potential of central approaches to treatment will not be realized until a better understanding of brain function is achieved.

The contribution of the central nervous system (CNS) to the development and maintenance of hypertension has long been the subject of speculation and investigation. While many early studies described the central actions of neurochemicals and their antagonists on blood pressure, the development of modern neurobiologic techniques has permitted substantive progress in recent years. The application to the study of cardiovascular function of neural pathway tracing techniques, immunocytochemistry, cellular electrophysiology, molecular biology, imaging, and other methods, have provided new insights into how the brain interacts with the cardiovascular system in pathophysiologic states.

The sympathetic nervous system is the principal effector system that mediates changes in blood pressure originating from the brain. The sympathetic nerves and the adrenal medulla comprise a powerful control mechanism that causes large rapid changes in arterial pressure. Complex interactive neural pathways regulate the sympathetic nervous system controlling cardiovascular function in response to internal and external stimuli. CNS pathways contributing to hypertension are activated in response to chemical (e.g., sodium), hormonal (e.g., angiotensin II [Ang II]) and neural stimuli (e.g., baroreceptor afferent nerves). These stimuli can act independently or in concert to stimulate

sympathetic nerve activity. In addition, hormones and neural reflex mechanisms can modulate normal or elevated levels of neural activity in the brain to further increase sympathetic nerve activity or release hormones from the brain that lead to hypertension. Dysfunction of these interactions contributes to the multifactorial nature of the hypertensive process.

While many questions remain to be answered concerning central neural mechanism triggering and maintaining the hypertensive state, much has been learned about the many stimuli that can activate (or inhibit) complex neural pathways and networks leading to hypertension. This chapter will review the anatomic pathways and neurotransmitters involved in blood pressure control, discuss some of the physiologic mechanisms that dysfunction to cause an elevated blood pressure, and then present the clinical implications of current therapeutic approaches.

ANATOMY AND BIOCHEMISTRY

Anatomy of central neural pathways

The influence of the brain on blood pressure is mediated through four principal effector systems. The first principal effector system is the sympathetic nervous system. Sympathetic preganglionic neurons originate from cell bodies in the intermediolateral column in the thoracolumbar region of the spinal cord to paravertebral and prevertebral ganglia and the adrenal medulla. The second effector system is the parasympathetic vagal control of the heart by two nuclei in the hindbrain—the dorsal motor nucleus and the nucleus ambiguus. The vagus exerts predominant neural control on heart rate in most species and is usually activated as a compensatory mechanism to increased blood pressure or is inhibited to enhance rises in arterial pressure. The third principal effector system is the posterior pituitary. Vasopressin released from the posterior pituitary can contribute to sodium-dependent hypertension.[1] Oxytocin, which is also released from the posterior pituitary, has been implicated in the hypertensive process as well. The final effector system is the anterior pituitary, which is responsible for the release of hormones such as adrenocorticotropic hormone (ACTH) that, in turn, stimulates the release of cortisol from the adrenal cortex. Glucocorticoids are known to have direct effects on vascular function, but appear also to have significant indirect actions in modulating brain function and fetal programming of hypertension.[2]

The foundation of understanding central nervous system control of blood pressure in hypertension is supported by our knowledge of the neural pathways that are involved in the maintenance of blood pressure. Observations by Strack and Lowey[3] first demonstrated the principal nuclei that project to the intermediolateral cell column of the spinal cord. Five areas of the brain were shown to project directly to the intermediolateral cell column of the spinal cord: hindbrain structures including the rostral ventrolateral medulla (RVLM), rostral ventromedial medulla (RVMM), and the raphe pallidus nucleus (caudal portion of the raphe); the midbrain A5 catecholamine cell bodies; and the hypothalamic paraventricular nucleus (PVN). Figure 25–1 provides an overview of the organization of the brain in influencing neural and hormonal outputs controlling blood pressure. Higher complex center function funnels into basic autonomic and hormonal mechanisms. The discussion below starts with the hindbrain and describes connections to higher centers.

Hindbrain

The RVLM has long been considered the principal part of the vasomotor center largely because of the significant fall in blood pressure associated with chemical inhibition or ablation of the area.[4] The vasomotor area includes the C1 epinephrine-containing cell bodies, as well as cell bodies in the surrounding area with different neurochemical phenotypes.[5] These neurons have been shown to have an intrinsic rhythm, they are modulated by the baroreflex, and they project to the preganglionic sympathetic neurons in the spinal cord. The RVMM and the raphe pallidus have also been shown to have direct connections to the intermediolateral cell column influencing

sympathetic preganglionic neurons. These areas do not possess intrinsic rhythms; however, one subpopulation of cells in these areas is important in cardiovascular function and is sensitive to baroreflex control. This group of neurons receives input from other brainstem areas such as the lateral tegmental area, which may be involved in mediating baroreflex control in some species.[6] Another subpopulation of neurons is insensitive to baroreflex control and has a less direct role in cardiovascular function regulating thermogenesis, lipolysis, and cutaneous circulation.

The glossopharyngeal nerve or cardiopulmonary receptors via the vagus terminate in the nucleus tractus solitarii (NTS) providing afferent input to the brain from the carotid and aortic arch high pressure baroreceptors. Second-order excitatory neurons from the NTS project to the caudal ventrolateral medulla, which contains GABAergic inhibitory neurons that limit sympathetic outflow and hypothalamic neuroendocrine mechanisms. Projections to the PVN and supraoptic nucleus (SON) modulate vasopressin and ACTH release while the pathway to the RVLM regulates sympathetic activity. The NTS also projects to the dorsal motor vagal nucleus and the nucleus ambiguus to influence vagal control of the heart rate. Other reflex afferent neurons project to the NTS and affect autonomic and cardiovascular regulation, including chemoreflexes, renal afferent nerves, skeletal muscle afferents, and gastrointestinal inputs. The NTS is also modulated by the area postrema (AP), a circumventricular organ that lacks a blood–brain barrier and permits access of peptides and other circulating chemicals to the NTS neurons to facilitate or diminish reflex function.[7]

Midbrain

Hindbrain sites receive direct projections from midbrain and hypothalamic areas. In the midbrain, the parabrachial nucleus serves as a relay station for projections to and from the forebrain. Afferent projections from the NTS to the parabrachial nucleus carry visceroreceptive, nociceptive afferents, respiratory, and cardiovascular information to the hypothalamus.[8] Descending projections to the parabrachial nucleus extend from the PVN, amygdala, and dorsomedial hypothalamic nuclei. The parabrachial nucleus relays information to the NTS and RVLM. Many descending pathways from the hypothalamus to the hindbrain and spinal cord pass through the periaqueductal gray. The area contains synapses as well as fibers of passage.[9] Another major midbrain site to receive projections from the hypothalamus is the A5 area. The A5 is one of the principal nuclei that projects to the preganglionic sympathetic neurons; it also projects to the RVLM and NTS. The A5 receives input from the PVN and other hypothalamic nuclei.

Hypothalamus

The hypothalamus serves as a higher level of integration for cardiovascular regulation. The principal nuclei integrating the hormonal and sympathetic neural responses in the hypothalamus are the paraventricular and dorsomedial nuclei. It appears, however, that these nuclei mediate different responses. The dorsomedial hypothalamus

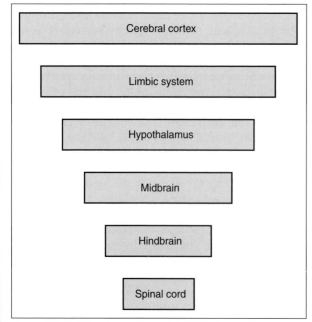

Figure 25–1. This schematic represents the layers of complexity of neural pathways contributing to the regulation of the autonomic function controlling the cardiovascular system.

(DMH) is more involved with stress-related stimuli while the PVN contributes to mechanisms maintaining overall body homeostasis. The PVN has received a great deal of attention in cardiovascular regulation because it sends direct excitatory projections to the intermediolateral column of the spinal cord, RVLM, and parabrachial nucleus, and an inhibitory projection to the NTS.[10,11] The DMH projects to the midbrain and hindbrain cardiovascular centers to modulate autonomic function including blood pressure and heart rate. The posterior hypothalamus is involved in sympathetic regulation as well, but appears to have a less pivotal role in blood pressure control than the PVN and DMH. Both the PVN and DMH receive innervation from the parabrachial nucleus. The PVN also receives input from the NTS and the CVLM as part of the cardiovascular baroreflex loop. Another potential projection in the reflex loop is to the anterior hypothalamic area (AHA). Increases in blood pressure stimulate catecholaminergic activity in the AHA.[12] The AHA sends a GABAergic projection to the PVN, which provides a significant amount of the GABA innervation in the PVN that can reduce sympathetic outflow.[13–15] Other input to the PVN and DMH from areas such as the lateral and ventromedial hypothalamic nuclei can also modulate cardiovascular function. These areas and others serve as relay stations carrying inputs from sensory areas in the hypothalamus and the hindbrain.

There are also sensory areas of the hypothalamus that can activate neural pathways influencing cardiovascular function. Two sites, the organum vasculosum of the lamina terminalis (OVLT) and the subfornical organ (SFO), are circumventricular organs like the AP where peptides can exert their actions. The OVLT and the SFO are both important for the central actions of Ang II, sodium, and cytokines that result in the activation of the PVN and descending autonomic pathways as well as the SON, PVN for neuroendocrine stimulation of vasopressin and oxytocin from the posterior pituitary, and ACTH from the anterior pituitary. The OVLT and SFO also converge on the nucleus medianus in the rostral portion of the third ventricular wall where they synapse with neurons projecting to the PVN and SON. The OVLT and the nucleus medianus are the principal structures of the anteroventral third ventricle region (AV3V) of the hypothalamus.[7] The arcuate nucleus is sensitive to circulating leptin, which is released by adipose tissue in obesity. Leptin activates proopiomelanocortin (POMC) pathways and inhibits neuropeptide Y (NPY) pathways to the DMH, PVN, and other areas of the hypothalamus to increase sympathetic outflow, decrease food intake, and stimulate lipolysis[16] (see Chapter 38). Other hormones and chemicals such as insulin, aldosterone, and free fatty acids stimulate the brain through these sites. Other sensory modalities also act through the hypothalamus. Light/dark balance, which acts through the suprachiasmatic nucleus, controls circadian rhythms and modulates cardiovascular and neuroendocrine function through the PVN, SON, and other nuclei.[17] Thermosensitive neurons in the medial preoptic area connect with the DMH to regulate sympathetic outflow to brown adipose tissue and the heart.[18]

Limbic system and cerebral cortex

Higher brain centers also influence neural and hormonal control of the circulation. The limbic system includes the limbic lobe of the cortex and deep-lying structures beneath the cortex that include the amygdala, fornix, hippocampus and other areas involved in behavioral responses composing the defense response or alerting behavior. The autonomic and hormonal systems linked to these areas permit the manifestation of responses associated with behavior. The amygdala is the principal structure that links the limbic system to the lateral hypothalamus, the parabrachial nucleus, the RVLM, vagal nuclei, and the NTS to evoke the autonomic components of the response.[19] The amygdala also receives projections from the NTS and the parabrachial nucleus. The limbic system drives acute cardiovascular responses associated with emotional behaviors; however, it also is involved in affective disorders such as depression that may contribute to the long-term control of blood pressure. Areas of the cerebral cortex have also been shown to modulate neurohumoral mechanisms controlling blood pressure. The insular cortex and the medial prefrontal cortex receive input from the NTS and parabrachial nucleus through projections that pass through the midbrain and the thalamus.[19,20] The somatic motor and sensory cortex receive projections from the limbs and viscera that are integrated in responses associated with exercise and cardiac pain. Descending projections extend to the hypothalamus and downstream sites in the midbrain and hindbrain that are associated with the integrated autonomic, hormonal, and motor responses. These areas are linked to cognitive behavioral influences on blood pressure and "central command" of cardiovascular function during exercise.

In summary, there a number of effector systems that influence and regulate blood pressure alterations and maintenance. These mechanisms involve numerous reciprocal projections between various structures throughout the brain. These interactions are responsible for the checks and balances that are typical in the maintenance in blood pressure. Figure 25–2 illustrates the intricate nature of the interactions in brain regions that are involved in blood pressure regulation. The complex nature of these networks contributes to the puzzle of neural pathways regulating cardiovascular control.

Biochemistry of neurotransmitters

The neurochemical control of blood pressure involves a wide range of neurotransmitter and neuromodulator systems. The same sequence of rapid to slower, more prolonged acting neurochemical mechanisms are involved in these pathways similar to other neuronal systems. In the brain, fast-acting amino acid neurotransmitters are important as both inhibitory and excitatory systems. The actions of the rapid systems are modulated by monoamine and cholinergic systems. Then peptides released by action potentials or formed in the extracellular fluid contribute a further level of modulation. Synapses are a complex organization of multiple inputs resulting in many different neurotransmitters that are actively released from both neurons and glia. The ultimate effect is a summation of

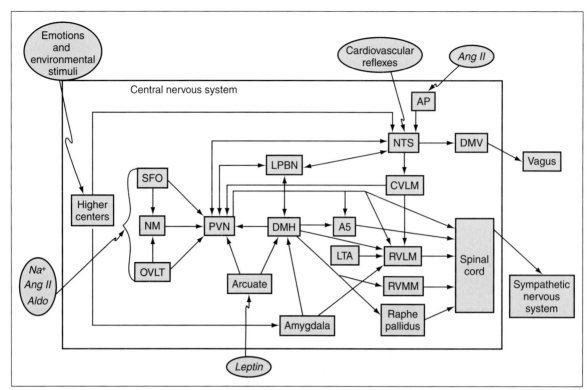

Figure 25–2. The schematic depicts the nuclei within the central nervous system (CNS) involved in the hypertensive process and their interconnections by neural pathways. Stimuli are represented in ovals, and their site of action is illustrated by the thickened arrows. Vagal and sympathetic nervous system outputs are shown outside the CNS.

chemical effects that will stimulate or inhibit the cell bodies or axons. Major neurotransmitter systems, the receptors they use, and the general signaling system are summarized in Table 25–1.

Amino acid neurotransmitters are fast-acting excitatory and inhibitory chemicals that include glutamate, γ-aminobutyric acid (GABA), glycine, and others. Glutamate and GABA are the principal neurotransmitters, and they act through specific receptors. Glutamate is used as the primary excitatory neurotransmitter in the CNS. The glutamate receptor is composed of two families of receptors: the first is the G-protein–coupled metabotropic glutamate receptors and the second is composed of the ionotropic glutamate receptors. The eight G-protein–coupled receptors belong to the seven transmembrane-spanning domain superfamily of receptors, and are comprised of three separate subgroups based on similarities in their amino acid sequences, second messengers, and their respective pharmacology.[21] The G-protein–coupled glutamate receptors are found throughout the CNS and are found post- and pre-synaptic. They are involved in the activation of signaling molecules, long-term potentiation, long-term depression, neuronal death, and synaptic plasticity.[22] The ion channel families of glutamate receptors are multimeric in composition and are comprised of three different subtypes based on pharmacologic structural similarities: N-methyl-D-aspartate (NMDA), α-amino-3-hydroxy-5-methylisoxazole-4-propionic acid (AMPA), and kainate. The NMDA receptors are localized postsynaptically and their activation leads to calcium influx into the post-

synaptic cells and they are known to regulate excitatory neurotransmission.[23] Neurotransmission occurs more slowly than that with AMPA receptors, but it lasts much longer. AMPA receptors are ubiquitously expressed throughout the CNS and mediate fast synaptic transmission in the CNS.[23] Kainate receptors are localized both pre- and post-synaptically, and due to lack of pharmacologic tools, their physiologic role is still not completely understood; however, it is suggested that they are involved in fast synaptic transmission, suppression of transmission (presynaptic), and synaptic plasticity.[23,24]

GABA is the main inhibitory neurotransmitter found in the CNS. It acts upon three different classes of receptors: $GABA_A$, $GABA_B$, and $GABA_C$. The $GABA_A$ and $GABA_C$ receptors are ionotropic, whereas the $GABA_B$ receptors are metabotropic. $GABA_A$ and $GABA_C$ are Cl^- channels that mediate fast synaptic inhibition; however, they differ biochemically, pharmacologically, and physiologically. $GABA_A$ receptors are the primary fast-acting inhibitory receptors in the CNS. $GABA_B$ receptors are G-protein coupled and activate second-messenger systems, phospholipase C and adenylate cyclase, as well as activate K^+ and Ca^{2+} ion channels. These receptors are localized both post- and pre-synaptically.[25] Synaptic activation of the $GABA_B$ receptor leads to a slow inhibitory postsynaptic potential unlike the fast inhibitory post-synaptic potential that is observed with $GABA_A$ receptors.[21] Glycine is another major inhibitory neurotransmitter in the CNS. It acts primarily at the glycine receptor, which is a ligand-gated Cl^- channel. It has both inhibitory postsynaptic function and can also

MAJOR NEUROTRANSMITTER SYSTEMS AND THEIR RECEPTORS, AND GENERAL SIGNALING SYSTEM		
Transmitter	**Receptors**	**G-Protein Coupled vs. Ionotropic**
GABA	GABA A	Ionotropic receptor
	α, β, γ, δ, σ isoforms	
	GABA B	G-protein coupled
	GABA C	Ionotropic receptor
Glutamate	AMPA	Ionotropic receptor
	KA	Ionotropic receptor
	GLU 1–4	
	NMDA	Ionotropic receptor
	NMDA 1,2$_{A-D}$	
	mGLU 1–7	G-protein coupled
Acetylcholine	Nicotinic	Ionotropic receptor
	Multiple α and β isoforms	
	Muscarinic	G-protein coupled
	M$_1$–M$_4$	
Norepinephrine	α_{1A-D}	G-protein coupled
	α_{2A-C}	G-protein coupled
	β_{1-3}	G-protein coupled
Dopamine	D1–D5	G-protein coupled
Serotonin	5-HT$_{1A-F}$	G-protein coupled
	5-HT$_{2A-C}$	G-protein coupled
	5-HT$_3$	G-protein coupled
	5-HT$_{4-7}$	G-protein coupled
Angiotensin II	AT1	G-protein coupled
	AT2	G-protein coupled
Ang 1–7	Mas	G-protein coupled

Table 25–1. Major Neurotransmitter Systems and Their Receptors, and General Signaling System

act as an excitatory neurotransmitter, by acting as a coagonist of the NMDA glutamate receptor. Several of the major excitatory and inhibitory neurotransmitters localized to the CNS have been discussed thus far.

Catecholaminergic pathways have also been studied extensively with regard to the CNS. Neurons projecting from cell bodies containing norepinephrine (A1, A2, A5, A6), epinephrine (C1, C2), and to a lesser extent dopamine (A13), significantly influence synaptic activity. There are multiple receptor subtypes that are activated by norepinephrine/epinephrine including, $\alpha1$, $\alpha2$, and β receptors. These receptors have multiple subtypes, are widely distributed, and can be found at both central and peripheral sites. These receptors are activated by norepinephrine released at synaptic terminals or epinephrine released from the adrenal medulla. $\alpha1$-Adrenoreceptor activation in the CNS generally results in depolarization and an increase in the firing rate; $\alpha2$-adrenoreceptor activation in the brainstem results in an inhibition of sympathetic outflow; and finally, prejunctional $\alpha2$-adrenoreceptor—activation and stimulation-evoked neurotransmitter release. These are just several of the actions mediated by these receptors. Serotonin (5-hydroxytryptamine; 5-HT) is another neurotransmitter that is found in the CNS that

is involved in blood pressure regulation. Serotonergic systems mainly originate from the raphe nuclei and have receptors that are localized in multiple brain regions. There are seven main types of 5-HT receptors, each with multiple subtypes that have a wide variety of endpoints. Activation of 5-HT receptors in the brain alters cardiovascular function by affecting autonomic outflow, as well as water and salt intake, reflexes, and more.

Amines can cause excitation or inhibition in synapses depending on the receptor subtype binding. They can also modulate sensitivity to other neurotransmitters and neuromodulators. Acetylcholine (Ach) is synthesized from acetyl coenzyme A and choline by acetyltransferase. Neuronal acetylcholinesterase quickly breaks down Ach in the brain. Ach acts on two main classes of receptors: nicotinic, which are ligand-gated cation channels, and muscarinic, which is G-protein coupled. Each receptor/subclass has different actions on neuronal activity.

In addition to the above mentioned neurotransmitters, there are numerous neuropeptides that are involved in blood pressure regulation. Angiotensin peptides represent a family of neuropeptides in that they have a role in the regulation of blood pressure. Ang II is the principal peptide that acts on two different receptor subtypes, the AT1 and AT2 receptors. The AT1 receptor has been localized in the hypothalamus, midbrain, and hindbrain. Additionally, Ang II has been found to be elevated in hypertensive models of hypertension.[26] Several angiotensin peptides have also been shown to act in the brain to increase blood pressure and stimulate thirst.[27,28] Ang 1–7, an angiotensin peptide, has been localized in the brain and is the product of angiotensin-converting enzyme 2 (ACE 2) on Ang II or endopeptidase on Ang I.[29,30] It acts through the mas receptor to cause a fall in arterial pressure. Other neuropeptides also act in areas of the brain to increase or decrease arterial pressure. This is just a very brief summary of the complex actions of numerous neurotransmitters that act in the brain and are involved in high blood pressure control.

GENETICS

Individual susceptibility to hypertension depends on multiple genetic and environmental factors affecting both physiologic and biochemical mechanisms that control blood pressure. As a result, determination of the genetic involvement in hypertension is a difficult endeavor. Since the development of the strain of rats developed by Smirk and Hall,[31] the use of genetic models that resulted from natural mutations has been a useful approach to understanding the pathophysiology of hypertension. So far it has not been apparent that any of these strains of rats or mice have developed hypertension as a result of a specific neural defect.

The polygenic, and therefore multifactorial, nature of the hypertensive process has been underscored by the investigation of these models over the years. However, it remains uncertain whether basic genetic defects in brain function of other genetic alterations leading to central neural dysfunction is the critical mechanism driving the hypertension in many of these models. One concern that has arisen is the lack of true controls for genetic strains; one example is the Wistar Kyoto (WKY) is commonly used as the control animal for the spontaneously hypertensive rat (SHR). The SHR is but one of several models that is used to examine the genetic role of blood pressure. It is commonly thought that changes between the models may be a result of strain differences or may be due to genetic drift.[32] Nevertheless, genetic alterations have been found in the brains of spontaneously hypertensive rats and Dahl salt-sensitive animals. For example, in the SHR, occurrence of NMDA-receptor splice variants NR2C and NR2D gene expression are significantly lower than in observed normotensive controls.[33] Receptor radioligand-binding studies have demonstrated increased numbers of angiotensin-binding sites in cardiovascular relevant brain areas of SHR.[34,35] In contrast, AT1 receptor mRNA levels are higher in the hypothalamus of the SHR compared to that of normotensive controls.[26] While genetic models have assisted further exploration of the genetic component of cardiovascular diseases, there are still many gaps in current knowledge. Many of the studies are observational versus descriptive; moreover, information on genetic involvement in CNS–cardiovascular disease interaction is still limited.

To investigate the potential of altered expression of neural genes to cause hypertension, overexpression of a specific gene candidate (transgenic) and deletion or knocking down of the genes are effective approaches. Overexpression of the gene assists in elucidating the normal tissue- and cell-specific expression patterns of a gene and can lead to information about the gene-specific physiologic changes that occur.[36] Deletion of the gene allows for interpretations of its function by examining physiologic response when the gene is missing.[36] With the identification of Ang II–immunoreactive fibers in specific brain regions,[37–41] a series of Ang II–related transgenic animals have been developed to investigate the role of the brain angiotensin system. Double-transgenic mice expressing human angiotensinogen (hAGT) or human renin (hREN) under the control of glial-specific glial fibrillary acidic protein (GFAP) promoter were developed and exhibited a modest Ang II type 1 receptor–dependent increase in blood pressure.[42,43] In addition, glial-specific deletion of AGT was performed in mice, and arterial pressure was found to be significantly lower in the overexpressors and unchanged from nontransgenic control mice. These results suggested a major contribution of glial AGT to the hypertensive state.[44]

In a transgenic mouse model with brain-restricted overexpression of Ang II 1a receptors (NSE-AT(1a)), mice underwent two-kidney/one-clip surgery to induce hypertension, which resulted in an early exacerbation of blood pressure increases.[45] A particularly interesting new transgenic model overexpresses a nonsecreted form of renin.[46] α2A-adrenergic receptors play a key role in cardiovascular regulation; moreover, they are widely expressed in the CNS. D79N mice, which lack functional α2A-adrenergic receptors, display no increase in blood pressure after injection with atrial natriuretic peptide (ANP) or α2 receptor agonists into the anterior hypothalamic nucleus. This result is unlike the changes observed in control C57BL/6 mice. These data support the concept that in the anterior hypothalamic nucleus of the mouse α2A-adrenergic receptors mediate both sympathoinhibitory responses to ANP and α2-adrenergic receptor agonists.[47] These are just a few examples in which brain-specific transgenic animals are used to understand the potential role of genetic influence in the CNS in the development of blood pressure. Investigators have used other genetic tools such as gene transfer and cre-lox systems to study timed gene expression in specific nuclei as well as the whole brain.

Another approach to examine genetic involvement in blood pressure is the use of gene arrays to examine gene expression profiles in hypertensive models. High-throughput gene profiling has permitted the examination of a large number of genes at one time, thus providing an opportunity to study changes in a large number of genes. While sequential and proximal gene effects may influence the results, potential intergene relationships can be studied using extensive software analysis. In addition, with the advent of proteomic technology, these strategies can be further exploited. Even these approaches are stymied by secondary effects such as the influence of elevated blood pressure causing baroreflex-related changes in gene expression rather than primary defective changes. Nevertheless, studies utilizing gene profiling in primary hypothalamic neuronal cultures have revealed differential expression of 299 genes and 109 expressed sequence tags (ESTs) between neuronal cultures treated with Ang II and control neurons. In addition, Ang II treatment resulted in the differential expression of 128 genes and 52 ESTs between WKY and SHR neurons.[48] These genes were involved in neurotransmission, signal transduction, ion transport, immune response/cytokines, proteolysis, and other areas.[48] This technique also assists in further elucidation of changes in underlying signaling in neurons that may influence changes in blood pressure. The information that the genetic profiling provides is useful; the challenge lies in determining the physiologic relevance of these genes. Hence the combination of the abovementioned techniques is required to fully evaluate the genetic involvement in the development and maintenance of hypertension.

PHYSIOLOGY

While many stimuli can cause an acute elevation in arterial pressure through central mechanisms, few stimuli are chronically activated, making it difficult to account for long-term control of blood pressure. For example, stressful situations can cause acute increases in sympathetic activity and hormonal responses; however, stressors are usually not sustained. Similarly, sodium and hormones can act on the brain to trigger increases in blood pressure, but these stimuli are linked to either the rhythmicity of hormone release or meal-associated increases in sodium.[49] The "error signal" for a stimulus to cause a sustained rise in blood pressure must be a result of a dysregulation of physiologic control and disposition of hormones and/or nutritional mediators or a neural memory mechanism that alters the sensitivity to the pressor stimuli. Of course, these mechanisms alone are not enough to result in the CNS drive because baroreflex mechanisms should restore excursions in blood pressure to normal. Hence, a further central dysregulation of volume and/or baroreflexes must occur for a long-term rise in blood pressure. The change in the "set point" for blood pressure during hypertension has been the focus of many studies and much speculation. Although the resetting of the baroreflex to a higher level and even a reduced sensitivity of the reflex has been demonstrated repeatedly for many years, the neural mechanism has been elusive. Recent work by Mifflin and colleagues[50] has suggested that an increase in presynaptic GABA$_B$ function in the NTS may contribute to the process of resetting blood pressure to a higher level.

Most evidence points to a dysfunction of the renin-angiotensin-aldosterone system as a major culprit in the hypertensive process. The peripheral vascular and renal actions of Ang II combined with the central actions of the hormones support the concept of hypertension as a multifactorial and multiple-organ dysfunction disease. The excitatory pathway cascade currently hypothesized in hypertension starts with circulating Ang II acting on the SFO and OVLT leading to the activation of the PVN, RVLM, and spinal cord preganglionic neurons, and thus leads to increased sympathetic outflow and ultimately elevation of blood pressure.[51] However, the physiology of CNS-mediated hypertension does not appear to be this straightforward because Ang II can also contribute to the hypertensive process through a number of other central mechanisms. Three examples of the complexity of Ang II will be discussed below to demonstrate principles brain involvement in hypertension. Included are the actions of Ang II working in concert with sodium and other circulating hormones to trigger the hypertensive process, evidence that Ang II synthesized in the PVN and RVLM that supports the role of a brain renin-angiotensin system, and the activation of cell signaling systems to mediating the actions of Ang II and modulating the function of other neurotransmitter systems.

Sodium-dependent hypertension is often associated with a dysregulation of the renin-angiotensin system. It has been suggested that the levels of Ang II and aldosterone are high in some forms of hypertension for the level of total body sodium.[52] The main Ang II- and sodium-sensitive region of the brain includes the SFO and the AV3V. The mechanisms of interaction of sodium and Ang II are not clear; however, the presence of sodium enhances the actions of Ang II. The presence of epithelial-like sodium channels and Ang II receptors in the OVLT and the SFO provide the structural machinery for them to work together to stimulate central neural pathways. Recent evidence has suggested that aldosterone may also be important in amplifying the actions of Ang II since mineralocorticoid receptors are also present in these areas.[53] Aldosterone antagonists also interfere with the pressor actions of sodium. While aldosterone can activate sodium channels to alter cell sodium content and sensitivity to Ang II, evidence is only starting to emerge to support the exact mechanisms. Another example of multiple stimuli acting centrally through merging pathways is in obesity. Obesity is associated with an increase in leptin, Ang II, and aldosterone.[54] The actions of Ang II on the forebrain were previously discussed.

Leptin also has a forebrain action through the arcuate nucleus to increase sympathetic nervous system activity. Liberated by adipose tissue, leptin activates excitatory melanocortin and inhibits NPY inhibitory pathways to the PVN to regulate feeding and sympathetic function. It is unknown whether the convergence of the SFO/OVLT and the arcuate pathways activate the same descending sympathoexcitatory mechanisms; however, the PVN plays a major role in mediating the responses.[16] Together these observations support the concept that multiple humoral systems are activated in hypertension, which can act at the same or different locations in the brain to stimulate the similar pathways.

The concept of a brain renin-angiotensin system has been discussed for many years. Confirmation of tissue-specific formation of Ang II has evolved rapidly with the advent of gene manipulation techniques. It is now clear that Ang II can be formed in the synapse and in some neurons.[44] Assay limitations make it difficult to actually measure the release of Ang II and satisfy the requirements for classification as a neurotransmitter. However, one of the interesting aspects of the brain Ang II system has been that sequential neural pathways were capable of using Ang II to mediate their activation.[38] Projections from the SFO to the nucleus medianus are stimulated by circulating Ang II and appear to use Ang II to, in turn, stimulate the projection to the PVN. As previously discussed, the PVN then sends more diffuse projections to activate the sympathetic nervous system. At least one of these projections to the RVLM also appears to use Ang II to mediate part of its actions.[55] As cotransmitters, peptides play important roles in enhancing and prolonging the actions of faster neurotransmitters like glutamate. The repeated occurrence of a peptide like Ang II in functional neural pathways presents a therapeutic opportunity to interfere with a pathophysiologic mechanism at more than one site of action.

In the brain, Ang II and glutamate use several cell-signaling systems to increase intracellular calcium levels and depolarize neurons. Among these systems is the nitric oxide/superoxide signaling system. Nitric oxide increases following Ang II stimulation as a compensatory mechanism to decrease the actions of Ang II. In contrast, both Ang II and glutamate activate the superoxide system to increase free radicals that work with other signaling systems to elevate calcium levels. The family of reactive oxygen species includes superoxide, hydroxyl ion, and the relatively stable and diffusible moiety, hydrogen peroxide, which is the product of superoxide dismutase. Superoxide also combines with nitric oxide to form peroxynitrites, which can bind to cellular proteins and alter their function. The formation of peroxynitrites also reduces the bioavailable concentration of nitric oxide limiting its activity. Components of the nitric oxide and superoxide systems act both intracellularly and extracellularly to alter neurotransmitter release. Nitric oxide has a paracrine function diffusing out of the cell and increasing the release of GABA from adjacent neurons.[56] Glutamate release can be altered by hydrogen peroxide. Thus, Ang II, working with glutamate, alters the balance between the nitric oxide and superoxide systems, and thus facilitates excitatory neurotransmission. Evidence suggests that this mechanism occurs in each of the sites where Ang II acts to stimulate a neural pathway.

The role of the underlying signaling processes and their involvement in neurotransmitter release and their involvement in blood pressure regulation has gained recent interest. Alterations in mitogen-activated protein (MAP) kinase and the phosphatidylinositol-3 kinase (PI3-kinase) families of proteins have been implicated in neuronal involvement in blood pressure regulation. MAP kinase has been found to be involved in Ang II–induced transcription of catecholamine-synthesizing enzymes.[57] Moreover, the PI3-kinase-Ang II signaling pathway has been observed in primary hypothalamic cell cultures from spontaneously hypertensive rats but not in cultures from control rats.[58] Inhibitors of these pathways when microinjected into the RVLM have demonstrated that the MAPK pathway contributes to resting arterial pressure, and the PI3-kinase pathway is important in maintaining the elevation in blood pressure observed in hypertensive animals.[59] In addition, elevated levels of PI3-kinase activity have been detected in brain areas involved in blood pressure control in the SHR.[48] Underlying signaling mechanisms have been of great interest in the periphery and have been found to play important roles in blood pressure regulation; however, the understanding of signaling mechanisms in the central control of blood pressure is in its infancy. Further research will add to the further understanding of the involvement of signaling processes in the brain and their involvement in hypertension.

The mechanisms involved in the long-term control of blood pressure are difficult to assess. In the study of factors contributing to increased arterial pressure, many different mechanisms have been investigated, but little has been done to determine the evolution of changes in factors sustaining blood pressure over time. No doubt environmental and dietary influences are major factors; however, compensatory mechanisms are also likely involved. Early studies by Bianchi, et al.[60] were among the first to indicate that when blood flow to the kidney is reduced, renin-angiotensin system activity is not sustained over a long period of time. Other work has suggested that even though the sympathetic nervous system may contribute to elevated blood pressure during the onset and maintenance phases of hypertension, different central mechanisms may be involved.[61,62] Decreases in GABAergic function in the PVN are decidedly reduced during the onset of renal wrap hypertension; however, chronic a functional GABA system is slightly increased in the PVN. These and other observations suggest that further work into mechanisms that cause these changes may lead to a clearer understanding of the hypertensive process as well as provide insights into the long-term control of blood pressure.

CLINICAL IMPLICATIONS AND PERSPECTIVES

The clinical relevance of understanding changes in the brain in hypertension extends beyond the role of potential causative mechanisms. Investigations into the central mechanisms of blood pressure control have been important in delineating the neural connections among specific nuclei. Studies related to the integration of peripheral stimuli by the brain, the pathways that the stimuli activate, and the physiologic responses that are elicited have also been critical for our understanding of how the brain processes information. The control of blood pressure is clearly linked to emotional and cognitive function in higher brain centers. Observations demonstrating impaired task performance and short-term memory in hypertensive patients suggest long-term patient impact other than peripheral end-organ failure and stroke.[63] Further, an association among depression, stress, and cardiovascular diseases including hypertension emphasizes the integrative relationship between the brain and blood pressure control mechanisms.[64–66] Understanding the cause–effect relationship between brain function and blood pressure regulation will be essential to the ultimate treatment of cardiovascular disease.

Although we have a working knowledge of the neuro-transmitters that mediate chemical neurotransmission, we know very little about how they interact in a synapse or how excitatory or inhibitory responses prevail. Further, the role of glia in regulating neurotransmission remains a looming question since glia around neurons and cerebral blood vessels performs a number of functions such as a chemical storage depot, barrier to chemicals, and cell-to-cell communication. The control of cellular and paracrine signal transduction systems are critical for the transmission of neural signals. Work aimed at understanding of how ion channels and signaling systems interact, and what determines the output signals from neurons and glia cells, has only begun. Then, of course, the roles of growth factors, neural regeneration, and apoptosis in the brain have received little attention. Similarly, the factors that determine gene expression and the ultimate phenotype of neurons determining the function and innervation patterns in the brain have only started to be explored. Finally, the integration of neural pathways to form circuits and interactions with other neural functions in the whole animal and patient will be the final pieces of the brain puzzle. Once these pieces have been put together, then we can develop better modes of treatment and intervention to lower blood pressure and improve lifestyle.

SUMMARY

The role of the brain in hypertension remains controversial. It is clear that neural pathways in the CNS are involved in blood pressure control. There is further evidence that specific stimuli such as reflex mechanisms, circulating hormones, and stressful behavioral situations can stimulate the brain to increase blood pressure. In addition, well-defined output systems such as the sympathetic and parasympathetic nervous systems and circulating hormones permit evaluation of the impact of stimuli to the brain. Evidence strongly points to a role for the renin-angiotensin-aldosterone system in stimulating central neural pathways and integrating responses to peripheral stimuli that lead to increased arterial blood pressure. However, the essential and complex integrative role that the brain plays also limits our ability to quantify the contribution of the CNS to blood pressure control. As our understanding of brain function and evolution of technology advances, the mysteries of how the brain works in many different circumstances will provide insights into blood pressure control and the hypertensive process.

REFERENCES

1. Hinojosa C, Shade RE, Haywood JR. Plasma vasopressin concentration in high sodium renal hypertension. *J Hypertens* 1986;4:529–34.
2. Scheuer DA, Mifflin SW. Glucocorticoids modulate baroreflex control of renal sympathetic nerve activity. *Am J Physiol Regul Integr Comp Physiol* 2001;280:1440–49.
3. Strack AM, Sawyer WB, Hughes JH, Platt KB, Loewy AD. A general pattern of CNS innervation of the sympathetic outflow demonstrated by transneuronal pseudorabies viral infections. *Brain Res* 1989;491:156–62.
4. Cochrane KL, Nathan MA. Cardiovascular effects of lesions of the rostral ventrolateral medulla and the nucleus reticularis parvocellularis in rats. *J Auton Nerv Syst* 1993;43:69–81.
5. Guyenet PA. The sympathetic control of blood pressure. *Nat Rev Neurosci* 2006;7:335–46.
6. Orer HS, Gebber GL, Phillips SW, Barman SM. Role of the medullary lateral tegmental field in reflex-mediated sympathoexcitation in cats. *Am J Physiol Regulatory Integrative Comp Physiol* 2004;286:451–64.
7. Johnson AK, Gross PM. Sensory circumventricular organs and brain homeostatic pathways. *FASEB J* 1993;7:678–86.
8. TL Krukoff TL, Morton TL, Harris KH, Jhamandas JH. Expression of c-fos protein in rat brain elicited by electrical stimulation of the pontine parabrachial nucleus. *J Neurosci* 1992;12:3582–90.
9. Farkas E, Jensen AS, Loewy AD. Periaqueductal gray matter input to

cardiac-related sympathetic premotor neurons. *Brain Res* 1997;764:257–61.
10. Coote JH. Cardiovascular function of the paraventricular nucleus of the hypothalamus. *Biol Signals* 1995;4:142–9.
11. Duan YF, Kopin IJ, Goldstein DS. Stimulation of the paraventricular nucleus modulates firing of neurons in the nucleus of the solitary tract. *Am J Physiol Regulatory Integrative Comp Physiol* 1999;277:403–11.
12. Peng N, Meng QC, King K, Oparil S, Wyss JM. Acute hypertension increases norepinephrine release in the anterior hypothalamic area. *Hypertension* 1995;25:828–33.
13. Roland BL, Sawchenko PE. Local origins of some GABAergic projections to the paraventricular and supraoptic nuclei of the hypothalamus in the rat. *J Comp Neurol* 1993;332:123–43.
14. Martin DS, Haywood JR. Hemodynamic responses to paraventricular nucleus disinhibition with bicuculline in conscious rats. *Am J Physiol Heart Circ Physiol* 1993;265:1727–33.
15. Akine A, Montanaro M, Allen AM. Hypothalamic paraventricular nucleus inhibition decreases renal sympathetic nerve activity in hypertensive and normotensive rats. *Auton Neurosci* 2003;108:17–21.
16. Bell ME, Bhatnagar S, Akana SF, Choi S, Dallman MF. Disruption of arcuate/ paraventricular nucleus connections changes body energy balance and response to acute stress. *J Neurosci* 2000;20:6707–13.
17. Hermes ML, Coderre EM, Buijs RM, Renaud LP. GABA and glutamate

mediate rapid neurotransmission from suprachiasmatic nucleus to hypothalamic paraventricular nucleus in rat. *J Physiol* 1996;496:749–57.
18. Morrison SF. Central pathways controlling brown adipose tissue thermogenesis. *News Physiol Sci* 2004; 19:67–74.
19. Loewy AD. Central autonomic pathways. In: Loewy AD, Spyer KM, eds. *Central Regulation of Autonomic Functions.* New York: Oxford University Press, 1990:208–223.
20. Neafsey EJ. Prefrontal cortical control of the autonomic nervous system: anatomical and physiological observations. In: Uylings HBM, Van Eden CG, De Bruin JPC, Corner MA, Feenstra MGP, eds. *Progress in Brain Research.* New York: Elsevier Science, 1990:147–166.
21. Watling KJ, ed. *The Sigma-RBI Handbook of Receptor Classification and Signal Transduction.* Natick MA: Sigma-Research Biochemicals Incorporated, 2001:36–41.
22. Pin JP, Duvosison R. The metabotropic glutamate receptors: structure and functions. *Neuropharmacology* 1995; 34:1–26.
23. Ozawa S, Kamiya H, Tsuzuki K. Glutamate receptors in the mammalian central nervous system. *Prog Neurobiol* 1998;54:581–618.
24. Chittajallu R, Braithwaite SP, Clarke VRJ, Henley JM. Kainate receptors: subunits, synaptic localization and function. *Trends Pharmacol Sci* 1999;20:26–35.
25. Chebib M, Johnston GAR. The 'ABS' of GABA receptors: a brief review. *Clin Exp Pharmacol Physiol* 1999;26:937–40.

26. Raizada MK, Sumners C, Lu D. Angiotensin II type 1 receptor mRNA levels in the brains of normotensive and spontaneously hypertensive rats. J Neurochem 1993;60:1949–52.

27. Wright JW, Harding JW. Important role for angiotensin III and IV in the brain renin-angiotensin system. Brain Res Rev 1997;25:96–124.

28. Fournie-Zaluski MC, Fassot C, Valentin B, Djordjijevic D, Reaux-Le Goazigo A, Corvol P, et al. Brain renin-angiotensin system blockade by systemically active aminopeptidase A inhibitors: a potential treatment of salt-dependent hypertension. Proc Natl Acad Sci U S A 2004;101:7775–80.

29. Moriguchi A, Tallant EA, Matsumura K, Reilly TM, Walton H, Ganten D, et al. Opposing actions of angiotensin-(1–7) and angiotensin II in the brain of transgenic hypertensive rats. Hypertension 1995;25:1260–65.

30. Campagnole-Santos MJ, Diz DI, Santos RA, Khosla MC, Brosnihan KB, Ferrario CM. Cardiovascular effects of angiotensin-(1–7) injected into the dorsal medulla of rats. Am J Physiol Heart Circ Physiol 1989;257:324–29.

31. Smirk FH, Hall WH. Inherited hypertension in rats. Nature 1958;182:727–28.

32. Rapp JP. Use and misuse of control strains for genetically hypertensive rats. Hypertension 1987;10:7–10.

33. Edwards MA, Loxley RA, Powers-Martin K, Lipski J, McKitrick DJ, Arnolda LF, et al. Unique levels of expression of N-methyl-D-aspartate receptor subunits and neuronal nitric oxide synthase in the rostral ventrolateral medulla of the spontaneously hypertensive rat. Molecular Brain Res 2004;129:33–43.

34. Gutkind JS, Kurihara M, Castern E, Saavedra JM. Increased concentration of angiotensin II binding sites in selected brain areas of spontaneously hypertensive rats. J Hypertens 1988;6:79–84.

35. Stamler JF, Raizada MK, Fellows RE, Phillips MI. Increased specific binding of angiotensin II in the organum vasculosum of the laminae terminalis area of the spontaneously hypertensive rat brain. Neurosci Lett 1980;17:173–77.

36. Cvetkovic B, Sigmund CD. Understanding hypertension through genetic manipulation in mice. Kidney Int 2000;57:863–74.

37. Tagawa T, Dampne RA. AT1 receptors mediate excitatory inputs to rostral ventrolateral medulla pressor neurons from hypothalamus. Hypertension 1999;34:1301–307.

38. Lind RW, Swanson LW and Ganten D. Angiotensin II immunoreactive pathways in the central nervous system of the rat: evidence for a projection from the subfornical organ to the paraventricular nucleus of the hypothalamus. Clin Exp Hypertens 1984;6:1915–20.

39. Fuxe K, Ganten D, Hoekfelt T, Bolme P. Immunohistochemical evidence for the existence of angiotensin II-containing nerve terminal in the brain and spinal cord in the rat. Neurosci Lett 1980;2:229–39.

40. Eshima K, Hirooka Y, Shigematsu H, Matsuo I, Kioke G, Sakai K, et al. Angiotensin in the nucleus tractus solitarii contributes to neurogenic hypertension caused by chronic nitric oxide synthase inhibition. Hypertension 2000;36:259–63.

41. Cato MJ, Toney GM. Angiotensin II excites paraventricular nucleus neurons that innervate the rostral ventrolateral medulla: an in vitro patch-clamp study in brain slices. J Neurophysiol 2005;93:403–13.

42. Morimoto S, Cassell MD, Beltz TG, Johnson AK, Davisson RL, Sigmund CD. Elevated blood pressure in transgenic mice with brain-specific expression of human angiotensinogen driven by the glial fibrillary acidic protein promoter. Circ Res 2001;89:365–67.

43. Morimoto S, Cassell MD, Sigmund CD. Glial- and neuronal-specific expression of the renin-angiotensin system in brain alters blood pressure, water intake, and salt preference. J Biol Chem 2002;277:33235–41.

44. Sherrod M, Davis DR, Xizhou Z, Cassell MD, Sigmund CD. Glial-specific ablation of angiotensinogen lowers arterial pressure in renin and angiotensinogen transgenic mice. Am J Physiol Regul Integr Comp Physiol 2005;289:R1763–69.

45. Lazartigues E, Lawrence AJ, Lamb FS, Davisson RL. Renovascular hypertension in mice with brain-selective overexpression of AT1a receptors is buffered by increased nitric oxide production in the periphery. Circ Res 2004;95:523–31.

46. Lavoie JL, Liu X, Bianco RA, Beltz TG, Johnson AK, Sigmund CD. Evidence supporting a functional role for intracellular renin in the brain. Hypertension 2006;47:461–66.

47. Peng N, Chambless BD. Oparil S, Wyss M. α2A-adrenergic receptors mediate sympathoinhibitory responses to atrial natriuretic pepetide in the mouse anterior hypothalamic nucleus. Hypertension 2003;41:571–75.

48. Veerasingham SJ, Yamazato M, Berecek KH, Wyss JM, Raizada MK. Increased PI3-kinase in presympathetic brain areas of the spontaneously hypertensive rat. Circ Res 2005;96:277–79.

49. Haywood JR, Hinojosa-Laborde C. Sexual dimorphism of sodium-sensitive renal-wrap hypertension. Hypertension 1997;30:667–71.

50. Mifflin SW. What does the brain know about blood pressure? News Physiol Sci 2001;16:266–71.

51. Ferguson AV, Washburn DL. Angiotensin II: a peptidergic neurotransmitter in central autonomic pathways. Prog Neurobiol 1998;54:169–92.

52. Brooks VL, Haywood JR, Johnson AK. Translation of salt retention to central activation of the sympathetic nervous system in hypertension. Clin Exp Pharmacol Physiol 2005;32:426–32.

53. Huang BS, Cheung WJ, Wang H, Tan J, White RA, Leenen FHH. Activation of brain renin-angiotensin-aldosterone system by central sodium in Wistar rats. Am J Physiol Heart Circ Physiol 2006;291:H1109–17.

54. de Paula RB, da Silva AA, Hall JE. Aldosterone antagonism attenuates obesity-induced hypertension and glomerular hyperfiltration. Hypertension 2004;43:41–47.

55. Dampney RA, Fontes MA, Hirooka Y, Horiuchi J, Potts PD, Tagawa T. Role of angiotensin II receptors in the regulation of vasomotor neurons in the ventrolateral medulla. Clin Exp Pharmacol Physiol 2002;29:467–72.

56. Horn T, Smith PM, McLaughlin BE, Bauce L, Marks GS, Pittman QJ, et al. Nitric oxide actions in paraventricular nucleus: cardiovascular and neurochemical implications. Am J Physiol Regul Integr Comp Physiol 1994;266:306–13.

57. Yang H, Lu D, Yu K, Raizada MK. Regulation of neuromodulatory actions of angiotensin II in the brain neurons by the Ras-dependent mitogen-activated protein kinase pathway. J Neurosci 1996;16:4047–58.

58. Yang H, Raizada MK. Role of phosphatidylinositol 3-kinase in angiotensin II regulation of norepinephrine neuromodulation in brain neurons of the spontaneously hypertensive rat. J Neurosci 1999;19:2413–23.

59. Seyedabadi M, Goodchild AK, Pilowsky PM. Differential role of kinases in brain stem of hypertensive and normotensive rats. Hypertension 2001;38:1087–92.

60. Bianchi G, Baer PG, Fox U, et al. Changes in renin, water balance, and sodium balance during development of high blood pressure in genetically hypertensive rats. Circ Res 1975;36:153–61.

61. Martin DS, Haywood JR. Reduced GABA inhibition of sympathetic function in renal-wrapped hypertensive rats. Am J Physiol Regulatory Integrative Comp Physiol 1998;275:1523–29.

62. Haywood JR, Mifflin SW, Craig T, Calderon A, Hensler JG, Hinojosa-Laborde C. γ-aminobutyric acid (GABA)-A function and binding in the paraventricular nucleus of the hypothalamus in chronic renal-wrap hypertension. Hypertension 2001;37:614–18.

63. Blumenthal JA, Madden DJ, Pierce TW, Siegel WC, Appelbaum M. Hypertension affects neurobehavioral functioning. Psychosom Med 1993;55:44–50.

64. Davidson K, Jonas BS, Dixon KE, Markovitz JH. Do depression symptoms predict early hypertension incidence in young adults in the CARDIA study? Arch Intern Med 2000;160:1495–500.

65. Scherrer JF, Xian H, Bucholz KK, Eisen SA, Lyons MJ, Goldberg J, et al. A twin study of depression symptoms, hypertension, and heart disease in middle-aged men. Psychosom Med 2003;65:548–57.

66. Räikkönen K, Matthews KA, Kuller LH. Trajectory of psychological risk and incident hypertension in middle-aged women. Hypertension 2001;38:798–802.

Chapter

26 Aldosterone and Other Steroids

John W. Funder

Definitions

- Aldosterone is a uniquely modified (18CHO) adrenal steroid, with a well-described physiologic action of promoting unidirectional transepithelial sodium transport.

- Mineralocorticoid receptors are high-affinity binding sites in epithelial and nonepithelial tissues for aldosterone and the physiologic glucocorticoids cortisol and corticosterone.

- 11β Hydroxysteroid dehydrogenase type 2 is a very efficient, operationally unidirectional enzyme catalyzing the metabolism on cortisol to cortisone (and corticosterone to 11-dehydrocorticosterone) in aldosterone target tissues. Thus, by lowering active glucocorticoid levels and increasing those of NADH, under physiologic conditions aldosterone selectively activates mineralocorticoid receptors in tissues expressing the enzyme.

Key Features

- Rare syndromes (glucocorticoid remediable aldosteronism, apparent mineralocorticoid excess, hypertension of pregnancy) have proven useful in establishing current (patho)physiology.

- Patients with hypertension (and heart failure) characteristically have plasma aldosterone concentrations in the normal range.

- Mineralocorticoid receptors can be activated by cortisol under conditions of 11β hydroxysteroid deficiency/blockade, or by redox change attendant on generation of reactive oxygen species.

Clinical Implications

- Mineralocorticoid receptor blockade is therapeutically beneficial regardless of aldosterone status in hypertension (and heart failure).

- If shown to be vascular protective in larger clinical trials, mineralocorticoid receptor blockade should be widely used in cardiovascular disease.

- Blockade may similarly be useful in other chronic inflammatory (e.g., autoimmune) disorders.

For over 50 years aldosterone excess has been known to raise blood pressure in humans (Conn's syndrome), and over 60 years ago the combination of deoxycorticosterone and salt was shown to do so in experimental animals. In both instances renal sodium and water retention was inculpated as the initial effector mechanism, with the resultant increase in circulatory volume followed by an

increased cardiac output, in turn normalized by elevation of blood pressure. Subsequently, steroids with predominantly glucocorticoid activity were also shown to raise blood pressure, an effect that was not blocked by spironolactone, thus presumably mediated via glucocorticoid rather than mineralocorticoid receptors, and which appears to be mediated by reduced nitric oxide availability.[1] In experimental animals, administration of high levels of testosterone causes hypertension, by blockade of the adrenal enzyme (CYP11B1) needed for glucocorticoid production, causing elevation of ACTH and deoxycorticosterone levels.

Although knowledge of the epithelial action of aldosterone, and that of glucocorticoids in decreased production/increased scavenging of nitric oxide, is far from complete, over recent years evidence has accrued for a range of other ways in which adrenal steroids may be/are involved in blood pressure regulation. The role of the specificity-conferring enzyme 11β hydroxysteroid dehydrogenase type II (11βHSD2) has been defined, at least in part, in allowing aldosterone selectively to activate mineralocorticoid receptors (MR) in epithelia.[2,3] MR have been demonstrated in nonepithelial tissues, in some of which (e.g., vascular wall, NTS, placenta) 11βHSD2 is also expressed[4–6]; in others (hippocampus, cardiomyocytes, AV3V neurons), the enzyme is at low levels or absent.[7,8] Regardless of whether 11βHSD2 is co-expressed, activation of MR in some of these sites (e.g., vascular smooth muscle cells [VSMC] and AV3V neurons) can have major effects on blood pressure. In terms of the genesis of steroid-induced hypertension, the focus has in many senses shifted from aldosterone acting at epithelia to mineralocorticoid receptor activation, by aldosterone or other steroids, in both epithelial and nonepithelial tissues. The sections of this chapter to follow attempt to illustrate this complexity, from basic biochemistry through physiology and pathophysiology to implications for clinical practice, focusing on aldosterone and other steroids that can activate MR, in classic mineralocorticoid target tissues and elsewhere, and the contexts in which this occurs to modulate blood pressure levels.

ANATOMY/BIOCHEMISTRY

Aldosterone and the physiologic glucocorticoids are classically produced in the zona glomerulosa of the adrenal cortex, under the stimulus of ACTH, and for aldosterone in addition (and predominantly) angiotensin II and plasma

[K$^+$]. Over the past decade there have been numerous reports of the ectopic synthesis of corticosteroids in general, and aldosterone in particular, in vasculature,[9] heart,[10] and brain.[11] In the glomerulosa cell the enzymes responsible for the biosynthesis of corticosteroids are exquisitely localized to particular intracellular compartments, allowing relatively confined distribution (and thus relatively high local concentration) of successive substrates. In the proposed sites of ectopic synthesis mRNA levels for the biosynthetic enzymes are reported to be 10^3- to 10^6-fold lower than in whole adrenal (of which glomerulosa cells are commonly only a very small minority in terms of number), with no evidence for intracellular compartmentalization; at such levels each enzymatic step would appear to be rate limiting, making substantial biosynthesis of the end-product problematic.

The claim of cardiac synthesis of aldosterone, stimulated by both angiotensin II and (counterintuitively) by raised sodium intake, caused considerable interest; this claim is not supported by studies on angiotensin II–infused rats on 0.9% NaCl solution, where the gross coronary/cardiac inflammatory response was abrogated by adrenalectomy as well as by systemic MR blockade.[12] Recent reexamination of cardiac mRNA levels for steroid biosynthetic enzymes has been interpreted as evidence against cardiac aldosterone synthesis.[13,14] The much more extenuated disappearance curve of aldosterone compared with corticosterone in the heart of rats post-adrenalectomy, and the findings of higher levels of aldosterone in the heart than plasma of intact rats, may reflect the sequestration of the noncyclized form of aldosterone ($\leq$1% of total), by adduct formation via the 18-aldehyde group.[14]

In terms of biochemistry, the biosynthesis of aldosterone from deoxycorticosterone in many species is effected by CYP11B2 (aldosterone synthase), which in a three-step process catalyzes the formation of 18-hydroxydeoxycorticosterone, 18-hydroxycorticosterone, and finally aldosterone. In other species, notably the bovine, the enzyme CYP11B1 (11β hydroxylase) is responsible for oxidation at both C11 and C18 to yield aldosterone. In terms of evolution, the primordial enzyme appears closer to CYP11B2 (which has 11β hydroxylase activity) than CYP11B1; this not withstanding, the ability to synthesize aldosterone appears routinely late in evolution, in terrestrial vertebrates. This contrasts with mineralocorticoid receptors, which are clearly present in fish,[15] prefiguring roles as high-affinity receptors, essentially always occupied by normal levels of glucocorticoids, in mammalian non-epithelial tissues, physiology poorly understood.

Aldosterone is unusual in that it is secreted in very low amounts, and circulates either free (40% to 50%) or loosely bound to albumin, so that its clearance is relatively rapid. The evolutionary gain in exploiting a pre-existing receptor, rendered aldosterone-selective by the co-expression of 11βHSD2, to regulate sodium flux in epithelia—rather than selecting for an inherently aldosterone-specific receptor—is not currently obvious. What is obvious, however, is that even modest elevations of aldosterone above the normal upper limit can be accompanied by markedly aggravated cardiovascular pathology, to an extent considerably greater than seen in uncomplicated essential hypertensives with the same blood pressure elevation. Both the very low plasma levels (1/1000 to 1/2000 those of glucocorticoids) and the rapid clearance may both thus reflect the potentially deleterious effects of inappropriate aldosterone for salt status, as seen in primary aldosteronism and various models of experimental hypertension.[16]

GENETICS

That hypertension may reflect a particular genetic makeup, external environment constant, is clear from both animal and human epidemiologic studies. Successive matings over 20 generations between rats registering higher blood pressures produced spontaneously hypertensive rats from the Wistar Kyoto breeding stock. In the clinic, three congenital conditions producing hypertension have proven prismatic—for aldosterone, for the selectivity-conferring enzyme 11βHSD2, and for the mineralocorticoid receptor—and will be illustrated in brief detail.

Glucocorticoid remediable aldosteronism (GRA), also known as glucocorticoid suppressible hypertension, was first described over 40 years ago, and its genetic basis reported in 1992.[17] The syndrome—of familial hypertension with elevated aldosterone levels, often at a relatively young age—reflects the operation of a chimeric steroid biosynthetic enzyme, in turn the product of a chimeric gene. The genes coding for CYP11B1 (11β hydroxylase, the signature enzyme for glucocorticoid activity) and for CYP11B2 (aldosterone synthase) lie adjacent on human chromosome 8, and show higher than 94% sequence identity. This high degree of homology is commonly construed as evidence for a relatively recent gene duplication event, consistent with the relatively recent (terrestrial) emergence of aldosterone; it also reflects an unequal crossing-over at meiosis, in the founder line, between the two genes to produce a chimeric gene—5′ CYP11B1, 3′ CYP11B2. Different pedigrees show different points of cross-over between exons 1–4, but all have the same net result—production of aldosterone in response to

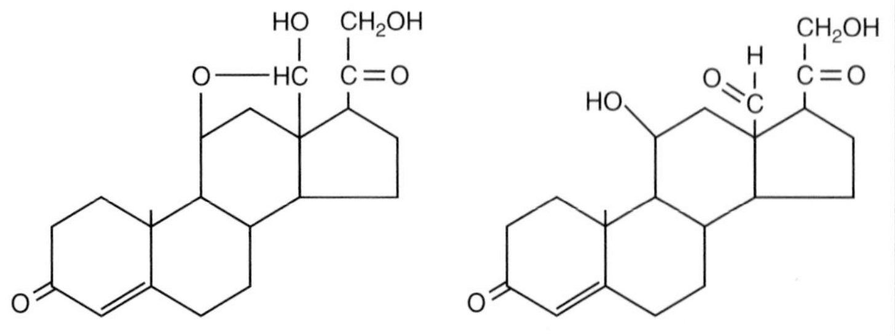

Figure 26–1. Molecular forms of aldosterone *in vivo*: (i) 11,18 hemiacetal, $\geq$99%; (ii) noncyclized form.

Aldosterone (i)   Aldosterone (ii)

ACTH, and throughout the adrenal cortex rather than confined to the glomerulosa.

Apparent mineralocorticoid excess (AME), as its name implies, is not a disorder of inappropriate aldosterone production, but rather one of inappropriate mineralocorticoid receptor activation reflecting deficient or absent action of the specificity-conferring enzyme 11βHSD2.[18] Unlike GRA, which is dominantly inherited, AME is recessive, and thus is less infrequently seen in offspring of consanguineous unions. When 11βHSD2 activity is deficient or absent, mineralocorticoid receptors (which in epithelial tissues are normally largely occupied[19] but not activated by normal circulating glucocorticoid levels) are both occupied and activated by glucocorticoids, to produce a syndrome of often severe juvenile hypokalemia, sodium retention, and hypertension.

Factitious AME can similarly follow enzyme blockade by glycyrrhizin/glycyrrhetinic acid, the active principle of licorice, widely used as a sweetener in confectionery. Its ability to raise blood pressure and circulatory volume had similarly been noted, well before the mechanism of AME was elucidated—which in turn proved to be a defining moment in establishing the physiology of aldosterone action in epithelia.

The final example that has proven illustrative is the S810L mutation of the human mineralocorticoid receptor, which produces juvenile hypertension very much exacerbated by pregnancy.[20] This rare mutation of a single nucleotide results in a receptor which is ~27% constitutively (absent steroid) active, and which sees progesterone and spironolactone as agonists, whereas they are antagonists of the wild-type human mineralocorticoid receptor. The aberrant pattern of activation reflects the altered geometry of the steroid binding cleft, and van der Waal's interactions between the leucine at residue 810 and the alanine at residue 773, which do not occur with the serine at residue 810 in the wild-type. The amino acid pairing in MR is quite distinct from that in closely related glucocorticoid/androgen/progesterone receptors, where the equivalent amino acids are methionine and glycine. In the S810L mutant, the leucine–alanine pairing is identical to that found in the more distantly related estrogen and retinoic acid receptors, and perhaps evidence for a primordial ancestry of MR in the MR/GR/AR/PR subfamily.[21]

PHYSIOLOGY AND PATHOPHYSIOLOGY

Classically, aldosterone was considered to raise blood pressure primarily by its effects on fluid and electrolyte retention in the kidney, and by central effects on mineralocorticoid receptors in the AV3V area of the brain.[22] More recently, aldosterone has been claimed to have direct deleterious effects in the heart, based on the undisputed therapeutic advantage conferred by MR blockade in progressive (RALES[23]) or post-infarct (EPHESUS[24]) cardiac failure. On the basis of current evidence, however, all these interpretations appear to be inadequate: renal effects do not appear to be the primary blood pressure drivers,[25] aldosterone under normal circumstances appears unable to access AV3V neuron mineralocorticoid receptors,[26] and finally, the steroid activating MR in cardiomyocytes in heart failure (or VSMC in hypertension) is almost certainly cortisol, not aldosterone.[27–29]

The case against a primarily renal action of aldosterone in elevating blood pressure is exemplified by a recent meta-analysis of clinical trials of the novel MR antagonist eplerenone in patients with essential hypertension.[25] In these trials patients were given eplerenone as monotherapy, with dosage titrated to effect (a diastolic blood pressure of <90 mmHg). After 4 weeks of treatment, of a total 397 patients started on 50 mg/day, just over 40% reached goal blood pressure at four weeks, and continued on this dose level, with the remainder up-titrated to 100 mg/day for weeks 5–8. On this dose a third (or 20% of the total) achieved goal diastolic blood pressure at the 100-mg dose. The remaining ~40% were further up-titrated to 200 mg/day for weeks 9–12, whereupon half reached goal blood pressure and half did not.

Table 26–1 shows the exact figures, and two unanticipated findings. First, at each dose the responders showed very large blood pressure reduction on average, and the nonresponders very little. The starkest comparison is at the 200-mg dose, where ~20% of the total cohort are

DOSE-TITRATION OF EPLERENONE AS MONOTHERAPY IN ESSENTIAL HYPERTENSIVE PATIENTS: EFFECTS ON ATTAINMENT OF GOAL (DIASTOLIC <90 MMHG) BLOOD PRESSURE, AND PLASMA [K⁺]						
Dose/Time	DBP	N	ΔSBP	ΔDBP	N	Δ[K⁺]
50 mg	<90	175	−15.9 (−17.8, −4.1)	−14.5 (−15.4, −13.6)	171	0.04 (−0.02, 0.09)
Week 4	≥90	222	−5.6 (−7.2, −4.0)	−3.3 (−4.0, −2.6)	218	0.09 (0.03, 0.15)
100 mg	<90	66	−19.9 (−22.4, −7.5)	−14.8 (−16.1, −13.6)	64	0.13 (0.05, 0.22)
Week 8	≥90	156	−4.6 (−6.7, −2.5)	−3.2 (−4.2, −2.3)	138	0.20 (0.13, 0.26)
200 mg	<90	75	−17.4 (−20.4, −4.4)	−14.6 (−15.7, −13.5)	72	0.20 (0.11, 0.30)
Week 12	≥90	81	−2.0 (−5.3, 1.3)	−1.4 (−3.0, 0.1)	45	0.19 (0.08, 0.30)

From Levy D, Rocha R, Funder JW. Distinguishing the antihypertensive and electrolyte effects of eplerenone. *J Clin Endocrinol Metab* 2004;89:2736–40. DBP, diastolic blood pressure; SBP, systolic blood pressure. Copyright 2004, The Endocrine Society.

Table 26–1. Dose-Titration of Eplerenone as Monotherapy in Essential Hypertensive Patients: Effects on Attainment of Goal (Diastolic <90 mmHg) Blood Pressure, and Plasma [K⁺]

essentially unresponsive to MR blockade. Second, at no dosage was there any sign of a correlation between responder/nonresponder status and change in plasma potassium values. These are not balance studies, but plasma [K$^+$] determination is the physician's yardstick for the obligate side effect of current anti-MR therapy; and there is no indication of any relationship between blood pressure and renal responses.

There is little doubt that in many species activation of MR in the AV3V region is followed by a rise in blood pressure. In rats, intracerebroventricular infusion of minute doses of aldosterone—at levels 100-fold lower than required systemically to raise blood pressure—raises blood pressure, an effect accelerated when the rats are maintained on 0.9% NaCl solution to drink.[30] Similarly, ICV infusion of RU28318, the water-soluble MR antagonist, completely blocks the rise in blood pressure that normally follows when salt-sensitive (jr/s) rats are placed on such a high salt intake.[31]

The evidence, however, is firmly against such blood pressure elevation being normally aldosterone-driven on several grounds. First, co-infusion of corticosterone, the physiologic glucocorticoid in rats, at doses one to two times those of aldosterone, progressively lowers the blood pressure response,[8] thus excluding the possibility of a "protected" (by 11β hydroxysteroid dehydrogenase) MR, and making selective aldosterone occupancy of the receptor in AV3V neurons highly improbable. Second, there appears to be no correlation between circulating aldosterone levels and the extent of AV3V MR activation: in rats on very low, normal, or very high salt diets, systemic aldosterone levels are very different, yet all respond to ICV infusion of RU28318 by a blood pressure fall of 20–30 mmHg, with no significant difference between groups.[26]

On this basis, it would appear that whereas experimentally administered aldosterone can elevate blood pressure via an AV3V involving pathway, *in vivo* AV3V MR are overwhelmingly always occupied by physiologic glucocorticoids.[32] The mechanisms whereby such glucocorticoid-occupied MR are activated, and the pathways involved, await exploration. These pathways presumably involve neural input, and it will be of considerable interest to see whether such input produces changes in intracellular redox change, as appears to be the case in the renal tubule and cardiomyocyte (see below) in response to 11β hydroxysteroid dehydrogenase deficiency[18] or reactive oxygen species generation.[33] The studies noted above, on exposing jr/s rats to salt, are consistent with inputs from the amygdala and the osmoreceptor area of the hypothalamus, and with possible vasopressinergic effects on AV3V neurons.

The third area—that of the presumed pathophysiologic role of aldosterone in hypertension and heart failure—has received considerably more attention over the past decade. The central issue is the assumption that the steroid-activating cardiomyocytes or vascular wall MR under such circumstances are aldosterone: the fact that baseline aldosterone levels in all three major trials of eplerenone (RALES, EPHESUS, 4E[34]) were in the low normal range, and sodium status unremarkable, is conveniently overlooked. This assumption is demonstrably not the case, witness the proven pathogenesis of apparent mineralocorticoid excess, where renal tubular MR are clearly cortisol-activated. The evidence that in VSMC and cardiomyocytes the pathophysiology is commonly driven by glucocorticoid-activated mineralcorticoid receptors is very strong.

In 11β hydroxysteroid dehydrogenase expressing tissues (which include VSMC), the enzyme normally protects against MR activation by normal levels of endogenous glucocorticoids,[4,19] but *not* (as was initially postulated, and still commonly assumed) glucocorticoid occupancy of such receptors. The enzyme is expressed at high levels in aldosterone target tissues, and has a remarkably low K$_m$ (high affinity) for the physiologic glucocorticoids. If, however, one does the mathematics[35]—or better still, the experiment[19]— the enzyme is clearly incapable of reducing intracellular glucocorticoid levels to an extent allowing selective aldosterone occupancy (and activation) of MR, in a renal principal cell for example. What the enzyme does is to debulk intracellular glucocorticoids by ~90%, which still leaves intracellular free glucocorticoid levels 10-fold or higher than those of aldosterone—and thus presumably, 90% of renal MR normally occupied but not activated by endogenous glucocorticoid hormones.

The other thing that the enzyme does is to convert cosubstrate NAD to NADH, stoichiometrically, one molecule of NADH for every molecule of cortisone generated. Normally NAD is at considerable excess, of the order of 600-fold; operation of the enzyme thus can generate steep increases in NADH product, with minimal depletion of substrate NAD levels. In other systems, NADH has been reported to activate co-repressors, and thus affect transcriptional regulation by nuclear trans-activating factors;[36] the mechanism whereby the resultant redox change activates glucocorticoid-occupied MR awaits exploration. In *Drosophila*, the E75 nuclear receptor was recently shown, for example, to have its binding cleft constitutively occupied by heme, and to be activated (or not) by redox state.[37]

The evidence for activation of MR by normal levels of endogenous glucocorticoids in the context of tissue damage and reactive oxygen species generation is both indirect and direct. In pigs subjected to experimental coronary angioplasty, eplerenone from day –5 until sacrifice at day 28 preserved luminal integrity compared with placebo-treated pigs. Neither group received administered mineralocorticoid or a high salt intake, raising the question (as in RALES, EPHESUS, and the 4E trials) of just what the antagonist was excluding from MR.[38] Second, uninephrectomized rats receiving deoxycorticosterone and maintained on 0.9% NaCl to drink responded by coronary inflammation and cardiac fibrosis, well established by 4 weeks, and thereafter modestly increasing by 8 weeks. If deoxycorticosterone is given for 8 weeks, but eplerenone given over weeks 5–8, then inflammation and fibrosis are reversed to baseline levels. In contrast, rats given deoxycorticosterone for 4 weeks, and then vehicle for weeks 5–8, showed coronary and cardiac pathology equivalent to that seen in rats killed immediately after 4 weeks of mineralo-corticoid exposure (i.e., substantially higher than controls). Our interpretation of these data is that the pathology is continued by continued activation of VSMC MR occupied by glucocorticoids in the context of established tissue damage.[39]

The direct demonstration of the bivalent nature of gluco-corticoids in MR is to date preliminary, and shown for a rapid nongenomic (and possibly nonphysiologic) effect of aldosterone via classical MR in rabbit cardiomyocytes.[33,40] Aldosterone at 15 minutes shows a 10-fold increase in pump current, reflecting a rapid direct effect on the $Na^+/K^+/2Cl^-$ cotransporter and subsequent activation of Na^+/K^+ ATPase by the increased intracellular $[Na^+]$. Cortisol at 100 nM alone has no effect, but co-administered with aldosterone stoichiometrically blocks its effect, evidence for a normal tonic inhibitory action of cortisol in MR. Oxidized glutathione (GSSG), administered alone via the broad-tipped pipette, has no effect. However, when cortisol is administered with GSSG, the latter to mimic reactive oxygen–species generation and redox change, cortisol becomes a MR agonist, mimicking the effect of aldos-terone and elevating pump current.

To deal with pathophysiology first, in a section on physiology and pathophysiology, may appear counter-intuitive—but in fact bears witness to the pathophysiologic and clinical studies having driven the reexamination of the biology of aldosterone (and MR) over the past decade. One element of physiology and one of pathophysiology remain unchallenged in the context of this reevaluation. In terms of physiology, the crucial role for MRs in epithe-lial sodium retention under conditions of limited sodium intake, has been reemphasized by the neonatal mortality in MR knock-out mice absent additional administered sodium.[41] One warning note, however, might be sounded by comparing the neonatal mortality (100%) in MR knock-out mice with that of "only" 30% in aldosterone synthase null mice, on a comparable (i.e., nonsupplemented) sodium intake.[42] In terms of pathophysiology, primary aldostero-nism (Conn's syndrome) is increasingly recognized as accounting for 8%–13% of unselected populations with essential hypertension[43]; importantly, the markedly higher risk of stroke, myocardial infarct, and associated cardiovascular pathology than in uncomplicated essential hypertension with equivalently elevated blood pressure is testament to the potentially deleterious effects of even modestly elevated aldosterone secretion in the context of a high (i.e., normal Western) sodium intake.[44]

If the primary mechanism of aldosterone action in terms of blood pressure control is neither renal nor via AV3V neuron stimulation, the question arises of its likely locus. More than two decades ago, the vascular wall was shown to express both MR and the protective enzyme 11 hydroxysteroid dehydrogenase, making it a candidate physiologic aldosterone target tissue.[5] In a variety of studies, this has been shown to be the case via both genomic and nongenomic mechanisms. Two illustrative examples of the latter, both human experiments, point to VSMC being the likely primary target for the blood pressure effects of aldosterone.

In the first, close intra-arterial infusion of aldosterone into the nondominant brachial artery, at a rate to mimic excursions in the physiological range and to cause no systemic rise in aldosterone levels, was shown to rapidly lead to vasoconstriction, with flow reduced to 60% of base-line levels, with an equally brisk return upon cessation of infusion.[45] In the second, aldosterone was shown to elevate intracellular pH in human uterine VSMC within 5 minutes; cortisol was without effect, until the 11β hydrogenase blocker carbenoxolone was introduced, when it mimicked aldosterone, with an identical dose–response curve and equivalently blocked by the MR antagonist RU28318.[4]

No consideration of the physiology of aldosterone can be complete without attention paid to the physiologic control of its secretion. Perhaps reflecting the undoubted clinical utility of angiotensin-converting enzyme inhibitors and angiotensin receptor blockers, most prominence has been given to angiotensin as the driver of aldosterone secretion in response to low salt intake. Studies on angiotensin knock-out mice would appear to dispute this emphasis, in that knock-out and wild-type mice raised their plasma aldosterone levels indistinguishably in response to 5 or 14 days low-sodium diet. The two groups, however, differed when given a diet low in both Na^+ and K^+ for 5 days: wild-type mice showed a muted response compared with low Na^+ alone, but knock-out mice aldosterone plasma levels were considerably lower than in wild-type mice.[46]

In evolutionary terms, the drivers of aldosterone secre-tion were arguably (1) acute volume depletion, following catastrophic diarrhea or blood loss, with sympathetic nervous system activation releasing renin to produce angiotensin, at once vasoconstrictor and salt-retaining (and thus volume-restoring) via increased aldosterone secretion; (2) chronic low-sodium/high-potassium intake to conserve sodium and unload potassium by the direct stimulatory effect of elevated plasma $[K^+]$ on aldosterone biosynthesis; and (3) orthostasis, a mechanism of aldos-terone elevation currently not completely clear, but consistent with the rapid vasoconstrictor role shown above, given the rapid elevation of aldosterone upon assuming the upright posture.

CLINICAL IMPLICATIONS AND PERSPECTIVES

A number of candidate agents are in use or have been proposed to reduce aldosterone action. These include renin antagonists, still under consideration but historically facing solubility problems; the commonly used angiotensin-converting enzyme inhibitors, which block the generation of angiotensin II; and angiotensin receptor blockers, which block its action on the adrenal glomerulosa (inter alia). Further down the pathway are aldosterone synthase inhibitors, currently in clinical trials, and MR antago-nists, both nonselective (spironolactone) and selective (eplerenone).

While it was commonly assumed that ACE inhibition/ AT_1R blockade would produce maintained low levels of plasma aldosterone, this has conclusively been shown not always to be the case for hypertensive patients, even on high-dose combination therapy.[47] Aldosterone synthase inhibition is at first sight an attractive concept, in the context of primary aldosteronism and the much reported possibility of ectopic aldosterone synthesis. Even in these circumstances, it appears to have no particular therapeutic advantage over MR blockade, and some considerable disadvantages.

The preference for MR blockade is that it blocks any agent from activating MR, and not just aldosterone. An experimental study in support of this—eplerenone from weeks 5–8 in rats receiving deoxycorticosterone completely reversing coronary inflammation and cardiac fibrosis, steroid withdrawal allowing inflammation and fibrosis to be maintained over weeks 5–8—has already been cited.[39] The clinical implications are thus clear—that MR blockade is the primary therapy for patients with Conn's syndrome (primary aldosteronism) not suitable for surgical intervention, and useful additional treatment in many patients with essential hypertension. This is particularly the case among patients with so-called resistant hypertension (blood pressure remaining elevated while on three or more antihypertensive agents), where the addition of low-dose spironolactone (12.5/25 mg) is reported to often be effective in causing blood pressure to fall.

Although extrapolation from animal studies to the clinic needs considerable caution, there are both animal and clinical studies supporting the utility of MR blockade even without blood pressure reduction. First, when stroke-prone spontaneously hypertensive rats are given an MR antagonist, they show dramatic falls in brain damage and proteinuria, with no change in the grossly raised blood pressure.[48] Clinically, when normotensives with familial hyperaldosteronism type 2 (inherited primary aldosteronism without the chimeric gene and enzyme characterizing glucocorticoid-remediable aldosteronism, FH1) are compared with age- and sex-matched controls, they show aldosterone-induced abnormalities in cardiac structure and function.[16] Even the 20% of essential hypertensives who did not respond in terms of blood pressure (SBP 2, DBP 1 mmHg fall) to 200-mg eplerenone[25] may thus be afforded vascular/renal/cardiac protection by MR blockade despite no fall in blood pressure.

Given experimental and clinical demonstrations that MR activation is proinflammatory in the context of inappropriate aldosterone for salt status, or by normal levels of endogenous glucocorticoids in the context of tissue damage/redox change, MR blockade may be efficacious in conditions other than frank aldosterone excess. These include cardiovascular disease where baseline aldosterone levels are commonly normal—for instance, the RALES/EPHESUS/4E trials—including heart failure, essential

hypertension, and atherosclerosis.[49] They may also include chronic inflammatory conditions of autoimmune or other provenance, quite distinct from hypertension or heart failure. The anecdotal success of adjuvant use of low-dose spironolactone in the treatment of the ptosis of myasthenia gravis, reported over 40 years ago, may represent one example of such a previously inexplicable therapeutic benefit.[50,51]

In terms of unanswered questions in hypertension, direct demonstration of vascular protection in humans following MR blockade, independent of effects on blood pressure, is central. If the question is answered in the affirmative, a good case can be made to generalize its use across the spectrum of hypertensive patients. This constitutes a clear future direction of research at the clinical level; at the basic level, the development of renal tubule–sparing MR antagonists, with less effectiveness in terms of raising plasma [K+], is a question currently being addressed to assuage fears of hyperkalemia, which has followed the careless use of spironolactone in very elderly patients with progressive cardiac failure.[52] Finally, a question yet to be systematically addressed at the basic or clinical level is the untapped potential of MR blockade to act as an anti-inflammatory therapy in conditions other than those affecting the cardiovascular system, ranging from cognitive disorders to autoimmune disease to premature labor.

SUMMARY

Whereas a decade ago it was taught that aldosterone normalized low blood pressure following volume loss by epithelial sodium and water retention, and that primary aldosteronism represented <1% of all hypertensives, from the vantage point of today neither of these appear correct. Over that decade a role for aldosterone in the pathophysiology of hypertension (and heart failure) was posited on the basis of experimental studies on inappropriate mineralocorticoid for salt status, and clinical studies using spironolactone and eplerenone. Subsequently, it appears that baseline levels of aldosterone, contrary to common assumptions, are usually low or normal in hypertension and heart failure, and that in these conditions, spironolactone/eplerenone are blocking the effect of ligands other than aldosterone (most probably cortisol) to activate MR in the context of redox change following tissue damage. The implications of this evolving pathophysiology are that MR blockade may be therapeutically useful in terms of end-organ protection in hypertension regardless of levels of aldosterone, and that such blockade may have a place in other conditions in which MR may be inappropriately activated in the context of tissue damage, for example, autoimmune disease.

REFERENCES

1. Li M, Wen C, Fraser T, Whitworth JA. Adrenocorticotrophin-induced hypertension: effects of mineralocorticoid and glucocorticoid receptor antagonism. *J Hypertens* 1999;17:419–26.

2. Funder JW, Pearce P, Smith R, Smith AI. Mineralocorticoid action: target-tissue specificity is enzyme, not receptor, mediated. *Science* 1988;242:583–85.

3. Edwards CR, Stewart PM, Burt D, et al. Localisation of 11 beta-hydroxysteroid dehydrogenase—tissue specific protector of the mineralocorticoid receptor. *Lancet* 1988;2:986–89.

4. Alzamora R, Michea L, Marusic ET. Role of 11beta-hydroxysteroid dehydrogenase on nongenomic aldosterone effects in human arteries. *Hypertension* 2000;35:1099–104.

5. Funder JW, Pearce PT, Smith R, Campbell J. Vascular type I aldosterone binding sites are physiological mineralocorticoid receptors. *Endocrinology* 1989;125:2224–26.

6. Funder JW. 15-Hydroxyprostaglandin dehydrogenase: Cinderella meets Prince Serendip. *J Clin Endocrinol Metab* 1999;84:393–94.

7. Qin W, Rudolph A, Bond B, et al. A transgenic model of aldosterone-driven cardiac hypertrophy and heart failure. *Circ Res* 2003;93:69–76.

8. Gomez-Sanchez EP, Venkataraman MT, Thwaites D, Fort C. ICV infusion of corticosterone antagonizes ICV-aldosterone hypertension. *Am J Physiol* 1990;258:E649–53.

9. Takeda Y, Miyamori I, Yoneda T, et al. Production of aldosterone in isolated rat blood vessels. *Hypertension* 1995;25:170–73.

10. Takeda Y, Yoneda T, Demura M, et al. Sodium-induced cardiac aldosterone synthesis causes cardiac hypertrophy. *Endocrinology* 2000;141:1901–94.

11. Gomez-Sanchez CE, Zhou MY, Cozza EN, et al. Aldosterone biosynthesis in the rat brain. *Endocrinology* 1997;138:3369–73.

12. Rocha R, Martin-Berger C, Yang P, et al. Selective aldosterone blockade prevents angiotensin II/salt-induced vascular inflammation in the rat heart. *Endocrinology* 2002;143:4828–36.

13. Ye P, Kenyon CJ, MacKenzie SM, et al. The aldosterone synthase (CYP11B2) and 11beta-hydroxylase (CYP11B1) genes are not expressed in the rat heart. *Endocrinology* 2005;146:5287–93.

14. Gomez-Sanchez EP, Ahmad N, Romero DG, Gomez-Sanchez CE. Origin of aldosterone in the rat heart. *Endocrinology* 2004;145:4796–802.

15. Greenwood A, Butler P, White R, et al. Multiple corticosteroid receptors in a teleost fish: distinct sequences. *Endocrinology* 2003;144:4226–36.

16. Stowasser M, Sharman J, Leano R, et al. Evidence for abnormal left ventricular structure and function in normotensive individuals with familial hyperaldosteronism type I. *J Clin Endocrinol Metab* 2005;90:5070–76.

17. Lifton R, Dluhy R, Powers M, et al. Hereditary hypertension caused by chimaeric gene duplications and ectopic expression of aldosterone synthase. *Nat Genet* 1992;2:66–74.

18. New MI, Levine LS, Biglieri EG, et al. Evidence for an unidentified steroid in a child with apparent mineralocorticoid hypertension. *J Clin Endocrinol Metab* 1977;44:924–33.

19. Funder JW, Myles K. Exclusion of corticosterone from epithelial mineralocorticoid receptors is insufficient for selectivity of aldosterone action: in vivo binding studies. *Endocrinology* 1996;137:5264–68.

20. Geller D, Farhi A, Pinkerton N, et al. Activating mineralocorticoid receptor mutation in hypertension exacerbated by pregnancy. *Science* 2000;289:119–23.

21. Hu X, Funder JW. The evolution of mineralocorticoid receptors. *Molecular Endocrinology* 2006;20:1471–78.

22. Gomez-Sanchez EP. What is the role of the central nervous system in mineralocorticoid hypertension. *Am J Hypertens* 1991;4:374–81.

23. Pitt B, Zannad F, Remme WJ, et al. The effect of spironolactone on morbidity and mortality in patients with severe heart failure. *N Engl J Med* 1999;341:709–17.

24. Pitt B, Remme W, Zannad F, et al. Eplerenone, a selective aldosterone blocker, in patients with left ventricular dysfunction after myocardial infarction. *N Engl J Med* 2003;348:1309–21.

25. Levy D, Rocha R, Funder JW. Distinguishing the antihypertensive and electrolyte effects of eplerenone. *J Clin Endocrinol Metab* 2004;89:2736–40.

26. Rahmouni K, Barthelmebs M, Grima M, et al. Influence of sodium intake on the cardiovascular and renal effects of brain mineralocorticoid receptor blockade in normotensive rats. *J Hypertens* 2002; 20:1829–34.

27. Funder JW. The role of mineralocorticoid receptor antagonists in the treatment of cardiac failure. *Expert Opin Investigational Drugs* 2003;12:1963–69.

28. Nagata K, Obata K, Xu J, et al. Mineralocorticoid receptor antagonism attenuates cardiac hypertrophy and failure in low-renin, low-aldosterone hypertensive rats. *Hypertension* 2006; 47:656–64.

29. Funder JW. Mineralocorticoid receptors and cardiovascular damage: it's not just aldosterone. *Hypertension* 47:634–35.

30. Gomez-Sanchez EP, Fort CM, Gomez-Sanchez CE. Intracerebroventricular infusion of RU28318 blocks aldosterone-salt hypertension. *Am J Physiol* 1990; 258:E482–84.

31. Gomez-Sanchez EP, Fort C, Thwaites D. Central mineralocorticoid receptor antagonism blocks hypertension in Dahl S/JR rats. *Am J Physiol* 1992; 262:E96–99.

32. Funder JW. How do central mineralocorticoid receptors modulate blood pressure? *Am J Physiol* 2005; 288:R356–57.

33. Funder JW. Is aldosterone bad for the heart? *Trends Endocrinol Metab* 2004; 15:139–42.

34. Pitt B, Reichek N, Willenbrock R, et al. Effects of eplerenone, enalapril, and eplerenone/enalapril in patients with essential hypertension and left ventricular hypertrophy: the 4E-left ventricular hypertrophy study. *Circulation* 2003;108:1831–38.

35. Funder J. Enzymes and receptors: challenges and future directions. *Steroids* 1994;59:164–69.

36. Fjeld C, Birdsong W, Goodman R. Differential binding of NAD⁺ and NADH allows the transcriptional corepressor carboxyl-terminal binding protein to serve as a metabolic sensor. *Proc Natl Acad Sci U S A* 2003;100:9202–207.

37. Reinking J, Lam MM, Pardee K, et al. The Drosophila nuclear receptor e75 contains heme and is gas responsive. *Cell* 2005;122:197–207.

38. Ward MR, Kanellakis P, Ramsey D, et al. Eplerenone suppresses constrictive remodeling and collagen accumulation after angioplasty in porcine coronary arteries. *Circulation* 2001;104:467–72.

39. Young MJ, Funder JW. Eplerenone, but not steroid withdrawal, reverses cardiac fibrosis in DOC/salt rats. *Endocrinology* 2004;145:3153–57.

40. Funder JW. RALES, EPHESUS and redox. *J Steroid Biochem Mol Biol* 2005;93:121–25.

41. Berger S, Bleich M, Schmid W, et al. Mineralocorticoid receptor knockout mice: pathophysiology of Na⁺ metabolism. *Proc Natl Acad Sci U S A* 1998;95:9424–29.

42. Lee G, Makhanova N, Caron K, et al. Homeostatic responses in the adrenal cortex to the absence of aldosterone in mice. *Endocrinology* 2005;146:2650–56.

43. Olivieri O, Ciacciarelli A, Signorelli D, et al. Aldosterone to renin ratio in a primary care setting: the Bussolengo study. *J Clin Endocrinol Metab* 2004;89:4221–26.

44. Rossi GP, Sacchetto A, Visentin PA, et al. Changes in left ventricular anatomy and function in hypertension and primary aldosteronism. *Hypertension* 1996;27:1039–45.

45. Romagni P, Rossi F, Guerrini L, et al. Aldosterone induces contraction of the resistance arteries in man. *Atherosclerosis* 2003;166:345–49.

46. Okubo S, Niimura F, Nishimura H, et al. Angiotensin-independent mechanism for aldosterone synthesis during chronic extracellular fluid volume depletion. *J Clin Invest* 1997;99:855–60.

47. McMahon EG. Recent studies with eplerenone, a novel selective aldosterone receptor antagonist. *Curr Opin Pharmacol* 2001;1:190–96.

48. Rocha R, Chander PN, Zuckerman A, Stier CT. Role of aldosterone in renal vascular injury in stroke-prone hypertensive rats. *Hypertension* 1999;33:232–37.

49. Takai S, Jin D, Muramatsu M, et al. Eplerenone inhibits atherosclerosis in nonhuman primates. *Hypertension* 2005;46:1135–39.

50. Gottlieb B, Laurent LPE. Spironolactone in the treatment of Myasthemia Gravis. *Lancet* 1961;II:528–29.

51. Cossa P. Le traitement des syndromes neuromusculaires par les spironolactones. *Gazz Med France* 1964;71:2685–91.

52. Juurlink DN, Mamdani MM, Lee DS, et al. Rates of hyperkalemia after publication of the Randomized Aldactone Evaluation Study. *N Engl J Med* 2004;351:543–51.

Chapter

27

The Renin-Angiotensin System in the Pathophysiology of Essential Hypertension

Robert M. Carey

Definitions

- The renin-angiotensin system (RAS) is a major hormonal regulatory system in the control of blood pressure (BP) and hypertension (HT).

- The primary means by which the RAS contributes to acute changes in extracellular fluid volume and BP homeostasis is by adjusting the level of renin in the circulation.

Key Findings

- Local tissue RASs, independently of the circulating RAS, also may play a role in the pathophysiology of HT.

- Several new components of the RAS have recently been identified, including a prorenin/renin receptor, angiotensin converting enzyme-2 (ACE-2), and angiotensin-1-7.

- Angiotensin II (Ang II), the major effector peptide of the RAS, binds to two major receptors, AT_1 and AT_2, which generally oppose each other.

- The RAS contributes to increased vascular resistance and remodeling in early HT; remodeling may be a cause and/or a consequence of HT.

- Major phenotypes of primary HT involving the RAS in humans include low-renin HT, nonmodulating HT, and salt-sensitive HT.

- Blockade of the RAS has been central to the treatment of hypertension, and its complications such as heart failure, atrial fibrillation, and coronary artery disease.

The renin-angiotensin system (RAS) is a major hormonal regulatory system in the control of blood pressure (BP) and the pathogenesis of hypertension (HT).[1] Because many new components of the RAS have been described during the past 5 years (Figure 27–1), the various RAS components and their actions initially will be discussed, followed by an analysis of the evidence for a role of the systemic and local tissue RAS in the pathophysiology of HT.

The traditional RAS begins with the biosynthesis of the glycoprotein hormone, renin, by the juxtaglomerular (JG) cells of the renal afferent arteriole. Renin is encoded by a single gene and renin mRNA is translated into preprorenin, containing 401 amino acids.[2] In the JG cell endoplasmic reticulum, a 20–amino-acid signal peptide is severed from preprorenin, leaving prorenin, which is packaged into secretory granules in the Golgi apparatus, where it is further processed into active renin by cleavage of a 46–amino-acid peptide from the N-terminal region of the molecule.

Mature, active renin is a glycosylated carboxypeptidase with a molecular weight of approximately 44 kDa. Active renin is released from the JG cell by an exocytotic process involving stimulus-secretion coupling. However, inactive prorenin is released constitutively across the cell membrane. Prorenin is converted to active renin by a trypsin-like activation step.[3]

In the past, renin has been considered to have no intrinsic biological activity, serving solely as an enzyme cleaving angiotensinogen (Agt), the only known precursor of Ang peptides, to form the decapeptide angiotensin I (Ang I). Liver-derived Agt provides the majority of systemic circulating Ang peptides, but Agt also is synthesized and constitutively released in other tissues, including heart, vasculature, kidney, and adipose tissue. Ang-converting enzyme (ACE), a glycoprotein (molecular weight 180 kDa) with two active carboxy-terminal enzymatic sites, hydrolyzes the inactive Ang I into biologically active Ang II.[4] ACE exists in two molecular forms, soluble and particulate. ACE is localized on the plasma membranes of various cell types, including vascular endothelial cells, the brush border (microvilli) of epithelial cells (e.g., renal proximal tubule cells), and neuroepithelial cells. In addition to cleaving Ang I to Ang II, ACE metabolizes bradykinin (BK), an active vasodilator and natriuretic autacoid, to BK-(1-7) an inactive metabolite.[5] ACE, therefore, increases the production of a potent vasoconstrictor, Ang II, while simultaneously degrading a vasodilator, BK.

Unlike renin and Agt, which have relatively long plasma half-lives, Ang II is degraded within seconds by peptidases, collectively termed angiotensinases, at different amino-acid sites, to form fragments, mainly des-aspartyl[1]-Ang II (Ang III), Ang-(1-7), and Ang-(3-8) (Ang IV). Ang II is converted to Ang III by aminopeptidase A and Ang III is converted to Ang IV by aminopeptidase N-(1).

The vast majority of cardiovascular, renal and adrenal actions of Ang II are mediated by the Ang type-1 (AT_1) receptor, a seven-transmembrane G protein–coupled receptor that is widely distributed in these tissues, is coupled positively to protein kinase C and negatively coupled to adenylyl cyclase.[6] AT_1 receptors mediate vascular smooth muscle cell contraction, aldosterone secretion, thirst, sympathetic nervous system stimulation, renal tubular Na^+ reabsorption, and cardiac ionotropic and chronotropic responses. Ang II also binds to another cloned receptor, the Ang type-2 (AT_2) receptor, but until recently the cell signaling mechanisms and functions of the AT_2 receptor were unknown.[6]

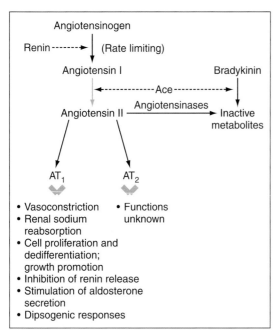

Figure 27–1. Schematic representation of the components of the RAS. (Adapted from Carey RM, Siragy HM. *Endocrinol Rev* 2003;24:261–71. Copyright 2003, The Endocrine Society.)

Biochemically, renin is the rate-limiting step in the RAS in most species, although angiotensinogen may be rate limiting in some species (e.g., mice) that have very high levels of renin.[3] The renal JG cell is probably the only source of circulating renin, because following bilateral nephrectomy renin quantitatively disappears from the circulation.[7] On the other hand, nephrectomy does not alter circulating levels of prorenin, indicating that nonrenal tissues not only produce prorenin but also secrete it into the circulation. In addition, many organs, such as the heart, can take up renin from the circulation by an unknown mechanism.[8]

The primary means by which the RAS contributes to acute changes in extracellular fluid volume and BP homeostasis is by adjusting the level of renin in the circulation. This process is mediated by active renin release from the secretory granules of JG cells. A primary mechanism of renin release is the afferent arteriolar baroreceptor, which increases renin release when arterial (and renal) perfusion pressure decreases, and vice versa. In addition, JG cells are innervated by sympathetic neurons, the activation of which stimulates norepinephrine release and subsequent stimulation of β_2-adrenergic receptors triggering renin release. JG cells also express both AT_1 and AT_2 receptors, and circulating Ang II participates in a short-loop negative feedback mechanism to inhibit renin release by binding to these two receptors.[9] Conversely, blockade of the RAS increases renin release and circulating renin levels. Indeed, chronic RAS blockade by AT_1 receptor antagonists or ACE inhibitors induces the recruitment of new renin-secreting cells in renal microvessels, further augmenting renin secretion.[10] Another renin secretory control mechanism resides in the *macula densa* segment of the early distal tubule, which relays a signal to the JG cell to increase renin release when a reduction in Na^+ and Cl^- in the distal tubule is detected.

Although renin has been considered as the enzyme responsible for cleaving the decapeptide Ang I from substrate Agt, and has been thought to have no direct biological actions, recent studies demonstrate that renin can bind to human glomerular mesangial cells in culture and that binding causes cell hypertrophy and increased levels of plasminogen-activator inhibitor.[11] The bound renin was not internalized or degraded. A renin receptor has now been cloned from mesangial cells, and its functional significance has been partially clarified.[12] The receptor is a 350–amino-acid protein with a single transmembrane domain that specifically binds both renin and prorenin.[12] Binding induces the activation of the extracellular signal-related mitogen-activated protein kinases (ERK 1 and ERK 2) associated with serine and tyrosine phosphorylation and a fourfold increase in the catalytic conversion of Agt to Ang I. The receptor is localized in renal mesangial cells and in the subendothelial layer of both coronary and renal arteries, associated with vascular smooth muscle cells, and co-localizes with renin.[12] Although recent data support the possibility of a direct functional role of renin and prorenin via the renin/prorenin receptor, the importance of this receptor in the biology of the RAS awaits further investigation.

ACE inactivates two vasodilator peptides, BK and kallidin. BK is both a direct and an indirect vasodilator via stimulation of NO and cGMP and also by release of the vasodilator prostaglandins, PGE_2, and prostacyclin.[13] Thus, when an ACE inhibitor is employed, not only is the synthesis of Ang II inhibited but also the formation of BK, NO and prostaglandin is facilitated. ACE inhibition induces cross-talk between the BK B_2 receptor and ACE on the plasma membrane, abrogating B_2 receptor desensitization, and potentiating both the levels of BK and the vasodilator action of BK at its B_2 receptor.[14]

Another ACE has recently been discovered. ACE-2 is a zinc metalloproteinase consisting of 805 amino acids with significant sequence homology to ACE.[15] Unlike ACE, however, ACE-2 functions as a carboxypeptidase rather than a dipeptidyl-carboxypeptidase. In contrast to ACE, ACE-2 hydrolyzes Ang I to Ang-(1-9), Ang II to Ang-(1-7) and BK to [des-Arg^9]-BK, an inactive metabolite. In marked contrast to ACE, ACE-2 does not convert Ang I to Ang II and its enzyme activity is not blocked with ACE inhibitors. Thus, ACE-2 is effectively an inhibitor of Ang II formation by stimulating alternate pathways for Ang I degradation. ACE-2 has been localized to the cell membranes of cardiac myocytes, renal endothelial and tubule cells and the testis. ACE-2 gene ablation does not alter BP, but impairs cardiac contractility and induces increased Ang II levels, suggesting that ACE-2 may at least partially nullify the physiologic actions of ACE.[16]

The heptapeptide fragment of Ang II, Ang-(1-7), has been discovered to have biological activity.[17] Ang-(1-7) can be formed directly from Ang I by a two-step process involving conversion to Ang-(1-9) by ACE-2 followed by conversion to Ang-(1-7) by endopeptidases. On the other hand, Ang-(1-7) can be formed directly from Ang II by the action of ACE-2. Interestingly, the major catabolic pathway for inactivation of Ang-(1-7) is by ACE, and ACE inhibitor administration markedly increases the level of Ang-(1-7).[18] The kidney is a major target organ for Ang-(1-7). The peptide is formed in the kidney, where it has specific actions via a non-AT$_1$ or -AT$_2$ receptor. These actions include increased GFR, inhibition of Na$^+$/K$^+$ATPase, vasorelaxation, and downregulation of AT$_1$ receptors, all of which are blocked by the specific Ang-(1-7) antagonist (D-Ala^7)-Ang-(1-7) and are mediated at least in part by NO and prostacyclin.[19] Most of these effects of Ang-(1-7) oppose those of Ang II via the AT$_1$ receptor. Although a specific Ang-(1-7) receptor has not been cloned, the peptide is an endogenous ligand for the *mas* oncogene, which mediates many of its actions.[20]

Ang II, the major effector peptide of the RAS, binds to two major receptors AT$_1$ and AT$_2$, that generally oppose each other.[6] The AT$_1$ receptor is widely distributed in the vasculature, heart and kidney.[21] Actions of Ang II mediated by the AT$_1$ receptor (Box 27–1) include vasoconstriction, sympathetic nervous system (SNS) activation, plasminogen activator inhibitor biosynthesis, platelet aggregation, thrombosis, cardiac contractility, superoxide formation, vascular smooth muscle cell growth, collagen formation, and aldosterone, vasopressin, and endothelin secretion. These actions are conducted by both G protein–coupled and –independent pathways and involve phospholipases C, A$_2$ and D activation, increased intracellular Ca^{++} and inositol (1,4,5)-triphosphate, activation of MAP kinases, ERKs and the JAK/STAT pathway, enhanced protein phosphorylation and stimulation of early growth response genes.[6] Tyrosine phosphorylation appears to be the major signaling pathway for AT$_1$ receptors.[22]

The AT$_2$ receptor is highly expressed in fetal tissues but regresses substantially in the postnatal period.[23] However, the AT$_2$ receptor is still expressed at low copy in the adult vasculature, especially in the endothelium and renal vasculature, JG cells, glomeruli, and tubules.[24] The AT$_2$ receptor

acts via the third intracellular loop by a G$_i$ protein–mediated process involving stimulation of protein tyrosine phosphatases and reduction of ERK activity.[25] The AT$_2$ receptor also induces sphingolipid and ceremide accumulation.[25] A major mechanism of action of AT$_2$ receptors is BK release (probably via kininogen activation through cellular acidification), with consequent NO and cGMP generation.[26,27] The AT$_2$ receptor mediates vasodilation, inhibition of cell growth, and possibly natriuresis.[28]

At least some of the actions of Ang II may be related to heterodimerization. If AT$_1$ and AT$_2$ receptors are expressed in the same cell, the physical association of these receptors on the cell membrane may inhibit the action of AT$_1$ receptors in a ligand-independent manner.[29] Similarly, there is evidence for AT$_1$ receptor and BK B$_2$ receptor heterodimerization resulting in increased AT$_1$ receptor effects via G-protein activation and AT$_2$-B$_2$ receptor heterodimerization resulting in increased cGMP formation.[30,31]

ROLE OF SYSTEMIC RAS IN THE PATHOPHYSIOLOGY OF HYPERTENSION

Demonstration that the RAS is activated and participates in the pathophysiology of human HT has been difficult. Past clinical studies classified patients with primary HT into three categories with respect to plasma renin activity (PRA), the standard clinical laboratory measurement of systemic RAS activity in humans. Of patients with primary HT, 60% have normal PRA, 15% have high PRA, and 25% have low PRA as compared with PRA measurements in the normotensive population[32] (Figure 27–2). Originally it was thought that the circulating renin classification would help define the role of the RAS in primary HT. Low-renin hypertensives were thought to have extracellular fluid volume expansion as a cause of their HT, possibly related to excess production of a "cryptic" mineralocorticoid other than aldosterone.[33,34] Indeed, BP in low-renin primary hypertension generally responded to mineralocorticoid receptor antagonist or diuretic therapy with normalization or near-normalization of BP.[35] However, studies failed to demonstrate excess of a nonaldosterone mineralocorticoid in low-renin primary HT,[36] and to date the pathophysiology of low-renin primary HT is unknown.[37] Possible causes of low circulating renin in HT are illustrated in Table 27–1. Similarly, high-renin primary HT was thought to be a disorder in which activation of the RAS was clearly involved in the pathogenesis of the HT, which could be reversed by lowering PRA using β-adrenergic antagonists, or blocking Ang II formation or action by ACE inhibitors or Ang receptor blockers, respectively.[33,35] Patients with HT and high circulating renin were demonstrated to have more severe HT than patients with normal or low PRA and increased prevalence of ischemic heart disease, cardiovascular morbidity, and mortality than patients with normal or low PRA.[38] However, multiple later studies demonstrated that this was not always the case, and "renin profiling" to study the pathophysiology, diagnosis, and treatment of HT has largely been abandoned.

In spite of the disappointment that the profiling of circulating renin yielded little useful information concerning

---

Box 27–1

Effects of Ang II via AT$_1$ Receptors

- Vasoconstriction
- Cardiac and vascular remodeling
- Activation of the sympathetic nervous system
- Superoxide anion production; nitric oxide destruction
- Aldosterone, vasopressin, and endothelin secretion
- Vascular smooth muscle hypertrophy, migration, proliferation, and growth
- Cardiac contractility
- Vascular remodeling and fibrosis
- Renin inhibition
- Decreased vascular compliance
- Sodium and water retention
- Collagen synthesis: fibrosis
- PA1-1 synthesis, platelet activation, aggregation and adhesion: thromobosis
- Activation of cytokine production by monocytes and macrophages: inflammation

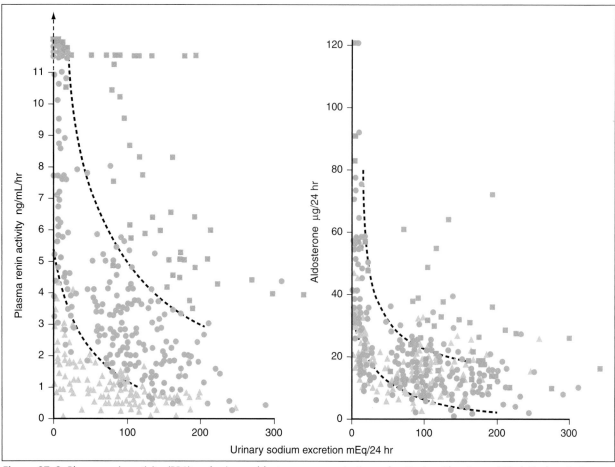

Figure 27–2. Plasma renin activity (PRA) and urinary aldosterone concentrations of patients with primary HT plotted against urinary Na+ excretion. Data for normal nonhypertensive subjects is plotted inside the dashed lines. (Adapted from Brunner HR, Laragh JH, Baer L, Newton MA, Goodwin FT, Krakoff LR, et al. *N Engl J Med* 1972;286:441–49. Copyright 1972 Massachusetts Medical Society.)

the pathogenesis of primary HT, the RAS has been implicated in the pathophysiology of the "nonmodulating" hypertensive phenotype. Nonmodulation, a disorder of renal vascular and adrenal aldosterone secretory responses to Ang II, occurs in approximately 40% of patients with primary HT. Nonmodulators are characterized as having abnormal (blunted) aldosterone responses to Ang II in subjects ingesting low dietary Na+ and abnormal (blunted) renal vasoconstriction to Ang II when they were placed on a high dietary Na+ intake.[39] Nonmodulators are unable to handle a Na+ load, have salt-sensitive HT, and have normal to high circulating renin levels. A striking family history of HT and concordance of responses to Ang II in sibling pairs suggested a genetic disorder. Agt gene polymorphisms were present in the nonmodulators and the HT was completely reversible with ACE inhibitor treatment.[39] The nonmodulating phenotype has been validated by a number of independent research groups. However, not all studies have confirmed the existence of nonmodulation, and further work is required to determine whether the nonmodulating phenotype is due to increased RAS activity alone or whether other mechanisms play a role. Furthermore, nonmodulation appears to be a quantitative rather than a qualitative trait, so that its pathophysiology may be complex.

Whereas it has been difficult to demonstrate *in vivo* activation of the RAS in early or established HT, there is no question that inhibition of the RAS is effective in lowering BP in patients with primary HT.[40] The results of multiple clinical trials demonstrate that blocking the RAS with ACE inhibitors or angiotensin receptor blockers (ARBs) demonstrate their beneficial effects to lower BP and reduce cardiovascular morbidity and mortality.[41–46] Not only does blocking the RAS lower BP, but also these interventions reduce BP variability, an independent risk factor for cardiovascular events and overall mortality.[47–50]

Perhaps the earliest pathophysiologic change demonstrable in primary HT is the process of vascular remodeling, a term employed to describe the functional, mechanical and structural changes in small resistance arteries (100 to 300 microns) that leads to reduction in lumen size and increased peripheral vascular resistance.[51,52] Increased peripheral vascular resistance is the hallmark of HT. However, even though vascular remodeling is already present in pre-HT or stage-1 HT, it is still unclear whether remodeling is a primary process that initiates HT or reflects early target organ damage as a result of the early increase in BP. Small resistance artery remodeling in HT is characterized by an increased media:lumen ratio that may derive from

CLINICAL CONDITIONS INFLUENCING PRA IN HUMANS	
Decreased PRA	**Increased PRA**
Expanded fluid volume	**Shrunken fluid volume**
Salt loads, oral or intravenous	Sodium restriction
Primary salt retention	Fluid losses
—Liddle's syndrome	—Diuretic induced
—Gordon's syndrome	—Gastrointestinal losses
Mineralocorticoid excess	—Hemorrhage
Primary aldosteronism	**Decreased effective plasma volume**
Cushing's syndrome	Upright posture
Congenital adrenal hyperplasia	Cirrhosis with ascites
Deoxycorticosterone (DOC), 18-hydroxy-DOC excess	Nephrotic syndrome
11β-hydroxysteroid dehydrogenase inhibition (licorice)	**Decreased renal perfusion pressure**
Sympathetic inhibition	Renovascular hypertension
Autonomic dysfunction	Accelerated-malignant hypertension
Therapy with adrenergic neuronal blockers	Chronic renal disease (renin dependent)
Therapy with β-adrenergic blockers	Juxtaglomerular hyperplasia
Hyperkalemia	**Sympathetic nervous system activation**
Decreased Agt	Therapy with direct vasodilators
Androgen therapy	Pheochromocytoma
Decrease in renal tissue mass	Stress: exercise, hypoglycemia
Hyporeninemic hypoaldosteronism	Hyperthyroidism
Chronic renal disease (volume dependent)	Sympathomimetic agents (caffeine)
Anephric state	**Hypokalemia**
Increasing age	**Increased Agt**
Unknown	Pregnancy
Low-renin primary hypertension	Estrogen therapy
African-American race/ancestry	**Decreased feedback inhibition**
Autonomous renin hypersecretion	Low Ang II levels (angiotensin-converting enzyme inhibitor [ACEI] therapy), AT$_1$ receptor blockers
Renin-secreting tumors	**Unknown**
Acute damage to juxtaglomerular cells	High-renin primary hypertension
Acute glomerulonephritis	

Table 27–1. Clinical Conditions Influencing PRA in Humans

a number of processes including vascular smooth muscle (VSM) cell growth (hyperplasia and hypertrophy), apoptosis, elongation of cells and altered biochemical composition of the extracellular matrix.[53,54] Ang II stimulates VSM cell hyperplasia, a process that increases VSM cell number accompanied by DNA synthesis.[55] Ang II also stimulates VSM cell hypertrophy by increasing protein synthesis and by activating transmembrane influx of ions and water. In experimental animal models of HT, both hyperplasia and hypertrophy contribute to vascular remodeling. In VSM cells from humans with primary HT, Ang II simulates both hypertrophy and hyperplasia to a greater extent than in cells from non-HT patients.[56] However, most of the *in vivo* studies showing this effect employed large, nonphysiologic concentrations of Ang II (e.g., 10^{-6} *M*). In mild primary HT, eutropic remodeling may also be a function of apoptosis. Inhibition of the RAS with ACE inhibitors or Ang receptor blockers may contribute to a growth imbalance by stimulating apoptosis.[57] Factors contributing to increased

vascular resistance in HT are depicted in (Figure 27–3). However, it must be kept in mind that much of the evidence suggests that the vascular remodeling observed in early HT is the consequence rather than the cause of increased BP.

In addition to the changes in lumen size typical of vascular remodeling, vascular injury in HT is characterized by inflammation.[51,52] Small arteries in HT have increased expression of surface adhesion molecules, inflammatory cell infiltration, cytokine production, chemokine release, and oxidative stress.[58–60] Indeed, evidence is present that vascular disease in HT is an inflammatory process and that chronic vascular inflammation may be a primary cause of HT.[52] The inflammatory process is composed of three components: increased vascular permeability, leukocyte extravasation (adhesion, migration, and chemotaxis) and tissue repair (cell growth and fibrosis).[52,60] Ang II is now recognized as a major inflammatory mediator in the vasculature, inducing its effects largely via oxidative stress.[61,62]

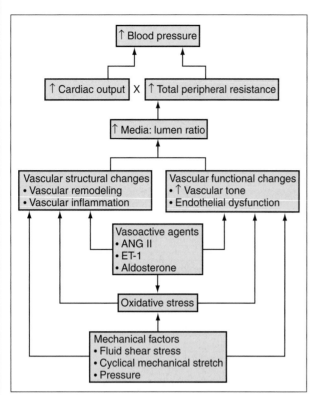

Figure 27–3. Blood pressure (BP) is the product of cardiac output and total peripheral vascular resistance. In general, increased vascular resistance is the major hemodynamic factor contributing to elevated BP in primary hypertension (HT). Flow diagram depicting vascular mechanisms contributing to increased vascular resistance, the hallmark of HT. Vasoactive agents, mechanical factors and oxidative stress interact to influence vascular structure and function. ↑, increase; ↓, decrease. (Adapted from Schiffrin EL, Touyz RM. *Am J Physiol Heart Circ Physiol* 2004;287:H435–46.)

The molecular and cellular mechanisms whereby Ang II influences vascular structure in HT are shown in Figure 27–4. Ang II via the AT_1 receptor induces vascular permeability and inflammation via stimulation of vascular endothelial growth factor (VEGF) in VSM[63] and endothelial cells.[64] Ang II upregulates VEGF expression through transcriptional regulation by redox-sensitive pathways.[65] VEGF is an important mediator of vascular inflammation because VEGF inhibition attenuates Ang II–induced vascular inflammation and remodeling without influencing BP.[56] Ang II also stimulates vascular production of prostaglandins, which can increase vascular permeability.[66]

Leukocyte adhesion, transmigration, and chemotaxis are important components of the inflammatory process. Ang II regulates multiple steps in leukocyte recruitment into the vessel wall. Ang II stimulates the production of a host of pro-inflammatory molecules—including growth factors, chemokines, cytokines, and other mediators (Box 27–2)—enhances the adhesion of leukocytes to endothelial cells, and induces trans-endothelial migration via chemokines and cytokines.[67] Ang II induces leukocyte rolling, adhesion, and migration in the absence of vasoconstriction, suggesting a BP-independent mechanism.[68] In cultured endothelial cells, Ang II increases expression of vascular cell adhesion

molecule-1 (VCAM-1), intracellular adhesion molecule-1 (ICAM-1), and E-selectin via generation of reactive oxygen species (ROS).[69,70] In VSM cells, Ang II via the AT_1 receptor stimulates the production of VCAM-1, the chemokine monocyte chemotactic protein-1 (MCP-1), and inflammatory cytokines and chemokines (IL-6, IL-8, and osteopontin).[71,72] Also, in whole animal studies, Ang II increases VCAM-1 and ICAM-1 expression in the vasculature. These processes are redox dependent and involve stimulation of MAP kinase. The role of Ang II in vascular inflammation has been confirmed by studies in apo E-deficient mice, whose increased MCP-1 expression was reversed by AT_1 receptor blockade.[73] Also, in hypercholesterolemic rabbits, AT_1 receptor blockade reduced neoinitimal proliferation and expression of P-selectin and MCP-1.[74] In mice lacking macrophage-colony stimulating factor, Ang II induced less vascular inflammation and remodeling than in wild-type controls.[75] In hypertensive patients, AT_1 receptor blockade decreased circulating MCP-1, tumor necrosis factor alpha (TNFα), and plasminogen activator inhibitor-1 (PAI-1).[59]

Vascular fibrosis is an important component of the reparative process in the setting of inflammation. Fibrosis involves the accumulation of extracellular matrix proteins, especially collagen and fibronectin, in the vascular media, resulting in structural remodeling. Ang II stimulates a number of fibrotic signaling pathways that increase the synthesis of collagen and fibronectin,[76,77] mitogenic factors such as transforming growth factor-β (TGF-β), platelet-derived growth factor (PDGF), and endothelin-1.[78] Ang II also promotes collagen degradation by reducing interstitial matrix metalloproteinase (MMP) and increasing a tissue inhibitor of MMP-1 production.[79] All of these mechanisms increase fibronectin, proteoglycans, and collagen deposition that contribute to vascular remodeling in HT.

Ang II mediates many of its cellular actions by stimulating the formation of intracellular reactive oxygen species (ROS), including superoxide anion (O_2^-), hydrogen peroxide (H_2O_2), hydroxyl free radical (OH^-), and peroxynitrite ($ONOO^-$).[80] Mediated by multiple redox-sensitive signaling pathways, ROS are involved in virtually every stage of the inflammatory process, including vascular cell permeability, leukocyte adhesion, transmigration, and chemotaxis, cell growth, and fibrosis. Although there are many potential sources of ROS (cyclooxygenase, lipoxygenase, hemeoxygenase, cytochrome P450 monooxygenase, xanthine oxidase, and leakage from the electron transport chain), membrane-bound nicotinamide adenine dinucleotide phosphate oxidase, reduced form (NAD[P]H oxidase) has been demonstrated to be of major critical importance in Ang II–induced vascular remodeling in HT.[73]

Ang II is a potent stimulator of vascular NAD(P)H oxidase[81] (Figure 27–5). Ang II increases the expression of NAD(P)H oxidase subunits, activates the enzyme, and increases the production of ROS both in cultured VSM cells and in intact arteries. Cell signaling pathways by which Ang II stimulates NAD(P)H oxidase include phospholipase D, phospholipase A_2 (PLA$_2$), protein kinase C (PKC), c-Src, PI-3 kinase, and Rac.[73] In HT, these processes are upregulated resulting in increased NAD(P)H oxidase activity and

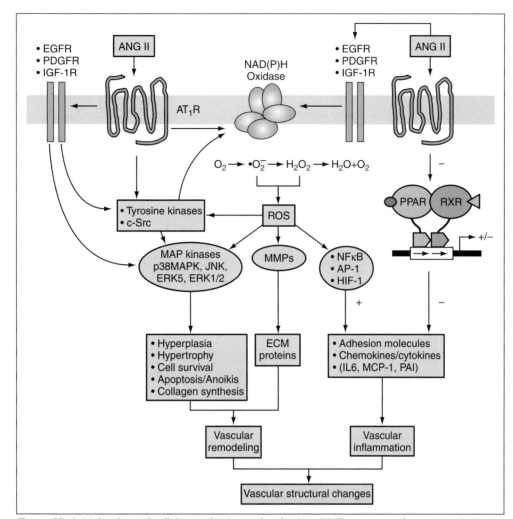

Figure 27–4. Molecular and cellular mechanisms whereby Ang II influences vascular structure in primary hypertension. Ang II binds to the AT_1 receptor leading to activation of receptor tyrosine kinases, such as the epidermal growth factor receptor (EGFR), platelet-derived growth factor receptor (PDGFR), and insulin-like growth factor-1 receptor (IGF-1R), and nonreceptor tyrosine kinases, such as c-Src. Ang II-AT_1 receptor binding also leads to activation of NAD(P)H oxidase, resulting in intracellular generation of ROS that influences redox-sensitive cell-signaling molecules such as mitogen-activated protein (MAP) kinases (p38 MAP kinase, JNK, ERK 1/2 and ERK5), transcription factors (NF-κB, AP-1, and hypoxia-inducible factor [H1F-1]) and matrix metalloproteinases (MMP). Ang II downregulates peroxisome proliferator activator receptors (PPARs), which have antiinflammatory effects, enhancing vascular inflammation. These cell-signaling events regulate VSM cell growth, extracellular matrix (ECM) formation, and inflammatory responses. In HT, altered Ang II signaling leads to altered vascular growth, fibrosis, and inflammation, which govern structural remodeling of HT. PAI, plasminogen activator inhibitor; RXR, retinoid X receptor. (Adapted from Schiffrin EL, Touyz RM. *Am J Physiol Heart Circ Physiol* 2004;287:H435–46.)

oxidative stress in the vasculature.[82] Vascular O_2^- and H_2O_2 function intracellularly as second messengers activating redox-sensitive signaling molecules, which induce VSM cell contraction, cell growth (hypertrophy and hyperplasia), apoptosis, and accumulation of extracellular matrix proteins.[83] In addition, some of the beneficial effects of ACE inhibitors and AT_1 receptor blockers in HT have been attributed to direct inhibition of NAD(P)H oxidase activity as well as to direct antioxidant actions of these blockers.[84]

In general, Ang II elicits enhanced vasoconstrictor responses in human primary HT (Figure 27–6). This action of Ang II may either be direct or indirect via stimulation of SNS activity. The augmented Ang II–induced VSM cell contraction is attributed to increased cytoplasmic free Ca^{++} concentration.[85] In addition, increased Ang II sensitivity of the VSM cell contractile machinery has been ascribed to RhoA/Rho kinase–dependent pathways.[86]

In terms of vascular growth, as well as contraction, c-Src has been identified as a critical kinase that is immediately phosphorylated in response to Ang II.[87] Ang II–induced activation of c-Src is augmented and is related to increased VSM cell growth in cells from hypertensive patients.[88] C-Src is a major cellular regulator of many cell signaling pathways, including PLC-β, Pyk2, FAK, JAK, Shc, MAP kinases, PI-3

Box 27–2

ANG II–Induced Proinflammatory Molecules and Markers

- Growth factors: TGF-β, PDGF, EGF
- Cytokines: interleukin-6, TNF-α
- Chemokines: MCP-1, RANTES
- Adhesion molecules: VCAM-1, ICAM-1, P-selectin
- Peptides: ET-1
- Lipids: Prostaglandins, PAF
- COX-2
- NO

COX-2, Cyclooxygenase 2; EGF, epidermal growth factor; ET-1, endothelin 1; ICAM-1, intercellular adhesion molecule-1; MCP-1, monocyte chemoattractant protein type 1; NO, nitric oxide; PAF, platelet activating factor; PDGF, platelet-derived growth factor; RANTES, regulated upon activation; normal T-cell expressed/secreted; TGF-β, transforming growth factor beta; TNF-α, tumor necrosis factor alpha; VCAM-1, vascular cell adhesion molecule-1.

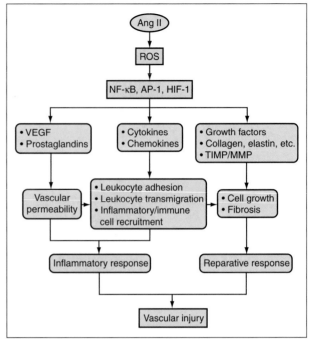

Figure 27–5. Ang II stimulates NAD(P)H oxidase to generate ROS, which activates redox-sensitive transcription factors (nuclear factor-κB [NF-κB], activating protein-1 [AP-1], hypoxia-inducible factor-1 [H1F-1]). These transcription factors release vascular endothelial growth factor (VEGF), prostaglandins, cytokines and chemokines, growth factors, matrix metalloproteinases (MMP), and tissue inhibitor of matrix metalloproteinase (TIMP). These signaling pathways lead to inflammatory and reparative processes inducing vascular injury. (Adapted from Touyz RM. *Curr Opin Nephrol Hypertens* 2005;14:125–31.)

kinase, and NAD(P)H oxidase.[89] These molecules affect cell survival, metabolism, cytoskeletal arrangement, and membrane trafficking processes that promote growth.[89]

In VSM cells, Ang II activates the MAP-kinase signaling pathways, including ERK 1/2, p38 MAP kinase, c-Jun NH2-terminal kinases (JNKs), and ERK 5.[90] These MAP kinases influence cell survival, apoptosis, differentiation, inflammation, and growth. In vascular tissue from rats and VSM cells from hypertensive patients, Ang II stimulation of MAP kinases is augmented[91,92] leading to VSM cell growth, inflammation, fibrosis, and increased contractility.

Ang II can also trans-activate receptor tyrosine kinases on the cell membrane, including the EGF, PDGF, and IGF-1 receptors.[93] Transactivation of these receptors may be mediated by activation of nonreceptor tyrosine kinases (Pyk2 and Src), redox-sensitive processes, and possibly mutation of MMPs releasing heparin-binding EGF.[93] Ang II also increases the production of vasoactive hormones and growth factors in HT, including endothelin-1, PDGF, TGF-β, basic FGF, and IGF-1, which could contribute to cell proliferation, protein synthesis, and fibrosis and, in turn, arterial remodeling.

Ang II activation of the AT_1 receptor is a major factor in eutropic inward remodeling observed in the earliest stages of HT. In patients with primary HT, AT_1 receptor blockade and β-adrenergic receptor inhibition both induce similar BP reduction, but only AT_1 receptor blockade corrects resistance arterial structure.[94] Also, in SHR either ACE inhibition or AT_1 receptor blockade normalizes resistance artery structure. Although it is now clear that Ang II plays a major role in vascular remodeling, it is still unclear whether Ang II has a primary initiating role in HT, or whether Ang II simply mediates the vascular damage, even at an early stage, resulting from a primary increase in BP due to other causes. These issues await future investigation.

ROLE OF LOCAL TISSUE RENIN-ANGIOTENSIN SYSTEMS IN THE PATHOPHYSIOLOGY OF HYPERTENSION

The circulating RAS is only one component of the overall RAS, and tissue RASs that can operate independently of the circulating RAS have been identified in brain, kidney, heart, blood vessels, and adrenal gland. While it is possible that tissue RASs are activated even when the circulating RAS is normal or suppressed, this has been difficult to establish in HT. In particular, it has been difficult to show the relative roles of the intrarenal RAS as opposed to the systemic RAS in the control of BP and HT. This issue has been considered important because the long-term regulation of BP has been thought to involve the kidney and the ability to sustain a hypertensive process chronically has been regarded as requiring renal Na^+ retention.[95] Indeed, the key sites that determine the level of BP could not be localized precisely utilizing AT_1 receptor blockers which inhibit the RAS in all tissues or by conventional gene targeting experiments.

Recently, however, the tissue sites whereby the RAS regulates BP have been clarified through a novel cross-transplantation approach in AT_{1A} receptor-deficient mice.[96] Rodents have two AT_1 receptors termed, AT_{1A} and AT_{1B}.

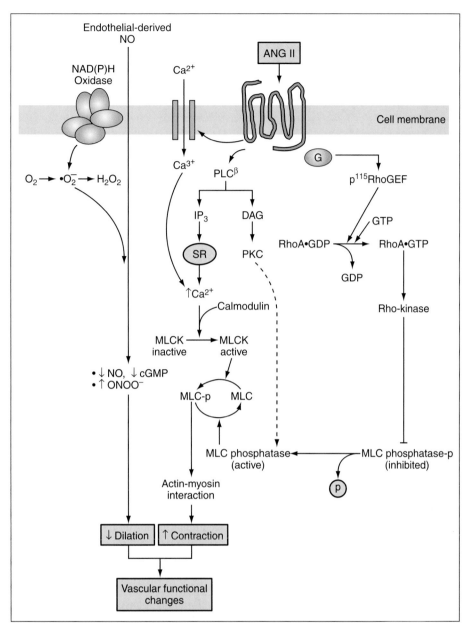

Figure 27–6. Molecular and cellular mechanisms whereby Ang II influences vascular function in HT. Ang II increases intracellular free Ca++ concentrations [Ca++]i) by stimulating Ca++ influx through mobilization from sarcoplasmic reticular (SR) stores, the latter in response to inositol (1,4,5)-triphosphate produced by activation of phospholipase C (PLC). Increased activity of RhoA/Rho kinase Ca++–sensing pathway and protein kinase C(PKC)–dependent pathways (dashed line) also influence vascular contractility. Ang II–induced stimulation of NAD(P)H oxidase generates superoxide (O_2^-) and hydrogen peroxide (H_2O_2) that quench NO formation, resulting in decreased cGMP and increased peroxynitrite formation compromising vasodilation. In HT, altered Ang-II signaling leads to contraction, reduced dilation, and consequent increased vascular tone. DAG, diacylglycerol; MLC, myosin light chain; GEF, guanine nucleotide exchange factor; p, phosphorylated; G,G protein; ↑, increase; ↓, decrease. (Adapted from Schiffrin EL, Touyz RM. *Am J Physiol Heart Circ Physiol* 2004;287:H435–46.)

The AT_{1A} receptor mediates the majority of actions of Ang II. In terms of expression, AT_{1A} receptors predominate in most organs except the adrenal gland and certain regions of the central nervous system (CNS), where AT_{1B} receptor expression is relatively more prominent. Absence of AT_{1A} receptors exclusively in the kidney, with normal receptors elsewhere, was sufficient to lower BP by about 20 mmHg[96]

(Figure 27–7). Thus, renal AT_1 receptors were deemed to have a unique and nonredundant role in the control of BP. As aldosterone levels were unaffected in these experiments, BP appears to be regulated by the direct action of AT_1 receptors on kidney cells, independent of mineralocorticoid secretion. However, in addition to the kidney, AT_1 receptors outside the kidney made an equivalent, unique, and

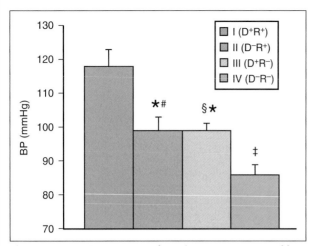

Figure 27–7. BP in cross-transplantation groups measured by radiotelemetry. *P<0.006 vs. group I; #P<0.02 vs. group IV; §P<0.002 vs. group IV; ≠P<0.00007 vs. group I (*n* = 6 per group). (Adapted from Crowley SD, Gurley SB, Oliverio MI, Pazmino AK, Griffiths R, Flannery PJ, et al. *J Clin Invest* 2005;115:1092–99.)

nonredundant contribution to BP control: animals with a full complement of AT$_1$ receptors in the kidney, but without AT$_1$ receptors in extrarenal tissues, also had BP reduction of about 20 mmHg[96] (Figure 27–7). This finding also was independent of aldosterone levels. Taken together, the new evidence suggests that AT$_1$ receptors either in the vasculature or the CNS mediate the component of BP control that is independent of the kidney. However, it is not completely clear that the extrarenal effects to increase BP do not ultimately influence kidney function. Indeed, pressure natriuresis is reset in these experiments. In addition, Ang II–induced HT has been shown not to occur in the absence of renal AT$_1$ receptors. Therefore, more work needs to be done to be certain that the RAS induces HT by renal-independent mechanisms.

It is clear that Ang I and II are synthesized in tissue sites. Indeed, most, if not all, tissue Ang II is synthesized locally from tissue-derived Ang I.[97] In addition, the beneficial actions of RAS blockers are most likely due to interference with tissue Ang II rather than Ang II in the circulation.[98] Although it was originally thought that the renin required for local Ang I synthesis was synthesized locally, studies in nephrectomized animal models proved that this was not the case.[99] In many tissues such as the heart and blood vessels, local Ang synthesis depends on tissue uptake of kidney-derived renin.[100] In other tissues such as the kidney, adrenal gland, and brain, renin is synthesized locally.[101] In addition, prorenin, the inactive precursor of renin, may contribute to Ang I generation at tissue sites.[102] This would require either activation of prorenin to renin following uptake from the systemic circulation or direct prorenin stimulation of the renin/prorenin receptor.

Intrarenal RAS in hypertension

The intrarenal RAS was first recognized when selective intrarenal inhibition of the RAS was demonstrated to increase GFR and renal Na$^+$ and water excretion.[103,104] Since that

time, the intrarenal RAS has increasingly been recognized a critical system in the regulation of Na$^+$ excretion and the long-term control of BP.[105] Indeed, there is growing recognition that inappropriate activation of the intrarenal RAS prevents the kidney from maintaining normal Na$^+$ balance at normal arterial pressures and is an important cause of HT.[105]

Several experimental models support an overactive intrarenal RAS in the development and maintenance of HT.[105] These include 2-kidney, 1-clip (2KIC) Goldblatt HT, Ang II–infused HT, transgenic rat (TGR) mRen2 HT with an extra renin gene, the remnant kidney HT model, and several mouse models over-expressing the renin or AGT gene. Indeed, there is increasing recognition that in many forms of HT development of renal function occurs that is due to inappropriate activation of the intrarenal RAS, which limits the ability of the kidney to maintain Na$^+$ balance when perfused at normal arterial pressure.[105] In addition to Na$^+$ and fluid retention and progressive HT, other long-term consequences of an inappropriately activated intrarenal RAS include renal vascular, glomerular and tubulointerstitial injury, and fibrosis.[106]

Evidence for over-activation of the intrarenal RAS in HT has accumulated for many of the components of the intrarenal RAS. In Ang II–dependent HT, renal vascular and glomerular AT$_1$ receptors are downregulated, but proximal tubule receptors are either upregulated or not significantly altered.[105] In some forms of HT (e.g., 2K1C Goldblatt HT, Ang II–induced HT and TGR [mRen2] HT), net intrarenal Ang II content is increased due to the intrarenal production of Ang II as well as increased uptake of the peptide from the circulation via an AT$_1$ receptor–mediated process.[105,107] Sustained increases in circulating Ang II cause progressive accumulation of Ang II within the kidney in these models. A substantial fraction of the increase in intrarenal Ang II is due to AT$_1$ receptor–mediated endocytosis.[105,108] In the 2K1C Goldblatt model, intrarenal Ang II was elevated in both the clipped and unclipped kidneys, both during the development phase (1 week) and up to 12 weeks following clipping.[109] These increases in intrarenal Ang II were present even in the absence of increases in plasma Ang II. Renal interstitial Ang II levels also are elevated in several Ang II–dependent models of HT, including the 2-kidney, 1-wrap (2K1W) Grollman model and the Ang II–infused HT model.[110,111] However, renal tubule fluid Ang II is similar in control and HT rats.[112] Because Ang II that binds to the AT$_1$ receptor is internalized by receptor-mediated endocytosis, endosomal accumulation of Ang II in renal cells has been studied in Ang II–infused HT. Endosomal Ang II was increased and the endosomal Ang II accumulation was blocked by an ARB.[108] At least some of the internalized Ang II remains intact and contributes to the increased total Ang II content as measured in renal cortical homogenates in this model.[108,113] The internalized Ang II could be recycled and secreted, being available to act at plasma membrane AT$_1$ receptors, or may act at cytosolic receptors, as has been described for VSM cells.[105,114] Another possibility is that Ang II could exert genomic effects in the nucleus as a part of an intracrine system.[115] Because Ang II may exert positive feedback stimulation of

Agt mRNA, intracellular Ang II may upregulate Agt or renin gene expression in renal proximal tubule cells.[116]

Agt is the only known precursor of Ang II, and most of the intrarenal Agt mRNA and protein is localized to proximal tubule cells, suggesting that intratubular Ang II is produced from locally formed Agt.[117] Both Agt and its metabolite Ang II derived from proximal tubule cells are secreted directly into the tubule lumen.[118] In response to a 2-week infusion of Ang II, intrarenal Agt mRNA and protein were upregulated.[117] Therefore, an intrarenal positive feedback loop may be present whereby increased Ang II stimulates its requisite precursor, leading to markedly increased Ang peptide levels in HT.[105] For confirmation, this needs to be demonstrated *in vitro* in a proximal tubule cell preparation.

Renin is not only synthesized and secreted in the JG cells of the afferent arteriole but also by connecting tubules, indicating that renin is probably secreted directly into distal tubule fluid.[118] Because intact Agt is present in urine, it is possible that some of the proximally formed Agt is converted to Ang II in the distal nephron.[118,119] Indeed, Ang II infusion significantly increased urinary Agt in a time- and dose-dependent manner associated with increased renal Ang II levels.[116,119] Furthermore, collecting duct renin is upregulated by Ang II via the AT_1 receptor.[120] Therefore, several intrarenal mechanisms seem to provide positive feedback control to enhance Ang II concentrations at both proximal and distal tubule sites, where Ang II has potent Na^+-retaining actions.[121] A schematic depiction of the intrarenal RAS is shown in Figure 27–8.

In addition to aforementioned work suggesting the pivotal role of kidney AT_1 receptors in the production of HT, recent studies have demonstrated that production of renin

and Agt in the proximal tubule can increase BP independently of the circulating RAS.[122] Transgenic mice expressing human Agt selectively in the proximal tubule via the kidney androgen-regulated protein (KAP) promoter, when bred with mice expressing human renin systemically, had a 20-mmHg increase in BP despite having normal circulating Ang II levels. The increase in BP could be abolished with AT_1 receptor blockade, indicating Ang II–dependent HT. This experiment constituted the first demonstration of systemic HT from isolated renal tissue activation of the RAS. Furthermore, when purely proximal tubule overexpression of both human renin and Agt was achieved, HT also was present, supporting the concept that intrarenal tubular RAS activation can induce HT. In these studies it is unclear whether Ang I was first generated within the proximal tubule cell from intracellular cleavage of Agt by renin or whether the renin and Agt interaction occurred in the tubule lumen after secretion. In addition, whether the HT is due to increased proximal or distal Na^+ reabsorption, or both, remains unanswered.

Brain RAS in hypertension

Although many tissues express all of the RAS components necessary for the biosynthesis and action of Ang II, the ability of the tissues to actually produce Ang II and the specific role of locally generated Ang II has only been proven for the kidney. An independently functioning RAS in the brain remains controversial because the level of the rate-limiting component, renin, is extremely low and difficult to detect. There is no question that acute administration of exogenous Ang II centrally increases BP, sympathetic outflow, vasopressin release, drinking behavior, and attenuation of baroreceptor reflex activity, and that these effects

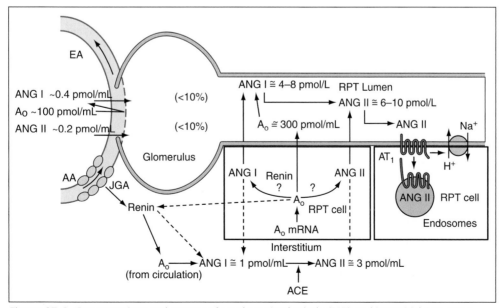

Figure 27–8. Concentrations and sources of renal proximal tubule (RPT) and interstitial Agt, Ang I, and Ang II. Ang II is internalized into endosomes via the AT_1 receptor. High interstitial Ang I and Ang II concentrations suggest local formation, but substrate may be from systemically delivered or locally produced Agt. AA, afferent arteriole; EA, efferent arteriole; JGA, juxtaglomerular cells. (Adapted from Navar LG, Harrison-Bernard LM, Nishiyama A, Kobori H. *Hypertension* 39(2 pt 2):316–22.)

are abolished by AT_1 receptor blockade.[123] In addition, specific brain nuclei clearly mediate Ang II responses, including the ventrolateral medulla (VLM), nucleus tractus solitarii (NTS), paraventricular nucleus (PVN), and subfornical organ (SFO), among several other nuclei.[124] Although all of the RAS components are present in various regions of the brain, renin expression in very low levels has been detected in the pituitary and pineal glands, choroids plexus, hypothalamus, cerebellum, and amygdala as well as other locations.[123] At the cellular level, renin has recently been detected in both neuronal and glial tissue.[125,126] If a neuronal source of renin is coupled with a glial source of Agt, Ang II could derive from secreted precursors in the extracellular space. However, recent studies have demonstrated colocalization of Agt with a novel nonsecreted form of renin, opening the door to intracellular Agt synthesis and possible action.[126]

Because brain renin levels are low, investigators have searched for a renin-independent Ang II–generating system in the brain. Many enzymes are present in brain which can generate Ang II either from Ang I or directly from Agt, including trypsin, tonin, elastase, cathepsin C, kallekrein, chymase, and chemostatin-sensitive Ang II–generating enzyme.[127]

In addition to nonrenin pathways, some investigators have suggested the involvement of non-Ang II peptides, including Ang III (des-Aspartyl¹-Ang II), Ang IV (Ang[3-8]), and Ang(1-7) as important regulators of BP.[128] In particular, Ang III appears to have a prominent role.[129] Aminopeptidase A (APA), which metabolizes Ang II to Ang III is present in the brain.[130] Ang II and Ang III are equally potent pressor substances when infused directly into the brain, and the pressor action of Ang II was abolished by pre-administration of an APA inhibitor, suggesting that conversion to Ang III may be required.[131,132] Ang II and Ang III have equal affinity for the AT_1 receptor and both also are agonists at the AT_2 receptor. However, the Ang III–mediated increase in BP appears to be mediated by the AT_1 receptor, as its action can be blocked with an AT_1 receptor blocker. In addition, inhibition of endogenous brain Ang III formation by intracerebroventricular, but not intravenous, APA inhibitor induced a large, dose-dependent reduction in BP in conscious SHR and the deoxycorticosterone acetate (DOCA)–salt rat, a RAS-independent model of HT.[131,132] On the other hand, administration of an inhibitor of aminopeptidase N (APN), which metabolizes Ang III to Ang IV, into the brain induces a pressor effect that is abolished with an AT_1 receptor blocker.[131] Thus, increasing endogenous brain Ang III levels increases BP via the AT_1 receptor. Moreover, the pressor action of an APN inhibitor could be blocked with an APA inhibitor, confirming the existence of an endogenous brain Ang III cascade in the control of BP.[131] Finally, work employing the nonmetabolizable peptide analogs, D-Asp¹-Ang II, and D-Asp¹-Ang III, demonstrated that Ang III is a centrally active agonist of the brain RAS.[130]

There is also evidence that Ang IV may be an endogenous ligand of the brain RAS. When Ang IV is over-expressed specifically in the brain, these transgenic mice developed HT that was abolished by an AT_1 receptor antagonist.[133]

The role of Ang-(1-7) as a counter-regulatory peptide to the pressor actions of Ang II is the subject of current studies.[127,128] These studies take on additional importance due to the recent discovery of ACE-2, which converts Ang II directly to Ang-(1-7) and the identification of the *mas* oncogene as a major Ang-(1-7) receptor.[20] With the cloning of the renin/prorenin receptor, which is highly expressed in brain,[12] it is possible that the renin receptor may enhance the formation of Ang peptides at selective neuronal sites within the CNS.

Vascular tissue RAS in hypertension

Evidence for local RASs have been found in the heart, large blood vessels, adrenal, uterus, ovaries, testes, placenta, and pancreas.[134,135] This evidence demonstrates that local systems may act independently of the circulatory system to produce Ang II. Within the vasculature, molecular expression of Agt has been found within the walls of large vessels, including the saphenous and umbilical vein and aorta.[136] Renin and Agt mRNA also have been detected within the aorta,[137] and in isolated small resistance arteries in skeletal muscle.[138] Microvessels also express AT_1 and AT_2 mRNA and protein.[139] There is functional evidence of a local vascular RAS,[140–142] and the concentration of Ang II within microvessels is much higher than in plasma.[138] Of note, renin or prorenin have been identified in fetal microvessels in the kidney[143] and in renal vessels of adult animals after ACE inhibition.[144,145] Thus, recent evidence would suggest the concept that renin is synthesized in vessels, even though this has been a topic of controversy. Since anephric patients and nephrectomized animals have undetectable circulating renin, local microvascular production of renin does not contribute to circulating renin.[146] Thus, the local vascular RAS is likely to act locally within the vessels. Whether the local vascular RAS contributes to vascular tone is currently unknown. However, some studies report an increase in the local microvessel concentration of renin and Ang II in SHR compared to Sprague-Dawley or WKY control rats,[137,141] suggesting the possibility of an overactive local vascular RAS that could play a pathophysiologic role in HT.

Cardiac RAS in hypertension

The importance of the cardiac renin-angiotensin-aldosterone (RAAS) is illustrated by the fact that blockade of the RAAS (with ACE inhibitors and angiotensin receptor blockers) has been central to treatment of HT, and its various complications such as heart failure, atrial fibrillation, and coronary artery disease.

Renin and its mRNA have been found in the heart.[147] Conclusive evidence exists that all of the necessary RAS components for synthesis of Ang II are present in the heart and that peptide formation does indeed occur.[135,148] Renin, Agt, ACE, and AT_1 and AT_2 receptors are present in the myocardium.[135] The majority of the Ang II localized in the heart derives from myocardial synthesis of Ang I and not from uptake into the myocardium from the systemic circulation.[149] The RAS components for Ang II biosynthesis are distributed among cardiomyocytes and myocardial fibroblasts as well as the endothelium and VSM of the coronary arteries and veins.[135] Although myocardial concentrations of renin and Agt are 1% to 4% those of plasma, cardiac interstitial fluid concentrations of Ang I and Ang II are greater than 100-fold those of plasma.[148] Cardiac interstitial fluid probably represents a separate tissue compartment from the systemic circulation, whereby Ang II may exert cell-to-cell (paracrine) actions. Intracardiac conversion of Ang I to Ang II may occur via chymase, which in contrast to ACE does not degrade BK.[150] In the human heart, chymase converts approximately 90% of Ang I to Ang II.[151]

Several recent studies have complicated the role of the intracardiac RAS in the pathophysiology of HT and cardiac hypertrophy. First, a cardiac renin receptor has been identified in cardiomyocytes that leads to the internalization of renin, the generation of Ang II in the cytoplasm and induces cardiac pathology.[152] Second, an alternative renin transcript that lacks the sequences encoding the secretory signal is retained in the intracellular space of the synthesizing cell. The product is in the active rather than the prorenin form. Upregulation of this form of renin has been observed in the left ventricle postmyocardial infarction.[153] Third, a novel intracrine mechanism has recently been described for Ang II–induced cardiac hypertrophy that does not require Ang II–AT_1 receptor interactions at the cell membrane.[154]

Although there is substantial evidence that all of the components of the RAS are present within the heart and that cardiac biosynthesis of Ang II occurs and is regulated, controversy remains as to whether Ang II synthesized in the heart acts as an autacrine/paracrine/intracrine regulator of cardiac function. However, the possible participation of the local cardiac RAS is suggested by transgenic animal studies showing that selective over-expression of Agt in the ventricles induces hypertrophy in the absence of HT.[135,155]

RAS AND ARRHYTHMIAS SUCH AS ATRIAL FIBRILLATION

Hypertension is frequently associated with atrial fibrillation, and increasing interest has been focused on the role of the RAS in atrial remodeling and arrhythmia.[156] Ang II is released from cardiomyocytes during atrial stretch and has been linked to atrial fibrosis. AT_1 receptors are upregulated in the atria of patients with atrial fibrillation and the ACE gene polymorphism is associated with both left ventricular hypertrophy and atrial fibrillation. Although these observations are intriguing, the role of the RAS in the pathophysiology of atrial fibrillation remains to be determined.

Perspectives

The RAS is a hormonal cascade of major critical importance to the control of BP and the pathophysiology of HT. Although this system has been carefully studied for many decades, its ultimate role in the etiology of HT and its target organ damage is still unclear. The recent discovery of several new components of the RAS coupled with the functional characterization of its previously known parts has opened the door to an understanding of the role of the RAS as a progenitor and effector of the HT disease process. Potential RAS therapeutic targets in HT now include the renin receptor, the enzymatic activity of renin, ACE-2, Ang(1-7), the *mas* oncogene, and the AT_2 receptor, among others. While the RAS is reasonably well understood at the cellular and molecular levels, its role in human primary HT remains largely enigmatic. Increased efforts in translational research, particularly the identification and characterization of phenotypes of human HT, will be required. Direct cellular studies in human tissues combined with molecular genetic approaches will create powerful leverage in dissecting the role of the RAS in this complex disease.

REFERENCES

1. Carey RM, Siragy HM. Newly recognized components of the renin-angiotensin system: potential roles in cardiovascular and renal regulation. *Endocr Rev* 2003;24:261–71.
2. Griendling KK, Murphy TJ, Alexander RW. Molecular biology of the renin-angiotensin system. *Circulation* 1993;87:1816–28.
3. Hsueh WA, Baxter JD. Human prorenin. *Hypertension* 1991;17:469–77.
4. Soubrier F, Wei L, Hubert C, Clauser E, Alhenc-Gelas F, Corvol P. Molecular biology of the angiotensin I converting enzyme. II. Structure–function. Gene polymorphism and clinical implications. *J Hypertens* 1993;11:599–604.
5. Erdos EG, Skidgel, RA. Metabolism of bradykinin by peptidases in health and disease. In: Farmer SC, ed. *The Kinin System: Handbook of Immunopharmacology.* San Diego, CA: Academic Press, 1993:112–41.
6. de Gasparo M, Catt KJ, Inagami T, Wright JW, Unger T. International

union of pharmacology. XXIII. The angiotensin II receptors. *Pharmacol Rev* 2000;52:415–72.
7. Sealey JE, White RP, Laragh JH, Rubin AL. Plasma prorenin and renin in anephric patients. *Circ Res* 1977;41:17–21.
8. Prescott G, Silversides DW, Reudelhuber TL. Tissue activity of circulating prorenin. *Am J Hypertens* 2002;15:280–5.
9. Siragy HM, Xue C, Abadir P, Carey RM. Angiotensin subtype-2 receptors inhibit renin biosynthesis and angiotensin II formation. *Hypertension* 2005;45:133–7.
10. Gomez RA, Lynch KR, Chevalier RL, Everett AD, Johns DW, Wilfong N, et al. Renin and angiotensinogen gene expression and intrarenal renin distribution during ACE inhibition. *Am J Physiol* 1988;254:F900–906.
11. Nguyen G, Delarue F, Berrou J, Rondeau E, Sraer JD. Specific receptor binding of renin on human mesangial cells in culture increases plasminogen

activator inhibitor-1 antigen. *Kidney Int* 1996;50:1897–903.
12. Nguyen G, Delarue F, Burckle C, Bouzhir L, Giller T, Sraer JD. Pivotal role of the renin/prorenin receptor in angiotensin II production and cellular responses to renin. *J Clin Invest* 2002;109:1417–27.
13. Linz W, Wiemer G, Gohlke P, Unger T, Scholkens BA. Contribution of kinins to the cardiovascular actions of angiotensin-converting enzyme inhibitors. *Pharmacol Rev* 1995;47:25–49.
14. Tschope C, Schultheiss HP, Walther T. Multiple interactions between the renin-angiotensin and the kallikrein-kinin systems: role of ACE inhibition and AT1 receptor blockade. *J Cardiovasc Pharmacol* 2002;39:478–87.
15. Tipnis SR, Hooper NM, Hyde R, Karran E, Christie G, Turner AJ. A human homolog of angiotensin-converting enzyme. Cloning and functional expression as a captopril-insensitive carboxypeptidase. *J Biol Chem* 2000;275:33238–43.

16. Crackower MA, Sarao R, Oudit GY, Yagil C, Kozieradzki I, Scanga SE, et al. Angiotensin-converting enzyme 2 is an essential regulator of heart function. *Nature* 2002;417:822–28.

17. Schiavone MT, Santos RA, Brosnihan KB, Khosla MC, Ferrario CM. Release of vasopressin from the rat hypothalamo-neurohypophysial system by angiotensin-1-7 heptapeptide. *Proc Natl Acad Sci U S A* 1988;85:4095–98.

18. Chappell MC, Allred AJ, Ferrario CM. Pathways of angiotensin-1-7 metabolism in the kidney. *Nephrol Dial Transplant* 2001;16(Suppl 1):22–26.

19. Diz DI, Chappell MC, Tallant EA, Ferrario CM. Angiotensin-1-7. *Hypertension* 2005;:100–10.

20. Santos RA, Simoes e Silva AC, Maric C, Silva DM, Machado RP, de Buhr I, et al. Angiotensin-1-7 is an endogenous ligand for the G protein–coupled receptor Mas. *Proc Natl Acad Sci U S A* 2003;100:8258–63.

21. Miyata N, Park F, Li XF, Cowley AW Jr. Distribution of angiotensin AT1 and AT2 receptor subtypes in the rat kidney. *Am J Physiol* 1999;277:F437–46.

22. Giasson E, Servant MJ, Meloche S. Cyclic AMP-mediated inhibition of angiotensin II–induced protein synthesis is associated with suppression of tyrosine phosphorylation signaling in vascular smooth muscle cells. *J Biol Chem* 1997;272:26879–86.

23. Ozono R, Wang ZQ, Moore AF, Inagami T, Siragy HM, Carey RM. Expression of the subtype 2 angiotensin (AT2) receptor protein in rat kidney. *Hypertension* 1997;30:1238–46.

24. Carey RM, Wang ZQ, Siragy HM. Role of the angiotensin type 2 receptor in the regulation of blood pressure and renal function. *Hypertension* 2000;35:155–63.

25. Berry C, Touyz R, Dominiczak AF, Webb RC, Johns DG. Angiotensin receptors: signaling, vascular pathophysiology, and interactions with ceramide. *Am J Physiol Heart Circ Physiol* 2001;281:H2337–65.

26. Siragy HM, Carey RM. The subtype-2 (AT2) angiotensin receptor regulates renal cyclic guanosine 3′, 5′-monophosphate and AT1 receptor-mediated prostaglandin E2 production in conscious rats. *J Clin Invest* 1996;97:1978–82.

27. Siragy HM, Carey RM. The subtype 2 (AT2) angiotensin receptor mediates renal production of nitric oxide in conscious rats. *J Clin Invest* 1997;100:264–69.

28. Carey RM. Cardiovascular and renal regulation by the angiotensin type 2 receptor: the AT2 receptor comes of age. *Hypertension* 2005;45:840–44.

29. AbdAlla S, Lother H, Quitterer U. AT1-receptor heterodimers show enhanced G-protein activation and altered receptor sequestration. *Nature* 2000;407:94–98.

30. AbdAlla S, Lother H, Abdel-tawab AM, Quitterer U. The angiotensin II AT2 receptor is an AT1 receptor antagonist. *J Biol Chem* 2001;276:39721–26.

31. Abadir PM, Periasamy A, Carey RM, Siragy HM. Angiotensin II type 2 receptor-bradykinin B2 receptor functional heterodimerization. *Hypertension* 2006;48:316–22.

32. Brunner HR, Laragh JH, Baer L, Newton MA, Goodwin FT, Krakoff LR, et al. Essential hypertension: renin and aldosterone, heart attack and stroke. *N Engl J Med* 1972;286:441–49.

33. Laragh JH, Letcher RL, Pickering TG. Renin profiling for diagnosis and treatment of hypertension. *JAMA* 1979;241:151–56.

34. Sennett JA, Brown RD, Island DP, Yarbro LR, Watson JT, Slaton PE, et al. Evidence for a new mineralocorticoid in patients with low-renin essential hypertension. *Circ Res* 1975;36:2–9.

35. Brunner HR, Sealey JE, Laragh JH. Renin subgroups in essential hypertension. Further analysis of their pathophysiological and epidemiological characteristics. *Circ Res* 1973;32:(Suppl 1):99–105.

36. Tan SY, Mulrow PJ. Low renin essential hypertension: failure to demonstrate excess 11-deoxycorticosterone production. *J Clin Endocrinol Metab* 1979;49:790–93.

37. Sealey JE, Gordon RD, Mantero F. Plasma renin and aldosterone measurements in low renin hypertensive states. *Trends Endocrinol Metab* 2005;16:86–91.

38. Alderman MH, Madhavan S, Ooi WL, Cohen H, Sealey JE, Laragh JH. Association of the renin–sodium profile with the risk of myocardial infarction in patients with hypertension. *N Engl J Med* 1991;324:1098–104.

39. Hollenberg NH, Williams, GH. Abnormal renal function, sodium-volume homeostasis and renin system behavior in normal-renin essential hypertension: the evalution of the non-modulator concept. Laragh JH, Brenner BM, eds. *Hypertension: Pathophysiology, Diagnosis and Management*. 2nd ed. 2 vols. New York: Raven Press, 1995:1837–56.

40. Dzau V. The cardiovascular continuum and renin-angiotensin-aldosterone system blockade. *J Hypertens Suppl* 2005;23:S9–17.

41. Sica DA. Combination angiotensin-converting enzyme inhibitor and angiotensin receptor blocker therapy: its role in clinical practice. *J Clin Hypertens (Greenwich)* 2003;5:414–20.

42. Julius S, Kjeldsen SE, Weber M, Brunner HR, Ekman S, Hansson L, et al. Outcomes in hypertensive patients at high cardiovascular risk treated with regimens based on valsartan or amlodipine: the VALUE randomised trial. *Lancet* 2004;363:2022–31.

43. Dahlof B, Devereux RB, Kjeldsen SE, Julius S, Beevers G, de Faire U, et al. Cardiovascular morbidity and mortality in the Losartan Intervention for Endpoint reduction in hypertension study (LIFE): a randomised trial against atenolol. *Lancet* 2002;359:995–1003.

44. ALLHAT Officers and Coordinators for the ALLHAT Collaborative Research Group. Major outcomes in high-risk hypertensive patients randomized to angiotensin-converting enzyme inhibitor or calcium channel blocker vs diuretic: the Antihypertensive and Lipid-Lowering Treatment to Prevent Heart Attack Trial (ALLHAT). *JAMA* 2002;288:2981–97.

45. Hansson L, Lindholm LH, Niskanen L, Lanke J, Hedner T, Niklason A, et al. Effect of angiotensin-converting-enzyme inhibition compared with conventional therapy on cardiovascular morbidity and mortality in hypertension: the Captopril Prevention Project (CAPPP) randomised trial. *Lancet* 1999;353:611–16.

46. Weber M. The telmisartan Programme of Research tO show Telmisartan End-organ proteCTION (PROTECTION) programme. *J Hypertens Suppl* 2003;21:S37–46.

47. Clement DL, De Buyzere ML, De Bacquer DA, de Leeuw PW, Duprez DA, Fagard RH, et al. Prognostic value of ambulatory blood-pressure recordings in patients with treated hypertension. *N Engl J Med* 2003;348:2407–15.

48. Muller JE, Tofler GH, Stone PH. Circadian variation and triggers of onset of acute cardiovascular disease. *Circulation* 1989;79:733–43.

49. Kario K, Pickering TG, Umeda Y, Hoshide S, Hoshide Y, Morinari M, et al. Morning surge in blood pressure as a predictor of silent and clinical cerebrovascular disease in elderly hypertensives: a prospective study. *Circulation* 2003;107:1401–406.

50. White WB, Lacourciere Y, Davidai G. Effects of the angiotensin II receptor blockers telmisartan versus valsartan on the circadian variation of blood pressure: impact on the early morning period. *Am J Hypertens* 2004;17:347–53.

51. Touyz RM. The role of angiotensin II in regulating vascular structural and functional changes in hypertension. *Curr Hypertens Rep* 2003;5:155–64.

52. Touyz RM. Molecular and cellular mechanisms in vascular injury in hypertension: role of angiotensin II. *Curr Opin Nephrol Hypertens* 2005;14:125–31.

53. Berk BC. Vascular smooth muscle growth: autocrine growth mechanisms. *Physiol Rev* 2001;81:999–1030.

54. Fukuda N. Molecular mechanisms of the exaggerated growth of vascular smooth muscle cells in hypertension. *J Atheroscler Thromb* 1997;4:65–72.

55. Gibbons GH, Pratt RE, Dzau VJ. Vascular smooth muscle cell hypertrophy vs. hyperplasia. Autocrine transforming growth factor-beta 1 expression determines growth response to angiotensin II. *J Clin Invest* 1992;90:456–61.

56. Touyz RM, He G, Deng LY, Schiffrin EL. Role of extracellular signal-regulated kinases in angiotensin II-stimulated contraction of smooth muscle cells from human resistance arteries. *Circulation* 1999;99:392–99.

57. Tea BS, Der Sarkissian S, Touyz RM, Hamet P, deBlois D. Proapoptotic and growth-inhibitory role of angiotensin II type 2 receptor in vascular smooth muscle cells of spontaneously hypertensive rats in vivo. *Hypertension* 2000;35:1069–73.

58. Tham DM, Martin-McNulty B, Wang YX, Wilson DW, Vergona R, Sullivan ME, et al. Angiotensin II is associated with activation of NF-kappaB-mediated genes and downregulation of PPARs. *Physiol Genomics* 2002;11:21–30.

59. Koh KK, Ahn JY, Han SH, Kim DS, Jin DK, Kim HS, et al. Pleiotropic effects of angiotensin II receptor blocker in hypertensive patients. *J Am Coll Cardiol* 2003;42:905–10.

60. Nathan C. Points of control in inflammation. *Nature* 2002;420:846–52.

61. Suzuki Y, Ruiz-Ortega M, Lorenzo O, Ruperez M, Esteban V, Egido J. Inflammation and angiotensin II. *Int J Biochem Cell Biol* 2003;35:881–900.

62. Dandona P, Kumar V, Aljada A, Ghanim H, Syed T, Hofmayer D, et al. Angiotensin II receptor blocker valsartan suppresses reactive oxygen species generation in leukocytes, nuclear factor-kappa B, in mononuclear cells of normal subjects: evidence of an antiinflammatory action. *J Clin Endocrinol Metab* 2003;88:4496–501.

63. Williams B, Baker AQ, Gallacher B, Lodwick D. Angiotensin II increases vascular permeability factor gene expression by human vascular smooth muscle cells. *Hypertension* 1995;25:913–17.

64. Chua CC, Hamdy RC, Chua BH. Upregulation of vascular endothelial growth factor by angiotensin II in rat heart endothelial cells. *Biochim Biophys Acta* 1998;1401:187–94.

65. Yamagishi S, Amano S, Inagaki Y, Okamoto T, Inoue H, Takeuchi M, et al. Angiotensin II–type 1 receptor interaction upregulates vascular endothelial growth factor messenger RNA levels in retinal pericytes through intracellular reactive oxygen species generation. *Drugs Exp Clin Res* 2003;29:75–80.

66. Harris RC, Zhang MZ, Cheng HF. Cyclooxygenase-2 and the renal renin-angiotensin system. *Acta Physiol Scand* 2004;181:543–47.

67. Ruiz-Ortega M, Lorenzo O, Suzuki Y, Ruperez M, Egido J. Proinflammatory actions of angiotensins. *Curr Opin Nephrol Hypertens* 2001;10:321–29.

68. Piqueras L, Kubes P, Alvarez A, O'Connor E, Issekutz AC, Esplugues JV, Sanz MJ. Angiotensin II induces leukocyte-endothelial cell interactions in vivo via AT[1] and AT[2] receptor-mediated P-selectin upregulation. *Circulation* 2000;102:2118–23.

69. Costanzo A, Moretti F, Burgio VL, Bravi C, Guido F, Levrero M, Puri PL. Endothelial activation by angiotensin II through NFkappaB and p38 pathways: involvement of NFkappaB-inducible kinase (NIK), free oxygen radicals, and selective inhibition by aspirin. *J Cell Physiol* 2003;195:402–10.

70. Ley K. The role of selectins in inflammation and disease. *Trends Mol Med* 2003;9:263–68.

71. Ito T, Ikeda U, Yamamoto K, Shimada K. Regulation of interleukin-8 expression by HMG-CoA reductase inhibitors in human vascular smooth muscle cells. *Atherosclerosis* 2002;165:51–55.

72. Funakoshi Y, Ichiki T, Shimokawa H, Egashira K, Takeda K, Kaibuchi K, et al. Rho-kinase mediates angiotensin II–induced monocyte chemoattractant protein-1 expression in rat vascular smooth muscle cells. *Hypertension* 2001;38:100–104.

73. Lassegue B, Clempus RE. Vascular NAD(P)H oxidases: specific features, expression, and regulation. *Am J Physiol Regul Integr Comp Physiol* 2003;285:R277–97.

74. Touyz RM, Chen X, Tabet F, Yao G, He G, Quinn MT, et al. Expression of a functionally active gp91phox-containing neutrophil-type NAD(P)H oxidase in smooth muscle cells from human resistance arteries: regulation by angiotensin II. *Circ Res* 2002;90:1205–13.

75. Rizzoni D, Porteri E, De Ciuceis C, Sleiman I, Rodella L, Rezzani R, et al. Effect of treatment with candesartan or enalapril on subcutaneous small artery structure in hypertensive patients with noninsulin-dependent diabetes mellitus. *Hypertension* 2005;45:659–65.

76. Ruperez M, Lorenzo O, Blanco-Colio LM, Esteban V, Egido J, Ruiz-Ortega M. Connective tissue growth factor is a mediator of angiotensin II–induced fibrosis. *Circulation* 2003;108:1499–505.

77. Zhao Q, Ishibashi M, Hiasa K, Tan C, Takeshita A, Egashira K. Essential role of vascular endothelial growth factor in angiotensin II-induced vascular inflammation and remodeling. *Hypertension* 2004;44:264–70.

78. Sarkar S, Vellaichamy E, Young D, Sen S. Influence of cytokines and growth factors in ANG II–mediated collagen upregulation by fibroblasts in rats: role of myocytes. *Am J Physiol Heart Circ Physiol* 2004;287:H107–17.

79. Castoldi G, Di Gioia CR, Pieruzzi F, D'Orlando C, Van De Greef WM, Busca G, et al. ANG II increases TIMP-1 expression in rat aortic smooth muscle cells in vivo. *Am J Physiol Heart Circ Physiol* 2003;284:H635–43.

80. Taniyama Y, Griendling KK. Reactive oxygen species in the vasculature: molecular and cellular mechanisms. *Hypertension* 2003;42:1075–81.

81. Griendling KK, Minieri CA, Ollerenshaw JD, Alexander RW. Angiotensin II stimulates NADH and NADPH oxidase activity in cultured vascular smooth muscle cells. *Circ Res* 1994;74:1141–48.

82. Suematsu M, Suzuki H, Delano FA, Schmid-Schonbein GW. The inflammatory aspect of the microcirculation in hypertension: oxidative stress, leukocytes/endothelial interaction, apoptosis. *Microcirculation* 2002;9:259–76.

83. Viedt C, Fei J, Krieger-Brauer HI, Brandes RP, Teupser D, Kamimura M, et al. Role of p22phox in angiotensin II and platelet-derived growth factor AA induced activator protein 1 activation in vascular smooth muscle cells. *J Mol Med* 2004;82:31–38.

84. Dohi Y, Ohashi M, Sugiyama M, Takase H, Sato K, Ueda R. Candesartan reduces oxidative stress and inflammation in patients with essential hypertension. *Hypertens Res* 2003;26:691–97.

85. Touyz RM, Schiffrin EL. Role of calcium influx and intracellular calcium stores in angiotensin II-mediated calcium hyper-responsiveness in smooth muscle from spontaneously hypertensive rats. *J Hypertens* 1997;15:1431–39.

86. Chitaley K, Weber D, Webb RC. RhoA/Rho-kinase, vascular changes, and hypertension. *Curr Hypertens Rep* 2001;3:139–44.

87. Touyz RM, Wu XH, He G, Salomon S, Schiffrin EL. Increased angiotensin II–mediated Src signaling via epidermal growth factor receptor transactivation is associated with decreased C-terminal Src kinase activity in vascular smooth muscle cells from spontaneously hypertensive rats. *Hypertension* 2002;39:479–85.

88. Touyz RM, He G, Wu XH, Park JB, Mabrouk ME, Schiffrin EL. Src is an important mediator of extracellular signal-regulated kinase 1/2-dependent growth signaling by angiotensin II in smooth muscle cells from resistance arteries of hypertensive patients. *Hypertension* 2001;38:56–64.

89. Saito Y, Berk BC. Angiotensin II–mediated signal transduction pathways. *Curr Hypertens Rep* 2002;4:167–71.

90. Meloche S, Landry J, Huot J, Houle F, Marceau F, Giasson E. p38 MAP kinase pathway regulates angiotensin II–induced contraction of rat vascular smooth muscle. *Am J Physiol Heart Circ Physiol* 2000;279:H741–51.

91. Frank GD, Eguchi S, Yamakawa T, Tanaka S, Inagami T, Motley ED. Involvement of reactive oxygen species in the activation of tyrosine kinase and extracellular signal-regulated kinase by angiotensin II. *Endocrinology* 2000;141:3120–26.

92. Wilkie N, Ng LL, Boarder MR. Angiotensin II responses of vascular smooth muscle cells from hypertensive rats: enhancement at the level of p42 and p44 mitogen activated protein kinase. *Br J Pharmacol* 1997;122:209–16.

93. Saito Y, Berk BC. Transactivation: a novel signaling pathway from angiotensin II to tyrosine kinase receptors. *J Mol Cell Cardiol* 2001;33:3–7.

94. Schiffrin EL, Park JB, Intengan HD, Touyz RM. Correction of arterial structure and endothelial dysfunction in human essential hypertension by the angiotensin receptor antagonist losartan. *Circulation* 2000;101:1653–59.

95. Hall JE, Brands MW, Henegar JR. Angiotensin II and long-term arterial pressure regulation: the overriding dominance of the kidney. *J Am Soc Nephrol* 1999;10(Suppl 12):S258–65.

96. Crowley SD, Gurley SB, Oliverio MI, Pazmino AK, Griffiths R, Flannery PJ, et al. Distinct roles for the kidney and systemic tissues in blood pressure regulation by the renin-angiotensin system. *J Clin Invest* 2005;115:1092–99.

97. van Kats JP, Schalekamp MA, Verdouw PD, Duncker DJ, Danser AH. Intrarenal angiotensin II: interstitial and cellular levels and site of production. *Kidney Int* 2001;60:2311–17.

98. van Kats JP, Duncker DJ, Haitsma DB, Schuijt MP, Niebuur R, Stubenitsky R, et al. Angiotensin-converting enzyme inhibition and angiotensin II type 1 receptor blockade prevent cardiac remodeling in pigs after myocardial infarction: role of tissue angiotensin II. *Circulation* 2000;102:1556–63.

99. Nussberger J. Circulating versus tissue angiotensin II. In: Epstein M, Brunner HR, eds. *Angiotensin II Receptor Antagonists*. Philadelphia: Hanley and Belfus, 2001.

100. Chai W, Danser AH. Is angiotensin II made inside or outside of the cell? *Curr Hypertens Rep* 2005;7:124–27.

101. Re RN. Tissue renin angiotensin systems. *Med Clin North Am* 2004;88:19–38.

102. Saris JJ, Derkx FH, Lamers JM, Saxena PR, Schalekamp MA, Danser AH. Cardiomyocytes bind and activate native human prorenin: role of soluble mannose 6-phosphate receptors. *Hypertension* 2001;37:710–15.

103. Kimbrough HM Jr, Vaughan ED Jr, Carey RM, Ayers CR. Effect of intrarenal angiotensin II blockade on renal function in conscious dogs. *Circ Res* 1977;40:174–78.

104. Levens NR, Freedlender AE, Peach MJ, Carey RM. Control of renal function by intrarenal angiotensin II. *Endocrinology* 1983;112:43–49.

105. Navar LG, Kobori H, Prieto-Carrasquero M. Intrarenal angiotensin II and hypertension. *Curr Hypertens Rep* 2003;5:135–43.

106. Wolf G. The renin-angiotensin system and progression of renal diseases. *Nephron Physiol* 2003;93:P3–13.

107. Ingert C, Grima M, Coquard C, Barthelmebs M, Imbs JL. Contribution of angiotensin II internalization to intrarenal angiotensin II levels in rats. *Am J Physiol Renal Physiol* 2002;283:F1003–10.

108. Zhuo JL, Imig JD, Hammond TG, Orengo S, Benes E, Navar LG. Ang II accumulation in rat renal endosomes during Ang II–induced hypertension: role of AT^1 receptor. *Hypertension* 2002;39:116–21.

109. Tokuyama H, Hayashi K, Matsuda H, Kubota E, Honda M, Okubo K, et al. Differential regulation of elevated renal angiotensin II in chronic renal ischemia. *Hypertension* 2002;40:34–40.

110. Siragy HM, Carey RM. Protective role of the angiotensin AT2 receptor in a renal wrap hypertension model. *Hypertension* 1999;33:1237–42.

111. Nishiyama A, Seth DM, Navar LG. Renal interstitial fluid concentrations of angiotensins I and II in anesthetized rats. *Hypertension* 2002;39:129–34.

112. Cervenka L, Wang CT, Mitchell KD, Navar LG. Proximal tubular angiotensin II levels and renal functional responses to AT1 receptor blockade in nonclipped kidneys of Goldblatt hypertensive rats. *Hypertension* 1999;33:102–107.

113. Chen R, Mukhin YV, Garnovskaya MN, Thielen TE, Iijima Y, Huang C, et al. A functional angiotensin II receptor-GFP fusion protein: evidence for agonist-dependent nuclear translocation. *Am J Physiol Renal Physiol* 2000;279:F440–48.

114. Haller H, Lindschau C, Erdmann B, Quass P, Luft FC. Effects of intracellular angiotensin II in vascular smooth muscle cells. *Circ Res* 1996;79:765–72.

115. Re RN, Cook JL. The intracrine hypothesis: An update. *Regul Pept* 2006;133:1–9.

116. Kobori H, Prieto-Carrasquero MC, Ozawa Y, Navar LG. AT1 receptor mediated augmentation of intrarenal angiotensinogen in angiotensin II–dependent hypertension. *Hypertension* 2004;43:1126–32.

117. Kobori H, Harrison-Bernard LM, Navar LG. Enhancement of angiotensinogen expression in angiotensin II–dependent hypertension. *Hypertension* 2001;37:1329–35.

118. Rohrwasser A, Morgan T, Dillon HF, Zhao L, Callaway CW, Hillas E, et al. Elements of a paracrine tubular renin-angiotensin system along the entire nephron. *Hypertension* 1999;34:1265–74.

119. Kobori H, Nishiyama A, Harrison-Bernard LM, Navar LG. Urinary angiotensinogen as an indicator of intrarenal angiotensin status in hypertension. *Hypertension* 2003;41:42–49.

120. Prieto-Carrasquero MC, Kobori H, Ozawa Y, Gutierrez A, Seth D, Navar LG. AT1 receptor–mediated enhancement of collecting duct renin in angiotensin II–dependent hypertensive rats. *Am J Physiol Renal Physiol* 2005;289:F632–37.

121. Komlosi P, Fuson AL, Fintha A, Peti-Peterdi J, Rosivall L, Warnock DG, et al. Angiotensin I conversion to angiotensin II stimulates cortical collecting duct sodium transport. *Hypertension* 2003;42:195–99.

122. Saccomani G. Angiotensin II stimulation of Na(+)H(+) exchange in proximal tubule cells. *Am J Phynol Renal Physiol* 1990;258:F1188–93.

123. Printz MP GD, Unger T, Phillips MI. The brain renin-angiotensin system. In: Ganten D, et al., eds. *The Renin-Angiotensin System in the Brain: A Model for Synthesis of Peptides in the Brain*. New York: Springer-Verlag, 2003.

124. Moulik S, Speth RC, Turner BB, Rowe BP. Angiotensin II receptor subtype distribution in the rabbit brain. *Exp Brain Res* 2002;142:275–83.

125. Lavoie JL, Cassell MD, Gross KW, Sigmund CD. Localization of renin expressing cells in the brain, by use of a REN-eGFP transgenic model. *Physiol Genomics* 2002;16:240–46.

126. Lavoie JL, Cassell MD, Gross KW, Sigmund CD. Adjacent expression of renin and angiotensinogen in the rostral ventrolateral medulla using a dual-reporter transgenic model. *Hypertension* 2004;43:1116–19.

127. Sakai K, Sigmund CD. Molecular evidence of tissue renin-angiotensin systems: a focus on the brain. *Curr Hypertens Rep* 2005;7:135–40.

128. Ferrario CM, Chappell MC. Novel angiotensin peptides. *Cell Mol Life Sci* 2004;61:2720–27.

129. Reaux-Le Goazigo A, Iturrioz X, Fassot C, Claperon C, Roques BP, Llorens-Cortes C. Role of angiotensin III in hypertension. *Curr Hypertens Rep* 2005;7:128–34.

130. Wright JW, Tamura-Myers E, Wilson WL, Roques BP, Llorens-Cortes C, Speth RC, et al. Conversion of brain angiotensin II to angiotensin III is critical for pressor response in rats. *Am J Physiol Regul Integr Comp Physiol* 2003;284:R725–33.

131. Reaux A, Fournie-Zaluski MC, David C, Zini S, Roques BP, Corvol P, et al. Aminopeptidase A inhibitors as potential central antihypertensive agents. *Proc Natl Acad Sci U S A* 1999;96:13415–20.

132. Fournie-Zaluski MC, Fassot C, Valentin B, Djordjijevic D, Reaux-Le Goazigo A, et al. Brain renin-angiotensin system blockade by systemically active aminopeptidase A inhibitors: a potential treatment of salt-dependent hypertension. *Proc Natl Acad Sci U S A* 2004;101:7775–80.

133. Lochard N, Thibault G, Silversides DW, Touyz RM, Reudelhuber TL. Chronic production of angiotensin IV in the brain leads to hypertension that is reversible with an angiotensin II AT1 receptor antagonist. *Circ Res* 2004;94:1451–57.

134. Danser AH. Local renin-angiotensin systems. *Mol Cell Biochem* 1996;157:211–16.

135. Dostal DE, Baker KM. The cardiac renin-angiotensin system: conceptual, or a regulator of cardiac function? *Circ Res* 1999;85:643–50.

136. Paul M, Wagner J, Dzau VJ. Gene expression of the renin-angiotensin system in human tissues. Quantitative analysis by the polymerase chain reaction. *J Clin Invest* 1993;91:2058–64.

137. Samani NJ, Swales JD, Brammar WJ. Expression of the renin gene in extra-renal tissues of the rat. *Biochem J* 1988;253:907–10.

138. Agoudemos MM, Greene AS. Localization of the renin-angiotensin system components to the skeletal muscle microcirculation. *Microcirculation* 2005;12:627–36.

139. Linderman JR, Greene AS. Distribution of angiotensin II receptor expression in the microcirculation of striated muscle. *Microcirculation* 2001;8:275–81.

140. Oliver JA, Sciacca RR. Local generation of angiotensin II as a mechanism of regulation of peripheral vascular tone in the rat. *J Clin Invest* 1984;74:1247–51.

141. Vicaut E, Hou X. Local renin-angiotensin system in the microcirculation of spontaneously hypertensive rats. *Hypertension* 1994;24:70–76.

142. Boddi M, Poggesi L, Coppo M, Zarone N, Sacchi S, Tania C, et al. Human vascular renin-angiotensin system and its functional changes in relation to different sodium intakes. *Hypertension* 1998;31:836–42.

143. Gomez RA, Lynch KR, Sturgill BC, Elwood JP, Chevalier RL, Carey RM, et al. Distribution of renin mRNA and its protein in the developing kidney. *Am J Physiol* 1989;257:F850–58.

144. Gomez RA, Chevalier RL, Everett AD, Elwood JP, Peach MJ, Lynch KR, et al. Recruitment of renin gene-expressing cells in adult rat kidneys. *Am J Physiol* 1990;259:F660–65.

145. Everett AD, Carey RM, Chevalier RL, Peach MJ, Gomez RA. Renin release and gene expression in intact rat kidney microvessels and single cells. *J Clin Invest* 1990;86:169–75.

146. Thurston H, Swales JD. Blood pressure response of nephrectomized hypertensive rats to converting enzyme inhibition: evidence for persistent vascular renin activity. *Clin Sci Mol Med* 1977;52:299–304.

147. Dzau VJ, Re RN. Evidence for the existence of renin in the heart. *Circulation* 1987;75:I134–36.

148. Dostal DE. The cardiac renin-angiotensin system: novel signaling mechanisms related to cardiac growth and function. *Regul Pept* 2000;91:1–11.

149. Dell'Italia LJ, Meng QC, Balcells E, Wei CC, Palmer R, Hageman GR, et al. Compartmentalization of angiotensin II generation in the dog heart. Evidence for independent mechanisms in intravascular and interstitial spaces. *J Clin Invest* 1997;100:253–58.

150. Urata H, Boehm KD, Philip A, Kinoshita A, Gabrovsek J, Bumpus FM, et al. Cellular localization and regional distribution of an angiotensin II–forming chymase in the heart. *J Clin Invest* 1993;91:1269–81.

151. Balcells E, Meng QC, Johnson WH Jr, Oparil S, Dell'Italia LJ. Angiotensin II formation from ACE and chymase in human and animal hearts: methods and species considerations. *Am J Physiol* 1997;273:H1769–74.

152. Peters J, Farrenkopf R, Clausmeyer S, Zimmer J, Kantachuvesiri S, Sharp MG, et al. Functional significance of prorenin internalization in the rat heart. *Circ Res* 2002;90:1135–41.

153. Sinn PL, Sigmund CD. Identification of three human renin mRNA isoforms from alternative tissue-specific transcriptional initiation. *Physiol Genomics* 2000;3:25–31.

154. Baker KM, Chernin MI, Schreiber T, Sanghi S, Haiderzaidi S, Booz GW, et al. Evidence of a novel intracrine mechanism in angiotensin II–induced cardiac hypertrophy. *Regul Pept* 2004;120:5–13.

155. Mazzolai L, Nussberger J, Aubert JF, Brunner DB, Gabbiani G, Brunner HR, et al. Blood pressure–independent cardiac hypertrophy induced by locally activated renin-angiotensin system. *Hypertension* 1998;31:1324–30.

156. Choudhury A, Varaghese GI, Lip GYH. Targeting the renin-angiotensin-aldosterone system in atrial fibrillation: shift from electrical to structural therapy? *Expert Opin Pharmacother* 2005;6:2193–207.

Chapter

28

The Endothelin System

Ernesto L. Schiffrin

Definition

■ Endothelins (ETs) are potent vasoconstrictor, growth-promoting, and proinflammatory peptides. In blood vessels the most abundant ET is ET-1.

Clinical Findings

■ Production of ET-1 is increased in the endothelium and the kidney in salt-dependent hypertension (e.g., deoxycorticosterone acetate–salt rats and Dahl salt-sensitive rats, in salt-loaded stroke-prone spontaneously hypertensive rats (SHRsp), in angiotensin II–infused and in diabetic rats).

■ ET receptor antagonism decreases blood pressure and vascular hypertrophic remodeling and corrects endothelial dysfunction in these hypertensive models.

■ Transgenic mice overexpressing human prepro-ET-1 in the endothelium develop hypertrophic vascular remodeling and endothelial dysfunction.

Clinical Implications

■ Patients with stage 2 essential hypertension have enhanced vascular expression of ET-1.

■ ET receptor antagonists lower blood pressure in hypertensive patients.

■ Side effects of ET receptor blockers have prevented their development for this indication. ET antagonists have only been approved for the treatment of primary pulmonary hypertension.

The 21–amino-acid peptide endothelin (ET) was isolated and cloned in 1985 by Yanagisawa et al.[1] ET-1 (Figure 28–1), -2 and -3 are isopeptides with different functions, and there are as well bigger 31- and 32-amino-acid peptides.[2] ET-1 is the most abundant ET produced in blood vessels and the kidneys, whereas ET-3 is mainly a neuropeptide. Endothelial cells are thus only one of the cell types that produce and release ETs. They secrete ET-1 toward underlying smooth muscle, with little spillover into the circulation (Figure 28–2).[3]

In endothelial and other cells, furin and other enzymes act on pro-ETs to generate 38– to 39–amino-acid peptides (big ETs) that are converted into mature 21–amino-acid ETs by zinc-dependent endoproteases, termed endothelin-converting enzymes (ECE-1 and 2). ECEs cleave big ET-1 at the Val[21]-Trp[22] bond, yielding the potent vasoconstrictor ET-1[1-21]. ECE-1, of which there are four differentially spliced isoforms encoded by a single

gene (ECE-1a, ECE-1b, ECE-1c, and ECE-1d) resulting from four alternative promoters, is present in endothelial cells.[4] The four isoforms of ECE-1 differ by their N-terminal amino-acid, which is responsible for their cellular localization. ECE-1a, -1c, and -1d are extracellular, whereas ECE-1b is an intracellular enzyme. ECE-1b heterodimerizes with other ECE-1 isoforms and regulates their activity.[5] ECE-2 is found on smooth muscle cells and converts big ET-1 to ET-1 in the vicinity of ET receptors, which may protect the peptide from degradation. There are other enzymes that generate ETs such as matrix metalloproteinase-2 that cleaves the Gly[32]-Leu[33] bond to generate ET-1[1-32],[2] chymase from mast cells that cleaves big ET-1 at the Tyr[31]-Gly[32] peptide bond, yielding ET-1[1-31], and neutral endopeptidase,[6] but their importance in this process is unclear. However, this suggests that there is differential expression of different pathways of activation of big ET-1, depending on the tissue localization of the activating protease.

ET production in blood vessels is modulated by inhibitors such as shear stress[7] and nitric oxide (NO), and agents that stimulate its production, such as epinephrine, thrombin, angiotensin II (Ang II), vasopressin, cytokines, insulin, growth factors (TGF-β1), and hypoxia. NO may be the mediator of the effect of increased shear stress on ET-1 generation.[8] Leptin stimulates ET-1 generation by endothelial cells,[9] which may be a mechanism involved in the link between ET-1 and obesity, thus contributing to the vascular injury, which is found in the metabolic syndrome and in type 2 diabetes mellitus. Peroxisome proliferator-activated receptor (PPAR) α activators (lipid-lowering fibrates) and γ agonists (insulin-sensitizing thiazo-lidinediones or glitazones) inhibit *in vivo* ET-1 production in deoxycorticosterone acetate (DOCA)–salt rats.[10]

ET-1 acts on ET_A and ET_B receptors. In the vascular wall, ET_A and ET_B receptors are present on smooth muscle cells, whereas endothelial cells only possess ET_B receptors. ET_A and ET_B receptors on vascular smooth muscle cells induce vasoconstriction and growth. They are present in systemic arteries, veins[11] and pulmonary vessels,[12-14] and in all vessels ET_A receptors predominate over ET_B. ET_B receptors on endothelial cells stimulate the production of nitric oxide (NO) and prostacyclin, exerting a vasodilator action. Whether physiologically ETs are vasoconstrictors or vasodilators remains unclear, but under pathophysiologic conditions when large amounts of ET-1 are produced by endothelial or smooth muscle cells, its effects appear to be mainly vasoconstrictor and mitogenic,

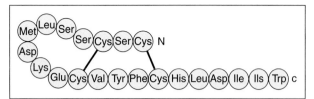

Figure 28–1. Molecular structure of ET-1, the major vascular member of the endothelin system. ET-2 and ET-3 exhibit two and five amino acid differences, respectively. ET-1[1-31] is an additional peptide of the system produced in the vasculature and the airway that functions as a vasoconstrictor of tracheal and vascular smooth muscle and could be involved in allergic inflammation. ET-1[1-32] is generated in the vascular wall by the action of matrix metalloproteinase-2. ET, endothelin.

inducing growth and inflammation. In other organs, the effect of ET receptors varies with the function of the organ. ET_A or ET_B receptors appear to predominate in the adrenal gland depending on the species. ET_A receptors predominate in the kidney. ET_B receptors appear to be the predominant ones in the brain.

EFFECTS OF PREPRO-ENDOTHELIN-1 OR ENDOTHELIN RECEPTOR GENE DELETION

Naturally occurring mutations or experimental deletion of ET peptide or receptor genes have demonstrated the importance of the system in development. Inactivation in

mice of the ET-1 gene or the ET_A receptor gene results in slight blood pressure (BP) elevation, which appears to be a consequence of abnormal craniofacial development that interferes with breathing and raises BP through anoxia.[15,16] The aorta exhibits as well developmental abnormalities, and consequently the phenotype resembles the Pierre Robin syndrome.

ET-3 is the cognate ligand of ET_B receptors and acts mainly on neural or neurally derived tissue. ET-3 regulates migration of neural crest cells. Mutations or gene inactivation of ET_B receptors induce aganglionic megacolon and pigmentary abnormalities.[17] Hereditary and sporadic human aganglionic megacolon (Hirschprung's disease) may result in many cases from mutations of the ET_B receptor gene. Heterozygous ET_B receptor knockout mice have slightly elevated BP, which supports the hypothesis that the physiologic action of ET_B receptors is vasodilatory.[18,19]

MECHANISM OF ACTION OF ENDOTHELINS

ET receptors mediate their actions through activation of phospholipase C, inositol trisphosphate generation, and calcium release. Activation of the calcium–calmodulin pathway, production of diacylglycerol, and stimulation of protein kinase C contribute to trigger vascular smooth muscle cell constriction. As well, the ras-raf-mitogen activated kinase (MAPK) cascade is stimulated and contributes to the growth-promoting action of ETs,

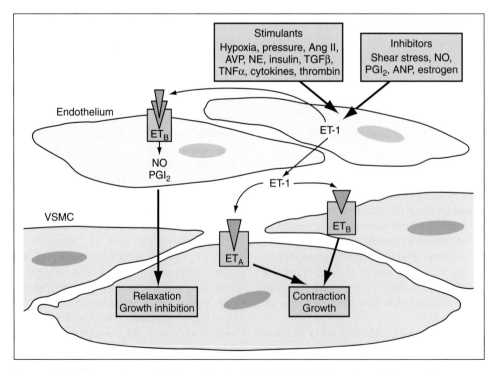

Figure 28–2. The vascular endothelin system is depicted. ET-1 is released mostly toward the underlying smooth muscle cells. Different agents stimulate or inhibit ET-1 release by the endothelium. ET-1 then acts on ET_A or ET_B smooth muscle receptors inducing contraction and growth. ET-1 acts as well as an autocrine or paracrine agent stimulating release of NO or PGI_2. It may thus induce relaxation and inhibition of growth. ANP, atrial natriuretic peptide; AVP, arginine-vasopressin; Ang II, angiotensin II; ET, endothelin; NO, nitric oxide; PGI_2, prostacyclin; VSMC, .

although p38MAPK does not appear to be activated by ET-1. Nonreceptor tyrosine kinases also participate in the intracellular cascade initiated by ET receptor stimulation.[20,21]

In DOCA-salt hypertensive rats, which have an important ET-1–dependent component,[22] enhanced generation of reactive oxygen species (ROS) has been well documented.[23,24] ROS are produced by reduced nicotinamide adenine dinucleotide phosphate (NAD(P)H) oxidase, xanthine oxidase, mitochondria, and uncoupled NO synthase.[25] Uncoupling of NO synthase is the result of low concentrations of folic acid–derived tetrahydrobiopterin. In contrast to angiotensin, which stimulates generation of ROS mostly from NAD(P)H oxidase, human smooth muscle cells stimulated by ET-1 generate superoxide principally from mitochondria, particularly complex III.[26] In rat vessels, xanthine oxidase and mitochondria also appear to be important sources of ROS.[27] In mice, superoxide stimulated by ET-1 is derived mainly from NA(D)PH oxidase.[28] ROS stimulated by ET receptor activation contribute to intracellular signaling via growth factor–receptor transactivation and MAPK activation.[21] As well, ROS are potent stimulators of ET-1 synthesis by endothelial cells,[29] which could participate in a dangerous positive feedback mechanism.

Through the mechanisms mentioned above, ET-1 induces vasoconstriction and remodeling. Inward remodeling of small arteries in organoid culture resulted from sustained contraction,[30] which may involve collagen reorganization through β_3-integrins. Indeed, an antibody to β_3-integrins blocked this remodeling. In small arteries in organoid culture, stimulation with ET-1 induced significant increase in c-fos mRNA that was inhibited by staurosporine and the calcium chelator BAPTA, but not by inhibitors of MAP kinases, protein kinase C, or tyrosine kinases, suggesting a role for intracellular calcium in ET-1–induced vascular remodeling.[31]

ET$_A$ receptors were found to induce both cell growth and apoptosis through NFκB activation.[32] ET$_B$ receptors may also have apoptotic effects on cells.[33] However, the final effect of ET-1 appears to be a survival effect as a consequence of reduced activation of caspase-3.[33,34]

PATHOPHYSIOLOGY OF ENDOTHELIN SYSTEM IN EXPERIMENTAL MODELS

The endothelin system plays a pathophysiologic role in hypertension, atherosclerosis, coronary artery disease, heart failure, subarachnoid hemorrhage and cerebral vasospasm, diabetes, primary pulmonary hypertension (the only approved indication of ET antagonists), pulmonary fibrosis, scleroderma, diabetic and nondiabetic renal disease, renal failure, hepatorenal syndrome, glaucoma, prostate cancer and its metastasis, and so on. Of these, only the role of endothelin in experimental and clinical hypertension will be discussed.

Vascular effects of endothelin-1 in experimental hypertension

Enhanced production of ET-1 in experimental hypertension[23] participates in the mechanisms that are respon-

sible for the remodeling of large and small arteries.[35,36] This occurs principally in salt-dependent models of experimental hypertension such as DOCA-salt hypertension or Dahl salt-sensitive rats, and in severe hypertension (Box 28–1). There appears to be little role of ETs in spontaneously hypertensive rats (SHR).[23,37] Nevertheless, in stroke-prone SHR (SHRsp), the endothelin system is activated and plays a role, particularly in salt-loaded rats,[38] or in SHRsp treated with the NO synthase inhibitor L-NAME.[39] In salt-loaded and low-renin models, hypertrophic remodeling of resistance arteries with increased cross-sectional area is found, rather than the "eutrophic" remodeling without true vascular hypertrophy more often found in essential hypertension and in SHR. This hypertrophic remodeling in hypertensive rats is shown to be ET dependent by the regression of these changes that occurs after treatment with ET antagonists.[35] Systolic BP, plasma ET, systemic oxidative stress, and vascular NADPH activity are increased in association with small-artery hypertrophic remodeling after infusion of aldosterone in place of aldosterone.[40] Increased vascular collagen, fibronectin, and intercellular adhesion molecule (ICAM-1) were decreased by ET$_A$ receptor antagonism, underlining the role of ET in these changes.

In a genetically engineered mouse that transgenically overexpresses human prepro-ET-1 in the endothelium by use of the endothelium-specific promoter Tie-2,[28] small-artery hypertrophic remodeling and endothelial dysfunction occurred despite the fact that BP was not elevated. This demonstrates the ability of ET-1 to induce BP–independent vascular remodeling.

Box 28–1

Activation of Endothelin System in Experimental Models of Hypertension

Experimental models in which endothelin system is activated
Deoxycorticosterone acetate (DOCA) salt
Spontaneously hypertensive rats-stroke prone (SHRsp)
DOCA–salt-treated SHR
Dahl salt-sensitive
Angiotensin II–infused
Female Tg Ren-2
Human Agt/human renin Tg
L-NAME–treated SHR
Fructose-fed
Streptozotocin treated
1-K, 1C Goldblatt
Chronic L-NAME induced

Experimental models in which endothelin system does not appear to be significantly activated
Tg Ren-2 (in some studies)
2-K, 1 C Goldblatt
SHR (in some studies)

Renal effects of endothelin-1 in experimental hypertension

Whereas salt loading stimulates ET-1 production, activation of renal ET_B receptors inhibits sodium reabsorption and helps to reestablish sodium balance.[41] Ang II infusion combined with high salt increased renal ET-1.[42] In transgenic rats overexpressing the ren2 gene (TGR(mRen2)27) treated with the selective ET_A receptor blocker darusentan or the ET_A/ET_B receptor antagonist LU420627,[43] BP and mortality, proteinuria and glomerulosclerosis, tubulointerstitial damage, and renal osteopontin mRNA expression were unchanged, suggesting that ET-1 does not play a role in renal damage in renin-dependent hypertension. However, in Ang II–infused mice the dual ET_A/ET_B receptor blocker bosentan partially prevented activation of the procollagen gene,[44] and rats overexpressing human angiotensinogen and human renin, which develop malignant hypertension, exhibited reduced renal and myocardial damage after treatment with bosentan.[45,46] The latter thus suggest that the endothelin system may mediate part of Ang II actions on the kidney as it does on the vasculature of Ang II–infused rats.[47] Whether ET-1 does or does not mediate actions of Ang II remains controversial.[48,49]

In salt-loaded SHRsp, in which the endothelin system is activated,[38] increased expression of ET-1 were associated with enhanced generation in the kidney of transforming growth factor (TGF)-β1, basic fibroblast growth factor (bFGF), procollagen I expression, and matrix metalloproteinase (MMP)-2 activity, and were reduced by a selective ET_A antagonist.[50] This demonstrates that ET-1 participates in renal fibrosis by initiating an inflammatory response and stimulation of growth factors.

Cardiac effects of endothelin-1 in experimental hypertension

TGF-β1 expression and collagen deposition in the heart of DOCA-salt hypertensive rats are increased, and may be prevented by ET_A blockade.[51] ET_A receptor antagonism also blocked the expression of inflammatory mediators (NFκB and adhesion molecules) and the antiapoptotic molecule X inhibitor of apoptosis peptide (xIAP).[52] Indeed, the antiapoptotic and hypertrophic actions of ET-1 on the heart were abrogated by inhibition of NFκB.[53] ROS generated by NAD(P)H oxidase and activation of MAPK contributed to ET-1's cardiac hypertrophic action.[54] The expression of ET-1 is stimulated in aldosterone-infused rats, and accordingly, ET_A receptor blockade prevented aldosterone-induced cardiac and fibrosis, which suggests that ET-1 mediates in part effects of aldosterone on the heart and blood vessels.[55,56]

Endothelin-1 in essential hypertension

In primary human hypertension, plasma concentrations of immunoreactive ET are normal in Caucasians,[57] but elevated in African Americans who have a volume-expanded low-renin form of hypertension.[58] High plasma ET levels may be related to subclinical renal dysfunction and smoking rather than hypertension.[59] However, vascular mRNA levels of prepro-ET are increased in stage

2 hypertension of the JNC 7 (Seventh Report of the Joint National Committee on Prevention, Detection, Evaluation, and Treatment of High Blood Pressure) classification[60] (Figure 28–3).

ET_A receptor antagonists caused greater vasodilatation in the forearm of hypertensive than normotensive subjects, suggesting that ET_A receptors play an important role in ET-1–dependent vascular tone in essential hypertension.[61] The ET_A antagonist BQ-123 improved the impaired vasodilation found in hypertensive patients. The ET_B blocker BQ-788 constricted forearm resistance arteries in normotensive subjects, which suggests that ET_B receptors are vasodilators in normotensive subjects.[62] BQ-788 dilated the forearm in hypertensive subjects, suggesting that ET_B receptors are vasoconstrictors in hypertensive patients.[62] An increase in vascular smooth muscle vasoconstrictor ET_B receptors has been documented in African-American hypertensive subjects.[63,64] Whereas in normotensive subjects, forearm blood flow response to BQ-123 was similar in white and black subjects, ET_A receptor blockade was a more potent vasodilator in blacks than in whites among hypertensive individuals.[65] However, ET-1 vasoconstricted equally in white and black hypertensive patients. Increased ET_A-mediated vasoconstriction may contribute to BP elevation in hypertensive blacks.

Intravenous infusion of Ang II increased BP and renal vascular resistance, and accordingly decreased renal plasma flow and glomerular filtration rate in humans, changes that were unaffected by ET_A receptor antagonism.[66] Thus, pressor responses to Ang II in humans were not mediated by ET-1, a point already discussed.[48] However, a lower BP increase or a decrease in renal blood flow and glomerular filtration with an ET_A receptor antagonist added to Ang II supports the opposite conclusion.[67]

ET-1 at concentrations of 10^{-11}mol/L may potentiate other vasoconstrictors (e.g., phenylephrine or serotonin).[68] This mechanism is under the influence of the *EDN1 K198N* polymorphism in the coding region of the prepro-ET-1 gene,[69] and could be enhanced in hypertension and contribute to BP elevation.[70]

Patients with essential hypertension, primary aldosteronism, or renovascular hypertension have enhanced ultrasound backscatter signals resulting from tissue heterogeneity in the myocardium, which correlates with plasma aldosterone and immunoreactive ET.[71] This finding suggests that as in experimental animal models, aldosterone and ET-1 contribute to myocardial fibrosis in human hypertension.[51,52,55]

Clinical trials have been performed with ET antagonists in human hypertension with the combined ET_A/ET_B antagonist bosentan and the ET_A antagonist darusentan. Bosentan lowered diastolic BP in essential hypertensive patients similarly to the ACE inhibitor enalapril.[72] Darusentan also reduced systolic BP.[73] However, bosentan may induce liver damage and liver enzyme elevation, which was not reported with darusentan.

ET receptor antagonists have not yet been approved for the treatment of essential hypertension and target organ damage associated with high BP because of side effects that include headache (an NO-related effect, therefore

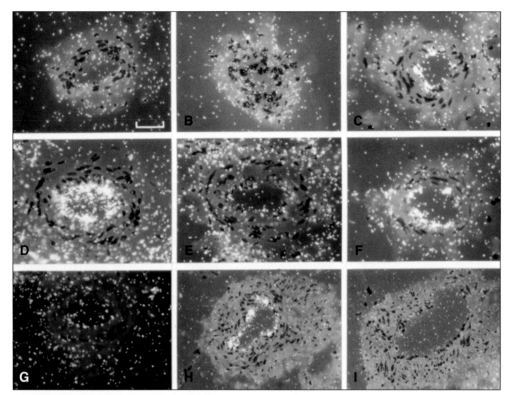

Figure 28–3. Representative microphotographs of *in situ* hybridization of gluteal subcutaneous fat biopsies from normotensive subjects, and mild and severe hypertensive patients, using human endothelin-1 cRNA probes. Original magnification of microphotographs shown was ×100, bar in *A* corresponds to 30 μm for all panels, except for panels *H* and *I*, for which original magnification was ×50, and bar in *A* represents 60 μm. **A,** Small artery from gluteal subcutaneous fat in normotensive subject. **B,** Small artery from gluteal subcutaneous fat in mild hypertensive patient. Small arteries of these subjects exhibit scant labeling when using the antisense endothelin-1 cRNA probe, similar to labeling found with the sense endothelin-1 cRNA probe (not shown). **C, D, F, H:** Small arteries from subcutaneous fat in biopsy material from severe hypertensive patients, hybridized with the endothelin-1 antisense probe, demonstrating increased density of labeling of the endothelium by specific grains. **E, G, I:** Increased density was not found with the sense endothelin-1 cRNA probe on adjacent sections of the same vessels. (From Schiffrin EL, Deng LY, Sventek P, Day R. *J Hypertens* 1997;15:57–63.)

interestingly lower in hypertensives who have impaired endothelial function than normotensives), and liver enzyme elevation, which make the use of these agents difficult in a chronic disease. However, there are ongoing trials of ET$_A$ antagonists in resistant hypertension.

MOLECULAR GENETICS OF ENDOTHELIN SYSTEM

A polymorphism (*EDN1 K198N*) in the coding region of the prepro-ET-1 gene has also been associated with hypertension in overweight individuals.[74] This is the same polymorphism associated with increased vasoreactivity.[66] *ECE1 C-388A* is a polymorphism present in the 5'-regulatory region of the ECE-1b gene that results in a binding site for the transcription factor E2F-2 and induces increased promoter activity. The A allele may raise expression of ECE-1b, with increased generation of ET-1. This polymorphism was found in untreated hypertensive German women in whom the A allele had a co-dominant effect on daytime and nighttime systolic and diastolic BP.[75] The association of BP and this polymorphism in the French epidemiologic study, Étude du Vieillissement Artériel, was found only in women,[76] suggesting that there may be a recessive effect of this variant in this cohort. The *EDN1 K198N* polymorphism of the prepro-ET-1 gene was not associated with BP values in either men or women in this study, but interacted with the *ECE1 C-338A* variant to influence systolic and mean BP levels in women. The *EDN1* variant did not correlate with BP, but the effect of the *ECE1 C-338A* variant on BP was only present in homozygous *EDN1* KK women. Stimulation of ET by androgens could explain the absence of effect in males.

SUMMARY

ET-1 is a potent vasoconstrictor that also promotes cardiac, vascular, and renal inflammation, hypertrophy, and fibrosis. ET-receptor antagonists could prevent some of the complications of hypertension, atherosclerosis, and diabetes, and it is possible that they could achieve BP-independent effects on cardiovascular pathology. However, because of side effects, their potential usefulness in hypertension, heart failure, atherosclerosis, chronic renal failure, and diabetes and other diseases cannot be currently exploited. The only approved indication to date of endothelin blockade is for the ET_A/ET_B receptor antagonist bosentan in primary pulmonary hypertension.

ACKNOWLEDGMENTS

This work was supported by the Canadian Institutes of Health Research (grant 37917 and Group Grant to Multidisciplinary Research Group on Hypertension).

REFERENCES

1. Yanagisawa M, Kurihara H, Kimura S, et al. A novel potent vasoconstrictor peptide produced by vascular endothelial cells. *Nature* 1988;332:411–5.
2. Fernandez-Patron C, Radomski MW, Davidge ST. Vascular matrix metalloproteinase-2 cleaves big endothelin-1 yielding a novel vasoconstrictor. *Circ Res* 1999;85:906–11.
3. Wagner OF, Christ G, Wojta J, et al. Polar secretion of endothelin-1 by cultured endothelial cells. *J Biol Chem* 1992;267:16066–8.
4. Valdenaire O, Lepailleur-Enouf D, Egidy G, et al. A fourth isoform of endothelin-converting enzyme (ECE-1) is generated from an additional promoter molecular cloning and characterization. *Eur J Biochem* 1999;264:341–9.
5. Muller L, Barret A, Etienne E, et al. Heterodimerization of endothelin-converting enzyme-1 isoforms regulates the subcellular distribution of this metalloprotease. *J Biol Chem* 2003;278:545–55.
6. D'Orléans-Juste P, Plante M, Honoré JC, et al. Synthesis and degradation of endothelin-1. *Can J Physiol Pharmacol* 2003;81:503–10.
7. Malek A, Izumo S. Physiological fluid shear stress causes downregulation of endothelin-1 mRNA in bovine aortic endothelium. *Am J Physiol* 1992;263:C389–96.
8. Boulanger C, Luscher TF. Release of endothelin from the porcine aorta. Inhibition by endothelium-derived nitric oxide. *J Clin Invest* 1990;85:587–90.
9. Quehenberger P, Exner M, Sunder-Plassmann R, et al. Leptin induces endothelin-1 in endothelial cells in vitro. *Circ Res* 2002;90:711–8.
10. Iglarz M, Touyz RM, Amiri F, et al. Effect of peroxisome proliferator-activated receptor-α and -γ activators on vascular remodeling in endothelin-dependent hypertension. *Arterioscl Thromb Vasc Biol* 2003;23:45–51.
11. Moreland S, McMullen DM, Delaney CL, et al. Venous smooth muscle contains vasoconstrictor ET_B-like receptors. *Biochem Biophys Res Commun* 1992;184:100–106.
12. Russell FD, Davenport AP. Characterization of endothelin receptors in the human pulmonary vasculature using bosentan, SB209670, and 97-139. *J Cardiovasc Pharmacol* 1995;26:S346–7.
13. Sato K, Oka M, Hasunuma K, et al. Effects of separate and combined ET_A and ET_B blockade on ET-1-induced constriction in perfused rat lungs. *Am J Physiol* 1995;269:L668–72.
14. Davie N, Haleen SJ, Upton PD, et al. ET(A) and ET(B)-receptors modulate the

proliferation of human pulmonary artery smooth muscle cells. *Am J Respir Crit Care Med* 2002;165:398–405.
15. Kurihara Y, Kurihara H, Suzuki H, et al. Elevated blood pressure and craniofacial abnormalities in mice deficient in endothelin-1. *Nature* 1994;368:703–10.
16. Clouthier DE, Hosoda K, Richardson JA, et al. Cranial and cardiac neural crest defects in endothelin-A receptor-deficient mice. *Development* 1998;125:813–24.
17. Hosoda K, Hammer RE, Richardson JA, et al. Targeted and natural (piebald-lethal) mutations of endothelin-B receptor gene produce megacolon associated with spotted coat color in mice. *Cell* 1994;79:1267–76.
18. Verhaar MC, Strachan FE, Newby DE, et al. Endothelin-A receptor antagonist-mediated vasodilatation is attenuated by inhibition of nitric oxide synthesis and by endothelin-B receptor blockade. *Circulation* 1998;97:752–6.
19. Goddard J, Johnston NR, Hand MF, et al. Endothelin-a receptor antagonism reduces blood pressure and increases renal blood flow in hypertension patients with chronic renal failure: a comparison of selective and combined endothelin receptor blockade. *Circulation* 2004;109:1186–93.
20. Schiffrin EL, Touyz RM. Vascular biology of endothelin. *J Cardiovasc Pharmacol* 1998;32:S2–13.
21. Ohanian J, Cunliffe P, Ceppi E, et al. Activation of p38 mitogen-activated protein kinases by endothelin and noradrenaline in small arteries, regulation by calcium influx and tyrosine kinases, and their role in contraction. *Arterioscler Thromb Vasc Biol* 2001;21:1921–7.
22. Larivière R, Thibault G, Schiffrin EL. Increased endothelin-1 content in blood vessels of deoxycorticosterone acetate-salt hypertensive but not in spontaneously hypertensive rats. *Hypertension* 1993;21:294–300.
23. Li LX, Fink GD, Watts SW, et al. Endothelin-1 increases vascular superoxide via endothelinA-NADPH oxidase pathway in low-renin hypertension. *Circulation* 2003;107:1053–8.
24. Callera GE, Touyz RM, Teixeira SA, et al. ET_A receptor blockade decreases vascular superoxide generation in DOCA-salt hypertension. *Hypertension* 2003;42:811–7.
25. Touyz RM, Schiffrin EL. Reactive oxygen species in vascular biology: implications in hypertension. *Histochem Cell Biol* 2004;122:339–52.
26. Touyz RM, Yao G, Viel E, et al. Angiotensin II and endothelin-1 regulate MAP kinases through different redox-dependent mechanisms in

human vascular smooth muscle cells. *J Hypertens* 2004;22:1141–9.
27. Viel EC, Amiri F, Touyz RM, Schiffrin EL. Evidence of mitochondrial involvement in vascular reactive oxygen species production in low-renin hypertension. *Can J Cardiol* 2004;19(Suppl. A):100D.
28. Amiri F, Virdis A, Fritsch Neves M, et al. Endothelium-restricted overexpression of human endothelin-1 causes vascular remodeling and endothelial dysfunction. *Circulation* 2004;110:2233–40.
29. Kahler J, Mendel S, Weckmuller J, et al. Oxidative stress increases synthesis of big endothelin-1 by activation of the endothelin-1 promoter. *J Mol Cell Cardiol* 2000;32:1429–37.
30. Bakker ENTP, Buus CL, VanBavel E, et al. Activation of resistance arteries with endothelin-1: From vasoconstriction to functional adaptation and remodeling. *J Vasc Res* 2004;41:174–82.
31. Buus CL, Kristensen HB, Bakker ENTP, et al. Force-independent expression of c-fos mRNA by endothelin-1 in rat intact small mesenteric arteries. *Acta Physiol Scand* 2004;181:1–11.
32. Mangelus M, Galron R, Naor Z, Sokolovsky M. Involvement of nuclear factor-kappaB in endothelin-A-receptor-induced proliferation and inhibition of apoptosis. *Cell Mol Neurobiol* 2001;21:657–74.
33. Shichiri M, Kato H, Marumo F, Hirata Y. Endothelin-1 as an autocrine/paracrine apoptosis survival factor for endothelial cells. *Hypertension* 1997;30:1198–203.
34. Diep QN, Intengan HD, Schiffrin EL. Endothelin-1 attenuates omega3 fatty acid-induced apoptosis by inhibition of caspase 3. *Hypertension* 2000;35:287–91.
35. Li JS, Larivière R, Schiffrin EL. Effect of a nonselective endothelin antagonist on vascular remodeling in deoxycorticosterone acetate-salt hypertensive rats. Evidence for a role of endothelin in vascular hypertrophy. *Hypertension* 1994;24:183–8.
36. Schiffrin EL. Endothelin: potential role in hypertension and vascular hypertrophy. *Hypertension* 1995;25:1135–43.
37. Li JS, Schiffrin EL. Effect of chronic treatment of adult spontaneously hypertensive rats with an endothelin receptor antagonist. *Hypertension* 1995;25(part 1):495–500.
38. Touyz RM, Turgeon A, Schiffrin EL. Endothelin-A-receptor blockade improves renal function and doubles the lifespan of stroke-prone spontaneously hypertensive rats. *J Cardiovasc Pharmacol* 2000;36(Suppl 1):S300–04.
39. Li JS, Deng LY, Grove K, et al. Comparison of effect of endothelin antagonism and angiotensin-converting enzyme inhibition on blood pressure and vascular structure in spontaneously

hypertensive rats treated with N^{ω}-nitro-L-arginine methyl ester. Correlation with topography of vascular endothelin-1 gene expression. *Hypertension* 1996;28:189–95.

40. Pu Q, Neves MF, Virdis A, et al. Endothelin antagonism on aldosterone-induced oxidative stress and vascular remodeling. *Hypertension* 2003;42: 49–55.

41. Plato CF, Pollock DM, Garvin JL. Endothelin inhibits thick ascending limb chloride flux via ET(B) receptor-mediated NO release. *Am J Physiol* 2000;279: F326–33.

42. Sasser JM, Pollock JS, Pollock DM. Renal endothelin in chronic angiotensin II hypertension. *Am J Physiol* 2002;283: R243–8.

43. Rothermund L, Kossmehl P, Neumayer H-H, et al. Renal damage is not improved by blockade of endothelin receptors in primary renin-dependent hypertension *J Hypertens* 2003;21: 2389–97.

44. Fakhouri F, Placier S, Ardaillou R, et al. Angiotensin II activates collagen type I gene in the renal cortex and aorta of transgenic mice through interaction with endothelin and TGF-beta. *J Am Soc Nephrol* 2001;12:2701–10.

45. Muller DN, Mervaala EM, Schmidt F, et al. Effect of bosentan on NF-kappaB, inflammation, and tissue factor in angiotensin II-induced end-organ damage. *Hypertension* 2000;36:282–90.

46. Muller DN, Mullally A, Dechend R, et al. Endothelin-converting enzyme inhibition ameliorates angiotensin II-induced cardiac damage. *Hypertension* 2002;40:840–6.

47. Rajagopalan S, Laursen JB, Borthayre A, et al. Role for endothelin-1 in angiotensin II-mediated hypertension. *Hypertension* 1997;30:29–34.

48. Schiffrin EL. The angiotensin-endothelin relationship: does it play a role in cardiovascular and renal pathophysiology? Editorial commentary. *J Hypertens* 2003;21:2245–7.

49. Li JS, Knafo L, Turgeon A, et al. Effect of endothelin antagonism on blood pressure and vascular structure in renovascular hypertensive rats. *Am J Physiol Heart Circ Physiol* 1996;40: H88–93.

50. Tostes RC, Touyz RM, He G, et al. Endothelin A receptor blockade decreases expression of growth factors and collagen and improves matrix metalloproteinase-2 activity in kidneys from stroke-prone spontaneously hypertensive rats. *J Cardiovasc Pharmacol* 2002;39:892–900.

51. Ammarguellat F, Larouche II, Schiffrin EL. Myocardial fibrosis in DOCA-salt hypertensive rats: effect of endothelin ET(A) receptor antagonism. *Circulation* 2001;103:319–24.

52. Ammarguellat FZ, Gannon PO, Amiri F, Schiffrin EL. Fibrosis, matrix metalloproteinases, and inflammation in the heart of DOCA-salt hypertensive rats: role of ET(A) receptors. *Hypertension* 2002;39:679–84.

53. Hirotani S, Otsu K, Nishida K, et al. Involvement of nuclear factor-kappaB and apoptosis signal-regulating kinase 1 in G-protein–coupled receptor agonist-induced cardiomyocyte hypertrophy. *Circulation* 2002;105:509–15.

54. Tanaka K, Honda M, Takabatake T. Redox regulation of MAPK pathways and cardiac hypertrophy in adult rat cardiac myocyte. *J Am Coll Cardiol* 2001;37:676–85.

55. Park JB, Schiffrin EL. Cardiac and vascular fibrosis and hypertrophy in aldosterone-infused rats: role of endothelin-1. *Am J Hypertens* 2002; 15:164–9.

56. Park JB, Schiffrin EL. ET(A) receptor antagonist prevents blood pressure elevation and vascular remodeling in aldosterone-infused rats. *Hypertension* 2001;37:1444–9.

57. Schiffrin EL, Thibault G. Plasma endothelin in human essential hypertension. Am *J Hypertens* 1991; 4:303–8.

58. Ergul S, Parish DC, Puett D, et al. Racial differences in plasma endothelin-1 concentrations in individuals with essential hypertension. *Hypertension* 1996;28:652–5.

59. Hirai Y, Adachi H, Fujiura Y, et al. Plasma endothelin-1 level is related to renal function and smoking status but not to blood pressure: an epidemiological study. *J Hypertens* 2004;22:713–8.

60. Schiffrin EL, Deng LY, Sventek P, Day R. Enhanced expression of endothelin-1 gene in resistance arteries in severe human essential hypertension. *J Hypertens* 1997;15:57–63.

61. Cardillo C, Kilcoyne CM, Waclawiw M, et al. Role of endothelin in the increased vascular tone of patients with essential hypertension. *Hypertension* 1999;33: 753–8.

62. Cardillo C, Campia U, Kilcoyne CM, et al. Improved endothelium-dependent vasodilation after blockade of endothelin receptors in patients with essential hypertension. *Circulation* 2002;105:452–6.

63. Ergul A, Tackett RL, Puett D. Distribution of endothelin receptors in saphenous veins of African Americans: implications of racial differences. *J Cardiovasc Pharmacol* 1999;34:327–32.

64. Grubbs AL, Anstadt MP, Ergul A. Saphenous vein endothelin system expression and activity in African American patients. *Arterioscler Thromb Vasc Biol* 2002;22:1122–7.

65. Campia U, Cardillo C, Panza JA. Ethnic differences in the vasoconstrictor activity of endogenous endothelin-1 in hypertensive patients. *Circulation* 2004;109:3191–5.

66. Bayerle-Eder M, Langenberger H, Pleiner J, et al. Endothelin ET_A receptor-subtype specific antagonism does not mitigate the acute systemic or renal effects of exogenous angiotensin II in humans. *Eur J Clin Invest* 2002;32: 230–5.

67. Montanari A, Biggi A, Carra N, et al. Endothelin-A receptors mediate renal hemodynamic effects of exogenous angiotensin ii in humans. *Hypertension* 2003;42:825–30.

68. Yang ZH, Richard V, von Segesser L, et al. Threshold concentrations of endothelin-1 potentiate contractions to norepinephrine and serotonin in human arteries. A new mechanism of vasospasm? *Circulation* 1990;2:188–95.

69. Iglarz M, Benessiano J, Philip I, et al. Preproendothelin-1 gene polymorphism is related to a change in vascular reactivity in the human mammary artery in vitro. *Hypertension* 2002;39:209–13.

70. Haynes WG, Hand MF, Johnstone HA, et al. Direct and sympathetically mediated venoconstriction in essential hypertension. Enhanced responses to endothelin-1. *J Clin Invest* 1994;94: 1359–64.

71. Kozàkovà M, Buralli S, Palombo C, et al. Myocardial ultrasonic backscatter in hypertension—relation to aldosterone and endothelin. *Hypertension* 2003;41: 230–6.

72. Krum H, Viskoper RJ, Lacourcière Y, et al. The effect of an endothelin-receptor antagonist, bosentan, on blood pressure in patients with essential hypertension. Bosentan Hypertension Investigators. *N Engl J Med* 1998;338: 784–90.

73. Nakov R, Pfarr E, Eberle S. Darusentan: an effective endothelin A receptor antagonist for treatment of hypertension. *Am J Hypertens* 2002;15:583–9.

74. Tiret L, Poirier O, Hallet V, et al. The Lys198Asn polymorphism in the endothelin-1 gene is associated with blood pressure in overweight people. *Hypertension* 1999;33:1169–74.

75. Funke-Kaiser H, Reichenberger F, Köpke K, et al. Differential binding of transcription factor E2F-2 to the endothelin-converting enzyme-1b promoter affects blood pressure regulation. *Hum Mol Genet* 2003; 12:423–33.

76. Funalot B, Courbon D, Brousseau T, et al. Genes encoding endothelin-converting enzyme-1 and endothelin-1 interact to influence blood pressure in women: the EVA study. *J Hypertens* 2004;22:739–43.

Chapter

29 Nitric Oxide

Marcela Herrera, Pablo A. Ortiz, Guillermo B. Silva, and Jeffrey L. Garvin

Definition

■ Nitric oxide (NO) is a reactive free radical produced by three gene products: NO synthase 1, 2, and 3.

Key Findings

■ Transcription and translation are differentially regulated. mRNA can be spliced alternatively.

■ The enzymes are regulated differently and have different patterns of expression in the kidney.

■ Although the half-life of NO is less than 30 seconds, it may diffuse more than 100 μm to affect processes distant from the site of production.

■ NO promotes renal excretion of salt and water and tends to lower blood pressure.

■ NO dilates renal vessels, increases glomerular filtration, inhibits salt and water absorption by the nephron, blunts pressure natriuresis, and can either inhibit or stimulate renin release.

■ Defects in production and/or actions of NO promote salt retention and contribute to salt-sensitive hypertension.

At the time of its discovery in 1980 by Furchgott and Zawadzki,[1] nitric oxide (NO) was referred to as endothelium-dependent relaxing factor. NO is a gaseous free radical, and as such is highly reactive. It is produced by a family of three different gene products originally referred to as neuronal, inducible, and endothelial NO synthase (NOS). As their names imply, neuronal NOS was first described in nervous tissue and endothelial NOS was first cloned from endothelial cells. Inducible NOS was first cloned from macrophages, and was referred to as inducible because its activity was originally thought to be regulated primarily by changes in transcription and translation rather than via allosteric modulation like the other two. With the discovery that neuronal and endothelial NOS are expressed in other tissues, and that inducible NOS can be allosterically regulated, the neuronal, inducible, and endothelial NOS isoforms are now generally referred to as NOS-1, -2, and -3, named for the order in which they were cloned.

NO is an extremely important regulator of blood pressure. Acute inhibition of NO production in animal models can increase blood pressure by more than 40 mmHg.[2] Its antihypertensive effects are due to actions on essentially every organ and tissue important to the regulation of blood pressure. NO is produced in neurons of the peripheral and central nervous systems, where it acts as a neurotransmitter.[3] It is produced by endothelial cells and diffuses to vascular smooth muscle cells, where it reduces total peripheral resistance by dilating the arteries.[4] In the heart, it acts as both a negative chronotropic and inotropic agent.[5] However, it is in the kidney where NO has perhaps its greatest and best described influences on blood pressure.

In the kidney, NO is produced by several different cell types and by various NOS isoforms. NO is produced by renal endothelial cells lining the vasculature. It can also be produced by mesangial and interstitial cells. Finally, it has been shown to be produced by the epithelial cells of nearly all segments of the nephron. NO production by each tissue is regulated by a unique set of humoral, chemical, and physical factors. In the kidney, NO can act as an autocrine or paracrine factor. Generally, renal NO induces natriuresis and diuresis through a variety of different mechanisms. However, there are instances in which the actions of NO appear contradictory, as is the case with its effects on renin release. The significance of the actions of NO in the kidney is best evidenced by the fact that inhibition of renal NO production causes salt-sensitive hypertension,[6] and defects in the production of or response to NO have been implicated in genetic models of hypertension.[7]

ANATOMY AND BIOCHEMISTRY

Nitric oxide production and regulation

The NOS family of enzymes is a group of dimeric proteins that catalyze the conversion of L-arginine and O_2 to citrulline and NO. All NOS family members contain oxygenase and reductase domains. The functional protein is a homo-dimer. Each monomer has binding sites for nicotinamide adenine dinucleotide phosphate (NADPH), flavin adenine dinucleotide (FAD), and flavin adenine mononucleotide (FMN) located in the reductase domain on the carboxy terminus. The oxygenase domain is on the amino terminus and has binding sites for L-arginine, tetrahydrobiopterin (BH_4), and iron protoporphyrin (Fe-PpIX). A calcium/calmodulin (Ca/CaM) binding site resides between the reductase and oxygenase domains (Figures 29–1 and 29–2).

Catabolism of L-arginine to citrulline and NO occurs in two cycles: mono-oxygenation I and II. L-arginine binds NOS only after dimer formation, near the BH_4 binding site and Fe-PpIX. Once L-arginine is bound, one electron

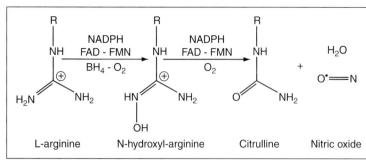

Figure 29–1. Linear order of binding domains of NOS. This is a schematic representation of NOS binding domains. In reality, they are not contiguous along the protein backbone. BH$_4$, 5,6,7,8-tetrahydrobiopterin; FAD, flavin adenine dinucleotide; FMN, flavin adenine mononucleotide; NADPH, nicotinamide adenine dinucleotide phosphate; NOS, nitric oxide synthase.

from NADPH is conducted by the FAD and FMN of one NOS monomer to the Fe^{3+}-PpIX of the second molecule of the dimer, reducing it to Fe^{2+}-PpIX. Electron transfer between NADPH and FAD/FMN requires a conformational change caused by Ca/CaM binding. Once Fe is reduced, O$_2$ then binds it, resulting in a ferric-superoxide complex. BH$_4$ donates a proton to the bound superoxide to form hydroperoxide. The hydroperoxide intermediate gains a second proton, cleaving the oxygen–oxygen bond to produce water and a ferryl-iron intermediate with a protein-bound cation radical. The cation radical is highly reactive and rapidly oxygenates arginine, resulting in N-hydroxy-L-arginine. The second round of mono-oxygenation begins with one electron from the reductase domain reducing Fe^{3+}-PpIX to Fe^{2+}-PpIX. Oxygen again binds to Fe, generating a ferrous-oxy complex that deprotonates N-hydroxy-L-arginine. The results are a hydroperoxy complex and a radical, arginine-O$^{.}$. After conformational rearrangement of unstable intermediates, NO and H$_2$O are generated and the oxygen atom originally bound to N-hydroxy-L-arginine is reduced, producing citrulline. Conformational changes occurring during the degradation

of unstable intermediates and the rearrangement of the atoms in order to produce NO, H$_2$O and citrulline also lead to re-oxidation of Fe-PpIX (Figure 29–3).

Under some circumstances, NOS can produce superoxide instead of NO. This is referred to as the "superoxide shunt." Superoxide production occurs in NOS mono-oxygenation I when the NOS dimer is not formed due to lack of cofactors needed for its formation and stability, such as BH$_4$. Superoxide formation by NOS is commonly called "NOS uncoupling."[8,9]

The activity of the various NOS isoforms can be regulated by post-translational modifications. These include phosphorylation, protein–protein interactions, and acylation. Phosphorylation may increase or decrease NOS activity by inducing conformational changes that affect the binding of cofactors, substrates, and protein regulators. These conformational changes may also increase or decrease the rate of electron transfer. Each of the NOS isoforms can be phosphorylated at different sites.

NOS-1 was originally shown to be phosphorylated by cAMP-dependent protein kinase, but changes in enzyme activity were not reported.[10] Subsequently it was shown that NOS-1 could be phosphorylated by Ca/CaM-dependent kinase isoforms Iα, IIα, and IV at serine position 847 (Ser[847]). In rat suprachiasmatic nuclei, NOS-1 phosphorylation causes activity to increase.[11] However, studies with a recombinant enzyme showed a decrease in activity when NOS-1 is phosphorylated at this site.[12] The explanation for this discrepancy is unclear. NOS-1 can also be phosphorylated at Ser[741] by Ca/CaM-dependent kinase I, which will inhibit enzyme activity.[13]

Scant information is available regarding NOS-2 phosphorylation. A study using phosphotyrosine antibodies in Raw 264.7 cells showed that after induction with LPS and interferon γ, NOS-2 is phosphorylated at tyrosine residues[14]; however, the effect on activity was not studied.

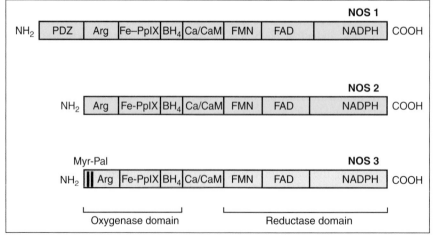

Figure 29–2. Generation of NO from L-arginine. Arg, L-arginine; BH$_4$, 5,6,7,8-tetrahydrobiopterin; Ca/CaM, calcium/calmodulin; FAD, flavin adenine dinucleotide; Fe-PpIX, iron protoporphyrin IX; FMN, flavin adenine mononucleotide; NADPH, nicotinamide adenine dinucleotide phosphate; NOS, nitric oxide synthase.

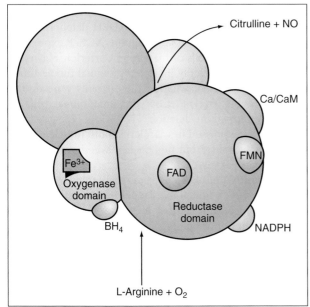

Figure 29–3. The functional NOS complex. Dimer formation is required for NOS activity. BH$_4$, 5,6,7,8-tetrahydrobiopterin; Ca/CaM, calcium/calmodulin; FAD, flavin adenine dinucleotide; Fe^{3+}, iron protoporphyrin IX; FMN, flavin adenine mononucleotide; NADPH, nicotinamide adenine dinucleotide phosphate; NOS, nitric oxide synthase.

The lack of data concerning NOS-2 phosphorylation may be a result of NOS-2 being regulated primarily by transcription and translation.

Phosphorylation is a major regulator of NOS-3 activity. Protein kinase B,[15,16] Ca/CaM-dependent kinase II,[17] and cAMP- and cGMP-dependent protein kinases[18,19] can phosphorylate NOS-3. All of these kinases have been shown to phosphorylate Ser[1177]; however, phosphorylation of this amino acid under physiologic circumstances is due primarily to activation of protein kinase B. Phosphorylation of Ser[1177] enhances NO production by increasing the affinity of the Ca/CaM binding site.[15] Under some circumstances, Ser[633] can also be phosphorylated by cAMP- and cGMP-dependent protein kinases.[18] This is also a positive regulatory site. In contrast, when Thr[495] is phosphorylated by protein kinase C[20] or AMP kinase, enzyme activity decreases and superoxide production may increase.[17,21] NOS-3 can also be phosphorylated at Ser[114]. This region of the enzyme contains a consensus sequence for ERK1/2 that may function as a switch between NO and superoxide production. However, this conclusion is based primarily on the proximity of the phosphorylation site to the BH$_4$ binding site.[22,23] Finally, phosphorylation of Ser[615] increases Ca/CaM affinity without altering maximum enzymatic activity.[24]

Our current understanding of NOS phosphorylation indicates that it is an important physiologic regulator of enzyme activity. As such, it is necessary to keep in mind that not only kinase but phosphatase activity is important for this process. Additionally, when considering the impact of phosphorylation/dephosphorylation of a given amino acid in any of the NOS family members, one must consider that the measured effect is a consequence of not only the phosphorylation of interest, but the state of other potential phosphorylation sites and interactions with regulatory proteins.

In addition to phosphorylation, NOS activity can be enhanced or diminished by interactions with other proteins. The first such interaction to be reported was binding of Ca/CaM. Ca/CaM is necessary for activation of NOS due to its induction of allosteric changes that modify the kinetics of the electron transfer in the flavin domains.[25] Originally, only the so-called constitutive NOS family members 1 and 3 were thought to bind Ca/CaM. However, it is now recognized that, in fact, NOS-1 and -3 have a significantly lower affinity for Ca/CaM than NOS-2. Consequently, an increase in intracellular Ca is required to elevate Ca/CaM concentrations sufficiently to bind NOS-1 and -3, and factors that change intracellular calcium levels are important regulators of NOS-1 and -3 activity.

In addition to Ca/CaM, NOS-1 binds a number of other proteins that alter its activity. Several studies demonstrated that heat shock protein 90 (HSP90), a multiclient chaperone protein, binds NOS-1, and that formation of the NOS-1-HSP90 complex increases NO production.[26] HSP90 may also increase NOS-1-Ca/CaM binding, thereby increasing NOS-1 function.[27] NOS-1 also binds proteins that inhibit its activity, including the membrane-scaffolding protein caveolin-3.[28] NOS-1 activity is regulated by the so-called protein inhibitor of NOS (PIN), which is expressed in the endothelial cells of the glomeruli, vasa recta, and luminal membranes of collecting ducts.[29,30] NOSIP (nitric oxide synthase interacting protein) co-localizes with NOS-1 and has recently been found to help regulate the activity and distribution of NOS-1. Studies both *in vitro* and *in vivo* show that NOS-1–NOSIP interaction decreases NOS-1 activity.[31,32]

Finally, NOS-1 interacts with a number of proteins whose effects on activity are unclear, primarily via PDZ domains. PSD-93, CAPON, and PSD-95 are proteins with PDZ domains that are reportedly associated with or serve as linkers in protein complexes with NOS-1.[33] In the macula densa, PSD-93 and NOS-1 have been found to be co-localized, presumably due to interactions of PDZ domains.[34]

Similar to NOS-1, NOS-2 interacts with a number of other proteins. NAP-10 is a protein expressed in macrophages that prevents dimerization of NOS-2 by binding to the amino terminal close to the active site. Interaction of NAP-10 and NOS-2 is thought to blunt NO production during inflammation. Kalirin also prevents NOS-2 dimerization.[35] Caveolin-1 binds to NOS-2, inducing proteolysis and decreased activity,[36] and caveolin-3 has a similar effect.[37] In apical membranes of proximal tubule cells, NOS-2 binds to EBP-50, possibly serving as an anchor to direct NO production in the regulation of ion transport.[38] PIN also binds NOS-2 and inhibits its activity as it does with other NOS family members, but this effect is small compared to its effect on NOS-1 or NOS-3.[39] Localization of NOS-2 within the cell is regulated by binding of Rac 1/2; however, they do not inhibit NOS-2 activity and in fact may play a role in its activation.[33,40]

NOS-3 activity is also regulated through a number of protein–protein interactions. HSP90 is involved in NOS-3 activation and translocation in endothelial cells[41] and thick ascending limbs[42] in the kidney. HSP90 interacts with Akt and NOS-3, forming a ternary complex that facilitates NOS-3 phosphorylation and thus increases its activity.[43,44] NOS-3 also binds dynamin-2, a GTPase that interacts with the FAD domain of NOS-3, enhancing electron transfer and NO production. Dynamin-2 is also involved in the correct targeting of NOS-3 to caveolin-enriched fractions in endothelial cells.[45,46]

In endothelial cells, but not thick ascending limb cells, NOS-3 binds caveolin-1, and this interaction inhibits NO production. However, when NOS-3 binds Ca/CaM, NOS-3 is released from caveolin-1.[47] Caveolin-3 has similar inhibitory properties.[37] NOS-3 activity is also suppressed when it forms a complex with NOSIP. NOSIP binds to the carboxy terminal region of NOS-3, inducing translocation from the plasma membrane to the cytoskeleton, and in the process inhibiting NO production. NOSIP is expressed in the kidney.[48] NOSTRIN, a NOS trafficking inducer, is also involved in NOS-3 translocation. This is a cytoskeleton-related protein that induces NOS-3 subcellular redistribution. Overexpression of NOSTRIN triggers NOS-3 redistribution and decreases NOS-3 activity.[49] Finally, *in vitro* studies demonstrate that in addition to NOS-1, PIN can also bind NOS-3 and disrupt its dimerization and L-arginine binding.[39]

NOS-3 is the only isoform known to contain acylation sites. Palmitic acid and myristic acid can be reversibly and irreversibly added, respectively.[9,50] There are two palmitoylation sites at Cys^{15} and Cys^{26}, but only one site for mirystoylation on an N-terminal glycine.[9] Both acylations are necessary for the trafficking and membrane binding of NOS-3.[51]

Nitric oxide synthase localization

Localization of specific NOS isoforms can be controversial, and one must exercise caution when judging published results. For instance, immunohistochemistry may not be sensitive enough to detect low levels of expression. In contrast, reverse transcriptase-polymerase chain reaction (RT-PCR) may detect a protein mRNA that has such a low copy number that it has no physiologic significance. Both antibodies and inhibitors may not be as selective as anticipated, or selectivity may change under certain conditions. Studies *in vivo* and *in situ* using knockout mice may be confounded by systemic effects of genetically deleting the protein of interest, or changes in physiology that mitigate the effect of the knockout. In the end, use of multiple techniques is required before one can state with any certainty whether a tissue expresses a given NOS isoform.

NOS-1 is distributed in a wide variety of tissues. It is expressed in both central and peripheral nerves and in the heart. In the kidney, NOS-1 is located in the neuronal somata of ganglionic nerves located around the interlobular artery and the wall of the renal pelvis, as well as the corresponding postganglionic fibers.[52] mRNA and immunocytochemical studies have shown that NOS-1 is expressed in principal cells of the collecting duct, but not

in intercalated cells.[53] It has also been found in the macula densa using several techniques. NADPH diaphorase and immunohistochemical assays support NOS-1 expression in the endothelial cells of the efferent arteriole.[54] Knockout of NOS-1 reportedly inhibited proximal tubule transport, but it is unclear whether these results were due to deletion of the enzyme from proximal tubule cells or systemic effects of the deletion.[55] NOS-1 has likewise been shown to be expressed in vascular smooth muscle cells of mesenteric vessels,[56] but it is unclear whether this is also true of renal vessels.[54]

NOS-2 mRNA has been detected in all tubular segments of the kidney.[57] Functional experiments using NOS-2 knockout mice indicate that NOS-2 is expressed in the proximal nephron,[58] but its physiologic significance in this segment is unclear because disparate effects have been reported.[59] mRNA for NOS-2 has been found in the outer medullary thick ascending limb,[57] but functional studies showed that inhibiting NOS-2 had no effect on NaCl absorption.[60] NOS-2 has also been found in the inner medulla by Western blot, but it is not clear which cell type(s) in this region was responsible. In the vasculature, significant amounts of NOS-2 have been detected in renal smooth muscle cells from patients with chronic allograft nephropathy,[61] but this is likely attributable to induction of the enzyme as the result of the disease.

NOS-3 is present in the endothelial cells along the entire vascular tree of the kidney, including the renal artery, interlobar artery, arcuate artery, afferent and efferent arterioles, glomerular capillaries, and vasa recta.[54] NOS-3 is also expressed in the proximal tubule, thick ascending limb, distal convoluted tubule, and collecting duct.[62]

GENETICS

NOS-1, -2, and -3 are encoded by different genes with a conserved sequence of 80% to 90% across various mammalian species. There is also strong similarity in the sequence and gene structure between the three NOS isoforms in terms of exon size and location of the intronic splice junctions. Despite these similarities in gene structure, transcriptional control of each NOS isoform is different and occurs in a cell- and tissue-specific manner, allowing specificity for NO signaling in physiologic and pathologic conditions.

The human NOS-1 gene has been mapped to chromosome 12, whereas homologous genes in the rat and mouse have been mapped to chromosome 12 and 5, respectively. Besides neuronal cells, NOS-1 is also expressed in the skeletal muscle, lung, kidney, testis, penis, and adrenal and pituitary glands. Its expression is regulated by a variety of physiologic stimuli such as oxygen tension and cellular stress as well as several hormones and neurotransmitters. However, regulation of NOS-1 expression is cell type-specific and extremely complex due to transcriptional variants of the NOS-1 gene as described below.

The human NOS-1 gene is present as a single copy in the human genome and is scattered over a region of approximately 200 kb. Potential sites for transcription factors upstream from the NOS-1 gene include AP-2, transcriptional enhancer factor-1/M-CAT binding factor, CREB, cFOS, Ets, nuclear factor-1, and NFκβ. The nucleotide sequence coding for the most abundant neuronal transcript is encoded in 29 exons, and the full open reading-frame codes for a protein of 1434 amino acids with a predicted mass of 161 kDa. This full-length (1–1434) NOS variant is usually called NOS-1α.

In addition to NOS-1α, multiple mRNA transcripts for NOS have been reported. They are produced by three different mechanisms: (1) use of multiple promoters and 5′ transcription start sites, (2) alternative splicing, and (3) use of alternative polyadenylation signals in exon 29. Alternative promoters in the various exon 1's result in different mRNAs containing alternative 5′ untranslated regions with varying translational efficiency. However, since all possible exon 1's are spliced to the same exon 2, only one protein is transcribed.

Alternative mRNA splicing of NOS-1 transcripts produces four splice variants called NOS-1-β, -γ, -μ and -2. In mice, alternative splicing of exon 2 produces the N-terminal truncated NOS-1 variants β (amino acids 236–1434) and γ (amino acids 336–1434) that lack the PDZ binding domain. In humans, an mRNA transcript similar to mouse NOS-1γ has been detected exclusively in testis Leydig cells, where its function is unknown. NOS-1μ is an extended splice variant detected in humans, rats, and mice that contains a 34–amino-acid insertion between the calmodulin- and flavin-binding domains. This splice variant is most highly expressed in skeletal muscle and the heart. Its kinetic parameters for NO production are similar to NOS-1α, but it has two important differences. First, the μ variant is degraded more slowly than NOS-1α, and it has a lower rate of NADPH oxidation.[63] Another NOS-1 alternative splice variant (NOS 1-2) has been detected in the mouse brain. This variant contains a 105–amino-acid in-frame deletion of residues 504–608. An opposing functional role of NOS-1 and NOS-1-2 has been proposed in morphine analgesia in mice. Finally, the human NOS-1 exon 29 contains three potential polyadenylation sites; however, the effect of these 3′-end variations on transcription of NOS-1 mRNA is unknown.

NOS-2 was originally cloned from mouse macrophages and from human macrophages and chondrocytes. The NOS-2 gene consists of 27 exons spanning a 40 kb genomic region located on human chromosome 17. The translation start codon is located on exon 2 and the stop codon on exon 27. The nucleotide sequence is 85% to 90% homologous among humans, rats, and mice. As an inducible enzyme, NOS-2 expression is tightly controlled at the transcriptional level by means of promoter regulation. It is also regulated by the stability of its mRNA.

In most cells, NOS-2 is induced by bacterial lipopolysaccharides (LPS) and cytokines such as interferon-γ and interleukins 1β and 6 among others. The NOS-2 promoter contains a TATA box 30 bp upstream from the transcription start site. The NOS-2 promoter contains binding sites for the transcription factors NF-κβ, IL6, activating protein-1 (AP-1), CCAAT-enhancer box binding protein/ EBP, cAMP-responsive element binding protein (CREB), interferon regulatory factor-1 (IRF-1), serum response factor (SRF), octamer factor-1 (Oct-1), and STAT 1α. Recent data indicate that NOS-2 promoter activity is inhibited under basal conditions by hypermethylation, which would explain the low basal expression of NOS-2 in most cells.

In addition to transcriptional regulation by promoter activation, NOS-2 expression is controlled by mRNA stability. Sequence analysis of NOS-2 mRNA showed that four sequence motifs (AUUUA) in the 3′-untranslated region confer destabilization of NOS-2 mRNA. Several RNA-binding proteins have been identified that bind the 3′ untranslated region of NOS-2 mRNA. Interaction of NOS-2 mRNA with some RNA-binding proteins, such as the embryonic lethal abnormal vision protein HuR, increases mRNA stability and augments cytokine-induced expression. In contrast, binding of NOS-2 mRNA to other proteins, such as hnRNP/AUF-1, decreases mRNA stability and diminishes NOS-2 expression. Since the discovery that NOS-2 mRNA stability plays a role in regulating expression, the number of proteins that bind the 3′ untranslated region of NOS-2 mRNA has grown steadily. Some new proteins of this family include tristetraprolin, the T-cell–restricted intracellular antigen-1–like (TIAR) protein, KH-type, splicing regulatory protein (KSRP), and the poly A tract binding protein (PABP).

Similar to NOS-1, the NOS-2 gene is also subject to alternative splicing. Alternative splice variants of NOS-2 mRNA have been detected in humans, rats, and mice. In addition, alternative splicing produces mRNA variants with deletions corresponding to exon 5; exons 8 and 9 ($_{8–9\ del}$); exons 9, 10, and 11 ($_{9–10–11\ del}$); and exons 15 and 16 ($_{15–16\ del}$).[64] The physiologic role of most of these NOS-2 variants is still unknown. The only variant studied in detail is NOS-2 $_{(-8–9)}$, which codes for a monomeric protein that does not produce NO, but retains NADPH diaphorase activity when expressed in cultured cells.[65] Recently a new splicing variant lacking exon 14 (NOS-2 $_{14del}$) has been detected in human B lymphocytes.[66]

NOS-3 was originally cloned from vascular endothelial cells. This enzyme is constitutively expressed in the vasculature and in many cell types including epithelial cells, cardiac and smooth muscle cells, fibroblasts, hepatocytes, platelets, lymphocytes, and some neuronal cells among others. The human NOS-3 mRNA is encoded by 26 exons spanning 22 kb of genomic DNA. The gene is present as a single copy in the human genome and has been localized to chromosome 7. Full-length NOS-3 cDNA encodes for a predicted 133-kDa protein. The nucleotide sequence for the NOS-3 gene is 90% conserved across mammalian species, with greater conservation (95%) in the amino acid sequence.

One important characteristic of the NOS-3 gene is that it is highly polymorphic. Single nucleotide polymorphisms have been observed in various vascular diseases ranging from hypertension to atherosclerosis and metabolic syndrome. The best-studied polymorphism is NOS-3 Glu298Asp, which appears to influence the blood pressure response to exercise. This variant is also associated with endothelial function and may be involved during the adaptive vascular changes of pregnancy, such that carriers of NOS-3 Asp298 may be at risk of developing preeclampsia. Most studies show that intact NOS-3 Asp298 has equivalent enzymatic activity to NOS-3 Glu298, but in some cells it undergoes selective proteolysis, increasing protein turnover rate and reducing active NOS-3. In addition, carriers of NOS-3 Asp298 may be at increased risk of developing atherosclerosis and cerebrovascular disease.

NOS-3 expression is regulated in a cell-type specific manner by a large array of physiologic factors; among the most important are shear stress, hypoxia, cell proliferation, estrogens, lipoproteins, glucose, angiotensin II, and cAMP. Analysis of the 5′-region indicates that the NOS-3 promoter does not have a TATA box, but shows proximal promoter elements of constitutively expressed genes like Sp1 and GATA binding motifs. It also contains consensus sequences for binding of transcription factors AP-1, AP-2, NF-1, nuclear factor IL6, NFκβ, PEA-3, heavy metal, shear stress, CREB, and sterol-regulatory *cis*-elements. In addition to promoter activity, NOS-3 expression is regulated by mRNA stability. For example, NOS-3 mRNA levels are approximately four- to six-fold higher in proliferating than in growth-arrested endothelial cells, a difference that cannot be explained by varying transcription rates. Hypoxia and cytokines, such as TNF, downregulate eNOS mRNA levels by decreasing the half-life of eNOS mRNA. NOS-3 mRNA half-life is regulated by a process involving the induction and expression of at least two cytosolic proteins (51 kDa and 60 kDa) that bind to a C-rich region within the 3′-untranslated region of NOS-3 mRNA. To date, there are no known alternative splice variants of NOS-3. However, polyadenyl 3′ tails of different lengths in NOS-3 mRNA have recently been shown in endothelial cells, where they affect mRNA stability and mediate the fast regulation of NOS-3 expression by shear stress.

PHYSIOLOGY AND PATHOPHYSIOLOGY

Nitric oxide produced within the kidney by the three NOS isoforms regulates many physiologic processes. Endothelial, epithelial, and other cells in the kidney can generate NO. Once produced, NO can act as either an autocrine or paracrine factor, regulating vascular tone, ion and solute transport along the nephron, pressure natriuresis, and tubuloglomerular feedback.[67–71] Because NO produced by different NOS isoforms has the same physiologic effect on all processes studied thus far (with the exception of renin release), it is easier to discuss the actions of NO according to physiologic effect rather than the isoform responsible for its production.

Renal vasculature

NOS-3, the endothelial isoform of NOS, is expressed in the glomerular arterioles as well as in the vasa recta, where it is functionally active and produces NO.[72] Increased luminal flow is the primary stimulator of NOS-3 in vascular endothelial cells.[71] Luminal flow activates phosphatidyl-inositol 3-OH kinase, although the exact mechanism is unknown. This enzyme generates phosphatidylinositol 3,4,5 trisphosphate, enhancing activity of phosphatidyl-inositol-dependent kinase, which in turn phosphorylates and stimulates protein kinase B. Protein kinase B then

phosphorylates and activates NOS-3. NO produced by NOS-3 in the endothelium of the afferent and efferent arterioles, the major resistance vessels in the kidney, diffuses to the vascular smooth muscle cells where it activates guanylate cyclase. This leads to generation of cGMP and activation of cGMP-dependent protein kinase I. cGMP-dependent protein kinase I phosphorylates inositol 1,4,5 triphosphate-receptor–associated protein kinase I substrate (IRAG) located at the endoplasmic reticulum membrane. cGMP-dependent phosphorylation of IRAG inhibits calcium release into the cytoplasm, decreasing intracellular calcium.[73] This decrease in calcium inactivates calcium-dependent myosin light chain (MLC) kinase and induces dephosphorylation of MLC by myosin phosphatase 1. Moreover, cGMP diminishes the sensitivity of the contractile machinery to calcium.[74]

In addition to NOS-3, NOS-1 may also regulate vascular tone in the kidney. NOS-1 is reportedly expressed in the endothelial cells of the efferent arteriole, but its functional significance is unknown. NOS-1 is also present in vascular smooth muscle cells of mesenteric resistance vessels, where it produces NO and directly affects vascular tone in an endothelium-independent fashion,[75] but it is unclear whether this occurs in the renal vasculature as well. NO-dependent vasodilatation increases blood flow to the glomeruli, which tends to raise the glomerular filtration rate.

NO production within the renal vasculature can be stimulated under physiologic situations by many factors. Systemic and intrarenal administration of the arginine analogues that inhibit NO production increased renal vascular resistance by 30% to 50%.[76] In addition, infusion of NO donors in the presence of NOS inhibition restored renal blood flow.[77] Thus *in vivo* and *in vitro* data from various species indicate that basal release of NO helps maintain the relative low vascular resistance that characterizes the renal circulation.[76] In addition to vascular NOS-3, NO can be produced by other structures located close to vascular cells, such as the tubular epithelium, and it is possible that NO produced by these structures also affects renal vascular tone.

In addition to NOS-3–derived NO, NO generated in the macula densa by NOS-1, the neuronal isoform of NOS, helps control glomerular hemodynamics via tubuloglomerular feedback and modulation of renin release.[78–80] Tubuloglomerular feedback is an important regulator of renal hemodynamics. When NaCl concentration in the lumen of the distal nephron rises, resistance of the afferent arteriole increases while resistance of the efferent arteriole decreases, a phenomenon known as tubuloglomerular feedback. This results in decreased glomerular filtration and increased sodium retention. Tubuloglomerular feedback starts at the macula densa. The macula densa plaque senses changes in luminal NaCl concentration via activation of luminal Na/K/2 Cl co-transport, setting in motion a number of signaling events that result in basolateral release of ATP and constriction of afferent arteriole diameter.[81,82] Increases in luminal NaCl also initiate a cascade that limits the magnitude of tubuloglomerular feedback. Increased NaCl enhances Na/H exchange in the macula densa, which raises intracellular pH. This in turn stimulates NOS-1 activity.[83] NO produced by NOS-1 in the macula densa attenuates tubuloglomerular feedback by increasing cGMP, activating cGMP-dependent protein kinase and inhibiting Na/K/2 Cl co-transport.[84]

The renin-angiotensin-aldosterone system plays an important role in blood pressure stabilization and electrolyte and fluid homeostasis. Angiotensin increases total peripheral resistance, reduces renal blood flow, enhances tubuloglomerular feedback and augments salt and water absorption primarily by the proximal nephron, while at the same time aldosterone increases salt absorption primarily by the distal nephron. The activity of the renin-angiotensin-aldosterone system in the circulation is mainly dependent on the protease renin, which is produced in the kidney by the juxtaglomerular granular cells. Their release of renin is influenced by NO produced by both NOS-3 from the afferent arteriole and NOS-1 from macula densa cells.[85,86]

The regulation of renin release is a unique case in which NO produced by different enzymes appears to have different effects on a physiologic process. Recent data suggest that the actions of NO on renin release depend critically on intracellular cAMP concentrations in the juxtaglomerular cells and thus the signaling cascades activated.[86] NO derived from the endothelial cells of the vasculature inhibits renin release via activation of soluble guanylate cyclase and cGMP-dependent kinase II. In contrast, NO derived from macula densa NOS-1 is thought to stimulate renin secretion via inhibition of phosphodiesterase 3 (which cleaves cAMP), increases in cAMP levels, and reductions in intracellular calcium (renin release is stimulated by reductions in calcium similar to parathyroid hormone). Whether the stimulatory or inhibitory effect of NO predominates is thought to depend on factors that alter intracellular cAMP or factors that stimulate cAMP, such as sympathetic nerve activity or prostaglandin production. However, additional research is required to fully understand how NO is involved in the regulation of renin release as well as its mechanisms of action.

Nephron transport

In addition to its actions in the renal vasculature, NO can induce natriuresis and diuresis without altering renal blood flow or glomerular filtration, suggesting that it regulates sodium and water reabsorption by the nephron.[69] NOS has been found in most tubular segments, implying that it can act as an autacoid to influence salt and water transport. However, NO produced by surrounding structures, such as the vasculature, can potentially affect transport as well.

In the proximal tubule, the data regarding the effect of NO on transport are controversial, with reports of inhibitory, stimulatory, and biphasic effects. *In vitro* and cell culture experiments have shown that NO inhibits both Na/H exchange (the primary route of Na entry into proximal tubule cells) and Na/K ATPase (the primary route of exit). In contrast, *in vivo* micropuncture experiments using knockout and wild-type mice and NOS inhibitors[58,87] indicate that NO acting as either an autocrine or paracrine factor stimulates transport in this segment. While

the resolution of these issues is uncertain, the micropuncture experiments may have been confounded by systemic effects of the knockout and effects of the inhibitors on surrounding tissues.

In the thick ascending limb, NO exogenously added by NO donors or produced endogenously inhibits NaCl absorption. This inhibition on its own would be expected to increase not only Na excretion but also urinary volume, due to reduction of the corticomedullary osmotic gradient. Suppression of net NaCl absorption is due to inhibition of Na entry via luminal Na/K/2 Cl co-transport and Na/H exchange. Na exit via Na/K ATPase does not appear to be affected. Reduction of both Na/K/2 Cl co-transport and Na/H exchange occurs via activation of soluble guanylate cyclase and increases in cGMP. However, the former is due to activation of cGMP-stimulated phosphodiesterase II, which in turn decreases cAMP levels, whereas the latter occurs via activation of cGMP-dependent protein kinase.[69] The NOS isoform responsible for producing NO in the thick ascending limb is NOS-3. L-arginine, the substrate for NOS, inhibits NaCl absorption by thick ascending limbs from wild-type, NOS-2 and NOS-1 knockout mice but not from NOS-3 knockout mice.[60] Furthermore, when NOS-3 is restored in thick ascending limbs from NOS-3 knockout mice, inhibition by L-arginine is also restored.[88] Acutely, NO production by this segment can be stimulated by factors that enhance NO production in endothelial cells, including endothelin, alpha 2 adrenergic agonists, and luminal flow.

Although NO has been reported to enhance luminal K channel activity, and K recycling across the luminal membrane is necessary for net NaCl absorption, the effect of NO on luminal K channels in the thick ascending limb does not result in enhanced NaCl absorption. The explanation may be that (1) actions of NO on K channel activity were measured by patch clamp, which does not take into account the full measure of cellular processes that may regulate an individual transporter; and/or (2) direct inhibition of luminal Na/K/2 Cl co-transport by NO may overwhelm the small stimulatory effect produced by activation of K channels.

In the collecting duct, exogenously added NO inhibits basal Na absorption and arginine vasopressin-stimulated sodium and water absorption. These actions on their own would tend to cause natriuresis and diuresis. As with the thick ascending limb, the effects of NO in the collecting duct are mediated via activation of cGMP-dependent protein kinase and cGMP-stimulated phosphodiesterase. Stimulation of these cGMP-dependent enzymes decreases both cAMP levels and cAMP-dependent protein kinase activity. Although NOS is highly expressed in the collecting duct, the contribution of endogenously produced NO within this segment to regulation of transport has not been elucidated to our knowledge.[69]

Pressure natriuresis

Pressure natriuresis is a process whereby increases in renal perfusion pressure result in enhanced Na excretion. A number of paracrine and/or autocrine factors have been suggested as mediators of pressure natriuresis, including

NO. Administration of NO synthase inhibitors via the renal artery suppresses pressure natriuresis.[89] Experiments in dogs have confirmed that there is a direct relationship between changes in arterial pressure and intrarenal NO activity as measured with NO-sensitive microelectrodes inserted in the cortical tissue. Changes in arterial pressure induced parallel alterations in intrarenal NO activity that correlated positively with the changes in sodium excretion rates.[90] Pretreatment with a NOS inhibitor decreased pressure natriuresis, and infusion of an NO donor reversed this process. However, although sodium excretion was enhanced by an NO donor, it failed to restore the slope of the curve relating arterial pressure to sodium excretion.[77] These data suggest that not only does NO at least partially mediate pressure natriuresis, but that changes in NO release accompany changes in pressure and that NO release is not static.

The site of action of NO in mediating pressure natriuresis is not clear. Originally, pressure natriuresis was thought to be due to inhibition of sodium transport in the distal nephron. This theory was supported by data showing that amiloride, an inhibitor of collecting duct sodium absorption, could prevent pressure natriuresis.[91] However, recent data indicate that pressure natriuresis may be due to inhibition of sodium absorption by the proximal tubule. Acute increases in renal perfusion pressure have been shown to inhibit Na/H exchange activity in this nephron segment, due to physical relocation of the transport proteins to the base of the brush-border microvilli.[92] However, there is general agreement that acute changes in arterial pressure alter intrarenal NO production, which inhibits tubular sodium reabsorption and causes pressure natriuresis.

Although NO is known to mediate pressure natriuresis, as far as we know the source(s) of NO have not been determined, nor precisely how the signal of increased perfusion pressure is translated into enhanced NO production. Although it is tempting to suggest that increases in flow through the renal vasculature accelerate NO production by NOS-3 in the endothelium, this seems unlikely. The kidney displays exquisite autoregulation of blood flow, indeed increasing renal perfusion pressure from 70 to 140 mmHg does not significantly increase renal blood flow due to heightened resistance of the afferent arteriole. It should be recognized, however, that this argument does not indicate that NOS-3 is not involved, only that luminal flow is not likely the signal for its activation. While the specific signaling mechanisms that lead to increased NO production are unclear, increases in renal perfusion pressure cause small changes in interstitial hydrostatic pressure (on the order of 4 to 5 mmHg). If the renal capsule is removed, increases in perfusion pressure no longer increase interstitial pressure and pressure natriuresis no longer occurs. How small changes in interstitial pressure lead to enhanced NO release is unknown.

Effect of high-salt intake on renal nitric oxide

The renal NO system is up-regulated in animals fed large amounts of salt, promoting sodium and water excretion. The importance of NO in maintaining blood pressure in the face of a high-salt diet is best evidenced by the fact that intrarenal infusion of L-NAME, a nonselective NOS inhibitor, causes hypertension in rats on high salt.[6] Expression of all three NOS isoforms is enhanced by high salt in the renal medulla, but they do not promote natriuresis equally. Conflicting reports concerning NOS-1 have been published. In one study selective inhibition of this enzyme caused salt-sensitive hypertension, while in another it did not. NOS-2 activity does not appear to be necessary for blood pressure homeostasis when animals are given high salt. Although these data suggest that NOS-3 is critical to promoting salt excretion when animals are on high salt, NOS-3 knockout mice are only very modestly salt-sensitive, if at all. However, this could be explained by adaptive mechanisms mitigating the effects of NOS-3 knockout.

The mechanism whereby high salt increases NOS expression has recently been delineated, but only for a single nephron segment. In the thick ascending limb, high salt increases NOS-3 expression and NO production.[93,94] The increase in NOS-3 expression is mediated via increases in medullary osmolality and release of endothelin-1 and activation of ET_B receptors on thick ascending limb cells.[95] In support of this, renal ET-1 production is augmented in parallel with sodium intake.[96] In addition, blockade of ET_B receptors leads to hypertension when rats are fed a high-salt diet, and ET_B-deficient rats display salt-sensitive hypertension. Studies in ET_B-deficient rats showed that the increase in renal NOS activity caused by high salt was diminished.[97]

Although NOS expression is enhanced by a high-salt diet, one cannot necessarily assume that this leads to sustained increases in NO production. In fact, the effect of salt on NOS expression is transient even though animals remain normotensive.[94] Furthermore, NO production declines faster than NOS expression.[94] Such data suggest that the response to a given amount of NO may be enhanced at later times.[93,94]

Hypertension

Defects in the renal NO system are associated with several models of experimental hypertension. This is not surprising because, by definition, pressure natriuresis must be shifted in order to maintain a hypertensive state, and it is at least partially mediated by NO. As discussed above, inhibition of renal NO production causes salt-sensitive hypertension. Defects in the response to or production of NO in the kidney also play a role in a genetic model of salt sensitivity, the Dahl salt-sensitive rat. The defect that causes hypertension in the Dahl rat has been localized to the kidney by cross-transplantation studies. When a kidney from a salt-sensitive animal was placed in a salt-resistant rat, it became salt-sensitive (and *vice versa*).[98] The renal defect appears to lie in the loop of Henle, because these rats display abnormal NaCl absorption by the loop of Henle, which includes the thick ascending limb and pressure natriuresis. L-arginine supplementation reduces blood pressure and restores pressure natriuresis to normal levels.[99]

Basal sodium reabsorption is enhanced in thick ascending limbs of Dahl salt-sensitive rats compared to normotensive salt-resistant controls. This is at least partially due to the fact that inhibition of sodium transport in response to NO is decreased in this segment.[100] Originally the reduced effects of NO in this model were attributed to decreased production of NO. However, linkage studies between blood pressure and NOS have been difficult to reproduce. Furthermore, recent data indicate that enhanced oxidative stress in this model may be responsible for decreased NO bioavailability. Scavengers of reactive oxygen species have been shown to blunt salt-sensitive hypertension significantly in this model.[101]

In the spontaneously hypertensive rat (SHR), NO production is normal or even increased. In this model, NO bioavailability within the kidney is reduced. The diminished actions of NO in this model have been studied primarily with regard to tubuloglomerular feedback and macula densa NO. Tubuloglomerular feedback is enhanced in SHR, but so is NOS-1 expression in the macula densa. However, when scavengers of O_2^- are infused, tubuloglomerular feedback is reduced in SHR but not in normotensive Wistar-Kyoto rats. Infusion of tempol, a superoxide dismutase mimetic, dramatically reduces blood pressure in SHR. These data suggest that increased renal oxidative stress is present in this model and blunts the effects of NO. Similar mechanisms may be involved in diabetes-induced hypertension.[102]

Pregnancy

Glomerular filtration rate and renal plasma flow are both increased by 50% to 60% during normal pregnancy via the vasoactive peptide endothelin-1, which, acting through ET_B receptors in the kidney, activates NOS to increase NO. Moreover, the hormone relaxin has recently been implicated in this mechanism. Relaxin is secreted by the corpus luteum during pregnancy and enhances metalloprotease activity, thus increasing cleavage of big endothelin to endothelin. Recent studies suggest that NO deficiency in pregnant rats may contribute to the pathogenesis of preeclampsia, in which renal plasma flow and glomerular filtration rate are decreased compared to normal pregnancy. Promoting NO production by administering L-arginine is known to attenuate pregnancy-induced hypertension.[103] This may be due to effects on the kidney, because large increases in NO that enhance renal blood flow occur during normal pregnancy.[104–106] The primary dysfunction in preeclampsia is a relative deficiency of available NO (secondary to oxidative degradation) and an excess of peroxynitrite ($ONOO^-$),[107] which together can directly or indirectly initiate the vast majority of physiologic and serologic changes associated with preeclampsia, such as increased blood pressure and glomerular filtration rate and proteinuria.

CLINICAL IMPLICATIONS AND PERSPECTIVES

The potential for the renal actions of NO to have great significance in human hypertension is clearly supported by an extensive literature based on experimental models. Human studies, although not as invasive (and therefore not as direct) as animal studies, show that the major actions of NO on renal function reported for animal models are also true in humans. L-arginine infusion decreases renal vascular resistance and increases glomerular filtration rate in normal subjects.[108] L-arginine infusion can increase urinary volume and sodium excretion without significant changes in glomerular filtration rate,[109] while inhibition of NO production decreases fractional sodium excretion.[110] Taken together, these data indicate that NO can directly inhibit sodium absorption along the nephron. Additionally, changes in the production or actions of NO are part of the adaptation to a high-salt diet.[111]

NO has also been shown to play a significant role in the development of human hypertension, and there is an extensive literature on this subject. However, while this is also true for NO in the kidney, the literature is not as extensive. This is partly due to the fact that the systemic actions of NO confound interpretation of the results, making it difficult if not impossible to study many aspects of renal function noninvasively.

In many forms of hypertension, NO production, bioavailability, or action is reduced in the systemic vasculature. NO production can be reduced by defects in the NOS enzyme, lack of cofactors, or insufficient substrate. Bioavailability can be reduced by increases in oxidative stress, while the actions of NO can be blunted by defects in signaling cascades. To date, all of the data concerning human hypertension associated with defects in the NO system involve either decreases in production or bioavailability.

L-arginine has been shown to decrease renal vascular resistance more dramatically in patients with essential hypertension than normotensive patients, while causing the same decrement in systemic vascular resistance. Thus either production of NO in the kidney at normal circulating L-arginine levels is deficient in essential hypertension[112] or else bioavailability of the NO that is produced is reduced. L-arginine infusion has been shown to increase urinary volume and sodium excretion with only modest changes in glomerular filtration rate in offspring from normotensive parents; however, these effects are mitigated in individuals with a family history of hypertension.[109] Such effects may be due to decreased NO production, because at least a subgroup of patients with essential hypertension has been shown to have decreased renal NO production.[113]

One of the more interesting developments in the field of renal NO and blood pressure regulation has been the discovery of natural circulating NOS inhibitors such as asymmetric dimethylarginine (ADMA). Acute infusion of ADMA in human volunteers can decrease urinary sodium excretion and increase renal vascular resistance via reductions in cGMP without changes in blood pressure.[114] These data suggest that NO produced in the kidney has similar functions in humans to those in animals, and that renal function may be more dependent on NO than cardiovascular function in general. Data showing that ADMA increases filtration fraction similar to L-NAME while decreasing urinary sodium excretion indicate that NO directly inhibits salt absorption along the nephron.[115] Thus the renal actions of ADMA may at least partially account for the hypertension seen in elderly patients with elevated ADMA.[116]

SUMMARY

NO is a highly reactive free radical produced by a family of enzymes, NOS-1, -2, and -3. NO production is regulated through both changes in enzyme expression and post-translational modifications. The latter include phosphorylation, interaction with other proteins, and acylation. NO production depends on a number of cofactors, including NADPH, FAD, FMN, BH$_4$, and Ca/CaM. L-arginine is the substrate for NO generation, producing citrulline in the same process. NO affects many physiologic processes in essentially all organs; however, its effects on the kidney have the greatest impact on regulation of blood pressure. Renal actions of NO include dilatation of the renal vasculature, inhibition of salt and water absorption along the nephron, and blunting of tubuloglomerular feedback. Renin release may either be inhibited or stimulated by NO depending on the conditions involved. Reductions in the production, bioavailability, or actions of NO have been shown to promote hypertension in both animal models and humans. Although we have come a long way in our understanding of the cardiovascular and renal actions of NO, a number of important questions remain.

REFERENCES

1. Furchgott RF, Zawadzki JV. The obligatory role of endothelial cells in the relaxation of arterial smooth muscle by acetylcholine. *Nature* 1980;288:373–6.
2. Lahera V, Salom MG, Miranda-Guardiola F, et al. Effects of NG-nitro-L-arginine methyl ester on renal function and blood pressure. *Am J Physiol* 1991;261:F1033–7.
3. Ott SR, Delago A, Elphick MR. An evolutionarily conserved mechanism for sensitization of soluble guanylyl cyclase reveals extensive nitric oxide-mediated upregulation of cyclic GMP in insect brain. *Eur J Neurosci* 2004; 20:1231–44.
4. Snyder SH, Bredt DS. Nitric oxide as a neuronal messenger. *Trends Pharmacol Sci* 1991;12:125–8.
5. Moncada S, Higgs EA. Endogenous nitric oxide: physiology, pathology and clinical relevance. *Eur J Clin Invest* 1991;21:361–74.
6. Salazar FJ, Alberola A, Pinilla JM, et al. Salt-induced increase in arterial pressure during nitric oxide synthesis inhibition. *Hypertension* 1993;22:49–55.
7. Ying WZ, Sanders PW. Dietary salt enhances glomerular endothelial nitric oxide synthase through TGF-beta1. *Am J Physiol* 1998;275:F18–24.
8. Alderton WK, Cooper CE, Knowles RG. Nitric oxide synthases: structure, function and inhibition. *Biochem J* 2001;357:593–615.
9. Govers R, Rabelink TJ. Cellular regulation of endothelial nitric oxide synthase. *Am J Physiol Renal Physiol* 2001;280:F193–206.
10. Brune B, Lapetina EG. Phosphorylation of nitric oxide synthase by protein kinase A. *Biochem Biophys Res Commun* 1991;181:921–6.
11. Hayashi Y, Nishio M, Naito Y, et al. Regulation of neuronal nitric-oxide synthase by calmodulin kinases. *J Biol Chem* 1999;274:20597–602.
12. Agostino PV, Ferreyra GA, Murad AD, et al. Diurnal, circadian and photic regulation of calcium/calmodulin-dependent kinase II and neuronal nitric oxide synthase in the hamster suprachiasmatic nuclei. *Neurochem Int* 2004;44:617–25.

13. Song T, Hatano N, Horii M, et al. Calcium/calmodulin-dependent protein kinase I inhibits neuronal nitric-oxide synthase activity through serine 741 phosphorylation. *FEBS Lett* 2004;570:133–7.
14. Pan J, Burgher KL, Szczepanik AM, Ringheim GE. Tyrosine phosphorylation of inducible nitric oxide synthase: implications for potential post-translational regulation. *Biochem J* 1996;314:889–94.
15. Dimmeler S, Fleming I, Fisslthaler B, et al. Activation of nitric oxide synthase in endothelial cells by Akt-dependent phosphorylation. *Nature* 1999; 399:601–5.
16. Fulton D, Gratton JP, McCabe TJ, et al. Regulation of endothelium-derived nitric oxide production by the protein kinase Akt. *Nature* 1999;399:597–601.
17. Fleming I, Fisslthaler B, Dimmeler S, et al. Phosphorylation of Thr(495) regulates Ca(2+)/calmodulin-dependent endothelial nitric oxide synthase activity. *Circ Res* 2001;88:E68–75.
18. Butt E, Bernhardt M, Smolenski A, et al. Endothelial nitric-oxide synthase (type III) is activated and becomes calcium independent upon phosphorylation by cyclic nucleotide-dependent protein kinases. *J Biol Chem* 2000;275:5179–87.
19. Chen ZP, Mitchelhill KI, Michell BJ, et al. AMP-activated protein kinase phosphorylation of endothelial NO synthase. *FEBS Lett* 1999;443:285–9.
20. Michell BJ, Chen Z, Tiganis T, et al. Coordinated control of endothelial nitric-oxide synthase phosphorylation by protein kinase C and the cAMP-dependent protein kinase. *J Biol Chem* 2001;276:17625–8.
21. Lin MI, Fulton D, Babbitt R, et al. Phosphorylation of threonine 497 in endothelial nitric-oxide synthase coordinates the coupling of L-arginine metabolism to efficient nitric oxide production. *J Biol Chem* 2003; 278:44719–26.
22. Fleming I, Busse R. Molecular mechanisms involved in the regulation of the endothelial nitric oxide synthase. *Am J Physiol Regul Integr Comp Physiol* 2003;284:R1–12.

23. Fulton D, Gratton JP, Sessa WC. Post-translational control of endothelial nitric oxide synthase: why isn't calcium/calmodulin enough? *J Pharmacol Exp Ther* 2001;299:818–24.
24. Michell BJ, Harris MB, Chen ZP, et al. Identification of regulatory sites of phosphorylation of the bovine endothelial nitric-oxide synthase at serine 617 and serine 635. *J Biol Chem* 2002;277:42344–51.
25. Lauf PK, McManus TJ, Haas M, et al. Physiology and biophysics of chloride and cation co-transport across cell membranes. *Fed Proc* 1987; 46:2377–94.
26. Bender AT, Silverstein AM, Demady DR, et al. Neuronal nitric-oxide synthase is regulated by the Hsp90-based chaperone system in vivo. *J Biol Chem* 1999;274:1472–8.
27. Song Y, Zweier JL, Xia Y. Heat-shock protein 90 augments neuronal nitric oxide synthase activity by enhancing Ca2+/calmodulin binding. *Biochem J* 2001;355:357–60.
28. Venema VJ, Ju H, Zou R, Venema RC. Interaction of neuronal nitric-oxide synthase with caveolin-3 in skeletal muscle. Identification of a novel caveolin scaffolding/inhibitory domain. *J Biol Chem* 1997;272:28187–90.
29. Jaffrey SR, Snyder SH. PIN: an associated protein inhibitor of neuronal nitric oxide synthase. *Science* 1996;274:774–7.
30. Roczniak A, Levine DZ, Burns KD. Localization of protein inhibitor of neuronal nitric oxide synthase in rat kidney. *Am J Physiol Renal Physiol* 2000;278:F702–7.
31. Dreyer J, Schleicher M, Tappe A, et al. Nitric oxide synthase (NOS)-interacting protein interacts with neuronal NOS and regulates its distribution and activity. *J Neurosci* 2004;24:10454–65.
32. Dreyer J, Hirlinger D, Muller-Esterl W, et al. Spinal upregulation of the nitric oxide synthase-interacting protein NOSIP in a rat model of inflammatory pain. *Neurosci Lett* 2003;350:13–6.
33. Kone BC, Kuncewicz T, Zhang W, Yu ZY. Protein interactions with nitric oxide synthases: controlling the right

time, the right place, and the right amount of nitric oxide. *Am J Physiol Renal Physiol* 2003;285:F178–90.

34. Tojo A, Bredt DS, Wilcox CS. Distribution of postsynaptic density proteins in rat kidney: relationship to neuronal nitric oxide synthase. *Kidney Int* 1999;55:1384–94.

35. Ratovitski EA, Alam MR, Quick RA, et al. Kalirin inhibition of inducible nitric-oxide synthase. *J Biol Chem* 1999;274:993–9.

36. Felley-Bosco E, Bender FC, Courjault-Gautier F, et al. Caveolin-1 down-regulates inducible nitric oxide synthase via the proteasome pathway in human colon carcinoma cells. *Proc Natl Acad Sci U S A* 2000;19; 97:14334–9.

37. Garcia-Cardena G, Martasek P, Masters BS, et al. Dissecting the interaction between nitric oxide synthase (NOS) and caveolin. Functional significance of the nos caveolin binding domain in vivo. *J Biol Chem* 1997;272:25437–40.

38. Glynne PA, Darling KE, Picot J, Evans TJ. Epithelial inducible nitric-oxide synthase is an apical EBP50-binding protein that directs vectorial nitric oxide output. *J Biol Chem* 2002; 277:33132–8.

39. Hemmens B, Woschitz S, Pitters E, et al. The protein inhibitor of neuronal nitric oxide synthase (PIN): characterization of its action on pure nitric oxide synthases. *FEBS Lett* 1998;430:397–400.

40. Kuncewicz T, Balakrishnan P, Snuggs MB, Kone BC. Specific association of nitric oxide synthase-2 with Rac isoforms in activated murine macrophages. *Am J Physiol Renal Physiol* 2001;281:F326–36.

41. Garcia-Cardena G, Fan R, Shah V, Sorrentino R, Cirino G, Papapetropoulos A, et al. Dynamic activation of endothelial nitric oxide synthase by Hsp90. *Nature* 1998; 392:821–4.

42. Ortiz PA, Hong NJ, Garvin JL. Luminal flow induces eNOS activation and translocation in the rat thick ascending limb. II. Role of PI3-kinase and Hsp90. *Am J Physiol Renal Physiol* 2004; 287:F281–8.

43. Fontana J, Fulton D, Chen Y, et al. Domain mapping studies reveal that the M domain of hsp90 serves as a molecular scaffold to regulate Akt-dependent phosphorylation of endothelial nitric oxide synthase and NO release. *Circ Res* 2002;90:866–73.

44. Sato S, Fujita N, Tsuruo T. Modulation of Akt kinase activity by binding to Hsp90. *Proc Natl Acad Sci U S A* 2000; 97:10832–7.

45. Chatterjee S, Cao S, Peterson TE, et al. Inhibition of GTP-dependent vesicle trafficking impairs internalization of plasmalemmal eNOS and cellular nitric oxide production. *J Cell Sci* 2003; 116:3645–55.

46. Cao S, Yao J, Shah V. The proline-rich domain of dynamin-2 is responsible for dynamin-dependent in vitro potentiation of endothelial nitric-oxide synthase activity via selective effects on reductase domain function. *J Biol Chem* 2003;278:5894–901.

47. Gratton JP, Fontana J, O'Connor DS, et al. Reconstitution of an endothelial nitric-oxide synthase (eNOS), hsp90,

and caveolin-1 complex in vitro. Evidence that hsp90 facilitates calmodulin stimulated displacement of eNOS from caveolin-1. *J Biol Chem* 2000;275:22268–72.

48. Dedio J, Konig P, Wohlfart P, et al. NOSIP, a novel modulator of endothelial nitric oxide synthase activity. *FASEB J* 2001;15:79–89.

49. Zimmermann K, Opitz N, Dedio J, et al. NOSTRIN: a protein modulating nitric oxide release and subcellular distribution of endothelial nitric oxide synthase. *Proc Natl Acad Sci U S A* 2002;99:17167–72.

50. Ortiz PA, Garvin JL. Trafficking and activation of eNOS in epithelial cells. *Acta Physiol Scand* 2003;179:107–14.

51. Liu J, Garcia-Cardena G, Sessa WC. Biosynthesis and palmitoylation of endothelial nitric oxide synthase: mutagenesis of palmitoylation sites, cysteines-15 and/or -26, argues against depalmitoylation-induced translocation of the enzyme. *Biochemistry (Mosc)* 1995; 34:12333–40.

52. Liu L, Liu GL, Barajas L. Distribution of nitric oxide synthase-containing ganglionic neuronal somata and postganglionic fibers in the rat kidney. *J Comp Neurol* 1996;369:16–30.

53. Wang X, Lu M, Gao Y, et al. Neuronal nitric oxide synthase is expressed in principal cell of collecting duct. *Am J Physiol* 1998;275:F395–9.

54. Bachmann S, Bosse HM, Mundel P. Topography of nitric oxide synthesis by localizing constitutive NO synthases in mammalian kidney. *Am J Physiol* 1995;268:F885–98.

55. Wang T, Inglis FM, Kalb RG. Defective fluid and HCO(3)(-) absorption in proximal tubule of neuronal nitric oxide synthase-knockout mice. *Am J Physiol Renal Fluid Electrol Physiol* 2000;279:F518–24.

56. Briones AM, Alonso MJ, Marin J, et al. Influence of hypertension on nitric oxide synthase expression and vascular effects of lipopolysaccharide in rat mesenteric arteries. *Br J Pharmacol* 2000;131:185–94.

57. Morrissey JJ, McCracken R, Kaneto H, et al. Location of an inducible nitric oxide synthase mRNA in the normal kidney. *Kidney Int* 1994;45:998–1005.

58. Wang T. Role of iNOS and eNOS in modulating proximal tubule transport and acid-base balance. *Am J Physiol Renal Fluid Electrol Physiol* 2002; 283:F658–62.

59. Wu XC, Harris PJ, Johns EJ. Nitric oxide and renal nerve-mediated proximal tubular reabsorption in normotensive and hypertensive rats. *Am J Physiol* 1999;277:F560–6.

60. Plato CF, Shesely EG, Garvin JL. eNOS mediates L-arginine–induced inhibition of thick ascending limb chloride flux. *Hypertension* 2000;35:319–23.

61. Romagnani P, Pupilli C, Lasagni L, et al. Inducible nitric oxide synthase expression in vascular and glomerular structures of human chronic allograft nephropathy. *J Pathol* 1999; 187:345–50.

62. Terada Y, Tomita K, Nonoguchi H, Marumo F. Polymerase chain reaction localization of constitutive nitric oxide synthase and soluble guanylate cyclase

messenger RNAs in microdissected rat nephron segments. *J Clin Invest* 1992; 90:659–65.

63. Laine R, de Montellano PR. Neuronal nitric oxide synthase isoforms alpha and mu are closely related calpain-sensitive proteins. *Mol Pharmacol* 1998;54:305–12.

64. Eissa NT, Strauss AJ, Haggerty CM, et al. Alternative splicing of human inducible nitric-oxide synthase mRNA. Tissue-specific regulation and induction by cytokines. *J Biol Chem* 1996; 271:27184–7.

65. Eissa NT, Yuan JW, Haggerty CM, et al. Cloning and characterization of human inducible nitric oxide synthase splice variants: a domain, encoded by exons 8 and 9, is critical for dimerization. *Proc Natl Acad Sci U S A* 1998;95:7625–30.

66. Tiscornia AC, Cayota A, Landoni AI, et al. Post-transcriptional regulation of inducible nitric oxide synthase in chronic lymphocytic leukemia B cells in pro- and antiapoptotic culture conditions. *Leukemia* 2004;18:48–56.

67. Navar LG, Inscho EW, Majid SA, et al. Paracrine regulation of the renal microcirculation. *Physiol Rev* 1996; 76:425–536.

68. Kone BC, Baylis C. Biosynthesis and homeostatic roles of nitric oxide in the normal kidney. *Am J Physiol* 1997; 272:F561–78.

69. Ortiz PA, Garvin JL. Role of nitric oxide in the regulation of nephron transport. *Am J Physiol Renal Physiol* 2002;282: F777–84.

70. Manning RD, Jr., Hu L. Nitric oxide regulates renal hemodynamics and urinary sodium excretion in dogs. *Hypertension* 1994;23:619–25.

71. Juncos LA, Garvin J, Carretero OA, Ito S. Flow modulates myogenic responses in isolated microperfused rabbit afferent arterioles via endothelium-derived nitric oxide. *J Clin Invest* 1995;95:2741–8.

72. Good DW. The thick ascending limb as a site of renal bicarbonate reabsorption. *Semin Nephrol* 1993; 13:225–35.

73. Ren Y, Arima S, Carretero OA, Ito S. Possible role of adenosine in macula densa control of glomerular hemodynamics. *Kidney Int* 2002; 61:169–76.

74. Nishimura J, van Breemen C. Direct regulation of smooth muscle contractile elements by second messengers. *Biochem Biophys Res Commun* 1989;163:929–35.

75. Sullivan JC, Giulumian AD, Pollock DM, et al. Functional NOS 1 in the rat mesenteric arterial bed. *Am J Physiol Heart Circ Physiol* 2002;283: H658–63.

76. Majid DS, Navar LG. Nitric oxide in the control of renal hemodynamics and excretory function. *Am J Hypertens* 2001;14:74S–82S.

77. Majid DS, Williams A, Kadowitz PJ, Navar LG. Renal responses to intra-arterial administration of nitric oxide donor in dogs. *Hypertension* 1993; 22:535–41.

78. Ren YL, Garvin JL, Ito S, Carretero OA. Role of neuronal nitric oxide synthase in the macula densa. *Kidney Int* 2001; 60:1676–83.

79. Beierwaltes WH. Macula densa stimulation of renin is reversed by selective inhibition of neuronal nitric oxide synthase. *Am J Physiol* 1997; 272:R1359–64.

80. Beierwaltes WH. Selective neuronal nitric oxide synthase inhibition blocks furosemide-stimulated renin secretion in vivo. *Am J Physiol* 1995;269:F134–9.

81. Schnermann J, Traynor T, Yang T, et al. Tubuloglomerular feedback: new concepts and developments. *Kidney Int Suppl* 1998;67:S40–5.

82. Bell PD. Luminal and cellular mechanisms for the mediation of tubuloglomerular feedback responses. *Kidney Int Suppl* 1982;12:S97–103.

83. Liu R, Carretero O, Ren YL, Garvin J. Increased intracellular pH at the macula densa activates nNOS during tubuloglomerular feedback. *Kidney Int* 2005;67:1837–43.

84. Kovacs G, Komlosi P, Fuson A, et al. Neuronal nitric oxide synthase: its role and regulation in macula densa cells. *J Am Soc Nephrol* 2003;14:2475–83.

85. Wagner C, Kurtz A. Regulation of renal renin release. *Curr Opin Nephrol Hypertens* 1998;7:437–41.

86. Sayago CM, Beierwaltes WH. Nitric oxide synthase and cGMP-mediated stimulation of renin secretion. *Am J Physiol Regul Integr Comp Physiol* 2001;281:R1146–51.

87. Wang T, Inglis FM, Kalb RG. Defective fluid and HCO(3)(-) absorption in proximal tubule of neuronal nitric oxide synthase-knockout mice. *Am J Physiol Renal Physiol* 2000;279: F518–24.

88. Ortiz PA, Hong NJ, Wang D, Garvin JL. Gene transfer of eNOS to the thick ascending limb of eNOS-KO mice restores the effects of L-arginine on NaCl absorption. *Hypertension* 2003; 42:674–9.

89. Majid DS, Williams A, Navar LG. Inhibition of nitric oxide synthesis attenuates pressure-induced natriuretic responses in anesthetized dogs. *Am J Physiol* 1993;264:F79–87.

90. Majid DS, Omoro SA, Chin SY, Navar LG. Intrarenal nitric oxide activity and pressure natriuresis in anesthetized dogs. *Hypertension* 1998;32:266–72.

91. Majid DS, Navar LG. Nitric oxide in the mediation of pressure natriuresis. *Clin Exp Pharmacol Physiol* 1997; 24:595–9.

92. Yang L, Leong PK, Chen JO, et al. Acute hypertension provokes internalization of proximal tubule NHE3 without inhibition of transport activity. *Am J Physiol Renal Physiol* 2002;282:F730–40.

93. Ortiz P, Stoos BA, Hong NJ, et al. High-salt diet increases sensitivity to NO and eNOS expression but not NO production in THALs. *Hypertension* 2003;41:682–7.

94. Herrera M, Garvin J. A high-salt diet dissociates NOS3 expression and NO production in the THAL. *Hypertension* 2006;47:95–101.

95. Herrera M, Garvin JL. A high-salt diet stimulates thick ascending limb eNOS expression by raising medullary osmolality and increasing release of endothelin-1. *Am J Physiol Renal Physiol* 2005;288:F58–64.

96. Sasser JM, Pollock JS, Pollock DM. Renal endothelin in chronic angiotensin II hypertension. *Am J Physiol Regul Integr Comp Physiol* 2002;283:R243–8.

97. Taylor TA, Gariepy CE, Pollock DM, Pollock JS. Gender differences in ET and NOS systems in ETB receptor-deficient rats: effect of a high salt diet. *Hypertension* 2003;41:657–62.

98. Dahl LK, Heine M. Primary role of renal homografts in setting chronic blood pressure levels in rats. *Circ Res* 1975;36:692–6.

99. Miyata N, Zou AP, Mattson DL, Cowley AW, Jr. Renal medullary interstitial infusion of L-arginine prevents hypertension in Dahl salt-sensitive rats. *Am J Physiol* 1998; 275:R1667–73.

100. Garcia NH, Plato CF, Stoos BA, Garvin JL. Nitric oxide-induced inhibition of transport by thick ascending limbs from Dahl salt-sensitive rats. *Hypertension* 1999; 34:508–13.

101. Manning RD Jr, Tian N, Meng S. Oxidative stress and antioxidant treatment in hypertension and the associated renal damage. *Am J Nephrol* 2005;25:311–7.

102. Dixon LJ, Hughes SM, Rooney K, et al. Increased superoxide production in hypertensive patients with diabetes mellitus: role of nitric oxide synthase. *Am J Hypertens* 2005;18:839–43.

103. Alexander BT, Llinas MT, Kruckeberg WC, Granger JP. L-arginine attenuates hypertension in pregnant rats with reduced uterine perfusion pressure. *Hypertension* 2004;43:832–6.

104. Alexander BT, Miller MT, Kassab S, et al. Differential expression of renal nitric oxide synthase isoforms during pregnancy in rats. *Hypertension* 1999; 33:435–9.

105. Sladek SM, Magness RR, Conrad KP. Nitric oxide and pregnancy. *Am J Physiol* 1997;272:R441–63.

106. Kassab S, Miller MT, Hester R, et al. Systemic hemodynamics and regional blood flow during chronic nitric oxide synthesis inhibition in pregnant rats. *Hypertension* 1998;31:315–20.

107. Granger JP, Alexander BT, Bennett WA, Khalil RA. Pathophysiology of pregnancy-induced hypertension. *Am J Hypertens* 2001;14:178S–185S.

108. Delles C, Jacobi J, Schlaich MP, John S, Schmieder RE. Assessment of endothelial function of the renal vasculature in human subjects. *Am J Hypertens* 2002;15:3–9.

109. Herlitz H, Jungersten LU, Wikstrand J, Widgren BR. Effect of L-arginine infusion in normotensive subjects with and without a family history of hypertension. *Kidney Int* 1999; 56:1838–45.

110. Haynes WG, Hand MF, Dockrell ME, et al. Physiological role of nitric oxide in regulation of renal function in humans. *Am J Physiol Renal Physiol* 1997;272:F364–71.

111. Barba G, Vallance PJ, Strazzullo P, MacAllister RJ. Effects of sodium intake on the pressor and renal responses to nitric oxide synthesis inhibition in normotensive individuals with different sodium sensitivity. *J Hypertens* 2000; 18:615–21.

112. Van Den Meiracker AH, van der Linde NA, Broere A, et al. Effects of L-arginine and L-NAME on the renal function in hypertensive and normotensive subjects. *Nephron* 2002;91:444–51.

113. Sierra M, Gonzalez A, Gomez-Alamillo C, et al. Decreased excretion of nitrate and nitrite in essential hypertensives with renal vasoconstriction. *Kidney Int Suppl* 1998;68:S10–3.

114. Kielstein JT, Simmel S, Bode-Boger SM, et al. Subpressor dose asymmetric dimethylarginine modulates renal function in humans through nitric oxide synthase inhibition. *Kidney Blood Press Res* 2004;27:143–7.

115. Kielstein JT, Impraim B, Simmel S, et al. Cardiovascular effects of systemic nitric oxide synthase inhibition with asymmetrical dimethylarginine in humans. *Circulation* 2004;109:172–7.

116. Kielstein JT, Bode-Boger SM, Frolich JC, et al. Asymmetric dimethylarginine, blood pressure, and renal perfusion in elderly subjects. *Circulation* 2003; 107:1891–5.

Chapter

30

Reactive Oxygen Species, Oxidative Stress, and Vascular Biology in Hypertension

Fatiha Tabet and Rhian M. Touyz

Definition

■ Reactive oxygen species (ROS) act as signaling molecules that play an important role in vascular (patho)biology.

Key Findings

■ All vascular cell types produce ROS, primarily via membrane-associated non-phagocytic NAD(P)H oxidase. Xanthine oxidase, uncoupled endothelial nitric oxide synthase, and mitochondrial enzymes also contribute to ROS generation in the vessel wall.

■ Since ROS are highly reactive biomolecules, the cellular redox state is carefully regulated by antioxidant systems to prevent the deleterious consequences of ROS excess. When this redox balance is perturbed, oxidants stress is increased in the vessel wall and, if not offset, vascular dysfunction and damage occurs. Factors that activate pro-oxidant enzymes remain poorly defined, but likely involve angiotensin II, mechanical stretch, and inflammatory cytokines.

■ ROS influence vascular function and structure by modulating cell growth, contraction/dilation and inflammatory responses, via redox-dependent signaling pathways. These processes are critically involved in cardiovascular pathologies and contribute to vascular remodeling associated with arteriosclerosis, diabetes and hypertension.

■ Oxidative stress has been demonstrated in experimental and human hypertension.

Clinical Implications

■ Therapies targeted against free radicals, by decreasing ROS generation and/or by increasing antioxidants, may be useful in minimizing vascular injury, and thereby preventing or regressing hypertension-associated target-organ damage.

Reactive oxygen species (ROS), such as superoxide anion ($\bullet O_2^-$), hydrogen peroxide (H_2O_2), hydroxyl anion (OH–), nitric oxide (NO), and peroxynitrite (ONOO–) are ubiquitous reactive derivatives of O_2 metabolism found in the environment and in all biological systems.[1] To protect against potentially damaging effects of ROS, cells possess several antioxidant enzyme systems, including superoxide dismutase (SOD) (which reduces $\bullet O_2^-$ to H_2O_2), catalase, and glutathione peroxidase (which reduces H_2O_2 to H_2O)[2,3] (Figure 30–1). Oxidative stress is defined as an imbalance between oxidant production and antioxidant capacity, and has been implicated in the vascular damage associated with

cardiovascular pathologies, such as atherosclerosis, diabetes, and hypertension.[4,5]

In the vasculature, ROS are produced primarily by non-phagocytic NAD(P)H oxidase. This enzyme is regulated by vasoactive peptides, such as angiotensin II (Ang II), growth factors, cytokines, and mechanical forces.[6,7] Vascular ROS can also be derived from mitochondrial enzymes, xanthine oxidase, nitric oxide synthase (NOS), cyclooxygenase, lipooxygenase, and heme oxygenases.[8] All vascular cell types, including endothelial, smooth muscle, and adventitial cells, produce ROS.[6,7,9–11] ROS act as intercellular and intracellular messengers that play an important (patho)physiologic role in vascular biology.[4,5] Under pathologic conditions associated with oxidative stress, increased ROS production leads to endothelial dysfunction, increased contractility, vascular smooth muscle cell (VSMC) growth and apoptosis, monocyte migration, lipid peroxidation, inflammation, and increased deposition of extracellular matrix proteins, all processes that are critically important in vascular changes associated with hypertension[12,13] (Figure 30–2).

Convincing evidence from experimental studies and clinical investigations indicates that oxidative stress is involved in the pathogenesis of many cardiovascular diseases including hypertension. In experimental models of hypertension, production of cardiac, renal, neural, and vascular ROS is increased.[14–16] In human hypertension, plasma and urine levels of thiobarbituric acid–reactive substances (TBARS) and 8-epi-isoprostane, markers of systemic oxidative stress, are elevated.[17,18] Furthermore, clinical studies have indicated that NAD(P)H oxidase activity/expression is increased, and antioxidant enzyme capacity is decreased in hypertensive patients.[19,20] The present chapter focuses on the importance of ROS in vascular (patho)biology and highlights the role of vascular oxidative stress in the development of hypertension. It should be stressed that the cardiac, renal, endocrine and nervous systems important in the pathogenesis of hypertension are also major targets for oxidative damage by ROS. However, these systems will not be discussed here, and the reader is referred to excellent reviews on these systems.[21]

VASCULAR PRODUCTION OF REACTIVE OXYGEN SPECIES

Although there are many pro-oxidant enzyme systems that can produce ROS in the vessel wall, four enzymes seem to predominate: non-phagocytic NAD(P)H oxidase,

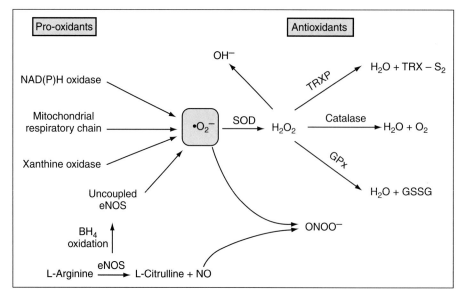

Figure 30–1. Pro-oxidant and antioxidant enzyme systems in the vessel wall. NAD(P)H oxidase is the primary source of vascular reactive oxygen species (ROS), although xanthine oxidase, mitochondrial enzymes, and uncoupled eNOS also play a role, particularly in pathologic conditions. Major enzymatic defense mechanisms against ROS accumulation are GPx, catalase, TRXP, and SOD. ROS are able to scavenge endothelium-derived NO to form ONOO-, and thereby contribute to impaired endothelium-dependent vasodilation. eNOS, nitric oxide synthase; GPx, glutathione peroxidase; NO, nitric oxide; ONOO-, peroxynitrite; SOD, superoxide dismutase; TRXP, thioredoxin peroxidase.

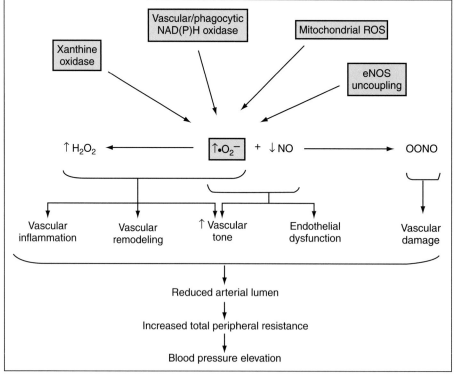

Figure 30–2. Possible role of reactive oxygen species in the pathogenesis of hypertension. Production of vascular reactive oxygen species leads to activation of multiple redox-dependent signaling pathways. These events contribute to vascular inflammation, growth, altered contraction/dilation (vascular tone) and endothelial dysfunction, which lead to vascular remodeling, arterial narrowing, increased peripheral resistance, and consequently to increased blood pressure.

xanthine oxidase, mitochondrial sources, and uncoupled NOS (Figure 30–1). Emerging evidence indicates that these systems interact such that activation of one enzyme system can influence another. This interplay amplifies ROS production contributing to further oxidative stress.[22]

NAD(P)H oxidase

NAD(P)H oxidase is a multisubunit enzyme that catalyzes the production of $\bullet O_2^-$ by the one electron reduction of oxygen using NAD(P)H as the electron donor: $2O_2+NAD(P)H \rightarrow 2O_2^- + NAD(P)^+ + H^+$.[23,24] The prototypical and best-characterized NAD(P)H oxidase is that found in phagocytes, which comprises at least five subunits: p47phox, p67phox, p40phox, p22phox, and gp91phox (phox for *ph*agocyte *ox*idase).[25] In resting cells, p40phox, p47phox, and p67phox exist in the cytosol, whereas p22phox and gp91phox are membrane associated, where they occur as a heterodimeric flavoprotein, cytochrome b558. Following activation, p47phox becomes phosphorylated, leading to the formation of a complex between the cytosolic subunits, which then translocates to the membrane and associates with cytochrome b558 to assemble the active enzyme.[26,27] In addition, free p47phox can translocate to the membrane by itself.[28,29] p47phox and p67phox are important in NAD(P)H oxidase assembly and play a critical role in oxidase activation and deactivation.[30]

Non-phagocytic NAD(P)H oxidase, analogous to the phagocytic oxidase, has been demonstrated in vascular cells[31,32] (Table 30–1). Vascular NAD(P)H oxidases possess most of the classical NAD(P)H oxidase subunits, but are structurally and functionally different from classical phagocytic oxidase, particularly with respect to gp91phox (Nox2, for NAD(P)H oxidase). Vascular cells possess Nox2 homologues, Nox1 and Nox4, which represent the catalytic subunit of NAD(P)H oxidase when Nox2 is absent. All Nox isoforms possess six transmembrane helices, conserved histidines and binding sites for NAD(P)H and FAD (Figure 30–3). Nox2 is expressed in endothelial cells and adventitial cells of large vessels and in VSMC from resistance arteries.[33–35] Constitutive Nox1 levels are low in vascular cells, but can be induced by stimuli, such as Ang II, PDGF, and serum.[33] Nox4 is constitutively expressed and constitutively active in VSMC and endothelial cells.[34] All Nox enzymes require p22phox, which functions as a

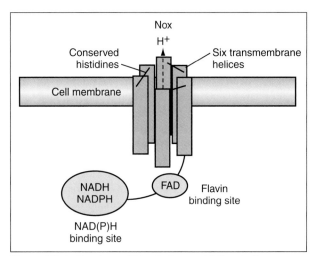

Figure 30–3. Structure of Nox isoforms. All Nox isoforms possess a six-transmembrane domain, conserved histidines, two hemes, and binding sites for NADPH/NADH and FAD. In the process of $\bullet O_2^-$ production, H^+ is formed. FAD, flavin adenine dinucleotide; NADPH, nicotinamide adenine dinucleotide phosphate.

scaffolding protein for other subunits and that stabilizes the Nox enzymes.[36] Nox1 activity requires p47phox and p67phox, regulated by NoxO1 (Nox organizer 1) and NoxA1 (Nox activator 1), respectively.[37,38] NoxO1 may be constitutively active with its SH3 domains always accessible for binding to Nox1.[38] NoxA1 seems to be expressed in a wider range of tissues than NoxO1.[39] The exact role of NoxO1 and NoxA1 in the vasculature remains to be clarified.

Enhanced activity of vascular NAD(P)H oxidase and increased expression of oxidase subunits have been demonstrated in spontaneously hypertensive rats (SHR) and in experimental models of hypertension.[40–42] In cultured VSMCs, cyclic stretch, Ang II, and growth factors increase NAD(P)H oxidase activity and expression, with enhanced effects in cells from hypertensive rats and humans.[43,44] To further support a role for NAD(P)H oxidase in Ang II–induced hypertension, mice deficient in p47phox, which have reduced oxidative stress, have lower blood pressures than wild-type counterparts.[45]

TABLE 30–1. DIFFERENCES BETWEEN PHAGOCYTIC AND VASCULAR NADPH OXIDASE

Characteristic	Phagocytic Oxidase	Vascular Oxidase
State of activity	Basal state inactive	Constitutively active
Mode of activity	Inducible	Inducible
Nox isoform	gp91phox (nox2)	gp91phox/Nox1/Nox4/Nox5
Pattern of $\bullet O_2^-$ release	Burst-like	Slow and sustained
Concentration released	High	Low (1%–10% of phagocytic)
Site of $\bullet O_2^-$ release	Extracellular	Intracellular
Substrate	NADPH	NADPH/NADH
Small G protein	Rac2	Rac1

Table 30–1. Differences Between Phagocytic and Vascular NADPH Oxidase

Xanthine oxidase

Xanthine oxidase (XO) generates $\bullet O_2^-$ by catalyzing the oxidation of xanthine and hypoxanthine during purine metabolism. XO reduces molecular oxygen, leading to the formation of $\bullet O_2^-$ and H_2O_2. In the vasculature XO can produce large amounts of ROS under pathophysiologic conditions, such as atherosclerosis and ischemia-reperfusion injury.[46] This enzyme is expressed not only in vascular and endothelial cells but also circulates in the plasma. Vascular XO activity is regulated by NAD(P)H oxidase, since NADPH-driven generation of H_2O_2 stimulates xanthine oxidase activity.[47] Hence cellular generation of ROS from one enzymatic source further generates ROS formation from another. A role for XO as a vascular source of ROS in hypertension was suggested on the basis of blood pressure-lowering actions of xanthine oxidase inhibitors, allopurinol and oxypurinol, and by the finding that oxidase activity is increased in SHR.[48–50] Vascular XO–derived ROS may be particularly important in conditions associated with endothelial dysfunction. Clinical studies demonstrated improved endothelial function by oxypurinol in patients with hypercholesterolemia but not in patients with hypertension.[51] Vascular XO activity correlates inversely with endothelial function in patients with heart failure and atherosclerosis.[52]

Mitochondrial respiratory electron transport chain enzyme

Mitochondria provide energy to the cell from adenosine triphosphate (ATP) through oxidative phosphorylation by the electron transport chain. Oxidative phosphorylation transfers electrons from NADH (and $FADH_2$) to O_2 to form H_2O. Mitochondria produce ROS either within the inner mitochondrial membrane by the electron transport chain or externally through the oxidation of monoamines by mitochondrial monoamine oxidase. The electron transport carrier is composed of four complexes: NADH-ubiquinone oxidoreductase complex I, succinate-ubiquinone oxidoreductase complex II, ubiquinol-cytochrome c oxidoreductase complex III, and cytochrome c oxidase complex IV. Only 1% to 2% of electrons leak out to form $\bullet O_2^-$, and this is scavenged by manganese SOD.[53] Under pathophysiologic conditions, the electron transport chain may become uncoupled, leading to increased $\bullet O_2^-$ production and spillover into the cytoplasm.[54] The precise contribution of mitochondrial-derived ROS to total ROS production in the vessel wall remains unclear, although it is evident that exposure of vascular cells to exogenous H_2O_2 or $ONOO^-$ leads to mitochondrial damage, which could contribute to vascular oxidative stress.[55,56] We recently demonstrated that in VSMCs endothelin-1 induces ROS production from mitochondrial sources.[57]

Uncoupled nitric oxide synthase

Under physiologic conditions, the oxidation of L-arginine by eNOS produces L-citrulline and NO, which scavenge ROS. Under certain conditions, eNOS can become uncoupled, such that it produces $\bullet O_2^-$ rather than NO[58] (Figure 30–4). Primary determinants for this uncoupling are the availability of the NOS substrate, L-arginine, or the cofactor 5,6,7,8-tetrahydrobiopterin (BH4).[59] If levels of L-arginine

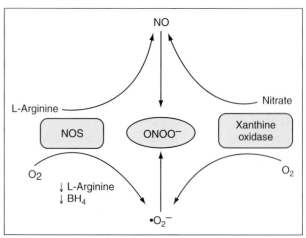

Figure 30–4. NOS and xanthine oxidase are able to produce either $\bullet O_2^-$ or NO. In the presence of adequate substrate L-arginine and O_2, NOS generates NO, whereas the same enzyme produces $\bullet O_2^-$ when L-arginine or co-factors, such as BH_4, are limited. Xanthine oxidase produces $\bullet O_2^-$ under pathologic conditions, such as in reperfusion post ischemia, whereas NO formation is preferred during hypoxia. BH4, 5,6,7,8-tetrahydrobiopterin; NO, nitric oxide; NOS, nitric oxide synthase.

or BH_4 are low, NOS is incapable of transferring electrons to L-arginine, and instead uses oxygen as a substrate for $\bullet O_2^-$ formation.[60] This phenomenon is called "uncoupling" of eNOS, and can produce large amounts of $\bullet O_2^-$ under pathophysiologic condition, especially in situations associated with underlying oxidative stress and in the presence of endothelial damage, such as diabetes, hypercholesterolemia, and hypertension.[61–63] Treatment of DOCA-salt hypertensive mice with BH_4 "re-couple" eNOS, leading to increased vascular NO production, reduced $\bullet O_2^-$ formation, and lowering of blood pressure,[64] suggesting that uncoupled eNOS is involved in blood pressure elevation. However, not all eNOS becomes uncoupled. Some of the enzyme continues to produce NO, favoring production of $ONOO^-$, which could further contribute to vascular damage.

Cytochrome P450 enzymes and other pro-oxidant enzymes

Cytochrome P450 enzymes are a large group of monooxygenase enzymes responsible for the metabolism of toxic hydrocarbons.[8,65] CYP2 and CYP4 families are expressed in VSMCs and endothelial cells and have been shown to generate ROS in vascular tissues.[66,67] The CYP2 family has been associated with endothelium-derived hyperpolarizing factor responses in some vascular beds.[8,65]

Other enzymatic sources capable of generating ROS in the vasculature are phagocyte-derived myeloperoxidases, cyclooxygenases, lipooxygenases, and heme oxygenases.

VASCULAR ANTIOXIDANT ENZYMES

Superoxide dismutase

Once generated, $\bullet O_2^-$ is dismutated to H_2O_2 by the activity of superoxide dismutase (SOD).[68,69] In vascular cells, the

SODs are a major cellular defense mechanism against increased $\bullet O_2^-$ production. Three different SOD isoforms have been identified: the mitochondrial manganese-containing SOD (Mn-SOD, SOD2), the cytosolic copper/zinc-containing SOD (Cu,Zn-SOD, SOD1), and the extracellular SOD (EC-SOD, SOD3).[3,70,71] SOD3 is a copper/zinc-containing SOD that is mainly produced and secreted by VSMCs, and binds to glycoaminoglycans in the vascular extracellular matrix on the endothelial cell surface. SOD3 is heavily expressed in the vascular interstitium and plays an important role in the regulation of the oxidant status in the vascular wall.[68,72] It serves to minimize the $\bullet O_2$–dependent inactivation of endothelial-derived NO.

Catalase

H_2O_2 that results from the action of SODs is reduced to water by catalase and the glutathione peroxidases (GPx).[73,74] Catalase is an antioxidant enzyme located mainly in cellular peroxisomes and to some extent in the cytosol. Catalase catalyzes the reaction of H_2O_2 to water and molecular O_2 in a two-step reaction involving compound I. The enzyme is especially important in the case of limited glutathione content or reduced GPx activity, and plays a significant role in the development of tolerance to oxidative stress in the adaptive response of cells.

Glutathione peroxidase

Glutathione peroxidase (GPx) is a selenium-containing antioxidant enzyme that effectively reduces H_2O_2 and lipid peroxides to water and lipid alcohols, respectively, and in turn oxidizes glutathione to glutathione disulfide. Reduced glutathione plays a major role in the regulation of the intracellular redox state of vascular cells by providing reducing equivalents for many biochemical pathways.[75,76] In the absence of adequate GPx activity or glutathione levels, hydrogen peroxide and lipid peroxides are not detoxified and may be converted to OH– radicals and lipid peroxyl radicals, respectively, by transition metals (Fe^{2+}). The GPx/glutathione system is thought to be a major defense in low-level oxidative stress. Four isoforms of GPx have been identified and characterized: GPx-1 (cellular GPx) is ubiquitous and reduces H_2O_2 and fatty acid peroxides, and has been inversely associated with increased cardio-vascular risk.[77] Esterified lipids are reduced by membrane-bound GPx-4 (phospholipids hydroperoxide GPx), which can use several different low-molecular-weight thiols as reducing equivalents. GPx2 (gastrointestinal GPx) is localized to gastrointestinal epithelial cells. GPx-3 (extra-cellular GPx) is the only member of the GPx family that exists in the extracellular compartment, and is believed to be the most important extracellular antioxidant enzyme in mammals.[78–80]

Thioredoxin reductase

Thioredoxin (TRX), via a series of coupled reactions catalyzed by thioredoxin reductase and NADPH, also functions as an antioxidant molecule in the cytosol of vascular endothelial and smooth muscle cells. The thioredoxin system (TRX, TRX reductase, and NADPH) reduces oxidized cysteine groups on proteins through an interaction with the redox-active center of TRX (cys-gly-pro-cys) to form a disulfide bond, which in turn can be reduced by TRX reductase and NADPH.[81] The enzyme regenerates reduced thioredoxin, which serves as reducing equivalent, and may also directly reduce lipid hydroperoxides. TRX plays an essential role in cell function by limiting oxidative stress directly via antioxidant actions,[82,83] and indirectly by protein–protein interactions with key signaling molecules, such as thioredoxin-interacting protein (TXNIP).[81] TRX is ubiquitously expressed in vascular endothelial and smooth muscle cells and protects cells from H_2O_2-induced cytotoxicity.[84] It is possible that the protective effects of TRX in endothelial cells are mediated in part through MnSOD, since induction of this enzyme by TRX is specific and because other antioxidant enzymes, including copper zinc SOD (Cu/Zn SOD) and catalase, are not induced by TRX.[85]

Thioredoxin function is altered in hypertension. In cardiac, aortic, and renal tissue from SHR and stroke-prone SHR-SP, increased oxidative stress is associated with TRX down-regulation.[86] In Ang II–infused rats, induction of TRX activity is impaired. Taken together these findings suggest that decreased TRX may contribute to hypertension and its sequelae.[81]

Genetic determinants of reduced antioxidant capacity and relation to hypertension

A number of heritable polymorphisms of antioxidant enzymes have been associated with hypertension. In an isolated Chinese population, a variant within the catalase promoter region has been associated with essential hypertension.[87] GPx-1 deficiency, associated with a polyalanine sequence polymorphism, is associated with endothelial dysfunction, heart failure, and abnormal structural changes in the vasculature and myocardium.[88] A promoter polymorphism of heme oxygenase-1 gene has been associated with hypertension in a population of Japanese women, but not men; women with the AA genotype had an increased frequency of hypertension and use of antihypertensive agents compared with those with the AT or TT genotype.[89] Glucose-6-phosphate dehydrogenase (G6PD), the major source of cytosolic reducing equivalents for thiol balance in all cells, is a highly polymorphic gene with many functional variants.[90] Recent studies demonstrated that individuals with G6PD deficiency have an increased risk of developing hypertension, diabetes, and endothelial dysfunction.[90,91] Glutathione S-transferase mu type 1, a protein involved in detoxification of reactive oxygen species, has recently been suggested as a positional and functional candidate gene linked to increased oxidative stress and hypertension.[92] Quantitative real-time polymerase chain reaction showed a highly significant, four-fold reduction of glutathione S-transferase mu type 1 mRNA expression in 5- and 16-week-old SHR-SP compared with the congenic and normotensive Wistar-Kyoto rats. mRNA expression changes were reflected at the protein level, with significant reductions in the SHR-SP glutathione S-transferase mu type, suggesting a pathophysiologic role of this protein in hypertension and oxidative stress.[93]

VASCULAR EFFECTS OF REACTIVE OXYGEN SPECIES

Molecular processes in which ROS influence vascular function and structure involve activation of redox-sensitive signaling pathways. Superoxide anion and H_2O_2 stimulate mitogen-activated protein (MAP) kinases, tyrosine kinases and transcription factors (NFκB, AP-1, and HIF-1), and inactivate protein tyrosine phosphatases.[94] ROS also increase $[Ca^{2+}]_i$ and upregulate proto-oncogene and proinflammatory gene expression.[95,96] These events occur through oxidative modification of proteins by altering important amino acid residues, inducing protein dimerization, and interacting with metal complexes such as Fe-S moieties. Changes in intracellular redox state through thioredoxin and glutathione systems may also influence signaling events.

It is important to emphasize that under physiologic conditions, ROS serve as integral components of cellular signaling pathways that contribute to normal vascular function. However, exposure to pathologic stimuli results in oxidant stress, which modifies biomolecules to modulate and alter vascular phenotype. It is becoming increasingly evident that increased ROS production may have minimal effects on vascular function and hemodynamics at baseline, but can augment the response to pathogenic stimuli. This is evidenced by recent studies,[97,98] where smooth muscle overexpression of p22phox or Nox1 resulted in increased ROS production without much effect on blood pressure or vascular reactivity and structure. However, exposure to Ang II resulted in augmented hypertension and vascular remodeling.

Vascular growth effects of reactive oxygen species

ROS play an important role in VSMC growth. During vascular damage in hypertension, when oxidative stress is increased, redox-sensitive growth processes may lead to accelerated proliferation and hypertrophy, further contributing to vascular injury and remodeling.[99] H_2O_2 induces a dual action on cell growth, depending on its cellular localization and intracellular levels. At high concentrations (>100 μM), H_2O_2 is proapoptotic and induces anoikis (cell detachment and shedding), whereas at lower concentrations it stimulates proliferation, hypertrophy, and differentiation.[100,101] The importance of ROS compartmentalization and spatial localization have recently been highlighted in studies examining VSMCs deficient in SOD1 (cytosolic SOD) or SOD2 (mitochondrial SOD). In SOD1-deficient VSMCs, proliferation and protein synthesis are enhanced through ERK1/2- and p38MAP kinase–dependent pathways, whereas in SOD2-deficient cells, growth is associated with preferential activation of the JAK/STAT pathway.[102] Whether these differential effects are due to increased $\bullet O_2^-$ or decreased H_2O_2 remains unclear. ROS also modulate vascular structure in hypertension by increasing deposition of extracellular matrix proteins, such as collagen and fibronectin and by modulating MMPs, particularly MMP2 and MMP9.[103] ROS mediate the proliferative response to agonists such as Ang II, platelet-derived growth factor (PDGF), epidermal growth factor (EGF), and thrombin.[104]

Vascular inflammation

ROS can promote a vascular proinflammatory state through direct activation of leukocyte adhesion molecule expression, by inducing proinflammatory gene activation and by reducing the availability of NO.[64] NO has many anti-inflammatory actions, including inhibition of VSMC proliferation and platelet aggregation.[64,105,106] The imbalance between ROS and NO in the vessel wall further contributes to inflammation by activation of the local renin-angiotensin system.[107] Ang II, which is systemically or locally elevated in various forms of hypertension, is a particularly potent mediator of ROS-dependent vascular inflammation.[64]

Many of the redox sensitive vascular changes that occur in hypertension also exist in atherosclerotic vessels. In VSMCs, Ang II and TNF-α induce proinflammatory genes through the activation of NF-κB in a ROS-dependent manner.[108,109] Increased activation of vascular NF-κB and AP-1 and associated inflammatory and mitogenic responses have been demonstrated in hypertensive rats.[110] These actions have been attributed, in part, to oxidative excess. Oxygen radicals induce endothelial permeability with extravasation of plasma proteins and other macromolecules, and the recruitment of inflammatory proteins and cells, which also impair endothelial function and aggravate vascular damage.[111,112] Peripheral polymorphonuclear leukocytes, which generate $\bullet O_2^-$, participate in the oxidative stress and inflammatory response in patients with hypertension.[113,114] Interactions between H_2O_2 and peroxidases, particularly myeloperoxidase, lead to the formation of oxidizing and nitrosating species that are proinflammatory and proatherogenic. The importance of Ang II in accelerating the development of atherosclerosis in the setting of hypertension was demonstrated in apo E–deficient mice infused with Ang II. Development of atherosclerosis in these mice was 4.5 times greater than in mice made hypertensive with norepinephrine.[115]

Vascular contraction/dilation and reactive oxygen species

The direct effect of ROS on VSMC contraction/dilation is controversial. ROS appear to elicit both contraction and dilation, depending on the vascular bed and type of species generated. Hydrogen peroxide causes vasodilation of pulmonary, coronary, and mesenteric arteries, and has been considered to be endothelium derived relaxing factor (EDRF).[116,117] In rat aorta, Ang II stimulates vasoconstriction via H_2O_2-dependent mechanisms,[118] whereas in human and porcine vessels, acute vasoconstriction by Ang II is not mediated via ROS.[95,119] In aortic and mesenteric arteries from SHR, hydrogen peroxide–mediated contractile effects are enhanced.[96,120] The apparent discrepancies may be due to the blood vessel studied, the presence or absence of the endothelium, the concentration and species of the free radical studied and the compartment in which $\bullet O_2^-$ and H_2O_2 predominate.[121]

Vascular cell migration and reactive oxygen species

Vascular smooth muscle cell migration is one of the major features of vascular injury. PDGF-induced VSMC chemotaxis is inhibited by catalase overexpression, NAC, DPI, ebselen, and dominant-negative Rac, suggesting that ROS production through NAD(P)H oxidase is critical for agonist-stimulated VSMC migration.[104,122]

REACTIVE OXYGEN SPECIES AND HYPERTENSION

Extensive experimental and clinical data implicate oxidative excess as being pathophysiologically important in hypertension. This is evidenced by findings that oxidative stress is increased in hypertension and that treatment with antioxidants or agents that inhibit NAD(P)H oxidase–driven generation of ROS reduces, and may even prevent, blood pressure elevation. Furthermore, because ROS serve as signaling molecules involved in VSMC growth and inflammation, they subserve a crucial role in mediating vascular remodeling and maintenance of hypertension.

Genetically hypertensive rats, such as SHR and SHR-SP, exhibit enhanced NAD(P)H oxidase–mediated $\bullet O_2^-$ generation in resistance arteries (mesenteric), conduit vessels (aorta), and kidneys.[123-128] Several polymorphisms in the promoter region of the p22^{phox} gene have been identified in SHR, which could contribute to enhanced NAD(P)H oxidase activity.[127,128] 8-hydroxy-2′-deoxyguanosine, a marker for oxidative stress-induced DNA damage, and protein carbonylation, a marker for oxidation status of proteins are enhanced in aorta, heart, and kidney, whereas endogenous antioxidants, including glutathione peroxidase and thioredoxin, are markedly suppressed in SHR and SHR-SP compared with normotensive Wistar-Kyoto rats (WKY).[96,128,129] Diminished NO bioavailability as a consequence of enhanced vascular $\bullet O_2^-$ generation may also contribute to oxidative stress in hypertension as evidenced in eNOS-deficient mice and in rats and humans after pharmacologic blockade of NOS.[130]

Oxidative excess has also been demonstrated in numerous models of experimental hypertension, including Ang II–induced hypertension,[131,132] Dahl-salt-sensitive hypertension,[133] lead-induced hypertension,[134] obesity-associated hypertension,[135] mineralocorticoid hypertension,[136,137] two-kidney, one-clip hypertension,[138] and in models of postmenopausal hypertension.[139] Enhanced activation of vascular and renal NAD(P)H oxidase and xanthine oxidase and uncoupling of eNOS have been implicated in enhanced $\bullet O_2^-$ generation in experimental hypertension.[140,141] Mitochondrial enzymes and xanthine oxidase may also contribute to oxidative excess in cardiovascular disease.[141,142] Inhibition of ROS production with apocynin (NAD(P)H oxidase inhibitor), allopurinol (xanthine oxidase inhibitor), quercetin (dietary flavonoid), and scavenging of free radicals with antioxidants or SOD mimetics, such as tempol, reduces oxidative stress, decreases blood pressure, and prevents development of hypertension in most models of experimental hypertension.[123,125,143-145] These antihypertensive actions have been attributed to improved endothelial function, regression of cardiovascular remodeling, improved renal function and reduced vascular, cardiac and renal inflammation.

Clinical studies have demonstrated that production of ROS is increased whereas levels/activity of antioxidant systems is decreased in hypertensive patients.[13,146-148] Oxidative excess has been shown in patients with essential hypertension, salt-sensitive hypertension, renovascular hypertension, malignant hypertension, and in preeclampsia.[149-155] Most of these findings are based on elevated levels of lipid peroxidation by-products, including plasma and urine TBARS, malondialdehyde and 8-epi-isoprostanes.[151,152] Increased plasma, platelet, and leukocyte $\bullet O_2^-$ and H_2O_2 concentrations have been demonstrated in hypertensive patients.[153,154] Treatment with the antioxidant vitamin, vitamin C, significantly reduced blood pressure in young hypertensive patients[156] and had a modest blood pressure–lowering effect in elderly patients.[157] The beneficial actions of vitamin C have been attributed in part to increased bioavailability of NO.

Studies in cultured VSMCs derived from resistance arteries of hypertensive patients revealed enhanced formation of ROS.[158] Increased levels/activity of vascular NAD(P)H oxidase has been implicated as the primary source of excess $\bullet O_2^-$ in essential hypertension.[159,160] Polymorphonuclear leukocytes, resident macrophages and platelets, all rich $\bullet O_2^-$ sources, further participate in vascular oxidative stress and inflammation in hypertensive patients.[161] Activation of the renin-angiotensin system has been proposed as a major mediator of NAD(P)H oxidase activation and ROS production in clinical hypertension.[162,163] Ang II is a potent stimulator of NAD(P)H oxidase and upregulates expression of NAD(P)H oxidase subunits in human VSMCs, fibroblasts, and endothelial cells.[4-7,164] Because of this interaction between Ang II and $\bullet O_2^-$–generating systems, it is not surprising that some of the therapeutic blood pressure–lowering actions of ACE inhibitors and AT$_1$ receptor blockers may be mediated by inhibiting NAD(P)H oxidase activity and reducing ROS production.[165,166]

Although experimental evidence and clinical studies provide compelling evidence that oxidative stress is important in the pathophysiology of hypertension, not all human hypertension is redox-dependent. Also, many large clinical trials on antioxidants failed to demonstrate beneficial therapeutic effects on blood pressure and cardiovascular outcomes.[167-171] Reasons for these discrepancies probably relate to the heterogeneous nature of hypertension and to the complexities of redox biology in the cardiovascular system. However, it is likely that ROS-dependent vascular remodeling and inflammation contributes to renal and cardiac end-organ damage.

SUMMARY

Reactive oxygen species are produced in the vasculature in a controlled and tightly regulated manner. Superoxide and H_2O_2 have important signaling properties, mainly through oxidative modification of proteins and activation of transcription factors that regulate vascular function. In hypertension, dysregulation of enzymes such as NAD(P)H oxidase, NOS, xanthine oxidase, mitochondrial enzymes, or SOD, altered thioredoxin and glutathione systems or reduced scavenging by antioxidants, results in increased formation of ROS, which have damaging actions on the vasculature. Factors that activate pro-oxidant enzyme systems remain poorly defined, but probably involve Ang II, mechanical stretch, and inflammatory cytokines.

Reactive oxygen species in hypertension contribute to vascular injury by promoting cell growth, extracellular matrix protein deposition, activation of matrix metalloproteinases, inflammation, endothelial dysfunction, and increased vascular tone. In experimental hypertension oxidative stress is increased and antioxidant levels/activity is decreased. Clinical data indicate that hypertensive patients exhibit oxidative excess. Although inconclusive at present, treatment strategies to alter ROS bioavailability by decreasing production and/or by increasing radical scavenging, may regress vascular remodeling, prevent further vascular injury, and reduce blood pressure in hypertensive patients. Because ROS, particularly H_2O_2, can diffuse from vascular to parenchymal cells in various organs, it is possible that vascular oxidative excess contributes to target-organ damage and that prevention of ROS formation will lead to end-organ protection in hypertension.

REFERENCES

1. Fridovich I. Superoxide anion radical (O2–), superoxide dismutases, and related matters. *J Biol Chem* 1997;272(30):18515.
2. Mueller CF, Laude K, McNally JS, Harrison DG. ATVB in focus: redox mechanisms in blood vessels. *Arterioscler Thromb Vasc Biol* 2005;25(2):274.
3. Mendez JI, Nicholson WJ, Taylor WR. SOD isoforms and signaling in blood vessels: evidence for the importance of ROS compartmentalization. *Arterioscler Thromb Vasc Biol* 2005;25(5):887.
4. Zafari AM, Ushio-Fukai M, Akers M, et al. Role of NADH/NADPH oxidase-derived H2O2 in angiotensin II–induced vascular hypertrophy. *Hypertension* 1998;32(3)4:88.
5. Touyz RM, Schiffrin EL. Reactive oxygen species in vascular biology: implications in hypertension. *Histochem Cell Biol* 2004;122(4):339.
6. Griendling KK, Sorescu D, Ushio-Fukai M. NAD(P)H oxidase: role in cardiovascular biology and disease. *Circ Res* 2000;86(5):494.
7. Touyz RM, Chen X, Tabet F, et al. Expression of a functionally active gp91phox-containing neutrophil-type NAD(P)H oxidase in smooth muscle cells from human resistance arteries: regulation by angiotensin II. *Circ Res* 2002;90(11):1205.
8. Fleming I, Michaelis UR, Bredenkotter D, et al. Endothelium-derived hyperpolarizing factor synthase (cytochrome P450 2C9) is a functionally significant source of reactive oxygen species in coronary arteries. *Circ Res* 2001;88(1):44.
9. Channon KM, Guzik TJ. Mechanisms of superoxide production in human blood vessels, relationship to endothelial dysfunction, clinical and genetic risk factors. *J Physiol Pharmacol* 2002;53(4 Pt 1):515.
10. Jones SA, O'Donnell VB, Wood JD, et al. Expression of phagocyte NADPH oxidase components in human endothelial cells. *Am J Physiol* 1996;271(4 Pt 2):H1626.
11. Rey FE, Pagano PJ. The reactive adventitia: fibroblast oxidase in vascular function. *Arterioscler Thromb Vasc Biol* 2002;22(12):1962.
12. Harrison DG. Cellular and molecular mechanisms of endothelial cell dysfunction. *J Clin Invest* 1997;100(9):2153.
13. Touyz RM. Reactive oxygen species, vascular oxidative stress, and redox signaling in hypertension: what is the clinical significance? *Hypertension* 2004;44(3):248.
14. Rajagopalan S, Kurz S, Munzel T, et al. Angiotensin II-mediated hypertension in the rat increases vascular superoxide production via membrane NADH/NADPH oxidase activation. Contribution to alterations of vasomotor tone. *J Clin Invest* 1996;97(8):1916.
15. Taylor NE, Cowley Jr AW. Effect of renal medullary H2O2 on salt-induced hypertension and renal injury. *Am J Physiol Regul Integr Comp Physiol* 2005;289:R277 (Epub ahead of print).
16. Welch WJ, Mendonca M, Blau J, et al. Antihypertensive response to prolonged tempol in the spontaneously hypertensive rat. *Kidney Int* 2005;68(1):179.
17. Fratta Pasini A, Garbin U, Nava MC, et al. Nebivolol decreases oxidative stress in essential hypertensive patients and increases nitric oxide by reducing its oxidative inactivation. *J Hypertens* 2005;23(3):589.
18. Manning Jr RD, Tian N, Meng S. Oxidative stress and antioxidant treatment in hypertension and the associated renal damage. *Am J Nephrol* 2005;25(4):311.
19. Sorescu D, Weiss D, Lassegue B, et al. Superoxide production and expression of nox family proteins in human atherosclerosis. *Circulation* 2002;105(12):1429.
20. Berry C, Hamilton CA, Brosnan MJ, et al. Investigation into the sources of superoxide in human blood vessels: angiotensin II increases superoxide production in human internal mammary arteries. *Circulation* 2000;101(18):2206.
21. Wilcox CS, Gutterman D. Focus on oxidative stress in the cardiovascular and renal systems. *Am J Physiol Heart Circ Physiol* 2005;288(1):H3.
22. Cai H. NAD(P)H oxidase-dependent self-propagation of hydrogen peroxide and vascular disease. *Circ Res* 2005;96(8):818.
23. Bokoch GM, Knaus UG. NADPH oxidases: not just for leukocytes anymore! *Trends Biochem Sci* 2003;28(9):502.
24. Babior BM, Lambeth JD, Nauseef W. The neutrophil NADPH oxidase. *Arch Biochem Biophys* 2002;397(2):342.
25. Gauss KA, Mascolo PL, Siemsen DW, et al. Cloning and sequencing of rabbit leukocyte NADPH oxidase genes reveals a unique p67(phox) homolog. *J Leukoc Biol* 2002;71(2):319.
26. Park JW, Ma M, Ruedi JM, et al. The cytosolic components of the respiratory burst oxidase exist as a M(r) approximately 240,000 complex that acquires a membrane-binding site during activation of the oxidase in a cell-free system. *J Biol Chem* 1992;267(24):17327.
27. Touyz RM, Yao G, Quinn MT, et al. p47phox associates with the cytoskeleton through cortactin in human vascular smooth muscle cells: role in NAD(P)H oxidase regulation by angiotensin II. *Arterioscler Thromb Vasc Biol* 2005;25(3):512.
28. el Benna J, Ruedi JM, Babior BM. Cytosolic guanine nucleotide-binding protein Rac2 operates in vivo as a component of the neutrophil respiratory burst oxidase. Transfer of Rac2 and the cytosolic oxidase components p47phox and p67phox to the submembranous actin cytoskeleton during oxidase activation. *J Biol Chem* 1994;269(9):6729.
29. Iyer SS, Pearson DW, Nauseef WM, et al. Evidence for a readily dissociable complex of p47phox and p67phox in cytosol of unstimulated human neutrophils. *J Biol Chem* 1994;269(35):22405.
30. Cross AR, Curnutte JT. The cytosolic activating factors p47phox and p67phox have distinct roles in the regulation of electron flow in NADPH oxidase. *J Biol Chem* 1995;270(12):6543.
31. Lassegue B, Clempus RE. Vascular NAD(P)H oxidases: specific features, expression, and regulation. *Am J Physiol Regul Integr Comp Physiol* 2003;285(2):R277.
32. Touyz RM, Yao G, Schiffrin EL. c-Src induces phosphorylation and translocation of p47phox: role in superoxide generation by angiotensin II in human vascular smooth muscle cells. *Arterioscler Thromb Vasc Biol* 2003;23(6):981.
33. Suh YA, Arnold RS, Lassegue B, et al. Cell transformation by the superoxide-generating oxidase Mox1. *Nature* 1999;401(6748):79.
34. Hilenski LL, Clempus RE, Quinn MT, et al. Distinct subcellular localizations of Nox1 and Nox4 in vascular smooth muscle cells. *Arterioscler Thromb Vasc Biol* 2004;24(4):677.
35. Ago T, Kitazono T, Ooboshi H, et al. Nox4 as the major catalytic component of an endothelial NAD(P)H oxidase. *Circulation* 2004;109(2):227.

36. Hanna IR, Hilenski LL, Dikalova A, et al. Functional association of nox1 with p22phox in vascular smooth muscle cells. *Free Radic Biol Med* 2004;37(10):1542.

37. Banfi B, Clark RA, Steger K, Krause KH. Two novel proteins activate superoxide generation by the NADPH oxidase NOX1. *J Biol Chem* 2003;278(6):3510.

38. Takeya R, Ueno N, Kami K, et al. Novel human homologues of p47phox and p67phox participate in activation of superoxide-producing NADPH oxidases. *J Biol Chem* 2003;278(27):25234.

39. Cheng G, Lambeth JD. Alternative mRNA splice forms of NOXO1: Differential tissue expression and regulation of Nox1 and Nox3. *Gene* 2005;356:118–26.

40. Bolterman RJ, Manriquez MC, Ortiz Ruiz MC, et al. Effects of captopril on the renin angiotensin system, oxidative stress, and endothelin in normal and hypertensive rats. *Hypertension* 2005;46:943 (Epub ahead of print).

41. Chen X, Touyz RM, Park JB, Schiffrin EL. Antioxidant effects of vitamins C and E are associated with altered activation of vascular NADPH oxidase and superoxide dismutase in stroke-prone SHR. *Hypertension* 2001;38(3 Pt 2):606.

42. Kobayashi N, Delano FA, Schmid-Schonbein GW. Oxidative stress promotes endothelial cell apoptosis and loss of microvessels in the spontaneously hypertensive rats. *Arterioscler Thromb Vasc Biol* 2005;25:2114.

43. Touyz RM, Schiffrin EL. Increased generation of superoxide by angiotensin II in smooth muscle cells from resistance arteries of hypertensive patients: role of phospholipase D-dependent NAD(P)H oxidase-sensitive pathways. *J Hypertens* 2001;19(7):1245.

44. Wassmann S, Wassmann K, Nickenig G. Modulation of oxidant and antioxidant enzyme expression and function in vascular cells. *Hypertension* 2004;44(4):381.

45. Landmesser U, Cai H, Dikalov S, et al. Role of p47(phox) in vascular oxidative stress and hypertension caused by angiotensin II. *Hypertension* 2002;40(4):511.

46. Harrison D, Griendling KK, Landmesser U, et al. Role of oxidative stress in atherosclerosis. *Am J Cardiol* 2003;91(3A):7A.

47. McNally JS, Saxena A, Cai H, et al. Regulation of xanthine oxidoreductase protein expression by hydrogen peroxide and calcium. *Arterioscler Thromb Vasc Biol* 2005;25(8):1623.

48. Berry CE, Hare JM. Xanthine oxidoreductase and cardiovascular disease: molecular mechanisms and pathophysiological implications. *J Physiol* 2004;555(Pt 3):589.

49. Suzuki H, DeLano FA, Parks DA, et al. Xanthine oxidase activity associated with arterial blood pressure in spontaneously hypertensive rats. *Proc Natl Acad Sci U S A* 1998;95(8):4754.

50. Minami M, Ishiyama A, Takagi M, et al. Effects of allopurinol, a xanthine oxidase inhibitor, on renal injury in hypercholesterolemia-induced hypertensive rats. *Blood Press* 2005;14(2):120.

51. Cardillo C, Kilcoyne CM, Cannon RO 3rd, et al. Xanthine oxidase inhibition with oxypurinol improves endothelial vasodilator function in hypercholesterolemic but not in hypertensive patients. *Hypertension* 1997;30(1 Pt 1):57.

52. Spiekermann S, Landmesser U, Dikalov S, et al. Electron spin resonance characterization of vascular xanthine and NAD(P)H oxidase activity in patients with coronary artery disease: relation to endothelium-dependent vasodilation. *Circulation* 2003;107(10):1383.

53. Fink BD, Reszka KJ, Herlein JA, et al. Respiratory uncoupling by UCP1 and UCP2 and superoxide generation in endothelial cell mitochondria. *Am J Physiol Endocrinol Metab* 2005;288(1):E71.

54. Ali MH, Pearlstein DP, Mathieu CE, Schumacker PT. Mitochondrial requirement for endothelial responses to cyclic strain: implications for mechanotransduction. *Am J Physiol Lung Cell Mol Physiol* 2004;287(3):L486.

55. Li N, Ragheb K, Lawler G, et al. Mitochondrial complex I inhibitor rotenone induces apoptosis through enhancing mitochondrial reactive oxygen species production. *J Biol Chem* 2003;278(10):8516.

56. Puddu P, Puddu GM, Galletti L, et al. Mitochondrial dysfunction as an initiating event in atherogenesis: a plausible hypothesis. *Cardiology* 2005;103(3):137.

57. Touyz RM, Yao G, Viel E, et al. Angiotensin II and endothelin-1 regulate MAP kinases through different redox-dependent mechanisms in human vascular smooth muscle cells. *J Hypertens* 2004;22(6):1141.

58. Xia Y, Dawson VL, Dawson TM, et al. Nitric oxide synthase generates superoxide and nitric oxide in arginine-depleted cells leading to peroxynitrite-mediated cellular injury. *Proc Natl Acad Sci U S A* 1996;93(13):6770.

59. Vasquez-Vivar J, Kalyanaraman B, Martasek P, et al. Superoxide generation by endothelial nitric oxide synthase: the influence of cofactors. *Proc Natl Acad Sci U S A* 1998;95(16):9220.

60. Vasquez-Vivar J, Kalyanaraman B, Martasek P. The role of tetrahydrobiopterin in superoxide generation from eNOS: enzymology and physiological implications. *Free Radic Res* 2003;37(2):121.

61. Dixon LJ, Hughes SM, Rooney K, et al. Increased superoxide production in hypertensive patients with diabetes mellitus: role of nitric oxide synthase. *Am J Hypertens* 2005;18(6):839.

62. Katusic ZS. Vascular endothelial dysfunction: does tetrahydrobiopterin play a role? *Am J Physiol Heart Circ Physiol* 2001;281(3):H981.

63. Landmesser U, Dikalov S, Price SR, et al. Oxidation of tetrahydrobiopterin leads to uncoupling of endothelial cell nitric oxide synthase in hypertension. *J Clin Invest* 2003;111(8):1201.

64. Landmesser U, Harrison DG. Oxidative stress and vascular damage in hypertension. *Coron Art Dis* 2001;12:455.

65. Fisslthaler B, Popp R, Kiss L, et al. Cytochrome P450 2C is an EDHF synthase in coronary arteries. *Nature* 1999;401(6752):493.

66. Puntarulo S, Cederbaum AI. Production of reactive oxygen species by microsomes enriched in specific human cytochrome P450 enzymes. *Free Radic Biol Med* 1998;24(7–8):1324.

67. Fleming I, Michaelis UR, Bredenkotter D, et al. Endothelium-derived hyperpolarizing factor synthase (Cytochrome P450 2C9) is a functionally significant source of reactive oxygen species in coronary arteries. *Circ Res* 2001;88(1):44.

68. Stralin P, Karlsson K, Johansson BO, Marklund SL. The interstitium of the human arterial wall contains very large amounts of extracellular superoxide dismutase. *Arterioscler Thromb Vasc Biol* 1995;15(11):2032.

69. Halliwell B. Antioxidant defence mechanisms, from the beginning to the end (of the beginning). *Free Radic Res* 31(4):261.

70. Faraci FM, Didion SP. Vascular protection: superoxide dismutase isoforms in the vessel wall. *Arterioscler Thromb Vasc Biol* 2004;24(8):1367.

71. Fukai T, Folz RJ, Landmesser U, Harrison DG. Extracellular superoxide dismutase and cardiovascular disease. *Cardiovasc Res* 2002;55(2):239.

72. Jeney V, Itoh S, Wendt M, et al. Role of antioxidant-1 in extracellular superoxide dismutase function and expression. *Circ Res* 2005;96(7):723.

73. Kirkman HN, Rolfo M, Ferraris AM, Gaetani GF. Mechanisms of protection of catalase by NADPH. Kinetics and stoichiometry. *J Biol Chem* 1999;274(20):13908.

74. Gaetani GF, Ferraris AM, Sanna P, Kirkman HN. A novel NADPH:(bound) NADP+ reductase and NADH:(bound) NADP+ transhydrogenase function in bovine liver catalase. *Biochem J* 2005;385(Pt 3):763.

75. Ulker S, McMaster D, McKeown PP, Bayraktutan U. Impaired activities of antioxidant enzymes elicit endothelial dysfunction in spontaneous hypertensive rats despite enhanced vascular nitric oxide generation. *Cardiovasc Res* 2003;59(2):488.

76. Schafer FQ, Buettner GR. Redox environment of the cell as viewed through the redox state of the glutathione disulfide/glutathione couple. *Free Radic Biol Med* 2001;30(11):1191.

77. Schnabel R, Lackner KJ, Rupprecht HJ, et al. Glutathione peroxidase-1 and homocysteine for cardiovascular risk prediction: results from the AtheroGene study. *J Am Coll Cardiol* 2005;45(10):1631.

78. Whitin JC, Bhamre S, Tham DM, Cohen HJ. Extracellular glutathione peroxidase is secreted basolaterally by human renal proximal tubule cells. *Am J Physiol Renal Physiol* 2002;283(1):F20.

79. Leopold JA, Loscalzo J. Oxidative enzymopathies and vascular disease. *Arterioscler Thromb Vasc Biol* 2005;25(7):1332.

80. Bierl C, Voetsch B, Jin RC, et al. Determinants of human plasma glutathione peroxidase (GPx-3) expression. *J Biol Chem* 2004;279(26):26839.

81. Yamawaki H, Berk BC. Thioredoxin: a multifunctional antioxidant enzyme in kidney, heart and vessels. *Curr Opin Nephrol Hypertens* 2005;14(2):149.

82. Nakamura H. Thioredoxin and its related molecules: update. *Antioxid Redox Signal* 2005;7(5–6):823.

83. Immenschuh S, Baumgart-Vogt E. Peroxiredoxins, oxidative stress, and cell proliferation. *Antioxid Redox Signal* 2005;7(5–6):768.

84. Okuda M, Inoue N, Azumi H, et al. Expression of glutaredoxin in human coronary arteries, its potential role in antioxidant protection against atherosclerosis. *Arterioscler Thromb Vasc Biol* 2001;21:1483.

85. Das KC, Lewis-Molock Y, White CW. Elevation of manganese superoxide dismutase gene expression by thioredoxin. *Am J Respir Cell Mol Biol* 1997;17(6):713.

86. Tanito M, Nakamura H, Kwon YW, et al. Enhanced oxidative stress and impaired thioredoxin expression in spontaneously hypertensive rats. *Antioxid Redox Signal* 2004;6(1):89.

87. Jiang Z, Akey JM, Shi J, et al. A polymorphism in the promoter region of catalase is associated with blood pressure levels. *Hum Genet* 2001;109(1):95.

88. Forgione MA, Weiss N, Heydrick S, et al. Cellular glutathione peroxidase deficiency and endothelial dysfunction. *Am J Physiol Heart Circ Physiol* 2002;282(4):H1255.

89. Ono K, Mannami T, Iwai N. Association of a promoter variant of the heme oxygenase-1 gene with hypertension in women. *J Hypertens* 2003;21:1497.

90. Gaskin RS, Estwick D, Peddi R. G6PD deficiency: its role in the high prevalence of hypertension and diabetes mellitus. *Ethn Dis* 2001;11(4):749.

91. Forgione MA, Loscalzo J, Holbrook M, et al. The A326G (A+) variant of the glucose-6-phosphate dehydrogenase gene is associated with endothelial dysfunction in African Americans. *J Am Coll Cardiol* 2003;41:249A.

92. McBride MW, Brosnan MJ, Mathers J, et al. Reduction of Gstm1 expression in the stroke-prone spontaneously hypertension rat contributes to increased oxidative stress. *Hypertension* 2005;45(4):786.

93. Dominiczak AF, Graham D, McBride MW, et al. Corcoran Lecture. Cardiovascular genomics and oxidative stress. *Hypertension* 2005;45(4):636.

94. Haddad JJ. Antioxidant and prooxidant mechanisms in the regulation of redox(y)-sensitive transcription factors. *Cell Signal* 2002;14(11):879.

95. Touyz RM, Cruzado M, Tabet F, et al. Redox-dependent MAP kinase signaling by Ang II in vascular smooth muscle cells: role of receptor tyrosine kinase transactivation. *Can J Physiol Pharmacol* 2003;81(2):159.

96. Tabet F, Savoia C, Schiffrin EL, Touyz RM. Differential calcium regulation by hydrogen peroxide and superoxide in vascular smooth muscle cells from spontaneously hypertensive rats. *J Cardiovasc Pharmacol* 2004;44(2):200.

97. Laude K, Cai H, Fink B, et al. Hemodynamic and biochemical adaptations to vascular smooth muscle overexpression of p22phox in mice. *Am J Physiol Heart Circ Physiol* 2005;288(1):H7.

98. Dikalova A, Clempus R, Lassegue B, et al. Nox1 overexpression potentiates angiotensin II-induced hypertension and vascular smooth muscle hypertrophy in transgenic mice. *Circulation* 2005;112:2668–76.

99. Griendling KK, Sorescu D, Lassegue B, Ushio-Fukai M. Modulation of protein kinase activity and gene expression by reactive oxygen species and their role in vascular physiology and pathophysiology. *Arterioscler Thromb Vasc Biol* 2000;20(10):2175.

100. Deshpande NN, Sorescu D, Seshiah P, et al. Mechanism of hydrogen peroxide–induced cell cycle arrest in vascular smooth muscle. *Antioxid Redox Signal* 2002;4(5):845.

101. Li AE, Ito H, Rovira II, et al. A role for reactive oxygen species in endothelial cell anoikis. *Circ Res* 1999;85(4):304.

102. Madamanchi NR, Moon SK, Hakim ZS, et al. Differential activation of mitogenic signaling pathways in aortic smooth muscle cells deficient in superoxide dismutase isoforms. *Arterioscler Thromb Vasc Biol* 2005;25:950.

103. Rajagopalan S, Meng XP, Ramasamy S, et al. Reactive oxygen species produced by macrophage-derived foam cells regulate the activity of vascular matrix metalloproteinases in vitro. Implications for atherosclerotic plaque stability. *J Clin Invest* 1996;98(11):2572.

104. Sundaresan M, Yu ZX, Ferrans VJ, et al. Requirement for generation of H2O2 for platelet-derived growth factor signal transduction. *Science* 1995;270(5234):296.

105. Khan BV, Harrison DG, Olbrych MT, et al. Nitric oxide regulates vascular cell adhesion molecule 1 gene expression and redox-sensitive transcriptional events in human vascular endothelial cells. *Proc Natl Acad Sci U S A* 1996;93:9114.

106. Alexander RW. Theodore Cooper Memorial Lecture. Hypertension and the pathogenesis of atherosclerosis. Oxidative stress and the mediation of arterial inflammatory response: a new perspective. *Hypertension* 1995;25(2):155.

107. Usui M, Egashira K, Tomita H, et al. Important role of local angiotensin II activity mediated via type 1 receptor in the pathogenesis of cardiovascular inflammatory changes induced by chronic blockade of nitric oxide synthesis in rats. *Circulation* 2000;101:305.

108. De Keulenaer GW, Ushio-Fukai M, Yin Q, et al. Convergence of redox-sensitive and mitogen-activated protein kinase signaling pathways in tumor necrosis factor-alpha–mediated monocyte chemoattractant protein-1 induction in vascular smooth muscle cells. *Arterioscler Thromb Vasc Biol* 2000;20(2):385.

109. Han Y, Runge MS, Brasier AR. Angiotensin II induces interleukin-6 transcription in vascular smooth muscle cells through pleiotropic activation of nuclear factor-kappa B transcription factors. *Circ Res* 1999;84(6):695.

110. Chen XL, Tummala PE, Olbrych MT, et al. Angiotensin II induces monocyte chemoattractant protein-1 gene expression in rat vascular smooth muscle cells. *Circ Res* 1998;83(9):952.

111. Li Q, Verma IM. NF-kappaB regulation in the immune system. *Nat Rev Immunol* 2002;2(10):725.

112. Kristal B, Shurtz-Swirski R, Chezar J, et al. Participation of peripheral polymorphonuclear leukocytes in the oxidative stress and inflammation in patients with essential hypertension. *Am J Hypertens* 1998;11(8 Pt 1):921.

113. Kim CH, Vaziri ND. Hypertension promotes integrin expression and reactive oxygen species generation by circulating leukocytes. *Kidney Int* 2005;67(4):1462.

114. Fortuno A, Olivan S, Beloqui O, et al. Association of increased phagocytic NADPH oxidase-dependent superoxide production with diminished nitric oxide generation in essential hypertension. *J Hypertens* 2004;22(11):2169.

115. Weiss D, Kools JJ, Taylor WR. Angiotensin II-induced hypertension accelerates the development of atherosclerosis in ApoE-deficient mice. *Circulation* 2001;103:448.

116. Yada T, Shimokawa H, Hiramatsu O, et al. Hydrogen peroxide, an endogenous endothelium-derived hyperpolarizing factor, plays an important role in coronary autoregulation in vivo. *Circulation* 2003;107(7):1040.

117. Matoba T, Shimokawa H, Nakashima M, et al. Hydrogen peroxide is an endothelium-derived hyperpolarizing factor in mice. *J Clin Invest* 2000;106(12):1521.

118. Torrecillas G, Boyano-Adanez MC, Medina J, et al. The role of hydrogen peroxide in the contractile response to angiotensin II. *Mol Pharmacol* 2001;59(1):104.

119. Schuijt MP, Tom B, de Vries R, et al. Superoxide does not mediate the acute vasoconstrictor effects of angiotensin II: a study in human and porcine arteries. *J Hypertens* 2003;21(12):2335.

120. Gao YJ, Lee RM. Hydrogen peroxide induces a greater contraction in mesenteric arteries of spontaneously hypertensive rats through thromboxane A(2) production. *Br J Pharmacol* 2001;134(8):1639.

121. Touyz RM. Activated oxygen metabolites: do they really play a role in angiotensin II–regulated vascular tone? *J Hypertens* 2003;21(12):2335.

122. Zhuang D, Ceacareanu AC, Lin Y, et al. Nitric oxide attenuates insulin- or IGF-I-stimulated aortic smooth muscle cell motility by decreasing H2O2 levels: essential role of cGMP. *Am J Physiol Heart Circ Physiol* 2004;286(6):H2103.

123. Park JB, Touyz RM, Chen X, Schiffrin EL. Chronic treatment with a superoxide dismutase mimetic prevents vascular remodeling and progression of hypertension in salt-loaded stroke-prone spontaneously hypertensive rats. *Am J Hypertens* 2002;15(1 Pt 1):78.

124. Nabha L, Garbern JC, Buller CL, Charpie JR. Vascular oxidative stress precedes high blood pressure in spontaneously hypertensive rats. *Clin Exp Hypertens* 2005;27:71.

125. Chabrashvili T, Tojo A, Onozato ML, et al. Expression and cellular localization of classic NADPH oxidase subunits in the spontaneously hypertensive rat kidney. *Hypertension* 2002;39(2):269.

126. Paravicini TM, Chrissobolis S, Drummond GR, Sobey CG. Increased NADPH-oxidase activity and Nox4 expression during chronic hypertension is associated with enhanced cerebral vasodilatation to NADPH in vivo. *Stroke* 2004;35(2):584.

127. Zalba G, San Jose G, Beaumont FJ, et al. Polymorphisms and promoter overactivity of the p22(phox) gene in vascular smooth muscle cells from spontaneously hypertensive rats. *Circ Res* 2001;88(2):217.

128. San Jose G, Moreno MU, Olivan S, et al. Functional effect of the p22phox-930A/G polymorphism on p22phox expression and NADPH oxidase activity in hypertension. *Hypertension* 2004;44:163.

129. Kumar U, Chen J, Sapoznikhov V, et al. Overexpression of inducible nitric oxide synthase in the kidney of the spontaneously hypertensive rat. *Clin Exp Hypertens* 2005;27:17.

130. Vaneckova I, Kramer HJ, Novotna J, et al. Role of nitric oxide and oxidative stress in the regulation of blood pressure and renal function in prehypertensive Ren-2 transgenic rats. *Kidney Blood Press Res* 2005;28(2):117.

131. Laursen JB, Rajagopalan S, Galis Z, et al. Role of superoxide in angiotensin II–induced but not catecholamine-induced hypertension. *Circulation* 1997;95:588.

132. Virdis A, Fritsch Neves M, et al. Spironolactone improves angiotensin-induced vascular changes and oxidative stress. *Hypertension* 2002;40(4):504.

133. Tojo A, Onozato ML, Kobayashi N, et al. Angiotensin II and oxidative stress in Dahl salt-sensitive rat with heart failure. *Hypertension* 2002;40(6):834–839.

134. Ding Y, Gonick HC, Vaziri ND, et al. Lead-induced hypertension. III. Increased hydroxyl radical production. *Am J Hypertens* 2001;14:169.

135. Dobrian AD, Davies MJ, Schriver SD, et al. Oxidative stress in a rat model of obesity-induced hypertension. *Hypertension* 2001;37:554.

136. Wu R, Millette E, Wu L, de Champlain J. Enhanced superoxide anion formation in vascular tissues from spontaneously hypertensive and desoxycorticosterone acetate-salt hypertensive rats. *J Hypertens* 2001;19(4):741.

137. Iglarz M, Touyz RM, Viel EC, et al. Involvement of oxidative stress in the profibrotic action of aldosterone. Interaction with the renin-angiotensin system. *Am J Hypertens* 2004;17(7):597.

138. Welch WJ, Mendonca M, Aslam S, Wilcox CS. Roles of oxidative stress and AT$_1$ receptors in renal hemodynamics and oxygenation in the postclipped 2K,1C kidney. *Hypertension* 2003;41(3 Pt 2):692.

139. Javeshghani D, Touyz RM, Sairam MR, et al. Attenuated responses to angiotensin II in follitropin receptor knockout mice, a model of menopause-associated hypertension. *Hypertension* 2003;42(4):761.

140. Hong HJ, Hsiao G, Cheng TH, Yen MH. Supplemention with tetrahydrobiopterin suppresses the development of hypertension in spontaneously hypertensive rats. *Hypertension* 2001;38(5):1044.

141. Kimura S, Zhang GX, Nishiyama A, et al. Mitochondria-derived reactive oxygen species and vascular MAP kinases: comparison of angiotensin II and diazoxide. *Hypertension* 2005;45(3):438.

142. Wallwork CJ, Parks DA, Schmid-Schonbein GW. Xanthine oxidase activity in the dexamethasone-induced hypertensive rat. *Microvasc Res* 2003;66(1):30.

143. Rodriguez-Iturbe B, Zhan CD, Quiroz Y, et al. Antioxidant-rich diet relieves hypertension and reduces renal immune infiltration in spontaneously hypertensive rats. *Hypertension* 2003;41(2):341.

144. Ratnayake WM, Plouffe L, Hollywood R, et al. Influence of sources of dietary oils on the life span of stroke-prone spontaneously hypertensive rats. *Lipids* 2000;35(4):409.

145. Dominiczak AF, Graham D, McBride MW, et al. Cardiovascular genomics and oxidative stress. *Hypertension* 2005;45:636.

146. Lacy F, Kailasam MT, O'Connor DT, et al. Plasma hydrogen peroxide production in human essential hypertension: role of heredity, gender, and ethnicity. *Hypertension* 2000;36(5):878.

147. Minuz P, Patrignani P, Gaino S, et al. Increased oxidative stress and platelet activation in patients with hypertension and renovascular disease. *Circulation* 2002;106(22):2800.

148. Stojiljkovic MP, Lopes HF, Zhang D, et al. Increasing plasma fatty acids elevates F2-isoprostanes in humans: implications for the cardiovascular risk factor cluster. *J Hypertens* 2002;20(6):1215.

149. Russo C, Olivieri O, Girelli D, et al. Anti-oxidant status and lipid peroxidation in patients with essential hypertension. *J Hypertens* 1998;16(9):1267.

150. Minuz P, Patrignani P, Gaino S, et al. Increased oxidative stress and platelet activation in patients with hypertension and renovascular disease. *Circulation* 2002;106:2800.

151. Redon J, Oliva MR, Tormos C, et al. Anti-oxidant activities and oxidative stress by-products in human hypertension. *Hypertension* 2003;41:1096.

152. Lip GY, Edmunds E, Nuttall SL, et al. Oxidative stress in malignant and non-malignant phase hypertension. *J Hum Hypertens* 2002;16(5):333.

153. Lee VM, Quinn PA, Jennings SC, Ng LL. Neutrophil activation and production of reactive oxygen species in pre-eclampsia. *J Hypertens* 2003;21(2):395.

154. Parslow RA, Sachdev P, Salonikas C, et al. Associations between plasma antioxidants and hypertension in a community-based sample of 415 Australians aged 60–64. *J Hum Hypertens* 2005;19(3):219.

155. Ward NC, Hodgson JM, Puddey IB, et al. Oxidative stress in human hypertension: association with antihypertensive treatment, gender, nutrition, and lifestyle. *Free Radic Biol Med* 2004;36:226.

156. Duffy SJ, Gokce N, Holbrook M, et al. Treatment of hypertension with ascorbic acid. *Lancet* 1999;354:2048.

157. Fotheby MD, Williams JC, Forster LA, et al. Effect of vitamin C on ambulatory blood pressure and plasma lipids in older patients. *J Hypertens* 2000;18:411.

158. Touyz RM, Schiffrin EL. Increased generation of superoxide by angiotensin II in smooth muscle cells from resistance arteries of hypertensive patients: role of phospholipase D-dependent NAD(P)H oxidase-sensitive pathways. *J Hypertens* 2001;19(7):1245.

159. Touyz RM, Tabet F, Schiffrin EL. Redox-dependent signalling by angiotensin II and vascular remodelling in hypertension. *Clin Exp Pharmacol Physiol* 2003;30(11):860.

160. Sagar S, Kallo IJ, Kaul N, et al. Oxygen free radicals in essential hypertension. *Mol Cell Biochem* 1992;111(1–2):103.

161. Minuz P, Patrignani P, Gaino S, et al. Determinants of platelet activation in human essential hypertension. *Hypertension* 2004;43:64.

162. Germano G, Sanguigni V, Pignatelli P, et al. Enhanced platelet release of superoxide anion in systemic hypertension: role of AT1 receptors. *J Hypertens* 2004;22(6):1151.

163. Rueckschloss U, Quinn MT, Holtz J, Morawietz H. Dose-dependent regulation of NAD(P)H oxidase expression by angiotensin II in human endothelial cells: protective effect of angiotensin II type 1 receptor blockade in patients with coronary artery disease. *Arterioscler Thromb Vasc Biol* 2002;22(11):1845.

164. Dechend R, Viedt C, Muller DN, et al. AT$_1$ receptor agonistic antibodies from preeclamptic patients stimulate NADPH oxidase. *Circulation* 2003;107(12):1632.

165. Welch WJ, Wilcox CS. AT$_1$ receptor antagonist combats oxidative stress and restores nitric oxide signaling in the SHR. *Kidney Int* 2001;59:1257.

166. Schiffrin EL, Touyz RM. Multiple actions of angiotensin II in hypertension: benefits of AT$_1$ receptor blockade. *J Am Coll Cardiol* 2003;42(5):911.

167. Vivekananthan DP, Penn MS, Sapp SK, et al. Use of antioxidant vitamins for the prevention of cardiovascular disease: meta-analysis of randomised trials. *Lancet* 2003;361(9374):2017.

168. Stephens NG, Parsons A, Schofield PM, et al. Randomised controlled trial of vitamin E in patients with coronary disease: Cambridge Heart Antioxidant Study (CHAOS). *Lancet* 1996;347(9004):781.

169. Salonen RM, Nyyssonen K, Kaikkomen J. Six year effect of combined vitamin C and E supplementation on atherosclerotic progression: the Antioxidant Supplementation in Atherosclerosis Prevention (ASAP) Study. *Circulation* 2003;107:947.

170. HOPE Investigators. Vitamin E supplementation and cardiovascular events in high-risk patients. *N Engl J Med* 2000;342:154.

171. HOPE-TOO Trial Investigators. Effects of long-term vitamin E supplementation on cardiovascular events and cancer. A randomized controlled trial. *JAMA* 2005;293:1338.

Chapter

31

Natriuretic Peptides

Jacob George and Allan D. Struthers

Definition

- Four members of the natriuretic peptide (NP) family are atrial natriuretic peptide (ANP), brain natriuretic peptide (BNP), C-type natriuretic peptide (CNP) and dendroaspis natriuretic peptide.

- Natriuretic peptide receptor (NPR) A and NPR B receptors mediate natriuretic peptide action by generating cGMP second messengers.

Key Findings

- NPs are eliminated by a clearance receptor NPR C or enzymatic degradation by neutral endopeptidase.

- Besides natriuresis, ANP, and BNP are antimitogenic and inhibit cardiac fibrosis.

- CNP acts in a paracrine manner in regulation of vascular tone and growth.

Clinical Implications

- ANP and BNP levels are elevated in many diseases such as hypertension and heart failure.

- BNP is useful as a rule-out test in the diagnosis of heart failure but not as a population screening tool.

- NP infusions improve hemodynamic parameters but a mortality benefit in heart failure is unproven.

- Safety concerns with BNP infusion due to increased short term mortality and worsening renal function.

- Neutral endopeptidase inhibitors are potent antihypertensives but increased incidence of angioedema.

Very few significant discoveries in medical research in the last 50 years have generated as much interest and debate as the natriuretic peptide system (NPS). As more information becomes available, we are slowly beginning to comprehend the importance of this system in the maintenance of cardiovascular health and also its role in redressing the balance when pathologic states predominate. The aim of this chapter is to provide an overview of the historical background, our current understanding of the physiology and pathophysiology, and the advances in translating the knowledge we have obtained into clinical application, both diagnostic and therapeutic.

Kisch[1] first observed small granules on electron microscope examination of guinea pig myocytes as early as 1956. Eight years later, Jamieson and Palade[2] made the discovery that these previously described granules were secretory in nature and found in mammalian atria but not

ventricles. The exact role of these atrial granules remained elusive until 1981, when de Bold et al.[3] published what was to become the seminal paper in the history of natriuretic peptides. They injected rat atrial extract into anaesthetized rats and observed a 30-fold increase in urinary sodium excretion, a 10-fold increase in urine volume, increased hematocrit and a sustained fall in arterial pressure. They repeated this with a ventricular extract but found no such effect. These results caused much interest in the scientific community and within 3 years, Kangawa and Matsuo[4] isolated the atrial natriuretic peptide (ANP) and determined its structure. The ANP gene was then located to the short arm of chromosome 1 and later sequenced.[5,6]

Brain Natriuretic Peptide (BNP) was then discovered by Sudoh et al.[7] in 1988 when they reported a peptide in porcine brain (hence the name) with a similar action to ANP. Subsequent studies have shown BNP to be secreted predominantly by ventricular myocardium. In contrast to ANP, which is stored in granules, BNP is constitutively released. The BNP mRNA expression is upregulated in various conditions that will be discussed later. There is a normal physiologic expression of both ANP and BNP in health that underlines the importance of the NPS in maintaining cardiovascular homeostasis.

C-natriuretic peptide (CNP) was then isolated from porcine brain by Sudoh et al. in 1990.[8] CNP has lower circulating levels than ANP or BNP, and is thought to act in a paracrine manner.[9] The latest member of the NPS is the dendroaspis natriuretic peptide (DNP) which was isolated by Schweitz et al.[10] from the green mamba snake (*Dendroaspis augusticeps*). It competes with ANP binding to its receptor and causes relaxation of cardiac muscles. There is very little data presently available on DNP and its precise role is still being defined.

The complete picture of the NPS with its receptors and second messengers is slowly emerging, including suggested relationships with osteoporosis and renal disease.[11]

BIOCHEMISTRY

Structure and synthesis

The three natriuretic peptides each have a 17–amino-acid ring structure that is linked by a disulfide bond between two cysteine residues. The cyclic moiety has an especially high amino acid–sequence homology. Unlike BNP, which shows great interspecies variability, the primary structure of ANP and CNP is conserved between species.

Atrial natriuretic peptide ANP

Pre-pro ANP is a 151–amino-acid precursor which contains a 25–amino-acid signal sequence. Removal of this signal peptide during synthesis gives rise to pro-ANP, also known as a-ANP, a 126–amino-acid peptide that is stored as membrane-bound granules in atrial cardiomyocytes.[12] This is the major storage form in atrial tissue, but humans differ from other species in having β-ANP, an antiparallel dimer of ANP present in atrial tissue of patients with heart failure.[13] β-ANP, like pro-ANP, has diuretic and natriuretic properties and a longer duration of action than ANP.[14]

Upon stimulation, these membrane-bound granules move to the cell surface and release stored pro-ANP,[15] which is cleaved by corin or pro-hormone convertase PCI/3, a transmembrane cardiac serine protease, to produce N-terminal ANP 1-98 (NT-ANP) and the biologically active ANP-28 (or ANP 99-126).[16] This processing probably occurs somewhere between secretion from atrial tissue and the entry of mature ANP into coronary sinus plasma.[18]

ANP-28, hereafter referred to simply as ANP, is a 28–amino-acid peptide with a 17–amino-acid ring structure closed by a disulfide bond between the two cysteine residues (see Figure 31–1). It is the major circulating form in humans and the amino acid sequence is highly conserved between species. All mammals have an identical sequence except for a single amino acid substitution.[17] It has a half-life of between 2 to 5 minutes, which is much shorter than the half-life of NT-ANP, which is between 40 to 60 minutes. This explains why plasma concentrations of NT-ANP are higher than ANP.[19] NT-ANP is raised more than ANP in patients with chronic renal failure and congestive cardiac failure.[20]

In most other hormone systems, the mature hormone is processed from the precursor before storage in granules. ANP is distinct from these systems in that it is stored in a pro-hormone form, and requires a processing mechanism during and after secretion.[17] Under normal conditions, ANP is mainly synthesized in the atria and released into the circulation via the coronary sinus. The quantity of ANP synthesized in the ventricles, under normal circumstances, is approximately 1% of total atrial secretion and the total ANP content of the ventricles is approximately $\frac{1}{30}$ that of the atria.[11] The ratios of relative abundance for ANP mRNA was 60:1 (atria–ventricles) and for BNP the corresponding ratio was 4:1.[21] These ratios alter dramatically in heart failure when synthesis and secretion of ANP in the ventricles markedly increases, equaling production levels in the atria.[22] ANP immunoreactivity is also seen in lung, aorta, adrenal, pancreas, kidney, thyroid, thymus, pituitary, salivary gland, skin, and corpus luteum tissue in rats.[23]

Brain natriuretic peptide

BNP is initially synthesized as a 134–amino-acid peptide called pre-pro BNP. The secondary cleaving of a 26–amino-acid signal peptide results in the formation of pro-BNP or BNP 1-108. This molecule is cleaved by furin, an endo-protease, into BNP 32 (Figure 31–1) and N-terminal BNP (NT-BNP 1-76).[24] Unlike ANP, there is a large biological variation of BNP homology between species. There is actually a greater homology between ANP and BNP within a species than between BNP molecules from different species.[25]

BNP mRNA and BNP have been well described in atrial myocytes[26] and the major storage form of BNP, which is found in atrial tissue is BNP-32. However, it must be remembered that the bulk of BNP secretion is expressed constitutively, and although BNP levels are higher in atrial than ventricular tissue, the greater mass of the ventricle means that a greater proportion (60%–80%) of plasma BNP originates from the ventricle.[27,28]

Like ANP, the biologic half life of BNP-32, hereafter referred to simply as BNP, is much shorter than that of NT–BNP (22 min vs. 120 min).[29] BNP is the biologically active hormone, and it is tightly regulated by precise endocrine control. NT-BNP is an inactive metabolite of pro-BNP, the blood concentrations of which do not influence the rate of myocardial hormonal secretion. Day-to-day NT-BNP levels, however, have been found to be more consistent suggesting that NT-BNP has more of an "averaging" effect, whereas BNP is more sensitive to acute changes in disease processes.[30]

Plasma BNP levels in normal subjects range from 0.6 pmol/L to 9.8 pmol/L (these are lower than concomitant ANP levels).[31] In all populations, women have higher BNP and NT-BNP levels than men.[29] In one study, women on hormone replacement therapy (HRT) had significantly higher levels than women not on HRT, suggesting that BNP production may be sensitive to estrogen regulation.[32] Obesity is not only linked to lower levels of plasma BNP, but also the attenuated release of BNP and/or increase in BNP clearance. Neither, however, has been proven.[33]

C-Type natriuretic peptide

CNP is mainly found in the vascular endothelium and central nervous system. It is the most prevalent natriuretic peptide in the central nervous system.[17] Prepro-CNP is a 126–amino-acid polypeptide which is processed into the 103–amino-acid polypeptide, pro-CNP. Further cleaving of pro-CNP by furin results in the biologically active CNP-22 and a larger biologically inactive CNP-53.[19] The predominant form of CNP in plasma is the inactive CNP-53. CNP-22, hereafter referred to simply as CNP (Figure 31–1), differs from the other natriuretic peptides in that it does not have a carboxy-terminal extension.

Dendroaspis natriuretic peptide

DNP is the latest member of the natriuretic peptide family to be identified. It is a 38–amino-acid peptide with a 17–amino-acid ring linked by a disulfide bond, similar to the other natriuretic peptides. DNP-like immunoreactivity is present in human plasma and atrial myocardium.[34] DNP levels are elevated in patients with heart failure and intravenous infusions of synthetic DNP are known to induce natriuresis and increase urinary cGMP in the canine coronary artery[35] and human internal mammary arteries.[36] However, there is not much more known about its role in cardiovascular hemodynamics, and therefore it will not be discussed further.

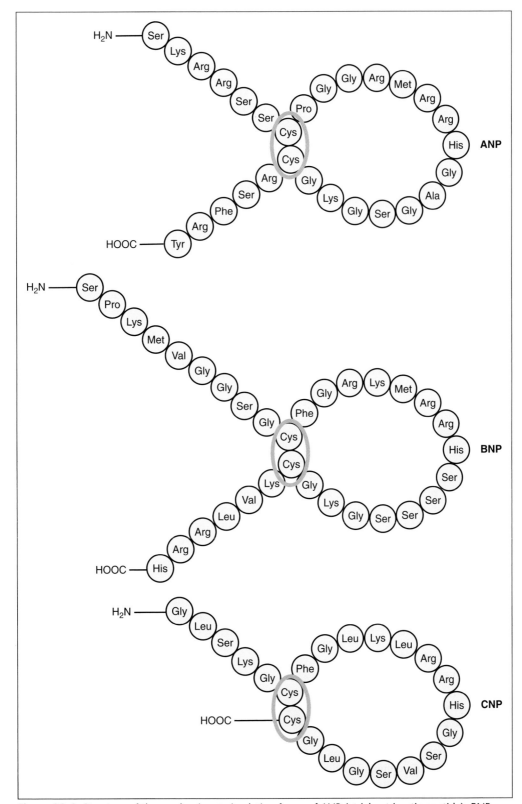

Figure 31–1. Structure of the predominant circulating forms of ANP (atrial natriuretic peptide), BNP (brain natriuretic peptide), and CNP (C-type natriuretic peptide).

GENETICS

Atrial natriuretic peptide

In humans the ANP and BNP genes are tandemly located on chromosome 1p36, only 8 kbp apart from each other.[11]

The ventricular myocytes are major sites of expression for both ANP and BNP in embryos,[37] but there is a rapid reduction in this expression after birth. In patients with left ventricular hypertrophy (LVH), there is a reversion to the fetal genotype with upregulation of the ANP gene in the ventricle.[19] The ANP gene is one of the most robust responders to diverse hypertrophic stimuli, with an increase in both ANP gene expression and the number of cells producing ANP.[38] In spontaneous hypertensive rat (SHR) models, both genes (ANP>BNP) were expressed in the left atrium and left ventricle, but not in the right atrium or ventricle.[39] Expression of the gene encoding ANP is considered a marker for hypertrophy. Other genes expressed in hypertrophic myocardium are a-myosin, β-myosin, and a-tubulin.[40]

ANP knockout mice exhibit a chronic salt-sensitive hypertension.[41] However, studies in humans have not revealed a similar relationship between ANP and salt sensitivity of blood pressure. One study investigated ethnic differences in restriction fragment–length polymorphisms for genes encoding for renin and ANP. The investigators looked for an association with blood pressure, and found that there was an association between blood pressure and the BgII and Taq1 polymorphisms for the renin gene but no association was found with the ANP gene.[42]

Brain natriuretic peptide

As stated earlier, ANP and BNP genes are tandemly located on chromosome 1p36, only 8 kbp apart from each other.[11] BNP appears to be an early-responsive gene that is upregulated at an early stage of pressure overload, well before the development of LVH.[43] In experimental rats, renal artery clipping produced BNP mRNA upregulation earlier than ANP mRNA but it is a transient phenomenon, indicating the difference between the gene expression of the two natriuretic peptides.[21] The elevation of BNP gene expression in response to mechanical loading appears to result from both transcriptional and post-transcriptional mechanisms that are very dependent on myocardial pre-load and after-load.[11] There is evidence that the mechano-transduction pathway for induction of BNP synthesis involves myocyte cell surface integrins,[44] protein kinase C, and tyrosine kinase,[45] but the exact signaling mechanism by which this hemodynamic overload induces a rapid (approximately within 2 hours) increase in BNP mRNA levels has not yet been elucidated.

C-Type natriuretic peptide

Like ANP, CNP is highly conserved between species, and CNP-22 is identical in rat, pig, and humans, whereas CNP-53 differs in only two amino acid positions between these species. The CNP gene is localized to chromosome 2q24.[11] It is thought that CNP is the ancestor gene that evolved into ANP and BNP.[11] There are four different subtypes of the CNP gene in the animal kingdom, and it is thought that a tandem duplication of CNP-3 gene before the evolutionary divergence of teleosts and tetrapods resulted in the generation of the ANP and BNP genes. The present CNP gene in mammals, however, is thought to have arisen from the CNP-4 gene.[46]

PHYSIOLOGY

The natriuretic peptides have a wide array of effects on cardiovascular hemodynamics. They exert their action by generation of intracellular cyclic guanosine 3′, 5′-monophosphate (cGMP) as second messengers. In this section, we will discuss the actions of the three main natriuretic peptides.

Atrial natriuretic peptide

Plasma ANP concentration is affected by dietary sodium intake, age, posture, and physical activity.[47] Physiologic maneuvers such as supine posture[48] and volume expansion[49] increase plasma ANP levels. Increased circulating levels are seen in congestive cardiac failure (CCF), chronic renal failure (CRF), and hypertension.

ANP mediates its effect over the short term by plasma sequestration and over the long term by promoting renal salt and water excretion as well as antagonizing the renin-angiotensin-aldosterone system (RAAS) at many levels. Both ANP and BNP antagonize the cardiac hypertrophic action of angiotensin II and continue working under conditions where endothelial nitric oxide synthase (eNOS) is compromised in conditions such as diabetes.[50] It also has inhibitory actions on the other aldosterone secretagogues such as potassium, ACTH, and metoclopramide.[28]

In vitro studies have shown that ANP inhibits sodium transport in the inner medullary collecting duct via the NPRA receptors and production of cGMP.[28] There is also evidence that the release of ANP may be under the control of a neuroendocrine reflex that acts via renal and sinoaortic baroreceptor input to the hypothalamic ANP neurons.[51,52] This release of intrahypothalamic ANP from the neuro-hypophysis activates the release of oxytocin, which in turn triggers the release of ANP from the heart using cardiac oxytocin receptors as effectors.[53] ANP has also been shown to be released from the olfactory bulb, but its function here is unclear. It has been suggested that it might produce an aversive effect on salt intake by altering salt taste.[53]

ANP has also shown to be antimitogenic. It attenuates the growth response to adrenergic stimuli and induces apoptosis by decreasing the [^{3}H] leucine incorporation.[54] This was shown by Klinger et al.[55] who demonstrated that transgenic overexpression of ANP in mice causes a decrease in heart weight and prevents right ventricular hypertrophy induced by pulmonary hypertension. The blockade of endogenous ANP also induces hypertrophy of cultured rat ventricular myocytes in a study by Horio et al.[56] This study also showed that endogenous ANP has a direct action on myocyte hypertrophy, which is independent of hemodynamic change. It is thought that ANP mediates its anti-hypertrophic action by a cGMP-dependent process that results in the activation of a cGMP-specific phospho-diesterase inhibitor that suppresses protein synthesis. It is also possible that ANP plays a role in regulation of myocardial growth during development in view of the fact that fetal and neonatal myocardium expresses the ANP gene and peptide even in normal development.[57]

ANP is thought to mediate its hypotensive effects by a combination of increased permeability of the vascular endothelium,[24] vasodilation, and increased salt and water excretion. In rats, ANP has been shown to cause dilatation of afferent arterioles and constriction of efferent arterioles within the kidney. This increases the rate of glomerular filtration and also the capillary pressure.[58] When the mechanism for arterial pressure control is impaired and body fluid volumes are elevated, such as in heart failure, large increases in atrial pressure and ANP secretion occur. The elevated plasma levels of ANP therefore are seen to exert a sustained natriuretic effect and chronically shift renal-pressure natriuresis to lower arterial pressures.[59]

ANP is generally believed to be released in response to atrial myocardial stretch. The precise mechanism for ANP release is not certain, but it is thought that stretch receptors on myocardial cells are responsible. ANP (but not BNP) levels rise in response to acute atrial or ventricular pacing.[60] It is known that pacing and tachycardia increases the frequency of depolarization and intracellular inflow of calcium ions, which in turn has the effect of promoting ANP release from secretory granules.[11] ANP is released within 2 minutes of stretching atrial and ventricular tissues. However, ventricular secretion wanes subsequently in contrast to atrial secretion which continues to increase.[61] In established heart failure, the ventricle becomes the major source of circulating ANP and it is thought that the presence of myocardial hypertrophy is a requirement for enhancing ventricular ANP gene expression.[28]

Brain natriuretic peptide

Like ANP, the actions of BNP are mediated by cyclic guanosine 3′, 5′-monophosphate (cGMP). Besides its diuretic action, BNP exerts its effect on fluid balance by causing a shift in intravascular fluid from the capillary bed into the interstitium and induces intravascular volume contraction.[62] The natriuretic and hypotensive effect of BNP is 2-3 times that of ANP but both peptides suppress the RAAS to a similar degree (approximately one-third fall in renin activity and plasma aldosterone).[63] Its biological action is mediated by the natriuretic peptide receptor-A (NPR-A) and its elimination is primarily by neutral endopeptidase (NEP) enzymes and the clearance receptor NPR-C, which will be discussed later in this chapter.

Studies have also shown that intravenous BNP inhibits vascular smooth muscle cell proliferation, reduces atheroma formation, and improves endothelial function.[64] There is also evidence that BNP suppresses cardiac sympathetic activity in humans and therefore shifts sympathovagal balance in a beneficial direction. These actions are mediated by guanylyl cyclase and NP receptors.[50]

All three natriuretic peptides have been shown to be capable of reducing thymidine incorporation in cardiac fibroblasts, which is an important step in the pathogenesis of cardiac fibrosis.[65] This effect is particularly pronounced with BNP infusions and mice lacking the BNP gene have been shown to develop extensive cardiac fibrosis.[66]

Plasma BNP levels are raised in a wide variety of states, both pathologic and nonpathologic, such as essential hypertension, LVH, chronic heart failure (CHF), right ventricular dysfunction, pregnancy-induced hypertension, aortic stenosis, with increasing age,[67] subarachnoid hemorrhage, cardiac allograft rejection, and cavo-pulmonary connections.[68] The rate and level of increase is more significant than ANP in the various cardiovascular

diseases.[60] BNP levels are also increased by drugs such as beta-blockers, cardiac glycosides, and vasopeptidase inhibitors.

C-Type natriuretic peptide

CNP is thought to play a paracrine role in regulation of vascular tone and growth.[69] However, the exact actions of CNP remain an area for future research. It has the potential to influence arterial pressure by altering autonomic regulation of vascular tone, but there has been little evidence to translate this to a relationship with human hypertension.

It has recently been suggested that CNP functions as an endothelium-derived hyperpolarizing factor (EDHF) in some vascular beds.[70] Recent evidence on porcine models suggest a dual role of inhibition of smooth muscle cell proliferation and simultaneous promotion of endothelial cell growth.[71] CNP mRNA expression in bovine endothelial cells is markedly enhanced by TGF-β, further raising the possibility of its role in vascular remodeling.[72] CNP is also known to possess antiatherogenic properties, as inflammatory cytokines such as IL-1β, TNF, and lipopolysaccharide are all known to stimulate the release of CNP from endothelial cells.[73] In addition to this, CNP also suppresses the production of proinflammatory cyclooxygenase-2 metabolites in isolated cells.[74] Thrombus formation and neointimal hyperplasia are also significantly suppressed by the presence of CNP, indicating that CNP alters leukocyte–endothelial interactions.[75]

Receptors

Most biologic effects of the natriuretic peptides result from stimulation of the second messenger, cyclic-GMP, linked receptors. In terms of cGMP generation by endocardial cells, CNP is the most potent stimulus for this. BNP is slightly less potent and ANP is the least potent cGMP-generator stimulus of the three natriuretic peptides.[76] However, CNP binding affinity and stimulatory effect on cGMP production is species dependent.[77] The natriuretic peptide receptor A (NPRA) preferentially binds ANP and BNP, whereas the natriuretic peptide receptor B (NPRB) preferentially binds CNP. NPRB is the predominant guanylate cyclase–coupled receptor in the ventricle and is downregulated in the presence of LVH.

The genes for NPRA are located on chromosome 1q21, for NPRB on chromosome 9p21, and for NPRC on chromosome 5p14. NPRA and NPRB are single transmembrane domain receptors with a very similar basic structure. The NPRA is a 115-kD glycoprotein with an intracellular protein kinase–like binding domain and a guanylate cyclase (GC) domain with enzymatic activity. Activated GC increases intracellular cGMP levels and modulates downstream proteins, such as phosphodiesterases, ion channels, and cGMP-dependent protein kinases.

Several transmembrane forms of guanylyl cyclase enzymes have been identified. They have a variable extracellular NP-binding domain, a single transmembrane domain, a more conserved intracellular kinase homology domain, and a catalytic domain.[78] The homology between the protein kinase–like domain of NPRA and NPRB is

63% and 88%, respectively, between the GC domains. The extracellular domains, however, only have a 44% homology.[11] The magnitude of biological activity of the natriuretic peptides depends greatly on their ligand selectivity. Kishimoto and Garbers[79] found that the ligand selectivity for NPRA is greatest for ANP followed by BNP, and much less for CNP. For NPRB, however, the selectivity is greatest for CNP followed by ANP and BNP. The ligand selectivity for NPRC is greatest for ANP followed by CNP and BNP.

ANP and BNP receptors have been found in the kidney, adrenal, vasculature, brain, gonads, and pituitary. Their actions at the latter two sites mainly alter steroidogenesis and pituitary hormone secretion.[80] Recent studies suggest that NP are also directly involved in moderating the cardiac growth response to hypertrophic stimuli as seen by growth inhibitory properties in noncardiac and cardiac cells in vitro.[81] The growth-regulating properties of the NPRA pathway appears to be distinct from the well-characterized MAP-kinase signaling cascade, which is the main effector of angiotensin II, endothelin-1, and a-agonists.[54] NPR knockout mice have an increased heart weight from birth that persists throughout life. The degree of cardiac hypertrophy in NPR-A–deficient mice is not decreased by normalizing blood pressure using four antihypertensive agents, which suggests that NPRA receptors regulate cardiac hypertrophy independent of blood pressure.[54]

However, there are other data that contradict this. In a series of experiments with transgenic mice, Oliver et al.[82,83] showed that overexpression of NPRA produced significantly lower blood pressure than wild-type mice, whereas NPRA knockout mice develop cardiac hypertrophy and experience sudden death. These studies show that genes for the NPS are closely involved in the mechanism of the development and progression of hypertension. They also show that mutations influencing their transcription activity, receptor binding, and cGMP-producing ability are sufficient to cause significant cardiac consequences.

The clearance receptor or natriuretic peptide receptor C (NPRC) is not linked to cGMP, and has a primary role, as its name suggests, in removal of the natriuretic peptides along with another enzyme, neutral endopeptidase (NEP). The NPRC is thought to act primarily as a clearance receptor and may also activate the phosphoinositol pathway,[84] inhibit cAMP production[85] and mediate ANP action on cell proliferation.[86] The natriuretic peptides are removed by endocytosis and lysosomal degradation.[24]

Neutral endopeptidase

Neutral endopeptidase (NEP) or endopeptidase 24.11 is a membrane-bound metallopeptidase ectoenzyme with zinc at its active site. It is connected through a single transmembrane segment to the extracellular domain containing the active site of the enzyme.[87,88] It is expressed in the brush border of the proximal tubule of the kidney, in vascular tissue (particularly of the lung and liver) and on vascular smooth muscle cells. It is also distributed throughout many tissues including the gastrointestinal (GI) system, lymph nodes, and pituitary.[89] Endopeptidase

24.11 is also involved in the degradation of AI, AII, bradykinin, adrenomedullin, endothelin, enkephalin, and gastrin. It inactivates the natriuretic peptides by opening their ring structure.[90] Kinetic studies show that CNP is the best substrate for NEP, followed by ANP and BNP.[91]

PATHOPHYSIOLOGY

The role of natriuretic peptides has been investigated in many conditions that impact cardiovascular disease either directly or indirectly. In this section, we will focus on its role in the two most studied areas, hypertension and heart failure.

Hypertension

There is a wide variation in NP levels in the population. Both ANP and BNP are elevated in hypertension with ANP:BNP ratios up to 3.8. In contrast, normal subjects have ANP:BNP ratios of 2.8, which suggest that ANP is increased to a greater level in hypertension.[92] Plasma concentration of ANP in patients with severe or complicated hypertension is elevated and well correlated with both systolic and diastolic arterial pressure,[47] and levels fall with effective treatment of high blood pressure.[93] The picture is not so clear in patients with mild and uncomplicated hypertension.[47] Most studies show that diuretics and angiotensin converting enzyme (ACE) inhibitors decrease ANP whereas β-blockers have the opposite effect.[94,95] The precise reason for this latter effect is unknown, although it is thought to be a compensatory mechanism to the central actions of these drugs.[47]

Obese patients have lower plasma BNP and NT-ANP compared to nonobese patients. Diabetic patients also have low plasma NP levels, and the negative effects of obesity and diabetes on NP levels are additive.[96] This may be part of the reason that obese patients are more likely to be hypertensive. A recent study[97] showed that in obese patients, ANP levels were mainly influenced by diastolic dysfunction, whereas BNP was influenced by both LVH and LV systolic dysfunction. The authors therefore suggest that ANP and BNP can be considered a useful marker of preclinical cardiac disease in obesity.

Impaired NP responses to dietary sodium may be an early step in the development of hypertension. Ferrier et al.[98] showed that normotensive offspring of hypertensive patients had impaired plasma ANP responses to dietary sodium. Widgren et al.[99] also showed that normotensive patients with positive family histories for hypertension had blunted plasma ANP responses to volume loading. Some studies have also shown that BNP is an independent predictor of future hypertension in males and females with a family history of hypertension,[100] while the Framingham Heart Study data suggest that this relationship is only seen in men.[101]

The etiology of hypertension seems to have an effect on the levels of various NP subsets. Patients with renovascular hypertension have higher NT pro-ANP and BNP levels compared to patients with essential hypertension despite similar blood pressure values, but plasma ANP rises progressively with increasing severity of hypertension in both renovascular and essential hypertension. However, these NPs are not suitable as screening tools for renovascular hypertension due to their low sensitivity in patients with this condition. NT pro-ANP seems to also be correlated with systolic blood pressure and the suggested cut-off value for hypertension is 530 pmol/L, which produces a sensitivity of 67% and a specificity of 86%.[101]

Plasma ANP and BNP have been found to positively correlate with the left ventricular mass index (LVMI)[97,103,104] and plasma BNP, as well as with interventricular septum thickness.[105] However, BNP seems to have a low discriminatory power to distinguish between normal and abnormal LVMI (area under receiver operating characteristic [ROC] curve 0.59–0.62 in various studies) showing that BNP was possibly not a good discriminator (and therefore not a useful screening test) to determine the presence or absence of LVH in hypertensive patients.[106–108] These data are contradicted by other studies which have shown that hypertensive patients with LVH have higher ANP and BNP levels compared to hypertensive patients without LVH.[103] This issue is further complicated by data from Murakami et al.,[104] who performed a stepwise multiple regression analysis and showed that it is atrial BNP, not ventricular BNP, which is an independent predictor of ventricular mass in patients with LVH.

It is thought that LV mass is not in itself the cause for elevated BNP levels. Although LVMI was significantly higher in athletes and hypertensive patients than in age-matched controls, plasma BNP levels were significantly higher in the hypertensive cohort compared to the athletes or age-matched controls who had similar BNP levels. This suggests that BNP is elevated in the presence of a pathologically (but not physiologically) increased LV mass.[109] There is a similar correlation between LV mass and the severity of aortic stenosis, suggesting that preoperative BNP level may help identify a subgroup of patients who are likely to have a worse outcome after valve replacement surgery.[110] Experimental evidence also suggests that induction of BNP gene expression is one of the earliest responses to hemodynamic pressure overload and occurs before the onset of LVH.[111]

Different patterns of LV hypertrophy seem to be related to specific natriuretic peptides. For example, there is evidence that patients with eccentric hypertrophy and concentric remodeling have raised ANP levels, but patients with concentric hypertrophy have raised levels of ANP and BNP.[112] This is further confirmed in patients with hypertrophic obstructive cardiomyopathy (HCM) in whom ANP mRNA is detected in significant quantities in the left ventricle myocytes.[113] Both ANP and BNP levels have been found to be higher in HCM patients with diastolic dysfunction compared to HCM patients without diastolic dysfunction.[114] There is evidence that reactivation of the whole embryonic repertoire (ANP, skeletal actin, β-myosin heavy chain) occurs in cardiac hypertrophy.[65] Of these, ANP gene reactivation is seen as one of the most sensitive markers of cardiac tissue hypertrophy.[115]

Patients with myocardial dysfunction seem to exhibit greater rises in BNP during exercise. Lim et al.[116] found that an exercise-induced BNP rise was a significant predictor of oxygen consumption as measured by VO$_2$max irrespective of the presence or absence of LVH. They have suggested that BNP may potentially act as a homeostatic mechanism that helps limit exercise incapacity in hypertensive patients.

Plasma BNP has also been shown to be an excellent marker for assessing functional impairment in patients with primary pulmonary hypertension as it is thought to parallel the extent of pulmonary hemodynamic changes and the degree of right heart failure.[117]

Heart failure

The role of BNP in heart failure (HF) diagnosis has been more extensively studied than the other peptides but there is clear evidence that both ANP and BNP are elevated in heart failure (Figure 31–2). Although CNP content in atrial and ventricular tissue is elevated in heart failure,[118] plasma CNP and DNP are not significantly elevated in patients with hypertension or heart failure.[34,119] In patients with congestive cardiac failure, each 1-mmHg rise in atrial pressure causes an approximate rise of 10 to 14 pmol/L in venous plasma ANP concentration.[120]

The natriuretic effects of ANP and BNP, however, are markedly blunted in HF patients.[19] Despite this, there is a significant correlation seen between NT-BNP and echocardiogram-derived LV ejection fraction.[121] BNP levels are seen to rise with increasing severity of HF and may equal or exceed ANP levels[31] (Figure 31–2). This pattern is also seen in right ventricular (RV) failure secondary to chronic obstructive pulmonary disease as well as patients with right ventricular dysfunction secondary to pulmonary emboli.[122,123] However, BNP levels do not show a consistent pattern in order to differentiate RV from LV dysfunction.[33]

Multivariate analyses of the FRESH-BNP study reveal that plasma NT-BNP and New York Heart Association (NYHA) classification, but not ejection fraction are inde-

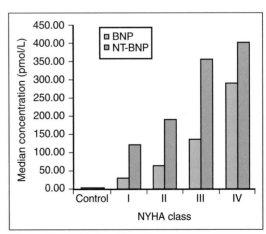

Figure 31–2. Relationship between BNP and NT-proBNP and the NYHA functional classification. BNP, B-type natriuretic peptide; NT-BNP, N-terminal-proBNP; NYHA, New York Heart Association. (Data from Roche Diagnostics, ProBrain Natriuretic Peptide package insert. Indianapolis, IN: Roche Diagnostics Inc., 2004; and Biosite, Triage BNP product insert. San Diego: Biosite Inc., 2000.)

pendent predictors of peak O_2 consumption (VO$_2$ max).[121] In a head-to-head comparison, BNP was found to be more accurate than NT-BNP in identifying patients with LV systolic dysfunction (area under ROC curve 0.83 vs. 0.79).[124] There are various strengths and weaknesses of measuring BNP or NT-BNP. On the one hand, BNP is available at the point of care, is less influenced by age and renal function and there is a single, approved cut-off point for HF diagnosis (100 pg/mL). On the other hand, the tight relation to renal function makes NT-BNP a better overall indicator of cardio-renal function and its use on large laboratory platforms makes it a much more economical test.[29] As many patients with HF have varying degrees of renal impairment, it must also be noted that BNP levels rise significantly in dialysis-dependent patients and does not always fall with dialysis.[125]

The role of NP is not as clear in patients with diastolic dysfunction. Some studies have indicated that BNP may not be useful in identifying diastolic dysfunction in the setting of a normal ejection fraction,[126] but this is contradicted by others[127] who have shown that the area under the ROC curve for BNP to detect diastolic dysfunction is as high as 0.92. Yancy[33] suggests that the presence of a normal RV and LV function with an elevated BNP should form a diagnostic tenet for diastolic dysfunction.

Although many patients with HF have chronic disease anemia, there is an association between lower hemoglobin levels and raised BNP that is independent of age, sex, serum creatinine, LV wall motion abnormalities, LVH, history of chronic heart failure, or atrial fibrillation.[128] There is also evidence to suggest that BNP (but not NT-BNP) is also an independent predictor of sudden death in patients with chronic HF.[129]

The role of BNP in heart failure seems to be as a rule-out tool as it has consistently shown to have a high negative predictive value for the diagnosis of LV dysfunction and HF.[33] The Breathing Not Properly study showed that incorporating BNP into the clinical evaluation of CHF raises diagnostic accuracy by 10% in patients whom emergency department physicians had a high confidence in the diagnosis of HF. The investigators reported 90% sensitivity and 76% specificity when 100 pg/mL was used as a cut-off for the diagnosis of HF.[130] This was also the finding of the REDHOT study,[131] and is consistent with European guidelines for the diagnosis and treatment of chronic HF, which have incorporated BNP as a diagnostic test for routine clinical practice along with echocardiography and a chest x-ray.[132] BNP testing is an economically feasible exercise as shown by the BASEL study. The investigators found that using BNP measurement in the initial diagnostic evaluation resulted in 26% lower costs from fewer admissions to the intensive care unit and a shorter overall stay.[133]

CLINICAL IMPLICATIONS

Natriuretic peptides as population screening tool

Tsutamoto et al.[134] found that BNP is superior to ANP in predicting mortality in patients with minimally sympto-

matic left ventricular dysfunction. They showed that each 10-pg/mL increase in plasma BNP associated with a 3% increase in cardiac death over the follow-up period of the study. A recent meta-analysis showed that BNP was a strong prognostic indicator for both asymptomatic patients and for patients with heart failure at all stages of disease.[135]

However, BNP testing is probably not appropriate for screening large asymptomatic populations for LV systolic dysfunction.[136] The pitfalls of BNP as a population screening tool is as predicted by Bayes theorem—the lower the prevalence of the condition screened for, the larger the false-positive rate, and hence the lower the positive predictive value.[19] McDonagh et al.[137] showed that using BNP to screen for LV dysfunction in the population yielded a high negative predictive value (97.5%), but a low positive predictive value (16%), further strengthening the case for BNP use as a rule-out test. This was further confirmed by Vasan et al.[138] using data from the Framingham Heart Study.

Natriuretic peptides as treatment modality

There are two ways in which NP levels can be raised: exogenous delivery and preventing degradation. Exogenous natriuretic peptides remain effective as a treatment modality even when endogenous peptide levels are raised.

Atrial natriuretic peptide

ANP infusions in patients with essential hypertension have been shown to induce a six-fold rise in natriuresis, enhance sodium excretion, and halve plasma aldosterone.[139] Almost 20 years ago, Weder et al.[140] showed that at low doses, ANP inhibits both renin and aldosterone, but at higher doses a substantial fall in blood pressure results in compensatory responses that abolish ANP's effect on renin and aldosterone. As intravenous ANP infusions are not a feasible long-term option, orally active NEP inhibitors that inhibit the breakdown of ANP are being investigated for its therapeutic potential.[141]

Brain natriuretic peptide

The therapeutic use of BNP is limited to in-hospital care as it is an orally inactivated peptide and delivery requires intravenous infusion. Richards et al.[142] demonstrated the effects of BNP infusions in patients with essential hypertension compared to normal controls. They showed an increase in plasma cGMP and also found that sodium excretion increased by 2.5-fold. Like ANP, plasma aldosterone levels were halved. Crucially, there were no changes to blood pressure or heart rate during the infusion, suggesting that the natriuretic response to BNP appears to be enhanced in hypertensive patients.

The main focus of research into the applicability of BNP infusions has been in the treatment of patients who are admitted to the hospital with acute decompensated heart failure. There is evidence that intravenous BNP infusions have a lusitropic but not a negatively inotropic effect on ventricular myocardium in normal and HF canine models.[143] Acute intravenous infusions of BNP lower mean systemic arterial pressure, pulmonary artery pressure (PAP), pulmonary capillary wedge pressure (PCWP), and systemic vascular resistance (SVR). It also increases plasma cGMP and levels of plasma ANP during the first hour of infusion. It has no direct effect of cardiac output or heart rate.[144]

In the Vasodilation in the Management of Acute Congestive Heart Failure (VMAC) study,[145] patients hospitalized with acute decompensated HF who were prescribed nesiritide, a recombinant form of human B-type natriuretic peptide, had significantly greater mean reduction in PCWP and fewer adverse events compared to nitroglycerin. However, there were no significant differences in 6-month mortality between the two groups, suggesting that the short-term intravenous BNP infusions may have a role as a first-time agent for hemodynamic and symptomatic improvements in the acute setting of decompensated HF. However, there have safety concerns with nesiritide recently. The PRECEDENT study looked at the safety of nesiritide, and found that intravenous BNP in patients with decompensated HF produced significantly more hypotension than dobutamine. On the positive side, unlike dobutamine, nesiritide had no effect on arrhythmias.[146] A recent meta-analysis of studies using nesiritide in acute decompensated heart failure[147] suggested that there is an increased short-term risk of death compared to non–inotrope-based therapy. There is also recent evidence that nesiritide significantly increases the risk of worsening renal function in the same population,[148] but the authors caution that further appropriately powered clinical trials are needed to determine whether the worsening renal function seen with nesiritide reflects the hemodynamic effect or renal injury.

Neutral endopeptidase inhibitors

Neutral endopeptidase (NEP) inhibitors prevent the breakdown of NP mainly in vascular tissue and the kidney. In addition to increasing ANP and BNP levels, they have the effect of increasing cGMP and natriuresis. Seymour et al.[149] showed that in spontaneously hypertensive rat (SHR) models, NEP inhibitors potentiated ANP-induced increases in sodium excretion and falls in blood pressure. Other groups have found that in order to achieve similar falls in blood pressure by means of exogenous ANP infusions, an eight-fold rise in plasma ANP was required.

Although single-dose or limited-dose studies using NEP inhibitors show enhanced natriuresis, increased plasma, and urinary cGMP and RAAS suppression, they have demonstrated little effect on blood pressure in either normotensive or hypertensive humans.[150] This is because reductions in blood pressure are offset by the fact that NEP inhibition also increases plasma angiotensin II, endothelin-1, and aldosterone. This is because those substances are also substrates for NEP.[151,152]

Studies on the effects of NEP inhibitors on BNP suggest that plasma BNP rises with a single dose of candoxatril (a novel oral neutral endopeptidase inhibitor).[47] The clinically important question of sustained inhibition is not fully known.

As NEP has been shown to be more effective in salt- and volume-dependent rather than renin-dependent hypertension, a combination with an ACE inhibitor has been effective in treating patients with hypertension and HF.[153–155] Other effects of this combination therapy include improved endothelial function,[156] increased cardiac output[157] and unlike single therapy with NEP, endothelin-1 levels were not increased.[158]

Recent trials on omapatrilat, a dual NEP and ACE inhibitor, have produced inconclusive safety data. The Omapatrilat versus Enalapril Randomized Trial of Utility in Reducing Events (OVERTURE) trial[159] showed non-inferiority of omapatrilat compared to enalapril with regard to risk of death and hospitalization in patients with chronic heart failure. There were similar rates of angioedema in the omapatrilat and enalapril groups (0.8 vs. 0.5%). However, in the recently reported Omapatrilat and Enalapril in Patients with Hypertension: The Omapatrilat Cardiovascular Treatment versus Enalapril (OCTAVE) trial,[160] despite greater reductions in blood pressure on the omapatrilat arm (especially seen in black patients), the relative risk of angioedema with omapatrilat compared to enalapril was 3.17. The authors conclude that the use of omapatrilat may be appropriate in patients with difficult-to-control hypertension and in patients with increased cardiovascular risk where the risk:benefit ratio may be more favorable.

Other peptides

There are two other peptides with natriuretic properties but that have mainly vasoactive action. Thus they have not been universally accepted as major players in the natriuretic peptide system. They are urodilatin and adrenomedullin. We will discuss these two peptides in brief.

Urodilatin

Urodilatin is a peptide consisting of amino acids 95–126 of pro-ANP, and is thought to be derived from pro-ANP by an alternative processing system. It was isolated in 1988 by Schulz-Knappe et al.[161] from human urine, and is not thought to circulate in plasma. Its actions are mediated by NPRA. It is inactivated by NPRC and by enzymatic degradation. Urodilatin is more resistant to NEP action when compared to ANP, and therefore has a more potent natriuretic than ANP.[162] Studies in healthy volunteers have shown that even small doses of urodilatin may decrease PCWP, SVR, stroke volume, and cardiac output without changes in plasma volume or blood pressure.[163] Other studies in healthy volunteers have shown a potent natriuretic response to urodilatin after 1-hour infusions. Higher doses elicit an increase in antidiuretic hormone/arginine vasopressin levels and therefore attenuate the diuresis. There is also evidence that it plays an important role in smooth muscle dilatation and immune defense.[164]

Adrenomedullin

Adrenomedullin (AM) was first discovered from human pheochromocytoma by Kitamura et al. in 1993.[165] The AM gene is found on chromosome 11, which encodes for prepro-AM, a 185–amino-acid peptide. This molecule is then cleaved into a 164–amino-acid peptide called pro-AM and a signaling molecule. Pro-AM is then processed to an immature and inactive molecule with a glycine extension, AM-Gly. The final AM molecule consists of 52 amino acids with an intramolecular disulfide bond forming a ring structure of six residues.[166] AM mRNA is expressed in all four compartments of the heart, but its main production site is vascular endothelium.[21] It is also found in the adrenals, kidneys, lungs, GI tract, and uterus.

Its major effect is on vasorelaxation but it has a potent inhibitory action on vascular proliferation.[167] Studies have shown it to be a potent vasodilator in both coronary and pulmonary arteries,[168,169] and a variety of experimental hypertensive rat models show an AM gene overexpression.[21] There is very little evidence of a role for AM in heart failure with suggestions of a link with diastolic but not systolic dysfunction.

AM produces marked natriuresis and diuresis in experimental animal models, particularly in the setting of heart failure.[170] There is contradictory data on its natriuretic effect in humans.[171,172] The effects of AM on other systems are beyond the scope of this chapter. For a thorough and excellent review on AM, see the review article by Bunton et al.[173]

SUMMARY

The concept of the heart as an endocrine organ and the subsequent discovery of the NPS have stimulated much research and debate into how clinicians can effectively use these peptides for diagnostic and therapeutic purposes. There may be other members of this family that are yet to be discovered, and therefore the complete picture of this complex regulatory system is yet to be seen.

As we have seen, the natriuretic and anti-mitogenic effects of the natriuretic peptides attempt to counterbalance pathologic fluid-balance dynamics and hypertensive changes seen in many different clinical conditions such as diabetes, pulmonary hypertension, pregnancy-induced hypertension, left ventricular hypertrophy, and heart failure. BNP also inhibits cardiac fibrosis by interfering with thymidine metabolism in fibroblasts. The paracrine role of CNP in vascular tone regulation, control of smooth muscle proliferation, and as an anti-inflammatory agent is slowly emerging with its recent identification as an endothelium-derived hyperpolarizing factor.

BNP and NT-BNP are generally regarded to have a higher diagnostic and prognostic accuracy than ANP and NT-ANP, but the use of BNP as a screening tool to detect left ventricular dysfunction in large asymptomatic populations is problematic. Its high negative predictive value does make it more useful as a rule-out test in symptomatic patients. However, as the Breathing Not Properly study[130] has shown, it may have a role in the evaluation of the acutely breathless patient in the emergency department setting and this has been incorporated into the latest European guidelines.[132]

The natriuretic peptides have been licensed in countries like Japan (ANP) and the United States (BNP) for treatment of acute heart failure. However, despite its beneficial effects on hemodynamic parameters as seen in the VMAC trial,[145] incorporating intravenous infusions of natriuretic peptides into the management of patients admitted with acute decompensated HF have not shown a significant mortality benefit. In addition to this, intravenous infusions are not a suitable long-term management option. Agents that prevent NP breakdown such as NEP inhibitors show much promise in this respect, especially in combination with ACE inhibitors.

The next few years should see further development of more cost-effective laboratory methods of measuring natriuretic peptides (especially BNP) on larger platforms. Newer and safer vasopeptidase/neutral endopeptidase inhibitors may also emerge.

REFERENCES

1. Kisch B. Electron microscopy of the atrium of the heart. I. Guinea pig. *Exp Med Surg* 1956;14:99.
2. Jamieson JD, Palade GE. Specific granules in atrial muscle cells. *J Cell Biol* 1964;23:151.
3. deBold AJ, Borenstein HB, Veress AT, Sonnenberg H. A rapid and potent natriuretic response to intravenous injection of atrial myocardial extract in rats. *Life Sci* 1981;28:89.
4. Kangawa K, Matsuo H. Purification and complete amino acid sequence of alpha-human natriuretic polypeptide (alpha hANP). *Biochem Biophys Res Commun* 1984;118:139.
5. Nakayama K, Ohkubo H, Hirose T, et al. mRNA sequence for human cardiolatin-atrial natriuretic factor precursor and regulation of precursor mRNA in rat atria. *Nature* 1984;310:699.
6. Seidman CE, Bloch KD, Klein KA, et al. Nucleotide sequence of the human and mouse atrial natriuretic factor genes. *Science* 1984;226:1206.
7. Sudoh T, Kangawa K, Minamino N, Matsuo H. A new natriuretic peptide in porcine brain. *Nature* 1988;332:78.
8. Sudoh T, Minamino N, Kangawa K Matsuo H. C-type natriuretic peptide (NP): a new member of the natriuretic peptide family identified in porcine brain. *Biochem Biophys Res Commun* 1990;168:863.
9. Wei C, Heublein DM, Perrella MA, et al. Natriuretic peptide system in human heart failure. *Circulation* 1993;88:1004.
10. Schweitz H, Vigne P, Moinier D, et al. A new member of the natriuretic peptide family is present in the venom of the green mamba (dendroaspis augusticeps). *J Biol Chem* 1992;267:13928.
11. Nakayama T. The genetic contribution of the natriuretic peptide system to cardiovascular disease. *Endocrine J* 2005;52(1):11.
12. Oikawa S, Imai M, Ueno A, et al. Cloning and sequence analysis of cDNA encoding a precursor for human atrial natriuretic polypeptide. *Nature* 1984;309:724.
13. Sugawara A, Nakao K, Morii N, et al. Synthesis of atrial natriuretic polypeptide in failing human hearts. Evidence of altered processing of atrial natriuretic polypeptide precursor and augmented synthesis of β-human ANP. *J Clin Invest* 1988;81:1962.
14. Itoh H, Nakao N, Shiono S, et al. Conversion of β-ANP in human plasma in-vitro. *Biochem Biophys Res Commun* 1987;143:560.
15. Klein RM, Kelley KB, Meriskoliversidge EM. A clathrin coated vesicle-mediated pathway in atrial natriuretic peptide (ANP) secretion. *J Moll Cell Cardiol* 1993;25:437.
16. Yan W, Wu F, Morser J, et al. Corin, a transmembrane cardiac serine protease, acts as a pro-atrial natriuretic peptide converting enzyme. *Proc Natl Acad Sci U S A* 2000;97:8525.
17. Yandle TG. Minisymposium: The natriuretic peptide hormones: biochemistry of natriuretic peptides. *J Intern Med* 1994;235:561.

18. Yandle T, Crozier I, Nicholls G, et al. Amino acid sequence of atrial natriuretic peptides in human coronary sinus plasma. *Biochem Biophys Res Commun* 1987;146:832.

19. Munagala VK, Burnett JC Jr, Redfield MM. The natriuretic peptides in Cardiovascular Medicine. *Curr Probl Cardiol* 2004;29:707.

20. Sundsford JA, Thiabult G, Larochelle P, Cantin M. Identification and plasma concentrations of the N-terminal fragment of pro-atrial natriuretic factor in man. *J Clin Endocrinol Metab* 1988; 66:605.

21. Wolf K, Kurtz A, Pfeifer M, et al. Different regulation of left ventricular ANP, BNP and adrenomedullin mRNA in the two-kidney, one-clip model of renovascular hypertension. *Eur J Physiol* 2001;442:212.

22. Saito Y, Nakao K, Arai H, et al. Augmented expression of atrial natriuretic polypeptide gene in ventricle of human failing heart. *J Clin Invest* 1989;83:298.

23. McKenzie JC, Tanaka I, Misono KS, Inagami T. Immunocytochemical localization of atrial natriuretic factor in the kidney, adrenal, pituitary and atrium rat. *J Histochem Cytochem* 1985;33:828.

24. Yap LB, Ashrafian H, Mukerjee D, et al. The natriuretic peptides and their role in disorders of right heart dysfunction and pulmonary hypertension. *Clin Biochem* 2004; 37:847.

25. Rosenweig A, Seidmen CE. Atrial natriuretic factor and related peptide hormones. *Ann Rev Biochem* 1991; 60:229.

26. Luchner A, Stevens TL, Borgeson DD, et al. Differential atrial and ventricular expression of myocardial BNP during evolution of heart failure. *Am J Physiol* 1998;274:H1684.

27. Ogawa Y, Nakao K, Mukoyama M, et al. Natriuretic peptides as cardiac hormones in normotensive and spontaneously hypertensive rats. The ventricle is a major site of synthesis and secretion of brain natriuretic peptide. *Circ Res* 1991; 69:491.

28. Espiner EA. Minisymposium: The natriuretic peptide hormones: physiology of natriuretic peptides. *J Intern Med* 1994;235:527.

29. McCullough PA Omland T, Maisel AS. B-type natriuretic peptide: a diagnostic breakthrough for Clinicians. Rev in Cardiovasc Med 2003;4(2):72.

30. Wu AHB, Smith A, Wieczorek S, et al. Biological variation for N-terminal pro- and B-type natriuretic peptides and implications for therapeutic monitoring of patients with congestive heart failure. *Am J Cardiol* 2003;92:628.

31. Mukoyama M, Nakao K, Hosoda K, et al. Brain natriuretic peptide as a novel cardiac hormone in humans—evidence for an exquisite dual natriuretic peptide system. *J Clin Invest* 1991;87:1402.

32. Redfield MM, Rodeheffer RJ, Jacobsen SJ, et al. Plasma brain natriuretic peptide concentration: impact of age and gender. *J Am Coll Cardiol* 2002; 40(5):976.

33. Yancy CW. Practical considerations for BNP use. *Heart Fail Rev* 2003;8:369.

34. Schirger JA, Heublein DM, Chen HH, et al. Presence of Dendroaspis natriuretic peptide-like immunoreactivity in human plasma and its increase during human heart failure. *Mayo Clin Proc* 1999;74:126–30.

35. Lisy O, Jougasaki M, Heublein DM, et al. Renal actions of synthetic dendroaspis natriuretic peptide. *Kidney Int* 1999;56:502.

36. Best PJ, Burnett JC, Wilson SH, et al. Dendroaspis natriuretic peptide relaxes isolated human arteries and veins. *Cardiovasc Res* 2002;55:375.

37. Ellmers LJ, Knowles JW, Kim HS, et al. Ventricular expression of natriuretic peptides in Npr1-/- mice with cardiac hypertrophy and fibrosis. *Am J Physiol Heart Circ Physiol* 2002;283:H707.

38. Lattion AL, Michel JB, Arnauld E, et al. Myocardial recruitment during ANF mRNA increase with volume overload in the rat. *Am J Physiol* 1986;251:H890.

39. Raizada V, Thakore K, Luo W, McGuire PG. Cardiac chamber specific alterations of ANP and BNP expression with advancing age and with systemic hypertension. *Moll Cell Biochem* 2001; 216(1–2):137.

40. Buttrick PM, Kaplan M, Leinwand LA, Scheuer J. Alterations in gene expression in the rat heart after chronic pathological and physiological loads. *J Mol Cell Cardiol* 1994;26:61–7.

41. John SW, Krege JH, Oliver PM, et al. Genetic decreases in atrial natriuretic peptide and salt-sensitive hypertension. *Science* 1995;267:679.

42. Barley J, Carter ND, Cruickshank JK, et al. Renin and atrial natriuretic peptide restriction fragment length polymorphisms: association with ethnicity and blood pressure. *J Hypertens* 1991;9:993.

43. Tokola H, Hautala N, Marttila M, et al. Mechanical load–induced alterations in B-type natriuretic peptide gene expression. *Can J Physiol Pharmacol* 2001;79:646.

44. Liang F, Kovacic-Milivojevic B, Chen S, et al. Signaling mechanisms underlying strain-dependent brain natriuretic peptide gene transcription. *Can J Physiol Pharmacol* 2001;79:640.

45. Magga J, Vuolteenaho O, Tokola H, et al. Involvement of transcriptional and post-transcriptional mechanisms in cardiac-overload induced increase of B-type natriuretic peptide gene expression. *Circ Res* 1997;81:694.

46. Inoue K, Naruse K, Yamagami S, et al. Four functionally distinct C-type natriuretic peptides found in fish reveal evolutionary history of the natriuretic peptide system. *Proc Natl Acad Sci U S A* 2003;100(17):10079.

47. Richards AM. Minisymposium: the natriuretic peptide hormones and hypertension. *J Intern Med* 1994; 235:543.

48. Solomon LR, Atherton JC, Bobinski H, Green R. Effect of posture on plasma immmunoreactive atrial natriuretic peptide concentrations in man. *Clin Sci* 1986;71:299.

49. Anderson JV, Donckier J, McKenna WJ, Bloom SR. The plasma release of atrial natriuretic peptide in man. *Clin Sci* 1986;71:151.

50. Woods RL. Cardioprotective functions of atrial natriuretic peptide and B-type natriuretic peptide: a brief review. *Clin Exp Pharmacol Physiol* 2004;31(11):791.

51. Carnio EC, Rettori V, Del Bel EA, et al. Hypertension induced by nitric oxide synthase inhibition activates the atrial natriuretic peptide (ANP) system. *Reg Peptides* 2004;117:117.

52. Antunes-Rodrigues J, Machado BH, Andrade HA, et al. Carotid-aortic and renal baroreceptors mediate the atrial natriuretic peptide release induced by blood volume expansion. *Proc Natl Acad Sci U S A* 1992;89:6828.

53. Gutkowska J, Antunes-Rodrigues J, McCann SM. Atrial natriuretic peptide in brain and pituitary gland. *Physiol Rev* 1997;77:465.

54. Knowles JW, Esposito G, Mao L, et al. Pressure-independent enhancement of cardiac hypertrophy in natriuretic peptide receptor A–deficient mice. *J Clin Invest* 2001;107(8):975.

55. Klinger JR, Petit RD, Curtin LA, et al. Cardiopulmonary responses to chronic hypoxia in transgenic mice that overexpress ANP. *J Appl Physiol* 1993; 75(1):198.

56. Horio T, Nishikimi T, Yoshihara F, et al. Inhibitory regulation of hypertrophy by endogenous atrial natriuretic peptide in cultured cardiac myocytes. *Hypertension* 2000;35:19.

57. Tsuchimochi H, Kurimoto F, Ieki K, et al. Atrial natriuretic peptide distribution in fetal and failed adult human hearts. *Circulation* 1988; 78:920.

58. Marin-Grez M, Fleming JT, Steinhausen M. Atrial natriuretic peptide causes pre-glomerular vasodilatation and post-glomerular vasoconstriction in rat kidney. *Nature* 1986;324:473.

59. Lohmeier TE, Mizelle HL, Reinhart GA. Role of atrial natriuretic peptide in long-term volume homeostasis. *Clin Exp Pharmacol Physiol* 1995;22(1):55–61.

60. Naruse M, Takeyama Y, Tanabe A, et al. Atrial and brain natriuretic peptides in cardiovascular diseases. *Hypertension* 1994;23(Suppl 1):I231.

61. Ruskoaho H. Atrial natriuretic peptide synthesis, release and metabolism. *Pharmacol Rev* 1992;44:479.

62. Hunt PJ, Espiner EA, Nicholls MG, et al. Differing biological effects of equimolar atrial and brain natriuretic peptide infusions in normal man. *J Clin Endocrinol Metab* 1996;81:3871.

63. Pidgeon GB, Richards AM, Nicholls MG, et al. Differing metabolism and bioactivity of atrial and brain natriuretic peptides in essential hypertension. *Hypertension* 1996;27(4):906.

64. Schirger JA, Grantham JA, Kullo IJ, et al. Vascular functions of brain natriuretic peptide: modulation by atherosclerosis and neutral endopeptidase inhibition. *J Am Coll Cardiol* 2000;35(3):796.

65. Cao L, Gardner DG. Natriuretic peptides inhibit DNA synthesis in cardiac fibroblasts. *Hypertension* 1995;25:227.

66. Tamura N, Ogawa Y, Chusho H, et al. Cardiac fibrosis in mice lacking brain natriuretic peptide. *Proc Natl Acad Sci U S A* 2000;97:4239.

67. Suzuki M, Hamada M, Yamamoto K, et al. Brain natriuretic peptide as a risk marker for incident hypertensive cardiovascular events. *Hypertens Res* 2002;25(5):669.

68. Doggrell SA. Brain natriuretic peptide: disease marker or more in cardiovascular medicine? *Drugs Today (Barc)* 2001; 37(7):463.

69. Komatsu Y, Nakao K, Itoh H, et al. Vascular natriuretic peptide. *Lancet* 1992;340:622.

70. Ahluwalia A, Hobbs AJ. Endothelium-derived C-type natriuretic peptide: more than just a hyperpolarizing factor. *Trends Pharmacol Sci* 2005; 26(3):162.

71. Pelisek J, Kuehnl A, Rolland PH, et al. Functional analyses of genomic DNA, cDNA and nucleotide sequence of the mature C-type natriuretic peptide gene in vascular cells. *Arterioscler Thromb Vasc Biol* 2004;24(9):1646.

72. Suga S, Nakao K, Itoh H, et al. Endothelial production of c-type natriuretic peptide and its marked augmentation by transforming growth factor β. Possible existence of a vascular natriuretic peptide system. *J Clin Invest* 1992;90:1145.

73. Suga S, Itoh H, Komatsu Y, et al. Cytokine-induced C-type natriuretic peptide (CNP) secretion from vascular endothelial cells—evidence for CNP as a novel autocrine/paracrine regulator from endothelial cells. *Endocrinology* 1993;133:3038.

74. Kiemer AK, Lehner MD, Hartung T, Vollmar AM. Inhibition of cyclo-oxygenase-2 by natriuretic peptides. *Endocrinology* 2002;143:846.

75. Ohno N, Itoh H, Ikeda T, et al. Accelerated reendothelialization with suppressed thrombogenic property and neointimal hyperplasia of rabbit jugular vein grafts by adenovirus-mediated gene transfer of C-type natriuretic peptide. *Circulation* 2002; 105:1623.

76. Kim SZ, Cho KW, Kim SH. Modulation of endocardial natriuretic peptide receptors in right ventricular hypertrophy. *Am J Physiol* 1999; 277:2280.

77. Koller KJ, Lowe DG, Bennett GL, et al. Selective activation of the BNP receptor by C-natriuretic peptide. *Science* 1991;252:120.

78. Tremblay J, Desjardins R, Hum D, et al. Biochemistry and physiology of the natriuretic peptide receptor guanyl cyclases. *Mol Cell Biochem* 2002; 230(1–2):31.

79. Kishimoto I, Garbers DL. Physiological regulation of blood pressure and kidney function by guanylyl cyclase isoforms. *Curr Opin Nephrol Hypertens* 1997;6:58.

80. Durocher D, Grepin C, Nemer M. Regulation of gene expression in the endocrine heart. *Recent Prog Horm Res* 1998;53:7.

81. Calderone A, Thaik CM, Takahashi N, et al. Nitric oxide, atrial natriuretic peptide and cyclic GMP inhibit the growth promoting effects of norepinephrine in cardiac myocytes and fibroblasts. *J Clin Invest* 1998; 101:812.

82. Oliver PM, John SW, Purdy KE, et al. Natriuretic peptide receptor 1 expression influences blood pressures of mice in a dose-dependent manner. *Proc Natl Acad Sci U S A* 1998; 95:2547.

83. Oliver PM, Fox JE, Kim R, et al. Hypertension, cardiac hypertrophy and sudden death in mice lacking natriuretic peptide receptor A. *Proc Natl Acad Sci U S A* 1997;94:14730.

84. Harata M, Chang CH, Murad F. Stimulatory effects of atrial natriuretic factor on phosphoinositide hydrolysis in cultured bovine aortic smooth muscle cells. *Biochem Biophys Acta* 1989;1010:346.

85. Anandsrivastava MB, Sairam MB, Cantin M. Ring-deleted analogs of atrial natriuretic factor inhibit adenylate cyclase cAMP system—possible coupling of clearance atrial natriuretic factor receptors to adenylate cyclase cAMP signal transduction system. *J Biol Chem* 1990;265:8566.

86. Levin ER. Natriuretic peptide C-receptor—more than a clearance receptor. *Am J Physiol* 1993;264:E483.

87. Greenwald JE, Needleman P, Siegel N, et al. Processing of atriopeptin prohormone by non-myocytic atrial cells. *Biochem Biophys Res Commun* 1992;188:644.

88. Roques BP, Noble F, Dauge V, et al. Neutral endopeptidase 24.11—structure, inhibition and experimental and clinical pharmacology. *Pharmacol Rev* 1993;45:87.

89. Gee NS, Bowes MA, Buck P, Kenny AJ. An immunoradiometric essay for endopeptidase 24.11 shows it to be widely distributed enzyme in pig tissues. *Biochem J* 1985;228:119.

90. Davidson NC, Struthers AD. Brain natriuretic peptide. *J Hypertens* 1994; 12:329.

91. Kenny AJ, Bourne A, Ingram J. Hydrolysis of human and pig brain natriuretic peptides, urodilation, C-type natriuretic peptide and some C-receptor ligands by endopeptidase 24.11. *Biochem J* 1993;291:83.

92. Buckley MG, Markandu ND, Miller MA, et al. Plasma concentrations and comparisons of brain and atrial natriuretic peptide in normal subjects and in patients with essential hypertension. *J Hum Hypertens* 1993; 7(3):245.

93. Richards AM, Tonolo G, Tillman D, et al. Plasma atrial natriuretic peptide in stable and accelerated essential hypertension. *J Hypertens* 1986;4:790.

94. Nakaoka H, Kitahara Y, Amano M, et al. Effect of β-adrenergic receptor blockade on atrial natriuretic peptide in essential hypertension. *Hypertension* 1987;10:221.

95. Kohno M, Yokokawa K, Yasunari K, et al. Changes in plasma cardiac natriuretic peptide concentrations during 1 year treatment with angiotensin converting enzyme inhibitor in elderly hypertensive patients with left ventricular hypertrophy. *Int J Clin Pharmacol Ther* 1997;35(1):38.

96. Wang TJ, Larson MG, Levy D, et al. Impact of obesity on plasma natriuretic peptide levels. *Circulation* 2004; 109(5):594.

97. Grandi AM, Laurita E, Selva E, et al. Natriuretic peptides as markers of preclinical cardiac disease in obesity. *Eur J Clin Invest* 2004;34(5):342.

98. Ferrier C, Weidmann P, Hollmann R, et al. Impaired response of atrial natriuretic factor to high salt intake in persons prone to hypertension. *N Engl J Med* 1988;319:1223.

99. Widgren BR, Hedner T, Hedner J, et al. Resting and volume-stimulated circulating atrial natriuretic peptide in young normotensive men with positive family histories of hypertension. *J Hypertens* 1991;9:139.

100. Pitzalis MV, Iacoviello M, Massari F, et al. Influence of gender and family history of hypertension on autonomic control of heart rate, diastolic function and brain natriuretic peptide. *J Hypertens* 2001;19(1):143.

101. Freitag MH, Larson MG, Levy D, et al. Plasma brain natriuretic peptide levels and blood pressure tracking in the Framingham Heart study. *Hypertension* 2003;41:978.

102. Mussalo H, Vanninen E, Ikaheimo R, Hartikainen J. NT-proANP and BNP in renovascular and in severe and mild essential hypertension. *Kidney Blood Press Res* 2003;26(1):34.

103. Yasumoto K, Takata M, Ueno H, et al. Relation of plasma brain and atrial natriuretic peptides to left ventricular geometric patterns in essential hypertension. *Am J Hypertens* 1999; 12:921.

104. Murakami Y, Shimada T, Inoue S, et al. New insights into the mechanism of the elevation of plasma brain natriuretic polypeptide levels in patients with left ventricular hypertrophy. *Can J Cardiol* 2002; 18(12):1294.

105. Sutovsky I, Katoh T, Ohno T, et al. Relationship between brain natriuretic peptide, myocardial wall stress and ventricular arrhythmia severity. *Jpn Heart J* 2004;45(5):771.

106. Almeida P, Azevedo A, Rodrigues R, et al. B-type natriuretic peptide and left ventricular hypertrophy in hypertensive patients. *Rev Port Cardiol* 2003;22(3):327.

107. Kohno M, Horio T, Yokokawa K, et al. Brain natriuretic peptide as a cardiac hormone in essential hypertension. *Am J Med* 1992;92:29.

108. Nishikimi T, Yoshihara F, Morimoto A, et al. Relationship between left ventricular geometry and natriuretic peptide levels in essential hypertension. *Hypertension* 1996;28:22.

109. Almeida SS, Azavedo A, Castro A, et al. B-type natriuretic peptide is related to left ventricular mass in hypertensive patients but not athletes. *Cardiology* 2002;98(3):113.

110. Vanderheyden M, Goethals M, Verstreken S, et al. Wall stress modulates brain natriuretic peptide production in pressure overload cardiomyopathy. *J Am Coll Cardiol* 2004;44:2349.

111. Marttila M, Hautala N, Paradis P, et al. GATA4 mediates activation of the B-type natriuretic peptide gene expression in response to haemodynamic stress. *Endocrinology* 2001;142:4693.

112. Kosmala W, Spring A. Plasma levels of atrial and brain natriuretic peptide and left ventricular geometry in patients with essential hypertension. *Pol Merkuriusksz Lek* 2003;14(81):216.

113. Takemura G, Fujiwara H, Mukoyama M, et al. Expression and distribution of human atrial natriuretic peptide in human hypertrophic ventricle of hypertensive hearts and hearts with hypertrophic cardiomyopathy. *Circulation* 1991;83:181.

114. Ogino K, Ogura K, Kinugawa T, et al. Neurohormonal profiles in patients with hypertrophic cardiomyopathy-differences to hypertrophic left ventricular hypertrophy. *Circ J* 2004; 68:444.

115. Day ML, Scwartz D, Wiegand RC, et al. Ventricular atriopeptin: unmasking of messenger RNA and peptide synthesis by hypertrophy or dexamethasone. *Hypertension* 1987; 9:485.

116. Lim PO, Donnan PT, Struthers AD, MacDonald TM. Exercise capacity and brain natriuretic peptide in hypertension. *J Cardiovasc Pharmacol* 2002;40(4):519.

117. Leuchte HH, Holzapfel M, Baumgartner RA, et al. Clinical significance of brain natriuretic peptide in primary pulmonary hypertension. *J Am Coll Cardiol* 2004;43:764.

118. Wei CM, Heublein DM, Perella MA, et al. Natriuretic peptide system in human heart failure. *Circulation* 1993;88:1004.

119. Cheung BM, Brown MJ. Plasma brain natriuretic peptide and C-type natriuretic peptide in essential hypertension. *J Hypertens* 1994; 12(4):449.

120. Raine AE, Erne P, Burgisser E, et al. Atrial natriuretic peptide and atrial pressure in patients with congestive cardiac failure. *N Engl J Med* 1986; 315:533.

121. Williams SG, Ng LL, O'Brien RJ, et al. Is plasma N-BNP a good indicator of functional reserve of failing hearts? The FRESH-BNP study. *Eur J Heart Fail* 2004;6(7):891.

122. Lang CC, Coutie WJ, Struthers AD, et al. Elevated levels of B-natriuretic peptide in acute hypoxaemic chronic obstructive pulmonary disease. *Clin Sci* 1992;83:529.

123. Tulevski II, Hirch A, Sanson BJ, et al. Increased brain natriuretic peptide as a marker for right ventricular dysfunction in acute pulmonary embolism. *Thromb Haemostasis* 2001;86:1193.

124. Hammerer-Lercher A, Neubauer E, Muller S, et al. Head-to-head comparison of N-terminal pro-brain natriuretic peptide, brain natriuretic peptide and N-terminal pro-atrial natriuretic peptide in diagnosing left ventricular dysfunction. *Clin Chim Acta* 2001;310:193.

125. Yandle TG, Richards AM, Gilbert A, et al. Assay of brain natriuretic peptide (BNP) in human plasma—evidence for high molecular weight BNP as a major plasma component in heart failure. *J Clin Endocrinol Metab* 1993;76:832.

126. Mottram PM, Leano R, Marwick TH. Usefulness of B-natriuretic peptide in hypertensive patients with exertional dyspnoea and normal left ventricular ejection fraction and correlation with new echocardiographic indexes of systolic and diastolic function. *Am J Cardiol* 2003;92:1434.

127. Lubien E, DeMaria A, Krishnaswamy P, et al. Utility of B-natriuretic peptide in detecting diastolic dysfunction: comparison with Doppler velocity recordings. *Circulation* 2002; 105(5):595.

128. Tsuji H, Nishino N, Kimura Y, et al. Haemoglobin level influences plasma brain natriuretic peptide concentration. *Acta Cardiol* 2004;59(5):527.

129. Berger R, Huelsman M, Strecker K, et al. B-type natriuretic peptide predicts sudden death in patients with chronic heart failure. *Circulation* 2002; 105:2392.

130. McCullough PA, Nowak RM, McCord J, et al. B-type natriuretic peptide and clinical judgement in emergency diagnosis of heart failure. Analysis from the Breathing Not Properly (BNP) multinational study. *Circulation* 2002;106:416.

131. Maisel A, Hollander JE, Guss D, et al. Primary results of the Rapid Emergency Department Heart Failure Outpatient Trial (REDHOT): a multicenter study of B-type natriuretic peptide levels, emergency department decision making, and outcomes in patients presenting with shortness of breath. *J Am Coll Cardiol* 2004;44(6):1328.

132. Remme WJ, Swedberg K. Guidelines for the diagnosis and treatment of chronic heart failure. *Eur Heart J* 2001;22:1527.

133. Mueller C, Scholer A, Laule-Killian K, et al. Use of B-type natriuretic peptide in the evaluation and management of acute dyspnoea. *New Engl J Med* 2004; 350:647.

134. Tsutamoto T, Wada A, Maeda K, et al. Plasma brain natriuretic peptide level as a biochemical marker of morbidity and mortality in patients with asymptomatic or minimally symptomatic left ventricular dysfunction. Comparison with plasma angiotensin II and endothelin-1. *Eur Heart J* 1999;20:1799.

135. Doust JA, Pietrzak E, Dobson A, Glasziou P. How well does B-type natriuretic peptide predict death and cardiac events in patients with heart failure: systematic review. *BMJ* 2005; 330(7492):625.

136. Cowie MR, Jourdain P, Maisel A, et al. Clinical application of B-type natriuretic peptide (BNP) testing. *Eur Heart J* 2003;24:1710.

137. McDonagh TA, Robb SD, Murdoch DR, et al. Biochemical detection of left-ventricular systolic dysfunction. *Lancet* 1998;351(9095):9.

138. Vasan RS, Benjamin EJ, Larson MG, et al. Plasma natriuretic peptides for community screening for left ventricular hypertrophy and systolic dysfunction: the Framingham Heart Study. *JAMA* 2002;288(10):1252.

139. Richards AM, Nicholls MG, Espiner EA, et al. Effects of alpha-human atrial natriuretic peptide in essential hypertension. *Hypertension* 1985; 7:812.

140. Weder AB, Sekkari MA, Takiyyudin M, et al. Antihypertensive and hypotensive effects of atrial natriuretic factor in men. *Hypertension* 1987;10:582.

141. Nicholls MG. Minisymposium: the natriuretic peptide hormones. Editorial and historical review. *J Intern Med* 1994;235:561.

142. Richards AM, Crozier IG, Holmes SJ, et al. Brain natriuretic peptide: natriuretic and endocrine effects in essential hypertension. *J Hypertens* 1993;11:163.

143. Lainchbury JG, Burnett JC Jr, Meyer DM, et al. Effects of the natriuretic peptides on load and myocardial function in normal and heart failure dogs. *Am J Physiol Circ Physiol* 2000; 278:H33.

144. Lainchbury JG, Richards AM, Nicholls MG, et al. The effects of pathophysiological increments in brain natriuretic peptide in left ventricular systolic dysfunction. *Hypertension* 1997;30(3):398.

145. Publication Committee for the VMAC Investigators. Intravenous nesiritide vs nitroglycerin for treatment of decompensated congestive heart failure: a randomized controlled trial. *JAMA* 2002;287:1531–40.

146. Burger AJ, Horton DP, LeJemtel T, et al. Effect of Nesiritide (B-type natriuretic peptide) and Dobutamine on ventricular arrhythmias in the treatment of patients with acutely decompensated congestive heart failure: the PRECEDENT Study. *Am Heart J* 2002;144:1102.

147. Sackner-Bernstein JD, Kowalski M, Fox M, Aaronson K. Short-term risk of death after treatment with Nesiritide for decompensated heart failure: a pooled analysis of randomized controlled trials. *JAMA* 2005; 293(15):1900.

148. Sackner-Bernstein JD, Skopicki HA, Aaronson KD. Risk of worsening renal function with Nesiritide in patients with acutely decompensated heart failure. *Circulation* 2005;111:1487.

149. Seymour AA, Swerdel JN, Fennell SA, et al. Potentiation of the depressor responses to atrial natriuretic peptides in consciuos SHR by an inhibitor of neutral endopeptidase. *J Cardiovasc Pharmacol* 1989;14:194.

150. Richards AM, Crozier IG, Espiner EA, et al. Acute inhibition of Endopeptidase 24.11 in essential hypertension: SCH34826 enhances atrial natriuretic peptide and natriuresis without lowering blood pressure. *J Cardiovasc Pharmacol* 1992;20:735.

151. Lefrancois P, Clerc G, Duchier J, et al. Antihypertensive activity of sinorphan. *Lancet* 1990;ii:307.

152. Corti R, Burnett JC Jr, Rouleau J, et al. Vasopeptidase inhibitors: a new therapeutic concept in cardiovascular diseases? *Circulation* 2001;104:1856.

153. Ruiloe LM, Palatini P, Grossman E, et al. Randomized double-blind comparison of Omapatrilat with Amlodipine in mild-to-moderate hypertension. *Am J Hypertens* 2000;13: S134.

154. Asmar R, Fredebohm W, Senftleber I, et al. Omapatrilat compared with lisinopril in treatment of hypertension as assessed by ambulatory blood pressure monitoring. *J Hypertens* 2000;18:S95.

155. McClean DR, Ikram H, Mehta S, et al. Omapatrilat Haemodynamic Study Group. Vasopeptidase inhibition with Omapatrilat in chronic heart failure: acute and long-term haemodynamic and neurohormonal effects. *J Am Coll Cardiol* 2002;19:2034.

156. d'Uscio LV, Quaschning T, Burnett JC Jr, Luscher TF. Vasopeptidase inhibition prevents endothelial dysfunction of resistance arteries in salt-sensitive hypertension in comparison with single ACE inhibition. *Hypertension* 2001;37(1):28.

157. Mc Clean DR, Ikram H, Garlick AH, et al. The clinical, cardiac, renal, arterial and neurohormonal effects of Omapatrilat, a vasopeptidase inhibitor, in patients with chronic heart failure. *J Am Coll Cardiol* 2000;36:479.

158. Rouleau J, Pfeffer M, Stewart D, et al. Comparison of vasopeptidase inhibitor, Omapatrilat, and Lisinopril on exercise tolerance and morbidity in patients with heart failure: IMPRESS randomised trial. *Lancet*;356(9230):615.

159. Packer M, Califf RM, Konstam MA, et al. Comparison of omapatrilat and enalapril in patients with chronic heart failure. the Omapatrilat versus Enalapril Randomized Trial of Utility in Reducing Events (OVERTURE). *Circulation* 2002; 106:920.

160. Kostis JB, Packer M, Black HR, et al. Omapatrilat and Enalapril in patients with hypertension: the Omapatrilat Cardiovascular Treatment vs Enalapril Octave Trial. *Am J Hypertens* 2004; 17:103.

161. Schulz-Knappe P, Forssmann K, Herbst F, et al. Isolation and structural analysis of urodilatin, a new peptide of the cardiolatin family, extracted from human urine. *Klin Wochenschr* 1988;66:752.

162. Hildebrant DA, Mizelle HL, Brands MW, Hall JE. Comparison of renal actions of urodilatin and atrial natriuretic peptide. *Am J Physiol* 1992;262:R395.

163. Bestle MH, Olsen NV, Christensen P, et al. Cardiovascular, endocrine and renal effects of urodilatin in normal humans. *Am J Physiol* 1999;276: R684.

164. Forssmann W-G, Meyer M, Forssmann K. The renal urodilatin system: clinical implications. *Cardiovasc Res* 2001; 51:450.

165. Kitamura K, Kangawa K, Ichiki Y, et al. Adrenomedullin- a novel hypotensive peptide isolated from human phaeochromocytoma. *Hypertension* 1993;22:448.

166. Kitamura K, Kato J, Kawamoto M, et al. The intermediate form of glycine-extended adrenomedullin is the major circulating form in human plasma. *Biochem Biophys Res Commun* 1998;244:551.

167. Cheung BM, Li CY, Wong LY. Adrenomedullin: its role in the cardiovascular system. *Semin Vasc Med* 2004;4(2):129.

168. Terata K, Miura H, Liu Y, et al. Human coronary arteriolar dilation to adrenomedullin: role of nitric oxide and K+ channels. *Am J Physiol* 2000; 279:H2620.

169. Feng CJ, Kang B, Kaye AD, et al. L-NAME modulates responses to adrenomedullin in the hindquarters vascular bed of the rat. *Life Sci* 1994; 55:L433.

170. Rademaker MT, Charles CJ, Lewis LK, et al. Beneficial haemodynamic and renal effects of adrenomedullin in an ovine model of heart failure. *Circulation* 1997;96:1983.

171. Lainchbury JG, Nicholls MG, Espiner EA, et al. Bioactivity and interactions of adrenomedullin and brain natriuretic peptide in patients with heart failure. *Hypertension* 1999; 34:70.

172. Nagaya N, Satoh T, Nishikimi T, et al. Haemodynamic, renal and hormonal effects of adrenomedullin infusion in patients with congestive cardiac failure. *Circulation* 2000;101:498.

173. Bunton DC, Petrie MC, Hillier C, et al. The clinical relevance of adrenomedullin: a promising profile? *Pharm Ther* 2004; 103:179.

Chapter

32

Other Peptide and Related Systems including Substance P, Calcitonin Gene-Related Peptide, and Serotonin

Adrian G. Stanley

Key Findings

- Substance P is a member of the tachykinin family and exhibits both vasoconstrictor and vasodilator properties. In humans, substance P can cause vasodilatation, and low levels have been observed in hypertensive subjects suggesting loss of a potential compensatory mechanism.

- Calcitonin gene-related peptide is a potent vasodilator and induces an enhanced vasodilator response in isolated arteries from human hypertensives.

- Serotonin (5-HT) has peripheral arterial vasoconstrictor properties and can trigger platelet aggregation. Any significant influence of 5-HT on blood pressure (BP) regulation is more dependent on 5-HT receptor/transporter expression, as free-circulating concentrations of 5-HT are very low.

- Adenosine is a potent vasodilator, and is released by vascular tissue in response to ischemic or hypoxic stimuli suggesting a compensatory autocrine/paracrine role.

- Enhanced neuropeptide Y activity in the brain results in hypotension, whereas its activity in peripheral resistance vessels is vasoconstricting and has synergistic effects with noradrenaline.

- Parathormone induces a vasodilator response when infused intravenously. Parathormone concentrations in humans are positively correlated with higher BP.

- Urotensin II is the most potent vasoconstrictor known. In some vascular beds, it stimulates nitric oxide synthesis and promotes vasodilatation.

The role of neurotransmitters and other peptides in the pathogenesis and regulation of blood pressure (BP) is highly complex, swamped by contradictory evidence, and rarely taught. At present, there are very few therapeutic agents that have been developed based on the understanding of neurotransmitter activity despite evidence that some play a significant role in BP regulation.

This review will describe each peptide in turn, highlighting its biochemistry before discussing the evidence supporting its role in BP regulation. For a detailed review of the central neurotransmitter activity and baroreceptor mechanisms, readers are directed to the review by Pilowsky and Goodchild.[1]

SUBSTANCE P AND OTHER TACHYKININS

Structure, genetics, and metabolism

The tachykinin family consists of substance P (SP), neurokinin A (NKA), neurokinin B (NKB), neuropeptide γ (NPγ), neuropeptide K (NPK), hemokinin 1 and endokinins A through D[2] and are characterized by a shared carboxyl terminal sequence, Phe-X-Gly-Leu-Met-NH2 (where X is an aromatic [Phe or Tyr] or hydrophobic [Val or Ile] residue).[3] These are deca- or undeca-peptides ranging in length between 9 and 42 amino acids and are derived from three preprotachykinin (PPT) genes: the PPT-A (now renamed TAC1) gene that contains four preprotachykinins (α-, β-, γ-, and δ-PPTA) encoding the sequence of SP, NKA, NPγ, and NPK, respectively; the PPT-B (TAC3) gene encoding the sequence of NKB[3]; and the PPT-C (TAC4) gene encoding hemokinin 1 and endokinins A through D.[2]

SP is an 11-amino acid peptide, and is predominantly synthesized in neuronal tissue.[4] The most significant areas of synthesis are the dorsal root ganglia (DRG) that innervate the blood vessels, viscera and sympathetic ganglia that are surrounded by a dense network of (SP)-immunoreactive fibers.[2]

SP activity is mediated via tachykinin receptors, which consist of seven hydrophobic transmembrane domains that are connected by extra- and intra-cellular loops and coupled to G-proteins.[5] There are three types of tachykinin receptors, namely, NK1, NK2, and NK3. Although SP's potency is greatest at NK1 (similarly, neurokinin A and neurokinin B at NK2 and NK3, respectively[6]), all tachykinins share a degree of activity with all receptors.[7] Calcitonin gene-related peptide (CGRP) is closely associated with SP and is often co-released in neuronal tissue.[8]

Tachykinins are degraded by tissue-specific peptidases.[9] SP is susceptible to peptidase activity from neprilysin, angiotensin-converting enzyme, dipeptidyl aminopeptidase IV, prolyl endopeptidase, and cathepsin D. The peptide products are inactive, except the neprilysin-generated fragment, which has tachykinin-like central nervous system activity.[10]

Generally the physiologic actions of SP include stimulation of salivary secretion, and both smooth muscle (SM) contraction and vasodilatation.[11]

Blood pressure regulation

There is direct and indirect evidence that tachykinins have a significant influence on BP regulation. Several studies have investigated the activity of SP and other tachykinins directly either by intravenous (IV) or intracerebroventricular (ICV) injection. Intravenous (IV) injection of exogenous SP resulted in a significant vasodilator response in salt-dependent hypertensive rats (SN [subtotal nephrectomy]-salt, DOC [deoxycortisosteroid]-salt rats),[12] the inbred genetically hypertensive strain (GH) of the Otago Wistar rat,[13] and normotensive Wistar-Kyoto rats (WKY).[14] In contrast, intravenous SP resulted in an increased BP in spontaneously hypertensive rats (SHR).[14]

Although the "peripheral" response to SP is predominantly vasodilator, ICV injection of tachykinins or selective NK-receptor agonists increases BP and heart rate in normotensive rats and SHRs,[15–18] and causes inhibition of renal salt and water excretion.[19] Similarly, tachykinin activity at NK3 receptors in the substantia nigra of SHRs results in a peripheral pressor effect,[20] and NK3 receptor activation promotes release of vasopressin from the hypothalamic paraventricular nucleus.[21,22]

SP induces the release of nitric oxide (NO) and a non-NO hyperpolarizing factor via stimulation of NK1 receptors in endothelial cells,[23] and its activity is dependent on an intact endothelium. Therefore, the vasodilator properties of tachykinins may be based on their ability to mediate their actions via the vasculature, superseding any pressor activity from enhanced central nervous system expression. In both human hypertensive subjects and spontaneously hypertensive rat-stroke prone (SHR-SP) rats, reduced levels of SP have been identified.[11] This suggests that SP might contribute to high BP because of insufficient synthesis, and/or release of what may be a counterregulatory hormone. Interestingly, and in contrast to the SHR-SP, the inbred genetically hypertensive strain (GH) of the Otago Wistar rat has greater levels of SP in superior cervical ganglia, and greater numbers of SP-containing sensory neurons compared to a normotensive strain. However, the primary defect causing hypertension in GH rats may be an abnormality in renal prostaglandin catabolism, and the higher SP levels observed in these rats may therefore be a compensatory mechanism.

Further evidence for SP acting as an antihypertensive compensatory mechanism is supported by studies in salt-dependent rat models of hypertension. SP antagonism by spantide-II (a potent NK1 receptor antagonist that crosses the blood–brain barrier) led to significant increases in BP in DOC-salt and SN-salt rats compared to controls.[8,11] In addition, the SN-salt rat does not have an increase in SP DRG mRNA or peptide synthesis,[8] suggesting that this SP-induced depressor effect may be mediated via increased vascular sensitivity (i.e., by increased endothelial NK1 receptor expression).

Tachykinin-induced pressor activity is mediated via stimulation of sympathetic ganglia. The pressor response in SHRs to SP is probably mediated by upregulation of ganglionic NK1 receptors. First, NK1 receptors are more abundant in the cervical ganglia of SHRs and NK1 receptor mRNA expression is increased compared to normoten-

sive rats. Second, the NK1 receptor antagonist GR-82334 blocks the pressor actions of the NK1 receptor agonist GR-73632, which acts on sympathetic ganglia in SHRs.[24] Third, greater depolarization has been observed in the superior cervical ganglionic cells within the SHRs compared to WKY rats in response to GR-73632.[25]

In summary, the role of SP in hypertension is contradictory. In acquired models of hypertension, namely salt-dependent hypertensive rats, SP may act as a compensatory mechanism to attenuate the increase in BP, in part, by an increase in endothelial sensitivity to SP. In contrast, in genetic models of hypertension, such as the SHR, there is evidence of a SP-induced pressor effect, which may be mediated by upregulation of NK1 sympathetic ganglionic receptors. However, low levels of SP have been observed in genetic hypertension, including human essential hypertension, and alternatively, this loss of SP antihypertensive activity would be a contributory factor in the development of high BP. The role of SP in human hypertension remains to be fully elucidated.

CALCITONIN GENE-RELATED PEPTIDE

Structure, genetics, and metabolism

CGRP is a 37–amino acid neuropeptide derived from tissue-specific splicing of the calcitonin (CT)/CGRP gene.[26] The two CGRP genes (rat α and β, and human I and II) differ in their protein sequences by one and three amino acids, respectively. The biological activity of both peptides is very similar, and *in vivo* and *in vitro* studies have shown that CGRP is a very potent vasodilator with 100 to 1000 times more potency than SP or adenosine.[27–29]

With similar properties to SP, CGRP synthesis is predominantly located in specific regions of neuronal tissue that innervate the vasculature and viscera (i.e., the DRG)[28,30,31]; however, CGRP is the predominant neurotransmitter in these capsaicin-sensitive sensory nerves.[32] Various stimuli (e.g., low pH, noxious heat, and tumor necrosis factor-α), can activate CGRP release.[33] Importantly, CGRP-specific receptors have been located in the media, intima, and endothelial layer of resistance blood vessels,[23,28,31,34] and a dense perivascular CGRP neural network is seen around the blood vessels in all vascular beds.[35] This suggests a potential role for CGRP in BP regulation.

CGRP is a potent endothelium-independent vasodilator with positive chronotropic and inotropic effects. *In vitro* studies of vascular SM cells have shown CGRP stimulation of cyclic AMP (cAMP) through activation of adenyl cyclase[36–38] and activation of KATP channels, resulting in enhanced vasodilatation secondary to membrane hyperpolarization[30] and activation of endothelium nitric oxide synthase (eNOS).[39]

Blood pressure regulation

Calcitonin gene-related peptide can selectively dilate multiple vascular beds,[27,40] particularly the coronary vessels, and systemic administration of CGRP has been shown to decrease BP in a dose-dependent manner in normotensive and hypertensive animals and humans.[41] The antihypertensive activity of CGRP is thought to be mediated either by upregulation of neuronal CGRP synthesis and release or by enhanced sensitivity of the vasculature to its dilator effects in a similar manner to SP,[41] with most of the evidence determined by animal models.

Synthesis and release of CGRP increases in acquired salt-dependent rat models of hypertension (DOC-salt,[42] two-kidney, one-clip,[43] and SN-salt rats[44]) and L-NAME–induced hypertension during pregnancy.[45] Although there is an increased neuronal expression of CGRP in DOC-salt rats, there is no change in neuronal expression of CGRP in the SN-salt model.[46,47] This would suggest that CGRP acts as compensatory vasodilator in an attempt to counteract the BP increase in these acquired forms of hypertension, and in DOC-salt rats this occurs via increased neuronal expression of CGRP.

In genetic animal models of hypertension, the neuronal expression of CGRP is decreased. Compared to age-matched normotensive WKY rats, CGRP mRNA levels in SHR dorsal root ganglia decreased with age, but CGRP activity in the atrium and mesenteric artery of older SHR is greater.[29] Similarly, in another genetic animal model of hypertension (Dahl salt-sensitive rats), lower CGRP levels in the DRG have also been observed.[6] Decreased neuronal CGRP content in the DRG, experimentally induced by capsaicin treatment in neonatal Wistar rats, ultimately leads to higher blood pressure, once these rats were fed a high-salt diet compared to non–capsaicin-treated Wistar rats. In addition, high-salt intake upregulated expression of mesenteric CGRP receptors in both treated and untreated rats without altering CGRP levels in plasma and DRG.[48,49] These latter experiments suggest that an increased expression of vascular CGRP receptors might play a counter-regulatory role in attenuating salt-induced and genetic models of high BP.

Further evidence for this enhanced vascular sensitivity has been demonstrated in rats influenced by factors affecting the renin-angiotensin system. Long-term intravenous angiotensin II (Ang II) resulted in an increase in CGRP-receptor expression in mesenteric arteries of Wistar rats, but CGRP plasma and DRG concentrations remained normal. The increase in mesenteric CGRP-receptor expression is pressure dependent and these animals exhibited an enhanced hypotensive response to infused exogenous CGRP, which suggests an adaptive functional response of the vasculature.[50]

As noted above, an age-related increase in mesenteric artery CGRP activity was found in SHRs, but not WKY rats. This decrease in CGRP nerve-fiber density was reversed in the mesenteric vessels of SHRs following treatment with temocapril or losartan, but not hydralazine despite similar and effective BP lowering.[51] This suggests that long-term inhibition of the renin-angiotensin system in SHR prevents remodeling of vascular CGRP nerve fibers, and loss of its compensatory function in genetic hypertension.

The interaction of CGRP and noradrenaline has also been explored. In models of phenol-induced hypertension, there is enhanced activity of sympathetic noradrenergic nerves associated with a decrease in the plasma concentration of CGRP, the content of DRG CGRP, and the density of CGRP nerve fibers in the mesenteric artery.[52,53] Noradrenaline is capable of inhibiting the neurotransmission in CGRP sensory nerves via a prejunctional mechanism,[54] and thus it is likely that the decreased activity of CGRP is secondary to increased sympathetic nerve activity.[52] How this interaction might explain the role of CGRP in human hypertension is not clear.

Few studies have explored the activity of CGRP in human essential hypertension. One study compared the response of isolated segments of small subcutaneous arteries to CGRP from patients with and without hypertension, and revealed an enhanced vasodilator response in the "hypertensive" vessels.[55] Although CGRP receptor density was not examined, it is possible that human arteries in hypertensive subjects have increased expression of vascular CGRP receptors as a compensatory mechanism similar to that described for genetic animal models of hypertension.

In summary, CGRP is a potent vasodilator. It is often co-expressed with SP in neuronal tissue, but in contrast to SP, there is no evidence of CGRP vasoconstrictor properties. Decreased CGRP neuronal activity has been identified in genetic models of animal hypertension, suggesting a possible role in the pathogenesis of hypertension. However, in most models of experimentally induced high BP, CGRP activity is enhanced. There are conflicting data regarding the exact nature of any compensatory CGRP activity, but there is a preponderance of evidence suggesting that vascular CGRP-receptor expression is either increased or its downregulation prevented.

SEROTONIN

Structure, genetics, and metabolism

Serotonin (5-hydroxytryptamine; 5-HT) is a vasoactive amine that was originally isolated from clotted blood.[56] It acts on multiple sites including the brain (influencing mood and sleep in addition to BP control), platelets (promoting platelet aggregation), the heart (positive chronotropy), and, of particular relevance to this chapter, blood vessels.

Ninety-five percent of circulating 5-HT originates from enterochromaffin cells in the intestine (via release into the portal circulation); the remainder originates from brain raphe nuclei and lung neuroendothelial cells.[57] 5-HT is synthesized from tryptophan by tryptophan hydroxylase (TPH) followed by decarboxylation.[57] Two genes code for TPH: TPH1 on chromosome 11[58] is preferentially expressed in peripheral tissues, and TPH2 is located on chromosome 12[59] and expressed predominantly in the brain.[60]

Most of the circulating 5-HT is inactivated by the liver in the portal circulation, or alternatively, a smaller quantity is degraded in pulmonary endothelial cells. The remainder is taken up by platelets and stored within dense granules.[61] Therefore, circulating levels of free 5-HT are usually low unless vascular damage promotes activation of platelets and thus 5-HT release. In turn, 5-HT can promote blood clotting and platelet aggregation through enhanced platelet

(5-HT$_{2A}$) receptor activation.[62] Importantly, 5-HT can interact with endothelial and SM cells in the vasculature.[63] Seven plasma-membrane 5-HT receptors are known. In vascular tissues, 5-HT$_{1B}$, 5-HT$_2$, 5-HT$_3$, 5-HT$_4$, and 5-HT$_7$ are influential,[62] particularly 5-HT$_2$, which is discussed in more detail below. In neuronal tissue, the lung and gastrointestinal tract, and now more recently peripheral arterial smooth muscle, a cellular 5-HT transporter (SERT) has been recognized. This is the site of action for selective serotonin re-uptake inhibitors (e.g., fluoxetine and citalopram) in the treatment of depression. This protein is localized to the cell membrane and transports 5-HT away from the cell surface for intracellular metabolism via monoamine oxidase-A forming 5-hydroxyindole acetic acid or for storage in vesicles.[64] In platelets, SERT facilitates the takeup, storage, and release of 5-HT.[62]

Blood pressure regulation

The exact role of 5-HT in the development and maintenance of essential hypertension is unclear. Some models of hypertension have been described as 5-HT dependent, including an erythropoietin-driven model[65] and cyclosporine-induced hypertension.[66]

Studies of genetic and experimental hypertension have met with equivocal and contrasting results, and clinical studies of human hypertension are few in number. In part, differences in the central compared to the peripheral action of 5-HT account for some of the uncertainty. Centrally, 5-HT has been shown to both increase and decrease BP.[62,67,68] However, the peripheral response to 5-HT is predominantly vasoconstrictor—evidence from the isolated blood vessels of hypertensive rat models and humans reveal hypersensitivity to the effects of 5-HT.[69–71]

In genetic rat models of hypertension, the central actions of 5-HT support the development and maintenance of hypertension. SHRs have higher levels of brain 5-HT than WKY,[62] and intracranial 5-HT injection in SHRs increases BP[68] via by stimulation of 5-HT$_3$ receptors in the nucleus tractus solitarius.[67] However, in cat and dog models, central 5-HT injections decrease BP,[68] and cranial (intra-cisternal) injections of a serotonergic toxin (5,6-dihydroxytryptamine) did not have any effect on BP in DOC-salt rats[72] and SHRs.[73]

As noted above, isolated peripheral vessels from hypertensive models demonstrate reactivity to 5-HT. Nevertheless, some investigators have questioned the importance of this peptide in BP regulation because of low circulating concentrations,[74] whereas others have advocated 5-HT receptor regulation as key to its pathophysiologic role.[64]

Studies to determine the activity of 5-HT on the vasculature by use of a specific 5-HT receptor antagonist, ketanserin (5-HT$_{2A/2C}$ inhibitor), have been SP inconclusive. Ketanserin lowered BP in normal and hypertensive subjects, including humans, but BP reduction was largely attributed to the α-1 adrenergic receptor blockade, rather than the 5-HT$_2$ receptor blockade.[75] Additional studies using 5-HT$_{2A}$ receptor antagonists that lacked affinity for the α-1 adrenergic receptor have been mixed: ritanserin did not lower BP in hypertensive humans[76] and in SHRs,[77] but sarpogrelate lowered BP in the rat.[78]

The differences in response to 5-HT receptor antagonism might be explained by changes in receptor expression in different disease states. In the normotensive rat, the 5-HT$_{2A}$ receptor mediates contraction to 5-HT in the aorta. However, in DOC-salt hypertensive rats, the 5-HT$_{2B}$ receptor is predominant. 5-HT has a 300-fold higher affinity for the 5-HT$_{2B}$ receptor compared with the 5-HT$_{2A}$ receptor.[62] Interestingly, the 5-HT$_{2A}$ receptor remains the primary contractile receptor in mesenteric resistance arteries,[62] and these resistance vessels likely exert a greater influence on BP regulation.

In addition to 5-HT receptors, the role of the 5-HT transporter (SERT) has been examined. The hypothesis that SERT may play a role in increasing peripheral concentrations of 5-HT is based on SSRI drugs such as fluoxetine, which have been associated with the "serotonin syndrome" and its use by some to treat orthostatic hypotension. SERT has recently been identified in endothelial cells and vascular SM cells from Sprague-Dawley rats,[64] suggesting that this may be an area for further investigation in the future.

In human studies, no differences were found in platelet-poor plasma or platelet 5-HT levels from hypertensive compared to normotensive subjects. In addition, no significant correlation was found between plasma or platelet 5-HT and BP. However, plasma 5-HT was associated with supine and standing pulse rates, predominantly in hypertensive individuals, but the significance of this is unclear.[79] In a study of essential hypertensive patients and matched normotensive healthy subjects, ranging from age 30 to 73 years, reduced uptake of 5-HT by blood platelets was evident in the hypertensive cohort. This decreased uptake was positively correlated with increasing blood pressure and age.[80] It is not possible to determine whether this finding in hypertensive individuals is in part compensatory, but may explain the higher risk of thrombo-embolism associated with hypertension.

In summary, 5-HT has the potential to cause peripheral vasoconstriction and elevation of BP. However, the exact nature of the relationship between this peptide and genetic hypertension is not clear, but any significant influence is more likely to be dependent on 5-HT receptor, SERT expression, or both, rather than circulating levels of 5-HT *per se.*

ADENOSINE

Structure, genetics, and metabolism

Adenosine (a purine nucleoside) is synthesized by both vascular (endothelial and SM) and cardiac (fibroblasts and cardiomyocytes) cells[81–85] in response to hypoxic and ischemic stimuli. It is formed by two distinct pathways involving two substrates, namely AMP and S-adenosylhomocysteine.[86] Hydrolysis of AMP by 5'-nucleotidase to adenosine occurs at both intra- and extra-cellular sites.[87] The second pathway, hydrolysis of S-adenosylhomocysteine by S-adenosylhomocysteine hydrolase provides a significant source of myocardial cytosolic adenosine.[88]

Four subtypes of adenosine receptors (A_1, A_{2A}, A_{2B}, and A_3) in mammalian cells have been characterized.[89,90] The vascular actions of adenosine are mediated by A_1 and A_2 receptors. Activation of A_1 receptors results in inhibition of adenylate cyclase and opening of potassium channels via G1 protein coupling. In contrast, A_2 receptor activation, similarly coupled to G1 proteins, leads to stimulation of adenylate cyclase.[91]

Adenosine exhibits properties that are protective against cardiovascular disease, including arterial vasodilatation,[92] inhibition of platelet aggregation,[93] stimulation of nitric oxide release from vascular endothelial cells,[94] and SM cells,[95] prevention of reactive oxygen species–induced damage,[96] reduction of Ang II and noradrenaline by inhibition of renin release,[97] activation of cellular antioxidants[98], and inhibition of vascular SM cell and cardiac fibroblast growth.[82]

Blood pressure regulation

The evidence supporting the role of adenosine in BP regulation is less ambiguous than has been described for other peptides. Arterial vasodilatation is predominately mediated via adenosine A_2 receptors,[99] and since A_2 receptor–mediated vasodilatation prevails over A_1 receptor–mediated vasoconstriction, adenosine lowers blood pressure when infused systemically.[100]

Interestingly, adenosine activity can result in both contraction and relaxation in pulmonary arterial vessels.[101] This dual activity seems to be dependent on the resting tone of the artery; when low, adenosine elicits a vasoconstrictor response mediated via A_1 receptors. At a higher tone, adenosine induces vasodilatation via A_2 receptors.[102] In the kidney, adenosine causes vasoconstriction, since A_1 receptor-mediated constriction of the afferent arterioles prevails over the A_2 receptor–mediated vasodilatation.[103]

Further evidence of the contrasting effects of A_1 and A_2 receptors has been identified in chronic and short-term treatment of normotensive rats with adenosine receptor antagonists. DPSPX (1,3-dipropyl-8-sulphophenylxanthine—a nonselective antagonist of adenosine receptors) given for 7 days leads to marked hyperplastic and hypertrophic alterations of the blood vessel walls and increase in blood pressure.[104,105] In contrast, specific A_1 antagonists KW- and FK-838 attenuated the development of hypertension in the Dahl salt-sensitive rat.[106,107]

The A_1 and A_2 receptors also differ in their diuretic and natriuretic properties. Selective A_1 receptor antagonists (such as 1,3-dipropyl-8-cyclopentylxanthine; DPCPX), but not selective A_2 receptor antagonists, produce diuresis and natriuresis in animal models including the SHR with a concomitant reduction in BP.[108]

An investigation of the role of nitric oxide (NO) in adenosine A_2 receptor–mediated vasodilatation in normotensive (WKY) and hypertensive (SHR) rat aortic ring preparations suggested adenosine A_2 receptor–mediated vasodilatation was in part endothelium dependent, possibly by releasing NO. Thus, endothelial dysfunction may be one of the factors leading to attenuation of adenosine receptor and receptor-mediated responses in SHR.[109] Increased adenosine deaminase activity may also be a factor. In aortic and renal afferent SM cell culture, increased adenosine deaminase activity led to decreased extracellular levels of adenosine in SHR SM cells compared to WKY rat cells; treatment with an adenosine deaminase inhibitor normalized these differences in extracellular adenosine levels and cell proliferation.[110]

Differences in the human adenosine receptor gene have been investigated after manipulation of the A_{2A} receptor (ADORA2A) gene was shown to increase blood pressure and heart rate in mice.[106] The results are not conclusive. In a human population of 249 unrelated hypertensive individuals and 249 normotensive control subjects, association analysis for both allele and genotype frequencies for the adenosine-receptor gene variants (ADORA1, ADORA2A, and ADA) did not reveal any significant differences.[111] In a Caucasian American population,[112] the A1 receptor (ADORA1) chromosome 1 band q was shown to have the highest logarithm of odds (LOD) score (2.96) linked to diastolic blood pressure.

The renin-angiotensin system may be involved in hypertension induced by nonselective adenosine receptor blockade (DPSPX). Plasma Ang II levels were higher, plasma renin activity increased,[113] and the maximum contractile effect of Ang II was lower in DPSPX-treated hypertensive rats compared with control rats.[114] Similarly, co-treatment of DPSPX-treated rats with captopril (angiotensin-converting enzyme inhibitor) or losartan (an angiotensin-II receptor antagonist) prevented DPSPX-induced hypertension and morphologic changes.[113,115] Atenolol (a β-adrenoceptor blocker) prevented the rise in blood pressure,[115] but not the morphologic changes.

In human studies, exogenous adenosine intravenous infusion into the left anterior descending coronary artery stimulates the release of renin and Ang II from the coronary arteries of essential hypertensive patients, but not normotensive control subjects. This observation was negated by angiotensin-converting enzyme inhibition.[116] In eight patients with essential hypertension, the administration a 100-mg single dose of FK453 (novel A_1 receptor antagonist) resulted in increased sodium excretion, decreased BP, and increased heart rate, the latter occurring once the natriuresis was complete. The natriuretic and BP-lowering actions of FK453 was short-lasting, as continued daily treatment of FK453 for 7 days did not reveal long-lasting effects.[117]

In summary, adenosine is synthesized by vascular tissue in response to hypoxic stimuli, and its activity on blood vessels is greatest at the A_2 receptor, which results in vasodilatation, suggesting a compensatory role. There is some evidence of synergism with NO and the renin-angiotensin system in experimental animal models and human hypertensive subjects. However, the role of adenosine in the pathogenesis of hypertension is not conclusive.

NEUROPEPTIDE Y

Structure, genetics, and metabolism

Neuropeptide Y (NPY) is a 36–amino acid peptide extensively expressed in the paraventricular nucleus, ventrolateral medulla, nucleus of tractus solitari, presynaptic bulbospinal neurons of the brain stem, and sympathetic fibers innervating blood vessels.[118] Four subtypes of NPY receptors have been identified in rat brains and five in mice (Y_1, Y_2, Y_4, Y_5, and Y_6 in mice),[119,120] but Y_1 predominates.[119] NPY receptors belong to the G-protein coupled-receptor family, and activation leads to inhibition of cAMP accumulation.[120]

This neuropeptide is an important cardiovascular neuromodulator and exhibits opposing properties. It co-localizes in neural tissue with noradrenaline. NPY is released on sympathetic nerve stimulation across mammalian species,[121] and in human disease, most notably heart failure.[122] NPY actions include vasoconstriction,[123] vasodilatation,[124] inhibition of noradrenaline release,[125,126] potentiation of other vasoconstrictors,[127] and stimulation of the mitogenesis of vascular SM cell growth[128] and angiogenesis.[129]

The human NPY gene is located on chromosome 7p15.1.[130] Genetic studies have highlighted a thymidine-to-cytosine polymorphism (T1128C), which results in a substitution of leucine to proline in the signal part of the preproNPY coding region.[131] A prospective study of 1032 hypertensive patients investigated T1128C polymorphism in the NPY gene and presentation of cardiac disease. The frequency of the NPY T1128C polymorphism was significantly higher in patients with a myocardial infarction or stroke, as compared to those who remained event-free (8.4% vs. 5.1%).[132] In population studies, the frequency of heterozygotes for NPY T1128C polymorphism ranges from 0% to 15%, the highest prevalence in Finns.[133]

Blood pressure regulation

The role of NPY in the regulation of BP needs to be evaluated in terms of its central and peripheral actions. Like other neurotransmitters, it is co-expressed with other neurohumoral factors and in the case of NPY, its activity is linked to the sympathetic nervous system. However, detailed investigation of the role of NPY in animal models has been limited due to the lack of specific NPY receptor agonists/antagonists.

In the brain, all NPY receptors are expressed, and thus specific activity against a particular receptor has not been identified. However, ICV infusion of NPY in normotensive rats results in hypotension and bradycardia,[134] and noncardiovascular features including increased feeding[135] and depressed spontaneous locomotor activity.[136] Similarly, in a transgenic rat model overexpressing NPY ameliorated L-NAME–induced hypertension, and ICV administration of a specific Y1 receptor antagonist (BIBP3226) blocked this effect.[126]

In peripheral resistant arteries, NPY nerve density is higher in the SHRSP than WKY rats, but no difference was found in cerebral arteries. Sympathectomy led to almost complete removal of NPY neuronal tissue in the peripheral vessels, but without an effect on the cerebral arteries.[137] Similarly, an increase in NPY is evident in the mesenteric vessels of SHRs, but in a rat model of hypertension induced by coarctation, there was no increase in mesenteric artery NPY content,[138] which suggests that this neurotransmitter may be influential in "genetic" but not acquired hypertension.

B_2-adrenergic receptor and neuropeptide Y are co-expressed in sympathetic neurons. The synergy between the sympathetic nervous system and NPY at a post-junctional nerve level allows NPY activity to increase noradrenaline-induced vasoconstriction.[139] In vessels such as the mesenteric artery, the direct constrictor action of NPY and the potentiation of noradrenaline are linked to Y1-receptor activation.[121] Further studies have suggested that NPY exerts vasoconstrictive effects by activation of postjunctional Y1 receptors and potentiation of tyramine and Ang II activity.[140]

In addition, noradrenaline and NPY have prejunctional inhibitory actions on sympathetic neurotransmission, and can negatively regulate their own expression as well as the expression of each other. As an example, NPY controls B_2-agonist–regulated lipolysis via sympathetic innervation of adipocytes[141] affecting energy balance, lipid mobilization, and circulating lipids. In a study of patients with essential hypertension, elevated LDL cholesterol was associated with polymorphisms of the B_2-adrenergic–receptor gene (Arg16Gly and Gln27Glu) and the NPY gene (Leu7Pro); however, all three polymorphisms were required for this relationship to exist.

In summary, NPY is expressed in the brain and with sympathetic neurons in peripheral blood vessels. In the brain, NPY activity results in hypotension, whereas its activity in peripheral resistance vessels is vasoconstrictor and has synergistic effects with noradrenaline. Genetic models of rat hypertension have increased mesenteric artery NPY content, but the exact role of NPY in the pathogenesis of hypertension is not clear.

PARATHORMONE AND PARATHORMONE-LIKE SUBSTANCES

Structure, genetics, and metabolism

Mammalian parathormone (PTH) is secreted by the parathyroid glands as a polypeptide containing 84 amino acids, and has a molecular weight of approximately 9.4 kDa. It is formed from preproparathyroid hormone (preproPTH), a 125–amino acid peptide encoded on chromosome 11.

PTH has a fundamental role in calcium and phosphorus metabolism. PTH regulates the conversion of 25-hydroxyvitamin D to the active metabolite $1,25(OH)_2D3$, and therefore stimulates and regulates bone remodeling, and influences the control of plasma calcium levels. In turn, $1,25(OH)_2D3$ causes marked suppression of both preproPTH mRNA and PTH secretion.[142]

The amino terminal region of PTH, which regulates mineral ion homeostasis, shows high sequence conservation with PTH-related peptide (PTHrP), but less homology in the middle and carboxyl terminal regions.

The single G-protein–coupled receptor, now referred to as the common PTH/PTHrP receptor or PTHR1, mediates most of the actions of PTH in mineral ion regulation and is critical to its actions on bone and kidney.[143] The gene encoding the PTHR1 is located on chromosome 3 in humans.[144] Activation of PTHR1 stimulates the production of intracellular cAMP and inositol 1,4,5-trisphosphate.[145] The carboxyl terminal PTH receptor may function as an antagonist of the actions of amino terminal PTH and PTHR1, but this is less well characterized.[144]

Blood pressure regulation

In experimental rat and rabbit models, infused PTH is a vasodilator, lowers blood pressure,[146-148] and attenuates noradrenaline and Ang II–induced BP increases in rats.[146,148] This vasodilator action may result from PTH ability to elevate intracellular cAMP via activation of adenylate cyclase[149] and/or inhibit calcium entry into vascular SM cells.[150,151]

However, chronic infusion of PTH into normal human subjects results in hypertension.[152] PTH has been implicated in the development of hypertension in humans and animal models of genetic hypertension. There are several studies to support this. Hypertension occurs more frequently in humans with primary hyperparathyroidism compared to those with normal parathyroid function.[153] In addition, excluding primary hyperparathyroidism, higher serum PTH levels correlate to higher BP in young hypertensive men,[154] young untreated hypertensives,[134] and both hypertensive and normotensive elderly persons.[155,156] However, the data are inconsistent in normotensive subjects: in younger study populations, one study demonstrated a positive correlation of serum PTH levels to clinic systolic BP and mean arterial pressure,[157] while another found no relationship.[134]

Whereas primary hyperparathyroidism results in high serum calcium levels, secondary hyperparathyroidism might reflect a reduced dietary calcium intake, and hypertensive individuals are more likely than normotensive subjects to be consuming low-calcium diets.[158] This is fundamental given that calcium regulation influences vascular SM contraction. Studies investigating the relationship of serum calcium to BP are also inconsistent: lower serum ionized calcium concentrations[159] and lower serum 1,25(OH)$_2$-vitamin D concentrations[160] have been observed in hypertensive compared to normotensive subjects. But other studies have not identified any relationship,[155,161] including a study of elderly subjects in which PTH levels, but not serum calcium and 1,25(OH)$_2$-vitamin D, correlated to ambulatory BP measurements.[155] A study of platelet intracellular calcium in primary hyperthyroid, hypertensive, and normotensive patients revealed that patients with essential hypertension had increased concentrations of platelet intracellular calcium and this correlated positively with BP level.[162]

Several reasons may account for the contradiction of a PTH-induced vasodilator response observed in experimental models and the finding of high PTH in hypertensive individuals. First, several studies have suggested PTH/PTHrp receptor adaptation (homologous desensitization or downregulation) to prolonged high concentrations of PTH.[163,164] Second, a parathyroid hypertensive factor (PHF) has been identified in both humans and SHRs.[165] PHF-like activity levels are elevated in hyper-

tensive individuals[166] and in normotensive rats; intravenous PHF induces a rise in BP.[167] Parathyroidectomy of hyperactive parathyroid glands in SHRs and humans with essential hypertension leads to lowering of BP and decreases the activity of PHF.[168-170] Interestingly, PHF, like PTH, is suppressed by high dietary calcium intake.[166]

In summary, there is a predominance of evidence that PTH is positively correlated with high BP, but the exact contribution of PTH, its related peptide PHF, and calcium metabolism in the pathogenesis of hypertension has not been fully elucidated.

UROTENSIN

Structure, genetics, and metabolism

Urotensin II (U-II) isopeptides have a cyclical structure and are 11 to 15 amino acids in length. The C-terminus ring structure is preserved, but the N-terminus tail varies in content and length.[171,172] Human U-II (hU-II) is an 11–amino acid peptide with its encoding gene, UTS2, located at 1p36. The spinal cord has the highest concentration of human prepro-U-II mRNA, but it has also been found in the brain, vascular and cardiac cells, kidney, liver, lung, pancreas, intestine, and other tissues.[173]

The receptor for hU-II is a G-protein–coupled receptor 14 (GPR14).[174,175] This receptor, now termed UT or sensory epithelia neuropeptide-like receptor, is a 389–amino acid, seven-transmembrane, G-protein–coupled receptor encoded on chromosome 17q25.3.[176] It shares 75% homology to rat GPR14, and is similar to the somatostatin receptor SST4 in structure.[174,175] The highest density of the UT receptor has been identified in the brain and skeletal muscle; other tissues include the spinal cord, cardiac and vascular cells, renal cortex, adrenal gland, and thyroid.[173]

Urotensin II is the most potent vasoconstrictor known,[174] mediated via UT. In addition to its vascular effects, U-II acts on the brain (stimulating prolactin and TSH release), kidney (increasing epithelial cell proliferation), and pancreas (inhibiting glucose-stimulated insulin secretion).[177]

Blood pressure regulation

There are epidemiologic data to support a relationship between U-II and human essential hypertension. In a study of 62 individuals with hypertension and 62 age-matched normotensive controls, plasma U-II levels were significantly higher in the hypertensive group and correlated positively with the systolic blood pressure.[178] Although no differences in mean plasma or cerebrospinal fluid U-II were observed in another study comparing 10 patients receiving long-term treatment for essential hypertension and 10 age-matched normotensive subjects, a positive correlation was noted for levels of cerebrospinal fluid U-II and BP.[179] In addition, U-II excreted in urine was significantly higher in patients with essential hypertension than in normotensives, and in patients with hypertensive renal disease compared to normotensive patients with renal disease.[180]

Urotensin II has predominantly peripheral vasculature effects and produces variable responses depending on species and vascular tissue.[181–183] In rats, U-II increased tone in isolated thoracic aorta with 10-fold greater efficacy than in abdominal aorta, in part as a consequence of thoracic membrane preparations exhibiting a greater expression of UT receptors.[184] Similarly, UT receptor mRNA is evident in rat arterial, but not venous SM cells, and a vasoconstrictor response to U-II was only found in arteries.[174,175] In humans, hU-II–induced vasoconstriction of coronary, mammary, and radial arteries is 50-fold more potent than endothelin-1 (ET-1). But a greater density of ET-1 receptors on coronary and mammary arteries results in a greater maximal response, as a third of these vessels exhibiting responses to ET-1 do not to respond U-II.[185]

In contrast, inconsistencies in human U-II biological activity have been highlighted by studies demonstrating a lack of response to hU-II in small muscular pulmonary arteries, abdominal resistance vessels, skeletal muscle resistance arteries, and small subcutaneous arteries and veins.[186,187] Interestingly, U-II causes relaxation in rat isolated small mesenteric arteries.[188] There is some evidence that U-II upregulates human[189] and rat[190] eNOS, which would suggest a hypothesis that U-II can cause arterial vasodilatation via NO, but causes vasoconstriction in diseased vessels without an intact endothelium.

The UT receptor is expressed extensively in the glial cells within the brain stem, hypothalamus, and thalamus,[191] and a central role for U-II has also been identified: ICV injections of U-II elicited a dose-dependent increase in blood pressure and heart rate in both SHR and normotensive WKY rats (greater in the SHR). Direct microinjection of U-II into the paraventricular nucleus of the hypothalamus and the arcuate nucleus also significantly increased BP and heart rate.[192] This U-II activity could be prevented by ganglion blockade, suggesting that it was, in part, mediated by the autonomic nervous system.[193]

In healthy sheep, an ICV infusion of U-II resulted in increased cardiac output and BP, but peripheral vasodilatation was noted in most vascular beds, suggesting that the increase in BP was dependent on the increased cardiac output,[194] rather than peripheral vasoconstriction.

In summary, U-II is a potent vasoconstrictor, but has some vasodilating properties in specific vascular beds, notably in nondiseased blood vessels via enhanced NO activity. The central action of U-II, in part mediated via the autonomic nervous system, leads to increased cardiac output and resultant higher BP.

VASOACTIVE INTESTINAL PEPTIDE

Structure, genetics, and metabolism

Vasoactive intestinal peptide (VIP) is a 28-residue peptide, derived by proteolytic cleavage from a 170–amino-acid precursor preproVIP[195] localized to chromosome 6.[196] This peptide is present in many tissues, including the brain, heart, intestine, lungs, thyroid, and kidney, and its actions include vasodilatation, bronchodilation, anti-inflammatory actions, immunosuppression, and SM relaxation. In the brain (cerebral cortex, hypothalamus, amygdala, hippocampus, corpus striatum, and medulla oblongata), VIP acts as a nonadrenergic, noncholinergic neurotransmitter.[197] In the heart, VIP immunoreactive nerve fibers are present in the epicardial coronary vessels, atria, ventricles, and conducting system (sinoatrial and atrioventricular nodes), and has 50 to 100 times more vasodilator potency than acetylcholine, with significant effects on coronary blood flow, cardiac contraction, and heart rate.[198]

Blood pressure regulation

The role of VIP in the development of hypertension has been explored in rat models. VIP nerve density is higher in the superior mesenteric arteries and veins of 6-month or older SHR-SP compared to WKY rats, and lower in the cerebral arteries of SHRSP than WKY. Sympathectomy reduced the density of these nerves in all peripheral vessels, but had little effect on the cerebral arteries.[137] However, concentration and peripheral release of VIP were lower in SHRSP at 8 to 48 weeks of age compared to WKY.[199] It is not certain whether this has any significance for human hypertension pathogenesis.

SUMMARY

The role of neurotransmitters and other peptide systems in the pathogenesis of hypertension is unclear, with differences in plasma levels of these substances and the target organ levels of their cognate receptors reported between hypertensive patients and normotensive subjects. Some of the published data are contradictory. However, some of these discrepancies may be resolved with further investigation of the physiologic regulation of these peptide systems in humans, especially with the advent of specific pharmacologic agonists and antagonists and the availability of genetic knock-out animal models.

REFERENCES

1. Pilowsky PM, Goodchild AK. Baroreceptor reflex pathways and neurotransmitters: 10 years on. J Hypertens 2002;20:1675–88.
2. Kurtz MM, Wang R, Clements MK, Cascieri MA, Austin CP, Cunningham BR, et al. Identification, localization and receptor characterization of novel mammalian substance P-like peptides. Gene 2002;296:205–12.
3. Pennefather JN, Lecci A, Candenas ML, Patak E, Pinto FM, Maggi CA. Tachykinins and tachykinin receptors: a growing family. Life Sci 2004;74:1445–63.
4. MacDonald M, Takeda J, Rice CM, Krause JE. Multiple tachykinins are produced and secreted upon post-translational processing of the three substance P precursor proteins, α-,
β- and γ-preprotachykinin. J Biol Chem. 1989;264:15578–92.
5. Nakanishi S. Mammalian tachykinin receptors. Annu Rev Neurosci 1991;14:123–36.
6. Regoli D, Boudon A, Fauchere JL. Receptors and antagonists for substance P and related peptides. Pharmacol Rev 1994;46:551–99.

7. Hardwick JC, Mawe GM, Parsons RL. Tachykinin induced activation of non-specific cation conductance via NK3 neurokinin receptors in guinea-pig intracardiac neurons. *J Physiol (Lond)* 1997;504:65–74.

8. Katki KA, Supowit SC, DiPette DJ. Substance P in subtotal nephrectomy-salt hypertension. *Hypertension* 2002; 39:389–93.

9. Turner AJ. Exploring the structure and function of zinc metallopeptidases: old enzymes and new discoveries. *Biochem Soc Trans* 2003;31:723–27.

10. Hall ME, Miley F, Stewart JM. The role of enzymatic processing in the biological actions of substance P. *Peptides* 1989;10:895–901.

11. Kohlmann O, Cesaretti ML, Ginoza M, Tavares A, Zanella MT, Ribeiro AB, et al. Role of substance P in blood pressure regulation in salt-dependent experimental hypertension. *Hypertension* 1997;29: 506–509.

12. Watson RE, Supowit SC, Zhao H, Katki KA, DiPette DJ. Role of sensory nervous system vasoactive peptides in hypertension. *Braz J Med Biol Res* 2002;35:1033–45.

13. Bakhle YS, Brogan JD, Bell C. Decreased vascular permeability response to substance P in airways of genetically hypertensive rats. *Br J Pharmacol* 1999;126:933–38.

14. Hancock JC, Lindsay GW. Enhancement of ganglion responses to substance P in spontaneously hypertensive rats. *Peptides* 2000;21:535–41.

15. Cellier E, Barbot L, Regoli D, Couture R. Cardiovascular and behavioural effects of intracerebroventricularly administered tachykinin NK3 receptor antagonists in the conscious rat. *Br J Pharmacol* 1997;122:643–54.

16. Cellier E, Barbot L, Iyengar S, Couture R. Characterization of central and peripheral effects of septide with the use of five tachykinin NK1 receptor antagonists in the rat. *Br J Pharmacol* 1999;127:717–28.

17. Couture R, Picard P, Poulat P, Prat A. Characterization of the tachykinin receptors involved in spinal and supraspinal cardiovascular regulation. *Can J Physiol Pharm* 1995;73:892–902.

18. Takano Y, Nagashima A, Hagio T, Tateishi K, Kamiya H-O. Role of central tachykinin peptides in cardiovascular regulation in rats. *Brain Res* 1990; 528:231–37.

19. Yuan Y-D, Couture R. Renal effects of intracerebroventricularly injected tachykinins in the conscious saline-loaded rat: receptor characterization. *Br J Pharmacol* 1997;120:785–96.

20. Lessard A, Campos MM, Neugebauer W, Couture R. Implication of nigral tachykinin NK3 receptors in the maintenance of hypertension in spontaneously hypertensive rats: a pharmacologic and autoradiographic study. *Br J Pharmacol* 2003;138:554–63.

21. Eguchi T, Takano Y, Hatae T, Saito R, Nakayama Y, Shigeyoshi Y, et al. Antidiuretic action of tachykinin NK-3 receptor in the rat paraventricular nucleus. *Brain Res* 1996;743:49–55.

22. Nakayama Y, Takano Y, Saito R, Kamiya H-O. Central pressor actions of tachykinin NK-3 receptor in the paraventricular nucleus of the rat

hypothalamus. *Brain Res* 1992; 595:339–342.

23. Marti E, Gibson SJ, Polak JM, Facer P, Springall DP, Aitchison M, et al. Ontogeny of peptide-and-amine-containing neurons in motor, sensory and autonomic regions of rat and human spinal cord, dorsal root ganglia and rat skin. *J Comp Neurol* 1987;226: 332–59.

24. Schoborg RV, Hoover DB, Tompkins JD, Hancock JC. Increased ganglionic responses to substance P in hypertensive rats due to upregulation of NK(1) receptors. *Am J Physiol Regul Integr Comp Physiol* 2000;279:R1685–94.

25. Tompkins JD, Hancock JC. Electrophysiological effects of tachykinin agonists on sympathetic ganglia of spontaneously hypertensive rats. *Auton Neurosci* 2002;97:26–34.

26. Rosenfeld MG, Mermod JJ, Amara SG, Swanson LW, Sawchenko PE, Rivier J, et al. Production of a novel neuropeptide encoded by the calcitonin gene via tissue-specific RNA processing. *Nature* 1983;304:129–35.

27. Brain SD, Williams TJ, Tippins JR, Morris JR, MacIntyre I. Calcitonin gene-related peptide is a potent vasodilator. *Nature* 1985;313:315–19.

28. DiPette DJ, Wimalawansa SJ. Cardiovascular actions of calcitonin generelated peptide. In: Crass J, Avioli L, eds. *Calcium Regulating Hormones and Cardiovascular Function.* Ann Arbor, NY: CRC Press, 1994:239.

29. Yamaga N, Kawasaki H, Inaizumi K, Shimizu M, Nakamura A, Kurosaki Y. Age-related decrease in calcitonin gene-related peptide mRNA in the dorsal root ganglia of spontaneously hypertensive rats. *Jpn J Pharmacol* 2001;86:448–50.

30. Bukoski RD, Kremer D. Calcium-regulating hormones in hypertension: vascular actions. *Am J Clin Nutr* 1991;54:220S–26S.

31. Wimalawansa SJ. Calcitonin gene-related peptide and its receptors: molecular genetics, physiology, pathophysiology, and therapeutic potentials. *Endocr Rev* 1996;17: 533–85.

32. Bell D, McDermott BJ. Calcitonin gene-related peptide in the cardiovascular system: characterization of receptor populations and their (patho)physiological significance. *Pharmacol Rev* 1996;48:253–88.

33. Opree A, Kress M. Involvement of the proinflammatory cytokines tumor necrosis factor-alpha, IL-1 beta, and IL-6 but not IL-8 in the development of heat hyperalgesia: effects on heat-evoked calcitonin gene-related peptide release from rat skin. *J Neurosci* 2000; 20:6289–93.

34. Breimer LH, MacIntyre I, Zaidi M. Peptides from the calcitonin genes: molecular genetics, structure and function. *Biochem J* 1988;255:377–90.

35. Wimalawansa SJ, MacIntyre I. Calcitonin gene-related peptide and its specific binding sites in the cardiovascular system of the rat. *Int J Cardiol* 1988;20:29–33.

36. Deng PY, Ye F, Cai WJ, Deng HW, Li YJ. Role of calcitonin gene-related peptide in the phenol-induced neurogenic hypertension in rats. *Regul Pept* 2004; 119:155–61.

37. Ohmura T, Nashio M, Kigoshi S, Muramatsu I. Electrophysiological and mechanical effects of calcitonin gene-related peptide on guinea-pig atria. *Br J Pharmacol* 1990;100:27–30.

38. Nelson MT, Huang Y, Brayden JE, Hescheler J, Standen NB. Arterial dilations in response to calcitonin gene-related peptide involve activation of K+ channels. *Nature* 1990;344: 770–73.

39. Yoshimoto R, Mitsui-Saito M, Ozaki H, et al. Effects of adrenomedullin and calcitonin gene-related peptide on contractions of the rat aorta and porcine coronary artery. *Br J Pharmacol* 1998;123:1645–54.

40. Asimakis GK, DiPette DJ, Conti VR, et al. Hemodynamic action of calcitonin gene-related peptide immunoreactivity in the spinal cord of man and eight other species. *Hypertension* 1978;9:142–46.

41. Supowit SC, Rao A, Bowers MC, Zhao H, Fink G, Steficek B, et al. Calcitonin gene-related peptide protects against hypertension-induced heart and kidney damage. *Hypertension* 2005;45:109–14.

42. Hokfelt T, Broberger C, Xu ZQ, Sergeyev V, Ubink R, Diez M. Neuropeptides: an overview. *Neuropharmacology* 2000;39: 1337–56.

43. Deng PY, Ye F, Zhu HQ, Cai WJ, Deng HW, Li YJ. An increase in the synthesis and release of calcitonin gene-related peptide in two-kidney, one-clip hypertensive rats. *Regul Pept* 2003; 114:175–82.

44. Supowit SC, Zhao H, Hallman DM, DiPette DJ. Calcitonin gene-related peptide is a depressor in subtotal nephrectomy hypertension. *Hypertension* 1998;31:391–96.

45. Gangula PR, Supowit SC, Wimalawansa SJ, Zhao H, Hallman DM, DiPette DJ, et al. Calcitonin gene-related peptide is a depressor in NG-nitro-L-arginine methyl ester (L-NAME)–induced preeclampsia. *Hypertension* 1997;29:248–53.

46. Supowit SC, Guraraj A, Ramana CV, Westlund KN, DiPette DJ. Enhanced neuronal expression of calcitonin gene-related peptide in mineralocorticoid-salt hypertension. *Hypertension* 1995; 25:1333–38.

47. Supowit SC, Zhao H, Hallman DM, DiPette DJ. Calcitonin gene-related peptide is a depressor of deoxycorticosterone-salt hypertension in the rat. *Hypertension* 1997;29: 945–50.

48. Li J, Wang DH. High-salt-induced increase in blood pressure: role of capsaicin-sensitive sensory nerves. *J Hypertens* 2003;21:577–82.

49. Wang DH, Li J, Qiu J. Salt-sensitive hypertension induced by sensory denervation: introduction of a new model. *Hypertension* 1998;32: 649–53.

50. Li J, Wang DH. Development of angiotensin II–induced hypertension: role of CGRP and its receptor. *J Hypertens* 2005;23:113–18.

51. Hobara N, Gessei-Tsutsumi N, Goda M, Takayama F, Akiyama S, Kurosaki Y, et al. Long-term inhibition of angiotensin prevents reduction of

periarterial innervation of calcitonin gene-related peptide (CGRP)–containing nerves in spontaneously hypertensive rats. *Hypertens Res Clin Exp* 2005; 28:465–74.

52. Deng PY, Yu J, Ye F, Li D, Luo D, Cai WJ, et al. Interactions of sympathetic nerves with capsaicin-sensitive sensory nerves: neurogenic mechanisms for phenol-induced hypertension in the rat. *J Hypertens* 2005;23:603–609.

53. Ye S, Zhong H, Duong VN, Campese VM. Losartan reduces central and peripheral sympathetic nerve activity in a rat model of neurogenic hypertension. *Hypertension* 2002; 39:1101–106.

54. Kawasaki H, Nuki C, Saito A, Takasaki K. Adrenergic modulation of calcitonin gene-related peptide (CGRP)–containing nerve-mediated vasodilation in the rat mesenteric resistance vessel. *Brain Res* 1990; 506:287–90.

55. Lind H, Edvinsson L. Enhanced vasodilator responses to calcitonin gene-related peptide (CGRP) in subcutaneous arteries in human hypertension. *J Hum Hypertens* 2002; 16:53–59.

56. Vanhoutte P, Amery A, Birkenhager W, et al. Serotoninergic mechanism in hypertension: focus on the effects of ketanserin. *Hypertension* 1988;11: 111–33.

57. Kuhn DM. Tryptophan hydroxylase regulation: drug-induced modifications that alter serotonin neuronal function. *Adv Exp Med Biol* 1999;467:19–27.

58. Craig SP, Boularand S, Darmon MC, Mallet J, Craig IW. Localization of human tryptophan hydroxylase (TPH) to chromosome 11p15.3-p14 by in situ hybridization. *Cytogenet Cell Genet* 1991;56:157–59.

59. Walther DJ, Peter JU, Bashammakh S, Hortnagl H, Voits M, Fink H, et al. Synthesis of serotonin by a second tryptophan hydroxylase isoform. *Science* 2003;299:76.

60. Zhang X, Beaulieu JM, Sotnikova TD, Gainetdinov RR, Caron MG. Tryptophan hydroxylase-2 controls brain serotonin synthesis. *Science* 2004;305:217.

61. Vanhoutte PM. Serotonin, hypertension and vascular disease. *Neth J Med* 1991;38:35–42.

62. Watts SW. Serotonin-induced contraction in mesenteric resistance arteries: signaling and changes in deoxycorticosterone acetate-salt hypertension. *Hypertension* 2002; 39:825–29.

63. Russell A, Banes A, Berlin H, Fink GD, Watts SW. 5-Hydroxytryptamine(2B) receptor function is enhanced in the N(omega)-nitro-L-arginine hypertensive rat. *J Pharmacol Exp Ther* 2002;303: 179–87.

64. Ni W, Thompson JM, Northcott CA, Lookingland K, Watts SW. The serotonin transporter is present and functional in peripheral arterial smooth muscle. *J Cardiovasc Pharmaco* 2004; 43:770–81.

65. Azzadin A, Mysliwiec M, Wollny T, Mysliwiec M, Buczko W. Serotonin is involved in the pathogenesis of hypertension developing during erythropoietin treatment in uremic rats. *Thrombosis Res* 1995;77:217–24.

66. Krygicz D, Azzadin A, Pawlak R, et al. Cyclosporine A affects serotonergic mechanisms in uremic rats. *Pol J Pharmacol* 1996;48:351–54.

67. Tsukamoto K, Kurihara T, Nakayama N, Isogai O, Ito S, Komatsu K, et al. Pressor responses to serotonin injected into the nucleus tractus solitarius of Sprague-Dawley rats and spontaneously hypertensive rats. *Clin Exp Hypertens* 2000;22:63–73.

68. Kuhn DM, Wolf WA, Lovenberg W. Pressor effects of electrical stimulation of the dorsal and median raphe nuclei in anesthetized rats. *J Pharmacol Exp Ther* 1980;214:403–409.

69. McGregor DD, Smirk FH. Vascular responses to 5-hydroxytryptamine in genetic and renal hypertensive rats. *Am J Physiol* 1970;219:687–90.

70. Nishimura Y, Suzuki A. Enhanced contractile responses mediated by different 5-HT receptor subtypes in basilar arteries, superior mesenteric arteries and thoracic aortas from stroke-prone spontaneously hypertensive rats. *Clin Exp Pharmacol Physiol* 1995;(Suppl 1):S99–101.

71. Dohi Y, Luscher TF. Altered intra- and extra-luminal effects of 5-hydroxytryptamine in hypertensive mesenteric resistance arteries: contribution of the endothelium and smooth muscle. *J Cardiovasc Pharmacol* 1991;18:278–84.

72. Myers MG, Reid JL, Lewis PJ. The effect of central serotonin depletion on DOCA-saline hypertension in the rat. *Cardiovasc Res* 1974;8:806–10.

73. Browning RA, Bramlet DG, Myers JH, Bundman MC, Smith ML. Failure to produce blood pressure changes following pharmacological or surgical depletion of brain serotonin in the spontaneously hypertensive rat. *Clin Exp Hypertens* 1981;3:953–73.

74. Martin GR. Vascular receptors for 5-hydroxytryptamine: distribution, function and classification. *Pharmacol Ther* 1994;62:283–324.

75. Watts SW. 5-HT in systemic hypertension: foe, friend or fantasy? *Clin Sci* 2005;108:399–412.

76. Stott DJ, Saniabadi AR, Hosie J, Lowe GD, Ball SG. The effects of the 5-HT2 antagonist ritanserin on blood pressure and serotonin-induced platelet aggregation in patients with untreated essential hypertension. *Eur J Clin Pharmacol* 1988;35:123–29.

77. Gradin K, Pettersson A, Hedner T, Persson B. Chronic 5-HT2 receptor blockade with ritanserin does not reduce blood pressure in the spontaneously hypertensive rat. *J Neural Transm* 1985;64:145–49.

78. Saini HK, Takeda N, Goyal RK, Kumamoto H, Arneja AS, Dhalla NS. Therapeutic potentials of sarpogrelate in cardiovascular disease. *Cardiovasc Drug Rev* 2004;22:27–54.

79. Missouris CG, Cappuccio FP, Varsamis E, Barron JL, Carr E, Markandu ND, et al. Serotonin and heart rate in hypertensive and normotensive subjects. *Am Heart J* 1998;135:838–43.

80. Fetkovska N, Amstein R, Ferracin F, Regenass M, Buhler FR, Pletscher A. 5-Hydroxytryptamine kinetics and activation of blood platelets in patients

with essential hypertension. *Hypertension* 1990;15:267–73.

81. Deussen A, Moser G, Schrader J. Contribution of coronary endothelial cells to cardiac adenosine production. *Pflugers Arch* 1986;406:608–14.

82. Dubey RK, Gillespie DG, Mi Z, Suzuki F, Jackson EK. Smooth muscle cell-derived adenosine inhibits cell growth. *Hypertension* 1996;27:766–73.

83. Dubey RK, Gillespie DG, Mi Z, Jackson EK. Exogenous and endogenous adenosine inhibits fetal calf serum-induced growth of rat cardiac fibroblasts: role of A2B receptors. *Circulation* 1997;96: 2656–66.

84. Meghi P, Holmquist CA, Newby AC. Adenosine formation and release from neonatal-rat heart cells in culture. *Biochem J* 1985;229:799–805.

85. Mullane K, Bullough D. Harnessing and endogenous cardioprotective mechanism: cellular sources and sites of action of adenosine. *J Mol Cell Cardiol* 1995;27:1041–54.

86. Sparks HV Jr, Bardenheuer H. Regulation of adenosine formation by the heart. *Circ Res* 1986;58:193–201.

87. Newby AC, Worku Y, Holmquist CA. Adenosine formation. Evidence for a direct biochemical link with energy metabolism. *Adv Mycardiol* 1985;6: 273–84.

88. Schutz W, Schrader J, Gerlach E. Different sites of adenosine formation in the heart. *Am J Physiol* 1981;240: H963–70.

89. Tucker AL, Linden J. Cloned receptors and cardiovascular responses to adenosine. *Cardiovasc Res* 1993;27: 62–67.

90. Fredholm BB, Arslan G, Halldner L, Kull B, Schulte G, Wasserman W. Structure and function of adenosine receptors and their genes. *Naunyn Schiemdebergs Arch Pharmacol* 2000; 362:364–74.

91. Biaggioni I. Contrasting excitatory and inhibitory effects of adenosine in blood pressure regulation. *Hypertension* 1992;20:457–65.

92. Headrick JP, Berne RM. Endothelium-dependent and -independent relaxations to adenosine in guinea pig aorta. *Am J Physiol* 1990;259:H62–67.

93. Cristalli G, Vittori S, Thompson RD, Padgett WL, Shi D, Daly JW, et al. Inhibition of platelet aggregation by adenosine receptor agonists. *Naunyn Schmiedebergs Arch Pharmacol* 1994; 349:644–50.

94. Vials A, Burnstock G. A2-purinoceptor-mediated relaxation in the guinea-pig coronary vasculature: a role for nitric oxide. *Br J Pharmacol* 1993;109: 424–29.

95. Dubey RK, Gillespie DG, Jackson EK. Cyclic AMP–adenosine pathway induces nitric oxide synthesis in aortic smooth muscle cells. *Hypertension* 1998;31:296–302.

96. Cornstein BN, Levin RI, Belanoff J, Weissmann G, Hirschhorn R. Adenosine: an endogenous inhibitor of neutrophil-mediated injury to endothelial cells. *J Clin Invest* 1986; 78:760–70.

97. Jackson EK. Adenosine: a physiological brake on renin release. *Annu Rev Pharmacol Toxicol* 1991;31:1–35.

98. Maggirwar SB, Dhanraj DN, Somani SM, Ramkumar V. Adenosine acts as an endogenous activator of the cellular antioxidant defense system. *Biochem Biophys Res Commun* 1994; 201:508–15.

99. Tabrizchi R. Effects of adenosine and adenosine analogues on mean circulatory filling pressure and cardiac output in anesthetized rats. *Naunyn Schiemdebergs Arch Pharmacol* 1997; 356:69–75.

100. Edlund A, Sollevi A, Linde B. Haemodynamic and metabolic effects of adenosine in man. *Clin Sci* 1990;79: 131–38.

101. Cheng DY, DeWitt BJ, Suzuki F, Neely CF, Kadowitz PJ. Adensoine A1 and A2 receptors mediate tone-dependent responses in feline pulmonary vascular bed. *Am J Physiol* 1996;270:H200–207.

102. Tabrizchi R, Bedi S. Pharmacology of adenosine receptors in the vasculature. *Pharmacol Ther* 2001;91:133–47.

103. Spielman WS, Arend LJ. Adenosine receptors and signaling in the kidney. *Hypertension* 1991;17:117–30.

104. Albino-Teixeira A, Matias A, Polonia J, Azevedo I. Blockade of adenosine receptors causes hypertension and cardiovascular structural changes in the rat. *J Hypertens* 1991;9 (Suppl.6):S196–97.

105. Guimaraes S, Morato M, Sousa T, Albino-Teixeira A. Hypertension due to blockade of adenosine receptors. *Pharmacol Toxicol* 2003;92:160–62.

106. Ledent C, Vaugeois JM, Schiffmann SN, Pedrazzini T, El Yacoubi M, Vanderhaeghen JJ, et al. Aggressiveness, hypoalgesia and high blood pressure in mice lacking the adenosine A2a receptor. *Nature* 1997;388:674–82.

107. Uehara Y, Numabe A, Hirawa N, Kawabata Y, Nagoshi H, Kaneko H, et al. A new adenosine subtype-1 receptor antagonist, FK-838, attenuates salt-induced hypertension in Dahl salt-sensitive rats. *Am J Hypertens* 1995;8:1189–99.

108. Kost CK Jr, Herzer WA, Li P, Jackson EK. Vascular reactivity to angiotensin II is selectively enhanced in the kidneys of spontaneously hypertensive rats. *J Pharmacol Exp Ther* 1994;269:82–88.

109. Fahim M, Hussain T, Mustafa SJ. Role of endothelium in adenosine receptor-mediated vasorelaxation in hypertensive rats. *Fundam Clin Pharmacol* 2001;15:325–34.

110. Dubey RK, Mi Z, Gillespie DG, Jackson EK. Dysregulation of extracellular adenosine levels by vascular smooth muscle cells from spontaneously hypertensive rats. *ArteriosclerThromb Vasc Biol* 2001;21:249–54.

111. Wright K, Tajouri L, Lea RA, Ovcaric M, Heux S, Morin F, et al. The role of adenosine-related genes variants in susceptibility to essential hypertension. *J Hypertens* 2004;22:1519–22.

112. Thiel BA, Chakravarti A, Cooper RS, Luke A, Lewis S, Lynn A, et al. A genome-wide linkage analysis investigating the determinants of blood pressure in whites and African-Americans. *Am J Hypertens* 2003; 16:151–53.

113. Sousa T, Morato M, Albino-Teixeira A. Angiotensin converting enzyme inhibition prevents trophic and hypertensive effects of an antagonist of adenosine receptors. *Eur J Pharmacol* 2002;441:99–104.

114. Morato M, Sousa T, Guimaraes S, Moura D, Albino-Teixeira A. The role of angiotensin II in hypertension due to adenosine receptors blockade. *Eur J Pharmacol* 2002;455:135–41.

115. Morato M, Sousa T, Guimaraes S, Moura D, Albino-Teixeira A. Losartan and atenolol on hypertension induced by adenosine receptor blockade. *Auton Autacoid Pharmacol* 2003;23:133–40.

116. Virdis A, Ghiadoni L, Marzilli M, Orsini E, Favilla S, Duranti P, et al. Adenosine causes the release of active renin and angiotensin II in the coronary circulation of patients with essential hypertension. *J Am Coll Cardiol* 1999; 33:1677–84.

117. van Buren M, Bijlsma JA, Boer P, van Rijn HJ, Koomans HA. Natriuretic and hypotensive effect of adenosine-1 blockade in essential hypertension. *Hypertension* 1993;22:728–34.

118. Dumont Y, Martel JC, Fournier A, St-Pierre S, Quirion R. Neuropeptide Y and neuropeptide Y receptor subtypes in brain and peripheral tissues. *Prog Neurobiol* 1992;38:125–67.

119. Chronwall BM, DiMaggio DA, Massari VJ, Pickel VM, Ruggiero DA, O'Donohue TL. The anatomy of neuropeptide-Y–containing neurons in rat brain. *Neuroscience* 1985;15: 1159–81.

120. Lin S, Boey D, Herzog H. NPY and Y receptors: lessons from transgenic and knockout models. *Neuropeptides* 2004; 38:189–200.

121. Donoso MV, Brown N, Carrasco C, Cortes V, Fournier A, Huidobro-Toro JP. Stimulation of the sympathetic perimesenteric arterial nerves releases neuropeptide Y potentiating the vasomotor activity of noradrenaline: involvement of neuropeptide Y-Y1 receptors. *J Neurochem* 1997;69: 1048–59.

122. Maisel AS, Scott NA, Motulsky HJ, Michel MC, Boublik JH, Rivier JE, et al. Elevation of plasma neuropeptide Y levels in congestive heart failure. *Am J Med* 1989;86:43–48.

123. Lundberg JM, Terenius L, Hokfelt T, Martling CR, Tatemoto K, Mutt V, et al. Neuropeptide Y (NPY)-like immunoreactivity in peripheral noradrenergic neurons and effects of NPY on sympathetic function. *Acta Physiol Scand* 1982;116:477–80.

124. Kobari M, Fukuuchi Y, Tomita M, Tanahashi N, Yamawaki T, Takeda H, et al. Transient cerebral vasodilatory effect of neuropeptide Y mediated by nitric oxide. *Brain Res Bull* 1993;31: 443–48.

125. Lundberg JM, Stjarne L. Neuropeptide Y (NPY) depresses the secretion of 3H-noradrenaline and the contractile response evoked by field stimulation, in rat vas deferens. *Acta Physiol Scand* 1984;120:477–79.

126. Michalkiewicz M, Zhao G, Jia Z, Michalkiewicz T, Racadio MJ. Central neuropeptide Y signaling ameliorates N([omega])-nitro-l-arginine methyl ester hypertension in the rat through a Y1 receptor mechanism. *Hypertension* 2005;45:780–85.

127. Edvinsson L, Ekblad E, Hakanson R, Wahlestedt C. Neuropeptide Y potentiates the effect of various vasoconstrictor agents on rabbit blood vessels. *Br J Pharmacol* 1984;83:519–25.

128. Erlinge D, Brunkwall J, Edvinsson L. Neuropeptide Y stimulates proliferation of human vascular smooth muscle cells: cooperation with noradrenaline and ATP. *Regul Pept* 1994;50:259–65.

129. Lee EW, Grant DS, Movafagh S, Zukowska Z. Impaired angiogenesis in neuropeptide Y (NPY)-Y2 receptor knockout mice. *Peptides* 2003;24: 99–106.

130. Baker E, Hort YJ, Ball H, Sutherland GR, Shine J, Herzog H. Assignment of the human neuropeptide Y gene to chromosome 7p15.1 by nonisotopic in situ hybridization. *Genomics* 1995; 26:163–64.

131. Karvonen MK, Pesonen U, Koulu M, Niskanen L, Laakso M, Rissanen A, et al. Association of a leucine(7)-to-proline(7) polymorphism in the signal peptide of neuropeptide Y with high serum cholesterol and LDL cholesterol levels. *Nat Med* 1998;4:1434–37.

132. Wallerstedt SM, Skrtic S, Eriksson A, Ohlsson C, Hedner T. Association analysis of the polymorphism T1128C in the signal peptide of neuropeptide Y in a Swedish hypertensive population. *J Hypertens* 2004;22:1277–81.

133. Helisalmi S, Valve R, Karvonen MK, Hiltunen M, Pirskanen M, Mannermaa A, et al. The leucine (7)-to-proline (7) polymorphism in the signal peptide of neuropeptide Y is not associated with Alzheimer's disease or the link apolipoprotein E. *Neurosci Lett* 2000; 287:25–28.

134. Hvarfner A, Bergstrom R, Morlin C, Wide L, Ljunghall S. Relationships between calcium metabolic indices and blood pressure in patients with essential hypertension as compared with a healthy population. *J Hypertens* 1987;5:451–56.

135. Clark JT, Kalra PS, Crowley WR, Kalra SP. Neuropeptide Y and human pancreatic polypeptide stimulate feeding behavior in rats. *Endocrinology* 1984;115:427–29.

136. Heilig M, Vecsei L, Widerlov E. Opposite effects of centrally administered neuropeptide Y (NPY) on locomotor activity of spontaneously hypertensive (SH) and normal rats. *Acta Physiol Scand* 1989;137:243–48.

137. Lee RM, Nagahama M, McKenzie R, Daniel EE. Peptide-containing nerves around blood vessels of stroke-prone spontaneously hypertensive rats. *Hypertension* 1988;11(Suppl I):117–20.

138. Morris MJ, Tortelli CF, Hart DP, Delbridge LM. Vascular and brain neuropeptide Y in banded and spontaneously hypertensive rats. *Peptides* 2004;25:1313–19.

139. Han S, Yang CL, Chen X, Naes L, Cox BF, Westfall T. Direct evidence for the role of neuropeptide Y in sympathetic nerve stimulation-induced vasoconstriction. *Am J Physiol* 1998; 274:H290–94.

140. Sun XY, Edvisson L, Hedner T. Effects of D-myo-inositoL-1,2,6-trisphosphate (PP56) on neuropeptide Y (NPY) induced potentiation of various vasoconstrictor agents in the rat. *J Pharmacol Exp Ther* 1992;261:1147–52.

141. Turtzo LC, Marx R, Lane MD. Cross-talk between sympathetic neurons and adipocytes in coculture. *Proc Natl Acad Sci U S A* 2001;98:12385–90.

142. Cantley LK, Russell JB, Lettieri DS, Sherwood LM. Effects of vitamin D3, 25-hydroxyvitamin D3, and 24,25-dihydroxyvitamin D3 on parathyroid hormone secretion. *Calcif Tissue Int* 1987;41:48–51.

143. Jüppner HW, Gardella TJ, Brown EM, et al. Parathyroid hormone and parathyroid hormone-related peptide in the regulation of calcium homeostasis and bone development. In: DeGroot LL, Jameson JL, eds. *Endocrinology*, 4th ed. Philadelphia: Elsevier, 2000:2:969–98.

144. Potts JT. Parathyroid hormone: past and present. *J Endocrinol* 2005;187: 311–25.

145. Abou-Samra A-B, Jüppner H, Force T, et al. Expression cloning of a parathyroid hormone/parathyroid hormone related peptide receptor from rat osteoblast-like cells: a single receptor stimulates intracellular accumulation of both cyclic AMP, and inositol triphosphate and increases intracellular free calcium. *Proc Natl Acad Sci U S A* 1992;89: 2732–36.

146. Nakamura R, Watanabe TX, Sokabe H. Acute hypotensive action of parathyroid hormone- (L-34) fragments in hypertensive rats. *Proc Soc Exp Biol Med* 1981;168:168–71.

147. Nickols GA, Nickols MA, Helwig JJ. Binding of parathyroid hormone and parathyroid hormone-related protein to vascular smooth muscle of rabbit renal microvessels. *Endocrinology* 1990;126:721–27.

148. Saglikes Y, Massry S, Iseki K, Nadler J, Campese V. Effect of PTH on blood pressure and response to vasoconstrictor agonists. *Am J Physiol* 1985;248: F674–81.

149. Nickols GA. Increased cAMP in cultured vascular smooth muscle cells and relaxation of aortic strips by parathyroid hormone. *Eur J Pharmacol* 1985;16:137–44.

150. Bukoski RD, Xue H, DeWan P, McCarron DA. Calciotropic hormones and vascular calcium metabolism in experimental hypertension. In: Halpern W, Pegram BL, Brayden JE, Mackey K, McLaughlin MK, Osol G, eds. *Resistance Arteries*. Ithaca, NY: Perinatology Press, 1988:320–28.

151. Schleiffer R, Helwig JJ, Pernot F, Gairard A. Vascular effects of calcitonin and parathyroid hormone. In: Doepfner W, ed. *Calcitonin 1984*. Amsterdam: Excerpts Medica, 1986: 15–24.

152. Hulter HN, Melby JC, Peterson JC, Cooke CR. Chronic continuous PTH infusion results in hypertension in normal subjects. *J Clin Hypertens* 1986;2:360–70.

153. Ljunghall S. Hypertension in primary hyperparathyroidism in relation to histopathology. *Eur J Surg* 1991; 157:457–59.

154. Young EW, McCarron DA, Morris CD. Calcium regulating hormones in essential hypertension. Importance of gender. *Am J Hypertens* 1990;3(Suppl): 161S–66S.

155. Morfis L, Smerdely P, Howes LG. Relationship between serum parathyroid hormone levels in the elderly and 24 h ambulatory blood pressures. *J Hypertens* 1997;15:1271–76.

156. St John A, Dick I, Hoad K, Retallack R, Welborn T, Prince R. Relationship between calcitrophic hormones and blood pressure in elderly subjects. *Eur J Endocrinol* 1994;130:446–50.

157. Brickman A, Nyby M, von Hungen K, Eggena P, Tuck M. Parathyroid hormone, platelet calcium, and blood pressure in normotensive subjects. *Hypertension* 1991;18:176–82.

158. McCarron DA, Morris CD, Henry HJ, et al. Blood pressure and nutrient intake in the United States. *Science* 1984;224:1392–98.

159. McCarron DA. Low serum concentrations of ionized calcium in patients with essential hypertension. *N Engl J Med* 1982;307:226–28.

160. Resnick LM, Laragh JH, Sealey JE, et al. Divalent cations in essential hypertension. Relations between serum ionized calcium, magnesium, and plasma renin activity. *N Engl J Med* 1983;309:888–91.

161. Buckley BM, Smith SC, Beevers M, et al. Lack of evidence of low ionized calcium levels in systemic hypertension. *Am J Cardiol* 1987;59:878–80.

162. Fardella C, Rodriguez-Portales JA. Intracellular calcium and blood pressure: comparison between primary hyperparathyroidism and essential hypertension. *J Endocrinol Invest* 1995; 18:827–32.

163. DiPette DJ, Christenson W, Nickols MA, Nickols GA. Cardiovascular responsiveness to parathyroid hormone (PTH) and PTH-related protein in genetic hypertension. *Endocrinology* 1992;130:2045–51.

164. Nyby MD, Hino T, Berger ME, Ormsby BL, Golub MS, Brickman AS. Desensitization of vascular tissue to parathyroid hormone and parathyroid hormone-related protein. *Endocrinology* 1995;136:2497–504.

165. Lewanczuk RZ, Resnick LM, Ho MS, Benishin CG, Shan J, Pang PKT. Clinical aspects of parathyroid hypertensive factor. *J Hypertens* 1994; 12:11–16.

166. Jorde R, Sundsfjord J, Haug E, Bonaa KH. Relation between low calcium intake, parathyroid hormone, and blood pressure. *Hypertension* 2000; 35:1154–59.

167. Lewanczuk RZ, Wang J, Zhang ZR, Pang PKT. Effects of spontaneously hypertensive rat plasma on blood pressure and tail artery calcium uptake in normotensive rats. *Am J Hypertens* 1989;2:26–31.

168. Lewanczuk RZ, Pang PKT. Expression of parathyroid hypertensive factor in hypertensive primary hyperparathyroid patients. *Blood Press* 1993;2:22–27.

169. Resnick LM, Muller FB, Laragh JH. Calcium-regulating hormones in essential hypertension. Relation to plasma renin activity and sodium metabolism. *Ann Intern Med* 1986; 105:649–54.

170. Mann JFE, Wiecek A, Bommer J, Ganten U, Ritz E. Effects of parathyroidectomy on blood pressure in spontaneously hypertensive rats. *Nephron* 1987;62:465–69.

171. Coulouarn Y, Lihrmann I, Jegou S, Anouar Y, Tostivint H, Beauvillain JC, et al. Cloning of the cDNA encoding the urotensin II precursor in frog and human reveals intense expression of the urotensin II gene in motoneurons of the spinal cord. *Proc Natl Acad Sci USA* 1998;95:15803–808.

172. Elshourbagy NA, Douglas SA, Shabon U, Harrison S, Duddy G, Sechler JL, et al. Molecular and pharmacological characterization of genes encoding urotensin-II peptides and their cognate G-protein coupled receptors from the mouse and monkey. *Br J Pharmacol* 2002;136:9–22.

173. Ong KL, Lam KS, Cheung BM. Urotensin II: its function in health and its role in disease. *Cardiovasc Drugs Ther* 2005;19:65–75.

174. Ames RS, Sarau HM, Chambers JK, Willette RN, Aiyar NV, Romanic AM, et al. Human urotensin II is a potent vasoconstrictor and agonist for the orphan receptor GPR14. *Nature* 1999; 401:282–86.

175. Liu Q, Pong SS, Zeng Z, Zhang Q, Howard AD, Williams DL Jr, et al. Identification of urotensin II as the endogenous ligand for the orphan G-protein coupled receptor GPR14. *Biochem Biophys Res Commun* 1999; 266:174–78.

176. Protopopov A, Kashuba V, Podowski R, Gizatullin R, Sonnhammer E, Wahlestedt C, et al. Assignment of the GPR14 gene coding for the G-protein-coupled receptor 14 to human chromosome 17q25.3 by fluorescent in situ hybridization. *Cytogenet Cell Genet* 2000;88: 312–13.

177. Douglas SA, Dhanak D, Johns DG. From "gills to pills": urotensin-II as a regulator of mammalian cardiorenal function. *Trends Pharmacol Sci* 2004; 25:76–85.

178. Cheung BM, Leung R, Man YB, Wong LY. Plasma concentration of urotensin II is raised in hypertension. *J Hypertens* 2004;22:1341–44.

179. Thompson JP, Watt P, Sanghavi S, Strupish JW, Lambert DG. A comparison of cerebrospinal fluid and plasma urotensin II concentrations in normotensive and hypertensive patients undergoing urological surgery during spinal anesthesia: a pilot study. *Anesth Analg* 2003;97:1501–503.

180. Matsushita M, Shichiri M, Imai T, Iwashina M, Tanaka H, Takasu N, et al. Co-expression of urotensin II and its receptor (GPR14) in human cardiovascular and renal tissues. *J Hypertens* 2001;19:2185–90.

181. Douglas SA, Sulpizio AC, Piercy V, Sarau HM, Ames RS, Aiyar NV, et al. Differential vasoconstrictor activity of human urotensin-II in vascular tissue isolated from the rat, mouse, dog, pig, marmoset and cynomolgus monkey. *Br J Pharmacol* 2000;131:1262–74.

182. Camarda V, Rizzi A, Calo G, Gendron G, Perron SI, Kostenis E, et al. Effects of human urotensin II in isolated vessels of various species;comparison with other vasoactive agents. *Naunyn-Schmiedebergs Arch Pharmacol* 2002; 365:141–49.

183. Russell FD, Molenaar P. Cardiovascular actions of human urotensin II—considerations for hypertension. *Naunyn-Schmiedebergs Arch Pharmacol* 2004;369:271–73.

184. Itoh H, McMaster D, Lederis K. Functional receptors for fish neuropeptide urotensin II in major rat arteries. *Eur J Pharmacol* 1988;149:61–66.

185. Maguire JJ, Kuc RE, Davenport AP. Orphan-receptor ligand human urotensin II: feceptor localization in human tissues and comparison of vasoconstrictor responses with endothelin-1. *Br J Pharmacol* 2000;131:441–46.

186. Hillier C, Berry C, Petrie MC, O'Dwyer PJ, Hamilton C, Brown A, et al. Effects of urotensin II in human arteries and veins of varying caliber. *Circulation* 2001;103:1378–81.

187. Stirrat A, Gallagher M, Douglas SA, Ohlstein EH, Berry C, Kirk A, et al. Potent vasodilator responses to human urotensin-II in human pulmonary and abdominal resistance arteries. *Am J Physiol Heart Circ Physiol* 2001;280:H925–28.

188. Bottrill FE, Douglas SA, Hiley CR, White R. Human urotensin-II is an endothelium-dependent vasodilator in rat small arteries. *Br J Pharmacol* 2000;130:1865–70.

189. Li L,Yuan WJ, Su DF. Effects of rat urotensin II on coronary flow and myocardial eNOS protein expression in isolated rat heart. *Acta Pharmacol Sin* 2004;25:1444–49.

190. Zhang AY, Chen YF, Zhang DX, Yi F-X, Qi J, Andrade-Gordon P, et al. Urotensin II is a nitric oxide-dependent vasodilator and natriuretic peptide in the rat kidney. *Am J Physiol Renal Physiol* 2003;285:F792–F98.

191. Lin Y, Tsuchihashi T, Matsumura K, Fukuhara M, Ohya Y, Fujii K, et al. Central cardiovascular action of urotensin II in spontaneously hypertensive rats. *Hypertens Res* 2003;26:839–45.

192. Lu Y, Zou C, Huang D, Tang C. Cardiovascular effects of urotensin II in different brain areas. *Peptides* 2002;23:1631–35.

193. Lin Y, Tsuchihashi T, Matsumura K, Abe I, Iida M. Central cardiovascular action of urotensin II in conscious rats. *J Hypertens* 2003;21:159–65.

194. Watson AM, Lambert GW, Smith KJ, May CN. Urotensin II acts centrally to increase epinephrine and ACTH release and cause potent inotropic and chronotropic actions. *Hypertension* 2003;42:373–79.

195. Itoh N, Obata KI, Yanaihara N, Okamoto H. Human preprovasoactive intestinal polypeptide contains a novel PHI-27-like peptide, PHM-27. *Nature* 1983;304:547–49.

196. Gozes I, Nakai H, Byers M, Avidor R, Weinstein Y, Shani Y, et al. Sequential expression in the nervous system of the VIP and c-myb genes located on the human chromosomal region 6q24. *Somat Cell Mol Genet* 1987;13:305–13.

197. Gozes I, Fridkin M, Hill JM, Brenneman DE. Pharmaceutical VIP: prospects and problems. *Curr Med Chem* 1999;6:1019–34.

198. Saetrum Opgaard O, Knutsson M, de Vries R, Tom B, Saxena PR, Edvinsson L. Vasoactive intestinal peptide has a direct positive inotropic effect on isolated human myocardial trabeculae. *Clin Sci* 2001;101:637–43.

199. Mori K, Asakura S, Ogawa H, Sasagawa S, Takeyama M. Decreases in substance P and vasoactive intestinal peptide concentrations in plasma of stroke-prone spontaneously hypertensive rats. *Jpn Heart J* 1993;34:785–94.

Chapter

33 Multiple Roles of Eicosanoids in Blood Pressure Regulation

John Quilley and John C. McGiff

Key Findings

- PGE$_2$ stimulates multiple receptor subtypes, including those of tubules that inhibit Na$^+$ transport and those of the renal vasculature that elicit dilation and increase medullary blood flow. In concert, they contribute to the diuresis–natriuresis in response to elevation of renal perfusion pressure and/or expansion of extracellular fluid volume.

- TxA$_2$ receptor stimulation contributes to angiotensin-dependent hypertension. Increased TxA$_2$ production participates in the elevation of blood pressure in young spontaneously hypertensive rats.

- Among the many properties of 20-hydroxyeicosatetraenoic acid (20-HETE), vasoactivity and modulation of transport in key nephron segments underlie its essential role in the regulation of the renal circulation (autoregulation and tubuloglomerular feedback) and electrolyte excretion (cotransporter and Na$^+$ pump inhibition), which impact directly on the regulation of blood pressure.

- The range and diversity of activity of 20-HETE also derive from cyclooxygenase-2–dependent transformation of 20-HETE in the renal vasculature to prostaglandin analogues.

- Production of antipressor epoxyeicosatrienoic acids (EETs) in rats by the cytochrome P450-arachidonic acid epoxygenase isoform 2C23 is stimulated by activating adenosine A$_{2A}$ receptors in response to salt loading; and inhibition of EET synthesis raises blood pressure in salt-loaded rats.

- 11,12-EET is the endogenous regulator of epithelial Na$^+$ channel in cortical collecting ducts; deficiency in 11,12-EET is a probable cause of a monogenic form of hypertension.

PROSTANOIDS

Prostaglandins are generally considered to be antihypertensive, although there is little doubt that PGH$_2$/TxA$_2$ contribute to the elevation of blood pressure in some forms of hypertension. The antihypertensive effects are based on the actions of prostaglandins that brake the vascular and renal tubular responses to stimulation of vasopressor systems and amplify the vasodilator and natriuretic effects of stimulation of vasodepressor systems. Thus prostaglandins moderate the effects of the renin-angiotensin system (RAS),[1] the sympathetic nervous system,[2] and vasopressin,[3] while enhancing the effects of the kallikrein-kinin system.[4]

Inhibition of cyclooxygenase (COX) increases vascular resistance and enhances vasoconstrictor responses to angiotensin II (Ang II) and other constrictor hormones.[1] Identification of the inducible form of COX, COX-2, and the development of specific inhibitors of each isoform and COX-1 and COX-2 knockout mice has enabled investigators to distinguish the functional consequences produced by inhibiting either the inducible COX-2 or the constitutive COX-1. COX-2 activates the RAS by initiating synthesis of PGI$_2$ (prostacyclin), the renin secretagogue. COX-2 in preglomerular microvessels (PGMVs) also has an important role in metabolizing and, thereby, moderating the pressor activity of 20-hydroxyeicosatetraenoic acid (20-HETE), the principal product of the cytochrome P450 (CYP) pathway of arachidonic acid (AA) metabolism (Figure 33–1).

DEFINING THE PHYSIOLOGIC ROLE OF PROSTAGLANDINS

Until recently, the definition of the role of prostaglandins in hypertension has defied rigorous analysis because of the lack of appropriate investigative tools. With the characterization of prostaglandin receptor subtypes and the development of receptor subtype knockout models and selective receptor agonists and antagonists, the role of individual prostaglandins in disease processes is becoming clearer. Conventionally, investigations relied on measurements of prostaglandins or metabolites in biological fluids as indices of renal or systemic production and on the effects of nonsteroidal anti-inflammatory drugs (NSAIDs) to inhibit synthesis. Both have severe limitations, the latter because both pro- and anti-hypertensive prostanoids will be affected, and the former because the sites of synthesis and action of prostaglandins may be limited to discrete cell types, thus limiting the value of measurements in biological fluids such as plasma and urine. Similar limitations are being re-experienced in investigations of the more recently discovered CYP-derived eicosanoids, epoxyeicosatrienoic acids (EETs), and HETEs, for which receptors have not been defined and where inhibitors of enzyme activity, epoxygenases, and ω/ω-1-hydroxylases may affect multiple isoforms and the formation of both pro- and anti-hypertensive products. This is apparent from the use of NSAIDs; depending on the form of hypertension and the predominance of pro- or anti-hypertensive prostanoids, NSAIDs may increase or decrease blood pressure.

As renin release is stimulated by PGI$_2$ and requires COX-2 expression, renin-dependent hypertension can be

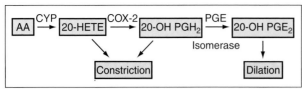

Figure 33–1. Schematic showing transformation of the vasoconstrictor, 20-HETE, by COX-2 and PGE$_2$ isomerase to 20-OH PGE$_2$, which produces vasodilation. 20-HETE, 20-hydroxyeicosatetraenoic acid; AA, arachidonic acid; COX-2, cyclooxygenase-2; CYP, cytochrome P450. (Redrawn from McGiff JC, Quilley J. *Am J Physiol Regal Integr Comp Physiol* 1999;277:R607–23. Used with permission.)

reduced by either COX inhibition or blockade of the IP receptor.[5,6] It is interesting to note that IP receptor deletion protects against renovascular hypertension by disengaging (uncoupling) RAS from the obligatory PGI$_2$ component that activates renin production/release.[6] Thus in wild-type mice, clipping of the left renal artery resulted in elevation of blood pressure that was associated with increased renal renin mRNA and plasma renin activity (PRA). In mice lacking the IP receptor, the elevations of blood pressure, PRA and renin mRNA were greatly reduced. This supports the earlier finding of Wang et al.[5] that inhibition of COX-2 lowered blood pressure in a model of renovascular hypertension, an effect associated with reduced renin. Presumably, the same mechanism accounted for the blood pressure lowering effect of aspirin in patients with renovascular hypertension.[7] However, most evidence suggests that prostaglandins subserve protective roles to limit the increase in blood pressure and maintain organ perfusion in response to activation of vasopressor systems; under such conditions, NSAIDs can precipitate acute renal failure and produce malignant hypertension.[8] Thus inhibition of prostaglandin synthesis may have no untoward effects under normal conditions but may have catastrophic effects in situations where prostaglandin synthesis is directed at maintenance of normal tissue function in the face of potentially detrimental stimuli. For example, in the anesthetized, surgically stressed dog, inhibition of prostaglandin synthesis resulted in a precipitous increase in renal vascular resistance (RVR) with elevation of blood pressure (Figure 33–2), whereas in resting animals, NSAIDs affected neither renal blood flow (RBF) nor blood pressure.[9]

The exhibition of fundamental properties of prostaglandins depends on the experimental conditions as seen in the effects of endogenous versus exogenous PGE$_2$ on pressor systems. In response to either Ang II or norepinephrine infused into the renal artery, activation of the antipressor PGE$_2$ was evident in its increased concentrations in venous effluents (Figure 33–3), coincident with reversal of the renal vasoconstrictor action of the pressor hormone. By way of contrast, infusion of PGE$_2$ into the renal artery of chronically instrumented dogs evoked elevation of blood pressure despite the accompanying diuresis.[10] The pressor response most likely was produced by activation of either EP$_1$ or EP$_3$ receptors (or both) that can elicit renal vasoconstriction with an attendant increase in blood pressure via activation of the RAS.

PROSTAGLANDIN RECEPTORS

There are five major types of receptors—EP, IP, DP, FP, and TP—that correspond to the various ligands produced by COX isoforms, namely, PGE$_2$, PGI$_2$, PGD$_2$, PGF$_{2\alpha}$, and PGH$_2$/TxA$_2$, respectively. The receptors are classical G protein–coupled receptors with seven transmembrane domains.[11] As FP and DP receptors are not involved to a major degree in cardiovascular control and hypertension, they will not be addressed. For a comprehensive review of prostaglandin receptors and the kidney, see Breyer and Breyer.[12]

EP receptors

There are four G-protein–coupled EP receptors. The vasodilator effects of PGE$_2$ are linked to activation of EP$_2$ and EP$_4$ receptors with increased cAMP. Activation of these receptors explains the acute hypotensive effect of PGE$_2$.[13] In EP$_2$ knockout mice, the hypotensive effect of exogenous PGE$_2$ was lost and converted to a pressor response, which was attributed to unmasking of the vasoconstrictor effects of PGE$_2$ that resulted from activation of EP$_1$ and EP$_3$ receptor subtypes. Thus activation of either the EP$_1$ or EP$_3$ receptor was associated with an increase in intracellular calcium [Ca^{2+}]$_i$ and vasoconstriction; deletion of the EP$_1$ receptor subtype in mice produced hypotension. Deletion of EP$_2$ receptors in mice elevated blood pressure when the mice were exposed to a high salt diet,[13] which indicates a role for this receptor subtype in the excretion of salt, although expression in the kidney is low under normal conditions.

The natriuretic and diuretic effects of PGE$_2$ have been attributed also to activation of EP$_1$ and EP$_3$ receptors, which are both expressed in the collecting duct while EP$_3$ is also abundant in the thick ascending limb (TAL). Stimulation of EP$_1$ receptors increases (Ca^{2+})$_i$ and inhibits Na$^+$ and water reabsorption in the collecting duct, whereas activation of EP$_3$ receptors inhibits cAMP formation and, thereby, may modulate the effect of vasopressin. Stimulation of the EP$_3$ receptor of parietal cells inhibits gastric acid secretion whereas the EP$_4$ receptor is involved in mucus secretion; these cytoprotective mechanisms can be negatively affected by NSAIDs, which may result in gastric ulceration.

IP receptors

Stimulation of IP receptors produces vasodilation, inhibition of platelet aggregation and vascular smooth muscle cell proliferation.[14] These effects result from activation of adenylate cyclase; antagonism or deletion of this receptor would be predicted to have deleterious cardiovascular effects, which may only be exhibited in disease states. Thus in IP knockout mice, blood pressure was unaffected although hypertension in response to renal artery constriction was blunted consistent with the role of PGI$_2$ as a renin secretagogue.[15] Of great concern was the observation that these same mice were more prone to thrombogenesis,[6] a finding that anticipated the proposed mechanism evoked by the increased incidence of thrombotic events in patients treated with COX-2 inhibitors.[16]

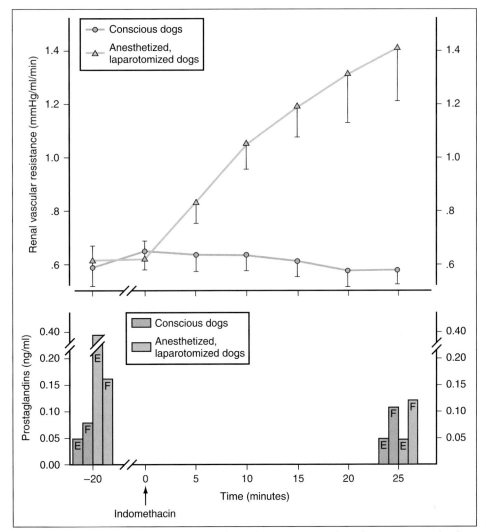

Figure 33–2. Effects of indomethacin on renal vascular resistance and renal venous prostaglandin concentrations (E=PGE$_2$, F=PGF$_{2\alpha}$) in conscious dogs and in those subjected to anesthesia and laparotomy. The vertical lines in the upper panel represent the standard error of the mean for the determination of vascular resistance. (Redrawn from Terragno NA, Terragno DA, McGiff JC. *Circ Res* 1977;40:590–5.)

TP receptors

These receptors can be activated by PGH$_2$ and TxA$_2$, as well as isoprostanes, all of which produce vasoconstriction.[17] Activation of TP receptors by either PGH$_2$ or TxA$_2$ contributes to hypertension of pregnancy[18] and to the elevation of blood pressure in some forms of experimental hypertension, particularly those that involve activation of the RAS. In the rat, coarctation of the aorta between the renal arteries resulted in hypertension that was associated with activation of the RAS for the first 2 to 3 weeks, during which time blockade of TP receptors lowered blood pressure.[19] The suggestion that TxA$_2$ contributes to the increase in blood pressure in response to stimulation of the RAS was confirmed by showing that TxA$_2$ was required for the full expression of the hypertensive response to Ang II.[20] In rats treated with an angiotensin-converting enzyme inhibitor to eliminate endogenous Ang II, the elevation of blood pressure to an infusion of Ang II for 7 days was reduced in animals given a Tx synthase inhibitor. Further confirmation came from TP receptor knockout mice in which the elevation of blood pressure in response to an infusion of Ang II was blunted.[21] Similar findings were reported by Kawada et al.[22] who concluded that TP receptor stimulation, via the AT1 receptor, mediated Ang II–induced increases in RVR, generation of reactive oxygen species and formation of pressor prostanoids (PGH$_2$/TxA$_2$). As COX-1 knockout mice also showed an attenuated pressor response to Ang II,[23] it seems likely that this COX isoform is responsible for the generation of PGH$_2$/TxA$_2$ in response to Ang II. In apparent conflict with the assigned role of COX-1 in the generation of pressor prostanoids, Wang et al.[24] provided evidence that in rabbits infused with Ang II, COX-2–derived PGH$_2$/TxA$_2$ mediated the enhanced constrictor effect of Ang II in microdissected afferent arterioles. However, species differences (rat vs. rabbit) and experimental conditions (isolated arterioles vs. whole animal) do not allow direct comparison of these studies. Nonetheless, under normal

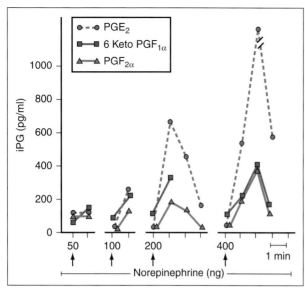

Figure 33–3. Line graphs showing norepinephrine-induced release of immunoreactive prostaglandins (iPG) from the rat isolated kidney. Norepinephrine, given by injection into renal artery at *arrows*, caused dose-related increases in perfusion pressure, from <10 mmHg to >100 mmHg (not shown). (Redrawn from Quilley J, McGiff JC. Eicosanoids. In: Swales ED, ed. *Textbook of Hypertension*. Oxford: Blackwell Scientific, 1994.)

conditions, TxA_2 does not contribute to the maintenance of blood pressure, as deletion of TP receptors in mice did not affect resting blood pressure but did increase the tendency for bleeding.[25]

A role for PGH_2/TxA_2 in the development of hypertension in spontaneously hypertensive rats (SHR) was suggested based on increased release of TxA_2 from kidneys of the young SHR.[26] Additionally, in the 6-week-old SHR, TP receptor antagonism reduced RVR and increased glomerular filtration rate (GFR).[27] In the young SHR (6 weeks), Tx synthase inhibitors either delayed or prevented the development of hypertension.[28] An aortic vasoconstrictor factor of endothelial origin generated by COX that acts through the TP receptor has been described in the SHR; it is released by acetylcholine (Ach) after inhibition of nitric oxide synthase (NOS).[29] As Tx synthase is a hemoprotein like CYP enzymes, it is vulnerable to catabolism by the inducible heme oxygenase (HO-1), which inactivates enzymes having a heme moiety.[30] Thus Sessa et al.[31] reported decreased Tx synthase activity in renal cortical microsomes from 7-week-old SHR treated with stannous chloride ($SnCl_2$) to induce HO-1 activity.

PREECLAMPSIA: RELATIVE DEFICIT OF PGI_2

An imbalance of anti- and pro-hypertensive prostanoids has been proposed to characterize toxemia of pregnancy; namely, a relative deficit in PGI_2 coupled with a relative excess of PGH_2/TxA_2.[32,33] In normal pregnancy, blood pressure is not elevated despite increased cardiac output, salt and water retention, and activation of the RAS because increased activity of antipressor systems including

prostaglandins, represented by PGE_2 and PGI_2, counter the responses to vasopressor hormones.[34] Thus the attenuated vasoconstrictor responses to Ang II in pregnancy can be reversed by inhibition of prostaglandin synthesis.[35,36]

Although TxA_2 is increased in pregnancy, the ratio of vasodilator to vasoconstrictor prostanoids remains higher in normal pregnancies than in those complicated by hypertension. A deficiency of PGI_2 precedes the elevation of blood pressure in pregnancy, and measurements of PGI_2 and TxA_2 metabolites may provide a useful index for women at risk of developing preeclampsia.[37] Under these conditions, low-dose aspirin improves the PGI_2/TxA_2 ratio and might be expected to counter the development of preeclampsia.[38,39] Thus low-dose aspirin gradually and irreversibly inhibits COX-1 of platelets, which cannot generate new enzyme while sparing vascular PGI_2, as endothelial cells retain the capacity to generate new enzymes. Similarly, inhibitors of Tx synthase or TP receptors might prove useful for the prevention of preeclampsia.[40] However, the promise of these therapies has not been fully realized in a clinical setting; for example, Duley et al.,[41] after examining results from 51 trials, concluded that low-dose aspirin produced small to moderate benefits in a small percentage of pregnant women considered to be at risk for preeclampsia.

It should be pointed out that other eicosanoids, namely EETs, have been implicated in cardiovascular regulation during pregnancy. Renal epoxygenase activity and expression of the major epoxygenase isoforms are increased during gestation in the rat.[42] These findings are consistent with an earlier report of increased urinary excretion of the major metabolites of EETs, dihydroxyeicosatrienoic acids (DHTs) in pregnant women.[43] In the rat, inhibition of epoxygenase activity for 4 days in the last third of gestation (21 days) resulted in an increase in blood pressure, reminiscent of preeclampsia.[42] Thus a relative deficit in EET formation may contribute to reduced intrauterine blood flow and preeclampsia. However, in women with pregnancy-induced hypertension, the excretion of 11,12-DHT was further increased.[43] This finding may not translate into increased EETs acting to lower blood pressure as 11,12-DHT is inactive and a product of metabolism of 11,12-EET by soluble epoxide hydrolase (sEH). The question that remains is whether catabolism to DHTs occurs before EETs exert their vasoactivity.

CYCLOOXYGENASE-2 INHIBITORS: NEGATIVE CARDIOVASCULAR CONSEQUENCES?

Interestingly, studies with COX knockout mice indicate that COX-2–derived prostaglandins counter the pressor effect of Ang II.[23] The latter is increased in COX-2 knockout mice as well as by selective inhibition of COX-2. In contrast, COX-1–derived prostanoids contribute to the pressor effect as COX-1 deletion reduced the pressor response to Ang II. The COX-1–derived mediators of the response are most likely PGH_2/TxA_2, consistent with studies cited earlier that support a role for TP receptor activation by Ang II in renin-dependent hypertension.[23]

Recently, there have been major concerns about the cardiovascular risks of long-term treatment with selective COX-2 inhibitors, which were developed with the view that these agents would be useful in the treatment of chronic inflammatory diseases without the adverse gastrointestinal effects[16] associated with removal of cytoprotective COX-1–derived prostaglandins. Thus nonselective NSAIDs are potent anti-inflammatory agents that are associated with gastric ulceration. A seminal finding to this discussion is based on the report by Gimbrone et al.[44] that endothelial COX-2, induced by shear stress, is the primary source of vascular PGI_2. The second finding of great import to reviewing the potential toxicity of selective inhibition of COX-2 is the clinical report by McAdam et al.[45] who showed that inhibition of COX-2 greatly reduced the excretion of a major PGI_2 metabolite, 2,3-dinor 6-ketoPGF$_{1\alpha}$, which is considered to reflect systemic generation of PGI_2. Inhibition of vascular PGI_2 that acts as an endogenous antiplatelet agent provides an explanation for the five-fold increase in the risk of myocardial infarction in patients taking rofecoxib to selectively inhibit COX-2 versus those taking the nonselective NSAID, naproxen.[46] Vascular PGI_2 synthesis would be reduced by selective COX-2 inhibitors, whereas platelet TxA_2 synthesis of COX-1 origin would be spared, predisposing to thrombogenesis. This is in direct opposition to the beneficial effects of low-dose aspirin, which gradually and irreversibly inhibits COX-1 of platelets, which cannot generate new enzyme, while sparing vascular PGI_2.[47] Consequently, low-dose aspirin is antithrombotic and is recommended to prevent myocardial infarction.

Like NSAIDs, selective COX-2 inhibitors can aggravate existing hypertension or impair the action of antihypertensive agents in susceptible individuals.[48] There is a tendency for all NSAIDs to increase blood pressure (Figure 33–4), which reflects their effects on salt/water excretion (retention) and vascular reactivity (increased).[49] In healthy individuals, COX-2 inhibitors do not elevate blood pressure. In the presence of systemic circulatory disorders such as congestive heart failure, hepatorenal syndrome, diabetes with nephropathy, and age-related declines in renal function, COX inhibitors will have adverse cardiovascular and renal effects with worsening of the underlying diseases. These include precipitating the onset of renal failure and compromising cardiac function. A recently recognized and potentially critical interaction involving inhibitors of COX relates to the disposition (metabolism) of the vasoconstrictor eicosanoid, 20-HETE, which is produced by and acts on PGMVs.[50] When the RAS is activated, 20-HETE is transformed by COX-2 and PGE_2 isomerase to 20-OH PGE_2, a dilator of renal resistance vessels.[51] The failure of this conversion, particularly in the face of increased activity of the RAS, can have dire consequences for renal function that is fully analyzed in the next section.

ARACHIDONATE METABOLITES ARISING FROM CYTOCHROME P450

In the first study that linked CYP-AA metabolites to blood pressure regulation, Sacerdoti et al.[52] demonstrated increased CYP-AA metabolism during the rapid phase of blood pressure elevation in the SHR. Between 5 and 20 weeks of age, systolic blood pressure of the SHR increased from 112 to 202 mmHg, the major increases occurring between 5 and 13 weeks, coincident with increased production of renal CYP-AA products which exceeded production by age-matched Wistar-Kyoto (WKY) rats (Figure 33–5). Once blood pressure levels were established in rats aged 13 weeks, total CYP-AA metabolism did not differ between SHR and WKY rats. However, as individual AA products were not measured and their sites of origin (nephron vs. renal vasculature) were not identified, aberrant CYP-AA metabolism by the adult SHR might have been overlooked. This distinction relative to individual eicosanoids and their sites of synthesis is critical to assigning decisive roles to single CYP-AA products in the pathogenesis of hypertension.[53] For example, deficient synthesis of 20-HETE by the TAL segment of the nephron has been proposed as the offending lesion responsible for blood pressure elevation

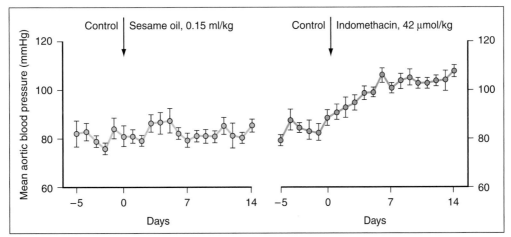

Figure 33–4. Mean arterial blood pressure in seven rabbits that received daily subcutaneous injections of indomethacin and in six that received only vehicle. (Redrawn from Colina-Chourio JA, McGiff JC, Nasjletti A. *Clin Sci* 1979;57:359–65.)

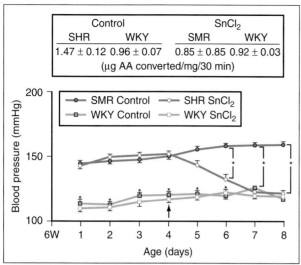

Figure 33–5. In response to SnCl$_2$ treatment beginning at 6 weeks, 4 days of age (at the *arrow*), BP showed a slow decline to normotensive levels by the 7th week coincident with a decline in CYP-dependent AA metabolism. In contrast, the BP and CYP-dependent AA metabolism in WKY rats were unaffected by SnCl$_2$ treatment. AA, arachidonic acid; BP, blood pressure; CYP, cytochrome P450; SHR, spontaneously hypertensive rats; WKY, Wistar-Kyoto rats.

in the salt-sensitive (SS) Dahl rat.[54] This singular finding would have escaped notice when using microsomal preparations derived from the renal cortex and medulla to assess aberrations in renal CYP-AA product synthesis.

The study by Sacerdoti et al.[52] anticipated future directions in this area of research—it identified two principal CYP-AA products, 11,12-EET and 20-HETE, that figure prominently in ongoing studies (Figure 33–6). For example, increased production of 20-HETE, which raises the tone of the afferent arteriole of the SHR,[55] has been shown to contribute to the rightward shift in the pressure–natriuresis curve, the hallmark of hypertension.[56] This effect of 20-HETE can be countered by the vasodilator action of 11,12-EET and served as a centerpiece to future studies of vascular mechanisms involving CYP-derived AA products having opposing effects on vascular tone and reactivity. Autoregulation of RBF has been examined by Imig et al.[57] with respect to the 20-HETE versus EETs paradigm; they demonstrated that the dynamic interactions of an EET and 20-HETE determine the autoregulatory response of RBF to changes in perfusion pressure.[57] We are now able to define the separate and opposing contributions of vasoactive epoxides (11,12- and 5,6-EETs) and 20-HETE to vascular mechanisms operating at the level of the intact renal vasculature as well as at the level of critical renal vascular segments, PGMVs. We owe these capabilities to J.R. Falck,[53,58] who has synthesized authentic standards of CYP-AA metabolites and selective inhibitors of each arm of CYP-dependent AA metabolism, the ω/ω-1-hydroxylases and epoxygenases. The critical role of 20-HETE in autoregulation of RBF was established by inhibiting ω-hydroxylases with either 17-ODYA or DDMS.[57,59] In response to inhibition of ω-hydroxylases, increased renal perfusion pressure was not countered by

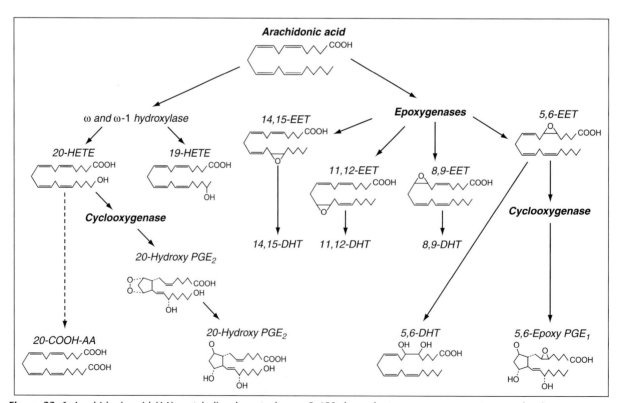

Figure 33–6. Arachidonic acid (AA) metabolism by cytochrome P-450-dependent monooxygenases to ω- and ω-1-hydroxyeicosatetraenoic acids (HETEs), epoxyeicosatrienoic acids (epoxides, EETS), and dihydroxyeicosatrienoic acids (diols, DHTs). 20-HETE and 5,6-EET can be converted by cyclooxygenase to analogues of prostaglandins. (Redrawn from McGiff JC, Quilley J. *Am J Physiol Regal Integr Comp Physiol* 1999;277:R607–23. Used with permission.)

increased RVR. Instead, a linear relationship obtained between RBF and perfusion pressure after inhibiting 20-HETE synthesis. In contrast, the autoregulatory response was exaggerated on eliminating the countering effect of 11,12-EET by inhibiting epoxygenases with MS PPOH.

Induction of heme oxygenase lowers blood pressure in spontaneously hypertensive rats

In the young (age 6–7 weeks) SHR, $SnCl_2$, an inducer of heme oxygenase-1 (HO-1), was used to deplete CYP enzymes and, thereby, reduce production of CYP-derived AA metabolites.[60] Induction of HO-1 depleted CYP enzymes, as HO-1 is the rate-controlling enzyme in heme catabolism that affects the availability of heme for hemoproteins such as CYP.[61] Catabolizing the heme moiety (catalytic center) of CYP enzymes, in response to $SnCl_2$ induction of HO-1, produces biliverdin and its product, bilirubin, as well as ferrous iron and carbon monoxide (CO). Elevated blood pressure of the SHR returned to normal levels in response to $SnCl_2$, coincident with natriuresis indicating restoration of the normotensive pressure-natriuresis curve[60] (Figure 33–7). Increased renal levels of CYP-AA metabolites in the SHR were reduced by $SnCl_2$ to levels found in the WKY rats, coincident with reduction of blood pressure to normotensive values. $SnCl_2$ treatment affected neither blood pressure nor renal CYP-AA metabolite levels in normotensive WKY rats (age 6–7 weeks) (Figure 33–5).

A study of consequence to the proposed prohypertensive action of CYP-derived AA metabolites was designed to determine whether either age or duration of treatment was critical to normalizing blood pressure in the male SHR[62] (Figure 33–8). The answer is "yes" on both counts. First, chronic treatment with $SnCl_2$, begun at age 5 weeks, prevented hypertension in the SHR. The age of initiation of $SnCl_2$ treatment is critical. In contrast to the 5-week-old SHR, blood pressure of the adult SHR (age 12–20 weeks) did not fall in response to $SnCl_2$. Second, suspension of $SnCl_2$ treatment at age 13 weeks in the SHR treated from 6 weeks of age did not result in the return of hypertension; that is, reduction of blood pressure was sustained through the duration of the study (ended at age 20 weeks). At the time of these studies, a selective inhibitor of ω-hydroxylase activity was not available for long-term use.

The products of heme catabolism can lower blood pressure. HO-1–derived vascular CO evoked by $SnCl_2$ treatment acts as an inhibitory modulator of the enhanced vascular reactivity produced by constrictors "via a mechanism that involves a TEA-sensitive K^+ channel."[63] Additionally, biliverdin as well as its product, bilirubin, are antioxidants, reducing oxidative injury to blood vessels, particularly the endothelium. These effects of the products of heme catabolism, which contribute to blood pressure reduction,[64] urge cautious interpretation when implicating diminished CYP-AA metabolite formation as the principal factor in the blood pressure–lowering response to induction of renal HO-1.

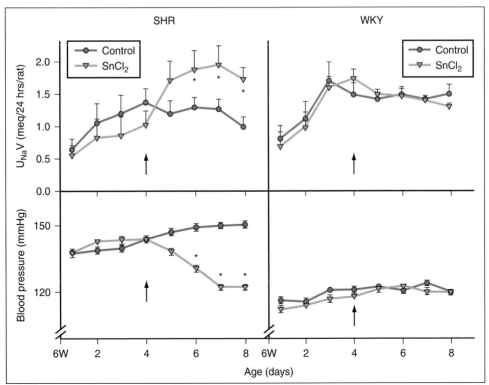

Figure 33–7. A decline in BP produced by $SnCl_2$ in the SHR (*left*) was associated with increased Na^+ excretion. $SnCl_2$, given between the 6th and 7th weeks on a daily basis (*arrow*), was without effect on BP and Na^+ excretion in WKY rats (*right*). *$p<0.05$ compared to control. BP, blood pressure; SHR, spontaneously hypertensive rats; WKY, Wistar-Kyoto rats.

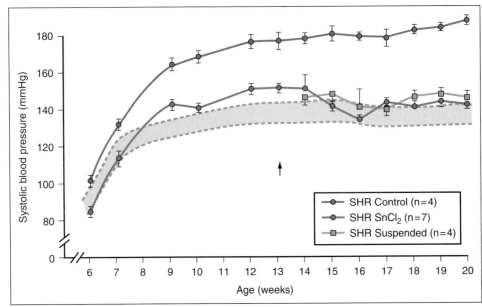

Figure 33–8. Line graph showing effect of chronic treatment of SHR with $SnCl_2$ (from age 5 to 20 weeks) on systolic BP (mean+SEM) compared with either untreated control SHR or SHR with $SnCl_2$ treatment suspended from age 13 to 20 weeks. Striped area represents the mean+1 SD of the systolic BP of control untreated and $SnCl_2$-treated WKY rats. BP, blood pressure; SD, standard deviation; SEM, standard error of the mean; SHR, spontaneously hypertensive rats; WKY, Wistar-Kyoto rats. (Redrawn from Escalante B, Sacerdoti D, Davidian MM, et al. *Hypertension* 1991;17:776–9.)

Cytochrome P450-Arachidonic acid metabolites: Pressor versus antipressor effects

Notwithstanding these concerns regarding collateral effects produced by the induction of HO-1, the proposed important role of 20-HETE in the development of hypertension in the SHR is supported by recent studies.

20-Hydroxyeicosatetraenoic Acid: Prohypertensive

1. Selective inhibition of ω-hydroxylase with 1-aminobenzo-triazole lowered blood pressure in the young SHR.[65,66]
2. Administration of CYP-4A antisense oligonucleotides to young SHRs decreased renal synthesis of 20-HETE accompanied by reduction of blood pressure.[67]
3. Inhibition of NO synthesis produced 20-HETE-dependent hypertension in rats by eliminating the tonic inhibitory effect that NO exerts on ω-hydroxylase activity.[68] L-NAME, an inhibitor of NO formation, produced precipitous elevations of blood pressure, rapid declines in RBF and GFR, and brisk diuresis that could be reversed by inhibition of 20-HETE synthesis.

Epoxyeicosatrienoic Acids: Antihypertensive

EETs participate in antipressor mechanisms counteracting vascular pressor mechanisms mediated by 20-HETE. EETs also inhibit Na^+ reabsorption at several sites in the nephron.[69,70]

1. Antagonism of the vasoconstrictor response to 20-HETE by EETs.[57]
2. Modulation by 5,6-EET of renal vascular reactivity,[71] and Na^+ reabsorption produced by Ang II in the proximal tubules.[70]

3. Inhibition by 5,6-EET of Na^+ transport in the rabbit cortical collecting ducts (CCD) via prostaglandin stimulation.[72] 11,12-EET is the endogenous inhibitor of the epithelial Na^+ channel (ENaC) in the rat CCD.[69]
4. 5,6- and 11,12-EETs are candidate endothelium-derived hyperpolarizing factors. They mediate NO and prostaglandin-independent vasodilator responses to Ach and bradykinin.[73–75]
5. EETs prevent elevation of blood pressure in response to high salt intake,[76] which has been related to stimulation of the adenosine A_{2A} receptor ($A_{2A}R$) in PGMVs of the rat.[77]
6. The antihypertensive potential of EETs is also displayed in the blood pressure lowering response to increasing tissue levels of EETs produced by inhibiting the principal enzyme, sEH, responsible for catabolism of EETs to DHTs.[78,79]

The cumulative import of these studies on 20-HETE *vis-a-vis* EETs supports both a prohypertensive and antihypertensive role for CYP-AA products. Further, the studies on 20-HETE indicate participation in both pressor and antipressor mechanisms, whereas EETs are likely exclusively antipressors.

20-Hydroxyeicosatetraenoic acid serves pressor and antipressor mechanisms

The assignment of a causative role to 20-HETE in the development of hypertension raises an apparent paradox, because both deficient[54] and excessive production of 20-HETE[60] by renal ω-hydroxylases have been linked to elevation of blood pressure. An attempt to explain these paradoxes requires some understanding of:

1. The diversity of ω-hydroxylase isoforms
2. Differences among ω-hydroxylases regarding localization in renal vasculature and nephron
3. Their individual regulation at the local and regional levels

There are four rat isoforms of ω- and ω-1-hydroxylases designated 4A1, 2, 3, and 4A8; these are distributed unevenly in the renal vasculature and nephron,[80,81] and are differentially regulated by circulating and local factors. Peroxisome proliferator-activated receptor-α (PPARα) has been assigned a pivotal role in the transcriptional regulation of CYP4A1 and 4A2/4A3 ω/ω-1-hydroxylase isoforms,[82] whereas expression of the CYP4A8 and 4A2 isoforms are regulated by androgens via a circuitous pathway.[83–85] The high sequence homology of CYP 4A2/4A3, 97% nucleotides and 96% amino acids,[86] makes differentiation of their individual effects and responses to regulators difficult to assess. This difficulty is indicated by 4A2/4A3 as opposed to these isoforms standing alone: 4A2 and 4A3. The CYP4A isoforms are variably affected by sex, age, hormones, and dietary influences.[87] The catalytic activities of the ω-hydroxylase isoforms vary by as much as 40-fold, with the 4A1 isoform having the highest catalytic efficiency.[88]

Androgen-sensitive cytochrome P4A isoforms

Either androgen receptor blockade or early castration acts as a brake on the development of hypertension in the male SHR.[89] An androgen-sensitive CYP4A isoform that causes hypertension has been identified.[84] Increased activity of the rat CYP4A8 ω-hydroxylase has been linked to an androgen effect. This linkage is based on a study in the mouse. Deletion of the mouse CYP4A14 isoform, the homologue of rat CYP4A2/4A3 ω-hydroxylases, enhanced expression and activity of the mouse CYP4A12 ω-hydroxylase, the homologue of the rat CYP4A8 ω-hydroxylase, via an androgen-dependent effect that produced increased 20-HETE generation. The study in mice has uncovered a "hitherto unrecognized regulatory loop" involving deletion of CYP4A14, a fatty acid hydroxylase, which elevates androgen levels that act on the CYP4A12 ω-hydroxylase isoforms, resulting in increased 20-HETE synthesis. Thus disruption of the CYP4A14 gene produced mice with hypertension that is androgen sensitive, mediated by 20-HETE, prevented by castration, and restored by androgen replacement. In a companion study in rats, the connection between androgen stimulation of the CYP 4A8 isoform and production of hypertension was established.[85] Treatment of normotensive rats with 5α-dihydro-testosterone produced hypertension, upregulation of the CYP4A8 gene and a four-fold increase in 20-HETE synthesis by renal microvessels.[85] Of note, AA epoxygenase activity was reduced "to a minimum." These findings provide a conceptual basis for evaluating and understanding gender-specific differences in blood pressure.

The above findings prompted examination of the CYP4A human homologue (CYP4A11) of the androgen-sensitive 4a12 (–/–) ω-hydroxylase isoform as a potential genetic determinant of hypertension in humans.[90] A functional variant of CYP4A11, which encodes a renal 20-HETE synthase, was identified that exhibited a thymidine-to-cytosine polymorphism at nucleotide 8590. This coding variant of the human CYP4A11 gene produced a CYP4A11 protein with diminished 20-HETE synthase activity that was more prevalent in hypertensive than normotensive white subjects. These findings suggest localization of the deficiency in 20-HETE production in these hypertensive subjects to one or more tubular segments because of the modulator action of 20-HETE on Na+ transport in key tubular segments and the pressor consequences of deletion of 20-HETE effects on tubular transport mechanisms. A comparable lesion, deficient 20-HETE synthesis in the TAL, has been described in the Dahl salt-sensitive hypertensive rat.[54]

Either deficiency or excess of 20-hydroxyeicosatetraenoic acid produces hypertension

Either increased or decreased synthesis of 20-HETE can result in an identical abnormality[75]—a rightward shift of the pressure-natriuresis curve that characterizes the hypertensive state.[56] Examples based on available evidence include increased 20-HETE synthesis in the SHR,[60,65] and second, decreased 20-HETE synthesis in the Dahl SS hypertensive rat.[54] Each has been described to produce hypertension. How does either increased or decreased production of an individual eicosanoid eventuate in hypertension? The answer, based on our present and incomplete understanding of this field of research (which needs maturation) may lie in the renal site involved—vascular[91] versus tubular[92]—and in the complex biological profile of 20-HETE, that is, constriction of renal microvessels (pressor effect) versus inhibition of renal tubular NaCl reabsorption (antipressor effect). Further, 20-HETE can be transformed by a COX-2–dependent step in PGMVs to a vasodilator analogue of PGE$_2$ when the RAS is activated by low salt.[51]

In the SHR, increased synthesis of 20-HETE by PGMVs constricts renal microvessels, having the greatest impact on the afferent arteriole.[55] 20-HETE acts as a second messenger to Ang II and endothelin ET-1 in both the vasculature and nephron.[53] A current interpretation of the consequences of increasing the resistance of PGMVs, particularly those of the juxtamedullary zone, is to decrease medullary blood flow and medullary interstitial pressure,[93] which—based on the interplay of Starling forces—facilitates the movement of tubular fluid into the interstitium and the vascular compartment, producing increased salt and water reabsorption with expansion of extracellular fluid volume and elevation of blood pressure.[53]

On the other hand, decreased production of 20-HETE by a critical tubular segment, the medullary TAL (mTAL), as proposed in the Dahl SS hypertensive rat,[54] will elevate blood pressure. Because 20-HETE reduces NaCl reabsorption in this segment by inhibiting the Na+-K+-2Cl− cotransporter[94] through its role as modulator, a deficiency of 20-HETE will promote Na+ reabsorption. In addition, decreased production of EETs by the Dahl SS rat will reinforce the elevation of blood pressure produced by mTAL 20-HETE deficiency.[76]

Epoxyeicosatrienoic acids–dependent renal vasodilatation: Activated by raising renal perfusion pressure

Additional evidence for an antihypertensive role for EETs has been uncovered in kidneys of normotensive rats: a dormant CYP-dependent vasodilator mechanism is activated by elevating perfusion pressure.[95] In addition, inhibition of prostaglandin synthesis eliminates a concurrent prostanoid vasoconstrictor response, allowing the epoxide-dependent vasodilator effect to be readily discerned.[96] When these conditions are met, AA dilates the renal vasculature. In their absence, AA constricts the renal vasculature on conversion to PGH_2 which activates the TP receptor. 5,6-EET is the putative EET mediator of the vasodilator effect of AA in the SHR,[71] as 5,6-EET possesses a four-fold greater renal vasodilator potency than 11,12-EET in the SHR. Based on these findings, we tested the hypothesis that the dormant EET-dependent renal vasodilator mechanism is attenuated/suppressed in the SHR.[96] Unexpectedly, the renal vasodilator response to AA was potentiated in the SHR. Moreover, in Ang II–induced hypertension (10-day infusion), the vasodilator response to AA was abolished,[96] a finding in keeping with the downregulation of renal CYP 2C23 epoxygenase mRNA and enzyme levels in rats given Ang II and a high-salt diet for several weeks.[97]

PREGLOMERULAR MICROCIRCULATION AND LIPID MEDIATORS

20-Hydroxyeicosatetraenoic acid: Basic mechanisms and activation by AT_2 receptors

The PGMVs—the arcuate and interlobular arteries and the afferent arterioles—occupy a key position in the regulation of the renal circulation.[98] Multiple signals feed into PGMVs from various sites including autonomic nerves, blood, renal tubules (macula densa) as well as those of autocrine and paracrine origin. These signals have the capacity to evoke lipid mediators, products of AA metabolism via COX, lipoxygenases (LOX), and CYP pathways. 20-HETE is an essential component of renal autoregulation[59] and tubuloglomerular feedback (TGF)[99] by virtue of its vasoconstrictor properties[53]; namely, 20-HETE serves as the final effector that constricts PGMVs. Production of 20-HETE by ω-hydroxylase increases as renal arterial diameter decreases.[100] The vascular segments, PGMVs, that contribute to the greatest degree in regulating RVR and GFR, particularly the afferent arterioles, are heavily invested with 20-HETE synthetic ability.[93]

20-HETE is released from PGMVs by Ang II via activation of AT_2 receptors[91] (Figure 33–9), an unexpected conjunction as AT_1, not AT_2, receptor stimulation is usually associated with activation of pressor mechanisms. However, the rat renomedullary circulation has been reported to react oppositely to the renal cortical circulation in

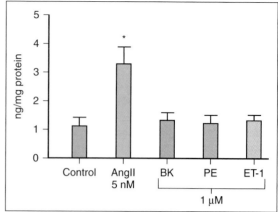

Figure 33–9. Release of 20-HETE following 5-minute incubation with vasoactive hormones. Incubates were extracted, HETEs purified, derivatized, and quantitated using GC-MS (mean±standard error of measurement). Ang II, angiotensin II; BK, bradykinin; ET-1, endothelin; PE, phenylephrine. *$p<0.05$. (Redrawn from Croft KD, McGiff JC, Sanchez-Mendoza A, Carroll MA. *Am J Physiol Renal Physiol* 2000;279:F544–51. Used with permission.)

response to stimulation of AT receptors[101]; namely, AT_1 receptor activation dilates medullary blood vessels which are antagonized by AT_2 receptor-mediated constriction. We interpret the AT_2 constrictor effect on medullary blood vessels to result from 20-HETE release from two possible sources that have been identified as synthesizing 20-HETE as a principal product: (1) the PGMVs of the juxtamedullary circulation,[102] which should facilitate entry of 20-HETE into the postglomerular circulation and the long loops of the *vasa rectae*; and (2) proximal tubules[103] and/or mTAL tubules[94] with release of 20-HETE into the medullary interstitium.

Pressure natriuresis and 20-hydroxyeicosatetraenoic acid

A related issue regarding the central role of 20-HETE in regulating renal hemodynamic and excretory function is the contribution of 20-HETE to pressure natriuresis. Pressure natriuresis, that is, increased Na^+ excretion in response to increased renal perfusion pressure, was identified by Guyton[56] as the central mechanism in the long-term regulation of extracellular fluid volume and blood pressure. Gross et al.[104] have demonstrated elevation of blood pressure with loss of pressure natriuresis in mice lacking the AT_2 receptor. This may be explained by the inability of PGMVs to generate 20-HETE consequent to deletion of AT_2 receptors,[91] thereby eliminating the candidate lipid mediator of pressure natriuresis. Further, 20-HETE, on release from PGMVs into the blood entering the glomerulus, may be filtered to act on the luminal surfaces of proximal tubules and TAL, the nephron segments mainly responsible for pressure natriuresis. This assumes that 20-HETE is not protein-bound in the vascular compartment, which has been subject to debate. Additionally, 20-HETE entering the postglomerular circulation on release from PGMVs[91] may act on the contraluminal surfaces of the nephron via diffusion into the interstitium.

20-HETE is also a principal product of AA metabolism in key tubular segments, the proximal tubules[103] and TAL,[105] at which sites locally generated 20-HETE can inhibit Na[+] transport. Proximal tubular 20-HETE satisfies major criteria for mediating pressure natriuresis as it inhibits Na[+]-K[+]-ATPase (the Na[+] pump) through activation of PKC[106] and produces internalization of the brush border Na[+]-H[+] exchanger (NHE$_3$).[107] A hormone-inducible inhibitor of the Na[+] pump was regarded as a feature of hypertension that accounts for the exaggerated natriuresis produced by volume expansion in clinical and experimental hypertension.[108]

In view of the multiple sources and sites of action of 20-HETE in the kidney, the coordinated response of three critical components—PGMVs, proximal tubules, and the TAL—each generating 20-HETE, can account for the cortical and juxtamedullary vascular and tubular components of pressure natriuresis. The renal medullary circulatory response to pressure natriuresis, increased medullary blood flow, also involves a prostaglandin-dependent mechanism.[109] Redistribution of RBF from the cortex to the medulla had been shown more than three decades ago to be effected by a PGE$_2$-dependent mechanism.[110,111]

20-Hydroxyeicosatetraenoic acid disposition

Tissue levels and biological activity of 20-HETE are greatly affected by incorporation into tissue phospholipids,[112] and by metabolism via COX to prostaglandin analogues that possess different biological properties from those of untransformed 20-HETE.[113] In addition, there are notable differences amongst species regarding disposition and metabolism of 20-HETE.[53] For example, in man, 20-HETE is excreted mainly as a glucuronide conjugate, there being negligible free urinary 20-HETE.[114,115] The principal route of efflux of renal 20-HETE in the rat isolated kidney is via the renal vein with little appearing in the urine (McGiff, personal observation). However, deterioration of renal function may promote 20-HETE excretion.[116] There is no universal agreement, however, on the paucity of urinary 20-HETE excretion in the rat, which probably reflects differences in the assay methods used to measure 20-HETE relative to their precision and sensitivity.

An eicosanoid conundrum: Excessive renal vascular 20-hydroxyeicosatetraenoic acid production without hypertension

The renal pathology in hepatic cirrhosis during the progression to hepatorenal syndrome is conspicuously innocuous, that is, "renal function progressively deteriorates without evidence of organic nephropathy."[117] Activation of the principal antidiuretic/antinatriuretic neurohumoral systems, the renin-angiotensin-adrenergic-aldosterone-ADH axis is a feature in patients with cirrhosis and ascites.[118] In patients with cirrhosis, urinary excretion of 20-HETE was selectively increased when compared to 16-, 17-, and 18-HETEs. Urinary excretion of 20-HETE exceeded by several-fold excretion of TxA$_2$, the principal prostanoid product in cirrhosis.

Of the eicosanoids, only excretion of 20-HETE correlated ($p<0.01$) with reductions in renal plasma flow in subjects with cirrhosis. These findings are compatible with assigning a significant role to 20-HETE in the progressive deterioration of renal function in patients with hepatic cirrhosis. However, they are in apparent conflict with those in experimental animals; namely, an established close relationship of 20-HETE production by PGMVs with the development of hypertension.[53] There are no easy answers to this conundrum. A selective stimulatory effect on a CYP4A isoform predominating in PGMVs such as 4A2, producing increased 20-HETE synthesis and restricted to renal microvessels, may explain the progressive renal functional abnormalities in hepatic cirrhosis. When inhibitors of ω-hydroxylase that pass Food and Drug Administration scrutiny for use in human studies become available, it will then be possible to test the following hypothesis: *Inhibition of renal ω-hydroxylase activity will reverse the renal hemodynamic abnormalities as well as the secondary salt and water retention that characterize hepatic cirrhosis with ascites.*

Angiotensin II interacts with products of all pathways of arachidonic acid metabolism

Arachidonate-derived products contribute to the regulation of tone and reactivity of the renal vasculature in general and PGMVs specifically,[102] and through these vascular effects contribute to maintaining normal renal function. AA metabolites interact, most strikingly, with Ang II and ET-1, serving as modulators and mediators of the actions of the peptides.[119] All species of eicosanoids, whether arising from COX, LOX, or CYP pathways, have been shown to interact with Ang II in the vasculature, acting either as second messengers (mediators) or modulators of the vascular effects of Ang II. Similar interactions involving Ang II and eicosanoids are evident in the nephron.[120] Species differences, as noted, in the renal circulatory responses to 20-HETE of the rat and rabbit can be striking.[113,119] Also, within a regional vasculature, large arteries versus small arteries/arterioles show major differences in the distribution of peptide receptors as well as in the localization of oxygenases.[53,121] Ang II–LOX product interactions have been demonstrated in responses of the vasculature of the intact kidney of the rat.[122] However, in the rat renal preglomerular microcirculation, as noted, 20-HETE predominated in response to stimulation of AT$_2$ receptors by Ang II.[91]

On reexamining the most important renal microvessels, the afferent arterioles, the operation of a LOX product was also uncovered; 12(S)-HETE was shown to act as a second messenger, contributing to the constrictor response to Ang II.[123] Expression of 12-LOX may be set in motion by tissue injury.[124] Whether this also obtains for renal microvessels has yet to be established. Renal microvascular 12(S)-HETE synthesis in the rat was increased by Ang II as was [Ca^{2+}]$_i$, the latter by four-fold. Blockade of L-type calcium channels abolished afferent arteriolar constrictor effects of Ang II. There is also definitive evidence noted above for recognizing the contribution of

20-HETE to the constrictor response of the afferent arteriole to Ang II.[55] How 20-HETE interacts, if it does, with 12-LOX or its product, 12-HETE, in the afferent arteriole is uncertain. A potential interaction described in platelets is based on 12-LOX metabolism of 20-HETE forming 12, 20-HETE,[125] a transformation that will most likely modify the vascular action of 20-HETE. Eicosanoid product formation in the vasculature differs substantially according to blood vessel size, the vascular bed under study and the presence of cardiovascular diseases. Species differences in eicosanoid synthesis are more likely to be quantitative rather than qualitative as observed in a classic study of nephron prostaglandin production by Bonvalet et al.[126] The rabbit nephron greatly exceeded that of the rat in prostaglandin production. However, the ratio of products formed was similar in both species: PGE_2 predominated; PGI_2 was much less than PGE_2 (1/20) and TxA_2 was vanishingly low when compared to PGE_2 synthesis (<1/100).

Cyclooxygenase-2 and transformation of 20-hydroxyeicosatetraenoic acid to 20-OH PGE$_2$

In the rabbit kidney, 20-HETE produces vasodilatation, an effect abolished by inhibition of COX which prevents conversion of 20-HETE to vasodilator prostaglandin analogues.[113] The putative mediator of this renal vasodilator response to 20-HETE is its COX metabolite, 20-OH PGE_2, which unlike untransformed 20-HETE, dilates renal blood vessels[51] (Figure 33–6).

Under conditions of low salt, mitigating factors can influence the outcome of the response of PGMVs to 20-HETE production via metabolism by COX-2 and membranal PGE_2 isomerase which are coexpressed in response to low salt.[127] Regional variations in the regulation of COX-2 expression in the kidney have been linked to salt intake[128]; low salt, as noted, induces COX-2 in the cortex, which impacts on control of the renal cortical circulation, whereas high salt activates COX-2 in the medulla, which is a key component via production of PGE_2 in salt and water excretory mechanisms. As Ang II releases 20-HETE in relative abundance from PGMV,[91] and as renal cortical COX-2 is expressed in response to low salt,[128] a study was designed in an attempt to forge a link between 20-HETE and COX-2 in terms of possible modification of the vascular effects of increased 20-HETE production by PGMVs.[127] Microdissected arteries of 6- to 7-week-old rats were used because 20-HETE formation has been described to peak at this age.[52] Interlobar arteries were separated from arcuate and interlobular arteries to discern segmental variations in production of CYP-derived AA metabolites. Because of the potential importance of COX-dependent transformation of 20-HETE,[129] vascular segmental changes in COX-1 and COX-2 expression were determined as well as those of ω/ω-1-hydroxylase CYP4A enzymes in interlobar arteries vis-a-vis arcuate and interlobular arteries. Low salt intake stimulated the RAS and activated renal cortical COX-2 expression. Low salt also increased 20-HETE production by PGMVs, a response greater in arcuate and interlobular than in interlobar

arteries[127] (Figure 33–10). However, inhibition of COX was required to demonstrate increased 20-HETE formation because of the avid metabolism of 20-HETE by COX-2.

The effects of low salt promoted conversion of 20-HETE via COX-2 to metabolites that have lost their ability to depress GFR.[51] This COX-dependent mechanism presumably serves a defensive function as its inhibition by NSAIDs may contribute to the adverse effects of aspirin-like drugs—increased RVR and reduced GFR with Na^+ retention—that result from the direct vasoconstrictor action of 20-HETE.[93] That is, during salt depletion as occasioned by diuretic therapy and when 20-HETE of renal vascular origin cannot be transformed to prostaglandin analogues because of concurrent treatment with a NSAID, the action of unconverted 20-HETE constricts PGMVs. In contrast, 20-HETE is converted by COX-2 and membranal PGE_2 isomerase to 20-OH PGE_2 when NSAIDs are withheld (Figure 33–6). Metabolism of 20-HETE by COX-

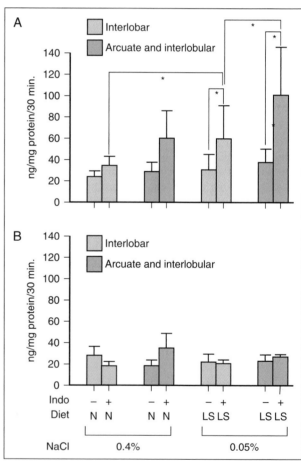

Figure 33–10. Release of 20-HETE (**A**) and epoxyeicosatrienoic acids (**B**) from arcuate and interlobular arteries and from interlobar arteries obtained from rats fed either a normal-salt (N) diet (0.4% NaCl, n=8) or low-salt (LS) diet (0.05% NaCl, n=8) for 10 days in the absence or presence of indomethacin (Indo, 10 μm) (mean±standard error of measurement). Arteries were incubated with 1 mM NADPH and 7 μM [14C] arachidonic acid for 30 minutes at 37°C. Samples were extracted and the supernates were separated by reverse-phase HPLC. *p<0.05. (Redrawn from Cheng MK, McGiff JC, Carroll MA. *Am J Physiol Renal Physiol* 2003;284:F474–9. Used with permission.)

2, we submit, represents an important regulatory mechanism in the PGMVs that governs tone and reactivity of these blood vessels and prevents precipitous falls in GFR in response to decreased salt intake.

Hydroxyeicosatetraenoic acid and salt-sensitive versus salt-resistant hypertensive humans

The principal tubular sites of 20-HETE production and activity, the proximal tubules and TAL, suggest a significant role for 20-HETE in the regulation of Na^+ excretion in humans. In particular, this area of research raises questions regarding whether abnormalities in 20-HETE–dependent mechanisms are discernible in hypertensive subjects. Laffer et al.[130] have addressed the relationship of urinary 20-HETE excretion (µg/h) to excretion of Na^+ ($U_{Na}V$ in mmol/h) in human essential hypertension under conditions of salt loading. Two groups of hypertensive subjects could be identified—salt-sensitive and salt-resistant—that were differentiated according to their ability to activate renal 20-HETE production, as reflected in urinary excretion of 20-HETE, when challenged with salt loading.[130] In salt-resistant hypertensive subjects, the relationship between excretion of 20-HETE and Na^+ in response to salt loading demonstrated a strong positive correlation. This relationship was absent in salt-sensitive hypertensive subjects. Instead, they demonstrated a relationship of Na^+ excretion to both blood pressure and degree of obesity. A subsequent study based on the exploration of the negative correlation between obesity as reflected in body mass index (BMI) and urinary 20-HETE excretion, disclosed a negative correlation between circulating insulin and 20-HETE excretion in obese hypertensive subjects, that is, "the higher the levels of serum insulin, the lower the levels of urine 20-HETE."[131] This association is also supported from a study in rats with streptozocin-induced diabetes. Insulin inhibited the activity of CYP4A isoforms isolated from both liver and kidney.[132]

PURINOCEPTORS

Recent studies have set the stage for viewing the preglomerular microcirculation, particularly the afferent arteriole, as sites in which 20-HETE and one or more EETs (likely 11,12-EET) act antagonistically in regulating arterial–arteriolar diameters in response to changes in renal perfusion pressure and salt intake.[57] These studies endorse an important concept; namely, that a counterpoised vascular mechanism in which products of CYP by each of its principal arms, epoxygenases and ω/ω-1-hydroxylases, operate in segments of the preglomerular vasculature. The resultant of the opposing effects of 20-HETE and 11,12-EET on tone and reactivity of PGMV, as noted, determines autoregulation of RBF. They are also involved in TGF[99] as their interactions determine the tone and reactivity of PGMV and, thereby, glomerular hemodynamics in response to the salt load presented to the macula densa. 20-HETE and 11,12-EET target the same effector mechanism, a K^+ channel.[133] That is, the outcome of EET–20-HETE interactions in determining renal vascular tone and reactivity is defined primarily by the resultant of their opposing effects on the open-state probability of the Ca^{2+}-activated K^+ channel of vascular smooth muscle.[74,134]

The most recent additions to CYP-derived eicosanoid mechanisms operating in the PGMVs are the purinergic portals: ATP-activated P_{2X} receptors[135] and adenosine-activated A_{2A} receptors ($A_{2A}R$),[50] producing 20-HETE and 11,12-EET, respectively. Inscho et al.[136] have identified and characterized the operation of the ATP-P_{2X} receptor—ω-hydroxylase–20-HETE vasoconstrictor limb; subsequently, Cheng et al.[50] identified an $A_{2A}R$–epoxygenase–11,12-EET vasodilator limb. A critical coupling between $A_{2A}R$ stimulation and CYP-related epoxygenase activity was uncovered; 11,12-EET is the likely candidate mediator of PGMV dilatation on adenosine activation of the $A_{2A}R$. Adenosine levels are increased by salt loading,[77,137,] as is the activity of renal epoxygenases that counteracts elevations in blood pressure produced by salt. Adenosine was identified as "the stimulus for increased renal epoxygenase activity in response to salt loading."[50,138] Blockade of the $A_{2A}R$ prevented stimulation of EET synthesis elicited by adenosine in rats on a high-salt diet, an effect that greatly increased RVR.[77]

TUBULAR TRANSPORT MECHANISMS: CYTOCHROME P450 PRODUCTS, TNF, AND CYCLOOXYGENASE-2

Medullary thick ascending limb

The TAL segment of the nephron occupies a pre-eminent position in the regulation of volume and composition of body fluids by virtue of its reabsorptive capacity, some 25% to 40% of filtered Na^+, and establishing the medullary osmolal gradient that determines the ability to excrete a concentrated urine.[139] The prevailing oxygenase in the mTAL that metabolizes AA under basal conditions as defined by studies in rats and rabbits is the CYP pathway, the principal product being 20-HETE, with lesser amounts of 19-HETE and a third product, 20-COOH AA, that resembles 20-HETE in its ability to inhibit Na^+-K^+-ATPase.[105] 19-HETE was not examined in terms of its impact on transport function. However, 19-HETE has been shown to counteract the inhibitory action of 20-HETE on transport in proximal tubules,[140] and to attenuate the ability of 20-HETE to elevate tone and reactivity of renal arteries.[141] As there has been no attempt thus far to assign a function to either 19-HETE or 20-COOH AA in the mTAL, experience dictates that future studies will require revising the paradigm at hand which is restricted to the effects of 20-HETE, namely (1) inhibition of the luminal cotransporter (Na^+-K^+-2Cl^-),[94] and (2) reducing the open state probability of the ROMK channel[142] (Figure 33–11), properties that summate to produce natriuresis and chloruresis. To date, the most compelling finding regarding blood pressure control that involved CYP-AA products in the mTAL, as noted, was deficient 20-HETE synthesis that produced hypertension in the Dahl SS rat by increasing the activity of the Na^+-K^+-2Cl^- cotransporter. When cor-

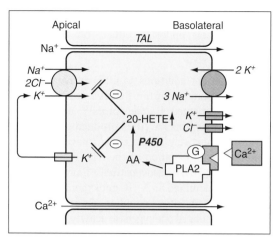

Figure 33–11. Modulation of Na$^+$-K$^+$-2Cl$^-$ cotransporter and K$^+$ channel activity by 20-HETE in the TAL. Changes in either extracellular calcium or Ang II can stimulate release of AA via receptor-coupled G-protein activation of phospholipase (PL) A$_2$. 20-HETE, 20-hydroxyeicosatetraenoic acid; AA, arachidonic acid; TAL, thick ascending limb. (Redrawn from McGiff JC, Quilley J. *Am J Physiol Regal Integr Comp Physiol* 1999;277:R607–23. Used with permission.)

rected by stimulation of 20-HETE synthesis, blood pressure was lowered.[54]

Furosemide also inhibits the TAL Na$^+$-K$^+$-2Cl$^-$ cotransporter, and has been shown to stimulate COX-2–dependent generation of PGE$_2$.[143] The functional consequences of this interaction have been demonstrated by blunting of the natriuretic action of furosemide in response to COX-2 selective inhibitors.[144] Because the target of furosemide, the cotransporter, is also the site of action of 20-HETE, Laffer et al.[130] examined a possible relationship between the natriuretic response to furosemide and urinary 20-HETE excretion in hypertensive patients classified as either salt sensitive or salt resistant. The natriuretic action of furosemide was shown to be modulated by 20-HETE in hypertensive subjects according to their sensitivity to salt, being impaired only in salt-sensitive patients.

An antipressor mechanism served by TNF: Angiotensin II activates this pathway

The discovery of TNF production by TAL cells and defining its essential role in the expression of COX-2 in this nephron segment impacts on blood pressure regulation.[145] Expression of COX-2 occurred within 3 hours of exposure of mTAL tubules to Ang II, COX-2 replacing CYP as the principal oxygenase[146]; production of TNF and PGE$_2$ were increased several-fold and ^{86}Rb uptake was inhibited significantly. TNF production was deemed essential to COX-2 expression in the mTAL because the inhibitory action of Ang II on ^{86}Rb uptake—which was COX dependent—was prevented by either TNF antisera or indomethacin.[146]

Acting through its effect on expression of COX-2 and PGE$_2$ synthesis, TNF serves an antipressor mechanism. TNF mediates a profound and irreversible hypotension, referred to as circulatory shock, in Gram-negative sepsis.

Under more contained conditions, however, in sublethal doses TNF caused diuresis that was prevented by inhibition of COX.[147] In view of the hypotensive-natriuretic effects of administered TNF and the ability of Ang II to increase TNF production, Ferreri et al.,[148] in an *in vivo* study, examined whether endogenous TNF mediated an antipressor effect as a response to an Ang II infusion. In an Ang II–dependent model of hypertension (10-day infusion), TNF antisera administered on day 10 increased rat mean aortic pressure by more than 20 mmHg. TNF antisera did not elevate blood pressure in sham-operated normotensive rats. In Ang II–infused and in control normotensive rats, mTAL tubules were obtained on day 10; TNF and PGE$_2$ production were increased by three-fold and four-fold, respectively, in rats receiving Ang II as compared to tubules of normotensive control rats. These findings suggest that TNF operates in an antipressor mechanism that acts through expression of COX-2 with production of PGE$_2$ that moderates the elevation of blood pressure in response to Ang II. A similar mechanism evoked by Ang II was demonstrated in mice rendered hypertensive by infusion of Ang II.[23] Either administration of an inhibitor of COX-2, or gene knockout of COX-2, potentiated the pressor response to the peptide, an effect attributed to eliminating synthesis of one or more antipressor prostanoids. An alternative explanation is based on unmasking Ang II–induced 20-HETE production by giving a NSAID which prevents 20-HETE metabolism by COX-2 and allows the vasoconstrictor action of 20-HETE to be asserted.[127]

Calcium receptor of thick ascending limb activates antipressor system

Increased Ca^{2+} intake can lower blood pressure by activating eicosanoid pathways similar to those recruited by Ang II.[146] In humans, raising serum ionized Ca^{2+} by 25% increases Na$^+$ excretion by 150%.[149] The antihypertensive mechanism evoked by increased extracellular ionized Ca^{2+} [Ca^{2+}]$_o$ was initiated by activation of a calcium-sensing receptor on the basolateral membrane of the mTAL[150] that, on long exposure (2–3 hours) like Ang II, induced via a TNF-dependent step, COX-2 expression, and PGE$_2$ synthesis (Figure 33–12). Stimulation of the calcium receptor (CaR) increased TNF synthesis by a mechanism that activated PKC with transcription of the TNF gene. Inhibition of PKC attenuated TNF production and prevented TNF activation of COX-2 expression in the mTAL. At this juncture, it is appropriate to review the temporal determinants of the pathways of arachidonate metabolism in the rat mTAL that regulate ion transport. Each pathway, CYP and COX, can be activated by either [Ca^{2+}]$_o$ or Ang II. The CYP pathway, which generates 20-HETE, represents a quick response (within 15 minutes), whereas the delayed response (2–3 hours), which requires expression of COX-2 and membranal PGE$_2$ isomerase, generates PGE$_2$. The natriuretic-chloruretic effect of 20-HETE, the mediator of the quick response, is based on inhibition of the Na$^+$-K$^+$-2Cl$^-$ cotransporter[94] and prevention of K$^+$ recycling[151] (Figure 33–11). The signaling mechanism evoking the quick response requires the participa-

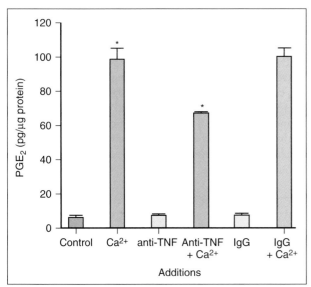

Figure 33–12. Effects of anti-TNF on Ca^{2+}-mediated PGE_2 production. mTAL cells were pretreated for 15 minutes with a neutralizing concentration of anti-TNF antibody and then treated with 1.2 mM of $CaCl_2$ for 9 hours. Addition of purified IgG (isotype control) had no effect on PGE_2 production by cells incubated in the absence or presence of Ca^{2+}. PGE_2 levels in supernatants were measured by ELISA. For each condition, an additional 0.42 mM of $CaCl_2$ were present in the media. *$p<0.05$, $n=3$. (Redrawn from Wang D, Pedraza AL, Abdullah HI, et al. *Am J Physiol Renal Physiol* 2002;283:F963–70. Used with permission.)

tion of phospholipase A_2; blockade of phospholipase C was without effect.[152] The delayed response evoked by either $[Ca^{2+}]_o$ or Ang II is based on the ability of PGE_2, the candidate mediator, to inhibit the Na^+ pump[153] and the intermediate conductance K^+ channel (ROMK).[142,146] These findings disclose a mechanism that reduces blood pressure in response to increasing Ca^{2+} intake. The development of clinically acceptable calcimimetics might serve as an ancillary measure in the management of hypertension by evoking expression of COX-2 and production of PGE_2, resulting in inhibition of mTAL ion transport analogous to the effects of "loop diuretics."

Proximal convoluted tubules: Interaction of 20-hydroxyeicosatetraenoic acid and endothelin-1

20-HETE serves as a second messenger for ET-1 in DOCA-salt hypertension.[116] A study was designed to examine whether 20-HETE also serves as a second messenger for ET-1 in the nephron.[154] The impetus for this study was the unique renal functional effects of both ET-1 and 20-HETE[154]; namely, diuresis despite renal vasoconstriction and depression of GFR, effects consonant with 20-HETE acting as a second messenger for the renal effects of ET-1.[68] Despite the negative effects of ET-1 on renal hemodynamics, release of CYP-AA metabolites by ET-1 increased Na^+ excretion in the anesthetized rat.[154]

The proximal tubules were selected to examine interactions of ET-1 and 20-HETE as this nephron segment is heavily invested with ω-hydroxylase forming 20-HETE as a principal eicosanoid.[155] ET-1 has also been shown to

inhibit proximal tubular ion transport.[156] Rat proximal tubular transport was examined in terms of 20-HETE acting as a mediator of the response to ET-1 by inhibiting ouabain-sensitive ^{86}Rb uptake.[103,156] Dibromo-dodecaenoic acid (DBDD), a specific inhibitor of ω-hydroxylase, abolished the inhibitory effect of ET-1 on ^{86}Rb uptake as did BMS 182874, an ETA-selective receptor antagonist. These findings support the proposed role of 20-HETE acting as a second messenger, mediating the effects of ET-1 on Na^+ transport in rat proximal tubules as has also been shown for the mitogenic response and renal injury produced by ET-1 in DOCA-salt hypertensive rats.[116]

Cortical collecting duct

EETs are involved in modulating Na^+ transport in the cortical collecting duct (CCD), a site responding to aldosterone-regulated Na^+ reabsorption.[69] The target of both aldosterone and AA is the ENaC on the luminal surface of the principal cells of the CCD.[157] ENaC is the principal pathway for Na^+ reabsorption in the CCD. Wei et al.[69] identified 11,12-EET as the mediator of the AA-induced inhibition of ENaC activity in the rat CCD. This conclusion was abundantly supported by abolishing the response to AA by inhibiting epoxygenases and then demonstrating inhibition of ENaC activity by 11,12-EET despite the presence of the epoxygenase inhibitor. The 11,12-EET action on ENaC was unique, as other EETs, including 5,6-EET, were without effect. Further, 11,12-EET was shown to be synthesized by CCDs based on GC-MS criteria. Confocal imaging identified the 2C23 epoxygenase isoform in CCD cells, the epoxygenase isoform responsible for the bulk of EET production in the rat and normalization of blood pressure when the animal is challenged with a salt load.[76] The contribution of ENaC to regulation of blood pressure has been stated emphatically by Lifton et al.[158]: "ENaC activity is absolutely required for normal salt homeostasis."

Sakairi et al.[72] demonstrated that 5,6-EET inhibits the Na^+/H^+ exchanger in the rabbit by increasing cytosolic Ca^{2+} concentration $[Ca^{2+}]_i$ associated with stimulation of prostaglandin synthesis in the CCD. The effect of 5,6-EET on Na^+ movement, as measured by electrogenic Na^+ reabsorption in the rabbit CCD, was blocked by inhibition of COX activity. The action of 5,6-EET was stereoselective and evoked by either luminal or basolateral application of 5,6-EET; the other EETs affected neither $[Ca^{2+}]_i$ nor Na^+ transport. This study confirms the earlier study of Jacobson al.[159] that identified 5,6-EET as an inhibitor of net Na^+ absorption by the rabbit CCD. Net potassium secretion was simultaneously reduced by 50%. Whether 5,6-EET serves as an endogenous mediator of Na^+ transport in the CCDs cannot be answered by these studies as the focus was on the response of Na^+ transport to exogenous 5,6-EET.

SUMMARY

The eicosanoids in their multiple forms act as mediators and modulators of blood pressure and can be involved in all phases of human hypertension, both primary and secondary forms, as well as their counterparts in experimental models of hypertension. 20-HETE is the dominant renal eicosanoid, overshadowing PGE_2. There are many opportunities for interactions of these pathways, particularly in renal arterioles and small arteries, as exemplified in the ready metabolism of 20-HETE by COX into products that are both pro- (20-OH PGH_2, 20-OH TxA_2) and antipressor (20-OH PGE_2, 20-OH PGI_2). A persuasive rationale exists for nominating the prostaglandin endoperoxide analogue of 20-HETE, 20-OH PGH_2, as the mediator of TGF.

In each of the two major pathways of AA metabolism, prostaglandins and CYP-AA metabolites, having opposing actions, affect circulatory responses and tubular function: PGE_2 and PGI_2 versus TxA_2 and PGH_2, 20-HETE versus 11,12-EETs, and 20-HETE versus 19-HETE. The linkage of specific prostaglandin synthases to COX isoforms determine: (1) vasodilator-diuretic responses on COX-2 activation via linkage to PGI_2 and PGE_2 synthases; and (2) pressor responses on activation of COX-1 via TxA_2 and PGH_2 synthesis. Examples follow: autoregulation of RBF represents the result of the interactions of 20-HETE-mediated vasoconstriction and 11,12-mediated vasodilatation; proximal tubular transport of Na^+ is inhibited by 20-HETE, the action of which is opposed by 19-HETE.

Eicosanoid research is in the logarithmic phase of its development, offering boundless opportunities to scientists in biomedical fields. The main objective has been summarized by Christiane Nüsslein-Volhard: "The most important thing is not any one particular piece but finding enough pieces and enough connections between them to recognize the whole picture."[160] We are still some distance from this objective.

ACKNOWLEDGMENTS

This review was made possible by National Institutes of Health grants (PPG HL-34300, RO1 HL-25394, RO1 HL-069061) and a grant from the American Diabetes Association. We are grateful to Melody Steinberg for editorial assistance and Chiara Kimmel-Preuss for help in manuscript preparation.

REFERENCES

1. Aiken JW, Vane JR. Intrarenal prostaglandin release attenuates the renal vasoconstrictor activity of angiotensin. *J Pharmacol Exp Ther* 1973;184:678–87.
2. Malik KU, McGiff JC. Modulation by prostaglandins of adrenergic transmission in the isolated perfused rabbit and rat kidney. *Circ Res* 1975;36:599–609.
3. Glanzer K, Prussing B, Dusing R, Kramer HJ. Hemodynamic and hormonal responses to 8-arginine-vasopressin in healthy man: effects of indomethacin. *Klin Wochenschr* 1982;60:1234–9.
4. McGiff JC, Terragno NA, Malik KU, Lonigro AJ. Release of a prostaglandin E-like substance from canine kidney by bradykinin. *Circ Res* 1972;31:36–43.
5. Wang JL, Cheng HF, Harris RC. Cyclooxygenase-2 inhibition decreases renin content and lowers blood pressure in a model of renovascular hypertension. *Hypertension* 1999;34:96–101.
6. Fujino T, Nakagawa N, Yuhki K, et al. Decreased susceptibility to renovascular hypertension in mice lacking the prostaglandin I2 receptor IP. *J Clin Invest* 2004;114:805–12.
7. Imanishi M, Kawamura M, Akabane S, et al. Aspirin lowers blood pressure in patients with renovascular hypertension. *Hypertension* 1989;14:461–8.
8. Strong CG, Romero JC. Effects of indomethacin in rabbit renovascular hypertension. *Clin Sci Mol Med Suppl* 1976;3:249s–51s.
9. Terragno NA, Terragno DA, McGiff JC. Contribution of prostaglandins to the renal circulation in conscious, anesthetized, and laparotomized dogs. *Circ Res* 1977;40:590–5.
10. Hockel GM, Cowley AW Jr. Prostaglandin E2-induced hypertension in conscious dogs. *Am J Physiol* 1979;237:H449–54.
11. Narumiya S, Sugimoto Y, Ushikubi F. Prostanoid receptors: structures, properties, and functions. *Physiol Rev* 1999;79:1193–226.
12. Breyer MD, Breyer RM. G protein-coupled prostanoid receptors and the kidney. *Annu Rev Physiol* 2001;63:579–605.
13. Kennedy CR, Zhang Y, Brandon S, et al. Salt-sensitive hypertension and reduced fertility in mice lacking the prostaglandin EP2 receptor. *Nat Med* 1999;5:217–20.
14. Moncada S, Vane JR. Prostacyclin and the vascular endothelium. *Bull Eur Physiopathol Respir* 1981;17:687–701.
15. Whorton AR, Misono K, Hollifield J, et al. Prostaglandins and renin release: I. Stimulation of renin release from rabbit renal cortical slices by PGI2. *Prostaglandins* 1977;14:1095–104.
16. FitzGerald GA. COX-2 and beyond: approaches to prostaglandin inhibition in human disease. *Nat Rev Drug Discov* 2003;2:879–90.
17. Audoly LP, Rocca B, Fabre JE, et al. Cardiovascular responses to the isoprostanes iPF(2alpha)-III and iPE(2)-III are mediated via the thromboxane A(2) receptor in vivo. *Circulation* 2000;101:2833–40.
18. Meagher EA, FitzGerald GA. Disordered eicosanoid formation in pregnancy-induced hypertension. *Circulation* 1993;88:1324–33.
19. Nasjletti A. The role of eicosanoids in angiotensin-dependent hypertension. *Hypertension* 1997;31:194.
20. Keen HL, Brands MW, Smith MJ Jr., et al. Thromboxane is required for full expression of angiotensin hypertension in rats. *Hypertension* 1997;29:310–4.
21. Francois H, Athirakul K, Mao L, et al. Role for thromboxane receptors in angiotensin-II–induced hypertension. *Hypertension* 2004;43:364–9.
22. Kawada N, Dennehy K, Solis G, et al. TP receptors regulate renal hemodynamics during angiotensin II slow pressor response. *Am J Physiol Renal Physiol* 2004;287:F753–9.
23. Qi Z, Hao CM, Langenbach RI, et al. Opposite effects of cyclooxygenase-1 and -2 activity on the pressor response to angiotensin II. *J Clin Invest* 2002;110:61–69.
24. Wang D, Chabrashvili T, Wilcox CS. Enhanced contractility of renal afferent arterioles from angiotensin-infused rabbits: roles of oxidative stress, thromboxane prostanoid receptors, and endothelium. *Circ Res* 2004;94:1436–42.
25. Thomas DW, Mannon RB, Mannon PJ, et al. Coagulation defects and altered hemodynamic responses in mice lacking receptors for thromboxane A2. *J Clin Invest* 1998;102:1994–2001.
26. Shibouta Y, Terashita ZI, Inada Y, et al. Enhanced thromboxane A2 biosynthesis in the kidney of spontaneously hypertensive rats during development of hypertension. *Eur J Pharmacol* 1981;70:247–56.
27. Shibouta Y, Terashita ZI, Inada Y, et al. Renal effects of pinane-thromboxane A2 and indomethacin in saline volume-expanded spontaneously hypertensive rats. *Eur J Pharmacol* 1982;85:51–9.
28. Stier CT JrJr, Itskovitz HD. Thromboxane A2 and the development of hypertension in spontaneously hypertensive rats. *Eur J Pharmacol* 1988;146:129–35.
29. Yang D, Feletou M, Levens N, et al. A diffusible substance(s) mediates endothelium-dependent contractions in the aorta of SHR. *Hypertension* 2003;41:143–8.

30. Botros FT, Laniado-Schwartzman M, Abraham NG. Regulation of cyclooxygenase- and cytochrome p450-derived eicosanoids by heme oxygenase in the rat kidney. *Hypertension* 2002;39:639–44.

31. Sessa WC, Abraham NG, Escalante B, Schwartzman ML. Manipulation of cytochrome P-450 dependent renal thromboxane synthase activity in spontaneously hypertensive rats. *J Hypertens* 1989;7:37–42.

32. Pedersen EB, Christensen NJ, Christensen P, et al. Preeclampsia—a state of prostaglandin deficiency? Urinary prostaglandin excretion, the renin-aldosterone system, and circulating catecholamines in preeclampsia. *Hypertension* 1983; 5:105–11.

33. Fitzgerald DJ, Entman SS, Mulloy K, FitzGerald GA. Decreased prostacyclin biosynthesis preceding the clinical manifestation of pregnancy-induced hypertension. *Circulation* 1987; 75:956–63.

34. Goodman RP, Killam AP, Brash AR, Branch RA. Prostacyclin production during pregnancy: comparison of production during normal pregnancy and pregnancy complicated by hypertension. *Am J Obstet Gynecol* 1982;142:817–22.

35. Gant NF, Daley GL, Chand S, et al. A study of angiotensin II pressor response throughout primigravid pregnancy. *J Clin Invest* 1973; 52:2682–9.

36. Everett RB, Worley RJ, MacDonald PC, Gant NF. Effect of prostaglandin synthetase inhibitors on pressor response to angiotensin II in human pregnancy. *J Clin Endocrinol Metab* 1978;46:1007–10.

37. Chavarria ME, Lara-Gonzalez L, Gonzalez-Gleason A, et al. Prostacyclin/thromboxane early changes in pregnancies that are complicated by preeclampsia. *Am J Obstet Gynecol* 2003;188:986–92.

38. Sanchez-Ramos L, O'Sullivan MJ, Garrido-Calderon J. Effect of low-dose aspirin on angiotensin II pressor response in human pregnancy. *Am J Obstet Gynecol* 1987;156:193–4.

39. Vainio M, Riutta A, Koivisto AM, Maenpaa J. Prostacyclin, thromboxane A and the effect of low-dose ASA in pregnancies at high risk for hypertensive disorders. *Acta Obstet Gynecol Scand* 2004;83:1119–23.

40. Seki H, Kuromaki K, Takeda S, et al. Trial of prophylactic administration of TXA2 synthetase inhibitor, ozagrel hydrochloride, for preeclampsia. *Hypertens Pregnancy* 1999;18:157–64.

41. Duley L, Henderson-Smart DJ, Knight M, King JF. Antiplatelet agents for preventing pre-eclampsia and its complications. *Cochrane Database Syst Rev* 2004;CD004659.

42. Zhou Y, Chang HH, Du J,, et al. Renal epoxyeicosatrienoic acid synthesis during pregnancy. *Am J Physiol Renal Physiol* 2005;288: F221–6.

43. Catella F, Lawson JA, Fitzgerald DJ, FitzGerald GA. Endogenous biosynthesis of arachidonic acid epoxides in humans: increased formation in pregnancy-induced hypertension. *Proc Natl Acad Sci U S A* 1990;87:5893–7.

44. Gimbrone MA Jr, Topper JN, Nagel T, et al. Endothelial dysfunction, hemodynamic forces, and atherogenesis. *Ann N Y Acad Sci* 2000; 902:230–9.

45. McAdam BF, Catella-Lawson F, Mardini IA, et al. Systemic biosynthesis of prostacyclin by cyclooxygenase (COX)-2: the human pharmacology of a selective inhibitor of COX-2. *Proc Natl Acad Sci U S A* 1999;96:272–77.

46. Bombardier C, Laine L, Reicin A, et al. Comparison of upper gastrointestinal toxicity of rofecoxib and naproxen in patients with rheumatoid arthritis. VIGOR Study Group. *N Engl J Med* 2000;343:1520–8.

47. Patrignani P, Filabozzi P, Patrono C. Selective cumulative inhibition of platelet thromboxane production by low-dose aspirin in healthy subjects. *J Clin Invest* 1982;69:1366–72.

48. Cheng HF, Harris RC. Does cyclooxygenase-2 affect blood pressure? *Curr Hypertens Rep* 2003; 5:87–92.

49. Harris RC Jr. Cyclooxygenase-2 inhibition and renal physiology. *Am J Cardiol* 2002;89:204–9.

50. Cheng MK, Doumad AB, Jiang H, et al. Epoxyeicosatrienoic acids mediate adenosine-induced vasodilation in rat preglomerular microvessels (PGMV) via A2A receptors. *Br J Pharmacol* 2004; 141:441–48.

51. Carroll M, Capparelli MF, Doumad AB, et al. Cyclooxygnease dependent transformation of 20-hydroxyeicosatetraenoic acid in renal microvessels during salt depletion. *Hypertension* 2001;38:P475.

52. Sacerdoti D, Abraham NG, McGiff JC, Schwartzman ML. Renal cytochrome P-450–dependent metabolism of arachidonic acid in spontaneously hypertensive rats. *Biochem Pharmacol* 1988;37:521–7.

53. McGiff JC, Quilley J. 20-HETE and the kidney: resolution of old problems and new beginnings. *Am J Physiol* 1999; 277:R607–23.

54. Ito O, Roman RJ. Role of 20-HETE in elevating chloride transport in the thick ascending limb of Dahl SS/Jr rats. *Hypertension* 1999;33:419–23.

55. Imig JD, Falck JR, Gebremedhin D, et al. Elevated renovascular tone in young spontaneously hypertensive rats. Role of cytochrome P-450. *Hypertension* 1993;22:357–64.

56. Guyton AC. Blood pressure control—special role of the kidneys and body fluids. *Science* 1991;252:1813–6.

57. Imig JD, Falck JR, Inscho EW. Contribution of cytochrome P450 epoxygenase and hydroxylase pathways to afferent arteriolar autoregulatory responsiveness. *Br J Pharmacol* 1999;127:1399–405.

58. Falck JR, Lumin S, Blair I, et al. Cytochrome P-450-dependent oxidation of arachidonic acid to 16-, 17-, and 18-hydroxyeicosatetraenoic acids. *J Biol Chem* 1990;265:10244–9.

59. Zou AP, Imig JD, Kaldunski M, et al. Inhibition of renal vascular 20-HETE production impairs autoregulation of renal blood flow. *Am J Physiol* 1994; 266:F275–82.

60. Sacerdoti D, Escalante B, Abraham NG, et al. Treatment with tin prevents the development of hypertension in spontaneously hypertensive rats. *Science* 1989;243:388–90.

61. Kappas A, Drummond GS. Control of heme metabolism with synthetic metalloporphyrins. *J Clin Invest* 1986; 77:335–9.

62. Escalante B, Sacerdoti D, Davidian MM, et al. Chronic treatment with tin normalizes blood pressure in spontaneously hypertensive rats. *Hypertension* 1991;17:776–9.

63. Zhang F, Kaide J, Wei Y, et al. Carbon monoxide produced by isolated arterioles attenuates pressure-induced vasoconstriction. *Am J PhysiolAm J Physiol Heart Circ Physiol* 2001;281:H350–8.

64. Yang L, Quan S, Nasjletti A, et al. Heme oxygenase-1 gene expression modulates angiotensin II-induced increase in blood pressure. *Hypertension* 2004;43:1221–6.

65. Su P, Kaushal KM, Kroetz DL. Inhibition of renal arachidonic acid omega-hydroxylase activity with ABT reduces blood pressure in the SHR. *Am J Physiol* 1998;275:R426–38.

66. Xu F, Straub WO, Pak W, et al. Antihypertensive effect of mechanism-based inhibition of renal arachidonic acid omega-hydroxylase activity. *Am J Physiol Regul Integr Comp Physiol* 2002; 283:R710–20.

67. Wang MH, Zhang F, Marji J, et al. CYP4A1 antisense oligonucleotide reduces mesenteric vascular reactivity and blood pressure in SHR. *Am J Physiol Regul Integr Comp Physiol* 2001; 280:R255–61.

68. Oyekan AO, McGiff JC. Functional response of the rat kidney to inhibition of nitric oxide synthesis: role of cytochrome p450-derived arachidonate metabolites. *Br J Pharmacol* 1998;125: 1065–73.

69. Wei Y, Lin DH, Kemp R, et al. Arachidonic acid inhibits epithelial Na channel via cytochrome P450 (CYP) epoxygenase-dependent metabolic pathways. *J Gen Physiol* 2004;124: 719–27.

70. Madhun ZT, Goldthwait DA, McKay D, et al. An epoxygenase metabolite of arachidonic acid mediates angiotensin II-induced rises in cytosolic calcium in rabbit proximal tubule epithelial cells. *J Clin Invest* 1991;88:456–61.

71. Pomposiello SI, Quilley J, Carroll MA, et al. 5,6-Epoxyeicosatrienoic acid mediates the enhanced renal vasodilation to arachidonic acid in the SHR. *Hypertension* 2003;42:548–54.

72. Sakairi Y, Jacobson HR, Noland TD, et al. 5,6-EET inhibits ion transport in collecting duct by stimulating endogenous prostaglandin synthesis. *Am J Physiol* 1995;268:F931–9.

73. Fulton D, McGiff JC, Quilley J. Pharmacological evaluation of an epoxide as the putative hyperpolarizing factor mediating the nitric oxide-independent vasodilator effect of bradykinin in the rat heart. *J Pharmacol Exp Ther* 1998;287:497–503.

74. Fisslthaler B, Popp R, Kiss L, et al. Cytochrome P450 2C is an EDHF synthase in coronary arteries. *Nature* 1999;401:493–7.

75. Quilley J, McGiff JC. Is EDHF an epoxyeicosatrienoic acid? *Trends Pharmacol Sci* 2000;21:121–4.

76. Holla VR, Makita K, Zaphiropoulos PG, Capdevila JH. The kidney cytochrome P-450 2C23 arachidonic acid epoxygenase is upregulated during dietary salt loading. *J Clin Invest* 1999;104:751–60.

77. Liclican EL, McGiff JC, Pedraza PL, et al. Exaggerated response to adenosine in kidneys from high salt-fed rats: role of epoxyeicosatrienoic acids. *Am J Physiol Renal Physiol* 2005; 289:F386–92.

78. Yu Z, Xu F, Huse LM, et al. Soluble epoxide hydrolase regulates hydrolysis of vasoactive epoxyeicosatrienoic acids. *Circ Res* 2000;87:992–8.

79. Imig JD, Zhao X, Capdevila JH, et al. Soluble epoxide hydrolase inhibition lowers arterial blood pressure in angiotensin II hypertension. *Hypertension* 2002;39:690–4.

80. Wang MH, Guan H, Nguyen X, et al. Contribution of cytochrome P-450 4A1 and 4A2 to vascular 20-hydroxyeicosatetraenoic acid synthesis in rat kidneys. *Am J Physiol* 1999; 276:F246–53.

81. Ito O, Alonso GM, Hopp KA, Roman RJ. Localization of cytochrome P-450 4A isoforms along the rat nephron. *Am J Physiol* 1998;274:F395–404.

82. Cowart LA, Wei S, Hsu MH, et al. The CYP4A isoforms hydroxylate epoxyeicosatrienoic acids to form high affinity peroxisome proliferator-activated receptor ligands. *J Biol Chem* 2002;277:35105–12.

83. Skott O. Androgen-induced activation of 20-HETE production may contribute to gender differences in blood pressure regulation. *Am J Physiol Regul Integr Comp Physiol* 2003;284:R1053–4.

84. Holla VR, Adas F, Imig JD, et al. Alterations in the regulation of androgen-sensitive Cyp 4a monooxygenases cause hypertension. *Proc Natl Acad Sci U S A* 2001;98: 5211–6.

85. Nakagawa K, Marji JS, Schwartzman ML, et al. Androgen-mediated induction of the kidney arachidonate hydroxylases is associated with the development of hypertension. *Am J Physiol Regul Integr Comp Physiol* 2003;284:R1055–62.

86. Kimura S, Hardwick JP, Kozak CA, Gonzalez FJ. The rat clofibrate-inducible CYP4A subfamily. II. cDNA sequence of IVA3, mapping of the Cyp4a locus to mouse chromosome 4, and coordinate and tissue-specific regulation of the CYP4A genes. *DNA* 1989;8:517–25.

87. Roman RJ. P-450 metabolites of arachidonic acid in the control of cardiovascular function. *Physiol Rev* 2002;82:131–85.

88. Nguyen X, Wang MH, Reddy KM, et al. Kinetic profile of the rat CYP4A isoforms: arachidonic acid metabolism and isoform-specific inhibitors. *Am J Physiol* 1999;276:R1691–700.

89. Reckelhoff JF. Gender differences in the regulation of blood pressure. *Hypertension* 2001;37:1199–208.

90. Gainer JV, Bellamine A, Dawson EP, et al. Functional variant of CYP4A11 20-hydroxyeicosatetraenoic acid synthase is associated with essential hypertension. *Circulation* 2005; 111:63–9.

91. Croft KD, McGiff JC, Sanchez-Mendoza A, Carroll MA. Angiotensin II releases 20-HETE from rat renal microvessels. *Am J Physiol Renal Physiol* 2000;279:F544–51.

92. Omata K, Abraham NG, Escalante B, Schwartzman ML. Age-related changes in renal cytochrome P-450 arachidonic acid metabolism in spontaneously hypertensive rats. *Am J Physiol* 1992;262:F8–16.

93. Imig JD, Zou AP, Stec DE, et al. Formation and actions of 20-hydroxyeicosatetraenoic acid in rat renal arterioles. *Am J Physiol* 1996; 270:R217–27.

94. Escalante B, Erlij D, Falck JR, McGiff JC. Effect of cytochrome P450 arachidonate metabolites on ion transport in rabbit kidney loop of Henle. *Science* 1991; 251:799–802.

95. Oyekan AO, McGiff JC, Quilley J. Cytochrome P-450-dependent vasodilator responses to arachidonic acid in the isolated, perfused kidney of the rat. *Circ Res* 1991;68:958–65.

96. Pomposiello SI, Carroll MA, Falck JR, McGiff JC. Epoxyeicosatrienoic acid-mediated renal vasodilation to arachidonic acid is enhanced in SHR. *Hypertension* 2001;37:887–93.

97. Zhao X, Pollock DM, Inscho EW, et al. Decreased renal cytochrome P450 2C enzymes and impaired vasodilation are associated with angiotensin salt-sensitive hypertension. *Hypertension* 2003;41:709–14.

98. Navar LG. Integrating multiple paracrine regulators of renal microvascular dynamics. *Am J Physiol* 1998;274:F433–44.

99. Zou AP, Imig JD, Ortiz de Montellano PR, et al. Effect of P-450 omega-hydroxylase metabolites of arachidonic acid on tubuloglomerular feedback. *Am J Physiol* 1994;266:F934–41.

100. Marji JS, Wang MH, Laniado-Schwartzman M. Cytochrome P-450 4A isoform expression and 20-HETE synthesis in renal preglomerular arteries. *Am J Physiol Renal Physiol* 2002;283:F60–7.

101. Duke LM, Widdop RE, Kett MM, Evans RG. AT(2) receptors mediate tonic renal medullary vasoconstriction in renovascular hypertension. *Br J Pharmacol* 2005;144:486–92.

102. Imig JD. Eicosanoid regulation of the renal vasculature. *Am J Physiol Renal Physiol* 2000;279:F965–81.

103. Escalante BA, McGiff JC, Oyekan AO. Role of cytochrome P-450 arachidonate metabolites in endothelin signaling in rat proximal tubule. *Am J Physiol Renal Physiol* 2002;282:F144–50.

104. Gross V, Schunck WH, Honeck H, et al. Inhibition of pressure natriuresis in mice lacking the AT2 receptor. *Kidney Int* 2000;57:191–202.

105. Carroll MA, Sala A, Dunn CE, et al. Structural identification of cytochrome P450-dependent arachidonate metabolites formed by rabbit medullary thick ascending limb cells. *J Biol Chem* 1991;266:12306–12.

106. Nowicki S, Chen SL, Aizman O, et al, et al. 20-Hydroxyeicosa-tetraenoic acid (20 HETE) activates protein kinase C. Role in regulation of rat renal Na+,K+-ATPase. *J Clin Invest* 1997;99:1224–30.

107. dos Santos EA, Dahly-Vernon AJ, Hoagland KM, Roman RJ. Inhibition of the formation of EETs and 20-HETE with 1-aminobenzotriazole attenuates pressure natriuresis. *Am J Physiol Regul Integr Comp Physiol* 2004;287:R58–68.

108. Postnov YU, Orlov S, Gulak P, Shevchenko A. Altered permeability of the erythrocyte membrane for sodium and potassium ions in spontaneously hypertensive rats. *Pflugers Arch* 1976; 365:257–63.

109. Roman RJ, Lianos E. Influence of prostaglandins on papillary blood flow and pressure-natriuretic response. *Hypertension* 1990;15:29–35.

110. McGiff JC, Itskovitz HD. Prostaglandins and the kidney. *Circ Res* 1973;33: 479–88.

111. Itskovitz HD, Terragno NA, McGiff JC. Effect of a renal prostaglandin on distribution of blood flow in the isolated canine kidney. *Circ Res* 1974; 34:770–6.

112. Carroll MA, Balazy M, Huang DD, et al. Cytochrome P450-derived renal HETEs: storage and release. *Kidney Int* 1997;51:1696–702.

113. Carroll MA, Garcia MP, Falck JR, McGiff JC. Cyclooxygenase dependency of the renovascular actions of cytochrome P450-derived arachidonate metabolites. *J Pharmacol Exp Ther* 1992;260:104–9.

114. Sacerdoti D, Balazy M, Angeli P, et al. Eicosanoid excretion in hepatic cirrhosis. Predominance of 20-HETE. *J Clin Invest* 1997;100:1264–70.

115. Prakash C, Zhang JY, Falck JR, et al, et al. 20-Hydroxyeicosatetraenoic acid is excreted as a glucuronide conjugate in human urine. *Biochem Biophys Res Commun* 1992;185:728–33.

116. Oyekan AO, McAward K, Conetta J, et al. Endothelin-1 and CYP450 arachidonate metabolites interact to promote tissue injury in DOCA-salt hypertension. *Am J Physiol* 1999; 276:R766–75.

117. Epstein M, Berk DP, Hollenberg NK, et al. Renal failure in the patient with cirrhosis. The role of active vasoconstriction. *Am J Med* 1970; 49:175–85.

118. Arroyo V, Planas R, Gaya J, et al. Sympathetic nervous activity, renin-angiotensin system and renal excretion of prostaglandin E2 in cirrhosis. Relationship to functional renal failure and sodium and water excretion. *Eur J Clin Invest* 1983; 13:271–8.

119. Oyekan A, Balazy M, McGiff JC. Renal oxygenases: differential contribution to vasoconstriction induced by ET-1 and ANG II. *Am J Physiol* 1997;273:R293–300.

120. Ferreri NR, McGiff JC, Carroll MA, Quilley J. Renal COX-2, cytokines and 20-HETE: tubular and vascular mechanisms. *Curr Pharm Des* 2004; 10:613–26.

121. Navar LG, Inscho EW, Majid SA, et al. Paracrine regulation of the renal microcirculation. *Physiol Rev* 1996; 76:425–536.

122. Bell Quilley CP, Lin YS, Hilchey SD, et al. Renovascular actions of angiotensin II in the isolated kidney

of the rat: relationship to lipoxygenases. *J Pharmacol Exp Ther* 1993;267: 676–82.

123. Yiu SS, Zhao X, Inscho EW, Imig JD. 12-Hydroxyeicosatetraenoic acid participates in angiotensin II afferent arteriolar vasoconstriction by activating L-type calcium channels. *J Lipid Res* 2003;44:2391–9.

124. Proctor KG, Shatkin S Jr, Kaminski PM, et al. Modulation of arteriolar blood flow by inhibitors of arachidonic acid oxidation after thermal injury: possible role for a novel class of vasodilator metabolites. *Circulation* 1988; 77:1185–96.

125. Hill E, Fitzpatrick F, Murphy RC. Biological activity and metabolism of 20-hydroxyeicosatetraenoic acid in the human platelet. *Br J Pharmacol* 1992; 106:267–74.

126. Bonvalet JP, Pradelles P, Farman N. Segmental synthesis and actions of prostaglandins along the nephron. *Am J Physiol* 1987;253:F377–87.

127. Cheng MK, McGiff JC, Carroll MA. Renal arterial 20-hydroxyeicosatetraenoic acid levels: regulation by cyclooxygenase. *Am J Physiol Renal Physiol* 2003;284:F474–9.

128. Yang T, Singh I, Pham H, et al. Regulation of cyclooxygenase expression in the kidney by dietary salt intake. *Am J Physiol* 1998;274:F481–9.

129. Carroll MA, Kemp R, Cheng MK, McGiff JC. Regulation of preglomerular microvascular 20-hydroxyeicosatetraenoic acid levels by salt depletion. *Med Sci Monit* 2001;7:567–72.

130. Laffer CL, Laniado-Schwartzman M, Wang MH, et al. 20-HETE and furosemide-induced natriuresis in salt-sensitive essential hypertension. *Hypertension* 2003;41:703–8.

131. Laffer CL, Laniado-Schwartzman M, Nasjletti A, Elijovich F. 20-HETE and circulating insulin in essential hypertension with obesity. *Hypertension* 2004;43:388–92.

132. Shimojo N, Ishizaki T, Imaoka S, et al. Changes in amounts of cytochrome P450 isozymes and levels of catalytic activities in hepatic and renal microsomes of rats with streptozocin-induced diabetes. *Biochem Pharmacol* 1993;46:621–7.

133. Zou AP, Fleming JT, Falck JR, et al. 20-HETE is an endogenous inhibitor of the large-conductance Ca(2+)-activated K+ channel in renal arterioles. *Am J Physiol* 1996;270:R228–37.

134. Campbell WB, Gebremedhin D, Pratt PF, Harder DR. Identification of epoxyeicosatrienoic acids as endothelium-derived hyperpolarizing factors. *Circ Res* 1996;78:415–23.

135. Inscho EW, Cook AK, Imig JD, et al. Physiological role for P2X1 receptors in renal microvascular autoregulatory behavior. *J Clin Invest* 2003;112: 1895–905.

136. Zhao X, Inscho EW, Bondlela M, et al. The CYP450 hydroxylase pathway contributes to P2X receptor-mediated afferent arteriolar vasoconstriction. *Am J Physiol Heart Circ Physiol* 2001; 281:H2089–96.

137. Siragy HM, Linden J. Sodium intake markedly alters renal interstitial fluid adenosine. *Hypertension* 1996;27: 404–7.

138. Makita K, Takahashi K, Karara A, et al. Experimental and/or genetically controlled alterations of the renal microsomal cytochrome P450 epoxygenase induce hypertension in rats fed a high salt diet. *J Clin Invest* 1994;94:2414–20.

139. Reeves WB, Winters CJ, Zimniak L, Andreoli TE. Medullary thick limbs: renal concentrating segments. *Kidney Int Suppl* 1996;57:S154–64.

140. Quigley R, Baum M, Reddy KM, et al. Effects of 20-HETE and 19(S)-HETE on rabbit proximal straight tubule volume transport. *Am J Physiol Renal Physiol* 2000;278:F949–53.

141. Zhang F, Deng H, Kemp R, et al. Decreased levels of cytochrome P450 2E1–derived eicosanoids sensitize renal arteries to constrictor agonists in spontaneously hypertensive rats. *Hypertension* 2005;45:103–8.

142. Wang W, Lu M. Effect of arachidonic acid on activity of the apical K+ channel in the thick ascending limb of the rat kidney. *J Gen Physiol* 1995; 106:727–43.

143. Kammerl MC, Nusing RM, Richthammer W, et al. Inhibition of COX-2 counteracts the effects of diuretics in rats. *Kidney Int* 2001; 60:1684–91.

144. Steinhauslin F, Munafo A, Buclin T, et al. Renal effects of nimesulide in furosemide-treated subjects. *Drugs* 1993;46(Suppl 1):257–62.

145. Macica CM, Escalante BA, Conners MS, Ferreri NR. TNF production by the medullary thick ascending limb of Henle's loop. *Kidney Int* 1994;46: 113–21.

146. Ferreri NR, Escalante BA, Zhao Y, et al. Angiotensin II induces TNF production by the thick ascending limb: functional implications. *Am J Physiol* 1998;274: F148–55.

147. van Lanschot JJ, Mealy K, Jacobs DO, et al. Splenectomy attenuates the inappropriate diuresis associated with tumor necrosis factor administration. *Surg Gynecol Obstet* 1991;172:293–7.

148. Ferreri NR, Zhao Y, Takizawa H, McGiff JC. Tumor necrosis factor-alpha-angiotensin interactions and regulation of blood pressure. *J Hypertens* 1997;15:1481–4.

149. McCarron DA. Diet and blood pressure—the paradigm shift. *Science* 1998;281:933–4.

150. Wang D, An SJ, Wang WH, et al. CaR-mediated COX-2 expression in primary cultured mTAL cells. *Am J Physiol Renal Physiol* 2001;281: F658–64.

151. Wang WH, Lu M, Hebert SC. Cytochrome P-450 metabolites mediate extracellular Ca(2+)-induced inhibition of apical K+ channels in the TAL. *Am J Physiol* 1996;271:C103–11.

152. Wang W, Lu M, Balazy M, Hebert SC. Phospholipase A2 is involved in mediating the effect of extracellular Ca2+ on apical K+ channels in rat TAL. *Am J Physiol* 1997;273:F421–9.

153. Wald H, Scherzer P, Rubinger D, Popovtzer MM. Effect of indomethacin in vivo and PGE2 in vitro on MTAL Na-K-ATPase of the rat kidney. *Pflugers Arch* 1990;415:648–50.

154. Oyekan AO, McGiff JC. Cytochrome P-450–derived eicosanoids participate in the renal functional effects of ET-1 in the anesthetized rat. *Am J Physiol* 1998;274:R52–61.

155. Omata K, Abraham NG, Schwartzman ML. Renal cytochrome P-450–arachidonic acid metabolism: localization and hormonal regulation in SHR. *Am J Physiol* 1992;262:F591–9.

156. Garvin J, Sanders K. Endothelin inhibits fluid and bicarbonate transport in part by reducing Na+/K+ ATPase activity in the rat proximal straight tubule. *J Am Soc Nephrol* 1991;2:976–82.

157. Kemendy AE, Kleyman TR, Eaton DC. Aldosterone alters the open probability of amiloride-blockable sodium channels in A6 epithelia. *Am J Physiol* 1992;263: C825–37.

158. Lifton RP, Gharavi AG, Geller DS. Molecular mechanisms of human hypertension. *Cell* 2001;104:545–56.

159. Jacobson HR, Corona S, Capdevila J, Chacos N, Manna S, Womack A, et al. Effects of epoxyeicostrienoic acids on ion transport in the rabbit cortical collecting tubule. In: Braquet P, et al., eds. *Prostaglandins and Membrane Ion Transport*. New York: Raven Press, 1984:311.

160. Nüsslein-Volhard C. Journey to the center of the egg. *New York Times Magazine*, October 12, 1997, 42–5.

Chapter

34

Role of Sex Steroids in Hypertension

Jane F. Reckelhoff, Licy L. Yanes, Radu Iliescu, Lourdes A. Fortepiani, and Julio C. Sartori-Valinotti

Key Findings

- Following menopause, blood pressure increases in women to levels even higher than in men.

- The roles that sex steroids play in mediating or protecting against cardiovascular disease (CVD) and hypertension are controversial. Men are at greater risk for cardiovascular and renal disease than are age-matched, premenopausal women.

- Animal studies have strongly implicated androgens as being mediators of CVD and hypertension, but human epidemiologic studies have shown that with chronic disease, including hypertension, serum testosterone levels are actually reduced. Whether androgens contribute to hypertension is not clear.

- Since premenopausal women are typically protected from CVD and hypertension compared to men, estradiol has been hypothesized to be protective against hypertension. However, the negative findings of recent studies on hormone replacement therapy in postmenopausal women have shaken our previous ideas.

SEX STEROIDS AND BLOOD PRESSURE IN HUMANS

Men are generally at greater risk for cardiovascular disease (CVD) and renal disease than are age-matched, premenopausal women. Studies using ambulatory blood pressure monitoring have demonstrated that blood pressure is higher in men than in women at similar ages.[1-5] For example, Wiinber et al.[6] studied 352 normotensive (for age) Danish men and women, aged 20 to 79 years, and found that blood pressure increased with aging in both groups, but that men had higher 24-hour blood pressure, by approximately 6 to 10 mmHg, than did women, until the age of 70 to 79 years when blood pressure was similar for men and women.[6] Khoury et al.[7] performed ambulatory blood pressure monitoring on 131 men and women, aged 50 to 60 years, and found that men had higher blood pressure than did women.[7] Findings were similar in a meta-analysis study performed by Staessen et al. In addition, NHANES III, the Third National Health and Nutrition Examination Survey, showed that in general, men had higher blood pressure than women through middle age.[9] Furthermore, the incidence of uncontrolled hypertension is also greater in men than women.

Following menopause, however, blood pressure increases in women as well. The data from NHANES III confirmed that by 60 to 69 years of age, Hispanic women and non-Hispanic black women developed higher blood pressure than men of similar ethnic background.[9] The mechanisms responsible for the hypertension in these populations are complicated by comorbid conditions of obesity and type II diabetes, which can also lead to increases in blood pressure. In the non-Hispanic white population, in which the incidence of obesity and type II diabetes with aging were not as high, blood pressure also increased after the average age of menopause (51.4 years). Thus by 60 to 69 years of age, non-Hispanic white women had similar prevalence of hypertension as men, and by 70 to 79 years of age, this population of women had higher prevalence than did men.

SEX STEROIDS AND BLOOD PRESSURE IN ANIMALS

Gender-associated differences in blood pressure observed in humans have also been documented in various animal models. In hypertensive rat models, many investigators have found that males have higher blood pressure than do females. For example, male spontaneously hypertensive rats (SHR) have higher blood pressure than do females of similar ages.[10] Similar gender differences in development of hypertension are also found in Dahl salt-sensitive rats,[11] deoxycorticosterone (DOC)-salt hypertensive rats,[12] and the New Zealand genetically hypertensive rat.[13] Therefore, as found in humans and hypertensive rat models, males have higher blood pressure than age-matched females.

Whether there are sex differences in blood pressure in normotensive rats, as found in humans, is not clear. Calhoun and Oparil[14] reported that 24-hour blood pressure measured at 12 weeks of age in male Wistar-Kyoto rats (WKY) was lower than in female WKY by approximately 9 mmHg (males, 96±3 mmHg; females, 105±1 mmHg).[14] However, by 14 weeks of age there was no difference in blood pressure over 24 hours between the genders (males, 101±3 mmHg; females, 106±1 mmHg). In any case, the issue could be resolved if blood pressure were measured over a prolonged period of time (months) by telemetry.

BIOCHEMISTRY

Synthesis of sex steroids

Sex steroids are produced mainly by the gonads, although the synthesizing machinery is present in other tissues. The enzymes involved in sex steroid synthesis are members of the cytochrome P450 (CYP) system. As shown in Figure 34–1, the rate-limiting step in sex steroid synthesis is the conversion of cholesterol to pregnenolone by the side-chain cleavage enzyme. Cholesterol is made available either from low-density lipoproteins in the extracellular fluid or from acetyl co-enzyme A in the cells. Pregnenolone is converted to progesterone or to dihydroepiandrostenedione (DHEA) by 17α-hydroxylase (also known as 17,20-desmolase). DHEA can be converted to either androstenedione by 3β-hydroxysteroid dehydrogenase or to androstenediol by 17β-hydroxysteroid dehydrogenase. Androstenedione and androstenediol can be converted to testosterone by 17β- or 3β-hydroxysteroid dehydrogenase, respectively. Testosterone is then converted either to dihydrotestosterone by 5α-reductase or to estradiol by CYP 19-aromatase.

Sex steroid receptors

The two estrogen receptors, ERα and ERβ, and the androgen receptor are typical nuclear receptors (reviewed in Black and Paschal[15] and Barkhem et al.[16]). Both estrogen and androgen receptors are present on many cell types in various tissues, including tissues involved in the cardiovascular system such as the vasculature, the heart, and the kidney.

PHYSIOLOGY AND PATHOPHYSIOLOGY

Evidence that sex steroids impact blood pressure: Role of androgens

Although the mechanisms responsible for the sex differences in blood pressure control are not clear, there is significant evidence that androgens, such as testosterone, play an important role in gender-associated differences in blood pressure regulation (Box 34–1). For example, studies using ambulatory blood pressure–monitoring techniques in children have shown that with increasing age, blood pressure increases in both boys and girls. However, after the onset of puberty, boys have higher blood pressure than do age-matched girls.[17,18] At ages 13 to 15 years, systolic blood pressure was approximately 4 mmHg higher in boys than girls and at ages 16 to 18 years, boys had higher systolic blood pressures than girls by 10 to 14 mmHg. The blood

pressure in postpubescent boys also does not dip as low at night as in girls. A reduction in nocturnal dipping is recognized as a hallmark of early dysfunction in blood pressure regulation. These data clearly show that with adolescence and puberty when androgen levels are increasing, blood pressure is higher in boys than girls. Increased androgens in adults are also associated with increased blood pressure. For example, women with polycystic ovary syndrome or adrenal virilizing tumors, which are characterized by elevated testosterone levels, experience hypertension.[19,20] Anabolic androgenic steroid use also leads to frank hypertension in borderline hypertensive men.

Another line of evidence that testosterone may impact blood pressure is found in rat studies. Castration at a young age (3 to 5 weeks) attenuates the development of hypertension in male SHR, Dahl salt-sensitive male rats, and male rats subjected to the two-kidney, one-clip (Goldblatt) maneuver or in male rats subjected to reduced renal mass.[21] Chronic blockade of the androgen receptor with the antagonist flutamide attenuates blood pressure in male SHR to the level found in females. Furthermore, testosterone and dihydrotestosterone are capable of increasing blood pressure in normotensive rats.[23,24]

Evidence that sex steroids impact blood pressure: Role of estrogens

Since male humans and rats have higher blood pressures than do females of both species, it is possible that female hormones may play a role in protecting females from developing higher blood pressures (Box 34–2). In women menopause is characterized by increases in blood pressure as determined by the NHANES III study and others.[9] Interestingly, blood pressure does not increase during the transitional phase from perimenopause to menopause,[25] but rather the increase in blood pressure following menopause takes an average of 5 to 20 years to develop, suggesting that lack of female hormones may not be the only contributing factor to elevated blood pressure. However, salt sensitivity of blood pressure has been shown to increase in women with age,[26] suggesting a role for the loss of estrogens in promoting salt-sensitive hypertension.

Animal studies suggest that estrogens may protect against hypertension. For example, Hinojosa-Laborde et al.[11,27] have reported using telemetry that ovariectomy results in

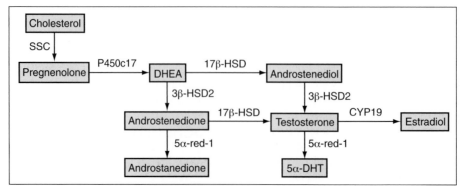

Figure 34–1. Synthesis of sex steroids. CYP19, aromatase; red, reductase; HSD, hydroxysteroid dehydrogenase; P450c17, 17α-hydroxylase; SSC, side chain cleavage enzyme.

Box 34–1

Mechanisms by Which Androgens Could Increase Blood Pressure

- Increase sodium and water reabsorption
- Activate the renin-angiotensin system
- Stimulate endothelin synthesis
- Stimulate oxidative stress

Box 34–2

Mechanisms by Which Estrogens Could Protect Against Hypertension

- Attenuate activation of renin-angiotensin system, reduce expression of AT1 receptors and converting enzyme, upregulate AT2 receptors
- Inhibit endothelin synthesis
- Act as an antioxidant; inhibit NADPH oxidase synthase, leading to reductions in oxidative stress

increased blood pressure in female Dahl salt sensitive rats whether on high- or low-salt diets. Ovariectomy of DOC-salt hypertensive rats also results in higher blood pressure than in intact females treated with DOC and salt.[12]

Abnormal pressure–natriuresis in hypertension: Impact of sex steroids

Substantial evidence supports the theory that some form of renal dysfunction plays a role in the development and maintenance of hypertension.[28] Many studies have demonstrated that "hypertension follows the kidney." For example, Curtis et al.[29] reported that blood pressure returns to normal in hypertensive patients who receive kidneys from normotensive donors. Animal studies have also confirmed that transplantation of the kidney from a hypertensive rat into a normotensive animal results in hypertension.[30] Similar results have been obtained in renal transplantation studies between Dahl salt-sensitive and salt-resistant rats. A common defect that has been characterized in several forms of hypertension is a shift in the pressure–natriuresis relationship. The pressure–natriuresis relationship refers to the fact that increased arterial pressure elicits a marked increase in sodium excretion by the kidney. According to the renal body fluid feedback concept,[28] a long-term increase in arterial pressure or hypertension occurs as a result of reduction in renal excretory function or a rightward shift in the pressure–natriuresis relationship.

Studies in animals have suggested that sex steroids can affect the pressure–natriuresis relationship. For example, the pressure–natriuresis relationship is blunted in male SHR compared to females.[10] Castration of the male SHR

restored the pressure–natriuresis relationship, whereas ovariectomy of female SHR had no effect. Testosterone treatment of ovariectomized female SHR resulted in an increase in blood pressure and a concomitant blunting of the pressure–natriuresis relationship. The androgen receptor is located predominantly in proximal tubule segments of the nephron, and treatment of normotensive rats with dihydrotestosterone increases blood pressure and proximal tubular sodium reabsorption.[24] These data provide initial support for the notion that androgens may have a direct effect on sodium reabsorption in the proximal nephron. Estrogen receptors have also been found in the kidney. Although no studies have been done to determine the biological significance of estrogen receptors in the tubular handling of sodium, it is tempting to speculate that perhaps estrogens may inhibit sodium reabsorption, either directly or via their effect on AT1 receptor expression.

When the kidney from male SHR was transplanted into females, there was not a significant rise in blood pressure, and female SHR with male kidneys had similar blood pressure as female SHR with female kidneys.[30] However, when the kidney from female SHR was transplanted into male SHR, blood pressure was not attenuated compared to blood pressure in a male SHR with male kidneys. These data indicate that the 25 to 30 mmHg higher blood pressure in the male SHR compared to the females is due to an extra-renal factor in the male that further increases blood pressure perhaps due to a reduction in pressure–natriuresis. Thus androgens may be this factor.

Mechanisms by which sex steroids could modulate blood pressure: Effect on renin-angiotensin system

The key system for controlling blood pressure and body fluid volume (i.e., pressure–natriuresis) is the renin-angiotensin system (RAS).[31] Angiotensin II (Ang II) increases proximal sodium reabsorption by the kidney by stimulating epithelial transport. In the event of abnormal Ang II levels for the level of volume in the body, the blood pressure will increase with abnormal sodium and water reabsorption leading to blunting of the pressure–natriuresis relationship. Similarly, if total body fluid volume levels are "perceived" incorrectly and thus Ang II levels do not respond appropriately, increases in blood pressure will also occur.

Sex steroids modulate components of the RAS that may play a role in the control of blood pressure. James et al.[32] measured plasma renin activity (PRA) in men and women over a 9-year period and documented that in this normotensive population, PRA was 27% higher in men than women regardless of age and ethnic heritage. Kaplan et al.[33] reported similar findings. Postmenopausal women also have higher PRA than premenopausal women do.

Estrogens have been shown to downregulate components of the RAS that could impact blood pressure. Ovariectomy of rats increases and estradiol repletion decreases the expression of AT1 receptors in vasculature and kidneys.[34,35] In addition, estradiol reduces the expression and activity of angiotensin I converting enzyme (ACE).[36,37] The reductions in both AT1 receptors and ACE should protect against activation of the RAS. However, estradiol also causes release of angiotensinogen substrate from the liver,[38] and this could offset any potential protective effect if renin enzyme is not working at Vmax, and thus renin activity is increased by increased angiotensinogen substrate leading to increased angiotensin II. However, if renin levels are lower in females than males as indicated by higher PRA in men than women, and since renin is the rate limiting step for Ang II production, females may be expected to have lower circulating and intrarenal Ang II production.

There is evidence that estradiol also affects AT2 receptors in the kidney. Silva-Antonialli et al.[39] reported that female SHR exhibited higher expression of AT2 receptors in the kidney than male SHR. There was no sex difference in expression of AT2 receptors in mesenteric arteries, however. Therefore, since AT2 receptors are thought to be linked to nitric oxide synthase, it is possible that estrogens could modulate blood pressure via AT2 receptor–mediated increases in nitric oxide production.

Animal studies have also supported a role for androgens in modulating components of the RAS. Male SHR have higher PRA than do females, testosterone treatment of ovariectomized female rats causes increases in PRA, and PRA decreases with castration in male rats.[21] Furthermore, there is a linear correlation between the level of serum testosterone and PRA in Sprague Dawley rats treated chronically (2 weeks) with increasing doses of testosterone. Data from two groups have independently shown in SHR and normotensive WKY rats that castration decreases and chronic testosterone treatment increases renal angiotensinogen mRNA.[40,41] Chronically increased renal angiotensinogen could increase renal tissue Ang II if renin enzyme is not working at Vmax, which has been reported in both humans and rats.[42] In support of this hypothesis, studies in mice have demonstrated that an increase in angiotensinogen gene copy numbers cause increases in blood pressure.[43]

The effect of androgens on expression of AT1 and AT2 receptors has not been studied as well as estrogens. However, Silva-Antonialli et al.[39] reported that male SHR had higher levels of AT1 receptors in aorta, mesenterics, and kidney vasculature, whereas AT2 receptor expression was lower in males than females. These data support the concept that androgens may stimulate expression of the vasoconstrictor AT1 receptors and downregulate the expression of the vasodilator AT2 receptors in the kidney.

The RAS has been shown to play an important role in mediating the sex difference in blood pressure in SHR. Chronic blockade with the Ang II–converting enzyme inhibitor enalapril resulted in normalized blood pressure regardless of gender.[23] In male SHR and ovariectomized female SHR treated with testosterone, in which blood pressure was elevated by 30 mmHg, blood pressure decreased by 65% with enalapril, whereas in female, castrated male, and untreated ovariectomized female SHR, blood pressure decreased by only 40%. These data suggest that the RAS plays an important role in mediating hypertension in SHR independent of the sex of the animal, but more importantly that the androgen-promoted exacerbation of the blood pressure in male and testosterone-treated ovariectomized female SHR is also mediated by the RAS.

Another component of the RAS is aldosterone, which is stimulated by Ang II and responsible for increasing sodium reabsorption in the distal nephron. Whether androgens can impact aldosterone synthesis is not clear. There are higher aldosterone levels in men than in women,[44] with a positive correlation between aldosterone levels, dehydroepiandrosterone sulfate (a metabolite of testosterone), and blood pressure in a population of hypertensive men.[45] However, testosterone replacement in castrated male rats decreased corticotropin-stimulated aldosterone release.[46] Whether sex steroids are capable of modulating synthesis of mineralocorticoid receptors is also not clear and will require further study.

Mechanisms by which sex steroids could modulate blood pressure: Effect on endothelin

Endothelin is another vasoconstrictor that has been shown to be affected by sex steroids. For example, in male-to-female transsexuals, estradiol therapy caused a significant reduction in serum endothelin.[47] In premenopausal women, a differential ratio of ET_A to ET_B receptors has also been found, favoring a vasodilator effect of endothelin via ET_B receptors.[48] In recent animal studies, estradiol or its metabolites have been shown to inhibit endothelin synthesis in endothelial cells,[49] and improve endothelial dysfunction in ovariectomized female SHR[50] and DOCA-salt hypertensive rats.[51] We found that postmenopausal SHR exhibit increased endothelin levels, and decreased ET_A and ET_B receptor mRNA in kidney cortex compared with young females.[52] Therefore, estrogens should be cardiovascular protective due to their positive effect on endothelin inhibition.

In contrast, androgens have been shown to cause an increase in endothelin in humans. Female-to-male transsexuals receiving large doses of testosterone have elevated levels of serum endothelin compared to untreated females.[47] Whether androgens affect expression of endothelin receptors is not clear. In any case, androgens could cause increases in blood pressure and endothelial dysfunction leading to CVD by increasing vasoconstrictors.

Mechanisms by which sex steroids could modulate blood pressure: Role in oxidative stress

Sex steroids have been shown to have an effect on oxidative stress either directly or indirectly. Estradiol is a mild antioxidant and protects against oxidative stress,[53] which is thought to be a causative factor in endothelial dysfunction associated with hypertension.[54] Lacy et al.[55] reported that women with essential hypertension had lower levels of plasma hydrogen peroxide than did men. Premenopausal women have also been shown to have lower levels of oxidative stress, as measured by F_2-isoprostanes, than do men[56] or postmenopausal women,[57] which suggests a role for estrogens in the lower levels of oxidative stress. In animal studies, Strehlow et al.[58] found that 17β-estradiol not only reduced Ang II–induced oxidative stress but increased expression of some of the isoforms of superoxide dismutase, an important antioxidant enzyme.

These data were also confirmed by Gragasin et al.[59] in cultured endothelial cells in which estradiol treatment reduced Ang II–mediated expression of NADPH oxidase and peroxynitrite production. The effect of estrogen was independent of the estrogen receptor, however.

There is also evidence that androgens may directly stimulate oxidative stress. Oxidative stress produced by renal intramedullary inhibition of superoxide dismutase has been shown to cause an increase in blood pressure in normotensive rats.[60] Our preliminary data suggest that treatment of mesangial cells from SHR with dihydrotestosterone at physiological doses increases oxidative stress and upregulates expression of $p47^{phox}$, a subunit of NADPH oxidase. $P47^{phox}$ expression is also attenuated in SHR subjected to castration, and NADPH oxidase activity and superoxide production are higher in intact males than castrated males. Furthermore, apocynin, the inhibitor of NADPH oxidase, reduces blood pressure in male SHR, but has no effect on castrated males (Iliescu and Reckelhoff, unpublished observations).

It is also possible that sex steroids could affect oxidative stress indirectly via the RAS. Both supraphysiologic and physiologic doses of Ang II can cause oxidative stress. For example, Rajagopalan et al.[61] found that pharmacologic doses of Ang II (0.7 mg/kg/d s.c. by minipump) increased blood pressure and superoxide levels in aortic segments of rats, while infusion of norepinephrine, which resulted in a similar increase in blood pressure as Ang II, had no effect on superoxide levels. In addition, these investigators found that increased superoxide levels could be normalized with losartan, the Ang II receptor antagonist, or with liposomes containing superoxide dismutase.[61] In further experiments, Ang II increased superoxide production via increased NAD(P)H oxidase activity.[62]

While supraphysiologic doses of Ang II can stimulate oxidative stress, chronic infusion of subpressor doses (i.e., doses that do not elicit an immediate blood pressure response) of Ang II (10 ng/kg/min) for 14 days into normotensive rats that were given enalapril to block endogenous Ang II formation, also result in the slow-onset development of hypertension and an increase in plasma F_2-isoprostanes, an indicator of oxidative stress.[63] It is possible that androgens could stimulate and estrogens could inhibit oxidative stress indirectly by their effect on the RAS.

Sex steroids could also affect oxidative stress indirectly by their effects on endothelin. Endothelin has been shown to cause oxidative stress by upregulating the subunits of NAD(P)H oxidase.[64] In addition, oxidative stress has been shown to upregulate endothelin.[65,66] This would set up a vicious cycle. Therefore, since estrogens have been shown to downregulate endothelin, they should protect against oxidative stress in this way. In contrast, androgens should promote oxidative stress via its effects to upregulate endothelin as described above.

Another effect of androgens is to upregulate thromboxane receptors.[67] Thromboxane receptor number has been shown to increase with testosterone treatment in aortic vascular smooth muscle cells.[67] One of the consequences of oxidative stress is the nonenzymatic synthesis of vasoconstrictor F_2-isoprostanes whose activity is mediated

via thromboxane receptors. F_2-isoprostanes in turn potentiate the vasoconstrictor effects of Ang II and stimulate endothelin production to increase blood pressure even further. Thus androgens could increase the number of thromboxane receptors by which the F_2-isoprostanes cause vasoconstriction. It is doubtful that thromboxanes themselves play any role in mediating higher blood pressure in male SHR, since we have found that male SHR excrete less thromboxane B_2, the stable metabolite of thromboxane A_2, than do females; blockade of the thromboxane receptors, but not thromboxane synthase, reduces blood pressure in male SHR but not in females.[68] Therefore, it is possible that the ligand for the thromboxane receptor in male SHR is F2-isoprostanes, which in turn would amplify the vasoconstrictor effects of Ang II and modulate endothelin synthesis to cause hypertension.

PERSPECTIVES

While there is significant evidence that sex steroids can modulate blood pressure, the mechanisms by which this occurs are not clear. Several clinical trials have shown that certain antihypertensive drugs have better efficacy in men than women and vice versa. For example, angiotensin-converting enzyme inhibitors have been shown to be more effective in men than women,[69] whereas, angiotensin receptor antagonists were more effective in women than men in the Antihypertensive and Lipid-Lowering Treatment to Prevent Heart Attack Trial.[70] Therefore, future clinical trials need to be powered to address sex differences in the responses to antihypertensive drugs in order to determine the most effective treatment for men and women.

Most clinical trials have not shown an antihypertensive effect of antioxidants, and this fact calls into question the role of oxidative stress in mediating hypertension in humans. However, as we have shown previously in hypertensive animals, males and females exhibit different depressor responses to antioxidants and clinical trials, to our knowledge, have not addressed different regimens of antioxidants depending on the sex of the participants. Therefore, future clinical trials will be necessary to determine what antioxidants are beneficial in reducing blood pressure in men compared to women and vice versa.

SUMMARY

This review has critically examined large numbers of fragmentary observations so as to create a coherent set of hypotheses (albeit complicated) by which the sex differences in blood pressure control could be explained. The hypotheses described in Figure 34–2 *A* represent the possible mechanisms by which androgens, mediated via Ang II, endothelin, and oxidative stress could mediate hypertension. As has been shown in animal studies, androgens could promote an increase in blood pressure in males by increasing renal angiotensinogen synthesis and thereby increasing intrarenal renin activity (and thus Ang II). Androgens may also affect the number and affinity of receptors for Ang II affecting sodium reabsorption and/or renal vasoconstriction. Ang II via AT1 receptors could directly cause renal vasoconstric-

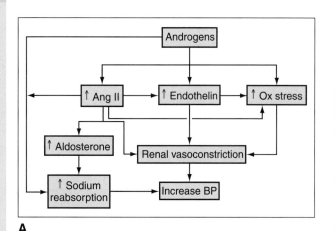

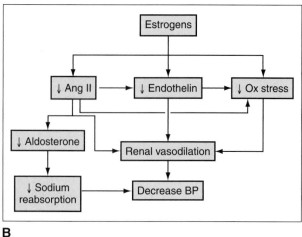

A

B

Figure 34–2. A, Possible mechanisms by which androgens could mediate increases in blood pressure in males. **B,** Possible mechanisms by which estrogens could protect against increases in blood pressure in females. BP, blood pressure; Ox, oxidative.

tion, and also stimulate proximal tubule sodium reabsorption and/or stimulate aldosterone-mediated distal tubule sodium reabsorption, blunt pressure–natriuresis, and increase blood pressure. Alternatively, Ang II could stimulate endothelin production and increase oxidative stress leading to renal vasoconstriction. Androgens may also directly stimulate sodium reabsorption, endothelin production, and/or oxidative stress. The combination of increased sodium reabsorption and renal vasoconstriction would lead to the increase in blood pressure.

As shown in Figure 34–2 *B*, in females, estrogens should inhibit renal Ang II production and AT1 receptor expression compared to males. The reduction in Ang II may decrease both endothelin synthesis and oxidative stress.

Alternatively, estrogens may directly inhibit endothelin synthesis and act as an antioxidant reducing oxidative stress. Another possibility is that estrogens may inhibit sodium reabsorption at the proximal tubule. The role that sex steroids play in control of blood pressure may potentially allow for sex-based treatment of hypertension and CVD in the future.

ACKNOWLEDGEMENT

The studies in this chapter were funded by National Institutes of Health (grants HL05197-11, HL69194, and HL66072).

REFERENCES

1. Liu P, Death A, Handelsman D. Androgens and cardiovascular disease. *Endocr Rev* 2003;24:313–40.
2. Herrington DM. The HERS trial results: paradigms lost? Heart and Estrogen/Progestin Replacement Study. *Ann Intern Med* 1999;131:463–6.
3. Grady D, Herrington D, Bittner V, et al. Cardiovascular disease outcomes during 6.8 years of hormone therapy: Heart and Estrogen/Progestin Replacement Study follow-up (HERS II). *JAMA* 2002;288:49–57.
4. Manson J, Hsia J, Johnson K, et al. Estrogen plus progestin and the risk of coronary heart disease. *N Engl J Med* 2003;349:523–34.
5. Burry KA. Risks and benefits of estrogen plus progestin in healthy postmenopausal women. Principal results from the Women's Health Initiative randomized controlled trial. *Curr Womens Health Rep* 2002;2:331–2.
6. Wiinber N, Hoegholm A, Christensen H, et al. 24-h Ambulatory blood pressure in 352 normal Danish subjects, related to age and gender. *Am J Hypertension* 1995;8:978–86.
7. Khoury S, Yarows, SA, O'Brien TK, Sowers JR. Ambulatory blood pressure monitoring in a nonacademic setting.

Effects of age and sex. *Am J Hypertension* 1992;5:616–23.
8. Staessen J, Fagard R, Lijnen P, et al. References values for ambulatory blood pressure: a meta-analysis. *J Hypertension* 1990;8:S57–64.
9. Burl VL, Whelton P, Roccella EJ, et al. Prevalence of hypertension in the US adult population. Results from the Third National Health and Nutrition Examination Survey, 1988–1991. *Hypertension* 1995;25:305–13.
10. Reckelhoff JF, Zhang H, Granger JP. Testosterone exacerbates hypertension and reduces pressure–natriuresis in male spontaneously hypertensive rats. *Hypertension* 1998;31:435–9.
11. Hinojosa-Laborde C, Lange DL, Haywood JR. Role of female sex hormones in the development and reversal of Dahl hypertension. *Hypertension* 2000;35:484–9.
12. Crofton JT, Share L. Gonadal hormones modulate deoxycorticosterone-salt hypertension in male and female rats. *Hypertension* 1997;29:494–9.
13. Ashton NB, Balment RJ. Sexual dimorphism in renal function and hormonal status of New Zealand genetically hypertensive rats. *Acta Endocrinol (Copenh)* 1991;124:91–7.

14. Calhoun DA, Oparil S. The sexual dimorphism of high blood pressure. *Cardiol Rev* 1998;6:356–63.
15. Black B, Paschal B. Intranuclear organization and function of the androgen receptor. *Trends Endocrinol Metab* 2004;15:411–7.
16. Barkhem T, Nilsson S, Gustafsson J. Molecular mechanisms, physiological consequences and pharmacological implications of estrogen receptor action. *Am J Pharmacogenomics* 2004;4:19–28.
17. Bachmann H, Horacek U, Leowsky M, Hirche H. Blood pressure in children and adolescents aged 4 to 18. Correlation of blood pressure values with age, sex, body height, body weight, and skinfold thickness. *Monatsschr Kinderheilkunde* 1987;135:128–34.
18. Harshfield GA, Alpert BS, Pulliam DA, et al. Ambulatory blood pressure recordings in children and adolescents. *Pediatrics* 1994;94:180–4.
19. Talbott E, Guzick D, Clerici A, et al. Coronary heart disease risk factors in women wih polycystic ovary syndrome. *Arterioscler Thromb Vasc Biol* 1995;15:821–6.
20. Mattson LAC, Hamberger L, Samsioe G, Silverstolpe G. Lipid metabolism in women with polycystic ovary syndrome:

possible implications for an increased risk of coronary heart disease. *Fertil Steril* 1984;42:579–84.

21. Reckelhoff JF. Gender differences in the regulation of blood pressure. *Hypertension* 2001;37:1199–208.

22. Reckelhoff JF, Zhang H, Srivastava K, Granger JP. Gender differences in hypertension in spontaneously hypertensive rats. Role of androgens and androgen receptor. *Hypertension* 1999;34:920–3.

23. Reckelhoff JF, Zhang H, Srivastava K. Gender differences in the development of hypertension in SHR: role of the renin-angiotensin system. *Hypertension* 2000;35:480–3.

24. Quan A, Chakravarty S, Chen J-K, et al. Androgens augment proximal tubule transport. *Am J Physiol Renal Physiol* 2004;287:F452–9.

25. Luoto R, Sharrett AR, Schreiner P, et al. Blood pressure and menopause transition: the Atherosclerosis Risks in Communities study (1987–1995). *J Hypertens* 2000;18:27–33.

26. Weinberger MH, Fineberg NS. Sodium and volume sensitivity of blood pressure. Age and pressure change over time. *Hypertension* 1991;18:67–71.

27. Hinojosa-Laborde C, Craig T, Zheng W, et al. Ovariectomy augments hypertension in aging female Dahl salt-sensitive rats. *Hypertension* 2004;44:405 (Epub ahead of print).

28. Guyton AC, Coleman TG, Cowley AW Jr, et al. Arterial pressure regulation: overriding dominance of the kidneys in long-term regulation and in hypertension. *Am J Med* 1972;52:584–94.

29. Curtis JJ, Luke HP, Dustan HP, et al. Remission of hypertension after renal transplantation. *N Engl J Med* 1983;309:1009–15.

30. Harrap SB, Wang BZ, MacClellan DG. Renal transplantation between male and female spontaneously hypertensive rats. *Hypertension* 1992;19:431–4.

31. Hall JE, Brands MJ, Henegar JR. Angiotensin II and long-term arterial pressure regulation: the overriding dominance of the kidney. *J Am Soc Nephrol* 1999;10:S258–65.

32. James GD, Sealey JE, Muller F, et al. Renin relationship to sex, race and age in normotensive population. *J Hypertens* 1986;4 (Suppl 5):S387-S389.

33. Kaplan NM, Kem DC, Holland OB. the intravenous furosemide test: a simple way to evaluate renin responsiveness. *Ann Intern Med* 1976;4: 639–45.

34. Nickenig G, Baumer AT, Grohe C, et al. Estrogen modulates AT1 receptor gene expression in vitro and in vivo. *Circulation* 1998;97:2197–201.

35. Harrison-Bernard L, Schulman I, Raij L. Postovariectomy hypertension is linked to increased renal AT1 receptor and salt sensitivity. *Hypertension* 2003;42:1157–63.

36. Dubey RK, Oparil S, Imthurn B, Jackson EK. Sex hormones and hypertension. *Cardiovasc Res* 2002;53:688–708.

37. Gallagher P, Li P, Lenhart J, et al. Estrogen regulation of angiotensin-converting enzyme mRNA. *Hypertension* 1999;33:323–8.

38. Stavreus-Evers A, Parini P, Freyschuss B, et al. Estrogenic influence on the regulation of hepatic estrogen receptor-alpha and serum level of angiotensinogen in female rats. *J Steroid Biochem Mol Biol* 2001;78:83–8.

39. Silva-Antonialli M, Tostes R, Fernandes L, et al. A lower ratio of AT1/AT2 receptors of angiotensin II is found in female than male spontaneously hypertensive rats. *Cardiovasc Res* 2004;62:587–93.

40. Ellison KE, Ingelfinger JR, Pivor M, Dzau VJ. Androgen regulation of rat renal angiotensinogen messenger RNA expression. *J Clin Invest* 1989;83:1941–5.

41. Chen Y-F, Naftilan AJ, Oparil S. Androgen-dependent angiotensinogen and renin messenger RNA expression in hypertensive rats. *Hypertension* 1992;19:456–63.

42. Johnston CL, Fabris B, Jandeleit K. Intrarenal renin-angiotensin system in renal physiology and pathophysiology. *Kidney Int* 1993;44 (Suppl 42):S59–63.

43. Smithies O. A mouse view of hypertension. *Hypertension* 1997;30:1318–24.

44. Miller JA, Anacta LA, Cattran C. Impact of gender on the renal response to angiotensin II. *Kidney Int* 1999;55:278–85.

45. Schunkert H, Hense HW, Andus T, et al. Relation between dehydroepiandrosterone sulfate and blood pressure levels in a population-based sample. *Am J Hypertens* 1999;12:1140–3.

46. Kau MM, Lo MJ, Wang SW, et al. Inhibition of aldosterone production by testosterone in male rats. *Metabolism* 1999;48:1108–14.

47. van Kesteren PJ, Kooistra T, Lansink M, et al. The effects of sex steroids on plasma levels of marker proteins of endothelial cell functioning. *Thromb Haemost* 1998;79:1029–33.

48. Ergul A, Shoemaker K, Puett D, Tackett RL. Gender differences in the expression of endothelin receptors in human saphenous veins in vitro. *J Pharmacol Exp Ther* 1998;285:511–7.

49. Dubey R, Jackson E, Keller P, et al. Estradiol metabolites inhibit endothelin synthesis by an estrogen receptor-independent mechanism. *Hypertension* 2001;37:640–4.

50. Widder J, Pelzer T, von Poser-Klein C, et al. Improvement of endothelial dysfunction by selective estrogen receptor-alpha stimulation of ovariectomized SHR. *Hypertension* 2003;42:991–6.

51. David FL, Carvalho MH, Cobra AL, et al. Ovarian hormones modulate endothelin-1 vascular reactivity and mRNA expression in DOCA-salt hypertensive rats. *Hypertension* 2001;38:692–6.

52. Yanes LL, Romero D, Cucchiarelli VE, et al. Role of endothelin in mediating postmenopausal hypertension in a rat model. *Am J Physiol Reg Integ Comp Physiol* 2005;288:R229–33.

53. Dantas A, Tostes R, Fortes A, et al. In vivo evidence for antioxidant potential of estrogen in microvessels of female spontaneously hypertensive rats. *Hypertension* 2002;39:405–11.

54. Hamilton C, Brosnan M, McIntyre M, et al. Superoxide excess in hypertension and aging: a common cause of endothelial dysfunction. *Hypertension* 2001;37:529–34.

55. Lacy F, O'Connor D, Schmid-Schonbein G. Plasma hydrogen peroxide is hypertensive and normotensive subjects at genetic risk of hypertension. *J Hypertension* 1998;16:291–303.

56. Ide T, Tsutsui H, Ohashi N, et al. Greater oxidative stress in healthy young men compared with premenopausal women. *Arterioscler Thromb Vasc Biol* 2002;22:1239–42.

57. Helmersson J, Mattsson P, Basu S. Prostaglandin F(2alpha) metabolite and F2-isoprostane excretion in migraine. *Clin Sci (Lond)* 2002;102:39–43.

58. Strehlow K, Rotter S, Wassmann S, et al. Modulation of antioxidant enzyme expression and function by estrogen. *Circ Res* 2003;93:170–7.

59. Gragasin F, Xu Y, Arenas I, et al. Estrogen reduces angiotensin-II–induced nitric oxide synthase and NAD(P)H oxidase expression in endothelial cells. *Arterioscler Thromb Vasc Biol* 2003;23:38–44.

60. Makino A, Skelton M, Zou A, et al. Increased renal medullary oxidative stress produces hypertension. *Hypertension* 2002;39:667–72.

61. Rajagopalan K, Kurz S, Munzel T, et al. Angiotensin II-mediated hypertension in the rat increases vascular superoxide production via membrane NADH/NADPH oxidase activation. Contribution to alterations of vasomotor tone. *J Clin Invest* 1996;97:1916–23.

62. Mollnau H, Wendt M, Szocs K, et al. Effects of angiotensin II infusion on the expression and function of NAD(P)H oxidase and components of nitric oxide/cGMP signaling. *Circ Res* 2002;90:E58–65.

63. Reckelhoff JF, Romero JC. Role of oxidative stress in angiotensin-induced hypertension. *Am J Physiol Regul Integr Comp Physiol* 2003;284:R893–912.

64. Duerrschmidt N, Wippich N, Goettsch W, et al. Endothelin-1 induces NAD(P)H oxidase in human endothelial cells. *Biochem Biophys Res Commun* 2000;269:713–7.

65. Kaehler J, Sill B, Koester R, et al. Endothelin-1 mRNA and protein in vascular wall cells is increased by reactive oxygen species. *Clin Sci (Lond)* 2002;103(Suppl 48):176S–8S.

66. Yura T, Fukunaga M, Kahn R, et al. Free-radical-generated F2-isoprostane stimulates cell proliferation and endothelin-1 expression on endothelial cells. *Kidney Int* 1999;56:471–8.

67. Masuda A, Mathur R, Halushka PV. Testosterone increases thromboxane A2 receptors in cultured rat aortic smooth muscle cells. *Circ Res* 1991;69:638–43.

68. Acosta Cazal MC, Fortepiani LA, Reckelhoff, JF. Gender differences in control of blood pressure: role of thromboxane receptors. *Gender Med* 2004;1:100–5.

69. Wing L, Reid C, Ryan P, et al. A comparison of outcomes with angiotensin-converting-enzyme inhibitors and diuretics for hypertension in the elderly. *N Engl J Med* 2003;348:583–92.

70. ALLHAT Officers and Coordinators for the ALLHAT Collaborative Research Group. Major outcomes in high-risk hypertensive patients randomized to angiotensin-converting enzyme inhibitor or calcium channel blocker vs diuretic: the Antihypertensive and Lipid-Lowering Treatment to Prevent Heart Attack Trial (ALLHAT). *JAMA* 2002;288:2981–97.

Chapter

35

Genetic Approaches to Hypertension: Relevance to Human Hypertension

Carlo Giansante and Nicola Fiotti

Key Findings

- Offspring of persons with hypertension have a 3.5-fold increased risk of having high blood pressure, and the risk is doubled when a sibling has hypertension.

- Hypertension is a multifactorial disease, in which a polygenic model interacts with the environment. A polygenic model is a model in which many small equal and additive loci would result in a Gaussian distribution for a phenotype.

- Mapping and candidate gene strategies do not show reproducible and consistent results in identifying the genes affecting hypertension.

- Several factors (such as polygenic inheritance, heterogeneity, epistasis, and developmental effects) hamper assessment of these genetic variants.

Clinicians have known intuitively for more than three decades that essential hypertension (EH) has a hereditary component. This intuitive knowledge was clinically demonstrated in the early 1990s. Ravogli et al., in a very small group of subjects (15 normotensive subjects whose parents were both hypertensive, 15 normotensive subjects with one hypertensive parent, and 15 normotensive subjects whose parents were not hypertensive), demonstrated that individuals whose parents were affected by hypertension had higher ambulatory blood pressure than those whose parents were not. The authors concluded that the higher blood pressure shown by individuals with a positive family history of parental hypertension reflected not a hyperreactivity to stress but rather an early permanent blood pressure elevation.[1]

A stronger demonstration was offered by Dekkers et al.[2], who in a longitudinal study explored the influence of genetic susceptibility to EH in youth. This study recruited 745 subjects (mean age 12 years; range 4.9 to 23.9 years) and followed them for a 10-year period with annual blood pressure measurements. Family history of EH was defined as the occurrence of EH in one or both biological parents. The results showed that compared to subjects without a family history for EH those with a family history developed hypertension earlier, had higher systolic blood pressure (SBP) readings from childhood to adulthood, and had a greater increase in SBP when growing older. The effect of genetic susceptibility to EH was independent of sex and ethnicity, being the same for African American and European American males and females. Such results, though convincing, suffer from both the rough definition of family history and the infeasibility of disaggregating family history from shared familial environments. The latter is one of the difficulties still encountered in assessing the genetic variations related to EH.

The identification of genes underlying Mendelian disorders has been enhanced significantly over the last decades by extraordinary achievements in gene mapping and the development of meticulous statistical methods. Such technological advances promoted several studies of EH, which is an important public health problem, with 25% of the adult population being affected in industrialized countries. Despite several years of meticulous and well-designed research, however, our knowledge about causes and mechanisms of EH is largely incomplete.

The aim of researching genetic variations related to hypertension goes beyond the better understanding of the pathophysiology of the disease. It involves several other relevant goals, such as the recognition of subjects at risk of developing EH before the onset of clinical symptoms, understanding the interaction between genes and environmental factors, and the customization of drug therapy according the specific genotype so that administration of available drugs can be tailored to the individual.

From the very beginning, genetic epidemiologic studies clearly indicated that a plain Mendelian pattern of inheritance (in which a single gene mutation causes early onset of hypertension) occurs only in rare familial syndromes, whereas the vast majority of cases of EH are due to several genetic variants. The contributions of genetic variants to the overall blood pressure levels in general population is really small. For example, apparent mineralocorticoid excess (AME) (hypertension, polydipsia/polyuria, severe hypokalemia, and metabolic alkalosis)—a syndrome attributable to the mutation in the gene encoding 11β-hydroxysteroid dehydrogenase type 2—has been diagnosed in only 40 patients worldwide in the past 20 years.[3]

The role of genes derives from the many and interrelated mechanisms accounting for the development of EH, such as salt sensitivity, fluid balance, impaired glucose tolerance, and obesity. If only a part of these mechanisms has a genetic regulation, a large number of genes (rather than a single gene) would be expected to explain the inheritability of this complex disease. In patients with hypertension, several patterns of genetic variations could then be found (compared to those without this condition)—making the interpretation of the results complex. Moreover, considering the interaction of many mechanisms it is also possible that the phenotypic effects of some genetic variations are concealed by some compensatory mechanisms.

With at least 30,000 genes in the human genome and the characterization of these genes in progress, the challenge is to break down the complexity of genetic disorders (e.g., diabetes, schizophrenia, and cancer), including hypertension.[4] This chapter reviews present identified genetic variations that may contribute to the onset of EH, with particular attention on search strategies and likely future developments. A glossary of terms is given in Box 35–1.

Box 35–1

Glossary of Terms

- *Allele:* One of the variant forms of a gene at a particular locus (location) on a chromosome.
- *Candidate gene:* A gene, located in a chromosome region suspected of being involved in a disease, whose protein product suggests that it could be the disease gene in question.
- *Domain:* A specific region or amino acid sequence in a protein associated with a particular function or corresponding segment of DNA.
- *Gene:* The functional and physical unit of heredity passed from parent to offspring.
- *Genetic code (ATCG):* The instructions in a gene that tell the cell how to make a specific protein. A, T, G, and C are the "letters" of the DNA code. They stand for the chemicals adenine, thymine, guanine, and cytosine, respectively, which make up the nucleotide bases of DNA. Each gene's code combines the four chemicals in various ways to spell out three-letter "words" that specify which amino acid is needed at every step in making a protein.
- *Haploid:* The number of chromosomes in a sperm or egg cell, half the diploid number.
- *Linkage:* The association of genes and/or markers that lie near each other on a chromosome. Linked genes and markers tend to be inherited together.
- *Locus:* The place on a chromosome where a specific gene is located; a type of address for the gene.
- *Mendelian inheritance:* Manner in which genes and traits are passed from parents to children.
- *Microsatellite:* Repetitive stretches of short sequences of DNA used as genetic markers to track inheritance in families.
- *Polymorphism:* A common variation in the sequence of DNA among individuals.
- *Promoter:* The part of a gene that contains the information to turn the gene on or off. The process of transcription is initiated at the promoter.
- *Substitution:* Replacement of one nucleotide in a DNA sequence by another nucleotide, or replacement of one amino acid in a protein by another amino acid.

GENETIC ANALYSIS OF BLOOD PRESSURE VARIABILITY: THE METHODS

Human DNA consists of a double string of three billion base pairs. They are organized in 23 pairs of chromosome within a 2-μm nucleus. The compacted DNA is 50,000 times shorter than its extended length. In the extended form, human genomic DNA would be a little over 6 feet long. If it were a ladder with each rung one foot apart, it would be 568,000 miles long. To view this in perspective, the distance between the earth and the moon is about 240,000 miles and the circumference of the earth at the equator is 25,000 miles. Within these 6 billion nucleotides there are approximately 30,000 to 40,000 protein-coding genes. The gene coding regions in the human actually make up less than 5% of the 6 billion nucleotides. The function of the remaining 95% of the DNA is not clear.

Alterations of DNA provide an important way of ensuring survival of populations in the event of environmental changes. Availability of genes with alternative products (so-called thrifty genes) within a population has been a resource for the species because it allows a reduction in food availability to be overcome, facilitating survival during environmental changes. This could lend an evolutionary advantage over other species and may help to colonize new environments. It is well demonstrated that genetic material of all species changes spontaneously and this leaves some mutated versions of the genes in the population. The pressure of selection can then act, expanding alleles beneficial for evolution or disposing of those hindering it.

Mutations are important because they are the major source of the genetic variation that fuels evolutionary change. As it is, replication errors by the cells' machinery tend to be fairly rare, occurring in only about 1 out of every 10^{-9} base-pair replications. From studies *in vivo* and other studies using human cells *in vitro*, the overall human mutation rate is estimated to be about 1×10^{-6} per gene per generation. This rate is similar to those measured in various prokaryotic and eukaryotic microorganisms. The estimated human mutation rate can be used to determine its impact on the likelihood of changes occurring in each generation. A rate of 1×10^{-6} mutations/gene $\times$ 3×10^{4} genes/haploid genome equals 3×10^{-2} mutations per gamete (=3/100 or 1/33). 1/33 $\times$ 2 gametes per zygote implies a 6/100 chance that each zygote carries a new mutation somewhere in the genome. This seems like a very high number, but one needs to remember that most mutations are recessive and thus will not be expressed in the heterozygous condition.

Changes within the human genome occur mainly for missense/nonsense mutations, deletions, splicing, insertion/duplication, and less frequent mutations that will be established within the genome of a population provided they are not a limitation for the carrier. Their prevalence is recognized as a mutation when its allelic frequency is less than 1% and a polymorphism when its prevalence is higher. An estimation of genome variability can come from the number of single nucleotide changes within the genome. In January of 2005, more than 5 million single-nucleotide polymorphisms (SNPs) have been submitted and validated at the Single Nucleotide Polymorphism NCBI database (*http://www.ncbi.nlm.nih.gov/SNP/snp_summary.cgi*). The data are constantly increasing. In 2001, the figure was about 2.1 million unique SNPs[5] and the public SNP consortium identified 1.4 million.[6] Marth et al.[7,8] report false-positive rates of 10 to 15%, although false negatives are of greater concern.[8] Fortunately, only a minor number of SNPs occur within genes and less than 1% in regulatory regions. In the human gene mutation database, 52,165 mutations within genes had been reported up to 2005. Identifying gene variants that contribute to hypertension may not only provide better understanding of the pathophysiology of the disease but elucidate the biochemical and pathophysiologic pathways that link various risk factors in hypertension.

Definition of the trait

Hypertension is defined as a clinical syndrome (a condition, not a pathologic identity) characterized by a stable increase of systolic and/or diastolic blood pressure above defined values. The blood pressure level used as a benchmark for a diagnosis of hypertension has changed in the last few years, making it somewhat awkward to analyze this trait as a discrete variable. Moreover, use of terms signifying different degrees of hypertension (borderline, mild, or severe) might further confuse the picture. The studies of genetic susceptibility to hypertension have to deal with an important issue, which is the precise definition of the condition.

During the 1960s, a heated debate between Sir George Pickering[9] and Sir Robert Platt[10] arose over the question of whether hypertension is a quantitative upper tail of a continuous distribution of blood pressure, and thus determined by a number of genes, or a qualitative trait due to an effect of a single major gene. At present, we can say that both Sir George and Sir Robert were right. Although several monogenic forms of hypertension have been clearly identified, EH is now understood as being a polygenic disease with complexities such as gene-gene and environment-gene interactions.

A careful definition of the condition sought is mandatory in avoiding contradictory and unsatisfactory results. The definition of hypertension established in May of 2005 by the American Society of Hypertension (*http://www.ash-us.org*) as a "progressive cardiovascular syndrome arising from complex and interrelated etiologies" is of little help in advancing comprehension, and from the research point of view confirms that genetic studies can be very complex and difficult. Lack of knowledge is reflected by a vague definition and the consequence is poor results. Two options in definition of the trait (qualitative and quantitative) are possible, but neither one perfectly reflects our definition of the condition as a pathophysiologic state—allowing us to recollect gene expression etiology and clinical conditions. Factors responsible for increased SBP might be different from those accounting for increased diastolic blood pressure. Even considering the mean blood pressure, other variables (e.g., heart rate) should be taken into account—thus complicating the overall picture. In turn, all factors (vessel compliance, vascular tone, baroceptor regulation, and so on) influencing each aspect of the trait (systolic or diastolic blood pressure) are subject to very strict regulation by environmental and genetic controls.

Even considering hypertension as a quantitative trait (i.e., high blood pressure), some problems could arise. In particular, analysis of genes involved in blood pressure regulation might encompass alleles involved in regulation within the physiologic range of pressure but not in extreme values.[11] Present data focus mainly on these definitions, although recently some other intermediate phenotypes (i.e., characteristics or features such as paradox hypertension, salt sensitivity, and postural changes) alleged to be more simply regulated have been published.

Investigative tools

Genetic epidemiology is a science born in the 1960s that encompasses classical epidemiology, statistics, and genetics. This science can answer several important questions about the genetic aspects of hypertension.

- Are there some genetic components influencing the presence of hypertension?
- What is the relative size of the genetic effect on hypertension, compared to nongenetically influenced effects (typically environmental)?
- What and where are the genetic components responsible?

Many studies have been published on these issues, each considering the effect of several biases and confounding factors (e.g., interaction of the phenotype with environment, genetic background, and other co-inheritable conditions such as type II diabetes and obesity). These variables require independent replication of the studies before a definite conclusion can be drawn. The types of studies used to answer to these three questions include genetic risk studies, segregation analysis, linkage studies, and association studies.

Genetic risk studies

These studies aim to assess the genetic components and distinguish between genetic and environmental factors. This task is particularly difficult to achieve for a condition such as hypertension, in which ethnic or genetic background could be linked to environmental factors. The typical approach is to study hypertension transmittance in families, siblings, or separately adopted twins.

Segregation analysis

After observing the risk of developing the condition due to genetic components, the next step is to assess its type (i.e., one gene with an important effect, few genes each with a moderate effect, many genes each with a small effect, or even a combination of these) and the transmission model of the genetic trait. For this step, multigenerational family trees are required to determine the type of inheritance. Segregation analysis is particularly useful when there are substantial numbers of affected subjects in each family.[12]

Linkage studies

These studies aim to detect where genetic components affecting hypertension are located within the human genome. This approach has been greatly helped by the recent completion of the map of human genome. The principle is the cosegregation of two genes/loci (one of which is the disease locus) with measurable genomic recombination between them. The method involves comparison of the genome of siblings and/or relatives. A statistical approach to the analysis of the linkage can consider some parameters (such as penetrance or disease allele frequency) of the inheritance, which is called parametric (and nonparametric when inheritance is not considered).

Association studies

Association studies analyze the allele associated with disease susceptibility, the principle being that the prevalence of a certain marker will be higher in affected compared to nonaffected individuals. Association studies may be family based (transmission/disequilibrium test, or TDT; also called transmission distortion test) or population based, such as the candidate gene approach. Alleles, haplotypes, or evolutionary-based haplotype groups may be used in association studies.

GENETIC RISK STUDIES

The relationship between genes and hypertension can be assessed in several ways. The first assessment is the degree of association in families and the eventual interferences played by the environment. These studies require nuclear families (index case and parents), affected relative pairs (siblings, cousins, any two members of the family), extended pedigrees, twins (monozygotic and dizygotic), and unrelated population samples. This type of approach is called familial aggregation (e.g., higher occurrence rates in siblings or offspring). Other traditional designs for distinguishing nongenetic shared family effects from genetic effects are the studies of twins.

Familial aggregation

Familial aggregation for a disease is measured by the relative recurrence risk (RRR) or familial risk ratio (FRR). These represent the probability that a particular type of relative (sibling, cousin, and so on) of an affected proband has a disease, divided by the prevalence of the disease in general population. These are quantities denoted by λ_R, where R denotes a relationship (S = siblings, O = offspring, DZ = dizygotic twin, and so on) and whose values are the risks of relatives of type R of affected individuals being themselves affected divided by the population prevalence.

In hypertension, RRR (i.e., λ_S) is ~3.5 (12), whereas λ_O is ~2. λ in other relatives is strongly influenced by ethnic and environmental confounding, making its estimation less reliable. No clear evidence on sex chromosomes has been gathered so far, nor has any for half-siblings. Therefore, although there is evidence of familial aggregation in hypertension it is not sufficient to infer the importance of genetic susceptibility because environmental and cultural influences can also aggregate in families—leading to family clustering and excess familial risk. A similar environment is a major confounding factor in familial aggregation.

Investigation into the environmental component of blood pressure regulation is far from over. Several factors hinder a precise estimate of family aggregation. They can be related to the timing of assessment or to strong interaction of blood pressure with the surrounding environment. Among the possible examples is the change in the rate of concordance and age of offspring. For DBP, an apparent reduction in heritability from 68 to 38% from young adulthood to middle age results from the increasing impact of individual environmental experience, with little or no influence from shared family environment.[13] A strong interaction between blood pressure and environment, also within the same family, is the conclusion of two studies[13,14] in which a significant correlation in blood pressure between spouses has been demonstrated even after standardization for important environmental variables such as education, socioeconomic status, smoking, exercise, age, and salt consumption.[13] Fava et al.[15] made the interesting and paradigmatic observation that although many intermediate phenotypes of hypertension could be inherited this is untrue for office measurements, the usual way of diagnosing hypertension.

Twin studies

The study of hypertension in two distinct individuals sharing the same genetic background is a valued opportunity to differentiate the effects of environment and genes. To estimate the genetic contribution to a trait, the comparison of monozygotic (MZ) pairs (who share all their genes) with dizygotic (DZ) twins (who share half their genes) has been traditionally used. The greater similarity of MZ twins compared to DZ twins is considered evidence of genetic factors. In theory, complete genetic determination of a disease would equate to MZ twins having 100% concordance and DZ twins having 50% concordance. The usual assumptions of a classic twin study are random mating, no interactions between genes and environment, and equivalent environments for MZ and DZ twins or the sharing to an equal extent of the environmental experiences of the two types of twins that are relevant for the development of the trait.

In studying a complex trait, phenotypic variance is divided into these components: inheritability, a component due to inherited genetic factors (A), a shared environmental component due to environmental factors common to both members of the pair of twins (C), and a nonshared environmental component due to environmental factors unique to each twin (E), being $1 = A^2 + C^2 + E^2$. All available data on these studies are subject to interethnic, age, and sex differences. A standard measure of similarity for a discrete variable used in twin studies is the concordance rate. This can be pairwise (Pr) or probandwise (Cc).[16] The Pr concordance is a descriptive statistic and simply gives the proportion of affected pairs that are concordant for the disease. It is calculated as the proportion of twin pairs (with both twins affected) of all ascertained twin pairs with at least one affected: Pr = C/(C+D), where C is the number of concordant pairs and D is the number of discordant pairs. The probandwise (Cc) concordance is the proportion of affected individuals among the co-twins of previously ascertained index cases. It allows for double counting of doubly ascertained twin pairs and has the advantage of being interpretable as the recurrence risk in a co-twin of an affected individual. The following formula is used in estimation: $Cc = 2C/(2C+D)$. Concordance rate in hypertension depends on categorizing hypertension as a dichotomous variable. In this case, however, the pairwise concordance rate was .36 and .08 in MZ and DZ twins, respectively, and probandwise concordance could be estimated as .53 and .07, respectively, in a Norwegian twin cohort.[17]

Other factors must be considered in this assessment as expressions of the increasing environmental role in blood pressure regulation (e.g., age at separation as an expression of increased influence of nonshared environmental component). An intrauterine environmental component such as the circulatory system might represent a first step in this evaluation. Chorionicity (i.e., the sharing of some circulatory system during intrauterine life) does not seem to influence blood pressure regulation in adult twins,[18] but in a Japanese twins cohort the intrapair concordance rate for blood pressure decreased from 0.78 (age of separation 26 and over) to 0.51 (age of separation 0 to 5) as the age of separation decreased.[19] Therefore, a unique and precise estimate of the rate of concordance is impossible to obtain. In spite of this, some other interesting data can be obtained comparing the correlation of blood pressure. Solid evidence exists showing that concordance (correlation) of SBP in MZ twins is ~0.8, whereas in DZ twins it is ~0.46 (19;20) or 0.60 and ~0.30 according to different studies[20–23] (Table 35–1).

One study in Caucasians has evaluated the effects of shared and nonshared environmental factors. Although the inheritability of hypertension in this study is about 50%, a larger proportion of nonshared environmental influences affect both systolic (.07 and .46 for shared and nonshared, respectively) and diastolic blood pressure (.08 and .41, respectively).[21]

Snieder et al. and others focused on inheritability of hypertension in African (AA) and European American (EA) twins. SBP levels were comparable in the two groups,

as was the estimated inheritability of about 57%. The environmental component accounted for the remaining 43%. Negligible differences could be detected after standardization for body mass index (BMI) and were equal in AAs and EAs. On the contrary, diastolic blood pressure was higher in AAs, compared to EAs with an increased estimated heritability: 0.58 in AAs and 0.45 in EAs.[22]

Migration studies

Although migration studies can be of interest in many diseases, in hypertension they have been controversial because blood pressure as a physiologic variable might change even with migration within the same environment (thus inducing an overestimation of the environmental effect). Although this might argue against a genetic control (showing an increase in blood pressure with no changes in genome), it should instead be seen as a typical gene/ environment interaction that reflects poorly the mechanisms of blood pressure regulation. One study showed an increase in blood pressure for both men and women. The previously cited differences were only partially explained by age, BMI, heart rate, smoking, and alcohol use. This study demonstrates an important effect of migration on the rise in blood pressure with age and on the prevalence of hypertension but is not of much help in evaluation of environmentally induced changes in hypertension.[24]

SEGREGATION ANALYSIS

After assessing and quantifying the genetic risk in hypertension (i.e., the role of genes in both blood pressure regulation and hypertension in families), the next step is to define its mode of inheritance. The previously cited RRRs within families may provide an estimation of the possible segregation modes, but only segregation analysis using maximum likelihood techniques are suitable in evaluating hypotheses representing different sources of genetic influence.

Segregation analysis aims to find a similar inheritance pattern among families by looking at multigenerational family data. Segregation analysis is suitable for revealing Mendelian inheritance patterns (autosomal or sex-linked and recessive or dominant), non-classical inheritance (mitochondrial diseases, genomic imprinting, parent of origin effect, genetic anticipation, and so on), or nonMendelian inheritance (no pattern). An important issue addressed by this analysis is about the number of genes affecting hypertension. Is it a single major gene (oligogene) or many genes of small effect (polygenes)? Further components of a genetic model (transmission probabilities, penetrance of each genotype, and allele frequencies in the population) might or might not be known. Accordingly, statistical methods can take into account or not (model free) frequencies and penetrance of disease. The methods usually look for segregation analysis in families, and large multigenerational families are of course more informative than small ones.

A potential pitfall is that segregation analysis is most useful in single-gene disorders due to a biallelic gene, but

CORRELATION COEFFICIENTS OF ARTERIAL OF BLOOD PRESSURE OF MONOZYGOTIC (MZ) AND DIZYGOTIC (DZ) TWINS		Systolic		Diastolic	
Study	Group	MZ	DZ	MZ	DZ
Luft [20]	Caucasians	0.82	0.46	N/A	N/A
Snieder [22]	Caucasians	0.59	0.42	0.44	–0.05
Snieder [22]	African Americans	0.65	0.35	0.61	0.40
McCaffery [21]	Caucasians	0.54	0.31	0.62	0.33
Tambs [23]	Caucasians	0.52	0.19	0.43	0.23
Average		0.62	0.35	0.53	0.23

Table 35–1. Correlation coefficients of arterial blood pressure of monozygotic (MZ) and dizygotic (DZ) twins.

when multiple loci with multiple alleles are involved (as in most complex diseases) it becomes less powerful and the results have to be cautiously interpreted. Moreover, there is a risk in analyzing families for complex traits such as hypertension of putting together different families with different origins for their conditions and thus obtaining a confused picture of inheritance. Segregation analysis is a prerequisite for linkage analyses. Development of more powerful and complete statistical packages might help in understanding the inheritance of the trait.

The most complete and recent study on essential hypertension comes from Crockford et al.[25] After Pickering, they performed the analysis considering segregation analysis under the liability model of hypertensive status as a qualitative trait and compared this with results using systolic blood pressure as a quantitative trait. Both analyses, qualitative (hypertension) and quantitative (systolic and diastolic blood pressure), identified models with major genes and polygenic components to explain the family aggregation of SBP. Neither one of the methods (qualitative or quantitative) estimated precisely the parameters, but both identified the most complicated model evaluated as the most accurate. The conclusion is that the true model is considerably more complicated than those available for the analysis. The important finding is that segregation analysis of hypertension using relatively simple models is unlikely to provide accurate parameter estimates because of polygenic components.

Forms of hypertension with a very clear inheritance pattern further complicate the scenario. These are called Mendelian forms of hypertension due to the clear pattern and are briefly reported in material following. As mentioned previously, the Mendelian forms are very rare. There are six single-gene (or Mendelian) forms of hypertension: Liddle syndrome, apparent mineralocorticoid excess (AME), glucocorticoid-remediable aldosteronism (GRA), mineralocorticoid-receptor-activating mutation (MRAM), and familial hyperaldosteronism types I (FH-I) and II (FH-II). We briefly overview the principal characteristics of such disorders. A detailed description is provided in Chapter 36.

Liddle Syndrome

In 1963, Grant Liddle (a physician at Vanderbilt University) found a Tennessee family in which several of the members had extremely high blood pressure and laboratory signs of hypokalemia, increased K^+ excretion and Na^+ retention, and reduced plasma renin activity, angiotensin II, and aldosterone. It is an autosomal dominant disorder that does not show any positive response to spironolactone administration. To date, 10 mutations have been identified on the *SCNN1B* and *SCNN1G* genes.[26]

Apparent mineralocorticoid excess

Patients affected by AME1, whose clinical features were previously cited, have a congenital deficiency of 11β-hydroxysteroid dehydrogenase type 2 that inactivates cortisol. Those affected by AME2 present a diminished function of the enzyme.

Mineralocorticoid-receptor-activating mutation

This disorder consists of a substitution, leucine for serine, at codon 810 (S810L). This substitution modifies the shape and specificity of the MR so that as opposed to normal subjects progesterone and spironolactone can activate the MR. The net result is the onset of early hypertension, particularly worse during pregnancy.[27]

Glucocorticoid-remediable aldosteronism or familial hyperaldesteronism type I

GRA, also called familial hyperaldosteronism type I, is inherited as an autosomal dominant trait. The syndrome consists of an early onset of hypertension, low renin values, and hyperaldosteronism (which can be counterbalanced with glucocorticoids). The syndrome is caused by a chimeric gene deriving from a crossing-over between the promoter of the 11β-hydroxylase (*CYP11B1*) and the coding of aldosterone synthase activities (*CYP11B2*).[28]

Pseudohypoaldosteronism type II or familial hyperaldosteronism type II (Gordon Syndrome)

Pseudohypoaldosteronism type II, also called Gordon syndrome,[29] is another rare Mendelian syndrome consisting of hypertension, hyperkalemia, hyperchloremia, and metabolic acidosis. It is counterbalanced with thiazide diuretics that inhibit the sodium chloride reabsorption in the kidney. The disorder is caused by mutations in two genes (WNK1 and WNK4) that encode the protein kinases.[30]

In conclusion, the genetic model best describing the transmission pattern of hypertension is called multifactorial (i.e., consisting of a polygenic model interacting with the environment). A polygenic model is a model in which many small equal and additive loci would result in Gaussian distribution for a phenotype whereas a few other loci might be responsible for rare forms of hypertension. This model applies to other complex diseases (such as diabetes, schizophrenia, or cancer) in which both multiple genes and environmental factors play a role in the development of the disease. Hypertension is presumed to result from additive effects of multiple genes with low penetrance and various, but generally weak, impact on phenotype. Individual mutations may not induce any particular phenotype but may produce a disease phenotype when they act in concert and in the presence of the necessary environmental conditions.

The last stage in genetic epidemiology of hypertension is the identification of the genes and of their variants modulating blood pressure and generating hypertension. No consensus has emerged about the best strategy for identifying complex disease genes.[31] The issues relate to the total number of SNPs or genetic variations in the human genome and to the subset of SNPs on which to focus in disease association studies. The enormous bulk of studies aiming at identifying these genes can be broadly grouped into two types of studies. In the terminology of Peltonen and McKusick[32] they can be defined as map based or sequence based.[33]

These two definitions relate to different questions: the first asks where the genes are that are associated with the condition and the second asks which are the genes associated with the condition. The tool applied in the map-based strategy is the recombination fraction, whereas linkage disequilibrium (LD) forms the basis of sequence-based studies. However, the two approaches proceed from a similar assumption: the genetic marker studied is close to the actual disease gene and this will result in an allelic association at the family or population level. Another critical assumption of both strategies is that there is little allelic heterogeneity within loci.

Two approaches to the map-based strategy have evolved for traits showing Mendelian and non-Mendelian segregation patterns: (1) those that require prior specification of mode of inheritance for the trait under study (model-based/parametric methods) and (2) those that do not assume a specific trait inheritance (model-free/nonparametric methods). The latter are useful for initial exploratory analysis, and the former for more detailed multivariate geometric analysis.

MAP-BASED STRATEGY

During meiosis, genetic material undergoes recombination. Thus, adjacent loci or alleles within two homologous but separate chromosomes can be recombined and segregated into the same chromosome. If two adjacent markers are close, there will not be much recombination between them and they will cosegregate. Markers adjacent to a locus carrying the condition will segregate more often with the condition than those far apart. The recombination fraction (denoted as θ and measured in Morgans or, more commonly, in centiMorgans, cM) between the known genetic locus (marker, or Aa) and the unknown disease locus (gene, or Bb) lies at the heart of map-based analyses. The Morgan unit expresses a genetic distance based on recombination, not a physical distance, although it can be estimated that 1 cM corresponds to about 1 million bases. If the two loci are far apart or are in different chromosomes, segregation of one locus will be independent of the other (they are equally likely to cosegregate as not to). At $\theta = 1/2$ (0.50) four types of gametes (AB, ab, Ab, and aB) two recombinant and two nonrecombinant for a total of four from a pair of homologous chromosomes are equally likely to be produced.

This ($\theta = 1/2$) is the baseline value in linkage studies where the proportion of gametes the person transmits in which a recombination has occurred is 50% (and the other 50% has no recombinants). Fifty percent is the possibility of two loci in two different chromosomes to cosegregate into a gamete. Linked loci are transmitted to the same gamete more than 50% of the time ($0 = \theta < 1/2$), and the "parental-type" gametes are more frequent than the "recombinant-type" gametes. Model-based linkage analysis is based on a likelihood ratio, and the logarithm to base 10 of this likelihood ratio is called a Logarithm Of oDds (LOD) score. This is the logarithm of the ratio of a particular value of the recombination fraction versus free recombination (i.e., $\theta = 0.5$). Obviously,

numerous LOD scores can be obtained for a range of θ values. Whichever θ maximizes the LOD score, this is the evidence for linkage with the particular recombination frequency {I}θ {/I} between the marker and the disease locus. LOD scores >1 are considered nominal evidence of linkage, LOD scores >2.2 as suggestive evidence, LOD scores >3.6 as genome-wide evidence, and LOD scores >5.4 as confirmed linkage. Linkage might lead to an association of a certain area with the condition, but this is usually intrafamilial. The association at the population level (linkage of genotype for a genetic marker to disease) might not be consistent.

The magnitude of linkage is affected by many factors, but if everything else is assumed to be equal the most important factor is the physical/genetic distance between the disease and marker alleles. The closer they are the lower the recombination frequency and the stronger the magnitude of linkage. This implies that close linkage between the marker and disease loci would result in longer periods of linkage disequilibrium within the population.

Within a model of multiple interacting loci, no single locus could account for more than a fivefold increase in the risk of first-degree relatives. Research strategies for detection of susceptibility genes in hypertension are important to be known, because some limitations might be important in understanding the disappointing results obtained thus far. Linkage studies aim to obtain a crude chromosomal location of the gene or genes associated with a phenotype of interest (e.g., a genetic disease or an important quantitative trait). Linkage is a phenomenon of cosegregating loci, not alleles, within families. Linkage studies are used for coarse mapping because they have a limited genetic resolution of about 1 cM. If two markers are close, there will not be much recombination between them and they will cosegregate. This results in a positive result in linkage analysis. This principle has been used in studies examining some areas of the genome, and in recent years (thanks to the completion of the human genome project and to technological advances) to the entire genome.

GENOME-WIDE SCAN

The genome-wide scan is best defined as a search for quantitative trait loci across the entire genome. The quantitative trait locus (QTL) is a chromosomal region containing a gene or genes that influence a trait of interest such as hypertension. This search is best performed comparing genomes of siblings or otherwise related subjects discordant for the trait or the disease. However, other study designs such as nuclear families, large pedigrees, and studies of normotensive sibling pairs have also been performed.[34] Genome-wide screens analyze hundreds of polymorphic markers, usually microsatellites, in a selected sample of individuals with or without a qualitative or quantitative trait. In contrast to candidate gene studies (see material following), a genome scan is designed primarily to detect genes not previously implicated in pathologic or physiologic regulation of blood pressure. The entire genome is

THE RESULTS OF GENOME-WIDE SCAN STUDIES						
Chrom.	Number of Loci	Lod Range Hypertens	Number of Loci	Lod Range Diastolic	Number of Loci	Lod Range Systolic
1	4	1,2–1,78	–	–	1	2,2
2p	3	1,2–4,21	1	1,3–3,92	4	1–2,28
2q	6	1,6–3,59	3	2,05–3,36	3	1,64–2,4
3	1	4,04	–	–	3	1,8–2,03
4	1	1,6	–	–	1	2,2
5	1	1,85	–	–	2	1–2,23
6	1	3,21	–	–	3	1–3,3
7	–	–	1	1,6	3	2,26–4,73
8	1	1,2	–	–	–	–
9	1	2,24	–	–	–	–
10	1	2,5	–	–	–	–
11	3	1,1–2	–	–	3	1,98–2,28
12	–	–	1	2,35	1	6,54
13	2	1,56–2	–	–	–	–
14	1	2,7	–	–	–	–
15	1	2	1	2,69	3	1–6,68
16	1	1,85	1	1,82	2	2,3–2,74
17	2	1,16–1,7	–	–	2	2,16–5,32
18	1	3,84	–	–	1	2,09
19	2	1,76–3,1	–	–	1	2,14
20	–	–	–	–	–	–
21	–	–	–	–	1	2,82
22	1	2,07	2	1,27–1,54	–	–
X	2	1,1–2,41	–	–	1	2,3
Y	–	–	–	–	–	–

Chrom. = chromosomes, number of loci = number of loci linked to the condition in the different studies, and lod range = range of lod scores measured within the chromosome and associated with hypertension and with diastolic and systolic blood pressure.

Table 35–2. The Results of Genome-Wide Scan Studies

screened with densely distributed microsatellite markers in order to detect linkage of groups of markers with the trait of interest. The density of markers and the throughput of marker genotyping have increased over the years, and the cost of marker genotyping has decreased, further facilitating QTL mapping by marker locus approach. Thus, availability of dense markers, high-throughput genotyping, and cost are no longer limiting factors for performing genome-wide scans for positional mapping of QTLs. The major problems at this time seem to be the difficulty of gathering high-quality phenotype data in a sample of adequate size using an appropriate study design and the analysis of these data using a method with high statistical power.

The locus approach, or whole-genome screening, due to availability of polymorphic markers and refinements of statistical methods is becoming very popular and several GWS have been published in the recent years (several reviews have focused on them).[35–37] Each genome scan published differs in the number of subjects studied, ethnicity, family types, design, and the phenotypic strategy, some considering hypertension as a discrete trait and some considering blood pressure as a continuous variable.

Out of 23 chromosomes, at least 21 have some identified loci in linkage with hypertension, and some have been found in more than one study. Of course, involvement of a chromosome is quite far from identification of a gene. Even if some of the loci are going to survive grid tightening and metanalysis,[35] inconsistency of the findings and lack of comparability with other strategies represent a poor result for such effort.

The main results are reported in Table 35–2. No agreement on the loci involved has been reached considering all studies performed thus far, but a separate metanalysis for Caucasians seems to identify certain QTL in chromosomes 2 and 3 as linked to hypertension.[35] The major effort for the future will be to try matching the loci identified with map-based strategies with those identified with candidate gene strategy.

ASSOCIATION STUDIES

Linkage analysis is not useful for finding so-called susceptibility loci (i.e., loci that are neither necessary nor sufficient for disease expression). Association studies evaluate and compare allelic genetic frequencies as well as haplotype in affected and nonaffected subjects. Association studies have some practical advantages over linkage studies. Knowledge about the mode of inheritance of the disease is not required and this type of study has the necessary statistical power in order to detect genes of weak effect. Reliability of the results of an association study are linked, independently, to the good number of patients studied, to the ethnic homogeneity of the population studied, to large data sets, to small P values, and (most important) to independent replication of results.

Association studies allow a fine mapping and identification of the genes. Association may be detected as direct involvement of the gene or as in linkage disequilibrium (LD) with the gene at the population level. The classical association study is the case control study or candidate gene approach. In the candidate gene approach (or association studies) genes codifying for proteins that are physiologically or biochemically relevant to the trait (defined candidate genes) are screened and the effects of variant alleles on the QT are investigated.

CANDIDATE GENE APPROACH

At present, association studies are the only means of confirming a functional role for a candidate gene in human populations. Even then, a confirmed association does not necessarily imply proof of cause. At best, it suggests a cause. This general limitation should be borne in mind among those who seek to unfold the pathophysiologic basis of hypertension in humans through genetic studies. The main concerns with this approach are as follows.

- The approach requires a good knowledge of the trait and of the related biochemical or physiological pathways, which rarely exists.

- The approach cannot lead to the detection of new QTLs.

- In theory, all genes could be analyzed. Further, every SNP or polymorphism should be analyzed, increasing enormously the risk of type I statistical error.

- Although this approach seems attractive, there is not yet sufficient evidence to support its general utility, at least not in human hypertension.

In spite of these limitations, this type of approach is the most used in the genetic assessment of hypertension. A bibliographical search offers more than 2,000 studies (discounting reviews; a listing can be found on the Web at *http://www.ncbi.nlm.nih.gov/entrez/dispomim.cgi?id= 145500*) (see Box 35–2).

Even if a generalization cannot be discerned, given the different role of each protein it must be recognized that discordant results are often published, and the more the research goes on with genetic polymorphisms the more the enthusiasm topples. A paradigmatic example is the angiotensinogen polymorphisms. The angiotensinogen gene (AGT) is a thrifty gene, which increases the risk for common disease with growth of civilization via sodium and body fluid retention. Four different polymorphisms [A(-20)C, G(-6)A, T174M, and M235T] have been described in this gene, and their effect on blood pressure is contradictory: a double heterozygosity for Thr235 and

---

Box 35–2

Studies of the Candidate Gene Approach

- Angiotensin-converting enzyme
- Type-2 angiotensin II receptor
- Atrial natriuretic factor precursor
- Natriuretic peptides B precursor
- C-type natriuretic peptide precursor
- Angiotensinogen precursor
- Atrial natriuretic peptide receptor A precursor
- Atrial natriuretic peptide receptor B precursor
- Adipocyte-derived leucine aminopeptidase precursor
- Bombesin receptor subtype-3
- Cytochrome P450 11B2, mitochondrial precursor
- Calcitonin gene-related peptide I precursor
- Chromogranin A precursor
- Atrial natriuteric peptide-converting enzyme
- Endothelin-1 precursor
- Fibrinogen (all subunits)
- Guanine nucleotide-binding protein G(I)/G(S)/G(T) beta subunit 3
- Glucagon receptor precursor
- Prostaglandin G/H synthase 1 precursor
- Prostaglandin G/H synthase 2 precursor
- SA protein precursor
- SA hypertension-associated homolog, isoform 2
- N-acylglucosamine 2-epimerase
- Renin precursor
- Solute carrier family 12, member 4
- Solute carrier family 12, member 6
- Urotensin-2 precursor
- Adducin
- Beta2-adrenergic receptor

Thr 174 increases by 10% the angiotensinogen plasma levels[38,39] and is a risk factor for hypertension, but only in males. Presence of the -6A allele or the AGT 235T allele was associated with the most pronounced SBP response to atenolol treatment (P = .001 when -6 AA+AG was compared with GG and P = .008 for presence of the 235T variant compared with 235 MM).[40] Moreover, M235T is in linkage disequilibrium with allelic variants of AGT such as A-6G and A-20C, which account for different expression of the protein.[41–44] In spite of all of this early evidence, two metanalyses[38,45] showed that allele 235T does increase the risk of hypertension, but only in Caucasians. The authors, however, raise much concern on publication bias and confounding, inviting a very cautious interpretation of the results. This skepticism has been confirmed in a recent large study (10,000 individuals), which did not reach any evidence of a role of these PM in blood pressure regulation, or incidence of vascular events.[46] For some authors, this was the final word on the angiotensinogen polymorphisms.[47]

Similarly, deletion insertion of 287 bp in intron 16 (D/I polymorphism) in ACE (on chromosome 17q23) showed some interesting data, but these results were not confirmed by other studies. A deletion seems associated to genetic risk for vascular disease but not for hypertension. Differences among subjects are ethnically related. Several studies have resequenced the gene and have shown more single-nucleotide polymorphisms in codifying and noncodifying regions;[48] but the conclusion should be that the D/I polymorphism has been demonstrated to affect plasma activity of ACE but not blood pressure or risk of vascular events.[49] Similarly, ACE I/D polymorphism is not a useful marker for predicting antihypertensive treatment response.[50]

The general picture obtained is frustrating: limited evidence of genetic variants that determine hypertension have so far been found from both genome-wide scan and from association studies. Moreover, genomic studies did not reach a consensus on the likely location of blood pressure genes. Many reasons have been put forward to explain these results. Causative genes are numerous, have small clinical impact, and are unevenly distributed among populations. However, the fact that in other diseases or conditions many polymorphisms in many diseases cannot be confirmed after the first publication[51] should induce researchers to revise the methodology applied thus far.

SUMMARY

Hypertension genetics still has many unexplored aspects, and many questions require further research. Genetic modeling of hypertension is enormously complex. Nevertheless, there is little doubt that hypertension is a multifactorial disease involving the interaction of the environment with several independent genetic variants. In rethinking approaches to genetics of hypertension it is helpful to consider that understanding the genetic aspects of multifactorial diseases has been a major challenge in other complex diseases—such as asthma, complex autoimmune diseases, cancer, and atherosclerosis, all of which have shared the same disappointing results. The lack of consistency between map- and sequence-based strategies might be due to inadequate statistical approaches or phenotypic characterization, but it is likely that more generalized problems vex the identification of genes underlying complex traits.[52,53] The most relevant of these are as follows.

- A number of genotypes or mutations/polymorphisms at different loci (which likely impact different physiological systems) must be transmitted to an individual before his/her system is sufficiently challenged to result in disease. Thus, despite the arbitrary nature with which blood pressure criteria are used to diagnose hypertension it may be necessary to have a number of genes before blood pressure will surpass these arbitrary thresholds. It may also be the case that number of genes must be had before additional pathologies associated with coronary heart disease (e.g., vascular damage) appear. This is called classical polygenic (or threshold) inheritance.

- Locus heterogeneity, in which defects in any of a number of genes or loci can confer disease susceptibility independently of each other. Thus, under heterogeneity individuals with similar phenotypic features or disease states may possess different genetic variants that lead to the disease.

- Gene interaction, in which the possession of a certain mutation or genotype will confer susceptibility to a degree dictated by the presence of other mutations or genotypes. This phenoemenon (called epistasis) reflects basic interactive effects of mutations, genotypes, and/ or their biological products.

- Gene/environment interactions occur when an allele or more alleles (haplotypes) have their deleterious effects only when the carrier is exposed to particular environmental stimuli.

- Time-regulated gene expression. A gene, whether in mutant/polymorphic form or not, has its most pronounced and deleterious effect at a certain developmental stage (e.g., puberty).

The possibility of having to deal with polygenic inheritance, heterogeneity, epistasis, and developmental effects in gene mapping and characterization studies is a major point for genetic epidemiologists and researchers. Traditionally, modeling and research have mainly focused on the testing of individual genes or genomic regions. Only recently have multiple genes or environmental factors been considered to influence particular traits. Available statistical models and methods are still not suitable for including so many variables and will probably need to accommodate an even wider array of complexities in the future in order to be realistic and useful.

REFERENCES

1. Ravogli A, Trazzi S, Villani A, et al. Early 24-hour blood pressure elevation in normotensive subjects with parental hypertension. *Hypertension* 1990; 16:491–97.

2. Dekkers JC, Treiber FA, Kapuku G, Snieder H. Differential influence of family history of hypertension and premature myocardial infarction on systolic blood pressure and left ventricular mass trajectories in youth. *Pediatrics* 2003;111:1387–93.

3. New MI, Geller DS, Fallo F, Wilson RC. Monogenic low renin hypertension. *Trends Endocrinol Metab* 2005;16:92–7.

4. Mein CA, Caulfield MJ, Dobson RJ, Munroe PB. Genetics of essential hypertension. *Hum Mol Genet* 2004; 13(Spec No 1):R169–75.

5. Venter JC, Adams MD, Myers EW, et al. The sequence of the human genome. *Science* 2001;291:1304–51.

6. Sachidanandam R, Weissman D, Schmidt SC, et al. A map of human genome sequence variation containing 1.42 million single nucleotide polymorphisms. *Nature* 2001; 409:928–33.

7. Marth G, Yeh R, Minton M, et al. Single-nucleotide polymorphisms in the public domain: How useful are they? *Nat Genet* 2001;27:371–72.

8. Botstein D, Risch N. Discovering genotypes underlying human phenotypes: Past successes for mendelian disease, future approaches

for complex disease. *Nat Genet* 2003; 33(Suppl S):228–37.

9. Pickering G. The inheritance of arterial pressure. In: Stamler J SRPT, ed. *The Epidemiology of Hypertension.* New York: Grune & Stratton, 1967: 18–27.

10. Platt R. The influence of heredity. In: Stamler J SRPT, ed. *The Epidemiology of Hypertension.* New York: Grune & Stratton, 1967:9–17.

11. Van Rooyen JM, Kruger HS, Huisman HW, et al. An epidemiological study of hypertension and its determinants in a population in transition: The THUSA study. *J Hum Hypertens* 2000;14:779–87.

12. Brown MJ. The causes of essential hypertension. *Br J Clin Pharmacol* 1996;42:21–7.

13. Sims J, Hewitt JK, Kelly KA, Carroll D, Turner JR. Familial and individual influences on blood pressure. *Acta Genet Med Gemellol (Roma)* 1986; 35:7–21.

14. Rice T, Vogler GP, Perusse L, Bouchard C, Rao DC. Cardiovascular risk factors in a French Canadian population: Resolution of genetic and familial environmental effects on blood pressure using twins, adoptees, and extensive information on environmental correlates. *Genet Epidemiol* 1989;6:571–88.

15. Fava C, Burri P, Almgren P, Groop L, Hulthen UL, Melander O. Heritability of ambulatory and office blood pressure phenotypes in Swedish families. *J Hypertens* 2004;22:1717–21.

16. McGue M. When assessing twin concordance, use the probandwise not the pairwise rate. *Schizophr Bull* 1992; 18:171–76.

17. Berg K. Twin studies of coronary heart disease and its risk factors. *Acta Genet Med Gemellol (Roma)* 1987;36:439–53.

18. Fagard RH, Loos RJ, Beunen G, Derom C, Vlietinck R. Influence of chorionicity on the heritability estimates of blood pressure: A study in twins. *J Hypertens* 2003;21:1313–18.

19. Hayakawa K, Shimizu T. Blood pressure discordance and lifestyle: Japanese identical twins reared apart and together. *Acta Genet Med Gemellol (Roma)* 1987;36:485–91.

20. Luft FC. Twins in cardiovascular genetic research. *Hypertension* 2001;37:350–56.

21. McCaffery JM, Pogue-Geile MF, Debski TT, Manuck SB. Genetic and environmental causes of covariation among blood pressure, body mass and serum lipids during young adulthood: A twin study. *J Hypertens* 1999; 17:1677–85.

22. Snieder H, Harshfield GA, Treiber FA. Heritability of blood pressure and hemodynamics in African- and European-American youth. *Hypertension* 2003;41:1196–1201.

23. Tambs K, Moum T, Holmen J, et al. Genetic and environmental effects on blood pressure in a Norwegian sample. *Genet Epidemiol* 1992;9:11–26.

24. He J, Klag MJ, Whelton PK, et al. Migration, blood pressure pattern, and hypertension: The Yi Migrant Study. *Am J Epidemiol* 1991;134:1085–1101.

25. Crockford GP, Bishop DT, Barrett JH. Segregation analysis comparing liability and quantitative trait models for hypertension using the Genetic Analysis Workshop 13 simulated data. *BMC Genet* 2003;4(Suppl 1):S79.

26. Swift PA, MacGregor GA. The epithelial sodium channel in hypertension: Genetic heterogeneity and implications for treatment with amiloride. *Am J Pharmacogenomics* 2004;4:161–68.

27. Geller DS, Farhi A, Pinkerton N, et al. Activating mineralocorticoid receptor mutation in hypertension exacerbated by pregnancy. *Science* 2000;289:119–23.

28. Jackson RV, Lafferty A, Torpy DJ, Stratakis C. New genetic insights in familial hyperaldosteronism. *Ann NY Acad Sci* 2002;970:77–88.

29. Gordon RD. Syndrome of hypertension and hyperkalemia with normal glomerular filtration rate. *Hypertension* 1986;8:93–102.

30. Wilson FH, Disse-Nicodeme S, Choate KA, et al. Human hypertension caused by mutations in WNK kinases. *Science* 2001;293:1107–12.

31. Risch NJ. Searching for genetic determinants in the new millennium. *Nature* 2000;405:847–56.

32. Peltonen L, McKusick VA. Genomics and medicine: Dissecting human disease in the postgenomic era. *Science* 2001;291:1224–29.

33. Majumder PP, Ghosh S. Mapping quantitative trait loci in humans: Achievements and limitations. *J Clin Invest* 2005;115:1419–24.

34. Dominiczak AF, Brain N, Charchar F, McBride M, Hanlon N, Lee WK. Genetics of hypertension: Lessons learnt from mendelian and polygenic syndromes. *Clin Exp Hypertens* 2004; 26:611–20.

35. Koivukoski L, Fisher SA, Kanninen T, et al. Meta-analysis of genome-wide scans for hypertension and blood pressure in Caucasians shows evidence of susceptibility regions on chromosomes 2 and 3. *Hum Mol Genet* 2004; 13:2325–32.

36. Liu W, Zhao W, Chase GA. Genome scan meta-analysis for hypertension. *Am J Hypertens* 2004;17:1100–06.

37. Samani NJ. Genome scans for hypertension and blood pressure regulation. *Am J Hypertens* 2003; 16:167–71.

38. Kunz R, Kreutz R, Beige J, Distler A, Sharma AM. Association between the angiotensinogen 235T-variant and essential hypertension in whites: A systematic review and methodological appraisal. *Hypertension* 1997;30:1331–37.

39. Sethi AA, Nordestgaard BG, Agerholm-Larsen B, Frandsen E, Jensen G, Tybjaerg-Hansen A. Angiotensinogen polymorphisms and elevated blood pressure in the general population: The Copenhagen City Heart Study. *Hypertension* 2001;37:875–81.

40. Kurland L, Liljedahl U, Karlsson J, et al. Angiotensinogen gene polymorphisms: Relationship to blood pressure response to antihypertensive treatment. Results from the Swedish Irbesartan Left Ventricular Hypertrophy Investigation vs Atenolol (SILVHIA) Trial. *Am J Hypertens* 2004;17:8–13.

41. Inoue I, Nakajima T, Williams CS, et al. A nucleotide substitution in the promoter of human angiotensinogen is associated with essential hypertension and affects basal transcription in vitro. *J Clin Invest* 1997;99:1786–97.

42. Ishigami T, Umemura S, Tamura K, et al. Essential hypertension and 5' upstream core promoter region of human angiotensinogen gene. *Hypertension* 1997;30:1325–30.

43. Jeunemaitre X, Inoue I, Williams C, et al. Haplotypes of angiotensinogen in essential hypertension. *Am J Hum Genet* 1997;60:1448–60.

44. Zhao YY, Zhou J, Narayanan CS, Cui Y, Kumar A. Role of C/A polymorphism at -20 on the expression of human angiotensinogen gene. *Hypertension* 1999;33:108–15.

45. Staessen JA, Kuznetsova T, Wang JG, Emelianov D, Vlietinck R, Fagard R. M235T angiotensinogen gene polymorphism and cardiovascular renal risk. *J Hypertens* 1999;17:9–17.

46. Sethi AA, Nordestgaard BG, Gronholdt ML, Steffensen R, Jensen G, Tybjaerg-Hansen A. Angiotensinogen single nucleotide polymorphisms, elevated blood pressure, and risk of cardiovascular disease. *Hypertension* 2003;41:1202–11.

47. Luft FC. Geneticism of essential hypertension. *Hypertension* 2004; 43:1155–59.

48. Rieder MJ, Taylor SL, Clark AG, Nickerson DA. Sequence variation in the human angiotensin converting enzyme. *Nat Genet* 1999;22:59–62.

49. Agerholm-Larsen B, Nordestgaard BG, Tybjaerg-Hansen A. ACE gene polymorphism in cardiovascular disease: Meta-analyses of small and large studies in whites. *Arterioscler Thromb Vasc Biol* 2000;20:484–92.

50. Arnett DK, Davis BR, Ford CE, et al. Pharmacogenetic association of the angiotensin-converting enzyme insertion/deletion polymorphism on blood pressure and cardiovascular risk in relation to antihypertensive treatment: The Genetics of Hypertension-Associated Treatment (GenHAT) study. *Circulation* 2005;111:3374–83.

51. Ioannidis JP, Ntzani EE, Trikalinos TA, Contopoulos-Ioannidis DG. Replication validity of genetic association studies. *Nat Genet* 2001;29:306–09.

52. Palmer LJ, Cookson WO. Using single nucleotide polymorphisms as a means to understanding the pathophysiology of asthma. *Respir Res* 2001;2:102–12.

53. Wandstrat A, Wakeland E. The genetics of complex autoimmune diseases: Non-MHC susceptibility genes. *Nat Immunol* 2001;2:802–09.

Chapter

36

Monogenic Forms of Human Hypertension

Beverley Burke, Johannie Gungadoo, Ana Carolina B. Marçano, Stephen J. Newhouse, Julian Shiel, Mark J. Caulfield, and Patricia B. Munroe

Definition

Monogenic forms of hypertension are rare inherited conditions with high blood pressure as part of the phenotype.

Key Findings

- The mutated gene product usually leads to incorrect electrolyte handling in the kidney.
- The phenotype of each condition can be variable.
- Key features of each include abnormal potassium levels (high or low), suppression of plasma renin, metabolic alkalosis or acidosis, abnormal aldosterone levels, and sodium retention.
- The ongoing elucidation of monogenic forms of hypertension is providing knowledge about new mechanisms of blood pressure control.

A monogenic disease can be defined as an inherited condition caused by a modification in a single gene. There are over 10,000 monogenic diseases that have been described, and although many are extremely rare they affect millions of people worldwide.[1] In the field of hypertension, there are 10 monogenic diseases that have high blood pressure as part of the phenotype. All diseases have now been defined at the molecular genetic level (Table 36–1). They include glucocorticoid remediable aldosteronism (GRA),[2] Liddle's syndrome,[3] pseudohypoaldosteronism type II (Gordon's syndrome),[4] congenital adrenal hyperplasia (CAH)-11β hydroxylase deficiency[5] and -17α hydroxylase deficiency, apparent mineralocorticoid excess,[7] the mineralocorticoid receptor in hypertension exacerbated in pregnancy,[8] hypertension with brachydactyly,[9] hypertension associated with peroxisome proliferator-activated receptor gamma mutations[10] and more recently hypertension, hypercholesterolemia, and

MONOGENIC FORMS OF HYPERTENSION			
Condition	Mode of Inheritance	Location	Gene and Reference
Glucocorticoid remediable aldosteronism	Autosomal dominant	8q24.3	11 β-hydroxylase/ aldosterone synthase (CYP11B1/CYP11B2) chimera[2]
Congenital adrenal hyperplasia with 11β-hydroxylase deficiency	Autosomal recessive	8q24.3	11 β-hydroxylase (CYP11B1)[5]
Congenital adrenal hyperplasia with 17α-hydroxylase deficiency	Autosomal recessive	10q24.32	17 α-hydroxylase (CYP17A1)[5]
Apparent mineralocorticoid excess	Autosomal recessive	16q22.1	11 β-hydroxysteroid dehydrogenase (HSD11B2)[7]
Gordon's syndrome	Autosomal dominant	12p, 17q, 1q	Protein kinase, lysine deficient 1 and 4 (WNK 1, WNK 4)[4]
Liddle's syndrome	Autosomal dominant	16q	Sodium channel nonvoltage-gated 1, β and γ subunits (SCNN1B, SCNN1G)[3]
Hypertension exacerbated by pregnancy	Autosomal dominant	4q31.23	Mineralocorticoid receptor (NR3C2)[8]
Hypertension associated with PPARγ mutations	Autosomal dominant	3p25	Peroxisome proliferator-activated receptor gamma (PPARγ)[10]
Hypertension and brachydactyly	Autosomal dominant	12p	Unknown[9]
Hypertension associated with mitochondrial mutations	Mitochondrial genome		Mitochondrial tRNA isoleucine gene[11]

Table 36–1. Monogenic Forms of Hypertension

hypomagnesia associated with mitochondrial gene mutations.[11] An interesting feature of most of these conditions is that the disease causing mutation directly affects salt/water homeostasis in the kidney.

Reabsorption of sodium and chloride from the bloodstream in the kidney is achieved through an integrated system of ion channels, exchangers, and transporters distributed throughout the length of the nephron (Figure 36–1).[12] The distal nephron consists of the distal convoluted tubule (DCT), the connecting tubule (CNT), and segments of the cortical collecting ducts (CCD). It is in the distal part of the nephron that the final adjustments to net renal sodium balance are achieved. In other words, the distal nephron is of critical importance in the maintenance of sodium homeostasis. The two main ion transport systems in this part of the nephron are the electroneutral apical thiazide-sensitive NaCl co-transporter (NCCT) and the renal

amiloride-sensitive epithelial sodium channel (ENaC).[13] In the late distal tubule, NCCT and ENaC expression overlap. Fine control of sodium reabsorption is provided by modulating the activity of NCCT and ENaC via aldosterone and the mineralocorticoid receptor (MR). In turn, this is under the influence of the renin-angiotensin-aldosterone system.[14] Sodium uptake in the distal tubule is closely linked to potassium and hydrogen ion secretion. Altered function in any of the ion transport proteins, or their regulators, participating in sodium reabsorption will affect blood pressure.

In this chapter we review the monogenic forms of hypertension caused by mutations in proteins now known to affect the regulation of salt/water homeostasis in the kidney: GRA, Liddle's syndrome, Gordon's syndrome, and two forms of CAH that have hypertension as part of the phenotype; namely, 11 β-hydroxylase deficiency

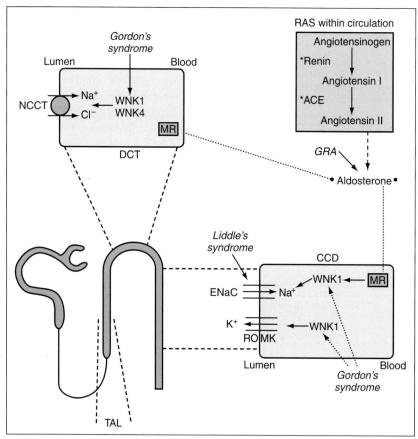

Figure 36–1. The major sites of sodium reabsorption in the mammalian kidney tubule. The distal nephron is of critical importance in the maintenance of sodium homeostasis. This diagram illustrates the structure of the nephron, indicating the location of the thick ascending limb of Henle (TAL), the distal convoluted tubule (DCT), and the cortical collecting duct (CCD). The key channels that regulate sodium homeostasis are the sodium chloride co-transporter (NCCT) and the epithelium sodium channel (ENaC). The renal outer medullary potassium channel (ROMK) is a key channel regulating potassium flux. The channels/hormones mutated in Gordon's syndrome, Liddle's syndrome, and GRA are indicated in italics. Also indicated is the renin-angiotensin system (RAS) because this is the major regulator of renal salt reabsorption. Other abbreviations: ACE (angiotensin-converting enzyme), MR (mineralocorticoid receptor), Na+ (sodium ion), Cl- (chloride ion), and K+ (potassium ion). (Modified from Cope et al. WNK kinases and the control of blood pressure. *Pharmacology & Therapeutics* 2005;106:221–31.)

(11-OHD) and 17 α-hydroxylase deficiency (17-OHD). Genetic, pathophysiologic, and clinical aspects are discussed for each disorder. The remaining five monogenic forms of hypertension are briefly discussed in the summary.

GLUCOCORTICOID REMEDIABLE ALDOSTERONISM

Definition

Glucocorticoid remediable aldosteronism (GRA), also known as familial hyperaldosteronism type I (OMIM: 103900), was first described in 1966.[15] It is an autosomal dominant condition characterized by elevated levels of circulating aldosterone (despite suppressed plasma renin levels), metabolic alkalosis, hypokalemia, hypertension, risk of stroke at a young age, and high levels of the adrenal steroids 18-hydroxycortisol and 18-oxycortisol. The symptoms of the disorder can be reversed by glucocorticoid (dexamethasone) administration.[16]

Genetics

Lifton and colleagues discovered the genetic mechanism causing GRA in 1992.[2,17] Analysis of one large multigenerational pedigree with GRA revealed a novel fragment of the 11β-hydroxylase gene, CYP11B1, to be present only in affected individuals. Linkage analysis using this fragment as a marker demonstrated complete linkage to GRA with a LOD score of 5.23. Subsequent investigations found this fragment to be part of a chimeric gene consisting of the 5′ tissue-specific and regulatory sequences of 11β hydroxylase (CYP11B1) and the coding sequence of aldosterone synthase (CYP11B2). The chimeric gene segregated with the disease phenotype and it was postulated that the gene product was the likely cause of GRA.[18] Eleven additional GRA kindreds were subsequently tested for the chimeric gene in order to prove this was the disease causing mutation.[17] Southern blot analysis revealed all affected individuals to have a chimeric gene. Sister and non-sister chromatid exchange was determined as the mechanism by which the chimeric gene was formed.[17]

The sequence 3′ of exon 5 in CYP11B2 is crucial for the preservation of the CYP11B2 activity,[19] and the sequence 5′ of intron 2 of CYP11B1 is thought to be sufficient to ensure expression in zona fasciculata and responsiveness to ACTH. The crossover site of the chimera therefore ranges from intron 2 to intron 4 of CYP11B1 in GRA. Since the cause of GRA was originally described, there have been several other reports of pedigrees with the CYP11B1/CYP11B2 chimeric gene from different ethnic groups.[20,21]

Physiology and pathophysiology

Aldosterone is a mineralocorticoid hormone expressed in the zona glomerulosa of the adrenal gland, and its production is regulated by angiotensin II and potassium. Its main function is to control salt/water homeostasis, blood pressure, and extracellular fluid potassium. Cortisol

is a glucocorticoid hormone, synthesized in the zona fasciculata of the adrenal gland. It is under the control of adrenocorticotrophic hormone (ACTH), and its function is to regulate the stress response, energy metabolism, and blood pressure control. The genes encoding CYP11B1 and CYP11B2, which are 95% identical, catalyze the final steps in the production of cortisol and aldosterone, respectively.[22] Cortisol and aldosterone have similar affinities for binding to the mineralocorticoid receptor (MR), which is responsible for the fine control of renal salt reabsorption (see Chapter 23). Plasma concentrations of cortisol are normally/physiologically 100 to 1000 times higher than aldosterone. Thus, it is aldosterone that regulates the MR, and therefore the amount of salt retained by the body, under normal circumstances.[23]

In GRA, the chimeric gene allows aldosterone to be ectopically expressed in the zona fasciculata while being regulated by ACTH. This increase in aldosterone production causes the MR to be hyperactivated, resulting in the retention of salt and water by the kidneys and therefore volume-expansion hypertension.[17] However, it appears that high blood pressure in GRA is caused not just by excess aldosterone secretion. Two biochemically unique "hybrid steroids" may also be important.[24] 18-oxocortisol and 18-hydroxycortisol are created by the exposure of cortisol and corticosterone to aldosterone synthase activity in the zona fasciculata. These compounds are thought to have mineralocorticoid receptor activity, thereby contributing to the salt retention and subsequent high blood pressure.[25]

Clinical implications and perspectives

The clinical phenotype of GRA is variable. Cerebrovascular complications (including hemorrhagic stroke) can occur at an early age, and the resultant ruptured intracranial aneurysms are significant events of mortality and morbidity.[26] The hypertension in GRA ranges from moderate to severe. However, it can be completely alleviated by suppressing steroid production in the inner cortical zones with a low-dose glucocorticoid such as dexamethasone. The administration of potassium-sparing drugs or mineralocorticoid receptor antagonists may be required instead of glucocorticoids to avoid disrupting growth in the young.[27]

Diagnosis of GRA is now primarily by genetic analysis using a long template PCR method or Southern blotting.[17,28] Previous diagnostic criteria (including measuring the urinary hybrid steroids 18-hydroxy/oxosteroids and the dexamethasone suppression test) have been shown to lack 100% specificity.[16,29]

Although all anomalies of GRA can be remedied by glucocorticoid administration, the phenotypic consequence of harboring the chimeric gene is yet to be fully understood. Blood pressure variation has been described between GRA patients within the same family, and recently normotensive individuals carrying the chimeric gene have been identified.[30] These latest findings raise the question of additional undetermined genetic and/or environmental factors being involved in regulating blood pressure in such individuals.

LIDDLE'S SYNDROME

Definition

Liddle's syndrome (pseudohypoaldosteronism, OMIM: 177200) was first described in 1963 in a single kindred.[31] It is an autosomal dominant disorder characterized by early onset hypertension, hypokalemic metabolic acidosis, and suppressed plasma renin and aldosterone levels.[32] All affected individuals respond well to triamterene or amiloride, which are specific inhibitors of the epithelial sodium channel (ENaC), suggesting that defects in this channel or its regulators may cause the condition.[3]

Genetics

In 1994, Shimkets and colleagues found mutations in the β subunit of ENaC to cause Liddle's syndrome.[3] Using Liddle's original kindred, complete genetic linkage was found with the gene encoding the β subunit of ENaC on chromosome 16, with a LOD score of 7.62. Mutation analysis revealed a novel variant to be present in affected individuals, but it was absent in the unaffected members of the family. Direct sequencing of this variant revealed a single base substitution, a C→T transition at the first nucleotide of codon Arg-564. This mutation was predicted to introduce a stop codon, causing 75 C-terminus amino acids to be deleted from the protein. Analysis of four further Liddle's kindreds found frameshift mutations or premature stop codons in the same region of this gene, confirming that mutations in the gene encoding the β subunit of ENaC caused Liddle's syndrome.[3]

Mutations were not found in the β subunit of ENaC in all families with Liddle's syndrome, suggesting the condition may be genetically heterogeneous. This was confirmed in 1995 when Hansson and colleagues discovered the β and γ subunits of ENaC to be closely linked on chromosome 16, and a nonsense mutation to be present in the γ subunit in affected members of a Liddle's kindred.[33] The single base substitution was at codon Trp-574, and this was predicted to lead to deletion of the last 76 amino acids of the protein. This mutation was in a location (i.e., the carboxy terminus of the protein) similar to those found in Liddle's patients with the β subunit mutations.

Thirteen mutations have now been reported in the gene encoding the β subunit (SCNN1B): missense, frameshift, and premature stop codons. Three mutations have been reported in the gene encoding the γ subunit (SCNN1G).[34,35]

Physiology and pathophysiology

The amiloride-sensitive epithelial sodium channel (ENaC) plays a critical role in controlling salt/water homeostasis, extracellular volume, and blood pressure and is regulated by the hormones aldosterone and vasopressin in the distal nephron of the kidney.[36] ENaC is a heterotrimer composed of three subunits (α, β and γ) in a ratio of 2:1:1. The subunits share 32 to 37% amino acid identity. Each subunit consists of a short intracellular amino terminus, a short carboxy terminus, two transmembrane regions, and an extracellular loop.[37] Studies in *Xenopus laevis* oocytes have demonstrated that the α subunit alone has the ability for sodium conductance, whereas the β and γ subunits augment the channels' activities.

Functional studies illustrating a potential mechanism by which mutations in the β and γ subunits of ENaC lead to Liddle's syndrome were published in 1995.[33,38] A mutated β subunit was coexpressed in *Xenopus laevis* oocytes with rat wild-type α and γ subunits. Similarly, a mutated γ subunit was coexpressed with rat wild-type α and β subunits. Analysis revealed marked increases in amiloride-sensitive sodium current (five- to sixfold) and increased numbers of ENaC channels at the cell surface (two- to threefold) of both mutants compared to the wild type. Increased activity of ENaC is predicted to lead to increased sodium reabsorption and hypertension, the primary clinical features observed in Liddle's syndrome.

The *Xenopus laevis* oocyte studies demonstrated that mutant ENaC have increased activity and numbers at the cell surface compared to wild-type receptors. However, the reasons were not determined. Since then, there have been a few other studies focusing on delineating the precise mechanism. All mutations causing Liddle's syndrome affect a conserved proline-rich sequence PPPXY (PY motif) present on β and γ subunits. Proline-rich motifs such as those observed in ENaC subunits are thought to be involved in protein-protein interactions.

Nedd 4 is a widely expressed ubiquitin-like ligase. In 1996 it was shown that WW domains of Nedd4 directly interact with the PY motif of ENaC.[39] As mutations in Liddle's patients disrupt the PY domain, a mechanism proposed to explain the increased numbers of ENaC receptors at the cell surface and hence overactivity of the channel is that ENaC is not being effectively removed via the ubiquination pathway from the cell surface.[40] More recently, a Nedd4-like protein has also been shown to directly interact via PY motifs in ENaC *in vitro*, suggesting that more than one pathway may be important for downregulation of ENaC.[41] One mechanism proposed to explain increased amiloride-sensitive sodium current in Liddle's patients is that mutant ENaC are not totally inhibited by intracellular sodium ions compared to wild-type ENaC, which is known to be downregulated by intracellular sodium levels.[42]

Clinical implications and perspectives

The clinical phenotype of Liddle's patients is variable and can also vary within families. However, the primary feature in most cases is hypertension. This is usually early-onset and severe, although there are also cases with mild hypertension.[3,33,43] Hypokalemia is found in most cases, but it is not always present.[43,44] Therefore, the diagnosis of Liddle's syndrome can be difficult, and it is best made by taking a full clinical history, checking for multiple family members with the condition, measurement of blood pressure and tests for hypokalemia, reduced plasma renin activity, and suppressed plasma aldosterone levels. Genetic screening is also useful because mutations causing Liddle's syndrome all cluster in the carboxy terminus of the protein, which enables easy screening by direct sequencing.

Administration of the ENaC antagonist amiloride or triamterene in combination with a low-salt diet corrects the abnormalities observed in Liddle's patients.[45] It has also been shown that small doses of amiloride can control blood pressure effectively in the long term, can correct plasma potassium, and can increase plasma renin. However, plasma aldosterone levels remain low.[46]

GORDON'S SYNDROME

Definition

Gordon's syndrome, also known as pseudohypoaldosteronism type II or PHA2 (OMIM: 145260), is an autosomal dominant disorder characterized by salt-dependent hypertension, hyperkalemia (despite normal glomerular filtration rate) due to impaired potassium excretion, and metabolic acidosis due to decreased urinary H+ excretion.[47] Suppressed plasma renin activity and hyperchloremia are variable associated findings.[48] The clinical features of PHA2 are chloride dependent and can be corrected with thiazide diuretics, which inhibit salt reabsorption in the distal nephron.[49,50] The thiazide diuretics are specific inhibitors of NCCT activity, and patients with PHA2 are extremely sensitive to these drugs. This suggested that increased NCCT activity could be responsible for some of the associated PHA2 phenotypes.

Genetics

PHA2 loci have been mapped in different families to chromosomes 1q31 to 1q42 (referred to as PHA2A), 17p11 to 17q21 (PHA2B), and 12p13.3 (PHA2C).[51,52] Not all PHA2 kindreds map to these regions, suggesting that at least one other (as yet unidentified) PHA2 locus may exist.[53] There are therefore at least four different genes that can cause PHA2. Wilson and colleagues discovered two PHA2 genes in 2001.[4] In their study, mutations in two members of a novel family of serine/threonine kinases—WNK1 (OMIM 605232, encoded by *WNK1*) and WNK4 (OMIM 601844, encoded by *WNK4*)—were shown to cause PHA2C and PHA2B.

Wilson et al. studied a PHA2C kindred that included 10 living members with typical features of PHA2.[4] Genome-wide linkage analysis in this pedigree revealed complete linkage of PHA2 to a locus at the telomeric segment of chromosome 12p, with a multipoint LOD score of 5.07. The affected family members had a deletion in the interval between markers D12S341 and D12S91. Closer examination of this region revealed affected family members having a 41-kb deletion within intron 1 of the newly discovered WNK1 gene.[4] Another PHA2C kindred had a 21-kb deletion in the same gene. These deletions were not detected in any unaffected family members, and no WNK1 coding mutations were identified in any of the affected members.

Using bioinformatics tools, a WNK1 paralog was discovered and was identified as the *WNK4* gene.[4] This gene mapped to chromosome 17q21, a region that had previously been linked to PHA2B. Examination of the *WNK4* gene in four PHA2B kindreds linked to chromosome 17q21 identified four missense mutations that cosegregated with the disease. All of the mutations result in a change of amino acid. Three of these mutations (Glu562Lys, Asp564Ala, and Gln565Glu) lie within exon 7 of the WNK4 gene—in a small

stretch of amino acids that is highly conserved among all members of the human WNK kinases, as well as their known orthologs in mouse and rat. The fourth mutation (Arg1185Cys) lies within exon 17 at a residue conserved between the WNK kinases in the second coiled-coil domain (see material following). None of these mutations was identified in any unaffected family members.[4] Since the discovery of mutations in WNK1 and WNK4 causing Gordon's syndrome, only one novel mutation in WNK4 has been reported. Golbang and colleagues (2005) recently reported a missense mutation in exon 7 (Asp564His) in another affected kindred.[54]

Physiology and pathophysiology
WNK kinases

The recently discovered WNK kinases comprise a small group of unique protein serine/threonine kinases.[55,56] Protein kinases are a superfamily of proteins that regulate the activity of other proteins by phosphorylating certain amino acid residues (serine, threonine, or tyrosine) in specific target proteins. Protein kinases play important roles in signal transduction pathways, activated in response to extracellular signals (e.g., cytokines and growth factors), to regulate almost every cellular function—including cell proliferation, apoptosis, metabolism, gene expression, cell-cell communication, and membrane transport.[57] Most serine/threonine kinases share a highly conserved catalytic domain of 250 to 300 amino acids subdivided into 12 domains, with several residues that are usually invariant.[58] One of these is a crucial lysine residue located in subdomain II that is involved in ATP binding and catalyzing phosphoryl transfer.[59] In the WNK kinases, this conserved lysine is replaced by a cysteine. Hence the acronym WNK, which stands for *With no K* (K = lysine). In WNK kinases, the catalytic lysine is found in subdomain I. Despite this novel substitution, the WNK kinases retain active kinase activity.[56]

The WNKs are widely expressed in many tissues and cell lines. Interestingly, however, both WNK1 and WNK4 are predominantly expressed in the kidney and are exclusively found in the DCT and CCD—sites involved in net renal salt reabsorption as well as net potassium and hydrogen excretion[4] (Figure 36–1). The identification of specific WNK1 and WNK4 mutations in patients with PHA2 proved these to be disease-causing genes. The mechanism by which they cause the phenotype of PHA2 has been shown to be via increased NCCT activity, due to either loss of normal inhibition or constitutive activation by mutant WNK1 or WNK4.[60,61]

PHA2 phenotype of hypertension

WNK4 is an effective inhibitor of the NCCT and this is dependent on its kinase function.[60–62] Mutant WNK4 proteins lacking kinase activity do not have this inhibitory effect. In addition, WNK4 proteins harboring the PHA2 missense mutations (Glu562Lys, Asp564Ala, or Gln565Glu) lose their ability to suppress NCCT activity. These observations demonstrate that WNK4 PHA2 mutations prevent inhibition of NCCT activity and imply that it is the unrestrained activity of this co-transporter that causes PHA2.

Yang et al. looked at the effects of WNK1 on NCCT activity.[61] They found that unlike WNK4 WNK1 did not directly affect NCCT activity. The WNK1 protein, however, was capable of suppressing the inhibitory effect WNK4, suggesting that both kinases act in the same signaling pathway. The effect of WNK1 on WNK4 had the net result of increasing NCCT activity. These findings revealed a previously unrecognized interaction between the two WNK kinases. It is important to note that the inhibition of WNK4 by WNK1 requires the full-length kinase active isoform (L-WNK1). In PHA2, overexpression of L-WNK1 inhibits WNK4 activity, leading to increased NCCT activity and thus increased sodium reabsorption and hypertension.

There are two main WNK1 transcripts expressed in the kidney—the full-length "long" isoform (L-WNK1) and the more abundant "short" kidney-specific isoform (KS-WNK1)—and until recently little was known about the role of KS-WNK1 in the regulation of renal ion transport. Recent work by Naray-Fejes-Toth et al. has suggested that KS-WNK1 might be an important regulator of ENaC activity.[63] They expressed functional mineralocorticoid receptors in a kidney cell line and demonstrated rapidly induced expression of KS-WNK1 but not L-WNK1 in response to aldosterone at physiologic concentrations. This overexpression of KS-WNK1 resulted in increased transepithelial sodium transport via ENaC, suggesting that KS-WNK1 might be part of the mechanism by which aldosterone regulates sodium reabsorption in the CCD. These observations suggest that WNK1 might play an important role in aldosterone-induced sodium retention and the development of hypertension. Thus, in PHA2 patients high aldosterone levels as a result of hyperkalemia (potassium ions are a strong stimulator of aldosterone) could contribute to increased sodium reabsorption and therefore to hypertension via aldosterone-induced WNK1 expression.

PHA2 phenotype and hyperkalemia

One of the major features of PHA2 is hyperkalemia, suggesting that the WNKs could have a direct effect on ROMK1—the major K^+ secretory channel in the distal nephron.[62] Using *Xenopus laevis* oocytes in expression studies, Kahle et al. demonstrated that wild-type WNK4 is also a potent inhibitor of ROMK1 activity. In contrast to NCCT inhibition, inhibition of ROMK1 activity by WNK4 is not dependent on its kinase function. Instead, inhibition is mediated by clathrin-dependent endocytosis of ROMK1 from cell surface membranes, a mechanism distinct from WNK4 inhibition of NCCT. In addition, WNK4 constructs carrying the PHA2 mutations Q565E or E562K increased inhibition of potassium current and surface expression of ROMK1. Thus, PHA2 mutations that increase NCCT activity act to decrease ROMK1 activity. This would result in increased sodium chloride reabsorption by NCCT and contribute to elevated blood pressure and reduced potassium reabsorption—leading to hyperkalemia as a result of ROMK1 inhibition. This would explain most of the physiologic abnormalities seen in PHA2 patients.

PHA2 and hyperchloremia

WNK4 is expressed predominantly in the tight junctions of the DCT and CCD in the kidney, suggesting that WNK4 may also have a role in regulating paracellular chloride flux in the distal nephron. The chloride dependence of PHA2 further supports this notion. Two independent studies have now shown that wild-type WNK4 increases paracellular ion conductance secondary to a twofold increase in absolute paracellular permeability to chloride ions.[64,65] This effect is kinase dependent, and is greatly enhanced by the WNK4 missense mutations that cause PHA2.[65,66] In addition, WNK4 was shown to physically interact with and phosphorylate claudins 1 through 4.[65] These are major tight-junction membrane proteins known to be involved in the regulation of paracellular ion permeability.[67] In support of the "chloride-shunt" hypothesis proposed by Schambelan et al., PHA2-mutant WNK4 demonstrated increased association with and increased phosphorylation of these tight-junction proteins—providing a possible mechanism for increased paracellular permeability to chloride ions in PHA2 patients.[50] These findings suggest that WNK4 regulates paracellular Cl^- transport by phosphorylating claudins.

Clinical implications and perspectives

The clinical symptoms of PHA2 vary from family to family. However, all affected individuals have sodium-dependent hyperkalemia and hypertension.[47] Hyperkalemia is the feature always present and is used to distinguish it from other monogenic forms of hypertension. The severity and age of onset of hypertension varies.[68]

After the discovery of mutations in WNK kinases causing Gordon's syndrome, genotype/phenotype comparisons were made. It has been observed that clinical symptoms differ between families with PHA2B or PHA2C. Patients with WNK1 mutations usually present with milder symptoms of the disease with a later age-of-onset of hypertension, normal calcium levels, and in some patients a milder degree of plasma renin suppression. In contrast, patients with WNK4 mutations develop hypertension at an earlier age, and have hypercalciuria and marked suppression of renin levels. Hyperkalemia is always present, but hypertension severity is variable even within families. This could be due to extrinsic factors such as low sodium intake.[49,68,69]

Diagnosis of PHA2 is a combination of taking a clinical history, measuring blood pressure, and analysis of urine, plasma, and serum. The transtubular potassium gradient is used to detect low potassium concentrations in the urine from affected subjects. The presence of low plasma renin and high serum aldosterone concentrations are indicative of the condition. Genetic diagnosis is possible through mutation screening. However, this is not used routinely.

Thiazide diuretics are an effective treatment for PHA2. They act by inhibiting NCCT activity and therefore preventing excess sodium reabsorption in the distal nephron.[70] However, the long-term use of these drugs leads to side effects (especially on glucose metabolism), with subsequent development of type II diabetes.[70] The recent discovery of mutations in WNK kinases causing PHA2 places them as putative targets for new drugs for the condition.[61,62,71] However, a more detailed understanding of WNK kinase functions and their interactions in various tissues will be required before any attempts should be made for their use as therapeutic agents.

CONGENITAL ADRENAL HYPERPLASIA

Definition

Congenital adrenal hyperplasia (CAH) is a term used to define a group of autosomal recessive conditions in which affected individuals have abnormal steroid hormone production. Two forms of CAH exhibit hypertension: 11 β-hydroxylase deficiency (11OHD, OMIM: 202110) and 17 α-hydroxylase deficiency (17OHD, OMIM: 202110). 11OHD only accounts for 5 to 8% of all CAH cases worldwide, whereas to date only 150 validated cases of 17OHD exist.[72,73]

Distinguishing clinical features of these two forms include cortisol deficiency, aldosterone suppression, high ACTH levels, adrenal cortex hyperplasia, hypokalemia, and hypertension. In 11OHD, the enzyme deficiency also results in androgen excess, whereas in contrast 17OHD patients suffer from signs of sex hormone deficiency.[74] The symptoms of CAH are treated with hormone replacement therapy and are aided by moderate dietary salt intake.

CAH due to 11OHD
Genetics

Mutations in the 11 β-hydroxylase gene CYP11B1 cause 11OHD.[5] A single point mutation in exon 8 (G448A) was found in 11 of 12 affected individuals from 6 Jewish families of Moroccan origin with 11OHD. The families were not related, but Moroccan Jews have a high prevalence of 11OHD and it is likely the mutations in this population result from a founder effect.[5]

Subsequent analysis of the CYP11B1 gene in other families with 11OHD has revealed mutations in all coding regions, but there is some clustering in exons 2, 6, 7, and 8.[75,76] To date, there have been over 30 reported mutations in CYP11B1 causing 11OHD, and they include premature termination codons, missense mutations, frameshift mutations, splice site changes, insertions, and deletions.[76–79] Most of the recorded mutations result in complete loss of enzymatic activity. However, partial impairment also occurs.[75,80]

Physiology and pathophysiology

11 β-hydroxylase is a mitochondrial cytochrome P450 enzyme that catalyzes the last step of glucocorticoid biosynthesis to produce cortisol and corticosterone (Figure 36–2). In 11OHD individuals, a deficiency of 11 β-hydroxylase leads to reduced cortisol and corticosterone biosynthesis. The reduced levels of cortisol trigger the ACTH-dependent feedback mechanism, resulting in the overproduction of steroid precursors within the adrenal cortex. In the case of 11OHD, the steroid precursors 11-deoxycortisol (S) and 11-deoxycorticosterone (DOC) accumulate. The accumulation of unwanted metabolites results in two principal clinical effects: (1) inappropriate

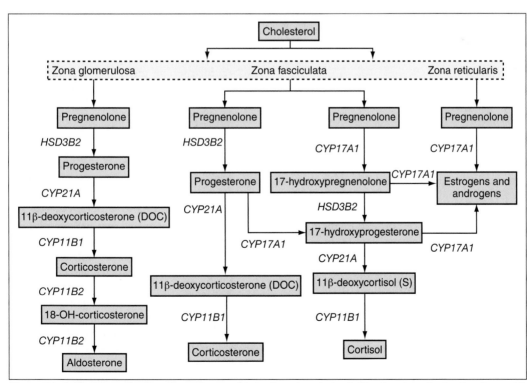

Figure 36–2. The biosynthetic pathway for steroids in the adrenal gland. The site of synthesis of each steroid and its precursor in the adrenal gland are shown in bold. The genes encoding enzymes in the pathway are indicated in italics. CYP11B1 encodes 11β-hydroxylase, which converts DOC to corticosterone and S to cortisol. This gene is mutated in 11OHD. CYP17A1 encodes an enzyme with two functions: (1) 17α hydroxylase activity (which catalyzes the initial step of cortisol synthesis) and (2) 17,20-desmolase activity, which is crucial for the production of sex hormones. This gene is mutated in 17OHD.

activation of the mineralocorticoid receptor, resulting in salt retention and hypertension, and (2) excessive production of androgens, resulting in the symptoms of androgenic excess.[27,81]

DOC is a potent mineralocorticoid of relative unimportance in healthy individuals. However, in 11 OHD patients excessive levels of DOC and its metabolites cause mineralocorticoid receptor hyperactivation and thus hypertension develops despite reduced aldosterone levels.[27]

The abnormalities in sex steroid synthesis arise as excess steroid precursors are shunted into the pathway of androgen biosynthesis. Thus, affected females present with masculinized external genitalia and males with hyperandrogenic symptoms such as acne, hyperpigmentation, and phallic enlargement.[82]

Despite the functional characterization of several mutations, at present no clear correlations between genotype and severity of hypertension or the degree of virilization have been made.[75,78] For reasons unknown, patients with identical CYP11B1 mutations demonstrate a range of different phenotypes.[76,83]

Clinical implications and perspectives

The clinical and biochemical phenotype of 11OHD is variable. Hypertension has been reported in 66% of 11OHD cases and usually develops late in childhood or in early adolescence.[74] Premature closure of the epiphyses leads to short stature in adulthood, despite rapid somatic growth and bone age acceleration in childhood.[27] The cortisol deficiency in 11OHD patients can expose affected individuals to frequent minor illnesses because they lack the ability to mount a stress response.[80] Rarely reported clinical features include dilated cardiomyopathy[84] and the development of a retroperitoneal mass,[85] both of which are alleviated by hydrocortisone therapy.

Multisteroid analysis after an ACTH-stimulation test reveals abnormal circulating DOC and S levels in 11OHD patients.[86] Confirmation by molecular genetic analysis using mutation screening is available but is not routinely used.

Initial treatment depends on the severity of the phenotype and actual metabolite levels, but the attenuation of symptoms is usually achieved by the administration of glucocorticoids such as hydrocortisone or dexamethasone. In general, hydrocortisone is the drug of choice because it is short acting, can be given in pulses that mimic natural cortisol secretion, and has a lower potential for growth retardation in children.[80]

Prenatal diagnosis, through the presence of elevated tetrahydro-S in the amniotic fluid or direct DNA sequence analysis from a chorionic villus sample, may be of significant use in populations with increased 11OHD prevalence, such as the Jewish families of North African origin.[76,87,88] Immediate prenatal therapy to prevent genital masculinization has been successfully achieved with the administration of dexamethasone.[89] In this instance, it is the preferred treatment because compared with other glucocorticoids it crosses the placenta more efficiently, has a longer half-life, and shows minimal unwanted side effects to the developing fetus.[90,91]

CAH due to 17OHD
Genetics

17OHD is an autosomal recessive disorder caused by mutations within the CYP17A1 gene. The CYP17A1 gene is located on chromosome 10q24.32 and encodes the 17 α-hydroxylase enzyme, which is expressed in adrenal gland and gonads.[92]

The molecular basis of 17OHD was discovered in 1988 when affected individuals were found to harbor mutations within exons 1 and 8 of the CYP17A1 gene.[6,93] Over 48 disease-causing mutations have since been described, including missense, nonsense, splice site, deletions, and insertions.[94–101] Enzymatic function can be completely or partially abolished by these mutations.[27] Most of the mutations are random and spontaneous. However, clusters of patients with the same mutation have been described in Dutch and Brazilian populations, suggesting a founder effect.[102,103]

Physiology and Pathophysiology

17 α-hydroxylase is also a member of the mitochondrial cytochrome P450 enzyme family. It has two distinct activities: 17 α-hydroxylation within the cortisol synthesis pathway and 17,20 desmolase activity within the sex steroid synthesis pathway (Figure 36–2). Thus, it is essential for the synthesis of cortisol and sex steroids.

Affected 17OHD individuals are unable to catalyze the 17α-hydroxylation of pregnenolone or progesterone, and/or to carry out the 17,20 desmolase reaction of 17-hydroxypregnenolone, resulting in reduced secretion of cortisol and/or androgenic steroids, respectively. Hypertension occurs when the action of 17α-hydroxylase is impaired. In this case, the excess pregnenolone is shunted down the corticosterone synthesis pathway, resulting in both corticosterone and DOC accumulation. Therefore, similar to 11OHD patients develop hypertension due to an excess of ligands for the MR.[93,104]

When 17,20 desmolase activity is abolished, individuals fail to synthesize adrenal androgens or gonadal steroids—resulting in hypogonadism in females and pseudohermaphroditism in males. Individuals with isolated 17,20 desmolase deficiency have normal blood pressure levels.[105]

Clinical implications and perspectives

17OHD was first reported in a patient with sexual infantilism and hypertension.[106] Previously thought to be extremely rare, the recent discovery of several novel CYP17A1 mutations suggests that the incidence rate of 17OHD is perhaps not as low as originally thought. In fact, 17OHD is relatively common in Dutch Mennonites[102] and Brazilians of Spanish/Portuguese origin.[103]

As with 11OHD, the phenotype of 17OHD varies considerably and depends on which of the enzyme's two activities is disrupted. Reasons for morbidity and mortality caused by 17α hydroxylase disruption include the delayed recognition of hypertension resulting in strokes, myocardial infarction, and chronic renal failure. Deficiencies in sex steroid synthesis can cause sexual ambiguity, infertility, and malignant degeneration of gonads.[73,107]

Similar to 11OHD, the ACTH stimulation test can be used to measure precursor/product ratios in 17OHD. In 17OHD, serum levels of DOC, corticosterone, 17-deoxysteroids, and progesterone rise to 5 to 10 times that of normal.[72] The condition can be further characterized by the reduction of urinary 17-hydroxysteroid-derived compounds, and by elevated circulating levels of follicle stimulating hormone (FSH) and luteinizing hormone (LH). Molecular genetic diagnosis by direct sequencing is the most sensitive diagnostic tool but is presently only available in research laboratory settings.[96]

Glucocorticoid replacement therapy is usually sufficient for normalizing the blood pressure of 17OHD individuals, but on occasion additional hypertensive drugs such as mineralocorticoid antagonist or calcium channel blocker may be required.[72] Surgery, including reconstruction of ambiguous genitalia and removal of testicles, may be required in cases where sex steroid synthesis/17,20 desmolase activity is severely disrupted.

SUMMARY

In this chapter we have reviewed five monogenic forms of human hypertension: GRA, Liddle's syndrome, Gordon's syndrome, and two hypertensive forms of CAH (11β-hydroxylase deficiency and 17α-hydroxylase deficiency). All of these have been characterized at the functional level and in all cases hypertension is due to increased renal sodium and water retention.

There are at least five other monogenic forms of hypertension (Table 36–1), some of which still remain to be fully characterized at the genetic and physiological level. These include apparent mineralocorticoid excess (AME) caused by mutations in 11β-hydroxysteroid dehydrogenase gene (11-HSD-2).[108] Mutations in 11-HDS-2 lead to cortisol binding to the mineralocorticoid receptor, and it is this inappropriate activation that disrupts renal electrolyte excretion and intravascular volume leading to hypertension.

Hypertension exacerbated by pregnancy is caused by mutations within the MR gene itself.[8] The mutant receptor has altered ligand specificity, allowing it to be activated by progesterone and other mineralocorticoids, which normally act as antagonists. Progesterone levels increase 100-fold in pregnancy, and therefore females with MR S810L mutation develop severe hypertension in pregnancy through MR hyperactivity.

Mutations within the peroxisome proliferator-activated receptor gamma (PPARγ) gene have recently been attributed to a rare monogenic syndrome, which displays hypertension as part of the phenotype (the underlying cause of which is currently not yet understood).[10] Further implications that PPARγ has an important role in blood pressure regulation come from the successful use of PPARγ agonists in the attenuation of hypertension.[109]

Recently, a mutation in the mitochondrial genome has been found to cause hypomagnesia, hypertension, and hypercholesterolemia.[11] The results from this paper suggest there may be links between the age-related loss of mitochondrial function and increases in both high blood pressure and cholesterol as people get older.

Finally, hypertension and brachydactyly type E, a condition which was first described in 1970s. The gene has yet to be found, and therefore the pathogenesis is not yet fully understood.[9,110] A recent description of neurovascular anomalies associated with the condition may prove significant in understanding its mechanism of hypertension.[111]

Since the discovery of the first gene causing a monogenic form of hypertension there has been a lot of excitement over the possibility that more subtle genetic variants in these genes may contribute to essential hypertension in the general population.[3] In support of this hypothesis, associations have now been reported between WNK1,[112] WNK4,[113,114] the β subunit of ENaC,[115] and CYP11B2[116] and essential hypertension in various populations. The discovery of novel mutations within these genes and their functional characterization may reveal some of the mechanisms leading to essential hypertension.

In summary, research into the causes of monogenic forms of hypertension has proved extremely successful, and we believe further studies in this area are likely to lead to the development of preclinical diagnostic tests and new therapeutic targets. These efforts might also shed light on the mechanisms causing essential hypertension.

REFERENCES

1. World Health Organization: Journal. http://www.who.int/genomics/public/geneticdiseases/en/index2.html

2. Lifton RP, Dluhy RG, Powers M, et al. A chimaeric 11 beta-hydroxylase/aldosterone synthase gene causes glucocorticoid-remediable aldosteronism and human hypertension. *Nature* 1992;355:262–65.

3. Shimkets RA, Warnock DG, Bositis CM, et al. Liddle's syndrome: Heritable human hypertension caused by mutations in the beta subunit of the epithelial sodium channel. *Cell* 1994;79:407–14.

4. Wilson FH, Disse-Nicodeme S, Choate KA, et al. Human hypertension caused by mutations in WNK kinases. *Science* 2001;293:1107–12.

5. White PC, Dupont J, New MI, et al. A mutation in CYP11B1 (Arg-448–His) associated with steroid 11 beta-hydroxylase deficiency in Jews of Moroccan origin. *J Clin Invest* 1991;87:1664–67.

6. Kagimoto M, Winter JS, Kagimoto K, et al. Structural characterization of normal and mutant human steroid 17 alpha-hydroxylase genes: Molecular basis of one example of combined 17 alpha-hydroxylase/17,20 lyase deficiency. *Mol Endocrinol* 1988;2:564–70.

7. Stewart PM, Krozowski ZS, Gupta A, et al. Hypertension in the syndrome of apparent mineralocorticoid excess due to mutation of the 11 beta-hydroxysteroid dehydrogenase type 2 gene. *Lancet* 1996;347:88–91.

8. Geller DS, Farhi A, Pinkerton N, et al. Activating mineralocorticoid receptor mutation in hypertension exacerbated by pregnancy. *Science* 2000;289:119–23.

9. Schuster H, Wienker TE, Bahring S, et al. Severe autosomal dominant hypertension and brachydactyly in a unique Turkish kindred maps to human chromosome 12. *Nat Genet* 1996;13:98–100.

10. Barroso I, Gurnell M, Crowley VE, et al. Dominant negative mutations in human PPARgamma associated with

severe insulin resistance, diabetes mellitus and hypertension. *Nature* 1999;402:880–83.

11. Wilson FH, Hariri A, Farhi A et al. A cluster of metabolic defects caused by mutation in a mitochondrial tRNA. *Science* 2004;306:1190–94.

12. Lote CJ, et al. *Principles of Renal Physiology, Third Edition.* New York: Chapman & Hall, 1994.

13. Loffing J, Kaissling B. Sodium and calcium transport pathways along the mammalian distal nephron: from rabbit to human. *Am J Physiol Renal Physiol* 2003;284:F628–43.

14. Goodman LS, Hardman JG, Limbird LE, Gilman AG. *Goodman & Gilman's The Pharmacological Basis of Therapeutics, Tenth Edition.* New York: McGraw-Hill, 2001.

15. Sutherland DJ, Ruse JL, Laidlaw JC. Hypertension, increased aldosterone secretion and low plasma renin activity relieved by dexamethasone. *Can Med Assoc J* 1966;95:1109–19.

16. Litchfield WR, New MI, Coolidge C, et al. Evaluation of the dexamethasone suppression test for the diagnosis of glucocorticoid-remediable aldosteronism. *J Clin Endocrinol Metab* 1997;82:3570–73.

17. Lifton RP, Dluhy RG, Powers M, et al. Hereditary hypertension caused by chimaeric gene duplications and ectopic expression of aldosterone synthase. *Nat Genet* 1992;2:66–74.

18. Lifton RP, Dluhy RG, Powers M, et al. A chimeric 11 beta-hydroxylase/ aldosterone synthase gene causes glucocorticoid-remediable aldosteronism and human hypertension. *Nature* 1992;355:262–65.

19. Pascoe L, Curnow KM, Slutsker L, et al. Glucocorticoid-suppressible hyperaldosteronism results from hybrid genes created by unequal crossovers between CYP11B1 and CYP11B2. *Proc Natl Acad Sci USA* 1992;89:8327–31.

20. Ding W, Liu L, Hu R, et al. Clinical and gene mutation studies on a Chinese pedigree with glucocorticoid-remediable aldosteronism. *Chin Med J (Engl)* 2002;115:979–82.

21. Yokota K, Ogura T, Kishida M, et al. Japanese family with glucocorticoid-remediable aldosteronism diagnosed by long-polymerase chain reaction. *Hypertens Res* 2001;24:589–94.

22. Lisurek M, Bernhardt R. Modulation of aldosterone and cortisol synthesis on the molecular level. *Mol Cell Endocrinol* 2004;215:149–59.

23. Odermatt A. Corticosteroid-dependent hypertension: Environmental influences. *Swiss Med Wkly* 2004;134:4–13.

24. Hall CE, Gomez-Sanchez CE. Hypertensive potency of 18-oxocortisol in the rat. *Hypertension* 1986;8:317–22.

25. Griffing GT, Dale SL, Holbrook MM, Melby JC. The regulation of urinary free 19-nor-deoxycorticosterone and its relation to systemic arterial blood pressure in normotensive and hypertensive subjects. *J Clin Endocrinol Metab* 1983;56:99–103.

26. Litchfield WR, Anderson BF, Weiss RJ, et al. Intracranial aneurysm and hemorrhagic stroke in glucocorticoid-remediable aldosteronism. *Hypertension* 1998;31:445–50.

27. White PC. Inherited forms of mineralocorticoid hypertension. *Hypertension* 1996;28:927–36.

28. Mulatero P, Veglio F, Pilon C, et al. Diagnosis of glucocorticoid-remediable aldosteronism in primary aldosteronism: Aldosterone response to dexamethasone and long polymerase chain reaction for chimeric gene. *J Clin Endocrinol Metab* 1998;83:2573–75.

29. Mosso L, Gomez-Sanchez CE, Foecking MF, Fardella C. Serum 18-hydroxycortisol in primary aldosteronism, hypertension, and normotensives. *Hypertension* 2001;38:688–91.

30. Stowasser M, Huggard PR, Rossetti TR, et al. Biochemical evidence of aldosterone overproduction and abnormal regulation in normotensive individuals with familial hyperaldosteronism type I. *J Clin Endocrinol Metab* 1999;84:4031–36.

31. Liddle GW, Bledsoe T, Coppage WS Jr. A familial renal disorder simulating aldosteronism but with negligible aldosterone secretion. *Trans Assoc Am Physicians* 1963;76:199–213.

32. Botero-Velez M, Curtis JJ, Warnock DG. Brief report: Liddle's syndrome revisited—a disorder of sodium reabsorption in the distal tubule. *N Engl J Med* 1994;330:178–81.

33. Hansson JH, Nelson-Williams C, Suzuki H, et al. Hypertension caused by a truncated epithelial sodium channel gamma subunit: genetic heterogeneity of Liddle syndrome. *Nat Genet* 1995;11:76–82.

34. Furuhashi M, Kitamura K, Adachi M, et al. Liddle's syndrome caused by a novel mutation in the proline-rich PY motif of the epithelial sodium channel beta-subunit. *J Clin Endocrinol Metab* 2005;90:340–44.

35. Stenson PD, Ball EV, Mort M, et al. Human Gene Mutation Database (HGMD): 2003 update. *Hum Mutat* 2003;21:577–81.

36. Rossier BC, Canessa CM, Schild L, Horisberger JD. Epithelial sodium channels. *Curr Opin Nephrol Hypertens* 1994;3:487–96.

37. Canessa CM, Schild L, Buell G, et al. Amiloride-sensitive epithelial Na+ channel is made of three homologous subunits. *Nature* 1994;367:463–67.

38. Schild L, Canessa CM, Shimkets RA, et al. A mutation in the epithelial sodium channel causing Liddle disease increases channel activity in the Xenopus laevis oocyte expression system. *Proc Natl Acad Sci USA* 1995;92:5699–703.

39. Staub O, Dho S, Henry P, et al. WW domains of Nedd4 bind to the proline-rich PY motifs in the epithelial Na+ channel deleted in Liddle's syndrome. *Embo J* 1996;15:2371–80.

40. Abriel H, Loffing J, Rebhun JF, et al. Defective regulation of the epithelial Na+ channel by Nedd4 in Liddle's syndrome. *J Clin Invest* 1999;103:667–73.

41. Harvey KF, Dinudom A, Cook DI, Kumar S. The Nedd4-like protein KIAA0439 is a potential regulator of the epithelial sodium channel. *J Biol Chem* 2001;276:8597–601.

42. Kellenberger S, Gautschi I, Rossier BC, Schild L. Mutations causing Liddle syndrome reduce sodium-dependent downregulation of the epithelial sodium channel in the Xenopus

43. Findling JW, Raff H, Hansson JH, Lifton RP. Liddle's syndrome: Prospective genetic screening and suppressed aldosterone secretion in an extended kindred. *J Clin Endocrinol Metab* 1997;82:1071–74.

44. Rayner BL, Owen EP, King JA, et al. A new mutation, R563Q, of the beta subunit of the epithelial sodium channel associated with low-renin, low-aldosterone hypertension. *J Hypertens* 2003;21:921–26.

45. Rodriguez JA, Biglieri EG, Schambelan M. Pseudohyperaldosteronism with renal tubular resistance to mineralocorticoid hormones. *Trans Assoc Am Physicians* 1981;94:172–82.

46. Jeunemaitre X, Bassilana F, Persu A, et al. Genotype-phenotype analysis of a newly discovered family with Liddle's syndrome. *J Hypertens* 1997;15:1091–1100.

47. Gordon RD. Syndrome of hypertension and hyperkalemia with normal glomerular filtration rate. *Hypertension* 1986;8:93–102.

48. Gordon RD, Geddes RA, Pawsey CG, O'Halloran MW. Hypertension and severe hyperkalaemia associated with suppression of renin and aldosterone and completely reversed by dietary sodium restriction. *Australas Ann Med* 1970;19:287–94.

49. Mayan H, Vered I, Mouallem M, et al. Pseudohypoaldosteronism type II: Marked sensitivity to thiazides, hypercalciuria, normomagnesemia, and low bone mineral density. *J Clin Endocrinol Metab* 2002;87:3248–54.

50. Schambelan M, Sebastian A, Rector FC Jr. Mineralocorticoid-resistant renal hyperkalemia without salt wasting (type II pseudohypoaldosteronism): Role of increased renal chloride reabsorption. *Kidney Int* 1981;19:716–27.

51. Mansfield TA, Simon DB, Farfel Z, et al. Multilocus linkage of familial hyperkalaemia and hypertension, pseudohypoaldosteronism type II, to chromosomes 1q31-42 and 17p11-q21. *Nat Genet* 1997;16:202–05.

52. Disse-Nicodeme S, Achard JM, Desitter I, et al. A new locus on chromosome 12p13.3 for pseudohypoaldosteronism type II, an autosomal dominant form of hypertension. *Am J Hum Genet* 2000;67:302–10.

53. Disse-Nicodeme S, Desitter I, Fiquet-Kempf B, et al. Genetic heterogeneity of familial hyperkalaemic hypertension. *J Hypertens* 2001;19:1957–64.

54. Golbang AP, Murthy M, Hamad A, et al. A new kindred with pseudohypoaldosteronism type II and a novel mutation (564D>H) in the acidic motif of the WNK4 gene. *Hypertension* 2005;46:295–300.

55. Verissimo F, Jordan P. WNK kinases, a novel protein kinase subfamily in multi-cellular organisms. *Oncogene* 2001;20:5562–69.

56. Xu B, English JM, Wilsbacher JL, et al. WNK1, a novel mammalian serine/threonine protein kinase lacking the catalytic lysine in subdomain II. *J Biol Chem* 2000;275:16795–801.

57. Pearson G, Robinson F, Beers Gibson T, et al. Mitogen-activated protein (MAP) kinase pathways: regulation and

physiological functions. *Endocr Rev* 2001;22:153–83.

58. Hanks SK. Genomic analysis of the eukaryotic protein kinase superfamily: A perspective. *Genome Biol* 2003;4:111.

59. Hanks SK, Hunter T. Protein kinases 6. The eukaryotic protein kinase superfamily: Kinase (catalytic) domain structure and classification. *Faseb J* 1995;9:576–96.

60. Wilson FH, Kahle KT, Sabath E, et al. Molecular pathogenesis of inherited hypertension with hyperkalemia: The Na-Cl cotransporter is inhibited by wild-type but not mutant WNK4. *Proc Natl Acad Sci USA* 2003;100:680–84.

61. Yang CL, Angell J, Mitchell R, Ellison DH. WNK kinases regulate thiazide-sensitive Na-Cl cotransport. *J Clin Invest* 2003;111:1039–45.

62. Kahle KT, Wilson FH, Leng Q, et al. WNK4 regulates the balance between renal NaCl reabsorption and K+ secretion. *Nat Genet* 2003;35:372–76.

63. Naray-Fejes-Toth A, Snyder PM, Fejes-Toth G. The kidney-specific WNK1 isoform is induced by aldosterone and stimulates epithelial sodium channel-mediated Na+ transport. *Proc Natl Acad Sci USA* 2004;101(50):17434–39.

64. Kahle KT, Wilson FH, Lalioti M, et al. WNK kinases: Molecular regulators of integrated epithelial ion transport. *Curr Opin Nephrol Hypertens* 2004; 13:557–62.

65. Yamauchi K, Rai T, Kobayashi K, et al. Disease-causing mutant WNK4 increases paracellular chloride permeability and phosphorylates claudins. *Proc Natl Acad Sci USA* 2004;101:4690–94.

66. Kahle KT, Macgregor GG, Wilson FH, et al. Paracellular Cl- permeability is regulated by WNK4 kinase: Insight into normal physiology and hypertension. *Proc Natl Acad Sci USA* 2004;101:14877–82.

67. Van Itallie CM, Anderson JM. The molecular physiology of tight junction pores. *Physiology (Bethesda)* 2004;19:331–38.

68. Mayan H, Munter G, Shaharabany M, et al. Hypercalciuria in familial hyperkalemia and hypertension accompanies hyperkalemia and precedes hypertension: Description of a large family with the Q565E WNK4 mutation. *J Clin Endocrinol Metab* 2004;89:4025–30.

69. Achard JM, Warnock DG, Disse-Nicodeme S, et al. Familial hyperkalemic hypertension: Phenotypic analysis in a large family with the WNK1 deletion mutation. *Am J Med* 2003;114:495–98.

70. Cope G, Golbang A, O'Shaughnessy KM. WNK kinases and the control of blood pressure. *Pharmacol Ther* 2005;106:221–31.

71. Zambrowicz BP, Abuin A, Ramirez-Solis R, et al. Wnk1 kinase deficiency lowers blood pressure in mice: A gene-trap screen to identify potential targets for therapeutic intervention. *Proc Natl Acad Sci USA* 2003;100:14109–14.

72. Uwaifo GI MD. C-17 Hydroxylase Deficiency, eMedicine.com 2005.

73. Zachmann M, Tassinari D, Prader A. Clinical and biochemical variability of congenital adrenal hyperplasia due to 11 beta-hydroxylase deficiency:

A study of 25 patients. *J Clin Endocrinol Metab* 1983;56:222–29.

74. Chemaitilly W, Wilson RC, New MI. Hypertension and adrenal disorders. *Curr Hypertens Rep* 2003;5:498–504.

75. Connell JM, Fraser R, Davies E. Disorders of mineralocorticoid synthesis. *Best Pract Res Clin Endocrinol Metab* 2001;15:43–60.

76. Curnow KM, Slutsker L, Vitek J, et al. Mutations in the CYP11B1 gene causing congenital adrenal hyperplasia and hypertension cluster in exons 6, 7, and 8. *Proc Natl Acad Sci USA* 1993; 90:4552–56.

77. Helmberg A, Ausserer B, Kofler R. Frame shift by insertion of 2 basepairs in codon 394 of CYP11B1 causes congenital adrenal hyperplasia due to steroid 11 beta-hydroxylase deficiency. *J Clin Endocrinol Metab* 1992;75:1278–81.

78. Krone N, Riepe FG, Gotze D, et al. Congenital adrenal hyperplasia due to 11-hydroxylase deficiency: Functional characterization of two novel point mutations and a three-base pair deletion in the CYP11B1 gene. *J Clin Endocrinol Metab* 2005;90:3724–30.

79. Lee HH, Won GS, Chao HT, et al. Novel missense mutations, GCC [Ala306]- > GTC [Val] and ACG [Thr318]- > CCG [Pro], in the CYP11B1 gene cause steroid 11beta-hydroxylase deficiency in the Chinese. *Clin Endocrinol (Oxf)* 2005;62:418–22.

80. Deaton MA, Glorioso JE, McLean DB. Congenital adrenal hyperplasia: Not really a zebra. *Am Fam Physician* 1999;59:1190–96.

81. Peter M. Congenital adrenal hyperplasia: 11beta-hydroxylase deficiency. *Semin Reprod Med* 2002;20:249–54.

82. White PC, Curnow KM, Pascoe L. Disorders of steroid 11 beta-hydroxylase isozymes. *Endocr Rev* 1994;15:421–38.

83. Zhu YS, Cordero JJ, Can S, et al. Mutations in CYP11B1 gene: Phenotype-genotype correlations. *Am J Med Genet A* 2003;122:193–200.

84. Al Jarallah AS. Reversible cardiomyopathy caused by an uncommon form of congenital adrenal hyperplasia. *Pediatr Cardiol* 2004;25:675–76.

85. Storr HL, Barwick TD, Snodgrass GA, et al. Hyperplasia of adrenal rest tissue causing a retroperitoneal mass in a child with 11 beta-hydroxylase deficiency. *Horm Res* 2003;60:99–102.

86. Sippell WG, Bidlingmaier F, Becker H, et al. Simultaneous radioimmunoassay of plasma aldosterone, corticosterone, 11-deoxycorticosterone, progesterone, 17-hydroxyprogesterone, 11-deoxycortisol, cortisol and cortisone. *J Steroid Biochem* 1978;9:63–74.

87. Rosler A, Leiberman E, Cohen T. High frequency of congenital adrenal hyperplasia (classic 11 beta-hydroxylase deficiency) among Jews from Morocco. *Am J Med Genet* 1992;42:827–34.

88. Rosler A, Weshler N, Leiberman E, et al. 11 Beta-hydroxylase deficiency congenital adrenal hyperplasia: update of prenatal diagnosis. *J Clin Endocrinol Metab* 1988;66:830–38.

89. Motaghedi R, Betensky BP, Slowinska B, et al. Update on the prenatal diagnosis and treatment of congenital adrenal hyperplasia due to 11 beta-

hydroxylase deficiency. *J Pediatr Endocrinol Metab* 2005;18:133–42.

90. Meyer-Bahlburg HF, Dolezal C, Baker SW, et al. Cognitive and motor development of children with and without congenital adrenal hyperplasia after early-prenatal dexamethasone. *J Clin Endocrinol Metab* 2004;89:610–14.

91. Travitz J, Metzger DL. Antenatal treatment for classic 21-hydroxylase forms of congenital adrenal hyperplasia and the issues. *Genet Med* 1999;1:224–30;quiz 231–32.

92. Voutilainen R, Miller WL. Developmental expression of genes for the stereoidogenic enzymes P450scc (20,22-desmolase), P450c17 (17 alpha-hydroxylase/17,20-lyase), and P450c21 (21-hydroxylase) in the human fetus. *J Clin Endocrinol Metab* 1986;63:1145–50.

93. Yanase T, Kagimoto M, Matsui N, et al. Combined 17 alpha-hydroxylase/ 17,20-lyase deficiency due to a stop codon in the N-terminal region of 17 alpha-hydroxylase cytochrome P-450. *Mol Cell Endocrinol* 1988;59:249–53.

94. Auchus RJ. The genetics, pathophysiology, and management of human deficiencies of P450c17. *Endocrinol Metab Clin North Am* 2001;30:101–19,vii.

95. Costa-Santos M, Kater CE, Auchus RJ. Two prevalent CYP17 mutations and genotype-phenotype correlations in 24 Brazilian patients with 17-hydroxylase deficiency. *J Clin Endocrinol Metab* 2004;89:49–60.

96. Di Cerbo A, Biason-Lauber A, Savino M, et al. Combined 17alpha-Hydroxylase/17,20-lyase deficiency caused by Phe93Cys mutation in the CYP17 gene. *J Clin Endocrinol Metab* 2002;87:898–905.

97. Katsumata N, Satoh M, Mikami A, et al. New compound heterozygous mutation in the CYP17 gene in a 46,XY girl with 17 alpha-hydroxylase/ 17,20-lyase deficiency. *Horm Res* 2001;55:141–46.

98. Lam CW, Arlt W, Chan CK, et al. Mutation of proline 409 to arginine in the meander region of cytochrome p450c17 causes severe 17 alpha-hydroxylase deficiency. *Mol Genet Metab* 2001;72:254–59.

99. Schwab KO, Moisan AM, Homoki J, et al. 17alpha-hydroxylase/17,20-Lyase deficiency due to novel compound heterozygote mutations: Treatment for tall stature in a female with male pseudohermaphroditism and spontaneous puberty in her affected sister. *J Pediatr Endocrinol Metab* 2005;18:403–11.

100. Takeda Y, Yoneda T, Demura M, et al. Genetic analysis of the cytochrome P-450c17alpha (CYP17) and aldosterone synthase (CYP11B2) in Japanese patients with 17alpha-hydroxylase deficiency. *Clin Endocrinol (Oxf)* 2001;54:751–58.

101. Yamaguchi H, Nakazato M, Miyazato M, et al. Identification of a novel splicing mutation and 1-bp deletion in the 17alpha-hydroxylase gene of Japanese patients with 17alpha-hydroxylase deficiency. *Hum Genet* 1998;102:635–39.

102. Imai T, Yanase T, Waterman MR, et al. Canadian Mennonites and

individuals residing in the Friesland region of The Netherlands share the same molecular basis of 17 alpha-hydroxylase deficiency. *Hum Genet* 1992;89:95–6.

103. Miller WL. Steroid 17alpha-hydroxylase deficiency—not rare everywhere. *J Clin Endocrinol Metab* 2004;89:40–2.

104. Goldsmith O, Solomon DH, Horton R. Hypogonadism and mineralocorticoid excess: The 17-hydroxylase deficiency syndrome. *N Engl J Med* 1967;277:673–77.

105. Geller DH, Auchus RJ, Mendonca BB, Miller WL. The genetic and functional basis of isolated 17,20-lyase deficiency. *Nat Genet* 1997;17:201–05.

106. Biglieri EG, Herron MA, Brust N. 17-hydroxylation deficiency in man. *J Clin Invest* 1966;45:1946–54.

107. Levran D, Ben-Shlomo I, Pariente C, et al. Familial partial 17,20-desmolase and 17alpha-hydroxylase deficiency presenting as infertility. *J Assist Reprod Genet* 2003;20:21–8.

108. Mune T, Rogerson FM, Nikkila H, et al. Human hypertension caused by mutations in the kidney isozyme of 11 beta-hydroxysteroid dehydrogenase. *Nat Genet* 1995;10:394–99.

109. Ryan MJ, Didion SP, Mathur S, et al. PPAR(gamma) agonist rosiglitazone improves vascular function and lowers blood pressure in hypertensive transgenic mice. *Hypertension* 2004;43:661–66.

110. Bilginturan N, Zileli S, Karacadag S, Pirnar T. Hereditary brachydactyly associated with hypertension. *J Med Genet* 1973;10:253–59.

111. Luft FC. Mendelian forms of human hypertension and mechanisms of disease. *Clin Med Res* 2003;1:291–300.

112. Newhouse SJ, Wallace C, Dobson R, et al. Haplotypes of the WNK1 gene associate with blood pressure variation in a severely hypertensive population from the British Genetics of Hypertension study. *Hum Mol Genet* 2005;14:1805–14.

113. Erlich PM, Cui J, Chazaro I, et al. Genetic variants of WNK4 in Whites and African Americans with hypertension. *Hypertension* 2003;41:1191–95.

114. Kokubo Y, Kamide K, Inamoto N, et al. Identification of 108 SNPs in TSC, WNK1, and WNK4 and their association with hypertension in a Japanese general population. *J Hum Genet* 2004;49:507–15.

115. Baker EH, Dong YB, Sagnella GA, et al. Association of hypertension with T594M mutation in beta subunit of epithelial sodium channels in black people resident in London. *Lancet* 1998;351:1388–92.

116. Lim PO, Macdonald TM, Holloway C, et al. Variation at the aldosterone synthase (CYP11B2) locus contributes to hypertension in subjects with a raised aldosterone-to-renin ratio. *J Clin Endocrinol Metab* 2002;87:4398–402.

Chapter

37

Therapeutic Potential of Systemic Gene Transfer Strategy for Hypertension and Cardiovascular Disease

Shant Der Sarkissian and Mohan K. Raizada

Definition

- Gene therapy is a strategy in which a vector is used to deliver beneficial genes, thereby changing the expression levels of that gene to correct the altered expression in the pathological state.

Key Findings

- The principal benefits of gene therapy over the use of traditional pharmacotherapy are as follows.
- Minimal side effects due to the specificity of gene therapy's mode of action
- Elimination of patient noncompliance problems
- May prove useful in the cure of certain diseases (e.g., hypertension) whose symptoms are only treatable with current pharmacotherapy

Clinical Implications

Cardiovascular gene therapy in humans is at an investigational phase. However, with the impressive results of preliminary studies and with the improvement of the tools and the knowledge in gene manipulation gene therapy may eventually become part of routine care for patients.

EPIDEMIOLOGY OF HYPERTENSION AND CARDIOVASCULAR DISEASE

Cardiovascular (CV) disease extends across all population segments and represents the leading cause of morbidity and mortality in industrialized nations.[1,2] A major risk factor for CV disease is arterial hypertension, which significantly increases the risk for peripheral artery disease, stroke, coronary artery disease, cardiomyopathies, and cardiac and renal failure.[1–5] Hypertension often goes undetected, and in those diagnosed with the disease only half receive adequate treatment and 70% of these patients do not fully comply with their treatment.[6] Thus, only about 10% of all hypertensives nationwide are adequately managed.

This escalation of the prevalence of CV disease and hypertension, even with the multitude of modern-day pharmaceuticals available for treatment, has led many to conclude that traditional pharmacotherapy has reached an intellectual plateau and that novel approaches for the treatment and control of CV disease and hypertension

must be explored. As a result, our efforts have been diverted to explore the use of gene transfer approaches for the long-term control of these diseases, and the experimental successes of our peers and of our group suggest that gene modification can work in preventing and reversing hypertension and CV diseases.

GENE THERAPY AS AN ALTERNATIVE APPROACH FOR THE TREATMENT OF HYPERTENSION AND CARDIOVASCULAR DISEASE

A recent report from the American Heart Association indicates that the incidence of hypertension has risen 30% in the last decade in spite of the availability of effective drug therapies. This increase has several causes. First, all of these drugs have short half-lives and repeat administration is necessary for the success of the treatments because the disease is generally reexpressed once therapy is discontinued. Second, the question of patient noncompliance is a critical issue because some patients have difficulty abiding by the daily requirement of the treatment, particularly in view of the fact that some of these drugs have intolerable side effects.[7,8] Third, because mild to moderate hypertension is usually asymptomatic patients often view pharmacotherapy as unnecessary and inconvenient. However, end-organ damage (a hallmark of the hypertensive state) may have already occurred once hypertension is diagnosed and unaware patients further precipitate the situation by not complying with their treatment regimen. Further drug development may yield more selective inhibitors with fewer side effects, but it seems unlikely that a cure for hypertension will come from pharmacologic intervention.

Gene therapy offers the possibility of producing long-term therapeutic effects with specificity tailored to a patient's own genetic profile. The benefits of this method over the use of traditional pharmacologic therapies are as follows.

- Compliance problems can be reduced or even eliminated because with GT a single injection can be effective for months, years, or even for the remainder of a patient's life.
- Side effects can be minimized because GT is very specific in its mode of action and specifically inhibits or enhances the expression of a particular gene.

- GT has the potential to maintain an optimally high and localized concentration of therapeutic genes over time, which may also reduce side effects.

The historic sequencing of the human genome, the advances in the understanding of CV biology and pathophysiology at the molecular level, and the improvements in gene targeting technologies and in tools for *in vivo* genetic manipulation and delivery have inspired active investigation into genetic treatments for hypertension and CV diseases. GT is an emerging field that offers targeted and time-controlled parameters especially relevant to CV diseases ranging from hypertension to ischemia to restenosis. Modification of gene expression offers a means to prevent, arrest, or reverse these pathophysiologic states. Moreover, the notion of treating localized disease with targeted therapy has emerged as one of the great promises of GT.[9]

The etiology of hypertension is poorly understood, with only a small percentage of sufferers demonstrating isolated genetic abnormalities. In the majority of cases, the cause of hypertension is unknown and falls into the category of primary hypertension. This has led many investigators to hypothesize that expression of the hypertensive phenotype is multigenetic and multifactorial,[10,11] and therefore not considered appropriate for GT because GT has tended to be limited to diseases resulting from single gene mutations or to life-threatening diseases for which few alternatives are available. Nevertheless, drug companies have for years made advances in the control of hypertension with single pharmaceutical targets. The most successful drugs developed to reduce hypertension have been designed to inhibit β- or α-adrenergic receptors, calcium channels, angiotensin-converting enzyme (ACE), and angiotensin-II AT_1 receptors (AT_1R). Based on this, GT for hypertension is feasible and for its success it is only necessary to analyze and target only those genes that have already been targeted by successful pharmacotherapy. Thus, it would be imperative to first provide proof of concept for GT with the use of these genes.

There are two critical issues that determine the success of GT: (1) selection of the targeted gene (one could target pressor genes to inhibit their expression, whereas genes relevant to vasodilation could be overexpressed) and (2) mode of gene transfer (i.e., selection of nonviral or viral vectors). Each of these issues must be considered based on the type of CV pathophysiologies to be targeted.

GENE DELIVERY VEHICLES

GT is a strategy in which a vector is used to deliver beneficial genes either systemically or directly into the tissue, thereby changing the expression levels of that gene to correct the altered expression in the pathologic state. The simplest way to deliver exogenous genes is by directly injecting naked plasmid DNA. This method can be used for localized delivery into a particular tissue. Naked DNA delivery has little or no toxic or adverse side effects.[12] Disadvantages of this technique include inefficient delivery, limited time for transgene expression, high levels of vector breakdown in circulation, and lack of chromosomal inte-

gration.[13] In fact, if naked plasmid DNA is in contact with cell membranes only a small amount will pass into the cell—leading to low gene transfer. Therefore, a carrier molecule or a viral vector is generally used to increase gene transfer efficiency. Each of these vehicles possesses its special characteristics, as well as advantages and disadvantages, which determine its use for a particular subset of CV diseases. For example, in hypertension research (where reversal and prevention is critical) long-term gene regulation is necessary, whereas in disorders such as ischemia or restenosis short-term gene control would prove more adequate. Currently, several methods are in use to facilitate the entry of nucleic acids into cells, and these can be divided into nonviral and viral vector-mediated systems. Table 37–1 summarizes the major pros and cons of different viral and nonviral gene delivery methods.

Nonviral mediated gene delivery

A wide variety of nonviral vector systems—such as synthetic cationic polymer carriers, liposomes, and hemagglutinating virus of Japan (HVJ-liposomes)—have been used to deliver genes *in vivo*.[14,15] Liposomes are the most often used method for the delivery of genes by nonviral means because they are nonpathogenic and easily produced and do not have a size constraint.[16] Liposomes increase infection efficiency over naked DNA delivery, minimize immunogenecity, and prevent DNA degradation in circulation. However, the inability of liposomal-delivered DNA to integrate into the recipient cell genome makes them less suitable in situations where long-term transgene expression is required (such as for the control of hypertension).[17,18] Consequently, liposomes remain an ideal choice for short-term transgene expression and have been used to deliver transgenes relevant in the inhibition of cell proliferation during restenosis.[19]

Viral-mediated gene delivery

Viral-mediated gene delivery is emerging as the preferred choice of gene delivery vehicles. For some viruses, integration into the host genome is required for transgene expression. Replacing genes required for viral replication with an expression cassette containing the therapeutic genes transforms the viruses into safe vectors. An ideal replication-deficient recombinant virus is able to efficiently infect quiescent cells, integrate into the host genome, mediate long-term and stable expression, and remain controllable with minimal nonspecific effects.

Several types of viral-mediated gene delivery systems exist, each having its own unique qualities. The major classes of viral vectors include the adenovirus, the adeno-associated virus, and the retrovirus (including the lentiviral vector).[20–22]

Adenovirus

Adenoviruses are large, linear double-stranded DNA viruses. Vectors derived from the human adenovirus serotypes 5 and 2 are commonly used for gene transfer, as these can be generated at high titers and express transgenes in both dividing and quiescent cells.[23] Other advantages of this vector include ease of manipulation, large insert capacity,

MAJOR ADVANTAGES AND DISADVANTAGES OF NONVIRAL VERSUS VIRAL GENE DELIVERY METHODS

Vehicle	Pros	Cons
Nonviral		
Oligonucleotide	Easy to produce; safe to handle	Lack of target specificity; transient expression pattern
Liposome	Easy to produce; safe to handle	Lack of target specificity; transient expression pattern
Viral		
Adenovirus	Infects dividing and nondividing cells; high titers	Immunogenic; transient expression; lack of integration
AAV	Nonpathogenic; specific integration site (wild-type); infects nondividing cells	Very small payload
Retrovirus	Stable long-term expression; large payload; relatively nonimmunogenic	Random integration; only infects dividing cells
Lentivirus	Stable long-term expression; large payload; infects dividing and nondividing cells; low immunogenicity	Random integration; safety concerns; low titers

Adapted from Katovich MJ et al., *Current and Future Novel Targets of Gene Therapy for Hypertension.*[173]

Table 37–1. Major Advantages and Disadvantages of Nonviral Versus Viral Gene Delivery Methods

and its extensive characterization.[24] Although adenoviral vectors have been readily used for studying various CV diseases, this vector has some drawbacks that may prevent its future use. First, most adenoviral vectors in their current form are episomal (i.e., they do not integrate into the host DNA and therefore only cause a transient transgene expression). Second, because most individuals have been exposed to natural adenovirus infections, immunologic responses may hamper gene transfer efficacy. In addition, because the adenoviral genes express hundreds of proteins adenoviruses stimulate the immune system and inflammatory responses. Newer second- and third-generation adenoviral vectors with many of the viral genes deleted have demonstrated significant improvements in terms of inflammation and immune response.[25] However, repeated gene transfer with this vector coupled with prior infection may still result in inflammatory responses with consequent tissue damage.[26] These limitations make current recombinant adenoviral vectors less than ideal for long-term GT in humans. Thus, the adenoviral vector remains a useful tool for gene transfer for experimental studies in animal models because it is easy to produce on a large scale.

Adeno-associated virus

The adeno-associated virus (AAV) has established its position as one of the most popular gene delivery systems. AAV has gained attention because of its safety, lack of immunogenic viral proteins, and efficient transgene expression in a very broad host range.[27] AAV infects all mammalian tissues tested,[28] and its ability to infect a large number of both dividing and nondividing cells makes it an appropriate vector for GT in adult tissues. However, the rate of transduction of nondividing cells remains much lower than for dividing cells.[29] AAV is not pathogenic and is not associated with disease, even though it has a broad range of infectivity. Upon infection, the AAV remains intact for long periods of time.

Upon infection of a human cell, the wild-type AAV integrates preferentially into chromosome 19,[24] although a low integration frequency in the region of active genes and frequent chromosomal deletions have been demonstrated in animal studies.[30] Although there are eight serotypes, most AAV vectors have been derived from AAV-2. AAV-2 is a small single-stranded DNA virus that can only package limited amounts of DNA (i.e., up to 4.4 kb of insert). Although this carrying capacity may limit the AAV to delivering large genes, it is amply suited to deliver small genes and particularly antisense cDNA. Another limitation of AAV is its production. Although it can be purified and concentrated, it has to be rendered free of adenovirus and this makes production more complicated than for other vectors. Therefore, many drawbacks must be overcome before this vector system can be an ideal vector for GT.

Retrovirus

The pioneering work on gene delivery *in vivo* was performed with retrovirus vectors, typically the Moloney murine leukemia virus (MLV). Retroviruses enter mammalian cells through specific surface receptors, which can limit their range of infectivity. Once inside cells, the RNA genome of the retrovirus is reverse transcribed by reverse transcriptase into a double-stranded DNA provirus that is incorporated into a pre-integration nucleoprotein complex (PIC). The PIC typically does not pass through intact nuclear membranes and therefore integration of the provirus requires breakdown of the nuclear envelope via mitosis.[31] Therefore, retroviruses are highly efficient in infecting dividing cells but have limited efficacy in nondividing cells. This raises the question of the suitability of retroviruses for the GT treatment of certain diseases such as adult hypertension, although retroviruses may be useful for other pathologies such as restenosis (where cells are actively dividing).

The retroviral DNA is integrated into the host genome, leading to gene expression for extended time periods. However, the integration is random, which raises concerns about safety. Another major limitation of the retrovirus is its low titers during production.[32–34] To overcome the cell-type range and titer limitations, retroviral vectors have been pseudotyped with envelope proteins from other viruses such as the G glycoprotein from vesicular stomatitis virus (VSV).[35] Vector development has been intense for retroviruses. New generations of the vector are less immunogenic, self-activating and inactivating vectors have been engineered,[36] and these newer vectors can integrate into specific locations in the host genome and have the improved ability to infect nondividing cells (which makes them ideal for hypertension therapy).[37]

Lentivirus

Although lentiviruses belong to the general category of retroviruses, their special features have made it appropriate to describe them separately. Many of the lentiviral vectors used in GT have been developed from primate lentiviruses, and most notably based on the human immunodeficiency virus type 1 (HIV-1).[38] In contrast to conventional retrovirus particles, lentiviral vectors form PICs that can pass through the pores of intact nuclear membranes and therefore can also infect nondividing cells.[39] HIV vectors can accommodate fairly large gene inserts and can provide long-term expression through chromosomal integration. Lenti-vectors have a capacity of ~10 kb for genetic material and sufficient amounts of high-concentration vector (10E8 to 10E9 infection units/mL) can easily be produced.

Despite these advantages, the limitations of using lentiviral vectors in clinical trials have been primarily related to the vector's HIV origin. However, over the years many modifications have been made to reduce the risk associated with the use of this gene delivery system. The necessary components for the production of the recombinant virus are segregated on three different plasmid constructs. Homologous sequences between these constructs have been reduced to the bare minimum to prevent recombination.[40,41] The transducing plasmid contains a functional cassette and viral long-terminal repeats (LTRs) containing self-inactivating (SIN) mutations that decrease the risk of replication-competent virus generation. As a result of these modifications, the lentivirus has become a safe, efficient, and well-characterized vector system that combines the advantages of retroviral and adenoviral vectors.

Although HIV based vectors have been extensively characterized, vectors based on nonprimate lentiviruses may be equally potent and more readily accepted by clinicians and patients. It is important to emphasize, however, that no data presently exist regarding the relative safety of primate versus nonprimate lentiviral vectors. Feline immunodeficiency virus (FIV) is one particularly

appealing nonprimate lentiviral vector. Phylogenetic analysis suggests that FIV is only distantly related to the primate lentiviruses,[42,43] and epidemiologic evidence indicates that there has been no occurrence of seroconversion in human populations.[44–46] FIV's low capacity for human cell infection is attributed to its envelope and low transcriptional activity in human cells.[47–51] Therefore, new generations of FIV have been developed[52] with modifications in order to overcome the low infection and transcriptional activity in human cells. Lentiviruses (including FIV) are among the most promising vehicles for gene transfer to the brain.[53,54] A recent series of studies involving FIV has targeted genes to sites and networks relevant to the brain renin-angiotensin system.[55]

An ideal vector

Major strides have been made in the last several years to develop both nonviral and viral vectors for GT. The choice of a gene delivery method is dependent on the needs of a given pathophysiologic condition. For example, an ideal vector for the control of hypertension would be one that could transduce nondividing and dividing cells with equally high efficiency, have a long-term transgene expression, and have a high capacity to introduce regulatory elements. At this time, the retrovirus family (particularly the lentiviruses) seems to fit these criteria (Figure 37–1). However, the adenoviral vector or HVJ-based naked DNA delivery may serve a prominent role in which transient expression of a given transgene is needed. In either case, for a GT vector to succeed it must have the following common characteristics: (1) the vector should not cause disease or elicit an immune or inflammatory response, (2) the vector should integrate into the genome in a desired site with no risk of disrupting other genes and cause mutations, (3) the virus needs to be replication deficient to prevent the spread to other tissues, and (4) the vector should be easy to produce on a large scale in a pure form and in high titer.

GENE THERAPY FOR CARDIOVASCULAR DISEASES

The increased understanding of CV biology and molecular pathophysiology has enabled the design and evaluation of gene-based therapies (for a variety of CV conditions) currently being successfully applied in both animal experiments and in human trials. In the following section, we summarize GT approaches in the treatment of a number of CV diseases.

Restenosis and bypass graft failure

Interventions such as balloon angioplasty and bypass grafts are highly effective for the treatment of stenosis and ischemic disease. However, in 20% of patients restenosis post-angioplasty leads to the obstruction of arteries within 6 months of the procedure.[56,57] Likewise, neointimal hyperplasia results in the re-occlusion of ~20% of peripheral arterial bypass grafts after the first year and of ~50% of coronary artery bypass grafts after 10 years. As a result, innovative gene transfer methods are being tried to inhibit restenosis post-angioplasty and in bypass grafts.

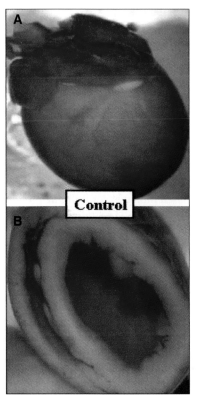

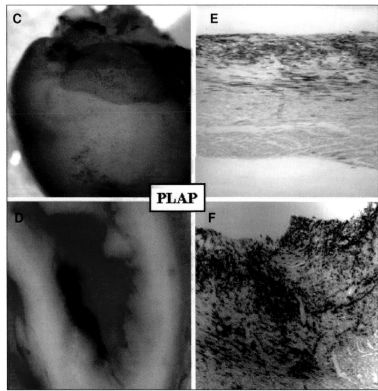

Figure 37–1. Lentiviral vector-mediated high-efficiency gene transfers in the myocardium. Lentiviral vector containing human placental alkaline phosphatase (PLAP) as a reporter gene was injected into the left ventricular cavity of the heart. Ten days following gene transfer, hearts were stained for PLAP. The control heart showed no staining (global view, panel A, and ventricular cross section, panel B). The lentivirus was able to efficiently transduce the entire heart (ventricles and atria, panel C, and magnified ventricular cross section, panel D). Histological sections of the ventricular wall reveals PLAP marker transduced with the lenti vector (panels E and F). Whole mount pictures were taken using a dissecting microscope and thin section pictures were taken at 10X objective magnification. (Reproduced by permission from [202].)

Intimal hyperplasia, which leads to vascular occlusion, develops in large part as a result of vascular smooth muscle cell (VSMC) proliferation and migration induced by a complex interaction of multiple growth factors (GFs) that are activated by injury. However, rapid regeneration of endothelial cells without replication of VSMC has also been hypothesized to modulate vascular growth. The process of VSMC proliferation is dependent on the coordinated activation of a series of cell cycle regulatory genes that result in mitosis. Therefore, GT strategies for restenosis have been largely directed toward the inhibition of VSMC migration and proliferation by targeting those specific genes.

The transition of G1 to S is a very important therapeutic target, and this checkpoint is regulated by the E2F family of transcription factors. The E2F transcription factor transactivates a variety of genes involved in cell cycle regulation. A synthetic DNA decoy has been used to sequester E2F and prevent gene transactivation, thereby arresting cells at the G1 checkpoint.[58] A proof-of-concept study, the Project in Ex-Vivo Vein Graft Engineering Via Transfection (PREVENT I), was the first study using genetic engineering techniques to inhibit cell cycle activation in vein grafts to treat peripheral arterial disease.[59] This study was followed with PREVENT II, the first randomized controlled trial of genetic suppression via transcription factor inhibition, which investigated the safety and feasibility of

E2F decoy oligodeoxynucleotides (ODNs) in preventing autologous vein graft failure after coronary artery bypass surgery. This trial demonstrated that E2F decoy was associated with a decreased vascular wall volume/index and a reduction of vein graft failure. Such strategy for the treatment of vascular occlusive disease has gained favor with several groups employing direct transduction of the vessel wall with genes designed to modulate cell cycle progression. Briefly, antisense or decoy ODN constructs against c-myb,[60] cdc-2,[61] cdk-2,[62] ras,[63] bcl-x,[64] and NFκB[65] have been tried. Expression of p21,[66] p27 and p16,[67] gax,[68] p53,[69] thymidine kinase,[70] cytosine deaminase,[71] fas ligand,[72] and retinoblastoma gene[73] have also been successfully investigated and have shown a decrease in the extent of intimal thickening in injury-mediated vascular proliferative disorders.

Other approaches limiting VSMC hyperplasia have involved the increase in local levels of nitric-oxide (NO). NO causes vasodilation, prevents cellular proliferation and clotting, acts as a scavenger of oxygen free radicals, and mitigates neointima formation. Finally, the *in vivo* transfer of plasmid DNA coding for endothelial NO synthase (eNOS: NO generating enzyme) in the rat carotid artery has improved vasomotor reactivity and has produced a 70% inhibition of neointima formation post angioplasty.[74] NOS transfection was also shown to produce a significant reduction in in-stent restenosis in pigs.[75]

Therapeutic angiogenesis

Substantial research has focused on the administration of angiogenic GFs to promote the development of supplemental collateral blood vessels that constitute bypass conduits around occluded arteries. This strategy is termed therapeutic angiogenesis, and is most used in patients suffering from critical limb ischemia (CLI) or chronic myocardial ischemia (MI) who are not good candidates for surgical revascularization.

GT might be the best way to produce therapeutic angiogenesis, in that sustained but transient expression of GFs is required for the formation of new blood vessels. In fact, GT has provided promising new approaches for the treatment of ischemia and for the protection of vessels and myocardium after injury.[76] Early phase 1 trials using many different angiogenic GFs to stimulate neovascularization have disclosed potentially favorable results in limb salvage in patients recommended for lower extremity amputation[77,78] and in reduced failure of lower extremity bypass grafts.[59] In addition, reduced angina, improved exercise tolerance, and improved myocardial perfusion have been reported in patients with coronary heart disease.[79–82]

Although many cytokines have angiogenic activity, vascular endothelial growth factor (VEGF) has been the best studied and the most widely used agent for therapeutic angiogenesis both in animal experiments and in clinical trials. The families of fibroblast growth factor (FGF)[83–85] and of hepatocyte growth factor (HGF)[86] have also been identified as factors that can induce angiogenesis *in vivo*. Other cytokines and GF, such as monocyte chemotactic protein-1[87] and platelet-derived growth factor (PDGF), may also indirectly increase angiogenesis by stimulating VEGF production.[88,89]

Critical limb ischemia

Critical limb ischemia (CLI) is estimated to develop in 500 to 1000 individuals per million per year and is considered as one of the most suitable diseases for GT. In a large proportion of these patients, the extent of the occlusive disease makes the patients unsuitable for surgical revascularization and amputation is often chosen. Therefore, the need for alternative treatment strategies in patients with CLI is compelling.

Initial preclinical studies established that the angiogenic activity of a single intra-arterial bolus injection of VEGF is sufficiently potent to achieve increase of collateral vessels and capillaries in rabbits with severe unilateral hindlimb ischemia.[90] Subsequently, other studies established meaningful biological outcomes following direct injection of naked plasmid VEGF DNA into skeletal muscle of ischemic rabbit hindlimbs[91] and AAV-mediated VEGF delivery into ischemic hindlimbs in diabetic mice.[92] Based on the successes of these and other preclinical studies demonstrating the efficacy of VEGF-induced angiogenesis in models of peripheral ischemia,[93] randomized trials have begun to evaluate the therapeutic potential of VEGF GT in patients with CLI.[77,78] These studies have shown that site-specific VEGF GT can achieve physiologically meaningful therapeutic angiogenesis in patients. Moreover, the safety and therapeutic efficacy of intramuscular

naked plasmid DNA encoding for FGF administered to patients with peripheral arterial disease has been reported,[94] and preclinical studies using HGF to stimulate angiogenesis in this disease model have also been undertaken.[95]

Myocardial ischemia

Health care projections suggest that by 2020 ischemic heart disease will be the most prevalent global cause of death and disability.[96,97] Recent advances in the understanding of the pathophysiology of ischemic heart disease coupled to improvements in GT offer the opportunity for the design of gene-based therapies for both the protection and rescue of the myocardium. GT strategies for ischemic heart disease have targeted angiogenesis and cytoprotection, as well as several different areas of cell function, including cell cycle progression and cell viability.

A human GT trial to treat coronary artery disease using the VEGF gene was initiated by late professor J. M. Isner.[81] His group performed injections of naked plasmid encoding VEGF gene into ischemic myocardium, and (similar to human trials in peripheral arterial disease) transfection of VEGF resulted in a marked increase in blood flow and improved clinical symptoms without apparent toxicity.[79] Moreover, in a phase I coronary artery disease study direct myocardial gene transfer of naked DNA-encoding VEGF reduced angina and sublingual nitroglycerin consumption in patients even at 1-year follow-up.[98,99] Several studies have also documented improved myocardial perfusion and functional recovery following GT for treatment of the ischemic myocardium using angiogenic GF other than VEGF such as FGF.[84,100,101] It is now established that the deleterious processes initiated by coronary ischemic events may be exacerbated by reperfusion, a phenomenon referred to as ischemia/reperfusion (I/R) injury, which is clinically manifested in patients suffering from acute coronary syndromes.[102–104]

Reoxygenation of the ischemic myocardium results in the formation of reactive oxygen species, leading to activation of the inflammatory cascade, myocyte injury, and endothelial dysfunction.[105,106] In time, repeated I/R injury leads to progressive impairment of contractile function and hemodynamic failure.[107] Therefore, a therapeutic approach aimed at potentiating endogenous antioxidant reserves could be used as a preventive measure against I/R-induced oxidative myocardial damage. A proof-of-concept study using an I/R model has been undertaken using direct injection of recombinant AAV for the delivery of human heme oxygenase (HO-1) gene into the rat myocardium.[108] The HO-1 gene conferred cytoprotective, anti-inflammatory, vasodilatory, and antioxidant properties. Moreover, the HO-1 gene transfer resulted in a significant reduction of the infarct size in treated animals as compared with untreated animals at 8 weeks post-GT.[108] Comparable findings were observed with extracellular superoxide dismutase (ecSOD),[109,110] an enzyme that converts superoxide anions to hydrogen peroxide, which breaks down into water and oxygen. Other groups have also demonstrated the feasibility of cardioprotective GT using alternative targets such as using decoy ODNs against NFκB, a pro-inflammatory transcription factor activated by oxidative stress,[111] or the overexpression of stress-induced heat shock proteins such as HSP-70,[112] survival genes such as Bcl-2,[113] and protein kinase B,[114] as well as immunosuppressive cytokines.[115,116]

GT is usually considered an acute intervention at the time of ischemia and/or reperfusion. However, problems lie in the delay in introducing the gene and the time for it to be transcribed and translated. Long-term use of GT ahead of the event is, however, a feasible option for myocardial protection because experimental and clinical findings suggest that novel preemptive gene transfer techniques may be beneficial for patients with (or who are at risk of developing) coronary ischemic events.

Heart failure

Rescue of contractile function in the failing myocardium is another major goal of myocardial GT. GT for heart failure (HF) is a promising alternative therapy because the targeted demographic of HF focuses on the elderly, who are generally not ideal candidates for heart transplant due to the increased surgical risk or to the limited availability of donor organs. The failing myocardium is characterized by alterations in calcium handling, decreased myofilament sensitivity, and adrenergic receptor downregulation and desensitization.[117] The sarcoplasmic reticulum calcium ATPase (SERCA2a) is an important protein involved in HF because a defect in SERCA2a results in contractile dysfunction leading to HF. The adenovirus-mediated GT of SERCA2a has been shown to improve contractility in aortic-banded rats.[118] In addition, the β2-adrenergic receptor has been used as a target for GT in HF. Activation of this receptor controls cathecholamine response through cAMP regulation, and a decrease in β2-adrenergic receptors causes a decrease in cardiac responses to catecholamines and leads to HF. Similarly, adenovirus-mediated intracoronary delivery of the β2-adrenergic receptor gene leads to improved contractility and hemodynamic function in an animal model.[119]

GENE THERAPY FOR HYPERTENSION

GT provides a powerful tool to influence the expression of a specific gene to compensate for the hypo- or hyperactivity of a defective gene. This can be achieved by overexpression of a normal gene or by suppression of a defective gene.

The preclinical GT studies for hypertension have adopted two approaches that represent the two sides to transferring DNA into cells. One is the sense approach (the normal DNA sequence direction), which consists of inserting extra copies of genes associated with ameliorating effects such as vasodilation and reduction of hypertrophy and proliferation. The other approach is the antisense approach (the opposite DNA sequence direction), which consists of silencing genes associated with exacerbating effects such as transmission of vasoconstrictor responses and growth promotion. Each of these approaches has advantages and disadvantages. As our knowledge of gene products involved in controlling the CV system expands,

GT for CV diseases (and hypertension in particular) presents several alternative choices of candidate genes to be targeted, which in return dictate the gene transfer approach to use in order to either increase or decrease the expression of the selected gene. Tables 37–2 and 37–3 summarize some of these studies.

Sense approach

Chao and associates have led the way in using the sense approach by overexpressing vasodilators such as kallikrein (kinin generating enzyme),[120,121] adrenomedullin (ADM),[122] atrial natriuretic peptide (ANP),[123] and eNOS[124] in several different experimental models of hypertension with measurable success at reducing high BP. Their studies have demonstrated that delivery of each gene, either by naked DNA or by using viral delivery, results in an impressive lowering of BP. This decrease in BP is accompanied by an attenuation of pathophysiology observed in major target organs of hypertension. For example, a single injection of plasmid containing human tissue kallikrein gene in adult or newborn spontaneously hypertensive rats (SHRs) effectively reduced BP for up to 10 weeks.[125] In salt-sensitive hypertensive rats, intravenous injection of adenovirus vector with kallikrein produced a transient reduction in BP and morphologic improvements in kidney and cardiac pathophysiology.[120,126] In addition, this group established that a single intramuscular injection of the same virus leads to a continuous supply of BP reducing kallikrein in the circulation.[127] Similarly, human eNOS gene reduced BP for 2 to 12 weeks in the SHR,[124] and overexpression of ADM using the adenoviral vector provided protection against hypertension, cardiac hypertrophy, and renal damage in both salt-sensitive and volume-dependent hypertension.[122,128] Even though the effects were not always very prolonged, reduction in end-organ damage was observed with these therapies.

Our group has used the sense approach to determine whether overexpression of the AT$_2$ receptor (AT$_2$R) reduces cardiac hypertrophy and cardiac fibrosis in two rat models of hypertension. In the first study, the AT$_2$R was overexpressed in 5-day-old SHR using a lentiviral vector. At 21 weeks following gene transfer, the lenti-AT$_2$R-treated SHR exhibited decreased left ventricular wall thickness and reduced heart/body weight ratio compared to normal animals. These beneficial outcomes were observed despite the elevated BP in these animals.[129] In another study, the AngII infusion rat model of hypertension was used to evaluate the role of AT$_2$R overexpression. Lenti-AT$_2$R overexpression resulted in the attenuation of left ventricular wall thickness, heart/body weight ratio, and decrease in myocardial fibrosis independently of high BP.[130] Together, both of these studies concluded that the AT$_2$R overexpression provides a cardioprotective effect against cardiac remodeling in both a genetic and non-genetic model of hypertension.

Recently, our group has begun using angiotensin-converting enzyme 2 (ACE2) as a potential target for GT. ACE2 is a newly discovered member of the renin-angiotensin system (RAS), which possesses 42% sequence homology with ACE[122,131,132] and is a central regulator of

INCREASED GENE EXPRESSION (SENSE APPROACH) FOR THE TREATMENT OF HYPERTENSION AND CARDIOVASCULAR DISEASES						
Transgene	Model	Vehicle	Delivery	Effect on BP	Comments	Ref.
Kallikrein	SHR	Adenovirus	IM	No effect	Increased capillary density in ischemic muscle	174
	SHR	Adenovirus	IM	Decreased		127
	Dahl-SS	Adenovirus	IV	Decreased	Reversed cardiac hypertrophy; fibrosis and renal damage	175
	Goldblatt-2K1C	Adenovirus	IV	Delay of onset	Reduced left ventricular mass; protection from renal dysfunction	176
	SHR	Adenovirus	IV	Decreased		177
	SHR	ODN	IV	Decreased	Decreased BP in adult but not in young SHR	178
	SHR	Plasmid DNA	IV	Decreased	Hypotensive effect reversed by kallikrein inhibitor	179
ADM	Goldblatt-2K1C	Adenovirus	IV	Delay of onset	Reduced left ventricular mass; decreased myocyte diameter; decreased myocardial fibrosis	180
	SHR	Plasmid DNA	IV	Decreased	Second injection further reduced BP	181
ANP	Dahl-SS	Adenovirus	IV	Decreased	Decrease in cerebral infarction; reduced thickness of arterial wall	182
	Dahl-SS	Adenovirus	IV	Decreased	Reduction in cardiac myocyte size; attenuation of glomerular sclerotic lesions	183
	SHR	Plasmid DNA	IV	Decreased	No effect on 12 week old SHR	123
NO	SHR	Adenovirus	ICV	Decreased	Depressor response in WKY but greater in SHR	184
	SHR-SP	Adenovirus	IV	No effect	Improved endothelial function	185
	SHR	Adenovirus	ICV	Decreased	Decrease in HR and BP reversed by microinjection of soluble guanylate cyclase inhibitor	186
SOD	SHR	Adenovirus	IV	Decreased	Effect greater in anesthetized compared with awake rats; improved endothelial function	187
	SHR-SP	Adenovirus	IV	No effect	Improved endothelial function	188
HO	SHR	Retrovirus	IC	Delay of onset		189
Adapted from Katovich MJ et al., *Current and Future Novel Targets of Gene Therapy for Hypertension.*[173]						

Table 37–2. Increased Gene Expression (Sense Approach) for the Treatment of Hypertension and Cardiovascular Diseases

angiotensin peptides. Most importantly, ACE2 shifts the balance in the formation of the vasoconstrictor and proliferative AngII toward the vasodilatory and anti-proliferative angiotensin 1-7 [(Ang (1-7)] fragment. Therefore, ACE2 is hypothesized to have beneficial effects in hypertension and CV diseases. Our group seized the opportunity to evaluate whether overexpression of ACE2 would protect the heart from hypertension-induced cardiac remodeling in an AngII-infused rat model. Lentiviral vector containing ACE2 sense sequence was injected in 5-day-old Sprague-Dawley (SD) rats in a single intracardiac injection, which resulted in a long-term expression of the ACE2 transgene. Infusion of AngII for 4 weeks in untreated SD resulted in an increase in BP, left ventricular wall thickness, heart/body weight ratio, and myocardial fibrosis. Cardiac transduction of ACE2 resulted in a profound attenuation in cardiac remodeling, and significant improvement in hypertrophy. However,

this was associated with only a little decrease in high BP.[133] Thus, our observations demonstrate that ACE2 overexpression holds great potential for GT against cardiac remodeling in hypertension. We are now evaluating the role of ACE2 overexpression in the prevention of cardiac remodeling post-MI. These consistent and impressive results provide conceptual support for the usefulness of the sense approach for the control of cardiac remodeling.

Antisense approach

The principle behind this approach for hypertension therapy is that antisense (AS) sequences target adverse genes and decrease their expression by blocking the formation of the targeted protein at the transcriptional and translational level. Many research groups, including our own, have been highly successful in using this AS approach to target members of the RAS. Our research group has selected the RAS as a target for AS therapy to

DECREASED GENE EXPRESSION (ANTISENSE APPROACH) FOR THE TREATMENT OF HYPERTENSION AND CARDIOVASCULAR DISEASES						
Transgene	Model	Vehicle	Delivery	Effect on BP	Comments	Ref.
AGT	SHR	ODN	IV	Decrease	Plasma AGT and AngII levels reduced	141
	SHR	ODN	IV	Decrease	AGT and AngII levels reduced	142
	SHR	ODN	ICV	Decrease	Decreased AT1R in PVN; decreased AngII in brainstem	190
	SHR	ODN	ICV	Decrease	Decreased AngII in brainstem	191
	SHR	AAV	IC	Decrease; delay of onset	Decreased left ventricular hypertrophy; decreased AGT	192
	SHR	AAV	IV	Decrease	Greater effect of AAV-plasmid vector with liposome	193
	Cold-induced SD	Liposome	IV	Decrease	Decreased spontaneous drinking response	145
	Goldblatt-2K1C	ODN	ICV	Decrease	Decreased the elevated hypothalamus AngII levels	194
ACE	SHR	Retrovirus	IC	Decrease	No effect on WKY	135
AT$_1$R	SHR	Retrovirus	IC	Decrease	Decreased AngII mediated responses in WKY and SHR but only decreased basal pressure in SHR	149
	SHR	Retrovirus	IC	Decrease	AngII-induced BP and dipsogenic responses attenuated	136
	Fructose-induced SD	Retrovirus	IC	Decrease	Prevented glucose intolerance	139
	SHR	Retrovirus	IC	Transient decrease	Repeated daily injections for 6 days	137
	SHR	AAV	ICV	Decrease	IC injection in 3 week old SHR also reduced BP	171
	SHR	ODN	ICV	Decrease		191
	LNAME SD	Retrovirus	IC	Decrease	Decreased left ventricular hypertrophy; endothelial dysfunction unchanged	195
	Renin transgenic	Retrovirus	IC	Decrease	Prevented cardiac hypertrophy	138
	AngII-induced SD	Retrovirus	IC	Decrease	Protected against AngII-induced increases in BP and cardiac hypertrophy	134
	Cold-induced SD	ODN	IC and/ or ICV	Decrease	Reduced spontaneous drinking response	145
	Goldblatt-2K1C	ODN	IV	Decrease		144
AT$_2$R	SD	ODN	SC	Increase	Increased pressor response to AngII	196
	SD	Retrovirus	IC	Increase	Increased pressor response to AngII	151
β-AR receptor	SHR	Liposome	IV	Decrease	No effect on HR	197
	SHR	Liposome	IV	Decrease	Decreased β1 but not β2 receptors; decreased plasma renin activity and AngII	198
EGFR	SHR	Liposome	IV	Decrease	Weekly injections for 2 months; decreasedleft-ventricular hypertrophy	199
	AngII-induced SD	ODN	IV	Decrease	Normalized left ventricular hypertrophy	200
FGFR	SHR	Liposome	IV	Acute decrease	Increases number of endothelial cells; ameliorated endothelial dependent response to vasoconstrictors	201
Adapted from Katovich MJ et al., Current and Future Novel Targets of Gene Therapy for Hypertension.[173]						

Table 37–3. Decreased Gene Expression (Antisense Approach) for the Treatment of Hypertension and Cardiovascular Diseases

provide proof-of-concept for hypertension GT for the following reasons: (1) the role of the RAS in hypertension is well established, (2) the RAS provides an ideal target for gene delivery because it is widely distributed, and (3) traditional pharmacologic agents that target the RAS are proven antihypertensive medications. For example, studies have shown that normotensive SD rats injected with AT$_1$ receptor (AT$_1$R)-AS virus are resistant to hypertension induced by chronic AngII infusion.[134] In addition, delivery of ACE-AS[135] or AT$_1$R-AS[136–138] prevents the development of both high BP and CV pathophysiology in the SHR. This observation was later extended to other genetic[136–138] and nongenetic models of hypertension.[139] These findings are the first of their kind and support the idea that genetic targeting of the RAS is conceptually sound and technically feasible in the prevention of hypertension.

Experiments with nonviral delivery methods

The first conceptual support that AS targeting of the RAS could be effective in the treatment of hypertension was derived from the experiments with the use of AS ODNs. Oligomers are designed to hybridize to the mRNA, and this complex prevents protein translation because it is unable to read through the ribosome. Effective AS ODN have been targeted to the mRNA from renin, AGT, ACE, and AT$_1$R and tested in three different models of hypertension—including the genetic model (SHR),[140–143] a surgical model [2-kidney, 1 clip hypertension (2K1C)],[144] and an environmental stress model (cold induced hypertension).[145] In each case, the BP-lowering effect was reproducible and persisted for days. Although these results are impressive, the antihypertensive effects seem to be of little improvement over traditional therapy. In contrast to vector delivery, ODNs can be used and understood as pharmaceutical agents because they act within a few hours, can be measured systemically, and have a dose-response relationship. However, long-term therapeutic potential of ODNs do not measure up to the vector delivery method.

Experiments with viral vectors

Our research group and that of Dr. Phillips' independently have built on these observations to establish experimental protocols for the systemic delivery of AS using viral vector gene delivery systems. The retroviral vector turned out to be an ideal vehicle for providing conceptual evidence for the AS GT based on the fact that one could produce large quantities of this vector with high titers and that the retroviral transgene has the ability to integrate into the genome for sustained antihypertensive effects.[146] We used a retroviral vector gene delivery system to produce lifelong transduction of the AT$_1$R-AS, resulting in permanent control of high BP and of both vascular and cardiac pathophysiology associated with hypertension.[7,136–138] The rationales for choosing the AT$_1$R as a target were several: (1) AT$_1$R antagonism is a proven traditional pharmacologic strategy for the control of hypertension, (2) a polymorphic substitution of adenine with cytosine in the AT$_1$R gene has been associated with severe hypertension,[147] and (3) interactions between ACE and AT$_1$R activity have been associated with the hypertensive state.[148]

In our experiments, a single intracardiac injection of a retroviral vector containing AT$_1$R-AS cDNA in 5-day-old SHR produced lifelong antihypertensive effects without any visible side effects. High BP was prevented from developing throughout life and was comparable with daily administration of losartan.[149] In addition, no BP-lowering effect was observed in the normotensive rat,[8,146] and this is consistent with pharmacotherapy in which both AT$_1$R antagonists and ACE inhibitors have little effect on normotensive individuals.[150] This leads us to propose that the expression of AT$_1$R-AS in the normal rat would only come into play when the RAS is challenged. In fact, our observations support this hypothesis in that AT$_1$R-AS expressing normotensive rats when challenged with chronic low-dose AngII are completely protected from developing hypertension.[134] In contrast to traditional AT$_1$R antagonist therapy, AT$_1$R-AS treatment does not increase plasma AngII levels,[149] and this may be an additional factor for the reduced side-effect profile of AT$_1$R-AS GT.

It is relevant to point out that the expression of the AT$_1$R-AS gene is associated with a 20- to 40% decrease in the numbers of AT$_1$R in tissues[145] and that this modest decrease is sufficient to provide comparable beneficial outcomes as those seen with traditional pharmacologic therapies. The lowered plasma AngII levels with GT as compared with traditional drugs may provide some explanation for this observation. Increased sensitivity to vasoconstrictors such as KCl, phenylephrine, and AngII (a hallmark of the SHR vasculature) was prevented by the AT$_1$R-AS, while correcting endothelial dysfunction. The delivery of the AT$_1$R-AS gene was also associated with the attenuation of cardiac pathophysiology, which includes the prevention of cardiac hypertrophy, perivascular and myocardial fibrosis, and inhibition of neointima formation in the coronary artery of SHR.[8,134,136,146,149]

These observations provide first proof-of-principle that AS GT may be feasible for hypertension. Further proof-of-concept was provided with the use of the AT$_2$R-AS. We argued that if the AT$_2$R is CV protective then its inhibition would increase BP in normotensive rats. A retroviral vector containing full-length AT$_2$R-AS cDNA was injected in 5-day-old normotensive SD rats to provide evidence for this hypothesis. Systolic BP in AT$_2$R-AS expressing normotensive rats was significantly increased compared to control rats. In addition, acute administration of AngII resulted in a significantly higher response in AT$_2$R-AS animals compared to controls.[151]

It is evident from the previous discussion that both sense and antisense strategies are technically sound and exciting approaches that offer innovative means for the long-term control of hypertension. Both approaches have their unique advantages and disadvantages. For example:

- The efficacy and efficiency of the AS strategy can be easily compared with the traditional pharmacologic approach. Such a comparison is difficult for the sense-based strategy because of the lack of an equivalent pharmacologic parallel.
- Introduction of a full-length gene in the sense approach that would result in a physiologically functional compensation would require a higher degree of transduction *in vivo*.
- Unlike with the AS approach, which can only attenuate gene expression in a cell that expresses it, the sense approach allows the transduction of genes in cells or tissues that do not normally express the therapeutic gene.

In the final analysis, we believe that the key to the success of GT with either of these strategies will be dependent on the availability of delivery vehicles that would be able to (1) transduce organs with high efficiency and specificity, (2) maintain long-term expression of a desired transgene, and (3) be regulated on demand. Development of such an ideal vector would be an important next step. Finally, for the sense and the antisense approach the outline of the GT development strategy used by our group remains the same as illustrated in Figure 37–2.

REGULATION OF GENE THERAPY

For GT to gain widespread consideration as a treatment alternative to pharmacotherapy a regulated system that exhibits cellular and tissue selectivity must first be developed. An ideal promoter driving the expression of a desired transgene that remains active for prolonged periods, that is switched on or off at will, and that is specific for a given tissue cell type such as cardiomyocytes or VSMC must be developed. This is crucial not only to control the degree of transgene expression (and thus the therapeutic response in the targeted cells) but to turn off expression if any unforeseen side effects occur. Temporal and quantitative control of transgene expression, which can minimize nonspecific or toxic effects, can be accomplished *in vitro* and *in vivo* using a regulatable "gene switch." A number of regulated gene expression systems that use exogenous ligands to control transgene expression have been developed in recent years. Among the different systems, the tetracycline-based activating ("tet-on") or repressible ("tet-off") systems—in which the delivery of the inducer drug (i.e., doxycycline) regulates gene expression—have been best characterized.[152,153] In addition, recent advances in the field have demonstrated the possibility of highly efficient transfections of tet-regulated genes using lentiviruses.[154]

Another emerging concept in GT for the regulation of gene expression is the use of physiologic signals to switch on therapeutic genes in chronic or life-threatening diseases. In this approach, a systemically injected "vigilant" (or conditional) vector awaits such signals as hypoxia to switch

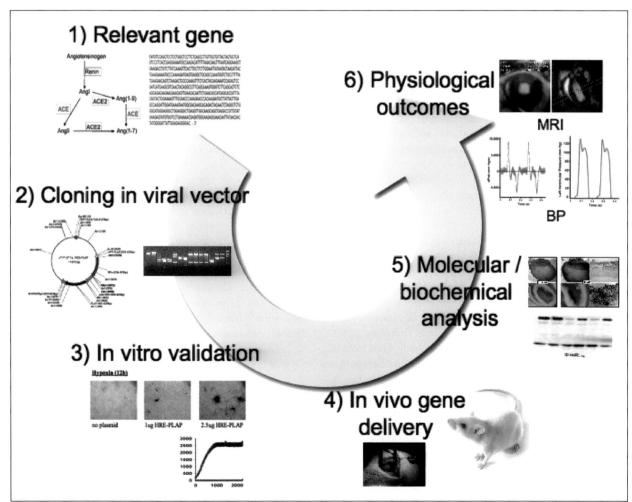

Figure 37–2. Outline of the gene therapy development strategy for cardiovascular diseases employed by Raizada et al. (1) Strategic identification of a relevant gene for investigation, (2) cloning of the gene in a viral vector of choice, (3) *in vitro* validation of the clone construct (immunohistochemistry, activity assay), (4) *in vitro* gene delivery (intracardiac injection in pups, direct tissue injection in adults), (5) molecular/biochemical analysis (immunohistochemistry, blots, and so on), and (6) measure of physiological outcomes (blood pressure, magnetic resonance imaging, and so on).

on genes that protect target tissues (such as the heart during MI) via high amplification of a protective gene.[155–157] Conditional promoters require several key components. The first is a safe and stable vector that can be administered by systemic injection and that expresses transgenes in both dividing and nondividing adult cells in a particular organ or tissue. The second component is a "gene switch" (biosensor) that can detect the specific physiologic signal (e.g., hypoxia response element, HRE, which can detect a decrease in O_2 levels in MI). The third is a tissue-specific promoter that restricts transgene expression to the tissue or organ of interest (e.g., MLC2v myocyte promoter[156] or Tie2 endothelial promoter[158,159]).

SAFETY ISSUES WITH GENE THERAPY

Safety of GT is of immense importance and has been a major concern. The first human trial in CV disease was started in 1994 to treat PAD using VEGF. Since then, many angiogenic GFs have been tested in clinical trials for different diseases, and the results seem to have exceeded expectations. These trials have shown that vascular gene transfer is safe and well tolerated, and whether using viral or nonviral vectors CV GT clinical trials have disclosed no evidence indicative of inflammatory or other complications, including death directly attributable to the vector used. However, a few incidents that have occurred during clinical trials have attracted renewed concerns about GT safety. For example, GT attempts to induce angiogenesis have raised appropriate concerns regarding the possibility of inducing pathological vessel growth. In fact, therapeutic angiogenesis has potential risks such as the production of nonfunctional vessels, stimulation of angiogenesis in tumors,[160] and hemorrhage or plaque rupture in atherosclerotic lesions.[161] It is important to mention that so far there have been no clinical reports of such complications, but ongoing surveillance will continue to inform us regarding their potential.

Safety of viral vectors should also be of great concern if it is to be a therapeutic method of choice. Traditional GT involves the delivery of transgenes by viral vectors and integration into the host genome for long-term expression.[162] However, insertion of foreign DNA can induce epigenetic changes[163] that may have implications in gene silencing or even tumor development. Therefore, it is imperative that the site of integration of the viral vector in the host genome and its influence on neighboring genes be established. Control of transgene expression also needs to be established with the use of vectors containing promoters that can be regulated. In addition, the vector must be free of immune and other adverse side effects. Deletion of unnecessary viral genes from vector constructs has significantly reduced cytotoxicity and immunogenicity and has prevented the generation of replication-competent particles and the spread of viral infections. Physiologic, pathophysiologic, and ethical aspects related to germ line transmission of the vector must also be evaluated by weighing the potential risks and benefits incurred by the treatment. This is particularly true with the improved transduction efficiency of newer viral vectors.

PERSPECTIVES

Nonviral delivery systems can be less immunogenic, easier to manufacture, and less costly. However, a major barrier has been the lack of genomic integration of the transgenes, which precludes long-term expression. The development of a nonviral transposon system ("Sleeping Beauty") has provided a significant advance in overcoming this barrier. The system uses a reconstructed transposase capable of excising a transgene from within the transposon and inserting it into the host genome without insertional mutagenesis.[164]

Another interesting approach that could lead to major advancement in GT has been the development of RNA interference (RNAi) technology, which was recently demonstrated to also induce stable gene silencing in mammalian cells.[165] Our research group has recently developed small interfering RNAs selectively silencing the AT$_{1a}$R as a first step toward this objective.[166]

Yet another alternative to traditional GT is gene repair, where nucleic acids have been designed to correct site-specific genomic mutations.[167] An advantage of this *in situ* repair method is that it allows the targeted gene to remain under the control of its endogenous regulatory elements.

The transfer of the AS or sense genes to somatic cells is achieved by an *in vivo* approach. It would be possible to use an *ex vivo* approach in which target cells are harvested and transduced, and then reimplanted as genetically modified autologous cells. This method has no clear applicability to hypertension, although it may offer an opportunity to treat many other disorders. In addition, the plasticity of stem cells to transdifferentiate into many different cell types, coupled with the possibility of gene correction, offers an immense opportunity to treat many diseases without the need to harvest cells for *ex vivo* repair. Stem cell therapy is likely to play a major role in treating disorders such as ischemic cardiac disease, cardiomyopathies, peripheral arterial disease, as well as the aging heart.[168,169] In fact, the possibility of correcting genetic defects in stem cells and then invoking their transdifferentiation into cardiac tissue may soon be possible. Finally, there are many diseases in which considerable damage occurs *in utero*, and the advent of *in utero* GT may offer substantial opportunities for prevention of damage and long-term cure of some of these disorders.[170]

CONCLUSIONS

At present, demonstration of the clinical utility of CV GT in humans is at an investigational phase. However, GT for CV disease now appears to be not far from reality. The improvement of vector design, the ability to link specific genes to disease, the technological advances in microarrays and proteomics, and the harnessing of the power of stem cells will undoubtedly advance the role of GT in CV disease. As the tools for *in vivo* genetic manipulation and delivery continue to improve it is possible that GT might eventually become a part of routine care for patients with established CV disease, especially those in whom conventional treatments have been exhausted.

As for the treatment of hypertension, although many excellent pharmacological agents are commercially available the incidence of this disease is on the rise and will continue to affect millions of people throughout the world if new approaches are not clinically investigated and implemented. Therefore, we need to develop ways that would improve high BP control by providing longer-lasting effects with a single therapeutic dose and by reducing side effects that lead to poor compliance. GT for hypertension is one such alternative that would give the patient continuous biological control over high BP with minimal or no side effects. Although a great deal more work in basic science needs to be done before GT for hypertension can be applied to humans, so far the results are encouraging. AAV and lentivirus-based vectors have shown great promise in preliminary experiments.[146] However, new viral vectors or variations of these that have higher transduction efficiency should be tried. Better routes of delivery of viral vectors also need to be established.

Safety is also a key issue and it is imperative that the genomic site of integration of the viral vector be well known and its influence on the neighboring genes established. Germ line transmission of transgenes by the vector must be determined, and tissue-specific targeting and the improvement of regulatable promoters must be continued. In addition, it would be interesting that other hypertension-related genes be targeted by GT; for example, Ca^{2+} channels, signaling-molecule-related genes, or genes relevant to matrix proteins. Finally, because prevention strategies for hypertension hold little promise for the treatment of humans due to lack of reliable genetic markers for early detection of the disease we must therefore determine whether the reversal strategy for established hypertension is a feasible option.

Our studies have established that genetic targeting of the RAS prevents hypertension for life in the SHR. These studies are consistent with data from other groups,[171,172] and it appears that the strategy could constitute the basis for further developments. Taken together, the GT strategy is an exciting therapeutic approach that holds great potential for permanent control of hypertension.

REFERENCES

1. www.americanheart.org/statistics/index.html.
2. Chronic disease notes and reports. Natl Ctrl for Chronic Disease Prevention and Health Promotion 1997;10:1–36.
3. Stamler J, Stamler R, Neaton JD. Blood pressure, systolic and diastolic, and cardiovascular risks: U.S. population data. Arch Intern Med 1993;153:598–615.
4. Jacobson EJ. Hypertension: Update on use of angiotensin II receptor blockers. Geriatrics 2001;56:20–1, 25–8.
5. Deshmukh R, Smith A, Lilly LS. Hypertension: Pathology of Heart Disease. Baltimore, MD: Williams & Wilkins 1998:267–68.
6. Burt VL, Whelton P, Roccella EJ, et al. Prevalence of hypertension in the US adult population. Results from the Third National Health and Nutrition Examination Survey, 1988–1991. Hypertension 1995;25:305–13.
7. Raizada MK, Katovich MJ, Wang H, Berecek KH, Gelband CH. Is antisense gene therapy a step in the right direction in the control of hypertension? Am J Physiol 1999; 277:H423–32.
8. Raizada MK, Francis SC, Wang H, Gelband CH, Reaves PY, Katovich MJ. Targeting of the renin-angiotensin system by antisense gene therapy: A possible strategy for the long-term control of hypertension. J Hypertens 2000;18:353–62.
9. Finkel T. Thinking globally, acting locally: The promise of cardiovascular gene therapy. Circ Res 1999;84: 1471–72.
10. Baxendale-Cox LM. An overview of essential hypertension in Americans as a multifactorial phenomenon: Interaction of biologic and environmental factors. Prog Cardiovasc Nurs 2000;15:43–9.
11. Hamet P, Pausova Z, Adarichev V, Adaricheva K, Tremblay J. Hypertension:

Genes and environment. J Hypertens 1998;16:397–418.
12. Phillips MI, Galli SM, Mehta JL. The potential role of antisense oligodeoxynucleotide therapy for cardiovascular disease. Drugs 2000; 60:239–48.
13. Nishikawa M, Huang L. Nonviral vectors in the new millennium: delivery barriers in gene transfer. Hum Gene Ther 2001;12:861–70.
14. Stephan DJ, Yang ZY, San H, et al. A new cationic liposome DNA complex enhances the efficiency of arterial gene transfer in vivo. Hum Gene Ther 1996;7:1803–12.
15. Turunen MP, Hiltunen MO, Ruponen M, et al. Efficient adventitial gene delivery to rabbit carotid artery with cationic polymer-plasmid complexes. Gene Ther 1999;6:6–11.
16. Romano G, Claudio PP, Kaiser HE, Giordano A. Recent advances, prospects and problems in designing new strategies for oligonucleotide and gene delivery in therapy. In Vivo 1998;12:59–67.
17. Harris JD, Lemoine NR. Strategies for targeted gene therapy. Trends Genet 1996;12:400–05.
18. Kaneda Y, Saeki Y, Morishita R. Gene therapy using HVJ-liposomes: The best of both worlds? Mol Med Today 1999;5:298–303.
19. Nikol S, Pelisek J, Engelmann MG, Rolland PH, Armeanu S. Prevention of restenosis using the gene for cecropin complexed with DOCSPER liposomes under optimized conditions. International Journal of Angiology 2000;9:87–94.
20. Verma IM, Somia N. Gene therapy: Promises, problems and prospects. Nature 1997;389:239–42.
21. Flotte TR, Carter BJ. Adeno-associated virus vectors for gene therapy. Gene Ther 1995;2:357–62.

22. Kovesdi I, Brough DE, Bruder JT, Wickham TJ. Adenoviral vectors for gene transfer. Curr Opin Biotechnol 1997;8:583–89.
23. Jaffe HA, Danel C, Longenecker G, et al. Adenovirus-mediated in vivo gene transfer and expression in normal rat liver. Nat Genet 1992; 1:372–78.
24. Samulski RJ, Zhu X, Xiao X, et al. Targeted integration of adeno-associated virus (AAV) into human chromosome 19. Embo J 1991; 10:3941–50.
25. Schiedner G, Morral N, Parks RJ, et al. Genomic DNA transfer with a high-capacity adenovirus vector results in improved in vivo gene expression and decreased toxicity. Nat Genet 1998; 18:180–83.
26. Tripathy SK, Black HB, Goldwasser E, Leiden JM. Immune responses to transgene-encoded proteins limit the stability of gene expression after injection of replication-defective adenovirus vectors. Nat Med 1996; 2:545–50.
27. Rabinowitz JE, Samulski J. Adeno-associated virus expression systems for gene transfer. Curr Opin Biotechnol 1998;9:470–75.
28. Lebkowski JS, McNally MM, Okarma TB, Lerch LB. Adeno-associated virus: A vector system for efficient introduction and integration of DNA into a variety of mammalian cell types. Mol Cell Biol 1988;8:3988–96.
29. Russell DW, Miller AD, Alexander IE. Adeno-associated virus vectors preferentially transduce cells in S phase. Proc Natl Acad Sci USA 1994; 91:8915–19.
30. Nakai H, Montini E, Fuess S, Storm TA, Grompe M, Kay MA. AAV serotype 2 vectors preferentially integrate into active genes in mice. Nat Genet 2003; 34:297–302.

31. Roe T, Reynolds TC, Yu G, Brown PO. Integration of murine leukemia virus DNA depends on mitosis. *Embo J* 1993;12:2099–108.

32. Morgan RA, Anderson WF. Human gene therapy. *Annu Rev Biochem* 1993; 62:191–217.

33. Nabel EG, Nabel GJ. Complex models for the study of gene function in cardiovascular biology. *Annu Rev Physiol* 1994;56:741–61.

34. Yla-Herttuala S, Luoma J, Viita H, Hiltunen T, Sisto T, Nikkari T. Transfer of 15-lipoxygenase gene into rabbit iliac arteries results in the appearance of oxidation-specific lipid-protein adducts characteristic of oxidized low density lipoprotein. *J Clin Invest* 1995;95:2692–98.

35. Burns JC, Friedmann T, Driever W, Burrascano M, Yee JK. Vesicular stomatitis virus G glycoprotein pseudotyped retroviral vectors: Concentration to very high titer and efficient gene transfer into mammalian and nonmammalian cells. *Proc Natl Acad Sci USA* 1993;90:8033–37.

36. Hu WS, Pathak VK. Design of retroviral vectors and helper cells for gene therapy. *Pharmacol Rev* 2000; 52:493–511.

37. Robbins PD, Ghivizzani SC. Viral vectors for gene therapy. *Pharmacol Ther* 1998;80:35–47.

38. Vigna E, Naldini L. Lentiviral vectors: Excellent tools for experimental gene transfer and promising candidates for gene therapy. *J Gene Med* 2000; 2:308–16.

39. Miller AD. *Development of Applications of Retroviral Vectors: Retroviruses.* Cold Spring Harbor (NY): Cold Spring Harbor Press 1997:437–73.

40. Chang LJ, Urlacher V, Iwakuma T, Cui Y, Zucali J. Efficacy and safety analyses of a recombinant human immunodeficiency virus type 1 derived vector system. *Gene Ther* 1999; 6:715–28.

41. Iwakuma T, Cui Y, Chang LJ. Self-inactivating lentiviral vectors with U3 and U5 modifications. *Virology* 1999;261:120–32.

42. Olmsted RA, Hirsch VM, Purcell RH, Johnson PR. Nucleotide sequence analysis of feline immunodeficiency virus: Genome organization and relationship to other lentiviruses. *Proc Natl Acad Sci USA* 1989; 86:8088–92.

43. Olmsted RA, Langley R, Roelke ME, et al. Worldwide prevalence of lentivirus infection in wild feline species: Epidemiologic and phylogenetic aspects. *J Virol* 1992;66:6008–18.

44. Donaldson LJ, Rankin J, Proctor S. Is it possible to catch leukaemia from a cat? *Lancet* 1994;344:971–72.

45. Nowotny N, Uthman A, Haas OA, et al. Is it possible to catch leukemia from a cat? *Lancet* 1995;346:252–53.

46. Yamamoto JK, Hansen H, Ho EW, et al. Epidemiologic and clinical aspects of feline immunodeficiency virus infection in cats from the continental United States and Canada and possible mode of transmission. *J Am Vet Med Assoc* 1989;194:213–20.

47. Ikeda Y, Tomonaga K, Kawaguchi Y, et al. Feline immunodeficiency virus

48. Miyazawa T, Kawaguchi Y, Kohmoto M, Tomonaga K, Mikami T. Comparative functional analysis of the various lentivirus long terminal repeats in human colon carcinoma cell line (SW480 cells) and feline renal cell line (CRFK cells). *J Vet Med Sci* 1994;56:895–99.

49. Sparger EE, Shacklett BL, Renshaw-Gegg L, et al. Regulation of gene expression directed by the long terminal repeat of the feline immunodeficiency virus. *Virology* 1992;187:165–77.

50. Tochikura TS, Tanabe-Tochikura A, Hayes KA, et al. Fusion activity dissociated from replication ability in feline immunodeficiency virus (FIV) in human cells. *J Acquir Immune Defic Syndr* 1993;6:1301–10.

51. Tomonaga K, Miyazawa T, Kawaguchi Y, Kohmoto M, Inoshima Y, Mikami T. Comparison of the Rev transactivation of feline immunodeficiency virus in feline and non-feline cell lines. *J Vet Med Sci* 1994;56:199–201.

52. Poeschla EM, Wong-Staal F, Looney DJ. Efficient transduction of nondividing human cells by feline immunodeficiency virus lentiviral vectors. *Nat Med* 1998; 4:354–57.

53. Alisky JM, Hughes SM, Sauter SL, et al. Transduction of murine cerebellar neurons with recombinant FIV and AAV5 vectors. *Neuroreport* 2000; 11:2669–73.

54. Kordower JH, Bloch J, Ma SY, et al. Lentiviral gene transfer to the nonhuman primate brain. *Exp Neurol* 1999;160:1–16.

55. Sinnayah P, Lindley TE, Staber PD, Cassell MD, Davidson BL, Davisson RL. Selective gene transfer to key cardiovascular regions of the brain: Comparison of two viral vector systems. *Hypertension* 2002;39:603–08.

56. Narins CR, Holmes DR Jr., Topol EJ. A call for provisional stenting: the balloon is back! *Circulation* 1998; 97:1298–305.

57. Bittl JA. Advances in coronary angioplasty. *N Engl J Med* 1996; 335:1290–302.

58. Morishita R, Gibbons GH, Horiuchi M, et al. A gene therapy strategy using a transcription factor decoy of the E2F binding site inhibits smooth muscle proliferation in vivo. *Proc Natl Acad Sci USA* 1995;92:5855–59.

59. Mann MJ, Whittemore AD, Donaldson MC, et al. Ex-vivo gene therapy of human vascular bypass grafts with E2F decoy: The PREVENT single-centre, randomised, controlled trial. *Lancet* 1999;354:1493–98.

60. Simons M, Edelman ER, DeKeyser JL, Langer R, Rosenberg RD. Antisense c-myb oligonucleotides inhibit intimal arterial smooth muscle cell accumulation in vivo. *Nature* 1992;359:67–70.

61. Morishita R, Gibbons GH, Ellison KE, et al. Single intraluminal delivery of antisense cdc2 kinase and proliferating-cell nuclear antigen oligonucleotides results in chronic inhibition of neointimal hyperplasia. *Proc Natl Acad Sci USA* 1993; 90:8474–78.

62. Morishita R, Gibbons GH, Ellison KE, et al. Intimal hyperplasia after vascular injury is inhibited by antisense cdk 2 kinase oligonucleotides. *J Clin Invest* 1994;93:1458–64.

63. Indolfi C, Avvedimento EV, Rapacciuolo A, et al. Inhibition of cellular ras prevents smooth muscle cell proliferation after vascular injury in vivo. *Nat Med* 1995;1:541–45.

64. Pollman MJ, Hall JL, Mann MJ, Zhang L, Gibbons GH. Inhibition of neointimal cell bcl-x expression induces apoptosis and regression of vascular disease. *Nat Med* 1998;4:222–27.

65. Morishita R, Sugimoto T, Aoki M, et al. In vivo transfection of cis element "decoy" against nuclear factor-kappaB binding site prevents myocardial infarction. *Nat Med* 1997; 3:894–99.

66. Chang MW, Barr E, Lu MM, Barton K, Leiden JM. Adenovirus-mediated over-expression of the cyclin/cyclin-dependent kinase inhibitor, p21 inhibits vascular smooth muscle cell proliferation and neointima formation in the rat carotid artery model of balloon angioplasty. *J Clin Invest* 1995;96:2260–68.

67. Tsui LV, Camrud A, Mondesire J, et al. p27-p16 fusion gene inhibits angioplasty-induced neointimal hyperplasia and coronary artery occlusion. *Circ Res* 2001;89:323–28.

68. Smith RC, Branellec D, Gorski DH, et al. p21CIP1-mediated inhibition of cell proliferation by overexpression of the gax homeodomain gene. *Genes Dev* 1997;11:1674–89.

69. Yonemitsu Y, Kaneda Y, Tanaka S, et al. Transfer of wild-type p53 gene effectively inhibits vascular smooth muscle cell proliferation in vitro and in vivo. *Circ Res* 1998;82:147–56.

70. Guzman RJ, Hirschowitz EA, Brody SL, Crystal RG, Epstein SE, Finkel T. In vivo suppression of injury-induced vascular smooth muscle cell accumulation using adenovirus-mediated transfer of the herpes simplex virus thymidine kinase gene. *Proc Natl Acad Sci USA* 1994;91:10732–36.

71. Harrell RL, Rajanayagam S, Doanes AM, et al. Inhibition of vascular smooth muscle cell proliferation and neointimal accumulation by adenovirus-mediated gene transfer of cytosine deaminase. *Circulation* 1997;96:621–27.

72. Sata M, Perlman H, Muruve DA, et al. Fas ligand gene transfer to the vessel wall inhibits neointima formation and overrides the adenovirus-mediated T cell response. *Proc Natl Acad Sci USA* 1998;95:1213–17.

73. Chang MW, Barr E, Seltzer J, et al. Cytostatic gene therapy for vascular proliferative disorders with a constitutively active form of the retinoblastoma gene product. *Science* 1995;267:518–22.

74. von der Leyen HE, Gibbons GH, Morishita R, et al. Gene therapy inhibiting neointimal vascular lesion: In vivo transfer of endothelial cell nitric oxide synthase gene. *Proc Natl Acad Sci USA* 1995;92:1137–41.

75. Muhs A, Heublein B, Schletter J, et al. Preclinical evaluation of inducible nitric oxide synthase lipoplex gene therapy for inhibition of stent-induced vascular neointimal lesion formation. *Hum Gene Ther* 2003;14:375–83.

76. Symes JF, Losordo DW, Vale PR, et al. Gene therapy with vascular endothelial growth factor for inoperable coronary artery disease. *Ann Thorac Surg* 1999; 68:830–36; discussion 836–37.

77. Baumgartner I, Pieczek A, Manor O, et al. Constitutive expression of phVEGF165 after intramuscular gene transfer promotes collateral vessel development in patients with critical limb ischemia. *Circulation* 1998;97: 1114–23.

78. Isner JM, Baumgartner I, Rauh G, et al. Treatment of thromboangiitis obliterans (Buerger's disease) by intramuscular gene transfer of vascular endothelial growth factor: preliminary clinical results. *J Vasc Surg* 1998;28:964–73; discussion 73–5.

79. Losordo DW, Vale PR, Symes JF, et al. Gene therapy for myocardial angiogenesis: Initial clinical results with direct myocardial injection of phVEGF165 as sole therapy for myocardial ischemia. *Circulation* 1998;98:2800–04.

80. Rosengart TK, Lee LY, Patel SR, et al. Angiogenesis gene therapy: phase I assessment of direct intramyocardial administration of an adenovirus vector expressing VEGF121 cDNA to individuals with clinically significant severe coronary artery disease. *Circulation* 1999;100:468–74.

81. Vale PR, Losordo DW, Milliken CE, et al. Left ventricular electromechanical mapping to assess efficacy of phVEGF(165) gene transfer for therapeutic angiogenesis in chronic myocardial ischemia. *Circulation* 2000;102:965–74.

82. Vale PR, Losordo DW, Milliken CE, et al. Randomized, single-blind, placebo-controlled pilot study of catheter-based myocardial gene transfer for therapeutic angiogenesis using left ventricular electromechanical mapping in patients with chronic myocardial ischemia. *Circulation* 2001; 103:2138–43.

83. Unger EF, Banai S, Shou M, et al. Basic fibroblast growth factor enhances myocardial collateral flow in a canine model. *Am J Physiol* 1994; 266:H1588–95.

84. Giordano FJ, Ping P, McKirnan MD, et al. Intracoronary gene transfer of fibroblast growth factor-5 increases blood flow and contractile function in an ischemic region of the heart. *Nat Med* 1996;2:534–39.

85. Lopez JJ, Edelman ER, Stamler A, et al. Angiogenic potential of perivascularly delivered aFGF in a porcine model of chronic myocardial ischemia. *Am J Physiol* 1998;274:H930–36.

86. Van Belle E, Witzenbichler B, Chen D, et al. Potentiated angiogenic effect of scatter factor/hepatocyte growth factor via induction of vascular endothelial growth factor: The case for paracrine amplification of angiogenesis. *Circulation* 1998;97:381–90.

87. Ito WD, Arras M, Winkler B, Scholz D, Schaper J, Schaper W. Monocyte chemotactic protein-1 increases collateral and peripheral conductance after femoral artery occlusion. *Circ Res* 1997;80:829–37.

88. Martins RN, Chleboun JO, Sellers P, Sleigh M, Muir J. The role of PDGF-BB on the development of the collateral circulation after acute arterial occlusion. *Growth Factors* 1994;10:299–306.

89. Waltenberger J. Modulation of growth factor action: Implications for the treatment of cardiovascular diseases. *Circulation* 1997;96:4083–94.

90. Takeshita S, Zheng LP, Brogi E, et al. Therapeutic angiogenesis. A single intraarterial bolus of vascular endothelial growth factor augments revascularization in a rabbit ischemic hind limb model. *J Clin Invest* 1994; 93:662–70.

91. Tsurumi Y, Takeshita S, Chen D, et al. Direct intramuscular gene transfer of naked DNA encoding vascular endothelial growth factor augments collateral development and tissue perfusion. *Circulation* 1996;94:3281–90.

92. Rivard A, Silver M, Chen D, et al. Rescue of diabetes-related impairment of angiogenesis by intramuscular gene therapy with adeno-VEGF. *Am J Pathol* 1999;154:355–63.

93. Witzenbichler B, Asahara T, Murohara T, et al. Vascular endothelial growth factor-C (VEGF-C/VEGF-2) promotes angiogenesis in the setting of tissue ischemia. *Am J Pathol* 1998;153:381–94.

94. Makinen K, Manninen H, Hedman M, et al. Increased vascularity detected by digital subtraction angiography after VEGF gene transfer to human lower limb artery: A randomized, placebo-controlled, double-blinded phase II study. *Mol Ther* 2002;6:127–33.

95. Taniyama Y, Morishita R, Aoki M, et al. Therapeutic angiogenesis induced by human hepatocyte growth factor gene in rat and rabbit hindlimb ischemia models: Preclinical study for treatment of peripheral arterial disease. *Gene Ther* 2001;8:181–89.

96. Murray CJ, Lopez AD. Alternative projections of mortality and disability by cause 1990–2020: Global Burden of Disease Study. *Lancet* 1997;349: 1498–504.

97. Murray CJ, Lopez AD. Mortality by cause for eight regions of the world: Global Burden of Disease Study. *Lancet* 1997;349:1269–76.

98. Lathi KG, Vale PR, Losordo DW, et al. Gene therapy with vascular endothelial growth factor for inoperable coronary artery disease: Anesthetic management and results. *Anesth Analg* 2001;92: 19–25.

99. Fortuin FD, Vale P, Losordo DW, et al. One-year follow-up of direct myocardial gene transfer of vascular endothelial growth factor-2 using naked plasmid deoxyribonucleic acid by way of thoracotomy in no-option patients. *Am J Cardiol* 2003;92:436–39.

100. Grines CL, Watkins MW, Helmer G, et al. Angiogenic Gene Therapy (AGENT) trial in patients with stable angina pectoris. *Circulation* 2002; 105:1291–97.

101. Grines CL, Watkins MW, Mahmarian JJ, et al. A randomized, double-blind, placebo-controlled trial of Ad5FGF-4 gene therapy and its effect on myocardial perfusion in patients with stable angina. *J Am Coll Cardiol* 2003;42:1339–47.

102. Rentrop KP. Thrombi in acute coronary syndromes: Revisited and revised. *Circulation* 2000;101:1619–26.

103. Yasue H, Kugiyama K. Coronary spasm: Clinical features and pathogenesis. *Intern Med* 1997;36:760–65.

104. Yeghiazarians Y, Braunstein JB, Askari A, Stone PH. Unstable angina pectoris. *N Engl J Med* 2000;342:101–14.

105. Seccombe JF, Schaff HV. Coronary artery endothelial function after myocardial ischemia and reperfusion. *Ann Thorac Surg* 1995;60:778–88.

106. Vanden Hoek TL, Shao Z, Li C, Zak R, Schumacker PT, Becker LB. Reperfusion injury on cardiac myocytes after simulated ischemia. *Am J Physiol* 1996;270:H1334–41.

107. Singal PK, Khaper N, Palace V, Kumar D. The role of oxidative stress in the genesis of heart disease. *Cardiovasc Res* 1998;40:426–32.

108. Melo LG, Agrawal R, Zhang L, et al. Gene therapy strategy for long-term myocardial protection using adeno-associated virus-mediated delivery of heme oxygenase gene. *Circulation* 2002;105:602–07.

109. Agrawal RS, Muangman S, Layne MD, et al. Pre-emptive gene therapy using recombinant adeno-associated virus delivery of extracellular superoxide dismutase protects heart against ischemic reperfusion injury, improves ventricular function and prolongs survival. *Gene Ther* 2004;11:962–69.

110. Li Q, Bolli R, Qiu Y, Tang XL, Guo Y, French BA. Gene therapy with extracellular superoxide dismutase protects conscious rabbits against myocardial infarction. *Circulation* 2001;103:1893–98.

111. Li N, Karin M. Is NF-kappaB the sensor of oxidative stress? *Faseb J* 1999;13:1137–43.

112. Okubo S, Wildner O, Shah MR, Chelliah JC, Hess ML, Kukreja RC. Gene transfer of heat-shock protein 70 reduces infarct size in vivo after ischemia/reperfusion in the rabbit heart. *Circulation* 2001;103:877–81.

113. Chen Z, Chua CC, Ho YS, Hamdy RC, Chua BH. Overexpression of Bcl-2 attenuates apoptosis and protects against myocardial I/R injury in transgenic mice. *Am J Physiol Heart Circ Physiol* 2001;280:H2313–20.

114. Miao W, Luo Z, Kitsis RN, Walsh K. Intracoronary, adenovirus-mediated Akt gene transfer in heart limits infarct size following ischemia-reperfusion injury in vivo. *J Mol Cell Cardiol* 2000; 32:2397–402.

115. Qin L, Chavin KD, Ding Y, et al. Retrovirus-mediated transfer of viral IL-10 gene prolongs murine cardiac allograft survival. *J Immunol* 1996; 156:2316–23.

116. Brauner R, Nonoyama M, Laks H, et al. Intracoronary adenovirus-mediated transfer of immunosuppressive cytokine genes prolongs allograft survival. *J Thorac Cardiovasc Surg* 1997;114:923–33.

117. Colucci WS. Molecular and cellular mechanisms of myocardial failure. *Am J Cardiol* 1997;80:15L–25L.

118. Miyamoto MI, del Monte F, Schmidt U, et al. Adenoviral gene transfer of SERCA2a improves left-ventricular function in aortic-banded rats in transition to heart failure. *Proc Natl Acad Sci USA* 2000;97:793–98.

119. Maurice JP, Hata JA, Shah AS, et al. Enhancement of cardiac function after adenoviral-mediated in vivo intracoronary beta2-adrenergic receptor gene delivery. *J Clin Invest* 1999;104:21–9.

120. Dobrzynski E, Yoshida H, Chao J, Chao L. Adenovirus-mediated kallikrein gene delivery attenuates hypertension and protects against renal injury in deoxycorticosterone-salt rats. *Immunopharmacology* 1999;44:57–65.

121. Jin L, Zhang JJ, Chao L, Chao J. Gene therapy in hypertension: Adenovirus-mediated kallikrein gene delivery in hypertensive rats. *Hum Gene Ther* 1997;8:1753–61.

122. Dobrzynski E, Wang C, Chao J, Chao L. Adrenomedullin gene delivery attenuates hypertension, cardiac remodeling, and renal injury in deoxycorticosterone acetate-salt hypertensive rats. *Hypertension* 2000; 36:995–1001.

123. Lin KF, Chao J, Chao L. Human atrial natriuretic peptide gene delivery reduces blood pressure in hypertensive rats. *Hypertension* 1995;26:847–53.

124. Lin KF, Chao L, Chao J. Prolonged reduction of high blood pressure with human nitric oxide synthase gene delivery. *Hypertension* 1997;30:307–13.

125. Wang C, Chao L, Chao J. Direct gene delivery of human tissue kallikrein reduces blood pressure in spontaneously hypertensive rats. *J Clin Invest* 1995; 95:1710–16.

126. Chao J, Zhang JJ, Lin KF, Chao L. Human kallikrein gene delivery attenuates hypertension, cardiac hypertrophy, and renal injury in Dahl salt-sensitive rats. *Hum Gene Ther* 1998; z9:21–31.

127. Zhang JJ, Wang C, Lin KF, Chao L, Chao J. Human tissue kallikrein attenuates hypertension and secretes into circulation and urine after intramuscular gene delivery in hypertensive rats. *Clin Exp Hypertens* 1999;21:1145–60.

128. Zhang JJ, Yoshida H, Chao L, Chao J. Human adrenomedullin gene delivery protects against cardiac hypertrophy, fibrosis, and renal damage in hypertensive dahl salt-sensitive rats. *Hum Gene Ther* 2000;11:1817–27.

129. Metcalfe BL, Huentelman MJ, Parilak LD, et al. Prevention of cardiac hypertrophy by angiotensin II type-2 receptor gene transfer. *Hypertension* 2004;43:1233–38.

130. Falcon BL, Stewart JM, Bourassa E, et al. Angiotensin II type 2 receptor gene transfer elicits cardioprotective effects in an angiotensin II infusion rat model of hypertension. *Physiol Genomics* 2004;19:255–61.

131. Tipnis SR, Hooper NM, Hyde R, Karran E, Christie G, Turner AJ. A human homolog of angiotensin-converting enzyme: Cloning and functional expression as a captopril-insensitive carboxypeptidase. *J Biol Chem* 2000;275:33238–43.

132. Turner AJ, Hooper NM. The angiotensin-converting enzyme gene family: Genomics and pharmacology. *Trends Pharmacol Sci* 2002;23:177–83.

133. Huentelman MJ, Grobe JL, Vazquez J, et al. Protection from Angiotensin II-induced cardiac hypertrophy and fibrosis by systemic lentiviral delivery of ACE2. *Exp Physiol* 90,783–790, 2005.

134. Pachori AS, Wang H, Gelband CH, Ferrario CM, Katovich MJ, Raizada MK. Inability to induce hypertension in normotensive rat expressing AT(1) receptor antisense. *Circ Res* 2000; 86:1167–72.

135. Wang H, Katovich MJ, Gelband CH, Reaves PY, Phillips MI, Raizada MK. Sustained inhibition of angiotensin I-converting enzyme (ACE) expression and long-term antihypertensive action by virally mediated delivery of ACE antisense cDNA. *Circ Res* 1999; 85:614–22.

136. Iyer SN, Lu D, Katovich MJ, Raizada MK. Chronic control of high blood pressure in the spontaneously hypertensive rat by delivery of angiotensin type 1 receptor antisense. *Proc Natl Acad Sci USA* 1996;93:9960–65.

137. Katovich MJ, Gelband CH, Reaves P, Wang HW, Raizada MK. Reversal of hypertension by angiotensin II type 1 receptor antisense gene therapy in the adult SHR. *Am J Physiol* 1999; 277:H1260–64.

138. Pachori AS, Numan MT, Ferrario CM, Diz DM, Raizada MK, Katovich MJ. Blood pressure-independent attenuation of cardiac hypertrophy by AT(1)R-AS gene therapy. *Hypertension* 2002; 39:969–75.

139. Katovich MJ, Reaves PY, Francis SC, Pachori AS, Wang HW, Raizada MK. Gene therapy attenuates the elevated blood pressure and glucose intolerance in an insulin-resistant model of hypertension. *J Hypertens* 2001; 19:1553–58.

140. Gyurko R, Tran D, Phillips MI. Time course of inhibition of hypertension by antisense oligonucleotides targeted to AT1 angiotensin receptor mRNA in spontaneously hypertensive rats. *Am J Hypertens* 1997;10:56S–62S.

141. Tomita N, Morishita R, Higaki J, et al. Transient decrease in high blood pressure by in vivo transfer of antisense oligodeoxynucleotides against rat angiotensinogen. *Hypertension* 1995;26:131–36.

142. Wielbo D, Simon A, Phillips MI, Toffolo S. Inhibition of hypertension by peripheral administration of antisense oligodeoxynucleotides. *Hypertension* 1996;28:147–51.

143. Makino N, Sugano M, Ohtsuka S, Sawada S. Intravenous injection with antisense oligodeoxynucleotides against angiotensinogen decreases blood pressure in spontaneously hypertensive rats. *Hypertension* 1998;31:1166–70.

144. Galli SM, Phillips MI. Angiotensin II AT(1A) receptor antisense lowers blood pressure in acute 2-kidney, 1-clip hypertension. *Hypertension* 2001;38:674–78.

145. Peng JF, Kimura B, Fregly MJ, Phillips MI. Reduction of cold-induced hypertension by antisense oligodeoxynucleotides to angiotensinogen mRNA and AT1-receptor mRNA in brain and blood. *Hypertension* 1998;31:1317–23.

146. Pachori AS, Huentelman MJ, Francis SC, Gelband CH, Katovich MJ, Raizada MK. The future of hypertension therapy: Sense, antisense, or nonsense? *Hypertension* 2001;37:357–64.

147. Szombathy T, Szalai C, Katalin B, Palicz T, Romics L, Csaszar A. Association of angiotensin II type 1 receptor polymorphism with resistant essential hypertension. *Clin Chim Acta* 1998; 269:91–100.

148. Hingorani AD, Jia H, Stevens PA, Hopper R, Dickerson JE, Brown MJ. Renin-angiotensin system gene polymorphisms influence blood pressure and the response to angiotensin converting enzyme inhibition. *J Hypertens* 1995;13: 1602–09.

149. Lu D, Raizada MK, Iyer S, Reaves P, Yang H, Katovich MJ. Losartan versus gene therapy: Chronic control of high blood pressure in spontaneously hypertensive rats. *Hypertension* 1997; 30:363–70.

150. Azizi M, Chatellier G, Guyene TT, Murieta-Geoffroy D, Menard J. Additive effects of combined angiotensin-converting enzyme inhibition and angiotensin II antagonism on blood pressure and renin release in sodium-depleted normotensives. *Circulation* 1995; 92:825–34.

151. Wang H, Gallinat S, Li HW, Sumners C, Raizada MK, Katovich MJ. Elevated blood pressure in normotensive rats produced by "knockdown" of the angiotensin type 2 receptor. *Exp Physiol* 2004;89:313–22.

152. Gossen M, Freundlieb S, Bender G, Muller G, Hillen W, Bujard H. Transcriptional activation by tetracyclines in mammalian cells. *Science* 1995;268:1766–69.

153. Baron U, Gossen M, Bujard H. Tetracycline-controlled transcription in eukaryotes: Novel transactivators with graded transactivation potential. *Nucleic Acids Res* 1997;25:2723–29.

154. Vigna E, Cavalieri S, Ailles L, et al. Robust and efficient regulation of transgene expression in vivo by improved tetracycline-dependent lentiviral vectors. *Mol Ther* 2002; 5:252–61.

155. Tang Y, Schmitt-Ott K, Qian K, Kagiyama S, Phillips MI. Vigilant vectors: Adeno-associated virus with a biosensor to switch on amplified therapeutic genes in specific tissues in life-threatening diseases. *Methods* 2002;28:259–66.

156. Phillips MI, Tang Y, Schmidt-Ott K, Qian K, Kagiyama S. Vigilant vector: Heart-specific promoter in an adeno-associated virus vector for cardioprotection. *Hypertension* 2002; 39:651–55.

157. Pachori AS, Melo LG, Hart ML, et al. Hypoxia-regulated therapeutic gene as a preemptive treatment strategy against ischemia/reperfusion tissue injury. *Proc Natl Acad Sci USA* 2004; 101:12282–87.

158. Korhonen J, Lahtinen I, Halmekyto M, et al. Endothelial-specific gene expression directed by the tie gene promoter in vivo. *Blood* 1995; 86:1828–35.

159. De Palma M, Venneri MA, Naldini L. In vivo targeting of tumor endothelial cells by systemic delivery of lentiviral vectors. *Hum Gene Ther* 2003;14: 1193–206.

160. Springer ML, Chen AS, Kraft PE, Bednarski M, Blau HM. VEGF gene delivery to muscle: Potential role for vasculogenesis in adults. *Mol Cell* 1998;2:549–58.

161. Moulton KS, Heller E, Konerding MA, Flynn E, Palinski W, Folkman J. Angiogenesis inhibitors endostatin or TNP-470 reduce intimal neovascularization and plaque growth in apolipoprotein E-deficient mice. *Circulation* 1999;99:1726–32.

162. Kay MA, Glorioso JC, Naldini L. Viral vectors for gene therapy: The art of turning infectious agents into vehicles of therapeutics. *Nat Med* 2001;7:33–40.

163. Muller K, Heller H, Doerfler W. Foreign DNA integration. Genome-wide perturbations of methylation and transcription in the recipient genomes. *J Biol Chem* 2001;276:14271–78.

164. Hackett PB, Ekker SC, Largaespada DA, McIvor RS. Sleeping beauty transposon-mediated gene therapy for prolonged expression. *Adv Genet* 2005;54: 189–232.

165. Paddison PJ, Caudy AA, Hannon GJ. Stable suppression of gene expression by RNAi in mammalian cells. *Proc Natl Acad Sci USA* 2002;99:1443–48.

166. Vazquez J, Correa de Adjounian MF, Sumners C, Gonzalez A, Diez-Freire C, Raizada MK. Selective silencing of angiotensin receptor subtype 1a (AT1aR) by RNA interference. *Hypertension* 2005;45:115–19.

167. Yanez RJ, Porter AC. Therapeutic gene targeting. *Gene Ther* 1998;5:149–59.

168. Sunkomat JN, Gaballa MA. Stem cell therapy in ischemic heart disease. *Cardiovasc Drug Rev* 2003;21:327–42.

169. Oh H, Bradfute SB, Gallardo TD, et al. Cardiac progenitor cells from adult myocardium: Homing, differentiation, and fusion after infarction. *Proc Natl Acad Sci USA* 2003;100:12313–18.

170. Zanjani ED, Anderson WF. Prospects for in utero human gene therapy. *Science* 1999;285:2084–88.

171. Phillips MI, Mohuczy-Dominiak D, Coffey M, et al. Prolonged reduction of high blood pressure with an in vivo, nonpathogenic, adeno-associated viral vector delivery of AT1-R mRNA antisense. *Hypertension* 1997;29: 374–80.

172. Phillips MI. Somatic gene therapy for hypertension. *Braz J Med Biol Res* 2000;33:715–21.

173. Katovich MJ, Grobe JL, Raizada MK. Current and future novel targets of gene therapy for hypertension. *Cardiovascular Genomics (Humana Press)* 2005;12:213–46.

174. Emanueli C, Salis MB, Stacca T, et al. Rescue of impaired angiogenesis in spontaneously hypertensive rats by intramuscular human tissue kallikrein gene transfer. *Hypertension* 2001; 38:136–41.

175. Chao J, Zhang JJ, Lin KF, Chao L. Adenovirus-mediated kallikrein gene delivery reverses salt-induced renal injury in Dahl salt-sensitive rats. *Kidney Int* 1998;54:1250–60.

176. Yayama K, Wang C, Chao L, Chao J. Kallikrein gene delivery attenuates hypertension and cardiac hypertrophy and enhances renal function in Goldblatt hypertensive rats. *Hypertension* 1998;31:1104–10.

177. Chen LM, Chao L, Chao J. Adenovirus-mediated delivery of human kallistatin gene reduces blood pressure of spontaneously hypertensive rats. *Hum Gene Ther* 1997;8:341–47.

178. Chao J, Jin L, Chen LM, Chen VC, Chao L. Systemic and portal vein delivery of human kallikrein gene reduces blood pressure in hypertensive rats. *Hum Gene Ther* 1996;7:901–11.

179. Xiong W, Chao J, Chao L. Muscle delivery of human kallikrein gene reduces blood pressure in hypertensive rats. *Hypertension* 1995;25:715–19.

180. Wang C, Dobrzynski E, Chao J, Chao L. Adrenomedullin gene delivery attenuates renal damage and cardiac hypertrophy in Goldblatt hypertensive rats. *Am J Physiol Renal Physiol* 2001; 280:F964–71.

181. Chao J, Jin L, Lin KF, Chao L. Adrenomedullin gene delivery reduces blood pressure in spontaneously hypertensive rats. *Hypertens Res* 1997; 20:269–77.

182. Lin KF, Chao J, Chao L. Atrial natriuretic peptide gene delivery reduces stroke-induced mortality rate in Dahl salt-sensitive rats. *Hypertension* 1999; 33:219–24.

183. Lin KF, Chao J, Chao L. Atrial natriuretic peptide gene delivery attenuates hypertension, cardiac hypertrophy, and renal injury in salt-sensitive rats. *Hum Gene Ther* 1998;9:1429–38.

184. Hirooka Y, Sakai K, Kishi T, Ito K, Shimokawa H, Takeshita A. Enhanced depressor response to endothelial nitric oxide synthase gene transfer into the nucleus tractus solitarii of spontaneously hypertensive rats. *Hypertens Res* 2003;26:325–31.

185. Alexander MY, Brosnan MJ, Hamilton CA, et al. Gene transfer of endothelial nitric oxide synthase but not Cu/Zn superoxide dismutase restores nitric oxide availability in the SHRSP. *Cardiovasc Res* 2000;47:609–17.

186. Tai MH, Hsiao M, Chan JY, et al. Gene delivery of endothelial nitric oxide synthase into nucleus tractus solitarii induces biphasic response in cardiovascular functions of hypertensive rats. *Am J Hypertens* 2004;17:63–70.

187. Chu Y, Iida S, Lund DD, et al. Gene transfer of extracellular superoxide dismutase reduces arterial pressure in spontaneously hypertensive rats: Role of heparin-binding domain. *Circ Res* 2003;92:461–68.

188. Fennell JP, Brosnan MJ, Frater AJ, et al. Adenovirus-mediated overexpression of extracellular superoxide dismutase improves endothelial dysfunction in a rat model of hypertension. *Gene Ther* 2002;9:110–17.

189. Sabaawy HE, Zhang F, Nguyen X, et al. Human heme oxygenase-1 gene transfer lowers blood pressure and promotes growth in spontaneously hypertensive rats. *Hypertension* 2001; 38:210–15.

190. Phillips MI, Wielbo D, Gyurko R. Antisense inhibition of hypertension: A new strategy for renin-angiotensin candidate genes. *Kidney Int* 1994; 46:1554–56.

191. Gyurko R, Wielbo D, Phillips MI. Antisense inhibition of AT1 receptor mRNA and angiotensinogen mRNA in the brain of spontaneously hypertensive rats reduces hypertension of neurogenic origin. *Regul Pept* 1993;49:167–74.

192. Kimura B, Mohuczy D, Tang X, Phillips MI. Attenuation of hypertension and heart hypertrophy by adeno-associated virus delivering angiotensinogen antisense. *Hypertension* 2001;37:376–80.

193. Tang X, Mohuczy D, Zhang YC, Kimura B, Galli SM, Phillips MI. Intravenous angiotensinogen antisense in AAV-based vector decreases hypertension. *Am J Physiol* 1999;277:H2392–99.

194. Kagiyama S, Varela A, Phillips MI, Galli SM. Antisense inhibition of brain renin-angiotensin system decreased blood pressure in chronic 2-kidney, 1 clip hypertensive rats. *Hypertension* 2001;37:371–75.

195. Reaves PY, Beck CR, Wang HW, Raizada MK, Katovich MJ. Endothelial-independent prevention of high blood pressure in L-NAME-treated rats by angiotensin II type I receptor antisense gene therapy. *Exp Physiol* 2003; 88:467–73.

196. Moore AF, Heiderstadt NT, Huang E, et al. Selective inhibition of the renal angiotensin type 2 receptor increases blood pressure in conscious rats. *Hypertension* 2001;37:1285–91.

197. Zhang YC, Bui JD, Shen L, Phillips MI. Antisense inhibition of beta(1)-adrenergic receptor mRNA in a single dose produces a profound and prolonged reduction in high blood pressure in spontaneously hypertensive rats. *Circulation* 2000;101:682–88.

198. Clare Zhang Y, Kimura B, Shen L, Phillips MI. New beta-blocker: Prolonged reduction in high blood pressure with beta(1) antisense oligodeoxynucleotides. *Hypertension* 2000;35:219–24.

199. Kagiyama S, Qian K, Kagiyama T, Phillips MI. Antisense to epidermal growth factor receptor prevents the development of left ventricular hypertrophy. *Hypertension* 2003; 41:824–9.

200. Kagiyama S, Eguchi S, Frank GD, Inagami T, Zhang YC, Phillips MI. Angiotensin II-induced cardiac hypertrophy and hypertension are attenuated by epidermal growth factor receptor antisense. *Circulation* 2002;106:909–12.

201. Cuevas P, Garcia-Calvo M, Carceller F, et al. Correction of hypertension by normalization of endothelial levels of fibroblast growth factor and nitric oxide synthase in spontaneously hypertensive rats. *Proc Natl Acad Sci USA* 1996;93:11996–2001.

202. Der Sarkissian S, Huentelman MJ, Stewart J, Katovich MJ, Raizada MK. ACE2: A novel therapeutic target for cardiovascular diseases. *Prog Biophys Mol Biol* 2006;91,163–198.

Chapter

38

Pathophysiology of Obesity-Induced Hypertension and Target Organ Damage

John E. Hall, Alexandre A. da Silva, Elizabeth Brandon, David E. Stec, Zhekang Ying, and Daniel W. Jones

Key Findings

- Excess weight gain, especially when associated with increased visceral adiposity, is a major cause of human primary (essential) hypertension, accounting for 65 to 75% of the risk for hypertension.

- Increased renal tubular sodium reabsorption and impaired pressure natriuresis play a major role in initiating obesity hypertension.

- Abnormal kidney function and hypertension in obesity are mediated by increased sympathetic nervous system (SNS) activity, activation of the renin-angiotensin-aldosterone system (RAAS), and physical compression of the kidneys by extrarenal fat and by increased intrarenal extracellular matrix.

- Obesity is a major risk factor for vascular, cardiac, and renal disease through diabetes and hypertension and perhaps other mechanisms such as "lipotoxicity" (ectopic lipid accumulation within organs).

- With prolonged obesity and development of target organ injury (especially renal injury), obesity-associated hypertension becomes more difficult to control, often requiring multiple antihypertensive drugs as well as pharmacological therapy of other risk factors, including dyslipidemia, insulin resistance and diabetes, inflammation, and hypercoagulation.

- Until effective anti-obesity drugs are developed, the impact of obesity on hypertension and related cardiovascular, renal, and metabolic disorders is likely to become even more important in the future as the prevalence of obesity continues to increase.

- More emphasis should be placed on prevention of obesity and on lifestyle modifications that help patients maintain a healthier weight.

Obesity is rapidly becoming the most important public health problem in industrialized countries. Surveys throughout the world have revealed dramatic increases in the prevalence of obesity in adults and children in many countries, and current estimates indicate that over 1 *billion* people in the world are overweight or obese.[1,2] In China alone, over 200 million people are overweight, and more than 20% of children in major Chinese cities are either clinically overweight or obese, compared to only a 1 to 2% prevalence in 1985.[3]

In the United States, over 64% of adults are overweight with a body mass index (BMI, kg weight/m^2 height) greater than 25 and almost one-third of the adult population is obese, with a BMI greater than 30.[4] The same trends toward increasing obesity have been reported in other industrialized countries and there appears to be no abatement of this worldwide "pandemic." Moreover, the rapid increase in obesity prevalence in young people, affecting at least 10% of children worldwide,[5] suggests that obesity-associated medical problems are likely to worsen in the future unless these trends can be attenuated or reversed.[6,7]

The global emergence of obesity has become a major economic challenge as well as the number one public health problem in many countries.[2] Excess weight gain is an important risk factor for many medical disorders, including osteoarthritis, sleep apnea, nonalcoholic fatty liver disease, gall bladder disease, diabetes, cerebrovascular disease, coronary heart disease, kidney disease, and several types of cancer (e.g., breast, colon, kidney, prostate). Table 38–1 shows the classification of overweight and obesity and the increasing risk for disease and premature mortality associated with increasing BMI.

The emerging epidemic of diabetes mellitus appears to be due largely to the increasing prevalence of overweight and obesity, with at least 60% of all cases of diabetes being directly attributable to excess weight gain.[8] According to the International Diabetes Federation, diabetes alone accounts for 5 to 10% of the total health care budget in many countries. The American Diabetes Association has estimated that the total cost of diabetes in the United States for 2002 was $132 billion, including direct and indirect costs. Total costs are predicted to rise even further, reaching $156 billion in 2010 and $192 billion in 2020.

Cardiovascular disease, occurring through multiple mechanisms (including hypertension, diabetes, dyslipidemia, and atherosclerosis) is another major consequence of excess weight gain (Figure 38–1). Many risk factors for cardiovascular disease are interdependent and are often grouped as the "metabolic syndrome."[9–11] However, excess weight gain (especially when associated with increased visceral adiposity) is the primary cause of each of these disorders in most patients.

Although obesity has not been widely recognized as an independent risk factor for renal disease, there is little doubt that excess weight gain is a major cause of the two main drivers of kidney disease: hypertension and type 2

CLASSIFICATION OF OVERWEIGHT AND OBESITY BY BMI, WAIST CIRCUMFERENCE, AND ASSOCIATED DISEASE RISK[a]				
Category	Class	BMI	Disease Risk[b] Men <40 in., Women <35 in.	Men >40 in., Women >35 in.
Underweight		<18.5	—	—
Normal		18.5-24.9	—	—
Overweight		25.0-29.9	Increased	High
Obesity	I	30.0-34.9	High	Very high
	II	35.0-39.9	Very high	Very high
Extreme obesity	III	>40	Extremely high	Extremely high

a. Source: NHLBI Expert Panel 1998.
b. Relative to normal weight and waist circumference.

Table 38–1. Classification of Overweight and Obesity by BMI, Waist Circumference, and Associated Disease Risk[a]

diabetes. Together, these two disorders account for approximately 70% of end-stage renal disease (ESRD). Accumulating evidence suggests, however, that obesity independently increases risk for kidney disease through mechanisms that are still somewhat obscure.[12] In this chapter we focus mainly on the pathophysiology of obesity-associated hypertension and target organ injury, recognizing that the metabolic, renal, and cardiovascular effects of obesity are closely intertwined.

Overweight and obesity as important causes of primary hypertension

Obesity is often considered a special form of hypertension rather than as a major cause of primary (essential) hypertension *per se*. Yet, excessive weight gain is the most common cause of human primary hypertension. Popu-

lation studies, for example, have shown that excess weight gain (as estimated by BMI, waist-to-hip ratio, abdominal diameter, and other indices of adiposity) is one of the best predictors for development of hypertension.[13–15]

The relationships between BMI and systolic and diastolic blood pressure appear to be nearly linear (Figure 38–2) in diverse populations throughout the world.[13–16] Moreover, the association between BMI and blood pressure occurs in non-obese normotensive subjects, as well as in hypertensive patients.[13,14] Thus, the relationship between BMI and blood pressure appears to be continuous, extending from the range of very lean to very obese.[14] The strength of the association between BMI and blood pressure, however, varies in different ethnic groups for reasons that are still poorly understood but may be related to differences in body fat distribution or other factors (genetic and environmental) that influence the susceptibility of blood pressure to increased adiposity.

The full impact of obesity on hypertension is difficult to assess with cross-sectional studies because the effects of excess weight gain on blood pressure are likely to worsen as obesity is sustained for many years and development of diabetes and target organ injury occurs. The time-dependent effects of obesity on diabetes have been clearly demonstrated (Figure 38–3). When obesity persists for more than five years, the adjusted relative risk for developing diabetes is 8.7 compared to 4.9 if a person has been obese for less than five years.[17] Thus, the health consequences of obesity (including hypertension) are likely to worsen the longer a person is obese, although this is often not considered in cross-sectional studies.

The presence of nonlinear synergistic relationships among the multiple effects of obesity (including hyperlipidemia, glucose intolerance, hypertension and renal injury) may also lead to underestimation of the importance of obesity in causing cardiovascular disease. These *interdependent* effects of obesity are difficult to assess in population studies that seek to establish "independent" risk factors. Yet, even with these caveats risk estimates from the Framingham Heart Study suggest that approximately 78% of primary hypertension in men and 65% in women can be ascribed to obesity.[15]

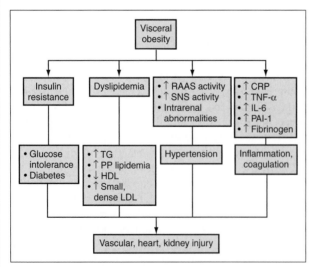

Figure 38–1. Cardiovascular, metabolic, and renal disease associated with visceral obesity. (Abbreviations: TG, triglycerides; PP, postprandial; HDL, high-density lipoprotein; LDL, low-density lipoprotein; RAAS, renin-angiotensin-aldosterone system; SNS, sympathetic nervous system; CRP, C-reactive protein; PAI, platelet activator inhibitor; TNF-α, tumor necrosis factor-α; and IL-6, interleukin-6.)

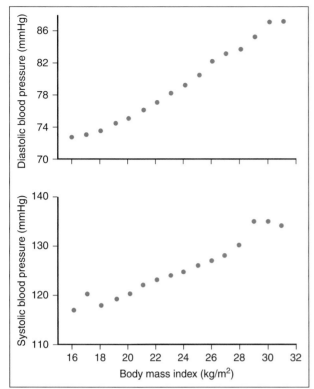

Figure 38–2. Relationship between body-mass index and systolic and diastolic blood pressures in 22,354 Korean subjects. (Redrawn from data in reference 14.)

Clinical studies also suggest that obesity is an important cause of increased blood pressure in most patients with primary hypertension, and the therapeutic value of weight loss in lowering blood pressure has been demonstrated in normotensive and hypertensive obese subjects.[13,18–20] Even modest weight loss of 5 to 10% often decreases blood pressure and may even reduce the need for anti-hypertensive medication.[19] Clinical trials have also demonstrated the effectiveness of weight loss in primary prevention of hypertension.[20]

Although weight loss does not always completely normalize blood pressure in obese hypertensive patients, this is perhaps not surprising in view of the many pathologic changes that occur when excess adiposity is maintained for long periods of time. For example, prolonged obesity may lead to glomerular injury, loss of functional nephrons, and resetting of renal-pressure natriuresis to higher blood pressures.[11,12] Some of these changes may not be easily reversible even with marked weight loss, and may make hypertension more difficult to control with antihypertensive medications.

Why are some obese persons not hypertensive?

One question that often crops up is why some overweight or obese persons are not hypertensive by the usual standards (i.e., blood pressure >140/90) if obesity is a major cause of hypertension? There are several potential explanations. First, it appears that blood pressure in "normotensive" obese people is higher than it would be at a lower body weight because weight loss often reduces their blood pressure. Excess weight gain shifts the frequency distribution of blood pressure toward higher levels, increasing the probability of a person's blood pressure registering in the hypertensive range (Figure 38–4).

Second, as discussed previously the length of time a person is obese likely has an impact on the blood pressure. Many obese persons who are not yet considered hypertensive may be "pre-hypertensive," a term recently introduced by the Seventh Report of the Joint National Committee on Prevention, Detection, Evaluation, and Treatment of High Blood Pressure (JNC 7).[21] It is increasingly recognized that reducing blood pressure in pre-hypertensive subjects may provide protection against future development of cardiovascular disease, especially when additional risk factors are present, as is the case for most obese subjects.

Third, the location of excess fat has a major impact on the blood pressure, with increased visceral adiposity carrying a much greater risk for hypertension and metabolic disorders compared to lower body or subcutaneous obesity.

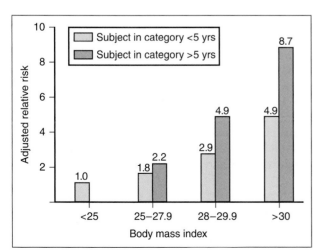

Figure 38–3. Time-dependent effect of obesity to increase risk of type 2 diabetes. (Redrawn from data in reference 17.)

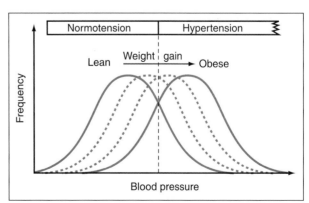

Figure 38–4. Effect of weight gain to shift the frequency distribution of blood pressure to higher levels. Not all obese subjects have blood pressures in the hypertensive range (>140/90 mmHg), but excess weight gain raises blood pressure above the baseline level for an individual.

In fact, there are many individuals (especially older sedentary people) who may have a normal BMI but are "metabolically obese" (with increased visceral adiposity and reduced muscle mass). Conversely, there are significant numbers of individuals (especially women) who have increased BMI and increased lower body (subcutaneous adiposity) but do not have substantial visceral obesity.

For reasons that are still unclear, increased amounts of subcutaneous adipose tissue do not appear to increase blood pressure or metabolic risk. For instance, removal of large amounts of subcutaneous fat by liposuction (an average of over 9 kg, or over 20 lb) did not significantly improve insulin sensitivity, did not reduce plasma levels of inflammatory cytokines, and did not reduce blood pressure.[22] These observations suggest that excess subcutaneous fat is not a major cause of insulin resistance, inflammation, or hypertension and reinforces the concept that the location of fat (i.e., visceral fat) is important in determining the blood pressure effects of increased adiposity.

HEMODYNAMIC AND HEART RATE CHANGES IN OBESITY HYPERTENSION

Studies in experimental animals have provided mechanistic insights into the cardiovascular and renal changes associated with excess weight gain. A highly reproducible rise in blood pressure is observed with weight gain induced by a high-fat diet in dogs and rabbits.[23-25] Moreover, the metabolic, endocrine, cardiovascular, and renal changes caused by dietary-induced obesity in experimental animals closely mimic the changes observed in obese humans[10,26] (Table 38–2).

Some of these changes occur rapidly after weight gain and later become obscured by pathologic changes. For example, glomerular hyperfiltration (characteristic of the early phases of obesity) subsides and may be replaced by a gradual decrease in glomerular filtration rate (GFR) as renal injury and nephron loss occur in association with prolonged obesity-induced hypertension and diabetes.

Obesity, blood flow, and cardiac output

Obesity is associated with expansion of extracellular fluid volume and blood volume and increased total tissue blood flow, thereby increasing venous return and cardiac output.[10-12,26,27] Part of the rise in cardiac output is due to increased blood flow in the extra adipose tissue, and in most studies cardiac output increases in direct proportion to increases in body weight.[23,24,26] However, much of the extra weight in obese persons is adipose tissue, and blood flow in adipose tissue is considerably lower than in many other tissues. Therefore, the rise in cardiac output in obesity is usually much greater than can be attributed to increased blood flow needed for the additional adipose tissue.

Studies in experimental animals and humans indicate that blood flow is increased in many tissues, including the heart, kidneys, gastrointestinal tract, and skeletal muscles.[23,24,27] Some of the increased blood flow is due to growth of tissues and organs in response to increased

workload and metabolic demands associated with obesity. However, prior to the onset of vascular disease blood flows in tissues such as the kidneys, skeletal muscle, and heart are increased in obese subjects even when flow is expressed per gram tissue weight.[23,24,27] Thus, it appears that obesity is associated with a functional vasodilation. The mechanisms responsible for obesity-induced vasodilation have not been fully elucidated but are probably due in part to increased metabolic rate, higher oxygen consumption, and accumulation of local vasodilator metabolites.

Despite higher resting blood flows in many tissues, there is reduced blood flow reserve during exercise or reactive hyperemia that occurs after briefly stopping tissue blood flow. This decreased blood flow reserve appears to be due in part to endothelial dysfunction, as discussed later in the chapter.

Obesity and heart rate

The elevated heart rate often found in obesity is mainly due to withdrawal of parasympathetic tone rather than increased sympathetic activity or increased intrinsic heart rate.[28,29] Increases in body weight are associated with decreases in parasympathetic tone, increases in average heart rate, and decreases in heart rate variability. Conversely, weight reduction increases parasympathetic tone and heart rate variability while decreasing the mean heart rate.[30] Although obesity increases sympathetic activity in many tissues (including the kidneys and skeletal muscles), cardiac sympathetic activity (as assessed by measurements of norepinephrine spillover) is usually normal or may even be reduced because of baroreflex inhibition of cardiac SNS activity.[31]

IMPAIRED RENAL-PRESSURE NATRIURESIS IN OBESITY-RELATED HYPERTENSION

Excess renal tubular sodium reabsorption appears to play a major role in initiating the rise in blood pressure associated with weight gain, and obese subjects require higher than normal arterial pressure to maintain sodium balance, indicating impaired renal-pressure natriuresis.[10,32] In the early phases of obesity, blood pressure is usually not very salt sensitive, so that the hypertension is not greatly exacerbated by high salt intake. With chronic obesity, increases in arterial pressure, glomerular hyperfiltration, neurohumoral activation, and metabolic changes may cause renal injury, further impairment of pressure natriuresis, increased salt sensitivity, and greater increases in blood pressure (Figure 38–5).

Three mechanisms appear to be especially important in mediating increased sodium reabsorption, impaired renal-pressure natriuresis, and hypertension associated with weight gain (Figure 38–1): (1) increased sympathetic nervous system (SNS) activity, (2) activation of the renin-angiotensin-aldosterone system (RAAS), and (3) physical compression of the kidneys by fat accumulation within and around the kidneys, and by increased abdominal pressure.

HEMODYNAMIC, NEUROHUMORAL, AND RENAL CHANGES IN EXPERIMENTAL OBESITY CAUSED BY A HIGH-FAT DIET AND IN HUMAN OBESITY

Model	Arterial Pressure	Heart Rate	Cardiac Output	Renal Sympathetic Activity	Plasma Renin Activity	Na+ Balance	Renal Tubular Reabsorption	GFR[a]	Insulin Resistance
Obese rabbits (high fat diet)	↑	↑	↑	↑	↑	↑	↑	↑	↑
Obese dogs (high fat diet)	↑	↑	↑	↑	↑	↑	↑	↑	↑
Obese humans	↑	↑	↑	↑	↑	↑	↑	↑	↑

Abbreviation: GFR, glomerular filtration rate.
a. The GFR changes refer to the early phases of obesity before major loss of nephron function has occurred.

Table 38–2. Hemodynamic, Neurohumoral, and Renal Changes in Experimental Obesity Caused by a High-fat Diet and in Human Obesity

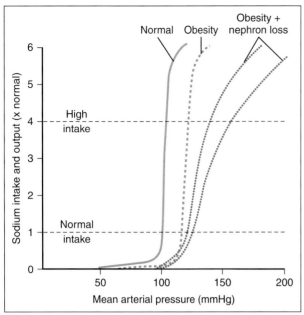

Figure 38–5. Effect of obesity to shift renal-pressure natriuresis curve to higher arterial pressure. With chronic obesity lasting for many years there may be a gradual loss of nephron function, further impairment of pressure natriuresis, increasing salt sensitivity, and higher blood pressures.

ROLE OF SYMPATHETIC NERVOUS SYSTEM IN OBESITY-RELATED HYPERTENSION

Several observations suggest that increased SNS activity impairs renal-pressure natriuresis and contributes to obesity hypertension:[10,11,32–34] (1) obese subjects have elevated SNS activity, especially in the kidneys and in skeletal muscle, as assessed by microneurography and tissue catecholamine spillover, (2) pharmacologic inhibition of adrenergic activity reduces blood pressure to a greater extent in obese than in lean subjects, and (3) renal denervation markedly attenuates renal sodium retention and the development of obesity hypertension associated with a high-fat diet in experimental animals.

SNS activation in obesity is differentially controlled in various tissues and depends on fat distribution

As discussed previously, cardiac sympathetic activity does not appear to be substantially elevated in most obese humans,[35,36] and the high heart rate observed in obese subjects appears to be related mainly to decreased parasympathetic activity.[28,29] In contrast, SNS activity is usually increased in skeletal muscle and kidneys of obese compared to lean subjects.[35–37,38]

SNS responses to weight gain may also vary depending on ethnicity and on other factors such as fat distribution. In Pima Indians, who have a high prevalence of obesity but a relatively low prevalence of hypertension, muscle SNS activity is lower than in whites and does not track well with adiposity.[39] In black men, SNS activity is higher,

and hypertension is more prevalent than in white men despite comparable levels of obesity.[40] In young, overweight black women adiposity is associated with high SNS activity.[40]

Although the mechanisms for ethnic differences in SNS responses to obesity are uncertain, differences in fat distribution may be important. For reasons that are still unclear, visceral obesity elicits greater SNS activation than lower body or subcutaneous obesity.[38,41] Unfortunately, the mechanisms responsible for the link between visceral obesity and SNS activation have not been widely studied, and in most human studies muscle SNS activity has been measured rather than renal SNS activity (the primary pathway by which the SNS causes chronic hypertension).[11] Because there is considerable heterogeneity in the control of autonomic outflow to different organs, measurements of muscle SNS activity may not necessarily reflect renal SNS activity. Thus far, a comprehensive analysis of the multiple factors that influence the relationships among visceral obesity, SNS activity, and hypertension in diverse populations has not been conducted.

Adrenergic blockade or renal denervation attenuates obesity hypertension

In experimental animals fed a high-fat diet, combined α- and β-adrenergic blockade markedly attenuates the rise in blood pressure during the development of obesity.[42] Clonidine, a drug that stimulates central α-2 receptors and reduces sympathetic activity, also prevents most of the rise in blood pressure in dogs fed a high-fat diet.[43] In obese hypertensive patients, combined α- and β-adrenergic blockade for one month reduced ambulatory blood pressure significantly more than in lean essential hypertensive patients.[44] These findings suggest that increased adrenergic activity contributes to the development and maintenance of obesity hypertension in experimental animals and in humans.

The renal sympathetic efferent nerves mediate most, if not all, of the chronic effects of SNS activation on blood pressure in obesity. In obese dogs fed a high-fat diet, bilateral renal denervation greatly attenuated sodium retention and hypertension.[45] Thus, obesity increases renal tubular sodium reabsorption, impairs pressure natriuresis, and causes hypertension—in large part by increasing renal SNS activity.

Mechanisms of SNS activation in obesity

Several potential mediators of SNS activation in obesity have been suggested, including (1) hyperinsulinemia, (2) increased levels of free fatty acids, (3) angiotensin II (Ang II), (4) impaired baroreceptor reflexes, (5) activation of chemoreceptor-mediated reflexes associated with sleep apnea, and (6) cytokines released from adipocytes (i.e., "adipokines"), such as leptin, tumor necrosis factor-α (TNF-α), and interleukin-6 (IL-6). Although these mechanisms have been reviewed previously,[46–49] there is scant evidence supporting cause-and-effect relationships for most of these factors and obesity-induced SNS activation.

Hyperinsulinemia does not mediate obesity hypertension in humans

Obesity is usually associated with fasting hyperinsulinemia and an exaggerated insulin response to glucose loads. The increased plasma insulin concentration occurs as a compensation for impaired metabolic effects of insulin, a condition known as insulin resistance. Some tissues such as the kidneys and SNS, however, are believed to remain sensitive to insulin and hypertension has been hypothesized to be one of the consequences of hyperinsulinemia.

Acute studies suggest that insulin infusion may cause modest sodium retention and increased SNS activity, and these observations have often been extrapolated to infer that hyperinsulinemia may be an important cause of obesity hypertension.[34] However, chronic hyperinsulinemia caused by insulin infusion or insulinoma in dogs and humans is associated with reduced, rather than increased, blood pressure due to the peripheral vasodilator effects of insulin.[47] Hyperinsulinemia also does not enhance the blood pressure or renal effects of other pressor substances such as norepinephrine or Ang II.[47] Moreover, hyperinsulinemia did not increase arterial pressure even in obese dogs that were resistant to the metabolic and vasodilator effects of insulin.[50] Thus, multiple studies indicate that hyperinsulinemia cannot explain SNS activation, increased renal tubular sodium reabsorption, impaired pressure natriuresis, or hypertension associated with obesity.

Do elevated fatty acids increase SNS activity and blood pressure in obesity?

Obese hypertensive patients have high fasting plasma non-esterified fatty acid (NEFA) concentrations and raising NEFA acutely increases vascular reactivity to α-adrenergic agonists.[51] High levels of NEFAs also enhance acute reflex vasoconstrictor responses in the peripheral circulation[51] and have been suggested to activate the SNS indirectly through hepatic afferent pathways.[52] However, chronic infusions of long-chain fatty acids for several days directly into the cerebral circulation[53], the portal vein (unpublished observations), or intravenously in dogs did not alter renal function or increase arterial pressure. Thus, the role of elevated fatty acids in linking obesity, SNS activation, and hypertension has not been clearly established.

Impaired baroreceptor reflexes in obesity

Studies in experimental animals and in humans suggest that obesity is associated with impaired ability of baroreceptor reflexes to suppress SNS activity during acute increases in blood pressure induced by pharmacologic agents.[46] Moreover, weight loss increases the sensitivity of the cardiovagal baroreflex in overweight and obese young and older men.[54] However, despite impaired baroreflexes in obesity there appears to be at least some sustained activation of the baroreflex that in turn acts as a compensatory response to attenuate (rather than stimulate) increases in SNS activity and hypertension.[55] Thus, it seems likely that the arterial baroreflexes act to buffer (rather than mediate) increases in SNS activity in obesity hypertension.

Obstructive sleep apnea and SNS activation in obesity

Obesity, especially when associated with increased visceral adiposity, is an important risk factor for obstructive sleep apnea (OSA). Associations between OSA and hypertension have been found in clinical and population studies and may contribute to hypertension in some obese individuals.[56,57] The factors linking OSA and hypertension are unclear but may include enhanced effects of obesity on SNS and RAAS activation.[58]

Patients with OSA have greater peripheral chemoreflex responses to hypoxia, including not only increased ventilation responses but enhanced muscle SNS responses.[59] Thus, when obesity is associated with OSA activation of the SNS and hypertension are likely to be more severe than in patients without OSA, and in general the effects of obesity and sleep apnea on blood pressure appear to be approximately additive.[57]

Leptin and hypothalamic melanocortins may contribute to obesity-induced SNS activation

Accumulating evidence suggests that leptin may be an important link between obesity and SNS activation[60] (Figure 38–6). Leptin is secreted by adipocytes in proportion to the degree of adiposity and crosses the blood/brain barrier via a saturable receptor-mediated transport system. Leptin binds to its receptors in various regions of the hypothalamus and activates signaling pathways in the hypothalamus and in the hindbrain (e.g., nucleus tractus solitarius) that regulate body weight by decreasing appetite and increasing energy expenditure.[61]

Evidence that leptin acts as a powerful controller of body weight comes from genetic studies of mice and humans that demonstrate that missense mutations of the leptin gene cause early onset of morbid obesity.[61] However, mutations of the leptin gene are very rare in humans and the importance of abnormalities of leptin production or sensitivity of leptin receptors in contributing to obesity in the general population is still unclear.

There is, however, substantial evidence that high levels of leptin, comparable to those found in severe obesity, can activate SNS activity and increase arterial pressure.[10,60,62,63] The rise in blood pressure with chronic hyperleptinemia is slow in onset and occurs over a period of several days despite decreased food intake, which would otherwise tend to lower blood pressure.[63] Moreover, the hypertensive effects of leptin are enhanced when nitric oxide synthesis is inhibited,[64] as often occurs in obese subjects with endothelial dysfunction. The chronic effects of leptin to raise arterial pressure are completely abolished by α- and β-adrenergic blockade, indicating that they are mediated by adrenergic activation.[65]

Another observation that points toward leptin as a potential link between obesity and hypertension is the finding that rodents with leptin deficiency or mutations

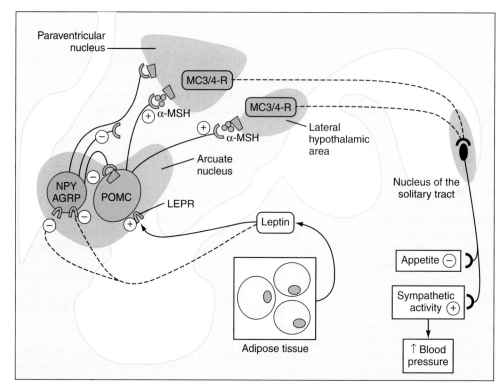

Figure 38–6. Possible links among leptin and its effects on the hypothalamus, sympathetic activation, and hypertension. Within the hypothalamus one of the key pathways of leptin's action on appetite, SNS activity, and blood pressure is stimulation of the pro-opiomelanocortin (POMC) neurons in the arcuate nucleus. These neurons send projections to the paraventricular nucleus and lateral hypothalamus, releasing α-melanocyte-stimulating hormone (α-MSH), which then acts as an agonist for melanocortin 3/4-receptors (MC3/4-R). These neurons then send projections to the nucleus of the solitary tract to effect changes in appetite, SNS activity, and blood pressure. Leptin also suppresses the NPY/AGRP neurons, but their role in controlling SNS activity and blood pressure is still unclear.

of the leptin receptor usually have little or no increase in arterial pressure despite severe obesity, insulin resistance, and dyslipidemia compared to their lean controls.[10,66]

Similar results have also been found in obese children with leptin gene mutations. For example, Ozata et al.[67] reported that four young patients with homozygous missense mutations of the leptin gene had early onset of morbid obesity but no indication of hypertension. Each of these children also had impaired SNS activity, postural hypotension, and attenuated RAAS responses to upright posture.[67] Moreover, the absence of hypertension occurred in spite of severe insulin resistance, hyperinsulinemia, and most other characteristics of the metabolic syndrome. These observations are consistent with those in leptin-deficient mice and suggest that the functional effects of leptin may be important in linking obesity with SNS activation and hypertension.

Leptin's stimulatory effect on SNS activity and blood pressure appear to be mediated mainly by activation of the hypothalamic pro-opiomelanocortin (POMC) pathway (Figure 38–6). Humans with POMC or melanocortin 4-receptor (MC4-R) mutations have early onset of morbid obesity and metabolic disorders similar to those observed in patients with leptin gene mutations. Chronic blockade

of the melanocortin 3/4 receptor (MC3/4-R) in rats also causes rapid weight gain, insulin resistance, and large increases in plasma leptin but no increase in arterial pressure and a decrease in heart rate.[69] As weight gain and hyperleptinemia usually raise blood pressure and heart rate, the possibility arises that a functional MC3/4-R is important in linking excess weight gain with increased SNS activity and hypertension. Moreover, antagonism of the MC3/4-R completely abolished leptin's acute effects on renal SNS activity[68] as well as the chronic hypertensive effects of leptin.[70]

The effects of leptin-POMC neuronal activation appear to be mediated mainly by the MC4-R, rather than the MC3-R, in that the chronic hypertensive effects of leptin are completely abolished in MC4-R knockout mice.[71] Although the importance of the POMC pathway and MC3/4-R in controlling appetite is well established their roles in regulating SNS activity and raising blood pressure in obese humans have to our knowledge not been investigated.

RENIN-ANGIOTENSIN-ALDOSTERONE SYSTEM ACTIVATION IN OBESITY

Obese subjects (especially those with visceral obesity) often have mild to moderate increases in plasma renin activity (PRA), angiotensinogen, angiotensin-converting enzyme (ACE) activity, Ang II, and aldosterone levels.[10,57,72] Activation of the RAAS in obese subjects occurs in spite of marked sodium retention, extracellular volume expansion, and hypertension—all of which would normally tend to suppress renin secretion, Ang II formation, and aldosterone secretion. Moreover, weight loss is usually associated with reductions in plasma renin activity and aldosterone.[57,73]

Potential mechanisms for increased renin secretion and Ang II formation include (1) increased loop of Henle sodium chloride reabsorption and reduced sodium chloride delivery to the macula densa and (2) activation of the renal sympathetic nerves. Increased angiotensinogen formation by adipose tissue has also been suggested to contribute to elevated Ang II levels in obesity,[72] although the importance of this pathway is still unclear. Regardless of the precise mechanisms involved, RAAS system activation appears to contribute to elevated blood pressure in obese subjects.

Role of Ang II in obesity hypertension

A significant role for Ang II in stimulating sodium reabsorption, impairing renal-pressure natriuresis, and mediating hypertension in obesity is supported by the finding that Ang II receptor blockade (ARB) or ACE inhibition blunts sodium retention, volume expansion, and increased arterial pressure in obese dogs.[74,75] ARB also reduced blood pressure to a greater extent in obese-prone compared to obese-resistant rats fed a high-fat diet.[76] In obese Zucker rats, there is increased sensitivity to the blood pressure effects of Ang II because RAAS blockade lowers blood pressure to a greater extent than in lean rats despite comparable (or perhaps even lower) PRA.[77]

Whether the effects of Ang II to raise blood pressure in obesity are due primarily to direct actions on the kidneys, to stimulation of aldosterone secretion, or to SNS activation is unclear. The direct renal sodium-retaining effects of Ang II are well known, as are the direct effects of Ang II to stimulate aldosterone secretion and to increase SNS activity in some conditions.[78]

Unfortunately, there have been no large-scale clinical studies comparing the effectiveness of RAS blockers in obese and lean hypertensive patients although smaller clinical trials have shown that both ARBs and ACE inhibitors are effective in lowering blood pressure in obese hypertensive patients, as discussed later in the chapter. Retrospective analysis of the Antihypertensive Lipid Lowering Heart Attack Trial (ALLHAT) data should also provide some useful information because there were many overweight and obese subjects in this trial and an ACE inhibitor was compared to other types of antihypertensive therapy.[79]

Activation of the RAAS may also contribute to the glomerular injury and nephron loss associated with obesity. By constricting efferent arterioles, increased Ang II formation exacerbates the rise in glomerular hydrostatic pressure caused by systemic arterial hypertension.[78] Studies in type 2 diabetic patients, who are usually over-weight or obese, clearly indicate that ACE inhibitors or ARB slow the progression of renal disease.[80–82] However, further studies are needed in nondiabetic obese subjects to determine the efficacy of RAAS blockers compared to other antihypertensive agents in treating hypertension and reducing the risk of renal injury.

Role of aldosterone and mineralocorticoid receptor activation in obesity hypertension

Studies in experimental animals and in humans have provided evidence that antagonism of mineralocorticoid receptors (MRs) may provide an important therapeutic tool not only for lowering blood pressure but for attenuating target organ injury in hypertension.[83,84] Antagonism of MRs in obese dogs markedly attenuated sodium retention, hypertension, and glomerular hyperfiltration (Figure 38–7).[85] Moreover, this protection against sodium retention and hypertension occurred despite marked increases in PRA, suggesting that combined blockade of MR and Ang II might be especially effective in preventing obesity-induced sodium retention and hypertension. The observation that MR antagonism attenuated glomerular hyperfiltration may have important implications for renal protection in obesity, although there are to our knowledge no studies that have tested this directly in obese humans.

There are few clinical studies that have tested the role of MR activation in obesity hypertension. Administration of the MR antagonist spironolactone, however, appears to provide significant antihypertensive benefit in resistant obese patients.[86] The reductions in blood pressure during MR antagonist occurred despite concurrent therapy with an ACE inhibitor or ARB, calcium channel blocker, and thiazide diuretic.[86] The observation that MR blockade lowered blood pressure when added to ACE inhibitors or ARB suggests that activation of the MR in obesity can occur independently of Ang-II-mediated stimulation of aldosterone secretion.

One question that emerges from these studies is why MR blockade is so effective in lowering blood pressure and altering renal function in obesity hypertension despite only mild increases, or even slight decreases (e.g., after administration of ACE inhibitors or ARB), in plasma aldosterone. One possible explanation is that enhanced sensitivity to the effects of aldosterone-mediated MR activation increases renal sodium reabsorption. For example, obesity-induced increases in the abundance of epithelial sodium channels (ENaCs), which limit the rate of sodium transport across the apical membrane of aldosterone-sensitive renal tubule epithelial cells, would tend to amplify the effects of MR activation to increase renal sodium reabsorption and blood pressure. Although increased abundance of the β subunit of ENaC in the renal cortex of obese Zucker rats[87] has been reported, it is unclear whether there is concomitant increase in the expression of the other subunits necessary to form functional ENaCs or whether such an increase plays a significant role in obesity hypertension.

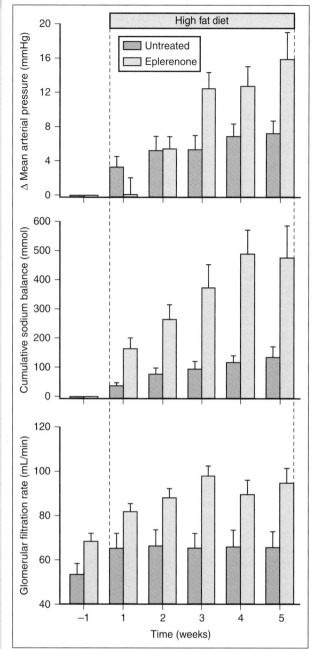

Figure 38–7. Changes (Δ) in mean arterial pressure (mmHg), cumulative sodium balance (mmol), and glomerular filtration rate (mL/min) in control, untreated dogs, and mineralocorticoid receptor antagonist (eplerenone) treated (10 mg/kg, twice daily) dogs fed a high-fat diet for five weeks to develop obesity. (Redrawn from data in reference 85.)

Do glucocorticoids activate the MR in obesity hypertension?

Another potential explanation for the marked effects of MR blockade to reduce blood pressure, despite normal or even reduced plasma aldosterone, is that the MR is activated by glucocorticoids in obesity hypertension. Normally, the renal tubular MR is "protected" from activation by glucocorticoids due to the action of 11β-hydroxysteroid dehydrogenase 2 (11β-HSD2), which converts active cortisol into inactive cortisone (see

Chapter 68). Deficient 11βHSD2 in the renal tubules leads to excessive activation of the MR by cortisol, causing sodium retention, hypokalemia, and hypertension[88] as occurs in the monogenic form of hypertension "apparent mineralocorticoid excess." Although some experimental models of hypertension (including the Dahl salt-sensitive rat) have reduced expression of 11β-HSD2 in the kidney, there are, to our knowledge, no studies that have assessed this mechanism in human obesity hypertension.

Obesity may also increase tissue levels of active glucocorticoids. Visceral obesity may be associated with increased adipocyte expression of 11β-HSD1, which converts inactive cortisone to active cortisol, and some investigators have suggested that central obesity may reflect "Cushing's disease of the omentum."[89] Support for the possibility that excess tissue 11β-HSD1 promotes hypertension comes from studies in transgenic mice that produce large amounts of 11β-HSD1 in adipocytes. When 11β-HSD1 cDNA was linked to the adipocyte fatty-acid-binding protein promoter, a sevenfold amplification of 11β-HSD1 occurred, leading to a phenotype of visceral obesity, insulin resistance, and hypertension.[90] However, the significance of these findings for understanding human obesity hypertension is unclear because other investigators have reported no change or even reduced adipose tissue 11β-HSD1 in obese compared to lean subjects.[88] Thus, the mechanisms responsible for the potent effects of MR blockade to reduce blood pressure in obesity hypertension are still unclear and await further investigation.

RENAL COMPRESSION CAUSED BY VISCERAL OBESITY

Visceral obesity initiates several changes that may lead to compression of the kidneys, increased intrarenal pressures, impaired pressure natriuresis, and hypertension.[10,11] For example, intra-abdominal pressure rises in proportion to sagittal abdominal diameter, reaching levels as high as 35 to 40 mmHg in some subjects.[91] In addition, retroperitoneal adipose tissue often encapsulates the kidneys and penetrates the renal hilum into the renal medullary sinuses, causing additional compression and increased intrarenal pressures.[10,11]

Obesity also causes increased formation of renal medullary extracellular matrix that could contribute to intrarenal compression and sodium retention.[10,11] Total glycosaminoglycan content and tissue hyaluronan, a major component of the renal medullary extracellular matrix, are markedly elevated in the inner medullae of obese dogs and rabbits compared with their lean controls (but not in the outer medulla or the cortex).[92,93] Although the cause of increased hyaluronan in the renal medulla is unknown, its accumulation is usually associated with increased interstitial fluid pressure, tissue edema, and inflammation.

Because the kidney is surrounded by a capsule with low compliance, increased extracellular matrix would raise interstitial fluid hydrostatic and solid tissue pressures and cause compression of the delicate loops of Henle and vasa recta. In support of this hypothesis, renal interstitial fluid hydrostatic pressure was elevated to 19 mmHg in obese dogs compared to only 9 to 10 mmHg in lean dogs.[94] Although small increases in interstitial fluid pressure may inhibit renal sodium reabsorption, large increases of the magnitude found in obese dogs would tend to reduce renal medullary blood flow, slow the flow rate in the renal tubules, and raise fractional sodium reabsorption, especially in the loop of Henle.[94]

Increased loop of Henle sodium chloride reabsorption caused by renal medullary compression could explain the renal vasodilation, glomerular hyperfiltration, and stimulation of renin secretion in obesity (Figure 38–8). Increased sodium chloride reabsorption in the loop of Henle would decrease sodium chloride delivery to the macula densa and cause (via tubuloglomerular feedback) reductions in afferent arteriolar resistance and increases in renal blood flow, GFR, and renin secretion.[78]

The increased GFR and elevated blood pressure would tend to return distal sodium chloride delivery toward normal in the face of increased loop reabsorption, and therefore help to restore sodium balance. Although these physical changes in the kidneys cannot account for the initial increase in arterial pressure that occurs with rapid weight gain, they may help explain why abdominal obesity is much more closely associated with hypertension than with lower body obesity.

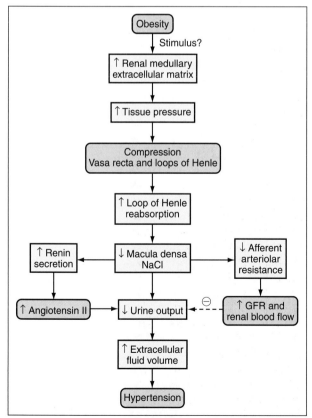

Figure 38–8. Possible mechanisms by which obesity-induced renal medullary compression may contribute to activation of the renin-angiotensin system, increased loop of Henle sodium reabsorption, volume expansion, and hypertension.

OBESITY AND TARGET ORGAN INJURY

Adipose tissue as source of inflammatory cytokines and hormones

Adipose tissue is believed to be a source of inflammatory cytokines such as TNF-α, interleukin-6 (IL-6), and C-reactive protein (CRP), and obesity has been suggested to be a state of low-grade inflammation.[95,96] Visceral fat is estimated to produce about three times more IL-6 than subcutaneous adipose tissue.[97] Although adipocytes themselves secrete IL-6, this accounts for only 10% of the total adipose tissue IL-6 production. Much of the IL-6 and TNF-α produced by adipose tissue appears to come from other cell types associated with adipocytes, including immune cells, monocytes, and fibroblasts.[97,98]

Adipose tissue also secretes non-cytokine substances that may increase cardiovascular risk[96,98] (Figure 38–9). For example, some studies suggest that adipose tissue hosts all of the components of the RAAS and secretes Ang II.[99] Adipose angiotensinogen mRNA expression may be higher in visceral than in subcutaneous adipose tissue, and weight loss reduces angiotensinogen in adipose tissue of obese humans.[99] However, the physiologic significance of the adipocyte RAAS and the mechanisms controlling its activity are still uncertain.

Although it is clear that adipocytes release many cytokines ("adipokines" or "adipocytokines") and hormones that are potential mediators of inflammation, direct cause-and-effect relationships for hypertension or target organ injury have not been well established for most of these factors. It is not known, for example, whether chronic treatment with aspirin or other nonsteroidal anti-inflammatory drugs reduces the level of inflammatory cytokines and cardiovascular disease in obese patients.

The picture is further complicated by the observation that visceral fat (rather than subcutaneous fat) confers

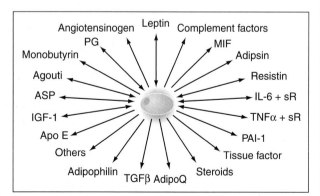

Figure 38–9. Hormones and cytokines ("adipokines") released from white adipose tissue. (Abbreviations: PG, prostaglandin; ASP, acylation-stimulating protein; IGF-1, insulin-like growth factor 1; apoE, apolipoprotein E; TGF-β, transforming growth factor-β; adipoQ, adipocyte complement-related protein of 30 kDa, also called Acrp30; PAI-1, plasminogen activator inhibitor-1; TNF-α, tumor necrosis factor-α; sR, soluble receptors; IL-6, interleukin-6; and MIF, macrophage migrating inhibitory factor.) (Redrawn from reference 98.)

most of the risk for cardiovascular and metabolic disorders associated with obesity even though subcutaneous fat also secretes many of the adipokines that have been hypothesized to cause inflammation, hypertension, and increased cardiovascular disease. Defining the importance of the many substances released by adipose tissue in cardiovascular regulation and in mediating target organ injury awaits further investigation.

Endothelial dysfunction, vascular stiffening, and injury of blood vessels

As discussed earlier in this chapter, obesity is associated with elevated resting blood flows in many tissues prior to the development of vascular damage. However, blood flow reserve during exercise or reactive hyperemia is reduced in obesity. For example, the reactive hyperemia and maximum blood flow observed after temporary occlusion of the brachial artery is reduced in obese compared to lean subjects.[100] This impaired flow reserve appears to be due in part to endothelial dysfunction. Obesity is associated with impaired endothelial-mediated vasodilation,[101] and weight reduction improves flow-mediated vasodilation in obese individuals.[102]

Accelerated arterial stiffening occurs in elderly, middle-aged, and even in young adults (20 to 40 years of age) who have excess adiposity as estimated by increased BMI, abdominal visceral fat, larger waist circumference, and increased waist/hip ratio.[103] Moreover, higher aortic pulse-wave velocity (a measure of aortic stiffness) strongly correlates with increases in BMI, waist circumference, and waist/hip ratio independent of systolic blood pressure, race, and sex.[103] Important effects of excess weight gain to impair vascular function may be apparent even in children.[104]

The mechanisms responsible for the deleterious effects of obesity on the vasculature are still poorly understood but are likely due to interactions of multiple disorders, including increased blood pressure, inflammation, hyperglycemia, lipotoxicity caused by excessive non-β-oxidative metabolism of fatty acids, oxidative stress, and activation of multiple neurohumoral systems. As discussed previously, there is evidence that excess visceral adipose tissue itself is an important source of cytokines and other factors that create a vascular milieu of inflammation and oxidative stress and that contribute to endothelial dysfunction, vascular stiffening, and eventually atherosclerosis.[105]

Even short-term increases in free fatty acid levels may impair endothelial-dependent vasodilation. For example, infusion of a mixture of several fatty acids for only two hours impaired the vasodilator response to methacholine chloride, an endothelial dependent vasodilator.[106] The mechanism for this effect is unclear, but may be related to a reduction in the cytosolic free coenzyme A (CoA) pool due to acylation of CoA by the increased free fatty acid.[106] Thus, infusion of carnitine (which plays a pivotal role in the metabolism of fatty acids by transporting activated acyl groups across membranes and buffering intracellular acyl-CoA pools) almost completely reversed the impairment of endothelial-dependent vasodilation caused by infusion of a mixture of fatty acids.[106]

With chronic increases in tissue fatty acid levels, accumulation of fatty acid metabolites (including acyl-CoA and ceramide) may in the tissues have deleterious effects such as increased formation of reactive oxygen species, endothelial dysfunction, and cell death.[107] However, the precise cellular pathways by which tissue accumulation of fatty acids causes endothelial dysfunction and tissue injury are still unclear and represent an important area for future investigation.

When obesity is sustained over many years and is associated with hypertension, glucose intolerance, and dyslipidemia, the vascular dysfunction becomes progressively worse and eventually manifests as atherosclerosis and injury to various organs throughout the body including the heart, brain, and kidneys. It is important to remember that obesity, especially when associated with increased visceral adiposity, is the main cause of the entire cascade of events that often culminates in vascular disease and target organ injury.

These risk factors for vascular disease interact in a manner that is more than additive. In the Prospective Cardiovascular Munster (PROCAM) study, for example, the risk for myocardial infarction was increased about twofold by hypertension and twofold by diabetes. When hypertension and diabetes occurred together, the risk was increased more than eightfold (Figure 38–10).[108] When hypertension, diabetes, and hyperlipidemia were all present (as occurs in many obese patients), the risk for myocardial infarction was increased almost twentyfold.[108]

Obesity is major risk factor for chronic renal disease

Obesity is not included as a cause of kidney failure in renal data registries, and has therefore not been widely recognized as a major risk factor for ESRD. However, the impact of obesity on renal disease is obvious considering

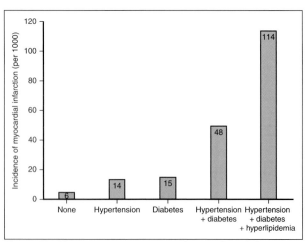

Figure 38–10. Interaction among cardiovascular risk factors in the Prospective Cardiovascular Munster (PROCAM) study. The incidence of myocardial infarction is shown in a group of 2,574 men with (1) no risk factors, (2) hypertension only, (3) diabetes only, (4) hypertension and diabetes, or (5) hypertension plus diabetes and hyperlipidemia. (Redrawn from data in reference 108.)

that diabetes and hypertension (both of which are closely associated with excess weight gain) account for more than 70% of ESRD. Moreover, the rapid rise in the prevalence of ESRD in the past two decades has paralleled increasing obesity and diabetes.[109] Most of the increasing prevalence of ESRD has been attributed to the increase in type 2 diabetes, although patients with type 2 diabetes are usually hypertensive and the increased blood pressure likely contributes to renal injury.

Population studies suggest that obesity is an important cause of renal disease even after adjustment for hypertension, diabetes, or preexisting renal disease.[110,111] In the Framingham Offspring cohort,[110] increased BMI was positively related to a low GFR in the fifth or lower percentile (≤59.25 mL/min per 1.73 m² in women, ≤64.25 mL/min per 1.73 m² in men) after long-term follow-up. In a retrospective analysis of 320,252 adults who were followed for 15 to 35 years, the rate of ESRD increased in a stepwise manner as BMI increased[111] (Figure 38–11). This relationship was not affected by blood pressure levels or diabetes, and the analysis was adjusted for age, sex, race, education level, smoking status, history of myocardial infarction, serum cholesterol level, proteinuria, hematuria, and serum creatinine level. Thus, observational studies suggest that obesity may be an important risk factor for renal disease through mechanisms other than hypertension and diabetes.

Obesity exacerbates development of nondiabetic renal diseases

Obesity also amplifies the effects of other primary renal insults, even those that are usually considered to be relatively benign, such as unilateral nephrectomy.[112] Retrospective analysis of patients who underwent unilateral nephrectomy (13.6 ±8.6 years previously) revealed that 62% of those with a BMI >30 developed proteinuria or renal insufficiency, whereas only 12% with a BMI <30 developed these disorders[112] (Figure 38–12).

Patients with immunoglobulin A (IgA) nephropathy and who were overweight (BMI >25) at the time of renal biopsy had more severe renal lesions and increased proteinuria (as well as a much faster decline of renal function and progression to chronic renal failure) compared to patients with IgA nephropathy and a BMI <25.[113] Moreover, moderate weight loss in overweight patients with chronic nondiabetic proteinuric nephropathies markedly reduced proteinuria, whereas in overweight subjects who did not lose weight renal function worsened with time.[114] These observations suggest that obesity greatly exacerbates the loss of renal function in patients with preexisting glomerulopathies, and that weight loss may lessen the impact of renal injury from other causes.

Early structural and functional renal changes in obese subjects

Even when there is no evidence of preexisting renal disease, excess weight gain causes early structural and functional changes in the kidneys that may eventually lead to more serious renal disorders. For example, structural changes in the kidneys were observed in dogs placed on a high-fat diet for only seven to nine weeks.[115] These changes included enlargement of Bowman's space, increased glomerular cell proliferation, increased mesangial matrix, thicker basement membranes, and increased expression of glomerular-transforming growth factor β.[115] Moreover, these early renal changes occurred with only modest hypertension, no evidence of diabetes, and only mild metabolic abnormalities.[115]

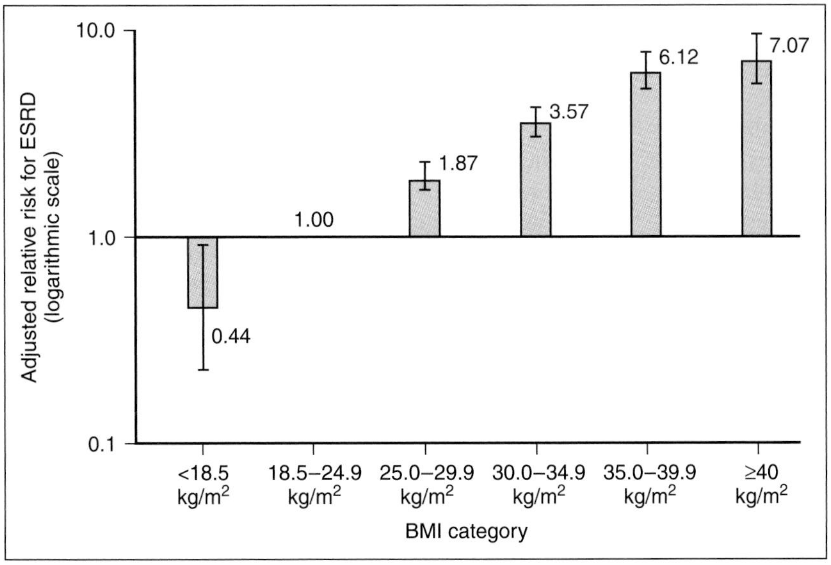

Obese humans often develop proteinuria, frequently in the nephrotic range, that may be followed by progressive loss of kidney function even in the absence of diabetes or severe hypertension.[114] The most common types of renal lesions observed in renal biopsies of obese subjects are focal and segmental glomerulosclerosis and glomerulomegaly.[116] A review of 6,818 biopsies indicated that the incidence of obesity-related glomerulopathy, defined as combined focal glomerulosclerosis and glomerulomegaly, rose tenfold from 1990 to 2000, coincident with the rapid increase in the prevalence of obesity during this period.[116]

The mechanisms of obesity-induced renal injury are not fully understood but likely involve a combination of hemodynamic and metabolic abnormalities. As discussed previously, obesity causes marked glomerular hyperfiltration and preglomerular

Figure 38–11. Adjusted relative risk for ESRD by BMI. In this retrospective cohort study of 320,252 adults followed for 15 to 35 years, the rate of ESRD increased in a stepwise manner as BMI increased. This relationship was not affected by blood pressure levels or diabetes. The model was adjusted for age, sex, race, education level, smoking status, history of myocardial infarction, serum cholesterol level, proteinuria, hematuria, and serum creatinine level (Redrawn from data in reference 111).

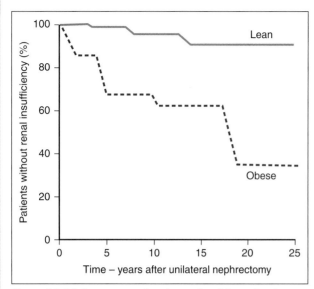

Figure 38–12. Percentage of patients who did not develop renal insufficiency after unilateral nephrectomy and who were lean (BMI <25, solid line) or obese (BMI >30, dashed line) at the time of unilateral nephrectomy. (Redrawn from data in reference 112.)

vasodilation that permit greater transmission of the increased arterial pressure to the glomerular capillaries.[117] These renal hemodynamic changes, along with metabolic abnormalities (such as hyperglycemia and hyperlipidemia) exacerbate the effects of increases in arterial pressure to cause renal injury. A synergistic relationship may exist between metabolic abnormalities and increased glomerular pressure in causing chronic renal vascular disease and nephron loss, similar to the synergistic effects of hypertension, diabetes, and dyslipidemia in increasing the risk for coronary artery disease and myocardial infarction.[108] However, there are no large-scale studies that have tested this idea.

Caloric restriction and weight loss may prevent or attenuate renal disease

There is compelling evidence in rodents that excess caloric intake causes progressive nephron loss and that caloric restriction protects against glomerular injury. Modest food restriction (8 to 18% below the usual *ad lib* amounts) in the obese Zucker rat, for instance, reduces renal injury and increases life span by approximately 30%.[118] Similar beneficial effects of food restriction have been observed in other models of obese and nonobese rodents, indicating that food restriction can largely prevent chronic renal disease in rats.

Short-term weight loss also reduces proteinuria in non-diabetic obese humans, even in overweight subjects with nephropathies caused by factors other than obesity.[114] The renal benefits of weight loss are evident regardless of whether they are induced by diet and exercise or by surgical methods (e.g., gastroplasty), although there have been no large studies directly comparing the effectiveness of different methods of weight loss on progression of renal dysfunction. Most of these studies have lasted only a few weeks or months.

Studies lasting for at least a year, however, have shown remarkable reductions in proteinuria (>80%) with a weight loss of about 12%.[119] Although the long-term consequences of weight loss in protecting against renal disease have not been rigorously tested in humans, there is little doubt that weight loss reduces hypertension and prevents or reverses the development of type 2 diabetes, the two main risk factors for development of ESRD.

Obesity causes of cardiac hypertrophy/ remodeling, impaired systolic and diastolic function, and increased risk for heart failure

Obesity is associated with eccentric and concentric cardiac hypertrophy.[120,121] Moreover, cardiac hypertrophy is more severe in obese than in lean subjects with comparable hypertension.[122] Because blood volume and venous return are increased, there is increased preload, cardiac dilation, and development of eccentric left ventricular hypertrophy in obese subjects. The rise in blood pressure also increases cardiac afterload, leading to increased left ventricular wall thickness. Thus, when obesity is combined with increased blood pressure cardiac workload is greatly amplified and marked left ventricular hypertrophy occurs. High sodium chloride intake often occurs concurrently with high caloric intake and exacerbates obesity-induced cardiac hypertrophy, even when the high-salt diet does not raise arterial pressure.[123]

Functional changes in the heart occur rapidly after excess weight gain. For example, in rabbits fed a high-fat diet for 12 weeks cardiac filling pressures were increased and diastolic dysfunction (associated with decreased left ventricular compliance) was evident even at this early stage of obesity.[124] Although left ventricular filling pressure in obese subjects may be within the upper limits of normal at rest, it increases disproportionately with increased venous return during exercise (often exceeding 20 mmHg). With longer durations of obesity, greater impairment of left ventricular diastolic function occurs and left ventricular systolic dysfunction may develop.[125]

The mechanisms responsible for cardiac diastolic and systolic dysfunction in obesity are not well understood but probably involve structural changes in the heart, such as increased TGF-β expression, fibrosis, and functional changes such as impaired β-adrenergic receptor signaling.[126,127] There may also be increases in intramyocellular lipids that lead to increased formation of reactive oxygen species, myocardial cell dysfunction, and apoptosis, a phenomenon known as "lipotoxicity."[128]

Although extreme obesity is widely recognized as a risk factor for heart failure, there is also evidence that overweight and lesser degrees of obesity pose a risk. For example, data from the Framingham study indicate that in obese subjects (BMI >30) the risk of heart failure was double that of subjects with a normal body-mass index.[129] A graded increase in the risk of heart failure was observed across categories of body-mass index even after adjustment for other established risk factors caused by obesity, such as hypertension and diabetes. These observations suggest that although obesity often accompanies other established heart failure risk factors (e.g., hypertension, left ventricular hypertrophy, and diabetes mellitus) there are other pathways by which excess adiposity may increase the risk of heart failure.

Established risk factors such as increased blood pressure, cardiac hypertrophy, and diabetes clearly play an important role in linking obesity to heart failure. Obesity markedly increases the workload on the heart, with attendant high cardiac output and high blood pressure, and could unmask latent ventricular dysfunction of other etiologies. The RAAS and SNS are activated in obesity, as discussed previously, and increased activity of these systems has been implicated in the pathophysiology of chronic heart failure.

As previously mentioned, lipid accumulation in and around myocytes may also contribute to cardiac cell death and eventually cardiomyopathy.[130] Although adipocytes have the capacity to store large amounts of excess free fatty acids in cytosolic lipid droplets, cells of non-adipose tissues such as the heart have a limited capacity for storage of lipids. When this capacity is exceeded, the excess lipid may lead to cell dysfunction or cell death. In addition, intramyocardial lipid accumulation can occur because of increased blood fatty acid levels and increased cellular uptake (as occurs in obesity) and/or because of mitochondrial dysfunction and decreased oxidation of fatty acids (as occurs in heart failure).

Heart failure patients with severe metabolic dysregulation have marked intramyocardial triglyceride accumulation,[131] and the lipid-overloaded human heart has a transcriptional profile similar to that of animal models of lipotoxicity and contractile dysfunction, suggesting that impaired fatty acid metabolism or excess fatty acid uptake may contribute to cardiac dysfunction.[131] In addition, chronic dependence on mitochondrial fatty acid oxidation for energy production (as occurs in the diabetic heart) may lead to cellular lipotoxicity, mitochondrial dysfunction, and cell death.

The gradual loss of cardiomyocytes may then impair cardiac function and increase the risk of heart failure. Although studies in obese rodents indicate that cardiac steatosis (lipid accumulation) can lead to lipotoxic cardiomyopathy,[128,130] the importance of this mechanism in causing cardiac dysfunction and heart failure in obese humans, and the cellular mechanisms involved, await further investigation.

Hypercoagulation and increased risk for thrombosis in obesity

Increased risk for thrombosis may also contribute to a higher incidence of target organ injury in obesity. Obesity is associated with polycythemia, and there is epidemiologic evidence that hypercoagulation and impaired fibrinolysis activity are related to BMI or waist-to-hip ratio.[132–134] For example, obese patients (especially those with increased visceral fat) have higher plasma concentrations of all pro-thrombotic factors (fibrinogen, von Willebrand factor, and factor VII) compared to nonobese controls.

Plasma concentration of plasminogen activator inhibitor-1 (PAI-1) is also higher in obese patients compared to nonobese controls and is directly correlated with visceral fat. The increased flux of free fatty acids in obesity may promote thrombosis by increasing protein C, PAI-1, and/or platelet aggregation. Adipose tissue production of leptin and other inflammatory mediators has also been suggested to be an important factor in causing increased thrombosis.[134]

TREATMENT OF OBESITY HYPERTENSION

Weight loss and lifestyle modification

Although obesity is rapidly becoming the most important and most prevalent health care problem of the modern world, few effective treatments are available to prevent or treat obesity. For morbidly obese patients (BMI >40) or for patients with a BMI >35 and co-morbid conditions, various surgical procedures (especially gastric bypass surgery) are becoming increasingly popular and usually produce significant weight loss. However, the long-term consequences of these procedures in reversing cardiovascular and renal disease and on overall mortality are still uncertain.

Only two drugs—sibutramine (a sympathomimetic that induces satiety and increases thermogenesis) and orlistat (a gastrointestinal lipase inhibitor)—are currently approved by the Food and Drug Administration (FDA) to promote weight loss. Both of these drugs have significant side effects that limit their use in many patients, and their long-term effects on morbidity and mortality are unknown.

Recently, another anti-obesity drug (rimonabant) has been tested in several clinical trials. Rimonabant, a selective blocker of the cannabinoid receptor type 1 (CB1), has been shown in several large trials to cause significant weight loss and reduction in waist circumference over a one-year period of treatment compared to placebo.[135] Therapy with rimonabant is also associated with favorable changes in serum lipid levels and an improvement in glycemic control in prediabetes patients and in type 2 diabetic patients. However, the long-term (over a period of many years) benefits of rimonabant, as well as other anti-obesity drugs, in maintaining weight loss and in reducing blood pressure and cardiovascular disease are uncertain.

Until more effective and safer pharmacologic treatments are available, voluntary weight loss initiated by lifestyle modification (including increased physical activity) is still the best option for most overweight patients.[136] Several studies have shown that weight loss lowers blood pressures in normotensive or hypertensive obese subjects,[137,138] and may prevent the development of hypertension in persons with "high normal" blood pressures.[137] Even modest (5 to 10%) weight reduction can improve control of blood pressure and reduce the amount of medication necessary to achieve goal blood pressures.[19,139,140] Weight loss is also effective in reducing other risk factors (e.g., blood glucose and lipids) for cardiovascular and renal disease in most hypertensive patients.

Current guidelines for achieving weight loss usually recommend the development of an individualized plan for lifestyle modification as a first step in reducing caloric intake and increase energy expenditure.[136] However, lifestyle modifications alone have not proved successful in producing significant long-term weight loss in most obese patients. One major challenge to successful prevention and treatment of obesity has been the lack of adequate involvement of health care professionals.

Less than half of obese adults report that their physicians advised them to lose weight.[141] On the other hand, patients whose physicians advised them to lose weight were three times more likely to attempt to lose weight as those who received no such advice from their physicians.[142] The successful management of obesity requires the same attention and planning for effective treatment as other important chronic medical conditions, such as hypertension.

Drug therapy of hypertension in obese patients

Until effective strategies for preventing and treating obesity are developed, the therapeutic strategy for managing most obese patients will continue to be aimed at treating the cardiovascular, metabolic, and renal consequences of obesity. Currently, there are no specific recommendations or treatment algorithms for obesity hypertension. Moreover, there are no specific treatment goals for obese hypertensive patients, although it has been suggested that goals for obesity hypertension should be similar to those recommended for other high-risk patients (e.g., diabetes, <130/80 mm Hg).[143] Other chapters in this book are devoted to drug therapy of hypertension and we will therefore provide only a brief summary of special considerations for the obese hypertensive patient.

Selection of specific drugs for antihypertensive therapy in obese subjects is often empiric or based on clinical experience and knowledge of the physiology of obesity hypertension.[144] The potential advantages and disadvantages of different antihypertensive drugs in obese patients have been previously reviewed and some of these are outlined in Table 38–3.[144,145] However, there have been no large clinical trials that have tested the effectiveness of different drugs in reducing blood pressure and in preventing cardiovascular and renal disease in obese compared with lean subjects.

The Antihypertensive Therapy and Lipid-Lowering Heart Attack Trial (ALLHAT), however, included many overweight subjects and provides useful information about the relative effectiveness of the four main classes of antihypertensive drugs tested: diuretics, β-adrenergic blockers, ACE inhibitors, and calcium antagonists.[146] In addition, some inferences may be drawn from randomized controlled clinical trials of drug therapy in essential hypertension patients because most of these trials have included many subjects who were overweight or obese.

Optimal blood pressure control

For many obese patients, the coexistence of additional risk factors such as hyperlipidemia, glucose intolerance or diabetes, and atherosclerosis strongly suggests that goal blood pressures should be lower than in lean hypertensive patients who do not have these risk factors. For patients with renal disease or diabetes, the blood pressure goal is <130/80 mmHg. Although overweight and obese individuals have increased risk for renal disease and diabetes, there have been no clinical trials assessing optimal blood pressure in obesity hypertension.

Recent recommendations stress that optimal blood pressure is <120/80 mmHg for all individuals, and this seems especially appropriate for obese hypertensive patients with multiple metabolic abnormalities. Because hypertension may be more difficult to control in obese subjects, combination drug therapy is often required to achieve goal blood pressures. As discussed previously,

ANTIHYPERTENSIVE THERAPY IN OBESITY HYPERTENSION: POTENTIAL BENEFITS AND ADVERSE EFFECTS		
Drug Class	**Potential Benefits**	**Potential Adverse Effects**
Diuretics	• Diuresis • Natriuresis	• ↓ Insulin sensitivity • ↑ LDL, triglycerides
Alpha blockers	• ↓ Total cholesterol • ↑ Insulin sensitivity • Vasodilation	• Orthostasis
ACE inhibitors	• ↑ Insulin sensitivity	• Cough
ARB	• ↓ Aldosterone • Natriuresis • ↑ Insulin sensitivity • ↓ Liver steatosis	• Angioedema
Beta blockers	• ↓ Heart rate • ↓ Renin release	• ↓ Insulin sensitivity • ↑ Triglycerides
Calcium channel blockers	• Natriuresis • Vasodilation	• Edema
Centrally acting sympatholytic agents	• ↓ Sympathetic activity	• Fatigue • Sedation • ↓ Fatty acid metabolism

Table 38–3. Antihypertensive Therapy in Obesity Hypertension: Potential Benefits and Adverse Effects

weight loss substantially reduces the number of medications needed to control blood pressure.

Diuretics

Because of their ability to reduce renal sodium and water reabsorption and decrease extracellular fluid volume, diuretics are useful in lowering blood pressure in many obese hypertensive patients.[147] Some clinicians prefer diuretics in obese patients because of the strong evidence from randomized controlled clinical trials indicating that reducing blood pressure with diuretics lowers cardiovascular morbidity and mortality.[21] However, because obese patients often have glucose intolerance and dyslipidemia some clinicians avoid diuretics, if possible, to prevent worsening these metabolic abnormalities.[148]

Although studies using high doses of diuretics have demonstrated significant adverse metabolic effects (e.g., increases in insulin resistance and plasma lipids), low doses of diuretics are less frequently associated with these effects, and, when used in combination with other agents, can be very useful in treating obesity hypertension.[21] However, because most clinical trials have been conducted over a relatively short period of time (five years or less) the overall impact of the potential adverse metabolic effects of diuretics in obese patients is still uncertain.

Beta-adrenergic blockers

In obese patients, β-blockers may be useful in counteracting some effects of obesity-induced sympathetic activation, such as stimulation of renin secretion. β-blockers are also especially beneficial in patients after myocardial infarction, and studies have demonstrated that these drugs decrease morbidity and mortality in diabetic patients (most of whom are overweight or obese).[149] However, β-blockers may make it more difficult for obese patients to lose weight. In addition, in some studies β-blockers are associated with worsening glucose control, higher lipid levels, and increased body weight.[144] Thus, although β-blockers may be indicated in obese hypertensive patients with ischemic heart disease and/or arrhythmias other drugs may be preferable for initial therapy in those who have no evidence of heart disease.

Angiotensin-converting enzyme (ACE) inhibitors

ACE inhibitors are useful in treating obesity hypertension. In a 12-week multicenter double-blind trial in which 77 obese patients were treated with lisinopril, 76 with hydrochlorothiazide (HCTZ), and 79 with placebo, findings suggested that ACE inhibition is effective in reducing blood pressure, particularly in young white patients, and may offer some advantages in patients with high risk of metabolic disorders.[150] The ability of ACE inhibitors to attenuate glomerular hyperfiltration and urinary protein excretion provides an advantage in managing blood pressure in obese patients prone to renal disease. Improved insulin sensitivity associated with ACE inhibitors is another advantage of these drugs.

One of the few randomized controlled trials in obese hypertensive patients included an ACE inhibitor. The Treatment of Obese Patients with Hypertension (TROPHY) study compared the blood pressure responses to the ACE inhibitor lisinopril and to the diuretic HCTZ in obese hypertensives.[150] Both agents effectively lowered systolic and diastolic blood pressure after 12 weeks of therapy. African Americans and older participants were more likely to respond favorably to the diuretic, whereas Caucasian and younger participants were more likely to respond to the ACE inhibitor.[150]

Studies in patients with hypertension and/or congestive heart failure have demonstrated that responses to ACE inhibitors depend on sodium intake and volume status. With high sodium intake, the effectiveness of ACE inhibitors is diminished. However, when these drugs are used in combination with diuretics they are effective even in patients who do not have elevated PRA.[21]

Angiotensin II receptor blockers (ARBs)

The effectiveness of ARBs has not been well characterized in obese hypertensive patients. In a study of 68 obese hypertensive patients treated with the ARB candesartan and 59 obese hypertensive patients treated with HCTZ, the ARB was found to have an antihypertensive effect similar to that of HCTZ.[151] Unlike diuretic treatment, however, ARB improved insulin sensitivity and appeared to exert a sympathoinhibitory effect in obese hypertensive patients.

Some ARBs are partial agonists for peroxisome proliferator activator receptor-gamma (PPARγ) and have been shown in rodents to reduce visceral fat accumulation and liver steatosis.[152] However, metabolic improvements, including increased insulin sensitivity, reduction in adipocyte cell size, and a trend toward reduction in intramyocellular lipids have also been reported with ACE inhibition in rodent models,[153] making it unclear whether the beneficial metabolic effects of ARBs are due to PPARγ activation or to Ang II blockade. Although these effects could be beneficial in obese patients, additional studies in obese hypertensive humans are needed.

Studies in patients with essential hypertension suggest that ARBs have blood-pressure-lowering effects very similar to those of ACE inhibitors.[21] There are some differences between these two drug classes (e.g., the effect of ACE inhibitors to increase kinin levels) that may be responsible for subtle differences in the incidence of complications such as angioedema and cough. It is likely that obese patients would have similar blood pressure responses to ACE inhibitors and ARB, although this has not, to our knowledge, been tested in a major clinical trial.

Extensive trials have been completed in hypertensive patients, including those with diabetes, to examine the effects of ARBs on cardiovascular morbidity and mortality and on progression of renal disease. Two different ARBs were demonstrated to prevent or decrease proteinuria in hypertensive patients with type 2 diabetes mellitus.[81,82,154] Thus, ARBs may be especially useful in obese patients with renal disease.

α1-adrenergic blocking agents

Results of ALLHAT suggest that α-adrenergic blockers as monotherapy are not as effective as thiazide diuretics in preventing heart failure and cardiovascular disease. Therefore, these drugs will likely be used less as monotherapy for patients with essential hypertension, including those who are obese. Because they lower plasma lipids, they may continue to play a role in combination therapy for managing obese hypertensive patients with dyslipidemia.[156] They may also be useful as part of a combination of medications in many patients with resistant hypertension, which is common in obese patients.[57,144]

Calcium channel blockers

These drugs are frequently used to treat obese hypertensive patients. Their effectiveness does not seem to depend much on sodium intake, the RAAS, or SNS activity. Because calcium channel blockers are effective in a broad range of hypertensive patients, including obese subjects, they have been widely used.[21] However, some studies suggest that calcium channel blockers are less effective in obese than in lean hypertensive patients.[146,157] The dihydropyridine calcium antagonists also have the potential disadvantage of further increasing heart rate in obese patients. The non-dihydropyridine calcium antagonists, in contrast, lower heart rate.[21]

It is obvious that randomized controlled clinical trials measuring morbidity and mortality as well as the physiologic consequences of different treatments would be helpful in guiding drug selection for obese hypertensive patients. In the absence of such trials (which are unlikely to be conducted in the near future), clinicians will need to make decisions based on their understanding of the pathophysiology of obesity hypertension and the characteristics of the individual patient. The overall therapeutic goal is, of course, to reduce morbidity and mortality by selecting pharmacologic therapy appropriate to control blood pressure, attenuate the development of cardiovascular and renal disease, and effectively treat the metabolic disorders associated with obesity.

Obstructive sleep apnea

Obstructive sleep apnea (OSA) is considered a cause of secondary hypertension but is usually associated closely with obesity.[49] Sleep apnea can exacerbate underlying disease or cause problems for those who are otherwise healthy. Although very common in obese subjects, this life-threatening disorder is often overlooked in the assessment and treatment of hypertensive patients. The association between sleep-disordered breathing and hypertension is seen in all gender, ethnic, and age groups.[158]

In the Wisconsin Sleep Cohort study, an independent relationship between sleep-disordered breathing and incident hypertension was seen in a four-year follow-up.[159] Individuals with mild to moderate OSA had a 42% greater chance of having hypertension than did persons with normal sleep patterns. Those with more severe OSA were two to three times more likely to develop hypertension compared to those without evidence of OSA.[160] Thus, there is a clear association between the severity of OSA and hypertension. In addition to daytime hypertension, OSA causes nocturnal surges in blood pressure.[49,159,161] OSA also causes pulmonary hypertension, increased sympathetic activity, hypoxia, cardiac arrhythmias (e.g., atrial fibrillation), and sleep disturbance.[161]

Increased sympathetic activity may be a key factor in mediating increased arterial pressure in OSA.[49,161] Impaired endothelial function and decreased release of nitric oxide may also play a role.[162] An understanding of the physiologic changes in OSA that cause hypertension may provide an opportunity to develop noninvasive treatments that improve blood pressure control in obese patients.

All patients with obesity hypertension should be questioned about symptoms of their sleep disturbance, including snoring, choking or gasping during sleep, daytime somnolence, and morning headaches. Treatment of OSA with continuous positive airway pressure (CPAP) decreases daytime and nocturnal blood pressures.[163] Identification of OSA and effective treatment with weight loss, continuous positive airway pressure, or surgical intervention may be necessary to achieve adequate blood pressure control in some obese patients. A reduction in hypertension and cardiovascular events and improvements in quality of life may result from management of this frequently overlooked disorder.

SUMMARY AND PERSPECTIVES

There has been an alarming increase in the prevalence of overweight and obesity in most industrialized countries and even in underdeveloped countries, resulting in a worldwide rise in diabetes mellitus, hypertension, and renal disease. Excess weight gain is the key risk factor for increased blood pressure in most patients with essential hypertension, and also appears to be a major cause of chronic renal disease. Obesity initially raises blood pressure by increasing renal tubular reabsorption, impairing pressure natriuresis, and causing volume expansion. These changes are due to activation of the SNS and RAAS and to physical compression of the kidneys when visceral obesity is present (Figure 38–13).

Sympathetic activation in obesity may in part be mediated by increased levels of leptin, acting via complex

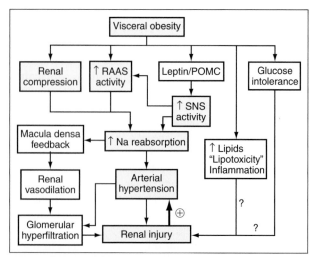

Figure 38–13. Summary of potential mechanisms by which obesity causes hypertension and renal injury.

hypothalamic pathways (especially stimulation of POMC neurons and subsequent activation of MC3/4R). Renal vasodilation, glomerular hyperfiltration, and increased blood pressure initially help to compensate for increased tubular reabsorption in obesity. However, the resultant increases in glomerular hydrostatic pressure and wall stress (along with activation of neurohumoral mechanisms, hyperlipidemia, and hyperglycemia) eventually cause glomerular injury and loss of nephron function. Blockade of the SNS and RAAS are therefore effective in reducing blood pressure in many obese patients. With prolonged obesity, there may be progressive renal dysfunction that worsens the hypertension. In some obese individuals, renal injury may progress to ESRD, especially if other preexisting glomerulopathies are present.

Weight reduction is an essential first step in the management of obesity-associated hypertension and renal disease. There are, however, few drugs available to produce significant long-term weight loss and few guidelines for treating obesity-associated hypertension other than the recommendation of reducing weight. Special considerations for the obese patient, in addition to controlling blood pressure, include correcting the metabolic abnormalities and protecting the kidneys from further injury. More emphasis should be placed on lifestyle modifications that help patients maintain a healthier weight and prevent obesity, and consequently hypertension and associated cardiovascular and renal disease. Efforts to prevent the development of obesity are critically needed in populations throughout the world.

ACKNOWLEDGMENTS

The authors' research was supported by a grant from the National Heart, Lung, and Blood Institute (P01 HL51971) and by the American Heart Association.

REFERENCES

1. World Health Organization. Controlling the obesity epidemic. Available at *http://www.who.int/nutrition/topics/obesity/en/*.

2. Yach D, Stuckler D, Brownell KD. Epidemiologic and economic consequences of the global epidemics of obesity and diabetes. *Nature Medicine* 2006;12:62–66.

3. Wang L, Kong, L, Wu, F, et al. Preventing chronic diseases in China. *Lancet* 2005;366:1821–24.

4. Flegal KM, Carroll MD, Ogden CL, Johnson CCL. Prevalence and trends in obesity among US adults 1999–2000. *JAMA* 2002;288:1723–27.

5. Lobstein T, Bauer L, Uauy R, IASO International Obesity Task Force. Obesity in children and young people: A crisis in public health. *Obes Rev* 2004;5(1):4–85.

6. Ogden CL, Flegal KM, Carroll MD, Johnson CL. Prevalence and trends in overweight among US children and adolescents. *JAMA* 2002;288:1728–32.

7. Sorof J, Daniels S. Obesity hypertension in children: A problem of epidemic proportions. *Hypertension* 2002; 40:441–47.

8. Zimmet P, Alberti KG, Shaw J. Global and societal implications of the diabetes epidemic. *Nature* 2001;414: 782–87.

9. Eckel RH, Krauss RM. American Heart Association call to action: Obesity as a major risk factor for coronary heart disease. *Circulation* 1998;97: 2099–2100.

10. Hall JE, Jones DW, Kuo JJ, et al. Impact of obesity on hypertension and renal disease. *Curr Hypertens Rep* 2003;5:386–92.

11. Hall JE. The kidney, hypertension, and obesity. *Hypertension* 2003; 41:625–33.

12. Hall JE, Henegar JR, Dwyer TM, Liu J, da Silva AA, Kuo JJ, Tallam L. Is obesity a major cause of chronic renal disease? *Advance Renal Replacement Therapy* 2004;11:41–54.

13. Alexander J, Dustan HP, Sims EAH, et al. Report of the Hypertension Task Force, US Department of Health, Education, and Welfare Publication 70-1631 (NIH). Washington, D.C.: U.S. Government Printing Office 1979:61–77.

14. Jones DW, Kim JS, Andrew ME, et al. Body mass index and blood pressures in Korean men and women: The Korean National Blood Pressure Survey. *J Hypertens* 1994;12:1433–37.

15. Garrison RJ, Kannel WB, Stokes J, et al. Incidence and precursors of hypertension in young adults: The Framingham Offspring Study. *Prev Med* 1987;16:234–51.

16. Cooper, RS, Potimi CN, Ward R. The puzzle of hypertension in African-Americans. *Sci Am* 1999;280:56–63.

17. Wannamethee, SG, Shaper GA. Weight change and duration of overweight and obesity in the incidence of type 2 diabetes. *Diabetes Care* 1999;22:1266–72.

18. Reisen E, Abel R, Modan M, et al. Effect of weight loss without salt restriction on the reduction of blood pressure in overweight hypertensive patients. *N Engl J Med* 1978;198:1–6.

19. Jones DW, Miller ME, Wofford MR, et al. The effect of weight loss interventions on antihypertensive medication requirements in the Hypertension Optimal Treatment (HOT) Study. *Am J Hypertens* 1999; 12:1175–80.

20. Stevens VJ, Obarzanek E, Cook NR, et al. Long-term weight loss and changes in blood pressure: Results of the Trials of Hypertension Prevention, phase II. *Ann Intern Med* 2001; 134(1):1–11.

21. Chobanian AV, Bakris GL, Black HR, et al. Joint National Committee on Prevention, Detection, Evaluation, and Treatment of High Blood Pressure. National High Blood Pressure Education Program Coordinating Committee. Seventh Report of the Joint National Committee on prevention, detection, evaluation, and treatment of high blood pressure. *Hypertension* 2003; 42:1206–52.

22. Klein S, Fontana L, Young VL, et al. Absence of an effect of liposuction on insulin action and risk factors for coronary heart disease. *N Engl J Med* 2004;350:2549.

23. Hall JE, Brands MW, Dixon WN, et al. Obesity-induced hypertension: Renal function and systemic hemodynamics. *Hypertension* 1993; 22:292–99.

24. Carroll JF, Huang M, Hester RL, et al. Hemodynamic alterations in obese rabbits. *Hypertension* 1995;26:465–70.

25. Rocchini AP, Mao HZ, Babu K, et al. Clonidine prevents insulin resistance and hypertension in obese dogs. *Hypertension* 1999;33:548–53.

26. Messerli FH, Christie B, DeCarvalho JG, et al. Obesity and essential hypertension: Hemodynamics, intravascular volume, sodium excretion and plasma renin activity. *Arch Intern Med* 1981;141:81–85.

27. Rocchini AP. The influence of obesity in hypertension. *News in Physiological Science* 1990; 5:245–49.

28. Van Vliet BN, Hall JE, Mizelle HL, et al. Reduced parasympathetic control of heart rate in obese dogs. *Am J Physiol* 1995;269:H629–37.

29. Arrone LJ, MacKintosh R, Rosenbaum M, et al. Autonomic nervous system activity in weight gain and weight loss. *Am J Physiol* 1995;269:222–25.

30. Hirsch J, Leibel, RL, Mackintosh R, Aguirre A. Heart rate variability as a measure of autonomic function during weight change in humans. *Am J Physiol* 1991;261:R1418–23.

31. Vaz M, Jennings G, Turner A, et al. Regional sympathetic nervous activity and oxygen consumption in obese normotensive human subjects. *Circulation* 1997;96:3423–29.

32. Hall JE. Mechanisms of abnormal renal sodium handling in obesity

hypertension. *Am J Hypertens* 1997; 10:s49–55.

33. Eslami P, Tuck M. The role of the sympathetic nervous system in linking obesity with hypertension in white versus black Americans. *Curr Hypertens Rep* 2003;5:269–72.

34. Landsberg L, Krieger DR. Obesity, metabolism, and the sympathetic nervous system. *Am J Hypertens* 1989;2:1255–1325.

35. Rumantir MS, Vaz M, Jennings GL, et al. Neural mechanisms in human obesity-related hypertension. *J Hypertens* 1999;17:1125–33.

36. Esler M. The sympathetic system and hypertension. *Am J Hypertens* 2000;13:99s-105s.

37. Grassi G, Servalle G, Cattaneo BM, et al. Sympathetic activity in obese normotensive subjects. *Hypertension* 1995;25:560–63.

38. Davy KP, Hall JE. Obesity and hypertension: Two epidemics or one? *Am J Physiol Regul Integr Comp Physiol* 2004;286:R803–13.

39. Weyer C, Pratley RE, Snitker S, et al. Ethnic differences in insulinemia and sympathetic tone as links between obesity and blood pressure. *Hypertension* 2000;36(4):531–37.

40. Abate NI, Mansour YH, Arbique D, et al. Overweight and sympathetic activity in black Americans. *Hypertension* 2001;38:379–83.

41. Alvarez GE, Beske SD, Ballard TP, Davy KP. Sympathetic neural activation in visceral obesity. *Circulation* 2002; 106:2533–36.

42. Antic V, Kiener-Belforti F, Tempini A, et al. Role of the sympathetic nervous system during the development of obesity hypertension in rabbits. *Am J Hypertens* 2000;13:556–59.

43. Rocchini AP, Mao HZ, Babu K, et al. Clonidine prevents insulin resistance and hypertension in obese dogs. *Hypertension* 1999;33:548–53.

44. Wofford MR, Anderson DC, Brown CA, et al. Antihypertensive effect of alpha and beta adrenergic blockade in obese and lean hypertensive subjects. *Am J Hypertens* 2001;14:164–68.

45. Kassab S, Kato T, Wilkins C, et al. Renal denervation attenuates the sodium retention and hypertension associated with obesity. *Hypertension* 1995;25:893–97.

46. Grassi G, Seravalle G, Dell'Oro R, et al. Adrenergic and reflex abnormalities in obesity-related hypertension. *Hypertension* 2000;36:538–42.

47. Hall JE. Hyperinsulinemia: A link between obesity and hypertension? *Kidney Int* 1993; 43:1402–17.

48. Narkiewicz K, Kato M, Pesek CA, et al. Human obesity is characterized by selective potentiation of central chemoreflex sensitivity. *Hypertension* 1999;33:1153–58.

49. Wolk R, Shamsuzzaman ASM, Somers VK. Obesity, sleep apnea, and hypertension. *Hypertension* 2003; 42:1067–74.

50. Hall JE, Brands MW, Zappe DH, et al. Hemodynamic and renal responses to chronic hyperinsulinemia in obese, insulin resistant dogs. *Hypertension* 1995;25:994–1002.

51. Stepniakowski KT, Goodfriend, Egan BM. Fatty acids enhance vascular

α-adrenergic sensitivity. *Hypertension* 1995;25:774–78.

52. Grekin RJ, Dumont CJ, Vollmer, AP, et al. Mechanisms in the pressor effects of hepatic portal venous fatty acid infusion. *Am J Physiol* 1997; 273:R324–30.

53. Hildebrandt DA, Kirk D, Hall JE. Renal and cardiovascular responses to chronic increases in cerebrovascular free fatty acids. *Fed Proc* 1999; 13:A780.

54. Alvarez GE, Davy BM, Ballard TP, et al. Weight loss increases cardiovagal baroreflex function in obese young and older men. *Am J Physiol Endocrinol Metab* 2005;289:E665–69.

55. Lohmeier TE, Warren S, Cunningham JT. Sustained activation of the central baroreceptor pathway in obesity hypertension. *Hypertension* 2003; 42:96–102.

56. Shamsuzzaman AS, Gersh BJ, Somers VK. Obstructive sleep apnea: Implications for cardiac and vascular disease. *JAMA* 2003;290:1906–14.

57. Goodfriend TL, Calhoun DA. Resistant hypertension, obesity, sleep apnea, and aldosterone: Theory and therapy. *Hypertension* 2004;43:518–24.

58. Wolk R, Shamsuzzaman AS, Somers VK. Obesity, sleep apnea, and hypertension. *Hypertension* 2003; 42:1067–74.

59. Narkiewicz K, van de Borne PJH, Cooley RL, et al. Sympathetic activity in obese subjects with and without obstructive sleep apnea. *Circulation* 1998;98:772–76.

60. Hall JE, Hildebrandt DA, Kuo JJ. Obesity hypertension: Role of leptin and sympathetic nervous system. *Am J Hypertens* 2001;14:103s-15s.

61. Jequier E. Leptin signaling, adiposity, and energy balance. *Ann NY Acad Sci* 2002;967:379–88.

62. Correia MLG, Morgan DA, Sivitz WI, et al. Leptin acts in the central nervous system to produce dose-dependent changes in arterial pressure. *Hypertension* 2001;27:936–42.

63. Shek EW, Brands MW, Hall JE. Chronic leptin infusion increases arterial pressure. *Hypertension* 1998; 31:409–14.

64. Kuo J, Jones OB, Hall JE. Inhibition of NO synthesis enhances chronic cardiovascular and renal actions of leptin. *Hypertension* 2001;37:670–76.

65. Carlyle M, Jones OB, Kuo JJ, Hall JE. Chronic cardiovascular and renal actions of leptin-role of adrenergic activity. *Hypertension* 2002; 39:496–501.

66. Mark AL, Shaffer RA, Correia ML, et al. Contrasting blood pressure effects of obesity in leptin-deficient ob/ob mice and agouti yellow mice. *J Hypertens* 1999;17:1949–53.

67. Ozata M, Ozdemir IC, Licinio J. Human leptin deficiency caused by a missense mutation: Multiple endocrine defects, decreased sympathetic tone, and immune system dysfunction indicate new targets for leptin action, greater central than peripheral resistance to the effects of leptin, and spontaneous correction of leptin-mediated defects. *J Clin Endocrinol Metab* 1999; 10:3686–95.

68. Haynes WG, Morgan DA, Djalali A, et al. Interactions between the

melanocortin system and leptin in control of sympathetic nerve traffic. *Hypertension* 1999;33:542–47.

69. Kuo JJ, Silva AA, Hall JE. Hypothalamic melanocortin receptors and chronic regulation of arterial pressure and renal function. *Hypertension* 2003; 41:768–74.

70. da Silva AA, Kuo JJ, Hall JE. Role of hypothalamic melanocortin 3/4 receptors in mediating the chronic cardiovascular, renal, and metabolic actions of leptin. *Hypertension* 2004;43:1312–17.

71. Tallam LS, da Silva AA, Hall JE. Melanocortin-4 receptor mediates chronic cardiovascular and metabolic actions of leptin. *Hypertension* 2006; 48:58–64.

72. Engeli S, Sharma AM. The renin angiotensin system and natriuretic peptides in obesity associated hypertension. *J Mol Med* 2001; 79:21–29.

73. Tuck ML, Sowers J, Dornfeld L, et al. The effect of weight reduction on blood pressure, plasma renin activity, and plasma aldosterone levels in obese patients. *N Engl J Med* 1981; 304: 930–33.

74. Hall JE, Henegar JR, Shek EW, et al. Role of renin-angiotensin system in obesity hypertension. *Circulation* 1997;96:I-33.

75. Robles RG, Villa E, Santirso R, et al. Effects of captopril on sympathetic activity, lipid and carbohydrate metabolism in a model of obesity-induced hypertension in dogs. *Am J Hypertens* 1993;6:1009–19.

76. Boustany CM, Brown DR, Randall DC, Cassis LA. AT1-receptor antagonism reverses the blood pressure elevation associated with diet-induced obesity. *Am J Physiol Regul Integr Comp Physiol* 2005;289:R181–86.

77. Alonso-Galicia M, Brands MW, Zappe DH, et al. Hypertension in obese Zucker rats: Role of angiotensin II and adrenergic activity. *Hypertension* 1996;28:1047–54.

78. Hall JE, Brands MW, Henegar JR. Angiotensin II and long-term arterial pressure regulation: The overriding dominance of the kidney. *J Am Soc Nephrol* 1999;10:s258–65.

79. Oparil S. Antihypertensive and Lipid-Lowering Treatment to Prevent Heart Attack Trial (ALLHAT): Practical implications. *Hypertension* 2003; 41:1006–09.

80. Ravid M, Lang R, Rachmani R, Lishner M. Long-term renoprotective effect of angiotensin-converting enzyme inhibition in non-insulin-dependent diabetes mellitus: A 7-year follow-up study. *Arch Intern Med* 1996;156:286–89.

81. Lewis EJ, Hunsicker LG, Clark WR, et al. Renoprotective effect of the angiotensive receptor antagonist irbesartan in patients with nephropathy due to type 2 diabetes. *N Engl J Med* 2001;345:851–60.

82. Brenner BM, Cooper ME, deZeeuw D, et al. Effects of losartan on renal and cardiovascular outcomes in patients with type 2 diabetes and nephropathy. *N Engl J Med* 2001;345:861–69.

83. Nishizaka MR, Zaman AM, Calhoun DA. Efficacy of low-dose spironolactone in

subjects with resistant hypertension. *Am J Hypertens* 2003;16:925–30.

84. Rocha R, Stier CT Jr. Pathophysiological effects of aldosterone in cardiovascular tissues. *Trends Endocrinol Metab* 2001;12:308–14.

85. de Paula RB, da Silva AA, Hall JE. Aldosterone antagonism attenuates obesity-induced hypertension and glomerular hyperfiltration. *Hypertension* 2004;43:41–47.

86. Goodfriend TL, Calhoun DA. Resistant hypertension, obesity, sleep apnea, and aldosterone: Theory and therapy. *Hypertension* 2004;43:518–24.

87. Bickel CA, Verbalis JG, Knepper MA, Ecelbarger CA. Increased renal Na-K-ATPase, NCC, and beta-ENaC abundance in obese Zucker rats. *Am J Physiol Renal Physiol* 2001; 281:F639–48.

88. Draper N, Stewart PM. 11beta-hydroxysteroid dehydrogenase and the pre-receptor regulation of corticosteroid hormone action. *J Endocrinol* 2005;186:251–71.

89. Bujalska IJ, Kumar S, Stewart PM. Does central obesity reflect "Cushing's disease of the omentum"? *Lancet* 1997;349:1210–13.

90. Masuzaki H, Paterson J, Shinyama H, et al. A transgenic model of visceral obesity and the metabolic syndrome. *Science* 2001;294:2166–70.

91. Sugarman HJ, Windsor ACJ, Bessos MK, et al. Intra-abdominal pressure, sagittal abdominal diameter and obesity co-morbidity. *J Intern Med* 1997;241:71–79.

92. Dwyer TM, Banks SA, Alonso-Galicia M, et al. Distribution of renal medullary hyaluronan in lean and obese rabbits. *Kidney Int* 2000; 58:721–29.

93. Alonso-Galicia M, Brands MW, Zappe DH, et al. Hypertension in obese Zucker rats: Role of angiotensin II. *Hypertension* 1996;28:1047–54.

94. Hall JE, Brands MW, Henegar JR. Mechanisms of hypertension and kidney disease in obesity. *Ann NY Acad Sci* 1999;892:91–107.

95. Neels JG, Olefsky JM. Inflamed fat: What starts the fire? *J Clin Invest* 2006;116:33–35.

96. Lyon CJ, Law RE, Hsueh WA. Adiposity, inflammation, and atherogenesis. *Endocrinology* 2003;144:2195–2200.

97. Fried SK, Bunkin DA, Greenberg AS. Omental and subcutaneous adipose tissues of obese subjects release interleukin-6: Depot difference and regulation by glucocorticoid. *J Clin Endocrinol Metab* 1998;83:847–50.

98. Fruhbeck G, Gomez-Ambrosi J, Muruzabal FJ, Burrell MA. The adipocyte: A model for integration of endocrine and metabolic signaling in energy metabolism regulation. *Am J Physiol Endocrinol Metab* 2001; 280:E827–47.

99. Engeli S, Negrel R, Sharma AM. Physiology and pathophysiology of the adipose tissue renin-angiotensin system. *Hypertension* 2000; 35:1270–77.

100. Rocchini AP, Moorehead C, Katch V, et al. Forearm resistance vessel abnormalities and insulin resistance in obese adolescents. *Hypertension* 1992; 19:615–20.

101. Steinberg HO, Chaker H, Learning R, et al. Obesity/insulin resistance is associated with endothelial dysfunction: Implications for the syndrome of insulin resistance. *J Clin Invest* 1996; 97:2601–10.

102. Raitakari M, Ilvonen T, Ahotupa M, et al. Weight reduction with very low-caloric diet and endothelial function in overweight adults: Role of plasma glucose. *Arterioscler Thromb Vasc Biol* 2004;24:124–28.

103. Wildman RP, Mackey RH, Bostom A, et al. Measures of obesity are associated with vascular stiffness in young and older adults. *Hypertension* 2003;42:468–73.

104. Tounian P, Aggoun Y, Dubern B, et al. Presence of increased stiffness of the common carotid artery and endothelial dysfunction in severely obese children: A prospective study. *Lancet* 2001; 358:1400–04.

105. Lyon CJ, Law RE, Hsueh WA. Adiposity, inflammation, and atherogenesis. *Endocrinology* 2003;144:2195–2200.

106. Shankar SS, Mirzamohammadi B, Walsh JP, Steinberg HO. L-carnitine may attenuate free fatty acid-induced endothelial dysfunction. *Ann NY Acad Sci* 2004;1033:189–97.

107. Unger R. Hyperleptinemia: Protecting the heart from lipid overload. *Hypertension* 2005;45:1031–34.

108. Assmann G, Schulte H. The prospective cardiovascular munster study (PROCAM): Prevalence of hyperlipidemia in persons with hypertension and/or diabetes mellitus and the relationship to coronary artery disease. *Am Heart J* 1988;1116:1713–24.

109. Hall JE, Crook ED, Jones DW, et al. Mechanisms of obesity-associated cardiovascular and renal disease. *Am J Med Sci* 2002;324(3):127–37.

110. Fox CS, Larson MG, Leip EP, et al. Predictors of new-onset kidney disease in a community-based population. *JAMA* 2004;291:844–50.

111. Hsu CY, McCulloch CE, Iribarren C, et al. Body mass index and risk for end-stage renal disease. *Ann Intern Med* 2006;144:21–28.

112. Praga M, Hernandez E, Herrero JC, et al. Influence of obesity on the appearance of proteinuria and renal insufficiency after unilateral nephrectomy. *Kidney Int* 2000; 58:2111–18.

113. Bonnet F, Deprele C, Sassolas A, et al. Excessive body weight as a new independent risk factor for clinical and pathological progression in primary IgA nephritis. *Am J Kidney Dis* 2001; 37:720–27.

114. Morales E, Valero MA, Leon M, et al. Beneficial effects of weight loss in overweight patients with chronic proteinuric nephropathies. *Am J Kidney Dis* 2003;41:319–27.

115. Henegar JR, Bigler SA, Henegar LK, et al. Functional and structural changes in the kidney in the early stages of obesity. *J Am Soc Nephrol* 2001;12:1211–17.

116. Kambham N, Markowitz GS, Valeri AM, et al. Obesity related glomerulopathy: An emerging epidemic. *Kidney Int* 2001;59:1498–1509.

117. Hall JE, Jones DW, Henegar J, et al. Obesity hypertension, and renal disease. In RH Eckel (ed), *Obesity: Mechanisms and Clinical Management*. Philadelphia: Lippincott, Williams & Wilkins, 2003:273–300.

118. Stern JS, Gades MD, Wheeldon CM, Borchers AT. Calorie restriction in obesity: Prevention of kidney disease in rodents. *J Nutr* 2001;131:913s-17s.

119. Praga M. Obesity: A neglected culprit in renal disease. *Nephrol Dial Transplant* 2002;17:1157–59.

120. Carroll JF, Braden DS, Cockrell K, et al. Obese rabbits develop concentric and eccentric hypertrophy and diastolic filling abnormalities. *Am J Hypertens* 1997;10:230–33.

121. Alpert MA. Obesity cardiomyopathy and the evolution of the clinical syndrome. *Am J Med Sci* 2001; 321:225–36.

122. Gottdiener JS, Reda DJ, Materson BJ, et al. Importance of obesity, race and age to the cardiac structural and functional effects of hypertension. *Journal of the American College of Cardiology* 1994;24:1492–98.

123. Carroll JF, Braden DS, Henegar JR, et al. Dietary sodium chloride (NaCl) worsens obesity-related cardiac hypertrophy. *FASEB J* 1998;12:A708.

124. Carroll JF, Summers RL, Dzielak DJ, et al. Diastolic compliance is reduced in obese rabbits. *Hypertension* 1999; 33:811–15.

125. Alpert MA, Lambert CR, Panayiotou H, et al. Relation of duration of morbid obesity to left ventricular mass, systolic function, and diastolic filling, and effect of weight loss. *Am J Cardiol* 1995;76:1194–97.

126. Philip-Couderc P, Smith F, Hall JE, et al. Kinetic analysis of cardiac transcriptome regulation during chronic high fat diet in dogs. *Physiol Genomics* 2004;19:32–40.

127. Carroll JF. Post-beta receptor defect in isolated hearts of obese-hypertensive rabbits. *Internat Journal of Obesity Related Metabolic Disorders* 1999; 23:863–66.

128. Unger RH. Weapons of lean body mass destruction: The role of ectopic lipids in the metabolic syndrome. *Endocrinology* 2003;144:5159–65.

129. Kenchaiah S, Evans JC, Levy D, et al. Obesity and the risk of heart failure. *N Engl J Med* 2002;347:305–13.

130. Zhou YT, Grayburn P, Karim A, et al. Lipotoxic heart disease in obese rats implications for human obesity. *Proc Natl Acad Sci USA* 2000;97:1784–89.

131. Sharma S, Adrogue JV, Golfman L, et al. Intramyocardial lipid accumulation in the failing human heart resembles the lipotoxic rat heart. *FASEB J* 2004; 18:1692–1700.

132. Chu NF, Spiegelman D, Hotamisligil GS, et al. Plasma insulin, leptin, and soluble TNF receptors levels in relation to obesity-related atherogenic and thrombogenic cardiovascular disease factors among men. *Atherosclerosis* 2001;157: 495–503.

133. Alessai MC, Morange P, Juhan-Vague I. Fat cell function and fibrinolysis. *Horm Metab Res* 2000;32:504–08.

134. Konstantinides S, Schafer K, Loskutoff DJ. The prothrombotic effects of leptin: Possible implications for the risk of cardiovascular disease in obesity. *Ann NY Acad Sci* 2001;947: 134–41.

135. Gelfand EV, Cannon CP. Rimonabant: A cannabinoid receptor type 1 blocker for management of multiple cardiometabolic risk factors. *J Am Coll Cardiol* 2006;47:1919–26.

136. National Institutes of Health Clinical guidelines on the identification, evaluation, and treatment of overweight and obesity in adults: The evidence report. National Heart, Lung, and Blood Institute and National Institute of Diabetes and Digestive and Kidney Diseases, Bethesda, MD, 1998. Available at *http://www.nhlbi.nih.gov/guidelines/index.htm*.

137. The Trials of Hypertension Prevention Collaborative Research Group. The effects of nonpharmacologic interventions on blood pressure of persons with high normal levels: Results of the Trials of Hypertension Prevention, Phase I. *JAMA* 1992; 267:1213–20.

138. Whelton PK, Appel LJ, Espeland MA, et al. (for the TONE Collaborative Research Group). Sodium reduction and weight loss in the treatment of hypertension in older persons: A randomized controlled trial of nonpharmacologic interventions in the elderly (TONE). *JAMA* 1998; 279:839–46.

139. Davis BR, Blaufoz MD, Oberman A, et al. Reduction in long-term antihypertensive medication requirements: Effects of weight reduction by dietary intervention in overweight persons with mild hypertension. *Arch Intern Med* 1993; 153:1773–82.

140. Imai Y, Sato K, Abe K, et al. Effects of weight loss on blood pressure and drug consumption in normal weight patients. *Hypertension* 1986;8:223–28.

141. Galuska DA, Will JC, Serdula MK, et al. Are health care professionals advising obese patients to lose weight? *JAMA* 1999;282:1576–78.

142. Serdula MK, Mokdad AH, Williamson DF, et al. Prevalence of attempting weight loss and strategies for controlling weight. *JAMA* 1999; 282:1353–58.

143. Sharma AM. Is there a rationale for angiotensin blockade in the management of obesity hypertension? *Hypertension* 2004;44:12–19.

144. Sharma AM, Pischon T, Engeli S, et al. Choice of drug treatment for obesity-related hypertension: Where is the evidence? *J Hypertens* 2001;19:667–74.

145. Zanella MT, Kohlmann O Jr., Ribeiro AB. Treatment of obesity hypertension and diabetes syndrome. *Hypertension* 2001;38:705–08.

146. Oparil S. Antihypertensive and lipid-lowering treatment to prevent heart attack trial (ALLHAT): Practical implications. *Hypertension* 2003; 41:1006–09.

147. Reisin E, Weed SG. The treatment of obese hypertensive black women: A comparative study of chlorthalidone versus clonidine. *J Hypertens* 1992; 10(5):489–93.

148. Bakris GL, Weir MR, Sowers JR. Therapeutic challenges in the obese diabetic patient with hypertension. *Am J Med* 1996;101(3A):33S-46S.

149. UK Prospective Diabetes Study Group. Efficacy of atenolol and captopril in reducing risk of both macrovascular and microvascular complications in type 2 diabetes (UKPDS 39). *BMJ* 1998;317:713–20.

150. Reisen E, Weir M, Falkner B, et al. Lisinopril versus hydrochlorothiazide in obese hypertensive patients: A multicenter placebo-controlled trial. *Hypertension* 1997;30:140–45.

151. Grassi G, Seravalle G, Dell'Oro R, et al. Comparative effects of candesartan and hydrochlorothiazide on blood pressure, insulin sensitivity, and sympathetic drive in obese hypertensive individuals: Results of the CROSS study. *J Hypertens* 2003;21:1761–69.

152. Sugimoto K, Qi NR, Kazdova L, Pravenec M, Ogihara T, Kurtz TW. Telmisartan but not valsartan increases caloric expenditure and protects against weight gain and hepatic steatosis. *Hypertension* 2006;47:1003–09.

153. Sharma AM. Telmisartan: The ACE of ARBs? *Hypertension* 2006;47:822–23.

154. Parving HH, Lehnert H, Brochner-Mortensen J, et al. The effect of irbesartan on the development of diabetic nephropathy in patients with type 2 diabetes. *N Engl J Med* 2001; 345:870–78.

155. Black HR. The addition of doxazosin to the therapeutic regimen of hypertensive patients inadequately controlled with other antihypertensive medications. *American Journal of Hypertension* 2000;13:468–74.

156. Stoa-Birketvedt G, Thom E, Aarbakke J, Florholmen J. Body fat as a prediction of the antihypertensive effect of nifedipine. *J Int Med* 1995; 237:169–73.

157. Kaplan NM. Obesity in hypertension: Effects on prognosis and treatment. *Journal of Hypertension* 1998; 16(1):S35–37.

158. Nieto FJ, Young TB, Lind BK, et al. Association of sleep-disordered breathing, sleep apnea, and hypertension in a large community-based study: Sleep Heart Health Study. *JAMA.* 2000;283:1829–36.

159. Peppard PE, Young T, Palta M, Skatrud J. Prospective study of the association between sleep-disordered breathing and hypertension. *N Engl J Med* 2000;342:1378–84.

160. Weiss JW, Remsburg S, Garpestad E, et al. Hemodynamic consequences of obstructive sleep apnea: State of the art review. *Sleep* 1996;19:388–97.

161. Caples SM, Gami AS, Somers VK. Obstructive sleep apnea. *Ann Intern Med* 2005;142:187–97.

162. Kanagy LK, Walker BR, Nelin LD. Role of endothelin in intermittent hypoxia-induced hypertension. *Hypertension* 2001;37:511–15.

163. Faccenda JF, Mackay TW, Boon NA, Douglas NJ. Randomized placebo controlled trial of continuous positive airway pressure on blood pressure in the sleep apnea-hypopnea syndrome. *Am J Respir Crit Care Med* 2001; 163:344–48.

Chapter

39 Exercise and Hypertension

Kevin P. Davy and Christopher L. Gentile

Key Findings

- Physical inactivity is a major risk factor for the development of hypertension.

- There is an inverse relation between the amount of physical activity and the level of arterial BP.

- Regular aerobic exercise training decreases systolic and diastolic BP in both normotensive and hypertensive individuals.

- The BP-lowering effect of regular aerobic exercise is independent of changes in total body adiposity. Whether reductions in abdominal visceral fat with exercise training contribute independently of total body adiposity is unclear.

- Consistent with public health recommendations, BP lowering can be achieved with as little as 30 minutes per day of moderate-intensity walking activity.

Physical inactivity is a major risk factor for cardiovascular diseases, including hypertension.[1] Regular physical activity has long been regarded as an effective means of reducing risk.[2] The results of numerous epidemiologic and experimental studies support the idea that physical activity plays an important role in the etiology, prevention, and treatment of hypertension. Thus, regular physical activity has been included in the broader recommendation of lifestyle modification to prevent and manage hypertension.[3]

ROLE OF PHYSICAL INACTIVITY IN THE ETIOLOGY OF HYPERTENSION

Physically inactive individuals demonstrate higher levels of blood pressure (BP) compared with their more active peers,[4] and there is an inverse relation between the amount of physical activity performed and both the level of BP and incidence of hypertension.[5] Furthermore, low levels of physical activity are associated with an increase in the incidence of hypertension.[6-10] Taken together, these facts indicate that physical inactivity appears to play an important role in the development of hypertension.

An observation that may cause some to discount physical inactivity as an important cause of hypertension is the fact that not all sedentary individuals have hypertension by clinical standards (i.e., 140/90 mmHg). However, it is also a possibility that most individuals experience an increase in BP with physical inactivity, but the baseline BP is variable. A person with a low baseline BP may not attain hyper-

tensive levels of BP with physical inactivity, but BP is higher than observed in the physically active state. On a population basis, physical inactivity likely shifts the frequency distribution of BP, so that a much greater fraction of sedentary individuals would be hypertensive compared with active subjects. This would be consistent with observations that regular aerobic exercise reduces BP in normotensive and hypertensive subjects,[11-13] as well as the observation that cessation of exercise training increases BP.[14] Furthermore, it is important to emphasize that the association between BP and cardiovascular mortality is evident at BPs as low as 120/80 mmHg[15] and perhaps lower. Thus, any elevation in BP above normal would be associated with an increased risk. In turn, any reduction in BP in individuals with elevated baseline levels should confer cardiovascular protection.

Obesity, particularly abdominal obesity, substantially increases the risk of developing hypertension.[16,17] Physically inactive individuals have higher levels of total body and abdominal visceral fat compared with their active peers.[4,18] Importantly, the scenario described previously does not preclude a role for other important factors such as obesity and weight gain in hypertension development.[16,17] Rather, physical inactivity and obesity interact to further increase BP and its cardiovascular sequelae.[9,19] Indeed, physical inactivity amplifies the risk of hypertension with weight gain,[9,19] particularly in those with an excess accumulation of abdominal visceral fat.[20]

ROLE OF PHYSICAL ACTIVITY IN THE TREATMENT OF HYPERTENSION

Regular physical activity is recommended for individuals with elevated BP.[3] The results of several meta-analyses on the topic have concluded that regular aerobic exercise lowers resting systolic (~4 to 7 mmHg) and diastolic (~2 to 6 mmHg) BP in hypertensive individuals.[12,13,21] The conclusion of more traditional literature reviews has been that regular aerobic exercise produces a much larger reduction in systolic (~11 mmHg) and diastolic (~8 mmHg) BP in hypertensives.[11] Importantly, the reduction in BP with exercise training is dependent on sustaining regular physical activity[14] because detraining is associated with a return in BP to its initial level.

There is increasing evidence that ambulatory BP is a stronger predictor of adverse outcomes[22-25] than resting BP. The results of randomized controlled studies suggest that regular aerobic exercise training reduces ambulatory BP, but the effect is generally smaller than observed for resting BP.[26] In addition, regular physical activity appears to exert a larger influence on daytime compared to nighttime BP. The reduction in daytime BP may be due to both a reduction in BP at rest as well as during submaximal activities of daily living.

Characteristics of the stimulus

The intensity, frequency, duration, and mode of the exercise stimulus all may influence the magnitude of reduction in BP (Box 39–1). The general characteristics of the exercise stimulus in previous studies vary considerably and range from an intensity of ~40 to 80% of maximal oxygen consumption 2 to 6 times per week for a duration lasting from 4 weeks to 1.5 years. Many modes of exercise have been studied, including walking, jogging/running, cycling, and swimming.[26]

The magnitude of BP lowering appears to be as great or greater with low- to moderate-intensity exercise (i.e., <70% of maximal aerobic capacity) compared with high intensity exercise (i.e., >70% maximal aerobic capacity).[11,13,26] This would seem important from a public health perspective because low to moderate intensities are recommended by the Institute of Medicine,[27] the American College of Sports Medicine, and the Centers for Disease Control and Prevention[28] and may be preferred by most individuals engaging in regular physical activity for the purposes of improving health.[29]

Neither the frequency nor duration of exercise training exerts any clear influence on the magnitude of BP lowering.[11,13,21,26] Most of the BP lowering is observed in the first 2 to 3 weeks of initiating exercise training, with little or no further reductions observed with time.[11,30]

Regular aerobic exercise involving walking, jogging/running, cycling, and swimming all appear to result in significant BP lowering.[26] Whether a particular mode has superior efficacy compared with other modes has not been directly tested.

The result of a recent meta-analysis suggests that strength training may lower systolic and diastolic BP by ~3 mmHg , although the efficacy of strength training for lowering BP in hypertensives remains unclear.[26] Strength training increases arterial stiffness in normotensive individuals.[31] However, whether this also occurs in hypertensive individuals is not

known. Taken together, these observations question the utility of resistance exercise as a sole therapeutic strategy for lowering BP in hypertensive individuals.

The relative benefit of intermittent compared with continuous physical activity on BP lowering has received little attention to date. Preliminary evidence suggests that reductions in BP may be observed when exercise is performed for 10 minutes 3 times a day (5 days/week) at a low to moderate intensity.[32] Whether this intermittent pattern of physical activity is more (or less) effective than continuous physical activity in sustaining the BP lowering is not at all clear.

Characteristics of the individual

There are numerous individual characteristics that have the potential to modify the magnitude of BP lowering with exercise training (Box 39–2). Of the characteristics studied, baseline BP appears to exert the most significant influence.[11,13,21,26] Individuals with the highest baseline BP generally demonstrate the largest reduction in BP with regular aerobic exercise. Therefore, regular aerobic exercise appears to be most beneficial for those in most need of its BP-lowering potential.

The prevalence of hypertension is similar in men and women and increases with advancing age in both genders. In this respect, middle-age and older individuals experience somewhat larger and more consistent reductions in BP with exercise compared with young individuals.[11,13,26] The effect of exercise on BP in children is less clear.[33] With regard to ethnicity, there are considerable differences in the prevalence of hypertension among ethnic groups. Despite these differences, exercise training appears to reduce BP in adult men and women of all ethnic groups studied to date,[11,13,21,26] including African Americans, the group with the highest prevalence of hypertension.

Obesity increases the risk of hypertension[16,34] and is considered by some to be a form of resistant hypertension.[35] However, the presence of obesity or the baseline level of total body adiposity (i.e., body mass index or body fat percentage) does not appear to predict the magnitude of BP lowering with exercise.[11,13,26]

There is considerable variability in the BP lowering observed with exercise training, suggesting that genetic variation may play a role.[11,26,36] Recent evidence suggests that hyper-

---

Box 39–1

Characteristics of the Exercise Stimulus That Could Affect the Blood Pressure Response

- Mode (walking/running, cycling, swimming, resistance)
- Intensity
- Duration
- Frequency
- Interaction with other interventions (e.g., weight loss, pharmacotherapy)
- Continuous versus intermittent

Box 39–2

Characteristics of the Individual That Could Affect the Blood Pressure Response

- Baseline BP
- Age
- Gender/menopausal status
- Genetics (e.g., gene polymorphisms)
- Ethnicity
- Obesity and fat distribution
- Aerobic fitness

tensives with one or both ACE I alleles demonstrate larger reductions in systolic BP with exercise training compared with individuals homozygous for the ACE D allele.[37] It is important to emphasize that although not all hypertensives may demonstrate BP lowering with exercise nonetheless exercise training may provide numerous other benefits (see material following). Importantly, the risk of mortality is reduced in physically active hypertensives.[38]

INFLUENCE OF REGULAR AEROBIC EXERCISE ON DISEASE RISK AND TARGET ORGAN DAMAGE IN HYPERTENSIVE INDIVIDUALS

Cardiovascular risk factors

Individuals with hypertension frequently exhibit a clustering of other cardiovascular and metabolic disease risk factors such as insulin resistance, glucose intolerance, dyslipidemia, impaired fibrinolysis, and low-grade inflammation.[39] In addition, hypertension and type 2 diabetes frequently coexist.[40] Regular exercise training is generally associated with increases in insulin sensitivity, glucose tolerance, and high-density lipoprotein cholesterol and with reductions in total cholesterol, low-density lipoprotein cholesterol, triglycerides, and markers of inflammation (e.g., c-reactive protein).[40] Thus, regular physical activity has the potential to markedly lower disease risk beyond BP lowering in hypertensive individuals.

Left ventricular mass and function

Left ventricular hypertrophy and ventricular dysfunction are associated with an increased risk of heart failure and are common consequences of hypertension. Thus, regression of left ventricular hypertrophy is an important goal of antihypertensive therapy and is frequently observed with BP lowering. Indeed, exercise training reduces left ventricular mass in hypertensive adults.[41,42] The magnitude of reduction in left ventricular mass appears to be most closely related to the magnitude of reduction in systolic BP.[42] The mechanism or mechanisms responsible for the reduction in left ventricular mass have not been determined. In contrast to that observed in normotensive older adults,[43,44] neither systolic nor diastolic function appears to improve with exercise training in hypertensives.[42]

Large artery stiffness

Large artery stiffening is independently associated with the development of hypertension.[45] In addition, arterial stiffness is an independent predictor of coronary events,[46] stroke,[47] and all-cause mortality[48] in individuals with hypertension. In contrast to observations in normotensive older adults,[49] the available evidence suggests that regular aerobic exercise is not effective in reducing large artery stiffness in adults with elevated BP.[50] However, the previous studies on this issue were relatively short in duration (i.e., 3 months), and the subjects did not experience weight loss. Whether longer-duration exercise training (with or without weight loss) is necessary to reduce large artery stiffness in this population is unknown.

Endothelial function

Endothelial dysfunction has been linked to several cardiovascular complications (e.g., arterial spasm, thrombosis, and myocardial infarction), which occur more frequently in hypertensive individuals.[1] Endothelial-dependent vasodilatation is impaired in hypertensive individuals, and the degree of impairment is influenced by the severity of hypertension[51,52] and by the presence of obesity.[53] Furthermore, the ability of the endothelium to release t-PA is also impaired in hypertensives.[54] Regular aerobic exercise enhances endothelium-dependent vasodilatation in hypertensive individuals.[55] The improvement appears to be due, at least in part, to enhanced nitric oxide production because the effect of physical activity is abolished following intra-arterial infusion of the nitric oxide synthase inhibitor NG-monomethyl-L-arginine.[56] Whether other mechanisms, such as reduced endothelin-mediated vasoconstriction and/or oxidative stress, contribute has not been determined. Regular exercise training increases endothelial t-PA release in nonobese and obese middle-age and older adults with normal BP,[57] although there is unfortunately no evidence in hypertensive individuals.

Kidney function

Prolonged hypertension is associated with an increase in urinary protein excretion and gradual loss of nephron function that worsens with time and aggravates hypertension. In addition, kidney disease progresses much more rapidly in the presence of hyperglycemia and dyslipidemia.[58] Unfortunately, little is known regarding the influence of regular exercise training on kidney function in hypertensive individuals. In general, lowering of BP and improvement in glucose and lipid metabolism would be expected to reduce kidney damage in hypertensive individuals. Certainly, regular physical activity would be expected to reduce kidney damage when accompanied by significant weight loss.[59]

MECHANISMS MEDIATING THE BP-LOWERING EFFECT OF ACUTE AND CHRONIC EXERCISE

In 1898, Hill[60] noted, perhaps for the first time on record, that "…after such exertion the pressure falls to normal far more rapidly than the pulse-frequency. The arterial pressure becomes depressed below the normal pressure after severe muscular work." Since that time, numerous studies have documented the phenomenon of postexercise hypotension.[26,61]

In normotensive individuals, moderate-intensity physical activity lasting 30 to 60 minutes may lower BP immediately postexercise ~5 to 10 mmHg in the supine posture for up to ~2 to 3 hours.[61] The postexercise hypotension (i.e., the reduction in BP after a single bout of exercise) may reach 16 to 20 mmHg in older hypertensive patients,[62] and may remain lower up to ~24 hours after exercise.[63] These reductions in BP following a single bout of exercise compare favorably with the reductions observed following exercise training. However, the degree to which the phenomenon of postexercise hypotension contributes to the lower BP observed following exercise training remains unclear.

It also is possible that the postexercise hypotension observed with acute exercise could be superimposed on the reduction in BP following exercise training. The duration of exercise necessary to elicit a significant postexercise hypotension is not known. If a significant postexercise hypotension were evident following, for example, 10 minutes of exercise a hypertensive patient might perform a vigorous 10-minute walk in the morning, afternoon, and evening.[64] As such, they might experience significant reduction in BP that would last every hour of the day. It is important to emphasize that the results of some previous studies suggest that the postexercise hypotension observed is sufficient in magnitude and duration to significantly lower the average 24-hour ambulatory BP level.[26]

The mechanisms responsible for postexercise hypotension are not clear. In young normotensive individuals the reduction in BP appears to be due to a pronounced fall in systemic vascular resistance that is not completely offset by an increase in cardiac output.[61,65,66] The significant vasodilatation does not appear limited to the previously active skeletal muscle but includes inactive regions as well.[61,65,66]

The postexercise hypotension observed in hypertensive patients is associated with a decrease in cardiac output and no change in system vascular resistance.[62,63] The factors contributing to the reduction in cardiac output may include a reduction in plasma volume, impaired diastolic filling, and/or reduced myocardial contractility. The reasons for the apparent difference in mechanisms contributing to postexercise hypotension in normotensive and hypertensive individuals remain unclear.

It is widely held that any long-term reductions in blood pressure, including those associated with exercise training, are due to alterations in kidney function. Although direct evidence for this notion is lacking, exercise training has been associated with reductions in muscle sympathetic nerve activity,[67] total and renal norepinephrine spillover,[68,69] plasma norepinephrine concentration,[26,70] and plasma renin activity.[71,72] These reductions in the activity of sympathetic nervous and renin-angiotensin systems and/or other factors (e.g., amelioration of oxidative stress, endothelin-1, and so on) could translate into an improvement in renal excretory function such that lower levels of BP are required to maintain sodium and water homeostasis following exercise training (Figure 39–1). However, the BP-lowering effect of regular physical activity has been observed in patients without functioning kidneys (i.e., end-stage renal disease patients undergoing dialysis),[73,74] suggesting that alterations in the kidney are not necessary for the BP-lowering effects of chronic physical activity. Alternatively, this observation may lend further merit to the notion that the BP-lowering effect of physical activity is not a chronic adaptation but is rather due primarily to the reduction in BP associated with the last bout of exercise (i.e., postexercise hypotension).

PHYSICAL ACTIVITY PER SE VERSUS WEIGHT LOSS?

Weight loss is generally associated with reductions in BP.[16,75,76] Thus, it is possible that the reductions in BP observed with exercise training could be due at least in part to weight loss. However, most studies have concluded that the reduction in BP with exercise training is independent of changes in whole-body adiposity.[11,13,26]

Regular aerobic exercise has been suggested to be an effective means of reducing abdominal visceral fat, and abdominal visceral fat has been more closely associated with BP and the presence of hypertension than measures of total adiposity.[77–83] There are several proposed mechanisms by which abdominal visceral fat might contribute to hypertension, including compression of the kidney, sympathetic neural activation, ectopic fat deposition, and local production of renin-angiotensin system components.[16] Whether the reductions in abdominal visceral fat with exercise training could be contributing to the observed reductions in BP through alterations in these or other factors is unclear (Figure 39–2).

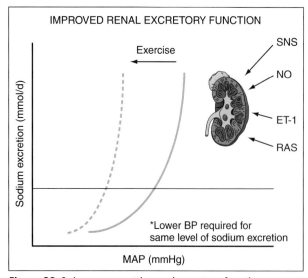

Figure 39–1. Improvement in renal excretory function following reductions in the activity of sympathetic nervous and renin-angiotensin systems.

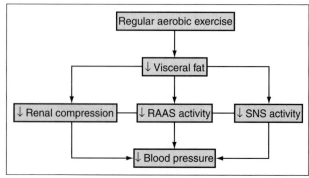

Figure 39–2. Mechanisms by which reduction in abdominal visceral fat might contribute to lower blood pressure.

REGULAR PHYSICAL ACTIVITY AND MULTIPLE LIFESTYLE INTERVENTIONS: ARE THE BP-LOWERING EFFECTS ADDITIVE?

The majority of studies suggest that regular aerobic exercise and weight loss produce similar or only slightly greater reductions in BP than either intervention alone.[84,85] Furthermore, the results of studies that combine multiple lifestyle interventions suggest that the magnitude of BP reduction is in the range of that observed with any single intervention (i.e., weight loss, sodium restriction, or exercise).[86]

Despite similar reductions in BP compared with a single intervention, there are benefits of combining therapies. For example, regular physical activity is one of the best predictors of weight maintenance.[87] Thus, improved weight maintenance and subsequent BP control may be one benefit of combining physical activity with weight loss. From a practical standpoint, some individuals may respond better to weight loss than regular physical activity (for example) and the benefits of these interventions extend beyond lowering BP. Although these issues require further study, they should be considered when implementing nonpharmacological interventions in hypertensive patients.

REGULAR AEROBIC AND MEDICATION REQUIREMENTS IN HYPERTENSION

Antihypertensive medications can be costly and are frequently associated with side effects in some individuals. As such, nonpharmacological therapy of hypertension should be effective in both lowering BP as well as in preventing or reducing the need for antihypertensive medication. In this regard, the antihypertensive effects of regular aerobic exercise can significantly reduce the amount of medication required to control BP.[41]

ROLE OF PHYSICAL ACTIVITY IN THE PREVENTION OF HYPERTENSION

There is no sign that the rising prevalence of obesity seen over the past two decades is dwindling,[88] and the prevalence of hypertension appears to be following closely behind.[89] The majority of the U.S. population is not engaged in adequate levels of physical activity to promote health[90] and is gaining weight at a rate of ~2 pounds per year.[91] Physical inactivity and weight gain are almost invariably associated with elevated BP, perhaps in an additive or synergistic manner. In addition, regular physical activity reduces the risk of weight gain.[87] Thus, physical activity and prevention of weight gain should be complementary therapeutic targets for reducing the problem of hypertension. This is particularly important among those with elevated BP or prehypertension because the risk of developing hypertension in the future is significant for these individuals.[92]

SUMMARY

Physical inactivity is a major risk factor for the development of cardiovascular diseases, including hypertension. There is extensive evidence supporting the favorable role of regular physical activity in the prevention and treatment of hypertension. The mechanisms responsible are unclear. Exercise training does appear to lower BP independently of changes in total body adiposity. However, it is not yet known whether reductions in abdominal visceral fat with exercise training contribute. In addition, BP can be lowered with a single bout of exercise. However, whether this phenomenon contributes to the BP lowering observed with exercise training is uncertain. Finally, the amount of physical activity necessary to lower BP may be as low as 30 minutes/day of continuous or intermittent low- to moderate-intensity exercise on most or all days of the week. The amount of physical activity necessary to prevent weight gain and hypertension may be greater.

REFERENCES

1. American Heart Association. Heart Disease and Stroke Statistics: 2005 Update. 2005.
2. Paffenbarger RS Jr., Blair SN, Lee IM. A history of physical activity, cardiovascular health and longevity: The scientific contributions of Jeremy N Morris, DSc, DPH, FRCP. Int J Epidemiol 2001;30:1184–92.
3. Chobanian AV, Bakris GL, Black HR, et al. The Seventh Report of the Joint National Committee on Prevention, Detection, Evaluation, and Treatment of High Blood Pressure: The JNC 7 report. J Am Med Assoc 2003;289:2560–72.
4. Montoye GJ, Metzner HL, Keller JB. Habitual physical activity and blood pressure. Med Sci Sports Exerc 1972;4:175–81.
5. Reaven PD, Barrett-Connor E, Edelstein S. Relation between leisure-time physical activity and blood pressure in older women. Circulation 1991;83:559–65.
6. Barengo NC, Hu G, Kastarinen M, et al. Low physical activity as a predictor for antihypertensive drug treatment in 25-64-year-old populations in eastern and south-western Finland. J Hypertens 2005;23:293–99.
7. Blair SN, Goodyear NN, Gibbons LW, Cooper KH. Physical fitness and incidence of hypertension in healthy normotensive men and women. J Am Med Assoc 1984;252:487–90.
8. Haapanen N, Miilunpalo S, Vuori I, et al. Association of leisure time physical activity with the risk of coronary heart disease, hypertension and diabetes in middle-aged men and women. Int J Epidemiol 1997;26:739–47.
9. Paffenbarger RS, Wing AL, Hyde RT, Jung DL. Physical activity and incidence of hypertension in college alumni. Am J Epidemiol 1983;117:245–57.
10. Pereira MA, Folsom AR, McGovern PG, et al. Physical activity and incident hypertension in black and white adults: The Atherosclerosis Risk in Communities Study. Prev Med 1999;28:304–12.
11. Hagberg JM, Park JJ, Brown MD. The role of exercise training in the treatment of hypertension: an update. Sports Med 2000;30:193–206.
12. Kelley GA, Kelley KA, Tran ZV. Aerobic exercise and resting blood pressure: A meta-analytic review of randomized, controlled trials. Prev Cardiol 2001; 4:73–80.
13. Whelton SP, Chin A, Xin X, He J. Effect of aerobic exercise on blood pressure: A meta-analysis of randomized, controlled trials. Ann Intern Med 2002;136:493–503.
14. Motoyama M, Sunami Y, Kinoshita F, et al. Blood pressure lowering effect of low intensity aerobic training in elderly hypertensive patients. Med Sci Sports Exerc 1998;30:818–23.
15. Domanski M, Mitchell G, Pfeffer M, et al. Pulse pressure and cardiovascular

disease-related mortality: follow-up study of the Multiple Risk Factor Intervention Trial (MRFIT). *J Am Med Assoc* 2002;287:2677–83.

16. Davy KP, Hall JE. Obesity and hypertension: Two epidemics or one? *Am J Physiol Regul Integr Comp Physiol* 2004;286:R803–13.

17. Hall JE. The kidney, hypertension, and obesity. *Hypertension* 2003;41:625–33.

18. Wong SL, Katzmarzyk P, Nichaman MZ, et al. Cardiorespiratory fitness is associated with lower abdominal fat independent of body mass index. *Med Sci Sports Exerc* 2004;36:286–91.

19. Paffenbarger RS, Hyde RT, Wing AL, and Hsieh CC. Physical activity and hypertension: An epidemiological view. *Annals of Medicine* 1991;23:319–27.

20. Lee S, Kuk JL, Katzmarzyk PT, et al. Cardiorespiratory fitness attenuates metabolic risk independent of abdominal subcutaneous and visceral fat in men. *Diabetes Care* 2005;28:895–901.

21. Fagard RH. Exercise characteristics and the blood pressure response to dynamic physical training. *Med Sci Sports Exerc* 2001;33:S484–92.

22. Hansen TW, Jeppesen J, Rasmussen S, et al. Ambulatory blood pressure and mortality: A population-based study. *Hypertension* 2005;45:499–504.

23. Kikuya M, Ohkubo T, Asayama K, et al. Ambulatory blood pressure and 10-year risk of cardiovascular and noncardiovascular mortality: The Ohasama study. *Hypertension* 2005;45:240–45.

24. Perloff D, Sokolow M, Cowan RM, Juster RP. Prognostic value of ambulatory blood pressure measurements: Further analyses. *J Hypertens Suppl* 1989;7:S3–10.

25. Verdecchia P, Porcellati C, Schillaci G, et al. Ambulatory blood pressure: An independent predictor of prognosis in essential hypertension. *Hypertension* 1994;24:793–801.

26. Pescatello LS, Franklin BA, Fagard R, et al. American College of Sports Medicine position stand. Exercise and hypertension. *Med Sci Sports Exerc* 2004;36:533–53.

27. Brooks GA, Butte NF, Rand WM, et al. Chronicle of the Institute of Medicine physical activity recommendation: How a physical activity recommendation came to be among dietary recommendations. *Am J Clin Nutr* 2004;79:921S–30S.

28. Pate RR, Pratt M, Blair SN, et al. Physical activity and public health: A recommendation from the Centers for Disease Control and Prevention and the American College of Sports Medicine. *J Am Med Assoc* 1995;273:402–07.

29. King AC, Taylor CB, Haskell WL. Effects of differing intensities and formats of 12 months of exercise training on psychological outcomes in older adults. *Health Psychology* 1993;12:292–300.

30. Seals DR, Silverman HG, Reiling MJ, Davy KP. Effect of regular aerobic exercise on elevated blood pressure in postmenopausal women. *Am J Cardiol* 1997;80:49–55.

31. Miyachi M, Kawano H, Sugawara J, et al. Unfavorable effects of resistance training on central arterial compliance: A randomized intervention study. *Circulation* 2004;110:2858–63.

32. Staffileno BA, Braun LT, Rosenson RS. The accumulative effects of physical activity in hypertensive post-menopausal women. *J Cardiovasc Risk* 2001;8:283–90.

33. Kelley GA, Kelley KS, Tran ZV. The effects of exercise on resting blood pressure in children and adolescents: A meta-analysis of randomized controlled trials. *Prev Cardiol* 2003;6:8–16.

34. Garrison RJ, Kannel WB, Stokes J III, Castelli WP. Incidence and precursors of hypertension in young adults: The Framingham Offspring Study. *Prev Med* 1987;16:235–51.

35. Goodfriend TL, Calhoun DA. Resistant hypertension, obesity, sleep apnea, and aldosterone: Theory and therapy. *Hypertension* 2004;43:518–24.

36. Rankinen T, Bouchard C. Genetics and blood pressure response to exercise, and its interactions with adiposity. *Prev Cardiol* 2002;5:138–44.

37. Hagberg JM, Ferrell RE, Dengel DR, Wilund KR. Exercise training-induced blood pressure and plasma lipid improvements in hypertensives may be genotype dependent. *Hypertension* 1999;34:18–23.

38. Blair SN, Kohl HW III, Barlow CE, Gibbons LW. Physical fitness and all-cause mortality in hypertensive men. *Ann Med* 1991;23:307–12.

39. Reaven G, Lithell H, Landsberg L. Hypertension and associated metabolic abnormalities: The role of insulin resistance and the sympathoadrenal system. *New Eng J Med* 1996;334:374–81.

40. Stewart KJ. Exercise training and the cardiovascular consequences of type 2 diabetes and hypertension: plausible mechanisms for improving cardiovascular health. *J Am Med Assoc* 2002;288:1622–31.

41. Kokkinos PF, Narayan P, Colleran JA, et al. Effects of regular exercise on blood pressure and left ventricular hypertrophy in African-American men with severe hypertension. *N Engl J Med* 1995;333:1462–67.

42. Turner MJ, Spina RJ, Kohrt WM, Ehsani AA. Effect of endurance exercise training on left ventricular size and remodeling in older adults with hypertension. *J Gerontol A Biol Sci Med Sci* 2000;55:M245–51.

43. Ehsani AA, Ogawa T, Miller TR, et al. Exercise training improves left ventricular systolic function in older men. *Circulation* 1991;83:96–103.

44. Levy WC, Cerqueira MD, Abrass IB, et al. Endurance exercise training augments diastolic filling at rest and during exercise in healthy young and older men. *Circulation* 1993;88:116–26.

45. Liao D, Arnett D, Tyroler H, et al. Arterial stiffness and the development of hypertension: The ARIC study. *Hypertension* 1999;34:201–06.

46. Boutouyrie P, Tropeano AI, Asmar R, et al. Aortic stiffness is an independent predictor of primary coronary events in hypertensive patients: A longitudinal study. *Hypertension* 2002;39:10–15.

47. Laurent S, Katsahian S, Fassot C, et al. Aortic stiffness is an independent predictor of fatal stroke in essential hypertension. *Stroke* 2003;34:1203–06.

48. Laurent S, Boutouyrie P, Asmar R, et al. Aortic stiffness is an independent predictor of all-cause and cardiovascular mortality in hypertensive patients. *Hypertension* 2001;37:1236–41.

49. Tanaka H, Dinenno FA, Monahan KD, et al. Aging, habitual exercise, and dynamic arterial compliance. *Circulation* 2000;102:1270–75.

50. Seals DR, Tanaka H, Clevenger CM, et al. Blood pressure reductions with exercise and sodium restriction in postmenopausal women with elevated systolic pressure: Role of arterial stiffness. *J Am Coll Cardiol* 2001;38:506–13.

51. Panza J, Garcia C, Kilcoyne C, et al. Impaired endothelium-dependent vasodilation in patients with essential hypertension: Evidence that nitric oxide abnormality is not localized to a single signal transduction pathway. *Circulation* 1995;91:1732–38.

52. Cardillo C, Campia U, Kilcoyne CM, et al. Improved endothelium-dependent vasodilation after blockade of endothelin receptors in patients with essential hypertension. *Circulation* 2002;105:452–56.

53. Higashi Y, Sasaki S, Nakagawa K, et al. Effect of obesity on endothelium-dependent, nitric oxide-mediated vasodilation in normotensive individuals and patients with essential hypertension. *Am J Hypertens* 2001;14:1038–45.

54. Jern S, Wall U, Bergbrant A, et al. Endothelium-dependent vasodilation and tissue-type plasminogen activator release in borderline hypertension. *Arterioscler Thromb Vasc Biol* 1997;17:3376–83.

55. Higashi Y, Sasaki S, Kurisu S, et al. Regular aerobic exercise augments endothelium-dependent vascular relaxation in normotensive as well as hypertensive subjects: Role of endothelium-derived nitric oxide. *Circulation* 1999;100:1194–202.

56. Higashi Y, Yoshizumi M. Exercise and endothelial function: role of endothelium-derived nitric oxide and oxidative stress in healthy subjects and hypertensive patients. *Pharmacol Ther* 2004;102:87–96.

57. Van Guilder GP, Smith DT, Hoetzer GL, et al. Endothelial T-PA release is impaired in overweight and obese adults but can be improved with regular aerobic exercise. *Am J Physiol Endocrinol Metab* 2005;289:E807–13.

58. Schrijvers BF, De Vriese AS, Flyvbjerg A. From hyperglycemia to diabetic kidney disease: The role of metabolic, hemodynamic, intracellular factors and growth factors/cytokines. *Endocr Rev* 2004;25:971–1010.

59. Chagnac A, Weinstein T, Herman M, et al. The effects of weight loss on renal function in patients with severe obesity. *J Am Soc Nephrol* 2003;14:1480–86.

60. Hill L. Arterial pressure in man while sleeping, resting, working, bathing. *J Physiol London* 1898;XXII:228.

61. Halliwill JR. Mechanisms and clinical implications of post-exercise hypotension in humans. *Exerc Sport Sci Rev* 2001;29:65–70.

62. Hagberg JM, Montain SJ, Martin WH III. Blood pressure and hemodynamic responses after exercise in older hypertensives. *J Appl Physiol* 1987;63:270–76.

63. Brandao Rondon MU, Alves MJ, Braga AM, et al. Postexercise blood pressure reduction in elderly hypertensive patients. *J Am Coll Cardiol* 2002;39:676–82.

64. Taylor-Tolbert NS, Dengel DR, Brown MD, et al. Ambulatory blood pressure

after acute exercise in older men with essential hypertension. *Am J Hypertens* 2000;13:44–51.

65. Wilkins BW, Minson CT, Halliwill JR. Regional hemodynamics during postexercise hypotension. II. Cutaneous circulation. *J Appl Physiol* 2004;97:2071–76.

66. Pricher MP, Holowatz LA, Williams JT, et al. Regional hemodynamics during postexercise hypotension. I. Splanchnic and renal circulations. *J Appl Physiol* 2004;97:2065–70.

67. Grassi G, Seravalle G, Calhoun DA, Mancia G. Physical training and baroreceptor control of sympathetic nerve activity in humans. *Hypertension* 1994;23:294–301.

68. Brown MD, Dengel DR, Hogikyan RV, Supiano MA. Sympathetic activity and the heterogenous blood pressure response to exercise training in hypertensives. *J Appl Physiol* 2002;92:1434–42.

69. Meredith TT, Friberg P, Jennings GL, et al. Exercise training lowers resting renal but not cardiac sympathetic activity in humans. *Hypertension* 1991;18:575–82.

70. Duncan JJ, Farr JE, Upton SJ, et al. The effects of aerobic exercise on plasma catecholamines and blood pressure in patients with mild essential hypertension. *J Am Med Assoc* 1985;254:2609–13.

71. Kohno K, Matsuoka H, Takenaka K, et al. Renal depressor mechanisms of physical training in patients with essential hypertension. *Am J Hypertens* 1997;10:859–68.

72. Dubbert PM, Martin JE, Cushman WC, et al. Endurance exercise in mild hypertension: Effects on blood pressure and associated metabolic and quality of life variables. *J Hum Hypertens* 1994;8:265–72.

73. Boyce ML, Robergs RA, Avasthi PS, et al. Exercise training by individuals with predialysis renal failure:

Cardiorespiratory endurance, hypertension, and renal function. *Am J Kidney Dis* 1997;30:180–92.

74. Hagberg JM, Goldberg AP, Ehsani AA, et al. Exercise training improves hypertension in hemodialysis patients. *Am J Nephrol* 1983;3:209–12.

75. Neter JE, Stam BE, Kok FJ, et al. Influence of weight reduction on blood pressure: A meta-analysis of randomized controlled trials. *Hypertension* 2003;42:878–84.

76. Staessen J, Fagard R, Amery A. The relationship between body weight and blood pressure. *J Hum Hypertens* 1988;2:207–17.

77. Barba G, Russo O, Siani A, et al. Plasma leptin and blood pressure in men: Graded association independent of body mass and fat pattern. *Obes Res* 2003;11:160–66.

78. Kanai H, Matsuzawa Y, Kotani K, et al. Close correlation of intra-abdominal fat accumulation to hypertension in obese women. *Hypertension* 1990;16:484–90.

79. Zhu S, Wang Z, Heshka S, et al. Waist circumference and obesity-associated risk factors among whites in the third National Health and Nutrition Examination Survey: Clinical action thresholds. *Am J Clin Nutr* 2002;76:743–49.

80. Siani A, Cappuccio FP, Barba G, et al. The relationship of waist circumference to blood pressure: The Olivetti Heart Study. *Am J Hypertens* 2002;15:780–86.

81. Doll S, Paccaud F, Bovet P, et al. Body mass index, abdominal adiposity and blood pressure: Consistency of their association across developing and developed countries. *Int J Obes Relat Metab Disord* 2002;26:48–57.

82. Ford ES, Giles WH, Dietz WH. Prevalence of the metabolic syndrome among US adults: Findings from the third National Health and Nutrition Examination Survey. *J Am Med Assoc* 2002;287:356–59.

83. Dyer AR, Liu K, Walsh M, et al. Ten-year incidence of elevated blood pressure and its predictors: The CARDIA study. Coronary Artery Risk Development in (Young) Adults. *J Hum Hypertens* 1999;13:13–21.

84. Hinderliter A, Sherwood A, Gullette EC, et al. Reduction of left ventricular hypertrophy after exercise and weight loss in overweight patients with mild hypertension. *Arch Intern Med* 2002;162:1333–39.

85. Dengel DR, Galecki AT, Hagberg JM, Pratley RE. The independent and combined effects of weight loss and aerobic exercise on blood pressure and oral glucose tolerance in older men. *Am J Hypertens* 1998;11:1405–12.

86. Miller ER III, Erlinger TP, Young DR, et al. Results of the Diet, Exercise, and Weight Loss Intervention Trial (DEW-IT). *Hypertension* 2002;40:612–18.

87. Jakicic JM. The role of physical activity in prevention and treatment of body weight gain in adults. *J Nutr* 2002;132:3826S–9S.

88. Hedley AA, Ogden CL, Johnson CL, et al. Prevalence of overweight and obesity among US children, adolescents, and adults, 1999–2002. *J Am Med Assoc* 2004;291:2847–50.

89. Fields LE, Burt VL, Cutler JA, et al. The burden of adult hypertension in the United States 1999 to 2000: A rising tide. *Hypertension* 2004;44:398–404.

90. Centers for Disease Control and Prevention. New physical activity measures include lifestyle activities-United States, 2001. *Morbidity and Mortality Weekly Reports* 2003;52:764–69.

91. Hill JO, Wyatt HR, Reed GW, Peters JC. Obesity and the environment: Where do we go from here? *Science* 2003;299:853–55.

92. Winegarden CR. From "prehypertension" to hypertension? Additional evidence. *Ann Epidemiol* 2005:15:720–25.

Chapter

40

Electrolyte Intake and Human Hypertension

Vamadevan S. Ajay, Dorairaj Prabhakaran, and Kolli Srinath Reddy

Key Findings

- Essential or primary hypertension is a sustained systolic blood pressure (BP) of greater than 140 mmHg or a diastolic BP of greater than 90 mmHg among adults of 18 years and above. Normal BP is systolic pressure of < 120 mmHg and a diastolic pressure of < 80 mmHg. Pre-hypertension is a systolic pressure of 130 to 139 mmHg or a diastolic pressure of 85 to 89 mmHg. Individuals with pre-hypertension (which is not a disease category) are at high risk for developing hypertension.

- Those in whom large changes in BP are caused by a severe abrupt change in salt intake or excretion are said to be sodium sensitive.

- Those in whom the least change in arterial pressure occurs after abrupt change in salt intake or excretion are said to be sodium resistant.

- BP may be affected by intake of electrolytes such as Na^+ and K^+, and possibly Ca^{2+} and Mg^{2+}.

- Renal mechanisms (including nephron heterogeneity, non-modulation, and altered pressure natriuresis) are involved in electrolyte-intake-related hypertension.

- From epidemiology and intervention studies, Na^+ or K^+ intake has been shown to elevate or lower (respectively) BP.

- Interventional studies with Ca^{2+} and Mg^{2+} supplementation have inconsistent effects on BP.

INTRODUCTION

Dietary electrolytes have an established relationship with human BP. Considerable evidence suggests a positive association between dietary sodium chloride (common salt) intake and BP.[1] In addition, dietary patterns associated with low intakes of potassium, calcium, and possibly magnesium are associated with higher levels of BP.[2]

An understanding of the association of the dietary electrolytes and BP has important implications not only for the prevention and treatment of hypertension but for developing population-based strategies to decrease cardiovascular disease risk by shifting the overall BP distribution toward lower levels. In this chapter we review the relationship of electrolyte intake and human hypertension.

SODIUM AND ESSENTIAL HYPERTENSION

The seventh report of the Joint National Committee on Prevention, Detection, Evaluation, and Treatment of High Blood Pressure defines *essential* or *primary hypertension* as a sustained systolic pressure of greater than 140 mmHg or a diastolic BP of greater than 90 mmHg among adults of 18 years and above.[3] Normal BP is systolic pressure of < 120 mmHg and a diastolic pressure of < 80 mmHg. *Pre-hypertension* is a systolic pressure of 130 to 139 mmHg or a diastolic pressure of 85 to 89 mmHg. Individuals with pre-hypertension (which is not a disease category) are at high risk for developing hypertension.

Those individuals in whom a severe abrupt change in salt intake or excretion induces large changes in BP are referred to as salt sensitive, whereas those in whom these maneuvers cause the least change in arterial pressure are termed salt resistant.[4] Weinberger defines salt sensitivity as a 10-mmHg or greater difference in mean BP between the level measured after 4 hours of infusion of 2 L normal saline compared to the level measured the morning after a day of a 10-mmol sodium diet, during which three oral doses of furosemide were given at 10 AM, 2 PM, and 6 PM.[5]

Changes in human dietary intake

Eaton and Konner have suggested that each species, including man, is genetically programmed to eat and metabolize specific foods (and that there is an optimum type and composition of food needed by them).[6] Therefore, whereas a lion or tiger is programmed to eat animal food exclusively, the cow or the deer is programmed to eat plant foods only. The nutrients provided by such food habits of these animals are believed to provide optimum nutrition to them. In wild animals, the genetic programming does not include any processing of food in the form of removal of or enrichment with any nutrient components.

Humans have the capacity to consume and metabolize both plant and animal food.[6,7] The human genetic program, which has remained essentially unchanged for the past 100,000 years, is most compatible with unprocessed mixed foods (that is, foods without removal of any nutrient components and without addition of any nutrients or other compounds). According to this theory, man-made changes in the composition of foods and diets would cause (or at least predispose man to) several pathological conditions (including elevated BP).[6,7]

One of the major reasons for the increased burden of hypertension worldwide is alteration in dietary habits and the way foods are being processed. Thus, a shift from simple foods to highly processed complex food (the preservation of which requires salt) has led to changes in the electrolyte consumption pattern of several populations. In addition, a shift to processed food results in lower consumption of fruits and vegetables (which are rich in dietary potassium and other micronutrients).

Evidence for the role of excess sodium intake in hypertension

Animal models

Animal models provide strong evidence for the link between high sodium intake and elevated BP. Experiments in chimpanzees, which are phylogenetically close to the human, show that the addition of NaCl (5, 10, and then 15 g/d) to the chimpanzee's usual diet (a fruit-and-vegetable diet low in NaCl and high in potassium) over 20 months results in significant and progressive elevations of BP.[8] After 84 weeks of added NaCl, the mean systolic and diastolic BPs increased by 33 mmHg and 10 mmHg (respectively) relative to both baseline values and a control group.

Within six months of cessation of the high-NaCl intake the elevated levels were completely reversed. In African green monkeys, a diet containing 6% salt for three months significantly increased the systolic and diastolic BP by 27 and 15 mmHg, respectively. Dahl salt-sensitive rats, a genetic animal model of hypertension, develop hypertension when they are fed a high-salt diet.[9] Hypertensive rats are also susceptible to salt-induced hypertension, although they exhibit hypertension and end-organ damage without high salt treatment.[10] Animal studies suggest that diets high in NaCl may also have deleterious cardiovascular consequences independent of BP (e.g., cerebral arterial disease and stroke, left ventricular hypertrophy, renal vascular disease, and glomerular injury).[11]

Human studies

Observational studies

The International Study of Salt and Blood Pressure (INTERSALT) evaluated both within-population and a cross population hypotheses on the relationship between BP and sodium excretion in more than 10,000 adults (aged 20 to 59 years) at 52 centers around the world.[1] In this study, the 24-hour sodium excretion was significantly related to median systolic and diastolic BP, the upward slope of systolic and diastolic BP with age, and the prevalence of high BP.[1] The within-population analyses demonstrated that for individuals the relationship between sodium excretion and BP was similar for nonhypertensive and all participants, indicating that varying degrees of salt sensitivity of BP occur throughout the population.

This study concluded that for individuals a difference of 100 mEq (6 g salt) per day of sodium intake is associated with an average difference of 3 to 6 mmHg in systolic BP. For populations a 100-mEq/day lower sodium intake is associated with reduction in the rise of systolic BP by 10 mmHg in persons aged 25 to 55 years. Another study,

Cardiovascular Diseases and Alimentary Comparison (CARDIAC), carried out in at least 3,681 men and 3,653 women aged 50 to 54 years from 60 centers in 25 countries worldwide examined the relationship between 24-hour sodium excretion and BP.[12]

This study showed that systolic BP and diastolic BP were positively associated with 24-hour sodium excretion. The cross-center correlation analyses indicated positive correlations between urinary salt excretion and systolic or diastolic BP in both men and women, although the association was significant only in the men (0.98 and 0.68 mmHg per urinary salt excretion (g/day) for systolic and diastolic BP, respectively).

Another example is a community-based program on prevention of hypertension from North Karelia, Finland, initiated in 1972. In this study from 1972 to 1977, BP levels improved among patients and eventually started to stabilize during 1977 to 1982, although only 10% of the population aged 35 to 64 years was treated with anti-hypertensive medication.[13] Upon exploring the factors contributing to the BP level, analyses confirmed that high sodium intake, high BMI, high fat intake, and alcohol drinking were significantly associated with BP both in the general population and in hypertensive persons. Furthermore, a high level of dietary sodium was also associated with unsatisfactory outcome of drug treatment among hypertensives. The North Karelia Salt Project also demonstrated that it is difficult to reduce salt intake at the community level during a short period and that a well-conceived program for a relatively long time period would be required to reduce the mean BP levels of the population.[13]

Intervention trials

The Dietary Approaches to Stop Hypertension (DASH) trial evaluated the effects on BP of three dietary patterns over eight weeks in 459 adults with high-normal BP or mild hypertension.[14] The dietary interventions included (1) a control diet with potassium, calcium, and magnesium levels close to the 25th percentile of U.S. consumption, (2) a diet rich in fruits and vegetables, and (3) a "combination" diet rich in fruits, vegetables, and fat-free or low-fat dairy products. Compared with the control diet, the intervention diets had a relatively higher content of potassium, calcium, magnesium, fiber, protein, carotenoid, and folate (whereas total fat, saturated fat, and cholesterol levels were lower).

NaCl content was equivalent in all three diets (7.5 g/d). Systolic and diastolic BPs were significantly reduced by a greater extent with the combination diet (–5.5/ –3.0 mmHg), followed by the diet enriched with fruits and vegetables (–2.8/–1.1 mmHg) among men and women and across all ethnic groups compared to the control diet group. BP reduction was more pronounced in hypertensive persons (–11.4/–5.5 mmHg), followed by normotensives (–3.5/–2.1 mmHg).

The DASH-II trial assigned individuals with BP ranging from 120/80 to159/95 to a control diet or the DASH combination diet randomized to one of three dietary sodium levels [high (150 mmol/d), intermediate (100 mmol/d), or low (50 mmol/d)] in a randomized crossover design.[15] The corresponding urinary sodium excretion values were 143 mmol/d on the high-, 107 mmol/d on the inter-mediate, and 66 mmol/d on the low-sodium diets (respec-tively), indicating a quite good adherence to the goal sodium intake. There was a graded reduction in BP with each level of reduced salt intake on both the control and DASH combination diets.

The mean difference in BP between those on the highest and lowest levels of sodium intake receiving the DASH diet was 12 mmHg (equivalent to that of potent antihypertensive drugs), substantiating that the DASH diet had a greater effect in reducing BP on the two higher levels of salt intake in comparison to the control diet. Among subgroups, African Americans had the greatest decrease in BP with dietary salt reduction. As in the earlier DASH trial, no adverse effects of dietary salt reduction were observed.

Evidence from ecological studies

Migration studies provide substantial evidence for the relationship between salt intake and BP. They primarily demonstrate acculturation of individuals from low-salt-eating countries whose BP rise with changes in their life-styles in the new environment, leading to increased consumption of salt. The seminal Kenyan Luo migration study carried out in a Kenyan agricultural community in which subsistence farmers traditionally ate a low-salt/high-potassium diet demonstrated the effect of migration on BP elegantly. Upon migration to an urban community their diet underwent marked changes.[16] Specifically, there was a substantial increase in salt intake coupled with low potassium intake similar to the diet in westernized societies. BP in these migrants rose after a few months (+6.9/6.2 mmHg for systolic and diastolic), whereas it did not increase in a control group who did not migrate (suggesting that some of the changes in BP are associated with urbanization, resulting in changes in dietary elec-trolyte consumption patterns).

Similarly the Yi Migrant Study from china demonstrated that changes in lifestyle, including higher intake of dietary sodium, contribute to a rise in BP.[17] The Yi people, an ethnic minority residing in a remote mountainous envi-ronment in southwestern China, consume a sodium-poor diet. Their BP rose very little with increasing age (0.13 and 0.23 mmHg/yr for systolic and diastolic, respec-tively). In contrast, Yi migrants who lived in urban areas who consumed a sodium-rich diet experienced a much greater increase in BP with progressive aging (0.33 and 0.33 mmHg/yr for systolic and diastolic, respectively).

Similar to Yi migrants, a significant positive relationship was found between sodium intake and BP among native (Han) men living in the urban areas. These findings support the role of environment in determining the dietary elec-trolytes intake and their impact on BP. Apart from these intra-country migrations, there are several examples of migration from one country to another leading to altera-tions in dietary practice with potential increases in sodium intake (resulting high BP in migrants compared to non-migrants).[18,19]

POTASSIUM AND ESSENTIAL HYPERTENSION

Introduction

Potassium (K) intake has been hypothesized to play an important role in determining BP levels, cardiac output, and peripheral vascular resistance (indirectly contributing to the epidemic of hypertension). Potassium acts indirectly be reducing body sodium levels. The excretion of excess sodium is markedly improved by increased intakes of potassium, calcium, and magnesium.[20]

Both in normal subjects and hypertensive subjects, BP is influenced by the dietary potassium intake.[21] In normal humans, dietary potassium depletion raises BP, and this is associated with a blunted ability to handle acute sodium load and sodium retention. A low-potassium diet (16 mmol/day) for 10 days increases systolic and diastolic pressures by 7 and 6 mmHg, respectively, relative to 10 days on a high-potassium diet (96 mmol/day) among the borderline hypertensive patients.[22] Dietary sodium excess increases urinary potassium excretion among normal human subjects. This is associated with a small fall in plasma potassium concentration. This effect can be attenuated by dietary potassium supplementation. This supplementation also attenuates the BP increase seen in diabetic children on a high-sodium diet.[22]

The BP-lowering effect of potassium involves several mechanisms, such as increased natriuresis, reduced sym-pathetic nervous activity, and decreased pressor response to noradrenaline and angiotensin II. Among hyperten-sives, an increase in the level of potassium intake by approximately 1.8 to 1.9 g a day lowers the BP of hyper-tensive subjects so that the average fall in systolic BP is approximately 4 mmHg and that of diastolic pressure about 2.5 mmHg.[20]

In addition, potassium may protect against stroke and other cardiovascular diseases by mechanisms unrelated to BP. Potassium is also linked to antiatherosclerotic proper-ties and is claimed to improve glucose tolerance.[20]

Thus, dietary supplementation of potassium can lower BP in normal and some hypertensive patients. Compared to NaCl restriction, the response to potassium supplemen-tation is slow to appear, taking approximately four weeks. Dietary potassium supplementation also reduces the need for antihypertensive medication and may even reduce organ system complications (e.g., stroke). Salt-sensitive hypertension responds to an extent because supplemen-tation with potassium increases the urinary excretion of sodium chloride.[22]

Pathogenetic mechanisms

The antihypertensive effect of dietary potassium supple-mentation involves several mechanisms. It is hypothe-sized that dietary potassium stimulates Na^+-K^+-ATPase in vascular smooth muscle cells and adrenergic nerve terminals, resulting in vasodilatation.[23,24] Further, dietary potassium supplementation also potentiates endothelium-dependent relaxation.[25] In later stages these changes may relate to more than a simple increase in turnover of Na^+-K^+-ATPase, resulting in a quasi-permanent increase in the number of enzyme molecules (termed *potassium adaptation*).

High intake of potassium over a long term induces an increased capacity for potassium secretion in the colon, as well as in a segment of the collecting duct of the kidney.[26] Aldosterone has been cited as the stimulus for both of these effects. Thus, long-term potassium loading and chronic hyperaldosteronism induce similar changes in epithelia in the colon and kidney, capable of potassium secretion. Apart from increased potassium secretion, these changes encompass an increase in the number of Na^+-K^+-ATPase pump sites, resulting in attenuation of the vasoconstriction seen in various hypertensive states. Increased turnover of the pumps (acute administration of K^+) or increased number of pumps (chronic administration of K^+) or both results in increased pumping.[22]

Potassium adaptation accounts for the stability of plasma potassium concentration in the face of altered potassium intake and for the delay in the antihypertensive response to dietary potassium supplementation in hypertensive subjects (the delay is more than four weeks versus one to two days in the case of sodium restriction). Hence, increased dietary potassium can lower BP in animals and humans, particularly if they have salt-sensitive hypertension (decreasing the need for antihypertensive medication).

Evidence for the role of potassium deficiency in hypertension
Animal models

There are several animal studies on the effect of potassium intake and changes in BP. Studies have documented reduction in BP in rats with reduced renal mass-saline hypertension after increased dietary potassium intake. Potassium intake significantly reduces arterial BP in the spontaneously hypertensive rat (SHR, a strain of rats generally used for studies in hypertension and cardiovascular research) through a phenomenon associated with a restoration of the endothelium-derived hyperpolarizing factor (EDHF)-mediated responses in the mesenteric vascular bed.[22,27]

It has been reported that the Dahl salt-sensitive rat receiving a 1% sodium chloride diet has a minimum BP when eating 1.6% KCl and responds to a reduction in KCl intake with an increase in BP.[22,28] Further, among rats a small increase in dietary potassium confers some protection against the effects of excess dietary sodium (attenuating the increase in pressure and increasing longevity, mainly by preventing strokes).[22]

Human studies
Observational studies

The international cooperative INTERSALT study (which explored the relationships among population mean sodium, potassium intake, and BP) showed that BP tends to be inversely related to urinary potassium excretion and directly related to the ratio of urinary sodium excretion to potassium excretion.[21] In this study, a significant positive association was found between 24-hour urinary sodium excretion and systolic BP as well as between the sodium/potassium ratio and systolic BP. It is reported that potas-

sium excretion of individuals was significantly and independently related inversely to their systolic BP.

Intervention trials

The DASH study demonstrated the role of dietary potassium in reducing BP. The DASH study has been discussed in detail in the section "Evidence for the Role of Sodium in Hypertension." Although the antihypertensive effect of DASH diet has been mainly attributed to a higher dietary potassium level (through consumption of fruits and vegetables), the contribution of potassium in the beneficial antihypertensive effect of the DASH diet is difficult to assess because multiple dietary changes occur at initiation of the diet.[22]

Ethnic differences

Several studies have showed that African American subjects consumed less potassium than Caucasian subjects and that high BP in African American subjects is associated with low potassium intake. The increased prevalence of high BP in the African American subjects may not to be related to greater dietary intake of sodium chloride, as the intake of sodium appears similar in African and Caucasian Americans and could be largely due to low-potassium diets.[22]

A study on effects of race and dietary potassium has demonstrated that in most normotensive black men, but not white men, salt sensitivity occurs when dietary potassium is even marginally deficient but is dose-dependently suppressed when dietary potassium is increased within its normal range. It is believed that such suppression might prevent or delay the occurrence of hypertension, particularly in the many blacks in whom dietary potassium is deficient.[29]

CALCIUM AND ESSENTIAL HYPERTENSION

Metabolic studies suggest that calcium may have a role in the regulation of BP. Elevated free calcium in the cytoplasm of smooth muscle cells of the vascular system creates an increased resistance in the small arterioles precipitating high BP. Several mechanisms have been invoked to explain the role of calcium in hypertension. Dietary components such as vitamin D and minerals (such as magnesium, sodium, potassium, and phosphorus) may modify calcium metabolism through alteration in the membrane pump, which controls the flow of calcium in and out of the cell. Vitamin D is essential for intestinal absorption of calcium and for the synthesis of calcium-binding protein, which serves as a carrier of calcium to the serosal side of the membrane (where calcium is actively transported out of the cell via the Na^+/Ca^{2+} exchanger). Thus, vitamin D deficiency will result in elevated free calcium in smooth muscle cells.[30] Cellular calcium metabolism may be partly mediated by calcium-regulating hormones that tend to be elevated in essential hypertension such as PTH and calcitriol.[31]

Recent studies using Na^+/Ca^{2+} exchange inhibitors and studies in mice demonstrate that salt-dependent hypertension is triggered by Ca^{2+} entry through Na^+/Ca^{2+} exchanger type 1 (NCX1) in arterial smooth muscle.[32] Endogenous cardiac glycosides (such as ouabain, marinobufagenin, proscillaridin A, and bufalin), which contribute to salt-dependent hypertension, seem to be necessary for NCX1-mediated hypertension. When cardiac glycosides inhibit Na^+, K^+-ATPase in arterial smooth muscle cells, the elevation of local Na^+ on the submembrane area is believed to facilitate Ca^+ entry through NCX1 (resulting in vasoconstriction).

Few epidemiological studies reported that people with a higher intake of calcium tend to have lower BP. A Cochrane review combining 13 RCTs found that participants receiving calcium supplementation compared to control found a significant reduction in systolic BP (mean difference of –2.5 mmHg) but not diastolic BP (mean difference of –0.8 mmHg).[33] The review concluded that due to the poor quality of trials and due to their heterogeneity the evidence in favor of causal association between calcium supplementation and BP reduction is weak and is probably due to bias. The review suggested the need for larger, longer-duration, and better-quality double-blind placebo controlled trials in assessing the effects of calcium supplementation on BP and cardiovascular outcomes.

MAGNESIUM AND ESSENTIAL HYPERTENSION

Magnesium homeostasis has important bearing on other cations, such as calcium and potassium. In humans, optimal BP depends on a balance of both Na:K and Mg:Ca ratios at both cellular and whole-body levels.[34] Dietary magnesium is directly proportional to dietary calcium. Magnesium deficiency can alter calcium metabolism even when calcium intake is adequate, resulting in a state of high intracellular calcium, low serum calcium, and low urinary calcium states. High intracellular calcium and high cellular Na:K ratio both occur when cellular magnesium ratio becomes too low and the Mg-ATP-driven sodium-potassium pump and calcium pump become functionally impaired. As discussed earlier, high intracellular calcium has several vasoconstrictor effects that lead to hypertension (an indirect result of low-magnesium status).

Hypertension occurs when cellular Na:K ratios become too high, a consequence of a high-sodium/low-potassium diet. Magnesium deficiency can precipitate a pseudo potassium deficit.[34] In addition, magnesium status has a direct relationship with the relaxation capability of vascular smooth muscle cells and cellular $Na^+:K^+$ ratio. As a result, nutritional magnesium has both direct and indirect impacts on the regulation of BP and hypertension. Magnesium supplementation above 15 mmol per day is required to normalize high BP in unmedicated hypertensive patients, while 15 mmol per day will lower high BP in patients treated with antihypertensive medications. The knowledge that low magnesium (impact of the Mg:Ca ratio) causes imbalance in both cellular and physiological calcium points toward the conclusion that hypertensives may have abnormal calcium metabolism.[34]

Even though metabolic and experimental studies suggest that magnesium may have a role in the regulation of BP, epidemiological evidence on the effects of magnesium on BP is inconsistent. A recently published Cochrane review evaluated 12 randomized control trials (RCTs) on the effects of magnesium supplementation as treatment for primary hypertension in adults.[35] The results of the individual trials were heterogeneous. Combining all trials, participants receiving magnesium supplements as compared to control did not significantly reduce systolic BP but did have a statistically significant reduction in diastolic BP. Due to the poor quality of trials and the heterogeneity among trials, the evidence in favor of a causal association between magnesium supplementation and BP reduction was weak.

DIETARY CHANGES FOR OPTIMAL ELECTROLYTE INTAKE

A transition toward modern diets has led to a substantial decline of K^+ intake compared with traditional (natural) food habits, and a large fraction of the population might now have suboptimal K^+ intake. A high K^+ intake has been reported to have protective effects against several conditions affecting the cardiovascular system, kidneys, and bones.[36] The levels of sodium, potassium, calcium, and magnesium provided by the typical current diet are significantly different in amounts and ratios than the natural diet. If a daily energy need of 2,100 kcal is satisfied by a natural diet composition, the daily intake of sodium is approximately 500 mg, that of potassium about 7,400 mg, that of calcium approximately 1,100 mg, and that of magnesium about 800 mg.

It is reported that in the average U.S. diet the energy-standardized intake (per 2,100 kcal) of sodium was about 3,000 mg a day (that is, approximately sixfold compared with the genetically programmed diet). The potassium intake was as low as 1,750 mg, which is only 24% of the amount provided by the natural diet. Further, the daily intake of calcium (about 440 mg) from modern diet is remarkably lower than that from the natural diet (approximately 40% only). Even the usual intake of magnesium (approximately 180 mg) is also very low (approximately 23% of the optimal requirement) compared with the amount provided by the natural diet.

The recommended dietary reference intake (DRI) for sodium is 1,500 mg a day, whereas 2,500 mg has been given as the maximum level of daily intake likely to pose no risk of adverse effects. The average current sodium intake of 3,000 to 4,500 mg a day in various westernized communities exceeds clearly even the highest sodium intake level, which has been estimated to be safe. The recommended intake of potassium for adolescents and adults is 4,700 mg/day. Recommended intake of potassium for children 1 to 3 years of age is 3,000 mg/day, for 4 to 8 years of age 3,800 mg/day, and for 9 to 13 years of age 4,500 mg/day. The DRI for calcium is 1,000 to 1,300 mg per day. The magnesium intake recommendation is 420 mg for adult men.[20,37]

SUMMARY

Electrolytes play an important role in determining the BP levels of both normotensive and hypertensive subjects. The mechanisms by which they influence BP are complex and involve the interplay of several factors. Simple alterations in the diet to enhance potassium intake and reduce sodium levels are extremely useful measures in reducing BP in individuals with hypertension and in maintaining "normotension" among individuals with normal BP.

REFERENCES

1. INTERSALT Cooperative Research Group. INTERSALT, An international study of electrolyte excretion and blood pressure: Results for 24 hour urinary sodium and potassium excretion. *BMJ* 1988;297:319–28.
2. Kotchen TA, McCarron DA. Dietary electrolytes and blood pressure: A statement for healthcare professionals from the American Heart Association Nutrition Committee. *Circulation* 1998; 98(6):613–17.
3. Chobanian AV, Bakris GL, Black HR, Cushman WC, Green LA, Izzo JL Jr., et al. Seventh report of the Joint National Committee on Prevention, Detection, Evaluation, and Treatment of High Blood Pressure. *Hypertension* 2003;42(6):1206–52.
4. Meneton P, Jeunemaitre X, de Wardener HE, MacGregor GA. Links between dietary salt intake, renal salt handling, blood pressure, and cardiovascular diseases. *Physiol Rev* 2005;85(2):679–715.
5. Weinberger MH, Miller JZ, Luft FC, Grim CE, Fineberg NS. Definitions and characteristics of sodium sensitivity and blood pressure resistance. *Hypertension* 1986;8(6/2):II127–34.
6. Eaton SB, Konner M. Paleolithic nutrition: A consideration of its nature and current implications. *N Engl J Med* 1985;312:283–89.
7. Eaton SB, Eaton SB III. Paleolithic vs modern diets: Selected pathophysiological implications. *Eur J Nutr* 2000;39:67–70.
8. Orlov SN, Adragna NC, Adarichev VA, Hamet P. Genetic and biochemical determinants of abnormal monovalent ion transport in primary hypertension. *Am J Physiol* 1999;276(3/1):C511–36.
9. Dahl LK, Heine M, Thompson K. Genetic influence of the kidneys on blood pressure: Evidence from chronic renal homografts in rats with opposite predispositions to hypertension. *Circ Res* 1974;40:94–101.
10. Ganguli M, Tobian L. Dietary K determines NaCl sensitivity in NaCl-induced rises of blood pressure in spontaneously hypertensive rats. *Am J Hypertens* 1990;3:482–84.
11. MacGregor GA. Salt: More adverse effects. *Am J Hypertens* 1997;10:37S–41S.
12. Yamori Y, Nara Y, Mizushima S et al. International cooperative study on the relationship between dietary factors and blood pressure: A report from the Cardiovascular Diseases and Alimentary Comparison (CARDIAC) Study. *J Cardiovasc Pharmacol* 1990;16:S43–47.
13. Tuomilehto J, Puska P, Nissinen A, Salonen J, Tanskanen A, Pietinen P, et al. Community-based prevention of hypertension in North Karelia, Finland. *Ann Clin Res* 1984;16(43):18–27.
14. Appel LJ, Moore TJ, Obarzanek E, Vollmer WM, Svetkey LP, Sacks FM, et al., for the DASH Collaborative Research Group. A clinical trial of the effects of dietary patterns on blood pressure. *N Engl J Med* 1997;336:1117–24.
15. Sacks FM, Svetkey LP, Vollmer WM, Appel LJ, Bray GA, Harsha D, et al., for the DASH-Sodium Collaborative Research Group. Effects on blood pressure of reduced dietary sodium and the Dietary Approaches to Stop Hypertension (DASH) diet. *N Engl J Med* 2001;344(1):3–10.
16. Poulter N, Khaw KT, Hopwood BE, Mugambi M, Peart WS, Rose G, et al. Blood pressure and associated factors in a rural Kenyan community. *Hypertension* 1984;6:810–13.
17. He J, Klag MJ, Whelton PK, Chen JY, Mo JP, Qian MC, et al. Migration, blood pressure pattern, and hypertension: The Yi Migrant Study. *Am J Epidemiol* 1991;134:1085–1101.
18. Patel JV, Vyas A, Cruickshank JK, Prabhakaran D, Hughes E, Reddy KS, et al. Impact of migration on coronary heart disease risk factors: Comparison of Gujaratis in Britain and their contemporaries in villages of origin in India. *Atherosclerosis* 2006;185(2):297–306.
19. Winkelstein W Jr., Kagan A, Kato H, Sacks ST. Epidemiologic studies of coronary heart disease and stroke in Japanese men living in Japan, Hawaii and California: Blood pressure distributions. *Am J Epidemiol* 1975;102(6):502–13.
20. Karppanen H, Karppanen P, Mervaala E. Why and how to implement sodium, potassium, calcium, and magnesium changes in food items and diets? *J Hum Hypertens* 2005;19(3):S10–19.
21. Stamler J, Rose G, Eliot P, Dyer A, Marmot M, Kesteloot H, et al. Findings of the international cooperative INTERSALT study. *Hypertension* 1991; 17(1):9–15.
22. Francis J. Haddy, Paul M. Vanhoutte, Michel Feletou. Role of potassium in regulating blood flow and blood pressure. *Am J Physiol Regul Integr Comp Physiol* 2006;290:R546–52.
23. Haddy FJ. Potassium effects on contraction in arterial smooth muscle mediated by Na+-K+-ATPase. *Fed Proc* 1983;42:239–45.
24. Haddy FJ. Ionic control of vascular smooth muscle cells. *Kidney Int* 1988; 346(25): S2–8.
25. Raij L, Luscher TF, Vanhoutte PM. High potassium diet augments endothelium-dependent relaxations in the Dahl rat. *Hypertension* 1988;12:562–67.
26. Hayslett J, Binder H. Mechanism of potassium adaptation. *Am J Physiol Renal Fluid Electrolyte Physiol* 1982; 243:F103–12.
27. Pamnani M, Chen S, Haddy F, Schooley F, Mo Z. Mechanism of the antihypertensive effect of dietary potassium in experimental volume expanded hypertension in rats. *Clin Exp Hypertens* 2000;22:555–69.
28. Manger WM, Simchon S, Stier CT Jr., Loscalzo J, Jan KM, Jan R, et al. Protective effects of dietary potassium chloride on hemodynamics of Dahl salt-sensitive rats in response to chronic administration of sodium chloride. *J Hypertens* 2003;21(12):2305–13.
29. Morris RC Jr., Sebastian A, Forman A, Tanaka M, Schmidlin O. Normotensive salt sensitivity: Effects of race and dietary potassium. *Hypertension* 1999; 33(1):18–23.
30. Ljunghall S, Hvarfner A, Lind L. Clinical studies of calcium metabolism in essential hypertension. *Eur Heart J* 1987;8(B):37–44.
31. Oshima T, Young EW. Systemic and cellular calcium metabolism and hypertension. *Semin Nephrol* 1995; 15(6):496–503.
32. Iwamoto T, Kita S. Topics on the Na(+)/Ca(2+) exchanger: Role of vascular NCX1 in salt-dependent hypertension. *J Pharmacol Sci* 2006; 102(1):32–6.
33. Dickinson HO, Nicolson DJ, Cook JV, Campbell F, Beyer FR, Ford GA, Mason J. Calcium supplementation for the management of primary hypertension in adults. *Cochrane Database Syst Rev* 2006;2:CD004639.
34. Rosanoff A. Magnesium and hypertension. *Clin Calcium* 2005;15(2):255–60.
35. Dickinson HO, Nicolson DJ, Campbell F, Cook JV, Beyer FR, Ford GA, et al. Magnesium supplementation for the management of essential hypertension in adults. Cochrane *Database Syst Rev* 2006;3:CD004640.
36. Demigne C, Sabboh H, Remesy C, Meneton P. Protective effects of high dietary potassium: Nutritional and metabolic aspects. *J Nutr* 2004;134: 2903–06.
37. U.S. Department of Health and Human Services and U.S. Department of Agriculture. Dietary Guidelines for Americans 2005 (*www.healthierus.gov/dietaryguidelines*).

Chapter 41

Alcohol Intake and Blood Pressure

Ian B. Puddey and Lawrence J. Beilin

Key Findings

- The regular consumption of alcohol directly elevates blood pressure. The effect is predominantly on systolic blood pressure with a predicted increase of approximately 1 mmHg for each 10 g of alcohol consumed per day.

- Precise mechanisms have not been elucidated but several aetiological factors have been implicated both centrally (altered sympatho-vagal balance, impaired arterial baroreceptor responses) and peripherally (effects on vascular membrane ion handling and reactivity).

- In communities that regularly consume alcohol, the population-attributable risk from alcohol consumption may be as high as 20 to 30%. The consumption of 3 to 5 drinks per day results in a twofold increase in the incidence of hypertension.

- Alcohol-related increases in blood pressure have implications for incidence of cerebral thrombosis, cerebral hemorrhage, left ventricular hypertrophy, and coronary artery disease.

Astute clinicians have noted an association between excessive alcohol intake and an increase in blood pressure since at least 1877, when Frederick Akbar Mahomed (using his sphygomograph) reported a high-tension pulse in so-called "alcoholists."[1] The relationship between regular alcohol consumption and an increase in blood pressure lay largely unexplored thereafter until Lian[2] (Figure 41–1) observed in 1915 among 150 42- to 43-year-old French soldiers serving on the Western front that there was a linear increase in the prevalence of hypertension with increasing alcohol consumption, with very heavy drinkers ("tres grand buveurs," >3 L of wine per day) having fourfold the prevalence of hypertension compared to those drinking 1 L of wine per day (intriguingly labeled "les sobres"). Subsequent reports were scattered and infrequent and relied on observations from case control comparisons of higher levels of blood pressure in alcoholics that fell upon detoxification and increased in those who resumed drinking.[3]

Heavy alcohol consumption was thought responsible for a number of early reports of an increase in the prevalence of abnormal liver function tests among hypertensives. In a Swedish study of patients with established hypertension, heavy drinking was also thought to underlie resistance to antihypertensive drug therapy, although poor compliance with treatment rather than alcohol *per se* was thought to be the major contributing factor.[4] Further circumstantial evidence for an association between heavy alcohol intake and blood pressure was implied from the observation of a positive association between death rates from stroke and cirrhosis in England and Wales.[5] A considerable body of epidemiological literature since these early studies has confirmed that in drinking communities alcohol consumption is a major lifestyle factor responsible for an increased prevalence and incidence of hypertension.

EPIDEMIOLOGY

Cross-sectional studies

The first large-scale cross-sectional definition of the relationship between alcohol consumption and the prevalence of hypertension was established by Klatsky and colleagues in 1977[6] in an analysis of the Kaiser Permanente Insurance data from over 80,000 contributors to a health insurance plan. This data showed a threshold relationship between alcohol and increased level of blood pressure in men, but a J-shaped relationship in women, with a clearcut increase in blood pressure in both from three or more drinks per day. These relationships were consistent in the three ethnic groups studied: whites, African Americans, and those of Asian origin (Figure 41–2). They were also similar in either smokers or nonsmokers or in obese compared to nonobese subjects. Those drinking three or more drinks a day had twice the prevalence of hypertension (defined as >160/90 mmHg) when compared to nondrinkers. Ex-drinkers had similar levels of blood pressure to abstainers, suggesting reversibility of any blood-pressure-elevating effect of alcohol.

Since this groundbreaking study, more than 100 cross-sectional population studies from nations on all five continents have confirmed the positive relationship between alcohol, increased blood pressure, and prevalence of hypertension. In the worldwide Intersalt study,[7] of the 48 centers in which some people reported consuming at least 240 g/week of alcohol (~3 or more drinks per day) 35 had positive regression coefficients linking heavy alcohol consumption to blood pressure. After account was taken of key confounders, men who drank 240 to 400 g alcohol/week had systolic/diastolic blood pressure on average 2.7/1.6 mmHg higher than nondrinkers, and men who drank ≥400 g alcohol/week had pressures of 4.6/3.0 mmHg higher. For women, heavy drinkers (≥240 g alcohol/week)

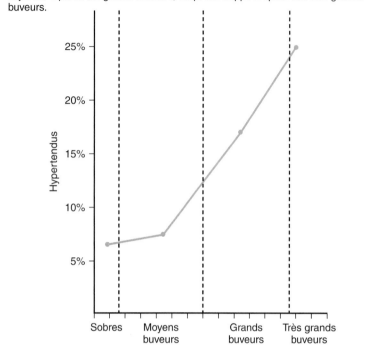

ALCOOLISME

Sobres,	16	sujets dont :	1	hypertendu	=	6,25% d'hypertendus.
Moyens buveurs,	53	–	4	hypertendus	=	7,54% –
Grands buveurs,	57	–	10	–	=	17,54% –
Très grands buveurs,	24	–	6	–	=	25,00% –

En d'autres termes, chez des territoriaux de quarante-deux à quarante-trois ans, l'hypertension artérielle n'est rencontrée que chez un sujet sur 16 parmi les sobres et chez un sujet sur 13 parmi les moyens buveurs, tandis qu'elle atteint 1 sujet sur 6 parmi les grands buveurs, et qu'elle frappe le quart des très grands buveurs.

Figure 41–1. Alcohol consumption and prevalence of hypertension in 150 French servicemen. (Reproduced with permission from Academic Nationale de Medecine.[2])

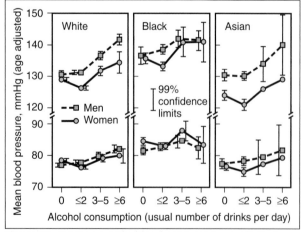

Figure 41–2. Mean systolic blood pressures (upper half of figure) and mean diastolic blood pressures (lower half of figure) of white, black, or Asian men and women with known drinking habits. Small circles represent data based on less than 30 persons. (Reproduced with permission from Klatsky et al.[6])

had blood pressures 3.9/3.1 mmHg higher than nondrinkers. In a recent systematic review of all studies from 1988 to 1999 of moderate alcohol consumption (<40 g/day) in relation to blood pressure, Burger et al.[8] concluded that there were linear blood pressure elevations at drinking levels of >20 g per day for women and >30 g per day for men.

These studies, however, have not clearly defined the effects of alcohol consumption on blood pressure at intakes below three drinks per day (30 g alcohol). Subsequent reports in which there has been more stringent evaluation of alcohol intake have since shown continuous positive relationships,[9,10] whereas a second Kaiser Permanente report nearly a decade after the first[11] (utilizing a more comprehensive alcohol database) found that even at 1 to 2 drinks per day there was a slight but significant increase in blood pressure in men. However, the curvilinear relationship observed in the original study in female participants with lower blood pressures at 1 to 2 drinks per day was still seen. However, there are many potential factors that could result in J-shaped or U-shaped relationships. These include differences among nondrinkers, light drinkers, and heavier drinkers in dietary habits, level of physical activity, prevalence of overweight, smoking habit, and socioeconomic background. They also include misclassification bias, with subjects underreporting their alcohol intake and being inappropriately included in a non or light drinker category or past heavy drinkers who have now given up drinking being mistakenly categorized as nondrinkers. In some studies, when these confounding influences have been carefully taken into account curvilinearity of the alcohol/blood-pressure relationship has been attenuated.

A consistent pattern of a stronger association of alcohol and blood pressure with aging has been reported in several cross-sectional studies, with the association of alcohol with blood pressure increasing with age at least up to the seventh decade.[12] In one study of elderly men and women 60 to 87 years of age,[13] alcohol intake was associated with higher blood pressure even when the mean background intake in men was only 12.5 g per day and in the women 5 g per day. At the other end of the spectrum, the alcohol/blood-pressure relationship has also been demonstrated surprisingly in teenage Argentinians[14] and Italian schoolchildren.[15]

Ambulatory blood pressure measurements have provided further insights into the relative effects of alcohol on blood pressure. The Harvest study[16] of 1100 Italians used ambulatory blood pressure to examine factors influencing the daily variation of blood pressure in hypertensive subjects aged 18 to 45 years. Alcohol intake was linearly related to daytime blood pressure, and heavier drinkers showed greater blood pressure variability. Alcohol intake influenced ambulatory blood pressures to a greater extent than its effect on office pressures.

Insights from more recent cross-sectional studies have concentrated on the relative effects on hypertension subtypes, the effects of drinking alcohol with or without food, and possible effects of individual alcoholic beverage preference. With respect to hypertension subtype, alcohol has generally been more strongly associated with increases in systolic rather than diastolic blood pressures. However, in a recent cross-sectional study that examined *a priori* the associations between alcohol intake and isolated systolic, combined systolic and diastolic and isolated diastolic hypertension in 5317 Chinese men it was found that those in the highest alcohol intake category (≥30 drinks/week) were twice as likely as nondrinkers to have any of these hypertensive subtypes—with population attributable risks of 13.9%, 13.4%, and 12.0%, respectively.[17] The consumption of alcohol with or without food was examined in a study of 2609 white men and women from western New York.[18] It was found that compared with lifetime abstainers participants reporting drinking mostly without food exhibited a 64% higher risk of hypertension.

When analyses were restricted to current drinkers, those consuming alcohol without food had a 41% higher risk of hypertension even after adjustment for the amount of alcohol consumed in the past 30 days. The relative effects of different types of alcoholic beverage on blood pressure remain controversial. The older Kaiser Permanente study[6] and a study from western New York[18] found no consistent beverage-specific associations with hypertension risk in North Americans drinking beer, wine, or spirits. On the other hand, in a recent Chinese study liquor drinking was associated with a higher odds ratio of isolated systolic hypertension, whereas combined systolic-diastolic hypertension and isolated diastolic hypertension did not differ by type of alcoholic beverage.[17] However, in that study liquor drinkers generally drank more alcohol. It is likely that this was the explanation for such findings given the results of a similar study in 4335 Japanese male workers,[19] which grouped subjects on the basis of their total consumption of beer, sake, shochu (traditional Japanese spirits), whiskey, or wine. Blood pressure was highest in the shochu group, but an analysis adjusting for total alcohol consumption resulted in disappearance of this difference.

There have also been consistent suggestions that wine drinking (especially red wine) is associated with smaller effects on blood pressure, an outcome attributed to its high content of potentially vasodilator flavonoids. In the Lipid Clinics Prevalence Study[20] there were significant positive regression coefficients for beer and spirits drinkers in relation to blood pressure but no significant relationship for wine drinkers. The PRIME study also found a weaker association for wine and blood pressure compared with beer.[21] Neither of these studies adjusted for diet, and given the now well recognized dietary differences among wine, beer, and spirits drinkers[22] this and other dissimilarities in lifestyle (as well as differences in the relative amounts and patterns of drinking) may account for such observations. This would appear a more likely explanation given the results of a 4-week crossover trial from Western Australia that compared effects of wine, dealcoholized red wine, beer, and water on 24-hour ambulatory blood pressure in 26 men. Similar increases in blood pressure were observed with either red wine or beer.[23] The effect of both of these alcoholic beverages was predominantly on awake systolic blood pressure, with increases of 2.9 mmHg for red wine and 1.9 mmHg for beer when compared to water (Figure 41–3).

Interaction with other lifestyle factors

If there is to be a balanced assessment of the overall clinical implications of alcohol-related hypertension, alcohol consumption cannot be considered in isolation from the effects on blood pressure of other lifestyle risk factors. Another study from Western Australia[9] focused on a younger population of working men, specifically evaluating the relative importance of the effects of alcohol on blood pressure in relation to other lifestyle factors. Careful evaluation of alcohol consumption in these 491 men aged 20 to 44 years revealed it to be linearly related to the prevalence of hypertension (>140 mmHg systolic and/or 90 mmHg diastolic) (Figure 41–4). The association was independent of smoking, physical activity, and tea and coffee consumption but additive to that of body mass index. The 50% of the men who averaged 3 or more standard drinks per day (1 standard drink equivalent to 10 g ethanol), principally as beer, had 3 to 4 times the prevalence of systolic hypertension (140 mmHg or more) compared with current nondrinkers. In multivariate analysis, alcohol consumption equated with body mass index in the magnitude of its contribution to the variance in blood pressure level, a reflection of the relatively high levels of alcohol drinking in this young to middle-age male population. In a recent meta-analysis, however (which quantified the contributions of body weight, physical inactivity, and dietary factors to the prevalence of hypertension in Finland, Italy, the Netherlands, the United Kingdom, and the USA),[24] the major impacts on population-attributable risk for hypertension were overweight, physical inactivity, high sodium intake, and low potassium intake—with the impact of alcohol consumption relatively small (2 to 3%).

Interactions of alcohol with other lifestyle effects on blood pressure also need to be considered. In one study,[25] salt intake was only found to be associated with increased blood pressure in subjects who consumed larger amounts of alcohol and simultaneously were characterized by a low calcium intake. However, an alcohol-salt interaction was not confirmed in a two-way factorial intervention study in which treated hypertensive drinkers reduced their alcohol intake, sodium intake, or both.[26] In this study, only alcohol restriction resulted in a fall in blood pressure. Population studies also indicate a potential interaction of physical activity and alcohol intake to determine level of blood pressure, with weaker alcohol/blood-pressure relationships in more active subjects.[27] In an intervention study in which sedentary drinkers were randomized to vigorous exercise, alcohol restriction, or both only alcohol restriction resulted in a fall in blood pressure.[28]

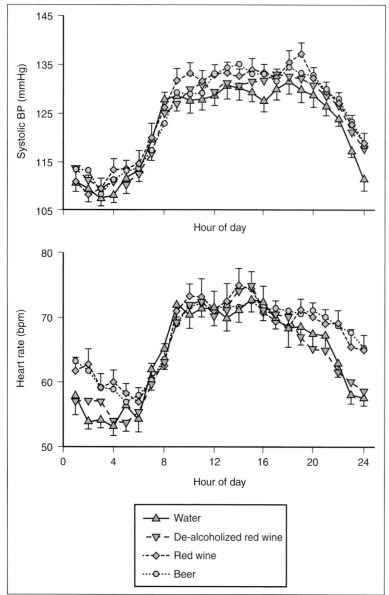

Figure 41–3. Top: 24-hour profile of systolic blood pressure following the four interventions. Compared to control/abstinence, both red wine and beer increased 24-hour and daytime systolic blood pressure (*p*<0.05). Bottom: 24-hour profile of heart rate (HR) following the four interventions. Compared to the control/abstinence, both red wine and beer increased HR for 8 to 10 hours after drinking (*p*<0.001). (Reproduced with permission from Zilkens et al.[23])

In contrast, the results from both population studies[6,9] and an intervention study[29] have been consistent in finding an additive effect of alcohol and obesity on blood pressure. In the intervention study, overweight drinkers who decreased their alcohol intake from approximately 5 to 1 standard drink per day and simultaneously followed a calorie-restricted diet decreased their weight by nearly 10 kg and experienced falls in systolic blood pressure of 10 to 14 mmHg after 16 weeks (Figure 41–5). Other reported interactions have been between alcohol and smoking (wherein those who both smoked and drank had the highest blood pressures)[30] and between alcohol and job strain, where regular heavy drinkers in high-strain jobs had higher blood pressure than those with low-strain jobs.[31]

Prospective studies

Prospective population studies have added strong support to the cross-sectional data implicating alcohol as a major risk factor for subsequent development of hypertension in both men and women. In 1999, a meta-analysis of the three prospective studies then available reported a 40% increase in the relative risk of developing hypertension in those drinking more than 25 g alcohol/day and over a fourfold increase in risk in those drinking more than 100 g a day.[32] Subsequently, large-scale prospective studies from Japan[33] and the USA[34] have reported up to a twofold increase in risk of hypertension with intakes of 30 to 50 g a day or more. In the ARIC study it was estimated that in subjects drinking 30 g/day or more one in five cases of hypertension could be attributed to alcohol consumption.[34] An effect with even lower levels of alcohol consumption has been reported in a native American population[35] in which in light to moderate drinkers (occasional drink up to 1 to 2 drinks a day) there were 1.24-fold and 1.53-fold increases in the incidence of hypertension in men and women, respectively. Similarly, in young middle-age Swedish males within a 6-year period of follow-up alcohol intake emerged as an important determinant of the development of hypertension.[36]

Randomized controlled trials

There have now been more than a dozen randomized controlled trials of the effects of alcohol on blood pressure. The consistent finding has been that that regular alcohol consumption directly elevates blood pressure. The first trial was carried out in community-based ambulatory subjects in Western Australia,[37] where normotensive drinkers reduced their alcohol consumption by drinking a low alcohol beer (0.9% ethanol) for 6 weeks before switching back to their usual alcohol intake, consuming a normal alcohol beer (5% ethanol) from which the low-alcohol beer had been distilled. This reduced their alcohol consumption by approximately 80% and was accompanied by a corresponding fall in blood pressure, increasing once again when normal intake was resumed. The main fall in blood pressure occurred within the first 1 to 2 weeks of switching to the low-alcohol beer but was still declining at 6 weeks (Figure 41–6). Similar effects of regular drinking have subsequently been shown to occur in both treated[38] (Figure 41–7) and untreated[39] hypertensives.

The first meta-analysis of all randomized controlled trials to 2000 of the effects of alcohol reduction on blood pressure[40] included 15 trials. The majority of these trials involved men, with three of the studies having included a

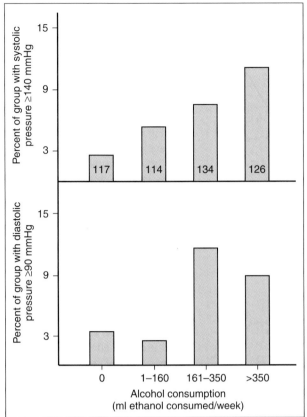

Figure 41–4. Percentage of each drinking category with systolic or diastolic hypertension. Numbers in columns refer to total in the population subgroup. The trend for systolic hypertension and alcohol consumption = 8.09, *p*<0.005; for diastolic hypertension, trend = 5.84, *p*<0.025. (Reproduced with permission from Arkwright et al.[9])

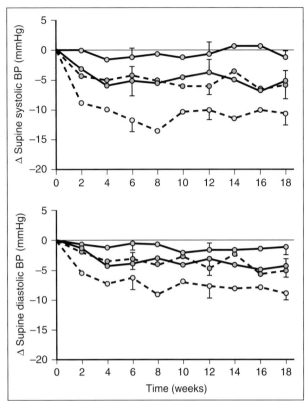

Figure 41–5. Line graphs show change in mean ± SEM systolic (top) and diastolic (bottom) blood pressure in four study groups. ○—○, normal alcohol intake/normal caloric intake (n=20); ○--○, normal alcohol intake/low caloric intake (n=22); ●—●, low alcohol intake/normal caloric intake (n=21); and ○--○ low alcohol intake/low caloric intake (n=23). (Reproduced with permission from Puddey et al.[29])

small number of women only. Seven studies included only hypertensive subjects: 6 normotensive subjects and 2 either normotensives or hypertensives. The hypertensives in six of these trials were taking blood-pressure-lowering medication. Subjects were studied for a median 8 weeks and reduced their alcohol consumption by a median 76% from baseline intakes of 3 to 6 standard drinks per day. The pooled effect estimates for the fall in systolic and diastolic blood pressure were 3.31 and 2.04 mmHg, respectively (Figure 41–8). These changes were similar in hypertensives and normotensives, and in treated versus untreated hypertensive subjects, with a dose response relationship between the falls in blood pressure and the drop in alcohol intake.

A further systematic review[41] focused primarily on studies that directly administered alcohol rather than the approach of Xin et al.,[40] which utilized randomized clinical trial data. It came to similar conclusions with estimates of a significant effect of alcohol restriction to reduce systolic and diastolic blood pressure by 2.7 mmHg and 1.4 mmHg, respectively. This meta-analytic review also compared data from studies that utilized conventional clinic or office review of blood pressure with those that incorporated ambulatory or home blood pressure monitoring and was able to highlight biphasic effects of alcohol on blood

pressure with an early presumably vasodilator effect of alcohol leading to a reduction in blood pressure (in the immediate hours after exposure) and a later effect (the next day) of raising blood pressure.

Gender effects

As discussed previously, cross-sectional studies have indicated that (similar to men) heavier drinking is associated with a higher prevalence of hypertension in women. However, with light to moderate drinking the nature of the relationship has been more controversial. First has been the persistent suggestion that the effects of alcohol on blood pressure may not be as substantial in women, with the NHANES III study[42] (which included over 9000 women) finding that associations between alcohol intake and blood pressure and pulse pressure were weaker in women than in men. This contrasts with a smaller Brazilian study,[10] which showed exactly the opposite. Second has been the suggestion that low-level alcohol intake may actually lower blood pressure in women, with the majority of cross-sectional studies suggesting lower blood pressures at lower levels of alcohol intake in women.[6,43] Moreover, in a meta-analysis of 11 population studies up to 1993[44] it was concluded that there was a decreased risk of hypertension in women with low-level alcohol intake.

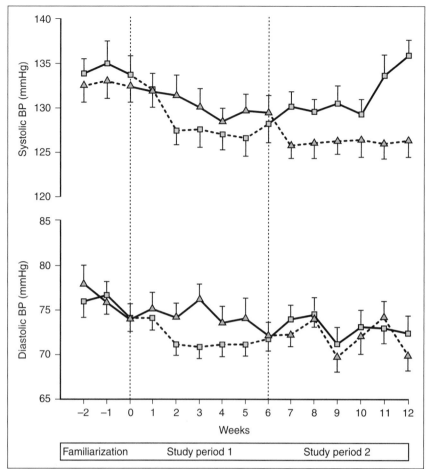

Figure 41–6. Line graphs show group systolic and diastolic blood pressure after 6 minutes of supine rest. Values are means ± SEM. Group 1 (closed squares) = low alcohol intake in period 1 (dotted line), normal alcohol intake in period 2 (solid line); group 2 (closed diamonds) = normal alcohol intake in period 1 (solid line), low alcohol intake in period 2 (dotted line). (Reproduced with permission from Puddey et al.[37])

largest was the Nurses Health Study[48] in women aged 25 to 42 at baseline. This found a biphasic effect of alcohol, with a 14% decrease in risk of developing hypertension in those consuming 2 to 3 drinks per week compared with nondrinkers and a 20% increase risk in those drinking more than 14 drinks a week. However, in the Atherosclerosis Risk in Communities Study[34] the relative risks for those drinking more than 210 g alcohol per week were increased similarly in men and women. As mentioned previously, randomized controlled trials have so far either been confined to men or contained too few women for assessment of a gender effect of alcohol on blood pressure.

A recently completed trial,[49] however, focused specifically on the blood pressure effects of alcohol in pre-menopausal women. Twenty-four normotensive women aged 25 to 49 were randomized to a three-period crossover study in which each evening they consumed either higher-volume red wine (146 to 218 g alcohol per week) or a lower-volume red wine (42 to 73 g ethanol/week) titrated against their alcohol intake at entry to the study. Dealcoholized red wine was consumed as a control for an identical period of 4 weeks. Ambulatory blood pressure and heart rate were monitored every 30 minutes for 24 hours at the end of each study period. With the higher-volume red wine there was a significant increase in 24-hour systolic and diastolic blood pressure relative to the dealcoholized red wine but no significant effect on blood pressure of the lower-volume red wine. The magnitude of the blood pressure elevation was similar to that reported in previous intervention studies in men (by 2.0/1.2 mmHg) but evident at even lower levels of intake, with no evidence provided for the contention that low levels of alcohol will lower blood pressure in women.

GENETICS

Given that there is already a wide acknowledgement of the genetic basis of both hypertension and predisposition to excessive alcohol consumption it should not be surprising if there is also a substantial genetic predisposition to alcohol-related hypertension. Research in this area is at an early stage, with the focus to date having been predominantly on a few functionally significant polymorphisms of genes integral to either alcohol metabolism or blood pressure regulation. A point mutation at –357 of the promoter region of the gene coding for the aldehyde

These results need to be interpreted, however, against those studies that have demonstrated a dose response relationship in women across the continuum of alcohol intake[10,45] that suggests unmeasured confounding as an explanation for the inconsistencies. They may, at least to some extent, be a consequence of gender-related differences in the accuracy of self-reporting of alcohol intake. In a cross-sectional survey of 19,000 subjects in the USA, women who reported a prior diagnosis of hypertension also reported drinking less alcohol than those not reporting hypertension,[46] whereas the opposite was true of hypertensive men. Other confounders may also be playing a role with differences in diet, drinking patterns, and other lifestyle parameters rarely or inadequately assessed in most studies. In this regard, a UK-based study of 14,000 female employees of the firm Marks and Spencer[47] noted that a finding of a decreased prevalence of hypertension with consumption of up to 14 drinks a week was no longer seen after accounting for age, BMI, physical activity, and family history of premature coronary artery disease.

The more stringent prospective population studies have also not been able to resolve the uncertainty as to gender differences in the alcohol/blood-pressure relationship. The

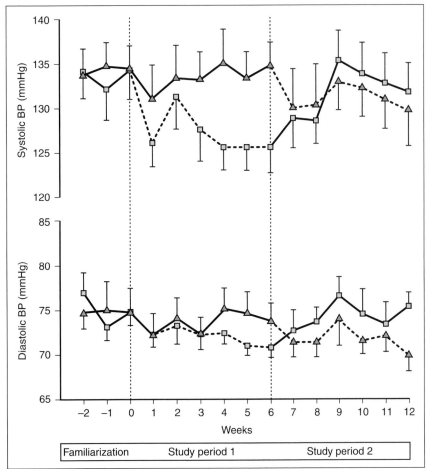

Figure 41–7. Line graphs show group systolic and diastolic blood pressure after 6 minutes of supine rest. Values are means ± SEM. Group 1 (closed squares) = low alcohol intake in period 1 (dotted line), normal alcohol intake in period 2 (solid line); group 2 (closed diamonds) = normal alcohol intake in period 1 (solid line), low alcohol intake in period 2 (dotted line). (Reproduced with permission from Puddey et al.[38] with permission from Elsevier.)

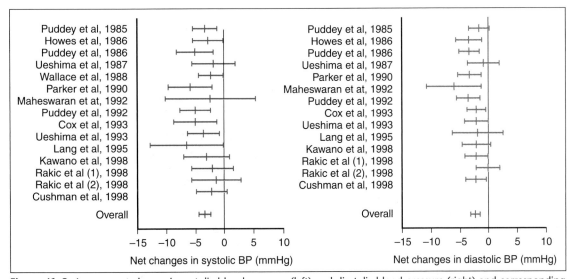

Figure 41–8. Average net change in systolic blood pressure (left) and diastolic blood pressure (right) and corresponding 95% CIs related to alcohol reduction intervention in 15 randomized controlled trials. Net change was calculated as the difference of the baseline minus follow-up levels of blood pressure for the intervention and control groups (parallel trials) or the difference in blood pressure levels at the end of the intervention and control treatment periods (crossover trials). The overall effect represents a pooled estimate obtained by summing the average net change for each trial, weighted by the inverse of its variance. (Reprinted with permission from Xin et al.[40])

dehydrogenase isozyme leads to a deficiency in metabolism of the major metabolite of ethanol (acetaldehyde), resulting in higher levels and a characteristic flushing and tachycardia after alcohol ingestion. This polymorphism has been well described in Japanese, Chinese, and Scandinavian populations, with speculation that it may predispose to alcohol-related hypertension.

The major problem in testing this hypothesis, however, is that those with the ALDH*2/2 genotype consume less alcohol because of the unpleasant symptoms and are therefore significantly less likely to be at risk of alcohol-related hypertension.[50] In one study in Japanese men and women,[51] after allowing for such lower levels of alcohol intake no causal relation between this mutation and the prevalence of hypertension could be seen. Another study, however (which included only subjects who consumed >300 g ethanol per week),[52] found increased odds for higher systolic blood pressure in those with the ALDH*2/2 genotype even after adjustment for alcohol consumption as well as other potential demographic and lifestyle confounders.

Polymorphisms of another important alcohol metabolizing enzyme, alcohol dehydrogenase, have been evaluated in the context of the alcohol/blood-pressure relationship. The wild-type ADH2^1/2^1 genotype has a substantially lower ethanol-oxidizing capacity compared to the mutant ADH2^1/2^2 and ADH2^2/2^2 genotypes, and is again more commonly seen in Japanese populations. Results have been inconsistent, however. This polymorphism has in one Japanese study[53] not predicted hypertension risk with alcohol, whereas in another after adjustment for alcohol consumption a significantly stronger alcohol blood pressure relationship was seen in men with the wild-type ADH2^1/2^1 genotype. Slow metabolism of alcohol due to presence of the alcohol dehydrogenase type 3 polymorphism has been associated with a decrease in risk of myocardial infarction in the Physicians' Health Study,[54] probably because of higher HDL-cholesterol levels. However, the implications of this polymorphism for alcohol-related hypertension have not yet been investigated. Alcohol metabolism also occurs through the hepatic mitochondrial cytochrome P450 oxidase pathway, especially following enzyme induction in high alcohol consumers. There is evidence that a genetic polymorphism of CYP2E1, the c2 allele, predisposes to higher blood pressure—possibly as a consequence of higher acetaldehyde levels.[53]

Apolipoprotein E polymorphisms have been proposed as determinants of alcohol-related hypertension in Finnish subjects.[55] Those with the E2/E3 and E3/E3 genotypes had a stronger alcohol/blood-pressure relationship than the E4/E3 genotype. However, in a Western Australian intervention study in regular drinkers no relationship between the apolipoprotein E genotype and the magnitude of the falls in blood pressure following alcohol restriction was seen.[56] In male Japanese workers, alcohol drinking has been associated with increased prevalence of high normal blood pressure in M allele carriers of angiotensinogen gene T174M polymorphism.[57] Other investigators have examined a possible role for polymorphisms in the beta-adrenoceptor (beta-AR)-stimulatory guanine nucleotide-binding (Gs) protein system.[58] They reported an interaction between the T393C polymorphism of the gene encoding the alpha-subunit of Gs proteins (GNAS1) and drinking status in the association with hypertension. The T allele carriers had a higher probability of hypertension than CC homozygotes in nondrinkers and light drinkers, whereas CC homozygotes had a higher probability of hypertension than T allele carriers in moderate to heavy drinkers. There was also a significant association between the T393C polymorphism and pulse pressure in moderate to heavy drinkers.

PHYSIOLOGY AND PATHOPHYSIOLOGY

Studies in animals

By far the majority of animal studies into the phenomenon of alcohol-related hypertension have been carried out in rats. The results have been inconsistent in relation to blood pressure outcomes, largely because of the use of different rat strains, the utilization of a variety of alcohol doses, and different routes of alcohol administration. The first such study surprisingly demonstrated no significant effects on blood pressure after chronic alcohol feeding to either normotensive Wistar Kyoto rats (WKY) or spontaneously hypertensive rats (SHR).[59] In fact, hypotensive effects of high-dose alcohol have been the usual finding in the SHR, stroke-prone SHR, and WKY rats. In these latter studies, falls in blood pressure were seen after feeding SHR rats 20% alcohol solutions for 16 weeks[60] (or there was a retardation of the rise in blood pressure normally seen with aging in both the SHR and the stroke-prone SHR).[61,62] In contrast, in the Wistar rat[63–65] and in experiments in WKY rats that used only low doses of alcohol (1, 5, and 10% alcohol v/v)[66–69] increases in blood pressure with alcohol have been consistently reported.

The unexpected finding of lower blood pressures following alcohol may have been due to depression of cardiac performance, a phenomenon known to be enhanced by alcohol in hypertensive rat strains.[70] The falls in blood pressure have occurred, however, despite enhanced vascular contractility[71] or heightened heart rate responses to stress.[72] Some of the differences between rat models may also have related to the timing of blood pressure measurement in relation to the last intake of alcohol. In the SHR, an increase in blood pressure lasting several days after sudden withdrawal of alcohol has been seen,[61] and similarly in Sprague-Dawley rats a hypertensive response has been reported 24 hours after cessation of alcohol feeding.[73] Such an acute increase in blood pressure is also characteristic of the alcohol withdrawal syndrome in man.

Utilizing radiotelemetry, hemodynamic effects of alcohol have once again been assessed more recently during chronic low-dose alcohol administration to SHRs and WKY controls (5% v/v for 12 weeks).[74] The advantage of such an approach is that it eliminates the potential stressful effects of other conventional techniques that attempt to measure rat-tail blood pressure after initial warming of the animals or the monitoring of intra-arterial blood pressure after anaesthesia. Again, alcohol had no effect on blood pressure in WKY rats but caused falls in blood pressure in the SHR, reaching a maximum at week 5 and remaining low thereafter.[74] Alcohol also caused reductions in the blood pressure variability and the circadian fluctuations in blood pressure in the SHR but not in WKY rats. Plasma norepinephrine levels were elevated by alcohol in WKY rats, but not in the SHR. The authors speculated that the absence of a fall in blood pressure in the WKY rats may have been related, at least in part, to the associated sympatho-excitation. Utilizing an identical telemetric approach, effects of alcohol on circadian haemodynamic rhythms were subsequently assessed. Alcohol resulted in a fall in blood pressure during both the day and night in the SHR. However, effects of alcohol to increase HR and decrease HR variability (consistent with inhibition of vagal tone) were only seen during the night.[75]

Some pathogenic insights into the mechanism of the pressor response to alcohol have been provided by those rat models that have consistently identified an increase in blood pressure with chronic alcohol feeding. In these studies alcohol was administered in the drinking water, gradually increased from 5 to 10% and then 20% v/v over 12 weeks.[63–65] Both a slight increase in calcium pump activity and a decrease in cell membrane cholesterol content were seen in association with the increase in blood pressure.[64] These changes were thought secondary to the known acute fluidizing effects of alcohol on cell membranes, with compensatory changes in lipid composition resulting in increased Ca^{2+}/Mg^{2+}-ATPase activity. Such an interpretation has been supported by observations in the same rat model of changes in the polyunsaturated to saturated fatty acid ratio in red cell membranes that were proportional to the magnitude of the alcohol-related rise in blood pressure.[76]

Increases in vascular smooth muscle calcium uptake together with an increase in blood pressure have also been seen in WKY rats chronically fed lower doses of alcohol (10% v/v in the drinking water).[66] After lowering the dose of alcohol even further to 5% v/v, renal vascular changes and increases in intracellular calcium in alcohol-fed rats have still been seen and could be reversed by either the calcium entry blocker verapamil[67] or by n-acetyl cysteine,[68] the latter suggesting a possible role for the metabolism of alcohol to acetaldehyde in the pathogenesis of alcohol-related hypertension. A pressor response to alcohol has even been seen with as little as 1% alcohol v/v in the drinking water over 14 weeks.[69] In that experiment, the administration of dietary vitamin B6 (which augments methionine metabolism to cysteine) decreased tissue acetaldehyde conjugates, prevented an increase in intracellular calcium levels, and counteracted both an increase in blood pressure and any renal arteriolar changes. Magnesium supplementation has also been reported to counteract the development of hypertension in Wistar rats chronically fed alcohol,[77] with the mechanism proposed that it possibly prevents an alcohol-induced increase in intracellular calcium and consequent suppression of sodium pump activity.

In combination, these studies highlight the potential for peripheral effects of alcohol on vascular membrane structure and function to ultimately influence resting vasomotor tone and vascular reactivity. In contrast, chronic alcohol administration to Sprague-Dawley rats raises the equally plausible possibility of centrally mediated effects. In these studies, alcohol attenuated acutely induced clonidine hypotension but augmented acutely induced hydralazine hypotension, suggesting opposite effects on centrally versus peripherally mediated hypotension.[78] This clonidine-alcohol interaction has only been seen with acute but not chronic clonidine administration.[79] Further experiments[80] indicate that acute hypotensive effects of rilmenidine or alpha-methyldopa are also significantly attenuated by ethanol feeding (2.5 or 5%) in a concentration-dependent manner. These findings have been interpreted as evidence that chronic ethanol attenuates both imidazoline I^1 receptor and alpha (2)-adrenoceptor-mediated hypotension.

Chronic alcohol administration to male Sprague-Dawley rats impaired arterial baroreceptor responses,[81] with the suggestion that such an effect could be an important prelude to subsequent increase in blood pressure. After 12 weeks of alcohol administration, this mechanism was also identified in Wistar rats,[82] although associated with only modest increases in blood pressure. Subsequent studies point to a centrally mediated action of alcohol in impairment of the arterial baro-receptor response. For example, acute exposure to ethanol decreased the sensitivity of the baroreceptor reflex, an effect seen in association with gamma-aminobutyric acid depletion in the brain stem.[83] Acute alcohol exposure has also been shown to exert a marked inhibitory action on glutamatergic pathways within the rostral ventrolateral medulla, leading to reduced baroreflex sensitivity.[84] A central effect has also been suggested by the observation in ethanol-fed rats (6.7% volume/volume for 28 days) that arterial blood pressure increased by 21% relative to pair-fed controls in association with simultaneous changes in the levels of both vasopressin and neuropeptide Y neurotransmitters in the neuronal pathways related to control of blood pressure.[85]

Studies in humans

Given the rapid onset and offset of alcohol-related hypertension evident in human intervention studies, effects of alcohol to elevate blood pressure are likely to be mediated at least in part by neuro-humoral mechanisms or by reversible effects on vascular tone, heart rate, or cardiac output. However, chronic effects of alcohol to alter vascular or cardiac structure are also implied from those studies where hypertension has persisted for months after alcohol cessation by alcoholics[86] and by evidence that suggests a link between at least heavy alcohol intake and hypertensive end-organ disease. This includes increased cardiovascular disease outcomes such as stroke[87] and myocardial infarction[88] together with surrogate markers such as increased intimal-medial thickness of carotid arteries,[89] increased vascular stiffness,[90] and increased left ventricular hypertrophy.[91] However, the contribution of alcohol-related hypertension to each of these endpoints has been largely undefined. Moreover, the precise mechanism for alcohol-related hypertension itself has not been characterized but is highly likely to be a multifactorial phenomenon.

In alcoholic subjects studied during detoxification, there is a relationship between level of blood pressure and the severity of alcohol withdrawal.[92] This has led to conjecture that the broader alcohol/blood-pressure relationship identified in population studies could also be caused by alcohol withdrawal. In some of these studies, level of blood pressure has been linked more closely to recent alcohol intake rather than to longer-term intake.[20,93] However, these comparative measures of recent and longer-term intake have been constructed from the same 7-day retrospective alcohol diary, raising the possibility that such results were influenced by recall bias, with more accurate recall of intake in the preceding 24 to 72 hours. Where longer-term and recent intake have been assessed with separate instruments, the relationship between longer-term intake and blood pressure has been predominant.[94]

In a Brazilian study[10] that measured the exact time since the last drink, blood pressure was lower in men who had consumed alcohol less than 3 hours before blood pressure measurement but higher in those who consumed alcohol 13 to 23 hours before measurement. As discussed previously, a number of intervention studies that used ambulatory blood pressure monitoring have reported a similar biphasic pattern following the acute ingestion of alcohol.[95] The early fall in blood pressure may reflect an initial vasodilator effect of alcohol, but the subsequent increase in blood pressure was not evident in one study until 7 days[95] and was therefore unlikely to have been due to alcohol withdrawal. Furthermore, the finding of an alcohol/blood-pressure association in population-based studies at relatively low levels (2 to 3 drinks per day) is also inconsistent with an alcohol withdrawal effect as the only explanation for a pressor effect of alcohol.

There is support, however, for a contribution of effects of alcohol withdrawal in heavier drinkers. In the British Heart Survey[96] of 7735 middle-age men, hypertension was more likely to be diagnosed on a Monday than on a Friday—the assumption being that heavy drinkers were exhibiting withdrawal pressor effects after heavy weekend drinking. Further support is provided by a comparative study of drinking and weekday blood pressure relationships in men from Northern Ireland versus France.[97] The Irishmen were characterized not only by weekend drinking but by blood pressures that were highest on Monday, whereas no weekday effect was seen in the French (whose alcohol consumption was more uniform throughout the week).

To shed further light on the relative effects of regular and intermittent drinking patterns on blood pressure, a randomized controlled crossover trial was conducted in Western Australia in 55 men, 14 of whom drank more than 60% of their alcohol on weekends (whereas the remainder were regular daily drinkers).[98] Baseline 24-hour blood pressures were higher on Mondays than on Thursdays in weekend but not daily drinkers, an effect lost after switching to low-alcohol beer. However, both groups showed a fall in 24-hour ambulatory blood pressure when changing from normal to low-alcohol beer—an effect evident after one week in the weekend drinkers but not until the fourth week in daily drinkers. This study indicated that there are contributing elements from both acute alcohol withdrawal and more sustained blood pressure elevation in weekend drinkers, whereas those who drink throughout the week show only a more sustained pressor response. Overall, the evidence suggests that consumption of alcohol averaged over a week or more is more important than pattern of intake with regard to alcohol-related blood pressure elevation.[94,99]

Hypertension is often part of a metabolic syndrome differentiated not only by an increase in blood pressure but by reduced insulin sensitivity, central adiposity, and a characteristic dyslipidaemia with a low HDL-cholesterol and high triglyceride levels and elevated uric acid. Alcohol has been linked not only to the increase in blood pressure but to several discrete elements of this syndrome, in particular the increase in triglyceride levels, central adiposity, and elevated uric acid. However, alcohol simultaneously acts to increase HDL-cholesterol levels[100] and thus whether it makes any significant contribution to the metabolic syndrome has remained controversial. This was highlighted in the 1998 Korean National Health and Nutrition Examination Survey,[101] in which drinking more than 30 g alcohol/day was associated with an increase in blood pressure in men, a high blood glucose in women, and higher triglycerides in both men and women. In addition, for both sexes and across all alcohol consumption categories there was a significant increase in HDL-cholesterol. Despite these contrasting effects on different components, overall there was a dose-response relationship between increasing alcohol intake and the odds of having the metabolic syndrome.

In contrast, another Korean study[102] found that although heavy consumption increased blood pressure and waist circumference there was no significant relationship between alcohol intake and the metabolic syndrome. This finding was thought to be a consequence of the corresponding higher HDL-C seen with increasing alcohol consumption. Similarly, in the smaller Alcohol and Insulin Resistance Study from Sweden[103] alcohol intake was positively related to triglyceride levels and blood pressure in men, but simultaneously linked to improved insulin sensitivity and higher HDL cholesterol levels so that overall there was no evidence of a significant difference in alcohol intake in those subjects with the metabolic syndrome compared to those without. These results contrast with those from a U.S. study on data from participants in the Third National Health and Nutrition Examination Survey,[104] in which alcohol consumption was significantly and inversely associated with the prevalence of at least three components of the metabolic syndrome: low serum HDL cholesterol, elevated serum triglycerides, and high waist circumference. It was also associated with hyperinsulinemia, leading to the conclusion that mild to moderate alcohol consumption was associated with a lower prevalence of the metabolic syndrome—a finding strongest among whites and among beer and wine drinkers.

The National Heart, Lung, and Blood Institute Family Heart Study has also indicated that alcohol consumption is associated with a lower prevalence of the metabolic syndrome but emphasised that this was irrespective of the type of beverage consumed.[105] Recent meta-analyses of the relationship between alcohol intake and incidence of new-onset diabetes mellitus in prospective population studies[106,107] have identified a biphasic relationship with a decrease in risk with low alcohol intake and an increase with heavy alcohol intake. The contrasting results from several different population studies therefore suggest that any overall effects of alcohol on the metabolic syndrome appear to be determined by a number of competing influences, including the volume and type of alcohol consumed, gender, race, and ethnicity. An effect of alcohol to impair insulin resistance as a primary pathogenic pathway for alcohol-induced hypertension therefore appears unlikely.

This conclusion is further supported by an intervention study from Western Australia,[108] in which a controlled decrease in alcohol intake by approximately 60 g per day had no effect on several indices of peripheral insulin sensitivity despite effects to decrease systolic and diastolic blood pressure by 5/4 mmHg and to decrease weight by 0.9 kg. An alternative causative pathway has been suggested by the finding in postmenopausal women that the ingestion of 15 to 30 g of alcohol per day increases serum leptin levels, suggesting that further investigations of the interrelationships among alcohol, central adiposity, and the metabolic syndrome need to consider a possible pathophysiologic role for leptin in alcohol-related hypertension—an increase in blood pressure now recognized as a correlate of chronic elevations of this hormone.[109]

There is some evidence that enhanced blood pressure sensitivity to sodium may participate in the pathogenesis of alcohol-related hypertension, at least in alcoholics. In a study of 30 alcoholics during detoxification[110] there was an abnormal response of both blood pressure and plasma renin activity to variations in salt intake, which was similar to that seen in sodium-sensitive hypertension. A subsequent study in 18 chronic alcoholics[111] demonstrated a persistence of this sodium sensitivity even after 1 year of abstinence, with the postulate that such sensitivity may be integral to the hypertensive response of alcoholics during withdrawal. These results contrast with those from an intervention study in moderately drinking ambulatory subjects who were all placed on a fixed intake of 160 mmol/day.[26] During a subsequent 4-week period of either a decrease in sodium intake or a decrease in alcohol intake (or both) only an effect of alcohol restriction to reduce blood pressure was seen. The absence of a fall in blood pressure with sodium restriction argues against enhanced sodium sensitivity to blood pressure in moderately drinking subjects.

Abnormal salt handling by the kidney has also been postulated to contribute to alcohol-related hypertension. In 6-week intervention studies in normotensive and treated hypertensive subjects from Western Australia no differences have been observed in 24-hour urinary excretion of sodium during periods of low versus high alcohol intake.[37,38] In contrast, in chronic alcoholics admitted for detoxification[112] there was evidence of altered renal sodium handling with lower fractional urinary sodium excretion in those subjects whose blood pressure was >160/95 mmHg upon admission. A study in Japanese males with hypertension, however, specifically investigated the effects of repeated alcohol intake (1 ml/kg per day) on blood pressure and sodium metabolism over 7 days.[113] Blood pressure, although falling initially, increased toward the end of the alcohol period. This corresponded with initial sodium retention and a subsequent return to baseline, with restoration of sodium balance after 7 days. The sodium retention during the early phase was thought secondary to the corresponding initial fall in blood pressure but could possibly have contributed to the subsequent increase in blood pressure.

It has been proposed that alcohol-related hypertension results from cellular magnesium deficiency in drinkers with inactivation of the sodium pump, an increase in intracellular sodium, and an increase in vascular tone. Such magnesium deficiency with chronic alcohol consumption may be secondary to reduced dietary magnesium intake or result from the combined effects of alcohol to induce both hypomagnesiumemia and magnesiumuria.[114] Support for this mechanism comes from the results of a Japanese study in hypertensive drinkers,[115] in which a fall in blood pressure during 4 weeks of alcohol restriction correlated with an increase in intra-erythrocyte magnesium and a decrease in intra-erythrocyte sodium. It has also been argued that intracellular free Mg^{2+} can act to maintain low resting levels of intracellular free Ca^{2+} and trigger muscle contraction or relaxation by competing with Ca^{2+} for membrane binding sites and by modulating Ca binding and release from the sarcoplasmic reticular membranes.[116] Decreasing Mg^{2+} levels may therefore increase resting vascular tone and level of blood pressure, and such a mechanism has been linked to alcohol-induced cerebrovascular spasm.[117]

Effects of alcohol on sympatho-vagal balance with either augmentation of sympathetic nervous system activity or dampening of parasympathetic tone (or both) have long been implicated in the genesis of alcohol-related hypertension. Effects on heart rate variability have been utilized as a surrogate for such effects, but reports of alcohol as an independent determinant of heart rate variability in cross-sectional population studies have not been consistent.[118,119] However, they appear likely given results from an intervention study in which 3 weeks of alcohol restriction in Japanese male drinkers produced reductions in ambulatory systolic blood pressure and heart rate and an index of sympatho-vagal balance with augmentations of parasympathetic indices of heart rate variability.[120] These findings suggest that drinking dampens vagal tone, with a corresponding relative increase in sympathetic tone.

An acute effect of alcohol to increase sympathetic tone has been demonstrated during skeletal muscle microneurography,[121] although in that study there was only an increase in heart rate but not blood pressure because of an initial acute vasodilator effect of alcohol. Acute intravenous infusion of alcohol rather than oral administration also caused sympathetic nerve activation as monitored by skeletal muscle microneurography,[122] but in this setting caused an increase in blood pressure that could be blocked by prior administration of dexamethasone. This was interpreted as evidence that alcohol was inducing a centrally mediated sympatho-excitatory effect mediated by release of corticotropin releasing hormone. Central autonomic effects of alcohol influencing blood pressure control have also been implied from the observation that acute ethanol ingestion leads to impaired baroreceptor function,[123] as well as from the finding in a cross-sectional study in healthy subjects that alcohol was an independent predictor of reduced baroreflex activity.[124]

Endothelial function is impaired in hypertensive subjects, and such impairment has been seen as an indication of subsequent risk for hypertension and vascular disease. An effect of alcohol to impair endothelial function has therefore been postulated to contribute to alcohol-related hypertension and the pathophysiological evidence for such an effect has been extensively reviewed.[125] The recent observation of increased plasma levels of asymmetric dimethylarginine, an endogenous nitric oxide synthase inhibitor, in male and female drinkers compared to abstainers[126] would be consistent with such a postulate. Furthermore, in a case control study in chronic alcohol abusers there was decreased flow mediated dilation (FMD) in the brachial artery after 3 months of abstinence as compared to non-drinking controls.[127] In contrast, in a study in Japanese males with coronary artery disease endothelial function of the brachial artery was less impaired in drinkers despite a worse coronary risk factor profile.[128]

The possibility of unaccounted confounding to account for these disparate results is likely given the finding in a randomized controlled crossover trial of reducing alcohol consumption from beer from 72.4 to 7.9 g/day in 16 healthy male drinkers of no changes in either FMD of the brachial artery or biomarkers of endothelial function.[129] This finding has since been repeated using a similar paradigm but with male subjects also drinking either red wine or dealcoholized red wine and again with no discernible effects on FMD.[23] Interestingly, in that study urinary endothelin-1 excretion was higher during alcohol administration, suggesting that this endothelially derived potent vasoconstrictor may have contributed to the blood pressure elevation seen with either red wine or beer consumption.

An impact of alcohol intake on not just endothelial function but on stiffness of the arterial wall may be relevant to the genesis of alcohol-related hypertension. Compliance and distensibility of arterial walls may play a role in subsequent genesis of hypertension, especially isolated systolic hypertension (which is characterized by a widened pulse pressure closely linked to the presence of stiff arteries). The overall effect of alcohol intake on arterial stiffness remains controversial. In an Irish study,[90] male heavy drinkers had higher aortic stiffness and aortic systolic blood pressure compared to lighter drinkers. However, the same authors found that when red wine containing alcohol (0.8 g/kg) was ingested it acutely

reduced arterial stiffness.[90] In a study of Japanese male office workers where the development of aortic stiffness was studied prospectively over 9 years,[130] aortic stiffness was observed to increase progressively with increasing alcohol intake. Another more recent Japanese study (131) of 1682 middle-age male workers with normal blood pressure also found that high alcohol intake (>60 g of ethanol/day) was associated with increased arterial stiffening, as reflected in an elevated brachial-ankle pulse wave velocity (an increase that remained significant after controlling for conventional cardiovascular risk factors).

A further recent report from the Atherosclerosis Risk in Young Adults study found that the heaviest drinkers (>3 glasses/day) had a significantly higher augmentation index, consistent with increased arterial stiffness.[132] In contrast to these reports, a Dutch study utilizing pulse wave velocity as a measure of arterial stiffness suggested a J-shaped relationship with alcohol intake, with a reduction in arterial stiffness with mild to moderate alcohol intake but a loss of this potential protective effect at higher intakes (>3 to 8 drinks per day).[133] This same group of authors reported a similar J-shaped relationship in a separate study in 371 healthy postmenopausal women aged 50 to 74 years.[134] More recently, in a cross-sectional analysis of data from a cohort study in men and women aged 28 years (240 men and 283 women) the same authors suggested that a moderate intake of alcohol may favorably affect vascular stiffness at a relatively early age, notably in women.[135]

A similar favorable association was reported in the Baltimore Longitudinal Study of Aging, in which a U-shaped relation was found between alcohol intake and stiffness index for the common carotid artery in those subjects >55 years old in 774 community-based subjects.[136] In contrast, the Atherosclerosis Risk in Community (ARIC) study did not find any effects of regular alcohol intake on arterial stiffness in subjects aged 45 to 64 years,[137] a finding similar to the finding in subjects <55 years old in the Baltimore Longitudinal Study of Ageing.[136] In summary, the more consistent observation appears to be of increased vascular stiffness with heavier drinking, whereas the improvements in compliance reported with lighter drinking have been dependent on age and gender. The question as to whether the increase in arterial stiffness with heavier drinking is a prelude to alcohol-related hypertension or a consequence requires further study.

Finally, given that in many different tissues the disease consequences of chronic and excessive alcohol consumption have been ascribed to its ability to increase oxidative stress the possibility that alcohol-related hypertension may also arise at least in part from such an effect needs to be discussed. By monitoring isoprostane levels (an *in vivo* marker of oxidative stress), alcohol has been shown to induce oxidative stress acutely[138] and is associated with other biomarkers of oxidative stress in population-based studies,[139,140] including gamma-glutamyl transpeptidase (γGT).[139] γGT is essential for the uptake of extracellular glutathione, which helps maintain intracellular glutathione levels and therefore oxidative balance. γGT has been consistently related to level of blood pressure in cross-sectional studies,[141] and to incidence of hypertension in longitudinal studies.[142] Higher γGT levels have also been related to poor blood pressure control in treated hypertensive drinkers.[4] Thus, an increase in γGT with increasing alcohol intake may indicate those subjects who develop increased oxidative stress with alcohol resulting in vascular wall nitric oxide depletion and increased susceptibility to development of alcohol-related hypertension. The finding in an intervention study that falls in blood pressure following a 4-week period of reduced alcohol intake were greatest in subjects who initially had the highest γGT levels[143] supports such a proposition.

CLINICAL IMPLICATIONS AND PERSPECTIVES

The mean 4/2 mmHg fall in systolic and diastolic blood pressure (respectively) predicted from a reduction in alcohol intake by the meta-analysis of Xin et al.[40] should translate into an 18% decrease in the incidence of death from stroke and a 12% decrease in that from coronary heart disease. However, the complicated and often biphasic effects of alcohol on multiple cardiovascular risk factors means that this simple equation has no correlate in epidemiologic reality. At the same time as increasing blood pressure, alcohol has a dose-dependent action to increase HDL-cholesterol, decrease fibrinogen levels, and reduce platelet adhesiveness. Effects to enhance fibrinolysis and decrease lipoprotein-a may also be relevant. At high levels of consumption, however, disadvantageous influences on cardiovascular risk are mediated not only by the increase in blood pressure but by higher triglyceride levels, increased plasma homocysteine, and increased risk of type 2 diabetes mellitus. These contrasting effects translate into complex relationships of alcohol to stroke and coronary heart disease outcomes.

The relationships of alcohol to stroke, for example, have recently been described as an epidemiological labyrinth[144]—predominantly due to the contrasting effects of light versus heavy alcohol consumption on the myriad of stroke outcomes (ischemic stroke, cardio-embolic stroke, hemorrhagic stroke, and so on). A comprehensive systematic review of the association between alcohol and stroke[145] suggests that for ischemic stroke there is a J-shaped relationship with a decrease in risk at light drinking and an increase in risk with heavier drinking. The evidence linking light drinking with a reduction in risk was considered inconsistent, whereas that linking increased consumption (especially recent consumption and binge drinking)[87] to increased risk of ischemic stroke was considered strong. Alcohol-induced hypertension is probably a mediator of this increase in ischemic stroke risk, although in some studies the increase in risk remains even after adjustment for level of blood pressure. Important further considerations may therefore be cardioembolic stroke in the setting of alcohol-related atrial fibrillation or after acute binge drinking a combination of dehydration, hypotension, and perhaps impaired fibrinolytic activity. For hemorrhagic stroke, systematic review[145] reveals only an increase in risk with increasing consumption—an outcome possibly dictated by an alcohol-related increase in blood pressure in combination with the antithrombotic actions of alcohol.

A recent meta-analysis of the risks for coronary artery disease with increasing alcohol consumption suggested a biphasic J-shaped curve similar to the relationship seen for ischemic stroke. The nadir of the curve was seen at 20 g ethanol per day, with a mean decrease in relative risk of 20%.[146] At the level of 72 g per day, any protective effect was lost. At intakes greater than 89 g per day there was a mean 5% increase in relative coronary risk. Loss of the protective effect and the increase in risk with heavy alcohol consumption may reflect, at least in part, an effect from alcohol-related hypertension—as well as the increased risk of cardiac arrhythmia (both atrial fibrillation and ventricular fibrillation) and sudden cardiovascular death known to attend heavy drinking. Several studies suggest that any protective effects for coronary artery disease and ischemic stroke are likely to be confined not only to older subjects but to those with other established risk factors for cardiovascular disease such as increased LDL-cholesterol,[147] smoking,[148] or preexisting vascular disease or with specific genetic predisposition (e.g., apoE4 polymorphism[149] or the ADH3 genotype[54]).

Any benefits of alcohol for protection against ischemic heart disease will also be correspondingly less in populations with a low risk of atherosclerosis. In this regard, an analysis from the landmark World Health Organization Global Burden of Disease 2000 Comparative Risk Analysis study[150] (which looked carefully at risks and benefits of alcohol by region and then globally) attributed 16% of all hypertensive disease to alcohol, as well as 10% of hemorrhagic stroke and 2% of coronary artery disease events. Any promulgation of alcohol drinking as a means of reducing coronary artery disease risk in specific populations needs to carefully consider a balance of risks and benefits that is highly dependent on the background prevalence of other cardiovascular risk factors or genetic predisposition to atherosclerotic vascular disease.

What are the implications of these interrelationships for those with established hypertension? There is evidence that hypertension and heavy drinking may act synergistically to increase the risk of both cerebral hemorrhage and infarction two- and threefold, respectively.[151] However, other studies (such as a British study of 10,000 attendees at a hypertension clinic)[152] found a 40% decrease in relative risk of stroke in drinkers, with the lowest risk of stroke mortality at intakes of 8 to 80 g alcohol per week. Similarly, a decrease in risk of ischemic heart disease mortality was seen, but this finding was confined to males only. The population, however, included few heavy drinkers and the beneficial effects of alcohol were offset at intakes >21 units/week by an increasing incidence of noncirculatory causes of death.

Age may be an important consideration in such studies, with any overall survival benefits being restricted to predominantly older subjects.[153] In the Physicians' Health Study cohort[104] a group of 14,125 men with a history of current or past treatment for hypertension who were free of myocardial infarction or stroke at baseline were assessed for incidence of cardiovascular disease mortality at follow-up. Among men with a systolic blood pressure of 140 mmHg or higher or a diastolic blood pressure of 90 mm Hg or higher (when compared with individuals who rarely or never drank alcoholic beverages), those who reported monthly, weekly, and daily alcohol consumption had multivariate adjusted relative risks for cardiovascular disease mortality of 0.82, 0.64, and 0.56, respectively. These results also suggested that light to moderate alcohol consumption might be associated with a reduction in risk of cardiovascular disease mortality in hypertensive men.[154] However, the mean age of participants was 60 years at baseline, alcohol intake and blood pressure measurement were both self-reported, there was only a single baseline measure of alcohol intake, and no measure of the pattern of alcohol intake.

More worryingly, the finding that consumption of as little as a single alcoholic drink monthly could reduce overall cardiovascular risk by 18% strongly suggests confounding from an unmeasured effect modifier with nondrinkers probably an inappropriate comparison group in this study. In this regard, results from the recent Behavioural Risk Factor Surveillance System Survey, a telephone survey of over 200,000 adults in the USA,[155] revealed that 27 of 30 cardiovascular-associated risk factors or groups of factors (demographic, behavioral, socioeconomic, health related) were significantly more prevalent in nondrinkers than in light to moderate drinkers. Such observations suggest caution in extrapolating risk estimates from population-based studies in which nondrinkers have been the only reference group, with the chances of confounding from unmeasured effect modifiers very likely to account for much of the observed cardiovascular protective effects.

Similar questions need to be asked of the results from a prospective cohort study of French middle-age men who attended the Center for Preventive Medicine.[156] In that study, in moderate wine drinkers (those who consumed <60 g alcohol/day and no beer) there was a decreased risk of cardiovascular death by 24% compared to abstainers. However, this was not observed in heavier wine drinkers or drinkers of beer and spirits. When broken down by quartiles of systolic blood pressure, it was also concluded that moderate wine drinkers who were hypertensive also had a decreased risk of mortality from all causes. The study ignored major dietary and drinking pattern differences that have been consistently reported in relation to predominant beverage choice (wine drinkers less likely to binge drink, more likely to drink with meals, and more likely to make healthier diet choices).[22,157] The most recent study measuring cardiovascular outcomes in drinking hypertensives compared to abstainers was in a cohort of subjects with not only hypertension but documented left ventricular hypertrophy: the LIFE study.[158] In that study, in drinkers (>8 drinks per week) there was no decrease in composite cardiovascular risk while being treated with losartan compared to atenolol because a decrease in the incidence of myocardial infarction in the drinkers was offset by an increase in the risk of stroke.

SUMMARY

Alcohol-related hypertension is now established as a distinct clinical entity. Similar to essential hypertension, its pathophysiologic basis is multifactorial and complex, with a high likelihood of a significant contribution from genetic predisposition. Unlike essential hypertension, there is a substantial degree of reversibility, with intervention studies suggesting that the majority of any fall in blood pressure will occur within 2 to 4 weeks of a reduction in alcohol intake. Therefore, given global estimates that the contribution of alcohol to the attributable risk of hypertension is 16% moderation of consumption must remain a major public health priority for prevention of hypertensive disease. The links between chronic heavy drinking, especially binge drinking, and adverse cardiovascular outcomes such as ischemic and hemorrhagic stroke are clear (although the role of alcohol-related hypertension in the causal pathway is not always as well defined).

Any benefits of alcohol for protection against ischemic heart disease and stroke appear confined to low levels of consumption and to individuals and populations at increased risk of atherosclerotic vascular disease. Subjects with established hypertension may similarly anticipate a decrease in risk with light drinking, although the magnitude of any benefit has probably been overestimated because of inability to control for important confounders. This has been recently reemphasized by Jackson et al.,[159] who hold that any benefits are likely to be outweighed by harmful effects (with the conclusion that there was "probably no free lunch"). In hypertensive subjects, from the point of view of cardiovascular benefits an intake averaging about 1 to 2 standard drinks a day in men (10 to 20 g alcohol) and up to one a day in women (10 g alcohol) would appear to offer the optimal level of consumption in terms of relative benefits and risks. In normotensive subjects, similar upper levels of intake would appear a sensible recommendation in terms of prevention of alcohol-related hypertension and its sequelae. Binge drinking (which poses a particularly high risk scenario for stroke, coronary events, arrhythmia, and sudden death) should be discouraged in all subjects.

REFERENCES

1. Mahomed FA. The sphygmographic evidence of arterio-capillary fibrosis. *Trans Path Soc* 1877;28:394–94.
2. Lian C. L'alcoolisme, cause d'hypertension arterielle. *Bull Acad Med* 1915;74:525–28.
3. Saunders JB, Beevers DG, Paton A. Alcohol-induced hypertension. *Lancet* 1981;2:653–56.
4. Henningsen NC, Ohlsson O, Mattiasson I, et al. Hypertension, levels of serum gamma glutamyl transpeptidase and degree of blood pressure control in middle-aged males. *Acta Med Scand* 1980;207:245–51.
5. Matthews JD. Alcohol use as a possible explanation for socio-economic and occupational differentials in mortality

from hypertension and coronary heart disease in England and Wales. *Aust NZ J Med* 1976;6:393–97.

6. Klatsky AL, Friedman GD, Siegelaub AB, Gerard MJ. Alcohol consumption and blood pressure: Kaiser-Permanente Multiphasic Health Examination Data. *N Engl J Med* 1977;296:1194–1200.

7. Marmot MG, Elliott P, Shipley MJ, et al. Alcohol and blood pressure: The INTERSALT study. *Br Med J* 1994; 308:1263–67.

8. Burger M, Bronstrup A, Pietrzik K. Derivation of tolerable upper alcohol intake levels in Germany: A systematic review of risks and benefits of moderate alcohol consumption. *Prev Med* 2004; 39:111–27.

9. Arkwright PD, Beilin LJ, Rouse I, et al. Effects of alcohol use and other aspects of lifestyle on blood pressure levels and prevalence of hypertension in a working population. *Circulation* 1982;66:60–6.

10. Moreira LB, Fuchs FD, Moraes RS, et al. Alcohol intake and blood pressure: The importance of time elapsed since last drink. *J Hypertens* 1998;16:175–80.

11. Klatsky AL, Friedman GD, Armstrong MA. The relationship between alcoholic beverage use and other traits to blood pressure: A new Kaiser Permanente study. *Circulation* 1986;73:628–36.

12. Krogh V, Trevisan M, Jossa F, et al. Alcohol and blood pressure: The effect of age, findings from the Italian Nine Communities Study. *Ann Epidemiol* 1993;3:245–49.

13. Burke V, Beilin LJ, German R, et al. Association of lifestyle and personality characteristics with blood pressure and hypertension: a cross-sectional study in the elderly. *J Clin Epidemiol* 1992; 45:1061–70.

14. Jerez SJ, Coviello A. Alcohol drinking and blood pressure among adolescents. *Alcohol* 1998;16:1–5.

15. Trevisan M, Strazzulo P, Cappuccio F, et al. Alcohol consumption and blood pressure in school children. *Int J of Pediat Nephrol* 1987;8:25–8.

16. Palatini P. Factors affecting the daily variation of blood pressure. The HARVEST study. *Cardiovascular Risk Factors* 1997;7:206–13.

17. Wildman RP, Gu DF, Muntner P, et al. Alcohol intake and hypertension subtypes in Chinese men. *J Hypertens* 2005;23:737–43.

18. Stranges S, Wu T, Dorn JM, et al. Relationship of alcohol drinking pattern to risk of hypertension: A population-based study. *Hypertension* 2004; 44:813–19.

19. Okamura T, Tanaka T, Yoshita K, et al. Specific alcoholic beverage and blood pressure in a middle-aged Japanese population: The High-risk and Population Strategy for Occupational Health Promotion (HIPOP-OHP) Study. *J Hum Hypertens* 2004;18:9–16.

20. Criqui MH, Wallace RB, Mishkel M, et al. Alcohol consumption and blood pressure: The Lipid Research Clinics Prevalence Study. *Hypertension* 1981;3:557–65.

21. Marques-Vidal P, Montaye M, Haas B, et al. Relationships between alcoholic beverages and cardiovascular risk factor levels in middle-aged men: The PRIME study. *Atherosclerosis* 2001; 157:431–40.

22. Tjonneland A, Gronbaek M, Stripp C, Overvad K. Wine intake and diet in a random sample of 48763 Danish men and women. *Am J Clin Nutr* 1999; 69:49–54.

23. Zilkens RR, Burke V, Hodgson JM, et al. Red wine and beer elevate blood pressure in normotensive men. *Hypertension* 2005;45:874–79.

24. Geleijnse JM, Kok FJ, Grobbee DE. Impact of dietary and lifestyle factors on the prevalence of hypertension in Western populations. *European J Pub Health* 2004;14:235–39.

25. Hamet P, Mongeau E, Lambert J, et al. Interactions among calcium, sodium, and alcohol intake as determinants of blood pressure. *Hypertension* 1991; 17:I150–54.

26. Parker M, Puddey IB, Beilin LJ, Vandongen R. Two-way factorial study of alcohol and salt restriction in treated hypertensive men. *Hypertension* 1990;16:398–406.

27. Hartung GH, Kohl HW, Blair SN, et al. Exercise tolerance and alcohol intake: Blood pressure relation. *Hypertension* 1990;16:501–07.

28. Cox KL, Puddey IB, Morton AR, et al. The combined effects of aerobic exercise and alcohol restriction on blood pressure and serum lipids: A two-way factorial study in sedentary men. *J Hypertens* 1993;11:191–201.

29. Puddey IB, Parker M, Beilin LJ, et al. Effects of alcohol and caloric restrictions on blood pressure and serum lipids in overweight men. *Hypertension* 1992; 20:533–41.

30. Keil U, Chambless L, Filipiak B, Hartel U. Alcohol and blood pressure and its interaction with smoking and other behavioural variables: Results from the MONICA Augsburg Survey 1984–1985. *J Hypertens* 1991; 9:491–98.

31. Schnall PL, Schwartz JE, Landsbergis PA, et al. Relation between job strain, alcohol and ambulatory blood pressure. *Hypertension* 1992;19:488–94.

32. Corrao G, Bagnardi V, Zambon A, Arico S. Exploring the dose-response relationship between alcohol consumption and the risk of several alcohol-related conditions: A meta-analysis. *Addiction* 1999;94:1551–73.

33. Nakanishi N, Yoshida H, Nakamura K, et al. Alcohol consumption and risk for hypertension in middle-aged Japanese men. *J Hypertens* 2001;19:851–55.

34. Fuchs FD, Chambless LE, Whelton PK, et al. Alcohol consumption and the incidence of hypertension: The Atherosclerosis Risk in Communities Study. *Hypertension* 2001;37:1242–50.

35. Saremi A, Hanson RL, Tulloch-Reid M, et al. Alcohol consumption predicts hypertension but not diabetes. *J Stud Alcohol* 2004;65:184–90.

36. Henriksson KM, Lindblad U, Gullberg B, et al. Development of hypertension over 6 years in a birth cohort of young middle-aged men: The Cardiovascular Risk Factor Study in southern Sweden (CRISS). *J Intern Med* 2002;252:21–6.

37. Puddey IB, Beilin LJ, Vandongen R, et al. Evidence for a direct effect of alcohol consumption on blood pressure in normotensive men: A randomized controlled trial. *Hypertension* 1985;7:707–13.

38. Puddey IB, Beilin LJ, Vandongen R. Regular alcohol use raises blood pressure in treated hypertensive subjects: A randomised controlled trial. *Lancet* 1987;1:647–51.

39. Ueshima H, Mikawa K, Baba S, et al. Effect of reduced alcohol consumption on blood pressure in untreated hypertensive men. *Hypertension* 1993; 21:248–52.

40. Xin X, He J, Frontini MG, et al. Effects of alcohol reduction on blood pressure: A meta-analysis of randomized controlled trials. *Hypertension* 2001; 38:1112–17.

41. McFadden CB, Brensinger CM, Berlin JA, Townsend RR. Systematic review of the effect of daily alcohol intake on blood pressure. *Am J Hypertens* 2005;18:276–86.

42. Hajjar IM, Grim CE, George V, Kotchen TA. Impact of diet on blood pressure and age-related changes in blood pressure in the US population: Analysis of NHANES III. *Arch Int Med* 2001;161:589–93.

43. Harburg E, Ozgoren F, Hawthorne V, Schork A. Community norms of alcohol usage and blood pressure: Tecumseh, Michigan. *Am J Pub Health* 1980;70:813–20.

44. Holman CDJ, English DR, Milne E, Winter MG. Meta-analysis of alcohol and all-cause mortality: A validation of NHMRC recommendations. *Med J Aust* 1996;164:141–45.

45. Cooke KM, Frost GW, Stokes GS. Blood pressure and its relationship to low levels of alcohol consumption. *Clin Exp Pharmacol Physiol* 1983; 10:229–33.

46. Laforge R, Williams GD, Dufour MC. Alcohol consumption, gender and self-reported hypertension. *Drug Alc Dependence* 1990;26:235–49.

47. Nanchahal K, Ashton WD, Wood DA. Alcohol consumption, metabolic cardiovascular risk factors and hypertension in women. *Int J Epidemiol* 2000;29:57–64.

48. Thadhani R, Camargo CA Jr., Stampfer MJ, et al. Prospective study of moderate alcohol consumption and risk of hypertension in young women. *Arch Int Med* 2002;162:569–74.

49. Puddey IB, Mori TA, Burke V, et al. The effects of red wine on ambulatory blood pressure in pre-menopausal women: A controlled intervention study. *J Hypertens* 2005;S99.

50. Tsuritani I, Ikai E, Date T, et al. Polymorphism in ALDH2-genotype in Japanese men and the alcohol-blood pressure relationship. *Am J Hypertens* 1995;8:1053–59.

51. Amamoto K, Okamura T, Tamaki S, et al. Epidemiologic study of the association of low-K-m mitochondrial acetaldehyde dehydrogenase genotypes with blood pressure level and the prevalence of hypertension in a general population. *Hypertension Research* 2002;25:857–64.

52. Hashimoto Y, Nakayama T, Futamura A, et al. Relationship between genetic polymorphisms of alcohol-metabolizing enzymes and changes in risk factors for coronary heart disease associated with alcohol consumption. *Clin Chem* 2002;48:1043–48.

53. Yamada Y, Sun F, Tsuritani I, Honda R. Genetic differences in ethanol metabolizing enzymes and blood pressure in Japanese alcohol consumers. *J Human Hypertens* 2002;16:479–86.

54. Hines LM, Stampfer MJ, Ma J, et al. Genetic variation in alcohol dehydrogenase and the beneficial effect of moderate alcohol consumption on myocardial infarction. *N Engl J Med* 2001;344:549–55.

55. Kauma H, Savolainen MJ, Rantala AO, et al. Apolipoprotein E phenotype determines the effect of alcohol on blood pressure in middle-aged men. *Am J Hypertens* 1998;11:1334–43.

56. Puddey IB, Rakic V, Dimmitt SB, et al. Apolipoprotein E genotype and the blood pressure raising effect of alcohol. *Am J Hypertens* 1999;12:946–47.

57. Takashima Y, Kokaze A, Matsunaga N, et al. Relations of blood pressure to angiotensinogen gene T174M polymorphism and alcohol intake. *J Physiol Anthropol Appl Human Sci* 2003;22:187–94.

58. Chen Y, Nakura J, Jin JJ, et al. Association of the GNAS1 gene variant with hypertension is dependent on alcohol consumption. *Hypertens Res* 2003;26:439–44.

59. Khetarpal V, Volicer L. Effects of ethanol on blood pressure of normal and hypertensive rats. *J Stud Alc* 1979; 40:732–36.

60. Sanderson JE, Jones JV, Graham DI. Effect of chronic alcohol ingestion on the heart and blood pressure of spontaneously hypertensive rats. *Clin Exp Hypertens* 1983;5:673–89.

61. Howe PRC, Rogers PF, Smith RM. Effects of chronic alcohol consumption and alcohol withdrawal on blood pressure in stroke-prone spontaneously hypertensive rats. *J Hypertens* 1989; 7:387–93.

62. Howe PR, Rogers PF, Smith RM. Antihypertensive effect of alcohol in spontaneously hypertensive rats. *Hypertension* 1989;13:607–11.

63. Chan TC, Sutter MC. The effects of chronic ethanol consumption on cardiac function. *Can J Physiol Pharmacol* 1982;60:777–82.

64. Chan TC, Sutter MC. Ethanol consumption and blood pressure. *Life Sci* 1983;33:1965–73.

65. Chan TC, Godin DV, Sutter MC. Erythrocyte membrane properties of the chronic alcoholic rat. *Drug Alc Dependence* 1983;12:249–57.

66. Vasdev S, Sampson CA, Prabhakaran VM. Platelet-free calcium and vascular calcium uptake in ehtanol-induced hypertensive rats. *Hypertension* 1991; 18:116–22.

67. Vasdev S, Gupta IP, Sampson CA, et al. Ethanol induced hypertension in rats: Reversibility and role of intracellular cytosolic calcium. *Artery* 1993; 20:19–43.

68. Vasdev S, Mian T, Longerich L, et al. N-acetyl cysteine attenuates ethanol induced hypertension in rats. *Artery* 1995;21:312–36.

69. Vasdev S, Wadhawan S, Ford CA, et al. Dietary vitamin B6 supplementation prevents ethanol-induced hypertension in rats. *Nutr Metab Cardiovasc Dis* 1999;9:55–63.

70. Jones JV, Raine AEG, Sanderson JE, et al. Adverse effect of chronic alcohol ingestion on cardiac performance in spontaneously hypertensive rats. *J Hypertens* 1988;6:419–22.

71. Hatton DC, Bukoski RD, Edgar S, McCarron DA. Chronic alcohol consumption lowers blood pressure but enhances vascular contractility in Wistar rats. *J Hypertens* 1992; 10:529–37.

72. Beilin LJ, Hoffmann P, Nilsson H, et al. Effect of chronic ethanol consumption upon cardiovascular reactivity, heart rate and blood pressure in spontaneously hypertensive and Wistar-Kyoto rats. *J Hypertens* 1992; 10:645–50.

73. Crandall DL, Ferraro GD, Lozito RJ, et al. Cardiovascular effects of intermittent drinking: Assessment of a novel animal model of human alcoholism. *J Hypertens* 1989; 7:683–87.

74. El Mas MM, Abdel-Rahman AA. Radiotelemetric evaluation of hemodynamic effects of long-term ethanol in spontaneously hypertensive and Wistar-Kyoto rats. *J Pharmacol Exp Ther* 2000;292:944–51.

75. El Mas MM, Abdel-Rahman AA. Autonomic modulation of altered diurnal hemodynamic profiles in ethanol-fed hypertensive rats. *Alcohol Clin Exp Res* 2005;29:499–508.

76. Puddey IB, Burke V, Croft K, Beilin LJ. Increased blood pressure and changes in membrane lipids associated with chronic ethanol treatment of rats. *Clin Exp Pharmacol Physiol* 1995; 22:655–57.

77. Hsieh ST, Sano H, Saito K, et al. Magnesium supplementation prevents the development of alcohol-induced hypertension. *Hypertension* 1992; 19:175–82.

78. El Mas MM, Abdel-Rahman AA. Contrasting effects of chronic ethanol feeding on centrally and peripherally evoked hypotension in telemetered female rats. *Vascul Pharmacol* 2004; 41:59–66.

79. El Mas MM, Abdel-Rahman AA. Chronic ethanol-clonidine hemodynamic interaction in telemetered spontaneously hypertensive rats. *Vascul Pharmacol* 2004;41:107–13.

80. El Mas MM, Abdel-Rahman AA. Chronic ethanol administration attenuates imidazoline I1 receptor- or alpha 2-adrenoceptor-mediated reductions in blood pressure and hemodynamic variability in hypertensive rats. *Eur J Pharmacol* 2004;485:251–62.

81. Abdel-Rahman A-RA, Dar MS, Wooles WR. Effect of chronic ethanol administration on arterial baroreceptor function and pressor and depressor responsiveness in rats. *J Pharmacol Exp Ther* 1984;232:194–201.

82. Abdel-Rahman AA, Wooles WR. Ethanol-induced hypertension involves impairment of baroreceptors. *Hypertension* 1987;10:67–73.

83. Varga K, Gantenberg NS, Kunos G. Endogenous gamma-aminobutyric acid (GABA) mediates ethanol inhibition of vagally mediated reflex bradycardia elicited from aortic baroreceptors. *J Pharmacol Expl Ther* 1994;268:1057–62.

84. Mao L, Abdel-Rahman AA. Blockade of L-glutamate receptors in the rostral ventrolateral medulla contributes to ethanol-evoked impairment of baroreflexes in conscious rats. *Brain Res Bull* 1995;37:513–21.

85. Silva TP, Silveira GA, Fior-Chadi DR, Chadi G. Effects of ethanol consumption on vasopressin and neuropeptide Y immunoreactivity and mRNA expression in peripheral and central areas related to cardiovascular regulation. *Alcohol* 2004;32:213–22.

86. York JL, Hirsch JA. Residual pressor effects of chronic alcohol in detoxified alcoholics. *Hypertension* 1996; 28:133–38.

87. Hansagi H, Romelsjo A, Gerhardsson de Verdier M, et al. Alcohol consumption and stroke mortality: 20-year follow-up of 15,077 men and women. *Stroke* 1995;26:1768–73.

88. Shaper AG, Phillips AN, Pocock SJ, Walker M. Alcohol and ischaemic heart disease in middle aged British men. *Br Med J* 1987;294:733–37.

89. Sutton-Tyrrell K, Alcorn HG, Wolfson SK Jr., et al. Predictors of carotid stenosis in older adults with and without isolated systolic hypertension. *Stroke* 1993;24:355–61.

90. Mahmud A, Feely J. Divergent effect of acute and chronic alcohol on arterial stiffness. *Am J Hypertens* 2002;15: 240–43.

91. Manolio TA, Levy D, Garrison RJ, et al. Relation of alcohol intake to left ventricular mass: The Framingham Study. *J Am Coll Cardiol* 1991;17: 717–21.

92. Potter JF, Beevers DG. The possible mechanisms of alcohol associated hypertension. *Ann Clin Res* 1984; 16(Suppl 43):97–102.

93. Maheswaran R, Gill JS, Davies P, Beevers DG. High blood pressure due to alcohol. A rapidly reversible effect. *Hypertension* 1991;17:787–92.

94. Puddey IB, Jenner DA, Beilin LJ, Vandongen R. An appraisal of the effects of usual vs recent alcohol intake on blood pressure. *Clin Exp Pharmacol Physiol* 1988;15:261–64.

95. Abe H, Kawano Y, Kojima S, et al. Biphasic effects of repeated alcohol intake on 24-hour blood pressure in hypertensive patients. *Circulation* 1994;89:2626–33.

96. Wannamethee G, Shaper AG. Alcohol intake and variations in blood pressure by day of examination. *J Hum Hypertens* 1991;5:59–67.

97. Marques-Vidal P, Arveiler D, Evans A, et al. Different alcohol drinking and blood pressure relationships in France and Northern Ireland: The PRIME Study. *Hypertension* 2001;38:1361–66.

98. Rakic V, Puddey IB, Burke V, et al. Influence of pattern of alcohol intake on blood pressure in regular drinkers: A controlled trial. *J Hypertens* 1998; 16:165–74.

99. Seppa K, Laippala P, Sillanaukee P. Drinking pattern and blood pressure. *Am J Hypertens* 1994;7:249–54.

100. Masarei JR, Puddey IB, Rouse IL, et al. Effects of alcohol consumption on serum lipoprotein-lipid and apolipoprotein concentrations: Results

from an intervention study in healthy subjects. *Atherosclerosis* 1986;60:79–87.

101. Yoon YS, Oh SW, Baik HW, et al. Alcohol consumption and the metabolic syndrome in Korean adults: The 1998 Korean National Health and Nutrition Examination Survey. *Am J Clin Nutr* 2004;80:217–24.

102. Lee WY, Jung CH, Park JS, et al. Effects of smoking, alcohol, exercise, education, and family history on the metabolic syndrome as defined by the ATP III. *Diab Res Clin Pract* 2005; 67:70–7.

103. Goude D, Fagerberg B, Hulthe J. Alcohol consumption, the metabolic syndrome and insulin resistance in 58-year-old clinically healthy men (AIR study). *Clin Sci* 2002;102:345–52.

104. Freiberg MS, Cabral HJ, Heeren TC, et al. Alcohol consumption and the prevalence of the metabolic syndrome in the US: A cross-sectional analysis of data from the Third National Health and Nutrition Examination Survey. *Diab Care* 2004;27:2954–59.

105. Djousse L, Arnett DK, Eckfeldt JH, et al. Alcohol consumption and metabolic syndrome: Does the type of beverage matter? *Obesity Res* 2004;12:1375–85.

106. Koppes LLJ, Dekker JM, Hendriks HFJ, et al. Moderate alcohol consumption lowers the risk of type 2 diabetes: A meta-analysis of prospective observational studies. *Diab Care* 2005; 28:719–25.

107. Howard AA, Arnsten JH, Gourevitch MN. Effect of alcohol consumption on diabetes mellitus: A systematic review. *Ann Intern Med* 2004;140:211–19.

108. Zilkens RR, Burke V, Watts G, et al. The effect of alcohol intake on insulin sensitivity in men: A randomized controlled trial. *Diab Care* 2003; 26:608–12.

109. Roth MJ, Baer DJ, Albert PS, et al. Relationship between serum leptin levels and alcohol consumption in a controlled feeding and alcohol ingestion study. *J Natl Cancer Inst* 2003;95:1722–25.

110. Di Gennaro C, Barilli A, Giuffredi C, et al. Sodium sensitivity of blood pressure in long-term detoxified alcoholics. *Hypertension* 2000; 35:869–74.

111. Di Gennaro C, Vescovi PP, Barilli AL, et al. Sodium sensitivity as a main determinant of blood pressure changes during early withdrawal in heavy alcoholics. *Alcohol Clin Exp Res* 2002;26:1810–15.

112. De Marchi S, Cecchin E. Alcohol withdrawal and hypertension: Evidence for a kidney abnormality. *Clin Sci* 1985;69:239–40.

113. Kawano Y, Abe H, Kojima S, et al. Effects of repeated alcohol intake on blood pressure and sodium balance in Japanese males with hypertension. *Hypertens Res* 2004;27:167–72.

114. Flink EB. Magnesium deficiency in alcoholism. *Alcohol Clin Exp Res* 1986;10:590–94.

115. Hsieh ST, Saito K, Miyajima T, et al. Effects of alcohol moderation on blood pressure and intracellular cations in mild essential hypertension. *Am J Hypertens* 1995;8:696–703.

116. Altura BM, Altura BT. Mechanisms of alcohol-induced-hypertension: Importance of intracellular cations and magnesium. In: *Alcohol and the Cardiovascular System. National Institute on Alcohol Abuse and Alcoholism*, Research Monograph 31, Bethesda, MD: NIH 1996:591–614.

117. Ema M, Gebrewold A, Altura BT, et al. Alcohol-induced vascular damage of brain is ameliorated by administration of magnesium. *Alcohol* 1998;15: 95–103.

118. Virtanen R, Jula A, Kuusela T, et al. Reduced heart rate variability in hypertension: Associations with lifestyle factors and plasma renin activity. *J Hum Hypertens* 2003; 17:171–79.

119. Stolarz K, Staessen JA, Kuznetsova T, et al. Host and environmental determinants of heart rate and heart rate variability in four European populations. *J Hypertens* 2003; 21:525–35.

120. Minami J, Yoshii M, Todoroki M, et al. Effects of alcohol restriction on ambulatory blood pressure, heart rate, and heart rate variability in Japanese men. *Am J Hypertens* 2002;15:125–29.

121. van de BP, Mark AL, Montano N, et al. Effects of alcohol on sympathetic activity, hemodynamics, and chemoreflex sensitivity. *Hypertension* 1997;29:1278–83.

122. Randin D, Vollenweider P, Tappy L, et al. Suppression of alcohol-induced hypertension by dexamethasone [see comments]. *N Engl J Med* 1995; 332:1733–37.

123. Abdel-Rahman A-RA, Merrill RH, Wooles WR. Effect of acute ethanol administration on the baroreceptor reflex control of heart rate in normotensive human volunteers. *Clin Sci* 1987;72:113–22.

124. Kardos A, Watterich G, de Menezes R, et al. Determinants of spontaneous baroreflex sensitivity in a healthy working population. *Hypertension* 2001;37:911–16.

125. Puddey IB, Zilkens RR, Croft KD, Beilin LJ. Alcohol and endothelial function: A brief review. *Clin Exp Pharmacol Physiol* 2001;28:1020–24.

126. Paiva H, Lehtimaki T, Laakso J, et al. Dietary composition as a determinant of plasma asymmetric dimethylarginine in subjects with mild hypercholesterolemia. *Metabolism* 2004;53:1072–75.

127. Maiorano G, Bartolomucci F, Contursi V, et al. Noninvasive detection of vascular dysfunction in alcoholic patients. *Am J Hypertens* 1999;12:137–44.

128. Teragawa H, Fukuda Y, Matsuda K, et al. Effect of alcohol consumption on endothelial function in men with coronary artery disease. *Atherosclerosis* 2002;165:145–152.

129. Zilkens RR, Rich L, Burke V, et al. Effects of alcohol intake on endothelial function in men: a randomized controlled trial. *J Hypertens* 2003; 21:97–103.

130. Nakanishi N, Kawashimo H, Nakamura K, et al. Association of alcohol consumption with increase in aortic stiffness: A 9-year longitudinal study in middle-aged Japanese men. *Ind Health* 2001;39:24–8.

131. Kurihara T, Tomiyama H, Hashimoto H, et al. Excessive alcohol intake increases the risk of arterial stiffening in men with normal blood pressure. *Hypertens Res* 2004;27:669–73.

132. van Trijp MJ, Beulens JW, Bos WJ, et al. Alcohol consumption and augmentation index in healthy young men: The ARYA study. *Am J Hypertens* 2005;18:792–96.

133. Sierksma A, Muller M, van der Schouw YT, et al. Alcohol consumption and arterial stiffness in men. *J Hypertens* 2004;22:357–62.

134. Sierksma A, Lebrun CE, van der Schouw YT, et al. Alcohol consumption in relation to aortic stiffness and aortic wave reflections: A cross-sectional study in healthy postmenopausal women. *Arterioscler Thromb Vasc Biol* 2004;24:342–48.

135. van den Elzen AP, Sierksma A, Oren A, et al. Alcohol intake and aortic stiffness in young men and women. *J Hypertens* 2005;23:731–35.

136. Hougaku H, Fleg JL, Lakatta EG, et al. Effect of light-to-moderate alcohol consumption on age-associated arterial stiffening. *Am J Cardiol* 2005; 95:1006–10.

137. Demirovic J, Nabulsi A, Folsom AR, et al. Alcohol consumption and ultrasonographically assessed carotid artery wall thickness and distensibility: The Atherosclerosis Risk in Communities (ARIC) Study Investigators. *Circulation* 1993;88:2787–93.

138. Meagher EA, Barry OP, Burke AP, et al. Alcohol-induced generation of lipid peroxidation products in humans. *J Clin Invest* 1999;104:805–13.

139. Ward NC, Puddey IB, Hodgson JM, et al. Urinary 20-hydroxyeicosatetraenoic acid excretion is associated with oxidative stress in hypertensive subjects. *Free Rad Biol Med* 2005; 38:1032–36.

140. Trevisan M, Browne R, Ram M, et al. Correlates of markers of oxidative status in the general population. *Am J Epidemiol* 2001;154:348–56.

141. Henningsen NC, Janzon L, Trell E. Influence of carboxyhemoglobin, gamma-glutamyl-transferase, body weight, and heart rate on blood pressure in middle-aged men. *Hypertension* 1983;5:560–63.

142. Nilssen O, Forde OH. Seven-year longitudinal population study of change in gamma-glutamyltransferase: The Tromso Study. *Am J Epidemiol* 1994;139:787–92.

143. Yamada Y, Tsuritani I, Ishizaki M, et al. Serum gamma-glutamyl transferase levels and blood pressure falls after alcohol moderation. *Clin Exp Hypertens* 1997;19:249–68.

144. Klatsky AL. Alcohol and Stroke: An Epidemiological Labyrinth. *Stroke* 2005;36:1835–6.

145. Mazzaglia G, Britton AR, Altmann DR, Chenet L. Exploring the relationship between alcohol consumption and non-fatal or fatal stroke: A systematic review. *Addiction* 2001;96:1743–56.

146. Corrao G, Rubbiati L, Bagnardi V, et al. Alcohol and coronary heart disease: A meta-analysis. *Addiction* 2000;95: 1505–23.

147. Hein HO, Suadicani P, Gyntelberg F. Alcohol consumption, serum low density lipoprotein cholesterol concentration, and risk of ischaemic heart disease: six year follow up in the Copenhagen male study. *Br Med J* 1996;312:736–41.

148. Manttari M, Tenkanen L, Alikoski T, Manninen V. Alcohol and coronary heart disease: The roles of HDL-cholesterol and smoking. *J Int Med* 1997;241:157–63.

149. Mukamal KJ, Chung H, Jenny NS, et al. Alcohol use and risk of ischemic stroke among older adults: The Cardiovascular Health Study. *Stroke* 2005;36:1830–34.

150. Rehm J, Room R, Monteiro M, et al. Alcohol as a risk factor for global burden of disease. *Eur Addict Res* 2003;9:157–64.

151. Kiyohara Y, Kato I, Iwamoto H, et al. The impact of alcohol and hypertension on stroke incidence in a general Japanese population: The Hisayama Study. *Stroke* 1995; 26:368–72.

152. Palmer AJ, Fletcher AE, Bulpitt CJ, et al. Alcohol intake and cardiovascular mortality in hypertensive patients: Report from the Department of Health Hypertension Care Computing Project. *J Hypertens* 1995;13:957–64.

153. Bulpitt CJ. How many alcoholic drinks might benefit an older person with hypertension? *J Hypertens* 2005; 23:1947–51.

154. Malinski MK, Sesso HD, Lopez-Jimenez F, et al. Alcohol consumption and cardiovascular disease mortality in hypertensive men. *Arch Int Med* 2004;164:623–28.

155. Naimi TS, Brown DW, Brewer RD, et al. Cardiovascular risk factors and confounders among nondrinking and moderate-drinking U.S. adults. *Am J Prev Med* 2005;28:369–73.

156. Renaud SC, Gueguen R, Conard P, et al. Moderate wine drinkers have lower hypertension-related mortality: A prospective cohort study in French men. *Am J Clin Nutr* 2004;80:621–25.

157. Burke V, Puddey IB, Beilin LJ. Mortality associated with wines, beers, and spirits: Australian data suggest that choice of beverage relates to lifestyle and personality. *Br Med J* 1995; 311:1166–66.

158. Reims HM, Kjeldsen SE, Brady WE, et al. Alcohol consumption and cardiovascular risk in hypertensives with left ventricular hypertrophy: The LIFE study. *J Human Hypertens* 2004;18:381–89.

159. Jackson R, Broad J, Connor J, Wells S. Alcohol and ischemic heart disease: Probably no free lunch. *Lancet* 2005;366:1911–12.

Chapter

42

Psychosocial Stress and Hypertension

Michael W. Brands and Dexter L. Lee

Key Findings

- A psychosocial stressor is a culturally or socially based situation to which an individual attaches enough meaning so that it is perceived as a challenge.

- Once perceived as a challenge, the sympathetic nervous system and the hypothalamic-pituitary-adrenocortical axis are activated, varying in relative strength depending on coping strategy. An active response to control the stressor drives the sympathetic system.

- Sympathetic-mediated hypertension is augmented, particularly with chronic stress, by components of the HPA-axis and is linked to angiotensin II and cytokines.

- Sustained exposure to a psychosocial stressor causes sustained hypertension in susceptible individuals, and such a response should be considered a risk factor for essential hypertension.

It is interesting, if not perplexing, that even though psychological factors have been implicated as causes of essential hypertension since at least the 1930s[1] (and there is current scientific acceptance[2–14] and a general perception in the lay public that psychological factors can increase blood pressure), proof that there can be a psychological basis for chronic hypertension is elusive.[10] One explanation for this may be that the studies in mice in the 1960s and 1970s by Henry et al.[15–17] that began to strengthen the case for psychosocial stress-induced hypertension were not readily reproducible in rats,[18] and it often is difficult to make the association between results from animal and human studies. Another factor, to be discussed later, is the time frame in which the hypertension is studied or defined. In addition, evidence from the Western Collaborative Group Study[19,20] and Framingham that began linking stress to coronary artery disease (CAD) may have caused a shift in emphasis in the cardiovascular literature.[21,22] Indeed, much of the clinical interest in stress-induced increases in blood pressure lies in its predictive value for CAD,[3,21–24] although the deleterious effects of hypertension on other aspects of the circulation are well established. However, regardless of the perception there is evidence that psychosocial stress can cause hypertension in humans.[11,14]

An extensive study by Schnall et al.[25] revealed a significant effect of job stress in increasing blood pressure, and that group later confirmed those findings using ambulatory blood pressure monitoring.[26] However, the effect of job stress in causing hypertension has not been demonstrated consis-

tently,[27,28] with analyses from the same patient studies even yielding conflicting results.[8,29] Inconsistent results linking job stress to hypertension have been attributed to methods for measuring blood pressure and to considerations of what factors interact with job stress.[10,30] For example, low socioeconomic status has been associated with higher blood pressure in several studies (including large clinical trials[31–35]) but the effect of job stress in increasing blood pressure has been linked to both low[35,36] and high[8,37] socioeconomic status. The contrasting findings may be because the ability of job stress to increase blood pressure has been linked to the workers' perception of their control over their job,[10,11,30,38] and workers of higher socioeconomic status may be more stressed by low job control compared to workers of lower socioeconomic status.[8,30,38]

The issue of control and the attempt to gain or maintain control is a fundamental concept in evaluating not only the blood pressure response to stress but in determining whether a given event or condition is even defined as a stressor. The next section, therefore, defines a stressor and what makes it capable of inducing a physiological response such as increased blood pressure.

ANATOMY OF A PSYCHOSOCIAL STRESSOR

We will define psychosocial stress as psychological stress in which the meaning attached to the stressor is dependent on the cultural context and social environment (e.g., socioeconomic status). A logical assumption would be that psychosocial stress is a subset of a more generalized umbrella or syndrome of stress, and with regard to hypertension has unique characteristics that define its effect on blood pressure versus the blood pressure effects of other stress subtypes. This is true to a great extent, but it implies a framework in which a well-defined syndrome of stress is neatly subdivided into various subtypes (each of which has its own characteristic causes and effects). However, perhaps the most uniform observation when delving into the stress-hypertension literature is the frustration authors express at the outset in attempting just to define "stress."

This frustration can be traced back even to the person recognized as the originator of the modern concept of stress, Hans Selye. Selye began writing in 1936 about what he called the General Adaptation Syndrome, which was the nonspecific response of the body to any demand.[39–41] Thus, his focus was on the response, and Dr. Selye has been noted as saying that he would have been remembered as the father of the "strain" concept had his knowledge of English been more precise at the time of his early writings.[42] The reference was to Hooke's law, in which stress is an external force that produces strain in a malleable metal, and Dr. Selye's comment serves to highlight the importance of distinguishing between the challenge versus the stress response.

Challenges, or stressors, range from physical (e.g., heat or infection) to emotional or psychological. Responses also cover the same range, with seemingly infinite possibilities for combinations and overlap depending on the stressor and other factors. For example, being hot can provide a psychological challenge in addition to its physical challenge, leading to emotional and/or physiological stress responses (and different stressors may activate the same neural or hormonal response systems). Therefore, we will not attempt an all-inclusive discussion of stress and cardiovascular disease, but will extract from this complex mosaic of causes and responses a specific challenge: psychosocial stress. We will first attempt to define psychosocial stress and illustrate the characteristics that identify it as a unique subtype of stress challenge. We then will describe the overall cardiovascular-related response to psychosocial stress and draw some parallels to what is observed in response to other stress challenges. The focus, however, will move to the blood pressure component of the response, and the remainder of our discussion will therefore be devoted to psychosocial-stress-induced hypertension.

Psychosocial stress challenge

A particularly appealing global definition of a stressor is an event, or challenge, that threatens the maintenance of homeostasis of an organism.[6,43] This defines stress in the combined contexts of Claude Bernard's description of the need for constancy of the internal environment[44] and Walter B. Cannon's description of the coordinated physical processes (or control systems) that maintain the steady state (i.e., homeostasis).[45] In this model, organisms are always under conditions of some stress and the issue really becomes one of how these stressors are recognized and handled. In fact, stress is not necessarily a bad thing even if there is a threat to homeostasis.[7] Stressors that threaten homeostasis can be physical (such as temperature challenges or infection, as noted previously) or perceived, which means that the significance attached to the stressor rather than the stressor itself causes the response.[46-48] One of the earliest examples of this can be found in the conclusion by Cannon, in 1914, that the "emergency function" of the adrenal medulla was to prepare the body for "flight" or "fight" responses through actions of adrenalin to ensure adequate glucose and blood flow for skeletal muscle, heart, lungs, and brain.[49] That, and his discussions in that same paper of the fear response of a cat to a barking dog, illustrate that the cause of the stress response under fight-or-flight conditions, in general, is the perceived threat.

Psychosocial stress builds on that principle, because the stressor is still external and the stress response also is dependent on the meaning attached to the stressor. Psychosocial stress can be viewed as a type of psychological stress, but it is important to understand the subtle distinction between the two—especially with regard to psychological

stress typified by the "Type A" nomenclature so often linked to risk for coronary artery disease. Friedman and Rosenman in 1959 reported on the increased coronary risk in patients in Group A in their study. Those patients exhibited a "behavior pattern primarily characterized by intense ambition, competitive drive, constant preoccupation with occupational deadlines, and a sense of time urgency."[50] Follow-up prospective studies confirmed the increased cardiovascular risk in persons they later labeled Type A,[19-21,51-53] and the stress in those individuals (although not universally linked to CAD[21,22,54]) has been attributed to their attempt to control uncontrollable events.[55,56] Thus, the ultimate cause of the stress response in both is the psychological meaning attached to an event. However, a key distinction between classic Type A psychological stress and psychosocial stress is that the meaning in the latter is derived from a cultural context and dependent on the social environment.

Attributing psychosocial stress to the meaning attached to a socially dependent stressor may not seem to fit with our working definition of a stressor as a threat to homeostasis, because the meaning attached to the way a person is treated based on social status may not evoke in the reader the same image as the meaning a cat might attach to a barking dog. However, the studies of Henry et al.[15-17] in mice provide clear evidence that challenges to social status can indeed provoke an intense fight-or-flight response. Thus, the stressor in psychosocial stress is the challenge to an individual's real or perceived social position. However, the stress response is dependent on the meaning the individual places on that challenge.[46-48]

Psychosocial stress response: when is a challenge sufficient to elicit a response?

A comprehensive presentation of stress response and coping patterns is not feasible in the context of this chapter, and indeed would require considerably more space to be fairly discussed. There are, of course, many conflicting theories. However, even when considering theories with similar fundamental roots there are a multitude of variations. We will propose, therefore, a general framework that is reasonably inclusive and that also will help us focus more specifically on the hypertensive psychosocial stress response.

With that as our goal, there is an urge to jump immediately to a discussion of the measurable cardiovascular responses to a psychosocial stressor (such as changes in sympathetic nervous system activity or blood pressure). However, it is essential to understand first that the meaning attached to the stressor determines whether there actually will be a stress response.[46-48] Thus, just as there is a threshold in a pain receptor that determines when an external stimulus will activate it and initiate a response, there also may be a psychological threshold that determines when the individual will consider the external stressor a significant threat.[12,13] Lazarus, Folkman, and colleagues used the terms *cognitive appraisal* for the process through which an encounter with the environment is evaluated to determine its relative threat to well-being or homeostasis.[46-48]

There can be considerable variation in cognitive appraisal with psychosocial stressors. Thus, although there would be fair uniformity in the psychological appraisal of the stressor potential (or perceived threat) of a fire alarm by most people the appraisal of a racial slur may not be as uniform. A mature individual with high self-esteem and secure in their social environment may, for example, be able to attribute the slur to problems within the person making the comment. The slur would therefore not reach the "threshold" to generate a stress response. The same situation may trigger a stress response in other individuals, which indicates that they have attached a level of significance to the event so as to make it a psychosocial stressor. The first step in triggering a psychosocial stress response, therefore, is the individual attaching significant meaning to the event.

Psychosocial stress response: How coping determines the response pattern

Once the cognitive appraisal has reached the "psychological threshold" to identify an event as a psychosocial challenge or stressor, the second step is how the organism or individual copes with the challenge.[4,38,46–48,57,58] This will have a major impact, in conjunction with the magnitude of the stressor, on determining which physiologic processes are initiated and by what mechanism. Cannon's fight-or-flight response describes the sympathetic-adrenal medullary system activation in response to an identified threat.[45,49] This initial rapid-onset response was termed the "alarm reaction" stage within the universal framework of coping that Selye later developed.[40,41] Sympathetic-driven acute increases in blood pressure were part of that response in both models, but during the maintained response to a continued stressor in Selye's scheme (termed the *resistance stage*) the hypothalamic-pituitary-adrenocortical (HPA) axis dominated the stress response and adrenal corticoids were thought to be responsible for sustained hypertension.[40,41]

Henry later hypothesized that these two systems were not linked in such a serial fashion, but that a perceived stimulus activated one of two coping patterns that alternatively activated one or the other system.[17,59,60] Active coping was focused on gaining control of the stressor and was driven by the sympathetic-adrenal medullary system, whereas passive coping was associated with defeat (or loss of control) and was driven by the HPA axis. Thus, the coping pattern was determined in part by the success of the animal or person in meeting the challenge to homeostasis. There could be genetic predisposition to respond immediately to a perceived threat with active or passive coping. Alternatively, continued challenge to control could eventually lead to a transition from active coping to the defeat reaction. Hypertension in that model was due to persistent, or repeated, activation of the sympathetic system during active coping in the attempt to retain or gain control.

There remains strong support for dual roles of the sympathetic and HPA mechanisms in coping with perceived psychosocial stimuli,[4,6,57,61–63] but Sapolsky[64] and others[61,63,65] have shown that the HPA axis (although not a direct cause or mediator of increased blood pressure) may be required for maximal sympathetic effectiveness during a stress response. Thus, a more integrated action of these two systems may occur even during the initial response to a perceived psychosocial challenge. Figure 42–1 depicts the framework we will use to explain how these systems are

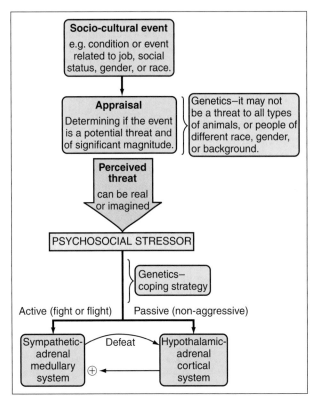

Figure 42–1. The framework to explain how the sympathetic-adrenal medullary and hypothalamic-adrenal cortical systems may be stimulated by psychosocial stress, and the potential different mechanisms for influence of genetic background on the response to a stress challenge.

stimulated by psychosocial stress. The figure also indicates the potential different mechanisms for influence of genetic background on the response to a stress challenge.

GENETICS

The role of genetics in psychosocial stress hypertension seems first to have been considered as an explanation for why the phenomenon appeared to be unique to mice, because there was difficulty in establishing the response consistently in rat studies.[18,66] However, psychosocial stress hypertension is not a uniform occurrence even in mice,[67] and the studies that have been done in rats actually can be used to support hypotheses for how genetics might help identify human subpopulations susceptible to psychosocial stress hypertension.[13]

Henry and colleagues reported that male mice housed in complex cage systems (which forced repeated exposure to challenges to social dominance) demonstrated sustained hypertension that was maintained even after removal from the social conflict caging system.[15–17] Later, Henry speculated that genetics and environmental factors must be coupled to the appropriate stress challenge to induce hypertension, and he tested that hypothesis in rats.[68] Although studies in the borderline hypertensive rat[69] and SHR[70] demonstrated the ability of the appropriate genetic background to enable acute stress to cause hypertension in rats, Henry and others showed that the ability of psychosocial stress to induce hypertension in rats was also significantly dependent on genetic background and propensity for fighting.[4,68]

However, the issue of genetics is not as simple as whether a given genetic background will or will not lead to hypertension under stressful conditions, and here it is important to define the time frame under which hypertension is considered. First, it must be established whether one is describing the ability of an acute stressor to cause an acute hypertensive response, the ability of repeated exposure to stress to cause sustained hypertension, or the establishment of chronic hypertension that is maintained even when the stress is removed. Rats, for example, can have significant acute increases in blood pressure caused by stress. However, strain differences appear to determine whether they do[4,68] or do not develop sustained hypertension.[18,66,70] Sustained stress-induced hypertension has been shown to lead to irreversible hypertension in mice,[16,71] but similar data are lacking in rats. On the other hand, Landbergis et al. reported inconsistent evidence that job strain caused rapid onset of significant sustained hypertension in humans and yet it was life-long job strain that was associated with higher blood pressure.[72] Most stress-hypertension data from human studies correlate baseline blood pressure with some measure of psychosocial stress derived from a survey or interview, often accompanied by measurement of the acute blood pressure response (or "reactivity") to a laboratory or real-life stressor. However, the predictive value of this acute blood pressure reactivity on long-term blood pressure is variable. The inconsistent results may be due to failure to consider positive family history of hypertension (i.e., genetics, along with environment and the acute stressor[12,13,17,68,73]).

Thus, whether one is considering the acute increase in blood pressure in response to a stressor or the ability of sustained stress to cause sustained hypertension, there can be a genetic component[73], and the tendency would be to explore genetic variation in blood pressure control systems. Although that has been a valid and fruitful approach,[73] it also is important to consider the role of genetics in determining whether the individual even considers a given psychosocial condition a stress challenge. Animals of different genetic backgrounds respond to the same psychosocial stimulus in a variety of ways, ranging from aggression, to fear, to nonresponsiveness—and even that can be modified by the animal's current social rank.[2,7,17,57] Therefore, when determining why there is a blunted or absent acute increase in blood pressure in response to a stressful event it is important to consider whether the subject even considers the event stressful before probing for physiologic explanations.

PHYSIOLOGY AND PATHOPHYSIOLOGY

As noted previously, most hypotheses for the integrated response to psychosocial stress continue to invoke activation of the sympathetic nervous system and the HPA axis—with responses that include increases in body temperature, blood pressure, heart rate, and plasma glucocorticoid concentration (interference with either system compromises the body's ability to respond to the stressor).[4,6,17,57,61,62,64,73–76] The HPA axis describes in general the stimulation of

corticotrophin-releasing hormone (CRH) synthesis and secretion from the paraventricular nucleus (PVN) of the hypothalamus, its stimulation of adrenocorticotropin hormone (ACTH) release from the anterior pituitary, and the effect of ACTH to increase glucocorticoid synthesis and secretion by the adrenal gland.[6,63,64,77–79] There are variations among hypotheses regarding how social rank and cognitive appraisal affect the time course and magnitude of activation of the sympathetic system and the HPA axis,[2,4,7,17,57,62,73,80] but this general paradigm is sound (Figure 42–2). However, there are important caveats to understand.

First, the long-standing belief that activation of the sympathetic nervous system was a global all-or-none response to stress[40,49] has given way to understanding that there is specific activation of selective sympathetic efferent pathways depending on the stimulus.[81] In addition, the classic negative feedback control of CRH and ACTH release by adrenal glucocorticoids now incorporates dose- and time-dependent interactions such as an effect of glucocorticoids under chronic stress to stimulate (or augment) CRH release.[63,64,77,79,82] There is also not a sharp distinction between the sympathetic system and the HPA axis centrally because CRH stimulates the locus ceruleus/norepinephrine nuclei of the brain stem and norepinephrine simulates the PVN.[6,63,77,79,83] Moreover, there are more central mediators involved than just the prototypical CRH and norepinephrine. Arginine vasopressin, for example, is secreted by the PVN along with CRH, and it acts synergistically with CRH to increase ACTH release and stimulates norepinephrine release from the locus ceruleus.[63,64,74,84,85]

ACTH is interesting because it is formed along with β-endorphin and α-melanocyte-stimulating hormone (α-MSH) from proopiomelanocortin (POMC) in the anterior pituitary.[74,86] Thus, in addition to the effects of glucocorticoids on food intake and metabolic rate, the interplay of melanocortins, insulin, and other central-acting satiety/metabolic regulators provides a link among stress, insulin resistance, and obesity.[79,82,87,88]

Mechanisms of hypertension

The considerable emphasis on the dual activation of the sympathetic nervous system and the HPA axis might seem misplaced given that increased blood pressure during stress is mediated by the sympathetic nervous system. Two points must be made in that regard. First is that hypertension is not necessarily a required or "programmed" response to all psychosocial stressors by animals or people of varied genetic backgrounds in various environments. For example, the defeat response (the perception of loss or lack of control that is not accompanied by attempts to regain or gain it) to long-term psychosocial stress is associated with long-term HPA-axis stimulation without hypertension, and we have just noted the multiple links between chronic activation of that system with regulation of food intake and metabolism that point to mechanisms linking psychosocial stress to obesity.[79,82,87,88] Responses of other animals or people (depending on the particular psychosocial stressor, the environment, and their genetic makeup) may be active and call upon the sympathetic nervous system,

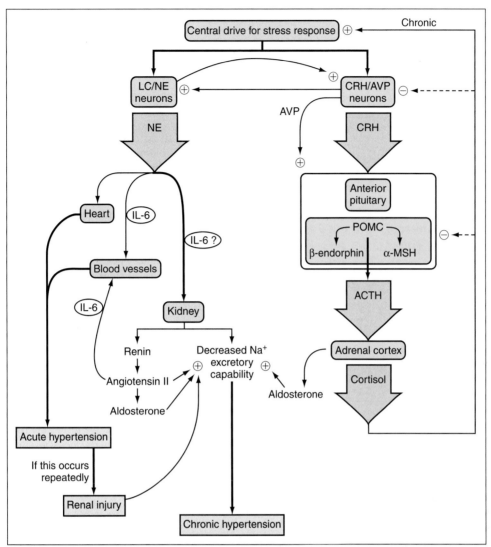

Figure 42–2. Potential mechanisms for how central activation of the sympathetic-adrenal medullary and hypothalamic-adrenal cortical systems may cause both acute and chronic hypertension.

acutely and perhaps long term. Thus, the second point to be made is to recall the previous discussion regarding the role of the HPA-axis (particularly with chronic stress) to amplify the stimulation and action of the sympathetic nervous system.[61,64]

Sympathetic nervous system: Renin angiotensin system

The sympathetic nervous system has well-described effects to increase blood pressure through vascular and cardiac actions, and Chapter 27 of this book covers those mechanisms in detail. We will explore its interaction with the renin-angiotensin system, because it is an important component of the integrated hypertensive effect of sympathetic activation that will also enable us to clarify the role of time in understanding psychosocial stress hypertension. In addition, the link between the sympathetic nervous system and angiotensin II provides a sound physiologic basis for understanding the potential role of inflammation in stress-induced hypertension.

The sympathetic nervous system stimulates renin secretion primarily through direct actions on juxtaglomerular cell beta-1 adrenoreceptors, but also through its effect on proximal tubular sodium reabsorption to decrease sodium delivery to the macula densa.[89–91] Angiotensin II, in turn, has rapid and direct vasoconstrictor actions[92,93] that enable it to contribute to the pressor response to activation of the sympathetic nervous system.[94] We recently tested the role of these two systems in the acute hypertensive response to a new model of psychosocial stress in mice.[95] The psychosocial stressor is a variation of cage-switch stress, in which a male mouse is placed into a cage that had been occupied by another mouse for 3 days. As shown in Figure 42–3, telemetry-measured mean arterial pressure (MAP) increases rapidly by approximately 40 mmHg and remains increased for over 90 minutes. Alpha-1-receptor blockade markedly blunted the initial increase in MAP with little effect after 20 minutes, whereas beta-receptor blockade had no effect on the initial increase in MAP but essentially eliminated the response after 20 minutes.

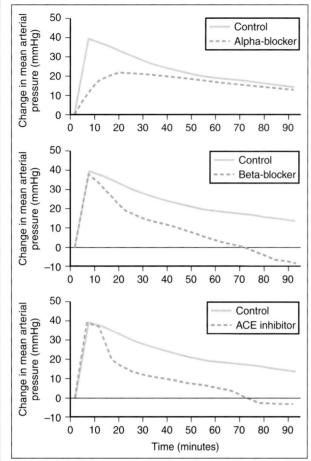

Figure 42–3. The roles of the sympathetic and renin-angiotensin systems in mediating the acute hypertensive response to psychosocial stress, as determined by administration of alpha blockers, beta blockers, and ACE inhibitors to mice undergoing cage-switch stress testing.

It was interesting that the beta-mediated effect was independent of an effect on heart rate, and we found in a third experiment that an ACE-inhibitor affected the MAP response virtually identically to that of the beta blocker. Not only does that provide evidence for a powerful role for AngII in the acute hypertensive response to psychosocial stress but suggests that the mechanism is through sympathetic beta-receptor-mediated stimulation of renin secretion. Plasma renin activity also is increased chronically in mice with sustained psychosocial hypertension,[96] and the hypertension is prevented by ACE inhibition.[97]

Stress and inflammation

It is an important new observation that both the sympathetic nervous system[98–106] and AngII[107–113] have been shown to increase production of the inflammatory cytokine interleukin-6 (IL-6). Approximately 25 years ago it became established that immunoregulatory cytokines, theretofore believed to be primarily autocrine/paracrine factors, had a powerful stimulatory effect on the HPA axis.[76,114,115] The stimulatory effect of cytokines on this system provided an important mechanism to link local inflammatory events with stress and stimulation of the HPA axis,[76,116,117] and the glucocorticoids in turn have been shown to have an important

function to prevent overshoot of the immune/inflammatory response and preserve the local specificity of the response.[74,76,118,119] An important consequence of the discovery and description of these negative feedback interrelationships between cytokines and the HPA axis is that classical hormonal modes of action, rather than only autocrine/paracrine functions, became increasingly ascribed to cytokines.

Armed with an appreciation for a physiologic role for circulating cytokines, new evidence that psychosocial stress triggers an inflammatory response[74,120–123] has raised the possibility that inflammatory mediators may mechanistically link stress to cardiovascular disease. This is bolstered by recent findings by Alexander et al.[124] that a twofold elevation in the plasma levels of tumor necrosis factor α (TNF-α) caused a significant increase in arterial pressure in pregnant rats (and by Orshal et al.,[125] who followed with a report infusing IL-6 in pregnant rats). IL-6 is particularly intriguing for the fact that of the three inflammatory cytokines IL-1β, TNF-α, and IL-6 only IL-6 typically increases significantly in the circulation, where it can act to stimulate CRH and ACTH release in addition to serving as the key trigger for the hepatic acute phase response and release of acute phase proteins such as C-reactive protein.[74,76,116,126,127] All three can act centrally to stimulate the HPA axis, but IL-6 inhibits production of IL-1β and TNF-α and is least sensitive to inhibition by the rise in glucocorticoids they stimulate.[74,76,116,127,128] Therefore, we tested the role of inflammatory cytokines in mediating psychosocial stress hypertension by subjecting IL-6 knockout mice to our cage-switch model.

Figure 42–4 shows the significant decrease in area under the MAP curve during stress in the IL-6 knockout versus wild-type mice. This was all the more interesting because there were no differences in the heart rate or activity responses, suggesting that the effect of IL-6 was not via central control of sympathetic outflow but perhaps at the level of the vasculature. The mechanism through which IL-6 may contribute to increased blood pressure during stress-induced activation of the sympathetic nervous system is

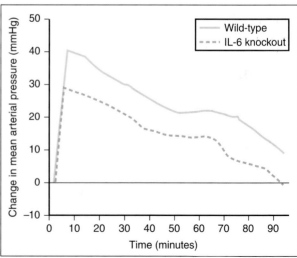

Figure 42–4. Changes in MAP during stress in the IL-6 knockout versus wild-type mice.

not known. Acute IL-6 infusion was shown not to increase blood pressure in dogs,[129] and the increased IL-6 that occurs with endotoxin shock, cirrhosis, or septic shock is associated with decreased blood pressure.[130–133] It appears, therefore, that IL-6 is not uniformly a vasoconstrictor or hypertensive factor, but because the sympathetic nervous system can increase IL-6 release from vascular smooth muscle cells[107–109] these observations together suggest that IL-6 (and perhaps other inflammatory cytokines) plays a role as permissive factor or amplifier of psychosocial stress hypertension.

CLINICAL IMPLICATIONS AND PERSPECTIVES

We raised the issue of time briefly in our discussion of genetics. Time is seldom addressed in reviews of the stress hypertension literature, and for that reason may be the biggest contributor to the confused perception of how stress affects blood pressure. When questioning whether a psychological stressor can cause hypertension, is the focus on the potential for an acute stress challenge to increase blood pressure acutely, on the ability of continued exposure to that stress to cause sustained increases in blood pressure, or on the establishment of permanent hypertension even after the stress has been removed? This may be apparent for a given experiment, but becomes a problem when attempting to reach a conclusion about whether stress causes hypertension: What is the time frame being considered?

By far, most of the experimental evidence in animals and humans for hypertension caused by psychosocial stress is for an acute increase in blood pressure when exposed to the stress challenge. In humans, this is most often expressed as blood pressure reactivity (i.e., the acute increase in blood pressure in response to stress). However, the acute stress actually might not be psychosocial in nature. Instead, chronic psychosocial stress (as determined by interview, for example) may be studied through its effect on blood pressure reactivity to other acute stressors. Nonetheless, overall there is strong support in animal and humans studies that acute exposure to psychosocial stress can cause an acute sympathetic-mediated increase in blood pressure. The only other point to make regarding acute pressor responses to acute psychosocial challenges is that not all stress is bad or causes blood pressure to rise. This is noted again to bring in the term *allostasis*, which was coined to avoid the negative connotation that accompanies the term *stress* and to describe the normal responses of the body to daily challenges to homeostasis.[80,134,135] In this context, the evolutionary value and benefit of increased blood pressure in response to an acute stressor (e.g., the flight-or-fight response) may be more evident.

To describe the negative consequences of a stress response, McEwen et al. developed the concept of allostatic load to quantify the impact of these responses, particularly with prolonged response to a given stressor.[7,80,135] Thus, although the activation of the sympathetic nervous system and increase in glucocorticoids (and perhaps inflammatory cytokines) are important in helping the animal or person meet and overcome what they have perceive as a significant stress challenge, continuing to respond to a stress challenge (e.g., loss of job and social position with no end in sight) in this manner can have pathologic consequences. Here is where the gray area regarding psychosocial stress hypertension develops.

From the literature reviewed here, there is good support for the hypothesis that psychosocial stress leads to (or at least contributes to) sustained irreversible hypertension in humans. The human data are correlational in that populations that score high on indexes of psychosocial stress tend to have higher baseline blood pressure. The attempts to use acute blood pressure reactivity as a predictor or gauge of this have yielded mixed results, but as noted previously this might be due to failure to consider genetic background and environment.[12] Thus, psychosocial stress could be viewed as a risk factor for essential hypertension.[10] The difficulty in making this link stronger is the lack of solid experimental evidence for mechanisms from animal studies. Animal studies have shown that sustained psychosocial stress can cause sustained hypertension as long as the stress is maintained in animals of certain genetic backgrounds. The two key questions are: What is the mechanism for the sustained hypertension and what mechanisms would be required for the hypertension to be maintained after the stimulus is removed?

The answer to these questions is rooted in hypotheses developed by Starling,[136] Borst,[137] and Guyton and Coleman [138] that the kidneys' ability to excrete sodium must be decreased in order for hypertension to be sustained chronically. This concept is discussed in detail in Chapter 23, but there is evidence for this mechanism to operate in psychosocial stress hypertension. First, if a person takes an active response to a psychosocial stressor the sympathetic nervous system will be activated. However, in addition to the acute effects on the heart and on blood vessels (also due in part to the stimulation of the renin-angiotensin system), continued high activity of the sympathetic system in a continued attempt to confront the stressor actively can shift the kidneys into a sodium-retaining state through effects on tubular sodium reabsorption, renal vascular resistance, and stimulation of the renin-angiotensin system.[73]

In fact, psychosocial stress has been shown to decrease urinary sodium excretion in dogs[139] and humans.[140] However, how could psychosocial stress cause a change in kidney function that would be maintained even after the stress is removed? This most likely would be related to some degree of glomerular injury, as seen with the mechanism for hypertension with progression of diabetic nephropathy, and studies in mice have shown that irreversible hypertension from psychosocial stress is associated with renal injury.[16,71] The probable mechanism would be repeated transmission of high systemic pressure to the glomeruli over many years due to the wide swings and high peaks in blood pressure associated with repeated sympathetic activation in response to repeated stress.[141–143] The difficulty in firmly linking psychosocial stress to sustained hypertension through that, or any quantifiable, mechanism is the basis for persistent questions about the "validity" of psychosocial stress hypertension.

SUMMARY

A psychosocial stressor is a culturally or socially based situation to which an individual attaches enough meaning so that it is perceived as a challenge. Once that has happened, there is activation of the sympathetic nervous system and the HPA axis. If the person chooses to confront the challenge directly and attempt to control it, the sympathetic nervous system predominates and causes an acute increase in blood pressure. Elements of the HPA axis and inflammatory cytokines may act centrally and at peripheral target tissues to augment the hypertensive actions of the sympathetic system.

Whether or not a person responds to a psychosocial stressor in this way is dependent not only on the stressor but on the environment and the family history of hypertension, and those factors also will determine whether sustained exposure to the stressor will cause a sustained hypertensive response. If that occurs, the focus must be on how the individual perceives the challenge and copes with it to prevent the hypertension—unless, of course, the stressor can be eliminated. Although there is no direct experimental support that long-term hypertensive responses to repeated psychosocial stressors can cause essential hypertension, correlational data from human populations and evidence that high blood pressure variability can lead to permanent renal injury suggest that acute psychosocial stress hypertension should be considered a risk factor for essential hypertension.

REFERENCES

1. Alexander FG. Emotional factors in essential hypertension. *Psychosomatic Medicine* 1939;1:175–9.
2. Sapolsky RM. The influence of social hierarchy on primate health. *Science.* 2005;308:648–52.
3. Ohlin B, Nilsson PM, Nilsson JA, Berglund G. Chronic psychosocial stress predicts long-term cardiovascular morbidity and mortality in middle-aged men. *Eur Heart J.* 2004;25:867–73.
4. Sgoifo A, Costoli T, Meerlo P, Buwalda B, Pico'-Alfonso MA, De Boer S, et al. Individual differences in cardiovascular response to social challenge. *Neurosci Biobehav Rev* 2005;29:59–66.
5. Schneider RH, Alexander CN, Staggers F, Rainforth M, Salerno JW, Hartz A, et al. Long-term effects of stress reduction on mortality in persons > or = 55 years of age with systemic hypertension. *Am J Cardiol* 2005;95:1060–64.
6. Rosmond R. Role of stress in the pathogenesis of the metabolic syndrome. *Psychoneuroendocrinology* 2005;30:1–10.
7. Korte SM, Koolhaas JM, Wingfield JC, McEwen BS. The Darwinian concept of stress: Benefits of allostasis and costs of allostatic load and the trade-offs in health and disease. *Neurosci Biobehav Rev* 2005;29:3–38.
8. Steptoe A, Willemsen G. The influence of low job control on ambulatory blood pressure and perceived stress over the working day in men and women from the Whitehall II cohort. *J Hypertens* 2004;22:915–20.
9. Treiber FA, Kamarck T, Schneiderman N, Sheffield D, Kapuku G, Taylor T. Cardiovascular reactivity and development of preclinical and clinical disease states. *Psychosom Med* 2003;65:46–62.
10. Esler M, Parati G. Is essential hypertension sometimes a psychosomatic disorder? *J Hypertens* 2004;22:873–76.
11. Pickering TG. Mental stress as a causal factor in the development of hypertension and cardiovascular disease. *Curr Hypertens Rep* 2001;3:249–54.
12. Light KC, Girdler SS, Sherwood A, Bragdon EE, Brownley KA, West SG, et al. High stress responsivity predicts later blood pressure only in combination with positive family history and high life stress. *Hypertension* 1999;33:1458–64.
13. Light KC. Hypertension and the reactivity hypothesis: The next generation. *Psychosom Med* 2001;63:744–46.
14. Kaplan MS, Nunes A. The psychosocial determinants of hypertension. *Nutr Metab Cardiovasc Dis* 2003;13:52–9.
15. Henry JP, Meehan JP, Stephens PM. The use of psychosocial stimuli to induce prolonged systolic hypertension in mice. *Psychosom Med* 1967;29:408–32.
16. Henry JP, Stephens PM, Santisteban GA. A model of psychosocial hypertension showing reversibility and progression of cardiovascular complications. *Circ Res* 1975;36:156–64.
17. Henry JP, Liu J, Meehan WP. Psychosocial stress and experimental hypertension. In: Laragh JH, Brenner BM (eds.) *Hypertension: Pathophysiology, Diagnosis, and Management, Second Edition.* New York: Raven Press 1995:905–21.
18. Harrap SB, Louis WJ, Doyle AE. Failure of psychosocial stress to induce chronic hypertension in the rat. *J Hypertens* 1984;2:653–62.
19. Rosenman RH, Friedman M, Straus R, Wurm M, Kositchek R, Hahn W, et al. A predictive study of coronary heart disease. *JAMA* 1964;189:15–22.
20. Rosenman RH, Brand RJ, Jenkins D, Friedman M, Straus R, Wurm M. Coronary heart disease in Western Collaborative Group Study: Final follow-up experience of 8 1/2 years. *JAMA* 1975;233:872–77.
21. Rozanski A, Blumenthal JA, Kaplan J. Impact of psychological factors on the pathogenesis of cardiovascular disease and implications for therapy. *Circulation* 1999;99:2192–217.
22. Bunker SJ, Colquhoun DM, Esler MD, Hickie IB, Hunt D, Jelinek VM, et al. "Stress" and coronary heart disease: Psychosocial risk factors. *Med J Aust* 2003;178:272–76.
23. Strike PC, Steptoe A. Psychosocial factors in the development of coronary artery disease. *Prog Cardiovasc Dis* 2004;46:337–47.
24. Hemingway H, Marmot M. Evidence based cardiology: Psychosocial factors in the aetiology and prognosis of coronary heart disease. Systematic review of prospective cohort studies. *BMJ* 1999;318:1460–67.
25. Schnall PL, Pieper C, Schwartz JE, Karasek RA, Schlussel Y, Devereux RB, et al. The relationship between "job strain," workplace diastolic blood pressure, and left ventricular mass index: Results of a case-control study. *JAMA* 1990;263:1929–35.
26. Schnall PL, Schwartz JE, Landsbergis PA, Warren K, Pickering TG. Relation between job strain, alcohol, and ambulatory blood pressure. *Hypertension* 1992;19:488–94.
27. Cesana G, Sega R, Ferrario M, Chiodini P, Corrao G, Mancia G. Job strain and blood pressure in employed men and women: A pooled analysis of four northern italian population samples. *Psychosom Med* 2003;65:558–63.
28. Friedman R, Schwartz JE, Schnall PL, Landsbergis PA, Pieper C, Gerin W, et al. Psychological variables in hypertension: Relationship to casual or ambulatory blood pressure in men. *Psychosom Med* 2001;63:19–31.
29. Carroll D, Smith GD, Shipley MJ, Steptoe A, Brunner EJ, Marmot MG. Blood pressure reactions to acute psychological stress and future blood pressure status: A 10-year follow-up of men in the Whitehall II study. *Psychosom Med* 2001;63:737–43.
30. Theorell T, Karasek RA. Current issues relating to psychosocial job strain and cardiovascular disease research. *J Occup Health Psychol* 1996;1:9–26.
31. Matthews KA, Kiefe CI, Lewis CE, Liu K, Sidney S, Yunis C. Socioeconomic trajectories and incident hypertension in a biracial cohort of young adults (CARDIA). *Hypertension* 2002;39:772–76.
32. Panagiotakos DB, Pitsavos CE, Chrysohoou CA, Skoumas J, Toutouza M, Belegrinos D, et al. The association between educational status and risk factors related to cardiovascular disease in healthy individuals: The ATTICA study. *Ann Epidemiol* 2004;14:188–94.
33. Din-Dzietham R, Couper D, Evans G, Arnett DK, Jones DW. Arterial stiffness is greater in African Americans than in whites: Evidence from the Forsyth County, North Carolina, ARIC cohort. *Am J Hypertens* 2004;17:304–13.

34. Gravlee CC, Dressler WW. Skin pigmentation, self-perceived color, and arterial blood pressure in Puerto Rico. *Am J Hum Biol* 2005;17:195–206.

35. Carroll D, Ring C, Hunt K, Ford G, Macintyre S. Blood pressure reactions to stress and the prediction of future blood pressure: Effects of sex, age, and socioeconomic position. *Psychosom Med* 2003;65:1058–64.

36. Landsbergis PA, Schnall PL, Pickering TG, Warren K, Schwartz JE. Lower socioeconomic status among men in relation to the association between job strain and blood pressure. *Scand J Work Environ Health* 2003;29:206–15.

37. Olatunbosun ST, Kaufman JS, Cooper RS, Bella AF. Hypertension in a black population: Prevalence and biosocial determinants of high blood pressure in a group of urban Nigerians. *J Hum Hypertens* 2000;14:249–57.

38. Light KC, Brownley KA, Turner JR, Hinderliter AL, Girdler SS, Sherwood A, et al. Job status and high-effort coping influence work blood pressure in women and blacks. *Hypertension* 1995;25:554–59.

39. Selye H. A syndrome produced by diverse nocuous agents. *Nature* 1936;138:32–6.

40. Selye H. The general adaptation syndrome and the diseases of adaptation. *Journal of Clinical Endocrinology* 1946;6:117–231.

41. Selye H. *The Stress of Life*. New York: McGraw Hill, 1956.

42. Rosch PJ. Reminiscences of Hans Selye, and the birth of "stress." *Int J Emerg Ment Health* 1999;1:59–66.

43. Chrousos GP, Gold PW. The concepts of stress and stress system disorders: Overview of physical and behavioral homeostasis. *JAMA* 1992;267:1244–52.

44. Bernard C. *An Introduction to the Study of Experimental Medicine*, trans. Henry Copley Green. New York: Dover Publications, Inc. 1957.

45. Cannon WB. *The Wisdom of the Body*. New York: Norton, 1932.

46. Folkman S, Lazarus RS, Dunkel-Schetter C, DeLongis A, Gruen RJ. Dynamics of a stressful encounter: Cognitive appraisal, coping, and encounter outcomes. *J Pers Soc Psychol* 1986;50:992–1003.

47. Lazarus RS, DeLongis A, Folkman S, Gruen R. Stress and adaptational outcomes: The problem of confounded measures. *Am Psychol* 1985;40:770–85.

48. Lazarus RS, Launier R. Stress-related transactions between person and environment. In: Pervin LA, Lewis M (eds.) *Perspectives in Interactional Psychology*. New York: Plenum Press, 1978:287–327.

49. Cannon WB. The emergency function of the adrenal medulla in pain and the major emotions. *Am J Physiol* 1914;33:356–72.

50. Friedman M, Rosenman RH. Association of specific overt behavior pattern with blood and cardiovascular findings: Blood cholesterol level, blood clotting time, incidence of arcus senilis, and clinical coronary artery disease. *J Am Med Assoc* 1959;169:1286–96.

51. Blumenthal JA, Williams RB Jr., Kong Y, Schanberg SM, Thompson LW. Type A behavior pattern and coronary atherosclerosis. *Circulation* 1978;58:634–39.

52. Jenkins CD. Psychologic and social precursors of coronary disease (first of two parts). *N Engl J Med* 1971;284:244–55.

53. Jenkins CD. Psychologic and social precursors of coronary disease. (II). *N Engl J Med* 1971;284:307–17.

54. Haynes SG, Levine S, Scotch N, Feinleib M, Kannel WB. The relationship of psychosocial factors to coronary heart disease in the Framingham study. I. Methods and risk factors. *Am J Epidemiol* 1978;107:362–83.

55. Glass DC. Stress, behavior patterns, and coronary disease. *Am Sci* 1977;65:177–87.

56. Glass DC. Psychological and physiological responses of individuals displaying type A behaviour. *Acta Med Scand Suppl* 1982;660:193–202.

57. Koolhaas JM, Korte SM, De Boer SF, Van Der Vegt BJ, Van Reenen CG, Hopster H, et al. Coping styles in animals: Current status in behavior and stress-physiology. *Neurosci Biobehav Rev* 1999;23:925–35.

58. Light KC. Young Psychophysiologist Award address, 1980. Cardiovascular responses to effortful active coping: Implications for the role of stress in hypertension development. *Psychophysiology* 1981;18:216–25.

59. Henry JP, Ely DL, Stephens PM. The role of psychosocial stimulation in the pathogenesis of hypertension. *Verh Dtsch Ges Inn Med* 1974;80:1724–40.

60. Henry JP, Cassel JC. Psychosocial factors in essential hypertension: Recent epidemiologic and animal experimental evidence. *Am J Epidemiol* 1969;90:171–200.

61. Tsigos C, Chrousos GP. Hypothalamic-pituitary-adrenal axis, neuroendocrine factors and stress. *J Psychosom Res* 2002;53:865–71.

62. Esch T, Stefano GB, Fricchione GL, Benson H. Stress in cardiovascular diseases. *Med Sci Monit* 2002;8:RA93–101.

63. Black PH. Central nervous system-immune system interactions: Psychoneuroendocrinology of stress and its immune consequences. *Antimicrob Agents Chemother* 1994;38:1–6.

64. Sapolsky RM, Romero LM, Munck AU. How do glucocorticoids influence stress responses? Integrating permissive, suppressive, stimulatory, and preparative actions. *Endocr Rev* 2000;21:55–89.

65. Seckl JR, Meaney MJ. Glucocorticoid programming. *Ann NY Acad Sci* 2004;1032:63–84.

66. Mormede P. Genetic influences on the responses to psychosocial challenges in rats. *Acta Physiol Scand Suppl* 1997;640:65–8.

67. Lockwood JA, Turney TH. Social dominance and stress-induced hypertension: Strain differences in inbred mice. *Physiol Behav* 1981;26:547–49.

68. Henry JP, Liu YY, Nadra WE, Qian CG, Mormede P, Lemaire V, et al. Psychosocial stress can induce chronic hypertension in normotensive strains of rats. *Hypertension* 1993;21:714–23.

69. Lawler JE, Barker GF, Hubbard JW, Schaub RG. Effects of stress on blood pressure and cardiac pathology in rats with borderline hypertension. *Hypertension* 1981;3:496–505.

70. Ely D, Caplea A, Dunphy G, Smith D. Physiological and neuroendocrine correlates of social position in normotensive and hypertensive rat colonies. *Acta Physiol Scand Suppl* 1997;640:92–5.

71. Henry JP, Meehan WP, Stephens PM. Role of subordination in nephritis of socially stressed mice. *Clin Exp Hypertens A* 1982;4:695–705.

72. Landsbergis PA, Schnall PL, Pickering TG, Warren K, Schwartz JE. Life-course exposure to job strain and ambulatory blood pressure in men. *Am J Epidemiol* 2003;157:998–1006.

73. Snieder H, Harshfield GA, Barbeau P, Pollock DM, Pollock JS, Treiber FA. Dissecting the genetic architecture of the cardiovascular and renal stress response. *Biol Psychol* 2002;61:73–95.

74. Black PH, Garbutt LD. Stress, inflammation and cardiovascular disease. *J Psychosom Res* 2002;52:1–23.

75. O'Connor TM, O'Halloran DJ, Shanahan F. The stress response and the hypothalamic-pituitary-adrenal axis: From molecule to melancholia. *QJM* 2000;93:323–33.

76. Turnbull AV, Rivier CL. Regulation of the hypothalamic-pituitary-adrenal axis by cytokines: Actions and mechanisms of action. *Physiol Rev* 1999;79:1–71.

77. Chrousos GP, Gold PW. A healthy body in a healthy mind, and vice versa: The damaging power of "uncontrollable" stress. *J Clin Endocrinol Metab* 1998;83:1842–45.

78. Rosmond R, Dallman MF, Bjorntorp P. Stress-related cortisol secretion in men: Relationships with abdominal obesity and endocrine, metabolic and hemodynamic abnormalities. *J Clin Endocrinol Metab* 1998;83:1853–59.

79. Dallman MF, Akana SF, Strack AM, Scribner KS, Pecoraro N, La Fleur SE, et al. Chronic stress-induced effects of corticosterone on brain: Direct and indirect. *Ann NY Acad Sci* 2004;1018:141–50.

80. McEwen BS, Stellar E. Stress and the individual: Mechanisms leading to disease. *Arch Intern Med* 1993;153:2093–101.

81. Morrison SF. Differential control of sympathetic outflow. *Am J Physiol Regul Integr Comp Physiol* 2001;281:R683–98.

82. Dallman MF, Pecoraro NC, la Fleur SE. Chronic stress and comfort foods: Self-medication and abdominal obesity. *Brain Behav Immun* 2005;19:275–80.

83. Sved AF, Cano G, Passerin AM, Rabin BS. The locus coeruleus, Barrington's nucleus, and neural circuits of stress. *Physiol Behav* 2002;77:737–42.

84. Volpi S, Rabadan-Diehl C, Aguilera G. Vasopressinergic regulation of the hypothalamic pituitary adrenal axis and stress adaptation. *Stress* 2004;7:75–83.

85. Volpi S, Rabadan-Diehl C, Aguilera G. Regulation of vasopressin V1b receptors and stress adaptation. *Ann NY Acad Sci* 2004;1018:293–301.

86. Coll AP, Challis BG, Lopez M, Piper S, Yeo GS, O'Rahilly S. Proopiomelanocortin-deficient mice are hypersensitive to the adverse metabolic effects of glucocorticoids. *Diabetes* 2005;54:2269–76.

87. Bjorntorp P, Holm G, Rosmond R, Folkow B. Hypertension and the metabolic syndrome: Closely related central origin? *Blood Press* 2000;9:71–82.

88. Black PH. The inflammatory response is an integral part of the stress response: Implications for atherosclerosis, insulin resistance, type II diabetes and metabolic syndrome X. *Brain Behav Immun* 2003;17:350–64.

89. DiBona GF. Nervous kidney. Interaction between renal sympathetic nerves and the renin-angiotensin system in the control of renal function. *Hypertension* 2000;36:1083–88.

90. Kopp UC, DiBona GF. Neural regulation of renin secretion. *Semin Nephrol* 1993;13:543–51.

91. Kirchheim H, Ehmke H, Persson PB. Sympathetic modulation of renal hemodynamics, renin release and sodium excretion. *Klin Wochenschr* 1989;67:858–64.

92. Carretero OA, Scicli AG. Local hormonal factors (intracrine, autocrine, and paracrine) in hypertension. *Hypertension* 1991;18(Suppl I):I58–69.

93. Laragh JH. The renin system and four lines of hypertension research. *Hypertension* 1992;20:267–79.

94. Reid IA. Actions of angiotensin II on the brain: Mechanisms and physiologic role. *Am J Physiol* 1984;246:F533–43.

95. Lee DL, Webb RC, Brands MW. Sympathetic and angiotensin dependent hypertension during cage-switch stress in mice. *Am J Physiol Regul Integr Comp Physiol* 2004;287:R1394–98.

96. Vander AJ, Henry JP, Stephens PM, Kay LL, Mouw DR. Plasma renin activity in psychosocial hypertension of CBA mice. *Circ Res* 1978;42:496–502.

97. Webb RC, Hamlin NM, Henry JP, Stephens PM, Vander AJ. Captopril, blood pressure and vascualr reactivity in psychosocial hypertension in mice. *Hypertension* 1986;8(Suppl I):I119.

98. Nakamura A, Kohsaka T, Johns EJ. Differential regulation of interleukin-6 production in the kidney by the renal sympathetic nerves in normal and spontaneously hypertensive rats. *J Hypertens* 1993;11:491–97.

99. Marz P, Cheng JG, Gadient RA, Patterson PH, Stoyan T, Otten U, et al. Sympathetic neurons can produce and respond to interleukin 6. *Proc Natl Acad Sci USA* 1998;95:3251–56.

100. Mohamed-Ali V, Flower L, Sethi J, Hotamisligil G, Gray R, Humphries SE, et al. Beta-adrenergic regulation of IL-6 release from adipose tissue: In vivo and in vitro studies. *J Clin Endocrinol Metab* 2001;86:5864–69.

101. Gornikiewicz A, Sautner T, Brostjan C, Schmierer B, Fugger R, Roth E, et al. Catecholamines up-regulate lipopolysaccharide-induced IL-6 production in human microvascular endothelial cells. *Faseb J* 2000;14:1093–100.

102. Song DK, Im YB, Jung JS, Suh HW, Huh SO, Park SW, et al. Differential involvement of central and peripheral norepinephrine in the central lipopolysaccharide-induced interleukin-6 responses in mice. *J Neurochem* 1999;72:1625–33.

103. Huang QH, Takaki A, Arimura A. Central noradrenergic system modulates plasma interleukin-6 production by

104. Burger A, Benicke M, Deten A, Zimmer HG. Catecholamines stimulate interleukin-6 synthesis in rat cardiac fibroblasts. *Am J Physiol Heart Circ Physiol* 2001;281:H14–21.

105. von Patay B, Kurz B, Mentlein R. Effect of transmitters and co-transmitters of the sympathetic nervous system on interleukin-6 synthesis in thymic epithelial cells. *Neuroimmunomodulation* 1999;6:45–50.

106. Papanicolaou DA, Petrides JS, Tsigos C, Bina S, Kalogeras KT, Wilder R, et al. Exercise stimulates interleukin-6 secretion: Inhibition by glucocorticoids and correlation with catecholamines. *Am J Physiol* 1996;271:E601–05.

107. Funakoshi Y, Ichiki T, Ito K, Takeshita A. Induction of interleukin-6 expression by angiotensin II in rat vascular smooth muscle cells. *Hypertension* 1999;34:118–25.

108. Han Y, Runge MS, Brasier AR. Angiotensin II induces interleukin-6 transcription in vascular smooth muscle cells through pleiotropic activation of nuclear factor-kappa B transcription factors. *Circ Res* 1999;84:695–703.

109. Kranzhofer R, Schmidt J, Pfeiffer CA, Hagl S, Libby P, Kubler W. Angiotensin induces inflammatory activation of human vascular smooth muscle cells. *Arterioscler Thromb Vasc Biol* 1999;19:1623–29.

110. Moriyama T, Fujibayashi M, Fujiwara Y, Kaneko T, Xia C, Imai E, et al. Angiotensin II stimulates interleukin-6 release from cultured mouse mesangial cells. *J Am Soc Nephrol* 1995;6:95–101.

111. Sano M, Fukuda K, Kodama H, Pan J, Saito M, Matsuzaki J, et al. Interleukin-6 family of cytokines mediate angiotensin II-induced cardiac hypertrophy in rodent cardiomyocytes. *J Biol Chem* 2000;275:29717–23.

112. Keidar S, Heinrich R, Kaplan M, Hayek T, Aviram M. Angiotensin II administration to atherosclerotic mice increases macrophage uptake of oxidized ldl: A possible role for interleukin-6. *Arterioscler Thromb Vasc Biol* 2001;21:1464–69.

113. Phillips MI, Kagiyama S. Angiotensin II as a pro-inflammatory mediator. *Curr Opin Investig Drugs* 2002;3:569–77.

114. Woloski BM, Smith EM, Meyer WJ III, Fuller GM, Blalock JE. Corticotropin-releasing activity of monokines. *Science* 1985;230:1035–37.

115. Besedovsky H, del Rey A, Sorkin E, Dinarello CA. Immunoregulatory feedback between interleukin-1 and glucocorticoid hormones. *Science* 1986;233:652–54.

116. Chesnokova V, Melmed S. Minireview: Neuro-immuno-endocrine modulation of the hypothalamic-pituitary-adrenal (HPA) axis by gp130 signaling molecules. *Endocrinology* 2002;143:1571–74.

117. van Enckevort FH, Sweep CG, Span PN, Demacker PN, Hermsen CC, Hermus AR. Reduced adrenal response to bacterial lipopolysaccharide in interleukin-6-deficient mice. *J Endocrinol Invest* 2001;24:786–95.

118. del Rey A, Besedovsky H, Sorkin E. Endogenous blood levels of corticosterone control the immunologic

119. Munck A, Guyre PM, Holbrook NJ. Physiological functions of glucocorticoids in stress and their relation to pharmacological actions. *Endocr Rev* 1984;5:25–44.

120. Steptoe A, Willemsen G, Owen N, Flower L, Mohamed-Ali V. Acute mental stress elicits delayed increases in circulating inflammatory cytokine levels. *Clin Sci (Lond)* 2001;101:185–92.

121. Takaki A, Huang QH, Somogyvari-Vigh A, Arimura A. Immobilization stress may increase plasma interleukin-6 via central and peripheral catecholamines. *Neuroimmunomodulation* 1994;1:335–42.

122. Goebel MU, Mills PJ, Irwin MR, Ziegler MG. Interleukin-6 and tumor necrosis factor-alpha production after acute psychological stress, exercise, and infused isoproterenol: Differential effects and pathways. *Psychosom Med* 2000;62:591–98.

123. LeMay LG, Vander AJ, Kluger MJ. The effects of psychological stress on plasma interleukin-6 activity in rats. *Physiol Behav* 1990;47:957–61.

124. Alexander BT CK, Massey MB, Bennett WA, Granger JP. Tumor necrosis factor-alpha-induced hypertension in pregnant rats results in decreased renal neuronal nitric oxide synthase expression. *Am J Hypertens* 2002;15:170–75.

125. Orshal JM KR. Reduced endothelial NO-cGMP-mediated vascular relaxation and hypertension in IL-6-infused pregnant rats. *Hypertension* 2004;43:434–44.

126. Spath-Schwalbe E, Hansen K, Schmidt F, Schrezenmeier H, Marshall L, Burger K, et al. Acute effects of recombinant human interleukin-6 on endocrine and central nervous sleep functions in healthy men. *J Clin Endocrinol Metab* 1998;83:1573–79.

127. Papanicolaou DA, Wilder RL, Manolagas SC, Chrousos GP. The pathophysiologic roles of interleukin-6 in human disease. *Ann Intern Med* 1998;128:127–37.

128. DeRijk R, Michelson D, Karp B, Petrides J, Galliven E, Deuster P, et al. Exercise and circadian rhythm-induced variations in plasma cortisol differentially regulate interleukin-1 beta (IL-1 beta), IL-6, and tumor necrosis factor-alpha (TNF alpha) production in humans: High sensitivity of TNF alpha and resistance of IL-6. *J Clin Endocrinol Metab* 1997;82:2182–91.

129. Preiser JC, Schmartz D, Van der Linden P, Content J, Vanden Bussche P, Buurman W, et al. Interleukin-6 administration has no acute hemodynamic or hematologic effect in the dog. *Cytokine* 1991;3:1–4.

130. Forfia PR, Zhang X, Ochoa F, Ochoa M, Xu X, Bernstein R, et al. Relationship between plasma NOx and cardiac and vascular dysfunction after LPS injection in anesthetized dogs. *Am J Physiol* 1998;274:H193–201.

131. Rees DD, Monkhouse JE, Cambridge D, Moncada S. Nitric oxide and the haemodynamic profile of endotoxin shock in the conscious mouse. *Br J Pharmacol* 1998;124:540–46.

132. Nakamura T, Ebihara I, Shimada N, Koide H. Changes in plasma erythropoietin and interleukin-6

peripheral interleukin-1. *Am J Physiol* 1997;273:R731–38.

cell mass and B cell activity in mice. *J Immunol* 1984;133:572–75.

concentrations in patients with septic shock after hemoperfusion with polymyxin B-immobilized fiber. *Intensive Care Med* 1998;24:1272–76.

133. Genesca J, Gonzalez A, Segura R, Catalan R, Marti R, Varela E, et al. Interleukin-6, nitric oxide, and the clinical and hemodynamic alterations of patients with liver cirrhosis. *Am J Gastroenterol* 1999;94:169–77.

134. Sterling P, Eyer J. Allostasis: A new paradigm to explain arousal pathology. In: Fisher S, Reason J (eds.) *Handbook of Life Stress, Cognition, and Health.* New York: John Wiley and Sons, 1988:629–49.

135. McEwen BS. Stress, adaptation, and disease. Allostasis and allostatic load. *Ann NY Acad Sci* 1998;840:33–44.

136. Starling EH. *The Fluids of the Body.* London: Archibald Constable & Co., 1909.

137. Borst JGG, Borst-De Geus A. Hypertension explained by Starling's theory of circulatory homeostasis. *Lancet* 1963;1:677–82.

138. Guyton AC, Coleman TG. Quantitative analysis of the pathophysiology of hypertension. *Circ Res* 1969;24:1–19.

139. Koepke JP, Light KC, Obrist PA. Neural control of renal excretory function during behavioral stress in conscious dogs. *Am J Physiol* 1983;245:R251–58.

140. Light KC, Koepke JP, Obrist PA, Willis PWt. Psychological stress induces sodium and fluid retention in men at high risk for hypertension. *Science* 1983;220:429–31.

141. Bidani AK, Hacioglu R, Abu-Amarah I, Williamson GA, Loutzenhiser R, Griffin KA. "Step" vs. "dynamic" autoregulation: Implications for susceptibility to hypertensive injury. *Am J Physiol Renal Physiol* 2003;285:F113–20.

142. Parati G, Ravogli A, Frattola A, Groppelli A, Ulian L, Santucciu C, et al. Blood pressure variability: Clinical implications and effects of antihypertensive treatment. *J.Hytertension* 1994;12(Suppl 5):S35–40.

143. Orfila C, Damase-Michel C, Lepert J-C, Montastruc J-L, Suc J-M, Montastruc P, et al. Renal morphological changes after sinoaortic denervation in dogs. *Hypertension* 1993;21:758–66.

CLINICAL APPROACHES

Ernesto L. Schiffrin and
Robert J. MacFadyen

Chapter

43

Overview of Assessment and Investigation of Hypertension: A Pragmatic Practical Approach

Judith A. Whitworth

Key Findings

- Focus on hypertension is shifting to focus on elevation of blood pressure as a risk for cardiovascular disease.

- "Hypertension should be defined in terms of blood pressure level above which investigation and treatment do more good than harm" (Evans and Rose 1971).

- Blood pressure levels at which treatment is recommended depend on overall cardiovascular risk.

- Evaluation of the hypertensive patient aims to confirm elevation of blood pressure, identify secondary causes, evaluate target organ damage, and identify other cardiovascular risks.

- A comprehensive clinical history is essential both for the information it elicits and establishment of the doctor/patient relationship, which is critical to ongoing management.

- Full physical examination is required.

- Routine investigation should include urinalysis and urine microscopy, measurement of potassium, creatinine, fasting glucose and total cholesterol, and electrocardiography.

- A WHO-CVD-Risk Management Package has been designed for feasible and affordable assessment in low- and medium-resource settings.

We are rapidly moving from a paradigm of dichotomous normotension and hypertension to one of blood pressure as a cardiovascular disease (CVD) risk factor.[1] To quote the 2002 WHO Report: "Increasingly, the very terms *hypertension*, *hyperglycemia*, and *hypercholesterolemia*

will probably disappear, as the focus moves from treating a theoretically decided cut-off point, towards managing continuous distributions of risks that intersect and interact with each other: blood pressure, blood sugar and blood cholesterol should be the focus of control."[2]

Nonetheless, the words of Evans and Rose remain valid: "Hypertension should be defined in terms of blood pressure level above which investigation and treatment do more good than harm."[3] It follows that any assessment of the hypertensive patient, or the patient in whom blood pressure is contributing to risk, must start with careful blood pressure measurement. This topic, and its extension ambulatory blood pressure monitoring, are covered in Chapters 44 and 45.

Once blood pressure is known, it is essential to assess target organ damage because its presence will determine the extent of overall CVD risk (Table 43–1)[4] and thus modify the blood pressure levels at which treatment is recommended. This section on clinical assessment and approaches is followed by an extensive section on target organ damage and assessment of heart, vessels, eye, and kidney. According to the 1999 WHO/ISH Guidelines,[5] "The clinical and laboratory evaluation of the hypertensive patient should be conducted with four aims in mind:

- To confirm a chronic elevation of blood pressure and determine its level.
- To exclude or identify secondary causes of hypertension.
- To determine the presence of target-organ damage and to quantify its extent.
- To search for other cardiovascular risk factors and clinical conditions that may influence prognosis and treatment."

WHO/ISH STRATIFICATION OF RISK			
BP (mmHg)	**Grade 1**	**Grade 2**	**Grade 3**
	140–159/90–99	160–179/100–109	≥180/≥110
Other risks			
Nil	Low	Medium	High
1–2	Medium	Medium	High
≥3 TOD/ACC	High	High	High

TOD (target organ damage); ACC (associated clinical conditions).
From World Health Organization (WHO)/International Society of Hypertension (ISH) statement on management of hypertension. *J Hypertens* 2003;21:1983–92.

Table 43–1. WHO/ISH Stratification of Risk

This chapter focuses on basic investigations for the hypertensive patient in both developed and developing countries. More specialized cardiologic investigations are considered in Chapter 46 and in various chapters under the topic "secondary hypertension." Thus, this chapter should be considered in this broader context of clinical history, physical examination, and core investigations in different global settings.

CLINICAL HISTORY

According to the 1999 WHO/ISH Guidelines,[5] "A comprehensive clinical history is essential and should include:

- family history of hypertension, diabetes, dyslipidemia, CHD, stroke or renal disease;
- duration and previous levels of high blood pressure, and results and side effects of previous antihypertensive therapy;
- past history or current symptoms of CHD and heart failure, cerebrovascular disease, peripheral vascular disease, diabetes, gout, dyslipidemia, bronchospasm, sexual dysfunction, renal disease, other significant illnesses and information on the drugs used to treat those conditions;
- symptoms suggestive of secondary causes of hypertension;
- careful assessment of lifestyle factors including dietary intake of fat, sodium and alcohol, quantitation of smoking and physical activity, and enquiry of weight gain since early adult life as a useful index of excess body fat;
- detailed enquiry of intake of drugs or substances that can raise blood pressure, including oral contraceptives, nonsteroidal anti-inflammatory drugs, liquorice, cocaine and amphetamines, and attention should be paid to the use of erythropoietin, cyclosporins or steroids for concomitant disorders; and
- personal, psychosocial and environmental factors that could influence the course and outcome of antihypertensive care, including family situation, work environment and education background."

In eliciting a history of high blood pressure, it is useful to enquire specifically whether blood pressure has been measured in the past (e.g., for a life insurance examination or preoperatively) and whether any comment was made or advice given at the time.[6] It is also useful to ascertain the patient's understanding of hypertension and cardiovascular risk, and in the light of increasing knowledge of the deleterious effects of obstructive sleep apnea specific enquiry should be made for sleep disturbance.[6]

Analgesic abuse is now a rarity in many countries where it was formerly a scourge, but the possibility should not be forgotten when a drug history is being elicited. The specific symptoms of underlying causes of hypertension are protean, which are considered under specific chapters later in this book. Symptoms that may suggest underlying causes include anxiety, tremor, sweating and palpitations (pheochromocytoma), muscle cramps or weakness (Conn's syndrome), daytime somnolence, obesity, snoring (sleep apnea), polyuria, nocturia, and thirst (diabetes or chronic renal disease) or hematuria or frothy urine (kidney disease). Comprehensive history taking is not only valuable for the information it elicits but for the establishment of a doctor/patient relationship, which is so critical in the ongoing effective management of a chronic asymptomatic condition.

PHYSICAL EXAMINATION

The 1999 WHO/ISH Guidelines[5] state that "A full physical examination is essential and will include careful measurement of blood pressure. Other important elements of the physical examination include:

- measurement of height and weight, and calculation of BMI (weight in kilograms divided by height in meters squared);
- examination of the cardiovascular system, particularly for heart size, for evidence of heart failure, for evidence of arterial disease in the carotid, renal and peripheral arteries for coarctation of the aorta;
- examination of the lungs for rales and bronchospasm and of the abdomen for bruits, enlarged kidneys and other masses; and
- examination of the optic fundi and of the nervous system for evidence of cerebrovascular damage."

Findings that may suggest an underlying cause include truncal obesity and striae (Cushing syndrome), tachycardia (pheochromocytoma or thyrotoxicosis), diminished femoral pulses (coarctation), renal bruit (renovascular disease), or palpable kidneys (polycystic disease).

LABORATORY INVESTIGATIONS

The 1999 WHO/ISH Guidelines[5] state that "In all regions of the world, routine investigations should include urinalysis for blood, protein and glucose, and microscopic examination of urine. Blood chemistry should include measurements of potassium, creatinine, fasting glucose and total cholesterol. An ECG should also be performed. In some regions of the world this list of routine investigations is frequently expanded. . . . The cost of investigations should be considered in the context of the needs of the individual patient and the availability of resources in the particular health system or region." Canadian recommendations for routine laboratory tests also include complete blood cell count, plasma sodium, HDL and LDL cholesterol, and triglycerides.[7] The Heart Foundation of Australia[8] adds hemoglobin, plasma sodium, uric acid, LDL and HDL cholesterol, and triglycerides.

Urinalysis and urine microscopy are particularly valuable in the diagnosis of renal disease, the most common cause of secondary hypertension. Proteinuria found on dipstick testing should be quantified by 24-hour urine collection. According to the Caring for Australians with Renal Impairment (CARI) guidelines, some proteins are normally excreted in the urine (about 80 mg/day). These include filtered plasma proteins (albumin and low-molecular-weight immunoglobulin) and secreted tubular proteins. The cutoff for abnormal is laboratory dependent, between 150 and 300 mg/day. Urine albumin excretion is normally some 10 mg/day. It is increased during exercise, fever, standing, and pregnancy. Microalbuminuria is 30 to 300 mg/day, and macroalbuminuria >300 mg/day. Urine protein/albumin can be assessed in "spot" urine samples by measuring urine concentration or the albumin/ creatinine ratio.

CARI suggestions for clinical care based on levels III and IV sources state that testing for proteinuria is preferred in patients with hypertension or known vascular disease, whereas in diabetes initial testing for albuminuria is preferred because it allows detection of early nephropathy. Microscopy may reveal excess numbers of red or white cells or casts. Urine abnormalities will usually precede significant renal functional impairment. Red cell casts signify glomerulonephritis, whereas white cell casts indicate pyelonephritis. Granular cases represent degenerated cellular casts and are indicative of renal disease. Waxy casts are a feature of chronic renal disease. Hyaline casts may be present in small numbers in normal urine, but large numbers indicate renal disease. Increased red cell excretion raises the possibility of glomerulonephritis, and excess white cells (with or without bacteria) suggest renal infection. Using phase-contrast microscopy, dysmorphic (i.e., morphologically variable) red blood cells are suggestive of glomerular bleeding (glomerulonephritis), whereas isomorphic (i.e., morphologically uniform) erythrocytes in the urine indicate nonglomerular bleeding.[10]

Box 43–1

Essential Investigations

To investigate cause:
- Urinalysis
- Urine microscopy
- Serum potassium
- Serum creatinine

To assess target organ damage and CVD risk factors:
- Urinalysis
- Serum creatinine
- Serum cholesterol
- Blood glucose
- ECG

Hyperkalemia is suggestive of primary or secondary hyperaldosteronism, but a normal serum potassium does not by any means exclude these diagnoses. Normokalemic hyperaldosteronism is well recognized.[11] Serum potassium concentration is also useful as a baseline prior to diuretic therapy. Creatinine is a crude measure of renal function

PREVALENCE (%) OF SECONDARY HYPERTENSION			
a. Population Screening			
	Berglund et al. (13)	Rudrick et al. (14)	Sigurdsson et al. (15)	Lewin et al. (16)
n	689 (male)	665	260 (female)	5485
Renoparenchymal	3.6	4.7	3.1	1.0
Renovascular	0.6	0.2	0.8	0.1
Primary aldosteronism	0.1	–	–	0.1
Pheochromocytoma	–	–	–	–
Cushing's syndrome	–	0.2	–	–
Coarctation	0.1	0.2	–	–
Contraceptive pill	–	0.2	0.8	0.1
Total secondary	5.8	5.7	4.6	1.1
b. Referred Patients			
	Gifford (17)	Ferguson (18)	Danielsou & Dammstrom (19)	Sinclair et al. (20)
n	4939	246	1000	3783
Renoparenchymal	5	2.4	2.4	5.6
Renovascular	4	2.8	1.0	0.7
Primary aldosteronism	0.5	0.4	0.1	0.3
Pheochromocytoma	0.2	–	0.2	0.1
Cushing's syndrome	0.2	–	0.1	0.1
Coarctation	1	0	0	0
Contraceptive pill	-	4.0	0.8	1.0
Total secondary	11	10.6	4.7	7.9
Modified from Lever and Swales.[12]			

Table 43–2. Prevalence (%) of Secondary Hypertension

because it is not elevated until creatinine glomerular filtration rate is significantly decreased, but creatinine remains the best simple measure of renal function.

Fasting glucose is an important investigation because diabetes is a major CVD risk factor, mandating aggressive blood pressure lowering.[4] Electrocardiography is important in detection of left ventricular hypertrophy (LVH), of itself a major risk factor, as well as evidence of ischemia. It is less sensitive than echocardiocardiography in detecting LVH but is much less expensive and thus more appropriate for routine use. Essential investigations are listed in Box 43–1.

It should be remembered that secondary hypertension is relatively uncommon. Hypertension is so prevalent that even in resource-rich settings investigation for secondary causes should be targeted to those most likely to benefit, e.g., younger people with suggestive symptoms or signs of severe or treatment-resistant hypertension.

The goals are to find a surgically curable cause or a condition for which a particular therapy is indicated (e.g., aldosterone antagonist for aldosteronism consequent on bilateral adrenal hyperplasia), to determine associated risk factors and target organ disease (which would influence therapy), to provide a baseline for assessing progress, and to identify conditions that of themselves require management (e.g., polycystic kidney disease). Lever and Swales[12] compared prevalence of secondary hypertension in referred patients and population studies and found that although it was more common (about twofold) in referred patients it was exceptional in both groups (Table 43–2). In population studies, renoparenchymal disease was by far the most common secondary cause, followed by renovascular disease. Other causes were rare. In referred patients the pattern was similar, although the prevalence of renovascular disease was higher. It should also be remembered that identifying secondary hypertension does not necessarily influence management, and where hypertension is long-standing even removal of the primary cause may not cure or even improve the elevated blood pressure.

Investigation should always be tailored to the likely clinical benefit to the patient, but often even basic tests are ignored. In a U.S. study of 249 patients with newly diagnosed hypertension in community-based primary care clinics, hypertension was staged initially on a single blood pressure recording in 85% of patients. No electrocardiogram was ordered for 89%, and other mandatory laboratory tests were ordered for about 50%.[21]

A group from the Italian Society of Hypertension studied 228 consecutive patients with recently diagnosed hypertension from six outpatient hypertension centers throughout Italy. A complete clinical and laboratory evaluation according to the minimum work-up suggested by the 1999 WHO/ISH guidelines had been carried out in only 10% of patients. A full physical examination had been performed in 60% of the patients, electrocardiogram in 54%, serum total cholesterol in 53%, glucose in 49%, creatinine in 49%, urine analysis in 46%, potassium in 42%, and fundus oculi in 19%.[22]

Box 43–2

WHO CVD-Risk Management Package

Scenario One: Protocol for CVD-Risk Assessment and Management
Resource availability
Human resources: Non physician health worker
Equipment: Stethoscope; Blood pressure measuring device; Measuring tape or weighing scale; Optional: test tubes, holder, burner, solution or test strips for checking urine glucose
Other facilities: Referral facilities; Maintenance and calibration of blood pressure measurement devices
Measure SBP in all adults
Take history of heart attack, angina, stroke, TIA, diabetes
Check urine sugar if facilities available
Scenario Two: Protocol for CVD-Risk Assessment
Resource availability
Human resources: Medical doctor or specially trained nurse
Equipment: Stethoscope; Blood pressure measurement device; Measuring tape or weighing scale; Test tubes, holder, burner, solutions or test strips for checking urine glucose and albumin
Other facilities: Referral facilities; Maintenance and calibration of equipment
If BP ≥140 or ≥90 after 5–10 minutes rest
Take history of heart attack/angina, stroke/TIA, cardiac failure, peripheral vascular disease, family history of premature CVD (first degree relatives <50 years), tobacco use, alcohol intake
Examine for heaving apex, evidence of cardiac failure
Measure BMI or waist circumference
Look for features of secondary hypertension by history and physical examination
Check urine sugar and urine albumin
Scenario Three: Protocol for CVD-Risk Assessment
Resource availability
Human resources: Medical doctor with access to full specialist care
Equipment: Stethoscope; Blood pressure measurement device; Measuring tape and weighing scale; Electrocardiograph; Ophthalmoscope; Urine analysis; Blood analysis: fasting blood sugar, electrolytes, creatinine, cholesterol and lipoproteins
Other facilities: Access to full specialist care; Maintenance and calibration of equipment
Measure BP in all adults
If BP ≥140 or ≥90 after 5–10 minutes rest
Take history of heart attack/angina, stroke/TIA, cardiac failure, peripheral vascular disease, family history of premature CVD (first degree relatives <50), tobacco use, alcohol intake
Examine for heaving apex, evidence of cardiac failure
Measure BMI or waist circumference
Look for features of secondary hypertension by history and physical examination
Examine fundus for hypertensive retinopathy (if BP >180 or >110)
Check urine albumin, serum creatinine and electrolytes, fasting blood sugar, ECG, Total cholesterol or LDL and HDL

Adapted from WHO, 2002.[24]

An interesting study from Brazil[23] looked at 145 patients in a general outpatient clinic and found that hypertension was not associated with a higher number of abnormal laboratory tests than normotension (hemoglobin, blood sugar, plasma uric acid, potassium, total and LDL cholesterol, triglycerides, calcium, and creatinine), but both hypertensives and normotensives who were obese had more diabetes and hyperlipidemia.

ASSESSMENT FOR LOW- AND MEDIUM-RESOURCE SETTINGS

The WHO CVD Risk Management Package was designed to make the assessment and management of cardiovascular risk feasible and affordable in low- and medium-resource settings. The package provides clinical protocols that can be applied in three scenarios,[24] with hierarchical resource levels adapted to diverse health care facilities. These characteristics are outlined in Box 43–2. The package focuses on treatment but does include initial assessment (as shown in Box 43–2) and a questionnaire for the presence of CVD (Box 43–3).

Barriers to management of CVD risk in a low-resource setting in Nigeria, using hypertension as an entry point, were examined by Mendis and colleagues from WHO.[25] They interviewed 1000 consecutive hypertensives and their health care providers across a range of facilities. Laboratory and other investigations to exclude secondary hypertension or assess target organ damage were not available in the majority of facilities. They concluded that if the absolute risk approach for assessment of risk and effective management of hypertension is to be implemented in low-resource settings appropriate policy measures need to be taken to improve the competency of health-care providers, to provide basic laboratory facilities, and to develop affordable financing mechanisms.

ACKNOWLEDGMENTS

Mrs. Amanda Jacobsen provided expert secretarial assistance.

Box 43–3

Questionnaire to Determine Probable Angina, Heart Attack, Stroke, and TIA

1. Have you ever had any pain or discomfort or any pressure or heaviness in your chest?
   ❑ Yes   ❑ No

If no go to Q8, if yes proceed to the next question:
2. Do you get the pain in the center of the chest or left chest or left arm?
   ❑ Yes   ❑ No

If no, got to Q8, if yes proceed to next question:
3. Do you get it when you walk at an ordinary pace on level or when you walk uphill or hurry?
   ❑ Yes   ❑ No

4. Do you slow down if you get the pain while walking?
   ❑ Yes   ❑ No

5. Does the pain go away if you stand still or if you take a tablet under the tongue?
   ❑ Yes   ❑ No

6. Does the pain go away in less than 10 minutes?
   ❑ Yes   ❑ No

7. Have you ever had a severe chest pain across the front of your chest lasting for half an hour or more?
   ❑ Yes   ❑ No

If the answer to questions 3 or 4 or 5 or 6 or 7 is yes patient may have angina or heart attack and needs referral.
Stroke and TIA
8. Have you ever had any of the following: difficulty in talking, weakness of arm and/or leg on one side of the body or numbness on one side of the body?
   ❑ Yes   ❑ No

If the answer to question 8 is yes the patient may have had a TIA or stroke and needs referral.
From World Health Organization 2002. WHO CVD-risk management package for low- and medium-resource settings. World Health Organization, Geneva.

REFERENCES

1. World Health Organization. Integrated management of cardiovascular risk: Report of a WHO meeting. Geneva, 9–12 July 2002.

2. *The World Health Report 2002: Reducing Risks, Promoting Healthy Life.* Geneva: World Health Organization, 2002.

3. Evans JG, Rose G. Hypertension. *Br Med Bull* 1971;27:37–42.

4. World Health Organization (WHO)/ International Society of Hypertension (ISH) statement on management of hypertension. *J Hypertens* 2003; 21:1983–92.

5. Guidelines subcommittee 1999 World Health Organization-International Society of Hypertension Guidelines for the Management of Hypertension. *J Hypertens* 1999;17:151–83.

6. Ball SG. Clinical assessment of the hypertensive patient. In: JD Swales (ed.) *Textbook of Hypertension.* Oxford: Blackwell, 1994:1009–14.

7. Hemmelgarn BR, Zarnke KB, Campbell NRC, et al. The 2004 Canadian Hypertension Education Program recommendations for the management of hypertension: Part 1 - Blood pressure measurement, diagnosis and assessment of risk. *Can J Cardiol* 2004;20:31–40.

8. Heart Foundation. *Hypertension Management Guide for Doctors.* 2004.

9. CARI (Caring for Australians with Renal Impairment) Guidelines: 1. Testing for proteinuria. *Nephrology* 2004;9: S3–7.

10. Birch DF, Fairley KF, Whitworth JA, Forbes I, Fairley JD, Cheshire GR, et al. Urinary erythrocyte morphology in the diagnosis of glomerular hematuria. *Clin Nephrol* 1983;20:78–84.

11. Gordon RD. Mineralocorticoid hypertension. *Lancet* 1994;344:240.

12. Lever AF, Swales JD. Investigating the hypertensive patient. In: Swales JD (ed.) *Textbook of Hypertension*. Oxford: Blackwell, 1026–30.

13. Berglund G, Andersson O, Wilhelmsen L. Prevalence of primary and secondary hypertension: Studies in a random population sample. *BMJ* 1976; 2:554–56.

14. Rudnick KV, Sackett DL, Hirst S, Holmes C. Hypertension in a family practice. *Can Med Assoc J* 1977; 117:492–97.

15. Sigurdsson JA, Bengtsson C, Tibblin E, Wojciehowski J. Prevalence of secondary hypertension in a population sample of Swedish women. *Eur Heart J* 1977; 4:424–31.

16. Lewin A, Blaufox D, Castle H, Entvisle G, Langford H. Apparent prevalence of curable hypertension in the Hypertension, Detection and Follow-up Program. *Arch Intern Med* 1985;145:424–27.

17. Gifford RW Jr. Evaluation of the hypertensive patient with emphasis on detecting curable causes. *Milbank Mem Fund Q* 1969;47:170–75.

18. Ferguson RK. Cost and yield of the hypertensive evaluation. *Ann Intern Med* 1975;82:761–65.

19. Danielson M, Dammstrom B-G. The prevalence of secondary and curable hypertension. *Acta Med Scand* 1981;209:451–55.

20. Sinclair AM, Isles CG, Brown I, Cameron H, Murray GD, Robertson JWK. Secondary hypertension in a blood pressure clinic. *Arch Intern Med* 1987;147:1289–93.

21. Spranger CB, Ries AJ, Berge CA, Radford NB, Victor RG. Identifying gaps between guidelines and clinical practice in the evaluation and treatment of patients with hypertension. *Am J Med* 2004;117:14–8.

22. Cuspidi C, Michev I, Lonati L, Vaccarella A, Cristofari M, Garavelli G, et al. Compliance to hypertension guidelines in clinical practice: A multicentre pilot study in Italy. *J Hum Hypertens* 2002;16:699–703.

23. Reis RS, Bensenor IJ, Lotufo PA. Laboratory assessment of the hypertensive individual. Value of the main guidelines for high blood pressure. *Arq Bras Cardiol* 1999;73:201–10.

24. World Health Organization 2002. WHO CVD-risk management package for low-and medium-resource settings. World Health Organization, Geneva.

25. Mendis S, Abegunde D, Oladapo O, Celletti F, Nordet P. Barriers to management of cardiovascular risk in a low-resource setting using hypertension as an entry point. *J Hypertens* 2004; 22:59–64.

Chapter

44

Blood Pressure Measurement

Thomas G. Pickering

Key Findings

- With the demise of the mercury sphygmomanometer, the oscillometric method of blood pressure measurement is becoming the most widely used method.

- Hybrid sphygmomanometers, in which an electronic transducer replaces the mercury column, have promise.

- Measurement from the upper arm is the preferred location, although wrist measurement may be appropriate in patients with very obese arms.

- Applanation tonometry is a promising technique for measuring the central aortic pressure, which may give a better prediction of risk than the brachial artery pressure.

- The traditional clinic or office measurement of blood pressure often significantly over- or underestimates the true blood pressure, which is conceived as the average blood pressure over time.

- When automated monitors are used, only validated devices should be chosen.

- It is important to choose cuffs of the appropriate size, particularly in children and obese subjects.

Although hypertension can only be identified by measuring the blood pressure, the conventionally used methods for its detection are notoriously unreliable. There are three main reasons for this: inaccuracies in the methods, some of which are avoidable; the inherent variability of blood pressure; and the tendency for blood pressure to increase in the presence of a physician (the so-called white-coat effect). For clinical practice, the gold standard has for many years been measurements made with the Korotkoff sound technique by a physician using a mercury sphygmomanometer. However, there is increasing evidence that this may lead to the misclassification of large numbers of individuals as hypertensive. In addition, mercury is being banned in many countries and there is still uncertainty as to what will replace it. Neither the distribution of blood pressure in the population nor the relationship between blood pressure and cardiovascular morbidity provide any justification for a rigid separation between normotension and hypertension,[1] but for clinical purposes a threshold level of blood pressure above which antihypertensive treatment is recommended needs to be established. Thus, the accurate measurement of blood pressure is of extreme importance.

There are two general reasons for measuring blood pressure. The first is as a "vital sign" when evaluating a critically ill patient, in which case the blood pressure at the time of measurement is of critical interest. Is it too high, normal, or too low? For the vast majority of measurements, however, we are not interested in the pressure at the time of measurement so much as its ability to estimate the average (or "true") level of blood pressure—which is generally assumed to be responsible for the adverse effects of high blood pressure on the circulation and for which the clinic or office blood pressure is taken as a surrogate measure.

CLASSIFICATION/SUBTYPES OF HYPERTENSION

JNC 7 Classification

The latest report of the Joint National Committee on Prevention, Detection, Evaluation and Treatment of High Blood Pressure (JNC 7)[2] has classified hypertension as outlined in Table 44–1. For adults age 18 or older, the cutoff point for defining hypertension continues to be 140/90 mmHg. The classification is based on the average of two or more seated blood pressures, properly measured with well-maintained equipment, at each of two or more visits to the office or clinic.

For patients with diabetes or chronic kidney disease, the cutoff point is 130/80 mmHg. The category of prehypertension has created some confusion, in that a "normal" blood pressure is defined as being less than 120/80 mmHg, leading many people to think that this is the target level of drug treatment. The intent of introducing the concept of prehypertension was to emphasize that people with this level of blood pressure are at increased risk of developing hypertension over the years and that lifestyle changes may help to modify this process.

Isolated systolic hypertension

After the age of 50, the systolic pressure tends to increase with age, and the diastolic to fall. An elevation of systolic pressure (>140 mmHg) together with a normal diastolic pressure <90 mmHg) is defined as systolic hypertension. The primary mechanism underlying this is increased stiffness of the central arteries. Patients with systolic hypertension over the age of 50 are at increased risk of cardiovascular disease. In the Framingham study, predictors of isolated systolic hypertension (ISH) included older age,

CLASSIFICATION OF HYPERTENSION (JNC7)		
BP Classification	SBP (mmHg)[a]	DBP (mmHg)[a]
Normal	<120	<80
Prehypertension	120–139	80–89
Stage 1 hypertension	140–159	90–99
Stage 2 hypertension	≥160	≥100
a. Classification determined by highest blood pressure category.		

Table 44–1. Classification of Hypertension (JNC7)

female sex, and increased body mass index (BMI) during follow-up.[3]

Isolated systolic hypertension of the young

Although it has been recognized for many years that elevation of systolic pressure with a normal diastolic may also occur in young people (below the age of 30), it is only recently that the phenomenon has been given recognition as a distinct entity. The mechanism is unclear, and has been attributed to a high stroke volume (it is common in athletes) and increased amplification of the pressure waveform in the peripheral circulation.[4,5] The prognosis is unknown.

Isolated diastolic hypertension

Isolated diastolic hypertension (IDH) is a condition that is also not uncommon in young people, and is defined as a diastolic pressure >90 mmHg together with a normal systolic (<140 mmHg). In some cases this may be the result of early disappearance of the Korotkoff sounds, such that the true diastolic pressure is lower.[6] Its prognostic significance remains uncertain,[7,8] but it may be a precursor of systolic and diastolic hypertension and has been related to weight gain in the Framingham Heart Study.[3]

Pseudohypertension

In some elderly people, the noninvasive methods using a sphygmomanometer cuff compressing the brachial artery may give a very exaggerated estimate of the blood pressure because the artery may be so stiff that it becomes incompressible. The only accurate known method of confirming the diagnosis is to record the pressure intra-arterially, but this is rarely done in practice. Osler's maneuver (the ability to palpate the brachial or radial artery when the cuff is inflated to above systolic pressure) is sometimes positive, but is not a very reliable guide.[9]

Orthostatic (postural) hypotension

Orthostatic (postural) hypotension is defined as a reduction of systolic blood pressure of at least 20 mmHg or 10 mmHg in diastolic blood pressure within three minutes of quiet standing.[10] It is common in elderly patients, and is typically the result of impaired autonomic control. Blood pressure measurement is a major issue because of the increased variability (the pressure may be very low when the patient is upright and high when supine, particularly during the night).

Situational hypertension

In some patients, the blood pressure may be high or low depending on the situation or circumstances of measurement. Although measurements taken in a medical setting are the gold standard for defining hypertension, there is increasing evidence that they may not be representative of the blood pressure levels prevailing at other times. There is also consensus that the overall average blood pressure level is what ultimately determines risk. These types of hypertension are discussed in greater detail in Chapter 45.

White-coat hypertension

White-coat hypertension is defined as a persistently high blood pressure taken in the clinic setting (>140/90 mmHg) together with a normal pressure occurring at other times, away from the clinic. To allow for the white-coat effect, the upper limit of normal (whether measured by home or ambulatory monitoring) is typically taken as 135/85 mmHg. Note that some patients can be normotensive and have white-coat hypertension when attending the doctor, whereas some known hypertensives who are normally well controlled with drug treatment can have raised blood pressures when attending the clinic (due to a white-coat effect).

Masked hypertension

Masked hypertension is the converse of white-coat hypertension, being defined as a persistently normal blood pressure in the clinic but an elevated pressure (>135/85 mmHg) outside it.

TECHNIQUES

The methods currently available for blood pressure measurement in clinical practice are listed in Box 44–1. There are two basic techniques: the auscultatory and oscillometric methods. The former can be done with mercury or aneroid sphygmomanometers, or the more recently introduced hybrid technique. Measurements are preferably taken from the upper arm, although the wrist and finger are alternative sites. In addition, measurements can be taken in the office, at home, or over 24 hours with ambulatory monitoring. The use of all three methods has been endorsed by the JNC 7 recommendations.[2] This chapter reviews the techniques of blood pressure measurement and their use in the clinic or office setting. Chapter 45 reviews the applications of measurement outside the clinic with home and ambulatory monitoring. Applanation tonometry is a new technique that enables the central aortic pressure to be estimated from recordings made in the peripheral arteries.

The auscultatory technique

It is surprising that nearly 100 years after it was first discovered, and the subsequent recognition of its limited accuracy, the Korotkoff technique for measuring blood pressure has continued to be used without any substantial improvement. The Korotkoff sound method tends to give values for systolic pressure that are lower than the intra-

Box 44–1

Techniques of Blood Pressure Measurement in Clinical Practice

Methodologies
- Auscultatory (K sound)
- Mercury
- Aneroid
- Hybrid
- Oscillometric
- Applanation tonometry

Locations
- Upper arm
- Wrist
- Finger

Situations
- Clinic
- Home
- Ambulatory

arterial pressure, and diastolic values that are higher, but there is no obvious superiority for phase 5 over phase 4.[11-13] The range of discrepancies is quite striking: one author commented that the difference between the two methods might be as much as 25 mmHg in some individuals.[14]

There is still no universal agreement as to which phase of the Korotkoff sounds should be used for recording diastolic pressure. The official recommendation of organizations such as the American Heart Association[15,16] and British Hypertension Society[17] is to use the fifth phase, except in children or other situations in which the disappearance of sounds cannot reliably be determined.[15] Most of the large-scale clinical trials that have evaluated the benefits of treating hypertension have used the fifth phase.

The oscillometric technique

This was first demonstrated by Marey in 1876,[18] and it was subsequently shown that when the oscillations of pressure in a sphygmomanometer cuff are recorded during gradual deflation the point of maximal oscillation corresponds to the mean intra-arterial pressure.[19,20] The oscillations begin well above systolic pressure and continue below diastolic (Figure 44–1), so that systolic and diastolic pressure can only be estimated indirectly according to some empirically derived algorithm.

One advantage of the method is that no transducer need be placed over the brachial artery, so that placement of the cuff is not critical. Other potential advantages of the oscillometric method for ambulatory monitoring (see Chapter 45) are that it is less susceptible to external noise (but not to low-frequency mechanical vibration) and that the cuff can be removed and replaced by the patient (for example, to take a shower). The main disadvantage is that

such recorders do not work well during physical activity, when there may be considerable movement artifact.

The oscillometric technique has been used successfully in ambulatory blood pressure monitors and home monitors. It should be pointed out that different brands of oscillometric recorders use different algorithms, and there is no generic oscillometric technique. However, comparisons of several different commercial models with intra-arterial and Korotkoff sound measurements have shown generally good agreement.[21-23]

Ultrasound techniques

Some devices use an ultrasound transmitter and receiver placed over the brachial artery under a sphygmomanometer cuff. As the cuff is deflated, the movement of the arterial wall at systolic pressure causes a Doppler phase shift in the reflected ultrasound, and diastolic pressure is recorded as the point at which diminution of arterial motion occurs.[24] Another variation of this method detects the onset of blood flow at systolic pressure, which has been found to be of particular value for measuring pressure in infants and children.[25] Such devices are rarely used in clinical practice, having been supplanted by oscillometric monitors.

In patients with very faint Korotkoff sounds (for example, those with muscular atrophy), placing a Doppler probe over the brachial artery may help to detect the systolic pressure (by the appearance of pulsatile sounds as the cuff is deflated). The same technique can be used for measuring the ankle/arm index, in which the systolic pressures in the brachial artery and the posterior tibial artery are compared to obtain an index of peripheral arterial disease.

The finger cuff method of Penaz

This method, developed by Penaz,[26] works on the principle of the "unloaded arterial wall." Arterial pulsation in a finger is detected by a photoplethysmograph under a pressure cuff. The output of the plethysmograph is used to drive a servo-loop which rapidly changes the cuff pressure to keep the output constant, so that the artery is held in a partially opened state. The oscillations of pressure in the cuff are measured, and have been found to resemble the intra-arterial pressure wave in most subjects.

This method gives an accurate estimate of the changes of systolic and diastolic pressure, although both may be underestimated (or overestimated in some subjects) when compared to brachial artery pressures[26] (the cuff can be kept inflated for up to two hours). It is now commercially available as the Finometer (formerly Finapres) and Portapres recorders, and has been validated in several studies against intra-arterial pressures.[27,28] The Portapres enables readings to be taken over 24 hours while the subjects are ambulatory, although it is somewhat cumbersome.[29]

Applanation tonometry

This is a technique rapidly gaining in popularity that enables the shape of the arterial pressure waveform to be recorded noninvasively from a handheld probe, usually at the wrist (Figure 44–2). The principle of this technique is

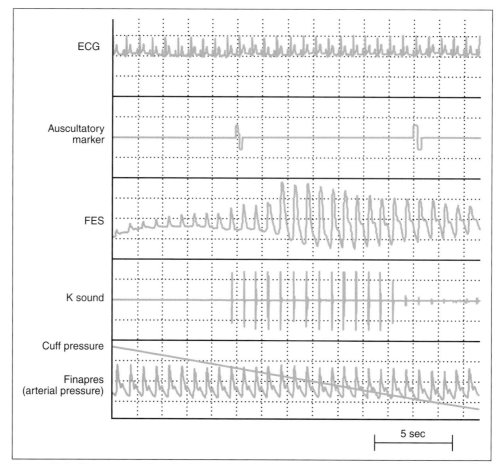

Figure 44–1. Changes occurring distal to a sphygmomanometer cuff during deflation. Upper trace (ECG), second trace (auscultatory marker when Korotkoff sounds were first and last heard), third trace (oscillations under cuff detected by foil electret sensor), fourth trace (Korotkoff sounds), and fifth trace (cuff pressure and arterial pressure, recorded noninvasively from other arm).

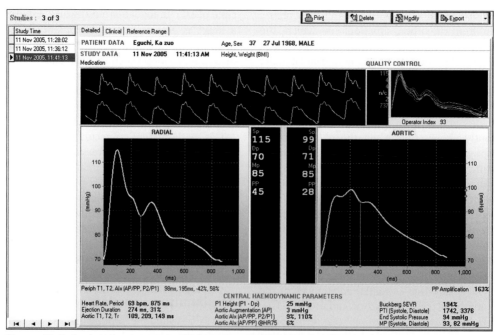

Figure 44–2. Applanation tonometry (Sphygmocor device). Upper left trace shows recordings of radial artery trace (10 pressure waves superimposed) made from a probe held on the radial artery. Upper right trace shows estimated central aortic pressure. Bottom right trace shows augmentation index.

that when an artery is partially compressed or splinted against a bone the pulsations are proportional to the intra-arterial pressure.[30] The objective of the technique is to be able to derive central aortic pressure, which is done by Fourier analysis of the waveform. This requires calibration of the recorded wave by taking the brachial artery pressure by the auscultatory or oscillometric technique. The rationale for performing the tests is that cardiovascular events and target organ damage may be more closely related to the central aortic pressure than to the peripheral pressure (as has been confirmed, for example, in the ASCOT CAFÉ study).[31]

Location of measurement

The standard location for noninvasive blood pressure measurement is the brachial artery, although there are several other sites where it can be done. Monitors that measure pressure at the wrist and fingers have become popular, but it is important to realize that the systolic and diastolic pressures vary substantially in different parts of the arterial tree. In general, the systolic pressure increases in more distal arteries, whereas the diastolic decreases. There is currently great interest in measuring the central aortic pressure, which can be derived indirectly from analyses of the blood pressure waveform recorded at more peripheral sites such as the radial artery using applanation tonometry (see material following). The rationale is that the central pressure may be more important in causing target organ damage.

Technical issues with measurement from the upper arm

There are important potential sources of error with measurements from the upper arm. These are discussed in the sections that follow.

Effects of posture

There is no consensus as to whether blood pressure should be routinely measured sitting or supine, although most guidelines recommend sitting.[15,32] In a survey of 245 subjects of different ages, Netea et al.[33] found that systolic pressures were the same in both positions, but there was a systematic age-related discrepancy for diastolic pressure

such that at the age of 30 the sitting diastolic was about 10 mmHg higher than the supine reading, whereas at the age of 70 the difference was only 2 mmHg.

Body position

Blood pressure measurements are also influenced by the position of the arm in relation to the position of the chest.[34,35] There is a progressive increase in the pressure of about 5 to 6 mmHg as the arm is moved down from the horizontal to vertical position. These changes are exactly what would be expected from the changes of hydrostatic pressure, and are even more pronounced when recording is made from the wrist (see material following). It is also important that the patient's back be supported during the measurement. If the patient is sitting bolt upright, the diastolic pressure may be 6.5 mmHg higher than if sitting back.[36] These differences are of critical importance for monitors that record blood pressure at the wrist (see Chapter 45).

Cuff size

The size of the cuff relative to the diameter of the arm is critical. The most common mistake is to use a cuff that is too small, which will result in an overestimation of the pressure.[37-39] In general, the error can be reduced by using a large adult-size cuff for all except the skinniest arms. The British Hypertension Society[17] recommends that if the arm circumference exceeds 33 cm a large adult cuff should be used (width 12.5 to 13 cm, length 35 cm). In the United States, the most widely advocated protocol for the selection of the appropriate cuff size is the one recommended by the American Heart Association (AHA),[16] outlined in Table 44–2.

There has been some controversy concerning the width of the largest cuff for use in very obese people (arm circumference more than 45 cm). The older guidelines recommended a maximum width of 22 cm, whereas the most recent AHA guidelines proposed a 16-cm-wide cuff (Table 44–2). The rationale for this was that 22 cm is longer than the upper arm in most people. Very few studies have systematically compared blood pressure measured with the two widths of cuffs in obese people, and where they have there is no consistent difference.[40]

1993 AND 2005 AMERICAN HEART ASSOCIATION RECOMMENDATIONS FOR CUFF SIZES IN OBESE AND OVERWEIGHT SUBJECTS				
Arm Circumference	Cuff	Year	Bladder Width	Bladder Length
22–26 cm	Small adult	1993/2005	10 cm	24 cm
27–34 cm	Adult	1993/2005	13 cm	30 cm
35–44 cm	Large adult	1993	16 cm	38 cm
		2005	16 cm	36 cm
45-52 cm	Adult thigh	1993	20 cm	42 cm
		2005	16 cm	42 cm

Table 44–2. 1993 and 2005 American Heart Association Recommendations for Cuff Sizes in Obese and Overweight Subjects

Blood pressure differences between the two arms

The standard recommendation in all guidelines is to measure the blood pressure in both arms when the patient is first seen, and then to use the arm with the higher pressure for subsequent measurements. In some studies of inter-arm differences, an average difference of more than 10 mmHg has been reported in as many as 20% of patients.[41] What is not clear from these studies is the extent to which the observed differences are reproducible, as opposed to random error. More recent work has shown that genuine differences that are clinically meaningful are very rare, and in the small number of patients who have such differences clinically overt vascular disease is usually present. There is, however, a consistent but small difference in the majority of patients, with the right arm being about 2 mmHg higher than the left arm.[42] This difference is more noticeable when the auscultatory technique is used, but is still detectable with oscillometric devices. To what extent it is due to handedness is not clear.

DEVICES

Devices for clinic and hospital measurement

Despite the increasing use and acceptance of out-of-office blood pressure measurement, readings taken in a clinic setting are still regarded as the standard by which blood pressure control is assessed. Traditionally, this was done using mercury sphygmomanometers, but these are rapidly disappearing from the clinical scene. They are being replaced by aneroid or hybrid devices (both of which use the auscultatory technique) and by oscillometric devices. As clinical measures of blood pressure and other variables become more widely used for the evaluation of physicians' performance and reimbursement, it is likely that there will be an increasing need for objective measures of clinic blood pressure that can be downloaded into electronic medical records (which at present can only be done with oscillometric devices).

Mercury sphygmomanometers

The mercury sphygmomanometer has always been regarded as the gold standard for clinical measurement of blood pressure, but this situation is rapidly changing (as discussed in material following). The design of mercury sphygmomanometers has changed little over the past 50 years, except that modern versions are less likely to spill mercury if dropped. In principle, there is less to go wrong with mercury sphygmomanometers than other devices, but this should not be any cause for complacency. One hospital survey found that 21% of devices had technical problems that would limit their accuracy,[43] whreas another found more than 50% to be defective.[44]

The future of mercury

A growing trend throughout the world is the removal of mercury-containing devices from hospitals. This has already happened with thermometers, and is now starting to happen with sphygmomanometers. The reason is not because any more accurate device has been developed but because there are concerns about the safety of mercury. In some European countries mercury has already been banned, and there is a growing tendency in the United States to replace mercury devices, although this is being resisted by organizations such as the Council for High Blood Pressure Research and the AHA.[45] The unresolved issue is what should replace mercury. Currently, the two alternatives are aneroid or electronic (oscillometric) devices, but neither is regarded as satisfactory. Hybrid devices (see material following) are another alternative.

Aneroid devices

The incipient demise of the mercury sphygmomanometer has placed new interest in alternative methods, of which aneroid devices are the leading contenders. Three surveys conducted in hospitals in the past 10 years have examined the accuracy of the aneroid dials. One was conducted in the University of Missouri hospitals, which found that 35% of monitors were in error. A second survey in the Hospital of the University of Sao Paolo in Brazil found 44% in error,[43] and the third in the Mayo Clinic Hospitals found only 1%.[46]

Hybrid devices

These devices combine the main advantages of the mercury technique while avoiding the use of mercury, by using an electronic transducer in place of the mercury column or aneroid scale (Figure 44–3). The blood pressure is recorded using the auscultatory technique.[47]

Automated devices for clinic use

The decline in the use of mercury, coupled with the ascendance of the oscillometric technique, has led to the introduction of automated oscillometric devices that can take a series of readings (typically three to five) in the clinic setting. These are usually lower than readings taken

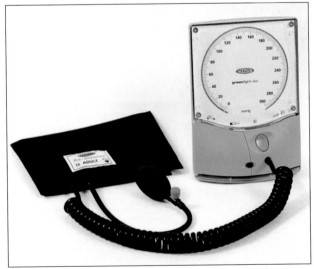

Figure 44–3. A hybrid sphygmomanometer (Accoson), which functions like an aneroid device except that the pressure is measured by an electronic transducer.

by physicians (and to a lesser extent nurses) and hence reduce but do not completely eliminate the white-coat effect.[48] Their use is likely to increase in the future.

Electronic monitors for clinic and home measurement of blood pressure

When home monitoring was first used, the majority of studies used aneroid sphygmomanometers.[49] Although inexpensive, such devices require a certain degree of training and dexterity on the part of the patient, and the dials are not always accurate. In one survey, 30% of aneroid dials had errors greater than 4 mmHg.[50] The mercury sphygmomanometer has never been considered very suitable for home use, partly because of its expense but also because of concerns about the toxicity of mercury.[51] In the past few years, automatic electronic devices have become increasingly popular.

Arm monitors

The standard type of monitor for home use is now an oscillometric device that records pressure from the brachial artery. Oscillometric monitors have the advantage of being easy to use because cuff placement is not as critical as with devices that use a Korotkoff sound microphone, and the oscillometric method has in practice been found to be as reliable as the Korotkoff sound method. The early versions were largely inaccurate,[52,53] but those currently available are often satisfactory.[54,55] Unfortunately, only a few have been subjected to proper validation tests such as the Association for the Advancement of Medical Instrumentation (AAMI) and British Hypertension Society (BHS) protocols.

The advantages of electronic monitors have begun to be appreciated by epidemiologists,[56] who have always been greatly concerned about the accuracy of clinical blood pressure measurement and who have paid much attention to the problems of observer error, digit preference, and the other causes of inaccuracy described previously. Cooper et al. have made the case that the ease of use of the electronic devices and the relative insensitivity to who is actually taking the reading can outweigh any inherent inaccuracy compared to the traditional sphygmomanometer method.[56] Electronic devices are now available that will take blood pressure from the upper arm, wrist, or finger. Although the use of the more distal sites may be more convenient, measurement of blood pressure from the arm (brachial artery) has always been the standard method and is likely to remain so for the foreseeable future.

Wrist monitors

Wrist monitors have the advantage of being smaller than arm devices, and they can be used in obese people because the wrist diameter is little affected by obesity. A potential problem with wrist monitors is the systematic error introduced by the hydrostatic effect of differences in the position of the wrist relative to the heart,[34] as shown in Figure 44–4. This can be avoided if the wrist is always at heart level when the readings are taken, but there is no way of knowing retrospectively whether this was complied with when a series of readings are reviewed.

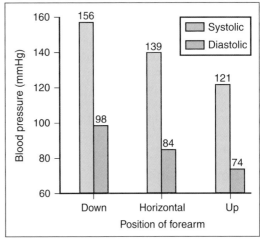

Figure 44–4. The effects of changes in the position of the forearm on the blood pressure recorded by a wrist monitor. Ten readings were taken in each of three positions: vertically down, horizontal, and vertically up. The average values are shown at the top of each bar.

Wrist monitors have potential, but need to be evaluated further.[57,58]

Finger monitors

Finger monitors are convenient, but so far have been found inaccurate. The pressure waveform in the finger is different from the brachial artery trace because of the effects of wave reflection. Thus, the systolic peak is shorter and higher, and hence finger monitors would be expected to overestimate the brachial artery systolic pressure by about 4 mmHg.[59] In practice, there may be little systematic disagreement between finger blood pressure measurement and conventional sphygmomanometry. However, the scatter of individual readings is excessively high.[60]

Choice of monitors

The standard recommendation for the use of automated monitors (whether they will be used for measurement in the clinic, for epidemiological studies, or by the patient at home) is for a device that records blood pressure from the upper arm and that has passed the standard validation tests. The results of validation studies that have been conducted according to these protocols are posted on two web sites: the dabl Educational Trust (*http://www.dableducational.org/*) and the British Hypertension Society (*http://www.bhsoc.org/ blood_pressure_list.htm*). Both of these sites are updated on a regular basis. One of the problems in choosing a monitor is that the manufacturers may change the brand number, making it difficult to know if the accuracy is the same as a similar model that has been validated. Manufacturers are being asked to post statements on these sites as to whether there has been any change in the measurement algorithm.

Ambulatory monitors

First developed more than 40 years ago, ambulatory blood pressure monitoring is only now beginning to find acceptance as a clinically useful technique. Technologic advances over the past few years have led to the introduction of monitors that are small, relatively quiet, and can take up to 100 readings of blood pressure over 24 hours while patients go about their normal activities. They are reasonably accurate while the patient is at rest, but less so during physical activity. The accuracy of the various devices can be found on the dabl and BHS web sites. The use of ambulatory and home monitors is discussed in Chapter 45.

Validation of monitors

The increasing use of electronic monitors for both self- and ambulatory monitoring has necessitated the development of standard protocols for testing them. The original two protocols that gained the widest acceptance were developed in the United States by the AAMI in 1987 and the BHS in 1990, with revisions to both in 1993. These required testing of a device against two trained human observers in 85 subjects, which made validations studies difficult to perform. One consequence of this has been that there are still many devices on the market that have never been adequately validated.

More recently, an international group of experts who are members of the European Society of Hypertension Working Group on Blood Pressure Monitoring have produced an international protocol[61] that should replace the two earlier versions and that is easier to perform. Briefly, it requires comparison of the device readings (four in all) alternating with five mercury readings taken by two trained observers. Devices are recommended for approval if both systolic and diastolic readings taken are at least within 5 mmHg of each other for at least 50% of readings.

One of the limitations of the validation procedures is that they analyze the data on a population basis, and pay no attention to individual factors. Thus, it is possible that a monitor will pass the validation criteria and still be consistently in error in a substantial number of individuals. For these reasons it is recommended that when large numbers of readings are going to be taken with an automated device in a particular patient (e.g., with an ambulatory or home monitor) the device be calibrated against a mercury sphygmomanometer.

Applanation tonometry

Devices using this technique are currently used mainly to record the arterial pressure wave at the radial artery, which is the most readily accessible peripheral artery. They may be handheld (using a pencil-shaped probe that is pressed onto the radial artery) or strapped around the wrist, with an array of transducers that ensures that at least one of them is optimally placed over the artery to record the pressure waveform. The basis of the technique is to identify the incident and reflected waves, and hence the augmentation index (a measure of the relative height of the reflected wave).[62] The results are expressed either as the augmentation index or the central aortic pressure. These devices are relatively expensive, and require some skill in their use.

MEASUREMENT OF BLOOD PRESSURE IN THE CLINIC

Although the mercury method is still considered the gold standard for measurement in the clinic, there is a huge gulf between the ideal measurements and those made in real life. The recent interest in alternative methods of measuring blood pressure has served to emphasize some of the potentially correctable deficiencies of its routine clinic measurement. By increasing the number of readings taken per visit, and the number of visits, as well as by attempting to eliminate sources of error such as terminal digit preference, the reliability of clinic pressure for estimating the true blood pressure and its consequences can be greatly increased. However, a number of factors relating to the physician, the patient, or their interaction may lead to either over- or under-estimation of the true blood pressure.

Patient preparation

The patient should be asked to remove all clothing that covers the location of cuff placement, and should be seated comfortably, with the legs uncrossed, and the back and arm supported, such that the middle of the cuff on the upper arm is at the level of the right atrium (the midpoint of the sternum). These requirements mean that blood pressure should not be measured while the patient is sitting on an exam table. The patient should be instructed to relax as much as possible, and not to talk during the measurement procedure; ideally 5 minutes should elapse before the first reading is taken. At the initial visit, blood pressure should be measured in both arms.

Sources of error with the auscultatory method

Some of the major causes of a discrepancy between the conventional clinical measurement of blood pressure and the true blood pressure are listed in Table 44–1. These include factors that apply whichever method of measurement is used, e.g., cuff size and posture of the patient (see Section IV), and those that are specifially prominent with the auscultatory method, which are described below. The measurement of blood pressure typically involves an interaction between the patient and the physician (or whoever is taking the reading), and factors related to both may lead to a tendency to either overestimate or underestimate the true blood pressure, or to act as a source of bi-directional error, as shown in Table 44–3. There may also be activities which precede or accompany the measurement that make it unrepresentative of the patient's "true" pressure. These include exercise and smoking before the measurement, and talking during it.

Observer error and observer bias are important sources of error when conventional sphygmomanometers are used. Differences of auditory acuity between observers may lead to consistent errors, and terminal digit preference is very common, with most observers recording a disproportionate number of readings ending in 5 or 0.[63] The average values of blood pressure recorded by trained individual observers have been found to vary by as much as 5–10 mmHg.[64] The level of pressure that is recorded

PATIENT- AND PHYSICIAN-RELATED FACTORS THAT LEAD TO A DISCREPANCY BETWEEN THE CLINIC AND TRUE BLOOD PRESSURE			
	Clinic BP Overestimates True BP	Bidirectional Error	Clinic BP Underestimates True BP
Physician	• Observer error • Cuff size too small	• Observer error	• Observer error • Cuff size too large
Patient	• Anxiety • Talking • Recent ingestion of pressor substances	• Spontaneous BP variability	• Smoker • Physically active during day • Stressful job
Physician-Patient Interaction	• White coat effect positive		• White coat effect negative
Possible Diagnosis	• White coat hypertension		• Masked hypertension

Table 44–3. Patient- and Physician-related Factors That Lead to a Discrepancy Between the Clinic and True Blood Pressure

may also be profoundly influenced by behavioral factors related to the effects of the observer on the subject, the best known of which is the presence of a physician. It has been known for more than 60 years that blood pressures recorded by a physician can be as much as 30 mmHg higher than pressures taken by the patient at home, using the same technique and in the same position.[65] Physicians also record higher pressures than nurses or technicians.[66,67] In a population of patients with mild hypertension (diastolic pressures between 90 and 104 mmHg), that approximately 20% may be expected to have "white-coat" hypertension, that is, pressures that are persistently high when in the presence of a physician, but normal at other times.[67] Other factors that influence the pressure that is recorded may include both the race and sex of the observer.[68,69] The extent to which inter-observer differences in blood pressure are due to differences in technique as opposed to the white-coat effect can be assessed by having two observers take simultaneous readings with a double-headed stethoscope.

The white-coat effect

One of the main reasons for the growing emphasis on blood pressure readings taken outside the physician's office or clinic is the white-coat effect, which is conceived as the increase of blood pressure that occurs at the time of a clinic visit, and dissipates soon thereafter. The mechanisms underlying the white-coat effect are not well understood, but may include anxiety, a hyperactive alerting response, or a conditioned response.[70] Recent evidence supports the idea that it is a conditioned anxiety response. Patients with a large white-coat effect do not appear to be more anxious than others in general, but do record higher levels during the actual blood pressure measurements,[71] and are much more likely to have been previously diagnosed as being hypertensive. The white-coat effect is seen to a greater or lesser extent in most if not all hypertensive patients, but is much smaller or absent in normotensive individuals. It has usually been defined as the difference between the clinic and daytime ambulatory pressure, which is certainly a convenient method of measurement, if not very precise scientifically.[72] A closely linked but discrete entity is white-coat hypertension, which refers to a subset of patients who are hypertensive according to their clinic blood pressures, but normotensive at other times. Thus white-coat hypertension is a measure of blood pressure levels, while the white-coat effect is a measure of blood pressure change. What distinguishes patients with white-coat hypertension from those with true or sustained hypertension is not that they have an exaggerated white-coat effect, but that their blood pressure is within the normal range when they are outside the clinic setting. White-coat hypertension is discussed in Chapter 45.

Stethoscope head

Some official recommendations have suggested that the bell of the stethoscope should be used rather than the diaphragm for taking blood pressure, but when it was systematically tested no difference was found between the readings taken with the bell or the diaphragm.[36]

Rate of cuff inflation and deflation

The rate of inflation has no significant effect on the blood pressure,[73] but with very slow rates (2 mmHg/sec or less) the intensity of the Korotkoff sounds is diminished, resulting in slightly higher diastolic pressures. This effect has been attributed to venous congestion reducing the rate of blood flow during very slow deflation.[74] The generally recommended deflation rate is 2 to 3 mmHg/sec.

Auscultatory gap

This can be defined as the loss and reappearance of Korotkoff sounds that occur between systolic and diastolic pressures during cuff deflation, in the absence of cardiac arrhythmias. Thus, if its presence is not recognized it may lead to the registration of spuriously high diastolic or low systolic pressures. It may occur because of phasic changes of arterial pressure or in patients who have faint Korotkoff sounds. The auscultatory gap may pose a problem for automatic recorders (which operate by the Korotkoff sound technique) and result in gross errors in the measurement of diastolic pressure.[75] Oscillometric devices are less susceptible to this problem.[75] Its presence is of clinical significance, because it is associated with an increased prevalence of target organ damage.[76]

Technical sources of error

There are also technical sources of error with the auscultatory method, although these are usually much less when a mercury column is used than with many of the semi-automatic methods (see material following). The mercury should read zero when no pressure is applied, and it should fall freely when the pressure is reduced (this may not occur if the mercury is not clean or if the pinhole connecting the mercury column to the atmosphere is blocked). It is essential that aneroid meters be checked against a mercury column both at zero pressure and when pressure is applied to the cuff. Surveys of such devices used in clinical practice have shown them to be frequently inaccurate.[50]

Training of observers

For the accurate measurement of blood pressure in the clinic setting, adequate training of the observers who will be taking the blood pressure is essential. This applies not only to the traditional auscultatory method but to the use of automated methods. Items such as the proper positioning of the patient (seated comfortably with the back supported, legs uncrossed, and not on an examination table) and the selection of the proper cuff size apply whichever method of measurement is used. When the auscultatory method is used, however, it is critical that the observers be trained in the detection of the Korotkoff sounds. The accuracy of observers' technique can be checked by the use of video recordings of a mercury column and Korotkoff sounds during cuff deflation. The training and certification of observers is described in more detail in the American Heart Association Guidelines.[16]

Measurement with automated devices

Although the standard method of clinic blood pressure measurement continues to be a physician or nurse using the auscultatory method, there is a trend to use automated devices, of which several models are now available. All are oscillometric devices that can be programmed to take a number of readings without a human observer present.

MEASUREMENT OF BLOOD PRESSURE IN SPECIAL POPULATIONS AND CIRCUMSTANCES

Infants and children

The Korotkoff sound technique is recommended as the standard for children above the age of one year, although it may give systematic errors in infants (where the sounds are very difficult to hear and the true systolic pressure may be underestimated).[25] In infants, the best indirect measurement technique is an ultrasonic flow detector.[77] A particular problem associated with blood pressure measurement in children of different ages is knowing which size of cuff to choose.

The recommended technique is to choose a cuff that has a bladder width that is approximately 40% of the upper arm circumference. This will usually be a cuff bladder with a length that will cover 80 to 100% of the circumference of the arm. The equipment necessary to measure blood pressure in children three years of age through adolescence includes pediatric cuffs of different sizes: for newborn/premature infants a cuff size of 4×8 cm is recommended; for infants, 6×12 cm; and for older children, 9×18 cm. A standard adult cuff, a large adult cuff, and a thigh cuff for leg blood pressure measurement and for use in children with very large arms (obese, muscular) should also be available. In children, particularly preadolescents, a difference of several millimeters of mercury is frequently present between the fourth Korotkoff sound, the muffling of Korotkoff sounds, and K5.[78] In some children, the Korotkoff sounds can be heard to 0 mmHg, which has limited physiologic meaning.

Blood pressure changes markedly with age, and the interpretation of blood pressure in children is very dependent on the child's height and weight. Tables are available that give the 95th percentile for age, sex, and height.[79]

White-coat hypertension (see Chapter 45) is well described in children, and may be diagnosed if either home or ambulatory monitoring shows normal daytime blood pressure values. Normal ranges for both types of monitoring have been published.[80,81] The use of both types of monitoring in children is increasing rapidly.

Pregnant subjects

In normal pregnancy there is a fall of blood pressure, together with an increase of cardiac output and a large decrease of peripheral resistance. As a result of this hyperkinetic state, Korotkoff-like sounds may occasionally be heard over the brachial artery without any pressure being applied to the cuff. These sounds are most probably due to turbulent flow in the artery. Consequently, the use of phase 4 has frequently been recommended for registering diastolic pressure in pregnant women, which may be 12 mmHg higher than phase 5.[82] The National High Blood Pressure Education Program (NHBPEP) Working Group report recommends recording both phases 4 and 5 throughout pregnancy.[83] However, in one study of 85 pregnant women phase 5 never approached zero, and phase 4 could be identified in only half, leading the authors to recommend phase 5.[84]

The International Society for the Study of Hypertension in Pregnancy currently recommends using K5 for the measurement of diastolic blood pressure in pregnancy.[85] Because blood pressure changes throughout the course of pregnancy, and the early detection of an increase may herald preeclampsia, a good case can be made for the wider use of home monitoring during pregnancy.[86]

Elderly subjects

In many older people there is an increase of systolic pressure without a corresponding increase of diastolic (systolic hypertension), which has been attributed to a diminished distensibility of the arteries with increasing age. They are also more likely than younger people to have white-coat hypertension (see Chapter 45) and pseudohypertension (see above—page 2 of this chapter).

Care should be taken to measure the seated blood pressure properly, two or more times at each visit, averaging the data. Blood pressure should be taken in the standing position routinely, because the elderly may have postural hypotension. Hypotension is more common in diabetic patients. It is frequently noticed by patients upon rising in the morning, after meals, and when standing quietly.

Obese subjects

It is well known that the accurate estimation of blood pressure using the auscultatory method requires an appropriate match between cuff size and arm diameter. In obese subjects, the regular adult cuff (12 × 23 cm) may seriously overestimate blood pressure.[87] The effects of arm circumference on the cuff method of measuring blood pressure were studied systematically by King.[38] Thus, it is essential to use a large cuff to obtain accurate readings (see Table 44–2). In very obese patients it may be difficult to wrap the cuff around the arm, and measurement at the wrist may be appropriate, either using an oscillometric device or with a stethoscope placed over the radial artery.

Exercise

During dynamic exercise, the auscultatory method may underestimate systolic pressure by up to 15 mmHg, whereas during recovery it may be overestimated by 30 mmHg.[88,89] Errors in diastolic pressure are unlikely to be as large, except during the recovery period, when falsely low readings may be recorded.[89] This is the reason the AHA recommends taking the fourth phase of the Korotkoff sound after exercise.[15]

Arrhythmias

When the cardiac rhythm is very irregular, such as in atrial fibrillation, the blood pressure varies greatly from beat to beat, leading to considerable error when the auscultatory method is used to measure blood pressure.[90] The best that can be done is to record blood pressure several times and use the average value. Automated devices using the oscillometric method are also often inaccurate, for example, in the presence of atrial fibrillation and should be validated in each subject before use.[91] However, ambulatory monitors have been found to provide data similar to that in subjects with normal cardiac rhythm.[92]

SUMMARY AND PERSPECTIVES

There is increasing attention being paid to small elevations of blood pressure, such as prehypertension, and to the poor state of hypertension control throughout the world. Both of these require that blood pressure be measured accurately and frequently. The traditional auscultatory method using a mercury sphygmomanometer or aneroid device has provided the basis for almost all of our knowledge about blood pressure in human subjects, but is prone to numerous errors (and mercury is being banned in most countries). It is being replaced by automated oscillometric devices, which while not as accurate in principle are less susceptible to faulty technique and can provide multiple readings.

For the foreseeable future, it is likely that measurements made in the clinic or office will continue to be the standard by which blood pressure control is judged. However, this is increasingly being done using automated devices, and there will continue to be greater reliance on out-of-office measurements for making clinical decisions.

REFERENCES

1. Pickering GW. *High Blood Pressure.* London: Churchill, 1968.
2. Chobanian AV, Bakris GL, Black HR, Cushman WC, Green LA, Izzo JL Jr., et al. The Seventh Report of the Joint National Committee on Prevention, Detection, Evaluation, and Treatment of High Blood Pressure: The JNC 7 report. *JAMA* 2003;289(19):2560–72.
3. Franklin SS, Pio JR, Wong ND, Larson MG, Leip EP, Vasan RS, et al. Predictors of new-onset diastolic and systolic hypertension: The Framingham Heart Study. *Circulation* 2005;111(9): 1121–27.
4. O'Rourke MF, Vlachopoulos C, Graham RM. Spurious systolic hypertension in youth. *Vasc Med* 2000;5(3):141–45.
5. Pickering TG. Isolated systolic hypertension in the young. *J Clin Hypertens (Greenwich)* 2004;6(1): 47–48.
6. Blank SG, Mann SJ, James GD, West JE, Pickering TG. Isolated elevation of diastolic blood pressure. Real or artifactual? *Hypertension* 1995; 26(3):383–89.
7. Pickering TG. Isolated diastolic hypertension. *J Clin Hypertens* 2003;5.

8. Franklin SS, Larson MG, Khan SA, Wong ND, Leip EP, Kannel WB, et al. Does the relation of blood pressure to coronary heart disease risk change with aging? The Framingham Heart Study. *Circulation* 2001;103(9):1245–49.
9. Belmin J, Visintin JM, Salvatore R, Sebban C, Moulias R. Osler's maneuver: Absence of usefulness for the detection of pseudohypertension in an elderly population. *Am J Med* 1995;98(1):42–49.
10. Consensus statement of the definition of orthostatic hypotension, pure autonomic failure, and multiple system atrophy. *J Neurol Sciences* 1996; 144:218–19.
11. Regan CBJ. The accuracy of clinical measurements of arterial blood pressure, with a note on the auscultatory gap. *Bull Johns Hopkins Hosp* 1941;69:504–28.
12. Roberts LN, Smiley JR, Manning GW. A comparison of direct and indirect blood-pressure determinations. *Circulation* 1953;8:232–34.
13. Holland WWHS. Measurement of blood pressure: Comparison of intra-arterial and cuff values. *Brit Med J* 1964; 2:1241–43.

14. Breit SN, O'Rourke MF. Comparison of direct and indirect arterial pressure measurements in hospitalized patients. *Aust N Z J Med* 1974;4(5):485–91.
15. Perloff D, Grim C, Flack J, Frohlich ED, Hill M, McDonald M, et al. Human blood pressure determination by sphygmomanometry. *Circulation* 1993;88(5/1):2460–70.
16. Pickering TG, Hall JE, Appel LJ, Falkner BE, Graves J, Hill MN, et al. Recommendations for blood pressure measurement in humans and experimental animals. Part 1: Blood pressure measurement in humans: A statement for professionals from the subcommittee of professional and public education of the american heart association council on high blood pressure research. *Circulation* 2005; 111(5):697–716.
17. Petrie JCOETLWADSM. British Hypertension Society Recommendations on Blood Pressure Measurement. *Brit Med J* 1986;293:611–15.
18. Marey EJ. Pression et vitesse du sang. Physiologie Experimentale (Paris). Pratique des hautes etudes de M Marey 1876.

19. Mauck GW, Smith CR, Geddes LA, Bourland JD. The meaning of the point of maximum oscillations in cuff pressure in the indirect measurement of blood pressure: Part II. *J Biomech Eng* 1980; 102(1):28–33.

20. Yelderman M, Ream AK. Indirect measurement of mean blood pressure in the anesthetized patient. *Anesthesiology* 1979;50(3):253–56.

21. Borow KM, Newburger JW. Noninvasive estimation of central aortic pressure using the oscillometric method for analyzing systemic artery pulsatile blood flow: Comparative study of indirect systolic, diastolic, and mean brachial artery pressure with simultaneous direct ascending aortic pressure measurements. *Am Heart J* 1982;103(5):879–86.

22. Wiinberg N, Hoegholm A, Christensen HR, Bang LE, Mikkelsen KL, Nielsen PE, et al. 24-h ambulatory blood pressure in 352 normal Danish subjects, related to age and gender. *Am J Hypertens* 1995;8(10/1):978–86.

23. Cates EM, Schlussel YR, James GD, Pickering TG. A validation study of the Spacelabs 90207 ambulatory blood pressure monitor. *J Ambul Monitor* 1990;3:149–54.

24. Ware RW, Laenger CJ. Indirect blood pressure measurement by Doppler ultrasonic kinetoarteriography. *Proc 20th Ann Conf Eng Med Biol* 1967; 9:27–30.

25. Elseed AM, Shinebourne EA, Joseph MC. Assessment of techniques for measurement of blood pressure in infants and children. *Arch Dis Child* 1973;48(12):932–36.

26. Penaz J. Photo-electric measurement of blood pressure, volume and flow in the finger. *Digest Tenth Int. Conf. Med. Biol. Eng.* (Dresden) 1973;104.

27. van Egmond J, Hasenbos M, Crul JF. Invasive v. non-invasive measurement of arterial pressure: Comparison of two automatic methods and simultaneously measured direct intra-arterial pressure. *Br J Anaesth* 1985;57(4):434–44.

28. Parati G, Casadei R, Groppelli A, Di Rienzo M, Mancia G. Comparison of finger and intra-arterial blood pressure monitoring at rest and during laboratory testing. *Hypertension* 1989; 13(6/1):647–55.

29. Imholz BPM, Langewouters GJ, van Montfrans GA, Parati G, van Goudoever J, Wesseling KH, et al. Feasibility of ambulatory, continuous 24-hour finger arterial presusure recording. *Hypertens* 1993;21:65–73.

30. O'Rourke MF. From theory into practice: Arterial haemodynamics in clinical hypertension. *J Hypertens* 2002;20(10):1901–15.

31. Williams B, Lacy PS, Thom SM, Cruickshank K, Stanton A, Collier D, et al. Differential impact of blood pressure-lowering drugs on central aortic pressure and clinical outcomes: Principal results of the Conduit Artery Function Evaluation (CAFE) study. *Circulation* 2006;113(9):1213–25.

32. Petrie JC, O'Brien ET, Littler WA, De Swiet M. Recommendations on blood pressure measurement. *Br Med J* (Clin Res Ed) 1986;293(6547):611–15.

33. Netea RT, Smits P, Lenders JW, Thien T. Does it matter whether blood pressure measurements are taken with subjects sitting or supine? *J Hypertens* 1998; 16(3):263–68.

34. Mitchell PL, Parlin RW, Blackburn H. Effect of vertical displacement of the arm on indirect blood-pressure measurement. *NEJM* 1964;271:72–74.

35. Webster JNDPJCLHG. Influence of arm position on measurement of blood pressure. *Brit Med J* 1984;228:1574–75.

36. Cushman WC, Cooper KM, Horne RA, Meydrech EF. Effect of back support and stethoscope head on seated blood pressure determinations. *Am J Hypertens* 1990;3(3):240–41.

37. Maxwell MH, Waks AU, Schroth PC, Karam M, Dornfeld LP. Error in blood-pressure measurement due to incorrect cuff size in obese patients. *Lancet* 1982; 2(8288):33–36.

38. King GE. Errors in clinical measurement of blood pressure in obesity. *Clin Sci* 1967;32:223–37.

39. Van Montfrans, Accuracy of auscultatory blood pressure measurement with a long cuff. *Brit Med J* 1987;295:354–55.

40. Pickering TG, Hall JE, Appel LJ, Falkner BE, Graves J, Hill MN, et al. Recommendations for blood pressure measurement in humans and experimental animals. Part 1: Blood pressure measurement in humans: Addendum. A statement for professionals from the subcommittee of professional and public education of the american heart association council on high blood pressure research. *Hypertens* 2006 (in press).

41. Lane D, Beevers M, Barnes N, Bourne J, John A, Malins S, et al. Inter-arm differences in blood pressure: When are they clinically significant? *J Hypertens* 2002;20(6):1089–95.

42. Eguchi K, Yacoub M, Jhalani J, Gerin W, Schwartz JE, Pickering TG. How consistent are blood pressure differences between the left and right arms? *Arch Int Med* (in press).

43. Mion D, Pierin AM. How accurate are sphygmomanometers? *J Hum Hypertens* 1998;12(4):245–48.

44. Markandu ND, Whitcher F, Arnold A, Carney C. The mercury sphygmomanometer should be abandoned before it is proscribed. *J Hum Hypertens* 2000;14(1):31–36.

45. Jones DW, Frohlich ED, Grim CM, Grim CE , Taubert KA. Mercury sphygmomanometers should not be abandoned: An advisory statement from the Council for High Blood Pressure Research, American Heart Association. *Hypertension* 2001; 37(2):185–86.

46. Canzanello VJ, Jensen PL, Schwartz GL. Are aneroid sphygmomanometers accurate in hospital and clinic settings? *Arch Intern Med* 2001;161(5):729–31.

47. Pickering TG. The case for a hybrid sphygmomanometer. *Blood Press Monit* 2002;6:177–80.

48. Myers MG, Valdivieso MA. Use of an automated blood pressure recording device, the BpTRU, to reduce the "white coat effect" in routine practice. *Am J Hypertens* 2003;16(6):494–97.

49. Kleinert HD, Harshfield GA, Pickering TG, Devereux RB, Sullivan PA, Marion RM, et al. What is the value of home blood pressure measurement in patients with mild hypertension? *Hypertension* 1984;6(4):574–78.

50. Burke MJ, Towers HM, O'Malley K, Fitzgerald DJ, O'Brien ET. Sphygmomanometers in hospital and family practice: Problems and recommendations. *Br Med J* 1982;285:469–71.

51. Langford NJ, Ferner RE. Toxicity of mercury. *J Hum Hypertens* 1999; 13:651–56.

52. Pickering TG, Cvetkovski B, James GD. An evaluation of electronic recorders for self monitoring of blood pressure. *J Hypertens* 1986;4(5):S328–30.

53. van Egmond J, Lenders JW, Weernink E, Thien T. Accuracy and reproducibility of 30 devices for self-measurement of arterial blood pressure. *Am J Hypertens* 1993;6(10):873–79.

54. Foster C, McKinlay S, Cruickshank JM, Coats AJS. Accuracy of the Omron HEM 706 portable monitor for home measurement of blood pressure. *J Hum Hypertens* 1994;8:661–64.

55. O'Brien E, Waeber B, Parati G, Staessen J, Myers MG. Blood pressure measuring devices: Recommendations of the European Society of Hypertension. *BMJ* 2001;322:531–36.

56. Cooper R, Puras A, Tracy J, Kaufman J, Asuzu M, Ordunez P, et al. Evaluation of an electronic blood pressure device for epidemiological studies. *Blood Pressure Monitoring* 1997;2:35–40.

57. Eckert S, Gleichmann S, Gleichmann U. Blood pressure self-measurement in upper arm and in wrist for treatment control of arterial hypertension compared to ABPM. *Z Kardiol* 1996; 85(3):109–11.

58. Wonka F, Thummler M, Schoppe A. Clinical test of a blood pressure measurement device with a wrist cuff. *Blood Press Monit* 1996;1(4):361–66.

59. Bos WJ, van Goudoever J, van Montfrans GA, van den Meiracker AH, Wesseling KH. Reconstruction of brachial artery pressure from noninvasive finger pressure measurements. *Circulation* 1996;94(8):1870–75.

60. Sesler JM, Munroe WP, McKenney JM. Clinical evaluation of a finger oscillometric blood pressure device. *DICP* 1991;25(12):1310–14.

61. O'Brien E, Pickering T, Asmar R, Myers M, Parati G, Staessen J, et al. Working Group on Blood Pressure Monitoring of the European Society of Hypertension International Protocol for validation of blood pressure measuring devices in adults. *Blood Press Monit* 2002;7(1):3–17.

62. O'Rourke MF, Staessen JA, Vlachopoulos C, Duprez D, Plante GE. Clinical applications of arterial stiffness: Definitions and reference values. *Am J Hypertens* 2002;15(5):426–44.

63. Padfield PL, Jyothinagaram SG, Watson DM, Donald P, McGinley IM. Problems in the measurement of blood pressure. *J Hum Hypertens* 1990;4(2):3–7.

64. Eilertsen E, Humerfelt S. The observer variation in the measurement of arterial blood pressure. *Acta Med Scand* 1968; 184(3):145–57.

65. Ayman P, Goldshine AD. Blood pressure determinations by patients with essential hypertension I: The difference between clinic and home readings before treatment. *Am J Med Sci* 1940; 200:465–74.

66. Mancia G, Bertini G, Grassi G, Gregorini L, Bertinieri G, Zanchetti A. Effects of blood pressure measurement by the doctor on patients' blood pressure and heart rate. *Lancet* 1983;2:695–97.

67. Pickering TG, James GD, Boddie C, Harshfield GA, Blank S, Laragh JH. How common is white coat hypertension? *JAMA* 1988;259:225–28.

68. Comstock GW. An epidemiologic study of blood pressure levels in a biracial community in the southern United States. *Am J Hygiene* 1957;65:271–315.

69. McCubbin JA, Wilson JF, Bruehl S, Brady M, Clark K, Kort E. Gender effects on blood pressures obtained uring an on-campus screening. *Psychosom Med* 1998;8.

70. Pickering TG. White coat hypertension. *Curr Opin Nephrol Hypertens* 1996; 5(2):192–98.

71. Jhalani J, Goyal T, Clemow L, Schwartz JE, Pickering TG, Gerin W. Anxiety and outcome expectations predict the white coat effect. *Blood Press Monit* 2005.

72. Verdecchia P, Schillaci G, Borgioni C, Ciucci A, Zampi I, Gattobigio R, et al. White coat hypertension and white coat effect: Similarities and differences. *Am J Hypertens* 1995;8(8):790–98.

73. King GE. Influence of rate of cuff inflation and deflation on observed blood pressure by sphygmomanometry. *Am Heart J* 1963;65:303–06.

74. Wilkins R, Bradley SE. Changes in arterial and venous blood pressure and flow distal to a cuff inflated on a human arm. *Amer J Physiol* 1946:l47:260–69.

75. Imai Y, Abe K, Sasaki S, Minami N, Munakata M, Sakuma H, et al. Clinical evaluation of semiautomatic and automatic devices for home blood pressure measurement: Comparison between cuff-oscillometric and microphone methods. *J Hypertens* 1989;7(12):983–90.

76. Cavallini MC, Roman MJ, Blank SG, Pini R, Pickering TG, Devereux RB. Association of the auscultatory gap with vascular disease in hypertensive patients. *Ann Intern Med* 1996;124(10):877–83.

77. Reder RF, Dimich I, Cohen ML, Steinfeld L. Evaluating indirect blood pressure measurement techniques: A comparison of three systems in infants and children. *Pediatrics* 1978; 62(3):326–30.

78. Sinaiko AR, Gomez-Marin O, Prineas RJ. Diastolic fourth and fifth phase blood pressure in 10–15-year-old children: The Children and Adolescent Blood Pressure Program. *Am J Epidemiol* 1990; 132(4):647–55.

79. National High Blood Pressure Education Program Working Group on Hypertension Control in Children and Adolescents. Update on the 1987 Task Force Report on High Blood Pressure in Children and Adolescents: A Working Group Report from the National High Blood Pressure Education Program. *Pediatrics* 1996;98:649–58.

80. Lurbe E, Redon J, Liao Y, Tacons J, Cooper RS, Alvarez V. Ambulatory blood pressure monitoring in normotensive children. *J Hypertens* 1994;12(12):1417–23.

81. Stergiou GS, Alamara CV, Kalkana CB, Vaindirlis IN, Stefanidis CJ, Dacou-Voutetakis C, et al. Out-of-office blood pressure in children and adolescents: Disparate findings by using home or ambulatory monitoring. *Am J Hypertens* 2004;17(10):869–75.

82. Villar J, Repke J, Markush L, Calvert W, Rhoads G. The measuring of blood pressure during pregnancy. *Am J Obstet Gynecol* 1989;161(4):1019–24.

83. Working group report on high blood pressure in pregnancy: National High Blood Pressure Education Program. NIH Publication No. 90–3029, 1990.

84. Shennan A, Gupta M, Halligan A, Taylor DJ, De Swiet M. Lack of reproducibility in pregnancy of Korotkoff phase IV as measured by mercury sphygmomanometry. *Lancet* 1996;347(8995):139–42.

85. Brown MA, Davis GK. Hypertension in pregnancy. In G Mancia, J Chalmers, S Julius, T Saruta, MA Weber, AU Ferrari, et al. (eds.), *Manual of Hypertension*. London: Harcourt, 2002:579–97.

86. Pickering TG. Reflections in hypertension: How should blood pressure be measured during pregnancy? *J Clin Hypertens* (*Greenwich*) 2005;7(1):46–49.

87. Nielsen PE, Janniche H. The accuracy of auscultatory measurement of arm blood pressure in very obese subjects. *Acta Med Scand* 1974;195(5):403–09.

88. Henschel A, De La Vega F, Taylor HL. Simultaneous direct and indirect blood pressure measurements in man at rest and work. *J Appl Physiol* 1954; 5:506–08.

89. Gould BA, Hornung RS, Altman DG, Cashman PM, Raftery EB. Indirect measurement of blood pressure during exercise testing can be misleading. *Br Heart J* 1985;53(6):611–15.

90. Sykes D, Dewar R, Mohanaruban K, Donovan K, Nicklason F, Thomas DM, et al. Measuring blood pressure in the elderly: Does atrial fibrillation increase observer variability? *BMJ* 1990; 300(6718):162–63.

91. Stewart MJ, Gough K, Padfield PL. The accuracy of automated blood pressure measuring devices in patients with controlled atrial fibrillation. *J Hypertens* 1995;13(3):297–300.

92. Lip GY, Zarifis J, Beevers M, Beevers DG. Ambulatory blood pressure monitoring in atrial fibrillation. *Am J Cardiol* 1996; 78(3):350–53.

Chapter

45

Out-of-Office Blood Pressure Monitoring

Thomas G. Pickering

Key Findings

- Self- (home) and ambulatory blood pressure (BP) monitoring are useful adjuncts to clinic or office measurements.

- BPs taken with these techniques are greatly influenced by the diurnal rhythm of BP and by the effects of physical and mental activity.

- In some patients, the normal dipping pattern of BP during sleep is lost or reversed, a phenomenon that can only be evaluated with ambulatory monitoring. The clinical significance of non-dipping is not clear.

- Two conditions detected by home and ambulatory monitoring are white coat hypertension (WCH; in which the clinic pressure is raised but the out-of-office BP is normal) and masked hypertension, which is the opposite situation. Thus, the clinic pressure overestimates risk in WCH and underestimates it in masked hypertension.

- Ambulatory monitoring provides the most reliable estimate of an individual patient's risk of cardiovascular events.

- The upper limit for normal daytime BP for both home and ambulatory monitoring is usually taken as 135/85 mmHg (to correspond with a clinic pressure of 140/90).

- Home monitoring is particularly well suited for monitoring changes of BP over time.

INTRODUCTION

The techniques for measuring BP in order to decide whether or not a patient is hypertensive have undergone considerable change in the past 20 years. Despite the fact that the bulk of our knowledge about the risks of hypertension and the benefits of treating it is based on the traditional method of taking a small number of readings using the auscultatory technique in a medical setting, there is increasing recognition that such measurements (while of enormous value on a population basis) may give a poor estimate of risk in an individual patient.

There are several reasons for this, which include poor observer technique such as terminal digit preference (the tendency to read to the nearest 10 mmHg), the white coat effect (the transient but variable elevation of BP in a medical setting), and the inherent variability of BP. Any clinical measurement of BP may be regarded as a surrogate measure for the patient's "true" BP, which may be conceived as the average level over prolonged periods of time.

Two techniques have been developed to improve the estimate of the true BP/ambulatory-BP monitoring (ABPM) and home (or self-) monitoring (HBPM), which may be subsumed under the title of "out-of-office monitoring" because they avoid many of the limitations of traditional clinic or office measurements described previously. The use of both techniques has been endorsed by national and international guidelines such as JNC 7[1] and the International Society of Hypertension (ISH).[2]

The first ambulatory monitor was developed by Dr. Maurice Sokolow in the 1960s.[3] This monitor required the patient to inflate the cuff manually, and thus only daytime readings could be obtained. Studies with this procedure established a number of important findings. First, there was enormous variability of BP during a normal day. Second, the agreement between the conventionally measured BP and the daytime average was relatively poor. Third, the relationships with the adverse effects of hypertension were stronger for the ambulatory measured BP. These early findings have been substantiated by numerous later studies, and form the basis for establishing ABPM as the gold standard for estimating BP-related risk in an individual patient.

Home (or self-) monitoring is much more widely used than ambulatory monitoring, and is gradually finding its way into routine care. Virtually all home monitors work on the oscillometric technique, and are valuable both for the initial diagnosis of hypertension and for monitoring the response to treatment.

Out-of-office monitoring has some distinct advantages over clinic BP measurement. These are (1) the ability to take larger numbers of readings, (2) the ability to make a better evaluation of "situational hypertension" (i.e., hypertension whose diagnosis depends on the circumstances of measurement, such as white coat and masked hypertension), and (3) the ability to assess nighttime BP, which at present can only be made with ABPM.

The relative values of the three methods of measuring BP are summarized in Table 45–1, and are described in more detail in material following. For the diagnosis of hypertension and the prediction of clinical outcomes, ABPM is usually regarded as the gold standard, although it has been suggested that any elevation of BP (whether measured in the office, at home, or by ABPM) carries an adverse prognosis.[4] It is important to recognize that the upper limits of "normal" BP are set lower for out-of-office measurements, to allow for the white coat effect. Home monitoring is particularly useful for assessing the

VALUE OF DIFFERENT METHODS OF BLOOD PRESSURE MEASUREMENT IN CLINICAL PRACTICE			
Utility	Method of Blood Pressure Measurement		
	Office	*Self*	*Ambulatory*
Predicts outcome	+	+	++
Diagnostic use	+	+	++
"Normal" limit	140/90	135/85	135/85 (day)
Evaluation of treatment	+	++	+
Improves adherence	−	+	−

Table 45–1. Value of Different Methods of Blood Pressure Measurement in Clinical Practice

effects of antihypertensive treatment, and for improving adherence. The major factor that distinguishes out-of-office BP measurements (both home and ambulatory) is that they are taken at different times of day and under different circumstances, and thus it is important to understand the effects of these on BP (as described in sections following).

FACTORS AFFECTING BLOOD PRESSURE DURING DAILY LIFE

Most biologic variables show a diurnal rhythm, and BP is no exception. This is determined by a combination of a built-in biologic clock and external influences such as the light/dark cycle. There are also changes of longer periodicity, such as the day of the week and the season of the year.

TEMPORAL INFLUENCES ON BLOOD PRESSURE

The diurnal rhythm of blood pressure

Evaluation of the time course of BP over 24 hours can only be achieved using ABPM. In normotensive subjects, there is a pronounced diurnal rhythm of BP[5] that falls to its lowest level during the first few hours of sleep. There is a marked surge in the morning hours coinciding with waking and getting out of bed. The average difference between the waking and sleeping BP is 10 to 20%.

Hypertensive patients usually show the same pattern, but the diurnal profile of BP is set at a higher level.[5] In some subjects, whether normotensive or hypertensive, the normal nocturnal fall of BP is diminished (<10%). This pattern is referred to as non-dipping, in contrast to the normal dipping pattern. A further classification that some authors have used is to identify people who show an excessive fall of pressure (the extreme dippers, whose nocturnal pressure falls more than 20%) or an actual increase (risers).[6]

Time of day

Studies using ABPM have generally shown that the highest BP is seen in the first few hours after waking. This is the so-called morning surge of BP, which is also the time of highest cardiovascular risk.[7,8] This can be attributed to the process of waking up and to increased physical activity.[9] However, this pattern is less readily discernible with self-monitoring. In studies where morning and evening measurements were both taken, the evening readings often tend to be higher for systolic pressure (by about 3 mmHg), although there are less consistent differences for diastolic pressure.[10,11] These differences may be more pronounced in hypertensive patients. In one study of untreated hypertensives,[12] the average home BP was 147/86 mmHg at 8 AM, 145/82 mmHg at 1 PM, and 152/86 mmHg at 10 PM. The differences between morning and evening pressures may be higher in men and in smokers.[11] The reason for the apparent discrepancy between morning and evening BP with the two techniques may be that self-monitored readings are taken under more standardized conditions.

The pattern of BP change over the day may vary considerably from one patient to another, depending on their daily routine. Antihypertensive treatment may also have a major influence.[11] For these reasons, it is generally recommended that patients should take readings in the early morning and at night.

Day of the week

There is relatively little information as to whether pressures recorded on non-workdays are the same as on workdays. In a study using ambulatory monitoring of BP, we found that the pressures in the middle of the day are higher if the subject is at work rather than at home, and the evening readings are also higher at home if the patient had gone to work earlier in the day.[13]

Season of the year

Home and ambulatory BP tend to be up to 5 mmHg higher in the winter than in the summer, at least in temperate climates.[14–16]

DEMOGRAPHIC FACTORS INFLUENCING HOME AND AMBULATORY BLOOD PRESSURE LEVELS

Gender

Home and ambulatory BP are generally lower in premenopausal women than men, as is true for office BP. This has been well documented by large epidemiologic studies.[17–20] However, the office/home differences are generally the same in men and women.

Age

Age influences out-of-office BP, with most studies that evaluated this (at least those in industralized societies) showing an increase. Many non-industrialized societies (e.g., primitive societies that have almost no obesity and low sodium intakes) have little or no increase in BP with aging.[21] In the largest population study to investigate this (conducted in Ohasama, Japan), the increase with age was surprisingly small. The average home BP was 118/71 mmHg for men aged 20 to 29 and 127/76 mmHg for men over 60.[19] The increase of ambulatory BP with age is also much smaller than the increase of office BP.[22]

The published results almost certainly underestimate the true changes, because subjects on antihypertensive medications were usually excluded and the prevalence of hypertension increases with age. Another age-related change is the increase of BP variability, as shown by the Ohasama study. The day-to-day variability of systolic pressure increases markedly with age in both men and women, whereas diastolic pressure is little affected and the variability of heart rate actually decreases.

ENVIRONMENTAL FACTORS INFLUENCING HOME AND AMBULATORY BLOOD PRESSURE LEVELS

As with any other measure of BP, the level of pressure recorded during out-of-office monitoring shows considerable variability and is likely to be influenced by several factors. These are summarized in the sections that follow.

Meals

In younger subjects, there is typically an increase of heart rate, a decrease of diastolic pressure, and little change of systolic pressure for up to three hours after a meal.[23] In older subjects, there may be a pronounced fall of both systolic and diastolic pressure after food. Thus, one study compared the effects of a breakfast of two eggs, two slices of toast, and orange juice in healthy elderly subjects (mean age 82 years) and controls aged 35 years.[24] The average fall of BP between 30 and 60 minutes after the meal was 16/10 mmHg in the elderly, but only 4/3 mmHg (not significant) in the young.

Alcohol

In people who drink alcohol regularly, it has been reported that evening BP is lowered by 7/6 mmHg and that there is also a smaller increase of morning BP (5/2 mmHg) that is only seen after a delay of two weeks.[25]

Caffeine

Drinking coffee increases BP, but not heart rate. The increase of BP begins within 15 minutes of drinking coffee, and is maximal in about one hour and may last for as much as three hours. Typical increases are between 5/9

and 14/10 mmHg.[26,27] Drinking decaffeinated coffee produces little or no change.[26] These changes are dependent on the level of habitual caffeine intake. BP changes are much greater in people who do not use caffeine regularly than in habitual users (12/10 versus 4/2 mmHg, respectively). Older subjects show greater increases of pressure than younger ones.[28] Caffeine also has an additive effect on the BP response to mental stress: higher absolute levels of pressure are achieved after caffeine, but the rise of pressure during the stressor is not affected.[29]

Smoking

Smoking a cigarette raises both heart rate and BP. In patients who were studied smoking in their natural environment during intra-arterial ambulatory BP monitoring, it was found that the BP increased by about 11/5 mmHg,[30] sometimes preceded by a transient fall of pressure. Changes were quantitatively similar in normotensives and hypertensives. The effect on BP is seen within a few minutes, and lasts about 15 minutes. Coffee and cigarettes are often taken together, and a study by Freestone and Ramsay showed that they may have an interactive effect,[31] which may raise BP for as long as two hours. Home BPs are usually lower than office BPs, but this difference is less in smokers,[32] presumably because they are likely to have smoked before taking the home readings.

ABP readings are typically higher during the day in smokers than in non-smokers, although office and night-time BPs tend to be the same. This can be explained by the fact that patients are unlikely to be smoking in the latter two situations.

Talking

Talking is a potent pressor stimulus that has both physical and psychological components. Reading aloud produces an immediate increase of both systolic and diastolic pressure (by about 10/7 mmHg in normotensive individuals) and of heart rate, with an immediate return to baseline levels once silence is resumed.[33] Reading silently, however, does not affect the pressure. Speaking fast produces a bigger increase than speaking slowly.[34]

Stress

Emotional stress can produce marked elevations of BP that can outlast the stimulus. In a study in which people were asked to recall a situation that made them angry, we found that the BP could increase by more than 20 mmHg, and was still elevated by more than 10 mmHg 15 minutes later.[35] In a survey of hypertensives who were monitoring their BP at the time of the Hanshin-Awaji earthquake in Japan in 1995, it was found that those who lived within 50 km of the epicenter showed an increase of BP of 11/6 mmHg (which took a week to wear off) on the day following the quake, whereas those living further away showed no change.[36]

After the terrorist attacks on the World Trade Towers in New York on 9/11/2001, we observed a 30-mmHg increase of home systolic pressure (which persisted for several days) in a patient whose office was immediately opposite one of the towers.[37] In a larger series of subjects monitoring their pressure using a teletransmission device (described in material following), in the months before and after 9/11/2001 in four sites in the United States we observed a 2-mmHg increase of systolic pressure.[38] This was not a seasonal effect, because comparable data were available for the same time during the previous year. Chronic stress, such as job strain, may elevate the BP throughout the 24 hours, thus resetting the diurnal profile of BP at a higher level.[39]

Exercise

Although BP rises markedly during physical exercise, it rapidly returns to its baseline level when the exercise is completed, and there may be a period of several hours after a bout of heavy exercise when the pressure may remain below the pre-exercise level (a phenomenon described as post-exercise hypotension).[40]

Bathing

Within about an hour after taking a bath, there is a modest fall of BP of 2 to 3 mmHg.[41]

AMBULATORY MONITORING

First developed more than 40 years ago, ambulatory BP monitoring is only now beginning to find acceptance as a clinically useful technique. Technological advances over the past few years have led to the introduction of monitors that are small, relatively quiet, and can take up to 100 readings of BP over 24 hours while patients go about their normal activities. They are reasonably accurate while the patient is at rest, but less so during physical activity. They can in theory provide information about the three main measures of BP: the average level, the diurnal variation, and short-term variability.

Because the currently available monitors take readings intermittently rather than continually, and are unreliable during exercise, they can only give a very crude estimate of the short-term variability of BP. Recordings in hypertensive patients show that in the majority of patients the average ambulatory pressure is lower than the office BP, and in some cases may be within the normal range, leading to a diagnosis of WCH (described in material following).

TECHNIQUES OF ABPM

The currently available ambulatory monitors are fully automatic, and can record BP for 24 hours or longer while patients go about their normal daily activities. Most use the oscillometric technique. The monitors measure about $4 \times 3 \times 1$ inches and weigh 4 pounds. They can be worn on a belt or in a pouch, and are a connected to a sphygmomanometer cuff on the upper arm by a plastic tube (Figure 45–1). They are typically programmed to take readings every 15 to 30 minutes throughout the day and night.

At the end of the recording period, the readings are downloaded into a computer. Subjects are asked to keep

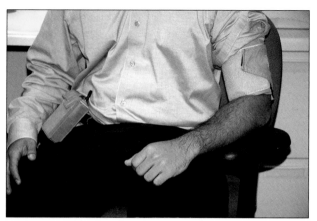

Figure 45–1. An ABPM device.

their arm still while the cuff is inflating, and to avoid excessive physical exertion. There are standard protocols for evaluating the accuracy of the monitors, and approved devices are usually accurate to within 5 mmHg of readings taken with a mercury sphygmomanometer. Some devices have been developed that can record 24-hour ECG, but they have not been widely used.

ADVANTAGES AND LIMITATIONS OF AMBULATORY MONITORING

ABPM can provide three types of information that is of potential value in the clinical field (Table 45–2). The first is an estimate of the true or average BP level, the second is the diurnal rhythm of BP, and the third is its variability. At the present time, there are clinical guidelines for only the first of these, and in principle the same information could be obtained by multiple office or home BP measurements. However, in many patients the white coat effect will lead to a distorted estimate. Evaluation of the time course of BP over 24 hours can of course only be achieved using ABPM. This may be of value in several ways. First, non-dippers may be at higher risk of cardiovascular events than dippers. Second, patients with an excessive morning surge of BP may also be at increased risk. Third, it is important to know if the patient's antihypertensive therapy is controlling BP throughout the 24 hours. The issue of BP variability is more complex.

It has frequently been suggested that increased variability of BP may be an independent risk factor for vascular damage, and there is some evidence that transient increases of BP provoked by mental or physical stress may trigger acute coronary events. There are many different ways of measuring variability, ranging from beat-to-beat variations to changes over weeks and months.

COMPARISON OF AMBULATORY AND OFFICE BLOOD PRESSURES

The correlation coefficient between ABP and office BP is usually about 0.5 to 0.7, but the slope is less than unity, such that at low levels of office BP the ABP is higher and at high levels the ABP is lower.[42] The daytime level of ABP

BLOOD PRESSURE PATTERN DATA THAT CAN BE OBTAINED BY ABPM AND OTHER METHODS			
Variable	ABPM	Office BP	Home BP
Average or true BP	Yes	Questionable	Yes
Diurnal BP rhythm	Yes	No	No
– Dipping status	Yes	No	No
– Morning surge	Yes	No	Questionable
– Duration of drug effects	Yes	No	Yes
BP variability	Yes	No	Questionable

Table 45–2. Blood Pressure Pattern Data That Can Be Obtained by ABPM and Other Methods

that corresponds to a office BP of 140/90 mmHg is usually taken to be 135/85 mmHg.[43]

REPRODUCIBILITY OF AMBULATORY READINGS

It was established many years go that office BP may vary by as much as 25 mmHg between successive visits without any intervention, a finding attributed to the small number of readings that could be taken.[44] Not surprisingly, therefore, both ambulatory and home BP levels are more stable when repeated over short periods of time such as two weeks.[45] It would be expected that longer time intervals between repeated measurements would give less agreement because there may be temporal trends related to the change of seasons, for example,[16] and this is indeed observed. However, the superiority of ABP over office BP in this respect is still seen.

In one study with an eight-month interval between measurements, the potential error (random change between the two occasions) was estimated to be as high as 38 mmHg for clinic pressure and 18 mmHg for ambulatory pressure.[46] A commonly used measure of the stability of a measure is the standard deviation of the difference (SDD) between successive readings. When a measure is reproducible, this number is low. In one study estimating the reproducibility over an interval of two years, this was reported to be 17/10 mmHg (systolic/diastolic) for clinic pressure and 10/5 mmHg for 24-hour pressure.[47]

AMBULATORY BLOOD PRESSURE IN NORMAL SUBJECTS

Because the distribution of BP in the population is continuous, with no natural separation between a normotensive and hypertensive group (and because the relationship between BP and risk of morbidity is also continuous), any division between "normal" and "abnormal" or "healthy" and "unhealthy" levels of BP must be arbitrary. This statement applies whichever measure of BP is used (office, ambulatory, or home readings). Both the JNC 7 and the WHO-ISH recommendations have accepted a clinic pressure of 140/90 mmHg as the threshold level for drug treatment in the majority of patients, and 130/85 mmHg for diabetics or patients with renal disease. They diverge

significantly, however, when it comes to ambulatory pressure.

JNC 7 is the same as the American Society of Hypertension (ASH) recommendations[48] for a daytime pressure of 135–140/85–90 mmHg, and a 24 hour pressure of 130–135/80–85 mmHg, whereas WHO-ISH recommends 125/80 mmHg as the upper limit of normal 24-hour pressure. The difference may seem small, but there are many millions of people who have pressures between these levels. In fact, using data obtained from population surveys of clinically normotensive people who underwent ambulatory monitoring it has been estimated that 45% of the population would be classified as being hypertensive by these criteria.[49] The JNC 7 and ASH criteria are closer to the levels identified in prospective studies as being associated with an increased risk of cardiovascular morbidity.

DIPPING AND NON-DIPPING

The normal pattern of the diurnal rhythm of BP is a decrease of about 10 to 20% during the night, which coincides with the hours of sleep, and is commonly referred to as dipping. This pattern is not universal, however, and in some people (about 25% of hypertensives) a non-dipping pattern is seen in which the normal nocturnal fall of pressure is absent. A further classification some authors have used is to identify people who show an excessive fall of pressure (the extreme dippers, whose nocturnal pressure falls more than 20%) or an actual increase (risers).

A major question at the present time is the pathologic significance of the differences in these patterns, and whether identification of them has clinical relevance. Several studies have indicated that non-dippers may be at higher risk of cardiovascular events than dippers. It is therefore worth discussing what factors influence dipping status. Of note, "reverse dipping" has also been reported (with high noctural BPs) in situations such as preeclampsia.[50]

Causes of non-dipping

Because all definitions of dipping and non-dipping rely on some measure of the differences between daytime and nighttime pressures, it is clear that both components will influence the classification. The nocturnal BP is mainly influenced by two factors: assuming the horizontal posture and going to sleep. Another factor that will affect nocturnal pressure is body position. When the patient is lying on one side, the BP recorded in the two arms will be different because of the effects of the hydrostatic pressure differences between the arm and the right atrium.

These differences can be 10 mmHg or more.[51] It is possible to record body position during ambulatory BP monitoring, and it has been reported that the non-dipping status may be influenced by the body position during sleep.[51] Changes of body position could thus be one reason for the relatively low reproducibility of dipping. The depth and quality of sleep may also affect dipping. Thus, in subjects who are kept awake during the first part of the night the BP remains high until they are allowed to go to sleep.[52] Normally, BP is at its lowest during the first few hours of sleep, when stage 4 sleep predominates. Therefore, one possible reason for non-dipping may be a diminished amount of stage 4 sleep.

One study found that non-dippers had a worse sleep profile than dippers (less stage 4 and less REM, and more micro-arousals).[53] In addition, non-dippers are likely to have some degree of sleep-disordered breathing (snoring and apnea), but the association between dipping and sleep apnea is not close.[54,55] Another factor affecting the dipping pattern is the volume and electrolyte status: sodium-sensitive subjects are more likely to be non-dippers than sodium-resistant subjects, and when the former are put on a low-sodium diet their BP tends to shift to a dipper pattern.[56]

Likewise, the daytime BP level will depend on posture and activity. This has been well illustrated in a two-day study combining activity monitoring and BP monitoring, when subjects were relatively active during one day and inactive during the other.[57] As expected, both the recorded activity levels and the daytime BPs were higher on the active day, and subjects were consequently more likely to be classified as dippers on the active day than on the inactive day.

Several studies have reported that African Americans are more likely to be non-dippers than whites. A recent meta-analysis of 18 such studies looked at American and non-American blacks separately and concluded that American blacks are more likely to be non-dippers than American whites, whereas this trend is not apparent in blacks studied outside the United States,[58] raising the possibility that the difference is of psychosocial rather than genetic origin.

The prevalence of the non-dipping pattern is increased in several disease states. These include diabetes, chronic kidney disease, congestive heart failure, and Cushing's disease.[59] Other conditions with "non-dipping" status include obesity, malignant hypertension, and preeclampsia.

Reliability of dipping status

If a classification such as dipping and non-dipping is to be clinically useful, it should be statistically reliable from one occasion to another. There has been considerable debate on this point, which is still unresolved. Thus, one study that performed three ABPM recordings in 79 untreated hypertensive and normotensive subjects at intervals of six months[60] found that only 54% of subjects were classified as dippers on all three occasions, leading the authors to conclude that the phenomenon was not a reliable one.

Others have obtained similar results.[61,62] Thus, the reproducibility of dipping status is limited, which means that it would be wrong to expect very close correlations between dipping and measures of target organ damage or clinical outcomes. It has been suggested that to get an accurate estimate of a patient's dipping status two ABP recordings should be made. This obviously is not practical for the majority of patients.

Does non-dipping predict clinical outcomes?

The big question here is whether the non-dipping pattern is related to a higher risk of cardiovascular events than dipping, independently of the 24-hour BP level. Although there have been several claims for this, the evidence is mixed. Three large-scale prospective studies have found that non-dipping is associated with a higher risk than dipping. The first was the Ohasama study, a population-based prognostic study of 1,542 Japanese who were followed for nine years, which found that dipping and BP level were independent predictors of the risk of cardio-vascular mortality. Compared with normotensive dippers, the relative risk in normotensive non-dippers was 2.35. In hypertensive dippers it was 2.67, and in hypertensive non-dippers it was 5.37.[63]

It is important to note that in both the normotensive and hypertensive groups the 24-hour average levels were the same in the dippers and non-dippers. The second study was the Italian PIUMA study, in which it was found that men and women who were non-dippers (defined in this case as the highest third of the distribution of the night/day ratio of BP) were at approximately double the risk of events as the dippers.[64] This was the case after controlling for the 24-hour level and diabetes. The third was the Syst-Eur study, a placebo controlled study of the treatment of isolated systolic hypertension, in which a subgroup were evaluated with 24-hour monitoring.[65] Office BP had a weak predictive value, but the 24-hour readings gave a much broader spread of risk because there were some patients at low risk (the white coat hyper-tensives) and others at much higher risk than predicted from the clinic pressures. The best predictor of risk was the night/day ratio, which was independent of BP level.

These three studies provide the strongest evidence for risk from the non-dipping pattern. Two other recent studies did not confirm these findings, however. One was a Japanese study of elderly patients, which reported that an exaggerated morning surge of BP (greater than 55 mmHg increase of systolic pressure from the lowest sleep level to the first two hours after waking) predicted risk independently of the BP level.[66] The people at the highest risk were thus those who showed a pronounced dipping pattern, and the non-dippers had a relatively small morning surge.

Another study by Bjorklund et al. performed in 872 elderly Swedish men found that nighttime BP and dipping were no better at predicting risk than the daytime pressure.[67] Another prospective study of treated hypertensives confirmed earlier reports that the ambulatory pressure was a better predictor of risk than the clinic pressure, but did not find any superior prediction of nighttime over daytime pressures.[68] One explanation for this finding may be the fact that the patients were on antihypertensive treatment when first studied, and it is well recognized that drug treatment may change the dipping pattern.

It has been proposed that the non-dipping pattern may be an independent risk factor for progression of renal damage. This is supported by results of a study by Timio and colleagues,[69] who conducted a three-year longitudinal study to test the hypothesis that an association exists between a reduced or absent nighttime fall in BP and a future decline of kidney function in renal hypertensive patients. After three years, non-dippers had a faster rate of decline in creatinine clearance compared with dippers (0.37 versus 0.27 mL/min/month). In addition, non-dippers had greater increases in proteinuria compared with dippers (993 versus 438 mg/24 h).

The authors recommended that proper nocturnal BP control should be an additional aim of antihypertensive therapy. In a second study of 95 patients with nondiabetic kidney disease, non-dipping at baseline was also associated with a faster rate of progression of renal disease during three years of follow-up.[70] However, in this study non-dipping was associated with a higher creatinine and greater proteinuria at baseline as well, making it difficult to determine what role, if any, non-dipping played in the progression of renal disease. Finally, in a study by Tripepi et al.[71] 168 dialysis patients without a history of diabetes, cardiovascular disease, or clinical evidence of heart failure were followed for 38 months. In a multiregression analysis model not including left ventricular hypertrophy (LVH), an association between the highest night/day BP tertile and increased cardiovascular and all-cause mortality was found.[71] In contrast, the pre-dialysis BP averaged over one month did not predict events.

MORNING SURGE OF BLOOD PRESSURE

Most cardiovascular events show a peak incidence during the morning hours, between 6 AM and noon,[72] and this coincides with the morning surge of BP. The increase of BP can be attributed both to waking up and to getting out of bed. Often these coincide, but when they are separated there is a rise of BP occurring with each of them.[9] The most direct evidence that there is a causal connection between the rise of BP and the occurrence of events comes from a study showing that patients with the greatest morning surge (defined as the difference in BP between the lowest level during sleep and the average during the first two hours after waking) were at increased risk of having a stroke during a four-year follow-up.[66]

Another prospective study concluded that this applied to hemorrhagic but not ischemic strokes.[73] Most antihypertensive medications have relatively little effect on the rate of rise of BP even if they are fully active throughout the 24 hours, although alpha-adrenergic blockade

may reduce it.[74] The morning surge can only be evaluated by 24-hour ambulatory monitoring, although comparisons of morning and evening BP measured by home monitoring have been proposed as a surrogate measure.[75]

AMBULATORY BLOOD PRESSURES, TARGET ORGAN DAMAGE, AND PROGNOSIS

The rationale for believing that ABPM gives a more valid estimate of an individual's true BP level than office measurements is that many studies have found that it correlates more closely with measures of BP-related target organ damage. More importantly, several prospective studies have shown that it predicts long-term clinical outcomes better. These are reviewed in material following.

Ambulatory blood pressure and target organ damage

A large number of predominantly cross-sectional studies have examined the correlations between ABP and target organ damage. Many of these compared office BP and ABP, but others have also looked to see which component of ABP (e.g., daytime versus nighttime BP) correlates best with target organ damage. The target organs that have been looked at include the heart (LVH), the kidney (microalbuminuria), the brain (magnetic resonance imaging, MRI), and the arteries (carotid ultrasound and measures of arterial stiffness).

LVH is the most frequently measured marker of hypertensive target organ damage. Even in asymptomatic hypertensive patients, those with LVH have a worse cardiovascular prognosis than those without it.[76,77] Although BP is certainly one of the major determinants of LVH, there is disagreement as to whether the daytime or nighttime pressure is more important. Some studies have shown that LVH is more pronounced in non-dippers,[20,78–80] whereas others have found no difference.[81–83]

In view of the fact that dipping has a relatively low reproducibility, the most rigorous test of the role of dipping on target organ damage is to look at the relationships in patients whose dipping status is derived by averaging the daytime and nighttime BPs measured on two separate occasions. This was done by Cuspidi et al., who compared left ventrical (LV) mass in 238 dippers with 117 non-dippers[84] and found an insignificantly higher LV mass in the non-dippers but a significantly higher prevalence of LVH. The overall (48-hour) average BP level was the same in the two groups, suggesting that there is indeed a modest effect of the non-dipping pattern on LVH.

Silent lacunar infarction can be detected by brain MRI in approximately 30 to 50% of asymptomatic elderly hypertensives,[85,86] and is a strong predictor of clinically overt stroke.[87] Its major determinants are aging and hypertension, but an abnormal diurnal BP pattern is also a factor and in elderly hypertensive patients non-dippers have more frequent lacunar infarcts than dippers.[85]

Microalbuminuria is thought to reflect the glomerular capillary leak, which is a consequence of endothelial cell dysfunction and increased intraglomerular pressure, both of which are partly determined by the systemic BP level.

The 24-hour ambulatory BP level is more closely related to microalbuminuria than office BP,[88,89] and thus white coat hypertensive patients are less likely to have microalbuminuria than patients with sustained hypertension.[90]

The arteries bear the brunt of the damage resulting from hypertension, and show major changes in their structure and function, which help to maintain the hypertension but also set in motion the processes that lead to its adverse consequences. Noninvasive measurements of arterial structure and stiffness are becoming very popular. Several studies have used carotid ultrasound and have shown that ABP relates more closely than office BP to carotid artery intimal-medial thickness.[90,91]

Ambulatory blood pressure and prognosis

A number of studies have compared conventional office BP measurements with ABPM for the prediction of cardiovascular events, and all have used some measure of the average level of ABP as the predictor variable.[63,65,67,68,92–98] These are summarized in Table 45–3. Most have included patients whose hypertension was untreated at the time of the initial measurements but who were treated during the follow-up period, in all cases according to the office BP. One trial included treated patients.[68] The follow-up period ranged from two to eight years.

There are now 12 major prospective studies comparing the prediction of cardiovascular events using office or ambulatory BP, and the overwhelming consensus is that ambulatory pressure is a better predictor of risk than office BP.[99] Thus, when the ambulatory pressure is low in comparison to the office BP (WCH) the prognosis is benign. This body of data was what led to the decision by the CMS (The Centers for Medicare and Medicaid Services) to approve ABPM for reimbursement in patients with suspected WCH, on the grounds that they are a low-risk group who do not necessarily need antihypertensive drug treatment.

One study looked at patients with refractory hypertension, defined as a diastolic pressure above 100 mmHg while on three or more antihypertensive medications.[100] Patients were classified in three groups according to their daytime ambulatory pressure. Those in the lowest tertile (below 88 mmHg) had a significantly lower rate of morbidity over the next four years, despite similar office BPs. An important study in this series was Syst-Eur, a large placebo-controlled study of the effects on cardiovascular morbidity of treating systolic hypertension of the elderly with a calcium channel blocker.

A sub-study of 808 patients used ABPM, and found that ABP was a much more potent predictor of risk than office BP.[65] This study is the only one that has examined the effects of treating patients with WCH, because there was a placebo group as well as an active treatment group. There was a significant reduction of events in the active treatment group in patients with sustained hypertension, but not in the group with WCH.

Which component of the 24-hour BP gives the best prediction of risk?

Although there is consensus that ABP is the best predictor of risk, it is uncertain which component of the diurnal pattern of BP is most important. The leading candidates are shown in Figure 45–2. The most widely used has been the average 24-hour level. There has been great interest in the role of the diurnal rhythm of BP, and many studies have compared the predictive value of the daytime versus the nighttime pressure. Many have found no difference,[67,96] although some recent studies have reported that the best prediction of risk comes from the nighttime BP.[65,94,97,98] A related method of analysis is to look at the dipping patterns, and there have been claims that non-dippers are at higher risk than dippers.[63] In addition, patients with an excessive morning surge of BP may also be at increased risk.[66]

PROSPECTIVE STUDIES COMPARING CLINIC AND AMBULATORY BLOOD PRESSURE FOR PREDICTING CLINICAL EVENTS				
Author	Year (Ref)	Population	N	Results
Perloff	1983	Referred	1076	Low risk if ABP < OBP
Verdecchia	1994	Referred	1187	WCH at low risk
Imai	1995	Population	1789	ABP and HBP predict, not OBP
Redon	1998	Refractory	86	Low risk if ABP < OBP
Khattar	1998	Referred	479	WCH at low risk
Staessen	1998	Syst-Eur	808	ABP gives best prediction
Fagard	2000	Syst-Eur	695	WCH at low risk
Kario	2001	Referred	958	WCH at low risk
Clement	2003	Referred	1963	ABP gives best prediction
Bjorklund	2004	Population	872	ABP gives best prediction
Sega	2005	Population	2051	Combination of ABP and OBP gives best prediction
Fagard	2005	Population	391	WCH at low risk
Abbreviations: ABP, ambulatory blood pressure; OBP, office blood pressure; WCH, white coat hypertension.				

Table 45–3. Prospective Studies Comparing Clinic and Ambulatory Blood Pressure for Predicting Clinical Events

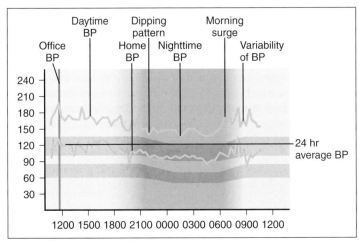

Figure 45–2. A 24-hour BP recording in a hypertensive patient. Yellow lines show systolic and diastolic pressure, and the gray zones indicate normal ranges. Light blue = day; dark blue = night. Boxes show various components of blood pressure that could be related to risk of events.

One study, using continuous intra-arterial BP monitoring,[101] found that BP variability was an independent predictor of increased LV mass seven years later, even after controlling for BP level. Another prospective study, using noninvasive monitoring, found that increased BP variability during the day did not predict cardiovascular events after controlling for factors known to be associated with increased variability (age, BP level, and diabetes).[102] It is quite conceivable that there is no single answer to this question, and that different components of the BP have different effects on risk. Nevertheless, the issue is important because antihypertensive drugs have different effects on different components of the diurnal BP profile and thus there is the possibility of more targeted treatment.

HOME MONITORING

The potential utility of hypertensive patients having their BPs measured at home, either by using self-monitoring or by having a family member make the measurements, was first demonstrated in 1940 by Ayman and Goldshine.[103] They found that home BPs could be 30 or 40 mmHg lower than the physicians' readings, and that these differences might persist over a period of six months. Home monitoring has the theoretical advantage of being able to overcome the two main limitations of office readings: the small number of readings that can be taken and the white coat effect. It provides a simple and cost-effective means of obtaining large numbers of readings, which are at least representative of the natural environment in which patients spend a major part of their day. Home monitoring has four practical advantages: it is helpful for distinguishing sustained from WCH, it can assess the response to antihypertensive medication, it may improve patient compliance, and it may reduce costs.

Home monitoring is now performed almost exclusively with automated oscillometric monitors, which are easy to use, relatively inexpensive, and readily available in drugstores and elsewhere. The latest generation of monitors has incorporated memory and the ability to calculate average levels of BP. A typical monitor is shown in Figure 45–3.

The limitations of home monitoring also need to be specified. First, readings tend to be taken in a relatively relaxed setting and thus may not reflect the BP occurring during stress. Second, patients may misrepresent their readings. Third, some patients may become more anxious as a result of home monitoring.

Although the technique has been readily available for many years, it is taking a surprisingly long time to find its way into general clinical practice. There has been a recent explosion in the sale of devices for home monitoring, few of which have been properly validated. Physicians are also endorsing the more widespread use of home monitoring, and national guidelines (such as produced by the American Society of Hypertension[48]) are beginning to appear. Patients are enthusiastic about home monitoring. In a survey of 855 treated hypertensive patients attending specialized clinics, 75% were using it regularly.[104]

COMPARISON OF HOME AND CLINIC PRESSURES

The original observation of Ayman and Goldshine[103] that home BPs are usually much lower than office BPs has been confirmed in a number of studies,[105,106] including the population surveys described previously (in which the vast majority of subjects were normotensive). In the Didima study of 562 normotensive subjects, home and office BPs were very similar (clinic SBP was 1 mm lower and DBP 1 mm higher).[10] Home BP was higher on day 1 of monitoring than on subsequent days. These differences may be more marked in older subjects.[107] The correlations between the office and home BP readings in the population studies were quite close, ranging from 0.73/0.64 (for systolic and diastolic pressures, respectively) in the PAMELA study[108] to 0.84/0.77 in PURAS.[107]

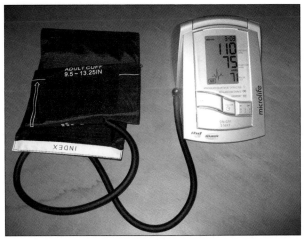

Figure 45–3. A typical digital home monitor.

In hypertensive subjects, the differences between office and home BPs are greater than in normotensive subjects, as shown in Figure 45–4. A notable exception to this was the HOT study, which included a sub-study of 926 treated hypertensives who had their BP evaluated by both office and home measurements using a semiautomatic device in both cases.[109] There were no differences between the two (the average levels of BP were 137/83 mmHg in the office and 137/83 at home). The probable explanation for this is that the readings were largely within the normal range, where differences are slight.

In patients with severe hypertension, office BPs may be 20/10 mmHg higher than home readings, and these clinic readings are also higher than readings taken in a hospital by a nurse.[110] The Ohasama study found that the correlations between home and office BP were stronger in untreated (r = 0.57 and 0.54 for SBP and DBP) than treated hypertensive subjects (r = 0.30 and 0.38).[11]

In some cases, home BPs may show a progressive decline with repeated measurement,[111] but this is by no means always seen.[106,112] Kenny et al. measured BP by four different techniques on three occasions separated by intervals of two weeks in 19 patients with borderline hypertension.[112] The techniques included conventional office measurement, basal BP (measured after lying for 30 minutes in a quiet room), daytime ambulatory pressure, and self-recorded home BP. None of the four measures showed any consistent change over the three study days, although there was an insignificant downward trend in all of them. For all three days, the office BPs were consistently higher than any of the other measures, but there were no significant differences between any of the other three measures. The average difference between office and home BPs was 9/4 mmHg.

That the office/home difference is due to the setting rather than the technique of BP measurement can be demonstrated by having patients take readings both at home and in the office. In the office, it may be found that the patients' and the physicians' readings are very similar and in both cases higher than the home readings. In 30 treated hypertensives who were evaluated with both office and home BP, clinic BPs were taken either by the physician or the patient using an electronic device and the BPs were the same.[113]

The discrepancy between home and office BPs raises the question of which is closer to the true pressure. As shown in Figure 45–5, the home BPs are closer to the 24-hour average than the office BPs.[106] Figure 45–5 also demonstrates the phenomenon seen in Figure 45–4; namely, that there is a progressively greater discrepancy between the clinic and the true pressure at higher levels of BP. Other studies have also found that the correlation between home and ambulatory pressure is closer than for either of them with clinic pressure.[114]

REPRODUCIBILITY OF HOME READINGS

Relatively little has been published on this issue, but it is important. In a study we performed some years ago comparing the reproducibility of home, clinic, and ambulatory readings (all measured twice separated by an interval of two weeks), we found that in hypertensive patients there was a significant decline of systolic pressure in the clinic over this period but the home and ambulatory pressures showed no significant change.[45] In normoten-

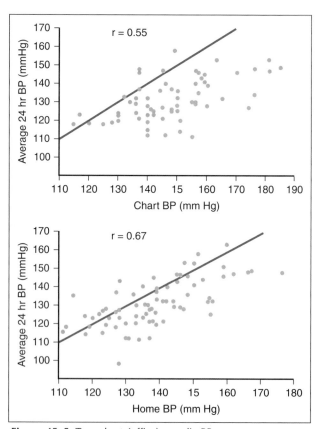

Figure 45–5. Top: chart (office) systolic BP versus average 24-hour BP. Bottom: home systolic pressure versus 24-hour average pressure. The lines are lines of identity. (Redrawn from Ayman P, Goldshine AD. Blood pressure determinations by patients with essential hypertension I: The difference between clinic and home readings before treatment. *Am J Med Sci* 1940;200:465–74.)

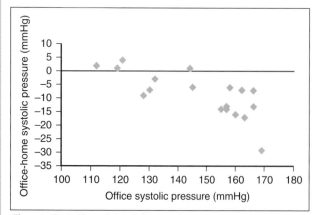

Figure 45–4. Plot of the difference between home and office BP as a function of BP level. Data from 18 studies published since 1992.

sive subjects, there was no consistent change in any of the three measures of BP.

In another study, Jyothinagaram et al. measured clinic and home BPs three times over a four-week interval in 17 hypertensive patients.[115] The clinic pressure fell from 181/97 to 162/93 mmHg, whereas the home BP showed no change (153/89 to 154/89 mmHg). The superior reproducibility of home and ambulatory measurements may be partly explained by the greater number of readings. These findings support the notion that the fall of office BP on successive visits is primarily due to habituation to the office setting or to regression to the mean.

In a typical study comparing the short-term reproducibility of the three measures of BP, the SDD for the home readings was 5.6/4.6 mmHg, which was similar to the SDD for ambulatory readings (5.3/5.4) and lower than for office readings (9.7/6.7).[45] The correlation coefficients for all three sets of measurements were very close (0.96/0.94 for home systolic and diastolic pressures, 0.93/0.87 for ambulatory, and 0.94/0.87 for office readings). Another study of 133 hypertensive subjects found that home BP gave the lowest SDD for systolic and diastolic pressures (6.9/4.7 mmHg), compared with 8.3/5/6 for ABP and 11.0/6.6 for office BP.[116] These studies thus show that the greater numbers of readings taken with home and ambulatory monitoring than with office measurement mean that the estimate of the true BP is much better.

The studies described previously investigated the reproducibility of home BPs over a period of weeks, and it might be expected that over longer periods of time the reproducibility would be lower. This is not necessarily the case, however. In the Ohasama study, 136 untreated subjects measured home BP for three days on two occasions one year apart.[117] The correlations between the two were high (r = 0.84 and 0.83 for SBP and DBP), and there were no consistent change over the year. In contrast, the office BPs declined 4/3 mmHg over the same period, and were less closely correlated (r = .69 for SBP and 0.57 for DBP). Thus, home BP appears to be relatively stable.

HOME BLOOD PRESSURE IN NORMAL SUBJECTS

As with ambulatory pressure, there is no universally agreed on upper limit of normal home BP, but there are several studies that have compared home and office levels of BP, and others which have described average levels in normal populations. There have been seven large epidemiologic studies of home BP, which have attempted to define normal ranges. These were the Tecumseh study,[118] the Dubendorf study,[18] the Ohasama study,[19] the Limbourg study,[119] the Didima study,[10] the PURAS study,[107] and PAMELA.[120,121] All seven studies found that home BPs were higher in men than in women (as has been shown for ambulatory pressures), and five of six studies (the Tecumseh Study could not evaluate this) found that home BPs increased with age.

The distribution of BP in the population is in the form of a skewed Gaussian or bell-shaped curve, which tails off at the higher end. Any division into "normal" and "high"

BP is thus arbitrary, and this applies whichever measure of BP is used. In practice, the need for such a dividing line is that it can be used as a treatment threshold. One common technique used to define the upper limit of a variable such as BP that is continuously distributed in the population is to take the 95th percentile, which defines the upper 5% as being "abnormal." A variation of this method is to use the mean plus 2 SD, which is very similar to the 95th percentile.

An obvious problem with this is that hypertension affects more than 5% of the population. Another is that hypertensive individuals are often excluded from population surveys. Thus, if in the population studies described previously the upper limit of normal home BP were defined as the 95th percentile the values would range from 137/86 to 152/99 mmHg, which are clearly too high. In a meta-analysis of 17 studies of home BPs in normotensive subjects, Thijs et al.[122] used a number of techniques to define the upper limit of normal. One was to use the 95th percentile, which gave a level of 135/86 mmHg. The mean plus 2 SD gave 137/89 mmHg.

An alternative method of defining the upper limit of normal home BP is to estimate the home BP equivalent to an office BP of 140/90 mmHg, as has also been done for ambulatory pressure. In the Thijs meta-analysis, two techniques were used to derive the home BP equivalent to 140/90 mmHg.[122] The first was to compute the linear regression between office and home readings, which gave a value for the home BP of 125/79 mmHg. The second was the percentile method, which calculated the percentile in the distribution of office BPs that corresponded to 140/90 mmHg, and used the same percentile for the distribution of the home BP. This gave a value of 129/84 mmHg. In the PAMELA study, the home BP equivalent to an office BP of 140/90 was 132/83 mmHg (calculated by the linear regression method).[123] The average values for home BP and the home BP estimated to be equivalent to 140/90 in the office for four of the studies are outlined in Table 45–4.

The ASH recommended that an appropriate level for the upper limit of normal home BP should be 135/85 mmHg.[48] This was based on the fact that home BPs tend to be somewhat lower than office BPs, and is in accord with the findings of several studies (as described previously). It is also consistent with the prospective findings of the Ohasama study, where home BPs above 138/83 mmHg were found to be associated with increased mortality.[124] The same value has been adopted by the JNC 7 recommendations[1] and by the American Heart Association.[125] As with office BP, a lower home BP goal is advisable for certain patients, including diabetics, pregnant women, and patients with renal failure. No specific limits have been set for these patients, however.

HOME BLOOD PRESSURES, TARGET ORGAN DAMAGE, AND PROGNOSIS

One of the factors that has limited the acceptance of home BP for clinical decision making has been the lack of prognostic data, but there are increasing numbers of

AVERAGE VALUES AND PROPOSED UPPER LIMITS OF NORMAL HOME BLOOD PRESSURE FROM POPULATION STUDIES					
Study	N	Average Values		Home BP Equivalent to 140/90 in Office	
		Clinic BP	Home BP	Percentile	Regression
PAMELA	1438	127/82	119/74	–	132/83
Didima	562	118/73	120/72	140/86	137/83
Dubendorf	503	130/82	123/77	133/86	–
PURAS	989	126/76	118/71	134/84	131/82

Table 45–4. Average Values and Proposed Upper Limits of Normal Home Blood Pressure from Population Studies

studies showing that self-measured BP predicts target organ damage and clinical outcomes better than traditional office BP. These are reviewed in material following.

Home blood pressure and target organ damage

In one of the first studies using home monitoring, it was reported that regression of LVH evaluated by the ECG correlated more closely with changes of home BP than with office BP following the initiation of antihypertensive treatment.[126] Several other studies have indicated that the correlation between echocardiographically determined LVH and BP is better for home than for office readings.[106,127,128] However, in one study of 84 previously untreated hypertensive patients home BP and clinic BP gave similar correlations with LVH (r = 0.31 and 0.32), but not as good as the correlation between ABP and LVH (r = 0.51).[12] In a study of treated hypertensives, home BP correlated with LVH but office BP did not.[129]

Home BP has also been related to other measures of target organ damage. It has been reported to correlate more closely than office BP with microalbuminuria[128,130] and with carotid artery intima-media thickness.[130,131]

Home blood pressure and prognosis

There are four studies that have compared the predictive value of office and home measurements, and all have shown that home measurements are potentially superior (see Table 45–4). In the first (conducted as a population survey in Ohasama, Japan), 1,789 people were evaluated with home, office, and 24-hour BP measurements.[132] Over a five-year follow-up it was found that the home BP predicted risk better than the office readings. For each measure of BP, the subjects were divided into quintiles. The survival rate was significantly lower for people whose initial home BP was above 138 mmHg systolic and 83 mmHg diastolic pressure.[133]

As also shown Figure 45–5, the consequences of a high clinic pressure were less clear. There was some suggestion from these data of a J-shaped curve, representing a paradoxical increase of mortality at low home BPs. The actual numbers were too small to be sure of this, however, and it was not observed for the screening BPs. A subsequent analysis over 10 years[134] found that the prediction of risk

became stronger with more home readings, up to a maximum of 25 measurements. There was no evidence of a threshold number. The second study (conducted in France) recruited 4,939 elderly hypertensives currently on treatment and found that morbid events observed over a 3.2-year follow-up period were predicted by the home BP at baseline but not by the clinic pressure.[135]

One particularly interesting aspect of this study was that patients who had normal office BPs but high home BPs were at increased risk, a phenomenon known as masked hypertension (see material following). It is not known if the variability of home BP readings is an independent predictor of events, although there is some evidence that the variability of daytime readings measured with ABPM may be.[136] The third study was an Italian population-based study[94] of 2,051 subjects who had one set of three clinic BP readings and two home BP readings (one in the morning and one in the evening) and who were followed for 11 years. Adding the data from a second office visit on the following day did not improve the prediction of cardiovascular events, whereas adding the home readings did. In the fourth study, Fagard et al. measured BP in the office, at home, and by ABPM in 391 elderly patients registered in family practices and followed them for 10 years. Office BP did not predict cardiovascular events, whereas home BP did[98] (Table 45–5).

A not uncommon finding is isolated diastolic hypertension, in which the systolic pressure is normal and the diastolic pressure is raised. There has been some controversy as to its prognosis, but the only report using home monitoring (the Ohasama study) concluded that it is benign.[137] The threshold values for defining it were a home systolic pressure <138 mmHg and a diastolic pressure >85 mmHg. In contrast, patients with isolated systolic hypertension were at increased risk.

There is also some evidence that self-monitored BP may predict the change of BP over time, as well as the decline of renal function in diabetics. In the Tecumseh study of 735 healthy young adults (mean age 32), home BP predicted future BP over three years better than clinic BP.[138] A prospective study of 77 hypertensive diabetic patients whose clinical course was followed over a six-year period using both clinic and home monitoring found that home BP predicted the loss of renal function (decrease of GFR) better than the office BP.[139]

PROSPECTIVE STUDIES COMPARING OFFICE AND HOME BLOOD PRESSURE FOR PREDICTING CLINICAL EVENTS				
Author	Year (ref)	Population	N	Results
Imai	1996	Population	1789	HBP better than OBP
Bobrie	2004	Clinic	4939	HBP better than OBP
Sega	2005	Population	2051	Combined HBP + OBP gives best prediction
Fagard	2005	Population	391	HBP better than OBP

Table 45–5. Prospective Studies Comparing Office and Home Blood Pressure for Predicting Clinical Events

CLINICAL APPLICATIONS OF OUT-OF-OFFICE MONITORING

In clinical practice, a patient's BP is typically characterized by a single value of the systolic and diastolic pressures, to denote the average level. Such readings are normally taken in an office setting, but there is extensive evidence that in hypertensive patients office BPs are consistently higher than the average 24-hour pressures recorded with ambulatory monitors.[140] This overestimation by office readings of the true pressure at high levels of pressure and underestimation at low levels has been referred to as the regression dilution bias, which refers to the fact that the slope of the line relating BP and cardiovascular morbidity should be steeper for the true BP than for the office BP.[141]

Thus, hypertension can be regarded as a disturbance of the set point or tonic level of BP with normal short-term regulation. Antihypertensive treatment reverses these changes, again by resetting the set point toward normal, with little effect on short-term variability. The normal diurnal rhythm of BP is disturbed in some hypertensive individuals, with loss of the normal nocturnal fall of pressure. This has been observed in a variety of conditions, including malignant hypertension, chronic renal failure, several types of secondary hypertension, preeclampsia, and conditions associated with autonomic neuropathy.[141]

For the foreseeable future, measurement of office BP by conventional sphygmomanometry will continue to be the principal method of clinical evaluation. A cardinal rule is that the closer the BP is to the threshold level at which treatment will be started the more readings should be taken over more visits before the decision is made. In patients who have persistently elevated office BP and evidence of BP-related target organ damage, it is usually unnecessary to supplement the office readings with other types of measurement before reaching a therapeutic decision.

When an elevated BP is the only detectable abnormality, however, the possibility that the office BP may overestimate the true pressure should be considered. This can be done either by home or ambulatory monitoring. A schema for the use of the different procedures for measuring BP when evaluating a newly diagnosed hypertensive patient is shown in Figure 45–6. If home monitoring is chosen and reveals pressures comparable to the office value, treatment may be appropriate. However, if the home readings are much lower than the office read-

ings it does not rule out the possibility that the BP may be elevated at work. This is the advantage of ambulatory monitoring, which gives the best estimate of the full range of BP experienced during everyday life.

CLASSIFICATION OF HYPERTENSION USING OUT-OF-OFFICE MONITORING

With the combined use of BP measurement in and out of the office, BP status can be classified differently from the traditional unidimensional method based solely on office BPs. As shown in Figure 45–7, the cutoff points for clinic and daytime ambulatory BPs are different: 140/90 mmHg for the former and 135/85 for the latter. There are four cells: true normotension (normotensive by both criteria), true hypertension (hypertensive by both), WCH (hypertensive by office criteria, normotensive by ambulatory), and masked hypertension (normotensive in the office and hypertensive during ambulatory monitoring). As also shown in the figure, current evidence indicates that the degree of cardiovascular risk goes with the ambulatory rather than the office BP.

There are several clinical situations in which out-of-office monitoring may help to establish the diagnosis of hypertension, as outlined in Table 45–6. These include suspected WCH, masked hypertension, or nocturnal hypertension (none of which can be diagnosed by exclusive reliance on office measurement), and others (labile

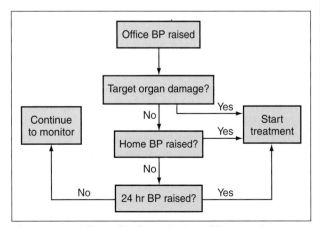

Figure 45–6. Schema for the evaluation of hypertensive patients using office and out-of-office measurement.

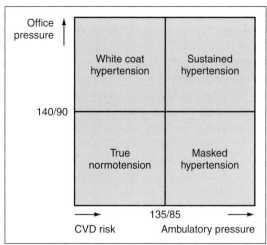

Figure 45–7. Classification of BP status according to office and out-of-office measurements.

CLINICAL SITUATIONS IN WHICH OUT-OF-OFFICE MEASUREMENT IS HELPFUL		
Clinical Situation	Home BP	ABP
White coat hypertension	+	++
Masked hypertension	+	++
Nocturnal hypertension	–	++
Labile blood pressure	+	+
Resistant hypertension	+	+
Autonomic insufficiency	+	++
Hypertension of pregnancy	++	+

Table 45–6. Clinical Situations in Which Out-of-Office Measurement Is Helpful

BP, resistant hypertension, autonomic insufficiency, and hypertension of pregnancy) in which out-of-office measurement greatly adds to the precision of the diagnosis.

White coat hypertension

This is the only indication that has been approved for reimbursement by the CMS in the United States. Suspected WCH is defined as a clinic BP above 140/90 mmHg on at least three occasions, with at least two sets of measurements below 140/90 mmHg out of the office plus an absence of target organ damage. The reason this diagnosis is important is that it is generally accepted that WCH is a relatively low-risk condition and that antihypertensive drug treatment is likely to be of no benefit.

There are two reasons for thinking this. First, several studies have shown that drug treatment of WCH reduces the clinic BP but has negligible effect on the ambulatory pressure, which by definition is normal to begin with.[142] Second, the only study to investigate the effects of treating WCH on morbid events found no significant benefit.[143] It is possible that some patients with WCH may go on to develop sustained hypertension[144] or masked

hypertension,[145] and there may be an increase in the risk of stroke after six years.[146] Therefore, long-term follow-up with repeated ABPM or home monitoring is essential.

WCH is defined as a persistently elevated clinic pressure (above 140/90 mmHg together with a normal daytime ambulatory pressure of 135/85 or less). It is important to emphasize that it requires several office visits to establish the diagnosis, because there may be a spontaneous decline of office BP with multiple visits. WCH is not a discrete entity because most hypertensive patients show a white coat effect. What distinguishes patients with WCH from those with true or sustained hypertension is not that they have an exaggerated white coat effect but that their BP is within the normal range when they are outside the office setting. Patients with WCH do not necessarily look anxious or have a tachycardia while in the office. Thus, it can only be diagnosed reliably by ambulatory monitoring. If patients with WCH are treated with antihypertensive drugs, there is typically a decline of office BP but little or no change of ambulatory pressure, which by definition is normal to start with.

The phenomenon of WCH (elevated office BP and normal out-of-office BP) is also observed in patients who are on antihypertensive treatment. In a survey of 3,303 treated Japanese patients, its prevalence was 19%.[147]

Masked hypertension

In the past few years there has been growing interest in the phenomenon of masked hypertension, defined as a normal office BP and high ambulatory BP (the obverse of WCH). The important point is that these are patients in whom the office BP underestimates the risk of cardiovascular events. A study of treated hypertensive patients[148] found that about a third of treated patients seen in a hypertension clinic had masked hypertension, and over a five-year follow-up their relative risk for cardiovascular events was 2.28 when compared with patients controlled by both office BP and ABP criteria.

Other studies have shown that masked hypertension in untreated and often undiagnosed patients is associated with an increase of target organ damage[149] and an adverse prognosis.[67] As with WCH, the condition may be suspected on the basis of high home BPs. One study has shown that masked hypertension diagnosed solely by home recordings is associated with increased mortality.[135] Not surprisingly, patients diagnosed with masked hypertension do not show complete concordance with those diagnosed using ABPM.[150]

The prevalence of masked hypertension may be as much as 10% in the general population, based on data from population studies in several countries.[67,151–153] As with WCH, masked hypertension is seen in treated hypertensive patients, and in one study its prevalence was 19%.[147]

Nocturnal hypertension

As described previously, BP may remain high or even increase during the night. At the present time there are no clear clinical indications for assessing this, but there are several conditions in which it is common, and in which its recognition might alter treatment regimens. These include diabetes, chronic kidney disease, and sleep apnea. There are also some studies (see previous material) that suggest that the nocturnal BP may give the best prediction of risk, but this is still controversial. Nevertheless, it has been clearly established that antihypertensive treatment can selectively lower nocturnal BP.

Labile hypertension

This title is something of a misnomer because all hypertension is labile. However, there are some patients who give a history of paroxysmal hypertension in whom ABPM may prove helpful. Pheochromocytoma may be suspected in some of these patients, but the hypertension in this condition is not always particularly labile.[154] A much more common cause of labile hypertension is panic attacks, which have been shown to be accompanied by surges of both BP and heart rate[155] and which may be detected by out-of-office monitoring. There are at present no norms for deciding if BP variability over 24 hours is greater than normal.

Resistant hypertension

In some patients whose clinic BP remains high despite being on three or more antihypertensive drugs, an exaggerated white coat effect may be suspected. Two prospective studies have shown that there is a subgroup of patients who have resistant hypertension by office BP criteria but whose ambulatory BP is normal and whose prognosis is benign.[100,148] However, it is probable that the two categories of resistant hypertension could be separated by home monitoring.

Autonomic insufficiency

This is a not uncommon finding in elderly patients who complain of dizziness when standing for long periods of time, and who may also have syncopal episodes. When they are supine, the BP may be quite high, particularly during the night.[156] Thus, their BP is unusually labile, depending on their body position. Treatment with pressor drugs and antigravity stockings is always a compromise between letting the BP go too low and making it go too high, and therefore ABPM is essential for evaluating the optimal BP control in these patients.

Hypertension of pregnancy

Hypertension of pregnancy is still one of the leading causes of maternal death, and is potentially preventable.[157] Close monitoring of BP is therefore essential. WCH is a significant problem, and can lead to unnecessary early terminations of pregnancy. There have been several attempts to detect preeclampsia in its early stages using ambulatory monitoring, and it was suggested that a loss of dipping might be an early sign. However, this has not been well substantiated. Home monitoring has more potential because it is well suited to detecting trends over time.[158] However, it has not been used very widely.[159]

EVALUATION OF THE BLOOD PRESSURE RESPONSE TO ANTIHYPERTENSIVE TREATMENT

Although still the gold standard for clinical practice and trials, the traditional method of evaluating the effects of antihypertensive treatment by the changes of office BP suffers from several major defects, which have become more apparent with the introduction of out-of-office monitoring. First is the well-known fact that the small number of readings that can be taken at a clinic visit may not be representative because of the inherent variability of BP. Second, readings are only taken at one time of day, and the effects of antihypertensive drugs are often not the same over 24 hours. In clinical trials, BP is typically measured at trough (just before the next dose is due), but this is rarely achieved in clinical practice. Third, there are variable changes in the white coat effect and thus the changes in office BP do not parallel the changes in the out-of-office BP. In principle, both methods of out-of-office monitoring can avoid these pitfalls.

ABPM is not commonly used in routine clinical practice for this purpose, mainly because of the cost and inconvenience of performing multiple ABP recordings However, changes in ABP correlate more closely than changes of office BP with regression of LVH during antihypertensive treatment.[160] Home BP monitoring is more practical. On the grounds that hypertension is usually characterized by a sustained increase of BP throughout the day and night, it seems reasonable to propose that the goal of antihypertensive drug treatment should be to lower the BP to the same extent during the day and night. Whether treatment should be directed to convert hypertensive non-dippers to normotensive dippers with treatment is unresolved, but certainly feasible.

Diuretics normalize the non-dipper pattern by lowering the nocturnal more than the daytime pressure.[161] In an analysis of the effects of doxazosin on dipping status, we found that non-dippers were likely to become dippers following treatment. The best explanation for this was that the effects of the drug on BP were proportional to the pretreatment level, such that the nighttime pressure is lowered more in non-dippers than dippers.[6] Similarly, studies with calcium channel blockers have found that the drugs lower daytime BP in both dippers and non-dippers, but nighttime BP more in non-dippers.[162]

The timing of antihypertensive drug dosing may also be factor. In patients with renal disease who were predominantly non-dippers, evening dosing of a calcium channel blocker (isradipine) lowered the nighttime pressure more than morning dosing.[163] However, it must be admitted that at the present time there is no evidence that selectively lowering the nighttime BP has any impact on clinical outcome.

Performing multiple ABP recordings to evaluate the effects of antihypertensive treatment may not be practical, but home monitoring is ideally suited to this task because it is easy to obtain serial measurements over long periods of time. Despite the general parallelism between office and home BPs during treatment, there may be considerable discrepancy between the two in individual patients. Other studies have shown that drug treatment lowers clinic BP more than home BP. In a study of 760 hypertensives treated with diltiazem 300 mg, the clinic BP fell by 20/13 mmHg and the home BP by 11/8 mmHg.[164]

In another study,[165] losartan lowered office BP by 17/13 mmHg and home BP by 7/5. Trandolapril lowered office BP by 17/13 and home BP by 7/5. Changes of ABP were closer to the changes of home BP. It is well recognized that drug treatment also lowers ambulatory BP less than office BP.[166] One study has looked at the effects of exercise training on office and home BP. Office BP fell by 13/8 in the experimental group and 6/1 mmHg in the controls, whereas home BPs fell by 6/3 and 1/-1, respectively.[167]

SELF-MONITORING FOR IMPROVING ADHERENCE TO ANTIHYPERTENSIVE TREATMENT

There is considerable interest in the use of home monitoring for improving BP control. The rationale is that patients who monitor their BP regularly are more likely to take their medications. A recent review of the effects of HBPM on adherence found 11 randomized trials, most of which used some additional interventions other than simple monitoring (such as counseling by nurses) to improve adherence.[168] The conclusion was that there was a modest improvement. There has also been a review of the effects of HBPM on BP control,[169] which found 18 randomized controlled trials and concluded that there was a 4/2 mmHg lower BP in the groups randomized to home monitoring as opposed to usual care.

ECONOMIC ISSUES AND REIMBURSEMENT

ABPM is not widely used at the present time in clinical practice, mainly because it is often not reimbursed by insurance companies. Medicare pays between $56 and $122 in different regions, but only for suspected WCH (defined as a high clinic BP, an absence of target organ damage, and evidence of normal BP outside the clinic). On the grounds that WCH does not warrant antihypertensive drug treatment, but that patients diagnosed with it undergo annual ABPM, it has been estimated that if all newly diagnosed hypertensive patients underwent ABPM

there would be a net saving of costs of managing hypertension if the average cost of drug treatment were $300 or higher.[170]

USE OF OUT-OF-OFFICE MONITORING IN CLINICAL TRIALS

ABPM is widely used for clinical trials of antihypertensive drugs, and to lesser extent for non-drug forms of treatment. The reduction of BP is almost always smaller for ABP than for clinic BP.[166] The potential advantages of ABPM for evaluating treatment effects in clinical trials include the evaluation of duration of action, analysis of the effects on nighttime BP, absence of a placebo effect, smaller sample size, and better correlation with clinical outcomes.[171] One of the goals of major outcome trials that have compared the effects of different drugs on cardiovascular morbidity has been to determine if there are effects on cardiovascular events that are independent of the drugs' effects on BP. Unfortunately, ABPM has often not been included. However, in one instance of it being included (the HOPE trial[172]) the BP changes recorded by ABPM were very different from the changes reported by office measurement.[173]

SUMMARY AND PERSPECTIVES

At the present time, ABPM is used only in the minority of patients but its use is gradually increasing. The monitors are reliable, reasonably convenient to wear, and generally accurate. ABPM can be regarded as the gold standard for BP measurement on the basis of prognostic studies showing that it predicts clinical outcome better than conventional measurements. Thus, a good case can be made for using it in all newly diagnosed hypertensive patients.

The procedure is relatively expensive in comparison with other methods of measuring BP, and many of the studies documenting its value were done without home monitoring. In contrast to ABPM, home monitoring has seen a dramatic growth in its clinical use over the past few years, and it remains to be seen to what extent it will be able to replace ABPM. It is likely that in the near future there will be a further decline in reliance on clinic BP measurements and an increased emphasis on out-of-office monitoring for the diagnosis and treatment of hypertensive patients.

REFERENCES

1. Chobanian AV, Bakris GL, Black HR, Cushman WC, Green LA, Izzo JL Jr., et al. The Seventh Report of the Joint National Committee on Prevention, Detection, Evaluation, and Treatment of High Blood Pressure: The JNC 7 report. JAMA 2003;289(19):2560–72.
2. 1999 World Health Organization/ International Society of Hypertension guidelines for the management of

hypertension. J Hypertens 1999; 17:151–83.
3. Sokolow M, Werdegar D, Kain HK, Hinman AT. Relationship between level of blood pressure measured casually and by portable recorders and severity of complications in essential hypertension. Circulation 1966; 34(2):279–98.
4. Mancia G, Facchetti R, Bombelli M, Grassi G, Sega R. Long-term risk of

mortality associated with selective and combined elevation in office, home, and ambulatory blood pressure. Hypertension 2006;47(5):846–53.
5. Pickering TG, Harshfield GA, Kleinert HD, Blank S, Laragh JH. Blood pressure during normal daily activities, sleep, and exercise: Comparison of values in normal and hypertensive subjects. JAMA 1982;247(7):992–96.

6. Kario K, Schwartz JE, Pickering TG. Changes of nocturnal blood pressure dipping status in hypertensives by nighttime dosing of alpha-adrenergic blocker, doxazosin: Results from the HALT study. *Hypertension* 2000; 35(3):787–94.

7. Muller JE, Stone PH, Turi ZG, Rutherford JD, Czeisler CA, Parker C, et al. Circadian variation in the frequency of onset of acute myocardial infarction. *N Engl J Med* 1985; 313(21):1315–22.

8. Elliott WJ. Circadian variation in the timing of stroke onset: A meta-analysis. *Stroke* 1998;29(5):992–96.

9. Khoury AF, Sunderajan P, Kaplan NM. The early morning rise in blood pressure is related mainly to ambulation. *Amer J Hypertens* 1992; 5:339–44.

10. Stergiou GS, Thomopoulou GC, Skeva II, Mountokalakis TD. Home blood pressure normalcy: The DIDIMA Study. *J Hypertens* 1999;17(3):S25.

11. Imai Y, Nishiyama A, Sekino M, Aihara A, Kikuya M, Ohkubo T, et al. Characteristics of blood pressure measured at home in the morning and in the evening: The Ohasama study. *J Hypertens* 1999;17(7):889–98.

12. Kok RH, Beltman FW, Terpstra WF, Smit AJ, May JF, de Graeff PA, et al. Home blood pressure measurement: reproducibility and relationship with left ventricular mass. *Blood Press Monit* 1999;4(2):65–69.

13. Pieper C, Warren K, Pickering TG. A comparison of ambulatory blood pressure and heart rate at home and work on work and non-work days. *J Hypertens* 1993;11(2):177–83.

14. Minami J, Kawano Y, Ishimitsu T, Yoshimi H, Takishita S. Seasonal variations in office, home and 24 h ambulatory blood pressure in patients with essential hypertension. *J Hypertens* 1996;14(12):1421–25.

15. Imai Y, Munakata M, Tsuji I, Ohkubo T, Satoh H, Yoshino H, et al. Seasonal variation in blood pressure in normotensive women studied by home measurements. *Clin Sci (Colch)* 1996;90(1):55–60.

16. Giaconi S, Palombo C, Genovesi-Ebert A, Marabotti C, Volterrani D, Ghione S. Long-term reproducibility and evaluation of seasonal influences on blood pressure monitoring. *J Hypertens* 1988;6(4):S64–66.

17. Mejia AD, Julius S, Jones KA, Schork NJ, Kneisley J. The Tecumseh Blood Pressure Study. Normative data on blood pressure self-determination. *Arch Intern Med* 1990;150(6): 1209–13.

18. Weisser B, Grune S, Burger R, Blickenstorfer H, Iseli J, Michelsen SH, et al. The Dubendorf Study: A population-based investigation on normal values of blood pressure self-measurement. *J Hum Hypertens* 1994;8(4):227–31.

19. Imai Y, Satoh H, Nagai K, Sakuma M, Sakuma H, Minami N, et al. Characteristics of a community-based distribution of home blood pressure in Ohasama in northern Japan. *J Hypertens* 1993;11:1441–49.

20. Staessen JA, Fagard R, Lijnen P, Thijs L, van Hulle S, Vyncke G, et al. Ambulatory blood pressure and blood pressure measured at home: Progress report on a population study. *J Cardiovasc Pharmacol* 1994;23(5): S5–11.

21. Henry JP, Cassel JC. Psychosocial factors in essential hypertension: Recent epidemiologic and animal experimental evidence. *Am J Epidemiol* 1969;90(3):171–200.

22. Aihara A, Imai Y, Sekino M, Kato J, Ito S, Ohkubo T, et al. Discrepancy between screening blood pressure and ambulatory blood pressure: A community-based study in Ohasama. *Hypertens Res* 1998;21(2):127–36.

23. Kelbaek H, Munck O, Christensen NJ, Godtfredsen J. Central haemodynamic changes after a meal. *Br Heart J* 1989; 61:506–09.

24. Peitzman SJ, Berger SR. Postprandial blood pressure decrease in well elderly persons. *Arch Intern Med* 1989; 149(2):286–88.

25. Kawano Y, Pontes CS, Abe H, Takishita S, Omae T. Effects of alcohol consumption and restriction on home blood pressure in hypertensive patients: Serial changes in the morning and evening records. *Clin Exp Hypertens* 2002;24(1/2):33–39.

26. Smits P, Thien T, Van't Laar A. Circulatory effects of coffee in relation to the pharmacokinetics of caffeine. *Am J Cardiol* 1985;56:958–63.

27. Robertson D, Frolich JC, Carr RK. Effects of caffeine on plasma renin activity, catecholamines and blood pressure. *NEJM* 1978;298:181–86.

28. Izzo JLJ, Ghosal A, Kwong T, Freeman RB, Jaenike JR. Age and prior caffeine use alter the cardiovascular and adrenomedullary responses to oral caffeine. *Am J Cardiol* 1983;52(7): 769–73.

29. Pincomb GA, Lovallo WR, Passey RB, Wilson MF. Effect of behavior state on caffeine's ability to alter blood pressure. *Am J Cardiol* 1988;61:798–802.

30. Cellina GU, Honour AJ, Littler WA. Direct arterial pressure, heart rate, and electrocardiogram during cigarette smoking in unrestricted patients. *Am Heart J* 1975;89(1):18–25.

31. Freestone S, Ramsay LE. Effect of coffee and cigarette smoking on the blood pressure of untreated and diuretic-treated hypertensive patients. *Am J Med* 1982;73(3):348–53.

32. Hozawa A, Ohkubo T, Nagai K, Kikuya M, Matsubara M, Tsuji I, et al. Factors affecting the difference between screening and home blood pressure measurements: The Ohasama Study. *J Hypertens* 2001;19(1):13–19.

33. Lynch JJ, Long JM, Thomas SA, Malinow KL, Katcher AH. The effects of talking on the blood pressure of hypertensive and normotensive individuals. *Psychosom Med* 1981; 43(1):25–33.

34. Friedmann E, Thomas SA, Kulick-Ciuffo D, Lynch JJ, Suginohara M. The effects of normal and rapid speech on blood pressure. *Psychosom Med* 1982;44(6):545–53.

35. Glynn LM, Christenfeld N, Gerin W. The role of rumination in recovery from reactivity: Cardiovascular consequences of emotional states. *Psychosom Med* 2002;64(5):714–26.

36. Minami J, Kawano Y, Ishimitsu T, Yoshimi H, Takishita S. Effect of the Hanshin-Awaji earthquake on home blood pressure in patients with essential hypertension. *Am J Hypertens* 1997;10(2):222–25.

37. Lipsky SI, Pickering TG, Gerin W. World Trade Center disaster effect on blood pressure. *Blood Press Monit* 2002;7(4):249.

38. Gerin W, Chaplin W, Schwartz JE, Holland J, Alter R, Wheeler R, et al. Sustained blood pressure elevation following an acute stressor: The effects of the September 11, 2001 attack on the New York City World Trade Center. *J Hypertens* 2005;23:279–84.

39. Schnall PL, Schwartz JE, Landsbergis PA, Warren K, Pickering TG. Relation between job strain, alcohol, and ambulatory blood pressure. *Hypertension* 1992;19(5):488–94.

40. MacDonald JR. Potential causes, mechanisms, and implications of post exercise hypotension. *J Hum Hypertens* 2002;16(4):225–36.

41. Kawabe H, Saito I. Influence of nighttime bathing on evening home blood pressure measurements: How long should the interval be after bathing? *Hypertens Res* 2006;29(3): 129–33.

42. Little P, Barnett J, Barnsley L, Marjoram J, Fitzgerald-Barron A, Mant D. Comparison of agreement between different measures of blood pressure in primary care and daytime ambulatory blood pressure. *BMJ* 2002; 325(7358):254–60.

43. Pickering TG, Hall JE, Appel LJ, Falkner BE, Graves J, Hill MN, et al. Recommendations for blood pressure measurement in humans and experimental animals. Part 1: Blood pressure measurement in humans: A statement for professionals from the subcommittee of professional and public education of the american heart association council on high blood pressure research. *Circulation* 2005;111(5):697–716.

44. Armitage P, Rose GA. The variability of measurements of casual blood pressure. I: A laboratory study. *Clin Sci* 1966;30(2):325–35.

45. James GD, Pickering TG, Yee LS, Harshfield GA, Riva S, Laragh JH. The reproducibility of average ambulatory, home, and clinic pressures. *Hypertension* 1988;11(6/1):545–49.

46. Musso NR, Lotti G. Reproducibility of ambulatory blood pressure monitoring. *Blood Press Monit* 1996;1(2):105–09.

47. Mansoor GA, McCabe EJ, White WB. Long-term reproducibility of ambulatory blood pressure. *J Hypertens* 1994; 12(6):703–08.

48. Pickering T. Recommendations for the use of home (self) and ambulatory blood pressure monitoring. American Society of Hypertension Ad Hoc Panel. *Am J Hypertens* 1996;9(1):1–11.

49. O'Brien E, Staessen J. What is hypertension? *Lancet* 1999;353: 1541–42.

50. Lip GY, Beevers DG. "Reverse dipping" on ambulatory blood pressure monitoring. *J Hum Hypertens* 1997; 11(12):821–22.

51. Cavelaars M, Tulen JH, Man in't Veld AJ, Gelsema ES, van den Meiracker AH. Assessment of body position to quantify its effect on nocturnal blood pressure under ambulatory conditions. *J Hypertens* 2000;18(12):1737–43.

52. Lusardi P, Mugellini A, Preti P, Zoppi A, Derosa G, Fogari R. Effects of a restricted sleep regimen on ambulatory blood pressure monitoring in normotensive subjects. *Am J Hypertens* 1996;9(5):503–05.

53. Pedulla M, Silvestri R, Lasco A, Mento G, Lanuzza B, Sofia L, et al. Sleep structure in essential hypertensive patients: Differences between dippers and non-dippers. *Blood Press* 1995; 4(4):232–37.

54. Portaluppi F, Provini F, Cortelli P, Plazzi G, Bertozzi N, Manfredini R, et al. Undiagnosed sleep-disordered breathing among male nondippers with essential hypertension. *J Hypertens* 1997;15(11):1227–33.

55. Hla KM, Young TB, Bidwell T, Palta M, Skatrud JB, Dempsey J. Sleep apnea and hypertension: A population-based study. *Ann Intern Med* 1994;120(5): 382–88.

56. Uzu T, Ishikawa K, Fujii T, Nakamura S, Inenaga T, Kimura G. Sodium restriction shifts circadian rhythm of blood pressure from nondipper to dipper in essential hypertension. *Circulation* 1997;96(6):1859–62.

57. O'Shea JC, Murphy MB. Nocturnal blood pressure dipping: A consequence of diurnal physical activity blipping? *Am J Hypertens* 2000;13(6/1):601–06.

58. Profant J, Dimsdale JE. Race and diurnal blood pressure patterns: A review and meta-analysis. *Hypertension* 1999; 33(5):1099–1104.

59. Pickering TG, Kario K. Nocturnal non-dipping: what does it augur? *Curr Opin Nephrol Hypertens* 2001;10(5): 611–16.

60. Manning G, Rushton L, Donnelly R, Millar-Craig MW. Variability of diurnal changes in ambulatory blood pressure and nocturnal dipping status in untreated hypertensive and normotensive subjects. *Am J Hypertens* 2000;13(9):1035–38.

61. Omboni S, Parati G, Palatini P, Vanasia A, Muiesan ML, Cuspidi C, et al. Reproducibility and clinical value of nocturnal hypotension: prospective evidence from the SAMPLE study: Study on Ambulatory Monitoring of Pressure and Lisinopril Evaluation. *J Hypertens* 1998;16(6):733–38.

62. Cuspidi C, Meani S, Salerno M, Valerio C, Fusi V, Severgnini B, et al. Reproducibility of nocturnal blood pressure fall in early phases of untreated essential hypertension: A prospective observational study. *J Hum Hypertens* 2004;18(7):503–09.

63. Ohkubo T, Hozawa A, Yamaguchi J, Kikuya M, Ohmori K, Michimata M, et al. Prognostic significance of the nocturnal decline in blood pressure in individuals with and without high 24-h blood pressure: The Ohasama study. *J Hypertens* 2002;20(11): 2183–89.

64. Verdecchia P, Schillaci G, Borgioni C, Ciucci A, Gattobigio R, Porcellati C. Nocturnal pressure is the true pressure. *Blood Press Monit* 1996;1(2):S81–85.

65. Staessen J, Thijs L, Fagard R, O'Brien E, Clement D, de Leeuw PW, et al. Predicting cardiovascular risk using conventional vs ambulatory blood pressure in older patients with systolic hypertension. *JAMA* 2000;282:539–46.

66. Kario K, Pickering TG, Umeda Y, Hoshide S, Hoshide Y, Morinari M, et al. Morning surge in blood pressure as a predictor of silent and clinical cerebrovascular disease in elderly hypertensives: A prospective study. *Circulation* 2003;107(10):1401–06.

67. Bjorklund K, Lind L, Zethelius B, Berglund L, Lithell H. Prognostic significance of 24-h ambulatory blood pressure characteristics for cardiovascular morbidity in a population of elderly men. *J Hypertens* 2004;22(9):1691–97.

68. Clement DL, De Buyzere ML, De Bacquer DA, de Leeuw PW, Duprez DA, Fagard RH, et al. Prognostic value of ambulatory blood-pressure recordings in patients with treated hypertension. *N Engl J Med* 2003;348(24):2407–15.

69. Timio M, Venanzi S, Lolli S, Lippi G, Verdura C, Monarca C, et al. "Non-dipper" hypertensive patients and progressive renal insufficiency: A 3-year longitudinal study. *Clin Nephrol* 1995;43(6):382–87.

70. Jacob P, Hartung R, Bohlender J, Stein G. Utility of 24-h ambulatory blood pressure measurement in a routine clinical setting of patients with chronic renal disease. *J Hum Hypertens* 2004;18(10):745–51.

71. Tripepi G, Fagugli RM, Dattolo P, Parlongo G, Mallamaci F, Buoncristiani U, et al. Prognostic value of 24-hour ambulatory blood pressure monitoring and of night/day ratio in nondiabetic, cardiovascular events-free hemodialysis patients. *Kidney Int* 2005;68(3): 1294–1302.

72. Johnstone MT, Mittleman M, Tofler G, Muller JE. The pathophysiology of the onset of morning cardiovascular events. *Am J Hypertens* 1996;9(4/3):22S-28S.

73. Metoki H, Ohkubo T, Kikuya M, Asayama K, Obara T, Hashimoto J, et al. Prognostic significance for stroke of a morning pressor surge and a nocturnal blood pressure decline: The Ohasama study. *Hypertension* 2006;47(2):149–54.

74. Kario K, Pickering TG, Hoshide S, Eguchi K, Ishikawa J, Morinari M, et al. Morning blood pressure surge and hypertensive cerebrovascular disease: Role of the alpha adrenergic sympathetic nervous system. *Am J Hypertens* 2004;17(8):668–75.

75. Ishikawa J, Hoshide S, Shibasaki S, Matsui Y, Kabutoya T, Eguchi K, et al. The Japan Morning Surge-1 (JMS-1) study: Protocol description. *Hypertens Res* 2006;29(3):153–59.

76. Levy D, Garrison RJ, Savage DD, Kannel WB, Castelli WP. Prognostic implications of echocardiographically determined left ventricular mass in the Framingham Heart Study. *N Engl J Med* 1990;322(22):1561–66.

77. Jeong D-U, Dimsdale JE. The effects of caffeine on blood pressure in the work environment. *Amer J Hypertens* 1990; 3:749–53.

78. Suzuki Y, Kuwajima I, Kanemaru A, Shimosawa T, Hoshino S, Sakai M, et al. The cardiac functional reserve in elderly hypertensive patients with abnormal diurnal change in blood pressure. *J Hypertens* 1992;10(2):173–79.

79. Verdecchia P, Schillaci G, Borgioni C, Ciucci A, Sacchi N, Battistelli M, et al. Gender, day-night blood pressure changes, and left ventricular mass in essential hypertension: Dippers and peakers. *Am J Hypertens* 1995; 8(2):193–96.

80. Mayet J, Shahi M, Hughes AD, Stanton AV, Poulter NR, Sever PS, et al. Left ventricular structure and function in previously untreated hypertensive patients: The importance of blood pressure, the nocturnal blood pressure dip and heart rate. *J Cardiovasc Risk* 1995;2(3):255–61.

81. Ferrara AL, Pasanisi F, Crivaro M, Guida L, Palmieri V, Gaeta I, et al. Cardiovascular abnormalities in never-treated hypertensives according to nondipper status. *Am J Hypertens* 1998;11(11/1):1352–57.

82. Roman MJ, Pickering TG, Schwartz JE, Cavallini MC, Pini R, Devereux RB. Is the absence of a normal nocturnal fall in blood pressure (nondipping) associated with cardiovascular target organ damage? *J Hypertens* 1997; 15(9):969–78.

83. Cuspidi C, Lonati L, Sampieri L, Macca G, Valagussa F, Zaro T, et al. Impact of nocturnal fall in blood pressure on early cardiovascular changes in essential hypertension. *J Hypertens* 2000;17:1339–44.

84. Cuspidi C, Michev I, Meani S, Severgnini B, Fusi V, Corti C, et al. Reduced nocturnal fall in blood pressure, assessed by two ambulatory blood pressure monitorings and cardiac alterations in early phases of untreated essential hypertension. *J Hum Hypertens* 2003;17(4):245–51.

85. Kario K, Matsuo T, Kobayashi H, Imiya M, Matsuo M, Shimada K. Nocturnal fall of blood pressure and silent cerebrovascular damage in elderly hypertensive patients: Advanced silent cerebrovascular damage in extreme dippers. *Hypertension* 1996; 27(1):130–35.

86. MacMahon S, Collins G, Rautaharju P, et al. Electrocardiographic left ventricular hypertrophy and effects of antihypertensive drug therapy in hypertensive participants in the Multiple Risk Factor Intervention Trial. *Am J Cardiology* 1989;63:202–10.

87. Kobayashi S, Okada K, Koide H, Bokura H, Yamaguchi S. Subcortical silent brain infarction as a risk factor for clinical stroke. *Stroke* 1997;28(10): 1932–39.

88. Palatini P, Canali C, Dorigatti F, Baccillieri S, Giovinazzo P, Roman E, et al. Target organ damage and ambulatory blood pressure in stage I hypertension: The Hypertension and Ambulatory Recording Venetia Study. *Blood Press Monit* 1997;2(2):79–88.

89. Bald M, Kubel S, Rascher W. Validity and reliability of 24hr blood pressure monitoring in children and adolescents using a portable, oscillometric device. *J Hum Hypertens* 1994;8:363–66.

90. Pierdomenico SD, Lapenna D, Guglielmi MD, Antidormi T, Schiavone C, Cuccurullo F, et al. Target organ status and serum lipids in patients with white coat hypertension. *Hypertension* 1995;26(5):801–07.

91. Cavallini MC, Roman MJ, Pickering TG, Schwartz JE, Pini R, Deveraux RB. Is white coat hypertension associated with arterial disease or left ventricular hypertrophy? *Hypertens* 1995;26: 413–19.

92. Perloff D, Sokolow M, Cowan RM, Juster RP. Prognostic value of ambulatory blood pressure measurements: Further analyses. *J Hypertens* Suppl 1989;7(3):S3–10.

93. Verdecchia P, Porcellati C, Schillaci G, Borgioni C, Ciucci A, Battistelli M, et al. Ambulatory blood pressure: An independent predictor of prognosis in essential hypertension. *Hypertension* 1994;24(6):793–801.

94. Sega R, Facchetti R, Bombelli M, Cesana G, Corrao G, Grassi G, et al. Prognostic value of ambulatory and home blood pressures compared with office blood pressure in the general population: Follow-up results from the Pressioni Arteriose Monitorate e Loro Associazioni (PAMELA) study. *Circulation* 2005;111(14):1777–83.

95. Kario K, Shimada K, Schwartz JE, Matsuo T, Hoshide S, Pickering TG. Silent and clinically overt stroke in older Japanese subjects with white-coat and sustained hypertension. *J Am Coll Cardiol* 2001;38(1):238–45.

96. Khattar RS, Senior R, Lahiri A. Cardiovascular outcome in white-coat versus sustained mild hypertension: A 10-year follow-up study. *Circulation* 1998;98(18):1892–97.

97. Dolan E, Stanton A, Thijs L, Hinedi K, Atkins N, McClory S, et al. Superiority of ambulatory over clinic blood pressure measurement in predicting mortality: The Dublin outcome study. *Hypertension* 2005;46(1):156–61.

98. Fagard RH, Van Den BC, De Cort P. Prognostic significance of blood pressure measured in the office, at home and during ambulatory monitoring in older patients in general practice. *J Hum Hypertens* 2005; 19(10):801–07.

99. O'Brien E, Asmar R, Beilin L, Imai K, Mancia G, Mengden T, et al. Practice Guidelines of the European Society of Hypertension for Clinic, Ambulatory, and Self Blood Pressure Measurement. *J Hypertens* 2005.

100. Redon J, Campos C, Narciso ML, Rodicio JL, Pascual JM, Ruilope LM. Prognostic value of ambulatory blood pressure monitoring in refractory hypertension: a prospective study. *Hypertension* 1998;31(2):712–18.

101. Frattola A, Parati G, Cuspidi C, Albini F, Mancia G. Prognostic value of 24-hour blood pressure variability. *J Hypertens* 1993;11:1133–37.

102. Verdecchia P, Borgioni C, Ciucci A, Gattobigio R, Schillaci G, Sacchi N, et al. Prognostic significance of blood pressure variability in essential hypertension. *Blood Press Monit* 1996;1(1):3–11.

103. Ayman P, Goldshine AD. Blood pressure determinations by patients with essential hypertension I: The difference between clinic and home readings before treatment. *Am J Med Sci* 1940;200:465–74.

104. Cuspidi C, Meani S, Lonati L, Fusi V, Magnaghi G, Garavelli G, et al. Prevalence of home blood pressure measurement among selected hypertensive patients: Results of a multicenter survey from six hospital outpatient hypertension clinics in Italy. *Blood Press* 2005;14(4):251–256.

105. Beckman M, Panfilov V, Sivertsson R, Sannerstedt R, Andersson O. Blood pressure and heart rate recordings at home and at the clinic: Evidence for increased cardiovascular reactivity in young men with mild blood pressure elevation. *Acta Med Scand* 1981; 210(1/2):97–102.

106. Kleinert HD, Harshfield GA, Pickering TG, Devereux RB, Sullivan PA, Marion RM, et al. What is the value of home blood pressure measurement in patients with mild hypertension? *Hypertension* 1984;6(4):574–78.

107. Divison JA, Sanchis C, Artigao LM, Carbayo JA, Carrion-Valero L, Lopez DC, et al. Home-based self-measurement of blood pressure: A proposal using new reference values (the PURAS study). *Blood Press Monit* 2004;9(4):211–18.

108. Mancia G, Sega R, Bravi C, De Vito G, Valagussa F, Cesana G, et al. Ambulatory blood pressure normality: Results from the PAMELA study. *J Hypertens* 1995;13(12/1):1377–90.

109. Kjeldsen SE, Hedner T, Jamerson K, Julius S, Haley WE, Zabalgoitia M, et al. Hypertension optimal treatment (HOT) study: Home blood pressure in treated hypertensive subjects. *Hypertension* 1998;31(4):1014–20.

110. Corcoran AC, Dustan HP, Page IH. The evaluation of antihypertensive procedures, with particular reference to their effects on blood pressure. *Ann Int Med* 1955;43:1161–77.

111. Laughlin KD, Fisher L, Sherrard DJ. Blood pressure reductions during self-recording of home blood pressure. *Am Heart J* 1979;98(5):629–34.

112. Kenny RA, Brennan M, O'Malley K, O'Brien E. Blood pressure measurements in borderline hypertension. *J Hypertens* 1987;5 (5):483–85.

113. Stergiou GS, Efstathiou SP, Alamara CV, Mastorantonakis SE, Roussias LG. Home or self blood pressure measurement? What is the correct term? *J Hypertens* 2003;21(12): 2259–64.

114. Mengden T, Schwartzkopff B, Strauer BE. What is the value of home (self) blood pressure monitoring in patients with hypertensive heart disease? *Am J Hypertens* 1998; 11:813–19.

115. Jyothinagaram SG, Rae L, Campbell A, Padfield PL. Stability of home blood pressure over time. *J Hum Hypertens* 1990;4(3):269–71.

116. Stergiou GS, Baibas NM, Gantzarou AP, Skeva II, Kalkana CB, Roussias LG, et al. Reproducibility of home, ambulatory, and clinic blood pressure: Implications for the design of trials for the assessment of antihypertensive drug efficacy. *Am J Hypertens* 2002; 15(2/1):101–04.

117. Sakuma M, Imai Y, Nagai K, Watanabe N, Sakuma H, Minami N, et al. Reproducibility of home blood pressure measurements over a 1-year period. *Am J Hypertens* 1997; 10(7/1):798–803.

118. Mejia AD, Julius S, Jones KA, Schork NJ, Kneisley J. The Tecumseh Blood Pressure Study: Normative data on blood pressure self-determination. *Arch Intern Med* 1990;150(6):1209–13.

119. Staessen J, Bulpitt CJ, Fagard R, Mancia G, O'Brien ET, Thijs L, et al. Reference values for the ambulatory blood pressure and the blood pressure measured at home: A population study. *J Hum Hypertens* 1991;5(5):355–61.

120. Sega G, Bravi C, Cesana G, Valagussa F, Mancia G, Zanchetti A. Ambulatory and home blood pressure normality: The Pamela Study. *J Cardiovasc Pharmacol* 1994;23(5):S12–15.

121. Mancia G, Sega R, Grassi G, Cesana G, Zanchetti A. Defining ambulatory and home blood pressure normality: Further considerations based on data from the PAMELA study. *J Hypertens* 2001;19(6):995–99.

122. Thijs L, Staessen JA, Celis H, de Gaudemaris R, Imai Y, Julius S, et al. Reference values for self-recorded blood pressure: A meta-analysis of summary data. *Arch Intern Med* 1998; 158(5):481–88.

123. Sega R, Cesana G, Milesi C, Grassi G, Zanchetti A, Mancia G. Ambulatory and home blood pressure normality in the elderly: Data from the PAMELA population. *Hypertension* 1997; 30(1/1):1–6.

124. Ohkubo T, Imai Y, Tsuji I, Nagai K, Ito S, Satoh H, et al. Reference values for 24-hour ambulatory blood pressure monitoring based on a prognostic criterion: The Ohasama Study. *Hypertension* 1998;32(2):255–59.

125. Pickering T.G., Hall JE, Appel LJ, Falkner B, Graves JW, Hill MN, et al. Recommendations for blood pressure measurement in humans: An AHA Scientific Statement from the Council on High Blood Pressure Research, Professional and Public Education Subcommittee. *Hypertension* 2005; 45:142–61.

126. Ibrahim MM, Tarazi RC, Dustan HP, Gifford RWJ. Electrocardiogram in evaluation of resistance to antihypertensive therapy. *Arch Intern Med* 1977;137(9):1125–29.

127. Verdecchia P, Bentivoglia M, Providenza M, Savino K, Corea L. Reliability of home self-recorded arterial pressure in essential hypertension in relation to the stage of the disease. In G Germano (ed.), *Blood Pressure Recording in the Clinical Management of Hypertension*. Rome: Ediziono Pozzi 1985:40–42.

128. Mule G, Caimi G, Cottone S, Nardi E, Andronico G, Piazza G, et al. Value of home blood pressures as predictor of target organ damage in mild arterial hypertension. *J Cardiovasc Risk* 2002; 9(2):123–29.

129. Cuspidi C, Michev I, Meani S, Salerno M, Valerio C, Fusi V, et al. Left ventricular hypertrophy in treated hypertensive patients with good blood pressure control outside the clinic, but poor clinic blood pressure control. *J Hypertens* 2003;21(8):1575–81.

130. Sakaguchi K, Horimatsu T, Kishi M, Takeda A, Ohnishi Y, Koike T, et al. Isolated home hypertension in the morning is associated with target organ damage in patients with type 2 diabetes. J Atheroscler Thromb 2005; 12(4):225–31.

131. Tachibana R, Tabara Y, Kondo I, Miki T, Kohara K. Home blood pressure is a better predictor of carotid atherosclerosis than office blood pressure in community-dwelling subjects. Hypertens Res 2004;27: 633–39.

132. Imai Y, Ohkubo T, Tsuji I, Nagai K, Satoh H, Hisamichi S, et al. Prognostic value of ambulatory and home blood pressure measurements in comparison to screening blood pressure measurements: A pilot study in Ohasama. Blood Press Monit 1996; 1(2):S51–58.

133. Tsuji I, Imai Y, Nagai K, Ohkubo T, Watanabe N, Minami N, et al. Proposal of reference values for home blood pressure measurement: prognostic criteria based on a prospective observation of the general population in Ohasama, Japan. Am J Hypertens 1997;10(4/1):409–18.

134. Ohkubo T, Asayama K, Kikuya M, Metoki H, Hoshi H, Hashimoto J, et al. How many times should blood pressure be measured at home for better prediction of stroke risk? Ten-year follow-up results from the Ohasama study. J Hypertens 2004; 22(6):1099–1104.

135. Bobrie G, Chatellier G, Genes N, Clerson P, Vaur L, Vaisse B, et al. Cardiovascular prognosis of "masked hypertension" detected by blood pressure self-measurement in elderly treated hypertensive patients. JAMA 2004;291(11):1342–49.

136. Kikuya M, Hozawa A, Ohokubo T, Tsuji I, Michimata M, Matsubara M, et al. Prognostic significance of blood pressure and heart rate variabilities: The Ohasama study. Hypertension 2000;36(5):901–06.

137. Hozawa A, Ohkubo T, Nagai K, Kikuya M, Matsubara M, Tsuji I, et al. Prognosis of isolated systolic and isolated diastolic hypertension as assessed by self-measurement of blood pressure at home: The Ohasama study. Arch Intern Med 2000;160(21): 3301–06.

138. Nesbitt SD, Amerena JV, Grant E, Jamerson KA, Lu H, Weder A, et al. Home blood pressure as a predictor of future blood pressure stability in borderline hypertension: The Tecumseh Study. Am J Hypertens 1997;10(11): 1270–80.

139. Rave K, Bender R, Heise T, Sawicki PT. Value of blood pressure self-monitoring as a predictor of progression of diabetic nephropathy. J Hypertens 1999;17(5): 597–601.

140. Pickering TG. Blood pressure variability and ambulatory monitoring. Curr Opin Nephrol Hypertens 1993;2(3):380–85.

141. Pickering TG. The ninth Sir George Pickering memorial lecture: Ambulatory monitoring and the definition of hypertension. J Hypertens 1992;10(5):401–09.

142. Pickering TG, Levenstein M, Walmsley P. Differential effects of doxazosin on clinic and ambulatory pressure according to age, gender, and presence of white coat hypertension: Results of the HALT Study. Hypertension and Lipid Trial Study Group. Am J Hypertens 1994; 7(9/1):848–52.

143. Fagard RH, Staessen JA, Thijs L, Gasowski J, Bulpitt CJ, Clement D, et al. Response to antihypertensive therapy in older patients with sustained and nonsustained systolic hypertension: Systolic Hypertension in Europe (Syst-Eur) Trial Investigators. Circulation 2000;102 (10):1139–44.

144. Verdecchia P, Reboldi GP, Angeli F, Schillaci G, Schwartz JE, Pickering TG, et al. Short- and long-term incidence of stroke in white-coat hypertension. Hypertension 2005;45(2):203–08.

145. Ugajin T, Hozawa A, Ohkubo T, Asayama K, Kikuya M, Obara T, et al. White-coat hypertension as a risk factor for the development of home hypertension: The Ohasama study. Arch Intern Med 2005; 165(13):1541–46.

146. Verdecchia P, Reboldi GP, Angeli F, Schillaci G, Schwartz JE, Pickering TG, et al. Short- and long-term incidence of stroke in white-coat hypertension. Hypertension 2005;45(2):203–08.

147. Obara T, Ohkubo T, Kikuya M, Asayama K, Metoki H, Inoue R, et al. Prevalence of masked uncontrolled and treated white-coat hypertension defined according to the average of morning and evening home blood pressure value: From the Japan Home versus Office Measurement Evaluation Study. Blood Press Monit 2005;10(6): 311–16.

148. Pierdomenico SD, Lapenna D, Bucci A, di Tommaso R, di Mascio R, Manente BM, et al. Cardiovascular outcome in treated hypertensive patients with responder, masked, false resistant and true resistant hypertension. Am J Hypertens 2005;.

149. Liu JE, Roman MJ, Pini R, Schwartz JE, Pickering TG, Devereux RB. Cardiac and arterial target organ damage in adults with elevated ambulatory and normal office blood pressure. Ann Intern Med 1999;131(8):564–72.

150. Stergiou GS, Salgami EV, Tzamouranis DG, Roussias LG. Masked hypertension assessed by ambulatory blood pressure versus home blood pressure monitoring: Is it the same phenomenon? Am J Hypertens 2005;18(6):772–78.

151. Imai Y, Tsuji I, Nagai K, Sakuma M, Ohkubo T, Watanabe N, et al. Ambulatory blood pressure monitoring in evaluating the prevalence of hypertension in adults in Ohasama, a rural Japanese community. Hypertens Res 1996;19(3):207–12.

152. Sega R, Trocino G, Lanzarotti A, Carugo S, Cesana G, Schiavina R, et al. Alterations of cardiac structure in patients with isolated office, ambulatory, or home hypertension: Data from the general population (Pressione Arteriose Monitorate E Loro Associazioni [PAMELA] Study). Circulation 2001;104(12):1385–92.

153. Kawabe H, Saito I, Saruta T. Status of home blood pressure measured in morning and evening: Evaluation in normotensives and hypertensives in Japanese urban population. Hypertens Res 2005;28(6):491–98.

154. Littler WA, Honour AJ. Direct arterial pressure, heart rate, and electrocardiogram in unrestricted patients before and after removal of a phaeochromocyoma. Q J Med 1974;43(171):441–49.

155. Shear MK, Polan JJ, Harshfield GA, Pickering TG, Mann JJ, Frances A, et al. Ambulatory monitoring of blood pressure and heart rate in panic patients. J Anxiety Dis 1992;6:213–21.

156. Mann S, Altman DG, Raftery EB, Bannister R. Circadian variation of blood pressure in autonomic failure. Circulation 1983;68(3):477–83.

157. Redman CW. Controlled trials of antihypertensive drugs in pregnancy. Am J Kidney Dis 1991;17(2):149–53.

158. Denolle T, Daniel JC, Calvez C, Ottavioli JN, Esnault V, Herpin D. Home blood pressure during normal pregnancy. Am J Hypertens 2005; 18(9/1):1178–80.

159. Pickering TG. Reflections in hypertension. How should blood pressure be measured during pregnancy? J Clin Hypertens (Greenwich) 2005;7(1):46–49.

160. Mancia G, Zanchetti A, Agabiti-Rosei E, Benemio G, De Cesaris R, Fogari R, et al. Ambulatory blood pressure is superior to clinic blood pressure in predicting treatment-induced regression of left ventricular hypertrophy: SAMPLE Study Group. Study on Ambulatory Monitoring of Blood Pressure and Lisinopril Evaluation. Circulation 1997;95(6):1464–70.

161. Uzu T, Kimura G. Diuretics shift circadian rhythm of blood pressure from nondipper to dipper in essential hypertension. Circulation 1999; 100(15):1635–38.

162. Kario K, Shimada K. Differential effects of amlodipine on ambulatory blood pressure in elderly hypertensive patients with different nocturnal reductions in blood pressure. Am J Hypertens 1997;10(3):261–68.

163. Portaluppi F, Vergnani L, Manfredini R, degli UE, Fersini C. Time-dependent effect of isradipine on the nocturnal hypertension in chronic renal failure. Am J Hypertens 1995;8(7):719–26.

164. Leeman MJ, Lins RL, Sternon JE, Huberlant BC, Fassotte CE. Effect of antihypertensive treatment on office and self-measured blood pressure: the Autodil study. J Hum Hypertens 2000; 14(8):525–29.

165. Ragot S, Genes N, Vaur L, Herpin D. Comparison of three blood pressure measurement methods for the evaluation of two antihypertensive drugs: feasibility, agreement, and reproducibility of blood pressure response. Am J Hypertens 2000; 13(6/1):632–39.

166. Mancia G, Parati G. Office compared with ambulatory blood pressure in assessing response to antihypertensive treatment: A meta-analysis. J Hypertens 2004;22(3):435–45.

167. Ohkubo T, Hozawa A, Nagatomi R, Fujita K, Sauvaget C, Watanabe Y, et al. Effects of exercise training on home blood pressure values in older adults: A randomized controlled trial. J Hypertens 2001;19(6):1045–52.

168. Ogedegbe G, Schoenthaler A. A systematic review of the effects of home blood pressure monitoring on medication adherence. *J Clin Hypertens (Greenwich)* 2006; 8(3):174–80.

169. Cappuccio FP, Kerry SM, Forbes L, Donald A. Blood pressure control by home monitoring: meta-analysis of randomised trials. *BMJ* 2004; 329(7458):145.

170. Krakoff LR. Cost-effectiveness of ambulatory blood pressure: A reanalysis. *Hypertension* 2006;47(1):29–34.

171. White WB. Advances in ambulatory blood pressure monitoring for the evaluation of antihypertensive therapy in research and practice. In WB White WB (ed.), *Blood Pressure Monitoring in Cardiovascular Medicine and Therapeutics*. Totowa, NJ: Humana Press 2005: 273–94.

172. Svensson P, de Faire U, Sleight P, Yusuf S, Ostergren J. Comparative effects of ramipril on ambulatory and office blood pressures: A HOPE Substudy. *Hypertension* 2001; 38(6):E28–32.

173. Effects of an angiotensin-converting-enzyme inhibitor, ramipril, on cardiovascular events in high risk patients: Heart Outcomes Prevention Evaluation Study Investigators. *NEJM* 2000;342:145–53.

Chapter

46 Cardiologic Investigation of the Hypertensive Patient

Robert J. MacFadyen

Key Findings

- Cardiological investigation in hypertension supplements blood pressure definition and management but does not supplant it.
- The sensitivity and specificity of many standard cardiologic investigations are fundamentally altered in hypertension.
- Although hypertension overlaps profoundly with coronary disease, not all patients with cardiac symptoms have coronary disease.
- Definitive assessment of cardiac status is critical in the definition and management of the risk of future occlusive vascular events in individual hypertensive patients and relies heavily on an integrated approach to cardiac test strategies.

The cardiologic investigation of a patient with hypertension is an important clinical topic with many relevant clinical lessons and a large amount of research to be considered, but this tends to get confused with the definition of a "new" disease (for example, coronary artery disease or valvular heart disease). This can lead to a misplaced focus on these linked pathologies at the expense of continuing emphasis on the definition and management of hypertension. Losing track of the importance of hypertension care while embarking on relevant cardiac investigation is a critical mistake that can nullify any benefits in subsequent cardiac management—whether by percutaneous interventional treatments or cardiac surgery.

Epidemiologic study reveals many independent statistical associations between hypertension and the evolution of a range of cardiac disease processes. Although it has been widely demonstrated that treating blood pressure alone can reduce the relative risk of future cardiac events,[1] it is essential that the many well-described aspects of cardiac structural and functional investigation are applied correctly in clinical practice. There is the necessity for individual physicians to appreciate the changes in sensitivity and specificity of cardiologic testing procedures that are applicable to the hypertensive patient. Indeed, it is important to apply appropriate testing patterns adjusted to the hypertensive patient wisely and without the need to apply every known test to every patient nor to over- or underinterpret the results obtained during these work-ups.

Myocardial ischemia

The relationship between coronary disease and hypertension is a complex one. The pathology of atherosclerosis and vascular degeneration is accelerated in the process of symptomatic and asymptomatic coronary artery disease, providing the link to both fatal and nonfatal coronary occlusive events. The definition of symptomatic coronary disease is confounded by the recognition of hypertension, which may have been present in the asymptomatic patient for some years. Thus, the diagnosis (or rather, recognition) of hypertension has a confounding association with the onset of symptomatic coronary artery disease. In a proportion of cases, death from a fatal first coronary occlusion can occur before hypertension is diagnosed or recognized as a primary factor in the development of coronary atherosclerosis in the index case. This is not a new association,[2] and the temporal sequence of these critical events has long been a source of concern.[3] Alternatively, the onset of ischemic symptoms in patients with hypertension is generally associated with fairly prompt testing to try to define the presence of myocardial ischemia and/or to exclude coronary disease.

Valvular function

It is generally appreciated that there are associations between hypertension and degenerative valvular heart disease. Specifically, these relate to left heart valve function and the aortic valve in particular. As with coronary artery atheroma, the coming together of degenerative changes in valve structure along with changes in vascular compliance and structure create increased pressure after load in the arterial system (a well-accepted detrimental phenomenon associated both with valvular stenosis and regurgitation in the aortic position). Valvular function in the mitral position can equally be affected by secondary myocardial remodeling of the left ventricle, which is common and may be severe in some hypertensive patients (see material following).

Restrictive myocardial changes and ventricular hypertrophy

Restrictive cardiac-filling abnormalities (primarily due to the myocardial hypertrophy associated with hypertension) are features that are often confused and that are to an increasing extent seen to overlap with hypertrophic myogenic or infiltrative cardiac disease. The range of hypertrophic cardiomyopathies in particular can be difficult to differentiate from hypertensive disease (e.g., clinically with restrictive changes in the pericardium). Definition of the myocardial geometry and the contractile and relaxing functions of the heart in hypertension is therefore essential. The linkage of these myogenic responses to the appearance of exercise limitation is important.

Ventricular function assessment

Net systolic contractility of the left ventricle is of great prognostic value and powerfully defines cardiac event rates in hypertensive patients. The evolution of hypertensive heart disease from the state of hypertrophic changes (with generally well-preserved systolic contractility) is a complex process (see other chapters), with progressive change through to a phase of ventricular dilatation and systolic impairment. These patients tend to have unrecognized, untreated, or persistently uncontrolled hypertension, and the progression to systolic impairment of the heart is not often recognized short of acute presentation of pulmonary edema. The widely cited but poorly analyzed association of arterial hypertension to systolic left ventricular impairment suggests the presence of such a progressive change regardless of the definition or recognition of intervening coronary occlusion and ventricular infarction.

Rhythm assessment

The primary changes in cardiac structure in hypertensive heart disease are also associated with changes in cardiac conduction and instability of cardiac rhythm. Similar to the situation with systolic ventricular impairment, these changes can occur with or without the impact of intervening intermittent cardiac ischemia or prior myocardial infarction. Much of the rhythm instability of hypertensive heart disease is asymptomatic until late in the disease, where there are major myocardial changes linked to hypertensive left ventricular hypertrophy and or ventricular infarction. Both resting conduction and ambulatory cardiac rhythm need to be considered.

SYMPTOMATIC STATE: SYMPTOMS IN HYPERTENSION

The investigation of the heart in hypertensive patients starts either at the detection of asymptomatic hypertension at chance screening or upon the presentation of linked or unlinked cardiac or general symptoms. The presence of symptomatic complaints among patients with hypertension is commonly the subject of population investigation. These do not often indicate a causal link, and separating these on the basis of clinical presentation alone can often be problematic.[4] In the interpretation of cardiac symptoms in hypertensive patients, similar problems apply.

A good example is the association between hypertension and headache. Although the association may be more direct in the case of patients with severe uncontrolled or untreated hypertension, most studies have conclusively shown that mild hypertension and headache are *not* causally associated. In a large sample of 1763 hypertensive patients, for example, intermittent headache was present in 903 subjects (51.3% of entire sample), and from these 378 of the patients (21.4%) were classified as having moderate to severe hypertension (stage III of the JNC-VI classification system). However, the diagnosis of moderate to severe hypertension was clearly not independently associated with headache (OR 1.02, 95% CI from 0.79 to 1.30) and arterial pulse pressure and headache were in fact *inversely* associated (OR 0.91, 95% CI from 0.86 to 0.97, for 10 mmHg).[5]

Many studies are directed at the impact of concomitant drug therapy on the symptomatic state of hypertensive patients. In this regard, the quality of life of untreated patients with hypertension is complex (dealt with elsewhere in this textbook). However, some symptoms due to treatment are of the orthostatic variety (dizziness, postural light-headedness, presyncope). Syncope is relatively rare, but among those with a documented episode of true syncope hypertension is a common co-morbidity, occurring in about 25% of patients.[6] There are simple biological links among syncope, hypertensive vascular disease, and cardiac function. For example, syncope is common among elderly hypertensive patients with preexisting or co-existent sinus node disease[7] and/or carotid sinus disease.[8] Furthermore, orthostatic symptoms are likely to be more common where patients have a white coat response yet normal ambulatory blood pressure (BP) and receive inappropriate hypotensive drug treatment. In addition, patients with neurodegenerative diseases affecting the dentato-rubro-spinothalamic pathways (which produce a spectrum of disorders from primary autonomic failure through to more mixed effects characterized by supine hypertension and orthostatic hypotension) are often grouped as neurocardiogenic syncope. The individual composition and origin of BP effects in these often elderly patients can be complex and require detailed assessment to define autonomic, arterial vasodilator, and/or cardiogenic (largely a vagal dromotropic response) elements.[9]

The link between chest pain symptoms and hypertension is probably the most important one for the average hypertensive patient and the responsible clinician. There is clearly a worsening outcome in terms of emergent cardiac events in patients with undiagnosed chest pain who have hypertension, and this is explained by the greater prevalence of coronary disease and underlying myocardial ischemia. There is a clear-cut profile of elevated risk of an acute cardiac event associated with an acute symptom onset[10] as opposed to patterns of undifferentiated chronic symptoms. In this regard, symptomatic presentation *alone* (regardless of its detailed characteristics) is a parameter neither sensitive nor specific enough to define the emergence of coronary disease in the hypertensive patient. For example, the electrocardiograph can contain many valuable observations but is at the same time inherently a very limited test strategy in the hypertensive patient.

THE INVESTIGATION OF THE HEART IN HYPERTENSIVE PATIENTS

The surface electrocardiograph (ECG/EKG) has been a fundamental part of basic cardiac assessment for over a century. Its utility comes from the ease of documentation and technical simplicity. Its value is amplified by repeated recordings made in a consistent fashion, and in particular where performed during a symptomatic episode (whether of pain, palpitation, or breathlessness). In hypertensive patients (as in other patient groups) its primary drawback (used at rest, continuously, or during exercise stress) is its demonstrably low sensitivity (failing to identify cardiac disease where this is present) and low specificity (suggesting cardiac disease when in fact none is present) to define even simple and common cardiac processes such as regional myocardial ischemia or global or regional ventricular hypertrophy. As the key aspects in the diagnostic management of hypertension are to assess reversible ischemia, evolving infarction, or patterns of cardiac hypertrophy, the ECG is clearly limited.

Rest ECG

The utility of the baseline electrocardiogram (ECG) has been defined in large population surveys. The prevalence of *any* electrocardiographic abnormality (regardless of significance) is increased in patients with hypertension compared to normotensive controls.

For example, in 1190 hypertensive patients from the WHO Community control program for Hypertension in Italy,[11] the overall prevalence of any 12-lead electrocardiographic abnormalities (i.e., all Minnesota codes) was 40.8%, with a slightly higher prevalence in males than in females (at 42.4 versus 39.4%). Electrocardiographic LVH (ECG-LVH; see material following) was more frequent in males (21.2%) than in females (14.5%), but not for ECG changes indicative of ischaemia (4:1 to 4:3 or 5:1 to 5:3). The prevalence of ECG abnormalities increased with age, with the exception of ECG-LVH. Predictably, younger males in the age class 20 to 29 years showed these more often (11.1 to 17.5% of the subjects, where these findings will often represent a false positive finding) than the oldest age group (60 to 64 years) where the prevalence of ECG-LVH ranged from 12.4–15.2%.

The prevalence of electrocardiographic abnormalities is in part due to the high rate of nonspecific false positive results (such as T wave changes or conduction defects) interpreted as evidence of ischemia, infarction, or hypertrophy without supporting evidence from more definitive studies (see material following).

P-wave changes in hypertension

P-wave morphology can in part clearly reflect atrial dimensions and structure.[12] It can therefore readily be seen as a reasonable point of interest on the surface ECG in hypertension—whether in sustained sinus rhythm or recorded in the phase before persistent atrial fibrillation is established in susceptible hypertensive patients. Studies in hypertension in general show a complex link between P-wave morphology on the rest ECG and cardiac structure. In several surveys of hypertensive patients, the most frequent rest ECG abnormality is an abnormal P-wave (duration or voltage; 23%). This compares with the much lesser prevalence of abnormal repolarization (10%), increased limb lead or chest lead QRS voltage (5.4%), and patterns of abnormal intraventricular conduction (10%).[13] In general, there is no simple correlation between abnormal P-wave and other ECG abnormalities, although patients with an abnormal P-wave are often shown to have higher systolic

blood pressure (SBP) and heart rate. The electrocardiographic findings are in general unresponsive to BP treatment, although this may simply be due to lack of sensitivity rather than to underlying structural change.

Genovesiebert et al.[14] explored the link between abnormal P-waves and structure in 53 untreated hypertensive patients. Although abnormal P-wave conformation was predictably common in their sample, they could not relate simple P-wave morphology (duration and voltage) to left atrial size or estimated LA volume as measured by echocardiography. However, they did show some relationship between abnormal P-wave morphology and trans-mitral Doppler indices of LV filling (see material following).[14] Thus, in patients with hypertension they suggest that simple P-wave changes indicative of LA abnormality were perhaps more likely to be indicative of increased left atrial work and mechanics, possibly secondary to an impaired ventricular filling rather than due to more simple left atrial enlargement.

To further address this lack of sensitivity of the P-wave in hypertension, some investigators have turned to the use of signal-averaging technology. This is similar in principle to the technology employed for many years in the assessment of ventricular conduction, defining the presence of after-potentials on repeatedly averaged and combined high-sensitivity ECG recordings and linking this to susceptibility to ventricular arrhythmia. In this setting studying a P-wave signal, averaged ECG (P-SAECG) has been analyzed in patients with hypertension. In 234 normotensive, 84 white hypertensive, and 34 black hypertensive patients undergoing P-SAECG analysis, Madu and colleagues[15] found that mean filtered P-wave duration and total P-wave time-voltage area for normotensives of either ethnic group were similar. However, hypertensive black patients had greater increase in P-wave duration (138 ±16 versus 132 ±12 ms; $p<0.01$) and total P-wave time-voltage area (922 ± 285 versus 764 ±198 µV.ms; $p<0.001$) than white hypertensive patients. In addition, the P-wave duration and total P-wave voltage integral increased with severity of hypertension.

Thus, the early stages of hypertension are associated with prolonged atrial conduction as defined using a resting P-SAECG and this index may better reflect the electrical remodeling of the atria. The changes seen in African American black hypertensive patients seem to be greater than those in white patients with hypertension and may link in with the greater cardiac structural changes seen in hypertension in black patients (see material following).

The role of the PR interval as an index of general autonomic tone reflecting atrial electrical conduction velocity has been confirmed in hypertensive patients.[16] However, the role of this simple measure in predicting (for example) the degeneration of sinus rhythm to either atrial fibrillation or atrioventricular block (both common features of electrophysiologic change in hypertension) has not yet been tested prospectively.

QT intervals and QT dispersion

Heart-rate-corrected QT interval is another important and well-studied general ECG marker of ventricular repolarization. It is generally susceptible to the prevailing level of autonomic tone, which is also the case in hypertensive patients. Prior to treatment, prolonged heart-rate-corrected QT interval is associated with higher risk of mortality in patients with coronary heart disease (CHD) and in the general population. Although unaffected by age, there is possibly a confounding effect of female gender[17] on the prognostic value of QT interval—and as with many ECG measures there is also some variance among patients of African descent (e.g., African American or Afro Caribbean).[18] Xiao and colleagues in a detailed, if small, cohort of hypertensive patients with pathologic ventricular hypertrophy (14/42 being due to the effects of hypertension, whereas the others had aortic valve disease or hypertrophic cardiomyopathy) suggested that QRS duration had a bimodal distribution and correlated with measured left ventricular mass only if the QRS duration was less than 135 msec.[19] In this study, the association of QRS duration and left ventricular mass was lost above a QTd figure of 135 msec, and perhaps predictably at these greater values correlated more with the onset of a proximal left bundle branch block and associated uncoordinated LV activation/contraction.

The presence of electrocardiographic intraventricular conduction delay and broad QRS duration are well documented in patients with hypertension. Although these are often automatically associated with the presence of epicardial coronary artery disease and prior infarction equally, they have been shown to have a strong association with hypertension *in the absence of CAD*[20] and more often reflect the impact of ventricular hypertrophy on intraventricular conduction.[21] Thus, the interpretation of these findings becomes more complex in separating structural change (hypertrophy) from functional changes (ischemia/infarction or intrinsic conduction disease), both of which obviously coexist in the hypertensive population (making conclusions from the individual ECG tracing of reduced value in the hypertensive population).

QT prolongation in the form of an analysis of the spatial dispersion of the QT interval (QT dispersion, corrected QT dispersion, or QT dispersion index) across the heart (most commonly a simple subtraction of maximal and minimal measured QT interval in msec across standard chest ECG leads) is a marker of adverse cardiac risk in hypertension,[22,23] in systolic heart failure,[24] in coronary artery disease, and even in the asymptomatic well general population.[25,26] The changes in QT dispersion again appear to track with changes in ventricular hypertrophy in hypertension (being elevated in untreated hypertrophy and at least in part reversed by management of ventricular hypertrophy), in the pressure overload of aortic stenosis, and in endurance athletes with exercise-related ventricular hypertrophy (the latter group being regarded as physiologic).[27] However, QT dispersion indices appear to be no better than simple voltage criteria at detecting left ventricular hypertrophy in the hypertensive patient.[28]

The relationship of variability in QT dispersion, as with RR interval, may be linked in part to autonomic tone in hypertension and in cases of pathological hypertrophic cardiomyopathy.[29] A recent small pilot study[30] has suggested that a minor adjustment to record QT interval to the peak T-wave voltage—rather than the asymptote of the T-wave

and the isoelectric line (a strategy previously well defined in the clinical pharmacology of antiarrhythmic drugs nearly 30 years previously)—should improve the sensitivity of QT interval measures to predict LVH calculations. Similarly, the use of time voltage area measures for the QRS complex in hypertension, particularly that derived from all 12 leads, might equally produce better sensitivity for the definition of LVH from the simple ECG.[31]

Ventricular hypertrophy definition using electrocardiography in hypertension

The electrocardiographic definition of ventricular hypertrophy has been well established for many decades and has been examined closely in population studies due to its ease of use, albeit with many and variable definitions.[32] Unfortunately, the patterns seen in hypertensive patients in the absence of other confounding disease are neither easily nor reliably distinguished from patients with coronary artery disease on the basis of the ECG appearance alone. This can be readily appreciated from studies completed in patients with normal coronary angiographic imaging yet marked LVH and strain patterns on the rest ECG.[33] Notwithstanding this difficulty in interpretation, there is no doubt about its linkage of electrocardiographic LVH to future vascular events in hypertensive patients.[34]

Electrocardiographic LVH as defined by the most widely used criteria (e.g., Sokolow Lyon = SV1 + RV5 or RV6 > or = 35 mm) have been reliably and independently related to untreated clinically measured BP levels, male gender, and Afro Caribbean racial origin and *inversely* associated with body mass index.[35] This latter relationship to generalized obesity, reducing the sensitivity of ECG detection of LVH in hypertension, is commonly ignored yet paradoxically becoming increasingly relevant to Westernized populations in which with each year there is evidence of a dramatically increased prevalence of obesity. Put simply, the ECG voltage is damped markedly by subcutaneous fat in the same way that this relationship is used to define body fat mass by bioimpedance frequency measures.

It is accepted that echocardiography and the rest ECG give different information with respect to the presence or absence of LVH. Their diagnostic reliability (sensitivity and specificity) is fundamentally different whether they are positive or negative. It is clear that ECG-defined LVH is significantly *less* sensitive than echocardiographic assessment of LV mass.[36] ECG-defined LVH is prone to being less specific, particularly in younger patients, and perhaps more importantly in nonwhite patients. In both of these settings, false positive results are more common.[37] Where increased body fat (in particular, subcutaneous fat, paradoxically less associated with increased cardiovascular risk) is associated with high electrical resistance, obesity markedly confounds the accuracy of surface ECG voltage and limits the ability of voltage-based criteria to reliably identify LVH.[38] A lack of specificity can be particularly problematic where a treatment decision is being made on the basis of elevated clinic BP readings and ECG-LVH might in many instances be taken as the sole confirmation of end-organ damage used to make a pharmacologic treatment decision.

A key finding is that the prevalence of ECG-LVH may be up to six times higher in African American patients with hypertension than in white patients, depending on the criteria used (given a range of 6 to 24% in blacks versus 1 to 7% in whites). However, this observation is due in part to a lack of specificity as the estimated difference in the prevalence of *echocardiographic* LVH appears less striking (26% in blacks versus 20% in whites; *p*>0.2). As can be seen, this is largely due to the underreporting of LVH (at least as defined by echocardiography) when defined by ECG in white patients with hypertension. However, the overall sensitivity of the rest ECG (generally low; range, 3 to17%) does not appear to differ significantly between African American and white patients for any of the conventional ECG-LVH criteria (Sokolow Lyon; Cornell adjusted score, and so on). Specificity indeed is lower in blacks for all criteria (range 73 to 94% versus 95 to 100% for whites; *p*=.0001 to .09). The predictive value of an ECG positive for LVH is therefore consistently lower in black subjects, even outside the U.S. African American population.[39] Black ethnic groups are indeed associated with the strongest independent predictor of a *decreased* ECG specificity in multiple logistic regression analysis factoring for age, gender, body mass index, left ventricular mass index, and smoking.[37]

Several attempts have been made to adjust the criteria used to define LVH on the basis of rest electrocardiography by modifying the voltage criteria[40] to account for the impact of obesity[41] and/or age.[42] In general, these can help improve sensitivity but still leave unacceptably low rates (missing cases affected by generally echocardiographically but occasionally MRI-defined LVH)—particularly in elderly or female patients.

In the CASTEL study of 447 subjects, the sensitivity, specificity, and positive and negative predictive values of the most commonly used ECG tests of LVH were calculated and compared. All ECG calculations and modifications or adjustments thereof had a very low sensitivity in the elderly.[43] Furthermore, except for the Cornell index and the Minnesota code, they were unable to demonstrate the higher prevalence of echocardiographic LVH in elderly females in comparison with males. In contrast, the predictive value of the rest ECG for echocardiographic LV mass appears consistently better in elderly males compared with females (whether negative or positive). Some criteria are more predictive in males, some more predictive in females, and others equally predictive in both sexes. Overall, Casiglia and colleagues reaffirmed general consensus that a rest ECG, regardless of how the voltage LVH calculation is derived, is *not* a reliable method for screening LVH in the elderly.

Exercise-based studies in hypertension

In the hypertensive population, diagnostic exercise stress testing gives important information from both the BP and electrocardiographic as well as symptomatic aspects of the response to exercise. The cardiac prognostic significance of exercise BP rise in the hypertensive population has been recognized for a long time.[44] Most recent exercise packages now incorporate automated or semiautomated oscillometric BP cuffs. To some extent this has helped reduce inadequate operator technique and number bias in the definition of exercise BP responses. Inadequate BP measurements in hypertensive patients off or on therapy are a totally unacceptable standard of practice whether as part of a screening test or part of a specific work-up for potential ischemia, which is directed more at the ECG and symptomatic response to exercise in routine practice.

Simplified submaximal exercises using step tests have been used in the assessment of hypertensive patients.[45] These have the value of added safety where an exercise-associated BP overshoot (occasionally of dramatic proportions) and may cause anxiety for patients or technicians supervising exercise tests and indeed appear to have some value in demonstrating associations with the presence of endothelial dysfunction[46] and levels of ambulatory blood pressure[47] and in predicting maximal QT interval dispersion on the rest ECG (see previous discussion). However, they are not predictive of echocardiographically or MRI-derived LV mass.[48] In one small study of maximal treadmill exercise testing, Gottdeiner and colleagues[49] from Washington suggested that they could demonstrate a correlation between echocardiographic LV mass and a BP overshoot on exercise testing (defined as measured SBP >210 mmHg) in normotensive male subjects. In all of the current studies of exercise BP response, there is a pathologic relationship to exercise BP loads for the heart both in persistent hypertension and in some prehypertensive states.[49] This alone underlines the general utility of exercise-based protocols and careful BP as well as other measurements in the hypertensive patient.

Many tests in hypertensive patients are performed to assess the possibility of myocardial ischemia in a hypertensive patient with either suspicious symptoms and/or minor nonspecific ECG changes on their rest ECG. With respect to the definition of myocardial ischemia in unselected subjects with a BP overshoot during a maximal exercise perfusion scintigram, Campbell and colleagues[50] found that their subjects with BP overshoot (peak systolic BP greater than or equal to 210 mmHg in men and greater than or equal to 190 mmHg in women) were in fact *less likely* to have a scintigraphic perfusion defect (transient, fixed, or reversible) rather than more likely. Importantly, over a 6-year prospective follow-up there were 283 deaths in this subset and reassuringly no association between the exercise BP overshoot and risk of mortality regardless of the BP ECG or symptomatic response. Thus, an exercise-induced BP rise was associated with a lower likelihood of myocardial perfusion abnormalities, and this was not associated with any increased mortality rate.

The limitations of exercise stress electrocardiography for the definition of myocardial ischemia in unselected patients are well recognized, and like the rest ECG is summarized as low sensitivity (false negative rates of >30%) and low specificity (false positive rates of >30%) in specific groups such as the elderly, women, and patients with diabetes. However, these figures are somewhat confounded by a requirement to exercise fully (which is essential in the interpretation of results and a valid definition of receiver operating characteristics for exercise stress). Notwithstanding this, there may be some value in submaximal exercise testing applied to the correct parameters (as discussed previously). There may be additional value derived from exercise tests and other aspects such as achieved work, cardiac rhythm, heart rate, and BP response. However, the key issue for most subjects remains the electrocardiographic response and whether this is indicative of myocardial ischemia.

In the hypertensive patient, the presence of electrocardiographic changes at rest (the strain pattern) would be expected to influence the predictive capacity of an exercise ECG test. However, Marwick et al. saw little impact (either positive or negative) on the *sensitivity* of exercise electrocardiography, although specificity was slightly reduced in the presence of ECG-LVH (74 versus 69%) in a group of 68 hypertensive patients.[51] Given the frequency of normal epicardial coronary angiographic studies in patients with a positive noninvasive testing for ischemia, it is often suggested that hypertension by its association with a poor coronary flow reserve (independent of epicardial coronary artery disease), left ventricular hypertrophy, and possibly microvascular coronary disease would indicate that different diagnostic strategies are required to define tissue ischemia in these patients compared to those with ischemia through epicardial flow-limiting stenoses.[52] Although stress-induced (physical, mental, or pharmacological) cardiac wall motion abnormalities (for example, detected at echocardiography) are generally highly specific for angiographic epicardial coronary disease, ST segment depression and/or scintigraphic myocardial perfusion abnormalities are often found in the presence of angiographically normal coronary arteries where there is coexistent hypertensive left ventricular hypertrophy and/or microvascular disease.

Given these findings, the value of exercise stress electrocardiography in hypertensive patients has been portrayed by some as its negative predictive value. This appears to be comparable in both normotensive and hypertensive patients. That is where the test is negative for inducible ischemia (it reliably defines an absence of epicardial coronary disease). Unfortunately, the overall negative predictive value of exercise electrocardiography in hypertensive patients remains poor, providing false negative rates in the region of 50% (low sensitivity) even with effective BP control.[69] Thus, whether an exercise-electrocardiography stress test is positive or negative or is uninterpretable or ambiguous generally another imaging stress test is warranted if there is a genuine high level of clinical suspicion of coronary artery disease, to suggesting a significant flow-limiting epicardial coronary disease and to justify targeted ischemia-guided revascularization.

Continuous ambulatory ECG studies in the definition of ischemia in hypertension

Despite its general utility in the definition of ambulatory ischaemia,[53] continuous ST segment monitoring has not been studied greatly in the assessment of patients with hypertension. Pringle et al. reported a detailed assessment of 90 hypertensive patients with left ventricular hypertrophy and abnormal 48-hour ambulatory ECG studies suggestive of ischemia.[54] From 68 men and 22 women (mean age 57; range 25 to 79) they completed 48-hour ambulatory ST segment monitoring (in all patients)—and addi-

tional exercise electrocardiography (n=79), stress thallium scintigraphy (n= 80), and coronary arteriography (n= 35)—to finalize diagnoses. They found that 48% of their sample (43 patients) had at least one episode of ST segment depression on ambulatory electrocardiographic monitoring. These were frequent (median number of episodes 16, range 1 to 84) and protracted (median duration of 8.6, range 2 to 17 minutes), but were in the vast majority *asymptomatic.* Twenty-six of the patients went on to show positive exercise electrocardiography, and 48 patients showed reversible stress thallium perfusion defects despite chest pain having occurred in only five of the patients during exercise. Eighteen of the 35 patients (20%) who progressed to coronary arteriography had clinically significant epicardial coronary artery disease. Of these, seven had no history of chest pain at any time.

Thus, symptomatic and asymptomatic myocardial ischemia are common in hypertensive patients with left ventricular hypertrophy, even in the absence of epicardial coronary artery disease. These patients could be reliably detected on Holter monitoring and continuous ECG analysis, yet this simple and effective technique remains poorly applied in the routine assessment of hypertensive patients. Unfortunately, this study did not define the false negative rate of this technique.

Similar studies by Asmar et al. studied unselected hypertensive patients for ambulatory ischemic changes, as defined by electrocardiographic criteria (a horizontal or down-sloping ST depression; >1 mm and >60 seconds). They found ST-segment depression together with concomitant BP and heart rate variations to be common and to follow a diurnal variation.[55] In 100 hypertensive patients (male/female ratio 1:1), 23 patients (15 men and 8 women) had 72 episodes of ST depression with 2 peaks: upon awakening and in the late afternoon periods. The mean ambulatory BP load was greater in the patients with than without ST-segment depression for both systolic and diastolic BP (135 +/- 14 versus 129 +/- 15 and 84 +/- 8 versus 79 +/- 10 mmHg, respectively; $p<0.01$). Plasma glucose (5.83 +/- 0.70 versus 5.46 +/- 0.71 mmol/L; $p=0.04$) and self-rated work-related stress levels (22% versus 13%; $p=0.03$) were also higher in patients with ambulatory ST-segment depression, regardless of symptoms suggestive of ischemia. There was no difference between the patient groups with or without ambulatory electrocardiographic ischemia on the basis of clinical parameters, left ventricular mass index, and other general cardiovascular risk factors (gender, smoking, lipids, and so on). This second study also suggested that 24-hour ambulatory ECG monitoring might have utility in defining ischemia in unselected hypertensive patients. They extended the analysis by suggesting that those hypertensive patients showing ambulatory ST depression episodes had a higher ambulatory BP load—and again by this technology electrocardiographic ischemic changes were common regardless of symptoms or the presence of LVH.

Finally, given the suggested role of potassium balance in ST segment interpretation Siegel and colleagues studied the role of diuretic-induced potassium depletion in the diagnostic utility of ambulatory ECG studies in 186 male hypertensive subjects. They treated their patients to ensure repletion of potassium following control of blood pressure using diuretic therapy. Siegel et al. found a 27% prevalence of silent ambulatory ST segment depression compatible with ischemia.[56] The episodes followed a pattern similar to that seen in the studies of both Asmar and Pringle, with peaks in the early morning hours between 0000 hr and 0600 hrs.

In summary, ambulatory ECG studies appear distinct from rest or exercise ECG testing in the hypertensive population and probably have a better diagnostic profile in the assessment of both symptomatic or asymptomatic hypertensive patients, regardless of the presence of either electrocardiographic or echocardiographic LVH. Why such simple and reliable technology remains generally infrequently applied in the routine assessment of hypertensive patients is unclear, but this may simply relate to the time and effort required to complete detailed analyses that cannot be easily automated.

Stress myocardial perfusion studies

As an initial investigation to supplement symptomatic clinical assessment, nuclear cardiac studies are generally accepted as more sensitive and specific than exercise electrocardiography in the definition of significant epicardial coronary artery disease. Symptom-limited bicycle exercise stress test in conjunction with technetium,[99] sestamibi, or tetrafosmin SPECT imaging provides similar levels of diagnostic accuracy; sensitivity, and specificity whether or not the patient is normotensive or hypertensive for the detection of fixed or reversible perfusion defects.[57] Abnormal cardiac function in patients with positive exercise electrocardiography yet normal coronary angiography is well recognized, and hypertension is a common finding.[58] Neither hypertension *per se* nor hypertensive left ventricular hypertrophy[59] (in the absence of coronary disease) increases the likelihood of perfusion abnormalities with a given level of cardiovascular risk.[60]

Comparative studies in hypertension generally show that the sensitivity of pharmacological stress perfusion is greater than that achieved by exercise stress electrocardiography and the specificity of results is improved.[61] The features of a false positive test (a perfusion study suggesting ischemia yet with a normal coronary angiography) may relate to the presence of small vessel coronary disease visualized as a slow angiographic runoff. Unfortunately, an optimal agent to provide flow/vasodilator or rate stress or the best perfusion tracer is not specifically identified for the assessment of hypertensive patients.

Stress echocardiography

In some studies of patients with hypertension there is evidence to suggest that the incidence of coronary artery disease can be overestimated not only by exercise stress electrocardiography (ECG) but by stress perfusion scintigraphy (symptomatic patients who have test results suggestive of epicardial coronary disease yet have unequivocally normal coronary angiography). Stress echocardiography has been suggested to be a more sensitive and specific technique than the previously cited testing modalities.

This strategy is particularly useful in patients who have limited exercise capacity or in those who cannot (or alternatively will not tolerate an adequate exercise stress work load) reach adequate levels of exercise stress to achieve a diagnostic outcome. Exercise echocardiographic technique is clearly more operator and subject dependent than electrocardiography or nuclear scintigraphy. This is because it is influenced by the echocardiographic image quality of the patient studied in order to achieve sufficient image quality for accurate definition of segmental ventricular wall motion.

A range of techniques similar to those used in nuclear cardiac scintigraphy can be used to place the heart under stress. The key differences are that imaging is generally completed at baseline and immediately after completion of physical exercise and that graded assessments during exercise are generally not possible. The exercise protocols used are generally similar to those used in exercise electrocardiography. Pharmacologic stress commonly using either dobutamine (with or without atropine), adenosine, dipyridamole, or a range of less commonly used agents has advantages in that patients are not physically moving and thus during these protocols graded imaging can be achieved during the infusion protocol.

The endpoint of analysis is the detection of stress-induced reversible wall motion impairment of contractility. Unlike exercise ECG studies, segmental wall motion analysis generally allows broad anatomical location of the ischemic response and the definition of these wall motion abnormalities has good prognostic validity in reliably predicting subsequent coronary events in that territory. Thus, anterior/LAD abnormalities are associated with a significantly increased risk of cardiac death and nonfatal infarction. This added prognostic risk of events is independent of the resting baseline LV ejection fraction and the perceived extent of wall motion abnormalities identified during stress echocardiography in hypertension.[62]

Echocardiographic imaging is normally acquired by the transthoracic route but can also be completed by the transesophageal route, where either a direct pacing stress or pharmacologic stress can be employed with reasonable comparability to pharmacologic transthoracic stress echocardiography.[63] Although pharmacological stress is generally preferred to minimize motion artifact during echocardiography, this is associated with some adverse effects on the patients studied. In some early studies, safety was a concern particularly for hypertensive patients for whom an abrupt pressor response is more often seen during pharmacologic stress protocols.[64,65] As with exercise electrocardiography, there are composite endpoints for the test (including symptoms, concomitant electrocardiographic changes, and most centrally the definition of reversible regional wall motion abnormalities), suggestive of flow-limiting myocardial ischemia.

Using an exercise echo technique (without electrocardiographic LVH) in hypertensive patients who had already undergone coronary angiography, Senior and colleagues from London showed improved sensitivity and specificity even in a relatively small sample of 43 patients (of whom only 29 had coronary disease).[66] Maltagliati et al. tested the role of exercise echocardiography as an alternative to exercise electrocardiography for the detection of epicardial coronary disease in hypertension, before and after adequate BP control.[67] In a parallel group case control study of 59 hypertensive and normotensive patients undergoing coronary angiography for chest pain, these investigators defined both upright bicycle exercise ECG and post-exercise stress echocardiographic results for each group. The hypertensive patients had repeated testing following BP control (in this study using sublingual nifedipine). Coronary artery disease (defined as >1 angiographic lumenal narrowing >50%) was found in 22 hypertensive and 41 normotensive patients. The sensitivity, specificity, and diagnostic accuracy of the two techniques were not statistically different (95%, 94%, 94%) in hypertensives or (82%, 77%, 83%) normotensives, but were significantly better than those seen on the bicycle exercise ECG test (68%, 70%, and 69%). BP lowering had little impact on exercise echocardiography, slightly decreasing sensitivity (91%)—whereas the sensitivity of exercise ECG decreased even more markedly (45%).

Elhendy et al. evaluated in 1164 hypertensive patients the hemodynamic profile, safety, and feasibility of combined dobutamine (up to 40 µg/kg per minute) and atropine (up to 1 mg) stress echocardiography in patients with "limited exercise capacity" (age, 60 +/- 12 years; 761 men). In this large study, 446 of the patients were known to have treated hypertension. The test protocol was defined using a limit of achieving 85% of age-predicted maximal heart rate and/or an ischemic endpoint (new or worsened wall motion abnormalities, ST segment depression, or angina). Predictably, dobutamine induced a significant increase of heart rate in patients with and without the presence of hypertension (59 +/- 25 and 63 +/- 23 beats per minute, respectively). A hypotensive response (>40 mmHg SBP drop) was more frequent in older hypertensive patients with higher baseline BP treated with calcium channel blockers (7% versus 4%). Protocol-related ventricular tachycardia occurred at a small but significant rate (4.1%) but was similar in normotensive or hypertensive patients and could be terminated promptly by intravenous metoprolol administration. This form of testing proved feasible in 91% of patients with and 92% of patients without hypertension. Therefore, they could reasonably conclude that this technology and protocol was safe, effective, and reliable in the assessment of hypertensive patients where evaluation for myocardial ischemia was indicated.

Perfusion imaging has been directly compared to stress echocardiography in other reports. Astarita et al. studied 53 patients with hypertension (29 males, aged 58 +/- 10 years) and with normal left ventricular systolic function and a positive exercise ECG test suggestive of ischemia. They further investigated these patients with dipyridamole-atropine stress echocardiography (DASE) and thallium-201 stress/rest myocardial single-photon emission computed tomography (SPECT).[68] All patients had additional coronary angiography. Coronary angiography was used to define the occurrence of >1 epicardial stenosis (>50%), which was present in 23 of the 53 patients (43%) who had a positive exercise ECG. The calculated sensitivity for detection of angiographic coronary artery disease was significantly higher

for perfusion scintigraphy compared to echocardiography (DASE = 78% versus SPECT = 100%, $p<0.05$), whereas specificity was higher for echo (DASE = 100% versus SPECT = 47%, $p<0.00001$). Diagnostic accuracy was also higher for echo (DASE = 91% versus SPECT = 70%, $p<0.01$). Thus, this group felt that in the further assessment of hypertensive patients with chest pain symptoms suggestive of ischemia and an exercise-induced ST segment depression both dipyridamole/atropine stress echo and SPECT perfusion scintigraphy were good diagnostic options. Dobutamine-atropine stress echo was characterized by a higher specificity but slightly lower sensitivity than stress perfusion SPECT.

In a later study, Elhendy et al. compared their pharmacologic stress echocardiography protocol with stress perfusion scintigraphy (this time using a sestamibi SPECT protocol and coronary angography) in hypertensive patients with or without LVH (where the presence of coronary stenoses at angiography was defined as more than one >50% lesion). From a sample of 88 patients where epicardial coronary disease was defined in 66, these two techniques were largely comparable without statistically significant differences in either sensitivity or specificity.[69] Both appeared to lack sensitivity compared with an angiographic standard (63% and 51%, respectively, for echocardiography and scintigraphy), but the presence of echocardiographic LVH had no impact on either technique.

Flow dilatation using dipyridamole in combination with echocardiography has similar value in the assessment of hypertensive patients with undiagnosed chest pain symptoms and appears to give reliable prognostic information. In a relatively small prospective study of 257 hypertensive patients with chest pain (110 men; age, 63 +/- 9 years), Cortigiani et al.[70] had no major complications with a stepped dipyridamole infusion protocol successfully completed in 98% of hypertensive patients symptomatic with chest pain. A positive echocardiographic response suggestive of ischemia was found in 72 patients: 27 during the low-dose (less than or equal to 0.56 mg/kg) and 45 during the high-dose (>0.56 mg/kg) dipyridamole infusion. During follow-up (32 ± 18 months), 27 cardiac events had occurred comprising 3 deaths, 8 myocardial infarctions, and 16 cases of admission with unstable symptoms. Twenty-seven patients underwent coronary revascularization. At multivariate analysis, the positive stress echocardiographic result [odds ratio (OR) = 5.5; 95% CI, 1.4 to 16.6] was the only predictor of subsequent major cardiac events (cardiac death or infarction). A positive stress echocardiographic study (OR, 4.2; 95% CI, 1.8 to 9.6) and family history of coronary disease (OR, 4.2; 95% CI, 1.5 to 6.9) were both independently associated with prognosis. The 5-year survival rates for the negative stress echo and the positive stress echo populations were, respectively, 97% and 87% ($p=0.0019$) for cardiac events.

In a more recent study, the same group assessed the relative value of dipyridamole stress echo or exercise electrocardiography in hypertensive patients with right-bundle branch block (35) or patients with right-bundle branch block and normal blood pressure (36). In this group (with right-bundle branch block) they found less concordance of testing in hypertension (69% cf 92%) compared to the normotensive patients, although overall the sensitivity of both techniques was similar. The accuracy of positive and negative predictive values was much higher with dipyridamole stress echocardiography (66, 61, and 75%, respectively, for exercise electrocardiography and 86, 87, and 84%, respectively, for dipyridamole stress echocardiography).[71]

However, this comparability of performance was not found in a further study in 101 patients with hypertension, chest pain, and positive exercise ECG.[72] This group completed an extensive comparison in their patient group using stress/rest SPECT with Tc^{99m}-MIBI, dipyridamole, and dobutamine stress echocardiography and coronary angiography in their patients, all of whom had normal global ventricular function (57 had preserved systolic function but echocardiographic LVH). They observed no side effects during perfusion scintigraphy but dose-limiting side effects in 5 patients during dipyridamole and 7 patients during dobutamine stress echo. The sensitivity, specificity, accuracy, and positive and negative predictive values for angiographic coronary disease were, respectively, 98%, 36%, 71%, 67%, and 94% for perfusion scintigraphy; 61%, 91%, 74%, 90%, and 64% for dipyridamole; and 88%, 80%, 84%, 85%, and 83% for dobutamine stress echocardiography. Thus, dipyridamole stress performed significantly less well in this series than dobutamine stress applied to symptomatic hypertensive patients for the definition of angiographic coronary disease.

In contrast to these isolated comparisons of the diagnostic performance of single-test strategies, Marwick et al.[75] published an important and more realistic stepwise analytical approach to define the added diagnostic value of stress echocardiographic assessment from a substantial study of 2363 hypertensive patients followed up for 10 years. Although the majority of their cohort had normal studies (63%), ischemia identified by stress echocardiography independently predicted mortality in those able to complete a treadmill exercise echo protocol (hazard ratio 2.21, 95% confidence intervals 1.10 to 4.43, $p=0.0001$) as well as those undergoing dobutamine echo (hazard ratio 2.39, 95% confidence intervals 1.53 to 3.75, $p=0.0001$). The other major predictors of events were age, the presence of resting LV systolic dysfunction, heart failure symptoms (regardless of systolic function), and the clinically derived Duke treadmill score. Using a stepwise model to replicate the sequence of clinical evaluation (applied after screening exercise electrocardiography), stress echocardiography added prognostic power to predictive models based on clinical and/or stress-testing variables. Thus, stress echocardiography (exercise or pharmacologic) were an independent predictor of cardiac death in hypertensive patients with known or suspected coronary artery disease, incremental to clinical risks and exercise ECG test results alone.[73]

Whether or not conduction defects influence stress echocardiography is not quite as straightforward as with stress perfusion scintigraphy. Hypertensive patients with resting conduction defects who undergo stress echocardiography and do not have studies indicative of ischemia (no regional wall motion abnormalities) are associated with low excess mortality. However, the specific combination of right-bundle branch block and anterior hemiblock has been associated with adverse outcomes, even where the stress echocardiographic study does not suggest coronary ischemia is present.[74] In a small sample of 161 hypertensive patients stratified on the basis of ventricular geometry, Yuda et al. suggested that the accuracy of dobutamine stress echocardiography is reduced in patients with concentric remodeling (61%) compared to hypertensive patients with normal geometry (85%, $p<0.05$) or concentric hypertrophy (86%, $p<0.05$). Accuracy with eccentric hypertrophy (64%, $p<0.05$) was lower than with concentric hypertrophy and similar to that found with concentric remodeling.[75]

Patients with chest pain symptoms and completely normal angiography often remain symptomatic and cause concern. However, Zouridalkis et al.[76] examined 33 such patients with exertional anginal chest pain, a positive exercise stress ECG, and a completely normal coronary arteriogram. All patients had normal left ventricular systolic function at rest and none fulfilled echocardiographic criteria for LVH, whereas 8 of the normotensive patients and 10 of the hypertensive patients had perfusion abnormalities on thallium SPECT ($p=0.61$). Dobutamine infusion reproduced anginal pain and ST segment changes in some patients, but none developed regional wall motion abnormalities indicative of ischemia. They concluded that the high prevalence of scintigraphic perfusion defects in both normotensive and hypertensive groups were probably false positive results or less likely that dobutamine stress echocardiography is insensitive to ischemia caused by microvascular dysfunction.

Coronary angiography

Coronary angiography is frequently performed in patients with hypertension due to the presence of equivocal or positive noninvasive testing for myocardial ischemia to define the nature of epicardial coronary flow. It is particularly appropriate in hypertension, where the implications of the presence (or indeed absence) of epicardial coronary disease are prognostically important.

Although the appearance at angiography is not equivalent to the absence of sub-intimal coronary atherosclerosis and does not guarantee absence of future coronary disease, there is general agreement that the presence of unequivocally normal coronary arteries is a useful prognostic indicator even in the presence of hypertension and or hypertensive LVH.[77] Although the morbidity of patients remains high (many have symptoms of chest pain both typical and atypical of inducible ischemia) mortality (in the absence of a documented myocardial infarction at any point[78]) is consistently low.

The prognostic significance of *nonobstructive* coronary disease seen at coronary angiography in hypertensive patients is less easy to predict. In unselected patients with noncritical lesions there is a significantly lower (albeit only slightly) 10-year survival rate (85.8%) than those with unequivocally normal coronary arteries (90.1%). The difference in survival rate in population studies of nonobstructive coronary atheroma detected at angiography is generally attributed to more advanced age, male gender, and a higher prevalence of cigarette smoking, diabetes, mellitus, and hypertension. However, it is also clear that the presence of noncritical coronary stenoses is *not* a statistically significant independent determinant of survival. Long-term survival rates of the patients with one or more critical lesions were in fact largely equivalent to those seen in patients with critical stenoses plus one or more noncritical lesions.[79] Thus, noncritical stenoses appear to be important only if they occur in conjunction with a critical flow-limiting stenosis.

In a relatively small comparative case control study using a positive treadmill exercise test involving 320 patients with hypertension and 320 patients without hypertension, De Cesare et al.[80] showed that *only in the sixth and seventh decade* did the patients with hypertension have a greater prevalence of triple vessel coronary disease (40 and 50% cf. 25 and 31%) than the normotensive comparator group. This appeared unrelated to standard cardiovascular risk factor distribution (age, gender, smoking, lipids, and so on) demographics. Thus, "diagnostic" exercise treadmill results suggestive or indicative of ischemia should be treated with some caution in patients with hypertension, as they need not reflect epicardial coronary stenoses with its attendant prognostic implications.

Vascular calcification and electron beam studies in hypertension

In the last 10 years, the long-standing association of vascular calcification with the process of endo-lumenal stenoses[81] has been explored using noninvasive electron beam tomography. The measurements have been applied to a variety of sites, but the most relevant to the heart of the hypertensive patient is in the assessment of the calcification occurring in the coronary circulation (CAC). The improving resolution and data interpretation of this noninvasive technology gives the technique some future potential. It has been suggested to provide independent predictive information on vascular occlusive event rates at least over and above that provided by a traditional demographic cardiovascular risk factor analysis.[82]

Although the technique appears to show an independent relationship to the severity of coronary stenosis, there are confounding associations with age, hyperlipidaemia, diabetes, smoking status, and gender. For example, African American ethnicity (and, interestingly, hypertension) does not appear to link coronary disease well with the appearance of coronary calcification using EBCT.[83] However, in the largest study so far (completed in 30,908 asymptomatic individuals undergoing EBCT), Hoff et al. report that for both men and women all conventional risk factors (including hypertension) were significantly associated with the presence of any detectable CAC, and the mean CAC score increased in proportion to the number of CAD risk factors. In age-adjusted (multivariable) logistic regression analysis, cigarette use, histories of hypercholesterolemia, diabetes, and hypertension were each significantly associated with mild to extensive CAC scores (greater than or equal to 10.0). Thus, they felt that CAC scores were associated with *presumed* higher atherosclerotic plaque burden in both men and women. Unfortunately, this association with risk factor scores is not an adequate definition of the presence or absence of coronary stenoses in these individuals, all of whom were ostensibly well.

In a relatively small early case control study, there was a relationship between the extent of coronary calcification scoring to the duration of high BP in a sample of 73 male hypertensive patients.[84] They found no association with the extent of BP elevation in this cohort but were able to suggest a weak link of CAC scores to age that was also demonstrable in asymptomatic normotensive subjects.[83] However, in some studies[85] and not in others[86] in angiographic coronary artery disease hypertension is less strongly linked to the extent of coronary calcification or stenosis scoring than are other generalized atherosclerosis risk factors.

Turner et al. have recently reexamined the relationship of BP to CAC in a sample of 298 hypertensive patients (male and female) using ambulatory BP recordings[87] and have found a link between ambulatory diastolic BP and CAC scoring. In a logistic regression analysis of CAC in the presence of hypertensive LVH, Altunkan et al. have suggested that body mass index and age were the main independent factors affecting the presence and amount of coronary calcification in patients with left ventricular hypertrophy.[88]

CARDIAC STRUCTURE AND FUNCTION IN HYPERTENSION

Valvular associations and hypertension

There are known associations between cardiac valvular dysfunction and hypertension, but these are confounded by the presence of concomitant disease. For example, secondary valvular dysfunction following ischemia or infarction with or without dilatation of the heart would be a well-accepted but separate pathologic process.

The coexistence of hypertension and stenosis of the aortic valve is well recognized and is a common clinical association in surveys of symptomatic aortic stenosis (32% of symptomatic cases of aortic stenosis in some series[89]). For example, hypertension is coexistent in 21% of patients with any grade of aortic stenosis, and aortic stenosis affects 1.1% of hypertensive patients.[90] Theoretically, the increased valve shear stress caused by hypertension may be a possible mediator (or at the very least an accelerating factor) in the development of aortic valve stenosis. However, the exact interrelationship of these two conditions is less clear.

Degenerative aortic valve disease is common in the elderly where hypertension is more prevalent. For example, in the 5201 subjects over 65 years of age enrolled in the Cardiovascular Health Study echocardiographic aortic valve sclerosis was evident in 26% and aortic valve stenosis in 2% of subjects. In those over 75 years of age, the prevalence of aortic sclerosis rose to 37% and aortic stenosis rose slightly (to 2.6%). Upon multiple logistic regression analysis, the independent predictors of this change somewhat predictably included age (twofold increased risk for each 10-year increase in age), male gender (twofold excess risk), smoking (35% increase in risk), and a history of hypertension (20% increase in risk).[91] Despite this association, hypertension does not appear to independently influence the natural course of aortic valve disease.[92] Although a higher left ventricular outflow tract velocity (common in hypertension in response to the changes associated with the hypertrophy remodeling of the hypertensive heart[93]) is associated with more rapid degeneration in aortic valvular stenosis, it is not a statistically independent predictor of progression.[94]

Studies in patients with both hypertension and aortic stenosis are limited, but recent reports suggest no significant differences between hypertensive and normotensive aortic stenosis patients with respect to age, gender, symptom class, ventricular function, or remodeling patterns. In hypertensive patients, symptoms tend to present with larger aortic valve areas and lower stroke work (i.e., less valvular stenosis).[91] This may be because of the additional overload due to hypertension or more practically due to simple earlier recognition by chance physical examination.

Data on the *spontaneous* detection of echocardiographic valvular regurgitation in patients with hypertension are not extensive, and examination of potential causal associations with arterial hypertension is scant. In the normal population, the presence of regurgitation at the mitral position has been shown to have a weak association with coexistent hypertension in the Framingham study. In 1696 men and 1893 women (preselected by those who had acceptable echocardiographic imaging), a multiple logistic regression analysis was used to define the association of clinical variables to mitral (MR) or tricuspid regurgitation (TR; more than or equal to mild severity) and aortic regurgitation (more than or equal to trace severity). MR of more than mild severity was seen in 19.0% of men and 19.1% of women, with AR of more than or equal to trace severity in 13.0% of men and 8.5% of women. The demographic associations with the finding of echocardiographic MR were increased age (OR = 1.3/9.9 years, 95% CI 1.2 to 1.5), hypertension (OR 1.6; 95% CI 1.2 to 2.0), and body mass index [OR 0.8/4.3 kg/m^2; 95% CI 0.7 to 0.9; i.e., less likely]. The determinants of AR were only age (OR 2.3/9.9 years; 95% CI 2.0 to 2.7) and male gender (OR 1.6; 95% CI 1.2 to 2.1).

In the hypertension genetic epidemiology study[95] conducted in 1496 hypertensive patients free of diabetes the occurrence of aortic and mitral regurgitation was 246/1496 (16.5%) and 75/1496 (5%), respectively. In short, the role of hypertension in the evolution of echocardiographic or symptomatic valvular regurgitation seems to be dependent on factors other than hypertension *per se*.

Ventricular function assessment
Role of rest echocardiography in routine management (asymptomatic)

Left ventricular function assessment is a crucial aspect of hypertension care. There are two key areas of interest: the definition of ventricular hypertrophy and the functional assessment of ventricular contraction and to some extent relaxation. By far the most widespread mode of diagnostic assessment is by use of transthoracic echocardiography. The definition of ischemia as a cause of symptoms or in the asymptomatic hypertensive patient can also be addressed (at least in part) by use of an echocardiographic technique (see previous material). There is little evidence to suggest

that ventricular function can be adequately addressed in isolation by a process of structured symptomatic enquiry (whether alone or supplemented by examination) or by employing basic tests such as electrocardiography or chest radiography[96] (which is *less likely* in hypertension given the more subtle nature of the changes involved in these patients, many of whom do not voice symptoms of any form).[97]

The use of a variety of technical assessments in hypertension is the subject of several regional and/or national guideline statements. In virtually all of these, echocardiography is not routinely recommended for all hypertensive subjects to stratify cardiovascular risk. However, the application of this technology *clearly* allows more precise definition of ventricular hypertrophy than would be possible on the basis of examination and routine chest X-ray and electrocardiography (see previous material).

For example, Cuspidi et al.[98] combined echocardiography with ultrasonographic carotid media thickness assessments (a similarly unclear clinical risk stratifier in hypertension) in 1074 hypertensive patients and were able to show reclassification of hypertensive patients as defined by population risk scoring alone. The proportion of patients (originally defined as low risk) decreased to 11.1%, and that of medium-risk patients also fell (to 35.7%). The largest change was that more than 50% of the patients previously classified at low or medium risk were deemed to be at high risk of subsequent vascular events following the addition of data from the use of these two ultrasonographic technologies (assessing LVH and IMT). A similar conclusion was reached by Schillaci et al. in their in reclassification of 792 untreated adult hypertensive patients with and without echocardiographic data.[99] Again, the main change in classification they saw was that a significant proportion of low-risk subjects that were reclassified as at higher vascular event risk and were now candidates for antihypertensive drug therapy (as opposed to BP monitoring or lifestyle interventions). Thus, although echocardiography appears to have a valuable role in the routine and *initial* assessment of hypertension it is clear that this data has not yet been incorporated into current national and international guidelines.

As indicated by Schillaci et al., echocardiographic assessments performed at the diagnostic phase of hypertension assessment may be of value in the classification of a white coat response and in the significance of white coat hypertension by putting blood pressure changes in the context of accurate end-organ assessments of the heart. Furthermore, the spectrum of ventricular change (which can be defined in hypertensive patients) can extend to the period *before* the appearance of fixed BP elevation. For example, echocardiographic indices of diastolic function appear to become abnormal when measured BP is within the normal range in the offspring of parents with hypertension. Indeed, Aeschbacher et al.[100] performed serial echocardiographic assessments in normotensive male offspring of hypertensive and normotensive parents. Over a 5-year period, although BP had not altered overall 5 offspring of hypertensive parents went on to develop mild sustained hypertension. Although overall LV mass was not different between the two groups at follow-up (92 ±17 versus 92 ±14 g/m²) and diastolic assessments had been similar at baseline, at follow-up mitral E-wave deceleration time and pulmonary vein reverse A-wave duration were both prolonged.

These changes were associated with significantly higher trans-mitral A-wave velocities (54 ± 7 versus 44 ±9 cm/sec, hypertensives versus normotensives, $p<0.05$), lower E/A ratio (1.31 ±0.14 versus 1.82 ± 0.48, $p<0.05$), increased systolic-to-diastolic pulmonary vein flow ratio (1.11 ± 0.3 versus 0.81 ± 0.16, $p<0.005$), longer myocardial isovolumic relaxation times (157 ± 7 versus 46 ± 12 msec, $p<.05$), and smaller myocardial E-wave velocity (10 ± 1 versus 13 ± 2 cm/sec, $p<.05$) and E/A ratio (1.29 ± 0.25 versus 1.78 ± 0.43, $p<.05$) despite similar LV mass (91 ± 16 versus 93 ± 18 g/m²). Thus, normotensive men with a moderate genetic risk for hypertension develop echocardiographic alterations of LV diastolic function before any appreciable rise in LV mass.

There is still some debate as to the best means of echocardiographic definition of diastolic relaxation in hypertension. Trans-mitral Doppler filling indices are commonly abnormal, but the independent relationship of these changes to hypertension and or ventricular remodeling (independent of aging) is not absolutely clear. It is clear that the aging process and the response to hypertension are different, dependent on gender. There is well-documented interest in the impact of hypertension on the systolic performance of the mid-wall of the left ventricle. Again distinct from symptoms, this echocardiographic analysis of LV systolic strain is suggested to be associated with a poorer cardio-vascular event rate. How this translates to overall systolic function defined by a volume technique such as MR or radionuclide ventriculography is less clear.

Recent investigations of the utility of ultrasonic tissue backscatter have shown some linkage to structure *in vivo* and have suggested that these relate to the abnormal restrictive filling patterns seen in hypertensive heart disease. Maceira et al.[101] defined real-time integrated backscatter analysis in 109 patients with essential hypertension. Backscatter cyclic variation and maximal intensity measured in 6 regions throughout the left ventricle were compared to trans-mitral filling patterns and subjects classified as showing normal BP and normal diastolic function (group 1, 29), hypertension with normal diastolic function (18, group 2) or hypertension with a delayed relaxation pattern (47, group 3). In addition, they found 11 hypertensives with a pseudo-normal filling pattern (group 4), and 4 hypertensives with a restrictive filling pattern (group 5). The highest cyclic variation was found in groups 1 and 2, the lowest in groups 4 and 5 (5.7 +/- 0.2 dB in group 1 and 5.7 +/- 0.2 dB in group 2 versus 2.9 +/- 0.3 dB in group 4 and 2.1 +/- 0.4 dB in group 5; $p<0.001$), with intermediate values within group 3 (5.2 +/- 0.2 dB). In correlation studies, left ventricular chamber stiffness was inversely related to the cyclic variation of backscatter signals ($p<0.05$) and directly correlated with mid-wall fractional shortening ($p<0.02$) in all patients with HBP. These results suggest a link between backscatter indices and diastolic function in hypertensive heart disease.

As an alternative, left atrial chamber dimensions or volume estimates can be readily defined using echocardiography.[102] As indicated previously, electrocardiographic indices of atrial conduction tend to link in best with simple diastolic filling parameters. Thus, atrial echocardiographic assessment might also hold useful indirect indices of diastolic function. Tsang et al. have shown that an echocardiographic atrial volume index has additional value in the retrospective cardiovascular event rate of elderly subjects referred within the Olmstead County survey.[103] A separate report from 140 subjects showed left atrial volume to correlate closely with age, ventricular dimensions, and mass in patients without evidence of atrial arrhythmia or valvular heart disease.[104] Thus left atrial volume appeared to be closely associated with the severity of a range of echocardiographic indices of diastolic dysfunction in these patients.

The white coat effect has little relationship to the structure or function of the left ventricle.[105] Although there are changes to trans-mitral flow reported in some series,[106] these are of uncertain clinical significance in the absence of ventricular hypertrophy or changes in systolic function despite signs of vascular dysfunction in these subjects.[107]

Studies in normotensive subjects also show small declines in resting LV systolic function and mid-wall contractility with aging. In a cross-sectional study of 272 asymptomatic adults (aged 25 to 80 years old) with untreated hypertension, Slotwiner et al.[108] found no change in endocardial or mid-wall stress-corrected left ventricular fractional shortening. Neither cardiac index nor total peripheral resistance changed with age in either gender because age-related increases in systolic pressure were offset by increased concentric remodeling in the female patients or enhanced systolic contractility in the males. Thus, in mild hypertension although cardiac index and peripheral resistance change with respect to age alone there are age-related increases in concentricity of ventricular geometry in women and increased ventricular performance indexes in hypertensive men.

Systolic function in patients with hypertension may also need more detailed assessment in hypertensive patients than in more straightforward studies designed to define contractility following infarction. Occult ischemia is a common cause of both systolic and diastolic impairment and may often be a cause of symptoms in the hypertensive population. Long-axis contraction of the left ventricle can be analyzed using a variety of echocardiographic techniques either using simple M-mode mitral annular movements alone or in conjunction with trans-mitral color flow studies or by tissue Doppler analyses.[109] The more recent application of myocardial tissue Doppler imaging can reveal subtle long-axis systolic ventricular impairment in patients previously presumed to have diastolic dysfunction.[111] The impact of hypertension is to change long-axis measures of contractility and these appear more sensitive in hypertensive patients than indices based on trans-mitral filling.[110] Clearly overall systolic contraction by a volume method might better appreciate such changes, but these are not often compared to purely echocardiographic indices.

The geometric pattern of ventricular remodeling seen in individual patients with hypertension can have an impact on cardiac function by influencing both systolic and diastolic mechanics differently at rest or during exercise. Stroke volume is higher in patients with eccentric hypertrophy (83 mL/beat) and lower in patients with concentric LVH (68 mL/beat) compared to matched normotensive adults (73 mL/beat).[111] In keeping with these changes, obviously cardiac output will then be higher in hypertensive patients with eccentric LV hypertrophy and lower in concentric LVH. These changes occur independently of achieved BP, although in multivariate analysis LV mass is predictably independently related to higher systolic pressure, older age, stroke volume, male gender, and body mass index. Stroke volume and cardiac output are lower in hypertensive patients with low stress-corrected mid-wall shortening.[112]

Role in symptomatic assessment

Although echocardiographic technology and image quality are constantly improving, the role of this investigation (echocardiography) in the routine assessment of symptomatic hypertensive patients has not been addressed in detail. It is feasible to complete rapid assessment at least of overall systolic function using portable machines. Using a handheld device and comparing this with a standard fully functional echocardiography platform, Senior and colleagues found a sensitivity of only 72% and positive and negative predictive values of 73 and 90% in 183 patients reviewed within a community systolic heart failure screening project.

Assessment of diastolic function in symptomatic patients

The subject of diastolic ventricular impairment in hypertension has been debated for many years. It has been marred largely by confusion over clinical definitions and importantly a failure to link many measurements to demonstrable exercise impairment in patients who voice heart failure symptoms. These are typically breathlessness upon exertion and/or undue fatigue, and they occur in patients who have normal systolic (generally short-axis contraction defined by echocardiography) ventricular function.

There is now general agreement that in the routine assessment of patients with heart failure symptoms (of whatever origin) many patients will have no demonstrable abnormality of systolic function, however this is assessed. Some may be accounted for by abnormal long-axis systolic function (although the significance of this phenomenon is as yet unclear where global volume ejection methods of stroke work are normal),[111] by valvular disease, by pulmonary hypertension, by intermittent occult arrhythmia (such as PAF common in conjunction with hypertension), or by parenchymal lung disease. Often the diagnosis of diastolic heart failure is arrived at by exclusion of other causes and the presence of indicators of impaired ventricular relaxation. A substantial proportion of these patients are female, many are overweight, and specifically there is often a clear association with hypertension and echocardiographic left ventricular hypertrophy.

In the Olmsted County survey, those patients (n=83) with a new clinical diagnosis of heart failure (i.e., a presentation of heart failure symptoms) and subsequent normal systolic function were generally very elderly (mean age 79 years) females (76%) who had defined histories of hypertension and/or coronary disease (85%).[113] Given the age range, it is perhaps not surprising therefore that the three-year mortality rate was high (60%). However, only half of these patients met broader ESC echocardiographic criteria for an association of the presenting symptoms with a diagnosis of *diastolic* heart failure.

Symptomatic heart failure without systolic contractile dysfunction remains an important, and for some observers even a dominant, form of heart failure presentation (particularly in the elderly).[114] The knowledge base regarding the epidemiology, pathophysiology, natural history, and therapy of these patients is still remarkably limited. There is a complex interaction with a number of age-related changes in the heart and vascular system that predispose to clinical presentation. Some population-based observational studies suggest that >50% of persons over 65 years who have heart failure symptoms will have normal LV systolic function. Of these, roughly half will have no other confounding variables (coronary, valvular, or pulmonary disease) and could meet suggested criteria for isolated DHF. This is substantially more common in older women than in men, and hypertension with echocardiographic left ventricular hypertrophy is almost invariably present. Although short-term mortality rates are about 50% lower than in systolic heart failure in stable patients, in acutely hospitalized or very elderly patients the mortality rate is similar in both systolic and potential diastolic heart failure. Furthermore, due to its higher prevalence the total mortality in the older population attributable to DHF in fact exceeds that of SHF. In the chronic setting, DHF patients can have severe exercise intolerance related to failure of the Frank-Starling mechanism with reduced peak cardiac output, heart rate, and stroke volume and increased LV filling pressure. DHF patients also appear to have increased vascular stiffness, accelerated systolic blood pressure response to exercise, neuro-endocrine activation, and reduced quality of life.

It is possible (and may be essential) to define diastolic heart failure by showing either impaired weight-corrected exercise capacity using expired gas analysis at cardiopulmonary testing,[115] or even elevated pulmonary wedge pressures at rest or during exercise in patients with symptomatic patients with echocardiographically normal systolic ventricular function.[116] Stress echocardiographic studies of potential diastolic filling abnormalities in hypertension (the difference between color tissue Doppler of myocardial segments at baseline and during pharmacological stress) show that hypertensive LVH is associated with reduced flow. In one survey of 30 patients free of epicardial coronary disease, and after adjusting for the LV mass and body mass, trans-mitral filling indices remained independently associated with impaired coronary flow reserve.[117] This may translate to impaired diastolic filling during subclinical (asymptomatic) myocardial ischaemia.

The role of transesophageal echocardiography (TOE) in the definition of diastolic relaxation is generally complementary to other techniques. Klein et al. have reported a large sample (n=181) from their practice where TEE was used primarily to assess for potential cause of diastolic dysfunction.[118] A large number in this selected group were found to have unsuspected restrictive cardiomyopathy (n=71), and a further substantial number (n=54) had features consistent with constrictive pericarditis, subsequently confirmed at surgery. Only a minority in this series (32%) had idiopathic diastolic dysfunction, and surprisingly only a very small number were found in association with hypertension (which would not be a general feature of these cases in most series).

There is no doubt that the technical assessment of diastolic filling has progressed rapidly in recent years since the clinical concept and significance of symptomatic isolated diastolic heart failure emerged. The population prevalence of this patient group is underrepresented by studies in hospital populations, which tend to be dominated by systolic ventricular dysfunction. In community-based surveys, prevalence figures as high as 15 to 20% are common in the elderly. Using only an echocardiographic point of analysis, Fischer et al. (examining the MONICA cohort in Augsburg) used the ESC definitions for diastolic heart failure, which are based on an age-dependent impairment of ventricular isovolumic relaxation time (95 to 105 ms) and early and late ventricular filling wave reversal (1 to 0.5). On this basis, they found a 15.8% prevalence of these characteristics in patients over 65 years of age from a sample of 1274 individuals. In this study, these echocardiographic abnormalities were more common in men than women, but were typically associated with hypertension, left ventricular hypertrophy, coronary artery disease, high body fat mass versus BMI, and diabetes. Abnormalities of diastolic filling were in fact rare (only 1 to 4% prevalence) in the absence of these features.[119]

Despite such surveys and prospective follow-up studies, there remains some debate as to the validity of diastolic filling abnormalities as the cause of heart failure symptoms in patients with normal systolic left ventricular ejection fraction, whether hypertensive or normotensive. The optimal means of the contribution of diastolic filling assessment to the definition of these patients remains somewhat controversial.

As with the assessment of coronary involvement and ischemia, invasive measures calculating the rate of decline in ventricular pressures in early diastole are often regarded as a gold standard by some cardiologists but in reality these can only reliably evaluate the active process of diastolic relaxation.[120] Changes in the more detailed end diastolic pressure volume filling loop are the most detailed physiological measure, but this these are generally approximated in clinical practice rather than measured directly.

Estimates of ventricular stiffness can be used as a surrogate for a pressure volume study, but this parameter is affected by any condition that will increase ventricular filling pressure. In addition, the assumption that ventricular hypertrophy is related to changes in passive diastolic filling is not entirely valid. For example, an acute ischemic stress will cause the upward shift in EDPV (end diastolic pressure volume) relationships, as will pericardial constriction and abnormal mechanical ventricular interaction. In some surveys of diastolic heart failure, EDPV curves are normal

both at rest and during exercise.[121] In others they are abnormal. This divergence of findings has further fueled questions as to the true nature of the abnormality in patients with heart failure symptoms and yet a preserved LV systolic ejection fraction.[122] The key issue is in the clinical definition of the patients themselves, and there is no doubt in almost every published survey in community or hospital clinic setting that these patients are predominantly older, female, hypertensive patients with echocardiographic ventricular hypertrophy.[123] The concomitant presence of obesity and hypertensive ventricular hypertrophy is common in many surveys. This simple association alone would seem logical, and many clinicians look to a cardiac cause for their symptoms, but it is still unclear if the linkage that so many feel is intuitive is indeed causal.

There is no doubt that echocardiographic parameters of diastolic filling and altered wall tension or echo backscatter are different between physiologic and pathologic hypertrophy. The latter is what is associated with isolated diastolic heart failure, whereas the former is associated with enhanced physical capacity and well being. In this respect, there is a lot of concern that the eccentric (predominantly septal) hypertrophic remodeling pattern of hypertensive heart disease should be differentiated from that seen with variants of genetic hypertrophic cardiomyopathy (HOCM). Although hypertensive eccentric hypertrophy is generally a less severe pattern than concentric remodeling in terms of its prognostic impact,[124] clearly HOCM has separate prognostic implications and differing molecular mechanisms that are not responsive to measures lowering BP that will predominantly reverse eccentric or concentric hypertensive ventricular remodeling.[125] The coexistence of hypertension and HOCM predictably causes confusion unless based on a molecular analysis. This is generally not available in routine practice, and it is clear that the linkage of many of these polymorphisms to outcome is still too complex to apply. The default position of some opinions is of course that all septal hypertrophy should be regarded as potentially malignant.[126]

Recent useful data looking at the value of BNP measurements confirm that this parameter (commonly seen as of diagnostic value in the definition of systolic dysfunction) is not in itself a good enough marker to allow reliable triage (at least of echocardiographic indices of diastolic ventricular function). In 72 hypertensive patients with heart failure symptoms, Mottram et al.[127] found that although BNP did relate independently to ventricular and atrial systolic parameters it was normally only within the high normal range in patients with echocardiographic diastolic dysfunction and therefore has limited positive diagnostic value in patients.

Contractile function and nonechocardiographic methods
MRI studies

The role of magnetic resonance and positron emission tomography studies in the assessment of the hypertensive patient continues to emerge. For example, Akinboboye et al. defined that myocardial oxygen demand in the hypertensive hypertrophied ventricle is best calculated using carbon-11 labeled acetate, and found that hypertensive LVH was most closely related to the physical wall stress as approximated by the stress mass heart rate product.[128]

The analysis of diastolic function by cardiovascular magnetic resonance can be completed to combine estimates of three-dimensional chamber volume, filling velocity, and flow, as well as myocardial strain and energy content.[129] These technologies can focus on specific regions of the myocardium (for example, a hypertrophied septum) and provide a real-time analysis of function applicable in clinical practice. Lamb and colleagues[130] from Leiden, using phosphorus[31] magnetic resonance spectroscopy, were able to readily define impaired LV filling in hypertension by an analysis of wall thinning (peak filling rates with normal systolic contractility). In association with these changes, atropine dobutamine stress levels of myocardial phosphocreatinine/ATP ratios were lowered from those values seen in normotensive controls. Although not all studies agree with these observations,[131] the accuracy of the technology and its ability to link energy metabolism with contractile function (as well as much more accurate morphological data than are possible with echocardiography)[132] might mean that this is the key area where the origins and significance of diastolic filling abnormalities in hypertension will finally be defined. Although echocardiographic measures are strongly correlated with MRI studies in selected echogenic patients, MR protocols still allow more accurate planimetry and variance in LV mass measurements are reduced about 40% (21% to 13%).[133] This reproducibility of assessment upon repeated measures is now widely accepted.

PET can similarly accurately map fatty acid oxidation and turnover in the heart. From a group based in St. Louis, data have been derived across a range of ventricular remodeling showing that myocardial fatty acid uptake, oxidation, and metabolism can be directly correlated to left ventricular mass in hypertension (as well as in other states such as ischemic cardiomyopathy).[134]

Coronary blood flow reserve (the maximal rise in coronary blood flow above its resting autoregulated values for a given perfusion pressure) can be accurately measured using N^{13}-labeled ammonia in hypertensive patients.[135] For example, the impact of BP-lowering therapy on the rest or stressed CFR of individual patients can be seen to be improved in response to treatment.[136] This type of study is regarded by some as the only truly quantitative noninvasive technique for the definition of coronary flow. These studies do not underestimate flow, as occurs with coronary sinus sampling.

PET studies

Gimelli et al.[137] used the flexibility of PET studies of N^{13} ammonia labeling (both at rest and following dipyridamole flow stress) to study the influence of ventricular hypertrophy on regional perfusion patterns in 50 hypertensive patients. Using this technology, they were able to show that patients with regional defects in perfusion were more likely to have ventricular hypertrophy but that overall myocardial blood flow was not simply related to total ventricular mass estimates. During pharmacologic stress, hypertensive patients who preserved a homogenous pattern of perfusion showed reduced coronary flow.

In the same way as MRI techniques have differentiated the stricture of the septum in HOCM from asymmetrical septal hypertrophy of hypertension, PET studies of glucose uptake show altered metabolism. F^{18}(2)-deoxy-glucose fractional uptake rations for the septum and posterior LV wall are similar in patients with HOCM or hypertensive heart disease but that the regional uptake is more heterogeneous in HOCM.[138]

CARDIAC RHYTHM IN HYPERTENSION

Assessment and relevance of arrhythmia in hypertension

The definition of cardiac arrhythmia in asymptomatic and symptomatic patients with hypertension is facilitated by ambulatory recordings either of a continuous or intermittent (where patients are symptomatic) nature. This allows a basic link to be made between patient symptoms (generally of palpitation but more realistically variably described) and rhythm. The key factor in hypertensive heart disease is an assessment of ventricular structure (generally echocardiographic) allowing both systolic and diastolic contractility; intercurrent valve function, and hypertrophy to be established. Although the presence of baseline conduction abnormalities has been alluded to previously, investigation of these generally relates to the linked processes of defining hypertrophy, ischemia, and valve function described previously. Two major areas require specific mention in the analysis of cardiac rhythm in hypertensive patients: atrial fibrillation and ventricular arrhythmia. Management of these conditions in hypertension is dealt with elsewhere in the text.

Atrial flutter-fibrillation

The etiological links among atrial fibrillation, hypertension, and stroke disease are important. As is now well appreciated, nonrheumatic atrial fibrillation is associated with an approximately fivefold increase in the risk of ischemic stroke and a 5 to 7% yearly increase in risk that increases with age. In addition, atrial fibrillation is associated with an increased incidence of clinically silent cerebral infarction and increased mortality. Treating hypertensive patients' stroke risk must take into account the definition of atrial fibrillation (and to a lesser extent atrial flutter coexistent with hypertension).

Unfortunately, few specific studies of atrial flutter and its association to hypertension have been completed. In patients with atrial flutter, there is a lesser prevalence of thromboembolic events. However, atrial flutter does *not* have a benign association where it occurs with concomitant hypertension. Using multivariate analysis, Seidl et al. (following only 191 patients with atrial flutter) found that the only independent risk factor on multivariate analysis for predicting thromboembolic events was a history of hypertension (OR = 6.5; 95% confidence intervals 1.5 to 45).[139] Atrial flutter cannot be ignored in the hypertensive patient, even if it is asymptomatic, and in contrast to many other clinical presentations should not be regarded as a benign feature.

In population studies, the relative risk ratio for acute atrial fibrillation is strongest at the onset of defined ischemic heart disease but diminishes in these patients over time. In contrast, the rate of atrial fibrillation is approximately 1.42 times increased in hypertensive men compared to normotensive men—and although congestive heart failure, valvular heart disease, and cardiomyopathy are important risk factors for the development of AF they are relatively uncommon in *known* AF patients.[140] Again, atrial fibrillation and hypertension are prevalent, and frequently coexistent, conditions in the elderly. The incidence of both *increases* with advancing age and independently they can both create significant burden of morbidity and mortality.[141] Although the interrelationship of these two conditions is long established,[142] the etiological details of this linkage are not yet well separated.

Hypertension is associated with left ventricular hypertrophy, impaired ventricular filling, left atrial enlargement, and a slowing of atrial conduction velocity. Such simple independent changes in cardiac structure clearly favor the loss of sinus rhythm and the development of atrial fibrillation. They also increase the risk of thromboembolic complications in both states. However, left atrial diameter (for example) determined by M-mode echocardiography does not predict stroke in patients with AF.[143] The pathological linkage of atrial fibrillation to hypertension is strong and simple, although dependent on a progression of several factors. Many factors contribute to changes in left atrial size, which in turn alters left atrial conduction and contributes to the promotion of paroxysmal atrial fibrillation. This links directly to the presence of increased left ventricular mass in hypertensive atrial fibrillation,[144] and as with ventricular arrhythmia is generally *unrelated* to concomitant epicardial coronary disease.[155] Thus, the important investigational issue is that in the hypertensive patient there should not be an immediate assumption that atrial fibrillation is a marker of coronary disease when in point of fact this is true only in the minority.

Verdecchia et al.[145] followed up 2482 hypertensive patients, all of whom were in sinus rhythm at presentation. Excluded were subjects with known valvular heart disease, CAD, ventricular arrhythmia, and thyroid or lung disease. This investigation reported that the incidence of a first episode of atrial fibrillation was 0.46 per 100 person-years (n=61). These affected patients at entry were older (59 versus 51 years), had higher office and 24-hour mean SBP (165 and 144 versus 157 and 137 mmHg, respectively), had a greater left ventricular mass {58 versus 49g/height[m](2.7)}, and echocardiographic left atrial diameter (3.89 versus 3.56 cm). In a multivariate logistic regression analysis, only age and left ventricular mass predicted the evolution of a first episode of atrial fibrillation in hypertension. They calculated that for every 1 standard deviation increase in left ventricular mass the risk of atrial fibrillation was increased 1.20 times (95% CI, 1.07 to 1.34). Interestingly, atrial fibrillation became chronic in only 33% of the subjects in the study during the follow-up period. Similarly, age, left ventricular mass, and left atrial diameter were independent predictors of chronic atrial fibrillation. The ischemic stroke rate was 2.7% and 4.6% per year for paroxysmal

and chronic atrial fibrillation, respectively. The interesting aspect of this study was that increased left atrial size predisposed to the degeneration of PAF to chronic or persistent AF. Thus, echocardiographic assessment may play a role in this hypertensive patient subgroup.

The general population prevalence of atrial fibrillation in the elderly is associated with clear structural changes in the heart definable at echocardiography. In the Framingham study, subjects routinely evaluated with M-mode echocardiography (n=1924 aged 59 to 90 years) provided data for analyzing the association of echocardiographic features with atrial fibrillation risk after adjustment for age, sex, hypertension, coronary heart disease, congestive heart failure, diabetes, and valvular heart disease.[146] Over a mean follow-up of 7.2 years, 154 subjects (8.0%) developed atrial fibrillation. Multivariable stepwise analysis identified left atrial size (hazard ratio [HR] per 5-mm increment, 1.39; 95% confidence interval [CI], 1.14 to 1.68), left ventricular fractional shortening (HR per 5% decrement, 1.34; 95% CI, 1.08 to 1.66), and sum of septal and left ventricular posterior wall thickness (HR per 4-mm increment, 1.28; 95% CI, 1.03 to 1.60) as independent echocardiographic predictors of atrial fibrillation. The likelihood of atrial fibrillation grew markedly when these changes occurred together, giving cumulative 8-year age-adjusted atrial fibrillation rates of 7.3 and 17.0%, respectively, when one and two or more highest-risk-quartile features were present compared with 3.7% when none was present. These echocardiographic precursors offer prognostic information beyond that provided by traditional clinical atrial fibrillation risk factors.

Although conventional therapy of atrial fibrillation has focused on interventions to control heart rate and/or rhythm and the prevention of stroke through the use of antithrombotic anticoagulant medications, in patients with hypertension and atrial fibrillation aggressive management of BP by reversing structural change in the heart can reduce the likelihood of thromboembolic complications and can retard or prevent the occurrence of atrial fibrillation.

The restoration of sinus rhythm by DC cardioversion is feasible in hypertensive atrial fibrillation, but the maintenance of sinus rhythm is lowest in patients with ventricular hypertrophy or concomitant ventricular dysfunction.[147] Such former strategies are currently being reevaluated because the benefits of rhythm control seem limited and the risks may outweigh benefit. The management issues will be dealt with elsewhere, but the key features for the development of atrial fibrillation are clear. The integrated risk of stroke in the hypertensive patient with atrial fibrillation is such that anticoagulation should be a priority.[148]

Ventricular arrhythmia

The presence of significant ventricular arrhythmia in hypertension is well established, as is the increased incidence of sudden death frequently assumed to represent serious ventricular arrhythmia. The key mediators are the involvement of ischemia (which can be clinically silent or symptomatic), prior infarction or left ventricular hypertrophy, and more rarely left ventricular systolic dysfunction.[149,150] However, there is often confusion over the sequence of events and the primary mediator in individual hypertensive patients. The links among serious arrhythmia, ventricular structural changes, arterial pressure/wall stress, ischemia, and sudden death are clearly complex and interdependent. The coincident occurrence of silent ischemia and LVH is a particularly powerful but independent (on population analyses) combination in hypertensive patients for future ventricular arrhythmia.[151]

Holter studies of the prevalence of ventricular arrhythmia show simple ectopy to be common (>70%), but this is confounded by age and many other factors—leading this feature to have little prognostic validity whether applied to uncomplicated or even symptomatic patients with hypertension. Complex ventricular arrhythmia is less frequent, is age and pressure dependent, and appears responsive in part to BP control.[152] Some studies suggest that the frequency of arrhythmia is graded and is related to the severity of LVH even in the absence of angiographic coronary disease.[153] In terms of prognosis for future cardiac or vascular events, the electrocardiographic definition of arrhythmia is perhaps less significant than the value of defining ventricular structure and/or the presence of inducible ischemia or systolic contractile function.

Prospective studies of arrhythmia and sudden death restricted to cases where hypertensive heart disease has been defined in detail are rare indeed. From the limited information available, there seems to be little evidence of a link between markers such as abnormal QT dispersion in LVH and the risk of serious arrhythmia in cases of hypertension.[154] This is despite well-documented investigation of the utility of QT dispersion in predicting sudden death or arrhythmia in unselected ischemic cardiomyopathy.[155] The impact and linkage of QT_c dispersion to ventricular arrhythmia may be stronger in nonischemic *dilated* cardiomyopathy than in hypertensive LVH.[156] The lack of association to LVH is similar to some studies in hypertension. Saadeh and Vann Jones prospectively found only LVH and documented Holter complex arrhythmia associated with sudden (presumed arrhythmic) death in a small cohort of hypertensive patients. They found only 6 sudden deaths from a long-term study of 54 hypertensive patients over nearly 10 years. Despite this, it remains a valuable if limited observation.

SUMMARY

There is little doubt that patients with hypertension present a particular challenge to completing effective diagnostic cardiac evaluation of symptoms or signs. Assessment must extend beyond the definition of BP alone, particularly in symptomatic patients. Although there is neither an excuse nor a justification for "scattergun" testing of asymptomatic patients, equally there is evidence that initial assessment of even asymptomatic hypertensive patients should encompass some routine cardiac assessment beyond the simplistic traditions of rest electrocardiography and chest radiology. A variety of factors affecting the hypertensive population (the impact of age, obesity, concomitant diabetes and vascular disease, drug therapy, and ethnicity) complicate coherent cardiac diagnostic evaluation by simple techniques alone. Although hypertensive patients are traditionally viewed as asymptomatic, sophisticated investigational assessment using both stress and rest studies are required to obtain a true overall cardiac risk assessment.

When hypertensive patients do start to present cardiac symptoms, their investigation is not often well served by relying solely on noninvasive or static evaluation techniques applied in an isolated fashion. As a good example, the definition of symptoms due to impaired diastolic relaxation are focused very clearly in the elderly hypertensive population in the community where purely echocardiographic definitions have little meaning unless accompanied by some reasonable quantification of what is often predictably poor exercise capacity and functional activity. The complexity of this patient group may be better analyzed using evolving MR-based technology even more so than invasive physiological measurements of intraventricular diastolic pressure wave forms applicable only to a tiny minority. Similarly, in the definition of myocardial ischemia the confounding impact of hypertension means that noninvasive testing protocols lag well behind a conventional approach of progressing rapidly toward invasive angiographic risk stratification, provided of course that BP control has been correctly achieved and that functional cardiac assessment is not ignored.

The investigation of the cardiac status of hypertensive patients remains a crucial aspect of clinical management in hypertension and cannot be abridged to simplistic BP control issues. Ultimately, many hypertensive patients pass on to be labeled "coronary" or "stroke" patients after surviving critical vascular events often where their systemic arterial BP cannot be sustained (through myocardial loss).

REFERENCES

1. Kannel WB. Some lessons in cardiovascular epidemiology from Framingham. *Am J Cardiol.* 1976;37(2):269–82.
2. Frank CW, Weinblatt E, Shapiro S, Sager RV. Prognosis of men with coronary heart disease as related to blood pressure. *Circulation* 1968 Aug;38(2):432–8.
3. Kuller L. Sudden death in arteriosclerotic heart disease: The case for preventive medicine. *Am J Cardiol* 1969;24(5):617–28.
4. Goyal D, MacFadyen RJ. Perception of symptoms in hypertensive patients and the relevance to the application of anti-hypertensive drug therapy. *Current Pharmaceutical Design* 2006;12: 1567–79.
5. Fuchs FD, Gus M, Moreira LB, Moreira, WD, Goncalves, SC, Nunes, G. Headache is not more frequent among patients with moderate to severe hypertension. *J Human Hypertension* 2003;17:787–90.
6. Sarasin FP, Louis-Simonet M, Carballo D, Slama S, Junod AF, Unger PF. Prevalence of orthostatic hypotension among patients presenting with

syncope in the ED. *Amer J Emerge Med* 2002;20:497–501.

7. O'Mahoney D. Pathophysiology of carotid sinus hypersensitivity in elderly patients. *Lancet* 1995;346:950–52.

8. Strasberg B, Sagie A, Erdman S, Kusniec J, Sclarovsky S, Agmon J. Carotid sinus hypersensitivity and the carotis sinus syndrome. *Progress in Cardiovascular Diseases* 1989;31:379–91.

9. Schutzman J, Jaeger F, Maloney J, Fouadtarazi F. Head up tilt and hemodynamic changes during orthostatic hypotension in patients with supine hypertension. *J Amer Coll Cardiol* 1994;24:454–61.

10. Gazes PC, Mobley EM Jr., Faris HM Jr., Duncan RC, Humphries GB. Preinfarctional (unstable) angina (a prospective study) ten year follow-up. Prognostic significance of electrocardiographic changes. *Circulation* 1973;48(2):331–37.

11. Zamboni S, Ambrosio GB, Stefanini MG, Urbani V, Dissegna L, Mazzucato L, et al. Electrocardiographic findings in hypertensive patients of a population sample: Role of sex, age, and antihypertensive treatment. *J Clin Hypertens* 1987;3:430–38.

12. Alpert MA, Munuswamy K. Electrocardiographic diagnosis of left atrial enlargement. *Arch Intern Med* 1989;149:1161–65.

13. Cristal N, Koren I. Evaluation of the electrocardiogram in hypertensive patients: The LOMIR-MCT-IL study experience. *Blood Press Suppl* 1994;1:43–7.

14. Genovesiebert A, Marabotti C, Palombo C, Ghione S. Electrocardiographic signs of atrial overload in hypertensive patients: Indexes of abnormality of atrial morphology or function. *Amer Heart J* 1991;121:1113–18.

15. Madu EC, Baugh DS, Gbadebo TD, Dhala A, Cardoso S. Phi-Res Multi-Study Group. Effect of ethnicity and hypertension on atrial conduction: Evaluation with high-resolution P-wave signal averaging. *Clin Cardiol* 2001;24(9):597–602.

16. Presciuttini B, Duprez D, De Buyzere M, Clement DL. How to study sympatho-vagal balance in arterial hypertension and the effect of antihypertensive drugs? *Acta Cardiologica* 1998;53:143–52.

17. Tran H, White CM, Chow MSS, Kluger J. An evaluation of the impact of gender and age on QT dispersion in healthy subjects. *Ann Noninvasive Electrocardiology* 2001;6:129–33.

18. Chapman N, Mayet J, Ozkor M, Foale R, Thom S, Poulter N. Ethnic and gender differences in electrocardiographic QT length and QT dispersion in hypertensive subjects. *J Human Hypertension* 2000;14:403–05.

19. Xiao HB, Brecker SJ, Gibson DG. Relative effects of left ventricular mass and conduction disturbance on activation in patients with pathological left ventricular hypertrophy. *Br Heart J* 1994;71:548–53.

20. Rotman M, Triebwasser JH. A clinical and follow-up study of right and left bundle branch block. *Circulation* 1975;51(3):477–84.

21. Sundstrom J, Lind L, Andren B, Lithell H. Left ventricular geometry and function are related to electrocardiographic characteristics and diagnoses. *Clin Physiol* 1998;18:463–70.

22. Clarkson PB, Naas AAO, McMahon A, MacLeod C, Struthers AD, MacDonald TMM. QT dispersion in essential hypertension. *QJM* 1995;88:327–32.

23. Mayet J, Shahi M, McGrath K, Poulter NR, Sever PS, Foale RA, et al. Left ventricular hypertrophy and QT dispersion in hypertension. *Hypertension* 1996;28:791–96.

24. Barr CS, Naas AAO, Freeman M, Lang CC, Struthers AD. QT dispersion and sudden unexpected death in chronic heart failure. *Lancet* 1994;343:327–29.

25. Elming H, Holm E, Jun L, Torp-Pedersen C, Kober L, Kirschoff M, et al. The prognostic value of the QT interval and QT interval dispersion in all-cause and cardiac mortality and morbidity in a population of Danish citizens. *Eur Heart J* 1998;19(9):1391–1400.

26. de Bruyne MC, Hoes AW, Kors JA, Hofman A, van Bemmel JH, Grobbee DE. QTc dispersion predicts cardiac mortality in the elderly: The Rotterdam Study. *Circulation* 1998;97:467–72.

27. Halle M, Huonker M, Hohnloser SH, Alivertis M, Berg A, Keul J. QT dispersion in exercise-induced myocardial hypertrophy. *Am Heart J* 1999;138(2 Pt 1):309–12.

28. Chapman N, Mayet J, Ozkor M, Lampe FC, Thom SAM, Poulter NR. QT intervals and QT dispersion as measures of left ventricular hypertrophy in an unselected hypertensive population. *Amer J Hypertension* 2001;14:455–62.

29. Piccirillo G, Germano G, Quaglione R, Nocco M, Lintas F, Lionetti M, et al. QT-interval variability and autonomic control in hypertensive subjects with left ventricular hypertrophy. *Clin Sci* 2002;102:363–71.

30. Wong KYK, Lim PO, Wong SYS, MacWalter RS, Struthers AD, MacDonald TM. Does a prolonged QT peak identify left ventricular hypertrophy in hypertension? *Int J Cardiol* 2003;89:179–86.

31. Okin PM, Roman MJ, Devereux RB, Pickering TG, Borer JS, Kligfield P. Time-voltage QRS area of the 12-lead electrocardiogram: Detection of left ventricular hypertrophy. *Hypertension* 1998;31:937–42.

32. Kannel WB, Gordon T, Offutt D. Left ventricular hypertrophy by electrocardiogram: Prevalence, incidence, and mortality in the Framingham study. *Ann Intern Med* 1969;71(1):89–105.

33. Huwez FU, Pringle SD, Macfarlane PW. Variable patterns of ST-T abnormalities in patients with left ventricular hypertrophy and normal coronary arteries. *Br Heart J* 1992;67:304–07.

34. Verdecchia P, Angeli F, Reboldi G, Carluccio E, Benemio G, Gattobigio R, et al. Improved cardiovascular risk stratification by a simple ECG index in hypertension. *Amer J Hypertension* 2003;16:646–52.

35. Antikainen R, Grodzicki T, Palmer AJ, Beevers DG, Coles EC, Webster J, et al. The determinants of left ventricular hypertrophy defined by Sokolow Lyon criteria in untreated hypertensive patients. *J Hum Hypertens* 2003;17:159–64.

36. Devereaux RB, Phillips MC, Casale PN, Eisenberger RR, Kligfeld P. Geometric determinants of electrocardiographic left ventricular hypertrophy. *Circulation* 1983;67:907–11.

37. Lee DK, Marantz PR, Devereux RB, Klingfield P, Alderman MH. Left ventricular hypertrophy in black and white hypertensives: Standard electrocardiographic criteria overestimate racial differences in prevalence. *J Amer Med Assoc* 1992;267:3294–99.

38. Tochikubo O, Miyajima E, Shigemasa T, Ishii M. Relation between body fat-corrected ECG voltage and ambulatory blood pressure in patients with essential hypertension. *Hypertension* 1999;33:1159–63.

39. Chapman JN, Mayet J, Chang CL, Foale RA, Thom SAM, Poulter NR. Ethnic differences in the identification of left ventricular hypertrophy in the hypertensive patient. *Amer J Hypertension* 1999;12:437–42.

40. Okin PM, Roman MJ, Devereux RB, Kligfield P. Electrocardiographic identification of increased left ventricular mass by simple voltage duration products. *J Amer Coll Cardiol* 1995;25:417–23.

41. Norman JE, Levy D. Adjustment of ECG left ventricular hypertrophy criteria for body mass index and age improves classification accuracy: The effects of hypertension and obesity. *J Electrocardiology* 1996;29(Suppl 5):241–47.

42. Okin PM, Roman MJ, Devereux RB, Kligfield P. Electrocardiographic identification of left ventricular hypertrophy: Test performance in relation to definition of hypertrophy and presence of obesity. *J Amer Coll Cardiol* 1996;27:124–31.

43. Casiglia E, Maniati G, Daskalakis C, Colangeli G, Tramontin P, Ginocchio G, et al. Left-ventricular hypertrophy in the elderly: Unreliability of ECG criteria in 477 subjects aged 65 years or more. The CArdiovascular STudy in the ELderly (CASTEL). *Cardiology* 1996;87:429–35.

44. Filipovsky J, Ducimetiere P, Safar ME. Prognostic significance of exercise blood pressure and heart rate in middle aged men. *Hypertension* 1992;20:333–39.

45. Jette M, Sidney K, Landry F, Quenneville J. Blood pressure responses to a progressive step test in normotensive males and females. *Can J App Physiol* 1994;19:421–31.

46. Lim PO, MacDonald TM. Non-invasive profiling of total peripheral vascular resistance using the Dundee step test. *Amer J Hypertension* 1999;12:173A.

47. Lim PO, Donnan PT, MacDonald TM. How well do office and exercise blood pressures predict sustained hypertension? A Dundee Step Test Study. *J Human Hypertension* 2000;14:429–33.

48. Lim PO, Rana BS, Struthers AD, MacDonald TM. Exercise blood pressure correlates with the maximum heart rate corrected QT interval in hypertension. *J Hum Hypertension* 2001;15:169–72.

49. Gottdiener JS, Brown J, Zoltick J, Fletcher RD. Left ventricular hypertrophy

in men with normal blood pressure: Relation to exaggerated blood pressure response to exercise. *Ann Int Med* 1990;112:161–66.

50. Campbell L, Marwick TH, Pashkow FJ, Snader CE, Lauer MS. Usefulness of an exaggerated systolic blood pressure response to exercise in predicting myocardial perfusion defects in known or suspected coronary artery disease. *Amer J Cardiol* 1999;84(II):1304–10.

51. Marwick TH, Torelli J, Harjai K, Haluska B, Pashkow FJ, Stewart WJ, et al. Influence of left ventricular hypertrophy on detection of coronary artery disease using exercise echocardiography. *J Amer Coll Cardiol* 1995;26:1180–86.

52. Picano E, Palinkas A, Amyot R. Diagnosis of myocardial ischemia in hypertensive patients. *J Hypertension* 2001;19:1177–83.

53. Jespersen CM, Rasmussen V. Detection of myocardial ischaemia by transthoracic leads in ambulatory electrocardiographic monitoring. *Brit Heart J* 1992;68:286–90.

54. Pringle SD, Dunn FG, Tweddel AC, Martin W, MacFarlane PW, McKillop JH, et al. Symptomatic and silent myocardial ischaemia in hypertensive patients with left ventricular hypertrophy. *Brit Heart J* 1992;67:377–82.

55. Asmar R, Benetos A, Pannier B, Agnes E, Topouchian J, Laloux B, et al. Prevalence and circadian variations of ST-segment depression and its concomitant blood pressure changes in asymptomatic systemic hypertension. *J Hypertens* 2001;19:1883–91.

56. Siegel D, Cheitlin MD, Seeley DG, Black DM, Hulley SB. Silent myocardial ischaemia in men with systemic hypertension and without clinical evidence of coronary artery disease. *Amer J Cardiol* 1992;70:86–90.

57. Elhendy A, van Domburg RT, Sozzi FB, Poldermans D, Bax JJ, Roelandt JRTC. Impact of hypertension on the accuracy of exercise stress myocardial perfusion imaging for the diagnosis of coronary artery disease. *Heart* 2001;85:655–61.

58. Berger HJ, Sands MJ, Davies RA, Wackers FJT, Alexander J, Lachman AS, et al. Exercise left ventricular performance in patients with chest pain ischemic appearing exercise electrocardiograms and angiographically normal coronary arteries. *Ann Int Med* 1981;94:186–91.

59. Cecil MP, Pilcher MP, Eisner RL, Chu TH, Merlino JD, Patterson RE. Absence of defects in SPECT Th-201 myocardial images in patients with systemic hypertension and left ventricular hypertrophy. *Amer J Cardiol* 1994;74:43–6.

60. Elhendy A, van Domburg RT, Bax JJ, Ibrahim MM, Roelandt JRTC. Myocardial perfusion abnormalities in treated hypertensive patients without known coronary artery disease. *J Hypertension* 1999;17:1601–06.

61. Schillaci O, Moroni C, Scopinaro F, Tavolaro R, Danieli R, Bossini A, et al. Technetium-99m sestamibi myocardial tomography based on dipyridamole echocardiography testing in hypertensive patients with chest pain. *Eur J Nuc Med* 1997;24:774–78.

62. Elhendy A, Mahoney DW, Khandheria BK, Paterick TE, Burger KN, Pellikka PA. Prognostic significance of the location

of wall motion abnormalities during exercise echocardiography. *J Amer Coll Cardiol* 2002;40:1623–29.

63. Lee CY, Pellikka PA, McCully RB, Mahoney DW, Seward JB. Non-exercise stress transthoracic echocardiography: Transoesophageal atrial pacing versus dobutamine stress. *J Amer Coll Cardiol* 1999;33:506–11.

64. Picano E, Mathias W, Pingitore A, Bigi R, Previtali M. Safety and tolerability of dobutamine atropine stress echocardiography a prospective multi centre study. *Lancet* 1994;344:1190–92.

65. Lee CY, Pellikka PA, Shub C, Sinak LJ, Seward JB. Hypertensive response during dobutamine stress echocardiography. *Amer J Cardiol* 1997;80:970–76.

66. Senior R, Basu S, Handler C, Raftery EB, Lahiri A. Diagnostic accuracy of dobutamine stress echocardiography for detection of coronary heart disease in hypertensive patients. *Eur Heart J* 1996;17:289–95.

67. Maltagliati A, Berti M, Muratori M, Tamborini G, Zavalloni D, Berna G, et al. Exercise echocardiography versus exercise electrocardiography in the diagnosis of coronary artery disease in hypertension. *Amer J Hypertension* 2000;13:796–801.

68. Astarita C, Palinkas A, Nicolai E, Maresca FS, Varga A, Picano E. Dipyridamole-atropine stress echocardiography versus exercise SPECT scintigraphy for detection of coronary artery disease in hypertensives with positive exercise test. *J Hypertension* 2001;19:495–502.

69. Elhendy A, Geleijnse ML, van Domburg RT, Bax JJ, Nierop PR, Beerens SAM, et al. Comparison of dobutamine stress echocardiography and technetium-99m sestamibi single-photon emission tomography for the diagnosis of coronary artery disease in hypertensive patients with and without left ventricular hypertrophy. *Eur J Nuc Med* 1998;25:69–78.

70. Cortigiani L, Paolini EA, Nannini E. Dipyridamole stress echocardiography for risk stratification in hypertensive patients with chest pain. *Circulation* 1998;98:2855–59.

71. Cortigiani L, Bigi R, Rigo F, Landi P, Baldini U, Mariani PR, et al. On behalf of the EPIC (Echo Persantine International Cooperative) Study Group. Diagnostic value of exercise electrocardiography and dipyridamole stress echocardiography in hypertensive and normotensive chest pain patients with right bundle branch block. *J Hypertens* 2003;21(11):2189–94.

72. Fragasso G, Lu CZ, Dabrowski P, Pagnotta P, Sheiban I, Chierchia SL. Comparison of stress/rest myocardial perfusion tomography, dipyridamole and dobutamine stress echocardiography for the detection of coronary disease in hypertensive patients with chest pain and positive exercise test. *J Amer Coll Cardiol* 1999;34:441–47.

73. Marwick TH, Case C, Sawada S, Vasey C, Thomas JD. Prediction of outcomes in hypertensive patients with suspected coronary disease. *Hypertension* 2002;39:1113–18.

74. Cortigiani L, Bigi R, Gigli G, Coletta C, Mariotti E, Dodi C, et al. Prognostic

implications of intraventricular conduction defects in patients undergoing stress echocardiography for suspected coronary artery disease. *Am J Med* 2003;115:12–18.

75. Yuda S, Khoury V, Marwick TH. Influence of wall stress and left ventricular geometry on the accuracy of dobutamine stress echocardiography. *J Amer Coll Cardiol* 2002;40:1311–19.

76. Zouridakis EG, Cox ID, Garcia-Moll X, Brown S, Nihoyannopoulos P, Kaski JC. Negative stress echocardiographic responses in normotensive and hypertensive patients with angina pectoris, positive exercise stress testing, and normal coronary arteriograms. *Heart* 2000;83:141–46.

77. Bory M, Pierron F, Panagides D, Bonnet JL, Yvorra S, Desfossez L..Coronary artery spasm in patients with normal or near normal coronary arteries: Long-term follow-up of 277 patients. *Eur Heart J* 1996;17:1015–21.

78. Da Costa A, Isaaz K, Faure E, Mourot S, Cerisier A, Lamaud M. Clinical characteristics, aetiological factors and long-term prognosis of myocardial infarction with an absolutely normal coronary angiogram: A 3-year follow-up study of 91 patients. *Eur Heart J* 2001;22:1459–65.

79. Crenshaw JH, Elezeky F, Zwaag RV, Sullivan JM, Ramanathan KB, Mirvis DM. The effect of non-critical coronary artery disease on long term survival. *Amer J Med Sci* 1995;310:7–13.

80. De Cesare N, Polese A, Cozzi S, Apostolo A, Fabbiocchi F, Loaldi A, et al. Coronary angiographic patterns in hypertensive compared with normotensive patients. *Am Heart J* 1991;21:1101–06.

81. Maher JE, Raz JA, Bielak LF, Sheedy PF, Schwartz RS, Peyser PA. Potential of quantity of coronary artery calcification to identify new risk factors for asymptomatic atherosclerosis. *Amer J Epidemiol* 1996;144:943–53.

82. Shaw LJ, Raggi P, Schisterman E, Berman DS, Callister TQ. Prognostic value of cardiac risk factors and coronary artery calcium screening for all-cause mortality. *Radiology* 2003;228:826–33.

83. Khurana C, Rosenbaum CG, Howard BV, Adams-Campbell LL, Detrano RC, Klouj A, et al. Coronary artery calcification in black women and white women. *Amer Heart J* 2003;145:724–29.

84. Megnien JL, Simon A, Lemariey M, Plainfosse MC, Levenson J. Hypertension promotes coronary calcium deposit in asymptomatic men. *Hypertension* 1996;27:949–54.

85. Schmermund A, Baumgart D, Gorge G, Gronemeyer D, Seibel R, Bailey KR, et al. Measuring the effect of risk factors on coronary atherosclerosis: Coronary calcium score versus angiographic disease severity. *J Amer Coll Cardiol* 1998;31:1267–73.

86. Guerci AD, Spadaro LA, Goodman KJ, Lledo-Perez A, Newstein D, Lerner G, et al. Comparison of electron beam computed tomography scanning and conventional risk factor assessment for the prediction of angiographic coronary artery disease. *J Amer Coll Cardiol* 1998;32:673–79.

87. Turner ST, Bielak LF, Narayana AK, Sheedy PF, Schwartz GL, Peyser PA. Ambulatory blood pressure and coronary artery calcification in middle-aged and younger adults. *Amer J Hypertension* 2002;15:518–24.

88. Altunkan S, Erdogan N, Altin L, Budoff MJ. Relation of coronary artery calcium to left ventricular mass and geometry in patients with essential hypertension. *Blood Pressure Monitoring* 2003;8:9–15.

89. Antonini-Canterin F, Huang GQ, Cervesato E, Faggiano P, Pavan D, Piazza R, et al. Symptomatic aortic stenosis: Does systemic hypertension play an additional role? *Hypertension* 2003;41:1268–72.

90. Pate GE. Association between aortic stenosis and hypertension. *J Heart Valve Disease* 2002;11:612–14.

91. Stewart BF, Siscovick D, Lind BK, Gardin JM, Gottdiener JS, Smith VE, et al. Clinical factors associated with calcific aortic valve disease. *J Amer Coll Cardiol* 1997;29:630–34.

92. Rosenhek R, Binder T, Porenta G, Lang I, Christ G, Schemper M, et al. Predictors of outcome in severe, asymptomatic aortic stenosis. *New Eng J Med* 2000;343:611–617.

93. Post WS, Larson MG, Levy D. Hemodynamic predictors of incident hypertension: The Framingham Heart Study. *Hypertension* 1994;24:585–90.

94. Palta S, Pai AM, Gill KS, Pai RG. New insights into the progression of aortic stenosis: Implications for secondary prevention. *Circulation* 2000;101:2497–502.

95. Palmieri V, Bella JN, Arnett DK, Oberman A, Kitzman DW, Hopkins PN, et al. Associations of aortic and mitral regurgitation with body composition and myocardial energy expenditure in adults with hypertension: The Hypertension Genetic Epidemiology Network study. *Amer Heart J* 2003;145:1071–77.

96. Thomas JT, Kelly RF, Thomas SJ, Stamos TD, Albasha K, Parrillo JE, et al. Utility of history, physical examination, electrocardiogram, and chest radiograph for differentiating normal from decreased systolic function in patients with heart failure. *Amer J Med* 2002;112:437–45.

97. Lim PO, MacFadyen RJ, Clarkson PBM, MacDonald TM. Impaired exercise tolerance in hypertensive patients. *Ann Int Med* 1996;124:41–55.

98. Cuspidi C, Ambrosioni E, Mancia G, Pessina AC, Trimarco B, Zanchetti A. Role of echocardiography and carotid ultrasonography in stratifying risk in patients with essential hypertension: The Assessment of Prognostic Risk Observational Survey. *J Hypertension* 2002;20:1307–14.

99. Schillaci G, de Simone G, Reboldi G, Porcellati C, Devereux RB, Verdecchia P. Change in cardiovascular risk profile by echocardiography in low- or medium-risk hypertension. *J Hypertension* 2002;20:1519–25.

100. Aeschbacher BC, Hutter D, Fuhrer J, Weidmann P, Delacretaz E, Allemann Y. Diastolic dysfunction precedes myocardial hypertrophy in the development of hypertension. *Amer J Hypertension* 2001;14:106–13.

101. Maceira AM, Barba J, Beloqui O, Diez J. Ultrasonic backscatter and diastolic function in hypertensive patients. *Hypertension* 2002;40:239–43.

102. Clarkson PBM, Wheeldon NM, Lim PO, Pringle SD, MacDonald TM. Left atrial size and function: Assessment using echocardiographic automated boundary detection. *Brit Heart J* 1995;74:664–70.

103. Tsang TS, Barnes ME, Gersh BJ, Takemoto Y, Rosales AG, Bailey KR, et al. Prediction of risk for first age related cardiovascular events in an elderly population: The incremental value of echocardiography. *J Amer Coll Cardiol* 2003;42:1199–1205.

104. Tsang TS, Barnes ME, Gersh BJ, Bailey KR, Seward JB. Left atrial volume as a morphophysiologic expression of left ventricular diastolic dysfunction and relation to cardiovascular risk burden. *Amer J Cardiol* 2002;15:1284–89.

105. Verdecchia P, Schillaci G, Borgioni C, Ciucci A, Zampi I, Gattobigio R, et al. White coat hypertension and white coat effect: Similarities and differences. *Amer J Hypertension* 1995;8:790–98.

106. Soma J, Wideroe TE, Dahl K, Rossvoll O, Skjaerpe T. Left ventricular systolic and diastolic function assessed with two-dimensional and Doppler echocardiography in "'white coat'" hypertension. *J Amer Coll Cardiol* 1996;28:190–96.

107. Glen SK, Elliott HL, Curzio JL, Lees KR, Reid JL. White-coat hypertension as a cause of cardiovascular dysfunction. *Lancet* 1996;348:654–57.

108. Slotwiner DJ, Devereux RB, Schwartz JE, Pickering TG, de Simone G, Roman MJ. Relation of age to left ventricular function and systemic hemodynamics in uncomplicated mild hypertension. *Hypertension* 2001;37:1404–09.

109. Poulsen SH, Andersen NH, Ivarsen PI, Mogensen CE, Egeblad H. Doppler tissue imaging reveals systolic dysfunction in patients with hypertension and apparent "isolated" diastolic dysfunction. *J Amer Soc Echocardiography* 2003;16:724–31.

110. Pela G, Bruschi G, Cavatorta A, Manca C, Cabassi A, Borghetti A. Doppler tissue echocardiography: Myocardial wall motion velocities in essential hypertension. *Eur J Echocardiog* 2001;2(2):108–17.

111. Bella JN, Wachtell K, Palmieri V, Liebson PR, Gerdts E, Ylitalo A, et al. Relation of left ventricular geometry and function to systemic hemodynamics in hypertension: The LIFE Study. *J Hypertension* 2001;19:127–34.

112. Desimone G, Devereux RB, Roman MJ, Ganau A, Saba PS, Alderman MH, et al. Assessment of left ventricular function by the mid wall fractionbal shortening end systolic stress relation in human hypertension. *J Amer Coll Cardiol* 1994;23:1444–51.

113. Chen HH, Lainchbury JG, Senni M, Bailey KR, Redfield MM. Diastolic heart failure in the community: clinical profile, natural history, therapy and impact of proposed diagnostic criteria. *J Cardiac Failure* 2002;8:279–87.

114. Kitzman DW. Diastolic heart failure in the elderly. *Heart Fail Rev* 2002;7(1):17–27.

115. Nodari S, Metra M, Dei Cas L. Beta blocker treatment of patients wit diastolic heart failure and arterial hypertension: A prospective randomised comparison of the long term effects of atenolol vs. nebivolol. *Eur J Heart Failure* 2003;5:621–27.

116. Clarkson PB, Wheeldon NM, MacFadyen RJ, Pringle SD, MacDonald TM. Effects of brain natriuretic peptide on exercise haemodynamics and neurohormones in isolated diastolic heart failure. *Circulation* 1996;93:2037–42.

117. Galderisi M, Cicala S, Caso P, de Simone L, D'Errico A, Petrocelli A, et al. Coronary flow reserve and myocardial diastolic dysfunction in arterial hypertension. *Amer J Cardiol* 2002;90:860–64.

118. Klein AL, Canale MP, Rajagopalan N, White RD, Murray RD, Wahi S, et al. Role of transesophageal echocardiography in assessing diastolic dysfunction in a large clinical practice: A 9 year experience. *Amer Heart J* 1999;138:880–89.

119. Fischer M, Baessler A, Hense HW, Hengstenberg C, Muscholl M, Holmer S, et al. Prevalence of left ventricular diastolic dysfunction in the community: Results from a Doppler echocardiographic based survey of a population sample. *Eur Heart J* 2003;24(4):320–28.

120. Weiss JL, Frederiksen JW, Weisfeldt ML. Hemodynamic determinants of the time course of fall in canine left ventricular pressure. *J Clin Invest* 1976;58:751–60.

121. Kawaguchi M, Hay I, Fetics B, et al. Combined ventricular and arterial stiffening in patients with heart failure and preserved ejection fraction: Implications for systolic and diastolic reserve limitations. *Circulation* 2003;107:714–20.

122. Burkhoff D, Maurer MS, Packer M. Heart failure with a normal ejection fraction: Is it really a disorder of diastolic function? *Circulation* 2003;107:656–58.

123. Angeja BG, Grossmann W. Evaluation and management of diastolic heart failure. *Circulation* 2003;107:659–63.

124. Shimizu M, Ino H, Okeie K, Emoto Y, Yamaguchi M, Yasuda T, et al. Cardiac sympathetic activity in the asymmetrically hypertrophied septum in patients with hypertension or hypertrophic cardiomyopathy. *Am J Hypertens* 1998;11:1171–77.

125. Takeda A, Takeda N. Different pathophysiology of cardiac hypertrophy in hypertension and hypertrophic cardiomyopathy. *J Mol Cell Cardiol* 1997;29:2161–65.

126. McKenna WJ, Elliott PM. Hypertrophic cardiomyopathy. *Evid Based Cardiovasc Med* 1998;2:89–91.

127. Mottram PM, Leano R, Marwick TH. Usefullness of B type natriuretic peptide in hypertensive patients with exertional dyspnea and normal left ventricular ejection fraction and correlation with new echocardiographic indices of systolic and diastolic function. *Amer J Cardiol* 2003;92:1434–38.

128. Akinboboye OO, Reichek N, Bergmann SR, Chou RL. Correlates of myocardial oxygen demand measured by positron emission tomography in the hypertrophied left ventricle. *Amer J Hypertension* 2003;16:240–43.

129. Paelinck BP, Lamb HJ, Bax JJ, Van der Wall EE, de Roos A. Assessment of diastolic function by cardiovascular magnetic resonance. *Amer Heart J* 2002;144:198–205.

130. Lamb HJ, Beyer bacht HP, van der Laarse A, Stoel BC, Doornbos J, van der Wall EE, et al. Diastolic dysfunction in hypertensive heart disease is associated with altered myocardial metabolism. *Circulation* 1999;99:2261–67.

131. Beer M, Seyfarth T, Sandstede J, Landschutz W, Lipke C, Kostler H, et al. Absolute concentrations of high-energy phosphate metabolites in normal, hypertrophied, and failing human myocardium measured noninvasively with P-31-SLOOP magnetic resonance spectroscopy. *J Amer Coll Cardiol* 2002;40:1267–74.

132. Missouris CG, Forbat SM, Singer DR, Markandu ND, Underwood R, MacGregor GA. Echocardiography overestimates left ventricular mass: a comparative study with magnetic resonance imaging in patients with hypertension. *J Hypertension* 1996;14:1005–10.

133. Germain P, Roul G, Kastler B, Mossard JM, Bareiss P, Sacrez A. Inter study variuability in left ventricular mass measurement: Comparison between M Mode echocardiography and MRI. *Eur Heart J* 1992;13:1011–19.

134. De las Fuentes L, Herrero P, Peterson LR, Kelly DP, Gropler RJ, Davila-Roman VG. Myocardial fatty acid metabolism: Independent predictor of left ventricular mass in hypertensive heart disease. *Hypertension* 2002;15:907–10.

135. Stauer BE, Schjwartzkopff B, Kelm M. Assessing the coronary circulation in hypertension. *J Hypertens* 1998;16(9):1221–33.

136. Masuda D, Nohara R, Tamaki N, et al. Evaluation of coronary flow reserve by 13N - NH3 positron emission tomography with dipyridamole in the treatment of hypertension with an ACE inhibitor. *Ann Nucl Med* 2000;14(5):353–60.

137. Gimelli A, Schneider-Eicke J, Neglia D, Sambuceti G, Gioretti A, Bigalli G, et al. Homogeneously reduced versus regionally impaired myocardial blood flow in hypertensive patients: Two different patterns of myocardial perfusion associated with degree of hypertrophy. *J Amer Coll Cardiol* 1998;31:366–73.

138. Shiba N, Kagaya Y, Ishide N, Takeyama D, Yamane Y, Chida M, et al. Myocardial glucose metabolism is different between hypertrophic cardiomyopathy and hypertensive heart disease associated with asymmetrical septal hypertrophy. *Tohoku J Exp Med* 1997;182:125–38.

139. Seidl K, Hauer B, Schwick NG, Zellner D, Zahn R, Senges J. Risk of thromboembolic events in patients with atrial flutter. *Amer J Cardiol* 1998;82:580–83.

140. Krahn AD, Manfreda J, Tate RB, Mathewson FAL, Cuddy TE. The natural history of atrial fibrillation: Incidence, risk factors and prognosis in the Manitoba Follow Up study. *Amer J Med* 1995;98:476–84.

141. Healey JS, Connolly SJ. Atrial fibrillation: Hypertension as a causative agent, risk factor for complications, and potential therapeutic target. *Am J Cardiol* 2003;22(Suppl 10A):9G–14G.

142. Benjamin EJ, Levy D, Vaziri SM, D'Agostino RB, Belanger AJ, Wolf PA. Independent risk factors for atrial fibrillation in a population based cohort: The Framingham Study. *J Amer Med Assoc* 1994;271:840–44.

143. Ezekowitz M, Laupacis A, Boysen G, Connolly S, Hart R, James K, et al. Echocardiographic predictors of stroke in patients with atrial fibrillation: A prospective study of 1066 patients from 3 clinical trials. *Arch Int Med* 1998;158:1316–20.

144. Hennersdorf MG, Hafke GJ, Steiner S, Dierkes S, Jansen A, Perings C, et al. Determinants of paroxysmal atrial fibrillation in patients with arterial hypertension. *Zeit fur Kardiol* 2003;92:370–76.

145. Verdecchia P, Reboldi G, Gattobigio R, Bentivoglio M, Borgioni C, Angeli F, et al. Atrial fibrillation in hypertension: Predictors and outcome. *Hypertension* 2003;41:218–23.

146. Vaziri SM, Larson MG, Benjamin EJ, Levy D. Echocardiographic predictors of non rheumatic atrial fibrillation: The Framingham Heart Study. *Circulation* 1994;89:724–30.

147. O'Toole L, Williams A, Shaw TRD, Starkey IR, Northridge DB. Hypertension strongly predicts early relapse after elective cardioversion of atrial fibrillation. *J Amer Coll Cardiol* 1998;31:195A.

148. Kerr C, Boone J, Connolly S, Greene M, Klein G, Sheldon R, et al. Follow-up of atrial fibrillation: The initial experience of the Canadian registry of atrial fibrillation. *Eur Heart J* 1996;17(Suppl C):48–51.

149. McLenachan JM, Henderson E, Morris KI, Dargie HJ. Ventricular arrhythmias in patients with hypertensive left ventricular hypertrophy. *New Eng J Med* 1987;317:787–92.

150. Haider AW, Larson MG, Benjamin EJ, Levy D. Increased left ventricular mass and hypertrophy are associated with increased risk for sudden death. *J Amer Coll Cardiol* 1998;32:1454–59.

151. Szlachcic J, Tubau JF, O'Kelly B, Ammon S, Daiss K, Massie BM. What is the role of siolent coronary artery disease and left ventricular hypertrophy in the genesis of ventricular arrhythmias in men with essential hypertension? *J Amer Coll Cardiol* 1992;19:803–08.

152. Schillaci G, Verdecchia P, Borgioni C, Ciucci A, Zampi I, Battistelli M, et al. Association between persistent pressure overload and ventricular arrhythmias in essential hypertension. *Hypertension* 1996;28:284–89.

153. Ghali JK, Kadakia S, Cooper RS, Liao Y. Impact of left ventricular hypertrophy on ventricular arrhythmias in the absence of coronary artery disease. *J Amer Coll Cardiol* 1991;17:1277–82.

154. Davey P, Bateman J, Mulligan IP, Forfar JC, Barlow J, Hart G. QT interval dispersion in chronic heart failure and left ventricular hypertrophy: Relation to autonomic nervous system and Holter tape abnormalities. *Brit Heart J* 1994;71:268–73.

155. Glancy JM, Garratt CJ, Woods KL, DeBono DP. QT dispersion and mortality after myocardial infarction. *Lancet* 1995;345:945–48.

156. Kluger J, Giedrimiene D, White CM, Verroneau J, Giedrimas E. A comparison of the QT and QTc dispersion among patients with sustained ventricular tachyarrhythmias and different etiologies of heart disease. *Ann Non Invasive Electrocardiology* 2001;6:319–22.

Chapter

47

The Effects of Hypertension on the Structure of Human Resistance Vessels

Enrico Agabiti Rosei and Damiano Rizzoni

Key Findings

- Hypertension is associated with changes in the structure of small arteries; namely, eutrophic remodeling (rearrangement of otherwise normal material around a narrowed lumen) or hypertrophic remodeling (vascular smooth muscle cell hypertrophy or hyperplasia).

- Essential hypertension is associated with eutrophic remodeling, whereas hypertrophic remodeling may be present in renovascular hypertension, acromegaly, and non-insulin-dependent diabetes mellitus.

- In arterioles and capillaries of patients with essential hypertension, a functional rarefaction (vessels temporarily not perfused) or a structural rarefaction (vessels actually missing) may be present.

- The presence of an increased media-to-lumen ratio of small-resistance arteries may amplify the effects of hypertensive stimuli, and may reduce organ flow reserve at maximum dilatation.

- In the genesis of eutrophic remodeling, changes in the extracellular matrix may play an important role. In the genesis of hypertrophic remodeling, growth factors, changes in wall stress, and impairment of myogenic response may have more relevant roles.

- Structural alterations in the microcirculation may possess a prognostic significance, in that they may predict the subsequent occurrence of cardiovascular events independently of other known risk factors.

- Hypertrophic remodeling seems to be associated with an even worse prognosis compared to eutrophic remodeling.

- Hypertensive treatment may induce a regression of vascular structural alterations in hypertensive patients. Some drugs (ACE inhibitors, angiotensin II receptor blockers, and calcium antagonists) may be more effective than others (β-blockers, diuretics) in this regard. It is possible that the beneficial effect is due to intrinsic properties of the drugs, more than to blood pressure reduction.

- It is not presently known whether regression of structural alterations of small arteries may improve prognosis *per se* in hypertensive patients, independently of blood pressure reduction.

- To answer this important question, the clinical application of noninvasive techniques of evaluation of vascular structure (presently under investigation) is needed.

Essential hypertension is often characterized by increased peripheral vascular resistance to blood flow, which occurs largely as a result of energy dissipation in arteries with a lumen diameter of 100 to 350 μm^2 and in smaller arterioles.[14] According to Poiseuille's law, flow resistance is inversely related to the fourth power of the vessel radius. Therefore, minor decreases in the lumen of resistance arteries may induce significant increase in resistance. It has therefore been proposed that this segment of the arterial tree may play an important role in the development of hypertension, and may contribute to its complications.

Vascular changes in resistance arteries may be structural, mechanical, or functional. In any case, a decrease in lumen size occurs.[1] It is now widely accepted that structural abnormalities of microvessels are common alterations associated with chronic hypertension.[1,5] An increase in arterial wall thickness together with a reduced lumen may play an important role in the increase of vascular resistance, and may be an adaptive response to an increased hemodynamic load. Alterations in the capillary structure and distribution may also be observed.

If structural changes in the resistance arteries are of hemodynamic importance, we have to face several issues, including the problem of how to appropriately measure vascular structure, how to meaningfully quantify or describe structural changes in hypertension, how to properly assess their pathologic role in terms of association with organ damage or cardiovascular events, and how to correct them. We address these issues in this chapter.

VASCULAR STRUCTURAL ALTERATIONS IN HYPERTENSION

Small resistance arteries

Resistance vessel structure is a difficult quantity to measure. *In vivo* studies of vascular resistance measured under conditions of complete relaxation provide a sensitive comparison of apparent resistance vessel diameter but are difficult to interpret because any difference could be due to alterations in vascular architecture rather than structure of the individual vessels.[4] *In vitro* studies of isolated resistance vessels have the advantage of precise measurements of vascular dimensions without fixation artifacts but suffer from the difficulty that there is no clear agreement as to the length to which vessels should be set.[4] Histologic studies have the advantage of allowing global analysis but may be compromised by unintended activation of vessels during fixation and lack of knowledge of the intravascular pressure during the process. Therefore, none of the methods is perfect, and it is unwise to draw strong conclusions on the basis of results from one method alone. Nevertheless, if measurements are confined to a comparison of the ratio of the wall thickness to the lumen diameter (wall:lumen ratio; or with measurements of tunica media thickness, the media:lumen, M/L, ratio)—ratios at a given lumen—there is general agreement that this parameter is increased in hypertension, at least in the more proximal resistance vessels.[4]

In the last two decades, the presence of structural alterations in subcutaneous and omental small resistance arteries dissected from biopsies performed in essential hypertensive patients has been confirmed with a direct investigation using the micromyographic method.[6–8] Patients with essential hypertension present an increased M/L ratio, without any relevant increase in the total amount of wall tissue as indicated by a media cross-sectional area similar to that observed in normotensive controls. Therefore, most of the structural changes observed in essential hypertension are the consequence of eutrophic remodeling (rearrangement of the same amount of wall material around a narrowed lumen)[9–12] without net cell growth (Figure 47–1). On the contrary, in patients with some forms of secondary hypertension (renovascular hypertension, primary aldosteronism) a more evident contribution of cell growth—leading to the development of hypertrophic remodeling (vascular smooth muscle cell hypertrophy or hyperplasia)—has been observed[13,14] (Figure 47–1).

In the development of hypertrophic remodeling, a relevant role is played by growth factors, especially endothelin-1 and angiotensin II (Figure 47–2). The mechanisms leading to eutrophic remodeling are less clear. The equivalence in media volume between hypertensive and normotensive blood vessels may be the result of media growth toward the lumen combined with enhanced apoptosis in the periphery of the vessel (Figure 47–2). According to Laplace's law, a smaller lumen decreases circumferential tension. Media stress diminishes due to increased media width, which protects the vessel wall from the effects of elevated

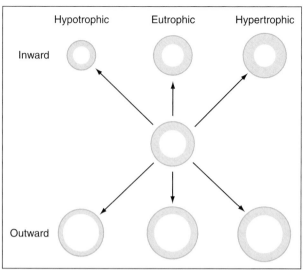

Figure 47–1. Types of vascular remodeling in hypertension. (Redrawn from Mulvany MJ, Aalkjaer C. Structure and function of small arteries. *Physiol Rev* 1990;70:921–71.)

blood pressure.[2] If hypertension is long-standing or severe, smooth muscle cell growth (in number or size) may predominate over apoptosis, and remodeling may be hypertrophic. As a consequence, this process leads to an increase in media cross-sectional area and in the M/L ratio. Both eutrophic and hypertrophic remodeling may be present to varying degrees and in different vascular beds in the same animal model or human beings.[2] It has also been suggested that the connections between vascular smooth muscle cells and the extracellular matrix proteins may be labile, allowing the vascular wall components to move relative to each other through a process that may be integrin mediated. It therefore seems likely that the remodeling process may be intimately connected with extracellular matrix protein activity, integrin α, V,[16] and tissue-type transglutaminase.[17]

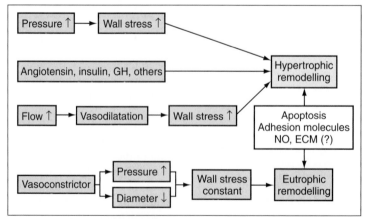

Figure 47–2. Some determinants of small artery remodeling. (Redrawn with modification from Mulvany MJ. Small artery remodeling and significance in the development of hypertension. *News Physiol Sci* 2002;17:105–109, and Mulvany MJ. Small artery remodeling in hypertension. *Curr Hypertens Rep* 2000;4:49–55.)

Among extracellular matrix proteins, matrix metallo-proteinases (MMPs) may have a prominent role in modulating remodeling of small arteries. MMPs are catabolic enzymes involved in the degradation of extracellular matrix proteins, and may be divided into three main groups: interstitial collagenases (MMP-1), which degrade type I and II native collagen; gelatinases (MMP-9, MMP-2), which act on elastin and type IV collagen; and stromelysins (MMP-3), which have specific proteolytic action toward proteoglycans, fibronectin, and laminin. The accumulation of collagen and other interstitial proteins in resistance arteries may be facilitated by diminished MMP activity. Changes in extracellular matrix are critically important to vascular remodeling (Figure 47–2). With chronic vasoconstriction (due to the influence of neurohumoral factors, the renin-angiotensin system, catecholamines, and other growth factors), vessels may become embedded in the remodeled extracellular matrix and not return to their more dilated state.[17] Some degree of cell migration, secretion of fibrillar and nonfibrillar components, and rearrangement of extracellular matrix/cell interactions may be involved. Collagen deposition is significantly enhanced in small arteries of spontaneously hypertensive rats (SHRs)[18] and in patients

with essential hypertension[19] (Figure 47–3) and may account for changes in compliance and stiffness.

Cell growth and extracellular matrix deposition may result from blood pressure elevation or from growth-promoting factors such as endothelin-1,[20] angiotensin II,[21] and catecholamines acting through α-adrenoreceptors.[22] Deposit of proteins (e.g., collagen) contributes to media thickening (in hypertrophic remodeling) and to the reorganization of vessel wall components, embedding the vessels in the chronically vasoconstricted state (in eutrophic remodeling). Increased extracellular matrix may also result from diminished activity of MMPs. Changes in MMP activity are particularly implicated in the accumulation of types IV and V collagen and of fibronectin in the extracellular matrix of resistance arteries. In hypertensive patients with augmented vascular type I collagen, serum concentrations of MMP-1 are reduced.[23] Finally, a possible stimulus for hypertrophic remodeling may be in increased wall stress, as a consequence of an impaired myogenic response (Figure 47–2). Myogenic response is a pressure-induced vasoconstriction, which is the key component in blood flow autoregulation and in the stabilization of capillary pressure. The loss of such a myogenic response

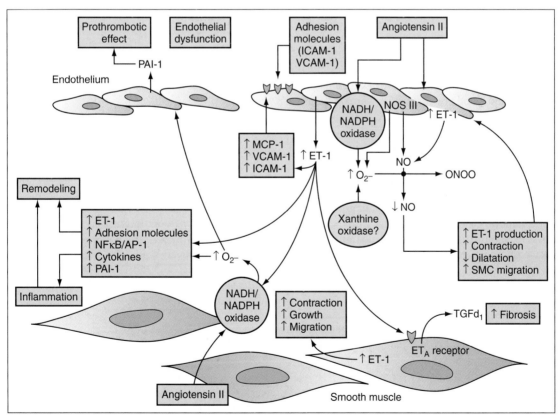

Figure 47–3. Cellular effects in the vascular wall associated with increased oxidative stress lead to cell growth and migration, upregulation of adhesion molecules, inflammation, endothelial dysfunction, and vascular damage. AP, activator protein; ET, endothelin; ICAM, intracellular adhesion molecule; MCP, monocyte chemoattractant protein; NADH, reduced nicotinamide adenine dinucleotide; NADPH, reduced nicotinamide adenine dinucleotide phosphate; NFκB, nuclear factor κB; NO nitric oxide; NOS, NO synthase; PAI-1, plasminogen activator inhibitor-1; SMC, smooth muscle cell; TGF, transforming growth factor; and VCAM, vascular adhesion molecule. (Redrawn from Schiffrin EL. Remodeling of resistance arteries in essential hypertension and effects of antihypertensive treatment. *Am J Hypertens* 2004;17:1192–1200.)

was previously observed in patients showing the presence of hypertrophic remodeling of small arteries.[24]

Time course of vascular structural alterations and blood pressure

The time course of the vascular structural changes in hypertension is not clear; nor is their role in promoting hypertension. Early detection of increased wall thickness, even in the pre-hypertensive phase of SHRs, may point toward a predominantly genetic mechanism for vascular structural changes. However, it is not clear whether vascular structural changes are an important factor in initiating hypertension in the SHR. If this is the case, the late increase of blood pressure (after the development of vascular structural changes) might be hypothetically explained by additional events such as a progressive increase of adrenergic activity or a progressive reduction of total vascular bed. In fact, it has been demonstrated that vascular structural abnormalities may act as an amplifier, able to increase the effect of any hypertensive stimulus (Figure 47–4).[25–27]

On the other hand, at least two findings would suggest that the influence of vascular structural changes on blood pressure is of minor importance at best: (1) the presence of an increased M/L ratio in 4-week-old pre-hypertensive SHRs as compared to Wistar-Kyoto normotensive controls[28] and (2) the persistence of a significant regression of vascular alterations in SHRs treated for a short period of time with nitrendipine from week 8 to week 12 (even at 38 weeks of age) in the presence of high pressure levels almost indistinguishable from those of untreated SHRs of the same age.[29] Similar dissociations between vascular structural alterations and blood pressure values were previously observed in one-kidney/one-clip rats after unclipping of the renal artery and in SHRs after withdrawal of a prolonged angiotensin II infusion. Both models showed a rapid decrease in blood pressure despite a persistent increase of the M/L ratio.[30]

Therefore, there is no clear evidence for the possible role of vascular structural changes in initiating hypertension. Neurohumoral or functional factors would play an important role, and the presence of a vascular amplifier of hypertensive stimuli is not enough for the induction of

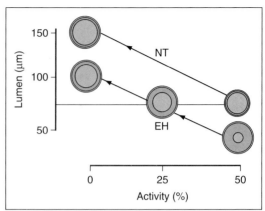

Figure 47–4. Relationships between percentage of contraction of vascular smooth muscle cells and lumen diameter in normotensive controls (NT) and in hypertensive patients (EH) with an increased media-to-lumen ratio. Structural alterations amplify vasoconstrictor stimuli (for any level of vascular contraction the lumen is smaller in hypertensive patients) and reduces flow reserve at maximum vasodilatation.

hypertension if the stimulus is lacking. Therefore, a complex interplay between vascular structure and function as well as neurohumoral factors may be postulated, and even the rebound effect of the increased hemodynamic load on vascular structure should be taken into account (Figure 47–5).[5,31] Figure 47–6 shows the evolution in time of the various changes that may occur in the vascular wall in hypertension, as suggested by Schiffrin.[2]

Arterioles and capillaries

Not only the diameter of individual vessels but the absolute number of perfused vessels contributes to total vascular resistance. Vascular rarefaction may be defined either as a functional rarefaction (when the vessels are temporarily not perfused or "recruited") or an anatomical rarefaction, when vessels are actually missing.[32,33] Many studies have reported microvascular rarefaction in some, but not all, vascular beds in hypertensive animals. Data available for humans are relatively scanty.[34,35] Greene et al.[36] calculated

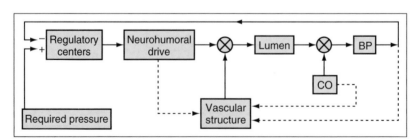

Figure 47–5. Role of resistance vessel structure in the control of blood pressure. Solid lines show fast processes; dashed lines show slow processes. ChrW(61636), multiplier. Increased blood pressure will tend to increase wall thickness; increased cardiac output (flow) will tend to increase vessel diameter. (Redrawn from Mulvany MJ. Small artery remodeling and significance in the development of hypertension. *News Physiol Sci* 2002;17:105–09, and Mulvany MJ. Small artery remodeling in hypertension. *Curr Hypertens Rep* 2000;4:49–55.)

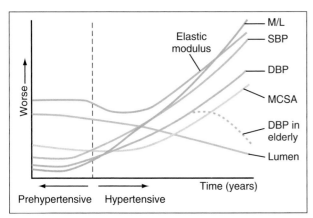

Figure 47–6. Changes in morphologic and mechanical aspects of resistance arteries as hypertension evolves in time. DBP, diastolic blood pressure; MCSA, minimal cross-sectional area; M/L, media:lumen ratio; and SBP, systolic blood pressure. (Redrawn from Schiffrin EL. Remodeling of resistance arteries in essential hypertension and effects of antihypertensive treatment. *Am J Hypertens* 2004;17:1192–1200.)

that a rarefaction of about 42% of third-order arterioles would increase tissue flow resistance by 21%.

A reduction of arteriolar [vessels smaller than 100 μm] and capillary number in skeletal muscle and other vascular beds of spontaneously hypertensive rats has been observed, together with a rarefaction of small vessels in the cremasteric muscle of renal hypertensive rats.[32,33] A reduction of arteriolar and capillary density in conjuntival microcirculation of hypertensive patients has been also detected by direct visualization *in vivo*.[37] In addition, Gasser et al.[38] observed a 20% reduction of capillary density in the nailfold capillaries using capillary microscopy *in vivo*.

A capillary rarefaction in the intestinal circulation,[39] in skeletal muscle,[40] in the myocardium, and in the stomach has been observed. However, because these are necropsy-derived data a main problem is a lack of healthy control data—the controls often being subjects with diseases that may impact on the microcirculation. Recently, some studies from Antonios et al.[34,35] using a direct technique have demonstrated the presence of capillary rarefaction in the skin of the fingers of patients with essential hypertension or borderline hypertension, and of normotensive offspring of patients with essential hypertension.

3-VASCULAR STRUCTURAL ALTERATIONS AND END-ORGAN DAMAGE

It has been proposed that structural alterations in the resistance vasculature may act as a "vascular amplifier" able to enhance the effects of any hypertensive stimulus[25,27] (Figure 47–4), but there is also some disagreement about this "amplifier hypothesis."[41,42] In any case, an important consequence of the presence of structural alterations in small resistance arteries and arterioles may be an impairment of vasodilator reserve.[43,44] In fact, remodeling of small resistance arteries is characterized by a narrowing of the lumen, which leads to an increase of flow resistance even at full dilatation (i.e., in the absence of vascular tone).

A significant correlation between coronary flow reserve and subcutaneous small resistance artery remodeling has been detected in hypertensive patients, suggesting that structural alterations in small resistance arteries may be present at the same time in different vascular districts (reflecting even clinically more important alterations in other vascular beds, including the coronary circulation).[45] A correlation between flow reserve in the foream and M/L ratio of subcutaneous vessels has been also observed.[8]

The extent of structural alterations in small resistance vessels is more pronounced in patients with both diabetes mellitus and hypertension, suggesting that clustering of risk factors may have synergistic deleterious effects on the vasculature.[24,46] Some data suggest that alterations in small resistance artery morphology may represent the most prevalent, and perhaps earliest, form of preclinical target organ damage in essential hypertension.[47] In addition, structural alterations in resistance arteries may be closely related to target organ damage, especially at the cardiac level. In fact, a linear relation between M/L ratio of subcutaneous small resistance arteries and left ventricular mass index or relative wall thickness has been detected in hypertensive patients. This relation with left ventricular geometry was more evident in patients with activation of the renin-angiotensin-aldosterone system.[48] Therefore, alterations in the microcirculation may play an important role in the development of target organ damage in hypertension.[49]

VASCULAR STRUCTURAL ALTERATIONS AND PROGNOSIS

It has been proposed that cardiovascular events are the consequence of vascular damage at both the macro- and microcirculatory level. Hence, the presence of structural alterations in the microcirculation may represent an important link between hypertension and ischemic heart disease, stroke, or renal failure. To evaluate the possible presence of a relationship between structural alterations in the subcutaneous small resistance arteries and the occurrence of cardiovascular events, 151 hypertensive and/or diabetic patients (together with some normal subjects) in whom a basal evaluation of small arteries morphology was available were evaluated.[50] All subjects were submitted to a biopsy of subcutaneous fat, and small resistance arteries were dissected and mounted on an isometric myograph. The tunica media to internal lumen ratio was measured. The subjects were reevaluated after an average follow-up time of 5.6 years. Thirty-seven subjects had a documented fatal or nonfatal cardiovascular event (5.32 events/100 patients/year), in that they suffered from ischemic heart disease, heart failure, cerebral ischemic attacks, and renal failure. Then, the subjects were subdivided according to the presence of an M/L ratio of small arteries greater or smaller than the mean and median value observed in the entire population.

Life table analyses showed a significant difference in event-free survival between the subgroups (Figure 47–7). Cox's proportional hazard model, considering all known cardiovascular risk factors, indicated that only pulse pressure ($p=0.009$) and M/L ratio ($p<0.0001$) were significantly associated with the occurrence of cardiovascular

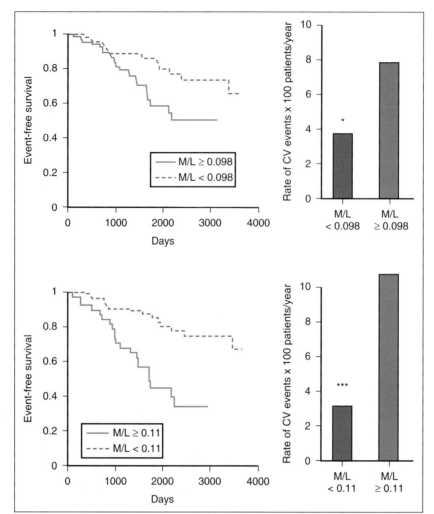

Figure 47–7. *Top left:* Event-free survival (Kaplan-Meier method) in group of patients with a media:lumen (M/L) ratio of subcutaneous small arteries ≥0.098 (mean and median values observed in whole population) (n=64, solid line) or <0.098 (n=64, dotted line). Mantel-Cox test between curves, *p*=0.015; Breslow test between curves, *p*=0.036. *Bottom left:* Event-free survival in group of patients with an M/L ratio of subcutaneous small arteries ≥0.11 (2 SD above mean value of our normal reference subjects) (n=36, solid line) or <0.11 (n=92, dotted line). Mantel-Cox test and Breslow test between curves, *p*=0.00001. *Top and bottom right:* Incidence of cardiovascular (CV) events in subgroups of patients. (Redrawn from Rizzoni D, Porteri E, Boari GEM, et al. Prognostic significance of small artery structure in hypertension. *Circulation* 2003;108:2230–35.)

events.[50] These results strongly indicate a relevant prognostic role of small resistance artery structural alterations in a high-risk population. More recently, we have reevaluated these data taking into account the chararacteristics of the vascular remodeling. For the same values of internal diameter, those subjects who suffered cardiovascular events had a greater media cross-sectional area in comparison to those without cardiovascular events[49] (Figure 47–8). Therefore, it seems that for the same size of vessels a more consistent cell growth (hypertrophic remodeling) means a worse prognosis. It has also been suggested that an impairment of myogenic response may have a relevant role in the development of hypertrophic remodeling in patients at high cardiovascular risk.[46,49]

The prognostic relevance of vascular structural alterations in the microcirculation has been partly confirmed in a different vascular territory (i.e., the retinal circulation). In fact, Wong et al.[51] observed that in a population-based cohort study of 9648 subjects [the Atherosclerosis Risk in Communities Study (ARIC) Study] retinal arteriolar narrowing (as evaluated by retinal photographs) was associated with a higher risk of coronary artery disease in women but not in men. In particular, for each decrease of one standard deviation of the retinal arteriole to venule ratio (AVR) a greater relative risk of coronary artery disease (1.37) and of myocardial infarction (1.50) occurs.

A similar evaluation was performed in another general population cohort of 4926 subjects in Wisconsin (Beaver

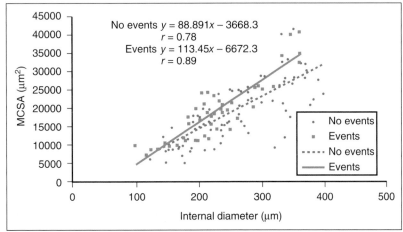

Figure 47–8. Medial cross-sectional area (MCSA) plotted against lumen diameter of the small arteries of patients with hypertension who have subsequently had a cardiovascular event (full squares) or who were event free (full circles) at the time of follow-up. The slopes of the two regression lines are significantly different (p=0.00009). (Redrawn from Izzard AS, Rizzoni D, Agabiti-Rosei E, Heagerty AM. Small artery structure and hypertension: Adaptive changes and target organ damage. *J Hypertens* 2005;23:247–50.)

Dam Study). In this study, no relation between smaller AVR and 10-year mortality was observed.[52] However, in the same cohort the presence of retinal disease (retinal micro-aneurysms, blot hemorrhages, cotton wool spots, hard exudates, venous beading, new vessels on the disk, and preretinal or vitreous hemorrhages) was associated with increased cardiovascular mortality, with an odds ratio of 1.8[53] and with a higher prevalence of cerebral white-matter lesions and stroke.[54] However, in another study lower grades of hypertensive retinopathy were not associated with a more prominent cardiac or extracardiac target organ damage.[55] Narrowed retinal arterioles, at least in women, may predict cardiovascular outcome. Therefore, data available suggest a prognostic role of structural changes of the subcutaneous microcirculation in patients with hypertension and other cardiovascular risk factors, probably because they are associated with similar changes in the coronary, renal, and cerebral microcirculation.

EFFECT OF ANTIHYPERTENSIVE TREATMENT

According to the previously mentioned observations, the possible regression of vascular alterations in small resistance arteries is an appealing goal of antihypertensive treatment. However, some years ago the first study employing a direct and reliable technique for the evaluation of structural alterations in the subcutaneous vascular bed[56,57] failed to observe a complete normalization of the vasculature during long-term antihypertensive treatment. In these studies, the patients were given diuretics, blockers, calcium antagonists, and angiotensin receptor blockers.

More recently, some studies have demonstrated an almost complete normalization of the structure of subcutaneous small resistance arteries with ACE inhibitors (cilazapril, perindopril).[58–61] On the contrary, the β blocker atenolol

was devoid of effects on resistance vessels, despite a blood pressure reduction similar to that observed with ACE inhibitors.[58–61]

We have also investigated the effects on vascular structure of treatment with the ACE inhibitor lisinopril for 3 years.[62] The M/L ratio in subcutaneous small resistance arteries was significantly lower in treated hypertensives than in well-matched untreated hypertensives. However, M/L ratio remained significantly higher than that observed in normotensive subjects. Because blood pressure values also remained higher in treated hypertensives than in normotensives, our data suggest that a persistent and complete normalization of blood pressure is probably mandatory in order to obtain a normalization of vascular structure.[62] A complete normalization of vascular structure of subcutaneous small resistance arteries was, however, also observed after effective treatment with the calcium antagonist nifedipine in an extended-release formulation.[63] It seems therefore probable that calcium entry blockers could share with ACE inhibitors the beneficial effect on vascular structure[2] (Figure 47–9).

On the contrary, diuretics seem to be less effective in terms of regression of vascular structural alterations.[64] Recently it has been demonstrated that the angiotensin II receptor blockers losartan and irbesartan are also quite effective in normalizing subcutaneous small resistance artery structure in hypertensive patients[65,66] (Figure 47–10).

The improved structure and function of resistance arteries during renin-angiotensin system blockade may be explained by several mechanisms, including vasodilation. Because angiotensin II induces oxidative stress and promotes inflammation as well as smooth muscle cell growth and migration, blockade of these actions (Figure 47–3) may also play a significant role.[2] Renin-angiotensin system blockade decreases reactive oxygen species and increases the bioavailability of nitric oxide, improving endothelial

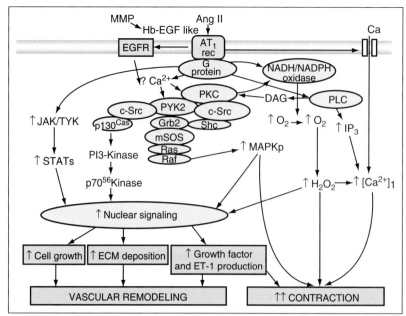

Figure 47–9. Signaling pathways of the AT_1 receptor and Ca^{2+} that participate in vascular remodeling. Blockade of these pathways explains some of the improvement in remodeling and endothelial dysfunction seen with antihypertensive treatment in hypertension. Ang II, angiotensin II; c-Src, normoreceptor tyrosine kinase; $[Ca^{2+}]_1$, intracellular (cytosolic) calcium; DAG, diacylglycerol; ECM, extracellular matrix; EGFR, epidermal growth factor receptor; ET-1, endothelin 1; Grb2, mSOS, Shc, adaptor proteins acting as scaffolding for signaling complex; Hb-EGF-like, heparin binding epidermal growth factor-like growth factor; IP_2, inositol triphosphate; JAK/TYK, Janus family kinases; MAPK, mitogen-activated protein kinase; MMP, matrix metalloproteinase; NADH, reduced nicotinamide adenine dinucleotide; NADPH, reduced nicotinamide adenine dinucleotide phosphate; p130[cas], docking protein; PKC, protein kinase C; PI3, phosphoinositide 3; PLC, phospholipase C; PYK2, calcium-dependent praline-rich tyrosine kinase-2; RAS, Raf, a mitogen-activated protein kinase kinase; and STATs, signal transducers and activators of transcription. (Redrawn from Schiffrin EL. Remodeling of resistance arteries in essential hypertension and effects of antihypertensive treatment. *Am J Hypertens* 2004;17:1192–1200 with permission from *The American Journal of Hypertension.*)

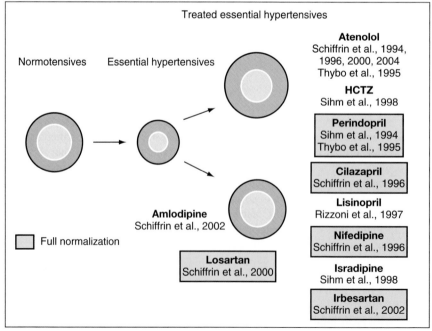

Figure 47–10. Effects of antihypertensive treatment on vascular structure.

function. Blockade of the renin-angiotensin system may also reduce collagen deposition and extracellular matrix remodeling induced by angiotensin II.[67,68]

Shargorodsky and co-workers[69] reported a significant increase in small artery elasticity ($p<0.01$) with valsartan during long-term treatment. Blood pressure was rapidly lowered, suggesting that improved elasticity was not directly related to the acute blood pressure effect of the drug. Treatment with perindopril also improved coronary reserve and significantly reduced pericoronary fibrosis in small vessels of hypertensive subjects.[70]

These findings may have clinical relevance. In fact, recently at least three studies (the LIFE, PROGRESS, and HOPE studies) have demonstrated that drugs able to inhibit the renin-angiotensin-aldosterone system (such as losartan, perindopril, and ramipril) may have some advantage over other drugs, beyond the decrease in blood pressure, in terms of reduced morbidity and mortality in high-risk hypertensive patients.[71] It is possible that their favorable effect on small resistance artery structure may partially explain the additional benefits observed. However, it should be emphasized that the prognostic impact of the regression of vascular structural alterations per se is still unknown, and prospective studies are needed to clarify whether structural alterations in small resistance arteries may be considered an "intermediate" endpoint in the evaluation of the effects of antihypertensive treatment.

CONCLUSIONS

Essential hypertension is associated with alterations in the resistance vasculature. In particular, an increased M/L ratio is almost uniformly detected. However, some methodologic problems in the evaluation of vascular structure in humans remain. In addition, it is not clearly established whether structural alterations in the microcirculation precede or are a consequence of hypertension. In particular, the causative role of vessel structure in hypertension is still a matter of debate, although vascular alterations may act as an amplifier of hypertensive stimuli.

Structural alterations in the microcirculation are associated with increased cardiovascular risk in hypertensive patients, perhaps as a consequence of an impaired vascular reserve in several vascular beds, including the coronary circulation. Structural alterations in different vascular regions are probably interrelated. It has been observed that the presence of an increase in wall:lumen ratio in the subcutaneous resistance arteries is associated with a worse prognosis in hypertensive patients, and that structural alteration in the microcirculation is probably the most potent predictor of cardiovascular events, together with pulse pressure. The characteristics of vascular remodeling might also be relevant in this context, in that hypertrophic remodeling seems to be associated with a worse prognosis.

The presence of structural alterations in the microcirculation may have an important role in the development of ischemic heart disease, heart failure, stroke, and renal failure. It is conceivable that vascular structural changes in small resistance arteries may be considered, in the future, as an important intermediate endpoint for evaluating the benefits of antihypertensive therapy, although this point needs to be demonstrated by specific intervention studies.

The current method for the evaluation of subcutaneous small artery structure is minimally invasive. Nevertheless, its invasiveness limits its application to large populations. It is possible that noninvasive techniques for investigation of the microcirculation presently under evaluation and validation (such as acoustic, confocal, fluorescence, and intravital microscopy) may in the near future provide important information in achieving a better diagnostic and therapeutic approach in hypertensive patients.

REFERENCES

1. Mulvany MJ, Aalkjaer C. Structure and function of small arteries. *Physiol Rev* 1990;70:921–71.
2. Schiffrin EL. Remodeling of resistance arteries in essential hypertension and effects of antihypertensive treatment. *Am J Hypertens* 2004;17:1192–1200.
3. Christensen KL, Mulvany MJ. Location of resistance arteries. *J Vasc Res* 2001;38:1–12.
4. Mulvany MJ. Structural abnormalities of the resistance vasculature in hypertension. *J Vasc Res* 2003;40:558–60.
5. Mulvany MJ. Small artery remodeling and significance in the development of hypertension. *News Physiol Sci* 2002;17:105–09.
6. Aalkjaer C, Haegerty AM, Petersen KK, et al. Evidence for increased media thickness, increased neural amine uptake, and depressed excitation-contraction coupling in isolated resistance vessels from essential hypertensives. *Circ Res* 1987;61(2):181–86.
7. Schiffrin EL, Deng LY, Larochelle P. Morphology of resistance arteries and comparison of effects of vasoconstrictors in mild essential hypertensive patients. *Clin Invest Med* 1993;16:177–86.
8. Agabiti-Rosei E, Rizzoni D, Castellano M, et al. Media:lumen ratio in human small resistance arteries is related to forearm minimal vascular resistance. *J Hypertens* 1995;13:341–47.
9. Baumbach GL, Heistad DD. Remodeling of cerebral arterioles in chronic hypertension. *Hypertension* 1989;13:968–72.
10. Heagerty AM, Aalkjaaer C, Bund SJ, et al. Small artery structure in hypertension: Dual process of remodeling and growth. *Hypertension* 1993;21:391–97.
11. Mulvany MJ, Baumbach GL, Aalkjaer C, et al. Vascular remodeling. *Hypertension* 1996; 28:505–06.
12. Bund SJ, Lee RMKW. Arterial structural changes in hypertension: A consideration of methodology, terminology and functional conseqences. *J Vasc Res* 2003;40:547–57.
13. Rizzoni D, Porteri E, Castellano M, et al. Vascular hypertrophy and remodeling in secondary hypertension. *Hypertension* 1996;28:785–90.
14. Rizzoni D, Porteri E, Guelfi D, et al. Cellular hypertrophy in subcutaneous small arteries of patients with renovascular hypertension. *Hypertension* 2000;35:931–35.
15. Heerkens EH, Shaw L, Izzard IS, et al. Integrins in hypertension mediate eutrophic remodeling of tgr(REN2)27 rat arteries. *Hypertension* 2004;44(4):49(abstract).
16. Bakker ENTP, Buus CL, Spaan JAE, et al. Small artery remodeling depends on tissue-type transglutaminase. *Circ Res* 2005;96:119–26.
17. Bakker ENTP, van der Meulen ET, van den Berg BM, et al. Inward remodeling follows chronic vasoconstriction in isolated resistance arteries. *J Vasc Res* 2002;39:12–20.

18. Intengan HD, Thibault G, Li JS, Schiffrin EL. Resistance artery mechanics, structure, and extracellular components in spontaneously hypertensive rats: Effects of angiotensin receptor antagonism and converting enzyme inhibition. *Circulation* 1999;100:2267–75.

19. Intengan HD, Deng LY, Li JS, Schiffrin EL. Mechanics and composition of human subcutaneous resistance arteries in essential hypertension. *Hypertension* 1999;33:569–74.

20. Park JB, Schiffrin EL. Cardiac and vascular fibrosis and hypertrophy in aldosterone-infused rats: Role of endothelin-1. *Am J Hypertens* 2002;15:164–69.

21. Touyz RM, He G, El Mabrouk M, Schiffrin EL. p38 MAP kinase regulates vascular smooth muscle cell collagen synthesis by angiotensin II in SHR but not in WKY. *Hypertension* 2001;37:574–80.

22. O'Callaghan CJ, Williams B. The regulation of human vascular smooth muscle extracellular matrix protein production by α and β-adrenoceptor stimulation. *J Hypertens* 2002;20:287–94.

23. Laviades C, Varo N, Fernández J, et al. Abnormalities of the extracellular degradation of collagen type I in essential hypertension. *Circulation* 1998;98:535–40.

24. Schofield I, Malik R, Izzard A, et al. Vascular structural and functional changes in type 2 diabetes mellitus: Evidence for the role of abnormal myogenic responsiveness and dyslipidemia. *Circulation* 2002;106:3037–43.

25. Lever AF. Slow pressor mechanisms in hypertension: A role for hypertrophy of resistance vessels? *J Hypertens* 1986;4:515–24.

26. Korner PI, Bobik A, Jennings GL, et al. Significance of cardiovascular hypertrophy in the development and maintenance of hypertension. *J Cardiovasc Pharmacol* 1991;17(Suppl 2):S25–32.

27. Schiffrin EL. Reactivity of small blood vessel in hypertension: Relation with structural changes. *Hypertension* 1992;19 (Suppl II):II1–19.

28. Rizzoni D, Castellano M, Porteri E, et al. Vascular structural and functional alterations before and after the development of hypertension in SHR. *Am J Hypertens* 1994;7:193–200.

29. Rizzoni D, Castellano M, Porteri E, et al. Delayed development of hypertension after short-term nitrendipine treatment. *Hypertension* 1994;24:131–39.

30. Mulvany MJ. Resistance vessel growth and remodelling: Cause or consequence in cardiovascular disease. *J Human Hypertens* 1995;9:479–85.

31. Mulvany MJ. Small artery remodeling in hypertension. *Curr Hypertens Rep* 2000;4:49–55.

32. Struijker Boudier HAJ. Microcirculation in hypertension. *Eur Heart J* 1999;1(Suppl L):L32–37.

33. Levy BI, Ambrosio G, Pries AR, Struijker-Boudier HAJ. Microcirculation in hypertension: A new target for treatment? *Circulation* 2001;104:735–40.

34. Antonios TF, Singer DR, Markandu ND, et al. Rarefaction of skin capillaries in borderline essential hypertension suggests an early structural abnormality. *Hypertension* 1999;34(4 Pt 1):655–58.

35. Antonios TF, Singer DR, Markandu ND, et al. Structural skin capillary rarefaction in essential hypertension. *Hypertension* 1999;33(4):998–1001.

36. Greene AS, Tonellato PJ, Lui J, et al. Microvascular rarefaction and tissue vascular resistance in hypertension. *Am J Physiol* 1989;256:H126–31.

37. Harper RN, Moore MA, Marr MC, et al. Arteriolar rarefaction in the conjunctiva of human essential hypertensies. *Microvasc Res* 1978;16:369–72.

38. Gasser P, Bühler FR. Nailfold microcirculation in normotensive and essential hypertensive subjects, as assessed by video-microscopy. *J Hypertens* 1992;10:83–6.

39. Short DS. Arteries of the intestinal wall in systemic hypertension. *Lancet* 1958;ii:1261–62.

40. Henrich HA, Romen W, Heimgartner W, et al. Capillary rarefaction characteristics of the skeletal muscle of hypertensive patients. *Klin Wochenschr* 1988;66:54–60.

41. Izzard AS, Heagerty AM, Leenen FHH. The amplifier hypothesis: Permission to dissent? *J Hypertens* 1999;17:1667–69.

42. Izzard AS, Heagerty AM, Leenen FH. The amplifier hypothesis: Persisting dissent. *J Hypertens* 2002;20:375–77.

43. Folkow B. Physiological aspects of primary hypertension. *Physiol Rev* 1982;62:347–504.

44. Sivertsson R. The hemodynamic importance of structural vascular changes in essential hypertension. *Acta Physiol Scand* 1970;343:14–9.

45. Rizzoni D, Palombo C, Porteri E, et al. Relationships between coronary vasodilator capacity and small artery remodeling in hypertensive patients. *J Hypertens* 2003;21:625–32.

46. Rizzoni D, Porteri E, Guelfi D, et al. Structural alterations in subcutaneous small arteries of normotensive and hypertensive patients with non insulin dependent diabetes mellitus. *Circulation* 2001;103:1238–44.

47. Park JB, Schiffrin EL. Small artery remodeling is the most prevalent (earliest ?) form of target organ damage in mild essential hypertension. *J Hypertens* 2001;19:921–30.

48. Muiesan ML, Rizzoni D, Salvetti M, et al. Structural changes in small resistance arteries and left ventricular geometry in patients with primary and secondary hypertension. *J Hypertens* 2002;20:1439–44.

49. Izzard AS, Rizzoni D, Agabiti-Rosei E, Heagerty AM. Small artery structure and hypertension: Adaptive changes and target organ damage. *J Hypertens* 2005;23:247–50.

50. Rizzoni D, Porteri E, Boari GEM, et al. Prognostic significance of small artery structure in hypertension. *Circulation* 2003;108:2230–35.

51. Wong TY, Klein R, Sharrett AR, et al. Retinal arteriolar narrowing and risk of coronary heart disease in men and woman: The Atherosclerosis Risk in Communities Study. *JAMA* 2002;287:1153–59.

52. Wong TY Knudtson MD, Klein R, et al. A prospective cohort study of retinal arteriolar narrowing and mortality. *Am J Epidemiol* 2004;159:819–25.

53. Wong TY, Klein R, Nieto FJ, et al. Retinal microvascular abnormalities and 10-year cardiovascular mortality: A population-based case-control study. *Ophtalmology* 2003;110:933–40.

54. Wong TY, Klein R, Sharrett AR, et al. Cerebral white matter lesions, retinopathy, and incident clinical stroke. *JAMA* 2002;288:67–74.

55. Cuspidi C, Meani S, Salerno M, et al. Retinal microvascular changes and target organ damage in untreated essential hypertensives. *J Hypertens* 2004;22:2095–102.

56. Aalkjaer C, Eiskjaer H, Mulvany MJ, et al. Abnormal structure and function of isolated subcutaneous resistance vessels from essential hypertensive patients despite antihypertensive treatment. *J Hypertens* 1989;7:305–10.

57. Heagerty AM, Bund SJ, Aalkjaer C. Effects of drug treatment on human resistance arteriole morphology in essential hypertension: Direct evidence for structural remodeling of resistance vessels. *Lancet* 1988;ii:1209–13.

58. Sihm I, Schroeder AP, Aalkjaer C, et al. Normalization of resistance artery structure and left ventricular morphology with a preindopril-based regimen. *Can J Cardiol* 1994;10(Suppl D):30D–32D.

59. Thybo NK, Stephens N, Cooper A, et al. Effect of antihypertensive treatment on small arteries of patients with previously untreated essential hypertension. *Hypertension* 1995;25(Part 1):474–81.

60. Schiffrin EL, Deng LY, Larochelle P. Effects of a β-blocker or a converting enzyme inhibitor on resistance arteries in essential hypertension. *Hypertension* 1994;23:8391.

61. Schiffrin EL, Deng LY, Larochelle P. Progressive improvement in the structure of resistance arteries of hypertensive patients after 2 years of treatment with an angiotensin I-converting enzyme inhibitor: Comparison with effects of a β-blocker. *Am J Hypertens* 1995;8:229–36.

62. Rizzoni D, Muiesan ML, Porteri E, et al. Effect of long-term antihypertensive treatment with lisinopril on resistance arteries in hypertensive patients with left ventricular hypertrophy. *J Hypertens* 1997;15:197–204.

63. Schiffrin EL, Deng LY. Structure and function of resistance arteries of hypertensive patients treated with a beta blocker or a calcium channel antagonist. *J Hypertens* 1996;14:1237–44.

64. Sihm I, Schroeder AP, Aalkjaer C, et al. Effect of antihypertensive treatment on cardiac and subcutaneous artery structure: A comparison between calcium channel blocker and thiazide-based regimens. *Am J Hypertens* 1998;11:263–71.

65. Schiffrin EL, Park JB, Integan HD, Toyuz RM. Correction of arterial structure and endothelial dysfunction in human essential hypertension by the angiotensin receptor antagonists losartan. *Circulation* 2000;101:1653–59.

66. Schiffrin EL, Park JB, Pu Q. Effect of crossing over hypertensive patients from a beta-blocker to an angiotensin receptor antagonist on resistance artery structure and on endothelial function. *J Hypertens* 2002;20:71–8.

67. Intengan HD, Thibault G, Li JS, Schiffrin EL. Resistance artery mechanics, structure, and extracellular components in spontaneously hypertensive rats: Effects of angiotensin receptor antagonism and converting enzyme inhibition. *Circulation* 1999;100:2267–75.

68. Touyz RM, Schiffrin EL. Signal transduction mechanisms mediating the physiological and pathophysiological actions of angiotensin II in vascular smooth muscle cells. *Pharmacol Rev* 2000;52:639–72.

69. Shargorodsky M, Leibovitz E, Lubimov L, et al. Prolonged treatment with the AT1 receptor blocker, valsartan, increases small and large artery compliance in uncomplicated essential hypertension. *Am J Hypertens* 2002;15:1087–91.

70. Schwartzkopff B, Brehm M, Mundhenke M, Strauer BE. Repair of coronary arterioles after treatment with perindopril in hypertensive heart disease. *Hypertension* 2000;36:220–25.

71. Guidelines Committee. 2003 European Society of Hypertension-European Society of Cardiology guidelines for the management of arterial hypertension. *J Hypertens* 2003;21:1011–53.

TARGET ORGAN DAMAGE : The Effects of Hypertension on the Structure of Human Resistance Vessels

Chapter

48 The Brain in Hypertension

Martin D. Fotherby, David J. Eveson, and Thompson G. Robinson

Key Findings

- Raised blood pressure (BP) has adverse consequences in causing brain diseases, including stroke and cognitive impairment/dementia.

- Lowering high BP will help protect the brain from developing these conditions, although optimal protection requires all relevant risk factors to be addressed in a holistic manner.

- Intervening to manage raised BP in mid-life may reduce the risk of cerebrovascular damage and cognitive impairment in later life.

- More than half of all strokes could be avoided if BP were optimized in all persons, as would a reduction in the development of dementias.

Hypertension is the most prevalent modifiable risk factor for both ischemic and hemorrhagic stroke, which is often associated with vascular cognitive impairment and dementia. Importantly, stroke and dementia are significant predictors of reduced total and disability-free life expectancy.[1] This chapter focuses on aspects of these clinical manifestations of hypertension-related brain target organ damage.

ANATOMY AND PATHOLOGY

Although the brain accounts for 2% of the body's weight, it receives 15% of the cardiac output at rest. The blood supply is via two pairs of arteries: the internal carotid arteries and the vertebral arteries (the latter joining to form the basilar artery). The arterial inflow joins in an anastomotic ring (the circle of Willis), from which three pairs of arteries arise on the external surface of the corresponding region of the cerebral cortex (Figure 48–1). Thereafter, these anterior, middle, and posterior cerebral arteries progressively divide into smaller perforating vessels to supply specific brain regions.

Hypertension is an important risk factor for the development of atherosclerotic changes in these vessels. The progression of atherosclerotic plaques in the larger extracerebral vessels (particularly at the carotid bifurcation) and in the medium-sized intracranial vessels (through a process of necrosis, ulceration, and thrombosis with complete or partial vessel occlusion or distal embolization) has been discussed in previous chapters. Furthermore, at the level of smaller arteries (such as the single deep-perforating end-arteries of the deep cerebral white matter) the process of vessel

occlusion by microatheroma and hypertensive lipohyalinosis has also been discussed.

The brain has important adaptive mechanisms to reduced inflow. The circle of Willis acts as a shunt, predominantly anterior to posterior, but also side to side. However, reduced collateral reserve (particularly in association with hypotension) will lead to border-zone or watershed infarction (for example, between anterior and middle, or middle and posterior, cerebral artery territories). There are also physiologic mechanisms to maintain cerebral blood flow (the process of cerebrovascular autoregulation, discussed in a later section). Nonetheless, the brain remains highly sensitive to changes in its blood supply. Loss or reduction of blood flow in a specific vascular territory results in stroke, producing specific pathologic changes related to the duration and degree of ischemia. Importantly, the time interval required to trigger irreversible injury (ischemic sensitivity) varies markedly among different regions. Nonetheless, focal ischemia of 30 to 60 minutes will result in a pannecrosis of all cell types (neuronal, glial, endothelial) within a vascular territory, surrounded by a transition zone of irreversibly injured neurones but preserved glial and endothelial cells (and then normal brain tissue).

Where stroke-related loss of brain tissue exceeds 50 to 100 mLs, dementia may result.[2] Vascular dementia (the cerebrovascular or cardiovascular-related loss of cognitive function secondary to ischemic, hypoperfusive, or hemorrhagic brain lesions) is the second most common cause of elderly dementia, after Alzheimer's disease. The term encompasses several clinico-pathologic subtypes. First, large-vessel disease may result in multiple large-vessel cortico-subcortical thrombotic or embolic strokes (multi-infarct) or in a single "strategic" stroke. Second, chronic, diffuse, partial, or occlusive small-vessel disease may result in predominantly subcortical white matter ischemia (Binswanger's disease) or frank lacunar infarction(s).[3]

PATHOPHYSIOLOGY

The pathophysiologic effects of hypertension on cerebral hemodynamics are considered in the following, as are changes in systemic and cerebral hemodynamics that occur in the most common hypertension-related brain injury (acute stroke).

Cerebral blood flow and cerebral autoregulation

The brain arterial blood supply has a low impedance, resulting in a high cerebral blood flow (CBF) of approximately

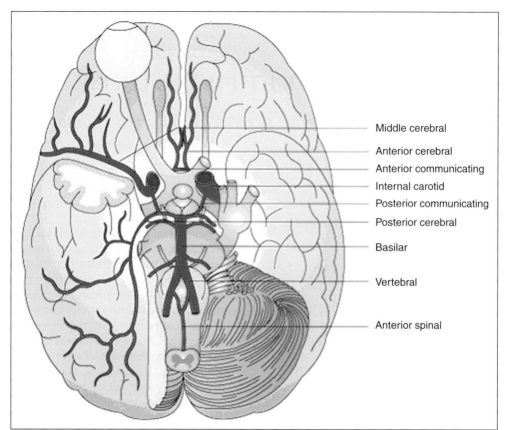

Figure 48–1. Anatomy of the blood supply to the brain. (From Instructor's Resource CD-ROM to accompany *Porth's Pathophysiology: Concepts of Altered Health States, Seventh Edition.* Philadelphia: Lippincott Williams & Wilkins, 2005, with permission.)

50 mL per 100 g per minute. The brain receives blood during both systole and diastole. In comparison to myocardium, which receives blood during diastole only, brain tissue may be more susceptible to the adverse effects of long-term changes in systolic and pulsatile pressure. CBF is closely coupled to the metabolic needs of brain tissue. For example, CBF is globally increased in epilepsy, anemia, and acidotic states and globally decreased in comatose states. Focal cerebral activation results in regional increases in CBF and oxygen consumption. The absolute level of CBF decreases with age but is similar in uncomplicated hypertensives and age-matched normotensive individuals. However, both aging and hypertension profoundly influence CBF regulation.

CBF is usually maintained at a near-constant level in the face of fluctuations in arterial BP levels across the physiological range by a process of cerebral autoregulation. This is mediated by changes in cerebrovascular resistance resulting from vasomotor changes at the arteriolar level. The mechanisms underlying cerebral autoregulation are as yet incompletely understood, but myogenic, metabolic, and neurogenic mechanisms have been postulated (including roles for nitric oxide, calcitonin gene-related peptide, endothelial-cell potassium channels, and the autonomic nervous system).[4] Cerebral autoregulation may be described in both static and dynamic terms. The ability of the brain to maintain CBF in response to a steady-state change in

cerebral perfusion pressure is described as *static* cerebral autoregulation (SCA), whereas the maintenance of CBF in response to transient changes in cerebral perfusion pressure (defined as >15 mmHg in <20 seconds) is the *dynamic* component (DCA). Noninvasive methods of measuring cerebral autoregulatory capacity in humans are described in a later section.

In normotensive subjects, when mean arterial pressure falls below approximately 60 mmHg (considered the lower limit of SCA) CBF decreases proportionally with BP (Figure 48–2). The upper limit in normotensive humans, above which CBF increases proportionally with BP, is untested but in primate models is between 120 and 150 mmHg. Chronic hypertension and aging result in a shift in the limits of SCA toward higher pressures in humans, through the induction of structural and functional changes in cerebral arteriolar walls. However, DCA appears to be unaffected by either chronic hypertension or aging.[5] Moderate BP reduction in chronic hypertension does not precipitate cerebral ischemia due to there being sufficient scope on the autoregulatory plateau to lower arterial pressure without affecting CBF and due to the ability of neuronal tissue to increase oxygen consumption.

In the longer term, sustained BP reduction results in a shift of the SCA curve to the left. Both SCA and DCA are impaired following stroke, in accelerated (malignant) hypertension, and following head injury, resulting in a pressure-

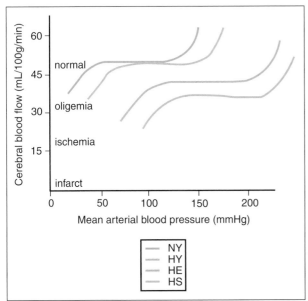

Figure 48–2. Curves depicting static autoregulation in normotensive young (NY), hypertensive young (HY), hypertensive elderly (HE), and hypertensive stroke (HS) subjects. Autoregulation is defined from the relationship between cerebral blood flow and mean arterial pressure.

passive relationship between BP levels and CBF.[6,7] BP reduction, particularly where this is rapid, may be deleterious in these situations. In addition, where there are established and widespread areas of small-vessel cerebrovascular disease (particularly in the very elderly patient in whom CBF is generally reduced and autoregulation impaired) BP reduction to usual target levels may in theory result in impairment of cerebral perfusion (although this has yet to be addressed by a randomized clinical trial).

The ischemic penumbra following acute stroke

During the first few hours following occlusion of a cerebral artery (and surrounding the dense core of infarcted tissue) is a zone of variable extent and distribution (the ischemic penumbra). The blood supply to the ischemic penumbra is reduced, abolishing electrical activity but not to sufficient levels to induce cell death. Neuronal cells appear to pass through two thresholds as CBF declines. Studies in humans have shown suppression of electrical activity to occur as flow falls below approximately 20 mL per 100 g/minute and irreversible loss of energy-dependent cellular ion gradients to occur at flow rates of approximately 10 mL per 100 g/minute, leading to cytotoxic edema and cell death. In theory, cells that have lost capacity for electrical activity but remain in a hibernated state have the capacity to be fully restored to normal with an increase in blood flow. The distribution and potential viability of the ischemic penumbra following a stroke is influenced by local metabolic activity, vascular anatomy, and the extent of collateral blood flow. The acute stroke phase presents additional challenges to penumbral viability due to relative oxygen deficiency, excitatory amino acid release, spreading waves of electrical depolarization, impaired autoregulation, and

increased BP variability. Methods of imaging the ischemic penumbra in the acute stroke phase are discussed later in the chapter.

Cardiovascular changes in the acute stroke phase

Although approximately two-thirds of the global stroke burden can be attributed to poorly controlled BP levels, a greater proportion of patients present with elevated BP levels immediately following a stroke. Over 80% of patients present with SBP >140 mmHg and 30% with SBP >180 mmHg within the first 48 hours of ischemic stroke, with levels even higher following hemorrhagic stroke. The mechanisms underlying the stroke-associated rise in BP levels are incompletely understood but include the stress of removal to hospital and alterations in autonomic nervous system activity with associated catecholamine, glucocorticoid, and mineralocorticoid release.

Many studies report a strong and independent relationship between the BP level in the acute stroke phase and short- and long-term outcomes, with most reporting a U-shaped relationship. For example, in the International Stroke Trial[8] for every 10 mmHg rise in SBP above 150 mmHg the risk of early death (by day 14) increased by 4%, and for each 10 mmHg decrease below this level the risk increased by 18%. In primary intracerebral hemorrhage, both the degree of hematoma expansion during the first few hours and patient outcome are related to the SBP level. The natural history of BP levels following stroke is for a spontaneous reduction to occur over a period of 4 to 10 days, with the greatest falls being associated with the highest baseline BP levels. However, no consistent data have emerged regarding the relationship between the magnitude or direction of the BP change in the acute stroke phase and stroke outcome. In addition to the absolute BP level, other abnormalities of cardiovascular function confer independent prognostic information in the acute stroke phase. For example, increases in beat-to-beat BP variability and decreases in cardiac baroreceptor sensitivity, coupled with impairment of autonomic reflexes, independently predict outcome in the short and longer terms.[9]

CLINICAL PRESENTATIONS

Some common clinical presentations of hypertension-related brain injury are considered in the following, with examples of stroke and dementia. Comprehensive details of acute and secondary stroke management are presented later in the chapter.

A case of lacunar stroke
History

An 80-year-old right-handed man presented to the emergency room with a speech disturbance and left arm and leg weakness. He awoke with these deficits and was last known to be symptom free when retiring to bed the previous evening 10 hours earlier. His past medical history was significant for hypertension and hyperlipidemia. He had no known history of myocardial infarction or stroke and no history of calf claudication. He was a life-long nonsmoker. His hypertension was being treated with a beta blocker and a diuretic, and his hyperchlolesterolemia with an HMG CoA-reductase inhibitor (statin). He had no known drug allergies. He had no family history of ischemic heart disease or stroke.

Physical examination

BP in both arms was elevated at 180/100, with a regular pulse of 90 bpm. Cardiovascular examination revealed a normally situated cardiac apex; a soft nonradiating systolic murmur at the cardiac base; no carotid, femoral, or supra-clavicular bruits; and palpable foot pulses. Respiratory examination was normal. Abdominal examination was normal without organomegaly or abdominal bruits.

Neurological examination

The patient was alert. He had dysarthria, but with no word-forming difficulties, neologisms, or paraphrasias. He was able to follow complex verbal instructions. Cognitive evaluation revealed a Mini-Mental State Examination score of 24/30. Cranial nerve examination confirmed a mild left lower facial paresis. Pupillary light reflexes, the visual fields, and the remainder of the cranial nerves were normal to examination. Funduscopic examination showed arteriolar narrowing, with arteriolar-venous nipping. Upon examination of the peripheral nervous system, there was diminished tone in the left arm and leg, 2/5 proximal and 2/5 distal strength in the left arm and leg, deep tendon reflex diminishment, and extensor left plantar response. Sensation to light touch was intact in the left arm and leg and there was a coordination deficit consistent with the level of motor weakness. Gait was not tested.

Initial investigations

The blood count, electrolytes, blood glucose, and renal function were normal. The activated partial thromboplastin and prothrombin times were normal. ECG fulfilled voltage criteria for left ventricular hypertrophy. An MRI brain scan was obtained (Figure 48–3, A).

Management

A diagnosis of right lacunar stroke was made using the OCSP classification (Table 48–1). Thrombolysis was not considered due to the onset of symptoms being beyond the 3-hour time window. The acute event was managed initially with aspirin, paracetamol, intravenous saline, and graduated compression stockings to reduce the venous thromboembolism risk. Early assessment and mobilization was initiated by the multidisciplinary team. Secondary preventative measures included the addition of dipyridamole, lipid-lowering therapy, and (2 weeks following the event) BP-lowering therapy with a combination of an ACE inhibitor and a thiazide diuretic. With a combination of hospital and community-based rehabilitation, the patient made a full recovery at 6 months (being independent in daily activities, with mild weakness of the left hand remaining).

Discussion

Classifying stroke events into stroke subtypes on the basis of clinical, neuroradiologic, and cardiovascular criteria confers several advantages (i.e., stratification of the possible etiologies of a stroke and associated risk factors, targeted and efficient use of appropriate investigations, and improved prognostication for survival and functional outcome). Classification systems are based on clinical, cardiovascular,

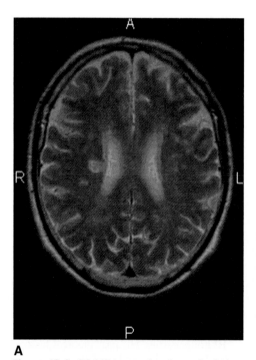
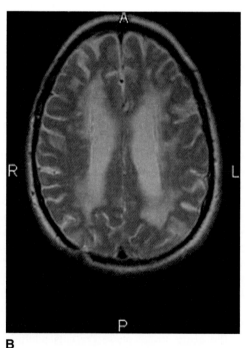

A **B**

Figure 48–3. (A) MR image showing a single lacunar infarct in the right hemisphere. (B) MR T2-weighted image of periventricular white matter hyperintensities resulting from cerebral small-vessel disease.

THE OXFORDSHIRE COMMUNITY STROKE PROJECT CLASSIFICATION			
Stroke Syndrome	Clinical Signs at Time of Maximum Deficit	Correlation with Neuroradiological Findings – CT or MRI (%)		Case Fatality at 30 Days, 6 Months, and 1 Year (%)
Total anterior circulation infarction (TACI)	■ Hemiplegia ■ Visual field defect ■ Disturbance of higher cerebral function	■ Cortical ■ Boundary zone ■ Lacunar ■ Posterior circulation ■ No lesion	96 2 0 2 0	39, 57, 60
Partial anterior circulation infarction (PACI)	■ Motor/sensory deficit + hemianopia or higher cerebral dysfunction ■ Higher cerebral dysfunction alone or with hemianopia ■ Motor/sensory deficit less extensive than for lacunar syndrome	■ Cortical ■ Boundary zone ■ Lacunar ■ Posterior circulation ■ No lesion	73 14 4 2 6	4, 11, 16
Lacunar infarction (LACI)	■ Pure motor stroke ■ Pure sensory stroke ■ Sensorimotor stroke ■ Ataxic hemiparesis	■ Cortical ■ Boundary zone ■ Lacunar ■ Posterior circulation ■ No lesion	11 16 68 1 5	2, 7, 11
Posterior circulation infarction (POCI)	■ Cranial nerve palsy with contralateral motor/sensory deficit ■ Bilateral motor/sensory deficit ■ Disorder of conjugate eye movement ■ Cerebellar dysfunction ■ Isolated hemianopia/cortical blindness	■ Cortical infarct ■ Boundary zone ■ Lacunar ■ Posterior circulation ■ No lesion	5 0 2 86 6	7, 14, 19
Primary intracerebral hemorrhage (PICH)	■ Any of above syndromes accounted for by primary intracerebral hemorrhage on neuroimaging			50, 58, 62
Data from the OCSP[11] and Tei.[82]				

Table 48–1. The Oxfordshire Community Stroke Project Classification

or neuroradiologic criteria or a combination of these. The TOAST classification of ischemic stroke, designed originally for use in a clinical trial,[10] organizes ischemic stroke according to origin: large-artery atherosclerosis, small-artery disease (lacunar) origin, and cardioembolic or other etiologies (e.g., carotid artery dissection, vasculitis, migraine). However, accuracy of the TOAST classification is dependent on comprehensive pre- and post-stroke investigations, which may not always be obtainable. Even when this information is available, approximately 40% of patients remain unclassified using this system. As a tool for predicting outcome (and with value in the acute stroke phase), most experience has been gained with the Oxford Community Stroke Project (OCSP) classification,[11] a system based solely on neurologic examination (Table 48–1)—with neuroimaging distinguishing between infarct and hemorrhage.

Lacunar stroke accounts for approximately 25% of acute ischemic stroke cases in Western populations and is most commonly caused by an occlusion of a deep perforating end artery, commonly through complex small-vessel disease and microatheroma. Embolism is an uncommon cause. Predisposing risk factors include hypertension, age, smoking, and diabetes. The risk of recurrent stroke is lower compared to other stroke subtypes (9% at one year compared to 17%

for PACI), and subsequent cardiovascular events may be reduced further with a combination of antiplatelet, antihypertensive, and lipid-lowering therapy.

A case of total anterior circulation infarction (TACI)
History
A 70-year-old right-handed woman was brought to the hospital with drowsiness, inability to speak, and weakness of the right arm and leg. She was accompanied by her husband, who reported that this had happened at breakfast (some 60 minutes earlier). Prior to this she had been symptom free. Her past medical history was significant for hypertension, hypercholesterolemia, myocardial infarction 2 years previously, and peripheral vascular disease giving rise to bilateral calf claudication. She had stopped smoking at the time of the myocardial infarction, having been a 20-cigarette-per-day smoker prior to this for most of her adult life. Her hypertension was being treated with a combination of an angiotensin-converting enzyme inhibitor and a diuretic. She was also receiving aspirin 75 mg daily and an HMG CoA-reductase inhibitor (statin). There was a family history of ischemic heart disease after the age of 50.

Physical examination

BP was 160/90 in both arms, and the pulse was 80 bpm and irregular. Her lungs were clear to auscultation. Cardiovascular examination showed a laterally displaced cardiac apex with irregular impulse and no added sounds. There were soft bilateral anterior cervical and femoral bruits. Femoral pulses were present, but dorsalis pedis and posterior tibial pulses were impalpable. Abdominal examination revealed no organomegaly or abdominal bruits.

Neurological examination

The patient was drowsy but rousable to voice. She spoke in abbreviated syllables insufficient to form words. She was unable to follow simple verbal commands. Further cognitive evaluation could not be performed because of the extent of the dysphasia. Cranial nerve examination revealed a right homonymous hemianopia, a preference for gaze to the right, a right lower facial paresis, a diminished right corneal reflex, and tongue deviation to the right. Pupillary light reflexes were normal. Funduscopic examination revealed arteriolar narrowing and tortuosity. Upon examination of the peripheral nervous system, there was hemiparesis of the right arm and leg (power 0/5 all groups), with hypotonia, diminished deep tendon reflexes, and an extensor right plantar response. Sensory examination was limited by language disturbance, but there appeared to be right-sided deficits to pinprick and light touch sensation.

Initial investigations

Full blood count, electrolytes, blood glucose, renal function, and clotting studies were unremarkable. ECG showed atrial fibrillation and evidence of an established anterior myocardial infarction. Neuroimaging showed early signs of infarction in the territory of the left MCA (Figure 48–4, A).

Management

A diagnosis of total anterior circulation infarction (TACI) was made (Table 48–1). The patient was considered for intravenous thrombolysis. Following discussion with the family, including explanation of the potential risks and benefits of treatment, she received intravenous r-tPA 120 minutes following symptom onset. During administration of the drug, stroke severity scores improved. She was admitted to the stroke unit. At discharge from the hospital on day 21 there was a partial right hemianopia but no sensory neglect, and although mild weakness of the right arm remained she returned home to an independent existence with help from her husband. Appropriate attention was paid to secondary prevention strategies, which included introduction of anticoagulation for permanent atrial fibrillation.

Discussion

TACI accounts for approximately 17% of acute ischemic strokes and is commonly caused by MCA occlusion by local disease or embolism from proximal arteries or the heart, or as a result of internal carotid artery occlusion. The risk of death or severe disability following TACI is high (Table 48–1). Intravenous thrombolysis with rtPA administered within 3 hours of the development of symptoms of ischemic stroke has been shown to reduce the risk of the combined endpoint of death or dependency at follow-up in all ischemic stroke subtypes (discussed further later in the chapter).

A case of cognitive decline due to cerebrovascular disease
History

An 80-year-old man was referred to his general practitioner by his wife, who had noticed he had become progressively more forgetful over the previous year. Initially, he had begun to lose his way while driving his car along previously familiar routes. He had become neglectful of his usual hobbies, and more recently had developed difficulty in

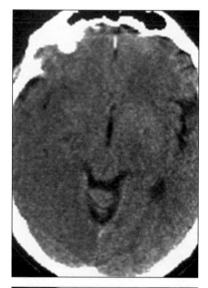

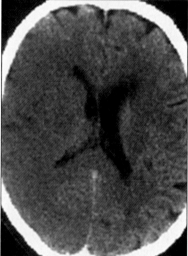

A

Figure 48–4. (A) CT of acute cerebral infarct (i) showing effacement of sylvian fissure "insular ribbon sign" and (ii) showing "dense MCA sign." (B) MR image showing an acute left middle cerebral artery infarct on T2-weighted imaging, apparent diffusion coefficient (ADC), and diffusion-weighted imaging (DWI) scans.

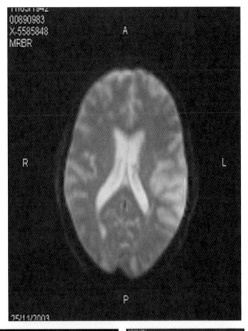

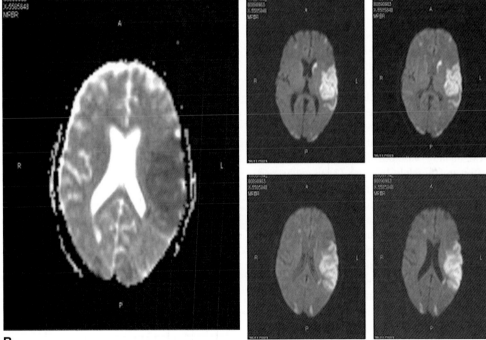

B
Figure 48–4.—cont'd

remembering the names of family members or close friends. Sleep had become fitful, and more recently he had developed periods of depression. His past medical history was significant for type II diabetes mellitus and hypertension, both diagnosed 12 years previously. His diabetes was treated with a combination of an oral biguanide and a sulphonylurea and his hypertension with a diuretic. The last glycated hemoglobin (HbA1c) level one year previously had been 9.0%.

Physical examination

BP was 170/100 in both arms, and the pulse was 70 bpm and regular. Cardiorespiratory examination revealed clear lung fields, a soft nonradiating systolic murmur at the cardiac base, no vascular bruits, and impalpable posterior tibial and dorsalis pedis pulses bilaterally. Bilateral corneal arcus was present. Abdominal examination was normal.

Neurological examination

The patient was alert but spoke with occasional paraphrasias. He was able to follow 3-step verbal instructions. A score of 16/30 was obtained on Mini-Mental State Examination. Cranial nerve examination revealed no abnormality, visual fields were intact, pupillary light reflexes were normal, and there was arteriolar narrowing and tortuosity upon funduscopy. Arm and leg tone were mildly increased, and there was global exaggeration of all deep tendon reflexes in the limbs (with no asymmetry). Both plantar responses were extensor. Sensory and cerebellar examinations were normal.

Investigations

Complete blood count, electrolytes, renal function, and clotting studies were normal. Random plasma glucose level was 11.0 mmol/L. An ECG fulfilled the voltage criteria for left ventricular hypertrophy. Referral was made to the memory clinic at the local hospital. There, detailed neuropsychologic testing was conducted—revealing deficits in episodic, semantic, and working memory (with relative preservation of personality). An MRI brain scan was performed (Figure 48–3, B). A diagnosis of vascular dementia was made. With liaison with primary care, a strategy for better control of his diabetes and BP was devised, aspirin commenced, and community mental health support accessed with appropriate caregiver support. A 3-month trial of an antidepressant was also commenced.

Discussion

Cognitive decline due to cerebrovascular disease encompasses a spectrum of underlying causes ranging from multiple cortical or subcortical infarcts to a single strategic infarct (e.g., genu of the internal capsule, thalamus) to ischemic demyelination of the white matter. Typical cases of vascular dementia have preexisting vascular risk factors, symptoms, and signs of cerebrovascular disease; undergo a step-wise deterioration; and unlike other forms of dementia usually preserve personality and insight until late in the disease. However, distinguishing vascular from other types of dementia is often not possible because (1) vascular risk factors are being increasingly recognized as independent risk factors for Alzheimer's pathology, (2) the classical step-wise deterioration in cognitive function with associated focal symptoms or signs of neurological disease does not always occur in vascular cases, and (3) frequently there is evidence of both vascular and Alzheimer's pathology. The evidence of vascular risk reduction on the progression of cognitive decline is discussed later in the chapter. Such a strategy may also reduce the incidence of subsequent macrovascular disease in these individuals.

DIAGNOSTIC TECHNIQUES

The discussion of investigational techniques for evaluating cerebrovascular disease will be limited to brain imaging techniques because these are of direct relevance to this chapter. Various imaging modalities have advanced the understanding of cerebrovascular disease (both acute and chronic) and the effect of BP and changes in blood flow on cerebral function. Indeed, results of imaging studies make a major contribution to the diagnosis and management of both chronic and acute cerebrovascular diseases.

Acute cerebrovascular disease

Computerized tomography (CT) remains the most commonly used imaging tool for the evaluation of suspected acute stroke. It can readily detect early hemorrhage, but

not all early infarcts. Magnetic resonance imaging (MRI) is becoming more commonly used in the investigation of acute stroke. It allows detection of intracranial hemorrhage within hours of stroke onset,[12] and unlike CT the presence of previous microhemorrhage (due to its breakdown product hemosiderin remaining) is easily visible. MR diffusion-weighted imaging readily reveals ischemic or infarcted tissue (within minutes of stroke onset) with better sensitivity and accuracy than CT[13] (Figure 48–4, B). Multimodal CT (perfusion CT and CT angiography) and multimodal MR imaging—diffusion-weighted imaging (DWI), perfusion-weighted imaging (PWI), fluid-attenuated inversion recovery (FLAIR), and MR angiography (MRA)—provide significantly more information useful in patient management. For example, abnormalities on DWI represent bioenergetic compromise and PWI abnormalities show areas of hemodynamic compromise. In an area of infarction, the diffusion abnormality has been taken to represent irreversibly damaged tissue and the surrounding region with abnormal perfusion represents damaged but potentially viable tissue (i.e., the penumbra). However, positron emission scanning studies reveal that the mismatch zone is only an approximation of the penumbra.[14] More sophisticated modeling allows more accurate representation of the penumbra, allowing patients with salvageable tissue to be selected for stroke treatments (e.g., thrombolysis).[15]

Cognitive impairment and dementia

Neuroimaging is recommended in the initial assessment of patients with dementia. CT and MRI can delineate structural brain changes associated with dementia (e.g., cortical atrophy with widening of cortical sulci and ventricular enlargement). Dementia type can be assessed from various imaging modalities. Indeed, guidelines for diagnosing vascular dementia include brain imaging to detect the presence of cerebrovascular disease. Compared to CT, white matter lesions are shown with greater sensitivity using MR techniques. Single-photon emission CT (SPECT) and positron emission tomography (PET) scanning (see material following) have been used to diagnose and differentiate dementias.[16]

Other techniques
Cerebral blood flow assessment

Numerous techniques are available for assessing cerebral blood flow and its abnormalities. These have recently been reviewed by Wintermark.[17]

Positron emission tomography

This is a noninvasive technique that can, using various positron emitting radioisotopes, measure not only regional cerebral blood flow, blood volume, metabolic rate of oxygen use, and oxygen extraction fraction (using $^{15}O_2$) but glucose consumption (using ^{18}F fluorodeoxyglucose) and neurotransmitter activity (using the appropriate isotope). PET can only be used in chronic conditions (e.g., chronic cerebrovascular disease and dementia). A further major drawback is the cost and requirement for a cyclotron to produce the very short-lived radiopharmaceuticals.

Single-photon emission CT

This uses radiopharmaceuticals that are more easily available (for example, based on 99 technetium or 133 xenon). Unlike PET scanning, this technique can be used in acute and chronic cerebrovascular disease and at the bedside. SPECT can determine relative changes in regional cerebral blood flow but does not provide quantitative data. It has clinical application in acute stroke and differential diagnosis of dementia.

Xenon-enhanced CT

Nonradioactive xenon is inhaled and rapidly dissolves in blood, acting as a contrast agent detected by the CT scanner. CT brain images allow blood flow data to be related to anatomy with a high degree of resolution, and quantitative assessment of regional cerebral blood flow to be undertaken. This technique can be used in acute and chronic cerebrovascular disease and can predict groups at high risk of stroke. Various CT and MR techniques with exogenous contrast and endogenous tracer using the patient's own blood (arterial spin labeling) allow investigation of perfusion abnormalities in acute and chronic stroke.

Doppler ultrasound

Doppler ultrasound techniques have long been able to measure blood flow velocity in the internal carotid artery and middle cerebral artery, but more recent developments (pulse wave digital doppler and dual-beam flow technology) allow estimation of blood flow volume. Differences in hemispheric blood flow can be compared, but although spatial resolution is limited temporal resolution is good and repeated measurements can follow dynamic blood flow changes.

MANAGEMENT

Stroke

Acute stroke is a medical emergency. Active management in the initial hours after stroke onset may save the ischemic brain from infarction (i.e., "time is brain"). A combination of public education and patient triage—by the use of the Face Arm Speech Test (FAST)[18] or Los Angeles Prehospital Stroke Screen (LAPSS)[19] by paramedical staff or the Recognition of Stroke In the Emergency Room (ROSIER) scale [Ford, Unpublished data] by Emergency Department Staff (Box 48–1)—can facilitate rapid access to stroke specialist care. Such organized care should be provided in a geographically identified unit by a coordinated multidisciplinary team with specialist expertise in stroke and rehabilitation,[20] supported by access to diagnostic services as outlined in the preceding section (although subsequently rehabilitation may be provided effectively by early supported discharge services).[21] The management of acute stroke is supported by a plethora of international and national guidelines established by such organizations as the American Stroke Association,[22] the European Stroke Initiative,[23] and the Royal College of Physicians.[24] Specific and general measures of acute ischemic and hemorrhagic stroke management drawn from these guidelines are summarized in the following.

Box 48–1

Pre-hospital Assessment Stroke Scales

Face Arm Speech Test (FAST)
- Speech impairment? Yes/No
- Facial palsy? Yes/No (affected side)
- Arm weakness? Yes/No (affected side)

Los Angeles Prehospital Stroke Screen (LAPSS)
- Age >45
- History of seizures or epilepsy absent
- Symptom duration less than 24 hours
- At baseline, patient is not wheelchair bound or bedridden
- Blood glucose between 60 and 400
- Examination: Look for obvious asymmetry
- Face smile/grimace (normal/droop)
- Grip (normal/weak grip/no grip)
- Arm strength (normal/drifts down/falls rapidly)

Recognition of Stroke in the Emergency Room (ROSIER) Scale
- Loss of consciousness or syncope?
  - Yes (-1)/No (0)
- Seizure activity?
  - Yes (-1)/No (0)
- New acute onset (or on awakening from sleep):
  - Asymmetric facial weakness: Yes (+1)/No (0)
  - Asymmetric arm weakness: Yes (+1)/No (0)
  - Asymmetric leg weakness: Yes (+1)/No (0)
  - Speech disturbance: Yes (+1)/No (0)
  - Visual field defect: Yes (+1)/No (0)

Stroke is likely if total score is >0

Specific measures

Major intracranial arterial thromboembolic occlusion is demonstrable in the majority of stroke patients, and therefore urgent reperfusion strategies are important. To date, only intravenous thrombolysis with recombinant tissue plasminogen activator (alteplase) has been approved for administration within 3 hours of acute ischemic stroke onset.[25] However, intra-arterial thrombolysis and mechanical clot disruption techniques continue to be studied.[26] Nonetheless, the short therapeutic window, the need to exclude hemorrhagic stroke, and the risk of precipitating hemorrhagic transformation limit the generalizability of this therapeutic modality (although the International Stroke Trial-3 aims to provide robust evidence of risks and benefits over a time window up to 6 hours to define more precisely which patients are most likely to benefit). (See *www.dcn.ed.ac.uk/ist3/*.) On the contrary, neuroprotection (the process of preventing ischemia and reperfusion-induced excitatory neurotransmitter, calcium channel, inflammatory, and free-radical-mediated cell death) might be more universally applicable. Unfortunately, no agent to date has proved efficacious, including multimodal physiologic magnesium.[27]

The use of anticoagulation in acute ischemic stroke has been studied for both unfractionated[28] and low-molecular-weight heparins.[29] There is no evidence to favor its routine use and it is associated with high risk of serious intracranial bleeding.[22,30] The early use of aspirin, however, is effective in reducing recurrent ischemic stroke, death, or dependency—with a small (but significant) risk of hemorrhagic transformation—but should be administered as soon as possible after the onset of stroke symptoms once a diagnosis of primary hemorrhage has been excluded at an initial dose of 300 mg.[31]

Specific treatments for patients with primary intracerebral hemorrhage are few. Although surgical intervention should be considered in patients with posterior fossa or cerebellar hemorrhage (and indeed infarction) without formal randomized trial evidence, its use in the management of supratentorial hemorrhage has been assessed in the Surgical Trial in Intra-Cerebral Hemorrhage (STICH). This trial compared immediate neurosurgical intervention within 72 hours (predominantly via craniotomy) with initial conservative management (although 26% progressed to neurosurgical intervention) and reported no significant benefit in favor of immediate intervention.[32] Medical treatment with recombinant activated factor VII has also been assessed within 3 hours of onset of intracerebral hemorrhage (in the Phase II NovoSeven Trial) and has been found to be associated with a significant reduction in hematoma expansion (although at the risk of increased thromboembolic complications).[33] Further trials are therefore needed.

General measures

Although early neuronal loss following acute stroke onset does occur, most patients have potentially viable "penumbral tissue" and measures that optimize perfusion and metabolism can be brought to bear and are important. As previously discussed, the process by which cerebral blood flow is maintained across a range of systemic BPs (cerebral autoregulation) is impaired following acute stroke, and flow becomes pressure dependent. Acute stroke is most commonly complicated by hypertension, although extremes of BP are associated with adverse prognosis (with a reported nadir of 150 mmHg).[8] Acute stroke BP management is an area of active clinical research, with few randomized controlled trials to inform the management of this common problem. Preliminary evidence supported the further assessment of angiotensin receptor blockade, combined alpha- and beta-adrenergic blockade, or nitrates for hypertensive patients—and volume expansion and phenylephrine or norepinephrine for relatively hypotensive patients.[34] Nonetheless, current consensus recommends the acute use of antihypertensive therapy for associated cardiac (acute myocardial infarction, severe left ventricular failure) or vascular urgencies (aortic dissection), hypertensive encephalopathy, acute renal failure, concurrent coagulant therapy (thrombolysis, intravenous heparin), or persistent BP elevation (with a threshold of >200/120 mmHg for

ischemic and >180/105 mmHg for hemorrhagic stroke).[22,23] For relatively hypotensive patients, the same guidelines recommend the exclusion of potential causes (for example, myocardial ischemia, cardiac failure, and sepsis). Thereafter, BP can be raised by adequate patient rehydration and due consideration to pressor therapy.[22,23]

However, a number of other general measures are also important. Maintaining adequate tissue oxygenation is vital—by maintaining the airway, monitoring respiration, preventing and treating aspiration pneumonia, and the empirical administration of supplemental oxygen. Acute coronary syndromes and arrhythmias are potential complications, and should be sought and appropriately managed. Pyrexia is associated with increased metabolic demand, enhanced neurotransmitter release, and increased free radical production. Therefore, infection should be sourced and actively managed—and antipyretics such as paracetamol considered,[35] although the use of therapeutic hypothermia is associated with serious adverse effects and lacks efficacy from clinical trials.[36] Abnormalities of glucose control are also common, and should be measured and treated. Hypoglycemia is an important stroke mimic, and untreated may lead to irreversible brain injury.

Hyperglycemia promotes increased tissue acidosis and blood/brain barrier permeability, and can be safely managed by a glucose-potassium-insulin infusion[37] (although the recently completed phase III Glucose Insulin in Stroke Trial (GIST) will further inform the efficacy of this approach). Under-nutrition is common in hospitalized stroke patients, being associated with increased risk of infection, greater difficulty with rehabilitation, and poor outcome. However, the FOOD trials (albeit underpowered) do not support a policy of routine oral supplementation in nondysphagic stroke patients,[38] report that early tube feeding in dysphagic patients may reduce case fatality at the expense of increasing the proportion of patients surviving with poor outcome, and do not support a policy of early percutaneous endoscopic gastrostomy (PEG) tube feeding.[39]

Finally, venothromboembolism presenting as deep vein thrombosis or pulmonary embolism is a complication of advanced age, immobility, severe or lower extremity paralysis, and atrial fibrillation (all common in acute stroke). Early mobilization is important. The effectiveness of graduated compression stockings is being assessed in the Clots in Legs or TEDs after Stroke (CLOTS) Trial (*www.clotstrial.com*), although routine use of prophylactic anticoagulation is associated with significant risk (as previously discussed).

Secondary prevention

Stroke patients remain at increased risk of recurrent stroke, and this may be as high as 15% within the first month for patients with transient ischemic attack (TIA). Therefore, a high priority should be attached to the delivery of an individualized strategy of evidence-based secondary prevention. First, the acute use of aspirin therapy has already been discussed, and this agent should be continued at a dose of 50 to 300 mg daily. However, it is also important to consider the role of other antiplatelet agents alone or in combination with aspirin. Dipyridamole acts to inhibit adenosine uptake into blood and vascular cells, and has both antiplatelet and vasodilator properties. The European Stroke Prevention Study 2 of modified-release dipyridamole reported risk reductions in recurrent vascular events when used in combination with aspirin compared to aspirin alone,[40] and the United Kingdom's National Institute for Health and Clinical Excellence recently recommended that patients following ischemic stroke or TIA be treated with combination therapy for a 2-year period before reverting to standard care.

Clopidogrel inhibits binding of adenosine phosphate to its platelet receptor. The Clopidogrel versus Aspirin in Patients at Risk of Ischemic Events (CAPRIE) study reported a significant reduction in composite vascular outcome with clopidogrel compared to aspirin, although this effect was not significant when only stroke patients were considered in an underpowered post-hoc analysis.[41] The Management of Atherothrombosis with Clopidogrel in High-Risk Patients with Recent Transient Ischemic Attack or Ischemic Stroke (MATCH) study also reported a significant reduction in composite vascular outcome with clopidogrel in combination with aspirin compared to clopidogrel alone, but at the expense of significant major bleeding complications.[42] Clopidogrel alone is therefore reserved for aspirin-intolerant stroke patients. However, there are a number of recently completed and ongoing trials (including CHARISMA, ESPRIT, and ProFESS) that will provide further information regarding which antiplatelet agent or combination is most effective. However, the recently published CHARISMA trial[G1][42a] suggested that clopidogrel plus aspirin was not significantly more effective than aspirin alone in reducing the rate of myocardial infarction, stroke, or death from cardiovascular causes (in 15,603 patients with either clinically evident cardiovascular disease or multiple risk factors). In subgroup analyses, benefit was found with clopidogrel treatment in patients with symptomatic atherothrombosis and a suggestion of harm in patients with multiple risk factors.

Second, statin treatment should be given to ischemic stroke and TIA patients with a total cholesterol >3.5 mmol/L unless contraindicated,[24] the subgroup of stroke patients treated with statin therapy within the Heart Protection Study having a significant reduction in subsequent major vascular events.[43] Finally, all patients should receive appropriate lifestyle advice on smoking cessation, regular exercise, appropriate diet, and the avoidance of excess alcohol.[24]

Two stroke patient subgroups demand specific treatment. Persistent or paroxysmal atrial fibrillation (valvular or nonvalvular) patients (following brain imaging to exclude hemorrhagic stroke and usually not until 14 days after stroke onset) should receive anticoagulation with a target International Normalized Ratio (INR) of 2.5 (range 2.0 to 3.0).[44] Carotid endarterectomy is highly beneficial in patients with 70% or more stenosis without near-occlusion, and of some benefit for 50 to 69% stenosis.[45] Benefit also depends on other clinical characteristics, including delay to surgery (which should ideally be undertaken within 2 weeks of last symptoms).[46]

Blood pressure and secondary stroke prevention

The reported association of BP or hypertension with recurrent stroke has not been consistent, some studies showing no association or a J-shaped relationship. However, data from the UK TIA Aspirin Trial (in which BP was measured prior to randomization in 2435 subjects with a history of minor stroke or TIA) demonstrated that a 10-mmHg lower systolic BP (SBP) was associated with a 28% lower risk of recurrent stroke.[47] This relationship between BP and stroke is similar to that seen in populations with no history of previous stroke.

Pharmacologic lowering of BP has long been known to be effective in the primary prevention of stroke. Other than a few small studies in hypertensive stroke survivors, there was little firm evidence on which to base clinical practice until 1995 (when the Chinese Post-Stroke Antihypertensive Treatment Study reported).[48] More than a month after episode, the diuretic Indapamide was compared to placebo in 5665 normotensive and hypertensive patients who had sustained a TIA, ischemic, or hemorrhagic stroke. Significant reductions in stroke recurrence (29%) and major cardiovascular events (23%) were reported. Since 2000, three further studies have reported on the effects of antihypertensive therapy in patients having had a history of stroke. The Heart Outcomes Prevention Evaluation (HOPE) study reported separately on 1013 subjects who had a history of stroke or TIA for which there was a nonsignificant 15% reduction in total stroke recurrence.[49] In the PROGRESS Trial, another ACE inhibitor (Perindopril, with or without Indapamide) was compared to placebo in 6105 normotensive and hypertensive patients with a history of ischemic or hemorrhagic stroke or TIA.[50] Active intervention reduced recurrent stroke by a significant 28%, and major vascular events by 26%, during 4 years of follow-up. The bulk of the benefit was seen in those patients who received both an ACE inhibitor and Indapamide where the BP reduction was the greatest. In those taking Perindopril only, compared to placebo only a 6% reduction in the risk of recurrent stroke was seen. The Perindopril and Indapamide combination, however, provided a 45% reduction. More recently, the Morbidity and Mortality after Stroke Eprosartan Study (MOSES) compared in hypertensive stroke survivors Eprosartan (an angiotensin receptor blocker) with Nitrendipine (a dihydropyridine calcium channel blocker).[51] For a similar fall in BP, there was a 21% risk reduction in the primary endpoint of all cardio and cerebrovascular events and a 25% reduction in recurrent cerebrovascular events in patients randomized to the Eprosartan-based regimen. The results from the PATS, HOPE, PROGRESS, and MOSES trials allow a number of issues to be considered.

Initial BP level

The initial BP level determines the need for commencing antihypertensive therapy in patients with a history of stroke. In the PATS, HOPE, and PROGESS studies, a similar benefit in stroke recurrence was seen regardless of BP level at entry (i.e., both normotensive and hypertensive patients appear to benefit from a further reduction in BP). However, whether all patients with cerebrovascular disease would benefit from a further reduction in BP regardless of their initial level is unclear. Concerns have been raised in two areas. First, it is unclear whether stroke survivors with severe carotid occlusion will develop impaired cerebral perfusion if BP is lowered too aggressively. In patients with bilateral carotid stenosis, Rothwell[52] found from a review of carotid endarterectomy studies an altered relationship between BP and stroke risk, suggesting that lowering BP in such patients aggressively may reduce cerebral perfusion and increase the risk of stroke. However, such severe bilateral carotid stenosis is uncommon and such concerns may be lessened following revascularization. The second area of concern is the effect on cognitive function of aggressive BP reduction in people with established cerebrovascular disease. This may be particularly relevant to those patients with cerebral small-vessel disease where cerebral blood flow is reduced (see material following). Further BP reduction may compromise cerebral perfusion, increasing the risk of cognitive decline and cerebrovascular disease progression.

Target BP level

No studies have addressed the issue of optimal BP to be attained, but in the PROGRESS Study a greater reduction in BP from baseline (even in normotensives) was associated with a greater reduction in stroke recurrence.

Effect of therapy in patients with different stroke subtype

In the PROGRESS Study, those with a hemorrhagic stroke had a relative risk reduction about twice as great as that for those with an ischemic stroke (49% versus 26%).[53] In the HOPE and PROGRESS studies, all ischemic stroke subtypes benefited from therapy to a similar extent. Overall, intervention with antihypertensive therapy reduced stroke recurrence regardless of stroke type.

Effect of type of antihypertensive therapy on outcome

Results of primary and secondary prevention trials suggest that for a similar reduction in BP different antihypertensive therapies vary in their effects on stroke outcome. In the MOSES Study, for a similar reduction in BP the angiotensin receptor blocker produced greater benefits in terms of stroke reduction than a calcium channel blocker. Primary prevention trials using an angiotensin receptor blocker have also suggested a preferential effect of angiotensin receptor blockers on stroke reduction compared to other therapies (e.g., β-blockers).[54] The ACE inhibitor Perindopril in PROGRESS reduced BP to an extent similar to that of Indapamide in PATS (5/2 mmHg), yet the latter reduced stroke incidence by 29% compared to no significant effect from Perindopril. It may not only be the extent to which BP is lowered but how it is lowered that achieves optimal benefits for stroke prevention.

Hypertension and cognitive impairment
Classification of cognitive impairment

Cognitive impairment spans the spectrum from mild cognitive impairment to dementia. Dementia affects about 3% of persons aged 65 to 74, but 28% of those over 85.

Traditionally, three main subtypes of dementia have been recognized: Alzheimer's disease (the most common; >50% of dementias), followed by vascular dementia (approximately 30% of dementias), and a small minority related to others such as Lewy Body disease. Alzheimer's disease, a neurodegenerative disorder characterized histologically by extracellular amyloid plaques and intracellular neurofibrillary tangles, has until recently been considered a separate entity from vascular dementia. More recently, evidence has accumulated to show associations between these two dementia subtypes; for example, with regard to shared risk factors (hypertension, diabetes mellitus, smoking, hypercholesterolemia) and proposed common pathologies.[55] Reduced cerebral blood flow and brain hypoperfusion secondary to atherosclerosis have also been associated with Alzheimer's disease.[56] Autopsy studies in patients with dementia frequently show features of both vascular dementia and Alzheimer's disease occurring together. These considerations have led to the concept of mixed dementia, perhaps the most common of all forms of dementia.[57]

Vascular cognitive impairment (VCI)

The narrow concept of vascular dementia caused by multiple infarcts has expanded to emphasize the role of cerebrovascular disease in general on cognitive function. Causes of VCI include post-stroke dementia, strategic infarcts, silent infarcts, and subcortical ischemic vascular dementia. Cerebrovascular damage leading to cognitive impairment can occur not only from atherothrombosis but through cerebral hemorrhage, hypoperfusion, and other arteriopathies. Hypertension, usually in the presence of other cardiovascular risk factors, plays a major role in promoting these pathologies.

Post-stroke dementia or cognitive decline occurs in up to one-third of patients within a year of stroke. Having a stroke may double the risk of dementia.[58] Patients with stroke may also have an earlier onset of Alzheimer's disease. In the presence of stroke, a smaller burden of Alzheimer's pathology is required to produce dementia. It is unclear whether stroke predisposes to Alzheimer's or both occur independently with additive effects.

Subcortical ischemic vascular disease primarily involves small-vessel disease, leading to lacunar infarcts and/or ischemia of the deep white matter (see Figure 48–3). The main cause of the small-vessel disease is hypertension, although other vascular risk factors play an important role (e.g., smoking, diabetes mellitus, and older age). The hypertensive arteriopathy leads to thrombotic occlusion or microaneurysm formation and hypertensive cerebral hemorrhage. Subcortical ischemic vascular dementia probably forms the bulk of vascular dementia subtypes. Major features include loss of executive functioning (attention, working memory, organization and constructional skills), motivation, and effects on mood and behavior. Gait disturbances (i.e., short stepped and wide based) and urinary problems are also common. White matter lesions are commonly seen on MRI brain scans in middle-age individuals but are not necessarily benign[59] and increase dramatically in the elderly where more than 70% of 70-year-olds are affected.[60]

Relationship of blood pressure to cognitive impairment

Epidemiological studies can broadly be divided into cross-sectional (which limit causal inference) and longitudinal, which if of sufficient follow-up allow the temporal relations between BP and cognition to be examined and causality inferred.

Cross-sectional studies

Cross-sectional studies have reported that low BP in older subjects is related to the prevalence of dementia.[61,62] In contrast, cognitive impairment (without dementia) has more commonly been associated with high BP. In the Atherosclerosis Risk in Communities study of 1384 persons aged 45 to 69, BP >160/95 mmHg was related to lower cognitive test scores.[63] Other smaller studies in young[64] and older subjects have shown similar associations.[65–67] An association of low BP with cognitive impairment, largely in studies of elderly groups (>75 years), has been reported in the Helsinki Aging Study, Honolulu-Asia aging study, and the Kungsholmen Project.[68–70] Overall, there is some indication that high BP is related to cognitive impairments. In older subjects a sufficient BP level is required to maintain cerebral perfusion to preserve optimum cognitive functioning.[71]

Longitudinal studies

High BP in middle age without or with other vascular risk factors has consistently been associated with cognitive decline and dementia of both vascular and Alzheimer type when assessed after follow-up periods of 10 to 25 years.[69,72,73] In contrast to studies undertaken in middle-age persons, follow-up of elderly cohorts has shown no consistent association of BP with cognition or dementia. As in younger groups, high BP in the elderly has been related to decline in cognitive performance.[71,74] However, in distinction from younger cohorts in the elderly low BP has in some studies been associated with the development of dementia.[75,76] Overall, these longitudinal studies strongly suggest an adverse effect of high BP in middle age (and perhaps also older age) on cognitive functioning. There is also an adverse effect of low BP in the elderly for the development of dementia. Follow-up studies examining the effect of BP on brain structural changes provide further evidence for the adverse effect of high BP on cognitive performance.[69,77]

Effect of treating hypertension on cognition and dementia

Several randomized controlled trials had as secondary objectives the assessment of antihypertensive therapy on changes in cognition or the development of dementia. These studies have mainly involved older participants followed up for a relatively short duration of 2 to 4 years.

The Medical Research Council Trial in older persons aged 65 to 74 years[78] and the Systolic Hypertension in the Elderly Programme (SHEP), using thiazide-based regimens, found no effect of active treatment on cognition (SHEP). The Study on Cognition and Prognosis in the Elderly (SCOPE) of hypertensives aged 70 to 89 years (whether analyzed with all participants or restricted to the subgroup randomized to candesartan versus placebo) found no difference on the Mini-Mental State Exam (MMSE).[79] In all of these studies, active therapy significantly reduced BP (and vascular events), with no apparent adverse effect on cognition.

The SYST-EUR Study of Nitrendipine versus placebo in subjects with systolic hypertension reported a 50% reduction in dementia incidence after 2 years, although the number of dementia cases was small.[80] Follow-up occurred for another 2 years, with all participants receiving active treatment. Compared to the original placebo group, the "active" treatment group (i.e., those treated the longest) had dementia risk reduced by half. In contrast to the previously cited studies, the HOPE Trial included normotensives randomized to Ramipril or placebo. Subjects who went on to develop stroke had less of a reduction in cognitive performance if they were taking Ramipril.[49]

Two studies have reported on the effect of antihypertensive therapy on cognitive function in patients who have previously suffered a stroke. In the PROGRESS study, therapy with an ACE inhibitor and Indapamide attenuated the decline in the MMSE and significantly reduced the risk of dementia with recurrent stroke by 34% and the risk of severe cognitive decline. In the MOSES study of two active treatments, Eprosartan and Nitrendipine, a similar and significant BP fall occurred in both groups without any change from baseline in MMSE or between active therapies.

So far, the controlled randomized intervention studies suggest no deterioration in cognitive performance with antihypertensive therapy in well elderly hypertensive patients, in those normotensive patients with vascular disease, or in hypertensive patients with a history of stroke. There is limited evidence from one study that antihypertensive therapy may reduce the incidence of dementia, although further confirmation of this effect is required.

PROGNOSIS

About a quarter of the world's population, or almost one billion, have hypertension. Two-thirds of these people are in the economically developing world and one-third in the developed world. In 20 years' time, over one-and-a-half billion people are expected to have hypertension. It will then be the most common risk factor for death and disability.

Stroke is the second leading cause of death worldwide, causing up to five million deaths per year. Another fifteen million stroke survivors add to the global burden of disability. By 2020, it is estimated that cerebrovascular diseases will become the second most prevalent cause of death and disability in developed countries, and will be ranked fifth in developing countries.

Dementia is also predicted to be in the top eight leading causes of death and disability in developed regions. Dementia is also one of the leading causes of death and disability in the older population. By 2020, it is predicted that worldwide there will be nearly 29 million people with dementia.[81]

SUMMARY

BP, as discussed earlier in this chapter, has a close relationship with stroke (especially in Asian populations). Over 50% of stroke deaths can be attributed to increased BP levels. A modest population-wide reduction in BP of 2% and a targeted approach in hypertensives could annually prevent about 20% of stroke deaths worldwide. Although high BP is the greatest population-attributable risk for stroke, other factors (e.g., high cholesterol, smoking, poor diet, and inactivity) also contribute. Removal of all of these risks could reduce global stroke burden by approximately 70%. Beneficial effects of modest BP reduction would also be seen not only in reduction of stroke-related dementia but likely in other dementia types (e.g., vascular, mixed, and Alzheimer's). Again, multiple vascular risk factor reductions could have greater benefits. Global management of hypertension has the potential for making a significant impact on reducing the burden from brain diseases.

REFERENCES

1. Spiers NA, Matthews RJ, Jagger C et al. Diseases and impairments as risk factors for onset of disability in the older population in England and Wales: Findings from the Medical Research Council Cognitive Function and Ageing Study. *J Gerontol A Biol Sci Med Sci* 2005;60:248–54.
2. Tomlinson BE, Blessed G, Roth M. Observations on the brains of demented old people. *J Neurol Sci* 1970;11:205–42.
3. Roman GC. Vascular dementia: Distinguishing characteristics, treatment, and prevention. *J Am Geriatr Soc* 2003; 51:S296–304.
4. Brian JE Jr., Faraci FM, Heistad DD. Recent insights into the regulation of cerebral circulation. *Clin Exp Pharmacol Physiol* 1996;23:449–57.
5. Lipsitz LA, Mukai S, Hamner J, et al. Dynamic regulation of middle cerebral artery blood flow velocity in aging and hypertension. *Stroke* 2000;31:1897–903.
6. Dawson SL, Blake MJ, Panerai RB, Potter JF. Dynamic but not static cerebral autoregulation is impaired in acute ischemic stroke. *Cerebrovasc Dis* 2000;10:126–32.
7. Immink RV, van den Born BJ, van Montfrans GA et al. Impaired cerebral autoregulation in patients with malignant hypertension. *Circulation* 2004;110:2241–45.
8. Leonardi-Bee J, Bath PM, Phillips SJ, Sandercock PA. Blood pressure and clinical outcomes in the International Stroke Trial. *Stroke* 2002;33:1315–20.
9. Colivicchi F, Bassi A, Santini M, Caltagirone C. Prognostic implications of right-sided insular damage, cardiac autonomic derangement, and arrhythmias after acute ischemic stroke. *Stroke* 2005;36:1710–15.
10. Adams HP Jr., Woolson RF, Biller J, Clarke W. Studies of Org 10172 in patients with acute ischemic stroke: TOAST Study Group. *Hemostasis* 1992; 22:99–103.
11. Bamford J, Sandercock P, Dennis M, et al. Classification and natural history of clinically identifiable subtypes of cerebral infarction. *Lancet* 1991;337:1521–26.
12. Fiebach JB, Schellinger PD, Gass A, et al. Stroke magnetic resonance imaging is accurate in hyperacute intracerebral hemorrhage: A multicenter study on the validity of stroke imaging. *Stroke* 2004;35:502–06.
13. Fiebach JB, Schellinger PD, Jansen O, et al. CT and diffusion-weighted MR imaging in randomized order: Diffusion-weighted imaging results in higher accuracy and lower interrater variability in the diagnosis of hyperacute ischemic stroke. *Stroke* 2002;33:2206–10.
14. Sobesky J, Zaro WO, Lehnhardt FG, et al. Does the mismatch match the penumbra? Magnetic resonance imaging and positron emission tomography in early ischemic stroke. *Stroke* 2005; 36:980–85.
15. Butcher KS, Parsons M, MacGregor L, et al. Refining the perfusion-diffusion mismatch hypothesis. *Stroke* 2005; 36:1153–59.
16. Silverman DH. Brain 18F-FDG PET in the diagnosis of neurodegenerative dementias: Comparison with perfusion SPECT and with clinical evaluations lacking nuclear imaging. *J Nucl Med* 2004;45:594–607.
17. Wintermark M, Sesay M, Barbier E, et al. Comparative overview of brain perfusion imaging techniques. *Stroke* 2005;36:e83–99.
18. Harbison J, Massey A, Barnett L, et al. Rapid ambulance protocol for acute stroke. *Lancet* 1999;353:1935.
19. Kidwell CS, Saver JL, Schubert GB, et al. Design and retrospective analysis of the Los Angeles Prehospital Stroke Screen (LAPSS). *Prehosp Emerg Care* 1998;2:267–73.
20. Stroke Unit Trialists' Collaboration. *Organised Inpatient (Stroke Unit) Care for Stroke (Cochrane Review)*. The Cochrane Library. Issue 1. Chichester, UK: John Wiley and Sons, 2004.
21. Langhorne P, Taylor G, Murray G, et al. Early supported discharge services for stroke patients: a meta-analysis of individual patients' data. *Lancet* 2005; 365:501–06.
22. Adams H, Adams R, Del Zoppo G, Goldstein LB. Guidelines for the early management of patients with ischemic stroke: 2005 guidelines update a scientific statement from the Stroke Council of the American Heart Association/American Stroke Association. *Stroke* 2005;36:916–23.
23. Hack W, Kaste M, Bogousslavsky J, et al. European Stroke Initiative Recommendations for Stroke Management: Update 2003. *Cerebrovasc Dis* 2003;16:311–37.
24. Royal College of Physicians. *National Clinical Guidelines for Stroke, Second Edition*. London: Royal College of Physicians, 2004.
25. Liu M, Wardlaw J. *Thrombolysis (Different Doses, Routes of Administration and Agents) for Acute Ischemic Stroke (Cochrane Review)*. The Cochrane Library. Issue 1. Chichester, UK: John Wiley and Sons, 2004.
26. Leary MC, Saver JL, Gobin YP, et al. Beyond tissue plasminogen activator: Mechanical intervention in acute stroke. *Ann Emerg Med* 2003;41:838–46.
27. Muir KW, Lees KR, Ford I, Davis S. Magnesium for acute stroke (Intravenous Magnesium Efficacy in Stroke trial): Randomised controlled trial. *Lancet* 2004;363:439–45.
28. International Stroke Trial Collaborative Group. The International Stroke Trial (IST): A randomised trial of aspirin, subcutaneous heparin, both, or neither among 19435 patients with acute ischemic stroke. *Lancet* 1997;349:1569–81.
29. Bath PM, Iddenden R, Bath FJ. Low-molecular-weight heparins and heparinoids in acute ischemic stroke: A meta-analysis of randomized controlled trials. *Stroke* 2000;31:1770–78.
30. Sandercock P, Mielke O, Liu M, Counsell C. *Anticoagulants for Preventing Recurrence Following Presumed Non-cardioembolic Ischemic Stroke or Transient Ischemic Attack (Cochrane Review)*. The Cochrane Library. Issue 1. Chichester, UK:.John Wiley and Sons, 2004.
31. Chen ZM, Sandercock P, Pan HC, et al. Indications for early aspirin use in acute ischemic stroke: A combined analysis of 40 000 randomized patients from the chinese acute stroke trial and the international stroke trial. On behalf of the CAST and IST collaborative groups. *Stroke* 2000;31:1240–49.
32. Mendelow AD, Gregson BA, Fernandes HM, et al. Early surgery versus initial conservative treatment in patients with spontaneous supratentorial intracerebral hematomas in the International Surgical Trial in Intracerebral Hemorrhage (STICH): A randomised trial. *Lancet* 2005;365:387–97.
33. Mayer SA, Brun NC, Begtrup K, et al. Recombinant activated factor VII for acute intracerebral hemorrhage. *N Engl J Med* 2005;352:777–85.
34. Eames PJ, Mistri AK, Shah N, Robinson TG. Acute stroke hypertension: Current and future management. *Expert Rev Cardiovasc Ther* 2005;3:405–12.
35. Dippel DW, van Breda EJ, van Gemert HM, et al. Effect of paracetamol (acetaminophen) on body temperature in acute ischemic stroke: A double-blind, randomized phase II clinical trial. *Stroke* 2001;32:1607–12.
36. Olsen TS, Weber UJ, Kammersgaard LP. Therapeutic hypothermia for acute stroke. *Lancet Neurol* 2003;2:410–16.

37. Scott JF, Robinson GM, French JM, et al. Glucose potassium insulin infusions in the treatment of acute stroke patients with mild to moderate hyperglycemia: The Glucose Insulin in Stroke Trial (GIST). *Stroke* 1999;30:793–99.

38. Dennis MS, Lewis SC, Warlow C. Routine oral nutritional supplementation for stroke patients in hospital (FOOD): A multicentre randomised controlled trial. *Lancet* 2005;365:755–63.

39. Dennis MS, Lewis SC, Warlow C. Effect of timing and method of enteral tube feeding for dysphagic stroke patients (FOOD): A multicentre randomised controlled trial. *Lancet* 2005;365:764–72.

40. Diener HC, Cunha L, Forbes C, et al. European Stroke Prevention Study. 2. Dipyridamole and acetylsalicylic acid in the secondary prevention of stroke. *J Neurol Sci* 1996;143:1–13.

41. CAPRIE Steering Committee. A randomised, blinded, trial of clopidogrel versus aspirin in patients at risk of ischemic events (CAPRIE). *Lancet* 1996;348:1329–39.

42. Diener HC, Bogousslavsky J, Brass LM, et al. Aspirin and clopidogrel compared with clopidogrel alone after recent ischemic stroke or transient ischemic attack in high-risk patients (MATCH): Randomised, double-blind, placebo-controlled trial. *Lancet* 2004;364:331–37.

42a. Bhatt DL, Fox KAA, Hacke W, Berger PB, Black HR, Boden WE, et al. Clopidogrel and aspirin versus aspirin alone for the prevention of atherothrombotic events. *N Engl J Med* 2006;354:1706–1717.

43. Collins R, Armitage J, Parish S, et al. Effects of cholesterol-lowering with simvastatin on stroke and other major vascular events in 20536 people with cerebrovascular disease or other high-risk conditions. *Lancet* 2004;363:757–67.

44. Koudstaal PJ. *Anticoagulants for Preventing Stroke in Patients with Non-rheumatic Atrial Fibrillation and a History of Stroke or Transient Ischemic Attacks (Cochrane Review).* The Cochrane Library. Issue 1. Chichester, UK: John Wiley and Sons, 2004.

45. Rothwell PM, Eliasziw M, Gutnikov SA, et al. Analysis of pooled data from the randomised controlled trials of endarterectomy for symptomatic carotid stenosis. *Lancet* 2003;361:107–16.

46. Rothwell PM, Eliasziw M, Gutnikov SA, et al. Endarterectomy for symptomatic carotid stenosis in relation to clinical subgroups and timing of surgery. *Lancet* 2004;363:915–24.

47. Rodgers A, MacMahon S, Gamble G, et al. Blood pressure and risk of stroke in patients with cerebrovascular disease: The United Kingdom Transient Ischemic Attack Collaborative Group. *BMJ* 1996;313:147.

48. PATS Collaborating Group. Post-stroke antihypertensive treatment study: A preliminary result. *Chin Med J (Engl)* 1995;108:710–17.

49. Bosch J, Yusuf S, Pogue J, et al. Use of ramipril in preventing stroke: Double blind randomised trial. *BMJ* 2002;324:699–702.

50. Progress Collaborative Group. Randomised trial of a perindopril-based blood-pressure-lowering regimen among 6,105 individuals with previous stroke or transient ischemic attack. *Lancet* 2001;358:1033–41.

51. Schrader J, Luders S, Kulschewski A, et al. Morbidity and Mortality After Stroke, Eprosartan Compared with Nitrendipine for Secondary Prevention: Principal results of a prospective randomized controlled study (MOSES). *Stroke* 2005;36:1218–26.

52. Rothwell PM, Howard SC, Spence JD. Relationship between blood pressure and stroke risk in patients with symptomatic carotid occlusive disease. *Stroke* 2003;34:2583–90.

53. Chapman N, Huxley R, Anderson C, et al. Effects of a perindopril-based blood pressure-lowering regimen on the risk of recurrent stroke according to stroke subtype and medical history: The PROGRESS Trial. *Stroke* 2004; 35:116–21.

54. Kjeldsen SE, Lyle PA, Kizer JR, et al. The effects of losartan compared to atenolol on stroke in patients with isolated systolic hypertension and left ventricular hypertrophy: The LIFE study. *J Clin Hypertens (Greenwich)* 2005;7:152–58.

55. de la Torre JC. Is Alzheimer's disease a neurodegenerative or a vascular disorder? Data, dogma, and dialectics. *Lancet Neurol* 2004;3:184–90.

56. Roher E, Esh C, Kokjohn TA, et al. Circle of willis atherosclerosis is a risk factor for sporadic Alzheimer's disease. *Arterioscler Thromb Vasc Biol* 2003; 23:2055–62.

57. Langa KM, Foster NL, Larson EB. Mixed dementia: Emerging concepts and therapeutic implications. *JAMA* 2004;292:2901–08.

58. Ivan CS, Seshadri S, Beiser A, et al. Dementia after stroke: The Framingham Study. *Stroke* 2004;35:1264–68.

59. Sachdev PS, Wen W, Christensen H, Jorm AF. White matter hyperintensities are related to physical disability and poor motor function. *J Neurol Neurosurg Psychiatry* 2005;76:362–67.

60. de Groot JC, de Leeuw FE, Oudkerk M, et al. Cerebral white matter lesions and subjective cognitive dysfunction: The Rotterdam Scan Study. *Neurology* 2001;56:1539–45.

61. Guo Z, Viitanen M, Fratiglioni L, Winblad B. Low blood pressure and dementia in elderly people: the Kungsholmen project. *BMJ* 1996;312:805–08.

62. Rockwood K, Lindsay J, McDowell I. High blood pressure and dementia. *Lancet* 1996;348:65–6.

63. Cerhan JR, Folsom AR, Mortimer JA, et al. Correlates of cognitive function in middle-aged adults: Atherosclerosis Risk in Communities (ARIC) Study Investigators. *Gerontology* 1998; 44:95–105.

64. Pavlik VN, Hyman DJ, Doody R. Cardiovascular risk factors and cognitive function in adults 30-59 years of age (NHANES III). *Neuroepidemiology* 2005;24:42–50.

65. Kilander L, Nyman H, Boberg M, et al. Hypertension is related to cognitive impairment: A 20-year follow-up of 999 men. *Hypertension* 1998;31:780–86.

66. Stewart R, Richards M, Brayne C, Mann A. Vascular risk and cognitive impairment in an older, British, African-Caribbean population. *J Am Geriatr Soc* 2001;49:263–69.

67. Kuo HK, Sorond F, Iloputaife I, et al. Effect of blood pressure on cognitive functions in elderly persons. *J Gerontol A Biol Sci Med Sci* 2004;59:1191–94.

68. Kahonen-Vare M, Brunni-Hakala S, Lindroos M, et al. Left ventricular hypertrophy and blood pressure as predictors of cognitive decline in old age. *Aging Clin Exp Res* 2004; 16:147–52.

69. Launer LJ, Masaki K, Petrovitch H, et al. The association between midlife blood pressure levels and late-life cognitive function: The Honolulu-Asia Aging Study. *JAMA* 1995;274:1846–51.

70. Guo Z, Fratiglioni L, Winblad B, Viitanen M. Blood pressure and performance on the Mini-Mental State Examination in the very old: Cross-sectional and longitudinal data from the Kungsholmen Project. *Am J Epidemiol* 1997;145:1106–13.

71. Waldstein SR, Giggey PP, Thayer JF, Zonderman AB. Nonlinear relations of blood pressure to cognitive function: The Baltimore Longitudinal Study of Aging. *Hypertension* 2005;45:374–79.

72. Elias MF, Wolf PA, D'Agostino RB, et al. Untreated blood pressure level is inversely related to cognitive functioning: The Framingham Study. *Am J Epidemiol* 1993;138:353–64.

73. Whitmer RA, Sidney S, Selby J, et al. Midlife cardiovascular risk factors and risk of dementia in late life. *Neurology* 2005;64:277–81.

74. Tzourio C, Dufouil C, Ducimetiere P, Alperovitch A. Cognitive decline in individuals with high blood pressure: A longitudinal study in the elderly. EVA Study Group. *Epidemiology of Vascular Aging Neurology* 1999;53:1948–52.

75. Morris MC, Scherr PA, Hebert LE, et al. Association of incident Alzheimer disease and blood pressure measured from 13 years before to 2 years after diagnosis in a large community study. *Arch Neurol* 2001;58:1640–46.

76. Verghese J, Lipton RB, Hall CB, et al. Low blood pressure and the risk of dementia in very old individuals. *Neurology* 2003;61:1667–72.

77. Goldstein IB, Bartzokis G, Guthrie D, Shapiro D. Ambulatory blood pressure and the brain: A 5-year follow-up. *Neurology* 2005;64:1846–52.

78. Prince MJ, Bird AS, Blizard RA, Mann AH. Is the cognitive function of older patients affected by antihypertensive treatment? Results from 54 months of the Medical Research Council's trial of hypertension in older adults. *BMJ* 1996;312:801–05.

79. Lithell H, Hansson L, Skoog I, et al. The Study on COgnition and Prognosis in the Elderly (SCOPE): Outcomes in patients not receiving add-on therapy after randomization. *J Hypertens* 2004;22:1605–12.

80. Forette F, Seux ML, Stessen JA, et al. Prevention of dementia in randomised double-blind placebo-controlled Systolic Hypertension in Europe (Syst-Eur) trial. *Lancet* 1998;352:1347–51.

81. Haan MN, Wallace R. Can dementia be prevented? Brain aging in a population-based context. *Annu Rev Public Health* 2004;25:1–24.

82. Tei H, Uchiyama S, Koshimizu K, et al. Correlation between symptomatic, radiological and etiological diagnosis in acute ischemic stroke. *Acta Neurol Scand* 1999;99:192–95.

Chapter

49

Kidney Disease and Hypertension

Panteleimon A. Sarafidis and George L. Bakris

Key Findings

- People with chronic kidney disease have a higher risk for cardiovascular events independent of elevated blood pressure.

- Presence of microalbuminuria (>30<300 mg/day) is a cardiovascular risk marker.

- Presence of macroalbuminuria (proteinuria) ≥300 mg/day indicates presence of kidney disease.

- Individuals with proteinuria and kidney disease must have both their blood pressure lowered to <130/80 mmHg and proteinuria reduced by at least 30%.

- Reductions in proteinuria of more than 50% following 6 months of treatment yields a 70% risk reduction for progression to end-stage renal disease at 5 years in nondiabetic kidney disease.

- Agents that block the renin-angiotensin system, either alone or combined, yield the greatest slowing of kidney disease progression (assuming blood pressure is reduced) in those with advanced disease and proteinuria.

- Combinations of ACE inhibitors with angiotensin receptor blockers or aldosterone receptor blockers may provide additional reductions in proteinuria independent of further blood pressure reductions.

below 89 mL/min/1.73 m^2 and is considered to be pronounced if the GFR is less than 60 mL/min/1.73 m^2 for more than 3 months.[1] In clinical terms, the latter is reflected in an elevation of serum creatinine levels above the normal range [=1.5 mg/dL (133 μmol/L) in men and =1.3 mg/dL (115 μmol/L) in women]. This decrease in renal function along with an increase in the presence of microalbuminuria (>30 mg/dL or <300 mg/dL) or development of albuminuria (>300 mg/dL) is a clear indication of the presence of renal dysfunction. Apart from the stage, diagnosis of the type of CKD based on etiology is also very important (Table 49–2). A definitive diagnosis could be assigned after biopsy or imaging studies, but in most patients well-defined clinical presentations and causal factors provide sufficient basis for a diagnosis without these procedures.[1]

During the past decades, CKD has grown to a worldwide public health problem. In the United States, about 20 million individuals are currently suffering from CKD.[2] Both the incidence and prevalence of kidney failure treated by dialysis and transplantation continue to increase, as shown in Figure 49–1.[3] In 2002, the number of patients with kidney failure rose to more than 430,000, and the incident rate of kidney failure has increased to 333 new cases per million people—a number almost four times higher than that in 1980.[3] The United States Renal Data System, taking into consideration the enormous growth of both the elderly and type 2 diabetic populations, estimates that by the year 2030 more than 2.2 million individuals will require treatment for end-stage renal disease (ESRD).[2] Among patients on dialysis, 5-year survival rates are extremely low (about 32%)—largely due to the parallel high prevalence of cardiovascular disease (CVD).[2] Moreover, the cost of treatment for ESRD is enormous and is expected to rise

Chronic kidney disease (CKD) is defined either as kidney damage, which is confirmed by kidney biopsy or markers of damage, or as the presence of glomerular filtration rate (GFR) under the level of 60 mL/min/1.73 m^2 for a period greater than 3 months.[1] The stage of CKD is based on the level of GFR, irrespective of the cause of kidney disease (Table 49–1). Decreased kidney function starts at a GFR

STAGES AND PREVALENCE OF CKD IN 2002				
Stage	Description	GFR (mL/min/1.73m²)	Prevalence N (1,000's)	(%)
1	Kidney damage with normal or ↑ GFR	≥90	5,900	3.3
2	Kidney damage with mild ↓ GFR	60–89	5,300	3.0
3	Moderate ↓ GFR	30–59	7,600	4.3
4	Severe ↓ GFR	15–29	400	0.2
5	Kidney failure	<15 of dialysis	300	0.1

Adapted from K/DOQI clinical practice guidelines on hypertension and antihypertensive agents in chronic kidney disease. *Am J Kidney Dis* 2004;43(5 Suppl 2):1–290 with permission from the National Kidney Foundation, Inc.

Table 49–1. Stages and Prevalence of CKD in 2002

MAJOR TYPES OF CKD AND PREVALENCE AMONG PATIENTS WITH END-STAGE RENAL DISEASE		
Disease	Major Types (Examples)	Prevalence Among Patients with ESRD (%)
Diabetic kidney disease	Type 1 and type 2 diabetes mellitus	33
Nondiabetic kidney diseases	Glomerular diseases	
	(autoimmune diseases, systemic infections, drugs, neoplasia)	19
	Vascular diseases	
	(hypertension, renal artery disease, microangiopathy)	21
	Tubulointerstitial diseases	
	(urinary tract infections, stones, obstruction, drug toxicity)	4
	Cystic diseases	
	(polycystic kidney disease)	6
Modified from K/DOQI clinical practice guidelines on hypertension and antihypertensive agents in chronic kidney disease. *Am J Kidney Dis* 2004;43(5 Suppl 2):1–290 with permission from the National Kidney Foundation, Inc.		

Table 49–2. Major Types of CKD and Prevalence Among Patients with End-stage Renal Disease

steeply. For example, Medicare costs associated with ESRD are projected to have increased from $12.7 billion in 1999 to $28.0 billion by the year 2010.[4] In contrast to this, several lines of evidence indicate that both establishment and progression of CKD as well as cardiovascular events can be delayed or avoided by several measures, among which achievement of hypertension control is the most important.

Goals of antihypertensive treatment in kidney disease

As shown in Table 49–2, hypertension represents an important cause of CKD but is also a consequence of it.[1] Several lines of evidence support the role of hypertension as a renal risk factor. In the Third National Health and Nutrition Examination Survey (NHANES III), 3% of the civilian population has been estimated to have elevated serum creatinine levels [=1.6 mg/dL (141 μmol/L) for men and =1.4 mg/dL (124 μmol/L) for women], and among those 70% also had hypertension.[5] In the Multiple Risk Factor Intervention Trial (MRFIT), which included 332,544 middle-age men, blood pressure was a strong predictor of the development of ESRD during the 16 years of follow-up.[6] In practical terms, the second most common cause of ESRD after diabetic nephropathy is hypertensive nephrosclerosis, which is typically represented by hyalinization and sclerosis of the walls of the afferent arterioles. On the other hand, many of the abnormalities present in an individual with CKD or certain agents used in the treatment of ESRD patients or graft recipients could be responsible for blood pressure elevation (Box 49–1).[7]

Apart from sex- and body-size-related variability, GFR varies according to age. Normally, age-related declines in GFR begin at about 50 years of age, at a rate of approximately 1 mL/min per year. However, this age-related loss of renal function is directly proportional to blood pressure level, and the rate of GFR decline can rise up to 4 to 8 mL/min per year if systolic blood pressure is elevated to a hypertensive level.[8] Interventions that lower blood pressure levels in patients with kidney disease have been consistently shown to slow down the progression of it. An analysis of long-term clinical trials in patients with diabetic or nondiabetic kidney disease clearly showed that lower blood pressures result in greater preservation of kidney function (Figure 49–2).[9]

Although GFR declines in varying rates depending on the type of underlying kidney disease, the impact of earlier blood pressure reduction is far more significant compared to later intervention, and therefore early treatment is invariably preferred.[10,11] Apart from the foregoing, hypertension has long been identified as one of the major independent risk factors for CVD,[12,13] and patients with kidney disease are at increased risk for cardiovascular events compared with patients with normal kidney function.[14–16] Therefore, according to the National Kidney Foundation (NKF)-Kidney Disease Outcomes Quality Initiative (KDOQI) Working Group guidelines, the goals of antihypertensive therapy in patients with CKD are to lower blood pressure, reduce the

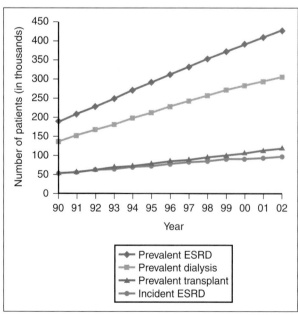

Figure 49–1. Incident and prevalent ESRD patient counts by modality. (Adapted from *Summary of Revisions for the 2004 Clinical Practice Recommendations. Diabetes Care* 2004;27(Suppl 1):S3.[11])

Box 49–1

Possible Mechanisms for BP Elevation in CKD

- Preexisting essential hypertension
- Extracellular fluid volume expansion
- Renin-angiotensin-aldosterone system stimulation
- Increased sympathetic activity
- Endogenous digitalis-like factors
- Prostaglandins/bradykinins
- Alterations in endothelium-derived factors (nitric oxide/endothelin)
- Increased body weight
- Erythropoietin administration
- Parathyroid hormone secretion/increased intracellular calcium/hypercalcemia
- Calcification of arterial tree
- Renal artery disease
- Chronic allograft dysfunction
- Cadaver allografts, especially from a donor with family history of hypertension
- Cyclosporine/tacrolimus/other immunosuppressive and corticosteroid therapy

Adapted from Mailloux LU, Levey AS. Hypertension in patients with chronic renal disease. *Am J Kidney Dis* 1998;32(5 Suppl 3):S120–41 with permission from The National Kidney Foundation, Inc.

risk of CVD in patients with or without hypertension, and slow the progression of kidney disease in patients with or without hypertension.[1]

Blood pressure goal

According to the Seventh Report of the Joint National Committee (JNC) 7, the blood pressure goal for a patient with hypertension is less than 140/90 mmHg.[17] Two multi-center outcome trials that randomized to different levels of blood pressure—the Hypertension Optimal Treatment

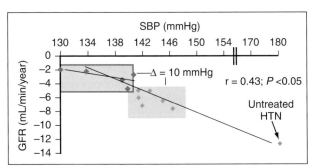

Figure 49–2. Relationship between achieved blood pressure control and declines in GFR in clinical trials of diabetic and nondiabetic kidney disease. (Adapted from Bakris GL, Williams M, Dworkin L, et al. Preserving renal function in adults with hypertension and diabetes: A consensus approach. National Kidney Foundation Hypertension and Diabetes Executive Committees Working Group. *Am J Kidney Dis* 2000;36(3):646–61.)

(HOT) trial[18] and the United Kingdom Prospective Diabetes Study (UKPDS) 38[19]—have shown a significant reduction in cardiovascular mortality in the groups of diabetic patients that achieved the lower levels of blood pressure and were the main reasons for setting a blood pressure goal of <130/80 for patients with diabetes in the JNC 7 report.[17] In particular, in the HOT trial (which included almost 19,000 hypertensive patients) the subgroup of diabetic patients randomized to the lowest diastolic blood pressure group (<80 mmHg) had the most significant reductions in cardiovascular events. This was not true, however, for the study as a whole. The same was found in the UKPDS 38 trial, which randomized 1148 patients with hypertension and type 2 diabetes to "tight blood pressure control" (<150/85 mmHg) and to "less tight control" (<180/105 mmHg). After 9 years of follow-up, those at the "tight blood pressure control" group (mean blood pressure achieved 144/82 mmHg) had far fewer cardiovascular events than those at the "less tight control" group (mean blood pressure achieved 154/87 mmHg) and medication selection did not affect clinical outcome.[19]

If CKD is present, JNC 7 also recommends a blood pressure goal of <130/80 mmHg.[17] The JNC 7 guidelines, however, are not the only to recommend this blood pressure goal. The evidence in favor of such a tight blood pressure control in order to reduce the rates of both kidney disease progression and cardiovascular events is so strong that all important international guidelines released during the past few years—including those from the JNC 7,[17] the European Society of Hypertension-European Society of Cardiology committee,[20] the NKF-KDOQI working group,[1] and the American Diabetes Association[11]—recommend a goal of <130/80 mmHg for patients with CKD and/or diabetes. Long-term clinical trials with primary renal outcomes in patients with or without diabetes, including those comparing intensive with regular blood pressure control, are summarized in Table 49–3.

The first trial to randomize individuals with advanced nephropathy to two different levels of blood pressure was the Modification of Diet in Renal Disease (MDRD) Study. In this study, patients with chronic kidney disease and high rates of protein excretion were randomly assigned to a low blood pressure group with a goal mean arterial pressure (MAP) <92 mmHg and a high blood pressure group (goal MAP <107 mmHg) for 4 years. At the end of the study, patients in the low target blood pressure group had a significantly slower reduction in GFR decline compared to patients assigned to the high target blood pressure group.[21] Moreover, an analysis of data obtained about 7 years after the end of the randomization trial revealed that the risks for kidney failure and the composite outcome of kidney failure and all-cause mortality were significantly lower in the low target blood pressure group.[22] In a meta-analysis of studies in nondiabetic kidney disease by the ACE Inhibition in Progressive Renal Disease (AIPRD) Study Group, a systolic blood pressure range of 110 to 129 mmHg was that associated with the lowest risk of kidney disease progression in patients with urine protein excretion >1 g/day (Figure 49–3).[23]

In patients with lower levels of urine protein excretion (i.e., <1 g/day), however, the evidence from the MDRD

LONG-TERM OUTCOME STUDIES WITH PRIMARY RENAL ENDPOINTS					
No Diabetes		**No. Patients**	**Baseline GFR**	**Follow-up**	**Favorable Therapy**
MDRD, 1993 (21)	Usual vs low blood pressure goal	840	40	2.2 years	Low blood pressure goal in patients with proteinuria
AIPRI, 1996 (96)	Benazepril vs placebo	583	52	3 years	Benazepril
REIN, 1997 (44)	Ramipril vs placebo	166	56 (39)	16 months	Ramipril
AASK, 2001 (24)	Metoprolol vs amlodipine vs ramipril	1094	46	3 - 6.4 years	Ramipril
	Low vs usual BP control				
COOPERATE, 2002 (47)	Losartan vs trandolapril vs combination	263	38	2.9 years	Combination
Diabetes					
Captopril Trial, 1993 (43)	Captopril vs placebo	409	68	3 years	Captopril
Bakris et al., 1996 (86)	Lisinopril vs nondihydropyridine CCB vs atenolol	52	59	6 years	Lisinopril and nondihydropyridine CCB
Bakris et al., 1997 (79)	Verapamil SR vs atenolol	34	62	54 months	Verapamil SR
ABCD, 2000 (97)	Moderate vs Intensive BP control	470	84	5 years	No difference
IDNT, 2001(28)	Irbesartan vs amlodipine vs placebo	1715	59	2.6 years	Irbesartan
RENAAL, 2001 (27)	Losartan vs placebo	1513	54	3.4 years	Losartan

Table 49–3. Long-Term Outcome Studies with Primary Renal Endpoints

trial in favor of such a low blood pressure goal is not as strong.[21] Another trial that did not show a benefit to a low blood pressure goal in patients with lower levels of proteinuria was the African-American Study of Kidney Disease and Hypertension (AASK), in which African-American patients with hypertensive kidney disease (GFR between 20 and 65 mL/min/1.73 m^2) and an average urine protein excretion <1 g/day were randomized to a low blood pressure goal (MAP=92 mmHg) or a usual one (MAP 102 to 107 mmHg). At the end of the study, no benefit of the lower blood pressure goal in reducing the decline in GFR compared to the usual goal was noted.[24] The mentioned above meta-analysis of the AIPRD Study Group further supports these findings, in that no significant relation between the level of systolic blood pressure and risk of kidney disease progression in patients with proteinuria <1 g/day was found (Figure 49–3).[23]

The percentage of hypertensive patients achieving the current blood pressure goals is rather disappointing. In the United States, estimates suggest that about 34% of the general hypertensive population and 36% of patients with diabetes manage to keep their blood pressure within recommended limits.[17,25] Data from NHANES III demonstrates that blood pressure control rates in patients with CKD are even lower, as only 11% of hypertensives with elevated serum creatinine levels had a blood pressure of less than 130/85 mmHg.[5] In clinical trials, the proportion of participants achieving such goals is roughly double that in routine clinical practice. However, in either setting no more than 75% of the total group achieve target blood pressure goal. In the Antihypertensive and Lipid-Lowering Treatment to Prevent Heart Attack Trial (ALLHAT), the mean number of medications needed to achieve the mean blood pressure (135/75 mmHg) in patients with stage 1 or 2 hypertension was 2.[26] In patients with kidney disease, achievement of blood pressure goals is more difficult and requires even more antihypertensive agents. In particular, to achieve these lower levels of blood pressure in people with renal insufficiency will require an average of 3.5 to 4.2 different antihypertensive agents in moderate to high doses, as shown in Figure 49–4.[24,27] For example, in the Irbesartan Diabetic Nephropathy Trial (IDNT)—which included subjects with diabetic nephropathy (median urine protein excretion of 2.9 g/day) and renal insufficiency (mean creatinine 1.65 to 1.69 mg/dL)—an average of 4.0 different antihypertensive medications (including the study medication) were required to reduce mean blood pressure from 159/87 mmHg at baseline to 140/70 mmHg at the end of the study.[28]

All agents that lower blood pressure are known to reduce cardiovascular risk, but certain antihypertensive compounds may have an advantage in reducing the rate of kidney disease progression in the presence of advanced nephropathy. Both JNC 7 and the KDOQI-blood pressure guidelines clearly state that there are compelling and specific indications for the use of ACE inhibitors or angiotensin receptor blockers (ARBs) in the armamentarium to lower blood pressure in individuals with either diabetes or kidney disease.[1,17] However, these reports also emphasize the fact that arterial pressure in such patients should be reduced to <130/80 mmHg, especially in the presence of proteinuria. It is therefore clear that once a person has established nephropathy the main factor that will slow its progression

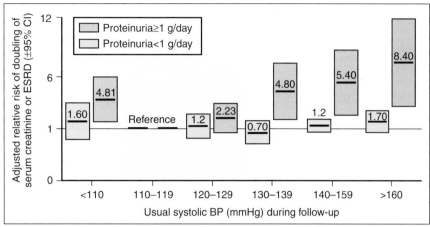

Figure 49–3. Relative risk for kidney disease progression based on current level of systolic blood pressure and urine protein excretion. Results based on a meta-analysis of 11 randomized controlled trials. The reference group for each is defined at a systolic blood pressure of 110 to 119 mmHg. (Adapted from Jafar TH, Stark PC, Schmid CH, et al. Progression of chronic kidney disease: The role of blood pressure control, proteinuria, and angiotensin-converting enzyme inhibition. A patient-level meta-analysis. *Ann Intern Med* 2003;139(4):244–52.)

is aggressive blood pressure reduction and that this will require multiple drug treatment.

Microalbuminuria

According to the NKF-KDOQI guidelines, microalbuminuria is defined as urine albumin excretion (UAE) between 30 and 300 mg/day if measured in a 24-hour urine collection or as 30 to 300 mg/g if measured by the preferred method of spot albumin to creatinine (Table 49–4).[1] The appearance of microalbuminuria is the earliest clinical sign of diabetic and hypertensive nephropathy.[1] A diabetic patient with microalbuminuria is considered to have incipient nephropathy, whereas the progression to UAE >300 mg/day or >300 mg/g is considered a sign of overt nephropathy.

Without specific interventions, about 80% of patients with type 1 and 20 to 40% of patients with type 2 diabetes and microalbuminuria will progress to overt nephropathy.

After the onset of overt nephropathy, about 75% of type 1 and 20% of type 2 diabetic patients will develop ESRD in a period of 20 years.[11] In addition to the previous, in several studies (either in the general population[29] or in individuals with other cardiovascular risk factors[5,30,31]) the presence of microalbuminuria was associated with an increased risk for cardiovascular events. As shown in Figure 49–5, higher levels of urinary albumin excretion are associated with increased risk for CVD outcomes.[5,29] Thus, in the JNC 7 guidelines microalbuminuria has been identified as an independent cardiovascular risk factor.[17]

Several lines of evidence support that reduction of microalbuminuria is best achieved with agents that block the renin-angiotensin-aldosterone (RAAS) system. In a previous study, Lebovitz et al. randomized patients with hypertension, type 2 diabetes, and GFR between 30 and 100 mL/min to enalapril or control treatment (not including an ACE-inhibitor) and followed them for 3 years. The change in UAE and rate of decline in GFR in both the albuminuria group and in the total study population favored use of the ACE inhibitor, but it did not reach statistical significance. In the group of patients with UAE <300 mg/day, significantly fewer patients progressed to overt nephropathy (7% versus 21%), and the rate of GFR decline was 0.20 versus –.33 mL/min/1.73 m²/month in the enalapril and the control group (respectively). However, these findings could not be conclusive, as mean blood pressure was 4.9 mmHg lower in the enalapril group.[32]

In the Irbesartan Microalbuminuria (IRMA 2) study, 590 patients with hypertension, type 2 diabetes, and GFR microalbuminuria (average range of UAE between 53.4 and 58.3 µg/min) were randomly

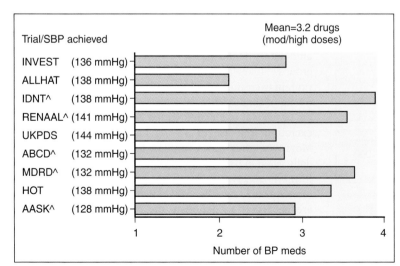

Figure 49–4. Number of blood pressure medications needed to achieve systolic blood pressure in large clinical trials (^ denotes trials with renal endpoints).

DEFINITIONS OF PROTEINURIA AND ALBUMINURIA				
	Urine Collection Method	Normal	Microalbuminuria	Albuminuria or Clinical Proteinuria
Total protein	24-hour excretion	<300 mg/d	NA	>300 mg/d
	Spot urine dipstick	<30 mg/dL	NA	>30 mg/dL
	Spot urine protein-to-creatinine ratio	<200 mg/g	NA	>200 mg/g
Albumin	24-hour excretion	<30 mg/d	30-300 mg/d	>300 mg/d
	Spot urine albumin-specific dipstick	<3 mg/dL	>3 mg/dL	NA
	Spot urine albumin-to-creatinine ratio	<30 mg/g	30-300 mg/g	>300 mg/g
	Spot urine albumin-to-creatinine ratio (gender-specific definition)	<17 mg/g (men)	17-250 mg/g (men)	>250 mg/g (men)
		<25 mg/g (women)	25–355 mg/g (women)	>355 mg/g (women)

Adapted from K/DOQI clinical practice guidelines on hypertension and antihypertensive agents in chronic kidney disease. *Am J Kidney Dis* 2004;43(5 Suppl 2):1–290 with permission from The National Kidney Foundation, Inc.

Table 49–4. Definitions of Proteinuria and Albuminuria

assigned to receive placebo or irbesartan 150 mg or 300 mg daily. The primary endpoint was the appearance of clinical nephropathy (i.e., albuminuria >200 µg/min) and at least a 30% increase from the baseline level. After 24 months of follow-up, the approach of the three groups to the endpoint was 14.9%, 9.7%, and 5.2% (respectively), which translates to a significant 68% reduction in progression to albuminuria between irbesartan 300 mg daily and placebo groups.[33] Whether reduction of microalbuminuria is linked with a reduction in cardiovascular endpoints is still uncertain. The LIFE trial, the only trial that prospectively measured microalbuminuria in a group of hypertensive patients with high CVD risk, demonstrated that the group with lowest cardiovascular event rate had the greatest reduction in microalbuminuria from baseline.[34]

In the Prevention of Renal and Vascular Endstage Disease Intervention Trial (PREVEND IT), 864 inhabitants of the city of Groningen in the Netherlands with microalbuminuria (UAE between 15 and 300 mg/day) were randomized to fosinopril 20 mg/day or matching placebo and pravastatin 40 mg/day or matching placebo.[35] Fosinopril reduced UAE by 26% during the mean follow-up of 46 months, but the reduction in cardiovascular mortality or cardiovascular hospitalization in patients treated with this agent showed only a trend toward statistical significance.[35] This study, however, was limited by the low overall number of cardiovascular events and by submaximal doses of ACE inhibitors.

In the IRMA 2 study, the higher dose of irbesartan (300 mg versus 150 mg/day) was clearly associated with improved kidney protection[33]—a finding indicating that the use of adequate dosages of agents that block the RAAS is necessary to provide maximal kidney protective effects. Recent studies support that ultra-high doses of ARBs can have even better renoprotective results. In one of these studies, 52 type 2 diabetic patients with microalbuminuria were randomized to 300, 600, and 900 mg of irbesartan daily for 2 months. All doses of irbesartan significantly reduced UAE, ambulatory blood pressure, and GFR from baseline, but the 900-mg dose provided an additional 15% reduction in UAE compared to the 300-mg dose. Reductions in ambulatory blood pressure were similar across the three groups.[36] Likewise, in a study in proteinuric subjects (mean protein excretion rate between 1 and 10 g/day), the use of 64 mg of candesartan daily for 4 weeks in patients already on 16 mg was associated with a 29% reduction in protein excretion. The use of 32 mg had no significant effect. Moreover, after down-titration of candesartan to 16 mg daily again in both groups proteinuria increased in patients formerly receiving 64 mg but remained stable in those formerly on 32 mg.[37] In view of these findings, further studies are necessary to delineate the optimal renal protective doses of ARBs.

Intervention with a RAAS blocker has been also shown to protect against the development of microalbuminuria in hypertensive patients with type 2 diabetes. In particular, in the Bergamo Nephrologic Diabetes Complications Trial

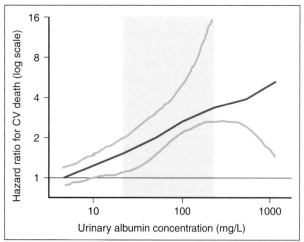

Figure 49–5. Albuminuria as a risk factor for CVD in individuals without diabetes. The adjusted effect of urinary albumin concentration (UAC) on hazard function in the Prevention of Renal and Vascular End Stage Disease (PREVEND) Study. (Adapted from Hillege HL, Fidler V, Diercks GF, et al. Urinary albumin excretion predicts cardiovascular and noncardiovascular mortality in general population. *Circulation* 2002;106(14):1777–82.)

(BENEDICT) 1204 patients with hypertension, type 2 diabetes, and normal UAE (median between 5.02 and 5.91 µg/min) were randomized to the non-dihydropyridine calcium-channel blocker (CCB) verapamil (240 mg per day), the ACE inhibitor trandolapril (2 mg per day), the combination of verapamil (180 mg per day), and trandolapril (2 mg per day) or to placebo.[38] After a median follow-up of 3.6 years, progression to microalbuminuria was significantly lower in the subjects treated with trandolapril or the combination (6.0 and 5.7%, respectively) compared to the subjects receiving verapamil or placebo (11.9 and 10.0%, respectively).[38]

Proteinuria

The NKF-KDOQI guidelines define albuminuria or clinical proteinuria as urinary albumin or protein excretion >300 mg/day if measured in a 24-hour urine collection (Table 49–5).[1] The presence of proteinuria and increased stage of kidney disease are associated with faster progression to kidney failure and increased risk of CVD.[1,14,15,39,40] Therefore, the goal of therapy in patients with proteinuria is to reduce rate of kidney disease progression and the risk of CVD.[1,40] Data from the MDRD study and the meta-analysis by the AIPRD Study Group show that reduction of blood pressure in patients with proteinuria slows the progression to kidney failure.[21,23] In addition, reductions in proteinuria correlate with preservation of kidney function, as well as with reductions in cardiovascular mortality.[41] It is interesting that the classes of drugs that fail to reduce proteinuria (i.e., dihydropyridine CCBs, alpha blockers, hydralazine, and minoxidil) have also failed to either slow progression of kidney disease or reduce mortality in the absence agents that reduce proteinuria.[42]

ACE inhibitors and ARBs are the antihypertensive agents that have most consistently been found to reduce proteinuria and the rate of renal function deterioration in diabetic and nondiabetic kidney disease. In a previous study, that of the Collaborative Study Group, 409 type 1 diabetic patients with overt nephropathy (UAE=0.5 g/day) and mild renal insufficiency (serum creatinine=2.5 mg/dL) were randomized to captopril or placebo. In the captopril-treated

group, a mean decrease of UAE of 0.3 g/day versus baseline was observed after a median follow-up of 3 years. In addition, patients treated with captopril had a 43% reduction in the primary endpoint of doubling of serum creatinine and a 50% reduction in the combined endpoints of death, need for dialysis, and transplantation in comparison with the placebo group.[43] The use of ACE inhibitors to reduce proteinuria in nondiabetic kidney disease is supported by the original REIN Study, the AASK trial, and the meta-analysis by the AIPRD Study Group. In the REIN study, nondiabetic patients with an average creatinine of 2.4 mg/dL and 24-hour urine protein excretion >3 g/day were randomized to ramipril 5 mg/day or placebo. The ramipril group presented a 55% reduction in median urine protein excretion from baseline and significant reductions in urine protein excretion and GFR decline compared to placebo.[44] In the AASK trial, African-American patients with hypertensive kidney disease, mean serum creatinine of 2.2 mg/dL, and 24-hour urine protein excretion of 0.6 g/day were randomized to ramipril, amlodipine, or metoprolol. Patients treated with ramipril had a 36% reduction in the secondary composite outcome of 50% reduction of GFR, ESRD, or death compared to amlodipine, and a 22% reduction compared to metoprolol.[24] The meta-analysis by the AIPRD Study Group in nondiabetic CKD showed that regimens including an ACE inhibitor were associated with a 31% reduction in progression to ESRD and a 30% reduction in the combined endpoint in doubling of serum creatinine or progression to ESRD.[45]

Two randomized controlled trials have shown that ARBs are effective in reducing proteinuria and in slowing the progression to kidney failure in nephropathy due to type 2 diabetes. In the Reduction in Endpoints in NIDDM with the Angiotensin II Antagonist Losartan (RENAAL) Study, 1513 type 2 diabetic patients with nephropathy (mean creatinine 1.9 mg/dL and median urine albumin-to-creatinine ratio 1237 mg/g) were randomized to losartan or placebo. Patients treated with losartan had a 35% reduction in the urinary albumin-to-creatinine ratio, whereas patients in the placebo group tended to have an increase. In addition, treatment with losartan resulted in a 16% reduction in

RECOMMENDATIONS ON HYPERTENSION AND ANTIHYPERTENSIVE AGENTS IN CHRONIC KIDNEY DISEASE			
Type of Kidney Disease	**Blood Pressure Target (mmHg)**	**Preferred Agents for CKD, with (or Without) Hypertension**	**Other Agents to Reduce CVD Risk and Reach Blood Pressure Target**
Diabetic kidney disease	<130/80	ACE inhibitor or ARB	Diuretic preferred, then BB or CCB
Nondiabetic kidney disease with spot urine total protein-to-creatinine ratio ≥200 mg/g	<130/80	ACE inhibitor or ARB	Diuretic preferred, then BB or CCB
Nondiabetic kidney disease with spot urine total protein-to-creatinine ratio <200 mg/g	<130/80	None preferred	Diuretic preferred, then ACE inhibitor, ARB, BB, or CCB
Adapted from K/DOQI clinical practice guidelines on hypertension and antihypertensive agents in chronic kidney disease. *Am J Kidney Dis* 2004;43(5 Suppl 2):1–290 with permission from The National Kidney Foundation, Inc.			

Table 49–5. Recommendations on Hypertension and Antihypertensive Agents in Chronic Kidney Disease

the primary endpoint of doubling of baseline serum creatinine, progression to ESRD, or death. The median rate of decline in estimated clearance was 4.4 and 5.2 mL/min/1.73 m²/ per year in the losartan and placebo groups, respectively.[27]

In the previously mentioned IDNT study, 1715 patients with diabetic nephropathy (mean creatinine 1.65 to 1.69 mg/dL and median urinary protein excretion 2.9 g/day) were randomized to 300 mg of irbesartan, 10 mg of amlodipine, or placebo. After a mean follow-up of 2.6 years, proteinuria was decreased by 33% in the irbesartan group versus 6% in the amlodipine group and 10% in the placebo group. Treatment with irbesartan also resulted in a 20% reduction compared to placebo and 23% reduction compared to amlodipine in the primary composite outcome of doubling of baseline serum creatinine, onset of ESRD, or death from any cause. The risk of a doubling of the serum creatinine concentration was 33% lower in the irbesartan group than in the placebo group, and 37% lower in the irbesartan group than in the amlodipine group. The mean rate of decline of creatinine clearance was –5.5, –6.8, and –6.5 mL/min/1.73 m² per year in the irbesartan, placebo, and amlodipine groups (respectively).[28]

The Diabetics Exposed to Telmisartan And enalaprIL (DETAIL) study more recently compared the long-term renoprotective effects of enalapril 10 to 20 mg and telmisartan 40 to 80 mg in 250 patients with type 2 diabetes, hypertension, and UAE between 11 and 999 μg/min.[46] After 5 years of follow-up, the change in the glomerular filtration rate (which was the primary endpoint) was –17.5 mL/min/1.73 m² in the telmisartan-treated subjects and –15.0/min/1.73 m² in the enalapril-treated subjects. The treatment difference was thus –2.6 mL/min/1.73 m², with 95 confidence interval (–7.1 to 2.0 mL/min/1.73 m²). Because the lower boundary of the confidence interval in favor of enalapril was greater than the predefined margin of –10.0 mL/min/1.73 m², statistical analysis revealed that telmisartan was not inferior to enalapril in preserving renal function. The effects of the two agents on the secondary endpoints of the annual changes in the glomerular filtration rate, serum creatinine level, UAE, blood pressure, end-stage renal disease, and cardiovascular events and the rate of death from all causes were not significantly different.[46]

Although kidney protection with dual blockade of the RAAS with the combined use of ACE inhibitors and ARBs has not been as extensively studied, preliminary data indicate that dual RAAS blockade can reduce proteinuria and slow kidney disease progression more effectively than either using ACE inhibitors or ARBs alone. In the COOPERATE trial, patients with nondiabetic kidney disease and mean urinary protein excretion of 2.5 g per day were randomized to trandolapril 3 mg daily, losartan 100 mg daily, or a combination of the two drugs at the same dosages.[47] After 3 years of follow-up, urinary protein excretion was reduced significantly more with combined therapy (75.6%) compared to trandolapril (44.3%) or losartan (44.1%) alone. Moreover, the group of patients treated with the combined therapy had a 60 to 62% reduction in the primary endpoint of time to doubling of serum creatinine concentration or ESRD compared to either trandolapril- or losartan-

treated group.[47] It is important to note that these findings were independent of blood pressure differences, as both the office and ambulatory blood pressure reductions were similar across all three groups.[48] However, because this trial included only 263 patients larger studies are needed to confirm these findings.

In addition, it has to be noted that recently published data from several of the previously cited renal outcome trials clearly show that the reported benefit on kidney disease progression with the use of an ACE inhibitor or an ARB could not be explained by blood pressure lowering alone and that reduction of proteinuria *per se* is a particularly important factor in retardation of kidney disease progression.[49-51] In particular, retrospective analyses of the AASK, RENAAL, and IDNT studies showed that a reduction in proteinuria of more than 35% with the use of an ACE inhibitor or an ARB resulted in a range of 39 to 72% risk reduction for dialysis at 3 to 5 years, identifying the change in the level of proteinuria as a strong predictor of subsequent progression of CKD.[49-51]

Further blockade of the RAAS with aldosterone receptor antagonists such as spironolactone and eplerenone in patients already on an ACE inhibitor or an ARB may also be beneficial. It has been shown that blockade of the RAAS with ACE inhibitors does not necessarily result in a maintained decrease in plasma aldosterone levels, which can either remain high or increase in the long run (aldosterone escape).[52,53] As far as ARBs are concerned, a preliminary study showed that hypertensive patients treated with losartan for 12 months had no change in plasma aldosterone levels.[54] Even in studies in which plasma aldosterone was decreased with RAAS blocking agents,[55] the reductions were small and therefore the action of this hormone was not fully suppressed. Plasma aldosterone levels are elevated in patients with chronic renal insufficiency and could play a role in kidney injury.[56,57] Several studies suggest that the addition of spironolactone in patients with proteinuric nephropathy already receiving an ACE or an ARB results in a reduction of urine protein excretion.[58-62] Eplerenone, the newer aldosterone receptor antagonist that lacks the side effect of gynecomastia,[63] has also been shown to further reduce urine albumin excretion in patients with hypertension and left ventricular hypertrophy when combined with an ACE inhibitor.[64] Future studies combining aldosterone blockade with the use of an ACE inhibitor or an ARB in larger populations of CKD patients are necessary to determine the effect of these combinations on kidney function preservation.

Cardiovascular disease

As mentioned previously, patients with decreased GFR have markedly increased risk of cardiovascular events compared to patients with normal kidney function, and this risk of cardiovascular events progressively increases as GFR declines.[14-16] Among patients in the Medicare database, 80% of those with CKD submitted CVD claims over a 2-year period compared with 45% of those without CKD and the prevalence of heart failure was four times higher in CKD patients compared to those without CKD.[2] In ESRD patients treated by dialysis, the risk of cardiovascular death increases further, with cardiovascular mortality rates approximately 5 to 500 times higher than age- and sex-matched controls in the general population.[1,65] This elevation of the risk for cardiovascular events and cardiovascular mortality with the progressive decrease of GFR has also been demonstrated in patients after a myocardial infarction.[66] Based on the NKF-KDOQI guidelines, patients with CKD can be considered in the highest risk category for CVD.[1]

Hypertension is one of the major independent risk factors for CVD,[12,13] and pharmacologic treatment of high blood pressure in hypertensive individuals has been shown beyond doubt to decrease the risk of a range of cardiovascular events.[67–69] Because of the slow rate of decline of kidney function and the high cardiovascular death rate associated with CKD, most individuals with CKD will not develop ESRD but instead die from an intercurrent cardiovascular event. Therefore, blood pressure control is imperative in the treatment of CKD not only to slow down the progression to ESRD but (perhaps most importantly) to deter cardiovascular morbidity and mortality. Apart from hypertension, there is a substantial overlap in the rest of the traditional risk factors for CVD and CKD.[8,70] Thus, the optimal therapeutic approach for CVD in patients with CKD requires a multi-intervention strategy with a coordinated effort by practitioners and apart from aggressive blood pressure control includes smoking cessation, management of diabetes, and lipid lowering with pharmacologic and lifestyle measures—as well as other interventions, from antiplatelet therapy (low-dose aspirin) to correction of anemia if present.[1,8]

Management of hypertension in kidney disease

As mentioned previously, the achievement of a goal blood pressure less than 130/80 mmHg in patients with kidney disease has been proven quite difficult and requires both lifestyle modifications (most important of which is sodium restriction due to the impaired salt excretion in CKD[7]) and multiple antihypertensive medications.[1,17] The selection of antihypertensive agents in CKD should be based on the pathophysiology of hypertension in kidney disease, which includes sodium and water retention and increased vasoconstriction due to activation of the RAAS and the sympathetic nervous system.[7] The combined use of agents that affect these mechanisms will counteract the effects of these pathophysiologic mechanisms, thereby helping blood pressure levels return to optimum and consequently providing a reduction in organ injury.

Several lines of evidence indicate that in various stages and types of CKD agents that block the RAAS should be the drugs of choice. Based on the results of IRMA 2 and PREVEND IT trials, adequate doses of an ARB or an ACE inhibitor should be preferentially used in patients with microalbuminuria in order to reduce UAE and to prevent the onset of overt nephropathy.[33,35] In patients with kidney disease and proteinuria, agents that block the RAAS (such as ACE inhibitors and ARBs) are also preferred as part of a regimen to achieve blood pressure control.[1] Based on the results of Captopril in Diabetic Nephropathy trial, ACE inhibitors should be the agents of choice in patients with proteinuria due to type 1 diabetes.[43] Patients with overt

nephropathy due to type 2 diabetes should be preferably treated with an ARB, based on the evidence from clinical trials such as IDNT an RENAAL—which both showed a regression in the decline in GFR as well as the onset of kidney failure with the use of ARBs.[27,28] However, the results of the DETAIL trial[46] suggest and the NKF-KDOQI guidelines indicate that either ACE inhibitors or ARBs can be used to manage blood pressure in people with type 2 diabetes to preserve kidney function.[1]

On the other hand, in patients with nondiabetic kidney disease and proteinuria ACE inhibitors should be preferred based on results from the REIN and AASK trials.[24,44] In addition to these quite similar renoprotective properties, ARBs and ACE inhibitors present other beneficial properties (i.e., they reduce the risk for new-onset diabetes[71] and reduce the incidence of recurrent stroke).[72,73] It must be noted, however, that ARBs are generally better tolerated than ACE inhibitors because they are associated with a lower incidence of cough, angioedema, and hyperkalemia.[74] Based on the previous, the NKF-KDOQI guidelines recommend the use of either an ACE inhibitor or an ARB (regardless of blood pressure) in all patients with diabetic kidney disease and in patients with nondiabetic kidney disease with a spot urine total protein-to-creatinine ratio =200 mg/g, as shown in Table 49–5.[1] In addition, the guidelines suggest that moderate to high doses (rather than low doses) of RAS-blocking agents be used to achieve additional benefits—according to the evidence that the use of higher doses of RAS-blocking agents may achieve greater reductions in microalbuminuria and proteinuria.

In spite of substantial evidence from long-term clinical trials demonstrating the renal protective effects of ACE inhibitors and ARBs for patients with CKD, there is general hesitancy among clinicians to prescribe these agents in patients with serum creatinine >1.4 mg/dL because serum creatinine often rises after an ACE inhibitor or an ARB is given. The most common cause of increased creatinine following blockade of the RAAS is from preexisting decreased arterial blood volume, often due to volume depletion or low cardiac output. With kidney dysfunction, the autoregulatory ability of the kidney to maintain intrarenal arterial pressure diminishes. This results in a direct relationship between systematic blood pressure and GFR. Therefore, an abrupt decrease in blood pressure often results in a pressure related drop in GFR, manifesting itself with an increase in serum creatinine levels. Analysis of long-term clinical trials has confirmed that ACE inhibitor induced reduction in kidney function plateaus within 2 months.[9]

If serum creatinine increases by >30% or continues to rise after 3 months of therapy with a RAAS-blocking agent, volume depletion, unsuspected left ventricular dysfunction, or bilateral renal artery stenosis should be considered.[9] In general, according to the JNC 7 and the NKF-KDOQI guidelines at serum creatinine values of <3.0 mg/dL and age <65 years a 30 to 35% increase in serum creatinine above the starting point is acceptable within the first 3 to 4 months of starting blood pressure treatment—as long as creatinine does not continue to rise and hyperkalemia does not occur.[1,17] Apart from this, ACE inhibitors and ARBs are often discontinued due to rises in serum potassium levels.

This should be worrisome only if serum potassium rises =0.5 mEq/L and the baseline level is already greater than 5 mEq/L. Otherwise, elevations in serum potassium can often be addressed by increasing the dose of appropriate diuretics, stopping agents known to increase potassium (such as nonsteroidal anti-inflammatory agents that decrease renal perfusion), and providing dietary education of potassium-containing foods.

In the COOPERATE trial, only 8% (7 out of 88 patients) of the patients on combination treatment with an ACE inhibitor and ARB developed hyperkalemia and were all successfully treated for it with dietary education or potassium binders.[47] Therefore, ACE inhibitors or ARBs should be withdrawn only when the rise of serum creatinine exceeds 30 to 35% above baseline within the first 3 to 4 months of therapy or when hyperkalemia (serum potassium >5.6 mEq/L) occurs.

Due to increased salt and water retention with kidney function deterioration, diuretics often need to be included in the antihypertensive regimen in patients with kidney disease. However, thiazide diuretics become less effective when GFR falls below 30 mL/min/1.73 m^2, because of the reduced renal blood flow and the accumulation of organic acid end products of metabolism that antagonize diuretics at the level of the secretion in the tubular fluid—which will require high doses of the drugs for an adequate amount to reach the tubular sites of action.[75] An adequate blood pressure control in patients with renal insufficiency is thus very likely to need a loop diuretic (furosemide, torsemide, bumetanide, and so on) as part of the blood-pressure-lowering regimen because these compounds have higher intrinsic efficacy compared to thiazides.[75] Potassium-sparing diuretics should be avoided in patients with preexisting hyperkalemia; that is, serum potassium more than 5.5 mEq/L from either diabetes or renal disease of other etiologies.

According to the previously cited data on the ability of aldosterone blockade to further reduce proteinuria in patients already receiving an RAAS blocking agent,[58-62] use of aldosterone receptor antagonists such as spironolactone and eplerenone in low doses may be indicated in patients with proteinuric CKD, especially if heart failure is present.[76] However, when using spironolactone or eplerenone serum potassium must be followed closely because levels rise in a dose-dependent fashion and a dose adjustment of the concomitant conventional diuretic therapy should always be considered.

It also has to be noted that although moderate to high doses of diuretics worsen insulin resistance and increase the risk for new onset diabetes, when currently recommended low doses of diuretics are taken in combination with an ACE inhibitor or ARB their effects on insulin sensitivity and other metabolic parameters are negligible.[77] Based on NKF/KDOQI guidelines, because combination of two or more antihypertensive agents are imperative to achieve the current blood pressure goal in most patients with CKD a diuretic should be the first agent added to the ACE inhibitor or the ARB regimen if necessary in all patients with diabetic kidney disease and in patients with nondiabetic kidney disease with spot urine total protein-to-creatinine ratio =200 mg/g (Table 49–5).[1] In addition, in patients with

nondiabetic kidney disease with spot urine total protein-to-creatinine ratio <200 mg/g a diuretic should be one of the initial choices to achieve blood pressure goal.[1]

The antihypertensive effects of conventional β-blockers, as well as their capability to reduce cardiovascular mortality in high-risk patients, have been well established.[69,78] However, there is no direct evidence that these agents provide additional renoprotective effects. Data regarding whether β-blockers are associated with increased risk of progression of kidney disease are conflicting. In a former study, type 2 diabetic patients with proteinuria were titrated to atenolol 100 mg/day versus sustained-release verapamil 480 mg/day. After 54 months of follow-up, patients treated with the non-dihydropyridine CCB had a significant reduction in creatinine rise and proteinuria compared to patients in the β-blocker group.[79] In the UKPDS 39 study, comparison of the effectiveness of captopril and atenolol as basic therapy in patients with type 2 diabetes with incipient nephropathy took place. Both study groups achieved the same levels of blood pressure with similar percentage of additional non-study drugs. The progress to overt nephropathy was 5% in the captopril group and 9% in the atenolol group at the end of the study, with no statistically significant difference between them. There was also no difference in the rate of plasma creatinine doubling or in plasma creatinine concentration between the two groups.[80]

These findings suggest that any renoprotective effect is due to lowering of blood pressure. It has to be noted, however, that a newer β-blocker with vasodilating properties (carvedilol) has a much better metabolic effect profile than conventional β-blockers[81] and has been shown to reduce the risk of microalbuminuria in patients with hypertension and diabetes[82] and mortality in people with ESRD.[83] Therefore, based on the NKF-KDOQI guidelines β-blockers should be normally used in patients with CKD when a combination of proper doses of an ACE inhibitor or an ARB regimen with a diuretic is not enough to low blood pressure levels below the goal of 130/80 mmHg.[1] The beneficial metabolic profile of carvedilol is an indication for preferable use of this β-blocker in such high-risk patients, whereas future studies should investigate the effect of this agent on renal function in patients with CKD.

Calcium channel blockers are effective antihypertensive agents in patients with kidney disease. However, within the class of CCBs the various agents have different effects on proteinuria beyond their blood-pressure-lowering effects due to differences in glomerular permeability.[84,85] As shown in Table 49–3, non-dihydropyridine CCBs (verapamil, diltiazem) have been shown to reduce proteinuria,[79,86] whereas dihydropyridine CCBs do not unless used in the presence of a RAAS blocker.[87,88] In addition, dihydropyridine CCBs are less efficacious in slowing kidney disease progression. As mentioned previously, the IDNT patients with proteinuria due to type 2 diabetes who were treated with irbesartan had a 23% reduction compared to amlodipine in the primary composite outcome of doubling of baseline serum creatinine, onset of ESRD, or death from any cause—as well as a significant reduction in urine protein excretion compared to amlodipine.[28] Similar findings with dihydropyridine CCBs have been observed in nondiabetic kidney disease with proteinuria. In the AASK trial, African-American patients with hypertensive nephrosclerosis treated with ramipril had a 36% reduction in the composite outcome of 50% reduction of GFR, ESRD, or death compared to patients treated with amlodipine.[24] Based on the previous, although dihydropyridine CCBs are effective in lowering blood pressure in patients with CKD they should not be used as monotherapy in diabetic or nondiabetic kidney disease with proteinuria but always in combination with an ACE inhibitor or an ARB if blood pressure is not adequately controlled.[1]

Recently published data from the second part of the Ramipril Efficacy in Nephropathy (REIN-2) study question the ability of dihydropyridine CCBs to help prevent renal function deterioration in proteinuric kidney disease even by means of blood pressure lowering. In this study, 335 patients with nondiabetic nephropathy and urine protein excretion >1 g/day who were already receiving background treatment with the ACE inhibitor ramipril (2.5 to 5 mg/day) were assigned to either conventional (diastolic blood pressure <90 mmHg) or intensified (systolic/diastolic blood pressure <130/80 mmHg)—with the addition of the dihydropyridine CCB felodipine (5 to 10 mg/day). After a median follow-up of 19 months and in spite of a difference of 4.1/2.8 mmHg in blood pressure levels throughout the study in favor of the intensified regimen, the cumulative incidence of end-stage renal disease, rate of GFR decline, and residual proteinuria were similar in the two arms.[89] These findings argue against the use of dihydropiridine CCBs in proteinuric nephropathies, but have to be further confirmed from other studies with longer follow-up periods.

Although combining effective blood pressure reduction[90] and a beneficial metabolic profile,[91,92] α-blockers have not been shown to slow renal disease progression or to reduce UAE in patients with type 2 diabetes and albuminuria.[93] Moreover, this class of agents also failed to reduce cardiovascular events in patients who have or develop heart failure—as evidenced by the results of the long-acting α-blocker arm of ALLHAT (which was stopped early due to increased incidence of heart failure[94]). Hence, this class should not be preferred as an initial or even secondary treatment for hypertension in patients with CKD but as third-line treatment, especially in older men with benign prostatic hypertrophy and urine flow problems.[95]

SUMMARY

As the prevalence of chronic kidney disease has grown dramatically during the past decades, slowing the decline in renal function to prevent kidney failure has become a therapeutic target of major importance. The goals of therapy in patients with CKD are to control blood pressure, reduce the risk of CVD, and slow the progression of renal dysfunction. There is now strong evidence that blood pressure levels should be reduced to less than 130/80 mmHg in patients with kidney disease, especially if proteinuria is present. There is also evidence that ACE inhibitors and ARBs are effective in reducing proteinuria and in slowing the progression of renal dysfunction. Based on these observations, hypertension in patients with CKD and proteinuria should be initially managed with an ACE inhibitor or an ARB, and if more antihypertensive agents are necessary to reach goal blood pressure initially a diuretic and then compounds from the other antihypertensive classes should be added.

REFERENCES

1. K/DOQI clinical practice guidelines on hypertension and antihypertensive agents in chronic kidney disease. *Am J Kidney Dis* 2004;43(5 Suppl 2):1–290.
2. USRDS-renal disease. 2005. Ref Type: Internet Communication.
3. Summary of Revisions for the 2004 Clinical Practice Recommendations. *Diabetes Care* 2004;27(Suppl 1):S3.
4. Mitch WE. Treating diabetic nephropathy: Are there only economic issues? *N Engl J Med* 2004;351(19):1934–36.
5. Coresh J, Wei GL, McQuillan G, et al. Prevalence of high blood pressure and elevated serum creatinine level in the United States: Findings from the third National Health and Nutrition Examination Survey (1988–1994). *Arch Intern Med* 2001;161(9):1207–16.
6. Klag MJ, Whelton PK, Randall BL, et al. Blood pressure and end-stage renal disease in men. *N Engl J Med* 1996; 334(1):13–18.
7. Mailloux LU, Levey AS. Hypertension in patients with chronic renal disease. *Am J Kidney Dis* 1998;32(5 Suppl 3):S120–41.
8. Bakris GL. Preventing hypertensive kidney disease: The critical role of combination therapy. *Am J Hypertens* 2005;18(4 Pt 2):93S–94S.
9. Bakris GL, Williams M, Dworkin L, et al. Preserving renal function in adults with hypertension and diabetes: A consensus approach. National Kidney Foundation Hypertension and Diabetes Executive Committees Working Group. *Am J Kidney Dis* 2000;36(3):646–61.
10. Abbott KC, Bakris GL. What have we learned from the current trials? *Med Clin North Am* 2004;88(1):189–207.
11. Clinical Practice Recommendations 2005. *Diabetes Care* 2005;28(Suppl 1):S1–79.
12. MacMahon S, Peto R, Cutler J, et al. Blood pressure, stroke, and coronary heart disease. Part 1, Prolonged differences in blood pressure: Prospective observational studies corrected for the regression dilution bias. *Lancet* 1990;335(8692):765–74.
13. Stamler J, Stamler R, Neaton JD. Blood pressure, systolic and diastolic, and cardiovascular risks: US population data. *Arch Intern Med* 1993;153(5):598–615.
14. Go AS, Chertow GM, Fan D, McCulloch CE, Hsu CY. Chronic kidney disease and the risks of death, cardiovascular events, and hospitalization. *N Engl J Med* 2004;351(13):1296–305.
15. Manjunath G, Tighiouart H, Ibrahim H, et al. Level of kidney function as a risk factor for atherosclerotic cardiovascular outcomes in the community. *J Am Coll Cardiol* 2003;41(1):47–55.
16. Sarnak MJ, Levey AS, Schoolwerth AC, et al. Kidney disease as a risk factor for development of cardiovascular disease: A statement from the American Heart Association Councils on Kidney in Cardiovascular Disease, High Blood Pressure Research, Clinical Cardiology, and Epidemiology and Prevention. *Hypertension* 2003;42(5):1050–65.
17. Chobanian AV, Bakris GL, Black HR, et al. Seventh report of the Joint National Committee on Prevention, Detection, Evaluation, and Treatment of High Blood Pressure. *Hypertension* 2003;42(6):1206–52.
18. Hansson L, Zanchetti A, Carruthers SG, et al. Effects of intensive blood-pressure lowering and low-dose aspirin in patients with hypertension: Principal results of the Hypertension Optimal Treatment (HOT) randomised trial. HOT Study Group. *Lancet* 1998;351(9118):1755–62.
19. Tight blood pressure control and risk of macrovascular and microvascular complications in type 2 diabetes: UKPDS 38. UK Prospective Diabetes Study Group. *BMJ* 1998;317(7160):703–13.
20. 2003 European Society of Hypertension-European Society of Cardiology guidelines for the management of

arterial hypertension. *J Hypertens* 2003;21(6):1011–53.

21. Peterson JC, Adler S, Burkart JM, et al. Blood pressure control, proteinuria, and the progression of renal disease. The Modification of Diet in Renal Disease Study. *Ann Intern Med* 1995;123(10):754–62.

22. Sarnak MJ, Greene T, Wang X, et al. The effect of a lower target blood pressure on the progression of kidney disease: Long-term follow-up of the modification of diet in renal disease study. *Ann Intern Med* 2005;142(5):342–51.

23. Jafar TH, Stark PC, Schmid CH, et al. Progression of chronic kidney disease: The role of blood pressure control, proteinuria, and angiotensin-converting enzyme inhibition: a patient-level meta-analysis. *Ann Intern Med* 2003;139(4):244–52.

24. Wright JT, Jr., Bakris G, Greene T, et al. Effect of blood pressure lowering and antihypertensive drug class on progression of hypertensive kidney disease: Results from the AASK trial. *JAMA* 2002;288(19):2421–31.

25. Saydah SH, Fradkin J, Cowie CC. Poor control of risk factors for vascular disease among adults with previously diagnosed diabetes. *JAMA* 2004;291(3):335–42.

26. Major outcomes in high-risk hypertensive patients randomized to angiotensin-converting enzyme inhibitor or calcium channel blocker vs diuretic: The Antihypertensive and Lipid-Lowering Treatment to Prevent Heart Attack Trial (ALLHAT). *JAMA* 2002;288(23):2981–97.

27. Brenner BM, Cooper ME, de Zeeuw D, et al. Effects of losartan on renal and cardiovascular outcomes in patients with type 2 diabetes and nephropathy. *N Engl J Med* 2001;345(12):861–69.

28. Lewis EJ, Hunsicker LG, Clarke WR, et al. Renoprotective effect of the angiotensin-receptor antagonist irbesartan in patients with nephropathy due to type 2 diabetes. *N Engl J Med* 2001;345(12):851–60.

29. Hillege HL, Fidler V, Diercks GF, et al. Urinary albumin excretion predicts cardiovascular and noncardiovascular mortality in general population. *Circulation* 2002;106(14):1777–82.

30. Gerstein HC, Mann JF, Yi Q, et al. Albuminuria and risk of cardiovascular events, death, and heart failure in diabetic and nondiabetic individuals. *JAMA* 2001;286(4):421–26.

31. Wachtell K, Ibsen H, Olsen MH, et al. Albuminuria and cardiovascular risk in hypertensive patients with left ventricular hypertrophy: The LIFE study. *Ann Intern Med* 2003;139(11):901–06.

32. Lebovitz HE, Wiegmann TB, Cnaan A, et al. Renal protective effects of enalapril in hypertensive NIDDM: Role of baseline albuminuria. *Kidney Int Suppl* 1994;45:S150–55.

33. Parving HH, Lehnert H, Brochner-Mortensen J, Gomis R, Andersen S, Arner P. The effect of irbesartan on the development of diabetic nephropathy in patients with type 2 diabetes. *N Engl J Med* 2001;345(12):870–78.

34. Ibsen H, Olsen MH, Wachtell K, et al. Reduction in albuminuria translates to reduction in cardiovascular events in hypertensive patients: Losartan intervention for endpoint reduction in hypertension study. *Hypertension* 2005;45(2):198–202.

35. Asselbergs FW, Diercks GF, Hillege HL, et al. Effects of fosinopril and pravastatin on cardiovascular events in subjects with microalbuminuria. *Circulation* 2004;110(18):2809–16.

36. Rossing K, Schjoedt KJ, Jensen BR, Boomsma F, Parving HH. Enhanced renoprotective effects of ultrahigh doses of irbesartan in patients with type 2 diabetes and microalbuminuria. *Kidney Int* 2005;68(3):1190–98.

37. Schmieder RE, Klingbeil AU, Fleischmann EH, Veelken R, Delles C. Additional antiproteinuric effect of ultrahigh dose candesartan: A double-blind, randomized, prospective study. *J Am Soc Nephrol* 2005;16(10):3038–45.

38. Ruggenenti P, Fassi A, Ilieva AP, et al. Preventing microalbuminuria in type 2 diabetes. *N Engl J Med* 2004;351(19):1941–51.

39. Culleton BF, Larson MG, Parfrey PS, Kannel WB, Levy D. Proteinuria as a risk factor for cardiovascular disease and mortality in older people: A prospective study. *Am J Med* 2000;109(1):1–8.

40. Gaede P, Vedel P, Larsen N, Jensen GV, Parving HH, Pedersen O. Multifactorial intervention and cardiovascular disease in patients with type 2 diabetes. *N Engl J Med* 2003;348(5):383–93.

41. Bakris GL, Weir MR, Sowers JR. Therapeutic challenges in the obese diabetic patient with hypertension. *Am J Med* 1996;101(3A):33S–46S.

42. Makrilakis K, Bakris G. Diabetic hypertensive patients: Improving their prognosis. *J Cardiovasc Pharmacol* 1998;31(Suppl 2):S34–40.

43. Lewis EJ, Hunsicker LG, Bain RP, Rohde RD. The effect of angiotensin-converting-enzyme inhibition on diabetic nephropathy. The Collaborative Study Group. *N Engl J Med* 1993;329(20):1456–62.

44. Randomised placebo-controlled trial of effect of ramipril on decline in glomerular filtration rate and risk of terminal renal failure in proteinuric, non-diabetic nephropathy. The GISEN Group (Gruppo Italiano di Studi Epidemiologici in Nefrologia). *Lancet* 1997;349(9069):1857–63.

45. Jafar TH, Schmid CH, Landa M, et al. Angiotensin-converting enzyme inhibitors and progression of nondiabetic renal disease: A meta-analysis of patient-level data. *Ann Intern Med* 2001;135(2):73–87.

46. Barnett AH, Bain SC, Bouter P, et al. Angiotensin-receptor blockade versus converting-enzyme inhibition in type 2 diabetes and nephropathy. *N Engl J Med* 2004;351(19):1952–61.

47. Nakao N, Yoshimura A, Morita H, Takada M, Kayano T, Ideura T. Combination treatment of angiotensin-II receptor blocker and angiotensin-converting-enzyme inhibitor in non-diabetic renal disease (COOPERATE): A randomised controlled trial. *Lancet* 2003;361(9352):117–24.

48. Nakao N, Seno H, Kasuga H, Toriyama T, Kawahara H, Fukagawa M. Effects of combination treatment with losartan and trandolapril on office and ambulatory blood pressures in non-diabetic renal disease: A COOPERATE-ABP Substudy. *Am J Nephrol* 2004;24(5):543–48.

49. Lea J, Greene T, Hebert L, et al. The relationship between magnitude of proteinuria reduction and risk of end-stage renal disease: Results of the African American study of kidney disease and hypertension. *Arch Intern Med* 2005;165(8):947–53.

50. De Zeeuw D., Remuzzi G, Parving HH, et al. Proteinuria, a target for renoprotection in patients with type 2 diabetic nephropathy: Lessons from RENAAL. *Kidney Int* 2004;65(6):2309–20.

51. Atkins RC, Briganti EM, Lewis JB, et al. Proteinuria reduction and progression to renal failure in patients with type 2 diabetes mellitus and overt nephropathy. *Am J Kidney Dis* 2005;45(2):281–87.

52. Sato A, Saruta T. Aldosterone escape during angiotensin-converting enzyme inhibitor therapy in essential hypertensive patients with left ventricular hypertrophy. *J Int Med Res* 2001;29(1):13–21.

53. Sato A, Saruta T. Aldosterone breakthrough during angiotensin-converting enzyme inhibitor therapy. *Am J Hypertens* 2003;16(9 Pt 1):781–88.

54. Grossman E, Peleg E, Carroll J, Shamiss A, Rosenthal T. Hemodynamic and humoral effects of the angiotensin II antagonist losartan in essential hypertension. *Am J Hypertens* 1994;7(12):1041–44.

55. Bakris GL, Siomos M, Richardson D, et al. ACE inhibition or angiotensin receptor blockade: Impact on potassium in renal failure. VAL-K Study Group. *Kidney Int* 2000;58(5):2084–92.

56. Epstein M. Aldosterone as a mediator of progressive renal disease: Pathogenetic and clinical implications. *Am J Kidney Dis* 2001;37(4):677–88.

57. Hollenberg NK. Aldosterone in the development and progression of renal injury. *Kidney Int* 2004;66(1):1–9.

58. Chrysostomou A, Becker G. Spironolactone in addition to ACE inhibition to reduce proteinuria in patients with chronic renal disease. *N Engl J Med* 2001;345(12):925–26.

59. Sato A, Hayashi K, Naruse M, Saruta T. Effectiveness of aldosterone blockade in patients with diabetic nephropathy. *Hypertension* 2003;41(1):64–8.

60. Rachmani R, Slavachevsky I, Amit M, et al. The effect of spironolactone, cilazapril and their combination on albuminuria in patients with hypertension and diabetic nephropathy is independent of blood pressure reduction: A randomized controlled study. *Diabet Med* 2004;21(5):471–75.

61. Rossing K, Schjoedt KJ, Smidt UM, Boomsma F, Parving HH. Beneficial effects of adding spironolactone to recommended antihypertensive treatment in diabetic nephropathy: A randomized, double-masked, cross-over study. *Diabetes Care* 2005;28(9):2106–12.

62. Schjoedt KJ, Rossing K, Juhl TR, et al. Beneficial impact of spironolactone in diabetic nephropathy. *Kidney Int* 2005;68(6):2829–36.

63. Sica DA. Current concepts of pharmacotherapy in hypertension. Eplerenone: A new aldosterone receptor antagonist-are the FDAs restrictions appropriate? *J Clin Hypertens (Greenwich)* 2002;4(6):441–45.

64. Pitt B, Reichek N, Willenbrock R, et al. Effects of eplerenone, enalapril, and eplerenone/enalapril in patients with essential hypertension and left ventricular hypertrophy: The 4E-left ventricular hypertrophy study. *Circulation* 2003;108(15):1831–38.

65. Sarnak MJ, Levey AS. Cardiovascular disease and chronic renal disease: A new paradigm. *Am J Kidney Dis* 2000;35(4 Suppl 1):S117–31.

66. Anavekar NS, Gans DJ, Berl T, et al. Predictors of cardiovascular events in patients with type 2 diabetic nephropathy and hypertension: A case for albuminuria. *Kidney Int Suppl* 2004; (92):S50–55.

67. Collins R, Peto R, MacMahon S, et al. Blood pressure, stroke, and coronary heart disease. Part 2, Short-term reductions in blood pressure: Overview of randomised drug trials in their epidemiological context. *Lancet* 1990; 335(8693):827–38.

68. MacMahon S, Rodgers A, Neal B, Chalmers J. Blood pressure lowering for the secondary prevention of myocardial infarction and stroke. *Hypertension* 1997;29(2):537–38.

69. Turnbull F, Neal B, Algert C, et al. Effects of different blood pressure-lowering regimens on major cardiovascular events in individuals with and without diabetes mellitus: Results of prospectively designed overviews of randomized trials. *Arch Intern Med* 2005;165(12):1410–19.

70. Fox CS, Larson MG, Leip EP, Culleton B, Wilson PW, Levy D. Predictors of new-onset kidney disease in a community-based population. *JAMA* 2004;291(7):844–50.

71. Pepine CJ, Cooper-Dehoff RM. Cardiovascular therapies and risk for development of diabetes. *J Am Coll Cardiol* 2004;44(3):509–12.

72. Randomised trial of a perindopril-based blood-pressure-lowering regimen among 6,105 individuals with previous stroke or transient ischaemic attack. *Lancet* 2001;358(9287):1033–41.

73. Schrader J, Luders S, Kulschewski A, et al. Morbidity and Mortality After Stroke, Eprosartan Compared with Nitrendipine for Secondary Prevention: Principal results of a prospective randomized controlled study (MOSES). *Stroke* 2005;36(6):1218–26.

74. Mangrum AJ, Bakris GL. Angiotensin-converting enzyme inhibitors and angiotensin receptor blockers in chronic renal disease: Safety issues. *Semin Nephrol* 2004;24(2):168–75.

75. Brater DC. Diuretic therapy. *N Engl J Med* 1998;339(6):387–95.

76. Pitt B, Williams G, Remme W, et al. The EPHESUS trial: Eplerenone in patients with heart failure due to systolic dysfunction complicating acute myocardial infarction. Eplerenone Post-AMI Heart Failure Efficacy and Survival Study. *Cardiovasc Drugs Ther* 2001;15(1):79–87.

77. Gress TW, Nieto FJ, Shahar E, Wofford MR, Brancati FL. Hypertension and antihypertensive therapy as risk factors for type 2 diabetes mellitus. Atherosclerosis Risk in Communities Study. *N Engl J Med* 2000;342(13):905–12.

78. Bakris GL. Role for beta-blockers in the management of diabetic kidney disease. *Am J Hypertens* 2003;16(9 Pt 2):7S–12S.

79. Bakris GL, Mangrum A, Copley JB, Vicknair N, Sadler R. Effect of calcium channel or beta-blockade on the progression of diabetic nephropathy in African Americans. *Hypertension* 1997;29(3):744–50.

80. Efficacy of atenolol and captopril in reducing risk of macrovascular and microvascular complications in type 2 diabetes: UKPDS 39. UK Prospective Diabetes Study Group. *BMJ* 1998; 317(7160):713–20.

81. Sarafidis PA, Bakris GL. Do the metabolic effects of β-blockers make them leading or supporting antihypertensive agents in the treatment of hypertension? *J Clin Hypertens* 2006;(in press).

82. Bakris GL, Fonseca V, Katholi RE, et al. Metabolic effects of carvedilol vs metoprolol in patients with type 2 diabetes mellitus and hypertension: A randomized controlled trial. *JAMA* 2004;292(18):2227–36.

83. Cice G, Ferrara L, D'Andrea A, et al. Carvedilol increases two-year survival in dialysis patients with dilated cardiomyopathy: A prospective, placebo-controlled trial. *J Am Coll Cardiol* 2003;41(9):1438–44.

84. Bakris GL, Weir MR, Secic M, Campbell B, Weis-McNulty A. Differential effects of calcium antagonist subclasses on markers of nephropathy progression. *Kidney Int* 2004;65(6):1991–2002.

85. Nathan S, Pepine CJ, Bakris GL. Calcium antagonists: effects on cardio-renal risk in hypertensive patients. *Hypertension* 2005;46(4):637–42.

86. Bakris GL, Copley JB, Vicknair N, Sadler R, Leurgans S. Calcium channel blockers versus other antihypertensive therapies on progression of NIDDM associated nephropathy. *Kidney Int* 1996;50(5):1641–50.

87. Smith AC, Toto R, Bakris GL. Differential effects of calcium channel blockers on size selectivity of proteinuria in diabetic glomerulopathy. *Kidney Int* 1998;54(3):889–96.

88. Bakris GL, Weir MR, Shanifar S, et al. Effects of blood pressure level on progression of diabetic nephropathy: Results from the RENAAL study. *Arch Intern Med* 2003;163(13):1555–65.

89. Ruggenenti P, Perna A, Loriga G, et al. Blood-pressure control for renoprotection in patients with non-diabetic chronic renal disease (REIN-2): Multicentre, randomised controlled trial. *Lancet* 2005;365(9463):939–46.

90. Achari R, Hosmane B, Bonacci E, O'Dea R. The relationship between terazosin dose and blood pressure response in hypertensive patients. *J Clin Pharmacol* 2000;40(10):1166–72.

91. Pollare T, Lithell H, Selinus I, Berne C. Application of prazosin is associated with an increase of insulin sensitivity in obese patients with hypertension. *Diabetologia* 1988;31(7):415–20.

92. Kasiske BL, Ma JZ, Kalil RS, Louis TA. Effects of antihypertensive therapy on serum lipids. *Ann Intern Med* 1995;122(2):133–41.

93. Rachmani R, Levi Z, Slavachevsky I, Half-Onn E, Ravid M. Effect of an alpha-adrenergic blocker, and ACE inhibitor and hydrochlorothiazide on blood pressure and on renal function in type 2 diabetic patients with hypertension and albuminuria. A randomized cross-over study. *Nephron* 1998;80(2):175–82.

94. Major cardiovascular events in hypertensive patients randomized to doxazosin vs chlorthalidone: The antihypertensive and lipid-lowering treatment to prevent heart attack trial (ALLHAT). ALLHAT Collaborative Research Group. *JAMA* 2000;283(15):1967–75.

95. Cooper KL, McKiernan JM, Kaplan SA. Alpha-adrenoceptor antagonists in the treatment of benign prostatic hyperplasia. *Drugs* 1999;57(1):9–17.

96. Maschio G, Alberti D, Janin G, et al. Effect of the angiotensin-converting-enzyme inhibitor benazepril on the progression of chronic renal insufficiency. The Angiotensin-Converting-Enzyme Inhibition in Progressive Renal Insufficiency Study Group. *N Engl J Med* 1996;334(15):939–45.

97. Estacio RO, Jeffers BW, Gifford N, Schrier RW. Effect of blood pressure control on diabetic microvascular complications in patients with hypertension and type 2 diabetes. *Diabetes Care* 2000;23(Suppl 2):B54–64.

Chapter

50 Hypertensive Heart Disease

Javier Díez

Definition

Hypertensive heart disease can be defined as the cardiomyopathy that results from the response of the myocardium to the biomechanical stress imposed on the left ventricle by progressively increasing arterial pressure.

Key Features

- Hypertensive heart disease is characterized by the presence of left ventricular hypertrophy in the absence of a cause other than arterial hypertension.

- Beyond macroscopic hypertrophy, complex changes in myocardial histological composition (which are responsible for the structural remodeling of the myocardium) develop in hypertensive heart disease.

- Hypertensive myocardial remodeling is the consequence of several pathologic processes mediated by mechanical, neurohormonal, and cytokine routes and occurring in the cardiomyocyte and the noncardiomyocyte compartments of the heart.

Clinical Implications

- Left ventricular hypertrophy represents not only an adaptation to increased pressure load but an independent risk factor and a marker of risk of cardiovascular complications in hypertensive patients.

- Hypertensive left ventricular hypertrophy is often associated with disturbances of cardiac function and electric activity, as well as with cardiac ischemia, heart failure, cardiac arrhythmias, and a higher incidence of stroke and sudden death.

- Concurrent atherosclerotic coronary disease and left ventricular hypertrophy in hypertensive patients increase the risk of all cardiovascular events.

- Left ventricular hypertrophy may be detected early and accurately in hypertensive patients by electrocardiography or echocardiography.

Therapy

- Effective long-term antihypertensive treatment is associated with regression of left ventricular hypertrophy.

- Regression of left ventricular hypertrophy by antihypertensive treatment is associated with improvement in outcome and with the decrease of the risk of cardiovascular morbidity and mortality.

In general, the cardiac complications of arterial hypertension can be considered as either atherosclerotic or hypertensive. The former have multiple causes and the latter are more directly caused by the increased blood pressure *per se*. In fact, because increased blood pressure is one of the major risk factors that facilitates atherosclerotic coronary artery disease, the prevalence of arterial hypertension is >60% in patients with chronic ischemic heart disease. On the other hand, hypertensive heart disease (HHD) can be defined as the response of the heart to the afterload imposed on the left ventricle by the progressively increasing arterial pressure and total peripheral resistance.[1]

HHD is characterized by increased left ventricular (LV) mass associated with left ventricular hypertrophy (LVH). Hypertension-induced LVH consists of a constellation of genetic, structural, and functional abnormalities of cardiac tissue that allow its differentiation as a separate entity, which has been recently referred to as a so-called "hypertensive cardiomyopathy."[2] LVH is associated with alterations of cardiac function, abnormalities of myocardial perfusion, and disturbances of cardiac rhythm in hypertensive patients. In addition, LVH is an independent risk factor associated with cardiovascular complications in these patients. The diagnostic methods such as electrocardiography and echocardiography that are used to define LVH are discussed elsewhere in this book. A number of studies have established that reduction of LV mass is achieved with effective antihypertensive treatment and that reversal of LVH by blood pressure control is associated with decreases in cardiovascular event rates in hypertensive patients. Therefore, there is an important need for physicians to recognize this entity, to understand its pathophysiology, and to become fluent in treatment options available.

STRUCTURAL AND MOLECULAR BASIS

The hypertrophy of the left ventricle

The essential anatomic criterion in defining HHD is the presence of LVH in the absence of a cause other than arterial hypertension. LV cavity dimension remains normal but LV mass is considerably increased due to increased wall thickness. Thus, HHD is generally characterized by a geometric pattern of concentric LVH (Figure 50–1).

LVH is mainly the result of cardiomyocyte growth in conjunction with changes in extracellular matrix and provides the adaptive response of the heart to pressure overload in an attempt to normalize systolic wall stress (as predicted by Laplace's law). The degree of cardiomyocyte hypertrophy to mechanical stress imposed by pressure overload is, however, inappropriate and the increase in LV mass is out of proportion to the hemodynamic stimulus.

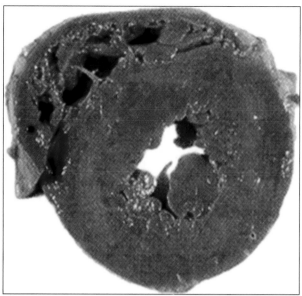

Figure 50–1. Macroscopic view of the typical geometric pattern of concentric left ventricular hypertrophy seen in hypertensive patients.

Recent data suggest that this exaggerated cardiomyocyte response is the result of the interaction between genetic (e.g., polymorphisms of the angiotensin-converting enzyme, ACE, gene) and environmental factors (e.g., obesity, excessive sodium intake). The growth of cardiomyocytes that follows mechanical loading of the LV is a true hypertrophic response (i.e., cardiomyocyte mass increases in the absence of an increase in cardiomyocyte number).

The hypertrophic response of cardiomyocytes can be categorized into several components:[3] (1) an increase in the transverse or longitudinal size (Figure 50–2) of the cell, (2) enhanced protein synthesis leading to the formation of new (sarcomeres that are added in parallel or in series) resulting in cardiomyocyte thickening and/or elongation, respectively, and (3) altered profile of gene expression linked to overexpression of several proto-oncogenes (i.e., c-fos, c-jun, and c-myc), mediating the expression of a range of gene transcripts that occur most often in embryonic but not adult ventricular myocardium

(i.e., skeletal α-actin and atrial natriuretic factor). A number of ultrastructural changes are also present in the hypertrophied cardiomyocyte, including polyploidization of nuclei with increased DNA content, decrease in the mitochondrial volume fraction with reduction of the ratio of mitochondrial to myofibrillar volume, increase of free polyribosomes, increase in the surface area of the T-tubules and smooth endoplasmic reticulum, and accumulation of Z-band material (which may serve as the locus of new sarcomere formation).

The remodeling of the myocardium

Beyond macroscopic and microscopic hypertrophy, however, complex changes in myocardial histological composition (responsible for the structural remodeling of the myocardium) develop in HHD (Box 50–1). Structural remodeling is the consequence of a number of pathologic processes mediated by mechanical, neurohormonal, and cytokine routes and occurring in the cardiomyocyte and the noncardiomyocyte compartments of the heart.

Cardiomyocyte apoptosis appears to be abnormally stimulated in the hypertrophied heart of hypertensive patients.[4] In addition, moderate cardiomyocyte loss has been demonstrated in long-term systemic hypertension. Interestingly, an association between increased apoptosis and diminished cardiomyocyte density has been reported in the human hypertensive heart; namely, when heart failure (HF) develops. Cardiomyocyte apoptosis has been proposed to occur as an excess of those factors that induce apoptotic cell death. Alternatively, it is possible that apoptosis reflects some abnormalities in those survival factors that act to determine the resistance of the cell to apoptosis.

Myocardial fibrosis secondary to an exaggerated accumulation of collagen type I and type III fibers within the interstitium and surrounding intramural coronary arteries and arterioles (Figure 50–3) is one of the key features of structural remodeling of the hypertensive left ventricle.[5] In fact, various studies performed in human heart postmortem specimens and endomyocardial human biopsy samples have shown that the fraction of myocardial volume occupied by collagen fibers (i.e., collagen volume fraction or CVF) is significantly increased in the heart of patients with HHD compared with that in normotensive popula-

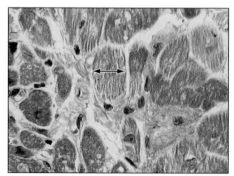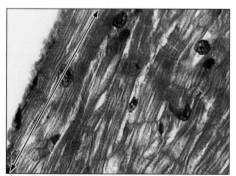

Figure 50–2. Microscopic view of the two patterns of cardiomyocyte growth present in the human hypertensive hypertrophied left ventricle. Left panel, transversal hypertrophy; right panel, longitudinal hypertrophy. (Sections were stained with hematoxylin-eosin.) (With permission from The American College of Cardiology Foundation.)

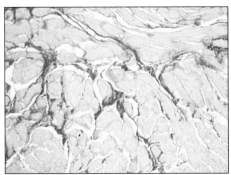
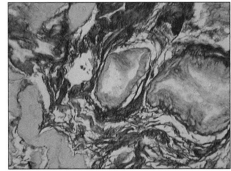

Figure 50–3. Microscopic view of the two topographical patterns of collagen deposition leading to myocardial fibrosis in the human hypertensive hypertrophied left ventricle. Left panel, interstitial fibrosis; right panel, perivascular fibrosis. (Sections were stained with picrosirius red and collagen fibers were identified in red.)

Box 50–1

Histologic Components of Structural Remodeling of the Myocardium in Hypertensive Heart Disease

At the parenchymal level:

- Cardiomyocytes: hypertrophy, increased apoptosis
- Fibroblasts: hyperplasia, phenotypic transformation to myofibroblasts
- Other cells: infiltration by monocytes/macrophages, proliferation of mast cells
- ECM: increased deposition of fibrillar collagen types I and III, increased deposition of fibronectin

At the microvascular level:

- Small arteries and arterioles: hypertrophy and/or hyperplasia of smooth muscle cells
- Disruption of the endothelial layer
- Increased wall deposition of ECM components
- Capillaries: diminished number

ECM means extracellular matrix.

---

tions. Excess of ventricular collagen seen in hypertension is suggested to be the result of both increased collagen synthesis by fibroblasts and phenotypically transformed fibroblast-like cells or myofibroblasts, as well as unchanged or decreased collagen degradation by matrix metalloproteinases. Hypertensive fibrosis is now considered to be the consequence of the loss of reciprocal regulation that normally exists at the myocardial level between profibrotic and antifibrotic molecules (Box 50–2).

Hypertensive patients with LVH present different structural alterations in the small coronary vessels.[6] On the one hand, hyperplasia and/or hypertrophy (and altered alignment of vascular smooth muscle cells leading to encroachment of the tunica media into the lumen) cause both an increase in the medial thickness/lumen ratio and

a reduction in the maximal cross-sectional area of intramyocardial arteries (Figure 50–4). In addition to mechanical factors, a number of local growth factors and vasoactive substances may directly stimulate proliferation and hyperplasia of vascular smooth muscle cells in the hypertensive heart. On the other hand, if the density of arterioles and capillaries is estimated as the vessel number per unit area there is a relative decrease in arteriolar and capillary density in LVH. This can be due to both capillary rarefaction (i.e., the vessels are actually missing or temporarily not perfused or "recruited") and inadequate vascular growth (i.e., impaired angiogenesis) in response to increasing muscle mass.

Box 50–2

Molecules That Regulate the Metabolism of Fibrillar Collagen in the Heart

Molecules favoring synthesis over degradation:

- Growth factors: transforming growth factor beta, connective tissue growth factor
- Cytokines: interleukin-6, cardiotrophin-1, osteopontin, thrombospondin
- Vasoactive substances: angiotensin II, norepinephrine, endothelin-1
- Adrenal steroids: aldosterone, deoxycorticosterone
- Other molecules: reactive oxygen species, plasminogen activator inhibitor 1

Molecules favoring degradation over synthesis:

- Cytokines: tumor necrosis factor alpha, interleukin-1 beta
- Vasoactive substances: bradykinin, prostaglandins, nitric oxide, natriuretic peptides
- Adrenal steroids: glucocorticoids
- Other molecules: N-acetyl-seryl-aspartyl-lysyl-proline, endogenous ligands of PPAR alpha, peroxisome proliferator-activated receptor

---

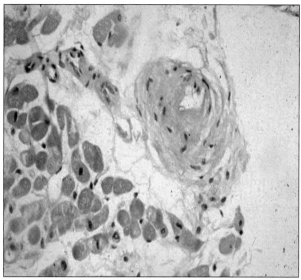

Figure 50–4. Microscopic view of an intramyocardial artery presenting thickening of the wall and narrowing of the lumen in a human hypertensive hypertrophied left ventricle.

PATHOPHYSIOLOGY

Mechanisms of LVH

It is well known that hypertension is the major factor involved in the development of LVH, but nevertheless the relationship is complex and simple linear correlation between the magnitude of the hypertrophy and measured arterial pressure is poor. In fact, in untreated patients with mild hypertension blood pressure levels (as assessed with clinical and ambulatory monitoring) explain at most approximately 40% of LV mass variability independent of demographics, nutrition, and lifestyle.[7] Thus, although hemodynamic mechanisms play a leading role in the development of LVH in hypertension this process reflects more than simple pressure or volume overload and other factors should be considered (Box 50–3).[8]

The occurrence of the different geometric forms of LVH is variable and is dependent on the hemodynamic and demographic characteristics of the population.[9–11] The prevalence of concentric hypertrophy is increased by greater severity of hypertension, advancing age, and higher peripheral resistance with normal intravascular volume. Eccentric hypertrophy is more common in young patients and in those with relative volume overload. The evolution of eccentric to concentric hypertrophy may be caused by the increase in peripheral resistance that occurs with aging. Ethnic differences in myocardial response to hypertension are clearly evident. Studies performed both in the United States and in the United Kingdom, comparing blacks and whites, concluded that African-American or Afro-Caribbean patients tend to have a greater prevalence of concentric LVH. Ventricular geometry and responses may also be influenced by gender. In the Framingham community survey, LV hypertrophy in the context of hypertension tended to be more often concentric in women and eccentric in men.

Whatever are the factors potentially responsible for the increase in LV mass in patients with hypertension, the signals for cardiomyocyte growth are multiple (generated both locally and systemically).[12] Such mediators include (1) mechanical stretch itself (which is communicated to both cardiomyocytes and non-cardiomyocytes) that may directly activate cell signaling, (2) autocrine factors (released by cardiomyocytes in response to stretch or growth factors), (3) paracrine factors (produced by cardiomyocytes or non-cardiomyocytes) that may be diffusible, matrix-bound, or mediated through cell-cell contact, and (4) endocrine factors (released in response to baroreceptor activation or renal hypoperfusion). Identification of specific growth signals involved in different types of hypertrophy, however, still remains an elusive goal and will probably require complex integrative systems for resolution.

Impact of myocardial remodeling on cardiac function

Myocardial fibrosis might contribute to the increased risk of HF and other adverse cardiac events in patients with HHD through different pathways (Figure 50–5). First, a linkage between fibrosis and LV systolic dysfunction may evolve over time.[13] Initially, the accumulation of collagen fibers compromises the rate of relaxation, diastolic suction, and passive stiffness, contributing to impaired diastolic function. This phase is often not recognized and may be asymptomatic. Continued accumulation of fibrotic tissue, accompanied by changes in the spatial orientation

---

Box 50–3

Factors with a Causal Role in Left Ventricular Hypertrophy

Factors with very strong supporting evidence:
- Increased blood pressure
- Obesity
- Excessive sodium intake

Factors with strong supporting evidence:
- Heritability
- Gender
- Black race
- Advanced age
- Stimulation of angiotensin II
- Insulin resistance
- Alterations of the GH/IGF-1 axis

Factors that need confirmation:
- Alcohol abuse
- Increased blood viscosity
- Excess of aldosterone
- Excess of parathormone
- Genetic polymorphisms

GH means growth hormone, IGF-1 insulin-like growth factor 1.

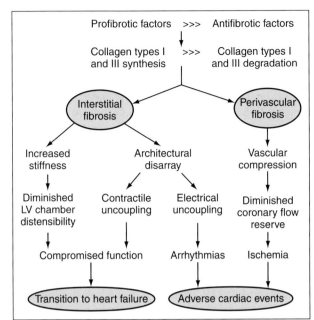

Figure 50–5. Potential consequences of myocardial fibrosis in hypertensive heart disease. (LV means left ventricle.)

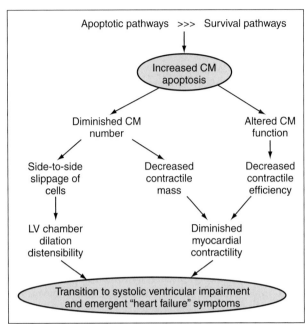

Figure 50–6. Potential consequences of cardiomyocyte apoptosis in hypertensive heart disease. (CM means cardiomyocyte, LV left ventricle.)

of collagen fibers, further impairs diastolic filling and may compromise transduction of cardiomyocyte contraction into myocardial force development. Thus, systolic performance may eventually be reduced. Second, impaired coronary flow reserve associated with HHD might be related to several factors, including perivascular fibrosis.[14] In fact, it has been demonstrated that perivascular CVF correlates inversely with coronary flow reserve in patients with HHD. Third, fibrosis may also contribute to the emergence of significant ventricular arrhythmia in patients with HHD.[15] It has been reported that patients with arrhythmia exhibit higher values of LV mass and CVF than patients without arrhythmia. The LV systolic ejection fraction (EF) and the frequency of coronary vessels with significant epicardial stenosis are similar in the two groups of patients. Perivascular and interstitial fibrosis induce conduction abnormalities to promote local reentry, and thereby cardiac arrhythmias.

Several observations suggest that apoptosis of cardiomyocytes may contribute to the transition from LVH to LV dilatation and failure of systolic contractions (Figure 50–6).[16] First, an association of increased cardiomyocyte apoptosis with diminished cardiomyocyte number has been found in the failing heart of hypertensive patients.[4] Thus, apoptosis may be one of the mechanisms involved in the loss of contractile mass and systolic contractile function in hypertensive cardiomyopathy. Second, impaired myocardial contractile function may reflect not only a decrease in the number of viable fully functional cardiomyocytes but a decrement in the function of viable cardiomyocytes, or a combination of these mechanisms. It has been reported recently that caspase-3 cleaved cardiac myofibrillar proteins resulted in an impaired force/Ca^{2+} relationship and myofibrillar ATPase activity.[17] Third, cytochrome c plays a major role in ATP production through

mitochondrial oxidative phosphorylation. Thus, it has been hypothesized that release of cytochrome c from mitochondria during the occurrence of the apoptotic process may interfere with cardiomyocyte energy production and lead to functional impairment.[18] Finally, severe cardiomyocyte apoptosis may lead to side-to-side slippage of cells, mural thinning, and chamber dilation.[19] Indeed, wall restructuring secondary to severe cardiomyocyte apoptosis may create an irreversible state of the myocardium, conditioning progressive dilatation and the continuous deterioration of cardiac hemodynamics and ventricular performance with time.

Alterations of coronary flow

As in other end organs of the hypertensive process, local regulation of blood flow is compromised in the heart. Thus, hypertensive LVH is associated with a profound impairment of coronary autoregulation.[20] In hypertensives with LVH, a shift of the pressure-flow autoregulatory relationship is evident, and coronary flow decreases progressively as coronary perfusion decreases below 90 mmHg. In hypertensives without LVH and in normotensive individuals, coronary flow is maintained down to a perfusion pressure of 60 mmHg.

On the other hand, hypertensive patients have frequently impaired coronary flow reserve (as estimated by the maximal increase in coronary flow above its resting level when the coronary vasculature is maximally dilated), even in the absence of LVH.[21] The decrease in coronary vasodilator response present in patients with HHD is accounted for by several changes in myocardial structure (perivascular fibrosis) and function (increase in left wall tension and oxygen consumption), as well as by structural alterations of intramyocardial arteries and/or changes in myocardial angiogenesis together with increased arteriolar tone, endothelial dysfunction, and extravascular systolic compression.

CLINICAL MANIFESTATIONS

Alterations of cardiac function

Epidemiological studies, such as the Framingham Heart Study, have suggested that hypertension is the most common etiological factor for congestive HF and is present in 50% of cases.[22] In addition to alterations of LV myocardium characteristic of HHD, hypertension may itself promote a systolic HF presentation linked to underlying coronary artery disease, as well as the evolution of arrhythmia (most commonly uncontrolled atrial fibrillation). Unlike HF presentations associated with coronary artery disease, in which systolic impairment may decline after a discrete event (myocardial necrosis and infarction) that damages the heart muscle, LV dysfunction/failure in the patient with HHD may evolve through several stages (Figure 50–7).

Alterations of diastolic function

The clinical presentation of diastolic dysfunction (an echocardiographic entity) in HHD is variable. It can be viewed as progressing from asymptomatic echocardiographic findings to symptomatic HF presentation, to congestive HF with generally normal systolic function (i.e., preserved radial systolic EF), to ultimately evolving systolic ventricular impairment. The prevalence of asymptomatic LV filling abnormalities in adults without hypertrophy and with ambulatory awake blood pressure greater than 130/85 mmHg may be as high as 33%.[22] These asymptomatic abnormalities may translate to a decrease in exercise EF when hemodynamically challenged by exercise or stress. In this regard, patients who had acute pulmonary edema and marked systolic hypertension were submitted to echocardiographic examination during the acute episode and after lowering treatment, and diastolic dysfunction was found to contribute to pulmonary edema in these hypertensive patients.[23] It has been estimated that 30 to 45% of hypertensive patients with chronic congestive HF symptoms present have diastolic dysfunction, with relatively normal normal systolic function.[24] Overall, the prognosis for patients with diastolic HF is poor, with survival rate at 3 months being 86%, at 1 year 76%, and at 5 years 48%.[25]

Alterations of systolic function

Most hypertensive patients have normal or supranormal conventional measures of LV systolic function, such as endocardial fractional shortening and EF. LV midwall shortening, in relation to stress, provides a different impression of the integrity of systolic performance. In fact, midwall shortening may be impaired in hypertensives with normal or supranormal EF and depressed midwall shortening has been shown to predict an adverse outcome in hypertensives, especially in the subgroup with LVH.[26]

However, depressed LV systolic function is the most potent risk factor for the development of overt congestive HF. In asymptomatic patients with abnormal LV systolic function, progression to ventricular dilatation appears to be slower—and clinical events, including death, are less common.[27] Nonetheless, in these patients survival at 2 years is significantly reduced (15 to 18%), compared with patients who have normal systolic function.

Development of LV dilatation is an indication of increased risk of major cardiac events and death.[28] In the hypertensive patient, the presence of LVH may lessen LV wall stress. However, at the expense of diastolic function systolic function is often preserved. However, the development of ventricular dilatation in the hypertensive patient with LVH, even if asymptomatic, is an ominous sign indicating that LVH is no longer able to maintain normal wall stresses. It may be hypothesized that with loss of the mechanical advantage conferred by LVH ventricular dilatation is the next compensatory response (through the Frank-Starling mechanism), which is invoked in an effort to restore normal LV systolic function. Any functional benefit derived, however, is at the cost of increased myocardial oxygen consumption, greater LV wall stress, and afterload mismatch.

Ischemic syndromes

Hypertensive patients with LVH frequently have signs and symptoms of myocardial ischemia due to a combination of microvascular disease, diminished coronary reserve, and atherosclerosis of epicardial vessels.[20] The reduction in dilating capacity of coronary flow is greater during exercise, when oxygen demand increases. In fact, under resting conditions the reduction in coronary flow reserve seen in hypertensive LVH may not have important consequences. However, in the presence of an exercise-induced increase in oxygen requirements it may become clinically relevant, producing the manifestations of myocardial ischemia and favoring the progression to LV systolic dysfunction.

There is a close relationship between hypertension and risk of coronary atherosclerotic disease. The risk for development of a cardiac ischemic event is approximately doubled in the hypertensive patient, and this is irrespective of sex or age, or whether systolic or diastolic blood pressure is increased.[29] Indeed, there is almost a "dose-response" relationship between coronary heart disease risk and increasing blood pressure, greater blood pressures being associated with greater risk. In patients with chronic angina pectoris, more than 50% have history of hypertension.[30] Furthermore, patients with hypertension have an increased incidence of unrecognized myocardial infarction, a greater likelihood of complications from acute

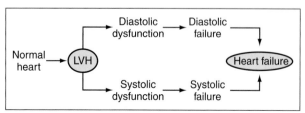

Figure 50–7. Stages in the clinical evolution of the heart in arterial hypertension (LVH means left ventricular hypertrophy.)

coronary syndromes, and compared with normotensive patients worse acute and 5-year survival after myocardial infarction.[31] However, many epidemiological reports of "silent" infarction in patients with hypertension are confounded by overinterpretation of nonspecific isolated ECG abnormalities (see Chapter 46).

Disturbances of cardiac rhythm

Hypertension is an important risk factor for the development of atrial and ventricular arrhythmias and sudden cardiac death.[32] Hypertension may play a direct part in the development of these rhythm disturbances by contributing to the development of LVH and myocardial remodeling, atherosclerotic disease, and microvascular abnormalities. The risk of arrhythmias is greatest with evidence of LVH and/or left atrial abnormality on echocardiography and electrocardiogram, even in patients with no clearly documented coronary artery disease.

Premature ventricular ectopy and complex ventricular tachyarrhythmias are more prevalent in patients with hypertension and LVH than in those without hypertrophy or in normotensive individuals.[33] However, electrophysiologic testing does not reveal an increased frequency of sustained ventricular tachycardia.

Atrial fibrillation is the most common and most serious of the atrial tachyarrhythmias, because of its association with fatal and nonfatal stroke and pulmonary edema. Indeed, hypertension and LVH account for more atrial fibrillation in the population than any other risk factor (Table 50–1).[34] In addition, hypertension is the only cardiovascular risk factor that independently predicts the development of atrial fibrillation, even after adjustment for age and associated co-morbidity.

Alterations of the aortic valve

Aortic valve sclerosis is defined by echocardiography as focal areas of increased echogenicity on aortic cusps not inducing stenosis. The prevalence of aortic sclerosis in hypertensive patients increases with age and with the presence of concentric LVH, and is associated with compromised diastolic function and mitral annular calcification.[35,36] The attention to this condition has been increased by the observation that aortic sclerosis is a marker for increased risk of cardiovascular events, even when the baseline cardiovascular factors are taken into account.[37]

It is known that hypertension predisposes to aortic root dilatation at sinuses of Valsalva and consequent aortic regurgitation. In fact, aortic root dilatation has been reported to be associated with higher LV mass (namely, eccentric LVH) and with lower systolic function in hypertensives.[38,39]

DIAGNOSTIC PROCEDURES

Physical examination

Hypertensive LVH may be associated with an absence of symptoms for many years before the development of congestive HF or unexpected sudden death. Nevertheless, physical examination may reveal some clues. One of the most important signs of LVH is a localized, sustained, and forceful apical impulse. This is best appreciated with the patient in the left lateral decubitus position. If the apical impulse in the supine position is laterally displaced, LV dilatation should be suspected.

The incidence of a fourth sound (S_4) in hypertensive patients has been estimated to be between 50 and 70%, especially in the presence of LVH. An S_4 is the auscultatory counterpart of a vigorous atrial contraction into a relatively noncompliant left ventricle. An S_4 may be associated with a palpable presystolic impulse or A-wave. The S4 is best appreciated when the patient is in the left lateral decubitus and the stethoscope is gently placed directly on the point of maximal apical impulse.

A systolic murmur can frequently be heard in hypertensive patients with LVH. This murmur is usually ejection in type, early in timing, and of low intensity (grade 1 or 2). This murmur can be heard at both the apex and the base. It most often represents aortic outflow turbulence related to a sclerotic aortic valve. An early diastolic

RISK FACTORS FOR DEVELOPMENT OF ATRIAL FIBRILLATION IN THE FRAMINGHAM HEART STUDY		
Risk Factors	Age-adjusted OR Men/Women	2-year Pooled Logistic Regression Men/Women
Smoking	1.0/1.4	$p < 0.05$
Diabetes mellitus	1.7/2.1	$p < 0.01 / p < 0.001$
Echo-LVH	3.0/3.8	$p < 0.001 / p < 0.001$
Hypertension	1.8/1.7	$p < 0.001 / p < 0.001$
Increased body mass index	1.03/1.02	– –
Alcohol abuse	1.01/0.93	– –
OR means odds ratio, Echo-LVH echocardiographic left ventricular hypertrophy. Adapted from Benjamin EJ, Levy D, Vaziri SM, D'Agostino RB, Belanger AJ, Wolf PA. Independent risk factors for atrial fibrillation in a population-based cohort. The Framingham Heart Study. *JAMA* 1994;271:840–44.		

Table 50–1. Risk Factors for Development of Atrial Fibrillation in the Framingham Heart Study

murmur of aortic regurgitation (secondary to dilatation of the aortic ring), which may be variable in intensity and duration, may occasionally be found in patients with HHD.

PROGNOSIS

LVH is an independent cardiovascular risk factor related to cardiovascular complications in hypertensive patients. In fact, considered as a categorical variable LVH significantly increases the risk of coronary artery disease, congestive HF, stroke, cardiac arrhythmia, and sudden death.[40] In addition, when LV mass is considered as a continuous variable a direct and progressive relationship exists between cardiovascular risk and the absolute amount of LV mass. During 4 years of follow-up in the Framingham Heart Study,[41] each 50-g/m^2 increase in LV mass was associated with a 1.49 increase in relative risk of cardiovascular disease for men and a 1.57 increase for women. The effect on cardiovascular mortality was even more striking, with a 1.73 and 2.12 relative risk for each 50 g/m^2 for men and women, respectively. More recently, it has been reported that the continuous relation between LV mass and cardiovascular risk in patients with essential hypertension remains significant after control for cardiovascular risk factors, including ambulatory blood pressure.[42]

The different patterns of ventricular shape and geometry are associated with markedly different risks for cardiovascular disease. A study performed with hypertensive patients followed up for 10 years reported that the incidence of cardiovascular events was 30% in subjects with concentric LVH, 25% in those with eccentric LVH, 15% in those with concentric remodeling, and 9% in those with normal LV mass.[43] Other reports have described associations between LV geometric pattern and extracardiac organ damage in essential hypertension, with hypertensives with concentric LVH having the most advanced funduscopic abnormalities, the greatest renal dysfunction,[44] and the most severe abnormalities of carotid artery structure and function.[45]

MANAGEMENT

Specific therapies

Antihypertensive therapy is effective in reducing LV mass. In fact, Mosterd et al.[46] analyzed data from 10,333 participants in the Framingham Heart Study and reported that the increasing use of effective antihypertensive therapy has caused a decrease in the prevalence of both high blood pressure and LVH in the general population. A large number trials and meta-analyses have attempted to compare the effects of different antihypertensive agents on LV mass, but flawed study designs and methodologic problems have limited the utility of these studies. Nevertheless, a recent meta-analysis by Kingbeil et al.[47]—including 80 double-blind randomized controlled trials with 146 active treatment arms (n=3767 patients) and 17 placebo arms (n=346 patients)—showed that after adjustment for treatment duration and change in diastolic blood pressure there was a significant difference ($p=0.004$) among medication classes. In fact, the decrease in LV mass indexed by surface area induced by the different classes was as follows: angiotensin II receptor antagonists > calcium antagonists > ACE inhibitors > diuretics > beta blockers (Table 50–2). In pairwise comparisons, angiotensin II receptor antagonists, calcium antagonists, and ACE inhibitors were more effective at reducing LV mass than were beta blockers and diuretics (all $p<0.05$ with Bonferroni correction).

A new generation of recent large well-designed trials support the notion that antihypertensive drugs need to be judged on their individual effects on LV mass in well-designed and adequately sized studies. In addition, extrapolation of the results of these studies in terms of class effects could be misleading and should be made with caution.

Outcomes

Different studies have examined the potential clinical prognostic benefit obtained from regression of LVH. Levy et al.[48] analyzed the data from 524 participants studied in the Framingham Heart Study, where LVH was measured according to electrocardiographic criteria. They reported that the decrease in electrocardiographic LVH toward normal, assessed using biannual serial examinations over a mean follow-up of 5 years, was associated with a reduction in cardiovascular risk. Recent data from the LIFE study have shown that a greater reduction of electrocardiographic LVH, after more than 4 years of treatment, with losartan than with atenolol was associated with higher reduction in the frequency of cardiovascular death, stroke, and myocardial infarction (Figure 50–8). Interestingly, there was substantial blood pressure reduction with both drugs with no significant differences between the two treatment groups (Figure 50–8).[49]

REDUCTION OF LEFT VENTRICULAR MASS INDEXED BY SURFACE AREA WITH DIFFERENT ANTIHYPERTENSIVE DRUGS					
	Angiotensin Receptor Antagonists	Calcium Antagonists	Angiotensin-converting Enzyme Inhibitors	Diuretics	Beta Blockers
Mean (%)	13	11	10	8	6
95% CI	8 to 18%	9 to 13%	8 to 12%	5 to 10%	3 to 8%
CI means confidence interval. Adapted from Kingbell AU, Schneider M, Martus P, Messerli FH, Schmieder RE. A meta-analysis of the effects of treatment on left ventricular mass in essential hypertension. Am J Med 2003;115:41–6.					

Table 50–2. Reduction of Left Ventricular Mass Indexed by Surface Area with Different Antihypertensive Drugs

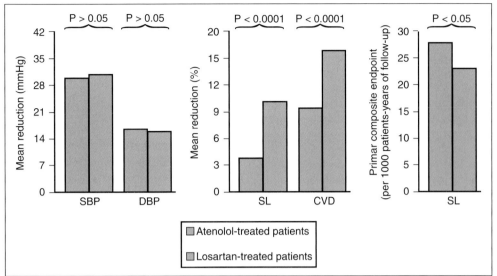

Figure 50–8. Despite a similar reduction in systolic and diastolic blood pressure (SBP and DBP, respectively) from baseline, the diminution in Sokolow-Lyon (SL) index and the Cornell voltage-duration product (CVD) from baseline was higher in hypertensive patients from the LIFE study treated with losartan than in hypertensive patients treated with atenolol. In addition, the primary composite endpoint (cardiovascular mortality, stroke, and myocardial infarction) occurred in fewer losartan-treated patients than atenolol-treated patients. (Adapted from Dahlöf B, Devereux RB, Kjeldsen SE, et al. Cardiovascular morbidity and mortality in the losartan intervention for endpoint reduction in hypertension study (LIFE): A randomised trial against atenolol. *Lancet* 2002;359:995–1003 with permission from Elsevier.)

Other studies have analyzed LV mass changes using echocardiography. In the study by Yurenev et al.,[50] 304 patients who all had LVH or high-normal LV mass at baseline echocardiographic examination were followed for 4 years and retrospectively divided into two groups, according to the presence or absence of cardiovascular complications. They reported that there was a strong relationship between LVH progression or regression and the probability of morbid events. In fact, there was only a significant reduction in LV mass in the group of patients without cardiac complications. Recently, Devereux et al.[51] published a substudy of the LIFE trial showing significant relative risk reductions in all-cause mortality, cardiovascular mortality, and the composite between those patients in whom LVH regressed by at least 25.3 g/m² compared with those who did not. These beneficial effects were independent of blood pressure lowering and other potential confounding factors, including age, smoking, diabetes, prior stroke, prior myocardial infarction, and baseline HF.

Collectively, these studies suggest that it is possible that treatment-induced LVH regression provides cardiovascular protection beyond blood pressure reduction. This can be related to the fact that reversing LVH has been shown to exert a beneficial influence on associated cardiac complications (i.e., improvement of diastolic and systolic function, amelioration of coronary reserve, and reduction of the incidence of cardiac arrhythmias).[52]

Preventive strategies

Although in most studies and meta-analyses the relationship between changes in blood pressure and LV mass was relatively weak (r<0.50), emerging evidence indicate that 24-hour monitoring of blood pressure may help to identify those hypertensive patients predisposed to develop LVH (i.e., patients with early morning rise in blood pressure and/or patients with a non-dipping profile) and more prone to benefit from the ability of some antihypertensive drugs to prevent LV growth.

LV mass is a complex phenotype influenced by the interacting effects of multiple genetic and environmental factors. Genetic variation probably contributes to inter-individual differences in the LV mass by virtue of effects on blood pressure level as well as via pathways that are not captured by measurements of blood pressure. It is possible that identification of genes that influence LV mass may enhance the ability to detect those patients who deserve early treatment to prevent the development of LVH. In this regard, a recent meta-analysis of case-control studies and association studies has shown that the D allele of the insertion/deletion (I/D) polymorphism of the ACE gene behaved as a marker for LVH in untreated hypertensive patients.[53]

Nonpharmacologic therapy may have some impact on the evolution of LVH, as some conditions that cause an increase in volume load (such as obesity and dietary sodium intake) also increase on LV mass. Results from the Treatment of Mild Hypertension Study (TOMHS)[54] reported that nutritional-lifestyle intervention with emphasis on weight reduction, restriction of salt, and alcohol intake and a physical exercise program was highly effective in both blood pressure and LV mass reduction.

Future perspectives

LVH that occurs as a consequence of pressure overload is termed *compensatory* on the premise that it facilitates ejection performance by normalizing systolic wall stress.

Recent experimental results, however, call into question the necessity of normalization of wall stress that results from hypertrophic growth of the heart. These findings, largely from studies in genetically engineered mice, raise the prospect of modulating hypertrophic growth of the myocardium to afford clinical benefit without provoking hemodynamic compromise.

To accomplish this goal, it is essential to identify molecular events involved in the hypertrophic process, and to identify commonalities and differences in the signaling systems that promote pathological hypertrophy versus physiological hypertrophy. Especially critical is elucidation of mechanisms underlying the maladaptive features of LVH, such as arrhythmogenicity, facilitation of ischemia, and transformation to HF. Observations from animal models and clinical trials identify signaling cascades that hold promise as potential targets for therapeutic interventions (Box 50–4).[55]

SUMMARY

HHD can be defined as the cardiomyopathy that results from the response of the heart to the stress imposed on the left ventricle by the progressively increasing arterial pressure. Clinically, HHD is characterized by LVH and its associated alterations, including disturbances of cardiac function and electric activity and coronary flow abnormalities. As a consequence, LVH is an independent cardiovascular risk factor related to cardiovascular complications in hypertensive patients. Therefore, early detection of LVH is mandatory in the clinical evaluation and risk stratification of these patients. In addition, LVH has become a validated surrogated endpoint for the treatment of hypertension and a decrease in LV mass is now considered a therapeutic goal in hypertensive patients. Most studies designed to evaluate the effect of treatment on patients with HHD conclude that if blood pressure decreases significantly there is LV mass reduction with most antihypertensive agents usually prescribed. Furthermore, a large number of studies have established that reversal of LVH decreases

---

Box 50–4

Pathways Investigated as Antihypertrophic Targets

- Ca^{2+}/calcineurin/nuclear factor of activated T cells
- G-protein-coupled receptors
- Phosphoinositide 3-kinase/serine-threonine kinase Akt/glycogen synthase kinase-3
- Myocyte enhancer factor-2/histone deacetylases
- Peroxisome proliferator-activated receptors
- Small G proteins
- Biomechanical sensors (stretch-activated ion channels and integrins)
- Na^+/H^+ exchanger
- Mitogen-activated protein kinase
- Glycoprotein130/janus kinase/signal transducer and activator of transcription

Adapted from Frey N, Katus HA, Olson EN, Hill JA. Hypertrophy of the heart: A new therapeutic target? *Circulation* 2004;109:1580–89.

---

the occurrence of adverse cardiovascular events in hypertensive patients.

Nevertheless, the time has come to revisit the current management of HHD simply focused on controlling blood pressure and reducing LV mass. In fact, it is necessary to develop new approaches aimed to repair myocardial structure and protect myocardial perfusion and function—and in so doing reduce in a more effective manner adverse risk associated with HHD. The development of noninvasive methods to assess those changes in the composition of myocardial tissue leading to structural remodeling of the myocardium, and the knowledge of those genes involved in both the process of LVH and its response to therapy, may be critical to advance in the development of these new approaches.

REFERENCES

1. Frohlich ED, Apstein C, Chobanian AV, et al. The heart in hypertension. *N Engl J Med* 1992;327:998–1008.
2. Lip GYH, Felmeden DC, Li-Saw-Hee FL, Beevers DG. Hypertensive heart disease: A complex syndrome or a hypertensive "cardiomyopathy"? *Eur Heart J* 2000; 21:1653–65.
3. Sadoshima J, Izumo S. The cellular and molecular response of cardiac myocytes to mechanical stress. *Annu Rev Physiol* 1997;59:551–71.
4. González A, Fortuño MA, Querejeta R, et al. Cardiomyocyte apoptosis in hypertensive cardiomyopathy. *Cardiovasc Res* 2003; 59:549–62.
5. Weber KT. Fibrosis and hypertensive heart disease. *Curr Opin Cardiol* 2000; 15:264–72.
6. Strauer BE, Schwartzkopff B. Left ventricular hypertrophy and coronary

microcirculation in hypertensive heart disease. *Blood Press* 1997; 2:6–12.
7. Armario P, Hernández del Rey R, Sánchez P, et al. Determinants of left ventricular mass in untreated mildly hypertensive subjects: Hospitalet Study in Mild Hypertension. *Am J Hypertens* 1999; 12:1084–90.
8. de Simone G, Pasanisi F, Contaldo F. Link of nonhemodynamic factors to hemodynamic determinants of left ventricular hypertrophy. *Hypertension* 2001;38:13–18.
9. Savage DD, Garrison RJ, Kannel WB, et al. The spectrum of left ventricular hypertrophy in a general population sample: The Framingham Study. *Circulation* 1987;75:126–33.
10. Krumholz HM, Larson M, Levy D. Sex differences in cardiac adaptation

to systolic hypertension. *Am J Cardiol* 1993;72:310–13.
11. Mayet J, Shabi M, Foale RA, et al. Racial differences in cardiac structure and function in essential hypertension. *BMJ* 1999;308:1011–4.
12. Hunter JJ, Grace A, Chien KR. Molecular and cellular biology of cardiac hypertrophy and failure. In: Chien KR (ed.) *Molecular basis of cardiovascular disease.* Philadelphia, PA: WB Saunders; 1999:211–50.
13. Díez J, López B, González A, Querejeta R. Clinical aspects of hypertensive myocardial fibrosis. *Curr Opin Cardiol* 2001;16:328–35.
14. Schwartzkopff B, Motz W, Frenzel H, Voght M, Knauer S, Strauer BE. Structural and functional alterations of the intramyocardial coronary arterioles in patients with arterial

hypertension. *Circulation* 1993;88: 993–1003.

15. McLenachan JM, Dargie JH. Ventricular arrhythmias in hypertensive left ventricular hypertrophy: Relation to coronary artery disease, left ventricular dysfunction, and myocardial fibrosis. *Am J Hypertens* 1990;3:735–40.

16. Fortuño MA, González A, Ravassa S, López B, Díez J. Clinical implications of apoptosis in hypertensive heart disease. *Am J Physiol Heart Circ Physiol* 2003;284:1495–506.

17. Communal C, Sumandea M, de Tombe P, Narula J, Solaro RJ, Hajjar RJ. Functional consequences of caspase activation in cardiac myocytes. *Proc Natl Acad Sci USA* 2002;99:6252–56.

18. Narula J, Arbustini E, Chandrashekhar Y, Schwaiger M. Apoptosis and systolic dysfunction in heart failure. Story of apoptosis interruptus and zombie myocytes. *Cardiol Clin* 2001;19:113–26.

19. Beltrami CA, Finato N, Rocco M, et al. The cellular basis of dilated cardiomyopathy in humans. *J Mol Cell Cardiol* 1995;27:291–305.

20. Kelm M, Strauer BE. Coronary flow reserve measurements in hypertension. *Med Clin N Am* 2004;88:99–113.

21. Scheler S, Motz W, Strauer BE. Mechanism of angina pectoris in patients with systemic hypertension and normal epicardial coronary arteries by arteriogram. *Am J Cardiol* 1994; 73:478–82.

22. Levy D, Larson MG, Vasan RS, Kannel WB, Ho KK. The progression from hypertension to congestive heart failure. *JAMA* 1996;275:1557–62.

23. Gandhi SK, Powers JC, Nomeir A-M, et al. The pathogenesis of acute pulmonary edema associated with hypertension. *N Engl J Med* 2001; 344:17–22.

24. Soufer R, Wohlgelernter D, Vita N, et al. Intact systolic left ventricular function in clinical congestive heart failure. *Am J Cardiol* 1985;55:1032–36.

25. Senni M, Tribouilloy CM, Rodeheffer RJ, et al. Congestive heart failure in the community. *Circulation* 1998;98: 2282–89.

26. de Simone G, Devereux RB, Koren MJ, et al. Midwall left ventricular mechanics: An independent predictor of cardiovascular risk in arterial hypertension. *Circulation* 1996; 93:259–65.

27. Vasan R, Larson MG, Benjamin E, Evans J, Levy D. Left ventricular dilatation and the risk of congestive heart failure in people without myocardial infarction. *N Engl J Med* 1997;336:1350–55.

28. Gaudron P, Eilles C, Kugler I, Erti G. Progressive left ventricular dysfunction and remodeling after myocardial infarction: Potential mechanisms and early predictors. *Circulation* 1993;87: 755–63.

29. Kannel WB. Coronary atherosclerotic sequelae of hypertension. In: S Oparil, Weber MA (eds.) *Hypertension*. Philadelphia: WB Saunders; 2000: 235–44.

30. Pepine CJ, Abrams J, Marks RG, Morris JJ, Scheidt SS, Handberg E, for the TIDES Investigators. Characteristics of a contemporary population with angina pectoris. *Am J Cardiol* 1994; 74:226–31.

31. Kannel WB, Abbott RD. A prognostic comparison of asymptomatic left ventricular hypertrophy and unrecognized myocardial infarction: The Framingham Study. *Am Heart J* 1986;111:391–97.

32. Kahan T, Bergfeldt L. Left ventricular hypertrophy in hypertension: Its arrhythmogenic potential. *Heart* 2005;91:250–56.

33. Pringle SD, Dunn FG, Macfarlane PW, McKillop JH, Lorimer AR, Cobbe SM. Significance of ventricular arrhythmias in systemic hypertension with left ventricular hypertrophy. *Am J Cardiol* 1992;69:913–17.

34. Benjamin EJ, Levy D, Vaziri SM, D'Agostino RB, Belanger AJ, Wolf PA. Independent risk factors for atrial fibrillation in a population-based cohort. The Framingham Heart Study. *JAMA* 1994;271:840–44.

35. Agno FS, Chinali M, Bella JN, et al. Aortic valve sclerosis is associated with preclinical cardiovascular disease in hypertensive adults: The HyperGen Study. *J Hypertens* 2005;23:867–73.

36. Olsen MH, Wachtell K, Bella JN, et al. Aortic valve sclerosis relates to cardiovascular events in patients with hypertension (a LIFE Substudy). *Am J Cardiol* 2005;95:132–38.

37. Gardin JM, McClelland R, Kitzman D, et al. M-Mode echocardiographic predictors of six to seven-year incidence of coronary heart disease, stroke, congestive heart failure, and mortality in an elderly cohort (the Cardiovascular Health Study). *Am J Cardiol* 2001;87: 1051–57.

38. Palmieri V, Bella JN, Arnett DK, et al. Aortic root dilatation at sinuses of Valsalva and aortic regurgitation in hypertensive and normotensive subjects: The Hypertension Genetic Epidemiology Network Study. *Hypertension* 2001;37:1229–35.

39. Bella JN, Wachtell K, Boman K, et al. Relation of left ventricular geometry and function to aortic root dilatation in patients with systemic hypertension and left ventricular hypertrophy (The LIFE Study). *Am J Cardiol* 2002; 89:337–41.

40. Levy D, Garrison RJ, Savage DD, et al. Prognostic implications of echocardiographically determined left ventricular mass in the Framingham Heart Study. *N Engl J Med* 1990; 322:1561–66.

41. Levy D, Anderson KM, Savage D, et al. Echocardiographically detected left ventricular hypertrophy: Prevalence and risk factors. The Framingham Heart Study. *Ann Intern Med* 1988;108:7–13.

42. Schillaci G, Verdecchia P, Porcellati C, et al. Continuous relation between left ventricular mass and cardiovascular risk in essential hypertension. *Hypertension* 2000;35:580–86.

43. Koren MJ, Devereux RB, Casale PN, et al. Relation of left ventricular mass and geometry to morbidity and mortality in uncomplicated essential hypertension. *Ann Intern Med* 1991; 114:345–52.

44. Shigematsu Y, Hamada M, Mukai M, Matsuoka H, Sumimoto T, Hiwada K. Clinical evidence for an association between left ventricular geometric adaptation and extracardiac target organ damage in essential hypertension. *J Hypertens* 1995;13:155–60.

45. Roman MJ, Pickering TG, Schwartz JE, Pini R, Devereux RB. Relation of arterial structure and function to left ventricular geometric patterns in hypertensive adults. *J Am Coll Cardiol* 1996;28: 751–56.

46. Mosterd A, D'Agostino RB, Silberschatz H, et al. Trends in the prevalence of hypertension, antihypertensive therapy, and left ventricular hypertrophy. *N Engl J Med* 1999;340:1221–27.

47. Kingbeil AU, Schneider M, Martus P, Messerli FH, Schmieder RE. A meta-analysis of the effects of treatment on left ventricular mass in essential hypertension. *Am J Med* 2003;115:41–6.

48. Levy D, Salomon M, D'Agostino R, et al. Prognostic implications of baseline electrocardiographic features and their serial changes in subjects with left ventricular hypertrophy. *Circulation* 1994;90:1786–93.

49. Dahlöf B, Devereux RB, Kjeldsen SE, et al. Cardiovascular morbidity and mortality in the losartan intervention for endpoint reduction in hypertension study (LIFE): A randomised trial against atenolol. *Lancet* 2002;359:995–1003.

50. Yurenev AP, Dyakonova HG, Novikov ID, et al. Management of essential hypertension in patients with different degrees of left ventricular hypertrophy: Multicenter trial. *Am J Hypertens* 1992; 5(6 Pt 2):182S–189S.

51. Devereux R, Wachtell K, Gerdts E, et al. Prognostic significance of left ventricular mass change during treatment of hypertension. *JAMA* 2004;292:2350–56.

52. Díez J, González A, López S, Ravassa S, Fortuño MA. Effects of antihypertensive agents on the left ventricle. Clinical implications. *Am J Cardiovasc Drugs* 2001;1:263–79.

53. Kuznetsova T, Staessen JA, Wang JG, et al. Antihypertensive treatment modulates the association between the D/I ACE gene polymorphism and left ventricular hypertrophy: A meta-analysis. *J Hum Hypertens* 2000;14: 447–54.

54. Liebson PR, Grandits GA, Dianzumba S, et al. Comparison of five antihypertensive monotherapies and placebo for change in left ventricular mass in patients receiving nutritional-hygienic therapy in the Treatment of Mild Hypertension Study (TOMHS). *Circulation* 1995; 91:698–706.

55. Frey N, Katus HA, Olson EN, Hill JA. Hypertrophy of the heart: A new therapeutic target? *Circulation* 2004; 109:1580–89.

Chapter

51 The Eye in Hypertension

Tien Yin Wong and Paul Mitchell

Key Findings

- Hypertensive retinopathy refers to a spectrum of microvascular signs in the retina pathophysiologically related to elevated blood pressure.

- Hypertensive retinopathy can be classified as mild (generalized and/or focal arteriolar narrowing, arterio-venous nicking, and arteriolar wall opacification), moderate (mild plus microaneurysms, hemorrhages, cotton wool spots, or hard exudates, in people without diabetes) or malignant (moderate plus optic disc swelling).

- Hypertensive retinopathy signs are strongly associated with elevated blood pressure, but inconsistently associated with cholesterol and other atherosclerosis risk factors.

- Data from recent prospective studies demonstrate that moderate hypertensive retinopathy predicts incident clinical stroke, congestive heart failure, and cardiovascular mortality, independent of blood pressure levels and other traditional vascular risk factors.

- A clinical assessment of retinopathy signs may provide information for risk stratification in persons with hypertension.

- Hypertension is also a known risk factor for other retinal vascular diseases, including diabetic retinopathy, retinal vein occlusion, artery occlusion, arteriolar emboli, and macroaneurysm.

Hypertension affects the eye in several ways. The retinal circulation undergoes a series of pathophysiologic changes in response to elevated blood pressure, resulting in a spectrum of clinical signs traditionally known as hypertensive retinopathy.[1] These signs include generalized arteriolar narrowing, focal arteriolar narrowing, arteriovenous (AV) nicking, retinal hemorrhages, microaneurysms, hard exudates, cotton wool spots, and rarely optic disc swelling.[2] With the exception of disc swelling, these signs can be detected frequently in adult persons, even in those without a known history of hypertension.[3]

In addition to hypertensive retinopathy, elevated blood pressure is also an important risk factor for the development of several retinal vascular diseases, such as retinal vein occlusion, artery occlusion, arteriolar emboli, and macroaneurysms (together with typical retinopathy in diabetes). These conditions, although less commonly seen than hypertensive retinopathy, are potentially blinding. Finally, elevated blood pressure has been implicated as a possible risk factor

for nonvascular conditions in the eye, such as glaucoma and age-related maculopathy.[4,5] This chapter focuses on hypertensive retinopathy and the common retinal vascular diseases associated with hypertension.

HYPERTENSIVE RETINOPATHY

Pathophysiology

Elevated blood pressure affects the retinal, optic nerve head, and choroidal circulations to produce three distinct manifestations: hypertensive retinopathy, hypertensive optic neuropathy, and hypertensive choroidopathy.[2] The initial response of the retinal circulation to a rise in blood pressure is vasospasm and an increase in vasomotor tone.[2] This response is reflected clinically as generalized retinal arteriolar narrowing. Persistently elevated blood pressure leads to more chronic "arteriosclerotic" changes, including intimal thickening, media wall hyperplasia, and hyaline degeneration. This is seen as more severe generalized arteriolar narrowing, arteriolar wall opacification, and focal areas of narrowing. Thickening of the retinal arteriolar wall by these arteriosclerotic processes may compress the venules at their common adventitial sheath, resulting in the clinical sign of AV nicking.

In the presence of more acute elevations in blood pressure, an "exudative" stage may develop, in which there is a breakdown of the blood/retinal barrier with necrosis of vascular smooth muscles and endothelial cells, exudation of blood and lipids, and retinal ischemia. These changes manifest as microaneurysms, hemorrhages, hard exudates, and cotton wool spots. Optic disc swelling and macular edema may occur at this stage, usually in the setting of severely elevated blood pressure, and represents malignant retinopathy. Optic disc swelling is believed to result from either elevated intracranial pressure from hypertensive encephalopathy or from ischemia to the optic nerve head.[2] The stages of hypertensive retinopathy so described are frequently not sequential, and retinopathy signs reflecting the "exudative" stage (e.g., retinal hemorrhages or microaneurysms) may be seen in eyes without features of the "arteriosclerotic" stage (e.g., AV nicking).

Classification and diagnosis

Marcus Gunn provided the first description of hypertensive retinopathy signs based on a series of patients with renal and cerebrovascular disease in the late nineteenth century.[6,7] The traditional classification of hypertensive retinopathy was developed based on work by Wagner and Barker in 1939.[8] Although many modern variations of this classification system bear their name, the original work was not an attempt to classify retinopathy signs but to show that severity of hypertension itself was predictive of mortality.[8] This classification typically includes four grades of retinopathy. "Mild" generalized retinal arteriolar narrowing is considered grade 1 retinopathy; "more severe" generalized narrowing, focal narrowing, and AV nicking are considered grade 2 retinopathy; the presence of retinal hemorrhages, microaneurysms, hard exudates, and cotton wool spots is considered grade 3 retinopathy; and grade 4 retinopathy, usually referred to as malignant retinopathy, consists of optic disc swelling and macular edema in the presence of signs in the preceding three grades.

Although widely used, one of the major limitations of this classification system is the difficulty in clinically distinguishing early retinopathy grades (e.g., grade 1 from grade 2).[2,3] Based on more recent data from prospective population-based studies, we propose a simple three-grade classification system (Table 51–1). Mild retinopathy consists of retinal arteriolar signs only, including generalized and focal arteriolar narrowing, arteriolar wall opacification, and AV nicking (Figure 51–1, A). Moderate retinopathy includes mild retinopathy changes plus the presence of microaneurysms, flame- or blot-shaped hemorrhages, cotton wool spots, and hard exudates (Figure 51–1, B). Malignant retinopathy includes moderate retinopathy changes plus optic disc and macular swelling.

It is important for the physician to be aware that some of these signs (particularly microaneurysms, hemorrhages and cotton wool spots) may also be found in many other systemic and ocular conditions (e.g., diabetic retinopathy, radiation retinopathy, retinopathy associated with anemia, leukemia, and other blood disorders, as well as trauma and human immunodeficiency virus and other infections). Thus, in atypical scenarios appropriate investigations may be necessary to rule out other important diseases.

Epidemiology

Until recently, there were few epidemiologic data on the prevalence of hypertensive retinopathy signs in the general population. In the Framingham Eye Study, only 0.8% of participants who had a dilated screening ophthalmoscopic examination were observed to have retinal hemorrhages or microaneurysms.[9] Prevalence of AV nicking and focal arteriolar narrowing were not reported.

Since the 1990s, there have been several population-based studies that have provided data on the prevalence and incidence of various hypertensive retinopathy signs as detected from retinal photographs.[10–17] These studies, summarized in Table 51–2, include the Beaver Dam Eye Study in Wisconsin,[10,11] the Blue Mountains Eye Study in Australia,[15,17] the Rotterdam Eye Study in Holland,[14] and two multicentered cohort studies of cardiovascular diseases in the United States [the Atherosclerosis Risk In Communities (ARIC) study[12] and the Cardiovascular Health Study].[16] Data from these studies have contributed to a greater understanding of the epidemiology, risk factors, and systemic associations of hypertensive retinopathy and other retinal vascular conditions.

In general, the prevalence of various hypertensive retinopathy signs, as detected from retinal photographs, ranges from 2 to 14% in the general adult population 40 years and older.[10–17] Data from the Beaver Dam Eye Study showed that the prevalence of focal arteriolar narrowing was 14%, AV nicking 2%, and retinal hemorrhages and microaneurysms 8%.[11] There are fewer studies on the incidence of new hypertensive retinopathy signs. In the Beaver Dam Eye Study, the 5-year incidence of focal arteriolar narrowing was 10%, AV nicking 7%, and retinal haemorrhages and microaneurysms 6%.[10]

Most of the studies to date have been conducted in white populations, and there are fewer data on the epidemiology of hypertensive retinopathy signs in non-white populations.[13] In the ARIC study, the prevalence of retinopathy signs was twice as high in blacks compared to whites.[18] However, after controlling for blood pressure levels and the severity of left ventricular hypertrophy the excess prevalence in blacks was reduced by 40%, suggesting that the higher frequency of these retinopathy signs in blacks may be related in part to poorer hypertension control.

Relationship with blood pressure

An abundance of data from clinical and population-based studies show a strong graded and consistent association of hypertensive retinopathy signs with blood pressure.[10–13,15–17] Figure 51–2 shows the strong relationship of blood pres-

CLASSIFICATION OF HYPERTENSIVE RETINOPATHY

Retinopathy Grade	Description	Systemic Associations
Mild	One or more of the following signs: generalized arteriolar narrowing, focal arteriolar narrowing, arteriovenous nicking, arteriolar wall opacity (silver-wiring)	Weak associations with stroke, coronary heart disease, and cardiovascular mortality
Moderate	Mild retinopathy with one or more of the following signs: retinal hemorrhage (blot, dot, or flame-shaped), microaneurysms, cotton wool spot, hard exudates	Strong association with stroke, congestive heart failure, renal dysfunction, and cardiovascular mortality
Malignant	Moderate retinopathy signs plus optic disc swelling and macular edema	Associated with mortality

Table 51–1. Classification of Hypertensive Retinopathy

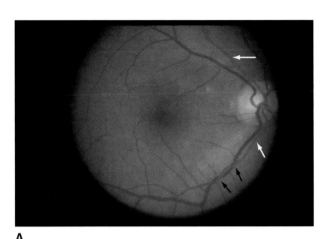
A

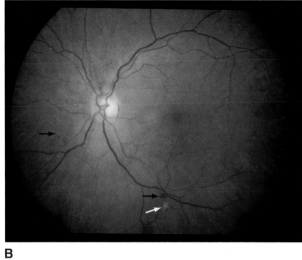
B

Figure 51–1. (A) Mild hypertensive retinopathy. Arteriovenous nicking (black arrows) and focal narrowing (white arrows). (B) Moderate hypertensive retinopathy. Retinal hemorrhages (black arrows), arteriovenous nicking (white arrow), and generalized retinal arteriolar narrowing. (From Wong TY, Mitchell P. Hypertensive retinopathy. *N Engl J Med* 2004;351(22):2310–17, with permission.)

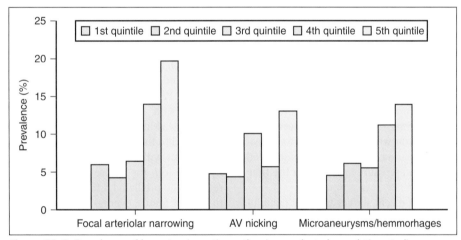

Figure 51–2. Prevalence of hypertensive retinopathy signs, selected population studies.

PREVALENCE OF HYPERTENSIVE RETINOPATHY: SUMMARY OF POPULATION-BASED STUDIES				
			Prevalence of Retinopathy Signs[a]	
Study	**Population**	**All Persons**	**Hypertensive Persons**	**References**
Beaver Dam Eye Study (BDES)	4926 persons aged 43 to 86 years, white ethnicity, Wisconsin	7.8 to 13.5%	2.8 to 19.4%	11
Blue Mountains Eye Study (BMES)	3654 persons aged 49 and older, white ethnicity, Australia	7.9 to 9.9%	6.8 to 15.4%	15,17
Atherosclerosis Risk in Communities (ARIC) Study	10,000+ persons aged 51 to 72 yrs, white and black ethnicity, four communities: North Carolina, Mississippi, Minneapolis, and Maryland	3.3 to 7.3%	5.0 to 11.9%	12
Cardiovascular Health Study (CHS)	2,400+ persons aged 69 to 97 yrs, white and black ethnicity, four communities: North Carolina, Pennsylvania, California, and Maryland	8.3 to 9.6%	9.0 to 12.3%	16
Rotterdam Eye Study	5674 persons aged 55 and older, white ethnicity, Holland	5%	—	14

a. Includes focal arteriolar narrowing, arteriovenous nicking, and retinal hemorrhages/microaneurysms/cotton wool spots in nondiabetic persons.

Table 51–2. Prevalence of Hypertensive Retinopathy: Summary of Population-based Studies

sure with focal arteriolar narrowing, AV nicking, and retinal hemorrhages/microaneurysms in the Cardiovascular Health Study.

In the Beaver Dam Eye Study, both the prevalence[11] and incidence of new hypertensive retinopathy signs[10] were strongly related to hypertension and elevated blood pressure. In that study, hypertensive individuals were 50 to 70% more likely to have retinal hemorrhages and micro-aneurysms, 30 to 40% more likely to have focal arteriolar narrowing, and 70 to 80% more likely to have AV nicking than normotensive people.[11] In addition, hypertensive persons whose blood pressure was still elevated despite use of antihypertensive medications (an indication of "poorer" control) were more likely to develop retinopathy than individuals whose blood pressure was controlled with medications. These findings were mirrored in data from the Blue Mountains Eye Study.[15,17]

To quantify generalized retinal arteriolar narrowing, recent population-based studies have employed computer-based imaging methods to measure retinal vascular diameters from photographs. These studies demonstrate that generalized retinal arteriolar narrowing, as indicated by narrower arteriolar diameters, is strongly associated with elevated blood pressure.[19–23]

The pattern of associations of blood pressure with specific hypertensive retinopathy signs varies. For example, generalized retinal arteriolar narrowing and AV nicking appear to be persistent markers of long-term hypertensive damage, and are independently associated with blood pressure levels measured up to 8 years prior to the retinal assessment.[21,22] In contrast, focal arteriolar narrowing, retinal hemorrhages, microaneurysms, and cotton wool spots appear to reflect more transient blood pressure changes and are associated only with concurrent blood pressure measured at the time of the retinal assessment.[21,22]

A new observation from recent studies was that generalized retinal arteriolar narrowing may predict the development of incident hypertension.[24–26] In the ARIC study, normotensive participants who had generalized arteriolar narrowing were 60% more likely to be diagnosed with hypertension within a 3-year period than those without arteriolar narrowing.[24] Thus, generalized retinal arteriolar narrowing, possibly reflecting systemic peripheral vasoconstriction, may be a preclinical marker of hypertension or moderate hypertension.[26]

Relationship with stroke

Because the retinal circulation is essentially an extension of the cerebral circulation (sharing similar anatomical, physiologic and embryological characteristics), numerous investigators have attempted to correlate retinal vascular changes with cerebrovascular diseases in both hypertensive and nonhypertensive populations.[27–32] As early as the 1970s, autopsy studies demonstrate similar histopathology changes in the retinal and cerebral arterioles among stroke decedents.[27] Functional studies show that retinal microcirculatory flow is reduced in persons with white matter lesions and lacunar infarction.[30]

The strongest evidence is based on the ARIC study, which showed that individuals with moderate hypertensive retinopathy signs (microaneurysms, retinal hemorrhages, cotton wool spots) were two to four times more likely to develop an incident clinical stroke event within three years—while controlling for the effects of age, gender, long-term blood pressure levels, cigarette smoking, lipids, and other risk factors.[33] Weaker associations with mild hypertensive retinopathy were also seen. In a related analysis, among the ARIC study participants without clinical stroke or transient ischaemic attacks hypertensive retinopathy signs were significantly related to changes in cognitive impairment (as defined from standardized neuropsychologic tests).[34] In a smaller subset of participants who also underwent cranial MRI, the study showed that hypertensive retinopathy signs were associated with presence and severity of cerebral white matter hyperintensity lesions[35] and cerebral atrophy.[36]

Relationship with coronary heart disease and heart failure

In contrast to stroke, there are fewer data on the association of hypertensive retinopathy signs with coronary heart disease and congestive heart failure. There have been reports of association of retinopathy signs with ischemic changes on electrocardiogram,[37] severity of coronary artery stenosis on angiography,[38] and with incident coronary heart disease and myocardial infarction in men[39] and women.[40]

In the ARIC study, controlling for predisposing risk factors persons with moderate hypertensive retinopathy were two times as likely to develop congestive heart failure as compared to those without retinopathy.[41] Even in low-risk individuals without preexisting heart disease, diabetes, or hypertension the presence of moderate hypertensive retinopathy predicted a threefold increased risk of congestive heart failure events. This may suggest that microvascular damage to the myocardium from hypertensive processes may play an important etiologic role in the development of heart failure.

Relationship with other systemic diseases and risk factors

In addition to stroke and heart disease, hypertensive retinopathy signs have been linked with a variety of systemic conditions and vascular risk factors. Hypertensive retinopathy signs have not been consistently associated with direct measures of subclinical atherosclerosis. In the ARIC study, while controlling for blood pressure generalized arteriolar narrowing was associated with carotid artery plaque but not intima-media thickness, AV nicking was associated with carotid artery intima-media thickness but not carotid artery plaque, and focal arteriolar narrowing was not related to either carotid artery measure.[12] In both the Rotterdam Eye Study and Cardiovascular Health Study, hypertensive retinopathy signs were not related to carotid artery disease.[16,18]

Similarly, most studies have not been able to demonstrate clear associations of hypertensive retinopathy with traditional atherosclerosis risk factors, including hyperlipidemia, cigarette smoking, or obesity.[19,42,43] There are several recent studies investigating associations with novel risk markers, such as biomarkers of inflammation (C-reactive protein, fibrinogen),[12,16,19] endothelial cell activation (von-Willebrand factor),[12] and angiogenesis (vascular growth endothelial factor,[44] adiponectin,[45] and leptin[46]). The significance of these associations remains to be determined.

Renal impairment is another marker of target organ damage in individuals with hypertension. The presence of microalbuminuria and renal impairment is often associated with concomitant hypertensive retinopathy.[47,48] In the ARIC study, individuals who developed renal dysfunction were more likely to have moderate retinopathy as compared to those without renal dsyfunction.[49] This association was independent of the shared risk factors and was seen in persons without diabetes or hypertension.

Cardiovascular mortality

Previous studies, largely conducted in the 1950s and 1960s, have shown that persons with hypertension and retinopathy are at increased risk of mortality.[8,50-52] However, inferences from many of these older studies are limited by the lack of data on the specific association between retinopathy severity and mortality, as well as inadequate control for potential confounders such as blood pressure and diabetes.

More recent studies provide stronger evidence that hypertensive retinopathy signs are independent predictors of mortality. In a nested case-control analysis of the Beaver Dam Eye Study, individuals who died from cardiovascular events were two times as likely to have hypertensive retinopathy sign controls after adjustment for age, gender, blood pressure, and other risk factors.[53]

Management

Data from recent studies support the hypertension guidelines regarding the prognostic significance of retinopathy signs.[54,55] These guidelines emphasize that retinopathy, along with left ventricular hypertrophy and renal impairment, may be considered an indicator of target organ damage and thus may represent a useful indication for physicians to consider a more aggressive approach in managing blood pressure in these patients.[7] Further, the information obtained from an assessment of the retinopathy status may be qualitatively different from that of measuring blood pressure, as the presence of retinopathy signs indicates susceptibility and the onset of preclinical systemic vascular disease.

Based on the simple three-grade classification system for hypertensive retinopathy shown in Table 51–1, a suggested management plan for patients with various retinopathy grades is shown in Figure 51–3. Patients with mild retinopathy signs will likely require routine care according to established guidelines. Patients with moderate retinopathy signs may benefit from further assessment of vascular risk (e.g., assessment of cholesterol levels), and if clinically indicated from appropriate risk reduction therapy (e.g., cholesterol lowering agents). Patients with malignant retinopathy will need urgent antihypertensive management.

There is, however, no convincing evidence that treatment of hypertension would reverse retinopathy changes, or that such reversal would result in a reduction in cardiovascular risk. A small number of experimental studies in animals[56,57] and clinical case series[58,59] have observed regression of some retinopathy signs (hemorrhages, cotton wool spots) but not others (AV nicking) with control of blood pressure. It is also unclear if specific antihypertensive medications such as those reported to have direct beneficial effects on microvascular structure (e.g., angiotension

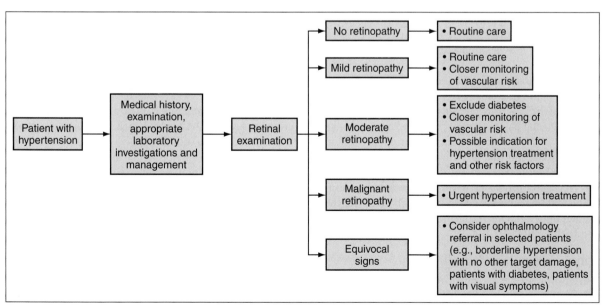

Figure 51–3. Evaluation and management of patients with hypertensive retinopathy.

converting enzyme inhibitors) would reduce retinopathy damage beyond the effects of lowered blood pressure alone. However, such agents may have added therapeutic value in preventing and treating cardiovascular diseases.

RETINAL VASCULAR CONDITIONS ASSOCIATED WITH HYPERTENSION

Retinal vein occlusion

Retinal vein occlusions are common potentially sight-threatening conditions frequently associated with hypertension. They are characterized clinically by dilated and tortuous retinal veins and the presence of retinal hemorrhages, cotton wool spots, and macular and optic disc edema. In central retinal vein occlusion (CRVO), these findings appear in all four quadrants, whereas branch retinal vein occlusion (BRVO) will manifest these findings in only one quadrant. Branch vein occlusion occurs at an arteriovenous crossing, typically affected by AV nicking. Approximately one-third of CRVOs are ischemic in nature and two-thirds nonischemic. Ischemic CRVO is typically associated with much poorer vision and visual prognosis.

There have been few population-based studies on the epidemiology and risk factors for retinal vein occlusions.[60–62] The Blue Mountains Eye Study reported the prevalence of BRVO at 1.1% and CRVO at 0.4%.[62] Slightly lower prevalence was found in the Beaver Dam Eye Study, with both prevalence and 5-year incidence of BRVO at 0.6%. For CRVO, the prevalence was 0.1% and 5-year incidence was 0.2%.[60] Most studies show a clear relationship between hypertension and risk of both CRVO and BRVO.[60–63] Hemispherical retinal vein occlusion typically involves an arteriovenous crossing at the optic disc rim, and is strongly associated with hypertension as well as glaucoma.[62] In both the Blue Mountains Eye Study and ARIC study, after adjusting for age retinal vein occlusion was associated with hypertension status, higher systolic blood pressure, and higher diastolic blood pressure.[62,63]

Management of patients with retinal vein occlusion should include a systemic evaluation and ophthalmologic follow-up to diagnose and prevent the two main complications: neovascularization and macular edema (both of which are potentially sight threatening). In relation to the prevention of neovascularization, randomized clinical trials have shown that prophylactic pan-retinal laser photocoagulation does not necessarily prevent neovascularization in ischemic vein occlusions, and that laser may be withheld until the patient develops ocular neovascularization.[64,65] Focal laser photocoagulation is useful in preventing visual loss in selected patients with macular edema from BRVO,[66] although this treatment does not appear to benefit macular edema associated with CRVO.[67]

Retinal arteriolar emboli

Hypertension is a risk factor for retinal arteriolar emboli, which are discrete plaque-like lesions lodged in the lumen of retinal arterioles.[68] Retinal emboli are pathologically heterogeneous, and are composed of cholesterol crystals (reflective or refractile emboli) or fibrin, platelets, calcium, and other materials (nonreflective emboli).

Data from epidemiologic studies suggest that retinal arteriolar emboli are seen in over 1% of adult persons 50 years and older.[69,70] Almost identical prevalences (1.3%, 1.4%) were reported from these two studies, and were strongly age related. The Beaver Dam Eye Study showed that the 5-year incidence of retinal emboli was 0.9%, but that up to 90% of eyes with retinal emboli at baseline were not present 5 years later (in keeping with observations that these emboli are transient retinal phenomena).[71] Indeed, it is likely that reported prevalences are underestimates.

Retinal emboli are associated with hypertension and other vascular risk factors, such as cigarette smoking and diabetes.[62,69,70] In both the Beaver Dam and Blue Mountains Eye studies, retinal emboli were associated with hypertension and cigarette smoking.[69,70] Furthermore, in the Blue Mountains Eye study population hypertensive persons who were cigarette smokers were six times as likely to have retinal emboli as normotensive persons who were not cigarette smokers.[69]

Like hypertensive retinopathy, the presence of retinal emboli is a poor prognostic marker.[72] In the ARIC study, participants with retinal arteriolar emboli were two times as likely to have prevalent coronary heart disease and four times as likely to have carotid artery plaque as those without emboli.[62] In the Beaver Dam Eye Study, retinal emboli at baseline was associated with a twofold higher risk of stroke mortality than persons without emboli (controlling for blood pressure and other risk factors).[70]

Management of patients with retinal emboli should include a thorough systemic evaluation, concentrating on modifiable risk factors such as the control of hypertension, dyslipidemia, and diabetes. Routine carotid ultrasonography for patients with asymptomatic retinal emboli detected incidentally remains controversial. Some studies suggest that between 60 and 80% of people with asymptomatic retinal emboli do not have significant carotid stenosis.[73] Furthermore, the benefits of carotid endarterectomy in asymptomatic patients with retinal emboli and significant carotid artery stenosis are unclear because this has not been systematically assessed.

Retinal artery occlusion

Elevated blood pressure is also a risk factor for retinal artery occlusion.[74,75] A central retinal artery occlusion (CRAO) is associated with a sudden painless unilateral loss of vision. A retinal embolus may be visible in the vessels at the optic disc, or downstream in branch retinal arterioles. A branch retinal artery occlusion (BRAO) is associated with a visual field defect, and central visual loss may be minimal—or when present have a good prognosis for recovery. CRAO is usually considered an ocular emergency, and attempts to dislodge the embolus within 3 hours after an occlusion has been suggested to restore ocular circulation and preserve vision. However, these methods (such as digital massage of the eyeball, paracentesis of anterior chamber fluid, breathing into a paper bag to induce carbon dioxide related vasodilation, and use of intraocular pressure-lowering agents) have not been proven to be effective in restoring vision, except in anecdotal cases.[76]

Retinal macroaneurysm

Retinal macroaneurysm, a fusiform or sacular lesion of the retinal arterioles, is a fairly common vascular condition seen almost always in patients with hypertension.[77–79] Approximately 20% of macroaneurysms are bilateral, and in 10% of cases multiple macroaneurysms can be found.[79] Macroaneurysms may be incidental findings in asymptomatic patients, but can present acutely with visual loss secondary to hemorrhage or exudation. Visual recovery occurs usually spontaneously with thrombosis of the macroaneurysm and resolution of the hemorrhage and exudate. Laser photocoagulation is useful in selected cases, particularly when exudation threatens or involves the macula.

CONCLUSIONS

Individuals with hypertension frequently develop typical retinal signs (termed *hypertensive retinopathy*) as well as other retinal vascular complications. Moderate hypertensive retinopathy (retinal hemorrhages, microaneurysms, and cotton wool spots) is associated with an increased risk of subclinical and clinical stroke, congestive heart failure, and cardiovascular mortality independent of traditional risk factors. Mild hypertensive retinopathy (generalized retinal arteriolar narrowing, focal arteriolar narrowing, and AV nicking) is less strongly associated with systemic outcomes. An assessment of hypertensive retinopathy signs may provide important information for prognostication and risk stratification. Conversely, patients with retinal vascular signs may need a careful review of their blood pressure and other cardiovascular risk factors.

REFERENCES

1. Wong TY, Mitchell P. Hypertensive retinopathy. N Engl J Med 2004;351:2310–17.
2. Tso M, Jampol LM. Pathophysiology of hypertensive retinopathy. Ophthalmology 1982;89:1132–45.
3. Wong TY, Klein R, Klein BEK, et al. Retinal microvascular abnormalities, and their relation to hypertension, cardiovascular diseases and mortality. Survey of Ophthalmology 2001;46:59–80.
4. Klein R, Klein BE, Jensen SC. The relation of cardiovascular disease and its risk factors to the 5-year incidence of age-related maculopathy: The Beaver Dam Eye Study. Ophthalmology 1997;104:1804–12.
5. Tielsch JM, Katz J, Sommer A, et al. Hypertension, perfusion pressure, and primary open-angle glaucoma: A population-based assessment. Arch Ophthalmol 1995;113:216–21.
6. Gunn RM. Ophthalmoscopic evidence of (1) arterial changes associated with chronic renal diseases and (2) of increased arterial tension. Trans Am Ophthalmol Soc 1892;12:124–25.
7. Gunn RM. On ophthalmoscopic evidence of general arterial disease. Trans Ophthalmol Soc UK 1898;18:356–81.
8. Keith NM, Wagener HP, Barker NW. Some different types of essential hypertension: Their course and prognosis. Am K Med Sci 1939;197:332–43.
9. Leibowitz HM, Krueger DE, Maunder LR, et al. The Framingham Eye Study monograph. Surv Ophthalmol 1980;24:335–610.
10. Klein R, Klein BEK, Moss SE. The relation of systemic hypertension to changes in the retinal vasculature. The Beaver Dam Eye Study. Trans Am Ophthalmol Soc 1997;95:329–50.
11. Klein R, Klein BEK, Moss SE, Wang Q. Hypertension and retinopathy, arteriolar narrowing and arteriovenous nicking in a population. Arch Ophthalmol 1994;112:92–8.
12. Klein R, Sharrett AR, Klein BEK, et al. Are retinal arteriolar abnormalities related to atherosclerosis? The Atherosclerosis in Communities Study. Arteroscler Thromb Vasc Biol 2000;20:1644–50.
13. Sharp PS, Chaturvedi N, Wormald R, et al. Hypertensive retinopathy in Afro-Caribbeans and Europeans: Prevalence and risk factor relationships. Hypertension 1995;25:1322–25.
14. Stolk RP, Vingerling JR, de Jong PT, et al. Retinopathy, glucose, and insulin in an elderly population. The Rotterdam Study. Diabetes 1995;44:11–5.
15. Wang JJ, Mitchell P, Leung H, et al. Hypertensive retinal vessel wall signs in the general older population: The Blue Mountains Eye Study. Hypertension 2003;42:534–41.
16. Wong TY, Klein R, Sharret AR, et al. The prevalence and risk factors of retinal microvascular abnormalities in older people. The Cardiovascular Health Study. Ophthalmology 2003;110:658–66.
17. Yu T, Mitchell P, Berry G, et al. Retinopathy in older persons without diabetes and its relationship to hypertension. Arch Ophthalmol 1998;116:83–9.
18. Wong TY, Klein R, Duncan BB, et al. Racial difference in the prevalence of hypertensive retinopathy. Hypertension 2003;41:1086–91.
19. Ikram MK, de Jong FJ, Vingerling JR, et al. Are retinal arteriolar or venular diameters associated with markers for cardiovascular disorders? The Rotterdam Study. Invest Ophthalmol Vis Sci 2004;45:2129–34.
20. Leung H, Wang JJ, Rochtchina E, et al. Relationships between age, blood pressure and retinal vessel diameters in an older population. Invest Ophthalmol Vis Sci 2003;44:2900–04.
21. Sharrett AR, Hubbard LD, Cooper LS, et al. Retinal arteriolar diameters and elevated blood pressure. The Atherosclerosis Risk in Communities Study. Am J Epidemiol 1999;150:263–70.
22. Wong TY, Hubbard LD, Klein R, et al. Retinal microvascular abnormalities and blood pressure in older people: The Cardiovascular Health Study. Br J Ophthalmology 2002;86:1007–13.
23. Wong TY, Klein R, Klein BEK, et al. Retinal vessel diameters and their associations with age and blood pressure. Invest Ophthalmol Vis Sci 2003;44:4644–50.
24. Wong TY, Klein R, Sharret AR, et al. Retinal arteriolar diameters and risk of hypertension. Ann Intern Med 2004;140:248–55.
25. Wong TY, Shankar A, Klein R, et al. Prospective cohort study of retinal vessel diameters and risk of hypertension. BMJ 2004;329:79–82.
26. Smith W, Wang JJ, Wong TY, et al. Retinal arteriolar narrowing is associated with 5-year incident severe hypertension. The Blue Mountains Eye Study. Hypertension 2004;44:442–47.
27. Goto I, Kimoto K, Katsuki S, et al. Pathological studies on the intracerebral and retinal arteries in cerebrovascular and noncerebrovascular diseases. Stroke 1975;6:263–69.
28. Aoki N. Epidemiological evaluation of funduscopic findings in cerebrovascular diseases. I. Funduscopic findings as risk factors for cerebrovascular diseases. Jpn Circ J 1975;39:257–69.
29. Tanaka H, Hayashi M, Date C, et al. Epidemiolgic studies of stroke in Shibata, a Japanese provincial city: Preliminary report on risk factors for cerebral infaction. Stroke 1985;16:773–80.
30. Schneider R, Rademacher M, Wolf S. Lacunar infarcts and white matter attenuation: Ophthalmologic and microcirculatory aspects of the pathophysiology. Stroke 1993;24:1874–79.
31. Nakayama T, Date C, Yokoyama T, et al. A 15.5-year follow-up study of stroke in a Japanese provincial city. The Shibata Study. Stroke 1997;28:45–52.
32. Kwa VI, van der Sande JJ, Stam J, et al. Retinal arterial changes correlate with cerebral small-vessel disease. Neurology 2002;59:1536–40.
33. Wong TY, Klein R, Couper DJ, et al. Retinal microvascular abnormalities and incident clinical strokes. The Atherosclerosis Risk in the Communities Study. Lancet 2001;258:1134–40.

34. Wong TY, Klein R, Sharret AR, et al. Retinal microvascular abnormalities and cognitive impairment in middle-aged persons: The Atherosclerosis Risk in Communities Study. *Stroke* 2002;33:1487–92.

35. Wong TY, Klein R, Sharret AR, et al. Cerebral white matter lesion, retinopathy and risk of clinical stroke: The Atherosclerosis Risk in the Communities Study. *JAMA* 2002;288:67–74.

36. Wong TY, Mosley TH, Klein R, et al. Retinal microvascular abnormalities and MRI signs of cerebral atrophy in healthy, middle-aged people. *Neurology* 2003;61:806–11.

37. Breslin DJ, Gifford RWJ, Fairbairn JFI. Essential hypertension: a twenty year follow-up study. *Circulation* 1966;33:87–97.

38. Michelson EL, Morganroth J, Nichols CW, MacVaugh H. Retinal arteriolar changes as an indicator of coronary artery disease. *Arch Intern Med* 1979;139:1139–41.

39. Duncan BB, Wong TY, Tyroler HA, et al. Hypertensive retinopathy and incident coronary heart disease in high risk men. *Br J Ophthalmology* 2002;86:1002–06.

40. Wong TY, Klein R, Sharret AR, et al. Retinal arteriolar narrowing and incident coronary heart disease in men and women: The Atherosclerosis Risk in the Communities Study. *JAMA* 2002;287:1153–59.

41. Wong TY, Rosamond W, Chang PP, et al. Retinopathy and risk of congestive heart failure. *JAMA* 2005;293:63–9.

42. van Leiden HA, Dekker JM, Moll AC, et al. Risk factors for incident retinopathy in a diabetic and nondiabetic population: The Hoorn study. *Arch Ophthalmol* 2003;121:245–51.

43. Wong TY, Duncan BB, Golden SH, et al. Associations between the metabolic syndrome and retinal microvascular signs: The Atherosclerosis Risk in Communities Study. *Invest Ophthalmol Vis Sci* 2004;45:2949–54.

44. Yilmaz MI, Sonmez A, Kilic S, et al. The association of plasma adiponectin levels with hypertensive retinopathy. *Eur J Endocrinol* 2005;152:233–40.

45. Tsai WC, Li YH, Huang YY, et al. Plasma vascular endothelial growth factor as a marker for early vascular damage in hypertension. *Clin Sci (Lond)* 2005 (in press).

46. Uckaya G, Ozata M, Sonmez A, et al. Is leptin associated with hypertensive retinopathy? *J Clin Endocrinol Metab* 2000;85:683–87.

47. Biesenbach G, Zazgornik J. High prevalence of hypertensive retinopathy and coronary heart disease in hypertensive patients with persistent microalbuminuria under short intensive antihypertensive therapy. *Clin Nephrol* 1994;41:211–18.

48. Pontremoli R, Sofia A, Ravera M, et al. Prevalence and clinical correlates of microalbuminuria in essential hypertension: The MAGIC Study. Microalbuminuria: A Genoa Investigation on Complications. *Hypertension* 1997;30:1135–43.

49. Wong TY, Coresh J, Klein R, et al. Retinal microvascular abnormalities and renal dysfunction in middle-aged people. *J Am Soc Nephrology* 2004;15:2469–76.

50. Breslin DJ, Gifford RWJ, Fairbairn JFI, Kearns TP. Prognostic importance of ophthalmoscopic findings in essential hypertension. *JAMA* 1966;195:335–38.

51. Frant R, Groen J. Prognosis of vascular hypertension: A nine year follow-up study of four hundred and eighteen cases. *Arch Intern Med* 1950;85:727.

52. Palmer RS, Loofbourow DCR. Prognosis in essential hypertension: Eight-year follow-up study of 430 patients on conventional medical treatment. *N Engl J Med* 1948;239:990.

53. Wong TY, Klein R, Nieto FJ, et al. Retinal microvascular abnormalities and ten-year cardiovascular mortality: A population-based case-control study. *Ophthalmology* 2003;110:933–40.

54. Williams B, Poulter NR, Brown MJ, et al. British Hypertension Society guidelines for hypertension management 2004 (BHS-IV): Summary. *BMJ* 2004;328:634–40.

55. Chobanian AV, Bakris GL, Black HR, et al. The Seventh Report of the Joint National Committee on Prevention, Detection, Evaluation, and Treatment of High Blood Pressure: The JNC 7 report. *JAMA* 2003;289:2560–72.

56. Ohta Y, Chikugo T, Suzuki T. Long-term therapeutic effects of ace inhibitor and calcium antagonists on hypertensive vascular lesions in M-SHRSP. *Clin Exp Pharmacol Physiol Suppl* 1995;22:S321–22.

57. Morishita R, Higaki J, Nakamura F, et al. Regression of hypertension-induced vascular hypertrophy by an ACE inhibitor and calcium antagonist in the spontaneously hypertensive rat. *Blood Press Suppl* 1992;3:41–7.

58. Bock KD. Regression of retinal vascular changes by antihypertensive therapy. *Hypertension* 1984;6:158–62.

59. Dahlof B, Stenkula S, Hansson L. Hypertensive retinal vascular changes: Relationship to left ventricular hypertrophy and arteriolar changes before and after treatment. *Blood Press* 1992;1:35–44.

60. Hayreh SS, Zimmerman B, McCarthy MJ, Podhajsky P. Systemic diseases associated with various types of retinal vein occlusion. *Am J Ophthalmol* 2001;131:61–77.

61. Klein R, Klein BE, Moss SE, Meuer SM. The epidemiology of retinal vein occlusion: The Beaver Dam Eye Study. *Trans Am Ophthalmol Soc* 2000;98:133–41.

62. Mitchell P, Smith W, Chang A. Prevalence and associations of retinal vein occlusion in Australia. The Blue Mountains Eye Study. *Arch Ophthalmol* 1996;114:1243–47.

63. Wong TY, Marino EK, Klein R, et al. Cardiovascular associations of retinal vein occlusion and arteriolar emboli: The Atherosclerosis Risk In Communities & Cardiovascular Health Studies. *Ophthalmology* 2005 (in press).

64. The Central Vein Occlusion Study Group N report: A randomized clinical trial of early panretinal photocoagulation for ischemic central vein occlusion. *Ophthalmology* 1995;102:1434–44.

65. Branch Vein Occlusion Study Group. Argon laser scatter photocoagulation for prevention of neovascularization and vitreous hemorrhage in branch vein occlusion: A randomized clinical trial. *Arch Ophthalmol* 1986;104:34–41.

66. Branch Vein Occlusion Study Group. Argon laser photocoagulation for macular edema in branch vein occlusion. *Am J Ophthalmol* 1984;98:271–82.

67. The Central Vein Occlusion Study Group M report: Evaluation of grid pattern photocoagulation for macular edema in central vein occlusion. *Ophthalmology* 1995;102:1425–33.

68. Wong TY, Klein R. Retinal arteriolar emboli: epidemiology and risk of stroke. *Curr Opin Ophthalmol* 2002;13:142–46.

69. Mitchell P, Wang JJ, Li W, et al. Prevalence of asymptomatic retinal emboli. *Stroke* 1997;28:63–6.

70. Klein R, Klein BE, Jensen SC, et al. Retinal emboli and stroke: The Beaver Dam Eye Study. *Arch Ophthalmol* 1999;117:1063–68.

71. Klein R, Klein BE, Moss SE, Meuer SM. Retinal emboli and cardiovascular disease: The Beaver Dam Eye Study. *Arch Ophthalmol* 2003;121:1446–51.

72. Bruno A, Jones WL, Austin JK, et al. Vascular outcome in men with asymptomatic retinal cholesterol emboli: A cohort study. *Ann Intern Med* 1995;122:249–53.

73. Sharma S, Brown GC, Pater JL, et al. Does a visible retinal embolus increase the likelihood of hemodynamically significant carotid artery stenosis in patients with acute retinal arterial occlusion? *Arch Ophthalmol* 1998;116:1602–06.

74. Mangat HS. Retinal artery occlusion. *Surv Ophthalmol* 1995;40:145–56.

75. Recchia FM, Brown GC. Systemic disorders associated with retinal vascular occlusion. *Curr Opin Ophthalmol* 2000;11:462–67.

76. Mueller AJ, Neubauer AS, Schaller U, Kampik A. European Assessment Group for Lysis in the Eye. Evaluation of minimally invasive therapies and rationale for a prospective randomized trial to evaluate selective intra-arterial lysis for clinically complete central retinal artery occlusion. *Arch Ophthalmol* 2003;121:1377–81.

77. Panton RW, Goldberg MF, Farber MD. Retinal arterial macroaneurysms: risk factors and natural history. *Br J Ophthalmol* 1990;74:595–600.

78. Brown DM, Sobol WM, Folk JC, Weingeist TA. Retinal arteriolar macroaneurysms: Long-term visual outcome. *Br J Ophthalmol* 1994;78:534–38.

79. Rabb MF, Gagliano DA, Teske MP. Retinal arterial macroaneurysms. *Surv Ophthalmol* 1988;33:73–96.

Chapter

52 Hypertension in Children and Adolescents

Joseph T. Flynn

Definition

- Hypertension in children and adolescents is defined as blood pressure persistently above the 95th percentile for age, gender, and height. New normative values and recommendations for evaluation and management have recently been published by the National High Blood Pressure Education Program.

Key Findings

- Less than 2% of children and adolescents have hypertension; however, the incidence is much greater in obese children.

- Hypertensive target-organ damage, including left ventricular hypertrophy and increased carotid intima-media thickness, occurs commonly in hypertensive children and adolescents.

- Causes of hypertension in children and adolescents are age-dependent, with secondary causes predominant in infants and younger children, and primary hypertension most common in adolescents.

Clinical Implications

- Treatment should include nonpharmacologic approaches in all patients, and antihypertensive medications if hypertensive target-organ damage, secondary hypertension or other compelling conditions are present.

- The special cases of hypertensive emergencies in children and adolescents and neonatal hypertension are addressed.

The lack of cardiovascular endpoints such as stroke and myocardial infarction in childhood means that definitions of normal and elevated blood pressure (BP) must be based upon statistical analyses of large-scale, cross-sectional studies of BP in normal children. Such analyses have been conducted under the auspices of the National Heart, Lung and Blood Institute, which has issued consensus guidelines with recommendations for identification and management of elevated BP in childhood have on four occasions over approximately the past 30 years. The most recent of these, "The Fourth Report on the Diagnosis, Evaluation, and Treatment of High Blood Pressure in Children and Adolescents"[1] is notable for its adaptation of terminology and staging criteria utilized in recent consensus guidelines for adult hypertension[2] to the problem of childhood hypertension, and for its emphasis on prevention of adult cardiovascular disease by early intervention in children and adolescents with elevated BP.

According to the Fourth Report,[1] normal BP in childhood is defined as systolic and diastolic BP below the 90th percentile for age, gender, and height, and hypertension is defined as systolic and/or diastolic BP equal to or higher than the 95th percentile on repeated measurement. BP percentile values for boys and girls aged 1 to 17 years can be found in Tables 52–1 and 52–2. Children with systolic or diastolic BP between the 90th and 95th percentiles, who in prior reports had previously been classified as having "high-normal" BP,[3] are now classified as "prehypertensive," in keeping with the terminology used for adults in the Seventh report of the Joint National Committee on Prevention, Detection, Evaluation, and Treatment of High Blood Pressure (JNC-7)[2]. Recognizing that the prehypertension cut-point of 120/80 used in adults begins to appear as the 90th percentile in children by the age of 12, the Fourth Report also recommends that adolescents with BP =120/80 be classified as having pre-hypertension.

The Fourth Report additionally provides guidelines for staging the severity of hypertension in children and adolescents, which can then be used clinically to guide evaluation and management[1] (Table 52–3). Stage 1 hypertension is defined as BP equal to or higher than the 95th percentile for age, gender, and height up to the 99th percentile plus 5 mmHg. This level of BP elevation is roughly similar to stage 1 hypertension in adults.[2] Stage 2 hypertension is any BP reading above the 99th percentile plus 5 mmHg. As will be discussed later, children or adolescents with stage 2 hypertension should be evaluated and treated more quickly and/or aggressively than those with less significant BP elevation.

PREVALENCE

Traditionally, hypertension has been considered to be an uncommon problem in childhood and adolescence. For example, a BP screening study conducted in Dallas in the late 1970s revealed that just 1.2% of eighth graders had persistent systolic hypertension and 0.37% diastolic hypertension.[4] Similarly, Sinaiko et al.[5] determined that the prevalence of hypertension in Minneapolis students aged 10 to 15 years was 0.3% for systolic and 0.8% for diastolic hypertension. A recent reanalysis of the Minneapolis data applying the normative values from the 1996 Working Group Report[6] resulted in a combined prevalence of systolic and diastolic hypertension of 1.2%.[7] These screening programs also demonstrated the importance of performing repeated measures of BP before labeling a child as hyper-

BLOOD PRESSURE LEVELS FOR BOYS BY AGE AND HEIGHT PERCENTILE

Age (Years)	BP Percentile ↓	Systolic BP (mmHg) ← Percentile of Height →							Diastolic BP (mmHg) ← Percentile of Height →						
		5th	10th	25th	50th	75th	90th	95th	5th	10th	25th	50th	75th	90th	95th
1	50th	80	81	83	85	87	88	89	34	35	36	37	38	39	39
	90th	94	95	97	99	100	102	103	49	50	51	52	53	53	54
	95th	98	99	101	103	104	106	106	54	54	55	56	57	58	58
	99th	105	106	108	110	112	113	114	61	62	63	64	65	66	66
2	50th	84	85	87	88	90	92	92	39	40	41	42	43	44	44
	90th	97	99	100	102	104	105	106	54	55	56	57	58	58	59
	95th	101	102	104	106	108	109	110	59	59	60	61	62	63	63
	99th	109	110	111	113	115	117	117	66	67	68	69	70	71	71
3	50th	86	87	89	91	93	94	95	44	44	45	46	47	48	48
	90th	100	101	103	105	107	108	109	59	59	60	61	62	63	63
	95th	104	105	107	109	110	112	113	63	63	64	65	66	67	67
	99th	111	112	114	116	118	119	120	71	71	72	73	74	75	75
4	50th	88	89	91	93	95	96	97	47	48	49	50	51	51	52
	90th	102	103	105	107	109	110	111	62	63	64	65	66	66	67
	95th	106	107	109	111	112	114	115	66	67	68	69	70	71	71
	99th	113	114	116	118	120	121	122	74	75	76	77	78	78	79
5	50th	90	91	93	95	96	98	98	50	51	52	53	54	55	55
	90th	104	105	106	108	110	111	112	65	66	67	68	69	69	70
	95th	108	109	110	112	114	115	116	69	70	71	72	73	74	74
	99th	115	116	118	120	121	123	123	77	78	79	80	81	81	82
6	50th	91	92	94	96	98	99	100	53	53	54	55	56	57	57
	90th	105	106	108	110	111	113	113	68	68	69	70	71	72	72
	95th	109	110	112	114	115	117	117	72	72	73	74	75	76	76
	99th	116	117	119	121	123	124	125	80	80	81	82	83	84	84
7	50th	92	94	95	97	99	100	101	55	55	56	57	58	59	59
	90th	106	107	109	111	113	114	115	70	70	71	72	73	74	74
	95th	110	111	113	115	117	118	119	74	74	75	76	77	78	78
	99th	117	118	120	122	124	125	126	82	82	83	84	85	86	86
8	50th	94	95	97	99	100	102	102	56	57	58	59	60	60	61
	90th	107	109	110	112	114	115	116	71	72	72	73	74	75	76
	95th	111	112	114	116	118	119	120	75	76	77	78	79	79	80
	99th	119	120	122	123	125	127	127	83	84	85	86	87	87	88
9	50th	95	96	98	100	102	103	104	57	58	59	60	61	61	62
	90th	109	110	112	114	115	117	118	72	73	74	75	76	76	77
	95th	113	114	116	118	119	121	121	76	77	78	79	80	81	81
	99th	120	121	123	125	127	128	129	84	85	86	87	88	88	89
10	50th	97	98	100	102	103	105	106	58	59	60	61	61	62	63
	90th	111	112	114	115	117	119	119	73	73	74	75	76	77	78
	95th	115	116	117	119	121	122	123	77	78	79	80	81	81	82
	99th	122	123	125	127	128	130	130	85	86	86	88	88	89	90
11	50th	99	100	102	104	105	107	107	59	59	60	61	62	63	63
	90th	113	114	115	117	119	120	121	74	74	75	76	77	78	78
	95th	117	118	119	121	123	124	125	78	78	79	80	81	82	82
	99th	124	125	127	129	130	132	132	86	86	87	88	89	90	90
12	50th	101	102	104	106	108	109	110	59	60	61	62	63	63	64
	90th	115	116	118	120	121	123	123	74	75	75	76	77	78	79
	95th	119	120	122	123	125	127	127	78	79	80	81	82	82	83
	99th	126	127	129	131	133	134	135	86	87	88	89	90	90	91
13	50th	104	105	106	108	110	111	112	60	60	61	62	63	64	64
	90th	117	118	120	122	124	125	126	75	75	76	77	78	79	79
	95th	121	122	124	126	128	129	130	79	79	80	81	82	83	83
	99th	128	130	131	133	135	136	137	87	87	88	89	90	91	91
14	50th	106	107	109	111	113	114	115	60	61	62	63	64	65	65
	90th	120	121	123	125	126	128	128	75	76	77	78	79	79	80
	95th	124	125	127	128	130	132	132	80	80	81	82	83	84	84
	99th	131	132	134	136	138	139	140	87	88	89	90	91	92	92

Age (Years)	BP Percentile ↓	Systolic BP (mmHg) ← Percentile of Height →							Diastolic BP (mmHg) ← Percentile of Height →						
		5th	10th	25th	50th	75th	90th	95th	5th	10th	25th	50th	75th	90th	95th
15	50th	109	110	112	113	115	117	117	61	62	63	64	65	66	66
	90th	122	124	125	127	129	130	131	76	77	78	79	80	80	81
	95th	126	127	129	131	133	134	135	81	81	82	83	84	85	85
	99th	134	135	136	138	140	142	142	88	89	90	91	92	93	93
16	50th	111	112	114	116	118	119	120	63	63	64	65	66	67	67
	90th	125	126	128	130	131	133	134	78	78	79	80	81	82	82
	95th	129	130	132	134	135	137	137	82	83	83	84	85	86	87
	99th	136	137	139	141	143	144	145	90	90	91	92	93	94	94
17	50th	114	115	116	118	120	121	122	65	66	66	67	68	69	70
	90th	127	128	130	132	134	135	136	80	80	81	82	83	84	84
	95th	131	132	134	136	138	139	140	84	85	86	87	87	88	89
	99th	139	140	141	143	145	146	147	92	93	93	94	95	96	97

BLOOD PRESSURE LEVELS FOR BOYS BY AGE AND HEIGHT PERCENTILE—cont'd

From National High Blood Pressure Education Program Working Group on High Blood Pressure in Children and Adolescents. *Pediatrics* 2004;114:555–76.
BP, blood pressure.
Note: To use the table, first plot the child's height on a standard growth curve (www.cdc.gov/growthcharts). The child's measured systolic BP and diastolic BP are compared with the numbers provided in the table according to the child's age and height percentile.

Table 52–1. Blood Pressure Levels for Boys by Age and Height Percentile

tensive: studies that used just one BP determination found significantly higher "prevalence" of hypertension than studies in which repeated screenings were performed[4,5,7–12] (Table 52–4).

Other studies, however, have suggested that this may be changing. Sorof et al.[12,13] conducted a screening study in the Houston public schools and found that 13% of adolescents had blood pressures persistently elevated above the 95th percentile for age, gender, and height, a significantly greater percentage than in the studies cited above. The children in this study also tended to be obese, with a mean BMI of 24 ± 6 kg/m^2, and hypertension was significantly more common among obese children. This is reflects the increasing prevalence of obesity among American children over the past decade: analyses of the 1999–2000 National Health and Nutrition Examination Survey (NHANES) data demonstrate a significantly greater prevalence of obesity in children of all ages and ethnic backgrounds compared to the NHANES III data from 1988 to 1994.[14]

ETIOLOGIES

In infants and preadolescent children, primary hypertension is exceedingly rare. In these age groups, secondary forms of hypertension are much more common (Table 52–5), with renal disease being the most common underlying cause. Especially in the young school-age child, the differential diagnosis of hypertension can be vast, necessitating a careful and thorough evaluation, as specific treatment of the underlying cause may result in "cure" of the child's hypertension. The reader interested in a detailed discussion of the causes of hypertension in infants and young children is encouraged to consult one of the recent comprehensive texts on pediatric hypertension.[15,16]

In adolescents, however, primary hypertension accounts for the majority of cases. An example of this can be seen in a 1992 study by Wyszynska et al.[17] of 1025 children referred to a Polish children's hospital for evaluation of hypertension (defined as blood pressure greater than the 95th percentile for age). Overall, 45% of their population had primary hypertension and 55% secondary hypertension. Adolescents (aged 15–18 years) comprised 60% of the study population, and 75% of the subjects in this age group had primary hypertension. The breakdown of causes of secondary hypertension (regardless of age) was comparable to the list of causes for younger children in Table 52–5.

Certain groups of children are at increased risk of developing primary hypertension in childhood, including children of hypertensive parents and obese children.[18–20] Along these lines, the recent increase in the prevalence of obesity among children in the United States will most likely be followed by an increased incidence of childhood hypertension in the next one to two decades.[21] The high frequency of obesity among children with primary hypertension is highlighted by two recent referral series, one consisting of primarily Caucasian children,[22] and the other consisting of primarily minority children.[23] In both of these series, primary hypertension was diagnosed after standardized evaluations for identifiable causes of hypertension. The mean age of the subjects in both series was approximately 14 years, and most had BMI's at or above the 95th percentile for age and gender. Isolated systolic hypertension was a common feature in both reports, and most of the adolescents had relatively mild hypertension, averaging 5% to 25% above the 95th percentile.[22,23] It is reasonable to assume, therefore, that most adolescents found to have sustained hypertension will have primary hypertension,

BLOOD PRESSURE LEVELS FOR GIRLS BY AGE AND HEIGHT PERCENTILE

Age (Years)	BP Percentile ↓	Systolic BP (mmHg) ← Percentile of Height →							Diastolic BP (mmHg) ← Percentile of Height →						
		5th	10th	25th	50th	75th	90th	95th	5th	10th	25th	50th	75th	90th	95th
1	50th	83	84	85	86	88	89	90	38	39	39	40	41	41	42
	90th	97	97	98	100	101	102	103	52	53	53	54	55	55	56
	95th	100	101	102	104	105	106	107	56	57	57	58	59	59	60
	99th	108	108	109	111	112	113	114	64	64	65	65	66	67	67
2	50th	85	85	87	88	89	91	91	43	44	44	45	46	46	47
	90th	98	99	100	101	103	104	105	57	58	58	59	60	61	61
	95th	102	103	104	105	107	108	109	61	62	62	63	64	65	65
	99th	109	110	111	112	114	115	116	69	69	70	70	71	72	72
3	50th	86	87	88	89	91	92	93	47	48	48	49	50	50	51
	90th	100	100	102	103	104	106	106	61	62	62	63	64	64	65
	95th	104	104	105	107	108	109	110	65	66	66	67	68	68	69
	99th	111	111	113	114	115	116	117	73	73	74	74	75	76	76
4	50th	88	88	90	91	92	94	94	50	50	51	52	52	53	54
	90th	101	102	103	104	106	107	108	64	64	65	66	67	67	68
	95th	105	106	107	108	110	111	112	68	68	69	70	71	71	72
	99th	112	113	114	115	117	118	119	76	76	76	77	78	79	79
5	50th	89	90	91	93	94	95	96	52	53	53	54	55	55	56
	90th	103	103	105	106	107	109	109	66	67	67	68	69	69	70
	95th	107	107	108	110	111	112	113	70	71	71	72	73	73	74
	99th	114	114	116	117	118	120	120	78	78	79	79	80	81	81
6	50th	91	92	93	94	96	97	98	54	54	55	56	56	57	58
	90th	104	105	106	108	109	110	111	68	68	69	70	70	71	72
	95th	108	109	110	111	113	114	115	72	72	73	74	74	75	76
	99th	115	116	117	119	120	121	122	80	80	80	81	82	83	83
7	50th	93	93	95	96	97	99	99	55	56	56	57	58	58	59
	90th	106	107	108	109	111	112	113	69	70	70	71	72	72	73
	95th	110	111	112	113	115	116	116	73	74	74	75	76	76	77
	99th	117	118	119	120	122	123	124	81	81	82	82	83	84	84
8	50th	95	95	96	98	99	100	101	57	57	57	58	59	60	60
	90th	108	109	110	111	113	114	114	71	71	71	72	73	74	74
	95th	112	112	114	115	116	118	118	75	75	75	76	77	78	78
	99th	119	120	121	122	123	125	125	82	82	83	83	84	85	86
9	50th	96	97	98	100	101	102	103	58	58	58	59	60	61	61
	90th	110	110	112	113	114	116	116	72	72	72	73	74	75	75
	95th	114	114	115	117	118	119	120	76	76	76	77	78	79	79
	99th	121	121	123	124	125	127	127	83	83	84	84	85	86	87
10	50th	98	99	100	102	103	104	105	59	59	59	60	61	62	62
	90th	112	112	114	115	116	118	118	73	73	73	74	75	76	76
	95th	116	116	117	119	120	121	122	77	77	77	78	79	80	80
	99th	123	123	125	126	127	129	129	84	84	85	86	86	87	88
11	50th	100	101	102	103	105	106	107	60	60	60	61	62	63	63
	90th	114	114	116	117	118	119	120	74	74	74	75	76	77	77
	95th	118	118	119	121	122	123	124	78	78	78	79	80	81	81
	99th	125	125	126	128	129	130	131	85	85	86	87	87	88	89
12	50th	102	103	104	105	107	108	109	61	61	61	62	63	64	64
	90th	116	116	117	119	120	121	122	75	75	75	76	77	78	78
	95th	119	120	121	123	124	125	126	79	79	79	80	81	82	82
	99th	127	127	128	130	131	132	133	86	86	87	88	88	89	90
13	50th	104	105	106	107	109	110	110	62	62	62	63	64	65	65
	90th	117	118	119	121	122	123	124	76	76	76	77	78	79	79
	95th	121	122	123	124	126	127	128	80	80	80	81	82	83	83
	99th	128	129	130	132	133	134	135	87	87	88	89	89	90	91
14	50th	106	106	107	109	110	111	112	63	63	63	64	65	66	66
	90th	119	120	121	122	124	125	125	77	77	77	78	79	80	80
	95th	123	123	125	126	127	129	129	81	81	81	82	83	84	84
	99th	130	131	132	133	135	136	136	88	88	89	90	90	91	92

Age (Years)	BP Percentile ↓	Systolic BP (mmHg) ← Percentile of Height →							Diastolic BP (mmHg) ← Percentile of Height →						
		5th	10th	25th	50th	75th	90th	95th	5th	10th	25th	50th	75th	90th	95th
15	50th	107	108	109	110	111	113	113	64	64	64	65	66	67	67
	90th	120	121	122	123	125	126	127	78	78	78	79	80	81	81
	95th	124	125	126	127	129	130	131	82	82	82	83	84	85	85
	99th	131	132	133	134	136	137	138	89	89	90	91	91	92	93
16	50th	108	108	110	111	112	114	114	64	64	65	66	66	67	68
	90th	121	122	123	124	126	127	128	78	78	79	80	81	81	82
	95th	125	126	127	128	130	131	132	82	82	83	84	85	85	86
	99th	132	133	134	135	137	138	139	90	90	90	91	92	93	93
17	50th	108	109	110	111	113	114	115	64	65	65	66	67	67	68
	90th	122	122	123	125	126	127	128	78	79	79	80	81	81	82
	95th	125	126	127	129	130	131	132	82	83	83	84	85	85	86
	99th	133	133	134	136	137	138	139	90	90	91	91	92	93	93

BLOOD PRESSURE LEVELS FOR GIRLS BY AGE AND HEIGHT PERCENTILE—cont'd

From National High Blood Pressure Education Program Working Group on High Blood Pressure in Children and Adolescents. *Pediatrics* 2004;114:555–76.
BP, blood pressure.
Note: To use the table, first plot the child's height on a standard growth curve (www.cdc.gov/growthcharts). The child's measured systolic BP and diastolic BP are compared with the numbers provided in the table according to the child's age and height percentile.

Table 52–2. Blood Pressure Levels for Girls by Age and Height Percentile

CLASSIFICATION OF HYPERTENSION IN CHILDREN AND ADOLESCENTS, WITH MEASUREMENT FREQUENCY AND THERAPY RECOMMENDATIONS

Classification	SBP or DBP Percentile[a]	Frequency of BP Measurement	Therapeutic Lifestyle Changes	Pharmacologic Therapy
Normal	<90th	Recheck at next scheduled physical examination.	Encourage healthy diet, sleep, and physical activity.	—
Prehypertension	90th to <95th or if BP exceeds 120/80 even if below 90th percentile up to <95th percentile[b]	Recheck in 6 months.	Counsel for weight management if overweight, and introduce physical activity and diet management.	Do not initiate therapy unless compelling indications exist, such as CKD, diabetes mellitus, heart failure, LVH.
Stage 1 hypertension	95th percentile to the 99th percentile plus 5 mmHg	Recheck in 1–2 weeks or sooner if the patient is symptomatic; if persistently elevated on two additional occasions, evaluate or refer to source of care within 1 month.	Counsel for weight management if overweight, and introduce physical activity and diet management.	Initiate therapy based on indications in Table 52–6 or if compelling indications as above.
Stage 2 hypertension	>99th percentile plus 5 mmHg	Evaluate or refer to source of care within 1 week or immediately if the patient is symptomatic.	Counsel for weight management if overweight, and introduce physical activity and diet management.	Initiate therapy.

From National High Blood Pressure Education Program Working Group on High Blood Pressure in Children and Adolescents. *Pediatrics* 2004;114:555–76.
BP, blood pressure; CKD, chronic kidney disease; DBP, diastolic blood pressure; LVH, left ventricular hypertrophy; SBP, systolic blood pressure.
[a]For sex, age, and height measured on at least three separate occasions; if systolic and diastolic categories are different, categorize by the higher value.
[b]This occurs typically at age 12 years for SBP and at 16 years for DBP.

Table 52–3. Classification of Hypertension in Children and Adolescents, with Measurement Frequency and Therapy Recommendations

PREVALENCE OF HYPERTENSION IN CHILDREN AND ADOLESCENTS						
Study Location	Number Screened	Age (years)	Number of Screenings	Threshold BP Value	Prevalence	Reference
Muscatine, IA, United States	1,301	14–18	1	140/90	8.9% sHTN 12.2% dHTN	Lauer et al., 1975[8]
Edmonton, Canada	15,594	15–20	1	150/95	2.2%	Silverberg et al., 1975[9]
Dallas, TX, United States	10,641	14	3	95th percentile	1.2% sHTN 0.4% dHTN	Fixler et al., 1979[4]
Minneapolis, MN, United States	14,686	10–15	1	1987 TF	4.2%	Sinaiko et al., 1989[5]
Tulsa, OK, United States	5,537	14–19	1	1987 TF	6.0%	O'Quin et al., 1992[10]
Buraidah, Saudi Arabia	3,299	3–18	1	1996 WG	10.6%	Soyannwo et al., 1997[11]
Minneapolis, MN, United States	14,686	10–15	2	1996 WG	0.8% sHTN 0.4% dHTN	Adrogue and Sinaiko, 2001[7]
Houston, TX, United States	5,102	12–16	3	1996 WG	4.5%	Sorof et al., 2002[12]

BP, blood pressure; dHTN, diastolic hypertension; sHTN, systolic hypertension; TF, Second Task Force Report[3]; WG, Working Group Report.[6]

Table 52–4. Prevalence of Hypertension in Children and Adolescents

CAUSES OF CHILDHOOD HYPERTENSION BY AGE GROUP (%)			
	Infants[a]	School-age	Adolescents
Primary/essential	<1	15–30	85–95
Secondary	99	70–85	5–15[b]
Renal parenchymal disease	20	60–70	
Renovascular	25	5–10	
Endocrine	1	3–5	
Aortic coarctation	35	10–20	
Reflux nephropathy	0	5–10	
Neoplastic	4	1–5	
Miscellaneous	20	1–5	

[a]Less than 1 year of age.
[b]Breakdown of causes is generally similar to that for school-age children.

Table 52–5. Causes of Childhood Hypertension by Age Group (%)

especially if the blood pressure elevation is not severe, or if diastolic hypertension is absent.

CONSEQUENCES OF CHILDHOOD HYPERTENSION

As noted previously, the long-term cardiovascular sequelae of hypertension seen in adults such as stroke and myocardial infarction do not occur in children. However, a large body of evidence has accumulated over the years documenting that persistent blood pressure elevation in children and adolescents can produce other target-organ effects that may be important to consider, especially when making treatment decisions.

Left ventricular hypertrophy (LVH) is probably the most common and most easily identified target-organ effect of hypertension in children and adolescents. It has been recognized as occurring commonly, even with mild blood pressure elevation, since the early 1980s.[24] More recent studies have established a prevalence of LVH in hypertensive children and adolescents of between 23% to 30%.[22,23,25] Abnormal left ventricular geometry has also been demonstrated, especially in those with more severe blood pressure elevation.[26] Although the adverse effects of LVH seen in adults such as sudden cardiac death[27] have not been proven to occur in hypertensive children, LVH is still considered an important cardiovascular risk factor in hypertensive children,[26] and treatment recommendations from consensus organizations have emphasized that if LVH is present, the child or adolescent should be aggressively treated with antihypertensive medications.[1]

Other vascular effects of hypertension have also been demonstrated in hypertensive children and adolescents, including retinal changes[28,29] and increased carotid intima-media thickness (cIMT).[30] Retinal changes, when systematically looked for, occur in a large number of hypertensive children and adolescents,[28] and in one study appeared more often in those with higher diastolic blood pressure.[29] Increased cIMT, which is well established as a correlate of atherosclerosis and increased cardiovascular risk in adults,[31,32] has recently been found to also occur in hypertensive children.[30,33,34] As in hypertensive adults, increased cIMT in the young is correlated with obesity[33] and left ventricular hypertrophy,[34] suggesting that this may someday be used as a marker of increased cardiovascular risk in hypertensive children and adolescents.

The other major target organ in hypertension is the kidney. In adults, hypertension is one of the most common causes of chronic kidney disease (CKD). According to the 2004 U.S. Renal Data Systems (USRDS) Annual Data Report, hypertension was the second leading cause of end-stage renal disease (ESRD) in adults in 2002, affecting approximately 125,000 individuals, or 24.4% of the entire ESRD population.[35] In children, on the other hand, it is not so clear if hypertension alone may result in ESRD. The North American Pediatric Renal Transplant Cooperative Study (NAPRTCS) dialysis, transplant, and chronic renal insufficiency registries do not list hypertension among the causes of CKD/ESRD in children.[36] However, close analysis of the USRDS data reveals that hypertension was reported as the cause of ESRD in over 150 children in 2002.[35] Hypertension was reported much less often than other forms of kidney disease in children, and was primarily reported as a cause of ESRD in children aged 10 years and older. Reconciling these two databases is difficult as they are derived from significantly different sources. Since hypertension was reported as a cause of ESRD mostly in older children, it is tempting to speculate that perhaps long-standing hypertension may indeed lead to CKD/ESRD in adolescents, adding further weight to recent recommendations advocating earlier use of antihypertensive medications in some children and adolescents.[1]

It is possible that hypertension may also have significant effects on mental function in children. In adults, it is well known that long-standing blood pressure elevation may cause impaired performance on neuropsychological testing,[37] with at least one study demonstrating an inverse relationship between blood pressure level and measures of attention and memory.[38] In children, only one study has examined the effects of elevated blood pressure on cognition. Lande et al.[39] examined data from the NHANES III, which included information on blood pressure as well as results of standardized neuropsychological testing (including tests of short-term memory, attention, concentration, and constructional skills). They found that children with blood pressure above the 90th percentile for age, gender, and height had decreased performance on the neuropsychological tests compared to control children with normal blood pressure. These findings are especially provocative given that only a single blood pressure measurement was made in the NHANES III. Further studies are clearly needed to examine the effects of sustained blood pressure elevation in childhood on mental function, as well as the potential effects of treatment on neuropsychological function in hypertensive children.

The final and perhaps most intriguing consequence of elevated childhood blood pressure is that it may predict the development of adult hypertension. This phenomenon, known as blood pressure "tracking," has been the subject of much study, with the overall conclusion in the literature being that BP does indeed track into adulthood,[40] especially in children with what used to be termed "high normal" blood pressure. Perhaps the most convincing of the avail-

able studies is the Muscatine study,[41] which enrolled schoolchildren aged 7 to 18 years in Muscatine, Iowa between 1971 and 1978. A subgroup (the "longitudinal cohort") was then recalled as young adults (aged 23–28 years). Subjects with systolic blood pressure in childhood higher than the 90th percentile were 3.9 times more likely than expected to develop adult hypertension, and subjects with diastolic blood pressure in childhood higher than the 90th percentile were 1.9 times more likely than expected to develop adult hypertension. The likelihood of developing adult hypertension increased with increasing numbers of childhood readings greater than the 90th percentile. In addition, the absence of abnormal readings in childhood was associated with a reduced risk of developing adult hypertension. Other important influences on adult blood pressure were ponderosity, change in ponderosity, and a positive family history of hypertension, which are all characteristics of primary hypertension in the young.[22] This phenomenon underscores the importance of detection and treatment of hypertension in childhood.

EVALUATION

Perhaps the most important step in evaluating a child or adolescent with elevated blood pressure is to confirm that the blood pressure is being measured correctly. As has been emphasized elsewhere,[1,42] proper cuff size is of paramount importance in accurately measuring blood pressure in the young. The bladder of the cuff should be long enough to encircle 80% to 100% of the arm circumference. If the cuff bladder has a 1:2 ratio of width:length, the cuff should be wide enough to obtain an accurate reading.[1] If the cuff dimensions differ from this standard, a larger/wider cuff may be needed for adolescents with long upper arms in order to avoid a falsely elevated reading due to a narrow cuff.

The method of blood pressure measurement is also important. While the use of oscillometric measurement devices has become widespread in pediatric settings,[43] these devices have inherent inaccuracies that make them suspect for diagnosing a child or adolescent with hypertension.[44,45] Furthermore, the normative blood pressure values published by the National Heart, Lung and Blood Institute are based on auscultated blood pressures.[1] Therefore, it is recommended that elevated BP readings obtained using oscillometric devices should be confirmed by auscultation. It is additionally recommended that the child or adolescent with elevated BP have this finding confirmed on at least three occasions before making a "diagnosis" of hypertension and embarking on a diagnostic evaluation.[1]

Once the child or adolescent has been confirmed to have hypertension, a diagnostic evaluation should be conducted to determine if an underlying cause can be identified. As discussed previously and as illustrated in Table 52–5, secondary causes of hypertension are common in younger children, so a comprehensive evaluation will need to be conducted in order to determine if there is an underlying cause. On the other hand, adolescents are likely to have primary hypertension, especially if obese and if there is a family history of hypertension,[22] so a less extensive work-up may suffice. The history and physical examination should focus on eliciting signs and symptoms of an underlying disorder; for example, a history of recurrent urinary tract infections in early childhood would be a clue to reflux nephropathy, while multiple café-au-lait spots and an epigastric bruit would be signs of renal artery stenosis in the setting of neurofibromatosis. Detailed discussions of the diagnostic approach to the hypertensive child or adolescent, including comprehensive tables of typical symptoms and physical exam findings, can be found elsewhere.[15,16,46]

In addition to determining whether the child or adolescent has an identifiable underlying cause for hypertension, evaluation should also include whether hypertensive target-organ damage is present, and whether any additional risk factors/comorbidities are present. As discussed earlier, many forms of hypertensive target organ damage have been shown to occur in children and adolescents. Since hypertension-related events such as stroke and myocardial infarction occur extremely rarely before adulthood, these other signs of hypertensive damage can be considered "surrogate endpoints" and if present, prompt aggressive treatment in order to prevent progression to more significant cardiovascular disease. Since left ventricular hypertrophy occurs commonly and is relatively easy to detect, it is recommended that echocardiography be performed at the time of diagnosis of hypertension and periodically thereafter in those with persistent hypertension.[1] Other examinations that may be considered include formal ophthalmologic exams to detect retinopathy, and urine testing for microalbuminuria (however, it must be stated that no clear recommendations currently exist for urine microalbumin testing in childhood).

Screening for the presence of other cardiovascular risk factors/comorbidities should also be performed as part of the evaluation of hypertensive children, particularly in obese adolescents. Currently, the best evidence supports testing for dyslipidemia and impaired glucose tolerance, both of which clearly increase cardiovascular risk in adults. It has long been known that dyslipidemia occurs commonly in children with elevated BP,[47] and recent case series confirm this association.[22] Impaired glucose tolerance also occurs frequently in obese hypertensive children, typically as part of the metabolic syndrome.[48] Other studies have demonstrated that these cardiovascular risk factors may be associated with the early development of atherosclerosis in the young.[49] It is therefore reasonable, as recommended by the Fourth Report,[1] to screen for these risk factors/comorbidities when evaluating hypertensive children and adolescents. Identification of multiple cardiovascular risk factors at an early age may in turn permit institution of measures aimed at prevention of adult cardiovascular disease.

THERAPY

In contrast to management of hypertension in adults, which is guided by evidence derived from the results of large-scale clinical trials, the management of hypertensive children and adolescents is still largely empiric. This is largely due to the lack of long-term outcome data regarding nonpharmacologic and pharmacologic approaches to treatment of hypertension in children and adolescents.[50] However, as some hypertensive children and adolescents will either have secondary hypertension or hypertensive target-organ damage, the practitioner caring for these patients should be familiar with appropriate treatment strategies, both pharmacologic and nonpharmacologic.

As discussed earlier, the Fourth Report from the National High Blood Pressure Education Program[1] recommends that, as in adults, elevated BP in children and adolescents be staged in order to help guide evaluation and management. Intervention is recommended even for children or adolescents with BPs that fall into the "prehypertension" range (Table 52–3). Such children should be counseled regarding lifestyle changes and should be seen within 6 months for a repeat BP measurement and assessment of how well they are adhering to the recommended lifestyle measures. At the other end of the scale, children or adolescents with stage 2 hypertension are candidates for immediate institution of pharmacologic therapy.

Nonpharmacologic management

Although the magnitude of change in BP may be modest, weight loss, aerobic exercise, and dietary modifications have all been shown to successfully reduce BP in children and adolescents, at least in research settings.

Studies in obese adolescents have demonstrated that modest weight loss not only decreases BP but also improves other cardiovascular risk factors such as dyslipidemia and insulin resistance.[51–54] In studies where a reduction in body mass index of about 10% was achieved, short-term reductions in BP were in the range of 8 to 12 mmHg. Unfortunately, weight loss is notoriously difficult and usually unsuccessful, especially in the primary care setting.[55] Additionally, even intensive efforts at weight loss in childhood may be followed by recidivism and an increased prevalence of adverse consequences of obesity in adulthood.[56] However, identifying a medical complication of obesity such as hypertension can perhaps provide the necessary motivation for patients and families to make the appropriate lifestyle changes.

Similarly, exercise training over 3 to 6 months has been shown to result in a reduction of 6 to 12 mmHg for systolic BP and 3 to 5 mmHg for diastolic BP.[57] However, cessation of regular exercise is generally promptly followed by a rise in BP to pre-exercise levels.[58] Aerobic exercise activities such as running, walking, or cycling are usually preferred to static forms of exercise in the management of hypertension.[59] Many children may already be participating in one or more appropriate activities, and may only need to increase the frequency and/or intensity of these activities to produce a reduction in their BP. Exercise should probably be combined with dietary changes such as those discussed later in this chapter for best results in terms of BP reduction.[60] The combination of dietary changes and exercise training may also restore vascular function in addition to reducing BP.[61]

Dietary modification in the management of hypertension in children and adolescents has received a fair amount of attention over the years. Nutrients that have been examined include the obvious, such as sodium, potassium, and calcium, as well as folate, caffeine, and other substances. Manipulation of sodium intake has received extensive study. Although it is controversial whether excessive sodium intake may cause hypertension,[62–64] once hypertension has been established, "salt sensitivity" becomes more common, and reduction in sodium intake is likely to be of benefit.[62,64–66] Trials of dietary sodium restriction in hypertensive children and adolescents have had mixed results, with some controlled studies showing no benefit,[67] and others showing a modest reduction in BP in obese adolescents but not lean adolescents.[68] Many authors have noted that the usual dietary sodium intakes of children and adolescents, at least in the United States, far exceed any nutritional requirement for sodium.[62,67] This suggests that dietary sodium restriction may have a role in those children with established hypertension, a substantial proportion of whom are likely to be salt-sensitive.

Other nutrients that have been examined in patients with hypertension include potassium and calcium, both of which have been shown to have antihypertensive effects.[66,67,69,70] A recent 2-year trial of potassium and calcium supplementation in hypertensive, salt-sensitive children demonstrated that this combination significantly reduced systolic BP.[70] Therefore, a diet that is low in sodium and enriched in potassium and calcium may be more effective in reducing BP than a diet that restricts sodium only. An example of such a diet is the so-called DASH (Dietary Approaches to Stop Hypertension) diet, which has been shown to have an antihypertensive effect in adults with hypertension, even in those receiving antihypertensive medication.[71] Although this diet has not been specifically studied in children or adolescents, the basic elements of the DASH eating plan are logical to apply the treatment of hypertensive children, especially if accompanied by counseling from a pediatric dietitian. The DASH diet also incorporates higher intake of such micronutrients as folate, which may have an antihypertensive effect,[72] as well as measures designed to reduce dietary fat intake, an important strategy given the frequent presence of both hypertension and elevated lipids in children and adolescents and the imperative to begin prevention of adult cardiovascular disease at as early an age as possible.[47,53,73]

Pharmacologic management

For many years, drug therapy of childhood hypertension relied upon either on trial-and-error, or on adapting efficacy data from studies conducted in adults.[74] Fortunately, this situation has changed because the number of antihypertensive medications that have been systematically studied in children has increased markedly over the past 7 to 8 years due to incentives provided to the pharmaceutical industry by the 1997 Food and Drug Modernization Act (FDAMA) and the 2002 Best Pharmaceuticals for Children Act (BPCA).[75,76] Thus, while the 2000 *Physicians Desk Reference* contained Food and Drug Administration (FDA)–approved pediatric dosing information for a minority of antihypertensive medications commonly used in children,[74] the 2004 Fourth Report[1] indicates that FDA-approved dosing information is now available for at least a dozen medications, including seven drugs for which pediatric trials have been conducted since 1999.

Experience in adults indicates that although some hypertensive patients may experience a decline in BP without treatment, in most it will likely persist and even progress over time.[77] This implies that once a hypertensive patient is started on medication, he or she is likely to remain on medication for the rest of his or her life. This is readily accepted for adults given the known long-term adverse consequences of untreated or undertreated hypertension.[2,79] However, since the long-term consequences of untreated hypertension in an asymptomatic, otherwise healthy child or adolescent remain unknown,[50] the decision to prescribe antihypertensive medications in a child or adolescent should not be made lightly. Furthermore, even the open-label extensions to pediatric clinical trials of antihypertensive medications will be insufficient to fully elucidate the long-term effects of antihypertensive medications on the growth and development of children. Therefore, a clear-cut indication for initiating pharmacologic therapy should be determined before a prescription is written.

Indications for use of antihypertensive medications in children and adolescents are listed in Box 52–1. These have been recommended by consensus organizations[1] because pharmacologic reduction of BP for hypertensive children who fall into one of these categories is likely to result in health benefit. This is especially true for children with secondary hypertension and diabetes, in whom the underlying/accompanying condition will probably be benefited by BP reduction. Not to be overlooked are children who fail a trial of nonpharmacologic measures; no matter whether the child's lifestyle has successfully been changed, if their BP remains persistently elevated, then pharmacologic treatment should be initiated. Since the long-term heath consequences (both good and bad) of using antihypertensive medications in childhood remain unknown, it is of paramount importance to ensure that there will be a potential health benefit before a prescription is written.

In hypertensive adults, recommendations for which antihypertensive medication to prescribe are based on the Antihypertensive and Lipid-Lowering Treatment to Prevent Heart Attack Trial (ALLHAT) and similar large-scale studies of hypertension treatment.[2,79] Many of these studies have compared the effects of various classes of antihypertensive agents on cardiovascular endpoints such as myocardial infarction and stroke. Since these events are exceedingly rare in the pediatric age group, it is unlikely that comparable studies will ever be conducted in children. Given this, the choice of

---

Box 52–1

Indications for Antihypertensive Medications in Children and Adolescents

Stage 2 hypertension
Symptomatic hypertension
Secondary hypertension
Hypertensive target-organ damage
Type 1 or 2 diabetes
Persistent hypertension despite nonpharmacologic measures

initial antihypertensive agent for use in children still remains up to the preference of the individual practitioner.

Diuretics and beta-adrenergic blockers, which were recommended as initial therapy in the First and Second Task Force Reports,[80,81] have a long track record of use in hypertensive children and are still appropriate choices. Newer classes of agents, including ACE inhibitors, calcium channel blockers, and angiotensin receptor blockers, have been shown to be safe and well tolerated (at least for short-term use) in hypertensive children in recent industry-sponsored trials.[82–86] A recent survey of current prescribing practices of North American pediatric nephrologists has demonstrated that these newer agents, particularly calcium channel blockers and ACE inhibitors, have become the most widely used initial agents in the pediatric age group, with diuretics and beta-adrenergic blockers being primarily used as add-on therapy when a second or third agent is required.[43] Current dosing recommendations for oral antihypertensive agents are given in Table 52–6.

Specific classes of antihypertensive medications should be prescribed in certain hypertensive children and adolescents with specific underlying or concurrent medical conditions. The best example of this would be the use of ACE inhibitors or angiotensin receptor antagonists in children with diabetes or proteinuric renal diseases, something that is already being done by many physicians who treat hypertensive children.[43] This parallels the approach outlined in the seventh report of the Joint National Committee on the Prevention, Detection, Evaluation, and Treatment of High Blood Pressure (JNC-7), which recommends that specific classes of antihypertensive agents be used in adults if compelling indications are present,[2] and is consistent with

RECOMMENDED DOSES FOR SELECTED ANTIHYPERTENSIVE AGENTS FOR USE IN HYPERTENSIVE CHILDREN AND ADOLESCENTS					
Class	Drug	Starting Dose	Interval	Maximum Dose[a]	Adverse Effects/Other Comments
Angiotensin-converting enzyme (ACE) inhibitors	Benazepril[b]	0.2 mg/kg/day up to 10 mg/day	QD	0.6 mg/kg/day up to 40 mg QD	1. Monitor serum chemistries shortly after initiating therapy and periodically thereafter.
	Captopril[b]	0.3–0.5 mg/kg/dose	BID–TID	6 mg/kg/day up to 450 mg/day	2. Contraindicated in patients with bilateral RAS or RAS in single kidney, and in pregnancy.
	Enalapril[b]	0.08 mg/kg/day	QD	0.6 mg/kg/day up to 40 mg/day	3. May cause cough and angioedema.
	Fosinopril	0.1 mg/kg/day up to 10 mg/day	QD	0.6 mg/kg/day up to 40 mg/day	4. Many ACEI are available in combination preparations containing a diuretic.
	Lisinopril[b]	0.07 mg/kg/day up to 5 mg/day	QD	0.6 mg/kg/day up to 40 mg/day	
	Quinapril	5–10 mg/day	QD	80 mg/day	
Angiotensin-receptor blockers	Candesartan	4 mg/day	QD	32 mg QD	1. Monitor serum chemistries shortly after initiating therapy and periodically thereafter.
	Irbesartan	75–150 mg/day	QD	300 mg/day	2. Contraindicated in patients with bilateral RAS or RAS in single kidney, and in pregnancy.
	Losartan[b]	0.75 mg/kg/day up to 50 mg/day	QD	1.4 mg/kg/day up to 100 mg/day	3. Many ARB are available in combination preparations containing a diuretic.
α- and β-adrenergic antagonists	Labetalol[b]	2–3 mg/kg/day	BID	10–12 mg/kg/day up to 1.2 g/day	1. Contraindicated in asthma, heart failure (labetalol only), and diabetes.
	Carvedilol	0.1 mg/kg/dose up to 12.5 mg BID	BID	0.5 mg/kg/dose up to 25 mg BID	2. Heart rate is dose-limiting. 3. May impair athletic performance. 4. Carvedilol beneficial in heart failure.
β-adrenergic antagonists	Atenolol	0.5–1 mg/kg/day	QD–BID	2 mg/kg/day up to 100 mg/day	1. Propranolol contraindicated in asthma and heart failure.
	Bisoprolol/HCTZ	2.5/6.25 mg/day	QD	10/6.25 mg qd	2. Heart rate is dose-limiting.
	Metoprolol	1–2 mg/kg/day	BID	6 mg/kg/day up to 200 mg/day	3. May impair athletic performance. 4. Should not be used in insulin-dependent diabetics.
	Propranolol	1 mg/kg/day	BID–TID	16 mg/kg/day up to 640 mg/day	5. Sustained-release formulations of propranolol and metoprolol are available that are dosed once daily.

RECOMMENDED DOSES FOR SELECTED ANTIHYPERTENSIVE AGENTS FOR USE IN HYPERTENSIVE CHILDREN AND ADOLESCENTS—cont'd

Class	Drug	Starting Dose	Interval	Maximum Dose[a]	Adverse Effects/Other Comments
Calcium channel blockers	Amlodipine[b]	0.06 mg/kg/day	QD	0.6 mg/kg/day up to 10 mg/day	1. Felodipine and extended-release nifedipine tablets must be swallowed whole.
	Felodipine	2.5 mg/day	QD	10 mg/day	2. May cause mild tachycardia, flushing, and headache.
	Isradipine[b]	0.05–0.15 mg/kg/dose	TID–QID	0.8 mg/kg/day up to 20 mg/day	3. Gingival hyperplasia may occur with prolonged use, especially in combination with calcineurin inhibitors.
	Extended-release nifedipine	0.25–0.5 mg/kg/day	QD–BID	3 mg/kg/day up to 120 mg/day	
Central α-agonists	Clonidine[b]	5–10 mcg/kg/day	BID–TID	25 mcg/kg/day up to 0.9 mg/day	1. May cause dry mouth and sedation.
	Methyldopa[b]	5 mg/kg/day	BID–QID	40 mg/kg/day up to 3 g/day	2. Clonidine also available in a transdermal preparation.
					3. Sudden withdrawal of clonidine may cause severe rebound hypertension.
Diuretics	Amiloride	5–10 mg/day	QD	20 mg/day	1. Electrolytes should be monitored shortly after initiating therapy and periodically thereafter.
	Chlorothiazide	10 mg/kg/day	BID	20 mg/kg/day up to 1.0 gram/day	2. All diuretics are best used as add-on therapy in combination with other classes of antihypertensives.
	Chlorthalidone	0.3 mg/kg/day	QD	2 mg/kg/day up to 50 mg/day	
	Furosemide	0.5–2.0 mg/kg/dose	QD–BID	6 mg/kg/day	
	HCTZ	0.5–1 mg/kg/day	QD	3 mg/kg/day up to 50 mg/day	3. Chlorothiazide and furosemide are commercially available as suspensions.
	Spironolactone[b]	1 mg/kg/day	QD–BID	3.3 mg/kg/day up to 100 mg/day	
	Triamterene	1–2 mg/kg/day	BID	3–4 mg/kg/day up to 300 mg/day	
Peripheral α-antagonists	Doxazosin	1 mg/day	QD	4 mg/day	1. All may cause first-dose hypotension.
	Prazosin	0.05–0.1 mg/kg/day	TID	0.5 mg/kg/day	
	Terazosin	1 mg/day	QD	20 mg/day	
Vasodilators	Hydralazine	0.25 mg/kg/dose	TID–QID	7.5 mg/kg/day up to 200 mg/day	1. Tachycardia and fluid retention are common side effects.
	Minoxidil	0.1–0.2 mg/kg/day	BID–TID	1 mg/kg/day up to 50 mg/day	2. Hydralazine can cause a lupus-like syndrome in slow acetylators.
					3. Prolonged use of minoxidil can cause hypertrichosis.

ACEI, angiotensin converting enzyme inhibitor; ARB, angiotensin receptor blocker; BID, twice daily; HCTZ, hydrochlorothiazide; QD, once daily; QID, four times daily; RAS, renal artery stenosis; TID, three times daily.
[a]The maximum recommended adult dose should never be exceeded.
[b]Information on preparation of a stable extemporaneous suspension is available for these agents.

Table 52–6. Recommended Doses for Selected Antihypertensive Agents for Use in Hypertensive Children and Adolescents

prior expert recommendations that the therapy of childhood hypertension should be tailored to the specific clinical status of the individual patient.[87]

For children with uncomplicated primary hypertension and no hypertensive target-organ damage, goal BP should be less than 95th percentile for age, gender, and height, whereas for children with secondary hypertension, diabetes, or hypertensive target-organ damage, goal BP should be less than 90th percentile for age, gender, and height.[1] These treatment goals are akin to current recommendations for therapy of hypertension in adults,[2] which are designed to achieve lower BPs in certain groups of patients in order to slow the progression of underlying renal disease, or reverse hypertensive target-organ damage.

Long-term issues in hypertension treatment

As in adults, treatment of hypertension in children and adolescents is a long-term proposition. Initially, medication doses should be adjusted until the desired goal BP is reached. After that, there should be ongoing monitoring of BP, surveillance for medication side effects, periodic moni-

RECOMMENDED DOSES FOR ANTIHYPERTENSIVE AGENTS USED FOR HYPERTENSIVE EMERGENCIES AND URGENCIES IN CHILDREN AND ADOLESCENTS				
Drug	Class	Dose	Route	Comments
Clonidine	Central α-agonist	0.05–0.1 mg/dose, may be repeated up to 0.8 mg total dose	Oral	Side effects include dry mouth and sedation.
Enalaprilat	ACE inhibitor	0.05–0.10 mg/kg/dose up to 1.25 mg/dose	IV bolus	May cause prolonged hypotension and acute renal failure.
Esmolol	β-blocker	100–500 mcg/kg/min	IV infusion	Very short-acting. May cause profound bradycardia.
Fenoldopam	Dopamine receptor agonist	0.2–0.8 mcg/kg/min	IV infusion	Less potent than nicardipine but may improve renal bloodflow in patients with acute renal failure.
Hydralazine	Vasodilator	0.2–0.6 mg/kg/dose	IV, IM	Should be given q 4 hours when given IV bolus.
Isradipine	Calcium channel blocker	0.05–0.1 mg/kg/dose	Oral	Stable suspension can be compounded.
Labetalol	α- and β-blocker	Bolus: 0.20–1.0 mg/kg/dose up to 40 mg/dose Infusion: 0.25–3.0 mg/kg/hr	IV bolus or infusion	Asthma and overt heart failure are relative contraindications.
Minoxidil	Vasodilator	0.1–0.2 mg/kg/dose	Oral	This drug is long-acting; most potent form is oral vasodilator.
Nicardipine	Calcium channel blocker	1–4 mcg/kg/min	IV infusion	May cause reflex tachycardia.
Sodium nitroprusside	Vasodilator	0.5–10 mcg/kg/min	IV infusion	Monitor cyanide levels with prolonged (>72 hours) use or in renal failure; or co-administer with sodium thiosulfate.

ACE, angiotensin-converting enzyme; IM, intramuscular; IV, intravenous.

Table 52–7. Recommended Doses for Antihypertensive Agents Used for Hypertensive Emergencies and Urgencies in Children and Adolescents

INTRAVENOUS ANTIHYPERTENSIVES FOR SEVERE HYPERTENSION IN INFANTS			
Drug	Dose/Interval	Route	Comments
Alpha- and Beta-Adrenergic Blocker			
Labetalol	Bolus: 0.2–1.0 mg/kg/dose, q 6–12 hours Infusion: 0.25–3.0 mg/kg/hr	Bolus injection or continuous infusion	Heart failure and lung disease are relative contraindications.
Angiotensin-Converting Enzyme Inhibitor			
Enalaprilat	15 ± 5 mcg/kg/dose, q 8–24 hours	Bolus injection	*Use with extreme caution.* May cause prolonged hypotension and acute renal insufficiency.
Beta-Adrenergic Blocker			
Esmolol	100–500 mcg/kg/min	Continuous infusion	Very short-acting; continuous infusion is necessary.
Calcium Channel Blocker			
Nicardipine	0.5–4 mcg/kg/min	Continuous infusion	May cause reflex tachycardia.
Vasodilators			
Hydralazine	0.15–0.6 mg/kg/dose q 4 hours	Bolus injection	Tachycardia is a common side effect. May also be given intramuscularly.
Sodium nitroprusside	0.3–10 mcg/kg/min	Continuous infusion	Thiocyanate toxicity can occur with prolonged (>72 hours) use or in renal failure.

Table 52–8. Intravenous Antihypertensives for Severe Hypertension in Infants

toring of electrolytes (in children treated with angiotensin-converting enzyme inhibitors or diuretics), counseling regarding other cardiovascular risk factors, and continued emphasis on nonpharmacologic measures, particularly weight loss and exercise. Home BP measurement has been found to be helpful in ensuring that BP control has been achieved.[43] Alternatively, repeat ambulatory BP monitoring may need to be performed in some patients, particularly if "resistant hypertension" appears to be present based on office BP measurements.[88] Hypertensive target organ damage such as left ventricular hypertrophy, if present, should be reassessed periodically.[1]

Withdrawal of antihypertensive medications may be considered in selected children and adolescents with hypertension. This involves an attempt at gradual reduction in medication after an extended course of good BP control, with the eventual goal of completely discontinuing drug therapy. Although no comparable studies have been performed in children, experience in adults suggests that a significant percentage of patients may remain normotensive, at least in the short-term, after withdrawal of active treatment.[77] Children with uncomplicated primary hypertension, especially obese adolescents who have successfully lost weight and remain compliant with recommendations for dietary modification and exercise, are probably the best candidates for medication withdrawal. These children should receive continued BP monitoring after drug therapy is withdrawn, as well as continued nonpharmacologic treatment.

HYPERTENSIVE EMERGENCIES AND URGENCIES IN CHILDREN AND ADOLESCENTS

The pathophysiology, management, and outcome of severe hypertension in children and adolescents have been comprehensively reviewed elsewhere.[89] Many aspects are similar to hypertensive emergencies and urgencies in adults as covered in Chapter 63. However, a few unique aspects merit consideration.

Underlying conditions that may produce a hypertensive emergency or urgency in a child or adolescent may

ORAL ANTIHYPERTENSIVES FOR CHRONIC HYPERTENSION IN INFANTS			
Drug	**Dose**	**Frequency**	**Comments**
Aldosterone Antagonist			
Spironolactone	0.5–1.5 mg/kg/dose Maximum 3.3 mg/kg/day	BID	This drug is potassium "sparing"; monitor electrolytes. It takes several days to achieve maximum effectiveness.
Angiotensin-Converting Enzyme Inhibitors			
Captopril	<3 months: 0.01–0.5 mg/kg/dose Maximum 2 mg/kg/day >3 months: 0.15–0.3 mg/kg/dose Maximum 6 mg/kg/day	TID	First dose in pre-term infants may cause rapid drop in BP; monitor serum creatinine and potassium.
Enalapril	0.08–0.6 mg/kg/day	QD or BID	Monitor serum creatinine and potassium.
Alpha- and Beta-Adrenergic Blocker			
Labetalol	0.5–1.0 mg/kg/dose Maximum 10 mg/kg/day	BID or TID	Monitor heart rate; avoid in infants with BPD or congestive heart failure.
Beta-Adrenergic Blocker			
Propranolol	0.5–1.0 mg/kg/dose Maximum 8–10 mg/kg/day	TID	Maximal dose depends on heart rate; avoid in infants with BPD or congestive heart failure.
Calcium Channel Blocker			
Amlodipine	0.05–0.17 mg/kg/dose Maximum 0.6 mg/kg/day	QD or BID	This drug is less likely to cause sudden hypotension than isradipine.
Isradipine	0.05–0.15 mg/kg/dose Maximum 0.8 mg/kg/day	TID or QID	In suspension, drug may be compounded; useful for both acute and chronic hypertension.
Central Alpha Agonist			
Clonidine	5–10 mcg/kg/day Maximum 25 mcg/kg/day	BID or TID	Rebound hypertension may occur with abrupt discontinuation.
Thiazide Diuretics			
Chlorothiazide	10–30 mg/kg/day	BID	Monitor electrolytes; in patients with renal disease,
Hydrochlorothiazide	1–3 mg/kg/dose	QD	thiazides may precipitate azotemia.
Vasodilators			
Hydralazine	0.25–1.0 mg/kg/dose Maximum 7.5 mg/kg/day	TID or QID	Suspension only stable for 1 week; tachycardia and fluid retention are common side effects.
Minoxidil	0.1–0.2 mg/kg/dose	BID or TID	Usually reserved for refractory hypertension.

BID, twice daily; BPD, bronchopulmonary dysplasia; QD, once daily; QID, four times daily; RAS, renal artery stenosis; TID, three times daily.

Table 52–9. Oral Antihypertensives for Chronic Hypertension in Infants

include acute or chronic renal disease, organ transplantation, renal artery stenosis, or congenital renal disease such as autosomal recessive polycystic kidney disease. Hypertensive encephalopathy is frequent, particularly in younger children with severe hypertension, emphasizing the need for slow, controlled reduction in BP to prevent complications arising through loss of normal autoregulatory processes.[89,90] Less severe symptoms may include nausea, vomiting, or unusual irritability; since these are somewhat nonspecific, a high degree of clinical suspicion must be maintained when evaluating such children.

Although evidence-based recommendations are lacking, the usual goal in treatment of a hypertensive emergency is to reduce the BP by no more than 25% over the first 8 hours, with a gradual return to normal/goal BP over 24 to 48 hours.[89,90] Treatment of most hypertensive emergencies in children should begin with a continuous infusion of an intravenous antihypertensive, with nicardipine and labetalol finding the greatest popularity in many centers.[89,91] The dopamine receptor agonist fenoldopam has also been reported effective,[92] although it is less potent than alternative agents, particularly nicardipine. For many hypertensive urgencies, or if the child's symptoms permit, oral antihypertensive agents can be administered. Recommended doses for intravenous and oral drugs used to treat severe hypertension in children and adolescents can be found in Table 52–7.

HYPERTENSION IN INFANTS

Neonatal hypertension is a problem primarily confined to infants admitted to neonatal intensive care units. Overall, the incidence of neonatal hypertension is low—from 0.2% in healthy newborns to 0.7% to 2.5% in high-risk infants. Those with indwelling umbilical catheters and those with chronic lung disease are at greatest risk.[93] Moreover, many of these infants have acute hypertension that resolves as the underlying condition improves. Those requiring chronic treatment generally have underlying renal disorders or persistent lung disease. The differential diagnosis for neonatal hypertension covers a wide spectrum of conditions, many of which are acute and resolve after prompt intervention (Box 52–2).

Proper identification of infants with hypertension can be problematic due to problems with BP measurement in the nursery, and also due to changes in BP that occur with maturation, especially in pre-term infants.[94] This topic is complex and beyond the scope of this chapter; the interested reader should consult other sources for detailed discussion of these issues.[93,95] Evaluation of infants with elevated BP, on the other hand, is usually fairly straightforward, and should begin with a targeted physical exam looking for signs of underlying renal disease or other easily identifiable conditions, followed by appropriate laboratory and imaging studies. Renal ultrasonography is the most important imaging modality as it will uncover a variety of the possible causes of elevated BP (Box 52–2); other techniques such as nuclear scans and angiography should only be performed in selected cases.[96]

Box 52–2

Causes of Hypertension in Infants

Renovascular

Thromboembolism
Renal artery stenosis
Aortic coarctation
Renal venous thrombosis
Compression of renal artery
Idiopathic arterial calcification
Congenital rubella syndrome

Renal Parenchymal Disease
Congenital
ARPKD
ADPKD
Multicystic-dysplastic kidney disease
Tuberous sclerosis
Ureteropelvic junction obstruction
Acquired
Acute tubular necrosis
Cortical necrosis
Hemolytic-uremic syndrome
Obstruction (stones, tumors)

Pulmonary

Bronchopulmonary dysplasia
Pneumothorax

Genetic
Single-gene disorders
Glucocorticoid-remediable aldosteronism
Liddle syndrome
Pseudohypoaldosteronism type II
Malformation syndromes
Williams syndrome
Turner syndrome
Neurofibromatosis
Cockayne syndrome

Endocrine

Congenital adrenal hyperplasia
Hyperaldosteronism
Hyperthyroidism

Medications/Intoxications
Infant
Dexamethasone, corticosteroids
Adrenergic agents
Vitamin D intoxication
Theophylline, aminophylline
Caffeine
Pancuronium
Phenylephrine eye drops
Maternal
Cocaine
Heroin

Neoplasia

Wilms' tumor
Mesoblastic nephroma
Neuroblastoma

Neurologic

Pain
Intracranial hypertension
Seizures
Opiate withdrawal

Box 52–2—cont'd

Causes of Hypertension in Infants—cont'd

Miscellaneous

Fluid overload
Closure of abdominal wall defect
Adrenal hemorrhage
Hypercalcemia
Traction
Birth asphyxia
Idiopathic

ADPKD, autosomal dominant polycystic kidney disease;
ARPKD, autosomal recessive polycystic kidney disease.

While an overriding priority in hypertensive neonates would seem to be quick, effective, and safe BP reduction, this is difficult because data regarding the use of antihypertensive agents in neonates are inadequate. Therefore, most treatment recommendations are empiric and based on expert opinion. Agents currently in use for acute, severe hypertension in infants are listed in Table 52–8, and oral agents for less severe neonatal hypertension are listed in Table 52–9. The management of neonatal hypertension requires experience and knowledge regarding the unique characteristics of neonatal renal physiology. For example, ACE inhibitors should be used with extreme caution in this age group due to the dependence of renal development on an intact renin-angiotensin system. The intravenous ACE inhibitor enalaprilat in particular may cause severe hypotension and persistent oliguric renal failure.

SUMMARY

Hypertension is an important pediatric problem that is growing in importance as a result of the childhood obesity epidemic. Cardiovascular risk factors, including hypertension, should be identified in children so that adult cardiovascular disease may be prevented. Evaluation and treatment of hypertension in children and adolescents should be guided by the likely etiology and should include evaluation for hypertensive target-organ damage and coexisting risk factors. Although the amount of information on antihypertensive agents for children and adolescents has increased, significant deficits remain, including data in neonates and data regarding the long-term risks and benefits of these drugs in this age group. Further research is needed to better define the optimal approach to the management of hypertensive children and adolescents.

REFERENCES

1. National High Blood Pressure Education Program Working Group on High Blood Pressure in Children and Adolescents. The Fourth Report on the Diagnosis, Evaluation, and Treatment of High Blood Pressure in Children and Adolescents. National Heart, Lung, and Blood Institute, Bethesda, Maryland. *Pediatrics* 2004;114:555–76.
2. Chobanian AV, Bakris GL, Black HR, et al. The seventh report of the Joint National Committee on Prevention, Detection, Evaluation, and Treatment of High Blood Pressure: the JNC 7 report. *Hypertension* 2003;42:1206–52.
3. Task Force on Blood Pressure Control in Children. Report of the Second Task Force on Blood Pressure Control in Children—1987. National Heart, Lung, and Blood Institute, Bethesda, Maryland. *Pediatrics* 1987;79:1–25.
4. Fixler DE, Laird WP, Fitzgerald V, et al. Hypertension screening in schools: results of the Dallas study. *Pediatrics* 1979;64:579–83.
5. Sinaiko AR, Gomez-Marion O, Prineas RJ. Prevalence of "significant" hypertension in junior high school-aged children: the Children and Adolescent Blood Pressure Program. *J Pediatr* 1989;114(4 Pt 1):664–9.
6. National High Blood Pressure Education Program Working Group. Update on the 1987 Task Force Report on High Blood Pressure in Children and Adolescents: a working group report from the National High Blood Pressure Education Program. *Pediatrics* 1996;98:649–58.
7. Adrogue HE, Sinaiko AR. Prevalence of hypertension in junior high school-aged children: effect of new recommendations in the 1996 Updated Task Force Report. *Am J Hypertens* 2001; 14(5 Pt 1):412–4.
8. Lauer RM, Connor WE, Leaverton PE, et al. Coronary heart disease risk factors in school children: the Muscatine study. *J Pediatr* 1975;86:697–706.
9. Silverberg DS, Nostrand CV, Juchli B, et al. Screening for hypertension in a high school population. *CMAJ* 1975;113:103–8.
10. O'Quin M, Sharma BB, Miller KA, Tomsovic JP. Adolescent blood pressure survey: Tulsa, Oklahoma, 1987 to 1989. *South Med J* 1992;85:487–90.
11. Soyannwo MAO, Gadallah M, Kurashi NY et al. Studies on preventative nephrology: Systemic hypertension in the pediatric and adolescent population of Gassim, Saudi Arabia. *Ann Saudi Med* 1997;17:47–52.
12. Sorof JM, Lai D, Turner J, et al. Overweight, ethnicity, and the prevalence of hypertension in school-aged children. *Pediatrics* 2004;113:475–82.
13. Sorof JM, Poffenbarger T, Franco K, et al. Isolated systolic hypertension, obesity, and hyperkinetic hemodynamic states in children. *J Pediatr* 2002; 140:660–6.
14. Ogden CL, Flegal KM, Carroll MD, Johnson CL. Prevalence and trends in overweight among US children and adolescents, 1999–2000. *JAMA* 2002;288:1728–32.
15. Feld LG, ed. *Hypertension in Children: A Practical Approach*. Boston, MA: Butterworth-Heinemann, 1997.
16. Portman RJ, Sorof JM, Ingelfinger JR, eds. *Pediatric Hypertension*. Totowa, NJ: Humana Press, 2004.
17. Wyszynska T, Cichocka E, Wieteska-Klimczak A, et al. A single center experience with 1025 children with hypertension. *Acta Paediatr* 1992; 81:244–6.
18. Luepker RV, Jacobs DR, Prineas RJ, Sinaiko AR. Secular trends of blood pressure and body size in a multi-ethnic adolescent population: 1986 to 1996. *J Pediatr* 1999;134:668–74.
19. Munger RG, Prineas RJ, Gomez-Marin O. Persistent elevation of blood pressure among children with a family history of hypertension: the Minneapolis children's blood pressure study. *J Hypertens* 1988;6:647–53.
20. Buonomo E, Pasquarella A, Palombi L. Blood pressure and anthropometry in parents and children of a southern Italian village. *J Hum Hypertens* 1996;10(Suppl 3):S77–9.
21. Daniels SR. Obesity in the pediatric patient: cardiovascular complications. *Prog Pediatr Cardiol* 2001;12:161–7.
22. Flynn JT, Alderman MH. Characteristics of children with primary hypertension seen at a referral center. *Pediatr Nephrol* 2005;20:961–6.
23. Sorof JM, Turner J, Martin DS, et al. Cardiovascular risk factors and sequelae in hypertensive children identified by referral versus school-based screening. *Hypertension* 2004;43:214–8.
24. Laird WP, Fixler DE. Left ventricular hypertrophy in adolescents with elevated blood pressure: assessment by chest roentgenography, electrocardiography,

and echocardiography. *Pediatrics* 1981;67:255–9.

25. Hanevold C, Waller J, Daniels S, et al. The effects of obesity, gender, and ethnic group on left ventricular hypertrophy and geometry in hypertensive children: a collaborative study of the International Pediatric Hypertension Association. *Pediatrics* 2004;113:328–33.

26. Daniels SR, Loggie JM, Khoury P, Kimball TR. Left ventricular geometry and severe left ventricular hypertrophy in children and adolescents with essential hypertension. *Circulation* 1998;97:1907–11.

27. Koren MJ, Devereux RB. Mechanism, effects, and reversal of left ventricular hypertrophy in hypertension. *Curr Opin Nephrol Hypertens* 1993;2:87–95.

28. Daniels SR, Lipman MJ, Burke MJ, Loggie JM. Determinants of retinal vascular abnormalities in children and adolescents with essential hypertension. *J Hum Hypertens* 1993;7:223–8.

29. Daniels SR, Lipman MJ, Burke MJ, Loggie JM. The prevalence of retinal vascular abnormalities in children and adolescents with essential hypertension. *Am J Ophthalmol* 1991;111:205–8.

30. Sorof JM, Alexandrov AV, Garami Z, et al. Carotid ultrasonography for detection of vascular abnormalities in hypertensive children. *Pediatr Nephrol* 2003;18:1020–4.

31. Bots ML, Hofman A, de Jong PTVM, Grobbee DE. Common carotid intima-media thickness as an indicator of atherosclerosis at other sites of the carotid artery: the Rotterdam Study. *Ann Epidemiol* 1996;6:147–53.

32. Cuspidi C, Mancia G, Ambrosioni E, Pessina A, et al. Left ventricular and carotid structure in untreated, uncomplicated essential hypertension: results from the Assessment Prognostic Risk Observational Survey (APROS). *J Hum Hypertens* 2004;18:891–6.

33. Oren A, Vos LE, Uiterwaal CS, Gorissen WH, et al. Change in body mass index from adolescence to young adulthood and increased carotid intima-media thickness at 28 years of age: the Atherosclerosis Risk in Young Adults study. *Int J Obes Relat Metab Disord* 2003;27:1383–90.

34. Sorof JM, Alexandrov AV, Cardwell G, Portman RJ. Carotid artery intimal-medial thickness and left ventricular hypertrophy in children with elevated blood pressure. *Pediatrics* 2003; 111:61–6.

35. U.S. Renal Data System. *USRDS 2002 Annual Data Report: Atlas of End-Stage Renal Disease in the United States.* Bethesda, MD: National Institutes of Health, National Institute of Diabetes and Digestive and Kidney Diseases, 2002.

36. Emmes Corporation. *North American Pediatric Renal Transplant Cooperative Study 2004 Annual Report.* Potomac, MD: Emmes Corporation, 2005.

37. Mazzucchi A, Mutti A, Poletti A, et al. Neuropsychological deficits in arterial hypertension. *Acta Neurol Scand* 1986;73:619–27.

38. Elias ME, Wolf PA, D'Agostino RB, et al. Untreated blood pressure level is inversely related to cognitive functioning: the Framingham study. *Am J Epidemiol* 1993;138:353–64.

39. Lande MB, Kaczorowski JM, Auinger P, et al. Elevated blood pressure and decreased cognitive function among school-age children and adolescents in the United States. *J Pediatr* 2003: 143:720–4.

40. Lever AF, Harrap SB. Essential hypertension: a disorder of growth with origins in childhood? *J Hypertension* 1992;10:101–20.

41. Lauer RM, Clarke WR. Childhood risk factors for adult blood pressure: the Muscatine Study. *Pediatrics* 1989;84:633–41.

42. Pickering TG, Hall JE, Appel LJ et al. Recommendations for blood pressure measurement in humans and experimental animals. Part 1: Blood pressure measurement in humans. A statement for professionals from the subcommittee of professional and public education of the American Heart Association Council on High Blood Pressure Research. *Hypertension* 2005;45:142–61.

43. WoronIecki RP, Flynn JT. How are hypertensive children evaluated and managed? A survey of North American pediatric nephrologists. *Pediatr Nephrol* 2005;20:791–7.

44. Kaufmann MA, Pargger H, Drop LJ. Oscillometric blood pressure measurements by different devices are not interchangeable. *Anesth Analg* 1996;82:377–81.

45. Park MK, Menard SW, Yuan C. Comparison of auscultatory and oscillometric blood pressures. *Arch Pediatr Adolesc Med* 2001;155:50–3.

46. Flynn JT. Evaluation and management of hypertension in childhood. *Prog Pediatr Cardiol* 2001;12:177–88.

47. Gidding SS. Relationships between blood pressure and lipids in childhood. *Pediatr Clin North Am* 1993;40:41–9.

48. Weiss R, Dziura J, Burgert TS, et al. Obesity and the metabolic syndrome in children and adolescents. *N Engl J Med* 2004;350:2362–74.

49. Berenson GS, Srinivasan SR, Bao W, et al. Association between multiple cardiovascular risk factors and atherosclerosis in children and young adults. *N Engl J Med* 1998;338:1650–6.

50. Kay JD, Sinaiko AR, Daniels SR. Pediatric hypertension. *Am Heart J* 2001;142:422–32.

51. Rocchini AP, Katch V, Anderson J, et al: Blood pressure in obese adolescents: effect of weight loss. *Pediatrics* 1988;82:16–23.

52. Figueroa-Colon R, Franklin FA, Lee JY, et al. Feasibility of a clinic-based hypocaloric dietary intervention implemented in a school setting for obese children. *Obes Res* 1996;4:419–29.

53. Williams CL, Hayman LL, Daniels SR, et al. Cardiovascular health in childhood: a statement for health professionals from the Committee on Atherosclerosis, Hypertension, and Obesity in the Young (AHOY) of the Council on Cardiovascular Disease in the Young, American Heart Association. *Circulation* 2002;106:143–60.

54. Reinehr T, Andler W. Changes in the atherogenic risk factor profile according to degree of weight loss. *Arch Dis Child* 2004;89:419–22.

55. Epstein LH, Myers MD, Raynor HA, et al. Treatment of pediatric obesity. *Pediatrics* 1998;101:554–70.

56. Togashi K, Masuda H, Rankinen T, et al. A 12-year follow-up study of treated obese children in Japan. *Int J Obes Relat Metab Disord* 2002;26:770–7.

57. Alpert BS. Exercise as a therapy to control hypertension in children. *Int J Sports Med* 2000;21(Suppl 2):S94–6.

58. Hagberg JM, Ehsani AA, Goldring D, et al. Effect of weight training on blood pressure and hemodynamics in hypertensive adolescents. *J Pediatr* 1984;104:147–51.

59. Alpert BS, Fox ME. Hypertension. In: Goldberg B, ed. *Sports and Exercise for Children with Chronic Health Conditions.* Champaign, IL: Human Kinetics, 1995:197–205.

60. Watts K, Jones TW, Davis EA, Green D. Exercise training in obese children and adolescents: current concepts. *Sports Med* 2005;35:375–92.

61. Ribeiro MM, Silva AG, Santos NS, et al. Diet and exercise training restore blood pressure and vasodilatory responses during physiological maneuvers in obese children. *Circulation* 2005;111:1915–23.

62. Falkner B, Michel S. Blood pressure response to sodium in children and adolescents. *Am J Clin Nutr* 1997;65(Suppl 2):618S–21S.

63. Chrysant GS, Bakir S, Oparil S. Dietary salt reduction in hypertension—what is the evidence and why is it still controversial? *Prog Cardiovasc Dis* 1999;42:23–38.

64. Hooper L, Bartlett C, Davey SG, Ebrahim S. Advice to reduce dietary salt for prevention of cardiovascular disease. *Cochrane Database Syst Rev* 2004;(1):CD003656.

65. Weinberger MH. Salt sensitivity of blood pressure in humans. *Hypertension* 1996;27:481–90.

66. Cutler JA. The effects of reducing sodium and increasing potassium intake for control of hypertension and improving health. *Clin Exp Hypertens* 1999;21:769–83.

67. Sinaiko AR, Gomez-Marin O, Prineas RJ. Effect of low sodium diet or potassium supplementation on adolescent blood pressure. *Hypertension* 1993;21:989–94.

68. Rocchini AP, Key J, Bondie D, et al. The effect of weight loss on the sensitivity of blood pressure to sodium in obese adolescents. *N Engl J Med* 1989;321:580–5.

69. Gillman MW, Oliveria SA, Moore LL, et al. Inverse association of dietary calcium with systolic blood pressure in young children. *JAMA* 1992;267:2340–3.

70. Mu JJ, Liu ZQ, Liu WM, et al. Reduction of blood pressure with calcium and potassium supplementation in children with salt sensitivity: a 2-year double-blinded placebo-controlled trial. *J Hum Hypertens* 2005;19:479–83.

71. Appel LJ, Moore TJ, Obarzanek E, et al. A clinical trial of the effects of dietary patterns on blood pressure. *N Engl J Med* 1997;336:1117–24.

72. Falkner B, Sherif K, Michel S, Kushner H. Dietary nutrients and blood pressure in urban minority adolescents at risk for hypertension. *Arch Pediatr Adolesc Med* 2000;154:918–22.

73. Kavey REW, Daniels SR, Lauer RM, et al. American Heart Association guidelines for primary prevention of atherosclerotic cardiovascular disease beginning in childhood. *Circulation* 2003;107:1562–6.

74. Flynn JT. Pediatric use of antihypertensive medications: much more to learn. *Curr Ther Res Clin Exp* 2001;62:314–28.

75. Wells TG. Trials of antihypertensive therapies in children. *Blood Press Monit* 1999;4:189–92.

76. Flynn JT. Successes and shortcomings of the FDA Modernization Act. *Am J Hypertens* 2003;16:889–91.

77. Kaplan NM. Primary hypertension: natural history and evaluation. In: Kaplan NM. *Kaplan's Clinical Hypertension*. 8th ed. Philadelphia: Lippincott Williams & Wilkins, 2002:136–75.

78. Klag MJ, Whelton PK, Randall BL, et al. Blood pressure and end-stage renal disease in men. *N Engl J Med* 1996;334:13–8.

79. ALLHAT Officers and Coordinators for the ALLHAT Collaborative Research Group. Major outcomes in high-risk hypertensive patients randomized to angiotensin-converting enzyme inhibitor or calcium channel blocker vs. diuretic: the Antihypertensive and Lipid-Lowering Treatment to Prevent Heart Attack Trial (ALLHAT). *JAMA* 2002;288:2981–97.

80. Blumenthal S, Epps RP, Heavenrich R, et al. Report of the task force on blood pressure control in children. *Pediatrics* 1977;59(Suppl 2):I–II, 797–820.

81. Task Force on Blood Pressure Control in Children. Report of the Second Task Force on Blood Pressure Control in Children—1987. National Heart, Lung, and Blood Institute, Bethesda, Maryland. *Pediatrics* 1987;79:1–25.

82. Soffer B, Zhang Z, Miller K, et al. A double-blind, placebo-controlled, dose-response study of the effectiveness and safety of lisinopril for children with hypertension. *Am J Hypertens* 2003;16:795–800.

83. Trachtman H, Frank R, Mahan JD, et al. Clinical trial of extended-release felodipine in pediatric essential hypertension. *Pediatr Nephrol* 2003;18:548–53.

84. Li JS, Berezny K, Kilaru R, et al. Is the extrapolated adult dose of fosinopril safe and effective in treating hypertensive children? *Hypertension* 2004;44:289–93.

85. Flynn JT, Newburger JW, Daniels SR, et al. A randomized, placebo-controlled trial of amlodipine in children with hypertension. *J Pediatr* 2004;145:353–9.

86. Shahinfar S, Cano F, Soffer BA, et al. A double-blind, dose–response study of losartan in hypertensive children. *Am J Hypertens* 2005;18:183–90.

87. Wells T, Stowe C. An approach to the use of antihypertensive drugs in children and adolescents. *Curr Ther Res Clin Exp* 2001;62:329–50.

88. Flynn JT. Value of repeat ambulatory blood pressure monitoring in children with hypertension. *Am J Hypertens* 2002;15(4, Pt 2):205A (abstract).

89. Adelman RD. Management of hypertensive emergencies. In: Portman R, Sorof J, Ingelfinger J, eds. *Pediatric Hypertension*. Totowa, NJ: Humana Press, 2004:457–70.

90. Deal JE, Barratt TM, Dillon MJ. Management of hypertensive emergencies. *Arch Dis Child* 1992;67:1089–92.

91. Flynn, JT, Mottes TA, Brophy PB, et al. Intravenous nicardipine for treatment of severe hypertension in children. *J Pediatr* 2001;139:38–43.

92. Strauser LM, Pruitt RD, Tobias JD. Initial experience with fenoldopam in children. *Am J Ther* 1999;6:283–8.

93. Flynn JT. Neonatal hypertension. In: Portman R, Sorof J, Ingelfinger J, eds. *Pediatric Hypertension*. Totowa, NJ: Humana Press, 2004:351–70.

94. Zubrow AB, Hulman S, Kushner H, et al. Determinants of blood pressure in infants admitted to neonatal intensive care units: a prospective multicenter study. *J Perinatol* 1995;15(6):470–9.

95. Nafday SM, Brion LP, Benchimol C, et al. Renal disease. In: MacDonald MG, Seshia MMK, Mullett MD, eds. *Neonatology: Pathophysiology and Management of the Newborn*. 6th ed. Philadelphia: Lippincott Williams & Wilkins, 2005:981–1065.

96. Roth CG, Spottswood SE, Chan JC, Roth KS. Evaluation of the hypertensive infant: a rational approach to diagnosis. *Radiol Clin North Am* 2003;41:931–44.

Chapter

53 Hypertension in the Elderly

Stanley S. Franklin

Key Findings

- The elderly, defined as 65 years of age and older, have a 90% lifetime risk of developing hypertension.

- Isolated systolic hypertension (ISH), once considered only an inconsequential part of the aging process, has become the predominant form of hypertension in the elderly.

- ISH—wide pulse pressure hypertension by definition—is a surrogate risk marker for increased arterial stiffness.

- ISH in the elderly is an independent risk factor for the development of coronary heart disease, heart failure, stroke, dementia, peripheral vascular disease, and renal failure.

Clinical Implications

- There is overwhelming evidence that effective pharmacologic treatment of both systolic–diastolic hypertension and ISH reduces cardiovascular events in the elderly.

- Treatment benefits of hypertension are greater in the old than in the young, but paradoxically, ISH in the elderly has the lowest rates of control; this occurs because ISH in the old is more difficult to treat to goal than diastolic hypertension in the young.

- The barriers to control of hypertension in the elderly can be overcome in part by an aggressive polytherapeutic approach to management that includes the use of a diuretic.

Approximately 65 million individuals in the United States and 1 billion worldwide are affected by hypertension.[1] With the aging of the population and the advent of effective antihypertensive therapy, there has been a shift toward a more slowly evolving form of hypertension that is predominately systolic in nature and affects middle-aged and older persons (Figure 53–1).[2] Indeed, the elderly, defined as persons 65 years of age and older, represent the fastest growing segment of the United States population with a 90% lifetime risk of developing hypertension.[3]

An age-associated rise in systolic blood pressure (SBP), occurring as a consequence of increased arterial stiffness, was once considered an inconsequential part of the aging process. Hypertension was largely defined using only the criterion of elevated diastolic blood pressure (DBP) until the 1990s. This slowly rising SBP with aging, out of proportion to the rise in DBP, is referred to as *isolated*

systolic hypertension (ISH). Previously, ISH was defined as an SBP ≥160 mmHg and a diastolic blood pressure (DBP) of <95 or <90 mmHg. With the recognition of its true cardiovascular risk, ISH was redefined as an SBP ≥140 and DBP <90 mmHg. Elderly individuals with ISH have at least a twofold increase in risk for cardiovascular disease events compared with younger individuals with systolic–diastolic hypertension. ISH is frequently associated with coronary heart disease (CHD), thrombotic and hemorrhagic stroke, dementia, peripheral vascular disease, and slowly progressive heart and renal failure; it has become the most common and the most difficult form of hypertension to treat successfully and hence a public health problem of major proportion. The purpose of this chapter is to provide a better understanding of hypertension in the elderly and how to treat it effectively.

EPIDEMIOLOGY

The U.S. Fourth National Health and Nutrition Examination Survey[4] (NHANES) recently showed an overall prevalence of hypertension (≥140 mmHg SBP or ≥90 mmHg DBP, or on antihypertensive medication) of 28.7% in 1999–2000, which varied from 7.2% in those aged 18 to 39 to 65.4% in those aged 60 and over, and which was greater in women (30.1%) than in men (27.1%). Noteworthy is the fact that since 1988–1991 the prevalence of hypertension has increased significantly in women and in all age groups, although most dramatically in those aged 60 and over who experienced an increase in prevalence from 57.9% in 1988–1991 to 65.4% in 1999–2000. Moreover, in the United States, prevalence of hypertension in the elderly is greatest among non-Hispanic blacks and lowest among Mexican Americans.[4] Compared to the United States, the prevalence of hypertension is similar in Canada, but is markedly higher in European countries (44% overall), being as high as 55% in Germany.[5]

ANATOMY AND PATHOLOGY

The elastic behavior of the arterial wall of the central blood vessels–the thoracic aorta and its branches–are profoundly affected by aging.[6,7] This process depends primarily on the composition and arrangement of the materials that make up the media of the arterial tree. In the media of the thoracic aorta and its immediate branches are large attachments of elastic lamellae to smooth muscle cells, constituting the contractile-elastic unit and

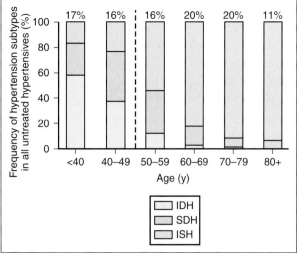

Figure 53–1. Frequency distribution of untreated hypertensive individuals by age and hypertension subtype. Numbers at the tops of bars represent the overall percentage distribution of all subtypes of untreated hypertension in the age group (National Health and Nutrition Examination Survey III [NHANES III], 1988 to 1994). IDH, isolated diastolic hypertension (SBP ≤140 mm Hg and DBP >90 mm Hg); ISH, isolated systolic hypertension (SBP >140 mm Hg and DBP ≤90 mm Hg); SDH, systolic–diastolic hypertension (SBP ≥140 mm Hg and DBP ≥90 mm Hg). (Adapted from Franklin SS, Jacobs MJ, Wong ND, et al. *Hypertension* 2001;37:869–74.)

arranged in an alternating oblique pattern, that exert maximum force in a circumferential direction. This arrangement is important for the balance of normal changes in intraluminal pressure and tension that occur during systole and diastole. The medial fibrous elements of the thoracic aorta contain a predominance of elastin over collagen, but as one proceeds distally along the arterial tree there is a rapid reversal favoring collagen over elastin in the peripheral, largely muscular arteries. Thus, the thoracic aorta and its immediate branches (such as carotid arteries) show maximum elasticity while more distal vessels become progressively stiffer.

Hypertension can produce arterial stiffness by both functional and structural mechanisms.[6,7] With the development of hypertension and increased distending pressure, the load-bearing elastic lamellae stretch and become stiffer on a functional basis. There are also longstanding struc-

tural changes with aging that cause increased stiffness of the thoracic aorta and its branches, but spare the more peripheral muscular arteries. Elastin, with a half-life of 40 years, is one of the most stable proteins in the body. Despite this stability, fatigue of elastin fibers and lamellae can occur by the sixth decade of life from the accumulated cyclic stress of more than 2 billion aorta expansions during ventricular contraction. Longstanding cyclic stress in the media of elastic-containing arteries produces fatigue and eventual fracturing of elastin along with structural changes of the extracellular matrix that include proliferation of collagen and deposition of calcium. This degenerative process, termed arteriosclerosis, is the pathologic process that results in increased central elastic arterial stiffness and the development of ISH in older age groups. Furthermore, hypertension left untreated may accelerate the rate of development of elastic artery stiffness; this, in turn, can perpetuate a vicious cycle of accelerated hypertension and further increases in stiffness.[6-8] Similarly, other disease processes such as type 1 and type 2 diabetes, obesity, hypercholesterolemia, generalized atherosclerosis, smoking, and chronic renal failure, can accelerate aging of central elastic arteries with earlier development of arterial stiffness and ISH.[6,7]

PATHOPHYSIOLOGY

Pulse pressure (PP) is determined not only by arterial stiffness, but also by stroke volume and to a lesser extent by the ejection rate of the left ventricle. In contrast, mean arterial pressure (MAP) is determined by cardiac output and total peripheral resistance. By definition, ISH is characterized by an increase in PP, but not necessarily by an increase in MAP, stroke volume, or ejection rate. Thus, in older subjects brachial PP is regarded as a surrogate measure of arterial stiffness.[6,7]

Both cross-sectional and longitudinal population studies show that SBP rises from adolescence, whereas DBP, although initially increasing with age, levels off at about age 50 and decreases after age 60.[8,9] Thus, PP begins to increase after age 50. The rise in SBP and DBP up to age 50 can best be explained by the dominance of peripheral vascular resistance (Table 53–1). The transition age of 50-60 years when DBP levels off constitutes a near balancing of increased resistance and increased thoracic aortic stiffness. By contrast, after age 60, the fall in DBP

HEMODYNAMIC PATTERNS OF AGE-RELATED CHANGES IN BLOOD PRESSURE					
Age (Years)	DBP (mmHg)	SBP (mmHg)	MAP (mmHg)	PP (mmHg)	Hemodynamics
30–49	↑	↑	↑	→↑	R>S
50–59	→	↑	→	↑↑	R=S
≥60	↓	↑	→↓	↑↑↑↑	S>R

From Franklin SS, Jacobs WJ, Wong ND, et al. *Circulation* 1997;96:308–15.
↑, increase, ↓decrease, →, no change; DBP, diastolic blood pressure; MAP, mean arterial pressure; PP, pulse pressure; R, small-vessel resistance, S, large-vessel stiffness; SBP, systolic blood pressure.

Table 53–1. Hemodynamic Patterns of Age-Related Changes in Blood Pressure

and the rapid widening of PP become surrogate indicators of central elastic arterial stiffening. Indeed, after age 60, central arterial stiffness, rather than peripheral vascular resistance, becomes the dominant hemodynamic factor in both normotensive and hypertensive individuals.

Arterial stiffness is also accompanied by the phenomenon of early wave reflection.[6,7] The central pressure waveform is produced by two major components: a forward-traveling wave generated by ventricular ejection, and a backward wave reflecting off of distal arteries at the branching origins of arterioles. In young subjects the reflected pressure waves return to the ascending aorta in diastole and serve to elevate mean DBP, thus boosting coronary artery perfusion. The summation of the incident pressure wave with the reflected wave in young adults produces a normal phenomenon of pressure amplification of PP and SBP from the aorta to the brachial artery. Between the ages of 20 and 70 years, as arteries stiffen, the pulse wave velocity doubles. In older individuals, the reflected pressure wave returns to the ascending aorta earlier during late systole and increases or "augments" the central SBP and PP, thus decreasing pressure amplification and simultaneously contributing to increased cardiac afterload.[6,7]

Paradoxically, the heart only "sees" SBP in the ascending aorta, and pressure wave amplification distorts the relationship between central and peripheral SBP, as measured at the brachial artery by the sphygmomanometer. Therefore, central and not peripheral SBP, regardless of age, determines cardiac afterload and hence cardiac risk. The changing pattern of age-related brachial artery blood pressure (BP) components that predict CHD risk results from altered peripheral resistance, aortic stiffness, and early wave reflection, all acting in concert to raise SBP, decrease DBP, and abolish pressure amplification; this leads to an age-related shift from sphygmomanometric-determined DBP to SBP and ultimately to ISH with wide PP as the predictors of cardiac risk (Figure 53–2).[10] These findings represent a significant paradigm

shift in our understanding of how we use brachial artery cuff BP components to predict cardiovascular risk.

In addition to arterial stiffening, the left ventricle itself becomes stiff, perhaps as an adaptation to facilitate cardiac ejection and maintain matched coupling of heart to arteries. This is particularly notable in hearts that develop left ventricular hypertrophy, a common occurrence in the elderly and particularly in those individuals with ISH. A stiffer left ventricular coupled to a stiffer arterial system can contribute to increased cardiovascular risk in several ways, as has been shown by the studies of Kass.[11] First, there is increased late-systolic wall stress, and the cardiac energy costs imposed on the heart. Second, the imposition of high late-systolic load that often rises markedly during stress demand slows cardiac relaxation rates, potentially leading to incomplete diastolic relaxation, elevated diastolic pressures, and compromised cardiac reserve. This appears to be a factor in patients with heart failure symptoms who have apparent preservation of left ventricular function. Third, loss of arterial distensibility appears to alter vascular mechano-signaling, so the normal augmentations of nitric oxide release and vasoprotective mechanisms are compromised. Lastly, increased pulsatile stress, secondary to the loss of the conduit artery cushioning function, can contribute to endothelial dysfunction, increased coronary atherosclerosis, rupture of unstable atherosclerotic plaques, and acute coronary heart syndromes.[12] Many of these disturbances in cardiovascular function characterize the elderly person with longstanding ISH and markedly elevated PP.

The conventional wisdom is that the reduction DBP that accompanies ventricular–arterial stiffening results in compromised coronary perfusion. Whereas reflected waves normally return during early diastole and thereby enhance coronary perfusion, this increased boost is absent in elderly persons with ISH[6,7]; the decline in DBP, however, rarely falls to the critical level (~50–60 mmHg) required to disturb coronary flow autoregulation.[13,14] Furthermore, cardiac ejection into the stiff arterial system results in more coronary perfusion during systole. This suggests that the frequent reduction in DBP that accompanies increased PP does not compromise coronary perfusion significantly. It is more likely that the reduction in DBP that occurs in most individuals with ISH is primarily a surrogate risk marker for ventricular–arterial stiffness.

In summary, *coupling disease* results from stiffness of both the heart and arteries interacting to produce diastolic dysfunction and heart failure; this results from the combination of an elevated cardiac afterload presented to a compromised left ventricle, which is unable to handle the load. Thus, cardiovascular risk of an increased PP is defined by (1) increased SBP, a marker of cardiac afterload, and by (2) discordant decreased DBP in association with an increased SBP, a marker of increased stiffness of the left ventricle and the proximal aorta.

As suggested by their age-dependent divergent patterns of onset, diastolic hypertension and ISH may be two distinct disorders with significant overlap. The conversion from diastolic hypertension to ISH in the older age group has been attributed to "burned-out" diastolic hypertension.

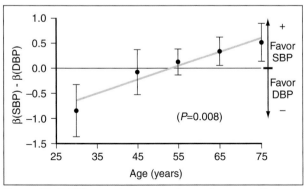

Figure 53–2. Difference in coronary heart disease prediction between SBP and DBP as function of age. Difference in β coefficients (from Cox proportional hazards regression) between SBP and DBP is plotted as function of age, obtaining the following regression line: β(SBP) – β(DBP) = –1.49848 + 0.0290 × age (p=0.008). DBP, diastolic blood pressure; SBP, systolic blood pressure. (Adapted from Franklin SS, Larson MG, Khan SA, et al. *Circulation* 2001;103:1245–9.)

While some people who have had untreated or poorly treated diastolic hypertension at a younger age develop ISH as they become older, data from the Framingham Study suggest that only about 40% of patients acquire ISH in this manner.[15] The majority of people who developed ISH do not go through a stage of diastolic hypertension (Figure 53–3).[15] The bias toward DBP over SBP by earlier generations of physicians may be, in part, due to the emphasis on hypertension as a young person's condition. However, with the aging of the population during the past half-century, hypertension has become largely a condition affecting older persons, that is, those with the ISH subtype.

Contrary to the conclusion of the Prospective Studies Collaboration (PSC)[16] and the Asian Pacific Cohort Studies Collaboration (APCSC)[17] that MAP is superior to PP as a predictor of future cardiovascular events in the elderly, the preponderance of evidence supports the opposite conclusion. PP is a surrogate risk marker for ventricular– arterial stiffness in the elderly, although at times an imperfect one. Moreover, PP is an independent risk factor for cardiovascular disease. Clearly, these findings call into question the belief that elevation of SBP and DBP contribute equally to cardiovascular risk in all age groups. However, there is as yet no evidence supporting the reduction of PP instead of SBP as a therapeutic goal. In addition, we have little information on the utility of using PP and SBP together, rather than SBP alone, to classify hypertensive risk. Since the majority of people with systolic hypertension are over 55 years of age and have ISH, the focus should be on high-risk systolic hypertension. From a practical viewpoint, effective antihypertensive therapy most often simultaneously lowers both SBP and PP. On the basis of prevailing data, it would be premature to modify current treatment guidelines that focus primarily on lowering SBP in middle-aged and the elderly for the prevention of cardiovascular events.

CLINICAL PRESENTATION AND EVALUATION

Hypertension in the elderly differs from younger individuals with essential hypertension in a number of ways (Table 53–2). Blood pressure fluctuates physiologically in response to changes in emotion, physical activity, and wakefulness. Furthermore, subjects with hypertension have more lability than do normotensive individuals. The higher the BP, the greater is the extent of lability. Aging is associated with disruption of normal baroreceptor reflex activity. In the absence of this stabilizing influence, it is not surprising that BP lability increases with age. Therefore, multiple measurements of BP on at least two separate visits may be necessary before labeling a patient as having hypertension.

The incidence of postural hypotension appears to increase with aging and especially after a meal. Indeed, orthostatic hypotension has been shown to be a powerful predictor of cardiovascular mortality in the Honolulu Heart Study.[18] Furthermore, the occurrence of postural hypotension may limit a person's ability to control supine and sitting SBP. Since BP recordings in the standing position disclose the presence and severity of orthostasis, it is imperative that these BP levels be used for defining pre-treatment levels and for determining the endpoint of therapy.

In patients with hypertension, a silent interval called the "auscultatory gap" may occur between the end of the first and the beginning of the third phases of Korotkoff sounds. In patients with geriatric hypertension, there appears to be a greater incidence and severity of an auscultatory gap.[19] Since the gap occurs only with auscultation, preliminary determination of SBP by palpation ensures the proper amount of cuff compression for the auscultatory technique and avoids the pitfall of beginning the evaluation of the Korotkoff sounds during the auscultatory gap. Without this maneuver, the auscultatory gap is not appreciated and erroneously low values of SBP can be recorded.

How well do indirect cuff blood pressure numbers correlate with direct intra-arterial BP values? With the most careful cuff measurements, true DBP is overestimated by 5 to 15 mmHg or more and true SBP is underestimated

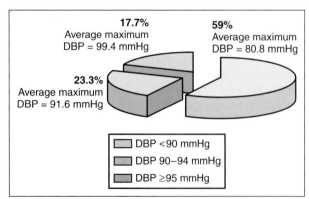

17.7%
Average maximum
DBP = 99.4 mmHg

59%
Average maximum
DBP = 80.8 mmHg

23.3%
Average maximum
DBP = 91.6 mmHg

☐ DBP <90 mmHg
▨ DBP 90–94 mmHg
▨ DBP ≥95 mmHg

Figure 53–3. Average maximum DBP reached prior to the development of isolated SBP for those who reached a DBP of <90 mmHg, from 90 to 94 mmHg, and ≥95 mmHg, respectively. DBP, diastolic blood pressure; SBP, systolic blood pressure. (Adapted from Franklin SS, Pio JR, Wong ND, et al. *Circulation* 2005;111:1121–7.)

SPECIFIC CHARACTERISTICS OF HYPERTENSION IN ELDERLY AND CLINICAL ASSESSMENT	
Characteristics	**Assessment**
Increased BP lability	Multiple measurements
Orthostatic hypotension	Sitting and standing BP
Post-prandial hypotension	Pre- and post-prandial BP
Ascultatory gap	Palpate radial pulse
Pseudohypertension	Pertains to DBP only
Increased % of RVHBP	Elevation of both SBP and DBP
BP, blood pressure; DBP, diastolic blood pressure; SBP, systolic blood pressure.	

Table 53–2. Specific Characteristics of Hypertension in Elderly and Clinical Assessment

by 0 to 5 mmHg or more compared with simultaneous intra-arterial pressure recordings.[20] Although the DBP artifact may be present regardless of age or BP level, this entity is found more frequently in elderly hypertensives with large artery stiffness. Moreover, correlation of pulse wave velocity with DBP cuff artifact suggests that increasing wall stiffness is responsible for erroneously high diastolic cuff values. The clinical importance of falsely over-estimating DBP in the geriatric hypertensive patient is that many elderly hypertensives who were previously classified with systolic–diastolic hypertension have, in reality, ISH or pseudo-diastolic hypertension. In contrast, the entity of pseudo-systolic hypertension in the elderly is a rare occurrence.

Although atherosclerotic renovascular hypertension is more common and often unrecognized in the elderly as compared to the younger person with hypertension, it is seldom cured and often not improved by angioplasty with stenting or by surgical intervention. Therefore, one can make a case for avoiding excessive evaluation, other than to assess other potential cardiovascular risk factors that coexist with hypertension. However, in the presence of severe systolic–diastolic hypertension in an elderly patient, one can be alerted to possible underlying renal artery stenosis. Other indications for proceeding with a workup for renal artery stenosis would be spontaneous or ACE inhibitor/angiotensin II inhibitor induced worsening of renal function, flash pulmonary edema, or drug-resistant hypertension.[21]

MANAGEMENT

Benefits of medical therapy

During the past few decades, the therapeutic approach in elderly hypertensive patients has changed markedly. In the early 1970s, prevailing wisdom questioned the benefit of antihypertensive agents in patients over 65 years of age. Beginning in the early 1990s, the publication of three major placebo-controlled studies that specifically addressed the treatment of ISH in older patients changed the perception of the significance of SBP control. In 1991, the landmark Systolic Hypertension in the Elderly Program (SHEP) study first established that older patients with ISH benefited from treatment.[22] The Syst-Eur[23] and the Syst-China[24] trials corroborated these findings.

Staessen et al.[25] conducted a meta-analysis of the 11,825 patients aged 60 years or older who participated in these three major trials (Figure 53–4). This analysis found that antihypertensive treatment significantly reduced fatal and nonfatal coronary events by 25%, fatal and nonfatal strokes by 37%, all cardiovascular events by 32%, cardiovascular mortality by 25%, and total mortality by 17%.[25] Additionally, a highly significant 49% reduction in fatal and nonfatal heart failure was reported from the SHEP study.[22] These studies negate prior assumptions that age-related changes in BP are benign, and reinforce the emerging paradigm that treatment will benefit patients with elevated SBP, even when they have normal or low DBP. Further-

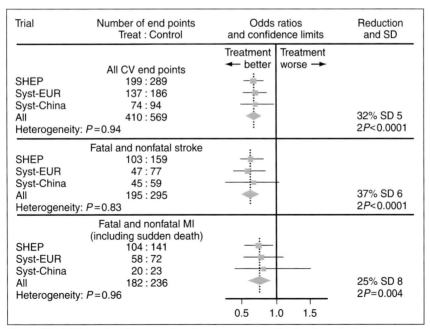

Figure 53–4. Effect of antihypertensive drug treatment on fatal and nonfatal cardiovascular endpoints in three outcome trials in older patients with isolated systolic hypertension. CV, cardiovascular; MI, myocardial infarct; SD, standard deviation; SHEP, Systolic Hypertension in the Elderly Program; Syst-China, Systolic Hypertension in China; Syst-EUR, European Trial on Isolated Systolic Hypertension in the Elderly. (Reprinted by permission from Macmillan Publishers Ltd: Staessen JA, Wang JG, Thijs L, Fagard R. *J Hum Hypertens* 1999;13:859-63.)

more, the benefit-to-risk ratio of antihypertensive therapy is higher in the elderly than in younger or middle-aged patients.

Currently life expectancy in the United States is 77 years, raising the question of the benefit of antihypertensive agents in patients over this age. A meta-analysis of six major trials that included 1670 patients aged 80 years or older suggested that even the very old may benefit from antihypertensive treatment (Figure 53–5).[26] In these patients, active treatment produced a 34% reduction in stroke (p=0.014), a 39% reduction in heart failure (p=0.01), and a 22% reduction in major cardiovascular events (p=0.01). The reduction in coronary events was not statistically significant and a nonsignificant 6% increase in mortality was observed.[26] Evidence from this meta-analysis was strong for older patients with SBP of at least 160 mmHg (stage 2 ISH); current data are weaker for treatment of stage 1 hypertension in the absence of target-organ damage.[27] Indeed, there is disagreement as to whether nonsustained systolic hypertension is innocuous compared with true normotension in the elderly patient. The Hypertension in the Very Elderly Trial,[28] a more definitive intervention study of the very old (age 80 or older) utilizing a randomized, double-blind, placebo-controlled protocol in 2100 subjects with ISH, is nearing completion. Until the results of this study are known, it would be inappropriate to withhold antihypertensive treatment in this age group. Even though we may not extend the lives of octogenarians, effective treatment of ISH may enhance the quality of their remaining years through prevention of strokes, heart failure, and major cardiovascular complications.

Therapeutic target goals

There are Joint National Committee (JNC-7)[29] and World Health Organization (WHO)[30] guidelines for the optimal reduction of BP to achieve maximum benefit from antihypertensive therapy that make no distinction between young and older adults. These guidelines, based on obser-

vational as well as on outcome data, suggest that low-risk patients be treated to a target goal of <140 SBP mmHg and <90 DBP mmHg. For high-risk subjects with diabetes, renal impairment, or heart failure, the therapeutic target goal is <130 SBP mmHg and <80 DBP mmHg. In patients with renal disease and at least 1 g of proteinuria per 24 hours, BP guidelines suggest that the BP treatment goal is <125/75.

Value of lifestyle intervention

A variety of lifestyle interventions have been shown to lower BP, with the most effective being successful weight reduction in overweight and obese hypertensives.[31] Reducing weight is of special importance if the elderly hypertensive has diabetes. Even a reduction of 10 to 15 pounds can have a significant benefit in lowering BP. Unfortunately, most patients are refractory to successful weight reduction, and even when partially successful, tend to have a high percentage of recidivism within a year of losing weight.

The older hypertensive patients are usually more salt-sensitive than the young, especially in persons with ISH.[32] However, successful salt restriction depends to a large extent on limiting milk, bread, and a variety of high salt-containing processed foods and substituting fruits, vegetables, and nuts. The more recent use of the Dietary Approaches to Stop Hypertension (DASH) diet,[33] rich in fruits, vegetables, high-calcium but low animal-fat foods, has been successful in reducing BP in older hypertensives even when they consume average salt intakes. Heavy alcoholic intake can precipitate or worsen hypertension in older patients, and is frequently refractory to usual drug therapy. Except for the unusual patient, lifestyle intervention is generally unsuccessful in correcting ISH fully. However, in addition to partial reduction in BP, lifestyle intervention may reduce the need for extensive antihypertensive therapy and minimize associated cardiovascular risk factors. It should be emphasized that lifestyle intervention is more likely to be successful in preventing rather than in reversing hypertension when initiated early at the high-normal BP level.[29]

Selection of antihypertensive drug therapy

The Blood Pressure Treatment Trialists Collaboration,[34] a meta-analysis of 29 trials involving 162,341 persons with a mean age of 65 years, concluded that all classes of commonly used antihypertensive agents were equally successful in reducing the risk of ischemic heart disease and stroke events. Moreover, the reduction in risk was directly proportional to the reduction in SBP. These conclusions were supported by the Antihypertensive and Lipid-Lowering Treatment to Prevent Heart Attack Trial (ALLHAT),[35] an outcome trial of over 42,000 high-risk subjects with a mean age of 67 years. The ALLHAT study showed that a thiazide-type diuretic (chlorthalidone) was equally effective in reducing the primary endpoints of nonfatal myocardial infarction and CHD deaths when compared to the calcium channel blocker amlodipine or the ACE inhibitor lisinopril.

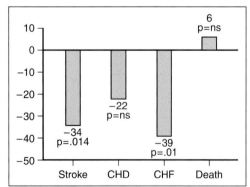

Figure 53–5. Effect of antihypertensive drug treatment in the very old (aged over 80 years) on cardiovascular endpoints in 1670 participants from five trials. CHD, coronary heart disease; CHF, congestive heart failure. (Adapted from Gueyffier F, Bulpitt C, Boissel J-P, et al. *Lancet* 1999;353:793–6, with permission from Elsevier.)

Perhaps beta-blockers represent an exception to the dictum that the benefit of an antihypertensive agent is directly proportional to its blood pressure lowering capability. This was shown in the Losartan Intervention for Endpoint Reduction (LIFE),[36] a trial of patients with hypertension and left ventricular hypertrophy, in which losartan (an angiotensin II receptor blocker [ARB]) was superior to atenolol (a beta-blocker) in preventing fatal and nonfatal strokes, independent of any significant difference in BP lowering between the two arms.[36] However, central BP may be more adversely affected by beta-blockade as compared to blockade of renin-angiotensin sytem.[37] It should be noted also that a diuretic was an add-on drug in more than 77% of both therapeutic arms, suggesting that the combination of a diuretic and ARB was an effective modality of treatment for stroke prevention in this high-risk group of older hypertensive patients. The LIFE study reinforces an earlier meta-analysis of 10 geriatric hypertension outcome studies that showed the inferiority of beta-blockers as compared to diuretics in reducing cardiovascular events.[38]

The question of which drug class is best suited to start first in patients with ISH may be a moot point. Although diuretics and calcium channel blockers have been shown to be most effective in decreasing BP and reducing cardiovascular events in the major geriatric hypertension intervention trials,[22–24] it should be remembered that reaching goal therapy is generally more difficult in geriatric ISH than in younger persons with systolic–diastolic hypertension. In practice, a combination of two or more drug classes will be necessary for BP control in the majority of patients with ISH.[39] The use of combination therapy generally increases BP reduction at lower doses of the component agents and often reduces adverse events when compared to higher-dose monotherapy.[40] Elevations in SBP by ≥ 20 mmHg and DBP by ≥ 10 mmHg above goal (the "20/10" rule)[29] will often require combination therapy from the start in order achieve goal therapy within a relatively short time and thereby minimize cardiovascular events.[41] Low-dose diuretics should almost always be part of combination therapy because of their efficacy in BP reduction, minimal adverse events, and low cost.

There are always potential dangers in reducing BP in the elderly, but the available evidence would suggest that adverse events are no more frequent in the elderly than in younger hypertensive subjects. However, it may be appropriate to start with lower doses of medication in the elderly and then titrate against response and symptoms. In addition, there are some potential hazards of combination therapy in the elderly. The combination of a beta-blocker and a nondihydropyridine calcium channel blockers may cause bradyarrhythmias. Alpha-blockers and calcium channel blockers may cause or exacerbate orthostatic hypotension. Ace inhibitors and potassium-sparing diuretics may cause or exacerbate hyperkalemia.

Optimal treatment of ISH should not only reduce peripheral vascular resistance, but also reduce large artery stiffness and the early wave reflection generated by that stiffness. Treatment approaches with the capability of minimizing arterial stiffness include a variety of approved agents. Most conventional antihypertensive drugs, however, fall short of optimally reducing age-related increases in PP.[42] Therapeutic benefit may result from at least five different mechanisms. First, reduction of peripheral resistance downstream will decrease large-artery stiffness upstream by a reduction in distending pressure that decreases the stretch on elastic arteries; a variety of antihypertensive agents that dilate arterials work in this manner.[6,7] Second, vasodilatation of small arteries and arterioles will shorten the artery reflection sites, decrease early wave reflection, decrease aortic late SBP peaking and hence decrease cardiac afterload without a structural decrease in arterial stiffness.[6,7] Nitrates, in doses that do not affect peripheral vascular resistance, have been shown to decrease early wave reflection, decrease central pulse pressure and hence lower left ventricular afterload—all without a significant change in arterial stiffness.[43] Third, long-term reduction in cardiac afterload will eventually result in regression of left ventricular hypertrophy, regression of vascular smooth muscle hypertrophy and remodeling of small blood vessels toward a normal wall to lumen ratio.[44] Indeed, the ability of angiotensin converting enzyme inhibitors and angiotensin receptor blockers to promote regression of LVH and arterial remodeling may have important long-term benefits in reducing arterial stiffness.[45] Fourth, therapy that blocks excessive aldosterone at the tissue level may over time result in regression of fibrosis in the heart, renal mesangium, and large blood vessels. Indeed, spironolactone and eplerenone may prove to be of value in reversing the stiffness of arteries in persons with ISH.[45] Fifth, some antihypertensive agents appear to possess properties that specifically influence arterial stiffness without affecting peripheral vascular resistance. In animal models, advanced glycation end product (AGE) cross-linking breakers have been shown to prevent arterial stiffening.[46] Although poorly understood, reduced-sodium diets to achieve negative salt balance, with or without the use of diuretics, can reduce arterial stiffness.[32] Other possible destiffening strategies include aerobic exercise, 3-hydroxy-methyglutaryl-coenzyme A reductase inhibitors (statins), antioxidants, and inhibiting of PDE5a with sildenafil.[11]

The optimal strategy in treating ISH is to maximize SBP reduction while minimizing the reduction in DBP. As was demonstrated by Koch-Weser in 1973[47] and recently confirmed by Wang et al.,[48] the higher the PP (in part, age related), the greater will be the fall in SBP as compared to the fall in DBP with conventional antihypertensive agents. Therefore, antihypertensive therapy will maximize the decrease in PP and minimize the further reduction in DBP, in direct proportion to the age of the patient and the extent of large artery stiffness.[48]

Achieving therapeutic goals

The realization that antihypertensive treatment of patients over age 60 to 65 correlates with improved outcomes makes awareness of hypertension and access to treatment important factors in achieving therapeutic goals. In recent decades awareness of hypertension has steadily increased. However, in the most recent U.S. NHANES survey

(1999–2000), awareness was approximately 70%, the same as in the previous NHANES survey, conducted approximately 5 years previously. Thus, a substantial proportion (30%) of hypertensive persons in the United States continue to be unaware of having hypertension, with nearly one-half of these persons over age 65.[49]

Furthermore, of the patients treated, many remain above recommended BP goals. Nearly 60% of hypertensive patients receive antihypertensive therapy, but a little more than 50% of those patients on therapy achieve the recommended SBP of 140 mmHg.[4] Not unexpectedly, the vast majority of treatment failures occur in patients over age 50 and especially in older women.[50] Only 14% of failures in NHANES III[2] occurred in patients under age 50, while 86% of treatment failures occurred in older individuals, most of whom had ISH, access to health care, and relatively frequent contact with physicians.[51] Analyzing treatment failures by age reveals the age-related discrepancy in the successful control of both SBP and DBP. Approximately 50% of younger patients who failed treatment had concordant SBP and DBP that were not at target goals. In contrast, older patients who failed to achieve treatment goals had discordant failure. Only 17% of patients aged 50 or over were above their DBP goal, but fully 82% were above their SBP target goal.[2]

The tendency toward failure to reach SBP treatment goal becomes more apparent with aging, as shown in the Framingham Heart Study by Lloyd-Jones et al.[52] More patients aged over 75 than under the age of 60 achieved their DBP goal (92% vs. 85%, respectively). In contrast, the SBP target progressively became more difficult to obtain: in patients aged less than 60, 69% reached their SBP target goal; in those aged 61 to 75 years, 48% of patients reached goal; and in those over the age of 75 years, only 34% reached goal.

That target SBP becomes more difficult to achieve with aging is best explained by age-related increasing arterial stiffness. Physician inertia and errors contribute greatly to inadequate control of ISH. In the past, treatment guidelines focused on the DBP, relegating the control of SBP to minimal importance. Some clinicians feared reaching excessively low DBP and, therefore, were fearful of lowering the SBP even at pressures above 150 or 140 mmHg as long as the DBP remained at or below its target. This fear of excessive therapeutic lowering of DBP-the so called "J curve phenomenon"—has been exaggerated. If there is any significant risk of precipitating an ischemic cardiac event with therapy-induced low BP, it would occur only with DBP reduction below 60 mmHg, as indicated in a post-hoc analysis of the SHEP study.[14] Failure to titrate medications upward, failure to use optimal polypharmacy, and, in particular, failure to incorporate diuretics as part of polypharmacy, may hamper the ability to control ISH. In addition, not treating to the lower target goals in high-risk patients with diabetes and with kidney disease likely further contributed to the disappointingly high incidence of treatment failures.

Patient noncompliance with antihypertensive medication contributes greatly to poor control of BP. Indeed, as many as 50% of individuals who start medications for hypertension discontinue their treatment within the first year. Achieving goal therapy is greatly facilitated by enlisting active patient participation in their care. This would include establishing treatment goals, home monitoring of blood pressure, simplifying treatment regiments, reviewing medications and refills on each visit, discussing realistic objectives for lifestyle modifications, and addressing potential drug side effects and cost issues.[53]

While several aspects involving treatment approaches may explain the failure to optimally control ISH overall, one must conclude that there exists a substantial number of patients with systolic hypertension that are truly resistant to currently available medications, even when used properly. Unrecognized conditions in the elderly that lead to poor BP control are the use of non steroidal anti-inflammatory agents for arthritis (especially with coexisting impaired renal function), occult alcoholism, undiagnosed sleep apnea, hypothyroidism, atherosclerotic renal artery disease, and recently described hyperaldosteronism associated with morbid obesity.[54]

SUMMARY

Once considered an inconsequential part of the aging process, the development of ISH represents a late manifestation of increased arterial stiffness in the middle-aged and elderly population. Its inherent increased risk for vascular events highlights the importance of its control. Furthermore, there is overwhelming evidence that pharmacologic treatment of ISH reduces cardiovascular events in the elderly. Paradoxically, ISH remains more difficult to control than diastolic hypertension and most middle-aged and elderly hypertensive patients fail to achieve recommended targets. Reaching target systolic pressure levels may require the use of polypharmacy that includes a diuretic, and perhaps includes future new agents that specifically and effectively target arterial stiffness.

REFERENCES

1. Fields LE, Burt VL, Cutler JA, et al. The burden of adult hypertension in the United States 1999 to 2000: a rising tide. *Hypertension* 2004; 44:398–404.

2. Franklin SS, Jacobs MJ, Wong ND, et al. Predominance of isolated systolic hypertension among middle-aged and elderly US hypertensives—analysis based on NHANES III. *Hypertension* 2001;37:869–74.

3. Vasan RS, Beiser A, Seshadri S, et al. Residual lifetime risk for developing hypertension in middle-aged women and women: the Framingham Heart Study. *JAMA* 2002;287:1003–10.

4. Hajjar I, Kotchen TA. Trends in prevalence, awareness, treatment, and control of hypertension in the United States, 1988–2000. *JAMA* 2003; 290:199–206.

5. Wolf-Maier K, Cooper RS, Banegas JR, et al. Hypertension prevalence and blood pressure levels in 6 European countries, Canada, and the United States. *JAMA* 2003;289:2363–9.

6. Nichols WW, O'Rourke MF. *Mc Donald's Blood Flow in Arteries.* 5th ed. London: Hodder Arnold, 2005.

7. Safar ME, Levy BI, Struijker-Boudier H. Current perspectives on arterial stiffness and pulse pressure in hypertension and cardiovascular diseases. *Circulation* 2003;107:2864–9.

8. Franklin SS, Gustin W, Wong ND, et al. Hemodynamic patterns of age-related changes in blood pressure. The Framingham Heart Study. *Circulation* 97;96:308–15.

9. Burt VL, Whelton P, Roccella EJ, et al. Prevalence of hypertension in the US adult population: results from the Third National Health and Nutrition Examination Survey, 1988–1991. *Hypertension* 1995; 25:305–13.

10. Franklin SS, Larson MG, Khan SA, et al. Does the relation of blood pressure to coronary heart disease risk change with aging? The Framingham Heart Study. *Circulation* 2001;103:1245–9.

11. Kass DA. Ventricular arterial stiffening. *Hypertension* 2005;46:185–93.

12. Lakatta EG, Levy D. Arterial and Cardiac Aging: major shareholders in cardiovascular disease enterprises. Part I. Aging arteries: a "set up" for vascular disease. *Circulation* 2003; 107:139–45.

13. Farhi ER, Canty JM, Klocke FJ. Effects of graded reductions in coronary perfusion pressure on the diastolic pressure-segment length relation and the rate of isovolumic relaxation in the resting conscious dog. *Circulation* 1989;80:1458–68.

14. Somes GW, Pahor M, Shorr RI, et al. The role of diastolic blood pressure when treating isolated systolic hypertension. *Arch Intern Med* 1991; 265:3255–64.

15. Franklin SS, Pio JR, Wong ND, et al. Predictors of new-onset diastolic and systolic hypertension. The Framingham Heart Study. *Circulation* 2005;111: 1121–7.

16. Prospective Studies Collaboration. Age-specific relevance of usual blood pressure to vascular mortality: a meta-analysis of individual data for one million adults in 61 prospective studies. *Lancet* 2002;360:1903–13.

17. Asia Pacific Cohort Studies Collaboration. Blood pressure indices and cardiovascular disease in the Asia Pacific Region. A pooled analysis. *Hypertension* 2003; 42:69–75.

18. Masaki KH, Schatz IJ, Burchfiel CM, et al. Orthostatic hypotension predicts mortality in elderly men: the Honolulu Heart Program. *Circulation* 1998;98: 2290–5.

19. Cavallini MC, Roman MJ, Blank SG, et al. Association of the auscultatory gap with vascular disease in hypertensive patients. *Ann Intern Med* 1996;124: 877–83.

20. Zweifler AJ, Shahab ST. Pseudohypertension: a new assessment. *J Hypertens* 1993;11:1–6.

21. Plouin PF, Rossignol P, Bobrie G. Atherosclerotic renal artery stenosis: to treat conservatively, to dilate, to stent, or to operate? *J Am Soc Nephrol* 2001;12:2190–6.

22. SHEP Cooperative Research Group. Prevention of stroke by antihypertensive drug treatment in older persons with isolate systolic hypertension: final results of the systolic hypertension in the elderly program (SHEP). *JAMA* 1991; 265:3255–64.

23. Staessen JA, Fagard R, Thijs L, et al. subgroup and per-protocol analysis of randomized European Trial on Isolated Systolic Hypertension in the Elderly. *Arch Intern Med* 1998;158:1681–91.

24. Liu L, Wang JG, Gong L, et al. comparison of active treatment and placebo in older Chinese patients with isolated systolic hypertension, Systolic Hypertension in China (SYST-CHINA) Collaborative Group. *J Hypertens* 1998; 16:1823–9.

25. Staessen JA, Wang JG, Thijs L, Fagard R. Overview of the outcome trials in older patients with isolated systolic hypertension. *J Hum Hypertens* 1999; 13:859–63.

26. Gueyffier F, Bulpitt C, Boissel J-P, et al. Antihypertensive drugs in very old people: a subgroup meta-analysis of randomized controlled trials. *Lancet* 1999;353:793–6.

27. Chaudhry SI, Krumholz HM, Foody JM. Systolic hypertension in older persons. *JAMA* 2004;292:1074–80.

28. Bulpitt CJ, Fletcher AE, Amery A, et al. The Hypertension in the Very Elderly Trial (HYVET). Rationale, methodology and comparison with previous trials. *Drugs Aging* 1994;5:171–83.

29. Chobanian AV, Bakris GL, Black HR, et al. The Seventh Report of the Joint National Committee on Prevention, Detection, Evaluation, and Treatment of High Blood Pressure: the JNC 7 report. *Hypertension* 2003;42:1206–52.

30. World Health Organization. 2003 World Health Organization (WHO)/International Society of Hypertension statement on the management of hypertension. *J Hypertens* 2003;21:1983–92.

31. Cushman W, Dubbert P. Nonpharmacologic approaches to therapy of hypertension. *Endocr Pract* 1997;3:106–11.

32. Feng J, Markandu ND, MacGregor GA. Modest salt reduction lowers blood pressure in isolated systolic hypertension and combined hypertension. *Hypertension* 2005;46:66–70.

33. Appel LJ, Moore TJ, Obarzanek E, et al. The effect of dietary patterns on blood pressure: results from the Dietary Approaches to Stop Hypertension (DASH) randomized clinical trial. *N Engl J Med* 1997;336:1117–24.

34. Blood Pressure Lowering Treatment Trialists' Collaboration. Effects of different blood-pressure-lowering regimens on major cardiovascular events: results of prospectively-designed overviews of randomized trials. *Lancet* 2003;362:1527–35.

35. ALLHAT Officers and Coordinators for ALLHAT Collaborative Research Group. Major outcomes in high-risk hypertensive patients randomized to angiotensin-converting enzyme inhibitor or calcium channel blockers vs diuretic. The Antihypertensive and Lipid-Lowering Treatment to Prevent Heart Attack Trial (ALLHAT). *JAMA* 2002;288:2981–97.

36. Dahlöf B, Devereux RB, Kjeldsen SE, et al. LIFE Study Group. Cardiovascular morbidity and mortality in the Losartan Intervention For Endpoint reduction in hypertension study (LIFE): a randomized trial against atenolol. *Lancet* 2002;359: 995–1003.

37. Hirata K, Vlachopoulos C, Adji A, O'Rourke MF. Benefits from angiotensin-converting enzyme inhibitor 'beyond blood pressure lowering': beyond blood pressure or beyond the brachial artery? *J Hypertens* 2005;23:551–6.

38. Messerli FH, Grossman E, Goldbourt U. Are beta-blockers efficacious as first-line therapy for hypertension in the elderly? A systematic review. *JAMA* 1998;279: 1903–7.

39. Kjeldsen SE, Dahlöf B, Devereux RB, et al. LIFE (Losartan Intervention for Endpoint Reduction) Study Group. Effects of losartan on cardiovascular morbidity and mortality in patients with isolated systolic hypertension and left ventricular hypertrophy: a Losartan Intervention for Endpoint Reduction (LIFE) substudy. *JAMA* 2002;288: 1491–8.

40. Law MR, Wald NJ, Morris JK, Jordan RE. Value of low dose combination treatment with blood pressure lowering drugs: analysis of 354 randomized trials. *BMJ* 2003;326:1427–34.

41. Julius S, Kjeldsen SE, Brunner HR, et al. Outcomes in hypertensive patients at high cardiovascular risk treated with regimens based on valsartan or amlodipine: the VALUE randomized trial. *Lancet* 2004; 363(9426):2022–31.

42. Mourad JJ, Blacher J, Blin P, Warzocha U. Conventional antihypertensive drug therapy does not prevent the increase of pulse pressure with age. *Hypertension* 2001;38:958–62.

43. Stokes GS, Bune AJ, Huon N, Arin ES. Long-term effectiveness of extended-release nitrate for the treatment of systolic hypertension. *Hypertension* 2005;45:380–4.

44. Schiffrin EL, Deng LY, Larochelle P. Progressive improvement in the structure of resistance arteries of hypertensive patients after 2 years of treatment with an angiotensin 1–converting enzyme inhibitor. Comparison with effects of a β-blocker. *Am J Hypertens* 1995;8:229–36.

45. Safar ME. Systolic hypertension in the elderly: arterial wall mechanical properties and the renin-angiotensin-aldosterone system. *J Hypertens* 2005; 23:673–81.

46. Vaitkevicius PV, Lane M, Spurgeon H, et al. A cross-link breaker has sustained effects on arterial and ventricular properties: I older rhesus monkeys. *Proc Natl Acad Sci U S A* 2002;98: 1171–5.

47. Koch-Weser J. Correlation of pathophysiology and pharmacotherapy in primary hypertension. *Am J Cardiol* 1973;32:499–510.

48. Wang JG, Staessen JA, Franklin SS, et al. Systolic and diastolic blood pressure lowering as determinants of cardiovascular outcome. *Hypertension* 2005;45:907–13.

49. Burt VL, Cutler JA, Higgins M, et al. Trends in the prevalence, awareness, treatment, and control of hypertension in the adult US population: data from the health examination surveys, 1960 to 1991. *Hypertension* 1995: 26:60–9.

50. Lloyd-Jones DM, Evans JC, Levy D. Hypertension in adults across the age spectrum. *JAMA* 2005;294:466–72.

51. Hyman DJ, Pavik VN. Characteristics of patients with uncontrolled hypertension in the United States. *N Engl J Med* 2001; 345:479–86.

52. Lloyd-Jones DM, Evans JC, Larson GM, et al. Differential control of systolic and diastolic blood pressure: factors associated with lack of blood pressure control in the community. *Hypertension* 2000;36:594–99.

53. Egan BM, Basile JN. Controlling blood pressure in 50% of all hypertensive patients: an achievable goal in the Healthy People 2010 Report? *J Investigative Med* 2003;51:373–95.

54. Goodfriend TL, Calhoun DA. Resistant hypertension, obesity, sleep apnea, and aldosterone: theory and therapy. *Hypertension* 2004;43:518–24.

Chapter

54 Hypertension in Pregnancy

Jason G. Umans

Definitions

■ Hypertension in pregnancy can be due to one of several distinct disorders, including pre-existing chronic hypertension, gestational hypertension, pre-eclampsia or pre-eclampsia superimposed on chronic hypertension.

■ Pre-eclampsia is a multisystem disorder that may present without proteinuria, and more severe phenotypes include central nervous system, hematologic, hepatic, and renal manifestations.

Clinical Implications

■ There are no formally established blood pressure (BP) targets in pregnancy, although BP is always controlled to less than 170/110, using drugs other than angiotensin-converting enzyme inhibitors or angiotensin II–receptor blockers.

■ Magnesium sulfate is the preferred agent for eclamptic seizures.

Hypertension is the most common medical complication of pregnancy, affecting 10% to 15% of all pregnancies in the developed world, where it is the second leading cause of maternal death and markedly increases the incidence of preterm birth, intrauterine growth restriction, placental abruption, and perinatal mortality. Its impact on maternal morbidity and mortality are even greater in the developing world. Hypertension in pregnancy includes several distinct disorders, whose differential diagnosis, although often difficult, is important because they differ in etiology and apparent mechanism, hemodynamics, clinical evolution, risks to mother and fetus, and long-term cardiovascular consequences. In addition, clinicians often fail to appreciate the presence or evolution of underlying hypertension as it may be obscured by the normal hemodynamic, renal, and biochemical adaptations to pregnancy.

In 2006, we are still without any evidence-based blood pressure (BP) treatment targets for hypertensive gravidas. Defining BP targets is even more difficult, because guidelines were developed using mercury sphygmomanometry, while practice has largely shifted to use of automated oscillometric BP devices, even though they often yield erroneous results in hypertensive pregnant women. Tight BP control appears not to benefit women without target-organ damage. Indeed, it is unclear which, if any, of the morbid complications of hypertensive pregnancy are prevented by varying degrees of BP control. However, all

agree that BP should not exceed either 170 mmHg systolic or 110 mmHg diastolic, since these high levels may lead to cerebrovascular catastrophe. Further, it remains important to recognize when hypertension is due to pre-eclampsia, as this disorder may evolve rapidly and unpredictably toward multiorgan failure and life-threatening complications. Antihypertensive therapy is limited by contraindications to the use of angiotensin-converting enzyme (ACE) inhibitors and AT_1 receptor blockers late in pregnancy and by a striking paucity of well-designed and adequately-powered studies to assess risks and benefits of other antihypertensive agents.

HEMODYNAMICS IN NORMAL AND HYPERTENSIVE PREGNANCY

Normal pregnancy strikingly alters systemic hemodynamics and renal function so as to impact our recognition of and approach to hypertension. Gestational decrements in systemic vascular resistance (SVR) are so profound that, despite an increase in cardiac output (CO) of nearly 50%, BP falls early in the first trimester.[1,2] Along with this microvascular vasodilation, there is a parallel adaptation of large artery function, with increased total arterial compliance early in pregnancy.[3] Paradoxically, the gestational hypotension is even more striking in women with underlying chronic hypertension, so that BP may fall by 30/15 mmHg, masking the recognition of pregestational hypertension when the patient is examined at her first prenatal visit.[4] Thus, a thorough history, review of records, funduscopic examination, and evidence of target-organ damage may be the only clues to chronic hypertension in the early phase of pregnancy; BP values of 120/80 during the first trimester may be abnormal and should lead to suspicion of underlying hypertension. The mechanisms of gestational vasodilation in women remain uncertain, but appear not to depend on either vasodilator prostaglandins or nitric oxide (NO).

Pregnancy alters every aspect of the renin-angiotensin-aldosterone system, markedly increasing levels of angiotensinogen, plasma renin activity, angiotensin II, Ang 1–7, and aldosterone.[5,6] However, there is a specific refractoriness to the AT_1 receptor–mediated effects of angiotensin, which manifests as decreased pressor response to infused angiotensin II and to blunted constriction of human resistance arteries *in vitro*. In addition, progesterone antagonizes the effects of aldosterone at mineralocorticoid receptors.[5,7]

Not only is there generalized systemic vasodilation, but pregnancy causes specific renal vasodilation and hyperfiltration. Afferent and efferent arteriolar vasodilation is balanced, so that renal plasma flow and glomerular filtration rate (GFR) increase in parallel.[2] In the same way that pregnancy may obscure the recognition of underlying essential hypertension, this gestational hyperfiltration may mask underlying renal insufficiency. A serum creatinine concentration of more than 0.8 mg/dL early in pregnancy should be viewed with suspicion. The mechanisms leading to gestational renal vasodilation have been elucidated in the rat and depend on a signaling cascade in which the ovarian hormone relaxin acts via gelatinase to cleave big endothelin (ET), resulting in ET_B receptor–mediated activation of NO synthase.[8] It appears that relaxin also underlies the increased arterial compliance and many of the systemic vascular changes of pregnancy in the rat; whether similar mechanisms occur in women is yet to be determined.[9]

Measuring blood pressure in pregnant women

Diagnosis of hypertension in pregnancy, defined as a BP greater than 140 mmHg systolic or greater than 90 mmHg diastolic occurring at any time during gestation,[10] depends, of course, on accurate BP measurement using standardized and validated techniques. Unfortunately, these validated techniques are rarely used in typical clinical practice. When possible, BP should be measured in the sitting position, with the arm supported, using an appropriately sized cuff, a mercury sphygmomanometer (or a recently calibrated aneroid device), and with diastolic BP defined by the fifth Korotkoff sound.[11] In bed-bound patients, many clinicians measure BP in the left lateral decubitus position so as to avoid spurious elevations, especially in late pregnancy, due to the mass effect of the gravid uterus when supine. This is a reasonable strategy as long as the clinician accounts for the artifactual lowering of BP if it is recorded from the right arm (inadvertently elevated relative to the heart). Most of the oscillometric devices now used routinely for home BP monitoring as well as for BP measurement in hospital clinics, on labor and delivery units, and even those devices which are integral to fetal monitoring devices, have not been validated in hypertensive pregnant women; nearly all depend on algorithms that provide erroneous values for diastolic BP. Because most guidelines for treatment of severe hypertension focus on diastolic values, all automated readings should be confirmed by auscultation when they might alter therapy.

Despite the possible inaccuracy of oscillometric devices in hypertensive gravidas, home BP monitoring can markedly improve the care of women at high risk for pre-eclampsia or with more severe underlying hypertension by detecting significant changes in systolic pressure, thus leading to earlier diagnosis of pre-eclampsia or to more careful titration of antihypertensive medications.[12] Similarly, there may be a role for ambulatory BP monitoring for risk assessment in pregnancy, although confirmatory and outcomes data remain lacking.[13]

DIAGNOSIS AND CLASSIFICATION OF HYPERTENSION IN PREGNANCY

Using a nomenclature endorsed by the International Society for the Study of Hypertension in Pregnancy, several national and international obstetrics groups, and by the National High Blood Pressure Education Program (NHBPEP) Working Group on Hypertension in Pregnancy,[10,11] we recognized four major hypertensive disorders of pregnancy. First, chronic hypertension (antedating pregnancy) may be either essential or secondary. Two disorders, gestational hypertension and pre-eclampsia, occur only in pregnancy. Finally, pre-eclampsia may be superimposed upon underlying chronic hypertension. Terms such as pregnancy-induced hypertension (PIH) may include a mix of disorders, with differing pathophysiology and risks, and should be abandoned.

Chronic hypertension

This is the most rapidly growing cause of hypertension in pregnancy, perhaps the combined result of several factors, including postponement of childbearing to more advanced age, and the epidemic of essential hypertension, often coupled with obesity and insulin resistance. Although less common than essential hypertension, three forms of secondary hypertension that affect young women deserve specific mention: pheochromocytoma, renovascular hypertension, and primary hyperaldosteronism.[4] Clinicians should have a low threshold for suspecting pheochromocytoma, despite its rarity, when hypertension is associated with classic signs and symptoms, since it may lead to hypertensive crisis during labor. Appropriate management, as in nonpregnant women, would include α-adrenoreceptor blockade and confirmatory measurements of catecholamines and their metabolites. There are several case reports of life-saving surgical management with proper pharmacologic blockade of pheochromocytoma during pregnancy.[14] Renovascular hypertension, most likely due to fibromuscular dysplasia or arteritis in women of childbearing age, so often leads to superimposed pre-eclampsia and poor pregnancy outcome that it should be corrected before or even during pregnancy. Diagnosis is difficult because usual measurements of renin activity are of little to no diagnostic utility during pregnancy; Doppler ultrasound measurements are often misleading, and radionuclide renal scans are avoided in pregnancy. Further, radiologists are often hesitant to perform magnetic resonance (MR) imaging or interventional procedures, even when indicated. Notwithstanding these obstacles, there are well-documented cases in which diagnosis by MR angiography and correction by angioplasty during pregnancy led to good maternal and neonatal outcomes.[15] Finally, hypertension due to primary hyperaldosteronism may have a variable and often mild course during pregnancy because high levels of progesterone during pregnancy can antagonize mineralocorticoid effects at the aldosterone receptor.[5,7] It is important to realize that serum and urinary aldosterone during normal pregnancy far exceeds levels usually observed in patients with a proven aldosteronoma.

In these cases, severe hypertension, hypokalemia, and suppression of endogenous plasma renin activity may only be unmasked postpartum.

Importantly, many apparently healthy young women have never had BP measurement (or any routine medical care) before conception. Normal gestational vasodilation and relative hypotension may then mask their underlying chronic hypertension, which can then be mistaken for either gestational hypertension or pre-eclampsia if it worsens later in pregnancy.

Gestational hypertension

Gestational hypertension is hypertension that occurs *de novo*, usually during the latter half of pregnancy in the absence of proteinuria and other signs or symptoms of pre-eclampsia (see below) and resolves postpartum. Although it may result in severe hypertension requiring treatment, its course is usually more benign than that of pre-eclampsia. It may recur in subsequent pregnancies and often predicts essential hypertension or, like pre-eclampsia, increased cardiovascular risk later in life.

Pre-eclampsia

Pre-eclampsia is characterized by *de novo* hypertension, usually during the latter half of pregnancy, although well-characterized cases have been reported as early as 16 weeks. However, it is a multisystem disorder, usually defined by proteinuria (>300 mg/day) and resolving postpartum. It occurs in ~6% of (usually primigravid) pregnancies. Its incidence falls dramatically in subsequent pregnancies, except when risk is increased by a persisting underlying medical disorder (see below), or when the subsequent pregnancy involves a new father. Risk factors, listed in Box 54–1, include a family history of pre-eclampsia, multifetal gestation, diabetes mellitus, renal or autoimmune diseases, and obesity with insulin resistance.

Box 54–1

Risk Factors for Pre-eclampsia

- Primigravida
- First pregnancy with this partner
- Family history of pre-eclampsia
- Multifetal pregnancy
- Pre-eclampsia in prior pregnancy
- IUGR, placental abruption, or fetal demise in prior pregnancy
- Obesity
- Renal disease of any cause or severity (including microhematuria or microproteinuria without specific etiologic diagnosis)
- Diabetes mellitus
- Chronic hypertension
- Connective tissue disease

In addition, a variety of unrelated genetic abnormalities, including mutations of angiotensinogen or NO synthase genes, seem to increase the risk of pre-eclampsia in some populations. Whereas clinically evident target-organ damage characterizes more severe disease, subtle symptoms or laboratory evidence of target-organ damage, including hyperuricemia, thrombocytopenia, and abnormalities of liver function or coagulation tests, are common. Because pre-eclampsia can have a variable course and explosive clinical evolution,[16] with real risks of maternal morbidity and mortality, one should err toward diagnosing pre-eclampsia, even in the absence of proteinuria (which can occur later in the evolution of the disorder), when hypertension is accompanied by abdominal pain, neurologic symptoms such as headache or blurred vision, or any evidence of thrombocytopenia or liver function or coagulation abnormalities.[11] Indeed, criteria advocated by the Australasian Society for the Study of Hypertension in Pregnancy (ASSHP) favor the diagnosis of pre-eclampsia, even in the absence of proteinuria, when hypertension is accompanied either by fetal growth restriction or by evidence of renal, hepatic, neurologic, or hematologic involvement.[17] This approach, which differs from the other consensus guidelines,[18] better identifies women at low risk for subsequent complications, labeling them as gestational hypertensives.

Pre-eclampsia can evolve rapidly to a convulsive and life-threatening phase, termed eclampsia. An especially threatening variant of pre-eclampsia is the HELLP (hemolysis, elevated liver enzymes, low platelets) syndrome, which may seem mild in its initial presentation, and then evolves over hours to microangiopathic hemolysis, severe thrombocytopenia, and hepatic necrosis with rupture.

It can be surprisingly difficult to distinguish pre-eclampsia from gestational hypertension by the detection of proteinuria or by hemodynamic assessment. Obstetricians in the United States typically screen for proteinuria using urine dipsticks, confirming positive (1+) results by 24-hour urine collection (using methods for quantitation of 24-hour urine protein that often vary from hospital to hospital, although with a fixed diagnostic threshold value of 300 mg/day). This "gold standard" case definition is based on historical studies of clearly defined cases before the availability of sensitive and specific methods for assessment of albuminuria, excretion of other specific urine proteins, or recent advances in our understanding of the pathophysiology of this disorder. Indeed, it is likely that these advances will eventually lead to new case definitions and diagnostic strategies that will then replace this "tarnished" standard. Many gravidas with proteinuria exceeding the 300 mg/day threshold will prove to have no glomerular protein leak; 500 mg/day proteinuria or some new definition of pathologic albuminuria may better predict morbid maternal and fetal outcomes.[19] Due mostly to variation in urinary concentration, the sensitivity of urine dipsticks and their prediction of 24-hour urine protein are both poor. This limitation may be overcome, in part, by efforts to standardize screening techniques based on measurement of albumin:creatinine ratios, correction for urine specific gravity, or use of automated point-of-care devices.[20,21] Beyond these minor technical considerations, it is now clear that the onset of proteinuria may lag, in some cases by many weeks, behind that of hypertension.[22] This asynchrony would lead to misdiagnosis of pre-eclamptic women as gestational hypertensives and would then support the notion that gestational hypertension could transform (or evolve) into pre-eclampsia in a subset of patients.

It is likely that markers such as sFlt-1 or AT_1 receptor autoantibodies or convenient noninvasive hemodynamic measurements may, in the future, allow for more certain differential diagnosis during pregnancy. While we await adequately powered prospective studies that link these markers to outcomes in women at normal and elevated risk for pre-eclampsia or superimposed pre-eclampsia,[23] the diagnosis of pre-eclampsia can only be made with real certainty in retrospect.

Superimposed pre-eclampsia

"Pure" pre-eclampsia complicates ~6% of (usually primigravid) pregnancies. It can, in addition, be superimposed on 20% to 40% of pregnancies in women with underlying chronic hypertension or other predisposing medical diseases, including even minor renal disease of any cause, such as early diabetic nephropathy, autoimmune disease, or even microscopic hematuria.[24,25] Superimposed pre-eclampsia tends to be more severe than pre-eclampsia without underlying medical disorders. Likewise, given the persistence of the underlying risk factor, it is not surprising that it is more apt to recur in subsequent pregnancies. Indeed, pre-eclampsia occurring in other than a first pregnancy with the same partner should lead the clinician to search for an underlying medical predisposition. Superimposed pre-eclampsia and progression to more severe hypertension represent the two major risks of chronic hypertension in pregnancy.

It is often difficult to decide when an already hypertensive or already proteinuric woman's course has worsened due to the onset of superimposed pre-eclampsia. Indeed, in a classic study using renal biopsies to verify diagnosis, while clinical diagnosis of pure pre-eclampsia was quite accurate in previously healthy primigravidae, a nephrologist and obstetrician were only able to correctly diagnose pre-eclampsia and distinguish it from competing disorders in 58% of parous women.[26] Since it is now known that sFlt-1 accounts for the typical renal lesion of "glomerular endotheliosis,"[27] we suspect that its diagnostic accuracy would be similarly discordant in parous women or in those with underlying disease, although this remains to be determined. Diagnosis of pre-eclampsia can be even more difficult in women with pregestational glomerular disease whose proteinuria usually worsens during pregnancy, often to nephrotic levels. In such complicated cases, we currently advocate a strategy of close monitoring, repeatedly re-establishing baseline data in order to detect interval changes in BP, proteinuria or albuminuria, symptoms, or blood test results that might suggest superimposed pre-eclampsia. This cumbersome strategy might be streamlined if ongoing studies of high-risk pregnancies confirm a role for routine diagnostic or predictive testing based on measurement of sFlt-1 or related proteins.[28]

PATHOPHYSIOLOGY OF PRE-ECLAMPSIA AND ECLAMPSIA

Molecular pathophysiology

Because pre-eclampsia may occur in molar pregnancy (i.e., without a fetus), resolves following delivery of the placenta, and seems uniformly associated with typical defects in placentation when it occurs in primigravid women without underlying risk factors, much attention has been focused on a pathophysiologic role of the placenta. It is widely believed that early defects in trophoblastic invasion and remodeling of spiral arteries may fail to decrease placental resistance appropriately, leading to focal ischemia in the placenta and elaboration of factors that may act on the maternal vasculature to result in pre-eclampsia. While it is unclear whether these placental abnormalities are specific to pre-eclampsia or occur similarly in pre-eclamptic women with either underlying risk factors or with later clinical onset of disease (i.e., nearer to term), a large literature seems to support this construct by demonstrating that experimental utero-placental hypoperfusion leads to hypertension in pregnant laboratory animals and, more recently, in primates.[29,30] In pre-eclamptic women, the placenta elaborates soluble fms-like tyrosine kinase-1 (sFlt-1), a soluble receptor for (and functional antagonist of) vascular endothelial growth factor (VEGF) and placental growth factor (PlGF).[8,27] Abnormalities of another angiogenic factor, angiopoietin-1 and its receptor, tie-2, are also evident in pre-eclampsia.[31] Abnormalities in the availability of these angiogenic factors may increase BP and almost certainly lead to proteinuria and to the renal biopsy lesion of glomerular endotheliosis, which is typical of pre-eclampsia.

The pre-eclamptic placenta also sheds soluble fragments of endoglin, a TGF_β co-receptor, which appears to act in concert with sFlt-1 to produce several of the more severe disease phenotypes, such as severe hypertension, nephrotic-range proteinuria, fetal growth restriction, and the HELLP syndrome.[32] In addition to their roles in the molecular pathophysiology of pre-eclampsia, these antiangiogenic proteins may have an important role in diagnosis or disease prediction,[28] their actual utility will depend on the results of adequately powered prospective studies, such as that being undertaken by the World Health Organization.

Sympathetic outflow is increased in women with pre-eclampsia, perhaps contributing to hypertension,[33] and preceding the onset of clinically evident disease.[34] Several studies have also demonstrated changes in angiotensin receptor expression and activity[35] or the occurrence of autoantibodies that activate AT_1 receptors in women with pre-eclampsia.[8,36] The former report noted the occurrence of (bradykinin) B_2-AT_1 receptor heterodimers in maternal resistance arteries from pre-eclamptic women; it is unknown whether these heterodimeric receptors reveal antigenic epitopes that then lead to the agonistic autoantibodies. The autoantibodies, which clear soon after delivery, may underlie not only vasoconstriction and hypertension, but also the oxidative stress (via AT_1 receptor activation of superoxide synthesis by NAD(P)H oxidase) and endothelial dysfunction that are characteristic of pre-eclampsia. The effect of these autoantibodies is inhibited *in vitro* by angiotensin receptor blockers (ARBs), but use of these agents, along with use of ACE inhibitors, is contraindicated in late pregnancy due to fetal toxicity.[37]

SYSTEMIC AND RENAL HEMODYNAMICS IN PRE-ECLAMPSIA

Pulmonary artery catheterization of untreated pre-eclamptic women reveals that hypertension in this disorder is due to systemic vasoconstriction associated with decreased CO and left ventricular filling pressures.[38] Paradoxically, early in pregnancy, prior to the onset of hypertension, CO is increased more in women who subsequently develop either gestational hypertension or pre-eclampsia than in those who go on to uneventful normotensive pregnancies, although not so reliably as to allow prediction of these disorders. Hemodynamics of these two disorders diverge when hypertension becomes manifest, with further increments of CO (and low SVR) in women with gestational hypertension and a "switch" to systemic vasoconstriction and low CO in women with pre-eclampsia.[39] Pre-eclampsia appears to reverse the increments in large-artery compliance that characterize normotensive pregnancy.[40] In addition, pulse wave analysis reveals marked increments of systolic augmentation index, determined by applanation tonometry, in women with pre-eclampsia. By contrast, the augmentation index is usually negative in normal gravidas and only modestly elevated in gravidas with chronic or gestational hypertension.[40–42]

Pre-eclampsia decreases GFR by ~33% and effective renal plasma flow by ~25%, consistent with selective afferent arteriolar renal vasoconstriction, and usually decreases renal uric acid clearance, elevating serum levels above the norms for pregnancy (2.8 to 3.2 mg/dL).[2] An older literature demonstrated striking parallels between the severity of hyperuricemia and either renal biopsy or clinical manifestations of pre-eclampsia.[43] Recent studies have revisited the clinical value of hyperuricemia, demonstrating that uric acid increases progressively before the onset of hypertension in women with pre-eclampsia and that hyperuricemia predicts fetal morbidity even in the absence of pre-eclampsia.[44,45] The proteinuria that characterizes pre-eclampsia is nonselective, with increased excretion of both albumin and nonalbumin proteins. Pre-eclampsia is the major cause of nephrotic-range proteinuria during pregnancy. The occurrence of edema (which is common even in normal pregnancy) is quite variable in pre-eclampsia; indeed, many women who present with eclamptic seizures may be free of edema.

Platelet abnormalities

Platelet activation is present in the hypertensive disorders of pregnancy, and platelets play a major role in the disease process.[46,47] In normal pregnancy, there is an increased platelet activation *in vivo*, which is usually accompanied by a limited decline in platelet numbers.[3,4] In pre-eclampsia, there is platelet consumption secondary to unchecked intravascular platelet activation and fibrin deposition, resulting in a progressive and marked decline in circulating platelets. Abnormal platelet activation and adhesion have also been shown.[48]

CEREBROVASCULAR ABNORMALITIES IN PRE-ECLAMPSIA

There has been long-standing controversy regarding the mechanisms that lead to eclamptic seizures and other central nervous system complications in pre-eclampsia. Some have viewed these as a form of hypertensive encephalopathy, while others, citing autopsy findings of hemorrhage and petechiae,[49] have suggested that brain injury is caused by focal ischemia due to vasoconstriction. The preponderance of recent studies, many using noninvasive Doppler and MR techniques, suggest a role for increased cerebral perfusion pressure or defective local autoregulation in most cases, supporting the former pathophysiologic construct.[50] Further, MR evidence associates cerebral edema and reversible posterior leukencephalopathy syndrome with even "minor" neurologic symptoms such as headache and blurred vision in pre-eclampsia. It is intriguing that anti-VEGF antibodies, which can mimic the effects of sFlt-1 on BP and proteinuria, also may lead to reversible posterior leukencephalopathy.[51,52] This cerebrovascular pathophysiologic construct leads to specific therapeutic strategies regarding selection of antihypertensive agents in pre-eclamptic women, since labetalol and magnesium (but not calcium channel blockers or other vasodilators) appear to decrease elevated cerebral perfusion pressure in these patients.[53,54]

PRE-ECLAMPSIA PREVENTION

Antihypertensive treatment and BP lowering *per se* fail to prevent pre-eclampsia.[55,56] Similarly, neither salt restriction nor prophylactic diuretics prevents pre-eclampsia, despite earlier claims to the contrary.[57] An extremely controversial literature has suggested that genetic thrombophilias, including the factor V Leiden and prothrombin gene mutations, may increase the risk of pre-eclampsia. Most recent studies appear to refute this association[58]; however, we are without a well-designed randomized trial of low-molecular-weight heparin in women at risk. Observations of hypocalciuria in pre-eclamptic women led to several large studies of calcium supplementation, which, however, failed to prevent pre-eclampsia.[59] By contrast, while there was still no effect on the incidence of pre-eclampsia, a randomized trial of calcium supplementation in 8325 nulliparous women with extremely low baseline dietary calcium decreased the incidence of eclampsia, severe gestational hypertension, and several composite measures of maternal morbidity.[60]

Observations consistent with an imbalance in arachidonic acid metabolism in pre-eclampsia that favored vasocontrictor thromboxanes over prostacyclin led to many primary prevention studies using low-dose (60 to 100 mg/day) aspirin. Many early small studies were extraordinarily promising; unfortunately, these results have not been confirmed in subsequent well-designed large trials that have included more than 25,000 women, demonstrating only trivial effects on maternal or fetal outcome or on the occurrence of pre-eclampsia.[61,62] Additional studies of women at high risk for recurrent or superimposed pre-eclampsia also failed to demonstrate meaningful prevention of proteinuric hypertension with aspirin. Although meta-analyses of trials that included more than 36,000 women have suggested some benefit (relative risk 0.81, confidence interval 0.75–0.88) of aspirin prophylaxis, this conclusion is not supported by any of the larger well-designed trials included within the meta-analysis and have failed to identify any aspirin-sensitive subgroups of women at risk.[63]

Evidence of placental, vascular, and systemic oxidative stress in pre-eclampsia along with plausible pathophysiologic schema relating oxidative stress to hypertension, renal dysfunction, and organ damage led to several large prophylactic studies using the antioxidant vitamins C and E. The Vitamins in Pre-eclampsia (VIP) trial showed no benefit in 2395 women at high risk for pre-eclampsia.[64] Indeed, vitamin supplementation in this study was surprisingly associated with more severe and earlier-onset pre-eclampsia, more severe hypertension, lower birth weight, and increased neonatal morbidity.[64,65] Vitamin supplementation resulted in neither benefit nor harm in a similarly large and well-conducted study of 1877 low-risk nulliparas (the Australian Collaborative Trial of Supplements).[66] An even larger trial is still ongoing in the United States.[65]

RISKS OF HYPERTENSION IN PREGNANCY AND GUIDELINES FOR EVALUATION AND MANAGEMENT

Chronic hypertension increases risks of several morbid pregnancy outcomes, including superimposed pre-eclampsia, preterm birth, intrauterine growth restriction, placental abruption, perinatal death, and accelerated hypertension threatening the mother.[67-69] Antihypertensive treatment fails to prevent these outcomes, except for the occurrence of more severe hypertension later in pregnancy. This remains important because adverse perinatal outcomes seem closely related to severity of maternal hypertension and because severe hypertension may be a major cause of both hospitalization and early delivery. Recognition of these risks and of clinical uncertainty regarding evaluation and treatment of hypertensive gravidas has led to updated guidelines by consensus groups in the United States, Canada, and Australia.[11,17,70]

All of the consensus groups agree, even without clear outcomes data, that BPs as low as 170/110 mmHg can lead to cerebrovascular hemorrhage during pregnancy, making control of such pressures a medical emergency. At the opposite extreme, it has been suggested, but not proven, that tight BP control may impair fetal growth.[71]

The ASSHP suggests maintaining BPs at less than 140/90 mmHg.[17] The Canadian Hypertension Society suggests similarly tight control only for some groups of women.[70] By contrast, the NHBPEP Working Group on Hypertension in Pregnancy suggests (re)instituting drug therapy at pressures of 150 to 160/100 to 110, targeting lower pressures in selected patients with target-organ damage or underlying renal disease.[11] Not only is there disagreement among national groups, but disagreement occurs even within a single system: a survey of Canadian practitioners with experience in the care of hypertensive pregnant women revealed no consensus regarding appropriate BP targets.[72] These uncertainties provide both the equipoise and impetus for adequately powered prospective trials to guide therapy, several of which are now planned or underway.

EVALUATION AND MANAGEMENT OF HYPERTENSION IN PREGNANCY

Ideally, evaluation of women with chronic hypertension or with a history of hypertension in a previous pregnancy should begin before conception. The clinician should focus on the possibility of secondary hypertension, assessment of renal function and hypertensive target-organ damage, detecting underlying diabetes or renal disease, and eliciting a family history of pregnancy complications. Proteinuria, *per se*, appears to increase pregnancy risk in hypertensive women. In addition, the obstetric history should focus on both maternal and neonatal outcome that includes premature birth, intrauterine growth restriction leading to small-for-gestational-age infants, placental abruption, fetal demise, neonatal morbidity and mortality, and the severity and timing of superimposed pre-eclampsia, because severe early-onset disease is more apt to recur.

Most women whose hypertension is well controlled using two or fewer antihypertensive drugs before conception will be able to discontinue therapy, due to the physiologic BP control effected by gestational vasodilation. Often, no antihypertensives will be required until later in pregnancy, obviating most concerns regarding drug safety in the first trimester. Women should have a baseline laboratory evaluation that includes urinalysis and urine culture, 24-hour urine for evaluation of creatinine clearance, protein and albumin excretion, comprehensive chemistry panel including measurement of hepatic transaminases, uric acid, and electrolytes, and complete blood count with platelets. Most clinicians would repeat these studies each trimester, in order to establish a new baseline to aid in the recognition of superimposed pre-eclampsia, although there are no prospective studies demonstrating benefit from this strategy. Women should then be seen every 2 to 3 weeks for measurement of BP and urine protein, and for fetal assessment as indicated.

Higher-risk chronic hypertensive women include those with advanced maternal age, long-standing hypertension, or any evidence of target-organ damage, diabetes mellitus, renal disease of any cause or severity, any connective tissue disease, cardiomyopathy, vascular malformation, previous history of fetal or perinatal loss, or worsened hypertension early in pregnancy. These women require closer observation, collaborative care with appropriate subspecialists, and probably tighter BP control to avoid progressive target-organ damage during pregnancy. Despite general agreement, there have been no studies that show benefit of tighter BP control in hypertensive gravidas with renal disease or other underlying medical disorders. Worsened hypertension or suspicion of superimposed pre-eclampsia will commonly lead to inpatient evaluation in order to ensure maternal and fetal well-being and titrate antihypertensive therapy, and to decide whether pregnancy may be prolonged safely with close monitoring.

Antihypertensive therapy remote from delivery

With some small differences, the American, Canadian, and Australasian consensus statements make note of the wealth of clinical experience that led to recognizing methyldopa as a preferred antihypertensive for use during pregnancy.[11,17,70] It is well tolerated, does not alter uteroplacental or fetal hemodynamics, and has the best long-term follow-up of childhood development following exposure *in utero*, albeit in an underpowered study.[73] Methyldopa-induced hepatitis is a rare adverse effect, and Coombs-positive hemolytic anemia is rare with short-term treatment. Many women are, however, unable to tolerate its more common adverse effects of drowsiness or dry mouth. A recent meta-analysis suggesting excess perinatal morbidity and mortality with methyldopa when compared with other antihypertensive drugs[56] should serve as impetus for further prospective studies rather than for abandonment of the long clinical experience and consensus support for use of methyldopa in pregnancy.

Beta-blockers are also widely used in pregnancy, have been assessed in several randomized trials, and are the subject of a Cochrane meta-analysis.[55] Early preclinical and clinical observations raised concerns of impaired uteroplacental perfusion, fetal growth restriction, and harmful cardiovascular effects on the fetus. Atenolol use early in pregnancy in one small trial led to striking fetal growth restriction, a conclusion supported by several reviews, retrospective series, and meta-analyses.[74–77] However, most prospective studies, focusing instead on β-blocker use during the third trimester, have shown effective BP control, prevention of more severe hypertension, and an absence of significant adverse effects, including bradycardia, on the fetus. A large single-center case series has noted superior perinatal outcome with β-blockers (primarily atenolol) compared with other agents (primarily nifedipine or methyldopa).[67] Further, a meta-analysis of several small trials suggested that β-blockers might decrease (and calcium channel blockers increase) the incidence of proteinuria or superimposed pre-eclampsia, perhaps by limiting abnormal elevations in cardiac output.[56,79] While many older studies focused on agents such as atenolol, the NHBPEP Working Group advocates labetalol (a combined α- and β-blocker) as an alternative to methyldopa, and the Australasian group advocates use of β-blockers with intrinsic sympathomimetic activity, such as oxprenolol or pindolol.[11,17]

Calcium channel blockers, principally extended-release nifedipine, are widely used, apparently safe, and effective in pregnancy.[11] Although data are limited, nifedipine is widely viewed as an acceptable alternative to methyldopa or β-blockers for chronic use during pregnancy. In the past, hydralazine was the most commonly used second-line agent, although its popularity has probably been exceeded by the calcium channel blockers. It is generally used in combination with either a β-blocker or methyldopa to limit reflex tachycardia. Alpha-adrenergic blockers are used seldom during pregnancy, although they remain first-choice agents in the rare setting of suspected pheochromocytoma. Diuretic use during pregnancy is controversial since they limit normal gestational volume expansion, and can decrease amniotic fluid volume and lead to electrolyte abnormalities. However, they do not seem to compromise fetal outcome.[57] Diuretics may be continued if they are crucial to BP control before conception, and may be combined with other agents, especially in patients with renal insufficiency or heart disease, or when clinical volume overload is a problem.[11] Diuretics are not used when pre-eclampsia is suspected, because its hemodynamics are characterized by decreased CO and primary systemic vasoconstriction.[1,38,39]

Increased circulating elements of the renin-angiotensin system during pregnancy and evidence for AT_1 receptor activation in pre-eclampsia might seem to support use of ACE inhibitors or ARBs in hypertensive gravidas. Indeed, many young women of childbearing age with either underlying diabetic nephropathy or proteinuric renal disease will be receiving these drugs for "renal protection" before conception. They are, however, frankly contraindicated during the latter half of pregnancy due to a specific fetopathy (including renal dysgenesis and calvarial hypoplasia) and the risk of (fatal) neonatal acute renal failure.[37,80,81] In addition, first trimester exposure now appears to convey some teratogenic risk as well. Using information from a Tennessee Medicaid database, Cooper et al.[82] identified 18 major congenital malformations in babies exposed to ACE inhibitors only during the first trimester. The risk of major malformation was ~2.7-fold greater than in unexposed infants and due primarily to a mixture of cardiovascular and central nervous system anomalies. It should be noted that many of these abnormalities were patent ductus arteriosus or septal defects that did not require surgical correction and that a previous unpublished study of first-trimester captopril exposure had failed to identify these risks.[83] Taken together, it would seem prudent to avoid ACE inhibitors and ARBs in women of childbearing potential for whom the only indication is essential hypertension that is easily controlled with other agents. By contrast, for women such as those with refractory hypertension, diabetes mellitus, or proteinuric renal disease, whose care may depend on these drugs, it would seem prudent to counsel them regarding these risks, discontinue their use when pregnancy is confirmed, and review fetal well-being with a detailed ultrasound examination at 18 weeks gestational age. Table 54–1 summarizes the agents most commonly used for chronic BP control in pregnancy.

ORAL ANTIHYPERTENSIVES USED COMMONLY IN PREGNANCY		
Drug (FDA risk[1,2])	Dose	Concerns or Comments
Most Commonly Used First Line Agents		
Methyldopa (B)	0.5-3.0g/d in 2-3 divided doses	Preferred agent of the NHBPEP working group; maternal side effects sometimes limit use.
Labetalol (C) or other β receptor antagonists	200-2400mg/d in 2-3 divided doses	Labetalol is preferred by NHBPEP working group as alternative to methlydopa. Atenolol most commonly used in Canada and β blockers with intrinsic sympathomimetic activity are preferred by some in Australia. May cause fetal growth restriction when started early
Nifedipine (C)	30-120mg/d of a slow-release preparation	Less experience with other calcium entry blockers.
Adjunctive Agents Hydralazine (C)	50-300mg/d in 2-4 divided doses	Few controlled trials, long experience; used only in combination with sympatholytic agent (eg methyldopa or a β blocker) to prevent reflex tachycardia.
Thiazide diuretics (C)	depends on specific agent	Most studies in normotensive gravidas.
Contraindicated ACE inhibitors and AT1 receptor antagonists (D[4])		Use after first trimester can lead to fetopathy, oligohydramnios, growth retardation, and neonatal anuric renal failure, which may be fatal.

[1] No antihypertensive has been proven safe for use during the first trimester (ie, FDA Category A).

[2] US Food and Drug Administrations classifies risk for most agents as C: either studies in animals have revealed adverse effects on the fetus (teratogenic or embryocidal effects or other) and there are no controlled studies in women, or studies in women and animals are not available. Drugs should only be given if the potential benefit justifies the potential risk to the fetus. This nearly useless classification unfortunately still applies to most drugs used during pregnancy.

Table 54–1. Oral Antihypertensives Used Commonly in Pregnancy

Antihypertensive therapy of more severe hypertension

Table 54–2 lists the antihypertensives most commonly used for urgent control of severe hypertension late in pregnancy. Parenteral labetalol, by continuous intravenous infusion or in repeated boluses, has replaced hydralazine at many centers and appears to have similar safety and efficacy, although comparative studies are few.[84–86] Hydralazine is used either in small (5 to 10 mg) repeated doses or as a continuous infusion, because larger doses or frequent dosing may lead to precipitous maternal hypotension and fetal distress. Despite its lack of approval by the U.S. Food and Drug Administration for the treatment of hypertension, the NHBPEP Working Group advocates oral (or sublingual) nifedipine as an acceptable alternative to hydralazine or labetalol for urgent BP control during pregnancy.[11] Its efficacy and safety, as well as that of parenteral nicardipine infused at 3 to 9 mg/h[87] appear similar to the other agents, while diazoxide and ketanserin seem inferior.[84] Concerns that dihydropyridine calcium channel blockers might accentuate adverse effects of magnesium sulfate in pre-eclamptic women seem unfounded.[88] Sodium nitroprusside remains a relatively contraindicated agent of last resort.[89] Finally, while there have been reports of ACE inhibitor use as "salvage therapy" during pregnancy,[90] there seems to be no justification for use of these agents or of angiotensin receptor blockers during the second or third trimester.

CLINICAL AND ADJUNCTIVE MANAGEMENT OF PRE-ECLAMPSIA

Suspicion of pre-eclampsia should lead to hospitalization and inpatient evaluation, although this might be undertaken in a day hospital or short-stay unit if available. Despite common practice, we still do not know if hypertensive gravidas benefit from bedrest.[91] Near to term (>34 weeks), if fetal maturity can be ensured, delivery is the preferred and definitive treatment for pre-eclampsia. Earlier in pregnancy, it may seem desirable to temporize, attempting to control BP, administer glucocorticoids to hasten fetal lung maturation, and monitor laboratory and clinical status closely so as to prolong pregnancy. The obstetric literature on such temporizing strategies often appears confusing and contradictory. Expectant management may result in a few days to, rarely, several weeks of additional fetal maturation; however, such strategies are best reserved to tertiary centers. Regardless of gestational age, consensus opinion currently suggests that any of the ominous signs or symptoms noted in Box 54–2 should lead to immediate delivery. Despite this widespread agreement, we caution that there are no prospective data to support the notion that our clinical definition of "severe" pre-eclampsia actually predicts morbid outcomes. Indeed, an ongoing multicenter prospective observational study in Canada, the United Kingdom, and New Zealand thus far suggests that only severe hypertension, throm-

ANTIHYPERTENSIVES USED COMMONLY FOR URGENT BP CONTROL		
Drug (FDA risk[1])	**Dose and Route**	**Concerns or Comments[2]**
Hydralazine (C)	5mg, iv or im, then 5-10mg every 20-40 min; or constant infusion of 0.5-10mg/hr	Higher doses or more frequent administration often precipitate maternal or fetal distress, which appear more common than with other agents.
Labetalol (C)	20mg iv, then 20-80 mg every 20-30 min, up to maximum of 300mg; or constant infusion of 1-2mg/min	Probably less risk of tachycardia and arrhythmia than with other vasodilators, likely less BP control than hydralazine.
Nifedipine (C)	5-10mg po, repeat in 30 min if needed, then 10-20mg every 2-6 hr	Oral and sublingual dosing are equivalent; neither is FDA-approved for hypertension treatment.
Nicardipine (C)	3-9 mg/h, iv, titrated to effect	Tachycardia more common than with labetalol.

[1] US Food and Drug Administration Class C, as noted in footnote to Table 54–1.

[2] Adverse effects for all agents, except as noted, may include headache flushing, nausea, and tachycardia (primarily due to precipitous hypotension and reflex sympathetic activation).

Table 54–2. Antihypertensives Used Commonly for Urgent BP Control

---

Box 54–2

Ominous Signs and Symptoms in Pre-eclampsia Suggesting Prompt Delivery

- Inability to control BP (systolic <160 mmHg or diastolic <105)
- Any evidence of acute renal failure or progressive oliguria
- Falling platelets or thrombocytopenia <105/mm^3
- Any evidence of microangiopathic hemolysis or coagulopathy
- Upper abdominal (epigastric or right upper quadrant) pain
- Headache, visual disturbance, or any CNS signs
- Retinal hemorrhage or papilledema
- Acute congestive heart failure or pulmonary edema

---

bocytopenia, elevated liver enzymes, chest pain, dyspnea, or right upper-quadrant abdominal pain might predict morbid outcomes strongly enough to justify delivery for maternal indications.[92] As noted earlier, accelerated hypertension should be treated at systolic levels of greater than 160 mmHg or diastolic of greater than 100 to 105 mmHg (Korotkoff 5), to avoid the cerebrovascular catastrophes that can occur at pressures of ≥170/110. We advocate treatment at these somewhat lower pressures due to increased BP lability and uncertainty in BP measurement in women with pre-eclampsia. Central nervous system signs or symptoms, including headache or blurred vision, should provoke treatment at even lower pressures. Despite findings from invasive hemodynamic studies, there appears to be no benefit from therapeutic volume expansion in addition to BP control.[93]

Parenteral magnesium sulfate has long been favored by North American clinicians for prevention or treatment of eclamptic seizures, which can occur antepartum (38% to 53% of cases), intrapartum (18% to 36% of cases), or postpartum (11% to 36% of cases).[94] Magnesium is superior to either phenytoin or diazepam in preventing recurrent seizures in women with eclampsia.[95,96] Several primary prevention trials in women with pre-eclampsia, including a placebo-controlled, double-blind study in over 10,000 women, demonstrated the efficacy of magnesium, without significant short-term adverse effects to mother or baby.[93,97] It remains unclear, however, which women with pre-eclampsia should be offered magnesium and how long treatment should continue if delivery is postponed. In most centers, treatment usually entails a loading dose of 4 to 6 g of MgSO$_4$ (infused over 10 minutes, never as a bolus), followed by continuous infusion of 1 to 2 g/h to achieve plasma levels of 5 to 9 mg/dL. Magnesium is then usually continued until the patient stabilizes or for 24 hours following delivery. Lower doses should be used, without continuous infusion, guided by serum levels, in women with any degree of renal insufficiency, as magnesium is excreted renally. Finally, a vial of calcium gluconate should always be kept at the bedside in case of magnesium toxicity.

Overall, our clinical approach to evaluation, management, and treatment of pregnant women with underlying hypertension is in accord with recommendations made by the NHBPEP Working Group,[11] although, as noted above, we favor the classification scheme of the Australasian group.[17] Our key objectives, to be carried out in close coordination with experienced high-risk obstetric colleagues, are to achieve BP control adequate to ensure maternal safety, to carefully and serially monitor maternal BP, well-being, and laboratory data in order to facilitate early recognition of superimposed pre-eclampsia, and to proceed to expeditious delivery (with or without magnesium prophylaxis) in the face of pre-eclampsia or accelerated hypertension when it presents a threat to maternal safety.

REFERENCES

1. McLaughlin MK, Roberts JM. Hemodynamic changes. In: Lindheimer MD, Roberts JM, Cunningham FG, eds. *Chesley's Hypertensive Disorders in Pregnancy*, 2nd ed. Stamford, CT: Appleton & Lange, 1999:69–102.

2. Conrad KP, Lindheimer MD. Renal and cardiovascular alterations. In: Lindheimer MD, Roberts JM, Cunningham FG, eds. *Chesley's Hypertensive Disorders in Pregnancy*, 2nd ed. Stamford, CT: Appleton & Lange, 1999:263–326.

3. Poppas A, Shroff SG, Korcarz CE, Hibbard JU, Berger DS, Lindheimer MD, et al. Serial assessment of the cardiovascular system in normal pregnancy. Role of arterial compliance and pulsatile arterial load. *Circulation* 1997;95:2407–15.

4. August P, Lindheimer MD. Chronic hypertension. Lindheimer MD, Roberts JM, Cunningham FG, eds. *Chesley's Hypertensive Disorders in Pregnancy*, 2nd ed. Stamford, CT: Appleton & Lange, 1999:605–33.

5. August PA, Seeley JE. The renin angiotensin system in normal and hypertensive pregnancy and in ovarian function. In: Laragh JH, Brenner BM, eds. *Hypertension: Pathophysiology, Diagnosis, and Management*, 2nd ed. New York: Raven Press, 1995:2225–44.

6. Merrill DC, Karoly M, Chen K, Ferrario CM, Brosnihan KB. Angiotensin-(1–7) in normal and preeclamptic pregnancy. *Endocrine* 2002;18:239–45.

7. Lindheimer MD, Richardson DA, Ehrlich EM, Katz AI. Potassium homeostasis in pregnancy. *J Reprod Med* 1987;32:517–32.

8. Davison JM, Homuth V, Jeyabalan A, Conrad KP, Karumanchi SA, Quaggin S, et al. New aspects in the pathophysiology of pre-eclampsia. *J Am Soc Nephrol* 2004;15:2440–48.

9. Debrah DO, Novak J, Matthews JE, Ramirez RJ, Shroff SG, Conrad KP. Relaxin is essential for systemic vasodilation and increased global arterial compliance during early pregnancy in conscious rats. *Endocrinology* 2006;147 (epub ahead of print doi:10.1210/en.2006-0567).

10. Brown MA, Lindheimer MD, DeSwiet M, et al. The classification and diagnosis of the hypertensive disorders of pregnancy: statement from the International Society for the Study of Hypertension in Pregnancy. *Hypertens Preg* 2001;20: IX–XIV.

11. NHBPEP. *Report of the National High Blood Pressure Education Project [NJHBPBP] Working Group on High Blood Pressure in Pregnancy*. Washington, DC: National Institutes of Health, NIH publication No. 00-3029, July 2000 (available at http://www.nhlbi.nih.gov/health/prof/heart/hbp_preg.htm).

12. Waugh J, Habiba MA, Bosio P, Boyce T, Shennan A, Halligan AW. Patient initiated home blood pressure recordings are accurate in hypertensive pregnant women. *Hypertens Pregnancy* 2003;22:93–97.

13. Hermida RC, Ayala DE. Prognostic value of office and ambulatory blood pressure measurements in pregnancy. *Hypertension* 2002;40:298–303.

14. Kamari Y, Sharabi Y, Leiba A, Peleg E, Apter S, Grossman E. Peripartum hypertension from pheochromocytoma: a rare and challenging entity. *Am J Hypertens* 2005;18:1306–12.

15. Le TT, Haskal ZJ, Holland GA, Townsend R. Endovascular stent placement and magnetic resonance angiography for management of hypertension and renal artery occlusion during pregnancy. *Obstet Gynecol* 1995;85:822–25.

16. Hauth JC, Cunningham FG. Pre-eclampsia-Eclampsia. In: Lindheimer MD, Roberts JM, Cunningham FG, eds. *Chesley's Hypertensive Disorders in Pregnancy*, 2nd ed. Stamford, CT: Appleton & Lange, 1999:169–99.

17. Brown MA, Hague WM, Higgins J, et al. The detection, investigation and management of hypertension in pregnancy: full consensus statement. *Aust N Z J Obstet Gynecol* 2000;40: 139–55.

18. Brown MA, Buddle ML. What's in a name? Problems with the classification of hypertension in pregnancy. *J Hypertens* 1997;15:1049–54.

19. Waugh J, Bell SC, Kilby MD, Lambert P, Shennan A, Halligan A. Urine protein estimation in hypertensive pregnancy: which thresholds and laboratory assays best predict clinical outcome? *Hypertens Pregnancy* 2005;24:291–302.

20. Meyer NL, Mercer BM, Friedman SA, Sibai BM. Urinary dipstick protein: a poor predictor of absent or severe proteinuria. *Am J Obstet Gynecol* 1994; 170:137–41.

21. Waugh JJ, Bell SC, Kilby MD, Blackwell CN, Seed P, Shennan AH, et al. Optimal bedside urinalysis for the detection of proteinuria in hypertensive pregnancy: a study of diagnostic accuracy. *BJOG Int J Obstet Gynaecol* 2005;112:412–17.

22. Wolf M, Shah A, Jimenez-Kimble R, Sauk J, Ecker JL, Thadhani R. Differential risk of hypertensive disorders of pregnancy among Hispanic women. *J Am Soc Nephrol* 2004;15:1330–38.

23. Williams WW Jr, Ecker JL, Thadhani RI, Rahemtullah A. Case records of the Massachusetts General Hospital. Case 38-2005. A 29-year-old pregnant women with the nephrotic syndrome and hypertension. *N Engl J Med* 2005; 353:2590–600.

24. Ekbom P, Damm P, Nogaard K, Clausen P, Feldt-Rasmussen U, Feldt-Rasmussen B, et al. Urinary albumin excretion and 24-hour blood pressure as predictors of pre-eclampsia in type I diabetes. *Diabetologia* 2000;43:927–31.

25. Stehman-Breen CO, Levine RJ, Qian C, Morris CD, Catalano PM, Curet LB, et al. Increased risk of pre-eclampsia among nulliparous pregnant women with idiopathic hematuria. *Am J Obstet Gynecol* 2002;187:703–708.

26. Fisher KA, Luger A, Spargo BH, Lindheimer MD. Hypertension in pregnancy: clinical-pathological correlations and remote prognosis. *Medicine* 1981;60:267–76.

27. Maynard SE, Min JY, Merchan J, Lim KH, Li J, Mondal S, et al. Excess placental soluble fms-like tyrosine kinase 1 (sFlt1) may contribute to endothelial dysfunction, hypertension, and proteinuria in pre-eclampsia. *J Clin Invest* 2003;111:649–58.

28. Levine RJ, Lam C, Qian C, Yu KF, Maynard SE, Sachs BPet al. Soluble endoglin and other circulating antiangiogenic factors in pre-eclampsia. *N Engl J Med* 2006;355:992–1005.

29. Khalil RA, Granger JP. Vascular mechanisms of increased arterial pressure in pre-eclampsia: lessons from animal models. *Am J Physiol* 2002; 283:R29–45.

30. Makris A, Thronton C, Thompson S, Thompson J, Martin R, McKenzie P, et al. Primate uteroplacental ischaemia results in proteinuric hypertension and elevated soluble Flt-1. *Hypertens Preg* 2006;25(Suppl 1):13, abstract.

31. Nadar S, Karalis I, Al-Yemeni E, Blann A, Lip GYH. Plasma markers of angiogenesis in pregnancy induced hypertension. *Thromb Haemost* 2005;94:1071–76.

32. Venkatesha S, Toporsian M, Lam C, Hanai J, Mammoto T, Kim YM, et al. Soluble endoglin contributes to the pathogenesis of pre-eclampsia. *Nat Med* 2006;12:642–49.

33. Schobel HP, Fischer T, Heuszer K, Geiger H, Schmieder RE. Pre-eclampsia—a state of sympathetic overactivity. *N Engl J Med* 1996;335:1480–85.

34. Fischer T, Schobel HP, Frank H, Andreae M, Schneider KT, Heusser K. Pregnancy-induced sympathetic overactivity: a precursor of pre-eclampsia. *Eur J Clin Invest* 2004;34:443–48.

35. AbdAlla S, Lother H, el Massiery A, Quitterer U. Increased AT(1) receptor heterodimers in pre-eclampsia mediate enhanced angiotensin II responsiveness. *Nat Med* 2001;7:1003–1009.

36. Wallukat G, Homuth V, Fischer T, Lindschau C, Horstkamp B, Jupner A, et al. Patients with pre-eclampsia develop agonistic autoantibodies against the angiotensin AT1 receptor. *J Clin Invest* 1999;103:945–52.

37. Serreau R, Luton D, Macher MA, Delezoide AL, Garel C, Jacqz-Aigrain E. Developmental toxicity of the angiotensin II type 1 receptor antagonists during human pregnancy: a report of 10 cases. *BJOG Int J Obstet Gynaecol* 2005;112: 710–12.

38. Visser W, Wallenburg HCS. Central hemodynamic observations in untreated preeclamptic patients. *Hypertension* 1991;17:1072–77.

39. Bosio PM, McKenna PJ, Conroy R, O'Herlihy C. Maternal central hemodynamics in hypertensive disorders of pregnancy. *Obstet Gynecol* 1999;94:978–84.

40. Hibbard JU, Korcarz CE, Nendaz GG, Lindheimer MD, Lang RM, Shroff SG. The arterial system in pre-eclampsia and chronic hypertension with superimposed pre-eclampsia. *BJOG Int J Obstet Gynaecol* 2005;112:897–903.

41. Spasojevic M, Smith SA, Morris JM, Gallery ED. Peripheral arterial pulse wave analysis in women with pre-eclampsia and gestational hypertension. *BJOG Int J Obstet Gynaecol* 2005;112:1475–78.

42. Elvan-Taspinar A, Franx A, Bots ML, Bruinse HW, Koomans HA. Central hemodynamics of hypertensive

disorders in pregnancy. *Am J Hypertens* 2004;17:941–46.

43. Pollak VE, Nettles JB. The kidney in toxemia of pregnancy: a clinical and pathologic study based on renal biopsies. *Medicine Baltimore* 1960;39:469–526.

44. Powers RW, Bodnar LM, Ness RB, Cooper KM, Gallaher MJ, Frank MP, et al. Uric acid concentrations in early pregnancy among preeclamptic women with gestational hyperuricemia at birth. *Am J Obstet Gynecol* 2006;194:160.e1–e8.

45. Roberts JM, Bodnar LM, Lain KY, Hubel CA, Markovic N, Ness RB, et al. Uric acid is as important as proteinuria in identifying fetal risk in women with gestational hypertension. *Hypertension* 2005;46:1263–69.

46. Whigham KA, Howie PW, Drummond AH, Prentice CR. Abnormal platelet function in pre-eclampsia. *Br J Obstet Gynaecol* 1978;85(1):28–32.

47. Nadar S, Lip GY. Platelet activation in the hypertensive disorders of pregnancy. *Expert Opin Invest Drugs* 2004;13:523–29.

48. Karalis I, Nadar S, Al-Yemeni E, Blann A, Lip GYH. Platelet activation in pregnancy-induced hypertension. *Thromb Res* 2005;116, 377–83.

49. Sheehan H, Lynch JB. *Pathology of Toxemia of Pregnancy*. London: Churchill, 1973.

50. Belfort MA, Varner MA, Dizon-Townson DS, Grunewald C, Nisell H. Cerebral perfusion pressure, and not cerebral blood flow, may be the critical determinant of intracranial injury in pre-eclampsia: a new hypothesis. *Am J Obstet Gynecol* 2002;187:626–34.

51. Fujiwara Y, Higaki H, Yamada T, Nakata Y, Kato S, Yamamoto H, et al. Two cases of reversible posterior leukoencephalopathy syndrome, one with and the other without pre-eclampsia. *J Obstet Gynaecol Res* 2005; 31:520–26.

52. Glusker P, Recht L, Lane B. Reversible posterior leukoencephalopathy syndrome and bevacizumab. *N Engl J Med* 2006;354:980–82.

53. Belfort MA, Saade GR, Yared M, Grunewald C, Herd JA, Varner MA, et al. Change in estimated cerebral perfusion pressure after treatment with nimodipine or magnesium sulfate in patients with pre-eclampsia. *Am J Obstet Gynecol* 1999;181:402–407.

54. Belfort MA, Tooke-Miller C, Allen JC Jr, Dizon-Townson DS, Varner MA. Labetalol decreases cerebral perfusion pressure without negatively affecting cerebral blood flow in hypertensive gravidas. *Hypertens Preg* 2002;21: 185–97.

55. Magee LA, Duley L. Oral beta blockers for mild to moderate hypertension during pregnancy. *Cochrane Database Syst Rev* 2003;(3):CD002863.

56. Abalos E, Duley L, Steyn DW, Henderson-Smart DJ. Antihypertensive drug therapy for mild to moderate hypertension during pregnancy. *Cochrane Database Syst Rev* 2001; 2:CD002252.

57. Collins R, Yusuf S, Peto R. Overview of randomised trials of diuretics in pregnancy. *BMJ* 1985;290:17–23.

58. Salomon O, Seligsohn U, Steinberg DM, Zalel Y, Lerner A, Rosenberg N, et al. The common prothrombotic

factors in nulliparous women do not compromise blood flow in the feto-maternal circulation and are not associated with pre-eclampsia or intrauterine growth restriction. *Am J Obstet Gynecol* 2004;191:2002–2009.

59. Levine RJ, Hauth JC, Curet LB, Sibai BM, Catalano PM, Morris CD, et al. Trial of calcium to prevent pre-eclampsia. *N Engl J Med* 1997;337:69–76.

60. Villar J, Abdel-Aleem H, Merialdi M, Mathai M, Ali MM, Zavaleta N, et al. World Health Organization randomized trial of calcium supplementation among low calcium intake pregnant women. *Am J Obstet Gynecol* 2006;194:639–49.

61. Sibai BM, Caritis SN, Thom E, Klebanoff M, McNellis D, Rocco L, et al. Prevention of pre-eclampsia with low-dose aspirin in healthy, nulliparous pregnant women. *N Engl J Med* 1993; 329:1213–18.

62. CLASP (Collaborative Low-Dose Aspirin Study in Pregnancy) Collaborative Group. CLASP: a randomised trial of low-dose aspirin for the prevention and treatment of pre-eclampsia among 9364 pregnant women. *Lancet* 1994;343: 619–29.

63. Duley L, Henderson-Smart DJ, Knight M, King JF. Antiplatelet agents for preventing pre-eclampsia and its complications. *Cochrane Database Syst Rev* 2004;(1):CD004659.

64. Poston L, Briley AL, Seed PT, Kelly FJ, Shennan AH, for Vitamins in Pre-eclampsia (VIP) Trial Consortium. Vitamin C and vitamin E in pregnant women at risk for pre-eclampsia (VIP trial): randomized placebo-controlled trial. *Lancet* 2006;367 (published online March 30, 2006, DOI:10.1016/ S0140-6736(06)68433-X).

65. Lindheimer MD, Sibai BM. Antioxidant supplementation in pre-eclampsia. *Lancet* 2006;367 (published online March 30, DOI:10.1016/ S0140-6736(06)68434-1).

66. Rumbold AR, Crowther CA, Haslam RR, Dekker GA, Robinson JS for ACTS Study Group. Vitamins C and E and the risks of pre-eclampsia and perinatal complications. *N Engl J Med* 2006; 354:1796–806.

67. Rey E, Couturier A. The prognosis of pregnancy in women with chronic hypertension. *Am J Obstet Gynecol* 1994;171:410–16.

68. Ferrer RL, Sibai BM, Mulrow CD, et al. Management of mild chronic hypertension during pregnancy: a review. *Obstet Gynecol* 2000;96:849–60 (full report available at http://www.ahcpr.gov/clinic/ evrptfiles.htm).

69. Sibai BM, Lindheimer M, Hauth J, Caritis S, VanDorsten P, Klebanoff M,. et al. Risk factors for pre-eclampsia, abruptio placentae, and adverse neonatal outcomes among women with chronic hypertension. *N Engl J Med* 1998;339:667–71.

70. Rey E, LeLorier J, Burgess E, et al. Report of the Canadian Hypertension Society consensus conference. 3. Pharmacologic treatment of hypertensive disorders in pregnancy. *CAMJ* 1997;157:1245–54.

71. von Dadelszen P, Ornstein MP, Bull SB, Logan AG, Koren G, Magee LA. Fall in mean arterial pressure and fetal growth

restriction in pregnancy hypertension: a meta-analysis. *Lancet* 2000;355:87–92.

72. Caetano M, Ornstein MP, Von Dadelszen P, Hannah ME, Logan AG, Gruslin A, et al. A survey of Canadian practitioners regarding the management of the hypertensive disorders of pregnancy. *Hypertens Preg* 2004;23:61–74.

73. Cockburn J, Moar VA, Ounsted M, Redman CW. Final report of study on hypertension during pregnancy: the effects of specific treatment on the growth and development of the children. *Lancet* 1982;1:647–49. (Earlier follow-up papers from this trial included Mutch, Moar, Ounsted, Redman, *Early Hum Dev* 1977;1:47–57, 1:59–67.)

74. Butters L, Kennedy S, Rubin PC. Atenolol in essential hypertension during pregnancy. *BMJ* 1990;301: 587–89.

75. Lip GY, Beevers M, Churchill D, Shaffer LM, Beevers DG. Effect of atenolol on birthweight. *Am J Cardiol* 1997;79: 1436–38.

76. Bayliss H, Churchill D, Beevers M, Beevers DG. Anti-hypertensive drugs in pregnancy and fetal growth: evidence for "pharmacological programming" in the first trimester? *Hypertens Preg* 2002; 21:161–74.

77. Lydakis C, Lip GY, Beevers M, Beevers DG. Atenolol and fetal growth in pregnancies complicated by hypertension. *Am J HypertensJ Hypertens* 1999;12:541–47.

78. Ray JG, Vermeulen MJ, Burrows EA, Burrows RF. Use of antihypertensive medications in pregnancy and the risk of adverse perinatal outcomes: McMaster outcome study of hypertension in pregnancy 2 (MOS HIP 2). *BMC Pregnancy Childbirth* 2001;1:6.

79. Easterling TR, Brateng D, Schmucker B, Brown Z, Millard SP. Prevention of pre-eclampsia;a randomized trial of atenolol in hyperdynamic patients before onset of hypertension. *Obstet Gynecol* 1999;93:725–33.

80. Sedman AB, Kershaw DB, Bunchman TE. Recognition and management of angiotensin converting enzyme inhibitor fetopathy. *Pediatr Nephrol* 1995;9:382–85.

81. Centers for Disease Control and Prevention. Postmarketing surveillance for angiotensin-converting enzyme inhibitor use during the first trimester of pregnancy—United States, Canada, and Israel, 1987–1995. *MMWR Morb Mortal Wkly Rep* 1997;46:240–42.

82. Cooper WO, Hernandez-Diaz S, Arbogast PG, Dudley JA, Dyer S, Gideon PS, et al. Major congenital malformations after first-trimester exposure to ACE inhibitors. *N Engl J Med* 2006;354:2443–51.

83. Briggs GG, Freeman RK, Yaffe ST. *Drugs in Pregnancy and Lactation: A Reference Guide to Fetal and Neonatal Risk*, 7th ed. Philadelphia: Lippincott Williams & Wilkins, 2005:212–17.

84. Duley L, Henderson-Smart DJ, Meher S. Drugs for treatment of very high blood pressure during pregnancy. *Cochrane Database Syst Rev* 2006;(3):CD001449.

85. Magee LA, Cham C, Waterman EJ, Ohlsson A, von Dadelszen P. Hydralazine for treatment of severe

hypertension in pregnancy: meta-analysis. *BMJ* 2003;327:955–60.

86. Vigil-De Gracia P, Lasso M, Ruiz E, Vega-Malek JC, de Mena FT, Lopez JC. Severe hypertension in pregnancy: hydralazine or labetalol: a randomized clinical trial. *Eur J Obstet Gynecol Reprod Biol* 2006 (online publication ahead of print, April 16).

87. Hanff LM, Vulto AG, Bartels PA, Roofthooft DW, Bijvank BN, Steegers EA, et al. Intravenous use of the calcium-channel blocker nicardipine as second-line treatment in severe, early-onset pre-eclamptic patients. *J Hypertens* 2005;23:2319–26.

88. Magee LA, Miremadi S, Li J, Cheng C, Ensom MH, Carleton B, et al. Therapy with both magnesium sulfate and nifedipine does not increase the risk of serious magnesium-related maternal side effects in women with pre-eclampsia. *Am J Obstet Gynecol* 2005;193:153–63.

89. Shoemaker CT, Meyers M. Sodium nitroprusside for control of severe hypertensive disease of pregnancy: a case report and discussion of potential toxicity. *Am J Obstet Gynecol* 1984;149:171–73.

90. Easterling TR, Carr DB, Davis C, Diederichs C, Brateng DA, Schmucker B. Low-dose, short-acting, angiotensin-converting enzyme inhibitors as rescue therapy in pregnancy. *Obstet Gynecol* 2000;96:956–61.

91. Meher S, Abalos E, Carroli G, Meher S. Bedrest with or without hospitalization for hypertension during pregnancy. *Cochrane Database Syst Rev* 2005; (4):CD003514.

92. Menzies J, Magee LA, Li J, MacNab YC, Douglas MJ, Gruslin A, et al. Current CHS and NHBEP criteria of "severe" pre-eclampsia do not uniformly predict adverse maternal outcomes. *Hypertens Pregnancy* 2006;25Suppl 1: 199 (abstract).

93. Ganzevoort W, Rep A, Bonsel GJ, Fetter WP, van Sonderen L, De Vries JI, et al. A randomized controlled trial comparing two temporizing management strategies, one with and one without plasma volume expansion, for severe and early onset pre-eclampsia. *BJOG Int J Obstet Gynaecol* 2005;112:1358–68.

94. Sibai BM. Diagnosis, prevention and management of eclampsia. *Obstet Gynecol* 2005;105:402–10.

95. The Eclampsia Collaborative Group. Which anticonvulsant for women with eclampsia? Evidence from the collaborative eclampsia trial. *Lancet* 1995;345:1455–63.

96. Lucas MJ, Leveno KJ, Cunningham FG. A comparison of magnesium sulfate with phenytoin for the prevention of eclampsia. *N Engl J Med* 1995;333: 201–205.

97. The Magpie Trial Collaborative Group. Do women with pre-eclampsia, and their babies, benefit from magnesium sulphate? The Magpie Trial: a randomised placebo-controlled trial. *Lancet* 2002;359:1877–79.

Chapter

55

Insulin Resistance and Diabetes in Hypertension

Maryann N. Mugo, Daniel Link, Craig S. Stump, and James R. Sowers

Key Findings

- In the United States, diabetes mellitus currently affects 18.2 million individuals and is the sixth leading cause of death.

- Coexistent hypertension contributes significantly to the development of cardiovascular disease and associated premature morbidity in these patients.

- "Prediabetic" states should be evaluated for hypertension as they are at increased risk for hypertension and cardiovascular disease.

- Genetic predisposition and acquired factors such as obesity and sedentary lifestyle result in insulin resistance, which is strongly associated with hypertension.

- The renin-angiotensin-aldosterone system plays a crucial role in the pathogenesis of both diabetes and hypertension and associated cardiovascular and renal disease.

Clinical Implications

- Several antihypertensive medications, including angiotensin-converting enzyme inhibitors and angiotensin receptor blockers, have beneficial effects in diabetes mellitus beyond blood pressure control, including reducing renal dysfunction, cardiovascular disease, and stroke.

- Some antihypertensive medications have been shown to decrease onset of diabetes mellitus when compared with placebo and others.

The rise in the prevalence of diabetes mellitus (DM) is a global phenomenon that is approaching epidemic proportions. It is currently estimated that approximately 300 million adults will be affected worldwide in the next few decades. In the United States alone, DM currently affects 6.3% of the adult population, or approximately 18.2 million individuals, and is the sixth leading cause of death.[1] Among adults over 60 years of age, 8.6 million are affected, representing 18.3% of this age group. The prevalence of DM is highest in persons above 65 years of age but adults under 45 years of age have shown the most striking rise in DM prevalence in the last decade.[2] Furthermore, ethnic groups other than Caucasians such as Hispanics, African Americans, and Native Americans are affected by DM at a rate two to four times that for Caucasian Americans.[3]

A notable rise in the prevalence of DM has occurred in children and adolescents primarily due to the rise in the prevalence of type 2 DM. The leading cause of premature

mortality in adults with DM is cardiovascular disease (CVD). Additionally, DM is now the leading cause of end-stage renal disease (ESRD) and nontraumatic amputations, both of which contribute to the higher rates of premature mortality. Coexistent hypertension contributes significantly to the development of CVD and renal disease in these patients.[4] In this chapter we review the pathophysiology of hypertension in DM—particularly type 2—clinical presentation, and treatment.

SPECTRUM OF INSULIN RESISTANCE, IMPAIRED GLUCOSE TOLERANCE, AND OVERT DIABETES MELLITUS TYPES 1 AND 2

Recently the recognition of "prediabetic" states such as impaired fasting glucose (IFG), impaired glucose tolerance (IGT), and the metabolic syndrome have expanded the spectrum of patients to be considered when approaching the management of hypertension in the DM population (Table 55–1).

First, it is important to make the distinction between type 1 (DM1) and type 2 diabetes mellitus (DM2) when tackling hypertension management. The most notable

TABLE 55–1. DEFINITIONS AND DIAGNOSIS	
State	**Characteristics**
Normal	FPG <100 mg/dL; 2-hour P <140 mg/dL (5.5 mmol/L)
"Prediabetes"	Impaired fasting glucose (IFG): ≥100 and <126 mg/dL (5.5–7.0 mmol/L)
	Impaired glucose tolerance (IGT): 2-hour post-75-g anhydrous glucose plasma glucose ≥140 mg/dL and <200 mg/dL (7.0–11.1 mmol/L)
Diabetes	FPG ≥126 mg/dL (7.0 mmol/L); fasting = no caloric intake for at least 8 hours
	Random glucose ≥200 mg/dL (11.1 mmol/L) without symptoms on two occasions *or* once with symptoms (*random glucose* means without regard to previous meal)
	2-hour post-75-g anhydrous glucose plasma glucose ≥200 mg/dL (11.1 mmol/L)
FPG, fasting plasma glucose.	

Table 55–1. Definitions and Diagnosis

differences are that DM1 patients form only 6% to 8% of the total population diagnosed with DM, are usually younger, and typically develop hypertension only after the onset of renal disease.[5] The onset of hypertension (HTN), however, accelerates the course of microvascular and macrovascular disease in this subgroup of patients.[4]

Most diabetic patients are in the DM2 group, and only a fraction of the population estimated to have DM2 have actually been diagnosed and treated despite more stringent diagnostic criteria. Many of these patients manifest the clustering of CVD risk factors described in the Framingham study and are at risk of developing DM2 and its attendant CVD complications.[6] In this subgroup of patients, HTN may precede the onset of DM2 or be present at the time of diagnosis, thus underscoring the importance of evaluating associated risk factors collectively in these patients.

The National Cholesterol Education Program (NCEP) Adult Treatment Panel III (ATP III) defined the metabolic syndrome as presence of any three or more of the following: blood pressure (BP) ≥130/85 mmHg, waist circumference >40 in in men or >35 in in women, triglycerides ≥150 mg/dL, HDL <40 mg/dL in men or <50 mg/dL in women, and fasting glucose ≥110 mg/dL (Table 55–2). The metabolic syndrome is a clustering of maladaptive characteristics that confers an increased risk of CVD.[3] A recent analysis of the National Health and Nutrition Examination Survey (NHANES 1999–2000) revealed that the overall prevalence of the metabolic syndrome is currently estimated at 26.7%, an increase from the NHANES III (1988–1994) survey estimate of 23.1%. Further, an age-dependent increase in prevalence is apparent in both men (10.7%, 33.0%, and 39.7%) and women (18.0%, 30.6%, and 46.1%) for ages 20 to 39, 40 to 59, and ≥60 years, respectively.[7] More recently, a new definition of metabolic syndrome has been proposed by the International Diabetes Federation[8] (Box 55–1) (Table 55–3).

Insulin resistance appears to play a key role in the pathophysiology of the metabolic syndrome and the associated cardiovascular risk.[9] These clustered risk factors provide the milieu for impaired glucose tolerance (IGT), impaired fasting glucose (IFG), and overt diabetes mellitus to increase cardiovascular risk.[9] IFG when associated with mild HTN (SBP 140–149) is independently associated with

---

Box 55–1

Metabolic Syndrome: International Diabetes Federation Definition

Central obesity
Waist circumference[a]—ethnicity specific (see Table 55–3)
Plus any two of the following:
Raised triglycerides
>150 mg/dL (1.07 mmol/L)
Specific treatment for this lipid abnormality
Reduced HDL cholesterol
<40 mg/dL (1.03 mmol/L) in men
<50 mg/dL (1.29 mmol/L) in women
Specific treatment for this lipid abnormality
Raised blood pressure
Systolic ≥130 mmHg
Diastolic ≥85 mmHg
Treatment of previously diagnosed hypertension
Raised fasting plasma glucose[b]
Fasting plasma glucose ≥100 mg/dL (5.6 mmol/L)
Previously diagnosed type 2 diabetes
If above 5.6 mmol/L or 100 mg/dL, oral glucose tolerance test is strongly recommended, but is not necessary to define presence of syndrome.

From Alberti KG, Zimmet P, Shaw J. *Lancet* 2005;366:1059–62 with permission from Elsevier.

[a]If body mass index is over 30 kg/m², central obesity can be assumed and waist circumference does not need to be measured.

[b]In clinical practice, impaired glucose tolerance is also acceptable, but all reports of prevalence of metabolic syndrome should use only fasting plasma glucose and presence of previously diagnosed diabetes to define hyperglycemia. Prevalences also incorporating 2-hour glucose results can be added as supplementary findings.

---

increased CVD mortality.[10] Obesity, specifically visceral obesity, has been associated with insulin resistance and premature CVD. A rising body mass index (BMI) is independently associated with a linear rise in systolic BP (SBP), diastolic BP (DBP), and pulse pressure.

PATHOPHYSIOLOGY

The rise in insulin resistance has paralleled the rise in obesity, and the two are strongly linked.[11] Obesity, defined in adults as a BMI greater than 30 kg/m², has also been associated with a higher incidence of HTN and DM2.[12] Excess abdominal adiposity is a hallmark of the metabolic syndrome, and imparts a higher risk than subcutaneous adiposity. Visceral adiposity tends to consist of large insulin-resistant adipocytes that have several metabolic abnormalities and are deficient in adiponectin. Insulin-mediated antilipolysis is decreased, and catecholamine-induced lipolysis is increased. Numerous adipocyte-derived cytokines (adipokines) produced by these viscerally located adipocytes mediate inflammation and insulin resistance. These cytokines include increased TNF-α, PAI-1, IL-6, and leptin.[3] Visceral adiposity is best measured in the clinical setting using waist circumference rather than weight alone. The parameters currently used are a waist circumference of >40 inches (102 cm) in men and >35 inches (88 cm) in women.

METABOLIC SYNDROME NCEP/ATP III GUIDELINES DEFINITION	
Risk Factor	**Levels**
Blood pressure	≥130/85 mmHg
Waist circumference	>40 in (men); >35 in (women)
Triglycerides	≥150 mg/dL
High-density lipoproteins	<40 mg/dL (men) and <50 mg/dL (women)
Fasting glucose	≥110 mg/dL

Note: Meeting any three of the above criteria qualifies for the patient for classification as metabolic syndrome.

Data from the National Cholesterol Program Adult Treatment Panel III, 2001.

Table 55–2. Metabolic Syndrome NCEP/ATP III Guidelines Definition

ETHNIC-SPECIFIC VALUES FOR WAIST CIRCUMFERENCE	
Ethnic Group	**Waist Circumference (Measure of Central Obesity)**
Europids[a]	
Men	>94 cm
Women	80 cm
South Asians	
Men	>90 cm
Women	>80 cm
Chinese	
Men	>90 cm
Women	>80 cm
Japanese	
Men	>85 cm
Women	90 cm
Ethnic South and Central Americans	Use South Asian recommendations until more specific data are available
Sub-Saharan Africans	Use European data until more specific data are available
Eastern Mediterranean and Middle East (Arab) populations	Use European data until more specific data are available

From Alberti KG, Zimmet P, Shaw J. *Lancet* 2005;366:1059–62 with permission from Elsevier.

Notes: Data are pragmatic cutoffs, and better data are required to link them to risk. Ethnicity should be the basis for classification, not country of residence.

[a]In the United States, Adult Treatment Panel III values (102 cm male, 88 cm female) are likely to continue to be used for clinical purposes. In future epidemiologic studies of populations of Europid origin (white people of European origin, regardless of where they live in the world), prevalence should be given, with both European and North American cutoffs to allow better comparisons.

Table 55–3. Ethnic-Specific Values for Waist Circumference

Decreased insulin action due to resistance and compensatory hyperinsulinemia may have adverse effects on the insulin signaling cascade.[13] Clinical consequences of these derangements include hypertension, DM2 and CVD.[14] Correspondingly, studies of patients with both DM2 and HTN show a causal role of insulin resistance and accompanying hyperinsulinemia.[14,15] Insulin resistance occurs in up to 50% of the 50 million patients with essential HTN in the United States.[16] Untreated patients with essential HTN have higher fasting and postprandial insulin levels than age- and sex-matched normotensive persons regardless of body mass.[17] Normotensive first-degree relatives of patients with HTN also have insulin resistance and dyslipidemia.[18] Genetic predisposition to both disorders tempered by the 21st-century environment (sedentary lifestyle, lack of exercise, poor dietary habits) are the link between HTN and insulin resistance, given that not all hypertensive patients have insulin resistance and hyperinsulinemia and, high insulin levels are not a feature of secondary hypertension.[19]

As noted, HTN in DM1 is usually a consequence of diabetic nephropathy. In contrast, HTN in patients with DM2, prediabetes, and metabolic syndrome is a much more complicated interplay of physiologic mechanisms.[20] Key players in this scenario include insulin resistance/hyperinsulinemia,[9] angiotensin II (Ang II), endothelin, and oxidative stress, all of which mediate endothelial and vascular dysfunction.[9,21] Other contributing factors are increased sympathetic nervous system (SNS) activity,[22] sodium retention, and renal dysfunction. Insulin resistance and hyperinsulinemia both play a crucial role in the pathogenesis of hypertension in diabetes mellitus, and obesity itself seems to contribute significantly. Hypertension is associated with hyperinsulinemia/insulin resistance in obese diabetic individuals, nondiabetic obese individuals, and in patients with essential hypertension.

Interestingly, the association among insulin resistance, obesity, and hypertension is absent in Pima Indians, who also have relatively lower muscle sympathetic nerve activity than obese insulin-resistant Caucasian males.[23] This suggests that the SNS may be a link among obesity, hyperinsulinemia, and hypertension in some populations.[22]

The mechanisms that are believed to be involved in the pathogenesis of diabetes-related hypertension are summarized in Figure 55–1.

Renin-angiotensin-aldosterone system

Ang II is a powerful vasoconstrictor and has a central role in blood pressure regulation. Studies have shown that Ang II infusion induces insulin resistance while blockade of Ang II results in increased insulin sensitivity.[24] Insulin is known to induce vasodilation *in vivo* but this ability of insulin is reduced in insulin-resistant

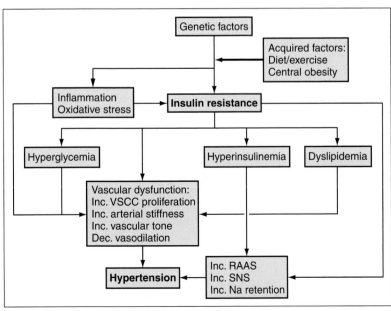

Figure 55–1. Interrelationship of the mechanisms contributing to hypertension in diabetes mellitus. Inc., increased; RAAS, renin-angiotensin-aldosterone system; SNS, sympathetic nervous system.

states and diabetes, potentially because of deranged endothelial synthesis combined with enhanced inactivation of nitric oxide (NO) via Ang II and other mechanisms.[19] Insulin increases the expression and activity of endothelial nitric oxide synthase (eNOS), which results in increased production of NO. NO plays a major role in endothelial vasodilation, and also inhibits the effects of vascular endothelial growth factor (VEGF) in promoting the expression of adhesion molecules such as intercellular adhesion molecule (ICAM) and vascular cellular adhesion molecule (VCAM). This in turn protects endothelial cells from interactions with circulating monocytes that are involved in the atherosclerotic process.

Initially recognized for its role in renal effect on salt and water metabolism, Ang II has been shown to have profound adverse effects on the endothelium.[25] For a long time, the most recognized effects of Ang II were mediated via the AT_1R receptor. More recently, Ang II has been shown to exert effects via the AT_1R and AT_2R receptors. Ang II has been shown to influence endothelial cell apoptosis and increase oxidative stress via the type 1 receptor (AT_1R). In contrast, the type 2 receptor (AT_2R) reduces reactive oxygen species (ROS) and increases nitric oxide (NO) production.[26] Other effects of Ang II on the endothelial cell have been discovered more recently. Uptake of oxidized LDL (oxLDL) by endothelial cells is mediated by the lectin-like oxLDL receptor-1 (LOX-1).[27] Ang II via the AT_1R has been shown to upregulate the effects of LOX-1, thereby enhancing the uptake of oxidized LDL into the endothelial cell, a key step in atherosclerosis. Ang II is a potent regulator of the prothrombotic plasminogen activator inhibitor type 1 (PAI-1). PAI-1 plays a key role in thrombosis, promotes atherosclerosis, and is the major physiologic inhibitor of plasminogen activator. Ang II has been shown to increase PAI-1 messenger RNA and protein in endothelial cells and this effect is mediated by AT_1R via a pathway that involves rho/rho kinase, cyclic adenosine monophosphate (AMP), and ROS.[28] Cyclooxygenase-2 (COX-2) activation plays a role in both angiogenesis and atherogenesis via synthesis of prostaglandins and thromboxane A2, thereby resulting in endothelial cell dysfunction. A different mechanism by which Ang II enhances angiogenesis is via the increased production of vascular endothelial growth factor (VEGF).[29] Increased endothelial cell VEGF may potentiate vascular remodeling, increased vascular permeability, and edema. The evidence implicating Ang II in the pathogenesis of HTN in diabetes mellitus is extensive[30] (Figure 55–2). Despite all this information, the precise mechanism by which insulin resistance interacting with Ang II results in hypertension still remains unknown and needs further investigation.

Several clinical studies using medications that interrupt the renin-angiotensin-aldosterone system (RAAS) have shown major benefit in decreasing incidence of stroke, diabetes mellitus and end-stage renal disease.[31] Ang II is synthesized from angiotensin I by angiotensin-converting enzyme. Angiotensin-converting enzyme inhibitors (ACEI) primarily block this conversion, thus preventing it from exerting its potent vasoconstrictor effect. Similarly, blockade of the AT_1R is the primary mechanism of action of

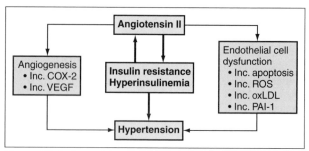

Figure 55–2. Potential pathways through which angiotensin II may contribute to hypertension in diabetes mellitus. COX-2, cyclooxygenase-2; ROS, reactive oxygen species; VEGF, vascular endothelial growth factor.

the angiotensin receptor blockers (ARBs), but they additionally activate multiple AT_1R independent pathways. These pathways include activation of eNOS by stimulation of a PI3-kinase/Akt pathway and activation of peroxisome proliferator-activated receptor.[27]

Reactive oxygen species

Under normal conditions, oxidant formation is balanced by the rate of oxidant removal.[19] An imbalance between pro-oxidants and antioxidants results in oxidative stress, which has adverse metabolic and clinical consequences. NAD(P)H oxidase is a major source of ROS, which under pathologic conditions play an important role in renal dysfunction and vascular damage. In the vasculature, ROS are derived from endothelial, adventitial, and smooth muscle cells. NAD(P)H oxidase, a multisubunit enzyme, catalyzes the production of oxygen free radicals from reducing oxygen using NAD(P)H as the electron donor.[32] Pathologically increased ROS result in endothelial dysfunction, increased contractility, VSMC proliferation, monocyte invasion, lipid peroxidation, inflammation, and deposition of extracellular matrix proteins, all of which may cause hypertension-associated vascular damage.[33] ROS are a strong link between insulin resistance and hypertension.[34]

Inflammation/Prothrombosis

Chronic inflammation may play a role in insulin resistance and may further aggravate vascular dysfunction, thus predisposing to atherosclerosis and CVD complications.[19] Adipose tissue is a key source of inflammatory cytokines (adipokines) and tumor necrosis factor-alpha (TNF-α) and interleukin-6 (IL-6) are important in this regard.

Cytokines are intercellular signaling polypeptides that regulate the hematopoietic, immune systems and also trigger the inflammatory cascade. Chronic upregulation of IL-6 may predispose to atherosclerosis via a direct effect on the atherosclerotic lesion.[35] TNF-α levels correlate with insulin resistance, and this occurs via its ability to serine phosphorylate insulin receptor substrate-1, thus decreasing the activity of the insulin receptor.[36] C-reactive protein (CRP) is increased in inflammatory states such as insulin resistance, DM2, and obesity, and is an independent predictor of cardiovascular events.[37] Patients with the metabolic syndrome also have increased plasma high-sensitivity CRP.[38] Collectively these increased cytokines contribute to CVD mortality, and HTN may be an additional risk factor in these patients.[19]

CLINICAL PRESENTATIONS

Stroke in patients with diabetes mellitus and hypertension

Patients with DM2 have a high incidence of stroke and poor outcomes. Although no clinical studies show a direct correlation between controlling glycemia and modification of stroke event rates, prevention of stroke in these patients is important due the poorer outcomes. Hypertension, heart failure, and cigarette and alcohol use are modifiable risk factors for stroke in patients with and without DM.[5] In 2002 there were 57 stroke-related deaths in the United States per 100,000 people. Stroke is currently ranked as the third leading cause of death in the United States. There are more than 700,000 strokes annually and more than 4.5 million stroke survivors.[39]

As the prevalence of DM increases, it has become a well-documented, independent, modifiable stroke risk factor. Indeed, the incidence of stroke among DM patients is up to three times that in the general population.[40] There is an increase in both short- and long-term mortality in patients with DM following stroke, and admission glucose levels are one predictor of poor outcomes in these patients.[41]

Numerous intervention trials have provided compelling support for intensive BP control in patients with DM to prevent stroke. In the UK Prospective Diabetes Study (UKPDS) for combined fatal and nonfatal stroke, achieving a mean BP of 144/82 mmHg resulted in a 44% relative risk reduction compared with the less-aggressive control group that had a mean BP of 154/87 mmHg.[42] Additional data from the Systolic Hypertension in Europe (Syst-Eur) trial, with nitrendipine-based antihypertensive therapy, showed that the excess risk of stroke associated with DM was abolished by antihypertensive treatment in older patients with DM2 and isolated HTN. In the microalbuminuria, Cardiac and Renal Outcomes in the Heart Outcomes Prevention Evaluation (MICRO-HOPE), 3577 patients with DM treated with ramipril showed a 25% reduction of primary combined endpoints of myocardial infarction, stroke, and CVD death, and a 33% stroke reduction.[43]

Recent studies have shown the beneficial effects of an ARB/diuretic or an ACEI/diuretic combination in reduction of primary and secondary strokes in high-risk patients, including those with DM.[44] The recent Antihypertensive and Lipid-Lowering Treatment to Prevent Heart Attack Trial (ALLHAT) also showed that treatments using a diuretic and lowering SBP were very important strategies to reduce stroke incidence in patients with DM.[45] These data support recent guidelines recommending a BP of less than 130/80 mmHg in patients with DM and HTN.[46] Further, early and aggressive attainment of BP less than 130/80 mmHg in these patients may help mitigate CVD risk and premature mortality.[47]

Renal dysfunction in patients with diabetes mellitus and hypertension

An estimated 35% of persons with DM will develop diabetic nephropathy characterized by proteinuria, decreased glomerular filtration rate, and increased BP, which has become the leading cause of ESRD in the United States. In patients with DM2, the incidence of nephropathy is approximately 20%. Nevertheless, because up to 95% of diabetic patients have DM2, more than half of ESRD cases in DM occur in patients with DM2. The prevalence and incidence of ESRD are approximately twice what they were 10 years ago, and if the trends of the past two decades persist, approximately 175,000 new cases of ESRD will be diagnosed in 2010. This is due in part to the expectation that the incidence of DM2 will double within the next 10 to 15 years, and the fact that patients with DM are living longer and are thus more likely to develop chronic problems, including ESRD. The cost associated with the management of ESRD, in the United States alone, is expected to exceed $28 billion per year by 2010.[48]

The appearance of clinically detectable, dipstick-positive proteinuria signals the onset of progressive diabetic nephropathy, which is typically followed by deterioration to ESRD over a period of 10 to 15 years. Microalbuminuria, which heralds the onset of nephropathy, is defined as albuminuria detected in urine at levels of 30 to 299 mg/day. Albumin excretion exceeding these parameters is macroalbuminuria or overt proteinuria. Both macro- and micro-albuminuria are major independent risk factors for CVD.[49]

Microalbuminuria predicts the development of CVD and stroke, in addition to progression of diabetic nephropathy. Microalbuminuria has been associated with insulin resistance/hyperinsulinemia, atherogenic dyslipidemia, the absence of a nocturnal drop in SBP and DBP, and salt sensitivity, and has been identified as a part of the cardiometabolic syndrome. For these reasons, it is not surprising that diabetic glomerulosclerosis parallels the process of diabetic atherosclerosis and is a powerful risk factor for CVD and stroke.[4] Even after adjustment for renal function, microalbuminuria remained a strong risk factor for CVD in a subanalysis of the HOPE trial.[50] In the HOPE trial, the presence of albuminuria doubled the risk for the composite endpoint of myocardial infarction, stroke, or CVD death, and all-cause mortality. The risk of clinical heart failure was 3.7 times greater in DM2 patients with microalbuminuria compared with those without albuminuria. Furthermore, these risks were significantly reduced with treatment with the ACE inhibitor, ramipril. Medications that interrupt the RAAS, such as ACEIs and ARBs, are increasingly important in reducing the progression of nephropathy in these patients. Chronic kidney disease and the presence of either microalbuminuria or proteinuria dictate lowering BP to a goal of <130/80 mmHg and reducing proteinuria by at least 30% to 50%.[51]

Other clinical considerations
Autonomic neuropathy

Autonomic neuropathy is common in diabetic patients, affecting 5% to 10% of long-term diabetic patients and as many as 35% of those patients with subclinical peripheral neuropathy. Autonomic neuropathy is usually manifested as orthostatic hypertension, sexual dysfunction, and abnormalities of gastrointestinal motility, among other symptoms. Once autonomic neuropathy becomes clinically apparent, it compromises BP regulation.[10] In patients with DM and autonomic dysfunction, excessive venous pooling can cause orthostatic or postural hypotension. Postural hypotension, a decrease in SBP >20 mmHg on standing from a supine position, is usually associated with hypo-adrenergic or hyperadrenergic signs and symptoms, such as lightheadedness, dizziness, dimming of vision, nausea, diaphoresis, and syncope. Because of the increased propensity of diabetic patients to manifest increased orthostatic BP changes, measurements should be performed in both the supine and standing positions.[51] Another effective tool is ambulatory BP monitoring, which can be useful in determining the presence of drug resistance, hypotensive symptoms, episodic HTN, or autonomic dysfunction. Autonomic neuropathy and the associated decrease in heart rate variability and increased electrocardiogram QT interval are in part a consequence of a reduced parasympathetic to sympathetic activity in diabetic patients. This abnormality contributes to the greatly increased risk of sudden death in diabetic patients.

Nondipping blood pressure/Pulse pattern

In normotensive and most hypertensive patients, the circadian BP rhythm demonstrates higher BP readings when patients are awake and lower BP readings when they are asleep. This is referred to as "dipping," and the expected drop is approximately 10% to 15%. "Non-dippers" have less than the usual 10% decline at night, a condition more frequent among diabetic patients, as demonstrated by ambulatory BP monitoring. Loss of nocturnal dipping of BP and heart rate are characteristics of HTN associated with DM. This loss of nocturnal dipping in BP and heart rate appears to be due, in part, to dysautonomia that is often present in diabetic patients.[27] The nondipping pattern of BP in diabetics is associated with microalbuminuria, proteinuria, and left ventricular hypertrophy, thereby conferring a higher CVD risk morbidity and mortality to patients who have it.[52] Reduced vascular compliance further contributes to elevations in systolic BP, increases in pulse pressure, and associated CVD risk.

Diabetic cardiomyopathy

Diabetic cardiomyopathy is increasingly being recognized as a specific entity in patients with DM2.[53] The development of diabetic cardiomyopathy is most likely multifactorial. Putative mechanisms include metabolic disturbances, such as defective glycolysis and glucose oxidation, myocardial fibrosis, small vessel disease and autonomic dysfunction. Abnormalities of calcium handling that can lead to subsequent diabetic cardiomyopathy have also been demonstrated. Existence of this condition in a diabetic patient may have several therapeutic implications including: improving glycemic control, earlier use of calcium channel blockers (CCBs), ACE inhibitors and ARBs, exer-

cise training, lipid-lowering therapy, and antioxidant and insulin-sensitizing drugs.[53] Calcium channel blockers may reverse the intracellular calcium defects and prevent DM-induced myocardial changes. Verapamil significantly improves the depressed rate of contraction and rate of relaxation, lowers peak LV systolic pressure, and elevates LV diastolic pressure.[54] ACE inhibitors may improve fibrosis in the myocardium and improve endothelial dysfunction.[53] Clinically, ACE inhibitors reduce CVD in diabetic patients, particularly diabetic patients with HTN. ARBs and aldosterone antagonists may also have effects similar to ACE inhibitors on myocardial fibrosis in diabetic patients.[3–5]

DIAGNOSTIC TECHNIQUES

Diagnosis of HTN in DM requires screening the population with risk factors such as central obesity, dyslipidemia, older age, sleep apnea, and any patient with a family history. Application of proper blood pressure measurement techniques in the office and in the ambulatory setting will lead to better identification of patients and early implementation of treatment. Accurate measurement in the supine and upright positions is recommended in diabetic patients. Both the Seventh Joint National Committee on the Prevention, Detection, Evaluation, and Treatment of High Blood Pressure (JNC-7) and the American Diabetes Association (ADA) have recommended targeting a blood pressure (BP) of 130/80 mmHg in diabetic patients. Generally this included the use of at least three antihypertensive agents that should encompass a diuretic and an inhibitor of the renin angiotensin system (RAS).[3–5]

MANAGEMENT: STRATEGIES TO REDUCE CARDIOVASCULAR RISK

The goal of HTN management in patients with DM is to reduce cardiovascular risk and prevent adverse cardiovascular events. Both pharmacologic and nonpharmacologic approaches to therapy are recommended. The JNC-7 emphasizes the need for the adoption of a healthy lifestyle, including aerobic exercise and a diet that is high in mineral and fiber content and relatively low in fat, refined carbohydrates, and salt content, for the prevention and treatment of HTN in all patients.[46] Aggressive nonpharmacologic interventions are not only pivotal but indispensable in the therapeutic outcome of all hypertensive populations.

Nonpharmacologic treatment
Diet and weight loss

Several randomized controlled trials have documented the value of modest weight loss in decreasing the risk of HTN and in some cases even obviates the need for antihypertensive medication.[51] The Dietary Approaches to Stop Hypertension (DASH) study, a diet abundant in fruits and vegetables, as well as low-fat dairy products, with or without sodium restriction, substantially reduced BP in hypertensive patients.[46] Overall, a diet that is high in fiber and potassium and lower in saturated fat, refined carbohydrates and salt can improve glycemic control, lipid profile, and BP.

Exercise

The Finnish Diabetes Prevention Study showed that overweight subjects with glucose intolerance randomized to intensified lifestyle intervention, consisting of diet and moderate exercise for at least 30 minutes per day, resulted in a marked reduction in the risk of developing DM2 and a significant drop in BP (4 mmHg for SBP and 2 mmHg for diastolic BP compared with control subjects).[55] A prospective study of 8302 Finnish men and 9139 women showed that regular physical activity was associated with a significantly reduced risk for HTN in men and women, independent of age, education, smoking habits, alcohol intake, and history of DM, BMI, and SBP at baseline.[56] Overweight and obesity were also associated with an increased risk of HTN, and the protective effect of physical activity was consistent in both overweight and normal-weight subjects. Further, exercise helps to accomplish weight loss. Most studies have shown that more benefit is derived from aerobic than nonaerobic exercise.[57] Data on effects of the intensity of physical activity on HTN, however, are conflicting. The most recent data show that high physical activity, defined as a combination of vigorous occupational activity more than 30 minutes daily and leisure-time physical activity more than 4 hours a week, is associated with a lower risk of HTN, independent of baseline BMI. Initiation of a graded exercise program is recommended in all hypertensive patients, including diabetics. Older diabetics may need to undergo cardiac assessment prior to initiating vigorous exercise programs. At the minimum, this requires a baseline electrocardiogram and exercise stress testing if there is clinical evidence for possible underlying ischemic heart disease.

Tobacco cessation

Smoking has been independently associated with enhanced risk of microvascular and macrovascular disease in diabetes. The synergistic effect results in an increased premature CVD mortality. Smoking-cessation strategies should be discussed with patients at each visit.[58]

Pharmacologic treatment

The choice of antihypertensive medications is wide and can be tailored to each specific patient. A key factor is consideration of comorbid conditions such as ischemic heart disease, chronic kidney disease, peripheral vascular disease, and dyslipidemia, as these all impact the choice of antihypertensive medication. On average, the diabetic patient will require at least three medications to reach the target blood pressure of BP <130/80 mmHg. The choice of medications includes medications that interrupt the RAAS (ACEIs and ARBs), thiazide diuretics, calcium channel blockers (CCBs), beta-blockers (BB), alpha-blockers, vasodilators and centrally acting medications such as clonidine. According to JNC-7, diabetes mellitus forms a compelling indication for consideration of specific medications as first-line therapy rather than using the currently recommended thiazide diuretic as first-line therapy (Table 55–4). Therapy should also include a RAS inhibitor. Once therapy is started, close monitoring and titration of medications to achieve goal BP is recommended.[47]

In addition, other interventions and medications that affect overall cardiovascular risk should be considered. These include aspirin (ASA), metformin, thiazolidinediones, sulphonylureas, and insulin to improve glycemic control and HMG-CoA inhibitors (statins) and fibrates to improve the lipid profile. These medications once initiated should be titrated until the targeted endpoint is attained (Figure 55–3).

EVIDENCE-BASED APPROACH: SPECIFIC PHARMACOLOGIC THERAPY

Angiotensin-converting enzyme inhibitors

The RAAS plays a role in almost every step in the progression of atherosclerosis and HTN. Multiple clinical trials have demonstrated the pleiotropic effects of the

ANTIHYPERTENSIVE MEDICATIONS USED IN TREATMENT OF DM-RELATED HYPERTENSION: "COMPELLING INDICATIONS" SPECIFIC TO DM HYPERTENSION		
Diagnosis	**Indication**	**Medication/Study**
Type 1 DM	Renal function deterioration	ACEI (CCSG)
Type 2 DM	Cardiovascular events	ACEI (MICRO-HOPE)
Type 2 DM	Renal function deterioration	ARB (IDNT/RENAAL)
Type 2 DM	Microalbuminuria progression	ACEI (MICROHOPE) ARB (IRMA-2)
ACEI, angiotensin converting enzyme inhibitors; ARB, angiotensin receptor blockers; CCSG, Captopril Cooperative Study Group; DM, diabetes mellitus; IDNT, Irbesartan Diabetic Nephropathy Trial; IRMA-2, Irbesartan Microalbuminuria Study; MICRO-HOPE, Microalbuminuria, Cardiovascular and Renal Outcomes substudy of the Heart Outcomes Prevention and Evaluation; RENAAL, Reduction of Endpoints in Noninsulin Dependent Diabetes Mellitus with the Angiotensin II Antagonist Losartan.		

Table 55–4. Antihypertensive Medications Used in Treatment of DM-Related Hypertension: "Compelling Indications" Specific to DM Hypertension

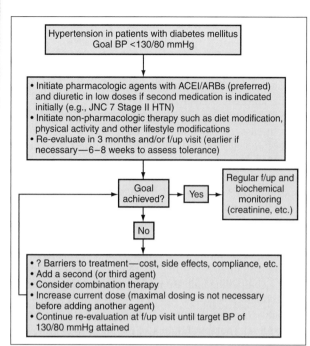

Figure 55–3. Suggested approach to treating hypertension in patients with diabetes mellitus. ACEI, angiotensin-converting enzyme inhibitor; ARB, angiotensin receptor blockers; BP, blood pressure; f/up, follow-up; HTN, hypertension; JNC-7, seventh report of Joint National Committee on the Prevention, Detection, Evaluation, and Treatment of High Blood Pressure.

ACE inhibitors. In addition to being an effective antihypertensive, the ACE inhibitors have been proven to offer additional benefits in patients with DM. The Heart Outcomes Prevention Evaluation (HOPE) trial studied 9541 patients, 3577 of whom were diabetic.[31] Ramipril use was associated with a significant 25% risk reduction in myocardial infarction, stroke, or cardiovascular death after a median follow-up period of 4.5 years. Furthermore, the MICRO-HOPE substudy also showed that ramipril treatment was associated with a decreased risk of development of proteinuria in type 2 DM patients with microalbuminuria.[59] Only 18 diabetics in MICRO-HOPE developed ESRD, but ramipril was associated with a non-significant 30% reduction in this important endpoint, possibly due to the small number of events.

In the Captopril Prevention Project (CAPP), of the 10,985 patients studied, 309 patients in the captopril group and 263 in the conventional therapy group were diabetic. Overall, captopril treatment markedly lowered the risk for fatal and nonfatal myocardial infarction, stroke, and cardiovascular deaths, compared to the conventional therapy group, which consisted of β-blocker or diuretic therapy. The effects of the two regimens in the diabetic subpopulation showed a clear difference in the risk of developing a primary endpoint in favor of a captopril-based regimen.[60]

In addition to lowering BP, ACE inhibitors also decrease the membrane permeability to albumin and decrease intra-glomerular pressure. By reducing microalbuminuria, ACE inhibitors can help prevent the progression to nephropathy. Meta-analyses have suggested that this anti-

proteinuric effect is independent of the changes in BP.[61] In type 1 diabetics, ACE inhibitors have been shown to prevent the progression of diabetic nephropathy to end-stage renal disease (ESRD), while in DM2 there is no clear evidence of this. One complication of therapy is a slight rise in serum creatinine, which is due to volume depletion and is usually reversible.[5,62] However, renal function should still be carefully monitored since a rise in serum creatinine by more than 30% or a continual rise during the first 2 months of therapy should alarm the physician to the possibility of renal artery stenosis or significant volume depletion. Interestingly, a recent meta-analysis of several long-term trials indicates that ACE inhibitors and ARBs, both of which inhibit the RAAS also reduce the incidence of new-onset diabetes[36] (Table 55–5).

Angiotensin receptor blockers

These agents specifically block the angiotensin II, subtype 1 (AT_1R) receptor, and offer effective blockade of the RAAS. ARBs have equivalent antihypertensive efficacy to ACE inhibitors, with fewer side effects, particularly cough and angioedema. This may clinically translate to improved adherence with an ARB compared to an ACE inhibitor. Similar to ACE inhibitors, the ARBs offer additional benefits in diabetic patients. Based on the current evidence and because of their tolerability, ARBs are recommended as first-line therapy for patients with DM, HTN, and significant proteinuria.[46]

The Losartan Intervention for Endpoint Reduction in Hypertension (LIFE) trial with losartan showed a significant 13% reduction in the composite primary endpoint (cardiovascular death, myocardial infarction, or stroke), most of which was due to a significant 25% reduction in stroke versus atenolol.[63] The diabetic patients in this study had an even more significant reduction (24%) in the primary endpoint, as well as in cardiovascular mortality (37%) and total mortality (39%), when compared to atenolol.

The Reduction of Endpoints in NIDDM with Angiotensin II Antagonist Losartan (RENAAL) and the Irbesartan Diabetic Nephropathy Trial showed that ARBs reduce proteinuria and the time to creatinine doubling, and slow the progression of renal disease.[64] The Irbesartan in Microalbuminuria (IRMA)-II trial also showed reduction in progression from microalbuminuria to proteinuria.[5] The beneficial effects of ARBs on nephropathy were said to be independent of the changes in BP.

In evaluating combination therapy, the Candesartan and Lisinopril Microalbuminuria (CALM) trial showed a numerically greater reduction in both BP and albuminuria when both ARB and ACE inhibitor were used in combination at half-maximal doses than when used alone.[65] In nondiabetic patients with hypertension and nephrotic syndrome, combination therapy has been shown to be more effective in reducing proteinuria than an ACE inhibitor or ARB alone. Furthermore, this antiproteinuric effect was not dependent on changes in BP or creatinine clearance. Although this appears promising, more data are needed before recommending the combination of these two agents to completely block the RAAS in patients with diabetes. Finally, both ACE inhibitors and ARBs have been

REDUCTION IN RISK OF DEVELOPING NEW-ONSET DIABETES MELLITUS BY ANTIHYPERTENSIVE MEDICATION					
Absolute Risk Reduction (%) (Decreasing Order)	Relative Risk Reduction (%)	Trial (*n*)	Demographics	Intervention Treatment	Control Treatment
16.5	74	Studies of Left Ventricular Dysfunction (SOLVD) (291)	LV dysfunction Men/women 18–80 years	Enalapril	Placebo
3.6	88	ALPINE (392)	Newly detected HTN Mostly women 18–75 years	Candesartan	HCTZ
3.5/1.7	30/17	Antihypertensive and Lipid-Lowering Treatment to Prevent Heart Attack Trial (15,573)	HTN and at risk for CVD Men/women ≥55 years	Lisinopril	Chlorthalidone or amlodipine
3.3	23	Valsartan Antihypertensive Long-Term Use Evaluation (10,419)	HTN and at risk for CVD Men/women ≥50 years	Valsartan	Amlodipine
2.0	39	CHARM (3023)	HF class II–IV Men/women >18 years	Candesartan	Placebo
2.0	25	Losartan Intervention for Endpoint Reduction (7998)	HTN and LVH Men/women 55–80 years	Losartan	Atenolol
1.8	33	Heart Outcomes Prevention Evaluation (9297)	CVD Men/women >55 years	Ramipril	Placebo
1.7	17	PEACE (6904)	Stable CVD Men/women >50 years	Trandolapril	Placebo
1.2	15	International Verapamil-Trandolapril Study (16,176)	HTN and CVD Men/women ≥55 years	Verapamil SR and then adding trandolapril and then HCTZ	Atenolol then adding HCTZ and then trandolapril
1.0	19	SCOPE (4330)	HTN Men/women 70–89 years	Candesartan	Placebo
0.8	11	Captopril Prevention Project (10,985)	Diastolic HTN Men/women 25–66 years	Captopril	Beta blocker

CVD, cardiovascular disease; HCTZ, hydrochlorthiazide; HF, heart failure; HTN, hypertension; LV, left ventricular; LVH, left ventricular hypertrophy.

Table 55–5. Reduction in Risk of Developing New-Onset Diabetes Mellitus by Antihypertensive Medication

shown to consistently reduce new onset diabetes in hypertensive patients, in part through reduction generation of reactive oxygen species that inhibit insulin signaling.

Thiazide diuretics

Although diuretics have the potential to worsen insulin resistance, perhaps via small reductions in potassium and magnesium, they have consistently demonstrated their ability to reduce the cardiovascular mortality in patients with DM. The ALLHAT, one of the largest antihypertensive trials, concluded that thiazide diuretics comparably reduced combined fatal and nonfatal coronary artery disease (CAD), and all-cause mortality when compared to an ACEI and CCB, and more importantly, prevented heart failure significantly better than any other initial therapy, in both diabetics and nondiabetics.[45]

ALLHAT and other studies have a follow-up period of less than 10 years, and the true impact of new onset

DM on cardiovascular outcomes may not be fully appreciated. In a recent analysis of an observational registry of morbidity and mortality in initially untreated individuals with essential HTN, patients who were treated with diuretics and β-blockers had an increased propensity to develop DM2.[66] The occurrence of new-onset DM in treated hypertensive patients carried a risk for subsequent CVD events that was not statistically different from those who already had DM and HTN at the onset of the study. However, both groups had a much higher risk than those who remained free of DM. Even though the electrolyte disturbances and the adverse effects on lipid and carbohydrate metabolism are uncommon with low dose thiazide therapy, these recent observations suggest that thiazide diuretics and β-blockers should be initiated cautiously in hypertensive patients with elevated fasting glucose levels, that is, above 100 mg/dL.[67] Nevertheless, diuretics continue to play an important role in the management of

HTN in patients with DM, especially as an adjunct to ACE inhibitors and ARBs. A recent review of long-term mortality data from the Systolic Hypertension in the Elderly Program (mean 14.3 years) showed that development of DM in patients treated with the diuretic chlorthalidone was not associated with increased cardiovascular or total mortality rates.[68] Moreover, diuretic treatment in diabetic subjects was strongly associated with lower long-term cardiovascular and total mortality rates. Further research is required to fully define the long-term risk/benefit profiles of commonly used thiazide diuretics in hypertensive patients with impaired fasting glucose levels, especially since hydrochlorothiazide has been more widely accepted in clinical practice than has chorthalidone. Finally, thiazide diuretics may loose their efficacy in lowering BP when creatinine exceeds 2.0 mg/dL.

Calcium channel blockers

At least 65% of hypertensive patients require two or more drugs to achieve BPs of less than 130/80.[69] Calcium channel blockers are effective antihypertensive agents but probably should be viewed as adjuncts to ACEIs, ARBs, and diuretics.[5] They not only lower BP effectively in diabetic patients, but they are intermediate in risk of new-onset diabetes between ACE inhibitors and ARBs (which reduce the risk of incidence DM) and thiazide diuretics or β-blockers (which increase it).[70] A post-hoc analysis of RENAAL suggested no difference in the primary renal endpoint between dihydropyridine and nondihydropyridine CCBs as second-line agents (after an ARB).[64] Additionally, the nondihydropyridine calcium antagonists, verapamil and diltiazem, can further reduce proteinuria when added to RAAS blocker therapy.[10] According to data from the Hypertension Optimal Treatment (HOT) study, dihydropyridine CCBs, which are often necessary for adequate BP control, are not contraindicated in patients with proteinuria and may be used as an adjunctive therapy.

The European Trial on Isolated Systolic Hypertension in the Elderly with nitrendipine (vs. placebo) demonstrated that intensive antihypertensive therapy for older patients with DM2 and isolated systolic HTN eliminated the additional risk for CVD events and stroke associated with DM.[71] However, in the ALLHAT study, an initial CCB had a significantly higher incidence of heart failure compared to an initial diuretic but fewer strokes than an ACE inhbitor.[45]

Beta-adrenergic blocking agents

The effectiveness of β-blockers in HTN, CAD, and heart failure management has been proven in multiple clinical trials.[51] Despite their adverse effects on glucose tolerance and the peripheral vasculature, β-blockers play a significant role in the management of HTN in diabetics, especially in those with associated micro- and macro-vascular complications. In the UKPDS, atenolol was comparable to captopril in reducing BP and CVD outcomes[49]; however, when comparing atenolol to other agents in many other trials, atenolol has been consistently and significantly worse than other therapies to which it has been compared.[72] Beta-blockers have adverse effects on glucose and lipid profiles and have also been implicated in new-onset DM in obese patients.[51] Beta-blockade may worsen the symptoms of peripheral vascular disease; however, clear evidence that this occurs in practice during controlled studies is lacking. Nonselective β-blockers, such as carvedilol, reduce CVD mortality and microalbuminuria without adversely affecting glucose or lipid profiles, although this may be a BP-lowering effect.[73] When used with RAS blockade, carvedilol and atenolol have also both been shown to reduce albuminuria.[74] In addition, carvedilol slows the progression of nephropathy and improves insulin sensitivity.[73] Therefore, these agents play a useful role in antihypertensive therapy of diabetic patients, specifically those with CAD and heart failure.

Alpha antagonists

The selective alpha-1-blockers, such as prazosin and doxazosin, are the only class of antihypertensive agents that may have the combined effect of lowering LDL cholesterol, raising HDL-cholesterol levels, and improving insulin sensitivity,[75] and they can be useful add-on drugs to reach target BP. Alpha-blockers, however, have relatively may produce orthostatic hypertension, especially in the elderly and those with diabetic neuropathy.[15] Thus, these agents are generally not part of first-line therapy in diabetic patients.[5]

In summary, there is considerable evidence that rigorous control of blood pressure in patients with diabetes reduces cardiovascular events, stroke, and progression of albuminuria and chronic renal disease. It usually requires at least three drugs accomplish goal blood pressure of 130/80 mmHg, and diuretics and RAS inhibitors should be a part of the antihypertensive regimen.

SUMMARY

Insulin resistance, DM, and HTN are closely linked. Genetic predisposition when combined with an enabling milieu (central obesity, inactivity, poor diet) can result in the synergistic occurrence of cardiovascular risk factors seen clinically. The approach to treatment entails consideration of the underlying pathophysiologic mechanisms understanding that insulin resistance is often a progressive state. The presence of peripheral vascular disease, heart failure, coronary artery disease, orthostatic hypotension, dyslipidemia, and diabetic nephropathy all influence the choice of antihypertensive therapy. Reversal of the essential condition with therapy would be ideal, and strategies such as interruption of the RAAS may have this effect. When this is not possible, an approach that targets specific complications, slows progression, or delays onset of target-organ damage should be used.

Quality of life, adverse effects of antihypertensive medications, and other comorbid conditions affect adherence to treatment regimens and the success of therapy. More importantly, the health care team should work closely with each individual patient to prudently, but aggressively, achieve and maintain the goal BP of less than 130/80 mmHg. Use of a statin and aspirin are also an integral part of the comprehensive care of the diabetic patient when aiming to reduce CVD risk, which is the ultimate goal of therapy.

REFERENCES

1. National Center for Chronic Disease Prevention and Health Promotion. National diabetes fact sheet: general information and national estimates on diabetes in the United States. Atlanta, GA: Centers for Disease Control, 003.

2. Healthy People 2010. Diabetes Progress Review, 2002 2005.

3. Mugo M, Sowers JR. Metabolic syndrome: implications of race and ethnicity. *Ethn Dis* 2004;14:S2–31.

4. Sowers JR, Epstein M, Frohlich ED. Diabetes, hypertension, and cardiovascular disease:an update. *Hypertension* 2001;37:1053–9.

5. Sowers JR. Treatment of hypertension in patients with diabetes. *Arch Intern Med* 2004:164:1850–7.

6. Ho KK, Anderson KM, Kannel WB, et al. Congestive heart failure/myocardial responses/valvular heart disease: survival after the onset of congestive heart failure in the Framingham Heart Study subjects. *Circulation* 1993;88(1): 107–15.

7. Ford ES, Giles WH, Mokdad AH. Increasing prevalence of the metabolic syndrome among U.S. adults. *Diabetes Care* 2004;27:2444–9.

8. Alberti KG, Zimmet P, Shaw J. IDF Epidemiology Task Force Consensus Group. The metabolic syndrome—a new worldwide definition. *Lancet* 2005; 366:1059–62.

9. McFarlane SI, Banerji M, Sowers JR. Insulin resistance and cardiovascular disease. *J Clin Endocrinol Metab* 2001; 86:713–8.

10. Tan AS, Kuppuswamy S, Whaley-Connell A, et al. Recommendations for special populations: the treatment of hypertension in diabetes mellitus. *Endocrinologist* 2004;14:368–81.

11. Sowers JR. Obesity as a cardiovascular risk factor. *Am J Med* 2003;115(Suppl 8A):37S–41S.

12. Aneja A, El-Atat F, McFarlane SI, Sowers JR. Hypertension and obesity. *Recent Prog Horm Res* 2004;59:169–205.

13. Wang CC, Goalstone ML, Draznin B. Molecular mechanisms of insulin resistance that impact cardiovascular biology. *Diabetes* 2004;53:2735–40.

14. Sowers JR. Insulin and insulin-like growth factor in normal and pathological cardiovascular physiology. *Hypertension* 1997;29:691–9.

15. Sowers JR. Insulin resistance and hypertension. *Am J Physiol Circ Physiol* 2004;286:H1597–602.

16. Lind L, Berne C, Lithell H. Prevalence of insulin resistance in essential hypertension. *J Hypertens* 1995;13: 1457–62.

17. Marigliano A, et al. Insulinemia and blood pressure. Relationships in patients with primary and secondary hypertension, and with or without glucose metabolism impairment. *Am J Hypertens* 1990;3:521–6.

18. Facchini FS, Chen YD, Clinkingbeard C. Insulin resistance, hyperinsulinemia and dyslipidemia in non-obese individuals with a family history of hypertension. *Am J Hypertens* 1992;5:694–9.

19. Sowers JR, Stump CS. Insights into the biology of diabetic vascular disease: what's new? *Am J Hypertens* 2004; 17:2S–6S.

20. Stas SN, El-Atat FA, Sowers JR. Pathogenesis of hypertension in diabetes. *Rev Endocrinol Metab Disord* 2004;5:221–5.

21. Pollock D. Endothelin, angiotensin and oxidative stress in hypertension. *Hypertension* 2005;45:477–80.

22. DiBona GF. The sympathetic nervous system and hypertension, recent developments. *Hypertension* 2004; 43:147–50.

23. Weyer C, et al. Ethnic differences in insulinemia and sympathetic tone as links between obesity and blood pressure. *Hypertension* 2004;36:531–7.

24. Ogihara T, Asano T, Ando K, et al. Angiotensin II enhanced insulin resistance is associated with enhanced insulin signaling. *Hypertension* 2002;40:872–9.

25. Sowers JR. Insulin resistance and hypertension. *Am J Physiol Heart Circ Physiol* 2004;286H1597–602.

26. Dimmeler S, Rippmann V, Weiland U, et al. Angiotensin II induces apoptosis of human endothelial cells. Protective effect of nitric oxide. *Circ Res* 1999; 81:970–6.

27. Watanabe T, Barker T, Berk B. Angiotensin II and the endothelium. *Hypertension* 2005;45:163–9.

28. Mehta JL, Li DY, Yang H, Raizada MK. Angiotensin II and IV stimulate expression and release of plasminogen activator inhibitor-1 in cultured human coronary artery endothelial cells. *J Cardiovasc Pharmacol* 2002;39:789–94.

29. Tamarat R, Silvestre JS, Durie M, Levy BI. Angiotensin II angiogenic effect in vivo involves vascular endothelial growth factor and inflammation related pathways. *Lab Invest* 2002;82:747–56.

30. Marrero MB, Fulton D, Stepp D, Stern DM. Angiotensin II–induced insulin resistance and protein tyrosine phosphatases. *Arterioscler Thromb Vasc Biol* 2004;24:2009–13.

31. Yusuf S, Sleight P, Pogue J, et al. Effects of the angiotensin converting enzyme inhibitor, ramipril, on cardiovascular events in high risk patients. The Heart Outcomes Prevention Evaluation Study Investigators. *N Engl J Med* 2000;342:145–53.

32. Lassegue B, Clempus RE. Vascular NAD(P)H oxidase: specific features, expression and regulation. *Am J Physiol Integr Comp Physiol* 2003;285:R277–97.

33. Touyz R. Reactive oxygen species, vascular oxidative stress, and redox signalling in hypertension: what is the clinical significance? *Hypertension* 2004; 44:248–52.

34. Sowers JR. Insulin resistance and hypertension. *Am J Physiol Heart Circ Physiol* 2004;286:H1597–602.

35. Huber SA, Sakkinen P, Conze D, et al. Interleukin-6 exacerbates early atherosclerosis in mice. *Arterioscler Thromb Vasc Biol* 1999;19:2364–7.

36. Hotamisligil GS, Peraldi P, Budavari A, et al. IRS-1 mediated inhibition of insulin receptor tyrosine kinase activity in TNF-alpha and obesity induced insulin resistance. *Science* 1996; 271:665–8.

37. Dandona P. A rational approach to pathogenesis and treatment of type 2 diabetes mellitus, insulin resistance, inflammation and atherosclerosis in diabetes. *Am J Cardiol* 2002;90: 27G–33G.

38. Libby P, Ridker PM. Inflammation and atherosclerosis: role of C-reactive protein in risk assessment. *Am J Med* 2004; 116(Suppl 1);9–16.

39. Sowers JR. Stroke in patients with diabetes. *J Clin Hypertens (Greenwich)* 2004;6:62–3.

40. Sacco RL. Reducing the risk of stroke in diabetes: what have we learned that is new? *Diabetes Obes Metab* 2002; 4(Suppl 1):S27–34.

41. Tuomilehto J, Rastenyte D. Diabetes and glucose intolerance as risk factors for stroke. *J Cardiovasc Risk* 1999; 6:241–9.

42. UK Prospective Diabetes Study Group. Tight blood pressure control and risk of macrovascular and microvascular complications in type 2 diabetes: UKPDS 38. *BMJ* 1998;317:703–13.

43. Heart Outcomes Prevention Evaluation Study Investigators. Effects of ramipril on cardiovascular and microvascular outcomes in people with diabetes mellitus: results of the HOPE study and MICRO-HOPE substudy. *Lancet* 2000; 355:253–9.

44. Lindholm LH, Ibsen H, Dahlof B, et al. Cardiovascular morbidity and mortality in patients with diabetes in the Losartan Intervention for Endpoint reduction in hypertension study (LIFE): a randomized controlled trial against atenolol. *Lancet* 2002;359:1004–10.

45. ALLHAT Officers and Coordinators for the ALLHAT Collaborative Research Group. Major outcomes in high-risk hypertensive patients randomized to angiotensin-converting enzyme inhibitor or calcium channel blocker vs. diuretic: the Antihypertensive and Lipid Lowering Treatment to Prevent Heart Attack Trial (ALLHAT). *JAMA* 2002; 288:2981–97.

46. Chobanian AV, et al. The Seventh Report of the Joint National Committee on Prevention, Detection, Evaluation, and Treatment of High Blood Pressure: the JNC 7 report. *JAMA* 2003;289: 2560–72.

47. Mugo MN, Sowers JR. Early and aggressive treatment of complex hypertension. *J Clin Hypertens (Greenwich)* 2005;7:8–10.

48. Bakris, G, Williams, M, Dworkin L, et al. Preserving renal function in adults with hypertension and diabetes: a consensus approach. National Kidney Foundation Hypertension and Diabetes Executive Committees Working Group. *Am J Kidney Dis* 2000;36:646–61.

49. Eknoyan, G., et al. Proteinuria and other markers of chronic kidney disease: a position statement of the national kidney foundation (NKF) and the national institute of diabetes and digestive and kidney diseases (NIDDK). *Am J Kidney Dis* 2003;42:617–22.

50. Gerstein HC, et al. Prevalence and determinants of microalbuminuria in high-risk diabetic and nondiabetic patients in the Heart Outcomes Prevention Evaluation Study. The HOPE Study Investigators. *Diabetes Care* 2000; 23(Suppl 2):B35–9.

51. Sowers JR, Haffner S. Treatment of cardiovascular and renal risk factors in the diabetic hypertensive. *Hypertension* 2002;40:781–8.

52. Ohkubo T, Hozawa A, Yamaguchi J, et al. Prognostic significance of the nocturnal decline in blood pressure in individuals with and without high 24-h blood pressure: the Ohasama study. *J Hypertens* 2002;20:2183–9.

53. Fang ZY, Prins JB, Marwick TH. Diabetic cardiomyopathy: evidence, mechanisms, and therapeutic implications. *Endocr Rev* 2004;25:543–67.

54. Frohlich ED., Sowers JR. Management of diabetic and hypertensive cardiovascular disease. *Curr Hypertens Rep* 2003;5:309–15.

55. Tuomilehto J, Lindstrom J, Eriksson JG, et al. Prevention of type 2 diabetes by changes in lifestyle among subjects with impaired glucose tolerance. *N Engl J Med* 2001;344:1343–50.

56. Hu G, Barengo NC, Tuomilehto J, et al. Relationship of physical activity and body mass index to the risk of hypertension: a prospective study in Finland. *Hypertension* 2004;43:25–30.

57. Whelton SP, Chin A, Xin X, et al. Effect of aerobic exercise on blood pressure: a meta-analysis of randomized, controlled trials. *Ann Intern Med* 2002;136:493–503.

58. Haire-Joshu D, Glasgow RE, Tibbs TL. Smoking and diabetes. *Diabetes Care* 2004;27(Suppl 1):S74–75.

59. Heart Outcomes Prevention Evaluation Study Investigators. Effects of ramipril on cardiovascular and microvascular outcomes in people with diabetes mellitus: results of the HOPE study and MICRO-HOPE substudy. *Lancet* 2000; 355:253–9.

60. Niskanen L, Hedner T, Hansson L, et al. Reduced cardiovascular morbidity and mortality in hypertensive diabetic patients on first-line therapy with an ACE inhibitor compared with diuretic/beta-blocker based regimen: a sub-analysis of the Captopril Prevention Project. *Diabetes Care* 2001;24:2091–6.

61. Bakris GL, Sowers JR. Microalbuminuria in diabetes: focus on cardiovascular and renal risk reduction. *Curr Diabetes Rep* 2002;2:258–62.

62. Bakris GL, Weir MR. Angiotensin-converting enzyme inhibitor-associated elevations in serum creatinine: is this a cause for concern? *Arch Intern Med* 2000;160:685–93.

63. Dahlof B, Devereux RB, Kjeldsen SE, et al. Cardiovascular morbidity and mortality in the Losartan Intervention for Endpoint reduction in hypertension study (LIFE): a randomized trial against atenolol. *Lancet* 2002;359:995–1003.

64. Bakris, G, Weir, M, Shanifar, S. Effects of blood pressure level on progression of diabetic nephropathy: results from the RENAAL study. *Arch Intern Med* 2003; 163:1555–65.

65. Mogensen CE Neldam S, Tiakkanen I, et al. Randomised controlled trial of dual blockade of renin-angiotensin system in patients with hypertension, microalbuminuria, and non-insulin dependent diabetes: the Candesartan and Lisinopril Microalbuminuria (CALM) study. *BMJ* 2000;321:1440–4.

66. Verdecchia P, Reboldi G, Angeli F. Adverse prognostic significance of new diabetes in treated hypertensive subjects. *Hypertension* 2004;43:963–9.

67. Bakris G, Sowers JR. When does new onset diabetes resulting from antihypertensive therapy increase cardiovascular risk? *Hypertension* 2004; 43:941–2.

68. Kostis JB, Lawrence-Nelson J, Ranjan R, et al. Association of increased pulse pressure with the development of heart failure in SHEP. Systolic Hypertension in the Elderly (SHEP) Cooperative Research Group. *Am J Hypertens* 2001;14:798–803.

69. McFarlane SI, et al. Control of cardiovascular risk factors in patients with diabetes and hypertension at urban academic medical centers. *Diabetes Care* 2002;25:718–23.

70. Pepine, C. J, Handberg EM, Cooper-DeHoff RM, et al. A calcium antagonist vs. non-calcium antagonist hypertension treatment strategy for patients with coronary artery disease. The International Verapamil-Trandolapril Study (INVEST): a randomized controlled trial. *JAMA* 2003;290:2805–16.

71. Birkenhager WH, Staessen JA, Gasowski J, et al. Effects of antihypertensive treatment on endpoints in the diabetic patients randomized in the Systolic Hypertension in Europe (Syst-Eur) trial. *J Nephrol* 2000;13:232–7.

72. Carlberg B, Samuelsson O, Lindholm LH. Ateolol in hypertension: is it a wise choice? *Lancet* 2004;354:1684–9.

73. Jacob S, Balletshofer B, Henriksen EJ, et al. Beta blocking agents in patients with insulin resistance: effects of vasodilating beta-blockers. *Blood Press* 1999;8:261–8.

74. Fassbinder W, Quarder O, Waltz A. Treatment with carvedilol is associated with a significant reduction in microalbuminuria: a multicenter randomized study. *Int J Clin Pract* 2005;53:519–22.

75. Khoury AF, Kaplan NM. Alpha-blocker therapy for hypertension. An unfulfilled promise. *JAMA* 1991;266:394–8.

Chapter

56 Hypertension in Renal Failure

Branko Braam and Hein A. Koomans

Definition

- Renal hypertension is blood pressure exceeding 140/90 mmHg, due to renal parenchymal disease, and occurring in approximately 40% to 70% of patients with chronic renal failure. Dialysis-associated hypertension is an ambulatory blood pressure or a week-average home blood pressure exceeding 140/90 mmHg in patients with end-stage renal disease (ESRD) on renal replacement therapy.

Key Features

- Structural and functional changes in the diseased kidney lead to (1) inadequate volume control with extracellular fluid volume (ECFV) expansion, (2) inappropriately high renin release, and (3) increased activity of the sympathetic nervous system.

- Furthermore, renal disease is associated with structural and functional changes in the vasculature, leading to reduced vascular compliance, which in turn will cause high systolic pressure load to the heart, low diastolic pressures with potential underperfusion of coronary and cerebral vessels, and high peak pressures in the vasculature leading to further vascular damage.

- Renal disease is associated with a very high prevalence of cardiovascular disease; hypertension further aggravates this risk.

- The "reverse epidemiology" reported for ESRD patients may well be due to the presence of different populations entering dialysis programs: a group with low blood pressure with previous phases of hypertension with cardiac damage and a group with still intact function, for which regular risk applies of high blood pressure.

Therapy

- Treatment of hypertension to levels of 130/80 is pursued by sequential interruption of all deranged axes: (1) normalize ECFV using diuretics or ultrafiltration, (2) inhibit the activity of the renin-angiotensin system using angiotensin-converting enzyme inhibitors or AT1 receptor antagonists, and (3) inhibit the activity of the sympathetic nervous system, primarily using beta receptor antagonists.

- Care should be taken with patients having high pulse pressures, indicating low vascular compliance. Here, blood pressure should be decreased, however, while avoiding excessively low diastolic blood pressure.

It is increasingly clear that chronic kidney disease (CKD) is extremely prevalent, and likely the most common form of secondary hypertension. Recent data collected in the United States indicates that ~4.7% of the overall population suffers from reduced glomerular filtration rate (GFR) (<60 mL/min).[1] Worldwide, the number of patients with end-stage renal disease (ESRD) (Stage 5 chronic kidney disease) approximates 0.03%.[2] CKD is strongly associated with hypertension. The prevalence of hypertension in ESRD approximates 80%.[3] Even in early CKD the prevalence of hypertension is increased threefold (Figure 56–1).

The prevalence of hypertension varies somewhat with the underlying disease, with an approximately 40% prevalence in chronic interstitial nephritis, IgA nephropathy, and minimal change disease, and 60% to 70% in diabetic nephropathy, adult-type polycystic kidney disease (ADPKD), and focal segmental glomerulosclerosis (FSGS).[4] In ESRD, systolic hypertension is more common than combined systolic and diastolic hypertension, and isolated diastolic hypertension is rare.[5,6]

Control of hypertension in the general population is poor, with only approximately 25% of the recognized hypertensive subjects being adequately controlled. Unfortunately, in patients with progressing CKD or ESRD this control is not better or even worse.[7–9] This is a serious problem, since it is clear that hypertension is a main factor driving progressive decline of kidney function in CKD, whereas adequate blood pressure control mitigates the rate of nephron loss in many patient groups and settings. Moreover, hypertension is one of the main causes of increased cardiovascular morbidity and mortality, hallmarks of patients with renal failure. Large population studies such as the Hypertension Detection and Follow-up Program (HDFP)[10] and the National Health and Nutrition Examination Survey (NHANES) I[11] demonstrated increased cardiovascular mortality in moderate renal failure. A recent meta-analysis of 85 reports covering over half a million patients showed that cardiovascular risk increases when GFR falls below ~75 mL/min.[2] The risk grows steeply with decreasing GFR and patients starting dialysis have a 5- to 10-fold increased mortality risk. The impact is tremendous in young subjects with ESRD, in whom cardiovascular risk is increased 100-fold.[12]

Hypertension is one risk factor among many others in CKD, such as dyslipidemia, insulin resistance, anemia, hyperhomocysteinemia, hyperphosphatemia, reduced nitric oxide availability, and chronic inflammation.[13] The presence of these additional factors increases with decreasing GFR[3] (Figure 56–2). Against that background, the added cardiovascular risk induced by high blood pressure is huge and, conversely, the impact of adequate

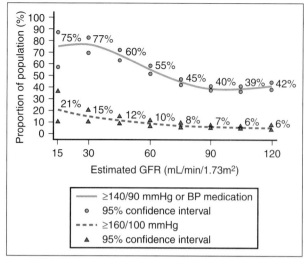

Figure 56–1. Prevalence of high blood pressure by level of GFR, adjusted to age 60 years in NHANES III. GFR was estimated using the abbreviated Modification of Diet in Renal Disease (MDRD) Study equation. Hypertension was defined as JNC Stage 1 (SBP=140 mmHg or DBP=90 mmHg, or taking medications for hypertension) or JNC=Stage 2 (SBP=160 or DBP=100 mmHg). Values are adjusted to age 60 years using a polynomial regression. Ninety-five percent confidence intervals are shown at selected levels of estimated GFR. DBP, diastolic blood pressure; GFR, glomerular filtration rate; JNC, Joint National Committee on Prevention, Detection, Evaluation and Treatment of High Blood Pressure; NHANES III, National Health and Nutrition Examination Survey III; SBP, systolic blood pressure. (Redrawn from National Kidney Foundation. *Am J Kidney Dis* 2002;39(2 Suppl 1):S1–266.)

blood pressure control on patient outcome can be huge. This is important, in part because currently available drugs and dialysis technology make adequate blood pressure control quite feasible. Many studies have shown

that antihypertensive drugs have beneficial effects on cardiovascular morbidity and patient outcome. Also, blood pressure reduction in ESRD by effective volume control during long or daily hemodialysis also improves survival.[14,15]

There are, however, questions specifically related to renal hypertension. Are blood pressure targets for the general population also applicable to CKD and ESRD patients? Is cardiovascular damage in CKD and ESRD patients typically the result of deficient systolic blood pressure or pulse pressure? Should we rely on predialysis or postdialysis blood pressure measurements? Should we apply 24-hour blood pressure measurements? Is blood pressure control enough, or should we target other properties of the vascular system to monitor and control cardiovascular risk such as pulse wave velocity? Are all drugs equally effective, or do we need a specific approach for this form of hypertension?

In this chapter we will focus on the pathophysiology of renal hypertension, and provide guidelines for management based on the available evidence. For the issue of protection against progression of renal failure, see Chapter 49. A central issue to be discussed in this chapter is the role of volume control, which is pivotal for the correction of renal hypertension.

PATHOPHYSIOLOGY

The mechanism of hypertension in renal failure involves volume overload and vasoconstriction. Volume overload is due to impaired renal sodium excretion, and vasoconstriction may be due to a host of factors related to renal parenchymal changes or renal failure. Volume overload and vasoconstriction are not mutually exclusive—in most patients both factors play a role.

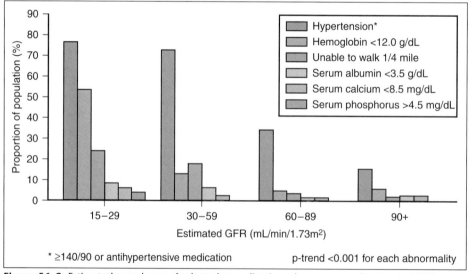

Figure 56–2. Estimated prevalence of selected complications, by category of estimated GFR, among participants aged 20 years in NHANES III, 1988 through 1994. These estimates are not adjusted for age, the mean of which is 33 years higher at an estimated GFR of 15 to 29 mL/min/ 1.73 m² than that at an estimated GFR 90 mL/min/1.73 m². GFR, glomerular filtration rate; NHANES III, National Health and Nutrition Examination Survey III. (Redrawn from National Kidney Foundation. *Am J Kidney Dis* 2002;39(2 Suppl 1):S1–266.)

Volume overload

Sodium (salt) balance plays a key role in the pathogenesis of renal hypertension. Maintenance of sodium balance (and thus volume balance) depends on excretion by the kidneys, which is impaired in renal failure. This implies that the pressure natriuresis curve is shifted to a higher blood pressure level. The tendency for sodium retention increases with decreasing GFR, and expanded blood and ECFV are found especially in patients with progressed renal failure. Indeed, the well-accepted "intact nephron hypothesis" implies that with declining fluid filtration, sodium balance can only be maintained at the cost of a changed environment, that is, hypervolemia and hypertension drive increased fractional sodium excretion. Many studies have showed direct correlations between blood volume and ECFV with blood pressure in patients with renal failure. However, these results were not consistently reported, perhaps due to variably successful "whole-body autoregulation," which tends to convert high-volume hypertension into vasoconstriction hypertension.

A strong argument for the role of impaired sodium excretion is the fact that a decreased GFR makes blood pressure more salt-sensitive: the lower the GFR, the more blood pressure tends to rise with an increase in salt intake. However, it is not only the decrease in GFR that makes patients salt-sensitive. When healthy persons are subjected to similar increments in sodium intake per GFR as patients with chronic renal failure, blood pressure does not increase as in patients with renal failure (Figure 56–3).[16] This confirms earlier observations that even extremes of sodium intake have relatively little effect on blood pressure when GFR (and the kidney) is normal. Probably absence of vasoconstrictive hyperactivity makes the difference. Healthy subjects on high sodium intake effectively suppress renin activity and sympathetic activity.

However, patients with kidney disease maintain relatively high renin activity and sympathetic activity, that is, for any ECFV, renin activity and sympathetic activity remain elevated (Figure 56–4).[16,17]

In some forms of renal parenchymal disease, sodium is retained even though GFR is still normal or only mildly impaired. For instance, accurate measurements of ECFV have shown modestly increased values together with modestly increased blood pressure also in early renal disease, such as in ADPKD.[18] In glomerular diseases, such as systemic lupus erythematosus, diabetic or IgA nephropathy sodium retention and hypertension also occur before GFR declines. In these conditions fractional sodium excretion is low, unless volume is retained and blood pressure is high.

The importance of increased intravascular volume rather than increased total ECFV for arterial hypertension becomes particularly clear when one compares patients with chronic renal failure with patients with the nephrotic syndrome: despite the same increase in total ECFV, patients with renal failure display much more increase in blood volume and blood pressure (Figure 56–5).[19] The difference results from the low protein mass in nephrosis, which mitigates the increase in blood volume.

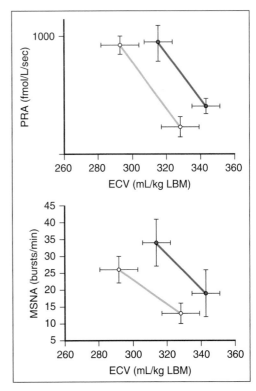

Figure 56–4. Plots of ECV, MSNA, and PRA in patients with chronic renal failure (*solid-fill circles*) in normovolemic and hypervolemic condition and in healthy volunteers (*hollow circles*) during use of low- and high-sodium diet. ECV, extracellular volume; MSNA, muscle sympathetic nerve activity; PRA, plasma renin activity. (Adapted from Koomans HA, Roos JC, et al. *Hypertension* 1985;7(5):714–21.)

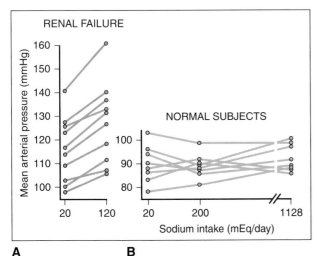

A   **B**

Figure 56–3. Mean arterial pressure on low (20 mmol/day) and high (120, 200, and 1128 mmol/day) sodium intake in patients with renal failure (**a**) and normal subjects (**b**). Note the consistent increase in mean arterial pressure in patients with renal failure and the absence of change in normal subjects even at extremes of sodium intake. (Redrawn from Koomans HA, Roos JC, et al. *Hypertension* 1985;7(5):714–21.)

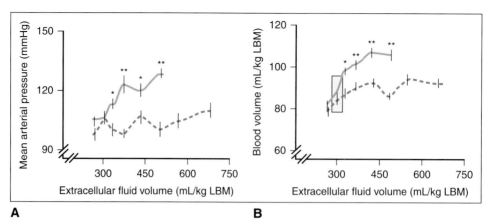

Figure 56–5. Dependence of extracellular fluid volume (per kilogram of lean body mass) on mean arterial pressure (**a**) and blood volume (**b**) in patients with nephrotic syndrome (*dashed curve*) and renal failure (*solid curve*). Note the marked increase of blood pressure in patients with renal failure compared with those with nephrotic syndrome. (*p < 0.05; **p < 0.01)

Theoretically, the body should correct a sustained hypervolemia and high cardiac output through autoregulation. By increasing peripheral vascular tone and blood pressure, the kidney is forced to restore the elevated blood volume, cardiac output and tissue supply of oxygen and nutrients to normal level. In practice, this concept appears very difficult to prove. Moreover, the gain of this mechanism may decrease when GFR is severely decreased. In fact, patients with ESRD often have a high cardiac output.[20] To a lesser extent, this is also the case in normotensive patients.[20] Therefore, other factors besides unsuccessful autoregulation may contribute to the persistence of high cardiac output. Anemia, commonly present in patients with ESRD, is associated with sustained high cardiac output to compensate for reduced oxygen delivery to the tissues. The presence of arteriovenous dialysis shunts also increases cardiac output, but tissue perfusion remains normal.

Vasoconstriction

Vasoconstrictive factors that are definitely or probably hyperactive in patients with renal failure are summarized in Box 56–1. Although the origin of these factors is mixed, it is clear the presence of abnormal kidneys plays a key role in their genesis: experimental and clinical data have shown that bilateral nephrectomy controls hypertension completely, as long as volume is also controlled.

Hyperactivity of renin angiotensin system

Studies from the 1970s showed that in about 20% of cases, hypertension of renal failure could not be corrected by treatment of the hypervolemia. Blood pressure became normal only after bilateral nephrectomy. This was attributed to hyperactivity of the renin angiotensin system (RAS) from the diseased kidneys, and it was concluded that in 80%, renal hypertension is based on volume overload, and in 20% on hyperactivity of the RAS. The advent of angiotensin-converting enzyme (ACE) inhibitors have changed this concept. Nearly all patients with renal hypertension have hyperactivity of the RAS relative to their volume status,[21] but in some cases the RAS is so hyperactive that blood pressure remains strongly elevated even after volume correction. In these cases blood pressure normalizes only with binephrectomy[22] or RAS blockade.[23] Nonetheless, correlation studies using the renin-volume product have suggested that other factors besides volume and the RAS also determine hypertension of CKD.[24]

The basis for RAS activation in CKD probably resides in patchy areas of underperfusion, leading to the situation that local activation of the RAS dictates sodium and fluid retention in other relatively healthy areas where perfusion is normal. This so-called nephron heterogeneity works as in two-kidney one-clip hypertension. In line with this hypothesis, RAS activation can occur in early-stage CKD when there is relatively much focal vascular damage, such as in nephrosclerosis, or when anatomic changes are prominent, such as in polycystic kidney disease,[25] reflux nephropathy[26] or (unilateral) hydronephrosis.[27] In the latter two situations, uninephrectomy can resolve the hypertension.[26,27]

Hyperactivity of sympathetic nervous system

It is increasingly clear that, besides RAS activity, sympathetic nervous activity is also high in hypertensive patients with CKD. First, ganglion blockade with debrisoquine

---

Box 56–1

Hyperactive Vasoconstrictors and Defective Vasodilators in Chronic Renal Failure

1. Whole-body autoregulation
2. Increased activity of the renin angiotensin system
3. Increased activity of the sympathetic nervous system
4. Diminished nitric oxide bio-activity (by increased asymmetric dimethylarginine [ADMA] levels)
5. Increased endothelin
6. Loss of renal vasodilator prostaglandins
7. Hypercalcemia
8. Decreased arterial compliance

was shown to lower blood pressure in hypertensive but not in normotensive patients with CKD.[28] Later, direct recordings of sympathetic activity with microneurography demonstrated sympathetic hyperactivity in patients with progressed CKD (Figure 56–6)[29] and ESRD.[30] On average, sympathetic activity was twice normal, similar as shown in the past for plasma catecholamine concentrations. Binephrectomy normalizes sympathetic activity,[30] showing that the kidneys are culprits of the sympathetic hyperactivity.

The afferent signal leading to increased sympathetic output from the CNS probably has a complex basis, involving both ischemia and local chemical factors in the kidney (Figure 56–7).[31] Unilateral clipping of the renal artery causes sympathetic activation, leading to vasoconstriction, salt retention by the contralateral kidney, and hypertension, effects that can be eliminated by cutting the afferent nerve of the clipped kidney.[32] In humans, angioplasty of unilateral renal artery stenosis that successfully lowered blood pressure and RAS activation also resolved the increased sympathetic nerve activity.[33] Therefore, a clear parallel exists with the pathophysiologic basis (and goal) of RAS hyperactivity. Hypertensive (but not untreated normotensive) patients with polycystic kidney disease and normal GFR also have increased sympathetic nervous activity,[34] suggesting that renal

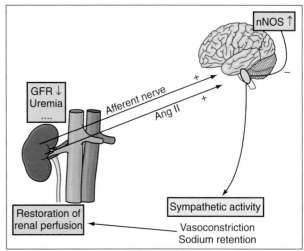

Figure 56–7. Sympathetic nervous system activity and renal disease. The diseased kidney sends signals to the brain, resulting in increased sympathetic output that will increase blood pressure. (Redrawn from Koomans HA, Blankestijn PJ, et al. *J Am Soc Nephrol* 2004;15(3):524–37.)

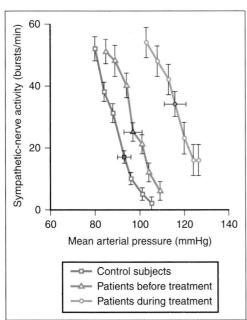

Figure 56–6. Baroreflex response to changes in mean arterial pressure in patients with chronic renal failure before and during long-term treatment with enalapril and in control subjects. Muscle sympathetic-nerve activity and heart rate were plotted against mean arterial pressures that were approximately 4, 8, and 12 mmHg below and 4, 8, and 12 mmHg above the resting levels (*solid symbols*). Tests were conducted before and during treatment with enalapril in 11 patients and 11 control subjects. Values are means plus or minus standard error.

parenchymal changes possibly associated with local ischemia activate the afferent signal. Besides renal afferent nerve activity, increased concentrations of angiotensin II may also increase sympathetic output through a direct effect on the brain stem. From clinical viewpoint this is important, since drugs that suppress RAS (hyper)activity automatically interfere with sympathetic (hyper)activity (Figure 56–6).[29] In fact, this characteristic of RAS blocking drugs may have caused that the role of sympathetic hyperactivity to remain somewhat underappreciated.

Nitric oxide

Studies with stable isotopes have shown decreased arginine-to-citrulline conversion in patients with pre-ESRD.[35] Others found evidence for approximately 40% reduction in NO production in hemodialysis patients.[36] Diminished NOS activity may be due to decreased renal clearance of the endogenous NOS inhibitor, asymmetric dimethylarginine, of which high concentrations haven been found even in early CKD,[37] or to decreased availability of NOS substrate L-arginine.[38] Patients with CKD also suffer from increased oxidative stress due to multiple reasons,[13] also reducing bio-availability of nitric oxide. As a consequence, endothelium-dependent vasodilation is diminished in patients with CKD.[39] However, it is not clear whether the reduced NO availability also participates in the hypertension, since we do not know whether restoration of normal nitric oxide balance in humans can attenuate renal hypertension. What we do know is that acute experimental inhibition of NOS activity in healthy humans to the level found in pre-ESRD patients or NOS inhibition in chronic studies in experimental animals[40] causes profound increase in blood pressure.[41] Experimental studies have further revealed that NOS inhibition increase renal and cardiac sensitivity to angiotensin II.[40]

Other pressors

For unknown reasons, plasma endothelin-1, a potent vasoconstrictor, is increased in patients with CKD.[42] However, the increase is modest, and the relevance for hypertension unclear. Acute blockade of endothelin-A receptor causes a greater blood pressure drop than in healthy controls,[43] but long-term studies are lacking. Erythropoietin and calcineurin inhibitors increase plasma endothelin concentrations, which may enhance the hypertensive effects of these substances. Hyperparathyroidism may increase blood pressure by increasing calcium content in smooth muscle cells. However, the effect on hypertension of PTH suppression by means of parathyroidectomy or vitamin D suppletion, if any, is modest.[44,45]

Depressor systems

The kidney also produces substances with depressor activity, such as prostaglandins, kallikrein, renomedullary lipids, and, as recently discovered, renalase.[46] These substances are involved in the maintenance of renomedullary perfusion, which from animal studies is known to be essential for normal blood pressure. Whether impaired release of renal depressor substances participates in human renal hypertension is not resolved. However, it is well known that patients with CKD are more sensitive to the hypertensive (and hyperkalemic) action of prostaglandin synthesis inhibitors.

Arterial stiffness

Compliance of large conduit vessels is reduced in patients with ESRD. This has been confirmed by many researchers, both directly as steep pressure–volume relationship of the carotid artery assessed with Doppler techniques,[47] and indirectly as high pulse wave velocity over the aorta assessed with applanation tonometry.[48] The effect is an increase in systolic pressure and decrease in diastolic pressure. Indeed, systolic pressure increases more than diastolic pressure in most patients with CKD.[5] As a result, afterload of the heart increases more than indicated by mean arterial pressure or diastolic pressure. Pathology and high-resolution ultrasonography studies confirm the structural basis involving arteriosclerosis and calcification.[49] However, there is also a functional component, since hypervolemia and neurohumoral factors such as angiotensin II, sympathetic activity, and endothelin also contribute to decreased arterial compliance.[50,51]

Besides these functional aspects, some insight has become available on the potential pathways mediating vascular stiffness, in particular on media calcification. On the one hand, dysregulation of calcium phosphate metabolism seems central in calcification, albeit that it is still under dispute whether phosphate levels, calcium-phosphate product or PTH is most important.[52] Besides, cells with osteoblast-like properties can be identified in the vascular wall in uremia,[53] and can be inhibited by bone morphometric protein 7 (BMP7). It is not completely clear whether these cells are vascular smooth muscle cells or bone progenitor cells. These cells can form intracellular phosphate deposits, which induce (intracellular) matrix vesicles, which in turn are involved in osteogenesis.

Interestingly, endogenous inhibitors of vascular calcification have been described, such as matrix Gla protein. MGP knockout mice develop severe media calcification[54]; deficiencies or diminished function of such factors may well contribute to vascular calcification in uremia. Taken together, vascular calcium regulation is a complex phenomenon involving differentiation of cells and seems to be well controlled; dysregulation in CKD is far from understood.

CLINICAL PRESENTATION

Patients with hypertension due to CKD often present with signs of volume excess but this is not necessarily so. Testing for the blood pressure–lowering effect of RAS blockade is helpful to disclose the "volume component" of the hypertension (see "Management" section). In dialysis patients, various other methods are in use to determine whether volume is excessive. There is evidence for reduced tissue compliance in patients with CKD, meaning that hypervolemia can occur in the absence of visible edema.

As mentioned, there is high prevalence of systolic hypertension in patients with CKD, and in particular in ESRD.[5,6] The prevalence of hypertension is estimated to be approximately 75%.[55,56] Diurnal blood pressure measurements have shown that the increase in 24-hour systolic pressure load is greater than in diastolic pressure load (Figure 56–8). These studies also showed a prevalence of non–dipping blood pressure profile (see Horl and Horl[57] for review). Less than 25% of patients with plasma creatinine of more than 600 µmol/L or on dialysis show a normal diurnal blood pressure rhythm.[58] Absence of nocturnal blood pressure–drop increases the more time has passed since the last dialysis (Figure 56–6), which suggests a role for hypervolemia. Both increased pulse pressure and non–dipping diurnal pressure rhythm predict for development of heart failure and increased cardiovascular mortality,[59] making this a poor combination.

About one-third of patients with moderate renal failure already have evidence for left ventricular hypertrophy (LVH), and this number increases to ~80% when patients

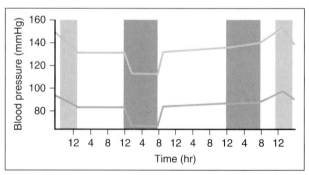

Figure 56–8. Schematic interdialytic blood pressure pattern. Blood pressure decreases during dialysis, is low during the postdialysis day, with an intact nocturnal dip, and then starts to increase. On Day 2 after dialysis, the nocturnal dip is absent, and blood pressure shows a steep increase just before the next dialysis session.

start hemodialysis.[60,61] In patients on dialysis, blood pressure correlates with LVH,[62,63] ventricular dilatation, and *de novo* heart failure,[60] and worsens the prognosis.[64]

Patients with CKD often present with clinically significant arteriosclerosis, with hypertension being a major risk factor. CT scans showed 92% incidence of coronary artery calcifications and significantly increased carotid artery intima media thickness (IMT) in young adults with childhood-onset CKD.[65] In the National Institutes of Health hemodialysis study, the prevalence of symptomatic cerebrovascular disease, peripheral artery disease, and coronary heart disease was 19%, 23%, and 40%, respectively.[66] Incidence of acute coronary syndromes is increased twofold in patients with GFR of less than 60 mL/min,[67] and 10-fold in patients with ESRD.[68] Brain-T2MR in predialysis patients has showed high intensity scores pointing to cerebrovascular disease in 75%, with a strong correlation with hypertension.[69] As many as 85% of patients with CKD and GFR of less than 40 mL/min show asymptomatic lacunar infarcts in association with hypertension.[70] The incidence of stroke is increased threefold in patients with GFR of less than 60 mL/min,[67] and 10-fold in patients on dialysis.[71] In dialysis patients, hypertension is a strong independent predictor of both hemorrhagic and ischemic stroke.[71,72] The prevalence of decreased ankle arm index is increased twofold in subjects with GFR lower than 40 mL/min.[73] In a large cohort of male patients presenting with advanced peripheral artery disease (rest pain, ulceration), the prevalence of moderate (GFR 30 to 60 mL/min) to severe (GFR <30 mL/min) CKD was 30% and 8%, respectively,[74] indicating a ~12-fold increased risk in CKD. Importantly, 90% of these subjects had or were treated for hypertension.

As discussed in Chapter 49, hypertension accelerates the decline of renal function in patients with chronic renal failure, and strict blood pressure control strongly reduces the rate of decline, especially in patients with proteinuria. The presence of cardiovascular disease shortens the time to ESRD,[68] pointing to a complex relation among hypertension, cardiovascular disease, and progression of CKD. The role of atherosclerotic renovascular disease in this process is unclear. The prevalence of severe renal artery stenosis in ESRD varies between 10% and 40% in adults, depending on measurement techniques. A recent study with CT-angiography in patients starting dialysis showed severe renovascular disease in 41%, the prevalence being extremely high in hypertensive subjects in whom the cause of the CKD was unknown.[75]

DIAGNOSTIC TECHNIQUES

Measurement of blood pressure: How and when?

For patients with chronic renal failure who are not on renal replacement therapy, assessment of blood pressure is not principally different from other hypertensive subjects, and precise instructions can be found in the K-DOQI guidelines[76] (see also "Management" section). Ambulatory blood pressure measurement (ABPM) is advised in case of suspected white coat hypertension, resistant hypertension, hypotensive symptoms while taking antihypertensive medications, episodic hypertension, or autonomic dysfunction.[76] Please note that 24-hour ABPM levels are somewhat lower than office measurements,[77–79] and boundaries are supplied in Table 56–1. It is becoming more and more clear that frequent home blood pressure measurement adequately reflects blood pressure, and leads to better blood pressure control.[80] In the absence of ABPM systems, frequent home measurements can be used as surrogates, although there is no proof yet of their ability to predict cardiovascular complications.

There is no consensus as to which blood pressure measurement most adequately reflects average pressure load and most accurately predicts the risk for cardiovascular disease in ESRD patients on hemodialysis. As mentioned, ABPM tracings illustrate that average pressure load is probably best assessed by average interdialytic blood pressure; the highest blood pressure and the blood pressure heart frequency product are reached just before the next hemodialysis session (Figure 56–6). Several studies have indicated that predialysis (or "dialysis center") blood pressure overestimates ambulatory blood pressure. In one study, predialysis systolic blood pressure exceeded the average of ABPM values in the 6 hours before arrival for dialysis by 25/13 mmHg in 40% of the patients.[81] Another report also indicates a strong overestimation of blood pressure by predialysis assessment and failed to show any good (Bland-Altman) agreement between predialysis blood pressure and ambulant blood pressure.[82] In both dialysis patients[82] and CKD patients[83] excellent agreement between ABPM and home blood pressure measurements has been reported. Taken together, these and other studies indicate that center blood pressure measurements are not likely to reflect interdialytic blood pressure, and either ABPM or home blood pressure measurements are preferred. Which blood pressure to take should, ultimately, be decided on a longitudinal

AMBULATORY BLOOD PRESSURE MEASUREMENT THRESHOLDS IN ADULTS			
	95th Percentile	Normotension	Hypertension
24 hour	132/82	≤130/80	≥135/85
Daytime	138/87	≤135/85	≥140/90
Nighttime	123/74	≤120/70	≥125/75
Source: Staessen JA, O'Brien ET. *Blood Press Monitoring* 1999;4(3–4):127–36.			

Table 56–1. Ambulatory Blood Pressure Measurement Thresholds in Adults

association with clinically relevant outcomes. A summary of 11 relevant studies suggests that, whereas predialysis (systolic and diastolic) blood pressure correlates with left ventricular mass, postdialysis (systolic and diastolic) blood pressure correlates with mortality (Table 56–2).[84] Studies of risk assessment based on ABPM are too scarce to allow a conclusion.

Assessment of pathophysiologic mechanism driving hypertension

Contributions of hypervolemia and vasoconstricting factors to the hypertension can often adequately be estimated with functional assessment of RAS activity using an ACE inhibitor test, by carefully assessing the volume status of the patient (edema, weight gain), and by using pulse rate as a reflection of sympathetic nervous system activity. Using these parameters and following a strict therapeutic approach (see "Management" section), measuring renin activity or sympathetic activity is rarely required or helpful. Only in special circumstances, particularly when blood pressure is low despite suspicion of volume excess, measurement of volume indicators such as brain natriuretic peptide, body composition assessed with bioelectric impedance, and vena cava index may be helpful to discern between hypovolemia or heart failure.

Consequences of hypertension

Left ventricular hypertrophy (or its absence) is easily assessed using electrocardiography; however, the ECG is not very sensitive, particularly in obese subjects.[85] Nevertheless, LVH indicated by ECG voltage criteria is a strong predictor of cardiovascular morbidity and mortality.[86] Echocardiography is much more sensitive and yields additional information, such as the type of LVH, potential diastolic dysfunction (which may complicate antihypertensive treatment) and valvular heart disease. It can be argued that informed management of hypertension without echocardiography is hardly possible.

There are currently two methods to assess vascular wall properties under research conditions that may well enter routine clinical use in the next few years: IMT assessment and pulse wave velocity (PWV). Carotid IMT correlates with cardiovascular mortality in hemodialysis patients, independent of blood pressure.[87] PWV has been shown to be a strong predictor of cardiovascular morbidity and mortality as well.[88] Interestingly, we have confirmed elevated PWV in hemodialysis patients and demonstrated that ACE inhibitor treatment and volume depletion additively reduced PWV to levels comparable with healthy controls.[89] This indicates that arterial wall characteristics are still modifiable.

MANAGEMENT

How to decrease blood pressure

It is important to manage both components of hypertension—hypervolemia and vasoconstriction—and to estimate the contribution of these factors in individuals. In patients with CKD who are not on dialysis, it is practical to start with an RAS blocker, which eliminates the vasoconstriction except structural vascular changes and some of the sympathetic hyperactivity.[29] Residual hypertension reveals the hypervolemia component, which can be treated next with diuretics (Figure 56–9). Preferably one should use loop diuretics, of which the dose should be increased to reach the high intratubular concentrations needed to further lower the (already low) fractional tubular sodium reabsorption.[90] Thiazide diuretics are often insufficient in CKD, but can still be very potent together with loop diuretics, since these shift sodium reabsorption to the thiazide-sensitive tubule segment. In some cases blood pressure remains high despite adequate suppression of the RAS and control of the hypervolemia. Residual vasoconstriction is mostly due to insufficiently suppressed sympathetic activity, to be distinguished from tachycardia. In those patients, addition of the central sympaticolytic drug moxonidine on top of RAS blockade can control both sympathetic hyperactivity and blood pressure.[91]

In patients with ESRD volume has to be controlled with ultrafiltration. Inadequate blood pressure control occurs more often in patients with large interdialytic weight increase,[92] pointing to the role of volume excess. Frequent (nocturnal) or long hemodialysis offers an alternative way to control blood pressure.[93–95] This method diminishes the need for drug therapy, suggesting that systematic and prolonged maintenance of normovolemia with slow

BLOOD PRESSURE IN END-STAGE RENAL DISEASE AND ESTABLISHED RISK FOR CARDIOVASCULAR DISEASE								
	Predialysis				Postdialysis			
	SBP	DBP	MAP	PP	SBP	DBP	MAP	PP
LVH	X	X	X					
Cardiovascular mortality					X	X		
AMI			X					
CVA	X							
PAD	?							
AMI, acute myocardial infarction; CVA, cerebrovascular accident; DBP, diastolic blood pressure; LVH, left ventricular hypertrophy; MAP, mean arterial pressure; PAD, peripheral arterial disease; PP, pulse pressure.								

Table 56–2. Blood Pressure in End-Stage Renal Disease and Established Risk for Cardiovascular Disease

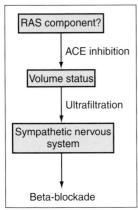

Figure 56–9. Schematic approach to treatment of hypertension in chronic kidney disease and end-stage renal disease. ACE, angiotensin-converting enzyme; RAS, renin angiotensin system.

ultrafiltration eliminates vasoconstrictive factors. The mechanism is unclear. In patients with CKD, it is often difficult to control blood pressure with diuretics alone because these drugs may evoke compensatory reactions of vasoconstriction.

Blood pressure control is important to retard progression of CKD and cardiovascular complications. There is some evidence that RAS blockade offers blood pressure independent protection against progression of CKD and also protects against development and progression of heart failure. Therefore, RAS blockade should be part of the antihypertensive regimen in CKD. Although sympatholytic drugs predictably will have additional value, this is less clear. A recent study showed that patients with CKD treated with RAS blockade showed better control of blood pressure and of renal function decline after addition of moxonidine compared to addition of nifedipine.[96] The strength of β-blockers in the prevention of coronary syndromes and heart failure is well appreciated in the general population with hypertension, yet their use is restricted to only 40% in patients with CKD and less than 20% in patients on hemodialysis.[97] This is difficult to understand since the mortality risk after myocardial infarction is extremely high in patients with renal disease. The mortality rate after MI is 14% and 21% in patients with moderate and advanced renal failure, respectively, and 30% with end-stage renal disease.[98]

Several practical problems arise with respect to blood pressure control in ESRD. First, antihypertensive medication is withheld in approximately 60% of patients on the day of dialysis.[92] Second, dietary sodium restriction, although seemingly trivial, often receives too little attention. This important measure requires careful explanation to the patient.[99]

Since the introduction of specific, high-affinity angiotensin AT1-receptor antagonists (ATRA), the interesting notion

developed that under certain conditions, combined treatment with ATRA and ACE inhibitors may have outcomes exceeding those of either compound alone. Specifically, additional reduction in proteinuria has been shown in diabetic[100] and nondiabetic[101] renal disease via RAS "double blockade" compared to ATRA or ACEi alone. Moreover, "double blockade" has been shown to be more effective as compared to single treatment in hypertensive diastolic heart failure[102] and improved cardiac output in another study on heart failure.[103] It is not clear whether such effects are due to residual Ang II activity or caused by high local activity of the renin angiotensin system,[104] or are due to actions of angiotensin AT2 receptors.[105] With respect to ESRD, little information is available, however, a recent report indicated that double blockade led to further regression of LVH in type 2 diabetic patients who recently started hemodialysis, an effect that was independent of blood pressure.[106] Thus, current data support the use of combined ATRA and ACE inhibitor therapy to minimize proteinuria and to optimize cardiac function in heart failure; however, there is no clear indication for combined treatment to further reduce blood pressure.

What is the blood pressure target?

In CKD, the Kidney Disease Outcomes Quality Initiative recommends the guidelines of the Joint National Committee on Prevention, Detection, Evaluation and Treatment of High Blood Pressure for patients with chronic renal failure (here defined as an estimated GFR <60 mL/min) and to reach less than 130/80 mmHg as target blood pressure.[107] The European Society of Hypertension Guidelines for Hypertension also recommends a target blood pressure of less than 130/80 mmHg in CKD and less than 125/75 mmHg if concomitant proteinuria of more than 1 g/L exists.[108]

In dialysis patients, determination of target blood pressure is more complicated. In contrast to large actuarial studies, several studies in hemodialysis patients have indicated that elevated blood pressure is not associated with increased cardiovascular mortality.[8,109] Investigators were urged to more precisely analyze this phenomenon; in effect, the absence of a relationship between blood pressure and mortality could be due to increased risk in patients with either low or high blood pressure. Indeed evidence for such a "J"-shaped relationship was derived from the observed increased cardiovascular (and noncardiovascular) mortality in dialysis patients with low predialysis blood pressure; predialysis hypertension was not associated with increased cardiovascular risk, although postdialysis hypertension was.[8] Others reported a positive association between an increased predialysis mean arterial pressure (MAP) and LVH, and *de novo* cardiac failure and *de novo* ischemic heart disease, but also that a low MAP was associated with increased mortality.[60] A recent study could not couple this "reverse epidemiology" of low predialysis blood pressure to the malnutrition–inflammation syndrome.[110]

More recently, serious concerns have emerged about the "J"-shaped relationship between blood pressure and mortality. One study showed that early mortality (3 to 4 years on dialysis) displayed a "U"-shaped relation with both low and high predialysis systolic and diastolic blood pressure; however, late mortality (>5 years) was associated with high blood pressures only.[111] Late more than early mortality was due to cardiovascular disease. Another study showed that hypertensive patients entering a dialysis program survived better when their systolic blood pressure was lowered to less than 160 mmHg, unless they also had ischemic heart disease.[112] The results of a large number of incident and prevalent cohorts were recently summarized. The incident cohorts seem to indicate that in dialysis populations with relatively little cardiovascular morbidity, hypertension presents itself as a risk factor. Inadequate designs may well have obscured the subgroup of patients with cardiac disease and other comorbidities; other problems with study design, such as erroneous measurements, lack of consideration of medication, inadequate sample size, and the presence of competing risk factors were also identified.[113] The term "reverse epidemiology" can only be justified when relationships are studied with adequate (prospective) designs, and studying relationships at the end of a disease spectrum may be inherently incorrect.[62]

In the absence of randomized controlled trials, recommendation of target blood pressure remains a matter of opinion. In agreement with recent expert reviews,[57,113–116] it seems reasonable to divide ESRD hypertension into classic systolic–diastolic and isolated systolic hypertension categories. In case of systolic–diastolic hypertension, it is reasonable to pursue a target of 130/80 mmHg (post-dialysis measurement confirmed by ambulatory or home measurements). These patients will be younger or have a shorter history of renal disease, or have been better protected with antihypertensive medication. In case of preferential systolic hypertension, it is probably better to keep diastolic pressure between 80 to 90 mmHg, and to accept systolic blood pressure levels between 150 to 160 mmHg, which concurs with the best prognosis in the "U" curve.[112] The latter patients will be older, have more LVH,[84] coronary insufficiency,[62] and less compliant aorta.[114] Further lowering of blood pressure in this group may lead to insufficient coronary perfusion in diastole.

Regarding the group with systolic hypertension, some specific points deserve attention. First, decreased aortic compliance often has a functional component induced by vasoconstrictor hyperactivity that can be eliminated by RAS blockade.[89] Therefore, we define systolic hypertension as systolic hypertension persisting despite RAS blockade. Second, overhasty blood pressure correction leading to dialysis instability or hypotension may well discourage doctor and patient from reaching optimal blood pressure control and should be avoided. Adaptations of large conduit vessels and smaller resistance vessels take time, as does whole-body autoregulation, and blood pressure correction after volume correction often follows a lag time.[14] Slow and long dialysis is probably the best way to correct blood pressure in these patients. Third, and this cannot be sufficiently stressed, preventing this condition is paramount by starting very strict blood pressure control in the earliest possible stage of CKD.

SUMMARY

Hypertension in CKD and ESRD is a serious threat for cardiovascular complications. Nevertheless, blood pressure is frequently inadequately controlled in these groups. Using overactivity of the RAS and of the sympathetic nervous system and ECFV expansion as pathophysiologic background, blood pressure can and should be well controlled. Few studies have systematically investigated the efficacy of various treatment strategies. Furthermore, prospective studies are needed to further determine optimal blood pressure in the ESRD population.

REFERENCES

1. Coresh J, Astor BC, et al. Prevalence of chronic kidney disease and decreased kidney function in the adult US population: Third National Health and Nutrition Examination Survey. *Am J Kidney Dis* 2003;41(1):1–12.
2. Vanholder R, Massy Z, et al. Chronic kidney disease as cause of cardiovascular morbidity and mortality. *Nephrol Dial Transplant* 2005;20(6):1048–56.
3. National Kidney Foundation. K/DOQI clinical practice guidelines for chronic kidney disease: evaluation, classification, and stratification. *Am J Kidney Dis* 2002;39(2 Suppl 1):S1–266.
4. Mailloux LU, Haley WE. Hypertension in the ESRD patient: pathophysiology, therapy, outcomes, and future directions. *Am J Kidney Dis* 1998; 32(5):705–19.
5. Raine AE, Margreiter R, et al. Report on management of renal failure in Europe, XXII, 1991. *Nephrol Dial Transplant* 1992;7(Suppl 2):7–35.
6. Agarwal R, Lewis RR. Prediction of hypertension in chronic hemodialysis patients. *Kidney Int* 2001;60(5):1982–9.
7. Schwenger V, Ritz E. Audit of antihypertensive treatment in patients with renal failure. *Nephrol Dial Transplant* 1998;13(12):3091–5.
8. Zager PG, Nikolic J, et al. U curve association of blood pressure and mortality in hemodialysis patients. Medical Directors of Dialysis Clinic, Inc. *Kidney Int* 1998;54(2):561–9.
9. Agarwal R, Nissenson AR, et al. Prevalence, treatment, and control of hypertension in chronic hemodialysis patients in the United States. *Am J Med* 2003;115(4):291–7.
10. Shulman NB, Ford CE, et al. Prognostic value of serum creatinine and effect of treatment of hypertension on renal function. Results from the hypertension detection and follow-up program. The Hypertension Detection and Follow-up Program Cooperative Group. *Hypertension* 1989; 13(5 Suppl):I80–93.
11. Garg AX, Clark WF, et al. Moderate renal insufficiency and the risk of cardiovascular mortality: results from the NHANES I. *Kidney Int* 2002; 61(4):1486–94.
12. Baigent C, Burbury K, et al. Premature cardiovascular disease in chronic renal failure. *Lancet* 2000;356(9224):147–52.
13. Himmelfarb J, Stenvinkel P, et al. The elephant in uremia: oxidant stress as a unifying concept of cardiovascular disease in uremia. *Kidney Int* 62(5): 1524–38.
14. Charra B, Calemard E, et al. Survival as an index of adequacy of dialysis. *Kidney Int* 1992;41(5):1286–91.
15. Woods JD, Port FK, et al. Clinical and biochemical correlates of starting daily

hemodialysis. *Kidney Int* 1999;55(6): 2467–76.

16. Koomans HA, Roos JC, et al. Sodium balance in renal failure. A comparison of patients with normal subjects under extremes of sodium intake. *Hypertension* 1985;7(5):714–21.

17. Klein IH, Ligtenberg G, Neumann J, et al. Sympathetic nerve activity is inappropriately increased in chronic renal disease. *J Am Soc Nephrol* 2003; 14:3239–3244.

18. Harrap SB, Davies DL, et al. Renal, cardiovascular and hormonal characteristics of young adults with autosomal dominant polycystic kidney disease. *Kidney Int* 1991;40(3):501–8.

19. Koomans HA, Braam B, et al. The importance of plasma protein for blood volume and blood pressure homeostasis. *Kidney Int* 1986;30(5): 730–5.

20. Lin YP, Chen CH, et al. Left ventricular mass and hemodynamic overload in normotensive hemodialysis patients. *Kidney Int* 2002;62(5):1828–38.

21. Beretta-Piccoli C, Weidmann P, et al. Blood pressure, circulating renin and the body sodium/volume state in patients with mild renal failure. *Proc Eur Dial Transplant Assoc* 1976; 12:2:291–8.

22. Lifschitz MD, Kirschenbaum MA, et al. Effect of saralasin in hypertensive patients on chronic hemodialysis. *Ann Intern Med* 1978;88(1):23–7.

23. Vaughan ED Jr, Carey RM, et al. Hemodialysis-resistant hypertension: control with an orally active inhibitor of angiotensin-converting enzyme. *J Clin Endocrinol Metab* 1979;48(5): 869–71.

24. Boer P, Koomans HA, et al. Renin and blood volume in chronic renal failure: a comparison with essential hypertension. *Nephron* 1987;45(1): 7–15.

25. Chapman AB, Johnson A, et al. The renin-angiotensin-aldosterone system and autosomal dominant polycystic kidney disease. *N Engl J Med* 1990;323(16):1091–6.

26. Gordon RD, Tunny TJ, et al. Unstimulated renal venous renin ratio predicts improvement in hypertension following nephrectomy for unilateral renal disease. *Nephron* 1987; 44(Suppl 1):25–8.

27. Wanner C, Luscher TF, et al. Unilateral hydronephrosis and hypertension: cause or coincidence? *Nephron* 1987; 45(3):236–41.

28. Schohn D, Weidmann P, et al. Norepinephrine-related mechanism in hypertension accompanying renal failure. *Kidney Int* 1985;28(5):814–22.

29. Ligtenberg G, Blankestijn PJ, et al. Reduction of sympathetic hyperactivity by enalapril in patients with chronic renal failure. *N Engl J Med* 1999; 340(17):1321–8.

30. Converse RL Jr, Jacobsen TN, et al. Sympathetic overactivity in patients with chronic renal failure. *N Engl J Med* 1992;327(27):1912–8.

31. Koomans HA, Blankestijn PJ, et al. Sympathetic hyperactivity in chronic renal failure: a wake-up call. *J Am Soc Nephrol* 2004;15(3):524–37.

32. Faber JE, Brody MJ. Afferent renal nerve-dependent hypertension following acute renal artery stenosis

in the conscious rat. *Circ Res* 1985; 57:676–88.

33. Miyajima E, Yamada Y, et al. Muscle sympathetic nerve activity in renovascular hypertension and primary aldosteronism. *Hypertension* 1991;17(6 Pt 2):1057–62.

34. Klein IH, Ligtenberg G, et al. Sympathetic activity is increased in polycystic kidney disease and is associated with hypertension. *J Am Soc Nephrol* 2001;12(11):2427–33.

35. Wever R, Boer P, et al. Nitric oxide production is reduced in patients with chronic renal failure. *Arterioscler Thromb Vasc Biol* 1999;19(5):1168–72.

36. Schmidt RJ, Baylis C. Total nitric oxide production is low in patients with chronic renal disease. *Kidney Int* 2000; 58(3):1261–6.

37. Kielstein JT, Boger RH, et al. Marked increase of asymmetric dimethylarginine in patients with incipient primary chronic renal disease. *J Am Soc Nephrol* 2002;13(1):170–6.

38. Bergstrom J, Alvestrand A, et al. Plasma and muscle free amino acids in maintenance hemodialysis patients without protein malnutrition. *Kidney Int* 1990;38(1):108–14.

39. van Guldener C, Lambert J, et al. Endothelium-dependent vasodilatation and distensibility of large arteries in chronic haemodialysis patients. *Nephrol Dial Transplant* 1997; 12(Suppl 2):2:14–8.

40. Verhagen AM, Braam B, et al. Losartan-sensitive renal damage caused by chronic NOS inhibition does not involve increased renal angiotensin II concentrations. *Kidney Int* 1999;56(1):222–31.

41. Dijkhorst-Oei LT, Boer P, et al. Nitric oxide synthesis inhibition does not impair water immersion-induced renal vasodilation in humans. *J Am Soc Nephrol* 2000;11(7):1293–302.

42. Lariviere R, Lebel M. Endothelin-1 in chronic renal failure and hypertension. *J PhysiolCan J Physiol Pharmacol* 2003; 81(6):607–21.

43. Goddard J, Johnston NR, et al. Endothelin-A receptor antagonism reduces blood pressure and increases renal blood flow in hypertensive patients with chronic renal failure: a comparison of selective and combined endothelin receptor blockade. *Circulation* 2004;109(9):1186–93.

44. Raine AE, Bedford L, et al. Hyperparathyroidism, platelet intracellular free calcium and hypertension in chronic renal failure. *Kidney Int* 1993;43(3):700–5.

45. Goldsmith DJ, Covic AA, et al. Blood pressure reduction after parathyroidectomy for secondary hyperparathyroidism: further evidence implicating calcium homeostasis in blood pressure regulation. *Am J Kidney Dis* 1996;27(6):819–25.

46. Xu J, Li G, et al. Renalase is a novel, soluble monoamine oxidase that regulates cardiac function and blood pressure. *J Clin Invest* 2005; 115(5):1275–80.

47. Blacher J, Guerin AP, et al. Arterial calcifications, arterial stiffness, and cardiovascular risk in end-stage renal disease. *Hypertension* 2001;38(4):938–42.

48. Blacher J, Safar ME, et al. Aortic pulse wave velocity index and mortality in end-stage renal disease. *Kidney Int* 2003;63(5):1852–60.

49. Amann K, Ritz E. Cardiovascular abnormalities in ageing and in uraemia—only analogy or shared pathomechanisms? *Nephrol Dial Transplant* 1998;13(Suppl 7):7:6–11.

50. Tycho Vuurmans JL, Boer WH, et al. Contribution of volume overload and angiotensin II to the increased pulse wave velocity of hemodialysis patients. *J Am Soc Nephrol* 2002;13(1):177–83.

51. Vuurmans TJ, Boer P, et al. Effects of endothelin-1 and endothelin-1 receptor blockade on cardiac output, aortic pressure, and pulse wave velocity in humans. *Hypertension* 2003;41(6):1253–8.

52. Floege J, Ketteler M. Vascular calcification in patients with end-stage renal disease. *Nephrol Dial Transplant* 2004;19(Suppl 5):V59–66.

53. Davies MR, Lund RJ, et al. BMP-7 is an efficacious treatment of vascular calcification in a murine model of atherosclerosis and chronic renal failure. *J Am Soc Nephrol* 2003; 14(6):1559–67.

54. Luo G, Ducy P, et al. Spontaneous calcification of arteries and cartilage in mice lacking matrix GLA protein. *Nature* 1997;386(6620):78–81.

55. Salem MM. Hypertension in the hemodialysis population: a survey of 649 patients. *Am J Kidney Dis* 1995; 26(3):461–8.

56. Rocco MV, Yan G, et al. Risk factors for hypertension in chronic hemodialysis patients: baseline data from the HEMO study. *Am J Nephrol* 2001; 21(4):280–8.

57. Horl MP, Horl WH. Hemodialysis-associated hypertension: pathophysiology and therapy. *Am J Kidney Dis* 2002;39(2):227–44.

58. Farmer CK, Goldsmith DJ, et al. An investigation of the effect of advancing uraemia, renal replacement therapy and renal transplantation on blood pressure diurnal variability. *Nephrol Dial Transplant* 1997; 12(11):2301–7.

59. Amar J, Vernier I, et al. Nocturnal blood pressure and 24-hour pulse pressure are potent indicators of mortality in hemodialysis patients. *Kidney Int* 2000;57(6):2485–91.

60. Foley RN, Parfrey PS, et al. Impact of hypertension on cardiomyopathy, morbidity and mortality in end-stage renal disease. *Kidney Int* 1996; 49(5):1379–85.

61. Levin A, CR Thompson, et al. Left ventricular mass index increase in early renal disease: impact of decline in hemoglobin. *Am J Kidney Dis* 1999; 34(1):125–34.

62. Foley RN. Cardiac disease in chronic uremia: can it explain the reverse epidemiology of hypertension and survival in dialysis patients? *Semin Dial* 2004;17(4):275–8.

63. Conlon PJ, Walshe JJ, Heinle SK, et al. Predialysis systolic blood pressure correlates strongly with mean 24-hour systolic blood pressure and left ventricular mass in stable hemodialysis patients. *J Am Soc Nephrol* 1996; 7(12):2658–63.

64. Silberberg JS, PE Barre, et al. Impact of left ventricular hypertrophy on survival in end-stage renal disease. *Kidney Int* 1989;36(2):286–90.

65. Oh J, Wunsch R, et al. Advanced coronary and carotid arteriopathy in young adults with childhood-onset chronic renal failure. *Circulation* 2002; 106(1):100–5.

66. Cheung AK, Sarnak MJ, et al. Atherosclerotic cardiovascular disease risks in chronic hemodialysis patients. *Kidney Int* 2000;58(1):353–62.

67. Weiner DE, Tighiouart H, et al. Chronic kidney disease as a risk factor for cardiovascular disease and all-cause mortality: a pooled analysis of community-based studies. *J Am Soc Nephrol* 2004;15(5):1307–15.

68. Levin A. Clinical epidemiology of cardiovascular disease in chronic kidney disease prior to dialysis. *Semin Dial* 2003;16(2):101–5.

69. Suzuki M, Wada A, et al. Cerebral magnetic resonance T2 high intensities in end-stage renal disease. *Stroke* 1997;28(12):2528–31.

70. Kobayashi S, Ikeda T, et al. Asymptomatic cerebral lacunae in patients with chronic kidney disease. *Am J Kidney Dis* 2004;44(1):35–41.

71. Seliger SL, Gillen DL, et al. Risk factors for incident stroke among patients with end-stage renal disease. *J Am Soc Nephrol* 2003;14(10):2623–31.

72. Iseki K, Fukiyama K. Predictors of stroke in patients receiving chronic hemodialysis. *Kidney Int* 1996; 50(5):1672–5.

73. Shlipak MG, Fried LF, et al. Cardiovascular disease risk status in elderly persons with renal insufficiency. *Kidney Int* 2002;62(3):997–1004.

74. O'Hare AM, Bertenthal D, et al. Impact of renal insufficiency on mortality in advanced lower extremity peripheral arterial disease. *J Am Soc Nephrol* 2005;16(2):514–9.

75. van Ampting JM, Penne EL, et al. Prevalence of atherosclerotic renal artery stenosis in patients starting dialysis. *Nephrol Dial Transplant* 2003;18(6):1147–51.

76. K/DOQI. K/DOQI clinical practice guidelines on hypertension and antihypertensive agents in chronic kidney disease. *Am J Kidney Dis* 2004;43(5 Suppl 1):S1–290.

77. Sega G, Bravi C, et al. Ambulatory and home blood pressure normality: the Pamela Study. *J Cardiovasc Pharmacol* 1994;23(Suppl 5):5:S12–5.

78. Ohkubo T, Imai Y, et al. Reference values for 24-hour ambulatory blood pressure monitoring based on a prognostic criterion: the Ohasama Study. *Hypertension* 1998;32(2):255–9.

79. Staessen JA, O'Brien ET. Development of diagnostic thresholds for automated measurement of blood pressures in adults. *Blood Press Monitoring* 1999; 4(3–4):127–36.

80. Cappuccio FP, Kerry SM, et al. Blood pressure control by home monitoring: meta-analysis of randomised trials. *BMJ* 2004;329(7458):145.

81. Mitra S, Chandna SM, et al. What is hypertension in chronic haemodialysis? The role of interdialytic blood pressure monitoring. *Nephrol Dial Transplant* 1999;14(12):2915–21.

82. Agarwal R. Role of home blood pressure monitoring in hemodialysis patients. *Am J Kidney Dis* 1999; 33(4):682–7.

83. Andersen MJ, Khawandi W, et al. Home blood pressure monitoring in CKD. *Am J Kidney Dis* 2005; 45(6):994–1001.

84. Lazar AE, Smith MC, et al. Blood pressure measurement in hemodialysis patients. *Semin Dial* 2004;17(4):250–4.

85. Okin PM, Roman MJ, et al. Electrocardiographic identification of left ventricular hypertrophy: test performance in relation to definition of hypertrophy and presence of obesity. *J Am Coll Cardiol* 1996;27(1):124–31.

86. Okin PM, Devereux RB, et al. Regression of electrocardiographic left ventricular hypertrophy during antihypertensive treatment and the prediction of major cardiovascular events. *JAMA* 2004;292(19):2343–9.

87. Nishizawa Y, Shoji T, et al. Intima-media thickness of carotid artery predicts cardiovascular mortality in hemodialysis patients. *Am J Kidney Dis* 2003;41(3 Suppl):S76–9.

88. Pannier B, Guerin AP, et al. Stiffness of capacitive and conduit arteries: prognostic significance for end-stage renal disease patients. *Hypertension* 2005;45(4):592–6.

89. Vuurmans TJL, Boer WH, et al. Contribution of volume overload and angiotensin II to the increased pulse wave velocity of hemodialysis patients. *J Am Soc Nephrol* 2002;13(1):177–83.

90. Fliser D, Schroter M, et al. Coadministration of thiazides increases the efficacy of loop diuretics even in patients with advanced renal failure. *Kidney Int* 1994;46(2):482–8.

91. Neumann J, Ligtenberg G, et al. Moxonidine normalizes sympathetic hyperactivity in patients with eprosartan-treated chronic renal failure. *J Am Soc Nephrol* 2004; 15(11):2902–7.

92. Rahman M, Dixit A, et al. Factors associated with inadequate blood pressure control in hypertensive hemodialysis patients. *Am J Kidney Dis* 1999;33(3):498–506.

93. Kooistra MP, Vos J, et al. Daily home haemodialysis in The Netherlands: effects on metabolic control, haemodynamics, and quality of life. *Nephrol Dial Transplant* 1998; 13(11):2853–60.

94. Laurent G, Charra B. The results of an 8 h thrice weekly haemodialysis schedule. *Nephrol Dial Transplant* 1998;(13 Suppl 6):6:125–31.

95. McCormick BB, Chan CT. Improved blood pressure control with nocturnal hemodialysis: review of clinical observations and physiologic mechanisms. *Curr Hypertens Rep* 2004;6(2):140–4.

96. Vonend O, Marsalek P, et al. Moxonidine treatment of hypertensive patients with advanced renal failure. *J Hypertens* 2003;21(9):1709–17.

97. U.S. Renal Data Systems. Medication use among dialysis patients in the DMMS. United States Renal Data System. Dialysis Morbidity and Mortality Study. *Am J Kidney Dis* 1998;32(2 Suppl 1):S60–8.

98. Wright RS, Reeder GS, et al. Acute myocardial infarction and renal dysfunction: a high-risk combination. *Ann Intern Med* 2002;137(7):563–70.

99. Dorhout Mees EJ. *Cardiovascular Aspects of Dialysis Treatment: The Importance of Volume Control.* New York: Springer, 2000.

100. Jacobsen P, Andersen S, et al. Additive effect of ACE inhibition and angiotensin II receptor blockade in type I diabetic patients with diabetic nephropathy. *J Am Soc Nephrol* 2003; 14(4):992–9.

101. Nakao N, Yoshimura A, et al. Combination treatment of angiotensin-II receptor blocker and angiotensin-converting-enzyme inhibitor in non-diabetic renal disease (COOPERATE): a randomised controlled trial. *Lancet* 2003;361(9352):117–24.

102. Yoshida J, Yamamoto K, et al. AT1 receptor blocker added to ACE inhibitor provides benefits at advanced stage of hypertensive diastolic heart failure. *Hypertension* 2004;43(3):686–91.

103. Gremmler B, Kunert M, et al. Improvement of cardiac output in patients with severe heart failure by use of ACE-inhibitors combined with the AT1-antagonist eprosartan. *Eur J Heart Fail* 2000;2(2):183–7.

104. Braam B, Mitchell KD, et al. Proximal tubular secretion of angiotensin II in rats. *Am J Physiol* 1993;264(5 Pt 2):F891–8.

105. Ruiz-Ortega M, Lorenzo O, et al. Angiotensin II activates nuclear transcription factor-kappaB in aorta of normal rats and in vascular smooth muscle cells of AT1 knockout mice. *Nephrol Dial Transplant* 2001;(16 Suppl 1):27–33.

106. Suzuki H, Kanno Y, et al. Comparison of the effects of angiotensin receptor antagonist, angiotensin converting enzyme inhibitor, and their combination on regression of left ventricular hypertrophy of diabetes type 2 patients on recent onset hemodialysis therapy. *Ther Apher Dial* 2004;8(4):320–7.

107. Chobanian AV, Bakris GL, et al. The Seventh Report of the Joint National Committee on Prevention, Detection, Evaluation, and Treatment of High Blood Pressure: the JNC 7 report. *JAMA* 2003;289(19):2560–72.

108. European Society of Hypertension. 2003 European Society of Hypertension-European Society of Cardiology guidelines for the management of arterial hypertension. *J Hypertens* 2003;21(6):1011–53.

109. Comorbid conditions and correlations with mortality risk among 3,399 incident hemodialysis patients. *Am J Kidney Dis* 1992;20(5 Suppl 2):32–8.

110. Kalantar-Zadeh K, Kilpatrick RD, et al. Reverse epidemiology of hypertension and cardiovascular death in the hemodialysis population: the 58th annual fall conference and scientific sessions. *Hypertension* 2005;45(4): 811–7.

111. Mazzuchi N, Carbonell E, et al. Importance of blood pressure control in hemodialysis patient survival. *Kidney Int* 2000;58(5):2147–54.

112. Tomita J, Kimura G, et al. Role of systolic blood pressure in determining prognosis of hemodialyzed patients. *Am J Kidney Dis* 1995;25(3):405–12.

113. Agarwal R. Hypertension and survival in chronic hemodialysis patients—past lessons and future opportunities. *Kidney Int* 2005;67(1):1–13.

114. London GM, Marchais SJ, et al. Blood pressure control in chronic hemodialysis patients. In: Horl WH, ed. *Replacement of Renal Function by Dialysis*. New York: Springer, 2004.

115. Dikow R, Wanner C, et al., eds. *Hypertension in the Patient with Uremia*. Oxford Textbook of Clinical Nephrology. Oxford and New York: Oxford University Press, 2005.

116. Kidney Disease Outcomes Quality Initiative. K/DOQI clinical practice guidelines for cardiovascular disease in dialysis patients. *Am J Kidney Dis* 2005;45(4 Suppl 3):S1–128.

Chapter

57

Hypertension in Racial and Ethnic Minorities

John M. Flack, Samar A. Nasser, Mark Britton, Anna B. Valina-Toth, Vineeta Ahooja, and Shannon M. O'Connor

Key Findings

- Although the prevalence of hypertension (HTN) differs among ethnic groups, there is little evidence that the relationship of blood pressure (BP) to target-organ injury differs substantively by race or ethnicity

- HTN control rates (<140/90 mmHg) are low among non-Hispanic blacks and non-Hispanic whites, and lowest among Mexican Americans. There is a high prevalence of treated but uncontrolled HTN in Asian Americans (33%), African Americans (35%), and Hispanics (32%) relative to Caucasians (24%). Less intensive antihypertensive pharmacologic treatment likely contributes to the lower BP control rates in African Americans compared to whites.

- There are insufficient data to support the thesis of the existence of unique risk factors for HTN across ethnic groups. However, some risk factors confer quantitatively different risks for HTN in various ethnic groups, in part, because the most pervasive risk factors for HTN—obesity, physical inactivity, dietary excesses/deficiencies—occur variably across racial and ethnic groups. The distribution of these risk factors is not homogenous within racial/ethnic groups as prevalence gradients have been noted across geographic and socioeconomic strata.

- Obesity contributes significantly to HTN risk in all populations and particularly in most racial and ethnic minorities manifesting disproportionate obesity. Obesity also appears to be an important mediator of chronic renal injury. In any population, weight loss and increased physical activity as well as potassium-rich, calcium-rich, and low-sodium diets should favor lower BP levels. An essential component of any HTN treatment regimen or HTN prevention strategy is comprehensive lifestyle modification to the greatest degree possible.

- The use of immutable characteristics to guide therapy for all members of various race/ethnicity groups will occur less frequently as we identify informative hemodynamic, genetic, and vascular markers that vary at the level of the individual.

Hypertension (HTN) is one of the most important and pervasive risk factors for virtually all forms of cardiovascular-renal disease. Although the prevalence of HTN differs among ethnic groups, there is little evidence that the relationship of blood pressure (BP) to target-organ injury differs substantively by race or ethnicity. This *assertion* is important for most non-African American and non-white populations because of the scarcity of longitudinal clinical trial outcomes data for these groups. Throughout this chapter, non-Hispanic whites will be used as a reference group for racial/ethnic contrasts of epidemiology, BP control, pathogenesis, pressure-related target-organ injury, and treatment outcomes.

EPIDEMIOLOGY

African Americans

The age-adjusted prevalence of HTN in the U.S. population aged 18 years and older is 28.7%. Non-Hispanic blacks have the highest HTN prevalence (33.5%), non-Hispanic whites are intermediate (28.9%), and Mexican Americans have the lowest at 20.7%. The excess prevalence of HTN in non-Hispanic blacks compared to whites is smaller in men (30.9% vs. 27.7%) than in women (35.8% vs. 30.2%). Over the last decade, HTN incidence and prevalence have risen in the major race/ethnicity groups, with the largest increases among women. Interestingly, adults in Spain, Germany, and Finland all have higher age-adjusted HTN prevalence than non-Hispanic blacks, while Nigerians have much lower HTN prevalence rates than U.S. whites.[1] One likely contributor to the lower prevalence of HTN is the much lower prevalence of obesity in Nigerians compared to either whites or African Americans in the United States.

Hispanic Americans

Hispanics are now the largest minority group in the United States. Even though the overall prevalence of HTN among Mexican Americans was similar in the 1982–1984 (Hispanic Health and Nutrition Examination Survey [HHANES]) and the 1988–1991 (NHANES III) timeframe, a slight reduction in population HTN burden (except among men aged 40 to 49 years) is suggested.[2]

Asian Americans

Asian Americans represent 4% of the U.S. population, although this percentage will increase to 9% by 2050.[3] In 2000, Kim and colleagues reported that the age-adjusted prevalence of HTN was 32% in Koreans, a burden that was higher than the prevalence of HTN in the general American population (24%). Hypertension was also more common among men (35%) than women (30%).[4] In the Multi-Ethnic Study of Atherosclerosis (MESA), the age-adjusted prevalence of HTN in Asian-American (Chinese) was 39%, which was similar to that of Caucasians (38%) and Hispanics (42%), but less than in African Americans (60%).[5]

Native Americans

Hypertension was relatively uncommon in the Native-American population until recently. The prevalence of HTN in Navajo Indians aged 19 years and older rose from 0.1% in 1937 to 4.7% in 1963.[6] By 1973, 20% of Papago (Tohono Oodham) Indians aged 15 years and older had HTN,[7] and by 1979 the prevalence of HTN in Navajo Indians aged 19 and older living on reservations was 17%.[6] However, the mean systolic and diastolic blood pressures in Navajo Indians did not show as great an increase with age as was seen in white and black Americans.

In 1991, 704 Cree and Ojibwa Indians ages 20 to 64 were surveyed in Canada, and only 27% had HTN. The Inter-Tribal Heart Project examined Chippewa and Menominee Indians over the age of 25 years, who were active users of the Indian Health Service clinics, and documented a 31% prevalence of HTN.[8] This high incidence of HTN among Native Americans was confirmed in the Strong Heart Study (SHS), the largest epidemiologic study of American Indians ever undertaken. The SHS data reported a HTN prevalence of 27% to 56% in both men and women aged 45 to 75 years.[9]

BLOOD PRESSURE AWARENESS, TREATMENT, AND CONTROL

Awareness

Over the past two decades, the number of Americans aware of their HTN has increased. In the NHANES III, HTN awareness was greater among non-Hispanic blacks (74%) and non-Hispanic whites (70%) compared to the Mexican American population (54%). Hispanic women are more aware of their HTN than men.[10]

Treatment

In the NHANES III (1999–2000), HTN pharmacologic treatment rates increased by 6.0% (*p*=0.007) between 1988 and 2000. The age-adjusted treatment rate was 63% for non-Hispanic blacks, 60.1% for non-Hispanic whites, and 40.3% for Mexican Americans.[11] There are, however, somewhat troubling data that hypertensive African Americans are less intensely treated than hypertensive whites. This occurs despite the fact that HTN is more severe and accompanied by more factors that confer resistance to the BP-lowering effects of pharmacologic treatment than in any other racial/ethnic group. Accordingly, in the Antihypertensive and Lipid-Lowering Treatment to Prevent Heart Attack Trial (ALLHAT),[12] African Americans, women, and older participants had lower BP control rates, and were less intensively treated than their comparator groups. The relatively high prevalence of nonbiomedical expectations (i.e., treatment can cure hypertension) in African Americans with HTN[13] also likely undermines good BP control.

In the Inter-Tribal Heart Project only 58% of hypertensive Indians took antihypertensive medication.[8] Fewer than 50% of Asian Americans with HTN were pharmacologically treated. Factors that may contribute to the low frequency of antihypertensive medication use and control of BP in the Asian-American population include inadequate understanding of medications used, economic difficulties, limited health care access, transportation issues, and lack of health insurance.[14]

Control

Hypertension control rates (<140/90 mmHg) are highest among non-Hispanic blacks and non-Hispanic whites, and lowest among Mexican Americans (25%, 24%, and 14%, respectively). Non-Hispanic black women have the highest levels of HTN awareness, treatment, and control (79%, 65%, and 29%, respectively). There is a high prevalence of treated but uncontrolled HTN in Asian Americans (33%), African Americans (35%), and Hispanics (32%) relative to Caucasians (24%).[5] Accordingly, in ALLHAT the largest difference in BP control was found in the black/nonblack group comparison, where blacks were 31% less likely to be controlled (odds ratio=0.69, 95% confidence interval [CI]=0.65–0.73) than nonblacks. Furthermore, between baseline and year 5, the highest control rate was in nonblack men (70.0%), while the lowest control rate was in black women (58.8%).[12] However, less intensive antihypertensive pharmacologic treatment likely contributes to the lower BP control rates in African Americans compared to whites.[15] Approximately 14% of Asian Americans appear to attain BP control with medication alone.[14] According to the Inter-Tribal Heart Project, of Indians who were hypertensive only 28% had blood pressures below recommended levels.[8]

PATHOPHYSIOLOGY

There are insufficient data to support the thesis of the existence of unique risk factors for HTN across ethnic groups. It is, however, accurate to say that some risk factors confer quantitatively different risks for HTN in various ethnic groups, in part, because the most pervasive risk factors for HTN—obesity, physical inactivity, dietary excesses/deficiencies—occur variably across racial/ethnic groups. Nevertheless, the distribution of these risk factors is not homogenous within racial/ethnic groups, as prevalence gradients have been noted across geographic and socioeconomic strata. Accordingly, some pathophysiologic mechanisms are sometimes more or less manifest in racial/ethnic groups. However, these are quantitative rather than qualitative differences. The subsequently discussed pathophysiologic perturbations are unlikely to be solely confined to any race/ethnicity group.

Obesity

Obesity is more common in both African Americans and Hispanics, particularly among women, compared to whites.[16] In African-American women the prevalence of extreme obesity (body mass index [BMI] >40 kg/m²) is almost 1 in 6, a prevalence that is three- to four-fold higher than that of either white or Hispanic women. There are marked ethnic and age-based differences in the rates of weight accumulation. Relative to white women (reference group), the onset of obesity was faster for African-American women and Hispanic women. Hispanic men also develop obesity at earlier ages than white men. After age 28, African-American men develop obesity more rapidly than white men.

Hayashi et al.[17] showed that visceral fat is an independent risk factor for the development of HTN in Japanese Americans. Additionally, high BP correlates well with obesity even in elderly Japanese Americans.[18] Obesity is also strongly associated with HTN in Native-American men and women. The increasing prevalence of obesity is of serious concern, particularly in young Native Americans. In 1992, a high proportion of Navajo adolescents were found to be overweight (33% of girls and 25% of boys).[19,20] In Native Americans, increasing BMI has been linked to higher systolic blood pressure (SBP) and diastolic blood pressure (DBP) in both boys and girls.[19]

Physical inactivity

Physical activity levels tend to decrease with advancing age and are also lower in women than men as well as in persons with lower levels of income and education. African-American women experience greater age-related decreases in the cross-sectional prevalence of physical activity than white women. Independent of social class, the prevalence of "no leisure-time physical activity" was much higher in non-Hispanic black men (24%) and black women (40%) compared to non-Hispanic white men (13%) and white women (23%).[21,22] Another study found that fewer than half of Asian and Pacific Islander women (42.6%) were sedentary, compared to 36.1% of white non-Hispanic women.[23]

MECHANISMS OF HYPERTENSION

Obesity

In all likelihood, obesity contributes significantly to HTN risk in all populations and particularly in most racial/ethnic minorities manifesting disproportionate obesity. Figure 57–1 displays a schematic that depicts how the myriad of metabolic, neurohumoral, and hemodynamic perturbations linked to obesity influence BP levels. There is a multiplicity of obesity-related physiologic effects that contribute to the intermediate BP phenotype, salt sensitivity,[24,25] as well as resistance to hypertensive drug therapy.[12,26] Additionally, obesity appears to be a plausible mediator of chronic renal injury.[27] Box 57–1 displays the known hemodynamic effects of obesity.

Physical activity

Physical activity lowers BP in hypertensive persons.[28,29] It is unlikely that the reduction of BP is race/ethnicity-specific. Physical activity improves endothelial function, primarily via the augmented release of nitric oxide (NO), less NO destruction attributable to lower levels of oxidative stress,[30–32] and greater release from the vascular endothelium. Renal sodium excretion also appears to increase after physical activity. Aerobic exercise reduces inflammation in persons with diabetes via augmentation of the cytoplasmic inhibitor of nuclear factor kappa beta (NF-κB), leading to decreased

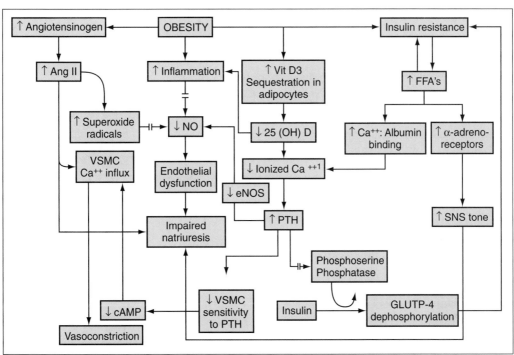

Figure 57–1. This figure provides an integrated schema for how obesity affects the renin-angiotensin system, nitric oxide synthesis, vitamin D, calcium, and PTH metabolism as well as insulin resistance. Persistently high PTH levels antagonize phosphoserine phosphatase, an enzyme that dephosphorylates GLUTP-4, rendering it an ineffective transporter of glucose across the cell membrane. [1]High dietary intake of sodium also promotes calciuria and plausibly contributes to lower circulating ionized calcium levels. Ang II, angiotensin II; FFAs, free fatty acids; Ca++, calcium; cAMP, cyclic adenosine 3′,5′ monophosphate; eNOS, endothelial nitric oxide; GLUTP-4, glucose transporter 4; NO, nitric oxide; PTH, parathyroid hormone; SNS, sympathetic nervous system; VSMC, vascular smooth muscle cell.

NF-κB activity and tumor necrosis factor alpha, an inflammatory cytokine.[33]

Diet

Long-term dietary patterns plausibly impact long-term trends in BP. Dietary sodium intake raises BP, at least in susceptible people, in the short term. There is also evidence that dietary sodium intake augments vascular angiotensin generation,[34] while in salt-sensitive persons, it reduces urinary NO metabolites.[35] Sodium also enhances urinary calcium excretion and may therefore contribute to reductions in ionized calcium that can upregulate parathyroid hormone (PTH) secretion (see Figures 57–2 and 57–3).

Dietary potassium intake has been shown to enhance renal natriuresis as well as to augment NO production. Increased dietary potassium intake has been shown to modestly lower BP as well as to augment the nocturnal fall in BP. Recent data documented that dietary potassium intake prevented the sodium-induced increase in circulating asymmetrical dimethyl arginine (ADMA), a known inhibitor of nitric oxide synthesis.[36]

African Americans consume less dietary calcium than whites, in part because of a much higher prevalence of lactose intolerance leading to lower consumption of calcium-rich dairy products. Lower dietary intake of calcium has been linked to HTN in African Americans. Calcium supplementation modestly lowers BP. It is, however, plausible to speculate that in persons at risk for vitamin D deficiency that low dietary calcium intake would further augment the physiologic signal to raise PTH levels (see Figures 57–2 and 57–3).

Thus, in any population, potassium-rich, calcium-rich, and low-sodium diets should favor lower BP levels. This type of diet would be rich in fresh fruits, vegetables, and dairy products, while simultaneously low in sodium.

Impaired diurnal blood pressure variability

Nocturnal BP levels are independently associated with end-organ damage, over and above the risk associated with daytime values. The attenuation of, or lack of, a nocturnal fall (nondipping) of BP has been associated with serious end-organ damage/dysfunction, such as left ventricular hypertrophy, microalbuminuria, cerebrovascular disease, more rapid loss of kidney function, and increased risk for heart failure.[37–42] Nocturnal decline in BP (daytime–nighttime difference) is approximately 10% to 20%. Obesity has been linked to nondipping of BP, and thus poses a plausible risk for end-organ damage via hemodynamic effects.[43] Furthermore, obesity is a risk factor for premature birth, which in turn, is a risk factor for elevated BP, decreased nephron number, and diabetes later in life.[44,45]

Hypovitaminosis D and secondary hyperparathyroidism

Vitamin D levels are maintained within the physiologic range, largely by conversion of 7-dehydrocholesterol to vitamin D3 after exposure to ultraviolet light. Figure 57–2 provides an overview of vitamin D metabolism. Dietary sources of vitamin D include fatty fish and fortified milk, although they are less important than exposure to ultraviolet light. In the United States, the prevalence of hypovitaminosis D (<37.5 nmol/L) is significantly more prevalent in African Americans than whites (42.4% vs. 4.2%).[46] A multiplicity of factors influences the striking excess preva-

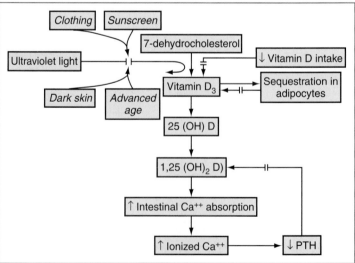

Figure 57–2. A simplified schematic of vitamin D metabolism is presented. Important factors that block the conversion of 7-dehydrocholesterol to vitamin D$_3$ are prominently displayed. Dark skin is an important factor in the high rates of hypovitaminosis D in African Americans and other dark-skinned populations. (Adapted in part from Yanoff LB, Parikh SJ, Spitalnik A, et al. The prevalence of hypovitaminosis D and secondary hyperparathyroidism in black Americans. *Clin Endocrinol* 2006;64:523; Liel Y, Ulmer E, Shary J, et al. Low circulating vitamin D in obesity. *Calcif Tissue Int* 1988;43:199; and Lips P. Vitamin D physiology. *J Prog Biophys Mol Biol* 2006;92:4.)

lence of hypovitaminosis D in African Americans than whites, including darker skin, higher prevalence of chronic kidney disease, and possibly more pervasive obesity.[47] However, the inverse relationship between body fat and 25(OH)D levels appears to be significantly more robust in white women compared to African-American women.[48] Vitamin D production in the skin in response to ultraviolet light is normal in obese persons; however, the significantly enhanced sequestration of vitamin D in adipocytes leads to reduced circulating levels.[49]

It is quite plausible that the physiologic perturbations caused by hypovitaminosis D are initiated by a transient fall in ionized calcium and lead to a reactive rise in PTH that maintains serum calcium levels within the physiologic range. Serum PTH levels begin to rise at 25(OH)D levels that are well above (~75 nmol/L) the deficiency threshold (<37.5 to 50 nmol/L). In a recent study of free-living African Americans living in the Washington, D.C. area, there was a high prevalence of hypovitaminosis D and secondary hyperparathyroidism; among individuals with BMI >35 kg/m^2, the prevalence of was 35.2% in African Americans and 9.7% in whites.[47] Intact PTH levels are also negatively correlated with vitamin D levels. Figure 57–3 displays the vascular and target-organ effects of PTH. These data suggest that hypovitaminosis D and secondary hyperparathyroidism are indeed highly prevalent in free-living African Americans, have biological effects that adversely affect vascular function and raise BP, and may be an important determinant in the burden of HTN and thus racial/ethnic disparities in the same. Accordingly, several studies have

shown reductions in BP in humans with elevated BP after supplementation with vitamin D[50,51] with a significant correlation between reduction in SBP and decline in serum PTH.[50]

Salt sensitivity

Salt sensitivity can be conceptualized as maintenance of intravascular volume homeostasis at the expense of higher blood pressure levels that augment pressure-induced renal natriuresis. Thus, in salt-sensitive persons consuming unrestricted amounts of sodium, steady state in–out volume homeostasis is maintained by raising BP, or, in drug-treated salt-sensitive hypertensives, the fall in BP is attenuated unless sodium intake is decreased. The sodium-linked attenuation of the BP-lowering effect varies by class of antihypertensive agent. Dietary sodium-induced attenuation of BP-lowering responsiveness appears to be greatest for angiotensin-converting enzyme (ACE) inhibitors (and possibly other renin-angiotensin system [RAS] antagonists) than for calcium antagonists[52,53] or diuretics.[52] Overall, salt sensitivity has also been linked to antihypertensive treatment resistance, target-organ injury, and nondipping of BP. Figure 57–4 displays a proposed mechanistic explanation for why salt-sensitivity undermines BP lowering in drug-treated hypertensives consuming a sodium-replete diet.

Multiple factors contribute to salt sensitivity including obesity,[54,55] NO deficient states,[56,57] psychosocial stressors,[58] low intake of dietary potassium,[59,60] advancing age, and reduced renal mass. Salt sensitivity has been documented in virtually every ethnic population that has been tested

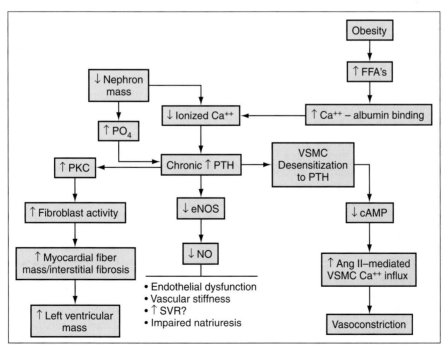

Figure 57–3. This figure displays the vascular and target-organ effects of parathyroid hormone. These effects will raise blood pressure and contribute to vascular injury/dysfunction and target-organ damage. Ang II, angiotensin II; Ca^{++}, calcium; cAMP, cyclic adenosine 3′,5′-monophosphate; eNOS, endothelial nitric oxide synthase; FFAs, free fatty acids; PO$_4$, phosphate; NO, nitric oxide; PKC, protein kinase C; PTH, parathyroid hormone; VSMC, vascular smooth muscle cell.

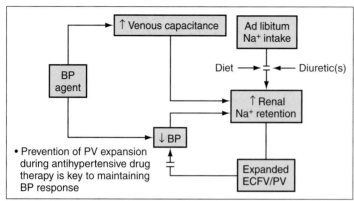

Figure 57–4. This figure displays a proposed mechanism through which antihypertensive drugs that expand venous capacitance (e.g., angiotensin-converting enzyme inhibitors) induce salt sensitivity. These agents expand venous capacitance, and therefore decentralize blood volume. In hypertensive (and obese) patients, venous capacitance vessels are constricted. When BP falls and venous capacitance expands, and blood volume is decentralized, renal sodium excretion increases. Sodium retention continues until the vascular system is "full" again. This expansion of extracellular fluid volume/plasma volume leads to diminution of the fall in BP unless the patient is given a diuretic and/or sodium intake is restricted to levels low enough to prevent plasma volume expansion. BP, blood pressure; ECFV, extracellular fluid volume; PV, plasma volume.

for it. Accordingly, African Americans,[61-63] whites,[53,64] Spaniards,[53,65] Caribbean Hispanics,[52] Venezuelans,[66,67] and Japanese[68,69] manifest salt sensitivity. And, although salt sensitivity has been found in both hypertensives and normotensives, the prevalence is usually higher in the former.[64,70,71] Moreover, salt sensitivity has often been found to be more prevalent in African Americans than in whites.[64,70,71]

Vascular function

Endothelium-dependent and endothelium-independent vascular responses have consistently been more abnormal in African Americans compared to whites.[72,73] There are data suggesting that bioavailable NO, the main determinant of endothelium-dependent vascular function, is lower in African Americans than whites, despite much higher levels of eNOS activity in the former.[74] It appears that the synthesis of oxygen radicals, mostly via uncoupled eNOS and lesser amounts via NADPH oxidase, raises levels of oxidative stress, accelerates NO destruction, and therefore leads to reduced NO bioavailability in African Americans.[74]

Endothelial dysfunction was linked to obesity in Hispanic women but not men who resided in northern Manhattan.[75] Impaired endothelial vasodilator function has also been linked to an exaggerated postexercise rise in blood pressure.[76] There are mixed data in regard to whether peripheral vascular resistance in higher in African Americans than whites.

Stress and hypertension

It has plausibly been speculated that persistent stress beyond the short term contributes to BP elevations.[77] Mental stress unequivocally raises BP in the short term, at least in part, via activation of the sympathetic nervous system. The

stress and HTN hypothesis may be of particular relevance to populations exposed chronically to persistently high environmental and psychosocial stressors. Although this thesis has not been proven, it is intuitively appealing and is under active investigation. Importantly, acute psychosocial stress (and increased SNS activity) activates NF-κB, an inflammatory transcription factor, that, in turn activates inflammatory cytokines as well as the hypothalamic-pituitary-adrenal axis.[78-81] The interrelation of the HPA, SNS, and NF-κB/inflammatory cytokines is displayed in Figure 57-5. NF-κB provides an important physiologic pathway through which high levels of stress that are characteristic of Western lifestyles, and especially in African Americans and other racial minorities, might contribute to systemic inflammation, oxidative stress, and vascular/hemodynamic perturbations such as endothelial dysfunction and elevated BP.

PRESSURE-RELATED TARGET-ORGAN INJURY

Albuminuria, chronic kidney disease, left ventricular hypertrophy, stroke, and heart failure predict an attenuated response to antihypertensive treatment.[15,82] One such example is microalbuminuria, which is associated with cardiovascular risk factors and is considered a marker for "resistance" to antihypertensive treatment.[15,83,84] Patients with microalbuminuria appear to progress more rapidly along the renal continuum to chronic kidney disease (CKD) (indicated by macroalbuminuria or proteinuria), increased serum creatinine concentration, and decreased GFR. With progressive CKD, single-nephron glomerular pressure increases, eventually leading to glomerulosclerosis.[85] In patients with early nephropathy, serum creatinine concentration and creatinine clearance is within normal limits, but microalbuminuria—the earliest clinical sign of nephropathy—is already present.[86] Mattix et al.[87] examined the distribution of urine albumin and creatinine concentrations measured in spot urine specimens in a nationally representative sample of men and women of various ethnicities. Overall, compared with non-Hispanic whites, non-Hispanic blacks had higher urinary albumin concentrations (21.4 vs. 13.6 μg/mL, $p<0.0001$). Mexican Americans did not have significantly different urine albumin concentrations compared with non-Hispanic whites. In this study, non-Hispanic black ethnicity remained independently associated with microalbuminuria even after adjusting for other risk factors, including age, diabetes, systolic and diastolic blood pressure, BMI, and smoking.

An additional detrimental consequence of pressure-related target-organ damage concerns the vascular tree. Arterial stiffness is similar to a double-edged sword, in that it is a cardiovascular disease (CVD) risk factor in itself, as well as a deleterious outcome of various diseases. Hypertension or increased luminal pressure stimulates excessive collagen production.[88] Furthermore, advanced glycation end-

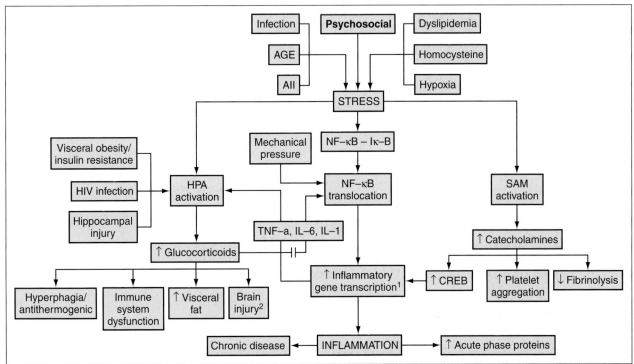

Figure 57–5. This schematic displays how a variety of stressors, including psychosocial stress, can activate NF-κB, causing separation from its cytoplasmic inhibitor, Iκ-B. Once NF-κB translocates to the nucleus, it can turn on inflammatory cytokines with NF-κB response elements. This leads to further upregulation of the hypothalamic pituitary adrenal axis. Increased glucocorticoids exert a mineralocorticoid effect and promote visceral fat deposition. Activation of the sympathetic nervous system also facilitates upregulation of inflammatory gene transcription. The net result is increased inflammation and oxidative stress. This will lead to decreased nitric oxide bioavailability. Thus, a plausible mechanism exists through which psychosocial stressors might plausibly cause chronic disease including hypertension. AGE, advanced glycation end products; AII, angiotensin II; CREB, cyclic AMP response element binding protein; HPA, hypothalamic-pituitary-adrenal axis; I κ-B, inhibitor kappa beta, an inhibitor of NF-κB; NF-κB , nuclear factor kappa beta; SAM, sympathetic adrenal medullary. [1]TNF-A, IL-1, IL-2, IL-6, interferon gamma, vascular cell adhesion molecule (VCAM)1, plasminogen activator inhibitor (PAI)-1, cyclooxygenase 2 (COX2), iNOS, and transforming growth factor (TGF)B. [2]Hippocampal atrophy and damage to frontal lobe neurons. 3C-reactive protein (CRP), fibrinogen, and cell adhesion molecules. (Adapted from Vale S. Psychosocial stress and cardiovascular diseases. *Postgrad Med J* 2005;81:429; Bierhaus A, Humpert PM, Nawroth PP. NF-kappaB as a molecular link between psychosocial stress and organ dysfunction. *Pediatr Nephrol* 2004;19:189; Padgett DA, Glaser R. How stress influences the immune response. *Trends Immunol* 2003;24:444; and Lemarie CA, Esposito B, Tedqui A, Lehoux S. Pressure-induced vascular activation of nuclear factor-kappaB: role in cell survival. *Circ Res* 2003;93:207.)

products (AGEs), which result from nonenzymatic protein glycation, form irreversible cross-links between these collagen proteins.[89] AGE may also affect endothelial cell function by inhibiting the bioavailability of NO.[90] The ability of the vascular endothelium to release NO in response to pulsatile blood flow during the cardiac cycle correlates inversely to the magnitude of arterial stiffness.

Pressure-induced target-organ damage and mortality are higher among African Americans than among white persons.[91] For example, compared to whites, African Americans have increased risk of many complications, including nonfatal stroke (1.3-fold), fatal stroke (1.8-fold), and end-stage renal disease (4.2-fold).[92] While African Americans have approximately twice the risk of first-ever stroke and a 1.8 times greater rate of fatal stroke, whites fare better than both Hispanics and African Americans, according to results of the Northern Manhattan Study.[93]

Asian Americans are believed to have a substantially lower mortality rate of CVD than African Americans. In addition, Asian Americans have a lower mortality rate from cerebrovascular disease in comparison to African Americans, but it is higher when compared to Caucasians.[94,95] Fang et al.[96] demonstrated that Asian Americans with a risk factor such as HTN were more likely to experience a lethal hemorrhagic stroke in comparison to Caucasians.[96] The prevalence of end-stage renal disease and other hypertension-related diseases are rising in the Asian-American population.[97] The cerebrovascular disease mortality rate is declining more rapidly in the general U.S. population than among Native Americans.

HYPERTENSION CLINICAL ENDPOINT STUDIES

AASK

Data from the African American Study of Kidney Disease (AASK)[98] confirmed that initial therapy with ramipril, an ACE inhibitor, slowed the progressive loss of kidney function, and lowered urinary protein excretion more effectively than amlodipine, a dihydropyridine calcium antagonist, in nondiabetic African Americans with depressed kidney function. There was a difference of less than 2 mmHg in blood pressure between the randomized treatment groups; both groups received the same number (mean 2.75) of antihypertensive drugs. The renoprotective effect of ACE inhibitors was most evident in patients with proteinuria. The AASK study confirmed the superiority of RAS system drugs in African Americans with nondiabetic kidney disease, as had previously been shown in non-African Americans with nondiabetic kidney disease.

ALLHAT

The Antihypertensive and Lipid-lowering Treatment to Prevent Heart Attack Trial (ALLHAT) was a 5-year clinical endpoint trial in high-risk hypertensives that sought to compare the effectiveness of various initial antihypertensive drug therapies for the prevention of CVD and overall mortality. The final study report was on 33,357 high-risk, stage-1 and -2 hypertensives aged 55 years and older with at least one other cardiovascular risk factor.[99,100] Eligible participants were randomized to chlorthalidone, amlodipine, or lisinopril, and were assigned a target BP of less than 140/90 mmHg. The primary outcome was the composite of fatal coronary heart disease and nonfatal myocardial infarction. In all three treatment arms, BP reductions in whites exceeded those of African Americans.[100] In African Americans relative to whites in the lisinopril group, the deficit in SBP response was –8.2, –6.8, and –4.9 mmHg lower, respectively, at the end of study years 1, 2, and 4. Achieving BP control at less than 140/90 mmHg was also higher in whites than African Americans in all randomized treatment arms. Over the course of the trial, SBP in African Americans was lowered ~1.5 to 2 mmHg more in the chlorthalidone compared to amlodipine treatment group. At baseline, 26% to 28% of BP levels in the randomized treatment groups were less than 140/90 mmHg. At year 4, control rates in the chlorthalidone, amlodipine, and lisinopril treatment arms were 63.4% versus 68.9%, 60.2% versus 68.6%, and 54.2% versus 67.4%, respectively. There were no differences among African-American ALLHAT participants randomized to the chlorthalidone and amlodipine treatment arms in the primary study endpoint or in any of the secondary outcomes. However, in the lisinopril compared to the chlorthalidone groups, African Americans experienced excess stroke (+40%) and combined CVD (+19%). Higher average blood pressure levels in the lisinopril group undoubtedly explained at least part of the excess risk.

INVEST

The International Verapamil sustained release/Trandolapril Study (INVEST) was a prospective, randomized, blinded endpoint study in patients with coronary artery disease and hypertension.[101] Study participants were randomized to either verapamil sustained release (SR), a rate-lowering calcium antagonist, or atenolol, a beta-blocker. A post-hoc analysis of 8045 Hispanic participants was made in comparison to 14,531 non-Hispanic participants. Treatment with either a verapamil SR or atenolol resulted in greater BP control in Hispanic compared to non-Hispanic partici-

pants. Hispanics were at significantly lower risk of experiencing a nonfatal myocardial infarction, nonfatal stroke, or death (hazard ratio [HR] 0.87, 95% CI=0.78–0.97) than non-Hispanics. Hispanic ethnicity was associated with a greater risk (HR=1.19, 95% CI=1.04–1.36) of new-onset diabetes. Randomization to the verapamil SR was associated with a decrease (HR=0.85, 95% CI=0.76–0.95) in the risk of new-onset diabetes. In Hispanic participants randomized to atenolol treatment, higher doses of atenolol and hydrochlorothiazide were associated with a higher risk of new-onset diabetes.

LIFE

A post-hoc analysis stratified by race/ethnicity of the Losartan Intervention for Endpoint Reduction (LIFE) trial[102] that enrolled hypertensives with left ventricular hypertrophy demonstrated that African Americans and whites experienced virtually identical levels of BP lowering. Nevertheless, in whites, losartan, an angiotensin receptor blocker, was superior to atenolol, a beta-blocker, in reducing the risk for the primary composite endpoint (cardiovascular death, stroke, myocardial infarction). Conversely, in African Americans atenolol was superior to losartan. There is no plausible explanation for these divergent results.

TREATMENT

Lifestyle modification

An essential component of any HTN treatment regimen or HTN prevention strategy is comprehensive lifestyle modification to the greatest degree possible. Dietary sodium intake to ~2 g/day or less, increased dietary potassium and calcium intake, avoidance of obesity, weight loss if already obese, and regular aerobic exercise (if feasible and appropriate) will lower blood pressure. In addition, these lifestyle changes will reduce antihypertensive medication requirements or allow attainment of lower blood pressure levels at any given dose of antihypertensive medication(s). Dietary practices not only vary among racial/ethnic groups, but vary substantially within these same groups along education, income, and geographic strata. Lifestyle modifications will likely vary more than pharmacologic therapeutic choices across ethnic groups due to different dietary preferences and prevailing cultural influences.

Pharmacologic treatment

There are several published HTN guidelines that provide guidance to practitioners regarding evidence-based therapeutic approaches.[103–105] Clearly there are differences in response to antihypertensive drugs by race/ethnicity. Nevertheless, as we[106] and Sehgal[107] have emphasized, the largest source of variation in blood pressure response, for example, to ACE inhibitors is within racial groups not between them. Furthermore, clinical trials showing these same differences have also highlighted that when treated with any single drug, the majority of hypertensives of all races/ethnicities tend to remain above the most conservative JNC 7 systolic blood pressure goal (<140 mmHg). Accordingly, drug therapy with multiple antihypertensive agents will be necessary to control BP. When multiple drugs are used, especially when the regimen contains either a diuretic or a calcium antagonist, racial/ethnic differences in response disappear. Thus, a major recommendation would be to avoid the use of race/ethnicity as the sole, or even major, criterion when selecting antihypertensive drugs. Of course, when a hypertensive patient of any race/ethnicity has an indication for a given antihypertensive drug class, by all means include an agent from that class in the antihypertensive regimen. A good rule of thumb is that when more than two antihypertensive drugs have been prescribed, at least one of them should be a diuretic appropriate to the level of kidney function. And, in some instances, one diuretic will not be enough to combat the expansion of the plasma volume caused by enhanced renal sodium reabsorption from drug-induced expansion of venous capacitance and subsequent fall in blood pressure.

Special considerations

The use of ACE inhibitors has been associated with a several-fold higher risk of angioedema in African Americans than in whites.[108] Nevertheless, until there are more individualized ways to determine who is at risk, it seems prudent to implement heightened vigilance in African Americans regarding angioedema, some of which may present only with cutaneous manifestations.

Most racial/ethnic minorities in the United States have a heightened risk of diabetes mellitus. The overwhelming preponderance of clinical trial data strongly infers that most of the risk reduction attributable to antihypertensive drug therapy is not class-specific. Many hypertensive patients who are racial/ethnic minorities will manifest either impaired fasting glucose or abnormal glucose tolerance. Thiazide diuretics[109] and beta-blockers increase the likelihood of developing diabetes. If diuretics are used, it is highly advisable to block the renin-angiotensin system with either an ACE inhibitor or an ARB to minimize the risk of diuretic-induced hypokalemia and worsening glucose tolerance. Renin-angiotensin system blockade has been shown to attenuate the diuretic-associated risk for diabetes mellitus. Alternatively, anchoring the antihypertensive regimen with a calcium antagonist or perhaps an aldosterone antagonist if kidney function is not depressed, is a reasonable strategy that provides a high likelihood of blood pressure control while avoiding impairment of glucose metabolism. Renin-angiotensin system blockade has been associated with a 14% to 34% reduction in new-onset diabetes.[110] Although the significance of this observation has been questioned, it seems reasonable to consider protection against diabetes as a desirable drug characteristic in diabetes-prone populations.

Treatment status of other cardiovascular risk factors such as dyslipidemia can influence BP responses and the likelihood of HTN control. Statins tend to be used less in African Americans than whites who qualify for treatment. Nevertheless, statins have been repeatedly shown to lower blood pressure.[111] Although only a small portion of these data were generated in African Americans or other racial/ethnic minorities, it seems inconceivable that the blood pressure–lowering effect would be limited to any racial/ethnic group. Accordingly, we have clear and convincing data in our largely African-American hypertensive patient population that statins lower blood pressure in persons with and without diabetes (unpublished observations). There are multiple plausible mechanisms that may explain how statins lower BP.[111] Pharmacologic treatment for diabetes mellitus also influences longitudinal BP levels. Specifically, thiazolidinediones lower BP in persons with diabetes.[112]

SUMMARY

Despite the fact that prevalence, treatment, and control rates vary among race/ethnicity groups, HTN remains a pervasive clinical and public health problem in virtually all groups. There do not appear to be any known risk factors that are unique solely to one race/ethnicity group, although established risk factors contribute variably to HTN risk because, in part, of their variable prevalence. It must be fully understood that the group characteristics or tendencies described in this chapter, including BP responses to antihypertensive agents, represent shifted, but largely overlapping distributions. The promise of molecular genetics is to develop accurate panels of genetic markers that predict risk of pressure-related complications, therapeutic responses to antihypertensive agents, and the likelihood of adverse drug side effects. Thus, use of immutable characteristics to guide therapy for all members of various race/ethnicity groups will occur increasingly less frequently as we identify informative hemodynamic, genetic, and vascular markers that vary at the level of the individual.

REFERENCES

1. Cooper RS, Wolf-Maier K, Luke A, et al. An international comparative study of blood pressure in populations of European vs. African descent. *BMC Med* 2005;3:2.
2. Centers for Disease Control and Prevention. Prevalence of selected cardiovascular disease risk factors among American Indians and Alaska Natives—United States, 1997. *MMWR Morb Mortal Wkly Rep* 2000;49:1.
3. Hughes DL. *Quality of Health Care for Asian-Americans*. New York: The Commonwealth Fund, 2002.
4. Kim MT, Kim KB, Juon HS, Hill MN. Prevalence and factors associated with high blood pressure in Korean Americans. *Ethn Dis* 2000;10:364.
5. Kramer H, Cong H, Post W, et al. Racial/ethnic differences in hypertension and hypertension treatment and control in the Multi-Ethnic Study of Atherosclerosis. *Am J Hypertens* 2004;17:963.
6. DeStefano F, Coulehan JL, Wiant MK et al. Blood pressure survey on the Navajo indian reservation. *Am J Epidemiol* 1979;109:335.
7. Strotz CR, Shorr GI. Hypertension in the Papago Indians. *Circulation* 1973;48:1299.
8. Welch VL, Casper ML, Rith-Nagarajan SJ. Correlates of hypertension among Chippewa and Menominee Indians, the Inter-Tribal Heart Project. *Ethn Dis* 2002;12:398.
9. Howard BV, Lee ET, Yeh JL. Hypertension in adult American Indians: the Strong Heart Study. *Hypertension* 1996;28:256.
10. Crespo CJ, Loria CM, Burt VL. Hypertension and other cardiovascular

disease risk factors among Mexican Americans, Cuban Americans, and Puerto Ricans from the Hispanic Health and Nutrition Examination Survey. *Pub Health Rep* 1996;111(2):7.

11. Hajjar I, Kotchen TA. Trends in prevalence, awareness, treatment, and control of hypertension in the United States, 1988–2000. *JAMA* 2003;290:199.

12. Cushman WC, Ford CE, Cutler JA, et al. Success and predictors of blood pressure control in diverse North American settings: the Antihypertensive and Lipid-Lowering Treatment to Prevent Heart Attack Trial (ALLHAT). *J Clin Hypertens* 2002;4:393.

13. Ogedegbe E, Mancuso CA, Allegrante JP. Expectations of blood pressure management in hypertensive African-American patients: a qualitative study. *J Natl Med Assoc* 2004;96:442.

14. Lau DS, Lee G, Wong CC, et al. Characterization of systemic hypertension in San Francisco Chinese community. *Am J Cardiol* 2005;96:570.

15. Cushman WC, Reda DJ, Perry HM Jr, et al. Department of Veterans Affairs Cooperative Study Group on Antihypertensive Agents. Regional and racial differences in response to antihypertensive medication use in a randomized controlled trial of men with hypertension in the United States. *Arch Intern Med* 2000;160:825.

16. Flegal KM, Carroll MD, Kuczmarski RJ, Johnson CL. Overweight and obesity in the United States: prevalence and trends, 1960–1994. *Int J Obes Relat Metab Disord* 1998;22:39.

17. Hayashi T, Boyko E, Leonetti DL, et al. Visceral adiposity is an independent predictor of incident hypertension in Japanese Americans. *Ann Intern Med* 2004;140:992.

18. Masaki KH, Curb JD, Chiu D, et al. Association of body mass index with blood pressure in elderly Japanese American men. *Hypertension* 1997;29:673.

19. Story M, Stevens J, Himes J, et al. Obesity in American-Indian children: prevalence, consequences, and prevention. *Prev Med* 2003;37(Suppl 1):S3.

20. Gilbert TJ, Percy CA, Sugarman JR, et al. Obesity among Navajo adolescents. Relationship to dietary intake and blood pressure. *Am J Dis Child* 1992;146:285.

21. Crespo CJ, Keteyian SJ, Heath GW, Sempos CT. Leisure-time physical activity among US adults. Results from the Third National Health and Nutrition Examination Survey. *Arch Intern Med* 1996;156:93.

22. Crespo CJ, Smit E, Andersen RE, et al. Race/ethnicity, social class and their relation to physical inactivity during leisure time: results from the Third National Health and Nutrition Examination Survey, 1988–1994. *Am J Prev Med* 2000;18:46.

23. National Center for Health Statistics (NCHS) Faststats. Overweight prevalence data for U.S. for 1999–2002. Available at: http://www.cdc.gov/nchs/faststats/overwt.htm (accessed 1/18/06).

24. Rocchini AP. Obesity hypertension, salt sensitivity and insulin resistance. *Nutr Metab Cardiovasc Dis* 2000;10:287.

25. Hall JE, Henegar JR, Dwyer TM, et al. Is obesity a major cause of chronic kidney disease? *Adv Ren Replace Ther* 2004;11:41.

26. Taler SJ. Treatment of resistant hypertension. *Curr Hypertens Rep* 2005;7:323.

27. Hsu CY, McCulloch CE, Iribarren C, et al. Body mass index and risk for end-stage renal disease. *Ann Intern Med* 2006;144:21.

28. Whelton SP, Chin A, Xin X, He J. Effect of aerobic exercise on blood pressure: a meta-analysis of randomized, controlled trials. *Ann Intern Med* 2002;136:493.

29. Hagberg JM, Montain SJ, Martin WH, Ehsani AA. Effect of exercise training on 60–69 year old persons with essential hypertension. *Am J Cardiol* 1989;64:348.

30. Galetta F, Franzoni F, Plantinga Y, et al. Endothelial function in young subjects with vaso-vagal syncope. *Biomed Pharmacother* 2006 (epub ahead of print).

31. Franzoni F, Ghiadoni L, Galetta F, et al. Physical activity, plasma antioxidant capacity and endothelium-dependent vasodilation in young and older men. *Am J Hypertens* 2005;18:510.

32. Rush JW, Denniss SG, Graham DA. Vascular nitric oxide and oxidative stress: determinants of endothelial adaptations to cardiovascular disease and to physical activity. *Can J Appl Physiol* 2005;30:442.

33. Sriwijitkamol A, Christ-Roberts C, Berria R, et al. Reduced skeletal muscle inhibitor of kappa B content is associated with insulin resistance in subjects with type 2 diabetes: reversal by exercise training. *Diabetes* 2006;55:760.

34. Boddi M, Poggesi L, Coppo M, et al. Human vascular renin-angiotensin system and its functional changes in relation to different sodium intakes. *Hypertension* 1998;31:836.

35. Cubeddu LX, Alfieri AB, Hoffmann IS, et al. Nitric oxide and salt sensitivity. *Am J Hypertens* 2000;13:973.

36. Fang Y, Mu J, He J, Wang S, Liu Z. Salt loading in plasma asymmetrical dimethylarginine and the protective role of potassium supplement in nomortensive salt-sensitive Asians. *Hypertension* 2006; 48:724.

37. Verdecchia P, Schillaci G, Guerrieri M, et al. Circadian blood pressure changes and left ventricular hypertrophy in essential hypertension. *Circulation* 1990;81:528.

38. Bianchi S, Bigazzi R, Baldari G, et al. Diurnal variations of blood pressure and microalbuminuria in essential hypertension. *Am J Hypertens* 1994;7:23.

39. O'Brien E, Sheridan J, O'Malley K. Dippers and non-dippers. *Lancet.* 1988;2:397.

40. Shimada K, Kawamoto A, Matsubayashi K, Ozawa T. Silent cerebrovascular disease in the elderly. Correlation with ambulatory blood pressure. *Hypertension* 1990;16:692.

41. Ingelsson E, Bjorkland-Bodegard K, Lind L, et al. Diurnal blood pressure pattern and risk of congestive heart failure. *JAMA* 2006;295:2859.

42. Farmer CK, Goldsmith DJ, Quin JD, et al. Progression of diabetic nephropathy-is diurnal blood pressure as important as absolute blood pressure level? *Nephrol Dial Transplant* 1998;13:635.

43. Antic V, Van Vliet BN, Montani JP. Loss of nocturnal dipping of blood pressure and heart rate in obesity-induced hypertension in rabbits. *Auton Neurosci* 2001;90:152.

44. Kumari AS. Pregnancy outcomes in women with morbid obesity. *Int J Gynaecol Obstet.* 2001;73:101.

45. Luyckx VA, Brenner BM. Low birth weight, nephron number, and kidney disease. *Kidney Int Suppl* 2005;(97):S68.

46. Nesby-O'Dell S, Scanlon KS, Cogswell ME et al. Hypovitaminosis D prevalence and determinants among African American and white women of reproductive age: third National Health and Nutrition Examination Survey, 1988–1994. *Am J Clin Nutr* 2002;76:187.

47. Yanoff LB, Parikh SJ, Spitalnik A, et al. The prevalence of hypovitaminosis D and secondary hyperparathyroidism in black Americans. *Clin Endocrinol* 2006;64:523.

48. Looker A. Body fat and vitamin D status in black versus white women. *J Clin Endocrinol Metab* 2005;90:635.

49. Liel Y, Ulmer E, Shary J, et al. Low circulating vitamin D in obesity. *Calcif Tissue Int* 1988;43:199.

50. Pfeifer M, Begerow B, Minne HW et al. Effects of a short-term vitamin D(3) and calcium supplementation on blood pressure and parathyroid hormone levels in elderly women. *J Clin Endocrinol Metab* 2001;86:1633.

51. Lind L, Lithell H, Skarfors E, et al. Reduction of blood pressure by treatment with alphacalcidol. A double-blind, placebo-controlled study in subjects with impaired glucose tolerance. *Acta Med Scand* 1988;223:211.

52. Laffer CL, Elijovich F. Essential hypertension of Caribbean Hispanics: sodium, renin, and response to therapy. *J Clin Hypertens (Greenwich)* 2002;4:266.

53. Weir MR, Chrysant SG, McCarron DA, et al. Influence of race and dietary salt on the antihypertensive efficacy of an angiotensin-converting enzyme inhibitor or a calcium channel antagonist in salt-sensitive hypertensives. *Hypertension* 1998;31:1088.

54. Flack JM, Grimm RH Jr, Staffileno BA, et al. New salt-sensitivity metrics: variability-adjusted blood pressure change and the urinary sodium-to-creatinine ratio. *Ethn Dis* 2002;12:10.

55. Rocchini AP, Key J, Bondie D, et al. The effect of weight loss on the sensitivity of blood pressure to sodium in obese adolescents. *N Engl J Med* 1989;321:580.

56. Kopkan L, Majid DS. Superoxide contributes to development of salt sensitivity and hypertension induced by nitric oxide deficiency. *Hypertension* 2005;46:1026.

57. Alvarez G, Osuna A, Wangensteen R, Vargas F. Interaction between nitric oxide and mineralocorticoids in the long-term control of blood pressure. *Hypertension* 2000;35:752.

58. Flack JM, Wiist WH. Epidemiology of hypertension and hypertensive target-organ damage in the United States. *J Assoc Acad Minor Phys* 1991;2:143.

59. Wilson DK, Sica DA, Miller SB. Effects of potassium on blood pressure in salt-sensitive and salt-resistant black adolescents. *Hypertension* 1999;34:181.

60. Coruzzi P, Brambilla L, Brambilla V, et al. Potassium depletion and salt sensitivity in essential hypertension. *J Clin Endocrinol Metab* 2001;86:2857.

61. Peters RM, Flack JM. Salt sensitivity and hypertension in African Americans: implications for cardiovascular nurses. *Prog Cardiovasc Nurs* 2000;15:138.

62. Watson K, Jamerson K. Therapeutic lifestyle changes for hypertension and cardiovascular risk reduction. *J Clin Hypertens (Greenwich)* 2003;5(Suppl 1):32.

63. Aviv A. Cellular calcium and sodium regulation, salt-sensitivity and essential hypertension in African Americans. *Ethn Health* 1996;1:275.

64. Wright JT Jr, Rahman M, Scarpa A, et al. Determinants of salt sensitivity in black and white normotensive and hypertensive women. *Hypertension* 2003;42:1087.

65. Malaga S, Diaz JJ, Arguelles J, et al. Blood pressure relates to sodium taste sensitivity and discrimination in adolescents. *Pediatr Nephrol* 2003;18:431.

66. Hoffman IS, Tavares-Mordwinkin R, Castejon AM, et al. Endothelial nitric oxide synthase polymorphism, nitric oxide production, salt sensitivity and cardiovascular risk factors in Hispanics. *J Hum Hypertens* 2005;19:233.

67. Castejon AM, Alfieri AB, Hoffmann IS, et al. Alpha-adducin polymorphism, salt sensitivity, nitric oxide excretion and cardiovascular risk factors in normotensive Hispanics. *Am J Hypertens* 2003;16:1018.

68. Katsuya T, Ishikawa K, Sugimoto K, et al. Salt sensitivity of Japanese from the viewpoint of gene polymorphism. *Hypertens Res* 2003;26:521.

69. Kato N, Sugiyama T, Nabika T, et al. Lack of association between the alpha-adducin locus and essential hypertension in the Japanese population. *Hypertension* 1998;31:730.

70. Peters RM, Flack JM. Salt sensitivity and hypertension in African Americans: implications for cardiovascular nurses. *Prog Cardiovasc Nurs* 2000;15:138.

71. Sullivan JM, Prewitt RL, Ratts TE. Sodium sensitivity in normotensive and borderline hypertensive humans. *Am J Med Sci* 1988;295:370.

72. Stein CM, Lang CC, Nelson R, et al. Vasodilation in black Americans: attenuated nitric oxide-mediated responses. *Clin Pharmacol Ther* 1997;62:436.

73. Houghton JL, Philbin EF, Strogatz DS, et al. The presence of African American race predicts improvement in coronary endothelial function after supplementary L-arginine. *J Am Coll Cardiol* 2002;39:1314.

74. Malinski T. Understanding nitric oxide physiology in the heart: a nanomedical approach. *Am J Cardiol* 2005;96(suppl):13i.

75. Pulerwitz T, Graham-Clarke C, Rodriguez CJ, et al. Association of increased body mass index and impaired endothelial function among Hispanic women. *Am J Cardiol* 2006;97:68.

76. Stewart KJ, Sung J, Hilber HA, et al. Exaggerated exercise blood pressure is related to impaired endothelial vasodilator function. *Am J Hypertens* 2004;17:314.

77. Steffen PR, Smith TB, Larson M, Butler L. Acculturation to Western society as a risk factor for high blood pressure: a meta-analytic review. *Psychosom Med* 2006;68:386.

78. Vale S. Psychosocial stress and cardiovascular diseases. *Postgrad Med J* 2005;81:429.

79. Bierhaus A, Humpert PM, Nawroth PP. NF-kappaB as a molecular link between psychosocial stress and organ dysfunction. *Pediatr Nephrol* 2004;19:189.

80. Padgett DA, Glaser R. How stress influences the immune response. *Trends Immunol* 2003;24:444.

81. Lemarie CA, Esposito B, Tedqui A, Lehoux S. Pressure-induced vascular activation of nuclear factor-kappaB: role in cell survival. *Circ Res* 2003;93:207.

82. Wright JT Jr, Dunn JK, Cutler JA, et al. ALLHAT Collaborative Research Group. Outcomes in hypertensive black and nonblack patients treated with chlorthalidone, amlodipine, and lisinopril. *JAMA* 2005;293:1595.

83. Dell'Omo G, Penno G, Giorgi D, et al. Association between high-normal albuminuria and risk factors for cardiovascular and renal disease in essential hypertensive men. *Am J Kidney Dis* 2002;40:1.

84. Duncan K, Ramappa P, Thornburg R, et al. The influence of urinary albumin excretion and estimated glomerular filtration rate on blood pressure response in drug-treated hypertensive patients in an academic hypertension clinic. *Am J Hypertens* 2001;14:493.

85. Weir MR. Diabetes and hypertension: blood pressure control and consequences. *Am J Hyperetens* 1999;12:170S.

86. Bakris GL. Microalbuminuria: what is it? Why is it important? What should be done about it? *J Clin Hypertens (Greenwich)* 2001;3:99.

87. Mattix HJ, Hsu C, Shaykevich S, Curhan G. Use of the albumin/creatinine ratio to detect microalbuminuria: implications of sex and race. *J Am Soc Nephrol* 2002;13:1034.

88. Xu C, Zarins CK, Pannaraj PS, et al. Hypercholesterolemia superimposed by experimental hypertension induces differential distribution of collagen and elastin. *Arterioscler Thromb Vasc Biol* 2000;20:2566.

89. Lee A, Cerami A. Role of glycation in aging. *Ann N Y Acad Sci* 1992;663:63.

90. Taddei S, Virdis A, Ghiadoni L, et al. Age-related reduction of NO availability and oxidative stress in humans. *Hypertension* 2001;38:274.

91. Jamerson K. The impact of ethnicity on response to antihypertensive therapy. *Am J Med* 1996;101(Suppl. 3A):22S.

92. American Heart Association. *2002 Heart and Stroke Statistical Update.* Dallas, TX: American Heart Association, 2001.

93. White H, Boden-Albala B, Wang C, et al. Ischemic stroke subtype incidence among whites, blacks, and Hispanics. The Northern Manhattan Study. *Circulation* 2005;111:1327.

94. Henderson SO, Phillip B, Henderson BE, Stram DO. Risk factors for cardiovascular and cerebrovascular death among African Americans and Hispanics in Los Angeles, California. *Acad Emerg Med* 2001;8:1163.

95. Mensah GA, Mokdad AH, Ford ES, et al. State of disparities in cardiovascular health in the United States. *Circulation* 2005;111:1233.

96. Fang J, Foo SH, Jeng JS, et al. Clinical characteristics among Chinese in New York City. *Ethn Dis* 2004;14:58.

97. Mau MK, West M, Sugihara J, et al. Renal disease disparities in Asian and Pacific-based population in Hawaii. *J Natl Med Assoc* 2003;95:955.

98. Wright JT Jr, Bakris G, Greene T, et al. African American Study of Kidney Disease and Hypertension Study Group. Effect of blood pressure lowering and antihypertensive drug class on progression of hypertensive kidney disease: results from the AASK trial. *JAMA* 200220;288:2421.

99. ALLHAT Collaborative Research Group. Major cardiovascular events in hypertensive patients randomized to doxazosin vs chlorthalidone: the antihypertensive and lipid-lowering treatment to prevent heart attack trial (ALLHAT). *JAMA* 2000;283:1967.

100. Wright JT Jr, Dunn JK, Cutler JA, et al. ALLHAT Collaborative Research Group. Outcomes in hypertensive black and nonblack patients treated with chlorthalidone, amlodipine, and lisinopril. *JAMA* 2005;293:1595.

101. Cooper-DeHoff RM, Aranda JM, Gaxiola E, et al. Blood pressure control and cardiovascular outcomes in high-risk Hispanic patients—findings from the International Verapamil SR/Trandolapril Study (INVEST). *Am Heart J* 2006;151:1072.

102. Kjeldsen SE, Dahlof B, Devereux RB, et al. Effects of losartan on cardiovascular morbidity and mortality in patients with isolated systolic hypertension and left ventricular hypertrophy: a Losartan Intervention for Endpoint Reduction (LIFE) substudy. *JAMA* 2002;288:1491.

103. Douglas JG, Bakris GL, Epstein M, et al. Management of high blood pressure in African Americans: consensus statement of the Hypertension in African Americans Working Group of the International Society on Hypertension in Blacks. *Arch Intern Med* 2003;163:525.

104. K/DOQI clinical practice guidelines on hypertension and antihypertensive agents in chronic kidney disease. Kidney Disease Outcomes Quality Initiative (K/DOQI). *Am J Kidney Dis* 2004;43(Suppl 1):S1.

105. Chobanian AV, Bakris GL, Black HR, Cushman, et al. The Seventh Report of the Joint National Committee on Prevention, Detection, Evaluation, and Treatment of High Blood Pressure: the JNC 7 report. *JAMA* 2003;289:2560–72.

106. Mowke E, Ohmit SE, Nasser SA, et al. Determinants of blood pressure response to quinapril in black and

white hypertensive patients: the Quinapril Titration Interval Management Evaluation trial. *Hypertension* 2004;43:1202.

107. Sehgal AR. Overlap between whites and blacks in response to antihypertensive drugs. *Hypertension* 2004;43:566.

108. Brown NJ, Ray WA, Snowden M, Griffin MR. Black Americans have an increased rate of angiotensin converting enzyme inhibitor-associated angioedema. *Clin Pharmacol Ther* 1996;60:8.

109. Zillich AJ, Garg J, Basu S, et al. Thiazide diuretics, potassium, and the development of diabetes: a quantitative review. *Hypertension* 2006;48:219.

110. Scheen AJ. Prevention of type 2 diabetes mellitus through inhibition of the renin-angiotensin system. *Drugs* 2004;64:2537.

111. Milionis HJ, Liberopoulos EN, Achimastos A, et al. Statins: another class of antihypertensive agents? *J Hum Hypertens* 2006;20:320.

112. Sarafidis PA, Nilsson PM. The effects of thiazolidinediones on blood pressure levels—a systematic review. *Blood Press* 2006;15:135.

Chapter

58 Hyperadrenergic and Labile Hypertension

Guido Grassi and Giuseppe Mancia

Definition

- The clinical condition, also called neurogenic, juvenile, labile, or borderline hypertension, is characterized by transient blood pressure elevation (and signs or symptoms of an adrenergic cardiovascular overdrive) that with time may become a stable hypertensive state.

Key Findings

- Frequently found in young subjects (40% of cases).
- Associated with resting tachycardia, palpitations, and generalized swelling.
- Not rarely associated with end-organ damage (cardiac, vascular, and/or renal).
- In some cases a differential diagnosis with pheochromocytoma may be required.

Clinical Implications

- Blood pressure monitoring, lifestyle measures, and correction of risk factors should be the cornerstones of therapeutic intervention, if cardiovascular risk profile is low.
- In the presence of stable blood pressure elevation or concomitant risk factors (smoking, overweight, or obesity), end-organ damage, diabetes or associated clinical conditions, a pharmacologic intervention is required.
- If cardiovascular risk profile is high or very high, pharmacologic treatment is necessary even when blood pressure is in the high-normal range.
- Antihypertensive compounds that actively interfere with the sympathetic nervous system (β-blockers, angiotensin-converting enzyme inhibitors, and angiotensin-II receptor blockers) should be the drugs of first choice.

The concept that sympathetic neural factors favor the development of transient blood pressure elevations that with time may progress to stable hypertensive forms dates back almost four decades.[1] Since then, however, some aspects concerning the definition of this clinical condition have been refined with the introduction of terms such as "juvenile hypertension," "hyperkinetic hypertension," and "borderline hypertension." All these definitions share at least three common features. First, is the fact that the occurrence of this clinical entity is prevalent in the young. Second, the evidence shows that at least in the earlier phases of the disease the abnormal blood pressure elevation can be intermittently detected over days, weeks, or months of observation. Third, based on clinical findings, this hypertensive state is usually associated with signs or symptoms suggestive of an activation of the sympathetic nervous system (SNS).

PATHOPHYSIOLOGY

The background for the hypothesis that abnormalities in sympathetic cardiovascular control may trigger transient elevations in blood pressure that with time may become stable hypertensive states is based on two main notions. First is the knowledge that the SNS exerts a pivotal role in blood pressure control by regulating cardiac output and peripheral vascular resistance. Second is the evidence that increases in cardiac output and elevation in peripheral vascular resistance represent fundamental hemodynamic features of this clinical condition.

Both notions stimulated studies designed to determine the SNS role in the pathogenesis of hypertension. In the following, I briefly review the evidence on this issue, as well as on the participation of the neuroadrenergic mechanisms at the development and progression of the target-organ damage that is frequently associated with the hypertensive state.

Sympathetic activation in early hypertensive phases: Indirect evidence

The early stages of hypertension are often characterized by a hyperkinetic circulation, that is, by an increase in cardiac output with a concomitant resting tachycardia. These findings, originally reported in the late 1950s,[1-2] have been confirmed by cross-sectional and longitudinal studies. For example, Brod et al.[3] demonstrated that early stages of human hypertension are characterized by an exaggerated hemodynamic response to mental stress that may mimic the so-called "defense reaction" described in experimental animals. Interestingly, in a longitudinal study the abnormal pressor responses to adrenergic stimuli have been associated with the future development of hypertension, a finding that for the first time has allowed researchers to link hyperactivity of the SNS to the occurrence of the high blood-pressure state.[4] This concept has been further strengthened by the observation, originally reported in 1945 and recently reproposed,[5,6] that a resting tachycardia (and thus an increase in cardiac sympathetic drive) may represent a marker of the future development of hypertension.

A further step forward in our understanding of the prohypertensive role of the SNS comes from a study by

Julius et al. showing that a consistent fraction (about 30% to 40%) of borderline hypertensive patients are characterized by an elevated cardiac output, a resting tachycardia, and elevated circulating levels of the main adrenergic neurotransmitter (i.e., norepinephrine) (Figure 58–1).[7] This finding, coupled with the evidence that the abovementioned hemodynamic abnormalities of border-line or juvenile hypertension are reversed by pharmacologic blockade of cardiac beta adrenergic receptors,[7] has strengthened the hypothesis that adrenergic neural factors are involved in the pathogenesis of the hyperkinetic state. Recently, this hypothesis has been confirmed by the evidence that blood pressure variability, that is, the blood pressure oscillations occurring during the daytime and nighttime periods and closely related to adrenergic drive,[8] are increased in young hypertensive patients as compared to normotensive ones.[9]

Sympathetic activation in early hypertension: Direct evidence

Interesting additional data on the neurogenic forms of hypertension have emerged through two approaches allowing direct assessment of sympathetic activity, that is, the intravenous tracer infusion of small doses of radiolabeled norepinephrine,[10] and the microneurographic recording of efferent postganglionic sympathetic nerve traffic.[10] By employing the first technique, it has been possible to demonstrate that the increased plasma norepinephrine levels characterizing young hyperadrenergic forms of hypertension depend on an increased norepinephrine release (norepinephrine spillover)[11] from adrenergic nerve terminals rather than on a reduced tissue clearance. This approach has also demonstrated that the hyperadrenergic state in labile hypertensive patients is particularly manifest at the level of the kidney and the heart, which are two organs of importance for blood pressure control (Figure 58–2).[11]

Direct measurement of efferent postganglionic sympathetic nerve traffic to the skeletal muscle district have further confirmed the abovementioned findings, by showing that patients with a borderline elevation in blood pressure display elevated central sympathetic neural outflow.[12] The finding that high blood pressure is characterized by a sympathetic overdrive has been confirmed throughout the years in mild and more severe stages of the disease,[13] and recently, has been found to characterize white-coat hypertension, that is, the clinical condition characterized by elevated office blood pressure values and by normal 24-hour ambulatory blood pressure profile.[14,15]

Mechanisms of sympathetic activation

Despite years of investigation, the origin of sympathetic activation in essential hypertension remains largely unknown. Several mechanistic hypotheses have been advanced (Figure 58–3). An attractive hypothesis, for example, is that this activation occurs because of an excessive number of, and/or reactivity to, stressful environmental stimuli that lead, through frequent transient blood pressure elevations, to a permanently hypertensive state. To date, however, this hypothesis has been confirmed only in animal studies, with controversial or circumstantial support in humans.[16]

Another attractive hypothesis (not exclusive of the previous one) is that the sympathetic activation originates from an impairment of the baroreflex, that is, of a main restraining mechanism of the sympathetic tone. This is supported by evidence that in congestive heart failure and other diseases, a sympathetic nerve traffic increase is related to reduced modulation of adrenergic tone by the baroreflex.[17] However, in hypertension, baroreflex impairment has been demonstrated for the heart rate, but not for the blood pressure component of the reflex.[18,19] Furthermore, recent findings by our group have shown that baroreceptor deactivation and stimulation by vasoactive drug-induced changes in blood pressure can affect sympathetic nerve traffic so that it remains unchanged as compared to normotension, at variance from the reduction in the heart rate alterations.[13]

Thus, the available evidence does not support the baroreflex as the origin of the sympathetic activation. These data, however, do not rule out the possibility that reflex cardiovascular regulation may contribute to this phenomenon. First, although unimpaired, the baroreflex is reset toward elevated blood pressure values in hypertension, which means that its influence preserves rather than suppresses the increased sympathetic drive. Second, the sympathoinhibitory influence of cardiac receptors is impaired in essential hypertension,

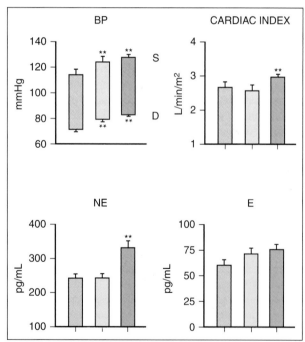

Figure 58–1. Blood pressure (BP), cardiac index, and plasma norepinephrine (NE) and epinephrine (E) values in normotensive subjects (gold bars), and in hypertensive patients without (green bars) and with (purple bars) hyperkinetic circulation. Note that only in the hyperkinetic hypertensive-state cardiac index and plasma norepinephrine are elevated. Asterisks refer to the statistical significance between groups. Values are shown as mean ± standard error of the mean. (Modified from Julius S, Conway J. Hemodynamic studies in patients with borderline blood pressure elevation. *Circulation* 1968;38:282–88.)

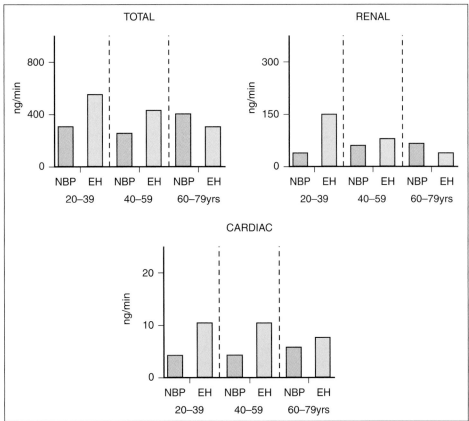

Figure 58–2. Systemic, renal, and cardiac norepinephrine spillover from adrenergic nerve terminals in young, middle-aged, and elderly normotensive (NBP) and hypertensive (EH) subjects. Only young hypertensive subjects display an increase in total, renal, and cardiac norepinephrine spillover, indicating the occurrence of systemic and regional sympathetic activation. (Modified from Esler M, Lambert G, Jennings G. Regional norepinephrine turnover in human hypertension. *Clin Exp Hypertens A* 1989;11(Suppl 1):75–89.)

although only when accompanied by left ventricular hypertrophy.[20] Thus, reflex mechanisms contribute to the sympathetic activation occurring in hypertension, although their effects appear to be late and nonspecific.

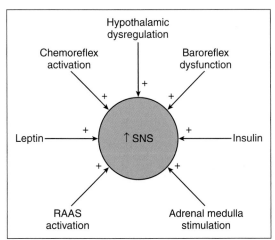

Figure 58–3. Scheme illustrating the possible mechanisms involved in activation of the sympathetic nervous system (↑SNS) in hypertension. RAAS, renin-angiotensin system.

A further hypothesis, which has been advanced in recent years, claims that the sympathetic activation seen in hypertension depends on a metabolic alteration (i.e., hyperinsulinemia and related insulin resistance) accompanying the hypertensive condition. This hypothesis comes from the evidence that in experimental animals and in humans acute infusions of insulin, without altering glycemic levels (the so-called euglycemic clamp infusion technique), markedly stimulate the SNS.[21,22] This finding is of particular relevance when one takes into account that a large proportion of hypertensive patients (>40%) display elevated insulin levels and an insulin-resistance state. This means that hyperinsulinemia and related insulin resistance may represent one of the mechanisms responsible for the sympathetic activation that characterizes essential hypertension, particularly in its earlier clinical phases. However, this effect is reciprocal, namely, that a state of sympathetic activation may cause insulin resistance as well.[23,24] A recent study performed in a large number of normotensive and hypertensive subjects, prospectively followed for a 10-year period,[25] indicates that sympathetic activation appears to precede the development of the hyperinsulinemic state and blood pressure elevation, a finding which supports the concept that the insulin-resistance state is a consequence rather than a cause of the adrenergic overactivity (Figure 58–4).

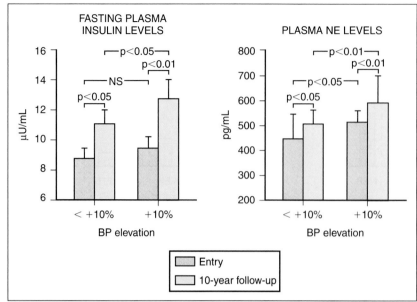

FASTING PLASMA
INSULIN LEVELS

PLASMA NE LEVELS

Figure 58–4. Values of fasting plasma insulin and plasma norepinephrine (NE) in subjects followed for a 10-year period in which blood pressure (BP) increased less or more than 10% of the baseline values. Note that subjects who will develop hypertension were characterized at baseline by elevated plasma norepinephrine but normal insulin values. Data are shown as mean ± standard error of the mean. (Modified from Masuo K, Mikami H, Ogihara T, Tuck ML. Sympathetic nerve hyperactivity precedes hyperinsulinemia and blood pressure elevation in a young, nonobese Japanese population. *Am J Hypertens* 1997;10:77–83.)

Cardiac and vascular consequences of sympathetic activation

A number of adverse cardiovascular effects have been reported to take place in experimental and clinical conditions characterized by a blood pressure elevation and an increase in sympathetic cardiovascular influence (Figure 58–5). For example, a direct pro-oscillatory effect of a hyperadrenergic

state on blood pressure profile and variability has been shown to be involved in the pathophysiology of major cardiovascular events as well as of the end-organ damage associated to high blood pressure. Evidence has been indeed provided that morning blood pressure rise is associated with a frequency of cardiac and cerebral ischemic episodes and with the occurrence of sudden death more closely than blood pressure values observed at other times of the day and night.[26] It has also been shown that the frequency of blood pressure peaks over a 24-hour period is significantly associated with the occurrence of left ventricular dysfunction.[27] Second, the increase in blood pressure during emotional stress at work or during physical exercise is more closely associated with the degree of left ventricular mass increase than resting or clinic blood pressure.[28] Third, the degree of blood pressure reduction during the night is inversely related to left ventricular mass.[29]

Although cross-sectional and indirect, these data support the notion that sympathetic neural factors may affect the cardiovascular system by increasing blood pressure variability. Other data, however, support the concept that a sympathetic activation may promote end-organ damage through more direct mechanisms. In the experimental setting this has been shown to occur for left ventricular hypertrophy, which can be promoted by infusion of suppressor doses of adrenergic

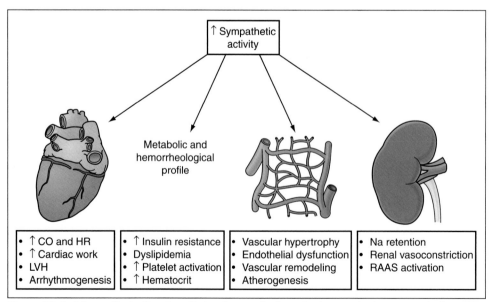

Figure 58–5. Scheme illustrating the effects of sympathetic activation on the heart, metabolic and hemorrheologic profile, and vascular and renal function. CO, cardiac output; HR, heart rate; LVH, left ventricular hypertrophy; RAAS, renin-angiotensin system.

agents (Figure 58–6) and prevented only if a blood pressure reduction is not accompanied by excessive reflex sympathetic stimulation.[30] It has also been shown to occur for arteriolar wall hypertrophy or remodeling, a structural vascular abnormality found at an early stage of hypertension.[31]

The involvement of adrenergic neural mechanisms in the hypertension-related vascular alterations is not limited, however, to development of structural changes of the vessel wall. Studies performed in recent years have indeed shown arterial distensibility to be also importantly modulated by sympathetic influences. Removal of adrenergic tone through anesthesia of the brachial plexus or the low spinal cord is accompanied by a marked increase in radial and femoral artery distensibility, respec-

tively (Figure 58–7).[32] Femoral artery distensibility also increases in patients with peripheral artery disease who have undergone lumbar sympathectomy.[32] This response may originate from abolition of smooth muscle contraction within the arterial wall, because the contracted vascular smooth muscle has an elastic modulus greater than the relaxed one. Such a response leads to the conclusion that sympathetic influences (as well as presumably other influences increasing vascular smooth muscle contraction, such as those elicited by angiotensin II and endothelin) may have a stiffening influence on arterial mechanical properties, particularly in vessels with muscular structure. This stiffening influence, however, may also involve large elastic arteries, because these arteries display smooth muscle tissue and sympathetic efferent innervation.

Functional modulation of arterial distensibility includes another variable that again is predominantly modulated by autonomic factors and, among them, by sympathetic cardiac drive, that is, heart rate.[33] In experimental animal models, a progressive increase in heart rate by pacing is accompanied by a progressive reduction of carotid artery distensibility.[34] This is the case in humans as well because in subjects with an implanted pacemaker, an increase in resting heart rate is accompanied by a reduction in carotid and radial artery distensibility.[34]

Finally, the importance of sympathetic neural factors in arrythmogenesis has been repeatedly confirmed, with the evidence that stimulation of cardiac sympathetic outflow reduces the myocardial arrythmogenic threshold and favors the development of

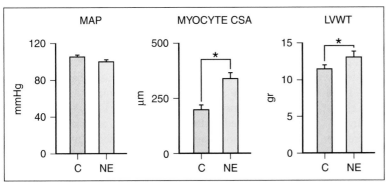

Figure 58–6. Effects of chronic administration of subpressor doses of norepinephrine (NE) on mean arterial pressure (MAP), myocyte cross-sectional area (CSA), and left ventricular wall thickness (LVWT) in experimental animals. Data are shown as mean ± SEM. Asterisks refer to the statistical significance with control values (C). (Modified from Sen S, Trazi RC, Khairallah P, Bumpus M. Cardiac hypertrophy in spontaneously hypertensive rats. *Circ Res* 1974;35:775–781.)

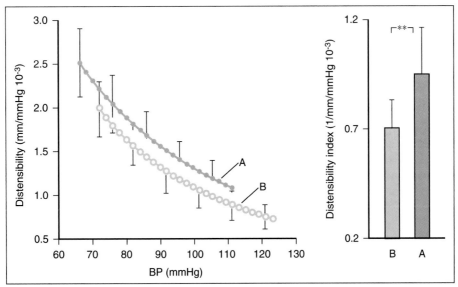

Figure 58–7. Effects of brachial plexus anesthesia on radial artery distensibility in humans. Note that removal of sympathetic vasoconstrictor influences on radial artery increase the vessel distensibility. B, control; A, after brachial plexus anesthesia; BP, blood pressure. Data are shown as mean ± SEM. (Modified from Failla M, Grappiolo A, Emanuelli G, et al. Sympathetic tone restrains arterial distensibility of healthy and atherosclerotic subjects. *J Hypertens* 1999;17:1117–23.)

ventricular tachycardia and fibrillation.[35] These effects may explain why sympathetic activation and mortality rate are closely and directly related to each other at least in congestive heart failure and in end-stage renal disease.[36,37] In the case of hypertension, the proarrythmogenic effects of the cardiac adrenergic overdrive appear to be potentiated by the presence of left ventricular hypertrophy and myocardial ischemia.

CLINICAL PRESENTATION AND DIAGNOSIS

The elevation in blood pressure values, particularly when as mild as occurs in labile or borderline hypertension, is usually a symptomless condition. In some instances, however, the clinical picture is characterized by manifestations related to a generalized adrenergic activation, such as tachycardia or palpitations at rest, anxiety, and excess sweating. Headache is generally of mild to moderate degree and frequently with a frontal or an occipital location.

The diagnosis is based on the presence of a blood pressure elevation, which is transient in nature and frequently associated with normal blood pressure values. With time, however, the periods characterized by blood pressure elevation become more frequent and a stable form of hypertension may subsequently develop. According to recent guidelines for the management of hypertension, jointly issued by the European Society of Hypertension and the European Society of Cardiology,[38] a close monitoring of blood pressure values is recommended in these clinical phases, particularly with the use of home and/or ambulatory blood pressure monitoring in order to avoid the occurrence of a blood pressure elevation due to the white-coat effect.[14]

In order to determine the cardiovascular risk profile of the patient, that is, a parameter representing the main indication for the therapeutic intervention (see below),[38] along with routine laboratory examinations (blood chemistry tests, urinanalysis, electrocardiogram), a number of recommended tests should be performed. These should include ultrasound examination of the heart, with particular focus on evaluation of left ventricular wall thickness, left ventricular end-diastolic diameter, and calculation of left

ventricular mass index; ultrasound investigation of the carotid arteries with the assessment of the intima-media complex thickness and detection of plaques; and finally, evaluation of renal function based on determination of serum creatinine, creatinine clearance and microalbuminuria. In some rare cases (particularly in young subjects without a family history of hypertension), the clinical picture may lead clinicians to suspect an adrenal or extradrenal pheochromocytoma. The differential diagnosis is based on the determination of catecholamines (norepinephrine and epinephrine) as well as of metanorepinephrine in several 24-hour urine samples as well as in venous blood. In most patients with pheochromocytoma, the urinary excretion of catecholamines as well as their plasma levels are so high (at least twice the normal values) as to avoid the need for complex further examinations (pharmacologic stress testing MRI examination of adrenal glands, metaiodiobenzylguanidine, or computer tomographic scans).[39]

THERAPEUTIC IMPLICATIONS

Based on the data discussed thus far, sympathoinhibition appears to be a key goal of the therapeutic approach to labile hypertension. Nonpharmacologic lifestyle interventions commonly used in clinical practice and capable of improving both the hemodynamic and the metabolic profile, such as energy-restricted diet or physical training, have been clearly shown to exert sympathoinhibitory effects.[40–42] Both these interventions are of particular relevance in the early phases of hypertension, given the evidence that frequently the patients display an overweight or a frank obese state of the central type. Interestingly, this sympathetic deactivation triggered by the two abovementioned nonpharmacologic approaches is usually paralleled by a clear-cut improvement in insulin sensitivity whose alteration represents a common hallmark of obesity.

Sympathetic deactivation should also be one of the goals of pharmacologic interventions based on the use of antihypertensive drugs (Boxes 58–1 and 58–2).[42] While diuretics appear to be clearly contraindicated due to their inability to counteract the sympathetic overactivity (and to their unfavorable effects on metabolic profile), beta-blockers (particularly those with vasodilating properties) are recommended in order to reduce the adrenergic overdrive to the heart and peripheral circulation. Other preferred antihypertensive drugs in the treatment of the disease appear

---

Box 58–1

Drugs Acting on Sympathetic Nervous System

- Ganglionic blockers
- Peripheral sympatholytics
- Alpha-1-blockers
- Alpha-beta blockers
- Beta blockers
- Central agents: imidazoline receptor agonists
- Angiotensin-converting enzyme inhibitors
- Angiotensin II–receptor antagonists

Box 58–2

Favorable Effects of Antihypertensive Drug-Induced Sympathoinhibition

$\downarrow$ in heart rate and myocardial oxygen demand
$\downarrow$ in blood pressure variability
$\uparrow$ in insulin sensitivity
$\uparrow$ in trough-to-peak ratio (measure of homogeneity of the antihypertensive effect of a given drug)
$\uparrow$ organ protection and organ damage regression

to be ACE inhibitors and angiotensin II antagonists.[42] These drugs are (1) effective in ensuring a blood pressure control over a 24-hour period, (2) lipid neutral, (3) capable of improving insulin sensitivity, and (4) exert sympathoinhibitory effects. Also, the new calcium channel blockers, such as cilnidipine and barnidipine, may exert inhibitory effects on adrenergic function,[43] unlike "classic" compounds, and the new central sympatholitic agents, such as imidazoline I_1 receptor agonists may trigger favorable metabolic and sympathoinhibitory effects.[44]

SUMMARY

Neurogenic or labile hypertension represents a clinical condition that requires careful examination and follow-up, given the evidence that it may be associated with end-organ damage and cardiovascular complications. The neuroadrenergic nature of the disease underlines the clinical usefulness of drugs capable of counteracting the sympathetic overdrive.

REFERENCES

1. Widinsky J, Fejfarova MD, Feifar Z. Changes of cardiac output in hypertension disease. *Cardiologia* 1957;31:381–389.
2. Widimsky K, Fejfarova MD, Feifar Z. High blood pressure in youth (in German). *Arch Kreislaufforschung* 1958;28:100–124.
3. Brod J, Fencl V, Hejl Z, Jyrka I. Circulatory changes underlying blood pressure elevation during acute emotional stress (mental arithmetic) in normotensive and hypertensive subjects. *Clin Sci* 1959;18:269–279.
4. Matthews KA, Woodall KL, Allen MT. Cardiovascular reactivity to stress predicts future blood pressure status. *Hypertension* 1993;22:479–85.
5. Levy RL, White PD, Stroud WD, Hillan CC. Transient tachycardia: prognostic significance alone and in association with transient hypertension. *JAMA* 1945;129:585–588.
6. Palatini P, Casiglia E, Pauletto P, et al. Relationship of tachycardia with high blood pressure and metabolic abnormalities: a study with mixture analysis in three populations. *Hypertension* 1997;30:1267–73.
7. Julius S, Conway J. Hemodynamic studies in patients with borderline blood pressure elevation. *Circulation* 1968;38:282–288.
8. Mancia G, Grassi G. Mechanisms and clinical implications of blood pressure variability. *J Cardiovasc Pharmacol* 2000;35:S15–9.
9. Mancia G. Ambulatory blood pressure monitoring: research and clinical applications. *J Hypertens Suppl* 1990;8:S1–13.
10. Grassi G, Esler M. How to assess sympathetic activity in humans. *J Hypertens* 1999;17:719–34.
11. Esler M, Lambert G, Jennings G. Regional norepinephrine turnover in human hypertension. *Clin Exp Hypertens A* 1989;11 Suppl 1:75–89.
12. Anderson EA, Sinkey CA, Lawton WJ, Mark AL. Elevated sympathetic nerve activity in borderline hypertensive humans. Evidence from direct intraneural recordings. *Hypertension* 1989;14:177–83.
13. Grassi G, Cattaneo BM, Seravalle G, et al. Baroreflex control of sympathetic nerve activity in essential and secondary hypertension. *Hypertension* 1998;3:68–72.
14. Grassi G, Turri C, Vailati S, et al. Muscle and skin sympathetic nerve

traffic during the "white-coat" effect. *Circulation* 1999;100:222–5.
15. Smith PA, Graham LN, Mackintosh AF, et al. Sympathetic neural mechanisms in white-coat hypertension. *J Am Coll Cardiol* 2002;40:126–32.
16. Folkow B. Physiological aspects of primary hypertension. *Physiol Rev* 1982;62:347–504.
17. Grassi G, Seravalle G, Cattaneo BM, et al. Sympathetic activation and loss of reflex sympathetic control in mild congestive heart failure. *Circulation* 1995;92:3206–11.
18. Mancia G, Grassi G, Ferrari AU. Reflex control of the circulation in experimental and human hypertension. In: Zanchetti A, Mancia G, eds. *Handbook of Hypertension*. Vol. 17. *Pathophysiology of Hypertension*. Amsterdam: Elsevier Science, 1997:586–601.
19. Mancia G, Ludbrook J, Ferrari A, et al. Baroreceptor reflexes in human hypertension. *Circ Res* 1978;43:170–7.
20. Grassi G, Giannattasio C, Cleroux J, et al. Cardiopulmonary reflex before and after regression of left ventricular hypertrophy in essential hypertension. *Hypertension* 1988;12:227–37.
21. Rowe JW, Young JB, Minaker KL, et al. Effect of insulin and glucose infusions on sympathetic nervous system activity in normal man. *Diabetes* 1981;30:219–25.
22. Anderson EA, Hoffman RP, Balon TW, et al. Hyperinsulinemia produces both sympathetic neural activation and vasodilation in normal humans. *J Clin Invest* 1991;87:2246–52.
23. Jamerson KA, Julius S, Gudbrandsson T, et al. Reflex sympathetic activation induces acute insulin resistance in the human forearm. *Hypertension* 1993;21:618–23.
24. Lembo G, Capaldo B, Rendina V, et al. Acute noradrenergic activation induces insulin resistance in human skeletal muscle. *Am J Physiol* 1994;266:E242–47.
25. Masuo K, Mikami H, Ogihara T, Tuck ML. Sympathetic nerve hyperactivity precedes hyperinsulinemia and blood pressure elevation in a young, nonobese Japanese population. *Am J Hypertens* 1997;10:77–83.
26. Rocco MB, Nabel EG, Selwyn AP. Circadian rhythms and coronary artery disease. *Am J Cardiol* 1987;59:13C–17C.
27. White WS, Dey HM, Sculman P. Assessment of the daily blood pressure

load as a determinant of cardiac function in patients with mild to moderate hypertension. *Am Heart J* 1989;118:782–95.
28. Devereux R, Pickering TG, Harshfiled GA, et al. Left ventricular hypertrophy in patients with hypertension: importance of blood pressure response to regularly recurring stress. *Circulation* 1983;68:470–76.
29. Verdecchia P, Schillaci G, Gatteschi C, et al. Blunted nocturnal fall in blood pressure in hypertensive women with future cardiovascular morbid events. *Circulation* 1993;88:986–92.
30. Sen S, Trazi RC, Khairallah P, Bumpus M. Cardiac hypertrophy in spontaneously hypertensive rats. *Circ Res* 1974;35:775–81.
31. Heagerty AM. Structural changes in resistance arteries in hypertension. In: Zanchetti A, Mancia G, eds. *Handbook of Hypertension*. Vol. 17. *Pathophysiology of Hypertension*. Amsterdam: Elsevier Science, 1997:426–37.
32. Failla M, Grappiolo A, Emanuelli G, et al. Sympathetic tone restrains arterial distensibility of healthy and atherosclerotic subjects. *J Hypertens* 1999;17:1117–23.
33. Mircoli L, Mangoni AA, Giannattasio C, et al. Heart rate-dependent stiffening of large arteries in intact and sympathectomized rats. *Hypertension* 1999;34:598–602.
34. Giannattasio C, Vincenti A, Failla M, et al. Effects of heart rate changes on arterial distensibility in humans. *Hypertension* 2003;42:253–56.
35. Meredith IT, Broughton A, Jennings GL, Esler MD. Evidence of a selective increase in cardiac sympathetic activity in patients with sustained ventricular arrhythmias. *N Engl J Med* 1991; 325:618–24.
36. Cohn JN, Levine TB, Olivari MT, et al. Plasma norepinephrine as a guide to prognosis in patients with chronic congestive heart failure. *N Engl J Med* 1984;31:819–23.
37. Zoccali C, Mallamaci F, Parlongo S, et al. Plasma norepinephrine predicts survival and incident cardiovascular events in patients with end-stage renal disease. *Circulation* 2002;105:1354–59.
38. 2003 European Society of Hypertension - European Society of Cardiology Guidelines for the management of arterial hypertension. Guidelines Committee. *J Hypertens* 2003;21:1011–53.

39. Bravo EL, Tagle R. Pheochromocytoma: state-of-the-art and future prospects. *Endocr Rev* 2003;24:539–53.

40. Grassi G, Seravalle G, Colombo M, et al. Body weight reduction, sympathetic nerve traffic, and arterial baroreflex in obese normotensive humans. *Circulation* 1998;97:2037–42.

41. Grassi G, Seravalle G, Calhoun DA, Mancia G. Physical training and baroreceptor control of sympathetic nerve activity in humans. *Hypertension* 1994;23:294–301.

42. Grassi G. Counteracting the sympathetic nervous system in essential hypertension. *Curr Opin Nephrol Hypertens* 2004;13:513–19.

43. Grassi G. Neuroadrenergic effects of calcium channel blockers: a developing concept. *J Hypertens* 2004;22:887–88.

44. van Zwieten PA. Centrally acting imidazoline I1-receptor agonists: do they have a place in the management of hypertension? *Am J Cardiovasc Drugs* 2001;1:321–26.

Chapter

59 Resistant Hypertension

William J. Elliott

Key Findings

■ Resistant hypertension (blood pressure [BP] ≥140/90 mmHg, despite three drugs at near maximal doses for perhaps 3 months) is an important public health problem because of the increased cardiovascular risk associated with uncontrolled hypertension.

■ The exact prevalence of resistant hypertension is uncertain.

■ At least one cause can be found in 90% to 95% of cases of resistant hypertension.

■ The most popular recent causes of resistant hypertension in tertiary hypertension clinics are a suboptimal medication regimen, sleep apnea, and mineralocorticoid excess states (perhaps related to obesity and sleep disorders). In primary care practice, nonadherence to prescribed therapy and white-coat hypertension are probably more common than in specialist clinics.

■ After a suitable evaluation, most patients with resistant hypertension achieve goal BP.

Many authors have offered various definitions of "resistant" or "refractory" hypertension; recent definitions are typically more stringent.[1–3] Since the late 1980s, a consensus definition might be, "Sustained blood pressure (BP) ≥140 mmHg systolic or ≥90 mmHg diastolic, despite prescription of a specific number (originally two, but now more commonly three) of appropriately selected antihypertensive drugs at near maximal doses." Some insist that at least one of the drugs should be a diuretic, while others require a specific duration (typically 3 months) for the drugs to be prescribed. Other authorities (typically from tertiary care centers) also suggest that a physician referral is necessary before the hypertension can truly be considered "resistant."

This definition obviously leaves open many opportunities for discussion. The setting of the measured BP is not specified; therefore individuals with BP that is uncontrolled sometimes (e.g., in the medical office) but controlled in others (e.g., at home) fit the definition. The fact that the medications are prescribed (as opposed to actually consumed) leaves open the possibility that some patients may not be adherent to the instructions about taking the prescribed pills as directed. What constitutes an "appropriately selected antihypertensive drug" is a matter of some debate, and is much less well studied than how medications are best combined to achieve BP goals. A

"near-maximal" dose for one patient may be a modest dose for another, particularly if the weight of the latter patient is twice that of the first.

SCOPE OF THE PROBLEM

Although hypertension has long been recognized as a major remediable risk factor for cardiovascular disease, the most common cause of death in most countries (including the United States), implementation of strategies to control hypertension continues to be suboptimal across the globe. Even in the United States, where public health authorities, pharmaceutical companies, and physicians have been in agreement for decades to reduce the proportion of uncontrolled hypertensives to 50%, current statistics indicate that 69% have BP of ≥140/90 mmHg.[3] Although this proportion was lower in 1999–2000 compared to previous years, the proportion in the 18- to 74-year-old age group improved only to 66% from 73%.[3] In other countries, uncontrolled hypertension is even more common than in the United States. It is more difficult to achieve the recently recommended lower BP targets for diabetics and those with chronic kidney disease, so larger segments of these high-risk subpopulations remain "uncontrolled."

How much the specific diagnosis of "resistant hypertension" contributes to population-based surveys of BP control is uncertain. No large national surveys have ascertained the proportion of hypertensives taking at least three medications daily, nor how many of these are uncontrolled. Nonetheless, the epidemiology of uncontrolled hypertension provides some clues to features of those who are more likely to have "resistant hypertension." The proportion of hypertensive patients with "resistant hypertension" varies from about 3% in worksite-based hypertension control programs that care for relatively healthy people to about 30% in some tertiary hypertension clinics.

EPIDEMIOLOGY OF UNCONTROLLED HYPERTENSION

Perhaps because hypertension prevalence increases with age, older Americans were less likely to have their BP controlled in either 1988–1994 or 1999–2000 (Figure 59–1).[4,5] Especially relevant to "resistant hypertension" are about 18 million individuals aged 60 years and older in the United States who are treated but uncontrolled (with BP ≥140/90 mmHg). No other subgroup of the population is as large as the treated but uncontrolled people

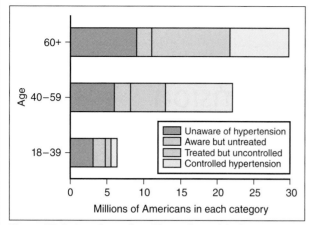

Figure 59–1. Prevalence (in millions of people) of various subtypes of hypertension in three age ranges in the United States, based on the 1999–2000 National Health and Nutrition Examination Survey,[5] and the 2000 US Census. The oldest age group (≥60 years) had the largest number (10.6 million) of Americans with treated, but uncontrolled hypertension (blue-green bars), which encompasses all patients with resistant hypertension.

over age 60 years. In the national survey of 1999–2002, fully 82.7% of Mexican-American hypertensives were uncontrolled, as opposed to 70.2% of either non-Hispanic white or African-American hypertensives. Treated but uncontrolled hypertension was present in 18.8% of the non-Hispanic whites, 25.8% of African Americans, and 17.6% of Mexican Americans. In 1988–1994, systolic BP elevations accounted for 66% of all BPs above threshold. On epidemiologic grounds, therefore, BP control would be expected to be less common among older minorities with systolic BP elevations.

RISKS OF UNCONTROLLED HYPERTENSION

A recent meta-analysis of 61 epidemiologic studies involving nearly 1 million people concluded that for every 20/10 mmHg of BP elevation, there is a twofold increase in the risk of cardiovascular mortality.[6] According to one interpretation of all clinical trials in hypertension, it matters more how much BP is lowered than which drug is used to begin the process. Over all clinical trials, a systolic BP difference of 10 mmHg translated to a 33% (95% confidence interval, 29% to 38%) reduction in cardiovascular events. Individuals with uncontrolled hypertension run an excess risk of cardiovascular events, as well as developing target organ damage.[7]

HYPERTENSION CONTROL RATES IN CLINICAL TRIALS

Under the best of circumstances (i.e., clinical trials), well-motivated physicians who treat carefully selected patients using free antihypertensive drugs, can achieve BP control rates in the 65% to 70% range. In all of these studies, a research protocol mandated an increase in the intensity of treatment for patients who did not achieve BP goal. These

data suggest an upper limit for the prevalence of "resistant hypertension" at no more than about 35% of hypertensive patients.

DIAGNOSTIC TECHNIQUES: DIFFERENTIAL DIAGNOSIS

After an appropriate evaluation, one or more reasons for resistant hypertension can be identified in about 90% to 95% of patients (Table 59–1).[8,9] The relative proportion of each of these diagnoses depends on the population studied. In primary care, nonadherence to prescribed drug therapy accounts for about 50% of patients not achieving BP goal, but in tertiary clinics, this proportion is typically only 5% to 10%. Secondary causes of hypertension display the opposite pattern, being 5 to 10 times more common in tertiary clinics (10%–20% of cases) than in primary care, where one is found in only 2% to 4% of cases.

Nonadherence to prescribed antihypertensive medications

Pharmacy refill data from the general population show that, in treatment of any chronic disease, including hypertension, about 50% of patients stop taking medication 1 year after the first prescription is filled.[10] In primary care, therefore, nonadherence is likely to be the most common cause of resistant hypertension, but this has been difficult to document. Simple, office-based methods to quantify pill consumption are inexact; one such study showed sensitivity of 10% and specificity of 86%.[11] Direct questioning of the patient about pill-taking behavior is probably the easiest approach. The best currently available method to document medication adherence is the use of pill containers fitted with electronic monitors that register the time and date of each opening of the bottle (which serves as a surrogate for pill consumption). When these monitors are used, however, many patients suddenly become much more adherent to their prescribed drugs, and improve their BPs.[12]

Two of three recent reports have challenged the long-held belief that nonadherence to prescribed medication is a common cause of resistant hypertension. In the most direct test of this hypothesis in a Swiss tertiary hypertension clinic, after informed consent, both electronic monitoring of pill containers for 4 weeks and ambulatory BP monitoring (ABPM) were performed for 103 patients. Among 49 patients with resistant hypertension, 82% were adherent to their therapy (defined as ≥80% of the expected number of container openings), as compared to 85% of treatment-responsive patients (*p*=0.33).[13] The authors therefore concluded that despite obvious limitations of their study, nonadherence to therapy is not more prevalent among resistant hypertensives. An uncontrolled Swiss study involving only 41 patients with treatment-resistant hypertension showed much-improved BPs after 2 months of electronic monitoring of adherence, and a further improvement when medications were changed, based on these results.[14] Patients with the lowest adherence rates (as determined by electronic monitoring) had the largest improvements in office BPs. These authors

CAUSES OF RESISTANT HYPERTENSION AND ESTIMATED PREVALENCE IN PRIMARY CARE VERSUS TERTIARY REFERRAL CENTERS		
Cause of Resistant Hypertension	**Estimated Prevalence in**	
	Primary Care (%)	*Tertiary Referral Centers (%)*
Nonadherence to prescribed medication	~50	10–20
Problems with blood pressure measurement		
Office resistance ("white-coat" hypertension)	~20–30	~10–20
Pseudohypertension or other technical problems	<1	<1
Drug-related problems		
Drug–drug interaction (especially NSAIDs)	~10	<5
Suboptimal antihypertensive drug regimens	~5	~30–50
Medication intolerance consistent with product labeling	<2	<2
Secondary hypertension		
Mineralocorticoid-excess states	<2	~1–10
Sleep apnea	<5	1–50
Renovascular hypertension	<2	2–15
Other known secondary causes of hypertension	<1	<1–3
Hypertension due to interfering (nondrug) substances		
Dietary or other exogenous sources of sodium	1–5	1–10
Excessive alcohol consumption	1–5	1–10
Other illicit substances	<1–2	<1–2
Psychological causes		
Anxiety, panic disorder, and related diagnoses	<1–2	<1–2
Medication intolerance inconsistent with product labeling	<1–2	<1–5
Adapted from Yakovlevitch M, Black HR. *Arch Intern Med* 1991;151:1786–92. NSAIDs, nonsteroidal anti-inflammatory drugs.		

Table 59–1. Causes of Resistant Hypertension and Estimated Prevalence in Primary Care versus Tertiary Referral Centers

therefore believe that electronic assessment of adherence is essential in evaluating resistant hypertension.[11] Lastly, a systematic review of 30 published studies concluded that there is insufficient evidence to implicate poor adherence (as objectively assessed by electronic monitors) as a cause of poor BP control.[15] However, adherence was significantly better with once daily (vs. twice daily) regimens, and declined as the duration of observation was increased.

The initial diagnostic strategy in primary care for all patients with resistant hypertension therefore involves questioning about pill-taking behaviors. A telephone call to the pharmacy about refill frequency can provide objective evidence of nonadherence. Electronic monitors can be rented for about $30 to $40/month, and although typically not reimbursed by insurance, provide the most precise and objective information about short-term (30-day) adherence to prescribed medications.

Problems with blood pressure measurement

In many individuals, BPs measured in the medical office may not be representative of those observed over the entire day. "White-coat hypertension" (office BP >10% higher than the daytime average, as assessed by 24-hour ABPM[16]) is found in about 20% to 25% of individuals with elevated office BP readings, whether referred from primary care offices or tertiary clinics.[17] Although its natural history and need for treatment are debated, most would agree that the "alerting effect" in these patients is seldom abrogated by therapy. In our clinic, the lowest prevalence of controlled hypertension during follow-up (average 1.6 years) was found among patients with nonadherence to prescribed medications (22%), followed by "white-coat hypertension" (25%).[9] Most physicians are content to diagnose the problem using ABPM, and recognize that, at best, only 75% to 80% of patients with resistant hypertension can be controlled.

"White-coat hypertensive" patients typically have much less target-organ damage than patients with other causes of resistant hypertension. In fact, in the United States, lack of target-organ damage is a prerequisite for ABPM to diagnose white-coat hypertension, its only Medicare-reimbursable indication. In an Italian study, patients with white-coat hypertension were slightly older and had slightly lower BPs at presentation,[18] but these differences are not very helpful with individual patients. In a study of 286 Brazilian patients with resistant hypertension, white-coat hypertension was found in 44% and was associated with a significantly larger nocturnal BP drop.[19] In our clinic, predictors of "white-coat hypertension" at the initial visit included admitting to "nervousness" or "worry" about office BP measurements, much lower BPs measurements at home with a calibrated device (compared to office BPs), and having a gradual decline in office BPs over 10 sequential readings. None of these, however, was sufficiently sensitive to obviate the need to confirm the diagnosis of white-coat hypertension with ABPM.

As a result, many authors now recommend ABPM routinely for evaluation of the "white-coat effect" as a contributor to resistant hypertension. Although the procedure is instrumental in making the diagnosis, its repeated use over time to monitor the patient's out-of-office BP is expensive, time consuming, and perhaps better done with home BP monitoring.

In many busy clinical settings, too little attention is paid to proper technique of BP measurement.[20] The three most common errors that result in erroneously high readings are using a cuff too small for the large arm, decreasing the cuff pressure more than 2 to 3 mmHg/s, and not having the patient rest comfortably for at least 5 minutes, with the back supported, without recent caffeine intake or smoking, before measuring BP.

A few patients with resistant hypertension have pseudohypertension, in which sclerotic arteries resist compression by an external BP cuff, resulting in much higher systolic BP readings than are obtained by intra-arterial measurement. Aortic and other arterial calcifications are often seen in x-rays of such patients. "Osler's maneuver" (palpation of a hard, nonpulsatile radial arterial when the BP cuff is inflated to obliterate the pulse, typically >200 mmHg) was originally proposed to screen for this condition,[21] but has since been found to be relatively imprecise. An even less common artifact is "cuff inflation hypertension," which can occasionally be observed when comparisons are made between traditional auscultatory and oscillometric BP measurements.[22]

Medication-related causes

There are three main causes of resistant hypertension that are directly related to medications used to treat it: drug–drug interactions, suboptimal antihypertensive drug regimens, and objective medication intolerance (i.e., when the ability to take a given drug is limited by a known side effect of that drug).

Drug–drug interactions

Antihypertensive drugs with important drug-drug interactions (e.g., propranolol, methyldopa, guanethidine) have generally decreased in prescription volume as other drugs have been introduced that did not have these potential problems. Nonetheless, many commonly used drugs can and do raise BP; some of these are available without a prescription and are therefore not identified by patients as being possible contributors to resistant hypertension.

Among the hypertensive population, nonsteroidal anti-inflammatory drugs (NSAIDs) are probably the most common agents that raise BP via a drug–drug interaction. About 36% of hypertensive Americans (~19 million people) have osteoarthritis, for which an NSAID is a treatment option. In addition, many more people take either an occasional or chronic NSAID for reasons unrelated to osteoarthritis. Meta-analyses published in the early 1990s indicated that NSAIDs increase BP by about 7–10/3–4 mmHg, with larger effects in hypertensive people, especially those treated with angiotensin-converting enzyme (ACE) inhibitors, beta-blockers, and diuretics. More recent data with NSAIDs selective for the second isoform of cyclooxygenase show similar results. Although acetaminophen is often recommended, many hypertensive patients find exercise (and even walking) without an NSAID difficult, if not impossible. In this setting, physicians tend to use more calcium antagonists and alpha-blockers for hypertension, rather than to prohibit NSAIDs altogether.

Many patients who are treated with cyclosporine, erythropoietin, or corticosteroids experience elevations in BP, but because these drugs are mandatory for their specific clinical condition, alterations are more commonly made to the antihypertensive treatment regimen than to these drugs. Oral contraceptive agents also occasionally raise BP, but because the risk of hypertension is so well known and reasonable alternatives exist, most women who develop hypertension with these agents have the offending agent stopped well before the hypertension becomes "resistant."

Some patients take drugs, but do not report their use (in addition to NSAIDs, previously discussed). Sympathomimetic drugs, typically found in nasal decongestants and "cold remedies" can raise both BP and pulse rates, especially when taken soon before a BP measurement. Some patients use cocaine and other stimulants, but seldom report this to a physician asked to assist with the BP elevations that these agents can cause. Monoamine oxidase inhibitors, which had been widely used some decades ago for depression, are making a comeback as treatments for dementia and other psychiatric disorders; these can interfere with agents that interfere with the sympathetic nervous system and ameliorate hypertension. Tricyclic antidepressants, which are less commonly used now than selective serotonin reuptake inhibitors, can also potentiate the BP-lowering properties of alpha-agonists (e.g., clonidine).

Suboptimal antihypertensive regimens

The definition of resistant hypertension mandates multidrug therapy, but the number of possible combinations of even the eight most commonly used drug classes is enormous. All meta-analyses since publication of the Antihypertensive and Lipid-Lowering to prevent Heart Attack Trial (ALLHAT) have indicated that no initial drug prevents coronary heart disease, cardiovascular events, or heart failure better than an initial diuretic. The question of what agent is best to add to the initial diuretic is largely left unanswered. Some combinations of commonly used antihypertensive agents are not very effective in lowering BP (ACE inhibitor plus angiotensin II receptor blocker [ARB], ACE inhibitor plus beta-blocker). In several tertiary clinics, suboptimal antihypertensive medication regimen was the most common of all the causes of resistant hypertension. Management of this problem is discussed in detail below.

Objective medication intolerance

Some patients with resistant hypertension have been previously treated with an antihypertensive agent that unfortunately caused intolerable side effects, resulting in discontinuation of the drug. When the specific side effect has already been reported, has a higher incidence with the drug than with placebo, and is included in the product label, the patient is said to have "objective medication intolerance." This situation is easier to associate with the drug than a similar one where the specific side effect has not previously been associated with the drug used (discussed below under "subjective medication intolerance"). "Objective medication intolerance" also includes situations during which specific drug therapies are contraindicated, such as a woman with hypertension treated with a diuretic, a calcium antagonist, and an ACE inhibitor, who becomes pregnant, and the ACE inhibitor must be at least temporarily discontinued for the duration of the pregnancy.

Secondary causes of hypertension

While most authors agree that a population of resistant hypertensives is enriched in cases of secondary hypertension, there is controversy about which specific cause is most common. In this context, chronic kidney disease is not usually numbered among the secondary causes of hypertension, as its treatment is similar to primary hypertension (with the exception of using loop diuretics and reducing the doses or frequency of administration of renally excreted drugs). In resistant hypertensives, primary hyperaldosteronism and sleep apnea are being more commonly reported as secondary causes of hypertension than renovascular disease, Cushing's syndrome, or pheochromocytoma, although some include obesity and insulin resistance as new and emerging secondary causes. Obesity is very important because higher doses of antihypertensive drugs are often required in obese patients to achieve the BP results seen routinely in patients of more desirable weight; in pediatrics and veterinary medicine, doses are calculated "per kilogram of body weight." Insulin-induced hypertrophy of vascular smooth muscle could account for resistant hypertension in patients with insulin resistance. Table 59–2 summarizes some of the currently recommended screening tests for the more common causes of secondary hypertension.

Interfering substances

Exogenous substances that are not usually prescription drugs are responsible for a small percentage of resistant hypertension. The BP-lowering effect of many antihypertensive drugs can be reduced, if not obliterated, by a high-sodium diet. This is particularly true among patients with "salt-sensitive hypertension," which is more common among blacks, the elderly, and those with chronic kidney disease. Recent data from a national survey suggest that dietary patterns (including a significantly higher salt intake) may account for some of the poor BP control in southern U.S. states (the "stroke belt").[23] Although patients may not be aware of their overconsumption of salt, a 24-hour urine is cheap and effective, but requires some education about proper timing and technique of collection.

The relationship of alcohol intake to hypertension and cardiovascular events is complex. Nonetheless, taking a proper history about alcohol consumption should be part of the initial evaluation of resistant hypertensive patients. Several studies have implicated heavy alcohol consumption with resistant hypertension; three have shown a graded (or dose–response) effect. The current recommendation of several authoritative bodies is to keep alcohol consumption to two or fewer drinks per day for men and one or fewer drinks per day for women.

Illicit substances such as cocaine, amphetamines, and anabolic steroids are typically not reported to the physician, and can raise BP and increase the risk of having resistant hypertension. Recent caffeine intake can also raise BP, as can prolonged high-dose intake. Using tobacco

COMMONLY RECOMMENDED SCREENING TESTS FOR SECONDARY HYPERTENSION		
Diagnosis	**Screening Test(s)**	**Other Tests**
Intrinsic renal disease	Serum creatinine ($15[a]), AM albumin/creatinine ratio ($20)	24-hour urine for creatinine clearance, protein, sodium, potassium ($40)
Mineralocorticoid excess states	24-hour urinary aldosterone during salt loading ($95), plasma aldosterone/renin ratio ($125)	Computed tomographic scan of adrenals ($1700)
Sleep apnea	Berlin Questionnaire (see text)	Formal sleep study ($900)
Renovascular hypertension	"Clinical prediction rule" (see text); followed by captopril scintigraphy ($300) if at moderate risk	Doppler ultrasound of renal arteries ($250), magnetic resonance angiography ($2900), renal angiogram ($8000)
Pheochromocytoma	24-hour urine for vanillylmandelic acid (VMA) and metanephrines ($175)	Plasma metanephrines ($250), plasma catecholamines ($250), T_2 weighted magnetic resonance imaging ($2750)
Cushing's Syndrome	8 AM plasma cortisol ($35)	Dexamethasone suppression test(s) ($120)
Hypothyroidism	Thyroid stimulating hormone (TSH, $55)	
[a]Costs vary over time and from institution to institution. These are approximate, as cited at Rush University Medical Center, Chicago, in July 2004.		

Table 59–2. Commonly Recommended Screening Tests for Secondary Hypertension

or other nicotine-containing products typically causes acute vasodilation and relative hypotension, but the effect is transient and usually followed by higher BPs than before the use. This pattern is occasionally seen on ABPM, and is the reason for prohibiting smoking within 30 minutes of a BP measurement.

Psychological causes

Some patients with resistant hypertension refuse to take specific antihypertensive medications, even though the drug may be useful in lowering BP, because they associate unusual symptoms to the drug. This situation is called "subjective medication intolerance" when these symptoms are not part of the known side-effect profile of the drug. This need not be a sign of psychological problems in the patient, as the first few cases of cough with an ACE inhibitor would have fit this scenario, and cough is now a well-established side-effect of these drugs. Nonetheless, some patients who report rare, unusual, and often incredible stories about their bad experiences with medications must be categorized somewhere, and this is the traditional place for them. The unusual details ("hair hurting, teeth itching") may be a useful clue in this setting.

Controversy exists about whether patients with resistant hypertension have a higher prevalence of panic disorder, anxiety attacks, or similar psychological diagnosis. Although it has been difficult to assemble a cohort of perfectly matched patients with and without these problems in a resistant hypertension clinic and study them carefully, some patients with resistant hypertension certainly have these problems. The most recent case–control study done in a tertiary clinic showed no difference in the frequency of panic disorder, anxiety, or depression among 136 cases of resistant hypertension, compared to 136 patients with controlled hypertension.[24] However, the proportion of patients who had experienced a panic attack (33% vs. 39%) or who fit criteria for current or previous diagnosis of panic disorder (12% vs. 14%) were higher than the authors expected.

MANAGEMENT

Nonadherence to chronic medications

Many simple measures to improve adherence to therapy have been advocated.[25] General health education, as well as drug-specific information, improve adherence, perhaps because patients better understand the medication and its intended benefit. Physicians can prescribe the minimum number of easy-to-swallow, once-daily combination pills that can be taken independently of food. Integrating pill taking into a schedule of other routine activities of daily living (e.g., when caring for teeth) regularizes the habit. Involving a significant other (in taking pills and measuring BPs at home) provides social support and a reminder of the importance of adherence. More extreme measures, including hospitalization or nursing home placement for supervised administration of prescribed medications, is seldom necessary.

Problems with blood pressure measurement

All patients should have BPs taken with appropriate technique,[20] although incorrect technique is probably not a common cause of resistant hypertension. For hypertensive patients without target organ damage, Medicare reimburses for ABPM to evaluate "white-coat hypertension." Optimal management of patients with white-coat hypertension is controversial, but all would agree that controlling BP when measured outside the medical office is advisable.

Medication-related causes
Drug–drug interactions

Few patients are currently prescribed the older antihypertensive medications that have serious drug–drug interactions with other medications. Few patients are willing to forego NSAIDs that make it possible to walk and perform other activities of daily living. Few doctors are willing to discontinue important therapies that increase BP (e.g., cyclosporine, erythropoeitin); instead higher doses of antihypertensive drugs are typically prescribed. More patients can stop sympathomimetic agents and avoid monoamine oxidase inhibitors, tricyclic antidepressants, and street drugs that raise BP.

Suboptimal drug regimens

The Seventh Report of the Joint National Committee on the Prevention, Detection, Evaluation, and Treatment of High Blood Pressure (JNC 7) has recommended a low dose of a thiazide-like diuretic as first-line therapy for uncomplicated hypertension, based on ALLHAT and other clinical trial data. Very few studies have provided information about what drug class is best as the next agent, so JNC 7 suggests an ACE inhibitor, ARB, beta-blocker, or calcium antagonist (in alphabetical order). A road map for treating resistant hypertension developed in our clinic is shown in Figure 59–2.

Like ALLHAT, the Systolic Hypertension in the Elderly Program, Treatment of Mild Hypertension Study, and the Hypertension Detection and Follow-up Program, we prefer the long-acting thiazide-like diuretic, chlorthalidone, to the much more popular hydrochlorothiazide (HCTZ). It has proven benefits in cardiovascular event reduction in many clinical trials, including the Multiple Risk Factor Intervention Trial. In this important study, the Steering Committee decreed that HCTZ should be replaced by chlorthalidone after 5 years of mean follow-up, because the former was associated with highly significant increases in all-cause and total mortality, when each diuretic-treated group was compared to its referred care group. After the change, the excess mortality disappeared. More recently, an indirect comparison of ALLHAT and the Second Australian Blood Pressure Trial showed that for all cardiovascular events, chlorthalidone was better than lisinopril (in ALLHAT), which is very similar chemically and pharmacologically to enalapril, which was more effective than HCTZ (in ANBP-2). Thus, if one ignores all other potentially substantive differences across these two trials, for cardiovascular risk, chlorthalidone is less than ACE

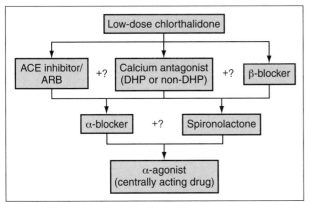

Figure 59–2. Road map for drug therapy of resistant hypertension, based on results at the Rush University Hypertension Center. Note that after chlorthalidone (for patients with estimated glomerular filtration rate of >40–45 mL/min), the second-line drug can be chosen from those on the second line, but the third-line drug should be adjacent to the second choice. Spironolactone can be added, for most patients, as the fourth-line drug, or introduced later. For patients with an estimated glomerular filtration rate of <40–45 mL/min, twice daily furosemide or another loop diuretic should be used, rather than a thiazide or thiazide-like diuretic. ARB, angiotensin II receptor blocker; DHP, dihydropyridine. (Adapted from Garg JP, Elliott WJ, Folker A, Izhar M, Black HR. *Am J Hypertens* 2005;18:619–26.)

inhibitor, which in turn is less than HCTZ. Unfortunately, chlorthalidone is available in the United States as 15-, 25-, and 50-mg pills, and in only three combination products, which just happen to be the ALLHAT second-step drugs (atenolol, reserpine, and clonidine). Those who practice evidence-based medicine should perhaps become more familiar with these three combination products, all of which are inexpensive and generically available.

Figure 59–2 gives a choice for second-line therapy: ACE inhibitor (or ARB, if cough or other adverse effect prevents use of an ACE inhibitor), calcium antagonist, or beta-blocker. In Figure 59–2, only second-line drugs that are adjacent to each other should be used in combination. This is consistent with ALLHAT, the "Birmingham square," and several studies of "renin profiling," all of which suggest that the combination of a beta-blocker + ACE inhibitor (the outside options in Figure 59–2) is less useful in hypertension than it is in systolic heart failure. After two or three drugs from the second-line selections, we and others find a long-acting alpha-blocker to be especially useful in lowering BP, especially when measured in the standing position.[9,26] Many physicians use clonidine as their usual fifth-line therapy, although its noxious side-effect profile at high doses can reduce adherence, and sudden withdrawal often leads to "rebound" hypertension. Reserpine and alpha-methyldopa have recently been recommended as inexpensive and effective medications that are well tolerated at low doses. Minoxidil, perhaps the most potent vasodilator drug, is particularly useful in men who are already treated with a diuretic (typically furosemide twice daily) and a beta-blocker.

Some authors recommend laboratory testing to more "physiologically" choose any but the initial antihyperten-

sive drug. This may be particularly useful when the patient's volume status and sodium balance are in question. The finding of a very low level of plasma renin activity despite a thiazide diuretic and an ACE inhibitor, for example, would suggest more (or a stronger) diuretic be added. Another approach, pioneered at the Mayo Clinic, is to perform noninvasive hemodynamic measurements by thoracic bioimpedance for patients with resistant hypertension, and then choose therapy intended to improve the profile. This approach led to significantly better control of hypertension (56% vs. 33%, *p*<0.05) than therapy directed by a certified hypertension specialist.[27] The authors believed their results were due to the bioimpedance measurements being able to detect occult volume expansion, which was followed by higher doses of diuretics.

The drug-related approach to resistant hypertension that is gathering the most attention in the recent medical literature is the use of spironolactone as an add-on drug. This practice is supported by several studies that reported a higher-than-expected prevalence of patients with presumed primary hyperaldosteronism, based on the ratio of plasma aldosterone/renin as a screening test. In addition, Nishizaka and Calhoun and Berecek et al.[28,29] have shown a good long-term BP-lowering response after adding spironolactone, first in patients with hypertension associated with obesity and the sleep apnea syndrome, and more recently in resistant hypertension (regardless of sleep apnea screening scores). Another study of 25 patients with resistant hypertension showed not only better BPs, but also a reduction in antihypertensive drug use when spironolactone was empirically added to the regimen.[30] These promising reports set the stage for a multicenter, randomized clinical trial of spironolactone (or a similar agent) in resistant hypertension.

Recent work from our clinic has indicated that 58% of 141 consecutive patients with physician-referred resistant hypertension had drug-related problems at referral; 94% of these were due to a suboptimal medication regimen.[9] After a small increase in the number of antihypertensive medications (3.7 ±0.9 to 4.1 ±1.0 per day, *p*<0.0001), 53% achieved their BP target during follow-up. The most common change (60 of 86 patients) that led to BP control involved a diuretic. Changing from a thiazide to a twice-daily loop diuretic (when the estimated glomerular filtration rate [*e*GFR] was <40–45 mL/min), or from a once daily loop diuretic to chlorthalidone if the *e*GFR was more than 50 mL/min, were successful in 21 patients. An increase in diuretic dose (often once daily to twice daily furosemide) was successful in 17 patients. Twelve patients had a diuretic added (as it was not part of the regimen on referral), 7 had the diuretic dose decreased, and only 3 had a diuretic discontinued. A summary of the other changes in medications from referral to successful BP control is shown in Figure 59–3. Significant increases in use of alpha-blockers, and calcium antagonists (especially dihydropyridine calcium antagonists) were accompanied by significant decreases in use of nonspecific vasodilators and beta-blockers. The many changes we observed are prioritized and summarized in Figure 59–2.

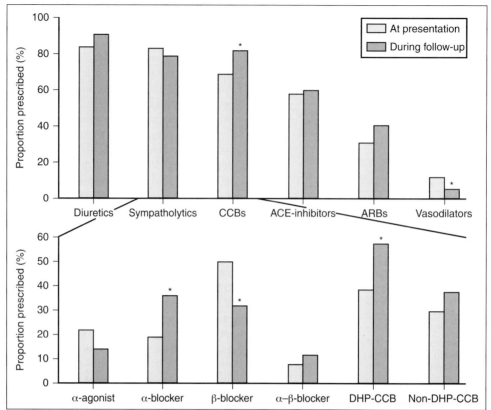

Figure 59–3. Proportion of patients receiving various pharmacologic classes (*top*) and subclasses (*bottom*) of antihypertensive drug therapy at presentation (*green bars*) and during follow-up (*blue bars*) (average 1.6 years) in a cohort of 141 physician-referred patients with resistant hypertension. During follow-up, the same percentage (53%) of all patients, and of those with a suboptimal medication regimen, achieved goal BP. * significant difference ($p<0.05$) at presentation versus during follow-up by chi-square test. (Data from Garg JP, Elliott WJ, Folker A, Izhar M, Black HR. *Am J Hypertens* 2005;18:619–26.)

Objective medication intolerance

Occasionally the problem with a specific medication can be overcome with the same drug supplied by a different delivery system. A good example is the flushing, headache, and tachycardia that commonly result with nifedipine capsules (typically given three to six times/day). These symptoms (but not the pedal edema) typically are much less common with the sustained-release form of the very same drug. A more common management strategy for objective medication intolerance is simply to avoid prescribing the implicated medication.

Secondary causes of hypertension
Mineralocorticoid excess states

As noted earlier, based on screening large populations with the plasma aldosterone renin ratio during a period of high-salt intake, several groups across the world have claimed that mineralocorticoid excess states account for 10% to 25% of resistant hypertension. Others note that these patients do not fulfill formal diagnostic criteria for primary hyperaldosteronism, and only very rarely have an adrenal adenoma; most may in fact simply have "low-renin essential hypertension." Currently, further investigation for primary hyperaldosteronism is warranted if the aldosterone to plasma renin activity ratio is more than

20 ng/dL per ng/mL/hour *and* the plasma aldosterone concentration is greater than 15 ng/dL.[31] These diagnostic cutpoints will soon require revision, since the direct renin assay has largely replaced the determination of peripheral renin activity in most clinical laboratories. Part of the reason for the increased interest in finding cases of primary hyperaldosteronism is that laparoscopic adrenalectomy is now widely available, at lower cost and probably a reduced risk of major complications, compared to traditional laparotomy. The recent introduction of eplerenone, a selective aldosterone blocker with much less estrogenic activity than spironolactone, may also make medical therapy of idiopathic hyperaldosteronism less troublesome.

Sleep apnea

Since about 1996 there has been an explosion of information about sleep apnea as a potential secondary cause of hypertension, perhaps because of the epidemic of obesity and its related disorders in the United States and much of the industrialized world.[32–34] The prevalence of previously unrecognized sleep apnea in resistant hypertensive patients has been reported to be as high as 83%.[35] In most studies, it is more common in obese (body mass index ~35 kg/m²) men at about age 60 years.[35,36] Many hypertensive patients with sleep apnea show little or no nocturnal drop in BP with ABPM, but this is not a very specific finding. The Berlin questionnaire, a very useful tool for screening for sleep apnea in primary care, has 86% sensitivity, 77% specificity, and 89% positive predictive value when evaluated in 744 patients subsequently formally evaluated with polysomnography.[37] The most specific screening questions appear to be loud snoring during sleep, daytime sleepiness/drowsiness (especially while driving), and (of greatest predictive value), observed episodes of irregular breathing and/or apneic periods during sleep. For individuals found on screening to be at high risk for sleep apnea, most specialists in sleep medicine routinely recommend a formal sleep study, followed by continuous positive airway pressure (CPAP) during sleep and a weight-loss regimen. This multidisciplinary approach has been shown to lower BP in the short term in refractory hypertensive patients who use the apparatus.[38] The stage is now set for a comparative clinical trial of CPAP versus spironolactone in patients with resistant hypertension who score highly on the Berlin Questionnaire.

Renovascular hypertension

The importance of renovascular disease as a common cause of resistant hypertension has been declining recently. Some of this may be due to the fact that renal artery stenosis is now diagnosed fairly often in patients who undergo angiography for other reasons (e.g., coronary or peripheral vascular disease evaluation), but there is uncertainty about the clinical consequences of the discovered stenoses. Similarly, since the publication of three trials comparing medical therapy and renal angioplasty showed few differences in BP control or renal function, enthusiasm for invasive approaches to open the renal arteries has waned.[39] In most centers, angiography and angioplasty (now usually with stenting) is reserved for patients who are likely to have fibromuscular dysplasia or atherosclerotic disease for which medical therapy does not control BP or leads to deteriorating renal function.[40] In the recent Dutch experience, resistant hypertension was found in 41% of patients at high risk for renovascular disease (based on their clinical prediction rule[41]), and 20% of these had renal artery stenosis. Initial therapy with enalapril was no more useful than amlodipine in identifying those with renal artery stenosis.[42]

Rarer causes of secondary hypertension

Because resistant hypertension has a higher prevalence of secondary hypertension than easily controlled hypertension, rare causes of hypertension are to be expected more commonly as well. Unusual aortic pathology and genetic mutations affecting sodium transport figure most prominently in the recent medical literature.

Interfering substances

Lifestyle modifications are the traditional recommended therapy for excessive dietary sodium intake, ethanol consumption, and illicit drug use. Short-term studies show an impressive reduction in BP with each, but longer-term clinical trials and everyday clinical practice are not as optimistic about the ability of many patients to adhere to these recommendations. For individuals whose 24-hour collection of urine contains more than 120 mEq of sodium, a visit with a nutritionist is recommended for the patient and the person from the same household who buys and prepares food. Reducing alcohol consumption has been followed by improved BP in some studies, but the large randomized clinical trial (performed in U.S. military veterans) comparing advice to reduce alcohol intake and usual care in heavy drinkers did not show a significant reduction in office BP, perhaps because all subjects decreased their reported intake between screening and randomization in the study.

Psychological causes

There are no clinical trial data to support a recommendation to send resistant hypertensive patients with psychological causes for counseling or psychiatric therapy, perhaps because this is a rare cause of resistant hypertension. Another option is to stimulate the peripheral nervous system to counter the perceived symptom; this may be the explanation why transcutaneous nerve stimulation was effective in lowering BP in 12 resistant hypertensive patients in a recent study.[43]

PROGNOSIS

Several series from tertiary centers that see many resistant hypertensive patients show that, after an appropriate evaluation and modification of drug therapy, the vast majority of patients can achieve goal BP.[8,9] Whether they have a higher risk of cardiovascular events, even after achieving goal BP, is unclear. However, several clinical trials (including the best example, the Valsartan Antihypertensive Long-Term Use Evaluation) have shown, as might be expected, that individuals with initially uncontrolled BP, do suffer more events in the short-term than those who achieve BP goals quite early after treatment is initiated. Insurance company databases show that treated hypertensives do not quite reduce their risk of death to that of similar individuals without hypertension, but those with uncontrolled hypertension fare much worse than those with controlled BP.

SUMMARY

Resistant hypertension (BP ≥140/90 mmHg, despite three drugs at near maximal doses for perhaps 3 months) is an important public health problem because of the increased cardiovascular risk associated with uncontrolled hypertension. Its exact prevalence is uncertain, but it accounts for perhaps 5% to 20% of referrals to most tertiary hypertension clinics. At least one cause of resistant hypertension can be found in 90% to 95% of cases; the most popular recent causes are a suboptimal medication regimen, sleep apnea, and mineralocorticoid excess states (perhaps related to obesity and sleep disorders). Nonadherence to prescribed therapy and white-coat hypertension are probably more common in primary care practice than in specialist clinics. After a suitable evaluation, most patients with resistant hypertension can and do achieve goal BP.

REFERENCES

1. Setaro JF, Black HR. Refractory hypertension. *N Engl J Med* 1992; 327:543–45.
2. Calhoun DA, Zaman MA, Nishizaka MK. Resistant hypertension. *Curr Hypertens Rep* 2002;4:221–28.
3. National High Blood Pressure Education Program Coordinating Committee. Seventh Report of the Joint National Committee on Prevention, Detection, Evaluation and Treatment of High Blood Pressure. *Hypertension* 2003;42:1206–52.
4. Hyman DJ, Pavlik VN. Characteristics of patients with uncontrolled hypertension in the United States. *N Engl J Med* 2001; 345:479–86.
5. Hajjar I, Kotchen TA. Trends in prevalence, awareness, treatment, and control of hypertension in the United States, 1988–2000. *JAMA* 2003; 290:199–203.
6. Prospective Studies Collaborative. Age-specific relevance of usual blood pressure to vascular mortality: a meta-analysis of individual data for one million adults in 61 prospective studies. *Lancet* 2002;360:1903–13.
7. Cuspidi C, Macca G, Sampieri L, et al. High prevalence of cardiac and extracardiac target organ damage in refractory hypertension. *J Hypertens* 2001;19:2063–70.
8. Yakovlevitch M, Black HR. Resistant hypertension in a tertiary care clinic. *Arch Intern Med* 1991;151:1786–92.
9. Garg JP, Elliott WJ, Folker A, Izhar M, Black HR. Resistant hypertension revisited: a comparison of two university-based cohorts. *Am J Hypertens* 2005;18:619–26.
10. McDonald HP, Garg AX, Haynes RB. Interventions to enhance patient adherence to medication prescriptions: scientific review. *JAMA* 2002;288: 2868–79.
11. Burnier M, Santschi V, Favrat B, Brunner HR. Monitoring compliance in resistant hypertension: an important step in patient management. *J Hypertens* 2003;21(Suppl. 2):S37–42.
12. Waeber B, Vetter W, Darioli R, Keller U, Brunner HR. Improved blood pressure control by monitoring compliance with antihypertensive therapy. *Int J Clin Pract* 1999;53:37–8.
13. Nuesch R, Schroeder K, Dieterle T, Martina B, Battegay E. Relation between insufficient response to antihypertensive treatment and poor compliance with treatment: a prospective case-control study. *BMJ* 2001;323:142–46.
14. Burnier M, Schneider MP, Chiolero A, Stubi CL, Brunner HR. Electronic compliance monitoring in resistant hypertension: the basis for rational therapeutic decisions. *J Hypertens* 2001;19:335–41.
15. Wetzels GWC, Nelemans P, Schouten JS, Prins MH. Facts and fiction of poor compliance as a cause of inadequate blood pressure control: a systematic review. *J Hypertens* 2004;22:1849–55.

16. Pickering TG. Ambulatory blood pressure monitoring. *Curr Hypertens Rep* 2000; 2:558–64.
17. Brown MA, Buddle ML, Martin A. Is resistant hypertension really resistant? *Am J Hypertens* 2001;14:1263–69.
18. Veglio F, Rabbia F, Riva P, et al. Ambulatory blood pressure monitoring and clinical characteristics of the true and white-coat resistant hypertension. *Clin Exp Hypertens* 2001;23:203–11.
19. Muxfeldt ES, Bloch KV, Nogueira AR, Salles GF. Twenty-four hour ambulatory blood pressure pattern of resistant hypertension. *J Hypertens* 2003;8:181–85.
20. Pickering TG, Hall JE, Appel LJ, et al. Recommendations for blood pressure measurement in humans and experimental animals. Part 1. Blood pressure measurement in humans: a statement for professionals from the Sub-committee of Professional and Public Education of the American Heart Association Council on High Blood Pressure Research. *Hypertension* 2005;45:142–61.
21. Messerli FH, Ventura HO, Amodeo C. Osler's maneuver and pseudohypertension. *N Engl J Med* 1985;312:1548–51.
22. Mejia AD, Egan BM, Schork NJ, Zweifler AJ. Artifacts in measurement of blood pressure and lack of target organ involvement in the assessment of patients with treatment-resistant hypertension. *Ann Intern Med* 1990; 112:270–77.
23. Hajjar I, Kotchen T. Regional variations of blood pressure in the United States are associated with regional variations in dietary intakes: the NHANES-III data. *J Nutr* 2003;133:211–14.
24. Davies SJC, Ghahramani P, Jackson PR, et al. Panic disorder, anxiety and depression in resistant hypertension: a case–control study. *J Hypertens* 1997; 15:1077–82.
25. Elliott WJ. Optimizing medication adherence in older patients with hypertension. *Int Urol Nephrol* 2003; 35:557–62.
26. Black HR, Sollins JS, Garofalo JL. The addition of doxazosin to the therapeutic regimen of hypertensive patients inadequately controlled with other antihypertensive medications: a randomized, placebo-controlled study. *Am J Hypertens* 2000;13:468–74.
27. Taler SJ, Textor SC, Augustine JE. Resistant hypertension: comparing hemodynamic management to specialist care. *Hypertension* 2002;39:982–88.
28. Nishizaka MK, Calhoun DA. Use of aldosterone antagonists in resistant hypertension. *J Clin Hypertens* 2004; 6:458–60.
29. Berecek KH, Farag A, Bahtiyar G, Rothman J, McFarlane SI. Adding low-dose spironolactone to multidrug regimens for resistant hypertension. *Curr Hypertens Rep* 2004;6:211–12.

30. Ouzan J, Pérault C, Lincoff AM, Carré E, Mertes M. The role of spironolactone in the treatment of patients with refractory hypertension. *Am J Hypertens* 2002; 15:333–39.
31. Young WF Jr. Minireview: primary aldosteronism—changing concepts in diagnosis and treatment. *Endocrinology* 2003;144:2208–13.
32. Silverberg DS, Oksenberg A, Iaina A. Sleep-related breathing disorders are common contributing factors to the production of essential hypertension but are neglected, underdiagnosed and undertreated. *Am J Hypertens* 1997; 10:1319–25.
33. Wolk R, Shamsuzzaman ASM, Somers VK. Obesity, sleep apnea and hypertension. *Hypertension* 2003; 42:1067–74.
34. Goodfriend TL, Calhoun DA. Resistant hypertension, obesity, sleep apnea and aldosterone: theory and therapy. *Hypertension* 2004;43:518–24.
35. Logan AG, Perlikowski SM, Mente A, et al. High prevalence of unrecognized sleep apnoea in drug-resistant hypertension. *J Hypertens* 2001; 19:2271–77.
36. Lavie P, Hoffstein V. Sleep apnea syndrome: a possible contributing factor to resistant hypertension. *Sleep* 2001;24:721–25.
37. Netzer NC, Stoohs RA, Netzer CM, et al. Using the Berlin Questionnaire to identify patients at risk for the sleep apnea syndrome. *Ann Intern Med* 1999;131:485–91.
38. Logan AG, Tkacova R, Perlikowski SM, et al. Refractory hypertension and sleep apnoea: effect of CPAP on blood pressure and baroreflex. *Eur Respir J* 2003;21:241–47.
39. Ives NJ, Wheatley K, Stowe RL, et al. Continuing uncertainty about the value of percutaneous revascularization in atherosclerotic renovascular disease: a meta-analysis of randomized trials. *Nephrol Dial Transplant* 2003; 18:298–304.
40. Textor SC. Managing renal arterial disease and hypertension. *Curr Opin Cardiol* 2003;18:260–67.
41. Krijnen P, van Jaarsveld BC, Steyerberg EW, et al. A clinical prediction rule for renal artery stenosis. *Ann Intern Med* 1998;129:738–40.
42. van Jaarsveld BC, Krijnen P, Derkx FH, et al. Resistance to antihypertensive medication as predictor of renal artery stenosis: comparison of two regimens. *J Hum Hypertens* 2001;15:669–76.
43. Jacobsson F, Himmelmann A, Bergbrant A, Svensson A, Mannheimer C. The effect of transcutaneous electric nerve stimulation in patients with therapy-resistant hypertension. *J Hum Hypertens* 2000;14:795–98.

Chapter

60 Perioperative Hypertension: Preparing the Hypertensive Patient for Anesthesia for Surgery

Pierre Foëx

Key Findings

- The presence of hypertensive disease increases the risk of cardiac complications of anesthesia and surgery.

- Hypertensive patients exhibit exaggerated cardiovascular responses to anesthesia and surgery.

- The risk of complications relates to the presence of target-organ damage more than to the level of hypertension.

- Empirical guidelines suggest that hypertension above 180/110 mmHg should be treated before elective surgery, preferably for several weeks. Treatment should also be considered for lower levels of blood pressure associated with target-organ damage.

- Treated hypertensive patients should be maintained on their medication throughout the perioperative period, although ACE inhibitors and angiotensin-receptor antagonists may need to be omitted on the day of surgery.

- Invasive monitoring of blood pressure is recommended for major surgery with active control of hypo- and hypertensive events.

The association between arterial hypertension and adverse cardiac outcome of anesthesia and surgery has been recognized for several decades. However, the level of blood pressure at which initiation or optimization of treatment is required to decrease the short-term risk of adverse events is not firmly established. Over the past decade this issue has become more complicated because the level of blood pressure requiring treatment in order to decrease the long-term risk of arterial hypertension has decreased. Therefore, those involved in the management of hypertensive patients presenting for elective surgery have to decide whether the guideline for reducing the long-term risk of adverse outcome should also be applied to the short-term outcome of patients subjected to the stress of surgery.

If values such as 140/80 mmHg were applied to all surgical patients, it follows that the number of cancellations or deferments would increase dramatically as many patients would present with "white coat" hypertension or exhibit an increase above their usual blood pressure level because they are apprehensive. Even fairly recently only 10% to 14% of treated hypertensive patients achieved the target of less than 140/80 mmHg.[1,2] As there is no evidence of threshold down to 115/75 mmHg,[3] 140/80 mmHg may

come to be regarded as "conservative" within a few years. This would make the question of deferment for treatment even more complicated than it is at present. Cancellations and deferments have significant implications for the patient and for healthcare systems. In order to reach a decision regarding the surgical patient, it is important to take into consideration not only the measured blood pressure but also the presence of target-organ damage and diabetes. However, admission for surgery could for some patients be an ideal opportunity to initiate long-term treatment. Whether this needs to be done before surgery or could be done after surgery is the central issue of this review.

EVOLUTION OF CONCEPTS AND PRACTICE

In 1929, Sprague[4] published important observations—in a series of 75 hypertensive patients, one-third died during the perioperative period, including 12 who died from cardiovascular complications. The introduction of antihypertensive drugs in the 1950s was initially regarded by anesthesiologists as creating a new hazard. It was thought that these drugs, because they interfere with the regulation of the circulation, increased the cardiovascular lability of patients. It became customary to stop antihypertensive medication 2 weeks before elective surgery. As this was not always practical, Dingle,[5] in 1966, proposed that hypertensive patients should undergo autonomic function testing before surgery. Evidence of impaired autonomic responses would indicate the need to stop the antihypertensive therapy several days before surgery and during the immediate perioperative period.[5]

The recommendation to stop treatment in hypertensive patients was still current in the early 1970s. A dramatic change occurred after Prys-Roberts et al.[6,7] published a series of observational studies of the interactions of anesthesia and hypertension. The first two studies compared the responses to induction of anesthesia, laryngoscopy and intubation, steady-state anesthesia, and awakening in three groups of patients: untreated hypertensives, treated hypertensives, and normotensive elderly patients. The studies showed that changes in blood pressure were greater in the untreated hypertensive patients than in the treated hypertensives or in elderly normotensives. On the basis of these observations, the authors concluded that treatment of hypertension should be maintained throughout the perioperative period as it would improve cardiovascular stability; this could only be regarded as beneficial.

At the same time the use of beta-blockers was causing great concern. The general consensus was that they should be stopped 2 weeks before surgery. A third observational study by the same group[8] showed that intravenous beta-blockade with practolol immediately after induction of anesthesia, or prior beta-blockade with oral practolol for 2 days before surgery, was well tolerated, did not reduce cardiac output more than anesthesia alone, and minimized the increase in blood pressure and heart rate seen after laryngoscopy and endotracheal intubation. More importantly beta-blocked patients did not develop ventricular arrhythmias or myocardial ischemia, unlike the non–beta-blocked patients. This could be regarded as a major benefit. The good tolerance of beta-blockade was confirmed by another study involving patients receiving up to 2000 mg of propranolol daily.[9]

Following these studies, the authors came to two conclusions: First, that treatment of hypertension, including beta-blockade, should be maintained; and second, that hypertensive patients should be treated and their blood pressure controlled before elective surgery. Over the next few years, these conclusions were generally adopted. However, almost 35 years later this issue has to be revisited in its current context. In the early 1970s, many hypertensive patients presented with very high blood pressures, well above 200 mmHg systolic and 110 mmHg diastolic. Today blood pressure above 140/80 mmHg is regarded as hypertension. Does it follow that patients with mild or moderate hypertension should be treated before surgery and their blood pressure brought to the currently accepted therapeutic goal to obtain some reduction of the immediate risk? The question becomes increasingly difficult as the seventh report of the Joint National Committee on Prevention, Detection, Evaluation, and Treatment of High Blood Pressure (JNC-7) does not make any differentiation between stages 2 and 3 hypertension.[10] Is there evidence that mild or moderate hypertension (stages 1 and 2 of the older classification) justifies postponement, while accepting that for the long term patients need to be treated?

HYPERTENSIVE DISEASE AND PERIOPERATIVE RISK

There is a definite association between arterial hypertension and perioperative adverse outcome. This has been established in a systematic review of observational studies published between 1971 and 2001.[11] The studies were concerned with the risk of major adverse event within 30 days of anesthesia and surgery. Studies examining stroke after coronary endarterectomy were excluded because they represent a specific population with a specific risk that relates directly to the operation itself. Eventually 30 studies satisfied the selection criteria. The total number of patients was 13,671, of which 5677 were hypertensive. The studies allowed odds ratios to be calculated and the pooled odds ratio was 1.31 (confidence interval [CI]=1.17–1.56, $p<0.001$). However, the test for heterogeneity between the studies was significant and the source of this variability was sought through a number of sensitivity analyses grouping the data by year of study and by

type of surgery. These analyses yielded little impact on the odds ratio, and heterogeneity among the studies included remains.

With a value of 1.31, the odds ratio is significant but relatively small. However, studies have almost never made any distinction among history of hypertension, treated and well-controlled hypertension, and uncontrolled hypertension. This may mean that some patients could be at high risk while others are a low risk. Patients with a higher blood pressure are likely to be at greater risk of short-term adverse outcome than those with moderately elevated blood pressure.

A number of cardiac risk indices have been developed to facilitate the assessment of surgical patients. These indices emphasized the major contribution of ischemic heart disease, heart failure, renal failure, and in earlier studies arrhythmias, all of which are frequently associated with hypertension. However, the studies did not identify hypertension itself as a significant determinant of adverse cardiac outcome.[12–16] This is not surprising because very few patients included in the populations examined to derive the risk indices had a blood pressure higher than 180/110 mmHg. Therefore, other cardiac disorders were playing a much greater role and could easily overshadow hypertension as a predictor of adverse outcome. Clearly, the possibility of organ damage must be borne in mind when evaluating hypertensive patients.[17,18]

ADMISSION BLOOD PRESSURE AND OUTCOME

If it is accepted that hypertension increases the risk of cardiovascular complications of anesthesia, is this the result of the presence of hypertensive heart disease or does it relate closely to the level of blood pressure at the time of admission for surgery? In 1979, Goldman and Caldera[19] examined patients with arterial hypertension who were included in their risk index.[12] No significant differences were found between patients who were hypertensive at the time of surgery and those who were normotensive, treated with diuretics, or hypertensive but relatively well controlled (blood pressure below 160/100 mmHg). The absence of difference may be ascribed to two factors: (1) the study did not have the statistical power to confirm or refute an association between hypertension and outcome, and (2) very few patients had blood pressures that could be classified as stage 3 hypertension. Indeed, only 5 of 196 patients had a diastolic blood pressure higher than 111 mmHg.[19] Other studies[20,21] also suffered a lack of statistical power. One study showed a clear association between hypertension and perioperative myocardial reinfarction.[22] Hypertension has also been shown to play a role in the risk of complications after coronary artery surgery.[23]

Two case-control studies[24,25] have examined the relationship between hypertension and cardiac death within 30 days of surgery with close matching for age, sex, and operation. There was no difference in the admission blood pressure between the patients who died and the survivors.[24] This was also true when both elective and emergency operations were considered, although there was a tendency for survivors to have a higher admission blood pressure.[25] While the studies suggest that high admission blood pressure does not correlate with postoperative cardiac death, the limitation of the studies, which also applies to most recent studies of hypertension in surgical patients, is that very few patients had stage 3 hypertension; most had stage 1 or 2 hypertension. Only older studies included many patients with stage 3 hypertension. In such patients cardiovascular lability is greatly increased, and there is a high risk of myocardial ischemia and ventricular arrhythmias if they are untreated.[7]

Today, the absence of a clear association between admission blood pressure and cardiac outcome of anesthesia and surgery may reflect changes in standards of perioperative care of these patients, changes in perioperative drug therapies, changes in standards of monitoring, or improvement in the standard of care of the hypertensive patient in the community leading to fewer patients exhibiting the complications of renal dysfunction, cerebrovascular disease, or other organ damage.

Medical patients with stage 3 hypertension are at a significantly increased risk of target-organ damage that is not always apparent. Unsurprisingly, a recent guideline recommends echocardiography for the detection of left ventricular hypertrophy, and carotid Doppler sonography to detect carotid artery disease,[26] as the presence of such target-organ damage increases the risk of perioperative cardiovascular complications.

With the increase in blood pressure there is an increased incidence of electrocardiographic abnormalities.[27,28] In hypertensive patients, there is evidence of an association between quality of blood pressure control and the occurrence of silent postoperative myocardial ischemia (a marker for postoperative cardiovascular complications).[29]

Most studies have not considered arterial pressure as a continuous variable, although it is well known that, in the long term, the risk of adverse outcome correlates with the severity of hypertension.[30] However, when blood pressure was considered as a continuous variable in surgical patients, it became apparent that the risk of perioperative myocardial ischemia increased with blood pressure: the odds ratio was 1.2 (CI=1.01–1.42) for each 10-mmHg increase in systolic pressure.[31] This observation indicates that in surgical patients, as in medical patients, the risk of adverse outcome increases with the level of hypertension.

ISOLATED SYSTOLIC HYPERTENSION

Isolated systolic hypertension (ISH), which accounts for the majority of hypertensive patients aged over 60 years, is a relatively new focus of interest. As a consequence of the increase in pulse pressure, ISH increases the cardiovascular risk.[32] It makes sense to consider that isolated systolic hypertension is also a risk factor for surgical patients. Studies that have included mostly elderly patients are likely to have included a high proportion of patients with isolated systolic hypertension.[20–22] As an association between high blood pressure and perioperative adverse outcome was found, these studies can be used to support the view that isolated systolic hypertension is a risk factor in surgical patients, and certainly where stage 3 is concerned.

More recently, the issue of isolated systolic hypertension has been examined in patients undergoing cardiac surgery in a large (more than 2400 patients) prospective multicenter study.[23] Isolated hypertension was defined as a systolic blood pressure above 140 mmHg with diastolic pressure less than 90 mmHg. Isolated systolic hypertension was associated with a statistically significant increase in the likelihood of perioperative cardiac complications (odds ratio 1.3, CI=1.1–1.6) but not mortality. Based on the findings of the Framingham population,[33] it can be assumed, as the average age of the patients was 65 years in this particular study,[23] that in most patients systolic pressure was considerably higher than the threshold for inclusion (i.e., 140 mmHg). In addition, a detailed study of patients with ISH has shown that, after correcting blood pressure, coronary blood flow was substantially lower than in normotensive patients.[34] This further supports the view that isolated systolic hypertension cannot be discounted as a risk factor for anesthesia and surgery.

WHITE-COAT HYPERTENSION

"White-coat hypertension" is particularly relevant to anesthesia and surgery as most patients admitted to hospital or attending an assessment clinic are anxious. As a result, their blood pressure may be repeatedly higher than it would be during ambulatory monitoring. White-coat hypertension seems to have a benign prognosis.[35] It is tempting to conclude that there is a low risk of organ damage and that, in the surgical setting, patients whose blood pressure settles to a level consistent with normotension are not at risk of short-term complications. However, this conclusion has not been tested in a scientific study. More importantly, these patients exhibit hyperreactivity to stress and reduced ability to control rapid increases in sympathetic activity.[36] This is potentially hazardous in surgical patients.

There is probably only one study that has examined the influence of labile hypertension on perioperative stability and myocardial ischemia.[37] The authors found that patients who were the most likely to develop arterial hypertension after endotracheal intubation often had elevated blood pressure at the time of hospital admission, even though they were normotensive while on the hospital ward. The need to intervene to control hypertensive episodes and myocardial ischemia demonstrates that labile hypertension can be regarded as a risk factor.

ANESTHESIA AND HYPERTENSIVE DISEASE

The risks of anesthesia and surgery relate to several factors: (1) the effect of hypertension on the heart as a target organ; (2) the association between hypertension, coronary artery disease, peripheral vascular disease, and diabetes; (3) the effect of hypertension on the cerebral and renal circulation; (4) the preoperative drugs and their interactions with anesthetic agents; (5) the possibility of undiagnosed diseases that cause hypertension; and (6) the need for life-saving procedures in patients with uncontrolled hypertension.[38] Although preoperative control of blood pressure is generally advocated, no guideline exists as to the level of blood pressure above which deferment of surgery for instituting treatment of hypertension is necessary.

Patients with arterial hypertension exhibit exaggerated hypotension following induction of anesthesia and excessive pressor response to stresses such as laryngoscopy, intubation, surgical incision, and extubation.[6,7] These changes reflect a large reduction in an otherwise elevated systemic vascular resistance in response to induction of anesthesia. Conversely, large increases in vascular resistance occur following sympathetic overactivity and are responsible for the large increases in blood pressure observed after laryngoscopy, during surgery, and on awakening. Indeed, in untreated hypertensive patients, large increases in norepinephrine and modest increases in epinephrine have been documented following laryngoscopy and intubation.[39] The exaggerated vascular responses are responsible for a pattern of blood pressure changes that has been termed "alpine anesthesia."[40] Hypertensive patients are also more prone to hypertensive responses (bladder distension, inadequate pain relief) postoperatively. Hypertensive episodes are often associated with arrhythmias and/or myocardial ischemia.[8] Hypo- and hypertension can cause cerebrovascular accidents. As vascular reactivity is increased in hypertensive patients,[41] the benefit of controlling their blood pressure preoperatively is to reduce this hyperreactivity and to improve their cardiovascular stability. Effective treatment of hypertension also brings cerebral autoregulation to more normal levels.[42]

Intraoperative hemodynamic abnormalities are associated with peri- and post-operative cardiovascular instability and, in some patients, cardiovascular events such as cardiac death, myocardial infarction, and stroke. In a study of 17,638 day-case patients, Chung et al.[43] observed an association between pre-existing arterial hypertension and intraoperative cardiovascular events (hypo- or hypertension, tachycardia). However, probably because most patients were undergoing relatively minor procedures, there were no deaths or perioperative myocardial infarctions. Another large study showed that hypertensive patients were more likely to require interventions for perioperative hypertension than their normotensive counterparts.[44] Reich et al.[45] have shown significant correlations among bradycardia, tachycardia, hypotension, hypertension (including pulmonary hypertension), and cardiovascular complications of coronary bypass surgery, confirming previous observations by Slogoff and Keats[46] regarding the adverse role of tachycardia and hypertension. More recently, Reich et al.[47] confirmed the association between tachycardia and hypertension and adverse cardiac outcome in patients undergoing prolonged operations.

Unsurprisingly, there is a relationship between the magnitude of changes in blood pressure and their duration and the risk of adverse events. Charlson et al.[48] found that patients with more than 1 hour of 20-mmHg or greater decreases in mean arterial pressure (MAP) or patients

with less than 1 hour of 20 mmHg or greater decreases and more than 15 minutes of greater than or equal to 20 mmHg increases were at highest risk for postoperative complications. As patients with uncontrolled hypertension are very likely to develop major hemodynamic abnormalities, these studies indirectly suggest that preoperative treatment of hypertension should be beneficial and that more extensive monitoring of the circulation is justified.

MANAGEMENT OF SURGICAL HYPERTENSIVE PATIENT

Ideally, all hypertensive patients should be treated because, in the long term, their prognosis is substantially improved. Hypertension discovered on the occasion of a surgical admission provides a unique opportunity to start antihypertensive therapy. However, such a policy, depending on the level of blood pressure at which treatment of hypertension is initiated, can lead to a very large number of cancellations or deferments. Currently, there is little scientific evidence that control of blood pressure has a significant impact on perioperative morbidity, at least in mild to moderate hypertension. Because no large randomized control trial has been undertaken, an empirical approach has developed.

PREOPERATIVE HYPERTENSION: IDEAL VERSUS EMPIRICAL APPROACHES

The difficulty in deciding which patients should be treated before anesthesia and surgery was highlighted in a survey of attitudes of anesthesiologists with respect to clinical scenarios involving hypertension. There was considerable variability as to which patients should have their procedures cancelled[49]; as a result, hypertension is the most common avoidable medical indication for deferring elective surgery.[50,51] In addition, in a short review published in 2005, Casadei and Abuzeid[36] stated, "Thus in the absence of controlled evidence, no firm recommendations can be made to improve patients' safety."

An empirical approach based on the severity of the hypertension may be helpful. Patients with severe hypertension (stage 3), defined as a systolic blood pressure of greater than 180 mmHg and/or a diastolic pressure greater than 110 mmHg, should be treated before elective surgery. They are at risk of life-threatening hypertensive crises likely to cause intracranial hemorrhage, ischemic stroke, acute left ventricular failure, ventricular arrhythmias, or renal failure. For patients with moderate hypertension (stage 2), with systolic pressure of 160 to 179 mmHg or diastolic pressure of 100 to 109 mmHg, preoperative treatment should be considered in patients with target-organ involvement. Finally, for those with mild hypertension (stage 1: 140–159/90–99 mmHg), treatment is regarded as optional.[52]

It can be argued that where blood pressure is consistently elevated to levels of 180 mmHg or greater but there is no target-organ damage, surgery can proceed if there is a strong indication for it. Care should be taken to ensure perioperative cardiovascular stability with administration of appropriate vasoactive agents. This requires invasive blood pressure monitoring not only during surgery but during the recovery period as well.

There are few substantive guidelines about which patients should be cancelled to allow treatment prior to surgery and for how long should such treatment be initiated before surgery. A recent American College of Cardiology/ American Heart Association guideline states that uncontrolled systemic hypertension appears to be a minor clinical predictor of increased perioperative cardiovascular risk.[18] The same guideline proposes that stage 3 hypertension (above 180/110 mmHg) should be controlled before surgery. Control "can be achieved over several days to weeks of preoperative outpatient treatment." However, "if surgery is more urgent, rapid-acting agents can be administered that allow effective control in a matter of minutes or hours." Among the agents available, "beta blockers appear to be particularly attractive."[18] If beta-blockers are used, it makes sense to titrate heart rate to below 60 beats per minute to ensure that beta-blockade is adequate.[53] The guideline emphasizes that "continuation of preoperative antihypertensive treatment throughout the perioperative period is critical."[18] A similar approach has been suggested by others for many years.[8,54]

In the surgical setting, the issue of white coat hypertension is particularly complex. As many repeat blood pressure measurements as possible must be obtained to inform any clinical decision. Even with this information there is a danger that usually normotensive patients suffering from white-coat hypertension may have their operation deferred and be started on therapy unnecessarily on the occasion of surgery.

Finally, if surgery is to be deferred to allow the blood pressure to be treated, it is unclear for how long treatment should be given before the patient returns. A recent editorial suggests a period of several weeks after therapy has been started.[55]

The major obstacle to the production of agreed guidelines is that no study has, as yet, conclusively shown that treatment of hypertension brings about a significant improvement in outcome in surgical patients. A possible explanation for the lack of clear evidence that treating hypertension prior to anesthesia and surgery is beneficial is that most studies of risk factors have not distinguished between treated and untreated hypertensive patients. Often patients with a history of hypertension have been included, whether or not they were currently hypertensive. No study has tried to divide the patients into subgroups as a function of the severity of their hypertension.

In the absence of strong evidence, patients have to be considered individually. A number of adverse factors (Box 60–1) are taken into consideration for the long-term treatment of hypertension.[56] It is legitimate to consider that patients with such adverse factors need particularly careful assessment of the risk of anesthesia and surgery and very careful monitoring during the perioperative period. They may need treatment even though their blood pressure does not reach stage 3 hypertension levels.

Box 60–1

Adverse Factors Relevant to Hypertensive Patients

Major Risk Factors

Smoking
Dyslipidemia (hypercholesterolemia >6.5 mmol/L)
Age >60 years
Male/postmenopausal female
Family history of cardiovascular events

Evidence of Target-Organ Damage

Left ventricular hypertrophy
Clinical ischemic heart disease
Heart failure
Stroke/transient ischemic attacks
Nephropathy
Peripheral vascular disease
Retinopathy

From The Sixth Report of the Joint National Committee on Prevention, Detection, Evaluation, and Treatment of High Blood Pressure. *Arch Intern Med* 1997;157:2413–46.

In view of the difficulty of defining the level of blood pressure at which patients should be treated before anesthesia and surgery, the question of regional anesthesia as an alternative to general anesthesia arises. Regional anesthesia based on epidural blockade is used extensively mostly because of excellent postoperative pain control. However, in untreated hypertensive patients, extradural blockade was found to be associated with severe hypotension and bradycardia requiring emergency treatment. Such complications were not observed in any of the treated hypertensive patients.[57] As a result, the need for preoperative treatment of hypertension is the same as that for patients presenting for general anesthesia.

THE PROBLEM WITH ATENOLOL

As many hypertensive patients receive the beta-blocker atenolol, or treatment with atenolol is initiated before surgery, recent findings concerning this particular beta-blocker need to be discussed. In 1997 Palda and Detsky,[58] in the American College of Physicians guideline for the management of surgical patients with coronary artery disease or risk factors for that condition, stated that these patients should be given atenolol. In the 2002 American College of Cardiology/American Heart Association guideline on the same topic, beta-blockade has been suggested for use in untreated hypertensive patients.[18] Atenolol is often the first beta-blocker that comes to mind. However, a systematic review has shown atenolol to lack protection in the long-term management of arterial hypertension.[59] This inefficacy has also been demonstrated in the Anglo-Scandinavian Cardiac Outcomes Trial study (ASCOT).[60] The atenolol-diuretic arm of the study had to be discontinued because of the poor protection offered by this treatment. However, there is little information on the efficacy of atenolol in the prevention of perioperative cardiac events in hypertensive patients, as opposed to their long-term event rate. In a randomized study of patients with coronary heart disease or risk factors for this condition, Mangano et al.[61] showed that atenolol given for 7 days reduced the risk of myocardial ischemia and improved the long-term prognosis. As early adverse events (i.e., those occurring while patients were in hospital) were not taken into consideration, the benefits of atenolol in the short term can be questioned.

PREOPERATIVE EVALUATION

There is a need to answer the following three questions:
1. Is hypertension primary or secondary? Although secondary hypertension is infrequent, pheochromocytoma, hyperaldosteronism, renal parenchymal hypertension, and renovascular hypertension must be considered because of their anesthetic and perioperative implications. This is of utmost importance because undiagnosed pheochromocytoma is likely to cause life-threatening cardiovascular complications on the occasion of even minor operations.
2. Is the hypertension severe? This requires multiple blood pressure readings to distinguish "white-coat" hypertension from sustained hypertension.
3. Are target organs involved? The presence of coronary or cerebrovascular disease, impairment of renal function, electrocardiographic and radiologic signs of left ventricular hypertrophy, or heart failure puts the patient in a high-risk category. Such patients may require further investigations and/or treatment of the underlying conditions as well as of hypertension.

The frequent use of diuretics in the management of arterial hypertension often results in hypokalemia—unless potassium supplements, ACE inhibitors, or potassium-sparing diuretics are used. Potassium-sparing diuretics may be superior to nonsparing diuretics.[62] The presence of chronic hypokalemia raises the question of preoperative potassium replacement. This is controversial as rapid normalization of plasma potassium may worsen the transmembrane K^+ gradient, thereby increasing rather than decreasing the risk of arrhythmias.[63] In the absence of arrhythmia and U waves, and with normal T waves, the transmembrane K^+ gradient is likely to be within acceptable limits (i.e., a 35-fold difference) and potassium supplements may not be needed. If there are electrophysiologic signs of hypokalemia, slow replacement over days rather than hours is indicated.

INTERACTIONS BETWEEN ANTIHYPERTENSIVE MEDICATION AND ANESTHESIA

While it was previously believed that antihypertensive drugs should be stopped before anesthesia and surgery, this is no longer accepted. For most drugs, treatment is continued throughout the perioperative period and drugs are given the morning of surgery. Because of the possibility of drug interactions, the influence of antihypertensive drugs on the hemodynamic response to anesthesia and surgery has been studied extensively.

Early studies showed that beta-adrenoceptor blockers were well tolerated and promoted hemodynamic stability.[8] Beta-blockade has been shown to prevent both hypertension and tachycardia in response to laryngoscopy and intubation and to decrease the risk of perioperative myocardial ischemia[64,65] and adverse cardiac outcome.[61,66] The evidence for improved outcome, however, is relatively weak as shown in a very recent systematic review of perioperative beta-blockade outside cardiac surgery.[67] By contrast, beta-blockade clearly reduces the relative risk of death after coronary artery bypass surgery.[68]

In patients with mild or moderate hypertension, chronic treatment with calcium channel blockers, ACE inhibitors, diuretics, and beta-blockers does not cause exaggerated hypotensive responses to induction of anesthesia.[69] However, ACE inhibitors have been reported to cause hypotension if they are given on the morning of surgery, especially if large doses are used. Some authors recommend omitting the morning dose of ACE inhibitors.[70] Refractory hypotension may require the administration of terlipressin where conventional drugs have failed to achieve an acceptable blood pressure.[71-73] In cardiac surgery, at least, the practice of stopping ACE inhibitors can increase the need for emergency treatment of hypertensive episodes.[74] It is generally recommended that administration of angiotensin II receptor antagonists be stopped the day before surgery because of the risk of refractory hypotension requiring angiotensin or terlipressin (a peptide similar to vasopressin) to restore an acceptable pressure.[72,73,75,76]

Studies in patients treated with alpha$_2$-adrenoceptor agonists have shown a decrease in sympathetic responses to noxious stimuli, decreased catecholamine release, and improved cardiovascular stability.[77,78] Premedication with alpha$_2$-adrenoceptor agonists may be useful but is not widely used. Clonidine provides hemodynamic stability and reduces the risk of myocardial ischemia by reducing sympathoadrenal activity.[79] In addition, clonidine causes anxiolysis and sedation, decreases the need for both inhalation and intravenous anesthetics, and improves the quality of regional anesthesia. However, at least in coronary artery surgery, these benefits may be offset by an increased need for vasoactive and inotropic drugs. The interest for clonidine is likely to increase because its perioperative administration for a short period has been recently shown to decrease the risk of adverse cardiac events.[80] Dexmedetomidine is more selective for alpha$_2$-receptors than clonidine. It attenuates both hemodynamic and stress responses to surgery but could cause coronary vasoconstriction.[81] Mivazerol, another alpha$_2$-adrenoceptor agonist, was shown to minimize the risk of adverse cardiac outcome in patients undergoing vascular surgery.[82] Because it was not efficacious in other types of surgeries, the development of this agent was discontinued.

PERIOPERATIVE INCIDENTS AND THEIR MANAGEMENT

Cardiovascular instability is the hallmark of untreated or poorly controlled hypertension. In order to make the management of hypertensive patients safer, invasive blood pressure monitoring for major surgeries is clearly indicated. Blood pressure can then be actively managed to prevent departure of the mean arterial pressure of greater than 20% from baseline. Monitoring should continue into the postoperative period until it is clear that the patient is cardiovascularly stable. It is now frequently suggested that in patients in whom there is no contraindication, perioperative beta-blockade is valuable.[18]

In hypertensive patients, induction of anesthesia is often associated with large reductions in arterial pressure. This may precipitate myocardial ischemia because the reduction in diastolic pressure reduces the coronary perfusion pressure. Cerebral ischemia can occur because of the reduction in mean arterial pressure in patients with a right shifted cerebral autoregulation. In these circumstances vasopressors may be indicated.

Laryngoscopy and intubation often cause large increases in blood pressure and heart rate. Laryngeal spraying with local anesthetics is generally ineffective in preventing this response which is due to sympathetic activation. Protection can be obtained with beta-blockers,[8] including labetalol[83] and intravenous bolus doses of esmolol.[84] Glyceryltrinitrate,[85] sodium nitroprusside,[86] prostaglandin E$_1$,[85] and fentanyl[87] have all been shown to minimize the increase in blood pressure. Deep anesthesia and the administration of droperidol, vasodilators such as hydralazine, and calcium channel blockers also minimize the rise in blood pressure. As hypertension associated with tachycardia can cause myocardial ischemia, prevention of the hypertensive response to laryngoscopy, intubation, and extubation is clearly advisable.[8,88]

Severe perioperative hypertension is a major threat to hypertensive patients, especially increases of blood pressure in excess of about 20% of the preoperative value. Consequences of pressure surges include bleeding from vascular suture lines, cerebrovascular hemorrhage, and myocardial ischemia/infarction. The mortality rate of such events may be as high as 50%.

With adequate blood pressure monitoring, many vasoactive agents can be used safely. The choice of the most appropriate antihypertensive therapy depends upon the clinical scenario (i.e., whether there is tachycardia, myocardial ischemia, cardiac failure, or renal functional impairment) (Table 60–1).

In the face of the most severe hypertensive crises, sodium nitroprusside may be needed; as tachycardia is likely to occur and compromise the coronary circulation, the addition of a beta-blocker may be required. Phentolamine can be given as boluses or continuous infusion. It also causes tachycardia. Nitroglycerine is often advocated. Although it is not a very potent arteriolar dilator, its anti-ischemic properties are useful. Esmolol has gained wide acceptance in the control of hypertension and tachycardia in surgical patients. Because of its short half-life, esmolol has the advantage that undesirable side effects or poor tolerance, if they occur, are only short-lived. A continuous infusion is necessary if prolonged beta-blockade is required.

Other vasodilators for severe hypertension include diazoxide and oral drugs such as prazosin, doxazosin, and terazosin.

Labetalol, a stronger beta- than alpha-blocker, is an effective antihypertensive agent. Its relatively weak peripheral vasodilatation potentiates the hypotensive action of beta-blockade.

DRUGS FOR PERIOPERATIVE MANAGEMENT OF HYPERTENSIVE EMERGENCIES		
Clinical Requirement	**Mechanism of Action**	**Drug of Choice**
Extremely severe acute hypertension	NO donor	Sodium nitroprusside
Hypertension plus ischemia	NO donor	Nitroglycerine infusion
Hypertension plus tachycardia and ischemia	Beta blocker	Esmolol, bolus or infusion
	Alpha and beta blocker	Labetalol, bolus or infusion
Hypertension plus heart failure	ACE inhibitor, inodilator, vasodilator	Dobutamine, dopexamine
Hypertension without cardiac complication	Vasodilator	Hydralazine
		Phentolamine
		Nifedipine
		Nicardipine
Hypertension and renal impairment		Fenoldopam
Hypertension caused by pheochromocytoma		Phentolamine
		Labetalol
		Doxazosin, prazosin, terazosin
ACE, angiotensin converting enzyme; NO, nitric oxide.		

Table 60–1. Drugs for Perioperative Management of Hypertensive Emergencies

Intravenous hydralazine is an old "stand-by" with a proven track record. Its disadvantage is that it can cause marked tachycardia, as well as flushing, headaches, and dizziness.

Sublingual nifedipine is effective[89] but the reduction of blood pressure may be excessive and tachycardia may facilitate the development of ischemia. The sublingual route is difficult to control.[90] Yet 10 mg of sublingual nifedipine has been advocated in the management of postoperative hypertension after carotid endarterectomy.[91] However, because of the variability of its effects, sublingual nifedipine cannot be recommended.

Intravenous fenoldopam, a dopaminergic$_1$-receptor agonist, has been specifically tested in the management of postoperative hypertension.[92,93] At variance with other vasodilators, fenoldopam causes a natriuresis rather than sodium retention. There is risk of tachycardia.

Intraoperative and postoperative management has become safer owing to better monitoring, better anesthetic agents, and better recovery facilities. Nevertheless, the availability of very effective drugs to control hypertensive crises should not be taken as indication that proper preoperative preparation is no longer necessary. Devastating elevations in blood pressure can develop over 5 to 10 cardiac cycles: no drug, even injected intravenously immediately, can act quickly enough. It is therefore essential to ensure that patients with severe hypertension are well controlled before anesthesia and surgery. Similarly, those with moderate hypertension and target-organ involvement should be controlled. This approach coupled with the availability of potent hypotensive agents to combat hypertensive crises and effective vasopressors to restore adequate perfusion pressure should make it possible to reduce the risk of cardiovascular complications in surgical hypertensive patients.

SUMMARY

More than 30 years after the first detailed studies of the responses to anesthesia of hypertensive patients, specific evidence-based guidelines for their preoperative management are still lacking. Indeed, in an editorial published in 2004, Spahn and Priebe[55] state: "Any recommendation to postpone elective surgery for the purpose of blood pressure control must be balanced against the urgency and benefit of the planned operation; must take into account that arterial blood pressure should be corrected slowly, and up to two months may be required to reverse some of the hypertension-induced cardiovascular changes...." This echoes the view expressed earlier by Fleisher[53]: "Clearly the practice of postponing surgery must be balanced against the urgency of surgery."

Nevertheless, it is generally agreed that patients with stage 3 hypertension should be treated preoperatively, and those with stage 2 hypertension should be considered for treatment if there is evidence of target-organ damage.

The preoperative evaluation of hypertensive patients presents us with two unique opportunities: (1) to detect the presence of target-organ damage with appropriate investigations, and (2) to initiate long-term treatment where immediate treatment is not regarded as essential before surgery but is necessary for the long-term protection of the patient.[53]

REFERENCES

1. Primatesta P, Brookes M, Poulter NR. Improved hypertension management and control: results from the health survey for England 1998. *Hypertension* 2001;38:827–32.
2. Walley T, Duggan AK, Haycox AR, Niziol CJ. Treatment for newly diagnosed hypertension: patterns of prescribing and antihypertensive effectiveness in the UK. *J R Soc Med* 2003;96:525–31.
3. Lewington S, Clarke R, Qizilbash N, Peto R, Collins R. Age-specific relevance of usual blood pressure to vascular mortality: a meta-analysis of individual data for one million adults in 61 prospective studies. *Lancet* 2002; 360:1903–13.
4. Sprague HB. Heart in surgery;analysis of results of surgery on cardiac patients during past 10 years at Massachussetts General Hospital. *Surg Gynecol Obstet* 1929;49:54–58.
5. Dingle HR. Antihypertensive drugs and anaesthesia. *Anaesthesia* 1966; 21:151–72.
6. Prys Roberts C, Meloche R, Foex P. Studies of anaesthesia in relation to hypertension. I. Cardiovascular responses of treated and untreated patients. *Br J Anaesth* 1971;43:122–37.

7. Prys Roberts C, Greene LT, Meloche R, Foex P. Studies of anaesthesia in relation to hypertension. II. Haemodynamic consequences of induction and endotracheal intubation. *Br J Anaesth* 1971;43:531–47.
8. Prys-Roberts C, Foex P, Biro GP, Roberts JG. Studies of anaesthesia in relation to hypertension. V. Adrenergic beta-receptor blockade. *Br J Anaesth* 1973; 45:671–81.
9. Prys-Roberts C. Interactions of anaesthesia and high pre-operative doses of beta-receptor antagonists. *Acta Anaesthesiol Scand Suppl* 1982; 76:47–53.
10. Chobanian AV, Bakris GL, Black HR, Cushman WC, et al. The Seventh Report of the Joint National Committee on Prevention, Detection, Evaluation, and Treatment of High Blood Pressure: the JNC 7 report. *JAMA* 2003;289:2560–72.
11. Howell SJ, Sear JW, Foex P. Hypertension, hypertensive heart disease and perioperative cardiac risk. *Br J Anaesth* 2004;92:570–83.
12. Goldman L, Caldera DL, Nussbaum SR, Southwick FS, et al. Multifactorial index of cardiac risk in noncardiac surgical procedures. *N Engl J Med* 1977; 297(16):845–50.

13. Detsky AS, Abrams HB, Forbath N, Scott JG, et al. Cardiac assessment for patients undergoing noncardiac surgery. A multifactorial clinical risk index. *Arch Intern Med* 1986;146(11):2131–4.
14. Goldman L. Multifactorial index of cardiac risk in noncardiac surgery: ten-year status report. *J Cardiothorac Anesth* 1987;1(3):237–44.
15. Goldman L. Cardiac risk in noncardiac surgery: an update. *Anesth Analg* 1995; 80(4):810–20.
16. Lee TH, Marcantonio ER, Mangione CM, Thomas EJ, et al. Derivation and prospective validation of a simple index for prediction of cardiac risk of major noncardiac surgery. *Circulation* 1999; 100(10):1043–9.
17. Chassot PG, Delabays A, Spahn DR. Preoperative evaluation of patients with, or at risk of, coronary artery disease undergoing non-cardiac surgery. *Br J Anaesth* 2002;89:747–59.
18. Eagle KA, Berger PB, Calkins H, Chaitman BR, et al. ACC/AHA guideline update for perioperative cardiovascular evaluation for noncardiac surgery— executive summary a report of the American College of Cardiology/ American Heart Association Task Force on Practice Guidelines (Committee to

Update the 1996 Guidelines on Perioperative Cardiovascular Evaluation for Noncardiac Surgery). *Circulation* 2002;105:1257–67.

19. Goldman L, Caldera DL. Risks of general anesthesia and elective operation in the hypertensive patient. *Anesthesiology* 1979;50(4):285–92.

20. Cooperman M, Pflug B, Martin EW Jr, Evans WE. Cardiovascular risk factors in patients with peripheral vascular disease. *Surgery* 1978;84:505–9.

21. Eerola M, Eerola R, Kaukinen S, Kaukinen L. Risk factors in surgical patients with verified preoperative myocardial infarction. *Acta Anaesthesiol Scand* 1980;24:219–23.

22. Steen PA, Tinker JH, Tarhan S. Myocardial reinfarction after anesthesia and surgery. *JAMA* 1978;239:2566–70.

23. Aronson S, Boisvert D, Lapp W. Isolated systolic hypertension is associated with adverse outcomes from coronary artery bypass graft surgery. *Anesth Analg* 2002;94:1079–84.

24. Howell SJ, Sear YM, Yeates D, Goldacre M, et al. Risk factors for cardiovascular death after elective surgery under general anaesthesia. *Br J Anaesth* 1998; 80(1):14–9.

25. Howell SJ, Sear JW, Sear YM, Yeates D, et al. Risk factors for cardiovascular death within 30 days after anaesthesia and urgent or emergency surgery: a nested case-control study. *Br J Anaesth* 1999;82(5):679–84.

26. 2003 European Society of Hypertension–European Society of Cardiology guidelines for the management of arterial hypertension. *J Hypertens* 2003;21:1011–53.

27. Liao YL, Liu KA, Dyer A, Schoenberger JA, et al. Major and minor electrocardiographic abnormalities and risk of death from coronary heart disease, cardiovascular diseases and all causes in men and women. *J Am Coll Cardiol* 1988;12:1494–500.

28. Stamler J, Dyer AR, Shekelle RB, Neaton J, et al. Relationship of baseline major risk factors to coronary and all-cause mortality, and to longevity: findings from long-term follow-up of Chicago cohorts. *Cardiology* 1993; 82:191–222.

29. Allman KG, Muir A, Howell SJ, Hemming AE, et al. Resistant hypertension and preoperative silent myocardial ischaemia in surgical patients. *Br J Anaesth* 1994;73:574–8.

30. Stamler J, Stamler R, Neaton JD. Blood pressure, systolic and diastolic, and cardiovascular risks. US population data. *Arch Intern Med* 1993;153:598–615.

31. Howell SJ, Hemming AE, Allman KG, Glover L, et al. Predictors of postoperative myocardial ischaemia. The role of intercurrent arterial hypertension and other cardiovascular risk factors. *Anaesthesia* 1997;52:107–11.

32. Franklin SS. Cardiovascular risks related to increased diastolic, systolic and pulse pressure. An epidemiologist's point of view. *Pathol Biol (Paris)* 1999;47:594–603.

33. Franklin SS, Gustin Wt, Wong ND, Larson MG, et al. Hemodynamic patterns of age-related changes in blood pressure. The Framingham Heart Study. *Circulation* 1997;96:308–15.

34. Tamborini G, Maltagliati A, Trupiano L, Berna G, et al. Lowering of blood pressure and coronary blood flow in isolated systolic hypertension. *Coronary Artery Dis* 2001;12:259–65.

35. Pickering TG, Coats A, Mallion JM, Mancia G, et al. Blood Pressure Monitoring. Task force V: white-coat hypertension. *Blood Press Monit* 1999; 4:333–41.

36. Casadei B, Abuzeid H. Is there a strong rationale for deferring elective surgery in patients with poorly controlled hypertension? *J Hypertens* 2005;23:19–22.

37. Bedford RF, Feinstein B. Hospital admission blood pressure: a predictor for hypertension following endotracheal intubation. *Anesth Analg* 1980;59: 367–70.

38. Estafanous FG. Hypertension in the surgical patient: management of blood pressure and anesthesia. *Cleve Clin J Med* 1989;56:385–93.

39. Low JM, Harvey JT, Prys-Roberts C, Dagnino J. Studies of anaesthesia in relation to hypertension. VII. Adrenergic responses to laryngoscopy. *Br J Anaesth* 1986;58:471–7.

40. Longnecker DE. Alpine anesthesia: can pretreatment with clonidine decrease the peaks and valleys? *Anesthesiology* 1987;67:1–2.

41. Folkow B. Structure and function of the arteries in hypertension. *Am Heart J* 1987;114:938–48.

42. Barry DI, Lassen NA. Cerebral blood flow autoregulation in hypertension and effects of antihypertensive drugs. *J Hypertens* 1984;2:S519–26.

43. Chung F, Mezei G, Tong D. Pre-existing medical conditions as predictors of adverse events in day-case surgery. *Br J Anaesth* 1999;83:262–70.

44. Forrest JB, Rehder K, Cahalan MK, et al. Multicenter study of general anesthesia. III. Predictors of severe perioperative adverse outcomes. *Anesthesiology* 1992; 76:3–15.

45. Reich DL, Bodian CA, Krol M, Kuroda M, et al. Intraoperative hemodynamic predictors of mortality, stroke, and myocardial infarction after coronary artery bypass surgery. *Anesth Analg* 1999;89:814–22.

46. Slogoff S, Keats AS. Does perioperative myocardial ischemia lead to postoperative myocardial infarction? *Anesthesiology* 1985;62:107–14.

47. Reich DL, Bennett-Guerrero E, Bodian CA, Hossain S, et al. Intraoperative tachycardia and hypertension are independently associated with adverse outcome in noncardiac surgery of long duration. *Anesth Analg* 2002;95:273–7.

48. Charlson ME, MacKenzie CR, Gold JP, Ales KL, et al. Intraoperative blood pressure. What patterns identify patients at risk for postoperative complications? *Ann Surg* 1990; 212:567–80.

49. Dix P, Howell S. Survey of cancellation rate of hypertensive patients undergoing anaesthesia and elective surgery. *Br J Anaesth* 2001;86:789–93.

50. Morrissey S, Alun-Jones T, Leighton S. Why are operations cancelled? *BMJ* 1989;299:778.

51. Wildner M, Bulstrode C, Spivey J, Carr A, et al. Avoidable causes of cancellation in elective orthopaedic surgery. *Health Trends* 1991;23:115–6.

52. Foex P. Hypertension in 2005: who should be cancelled? *Acta Anaesthesiol Scand* 2005;49(Suppl. 117):140–2.

53. Fleisher LA. Preoperative evaluation of the patient with hypertension. *JAMA* 2002;287:2043–6.

54. Prys-Roberts C. Systolic hypertension. A reply. *Anaesthesia* 2002;57:606–7.

55. Spahn DR, Priebe HJ. Editorial II. Preoperative hypertension: remain wary? "Yes"—cancel surgery? "No." *Br J Anaesth* 2004;92:461–4.

56. The sixth report of the Joint National Committee on prevention, detection, evaluation, and treatment of high blood pressure. *Arch Intern Med* 1997; 157:2413–46.

57. Dagnino J, Prys-Roberts C. Studies of anaesthesia in relation to hypertension. VI. Cardiovascular responses to extradural blockade of treated and untreated hypertensive patients. *Br J Anaesth* 1984;56:1065–73.

58. Palda VA, Detsky AS. Perioperative assessment and management of risk from coronary artery disease. *Ann Intern Med* 1997;127:313–28.

59. Carlberg B, Samuelsson O, Lindholm LH. Atenolol in hypertension: is it a wise choice? *Lancet* 2004;364:1684–9.

60. ASCOT Study Investigators. *Anglo-Scandinavian Cardiac Outcomes Trial Study (ASCOT).* Available at: www.ascotstudy.org.

61. Mangano DT, Layug EL, Wallace A, Tateo I. Effect of atenolol on mortality and cardiovascular morbidity after noncardiac surgery. Multicenter Study of Perioperative Ischemia Research Group. *N Engl J Med* 1996;335(23):1713–20.

62. Hoes AW, Grobbee DE, Lubsen J, Man-in-'t-Veld AJ, et al. Diuretics, beta-blockers, and the risk for sudden cardiac death in hypertensive patients. *Ann Intern Med* 1995;123:481–7.

63. Wong BI, McLean RF, Fremes SE, Deemar KA, et al. Aprotinin and tranexamic acid for high transfusion risk cardiac surgery. *Ann Thorac Surg* 2000;69:808–16.

64. Stone JG, Foex P, Sear JW, Johnson LL, et al. Myocardial ischemia in untreated hypertensive patients: effect of a single small oral dose of a beta-adrenergic blocking agent. *Anesthesiology* 1988; 68:495–500.

65. Wallace A, Layug B, Tateo I, Li J, et al. Prophylactic atenolol reduces postoperative myocardial ischemia. McSPI Research Group. *Anesthesiology* 1998;88:7–17.

66. Poldermans D, Boersma E, Bax JJ, Thomson IR, et al. The effect of bisoprolol on perioperative mortality and myocardial infarction in high-risk patients undergoing vascular surgery. *N Engl J Med* 1999;341:1789–94.

67. Devereaux PJ, Beattie WS, Choi PT, Badner NH, et al. How strong is the evidence for the use of perioperative beta blockers in non-cardiac surgery? Systematic review and meta-analysis of randomised controlled trials. *BMJ* 2005; 331:313–21.

68. Weightman WM, Gibbs NM, Sheminant MR, Whitford EG, et al. Drug therapy before coronary artery surgery: nitrates are independent predictors of mortality and beta-adrenergic blockers predict survival. *Anesth Analg* 1999;88:286–91.

69. Sear JW, Jewkes C, Tellez JC, Foex P. Does the choice of antihypertensive therapy influence haemodynamic

responses to induction, laryngoscopy and intubation? *Br J Anaesth* 1994; 73:303–8.

70. Coriat P, Richer C, Douraki T, Gomez C, et al. Influence of chronic angiotensin-converting enzyme inhibition on anesthetic induction. *Anesthesiology* 1994;81:299–307.

71. Eyraud D, Brabant S, Nathalie D, Fleron MH, et al. Treatment of intraoperative refractory hypotension with terlipressin in patients chronically treated with an antagonist of the renin-angiotensin system. *Anesth Analg* 1999;88:980–4.

72. Boccara G, Ouattara A, Godet G, Dufresne E, et al. Terlipressin versus norepinephrine to correct refractory arterial hypotension after general anesthesia in patients chronically treated with renin-angiotensin system inhibitors. *Anesthesiology* 2003; 98:1338–44.

73. Meersschaert K, Brun L, Gourdin M, Mouren S, et al. Terlipressin-ephedrine versus ephedrine to treat hypotension at the induction of anesthesia in patients chronically treated with angiotensin converting-enzyme inhibitors: a prospective, randomized, double-blinded, crossover study. *Anesth Analg* 2002;94:835–40.

74. Pigott DW, Nagle C, Allman K, Westaby S, et al. Effect of omitting regular ACE inhibitor medication before cardiac surgery on haemodynamic variables and vasoactive drug requirements. *Br J Anaesth* 1999; 83:715–20.

75. Brabant SM, Eyraud D, Bertrand M, Coriat P. Refractory hypotension after induction of anesthesia in a patient chronically treated with angiotensin receptor antagonists. *Anesth Analg* 1999;89:887–8.

76. Bertrand M, Godet G, Meersschaert K, Brun L, et al. Should the angiotensin II

antagonists be discontinued before surgery? *Anesth Analg* 2001;92:26–30.

77. Quintin L, Roudot F, Roux C, Macquin I, et al. Effect of clonidine on the circulation and vasoactive hormones after aortic surgery. *Br J Anaesth* 1991; 66:108–15.

78. Stuhmeier KD, Mainzer B, Cierpka J, Sandmann W, et al. Small, oral dose of clonidine reduces the incidence of intraoperative myocardial ischemia in patients having vascular surgery. *Anesthesiology* 1996;85:706–12.

79. Nishina K, Mikawa K, Uesugi T, Obara H, et al. Efficacy of clonidine for prevention of perioperative myocardial ischemia: a critical appraisal and meta-analysis of the literature. *Anesthesiology* 2002;96:323–9.

80. Wallace AW, Galindez D, Salahieh A, Layug EL, et al. Effect of clonidine on cardiovascular morbidity and mortality after noncardiac surgery. *Anesthesiology* 2004;101:284–93.

81. Jalonen J, Halkola L, Kuttila K, Perttila J, et al. Effects of dexmedetomidine on coronary hemodynamics and myocardial oxygen balance. *J Cardiothorac Vasc Anesth* 1995;9:519–24.

82. Oliver MF, Goldman L, Julian DG, Holme I. Effect of mivazerol on perioperative cardiac complications during non-cardiac surgery in patients with coronary heart disease: the European Mivazerol Trial (EMIT). *Anesthesiology* 1999;91:951–61.

83. Chung KS, Sinatra RS, Chung JH. The effect of an intermediate dose of labetalol on heart rate and blood pressure responses to laryngoscopy and intubation. *J Clin Anesth* 1992;4:11–5.

84. Figueredo E, Garcia Fuentes EM. Assessment of the efficacy of esmolol on the haemodynamic changes induced by laryngoscopy and tracheal intubation: a meta-analysis. *Acta Anaesthesiol Scand* 2001;45:1011–22.

85. van den Berg AA, Savva D, Honjol NM. Attenuation of the haemodynamic responses to noxious stimuli in patients undergoing cataract surgery. A comparison of magnesium sulphate, esmolol, lignocaine, nitroglycerine and placebo given i.v. with induction of anaesthesia. *Eur J Anaesthesiol* 1997; 14:134–47.

86. Sklar GS, Oka Y. Sodium nitroprusside and the pressor response to laryngoscopy and intubation. *Mt Sinai J Med* 1979; 46:384–7.

87. Adachi YU, Satomoto M, Higuchi H, Watanabe K. Fentanyl attenuates the hemodynamic response to endotracheal intubation more than the response to laryngoscopy. *Anesth Analg* 2002; 95:233–7.

88. Hartley M, Vaughan RS. Problems associated with tracheal extubation. *Br J Anaesth* 1993;71:561–8.

89. Adler AG, Leahy JJ, Cressman MD. Management of perioperative hypertension using sublingual nifedipine. Experience in elderly patients undergoing eye surgery. *Arch Intern Med* 1986;146:1927–30.

90. Grossman E, Messerli FH. Effect of calcium antagonists on plasma norepinephrine levels, heart rate, and blood pressure. *Am J Cardiol* 1997; 80:1453–8.

91. Retamal O, Coriat P, Pamela F, Godet G, et al. Prevention of hypertensive attacks after carotid surgery. The value of nifedipine and diltiazem. *Ann Fr Anesth Reanim* 1986;5:278–86.

92. Murphy MB, Murray C, Shorten GD. Fenoldopam: a selective peripheral dopamine-receptor agonist for the treatment of severe hypertension. *N Engl J Med* 2001;345:1548–57.

93. Yakazu Y, Iwasawa K, Narita H, Kindscher JD, et al. Hemodynamic and sympathetic effects of fenoldopam and sodium nitroprusside. *Acta Anaesthesiol Scand* 2001;45:1176–80.

Chapter

61

Hypertension in the Context of Acute Myocardial Infarction and Percutaneous Coronary Interventions

Rumi Jaumdally and Gregory Y. H. Lip

Key Findings

- Reduction of blood pressure should be gradual to avoid end-organ hypoperfusion.
- Adequate analgesia and an anxiolytic if indicated should be prescribed.
- First-line treatment should include intravenous nitrates or beta blocker with sodium nitroprusside, and/or a calcium antagonist as alternatives, in severe hypertensive emergencies.
- Primary angioplasty is an option if thrombolytic therapy is unacceptable and such service is available.
- In the long-term postcoronary event, beta-blockers and angiotensin-converting enzyme inhibitors are the mainstays of treatment with convincing mortality benefits. In cases with clear contraindications or intolerance to the former, a calcium antagonist, such as verapamil or diltiazem, may be used as an alternative in patients with good left ventricular function.

Clinical Implications

- Thrombolytic therapy and glycoprotein IIb/IIIa inhibitor use may be delayed or contraindicated due to higher risk of cerebral hemorrhage with uncontrolled hypertension.
- Abnormal baseline electrocardiography may cause diagnostic uncertainty and mask ongoing ischemia.
- Left ventricular hypertrophy results in more cardiac complications or sudden cardiac death.
- Secondary causes of severe hypertension should be considered (e.g., aortic dissection, renal artery stenosis, pheochromocytoma).
- Risk of catheter-induced dissection of the aorta or coronary artery is higher in association with uncontrolled hypertension.

During sleep, blood pressure (BP) in most people is between 10% and 20% lower than the mean daytime value. On arousal and the start of day-to-day activities, there is a surge in BP that may last for 4 to 6 hours. Indeed, cardiovascular events, such as MI, cardiac ischemia, and stroke are more frequent in the morning hours soon after waking compared to other times of day.

For any given level of BP, mortality rates from coronary heart disease vary among different populations and ethnic groups. In the Seven Countries study,[3] for example, the absolute risk was much higher in the United States and Northern Europe compared to Japan and Mediterranean populations with similar BP. Indo-Asians appear to have a higher complication rate than white Europeans for equivalent BP elevations.[4,5] Indo-Asians also tend to experience cardiovascular events at a younger age, but have a lower rate of self-reported hypertension.[6,7] Afro-Caribbean patients with hypertension are also at greater risk of developing cardiovascular complications compared to white Europeans.[8]

As increased sympathetic nervous system activity has been implicated in the pathophysiology of high BP, a heightened pain exposure response to physical and psychosocial stress can result in high BP levels being recorded in patients undergoing PCI or with an AMI, who are not known to have precedent or antecedent hypertension. Rarely, accelerated or malignant phase hypertension can present with an AMI, as can illicit drug use. For example, MI remains the most frequent, single reported cardiac complication of cocaine use, which itself predisposes to hypertension and left ventricular hypertrophy (LVH).[9] Systemic causes of arteritis, such as lupus erythematosus and arch aortitis, can also present with a combination of hypertension and AMI.

CLINICAL ASSESSMENT

In addition to a clear and detailed history pertaining to coronary disease, patients should be asked specifically about the initial diagnosis of high BP, the duration of therapy, compliance, and drug type. Other clinical features such as ethnicity, time of presentation, and noninvasive investigations should be noted.

In patients with poorly controlled hypertension, the baseline 12-lead electrocardiogram (ECG) is frequently

Hypertension commonly coexists in patients presenting with acute myocardial infarction (AMI) or undergoing percutaneous coronary interventions (PCIs), often in association with hyperlipidemia and diabetes mellitus. Given the exaggerated coronary event rate in a diabetic cohort, up to 75% of these complications may be attributable to coexisting hypertension.[1] Effective treatment of hypertension leads to substantial reductions in stroke, coronary events, and cardiovascular mortality.[1,2]

abnormal with lateral ST-T segment depression and left bundle branch block, often in association with LVH.[10] As such changes mimic those of cardiac ischemia and infarction, unnecessary delay and confusion may arise in diagnosis, with further problems in recognizing ongoing cardiac ischemia or even re-infarction (Box 61–1).

THERAPEUTIC STRATEGIES

Once the diagnosis of acute coronary occlusion is made, patients with a very high BP present a clinical dilemma. Uncontrolled BP may contribute to a risk of bleeding with thrombolytic therapy for acute MI, or with the multiple antithrombotic drugs (aspirin, clopidogrel, glycoprotein IIb/IIIa inhibitors) used during PCI. Poorly controlled BP may also increase the risk of procedural blood loss during PCI maneuvers.

While use of thrombolytic agents is contraindicated in the presence of very high BP (>180/110 mmHg),[11] intravenous drug infusions to achieve adequate BP control may delay and exacerbate myocardial perfusion. Care should be taken to avoid an abrupt reduction of pressure with consequent loss of vasomotor autoregulation.[12] The effects may manifest as cerebral "watershed" infarction, acute tubular necrosis, and even more subendocardial ischemia. The aim, therefore, should be to lower the BP using intravenous drugs infused slowly, with stringent clinical assessment of the patient (Table 61–1).

Nitrates

Nitroglycerine (GTN) infusion probably has the safest profile, and thus is recommended as first-line treatment to lower BP in the acute setting. Nitrates lower the cardiac venous return at low doses with arteriolar (including coronary arteriolar) dilatation, thus improving both heart

failure and myocardial perfusion. In those patients with marked coronary spasm presenting with or exacerbating acute infarction, nitrate-induced vasodilatation may also be of particular benefit. A useful regimen of 5 to 10 mcg/minute with increases of 5 to 20 mcg/minute until symptoms are relieved or mean arterial BP is reduced by up to 30% for hypertensive patients has been suggested. Alternatively, sodium nitroprusside results in a reduction of both pre- and after-load in patients with BP in excess of 180/110 mmHg. In the context of AMI and PCI, nitrates have the advantage of prompt resolution (within

DRUGS FOR HYPERTENSIVE EMERGENCIES DURING AMI AND PERCUTANEOUS CORONARY INTERVENTION		
	Indication	Caution
Benzodiazepine	Anxiety / Drug abuse	Respiratory depressant
Morphine	Analgesia	Confusion state
ACE inhibitors	Heart failure / Diabetes	Aortic valve and renovascular disease / Volume depletion
Beta-blocker	AMI / Angina	Peripheral and pulmonary disease / Heart failure and block / Cocaine use
Calcium antagonist (dihydropyridine)	Isolated systolic hypertension in the elderly	Sublingual short-acting nifedipine should not be used
Calcium antagonist (rate limiting, nondihydropyridine)	Angina / AMI	Heart failure and block / Recent beta-blocker use
Nitrates or sodium nitroprusside	All	Concomitant use of sildenafil / Dehydration / Right ventricular AMI

AMI, acute myocardial infarction; ACE, antiotension-converting enzyme.

Table 61–1. Drugs for Hypertensive Emergencies during AMI and Percutaneous Coronary Intervention

minutes) of BP after intravenous cessation but reflex tachycardia remains an undesirable feature.

Pooled analyses of clinical trials have suggested a modest mortality benefit from nitrate-like preparations used acutely in AMI, with possibly three to four fewer deaths for every 1000 patients treated.[13] Thus, nitrates should be used if hypotension limits the administration of beta-blockers, which may exert more beneficial effects. Care should be employed if the systolic pressure drops below 90 mmHg in patients with suspected tachycardia or right ventricular wall ischemia or infarction.

Beta-blocker

In the absence of contraindications such as acute heart failure, conduction defects, advanced peripheral artery disease, and pulmonary disease, beta-blockers should be considered as first-line therapy particularly in the first few hours of AMI. Beta-blockers can be administered either orally or by infusion, and intravenous agents such as esmolol and metoprolol have a short half-life, with fast onset and offset of action.

These drugs are effective at lowering BP, and have beneficial cardiac effects by lowering the heart rate, myocardial oxygen demand, wall stress, ventricular arrhythmias, and cardiac output.[14] Furthermore, there is compelling evidence that beta-blockers as acute secondary prevention reduce the risk of all-cause mortality, coronary mortality, recurrent nonfatal MI, and sudden death in these patients.[15]

Following fibrinolytic therapy, intravenous metoprolol was associated with a diminished incidence of subsequent nonfatal reinfarction and recurrent ischemia, together with lowered rate of re-infarction or death if given early (<2 hours).[16] Such an effect appears in patients who are not receiving thrombolysis, with early studies suggesting a modestly favorable influence on infarct size and mortality benefit as well.[17,18] However, caution should be observed in patients with AMI precipitated by cocaine use because of the risk of exacerbating coronary spasm.[19]

Randomized trials of beta-blocker therapy in patients undergoing primary PCI have not been performed. However, for those with transient or sustained LV dysfunction, beta-blocker use has been associated with a reduction in composite endpoint of all-cause and cardiovascular mortality, and recurrent nonfatal MIs, whether patients had thrombolysis or PCI for AMI.[20] In the context of primary PCI,[21] beta-blockers can reduce malignant ventricular tachycardia[22] and minimize myocyte necrosis, as assayed using periprocedural creatinine kinase release.[23,24] Pre-treatment may also reduce mortality within the hospital and at a year.[25] As potential inhibitor of vascular smooth muscle–cell migration and proliferation,[26] some data even suggest that beta-blockers may lower clinical restenosis following PCI.[27]

Calcium channel antagonists

The calcium antagonists are effective antihypertensive drugs. Short-acting dihydropyridine calcium antagonists (in particular, sublingual nifedipine) can induce reflex tachycardia and dose-related BP fluctuations that may be detrimental in the setting of an acute MI. Trials in the 1980s of early or late use of nifedipine in patients with AMI have yielded no clear benefit, with the potential for exacerbating ischemia or re-infarction. It appears that there is no role for sublingual or oral nifedipine preparation in treating high BP during AMI. Long-acting dihydropyridine such as amlodipine and nisoldipine have also been studied following PCI. However, randomized controlled trials using the stent procedure showed no reduction in luminal loss following PCI.[28,29]

Rate-limiting calcium antagonists (verapamil and diltiazem) may be useful in the absence of heart failure or LV dysfunction, especially if beta-blockers are contra-indicated and atrial tachyarrhythmias are present. In cases of balloon angioplasty, a meta-analysis of calcium channel blocker use in five trials has shown a reduction in angiographic restenosis.[30] In the Verapamil Slow-Release for Prevention of Cardiovascular Events after Angioplasty (VESPA) Trial, the use of verapamil within 30 minutes of PCI and bare metal stent implantation gave broadly similar results.[31] Thus, the use of rate-limiting calcium antagonist may potentially help in reducing coronary spasm and flow during PCI.

Angiotensin-converting enzyme inhibitors and angiotensin receptor blockers

Angiotensin-converting enzyme (ACE) inhibitors are potent antihypertensive drugs via their vasodilator, neuro-hormonal, sympathetic, and renal effects. All the trials investigating oral ACE inhibitor prescription within 24 hours of AMI have shown beneficial results. In a large meta-analysis of more than 100,000 patients randomized following AMI, prescription of ACE inhibitors was linked with a reduction of about 7% in mortality. Patients, who seem to have the highest benefit belong to the 55- to 75-year age group, had anterior territory infarct, and had features of heart failure.[32] However, data from the Cooperative New Scandinavian Enalapril Survival Study (CONSENSUS) pointed to an increase in adverse clinical effects in the group treated with intravenous ACE inhibitor. This outcome seems to be related to inducing hypotension in an older cohort within the trial.

Data for the angiotensin receptor blockers (ARBs) also appear encouraging, suggesting that they may be comparable to ACE inhibitors. In the two trials comparing ARBs (losartan and valsartan) with captopril,[33,34] no difference in mortality was found at follow-up between the two drugs. Thus, ARBs could be considered in patients with AMI who are intolerant of ACE inhibitors, especially in the setting of LV dysfunction.

For patients undergoing PCI electively, oral ACE inhibitors remain the drug of choice. In the longer term, ACE inhibitor treatment is effective in cardiovascular prevention among patients with coronary artery disease, with particular benefits for those with LV dysfunction and diabetes.[35,36] There are no randomized trials looking at its systemic use in acute primary PCI. Several groups have investigated possible benefits of ACE inhibitors on secondary endpoints following PCI. Although ACE inhibitor therapy before PCI may lead to a reduction in the requirement for revascularization after coronary stent deployment,[37] randomized clinical trials have failed to show any significant reduction in coronary events[38] or instent restenosis.[39,40]

SUMMARY

In patients with AMI and those undergoing PCI, underlying secondary causes of hypertension should be excluded. Adequate analgesia and an anxiolytic if indicated should be prescribed.

In the majority of patients with AMI or undergoing PCI, treatment should be aimed at optimizing and restoring blood flow to viable but ischemic myocardial tissue, minimizing drug side effects and reducing mortality. Reduction of BP should be gradual to avoid end-organ hypoperfusion. Recommended strategies could include a regimen leading to a 30% reduction of BP gradually over minutes without inducing a drop to a systolic of less than 90 mmHg. First-line intravenous treatment should include a beta-blocker, failing which intravenous nitrates or sodium nitroprusside can be used. As for initiation of oral therapy within hours of AMI and PCI, beta-blockers and ACE inhibitor remain the drugs of choice. In all cases, contraindications to these drugs should be carefully screened for, with careful monitoring of vital signs during drug administration. Primary angioplasty is an option if thrombolytic therapy is unacceptable and such a service is available. An approach to the patient with AMI and severe hypertension is summarized in Figure 61–1.

In the long-term postcoronary event and or procedure, beta-blockers and ACE inhibitors are the mainstays of treatment with convincing mortality benefit. In cases with clear contraindications or intolerance to the former, ARBs may be used as an alternative. In patients withgood LV function, the rate-limiting calcium antagonists are an option.

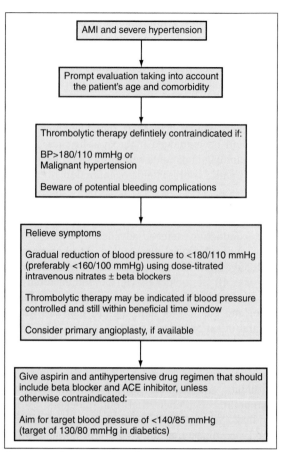

Figure 61–1. Approach to the patient with acute myocardial infarction and severe hypertension.

REFERENCES

1. Lakka HM, Laaksonen DE, Lakka TA, Niskanen LK, Kumpusalo E, Tuomilehto J, et al. The metabolic syndrome and total and cardiovascular disease mortality in middle-aged men. *JAMA* 2002;288:2709–16.
2. He FJ, MacGregor GA. Cost of poor blood pressure control in the UK: 62,000 unnecessary deaths per year. *J Hum Hypertens* 2003;17:455–7.
3. Van den Hoogen PC, Feskens EJ, Nagelkerke NJ, Menotti A, Nissinen A, Kromhout D. The relation between blood pressure and mortality due to coronary heart disease among men in different parts of the world. Seven Countries Study Research Group. *N Engl J Med* 2000;342:1–8.
4. Miller GJ, Kirkwood BR, Beckles GL, Alexis SD, Carson DC, Byam NT. Adult male all-cause, cardiovascular and cerebrovascular mortality in relation to ethnic group, systolic blood pressure and blood glucose concentration in Trinidad, West Indies. *Int J Epidemiol* 1988;17:62–9.

5. Khattar RS, Swales JD, Senior R, Lahiri A. Racial variation in cardiovascular morbidity and mortality in essential hypertension. *Heart* 2000;83:267–71.
6. Saleheen D, Frossard P. CAD risk factors and acute myocardial infarction in Pakistan. *Acta Cardiol* 2004;59:417–24.
7. Yusuf S, Hawken S, Ounpuu S, Dans T, Avezum A, Lanas F, et al. INTERHEART Study Investigators. Effect of potentially modifiable risk factors associated with myocardial infarction in 52 countries (the INTERHEART study): case-control study. *Lancet* 2004;364:937–52.
8. Hammond IW, Devereux RB, Alderman MH, Lutas EM, Spitzer MC, Crowley JS, et al. The prevalence and correlates of echocardiographic left ventricular hypertrophy among employed patients with uncomplicated hypertension. *J Am Coll Cardiol* 1986;7:639–50.
9. Brickner ME, Willard JE, Eichhorn EJ, Black J, Grayburn PA. Left ventricular hypertrophy associated with chronic cocaine abuse. *Circulation* 1991;84:1130–5.

10. Kannel WB, Gordon T, Castelli WP, et al. Electrocardiographic left ventricular hypertrophy and risk of coronary heart disease: the Framingham study. *Ann Intern Med* 1970;72:813–22.
11. Gurwitz JF, Gore JM, Goldberg RJ, et al. Risk for intracranial haemorrhage after tissue plasminogen activator treatment for acute myocardial infarction. Participants in the National Registry of Myocardial Infarction 2. *Ann Intern Med* 1998;129:597–604.
12. Prisant LM, Carr AA, Hawkins DW. Treating hypertensive emergencies. Controlled reduction of blood pressure and protection of target organs. *Postgrad Med* 1993;93:92–110.
13. ISIS-4 (Fourth International Study of Infarct Survival) Collaborative Group. ISIS-4: a randomised factorial trial assessing early oral captopril, oral mononitrate, and intravenous magnesium sulphate in 58,050 patients with suspected acute myocardial infarction. *Lancet* 1995;345:669–85.

14. Lip GYH, Lydakis C, Beevers DG. Management of patients with myocardial infarction and hypertension. *Eur Heart J* 2000;21:1125–34.

15. Teo KK, Yusuf S, Furberg CD. Effects of prophylactic antiarrhythmic drug therapy in acute myocardial infarction. *JAMA* 1993;270:1589–95.

16. The TIMI Study Group. Comparison of invasive and conservative strategies after treatment with intravenous tissue plasminogen activator in acute myocardial infarction: results of the thrombolysis in myocardial infarction (TIMI) phase II trial. *N Engl J Med* 1989;320:618–27.

17. First International Study of Infarct Survival Collaborative Group. Randomised trial of intravenous atenolol among 16 027 cases of suspected acute myocardial infarction: ISIS–1. *Lancet* 1986;2:57–66.

18. Yusuf S, Peto R, Lewis J, Collins R, Sleight P. Beta blockade during and after myocardial infarction: an overview of the randomized trials. *Prog Cardiovasc Dis* 1985;27:335–71.

19. Kloner RA, Hale S. Unraveling the complex effects of cocaine on the heart. *Circulation* 1993;87:1046–7.

20. Dargie HJ. Effect of carvedilol on outcome after myocardial infarction in patients with left-ventricular dysfunction: the CAPRICORN randomised trial. *Lancet* 2001;357:1385–90.

21. Halkin A, Grines CL, Cox DA, Garcia E, Mehran R, Tcheng JE, et al. Impact of intravenous beta-blockade before primary angioplasty on survival in patients undergoing mechanical reperfusion therapy for acute myocardial infarction. *J Am Coll Cardiol* 2004;43: 1780–7.

22. Mehta RH, Harjai KJ, Grines L. Sustained ventricular tachycardia or fibrillation in cardiac catheterization laboratory among patients receiving primary percutaneous coronary intervention: incidence, predictors and outcomes. *J Am Coll Cardiol* 2004;43:1765–72.

23. Sharma SK, Annapoorna K, Marmur J, Fuster V. Cardioprotective effect of prior beta-blocker therapy in reducing creatine kinase-MB elevation after coronary intervention. *Circulation* 2000; 102:166–72.

24. Wang FW, Osman A, Otero J, Stouffer GA, Waxman S, Afzal A, et al. Distal myocardial protection during percutaneous coronary intervention with an intracoronary beta-blocker. *Circulation* 2003;107:2914–9.

25. Harjai KJ, Stone GW, Boura J, Grines Li, Garcia E, Brodie B, et al. Effects of prior beta-blocker therapy on clinical outcomes after primary coronary angioplasty for acute myocardial infarction. *Am J Cardiol* 2003;91: 6:655–60.

26. Sung CP, Arleth AJ, Eichman C, Truneh A, Ohlstein EH. Carvedilol, a multiple-action neurohumoral antagonist, inhibits mitogen-activated protein kinase and cell cycle progression in vascular smooth muscle cells. *J Pharmacol Exp Ther* 1997;283:910–7.

27. Jackson JD, Muhlestein JB, Bunch TJ, Bair TL, Horne BD, Madsen TE, et al. Intermountain Heart Collaborative Study Group. Beta-blockers reduce the incidence of clinical restenosis: prospective study of 4840 patients undergoing percutaneous coronary revascularization. *Am Heart J* 2003; 145:875–81.

28. Dens JA, Desmet WJ, Coussement P, De Scheerder IK, Kostopoulos K, Kerdsinchai P, et al. Usefulness of Nisoldipine for prevention of restenosis after percutaneous transluminal coronary angioplasty (results of the NICOLE study). Nisoldipine in Coronary artery disease in Leuven. *Am J Cardiol* 2001;87:28–33.

29. Jorgensen B, Simonsen S, Endresen K, Forfang K, Vatne K, Hansen J, et al. Restenosis and clinical outcome in patients treated with amlodipine after angioplasty: results from the Coronary AngioPlasty Amlodipine REStenosis Study (CAPARES). *J Am Coll Cardiol* 2000;35:592–9.

30. Hillegass WB, Ohman EM, Leimberger JD, et al. A meta-analysis of randomised trials of calcium antagonists to reduce restenosis after coronary angioplasty. *Am J Cardiol* 1994;73:835–9.

31. Bestehorn HP, Neumann FJ, Buttner HJ, Betz P, Sturzenhofecker P, von Hodenberg E, et al. Evaluation of the effect of oral verapamil on clinical outcome and angiographic restenosis after percutaneous coronary intervention: the randomized, double-blind, placebo-controlled, multicenter Verapamil Slow-Release for Prevention of Cardiovascular Events After Angioplasty (VESPA) Trial. *J Am Coll Cardiol* 2004;43:2160–5.

32. Pfeffer MA, Braunwald E, Moye LA, Basta L, Brown EJ Jr, Cuddy TE, et al. Effect of captopril on mortality and morbidity in patients with left ventricular dysfunction after myocardial infarction. Results of the survival and ventricular enlargement trial. The SAVE Investigators. *N Engl J Med* 1992;327:669–77.

33. Dickstein K, Kjekshus J, OPTIMAAL Steering Committee of the OPTIMAAL Study Group. Effects of losartan and captopril on mortality and morbidity in high-risk patients after acute myocardial infarction: the OPTIMAAL randomised trial. Optimal Trial in Myocardial Infarction with Angiotensin II Antagonist Losartan. *Lancet* 2002;360:752–60.

34. Pfeffer MA, McMurray JJ, Velazquez EJ, Rouleau JL, Kober L, Maggioni AP, et al. Valsartan in Acute Myocardial Infarction Trial Investigators. Valsartan, captopril, or both in myocardial infarction complicated by heart failure, left ventricular dysfunction, or both. *N Engl J Med* 2003;349:1893–906.

35. Yusuf S, Sleight P, Pogue J, Bosch JDR, Dagenais G. Effects of an angiotensin-converting-enzyme inhibitor, ramipril, on cardiovascular events in high-risk patients. The Heart Outcomes Prevention Evaluation Study Investigators. *N Engl J Med* 2000;342:145–53.

36. Fox KM. EURopean trial On reduction of cardiac events with Perindopril in stable coronary Artery disease Investigators. Efficacy of perindopril in reduction of cardiovascular events among patients with stable coronary artery disease: randomised, double-blind, placebo-controlled, multicentre trial (the EUROPA study). *Lancet* 200; 362:782–8.

37. Ellis SG, Lincoff AM, Whitlow PL, Raymond RE, Franco I, Schneider JP, et al. Evidence that angiotensin-converting enzyme inhibitor use diminishes the need for coronary revascularization after stenting. *Am J Cardiol* 2002;89:937–40.

38. The MARCATOR Study Group. Does the new angiotensin converting enzyme inhibitor cilazapril prevent restenosis after percutaneous transluminal coronary angioplasty? Results of the MERCATOR study: a multicenter, randomised, double-blind, placebo-controlled trial. *Circulation* 1992; 86:100–10.

39. Meurice T, Bauters C, Hermant X, Codron V, VanBelle E, Mc Fadden EP, et al. Effect of ACE inhibitors on angiographic restenosis after coronary stenting (PARIS): a randomised, double-blind, placebo-controlled trial. *Lancet* 2001;357:1321–4.

40. Ribichini F, Wijns W, Ferrero V, Matullo G, Camilla T, Feola M, et al. Effect of angiotensin-converting enzyme inhibition on restenosis after coronary stenting. *Am J Cardiol* 2003;91:154–8.

Chapter

62

Hypertension in Patients with Concomitant Cardiac Disorders

Hung-Fat Tse

Key Findings

- In a significant proportion of patients, hypertension directly contributes to or is accompanied by a range of concomitant cardiac disorders, including heart failure, atrial fibrillation, and coronary heart disease.

- Numerous clinical trials have demonstrated that adequate blood pressure control, rather than the types of agents used, is essential in preventing those cardiac diseases in hypertensive patients.

Clinical Implications

- The treatment of hypertension in patients with concomitant cardiac diseases often requires multiple pharmacologic agents with additive or synergistic agents for the compelling indications to achieve acceptable blood pressure control and to improve the tolerability of treatment.

The management of hypertensive patients with concomitant cardiac disorders is important and challenging. In most patients, hypertension is accompanied by a range of concomitant cardiac disorders that can contribute to target-organ damage and have a key role in their progression and response to treatment. On the other hand, hypertension also contributes pathophysiologically to the development of these cardiac diseases. Therefore, adequate blood pressure control is particularly essential in those patients, and their blood pressure goals of drug therapy are substantially lower than those patients without cardiovascular diseases (Table 62–1).[1–4] Unfortunately, recent studies have shown that hypertension remains poorly controlled in a significant proportion of patients.[5] In the majority of patients with concomitant cardiac diseases, combinations of multiple antihypertensive agents with additive or synergistic are required to improve the efficacy of blood pressure control and tolerability of treatment. Congestive heart failure and atrial fibrillation have been described as two emerging epidemics of cardiovascular disease associated with an ageing population. Coronary heart disease remains the major cause of morbidity and mortality in developing countries. This chapter is intended to provide a comprehensive overview on the management of hypertension in patients with concomitant cardiac disorders, including heart failure, atrial fibrillation, and stable coronary heart disease.

ANATOMY AND PATHOLOGY

An excessive increase in afterload imposed by hypertension leads to cardiac compensation with progressive thickening of the left ventricular wall to cause concentric left ventricular hypertrophy (LVH). However, prolonged pressure overloading due to uncontrolled hypertension can eventually result in progressive deterioration in contractile pumping (systolic) function and the left ventricular cavity becoming dilated. An increase in left ventricular filling pressures due to impairment of left ventricular systolic and/or diastolic function can lead to left atrial enlargement. In patients with hypertension, left atrial enlargement may develop early in the course of disease, and is independent of the presence of LVH and atrial fibrillation.[6] However, the prevalence of left atrial enlargement increases with the development of LVH, and correlates with the degree of hypertension.[7] Both left atrial enlargement and LVH play an important role in the development of atrial fibrillation in patients with hypertension.[6] In addition to coronary microvascular disease, hypertension also contributes to the development of atherosclerotic coronary artery disease.

PATHOPHYSIOLOGY

The pathophysiologic interaction between hypertension and other concomitant cardiac diseases is summarized in Figure 62–1. Even before impairment of systolic function, the stiffness of the left ventricular wall can be increased by the myocardial fibrosis associated with LVH, and myocardial ischemia due to ischemic heart disease. Both of them contribute to the impairment of the filling (diastolic) function of the left ventricle. Ischemic heart disease may also occur because of the combination of hypertensive microvascular disease, concomitant atherosclerotic coronary artery disease in association with other coronary artery risk factors, and increased myocardial oxygen requirements as a consequence of LVH. The combination of decreased oxygen supply in the setting of increased oxygen demand with LVH explains why patients with hypertension have a higher risk of myocardial infarction or other major coronary events, and at higher mortality with acute myocardial infarction.[8]

Furthermore, hypertension is associated with structural changes in the left atrium that can contribute to the development of atrial fibrillation. The structural changes include left atrial enlargement and impairment of left

TARGET BLOOD PRESSURE FROM CLINICAL GUIDELINES				
	Overall	DM	Renal Diseases	CVS Diseases
JNC-7	<140/90	<130/80	<130/80	—
BHS IV	<140/90	<130/80	<130/80	<130/80
WHO/ISH	SBP <140	<130/80	<130/80	<130/80
ESH/ESC	<140/90	<130/80	—	—

BHS IV, British Hypertension Society, IV revision; CVS, cardiovascular; DM, diabetes mellitus; ESH/ESC, European Society of Hypertension/European Society of Cardiology; JNC-7, Joint Committee on Prevention, Detection, Evaluation, and Treatment of High Blood Pressure, seventh report; SBP, systolic blood pressure; WHO/ISH, World Health Organization/International Society of Hypertension.

Table 62–1. Target Blood Pressure from Clinical Guidelines

atrial mechanical function that subsequently lead to alteration of left atrial electrophysiology, and increased atrial ectopic activity that triggers the initiation of atrial fibrillation.[6] Finally, persistent uncontrolled blood pressure, tachycardia-induced cardiomyopathy associated with atrial fibrillation,[9] and the development of myocardial infarction can eventually lead to progressive deterioration of left ventricular systolic function that causes heart failure.

CLINICAL PRESENTATIONS

In patients with blood pressure higher than 160/90 mmHg, the lifetime risk of developing congestive heart failure is two times higher than those with blood pressure lower than 140/90mmHg.[10] The risk of coronary artery disease increases with blood pressure, and the risk of a recurrent coronary event in patients with coronary heart disease is also significantly affected by the blood pressure level.[11] Effective treatment of hypertension preventing the development of coronary heart disease and heart failure provides further evidences to support a major contribution of elevated blood pressure to the onset and progression of both conditions.[12–15] However, there are conflicting data regarding the prevalence of hypertension in patients with heart failure due to the difference in study design and population.[16] These studies have reported that hypertension is a comorbidity in up to 26% to 45% of patients with congestive heart failure. Although hypertension is considered to be the primary etiological factor for heart failure in only 7% of patients, the contribution of hypertension to heart failure is likely to be underappreciated. In patients with hypertension and coronary heart disease who develop heart failure, hypertension is usually regarded as secondary rather than primary cause of heart failure. Furthermore, blood pressure falls as progressive systolic left ventricular dysfunction develops in some patients with hypertension. Impairments of both systolic and diastolic dysfunction of left ventricle associated with hypertension can contribute to symptoms and signs of heart failure. On the other hand, patients with hypertension may also suffer from other primary or concomitant causes for impairment of left ventricular function, such as ischemic and dilated cardiomyopathy, valvular dysfunction, and atrial fibrillation.

Although the relative risk of developing atrial fibrillation in patients with hypertension is lower than other cardiovascular diseases, such as heart failure and myocardial infarction,[17,18] hypertension remains the most common causes of atrial fibrillation due to its high prevalence in the general population. Indeed, previous cohort studies in United Status have demonstrated that hypertension was present in up to half of patients with atrial fibrillation.[17–19] Although in these cases, hypertension was considered as causative for atrial fibrillation in ~15% of patients, the actual incidence remains unclear. One of the major complications of both hypertension and atrial fibrillation is stroke. As compared to general population, atrial fibrillation increases the risk of stroke by three- to six-fold and accounts for at least 15% of strokes.[20] The presence of hypertension further increase the risk of stroke associated with atrial fibrillation by an additional two- to three-fold.[21]

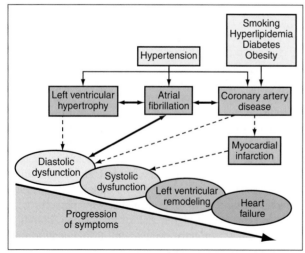

Figure 62–1. Complex pathophysiologic interactions between hypertension and progression to other concomitant cardiac diseases via the development of left ventricular hypertrophy, coronary artery disease, and left ventricular systolic and diastolic dysfunction.

DIAGNOSTIC TECHNIQUES

Rational approaches for treatment in those patients need detailed delineation of the pattern of left ventricular dysfunction and documentation of the arrhythmia in relation to symptoms. The symptoms and signs of heart failure in patients with systolic and diastolic ventricular dysfunction are very similar, and it is difficult to differentiate between them clinically, especially in elderly patients. Furthermore, typical symptoms and signs of heart failure may be absent in patients with early left ventricular systolic dysfunction, even when it is significant. On physical examination, the heart is enlarged and has a prominent left ventricular impulse. A fourth heart sound is frequently observed in hypertensive heart disease, and a third heart sound or gallop rhythm may be present. Electrocardiogram (ECG) may show LVH, evidence of myocardial ischemia or infarction, and the presence of atrial fibrillation. However, as atrial fibrillation can be paroxysmal and frequently asymptomatic in a significant proportion of patients, a 12-lead ECG has limited sensitivity for diagnosis of atrial fibrillation. The use of ECG monitoring with a Holter or loop recorder can improve the detection rate for atrial fibrillation. Measurement of the plasma levels of B-type natriuretic peptide (BNP) may be used to facilitate the initial screening for left ventricular dysfunction in patients with hypertension.[22,23] Both a BNP level of 35 pg/mL and N-terminal pro-BNP level of 235 pg/mL show a moderately high positive predictive value (82% to 89%) in predicting heart failure in patients with hypertension.[22]

Transthoracic echocardiography can be used to evaluate the left atrial size, LVH, and left ventricular function in patients with hypertension. The frequency of LVH detected by echocardiogram is higher than observed with ECG. Doppler assessment of mitral and pulmonary venous flow as well as tissue Doppler are very sensitive methods for detecting changes in left atrial function and left ventricular diastolic function. Analysis of the pulse-wave Doppler signal of the mitral inflow during diastole and the waveform analysis of pulmonary vein flow are common methods used to detect diastolic dysfunction. Based on the mitral and pulmonary Doppler flow, four stages of diastolic dysfunction have been described. In the first stage, the early mitral inflow (E wave) is less than the late mitral inflow due to atrial contraction (A wave). As a result, there is a reversal of E/A ratio (<1.0) and prolongation of deceleration time (>200 ms) of the E wave. In the second stage, pseudonormalization of the mitral Doppler flow with normal E/A ratio and deceleration time are observed, but the pulmonary venous flow is reversed due to elevated left atrial pressure. In the third stage, a restrictive filling pattern with an increased E/A ratio (>2) and a short deceleration time (<150 ms) occur, which can be normalized by Valsalva maneuver. In the fourth stage, this restrictive pattern can not be normalized by Valsalva maneuver.

However, one of the potential limitations of these Doppler indices is they are preload dependent. Tissue Doppler is a new technique that is used to directly measure the velocity of myocardial displacement at the mitral annulus as the left ventricle expands in diastole. These tissue velocities measured during early filling and after atrial contraction are termed E' and A', respectively. The ratio of E/E' is frequently used as an index diastolic dysfunction. In contrast, this tissue Doppler index is a minimally load-dependent measurement that can further increase the sensitivity and specificity of diastolic dysfunction detection. Furthermore, impaired left atrium and left ventricular diastolic function and the presence of LVH can predict the development of atrial fibrillation in patients with hypertension.

Diagnosis of coronary artery disease in patients with hypertension is important but can be difficult due to the presence of LVH. As a result, routine exercise stress ECG testing in hypertensive patients is associated with a high false-positive (62%) and -negative rate (53%). Exercise or pharmacologic SPECT thallium or sestamibi tests are more useful noninvasive tests in patients with hypertension. The negative predictive value of these tests is 94% to 98% with an overall accuracy of 70%.[24] Although the latest advances in multidetector computed tomography allow visualization of the coronary artery, coronary angiography still remains the gold standard for the diagnosis of coronary artery disease.

MANAGEMENT

Prevention

Adequate blood pressure control through lifestyle modification and antihypertensive therapy can directly prevent heart failure by reducing the left ventricular workload and indirectly via regression of LVH and prevention of ischemic heart diseases. As compared with placebo, previous clinical studies have demonstrated that blood pressure lowering with antihypertensive agents prevents coronary heart disease and heart failure in patients with diastolic or systolic hypertension.[13–16] Several meta-analyses have been performed to address the differences between regimens based on different drugs in their effects on prevention of heart failure and coronary heart disease.[25,26] These analyses demonstrate that regimens based on diuretics, angiotensin-converting enzyme (ACE) inhibitors or β-blocker are more effective at preventing heart failure than those regimens based on calcium channel blockers. For prevention of coronary heart diseases, meta-analyses show no clear difference between diuretic, ACE inhibitors, β-blocker, and calcium channel blockers. Treatment regimens based on angiotensin-receptor blockers (ARB) also appear to be useful in reducing heart failure, but not coronary heart disease. Thus these meta-analyses indicate that blood pressure lowering rather than the use of specific agents makes the difference in outcome.

Indeed, current evidence[27–32] confirms that the level of blood pressure lowering is important in reducing cardiovascular events. In the Heart Outcomes Prevention Evaluation (HOPE) trial, a small reduction in blood pressure with the ACE inhibitor ramipril in high-risk patients significantly reduced the risk of coronary heart disease and heart failure.[27] However, there are conflicting data on the specific benefits of various medications over and above the effects of blood pressure lowering. In the Antihypertensive and Lipid-Lowering Treatment to Prevent Heart Attack Trial (ALLHAT),[28] the incidence of fatal and nonfatal coronary artery disease were similar between patients treated with a diuretic, ACE inhibitor, or calcium channel blocker based treatment regimen. Further analysis showed that the blood pressure control was better in the diuretic group than the ACE inhibitor group, and the risk for development of heart failure was significantly lower in the diuretic group. In the Valsartan Antihypertensive Long-Term Use Evaluation (VALUE) study, there was no significant difference in the overall risk for fatal and nonfatal heart failure, but the risk of myocardial infarction was increased in patients treated with valsartan.[29] However, the risk of heart failure hospitalization was significantly reduced by 36% in patients with controlled blood pressure (systolic <140 mmHg) compared to those without blood pressure control, independent of drug type used.[30] In the Losartan Intervention for Endpoint Reduction in Hypertension (LIFE) studies, there was no significant difference in the risk of heart failure between treatments with an ARB versus β-blocker.[31] Finally, in the Anglo-Scandinavian Cardiac Outcomes Trial-Blood Pressure Lowering Arm (ASCOT-BPLA) trial,[32] a calcium channel blocker (plus an ACE inhibitor) regimen was compared with a β-blocker (plus a diuretic) regime. Although the former regimen reduced mortality, total coronary events and stroke, there was no difference between the two regimens in the primary endpoint of fatal and nonfatal myocardial infarction. Further analysis suggested that even after adjusting for the blood pressure difference; the calcium channel blocker-based regimen contributed significant effects in decreasing total coronary events and strokes.[33] Based on these findings, newer agents (ACEI inhibitor and calcium channel blocker) appear to be slightly better than older agents (β-blocker and diuretic) in reducing cardiovascular events; however, multiple medications are necessary to achieve blood pressure control and to reduce cardiovascular events.

Optimal blood pressure level

The optimal blood pressure targets in hypertensive patients with concomitant heart failure, atrial fibrillation, and coronary heart disease have not been defined. Despite the importance of hypertension in the development of these concomitant cardiac diseases and their complications, limited data are available on their prevention and treatment in patients with hypertension. Although the optimal blood pressure target in these patients with hypertension remains unclear, aggressive treatment of blood pressure in those patients is recommended.

In the Hypertension Optimal Treatment (HOT) study and INdividual Data ANalysis of Antihypertensive intervention (INDANA) database, there was no evidence of a J-shaped curve to suggest that blood pressure lowering had harmful effects in patients with coronary heart disease.[34,35] Furthermore, effective treatment of heart failure frequently requires lowering the blood pressure to values below current recommended target in patients with cardiovascular diseases (Table 62–1).

Antihypertensive therapy has been shown to reverse some of the structural changes, such as LVH and left atrial enlargement, that are associated with the development of these concomitant cardiac diseases in hypertension. In patients with hypertension, blood pressure lowering with antihypertensive agents results in regression of ventricular hypertrophy. However, certain new antihypertensive agents, such as calcium antagonists, ACE inhibitors, and ARBs, may result in more LVH regression, independent of the magnitude of blood pressure reduction.[25,26] The effect of antihypertensive therapy on regression of left atrial enlargement is less clear. In a comparison study, diuretic therapy appears to be more effective than other classes of agents, including clonidine, atenolol, diltiazem, prazosin, and captopril—in reduction of left atrial size, independent of blood pressure lowering and baseline left ventricular mass.[36] Although the clinical implications of these structural changes with antihypertensive treatment on the development of atrial fibrillation remain unclear, appropriate treatment of hypertension, even without atrial fibrillation, results in a significant reduction in mortality and strokes.[25,26]

Heart failure

In patients with systolic heart failure, ACE inhibitors[37] and β-blockers[38] are well-established treatment regimens to reduce cardiovascular morbidity and mortality. Current data suggested the use of bisoprolol fumarate, metoprolol succinate, and carvedilol, but not metoprolol tartrate or atenolol in patients with heart failure.[39] As shown in Table 62–2, initial treatment of hypertension in patients with systolic heart failure should include ACE inhibitors and β-blockers.[1-4] Diuretic therapy alone should not be the initial treatment in patients with established heart failure. However, diuretic therapy is an effective adjunct to ACE inhibitors and β-blockers for blood pressure control, and to relieve congestive symptoms of heart failure. In patients with advanced heart failure, antialdosterone therapy with spironolactone reduced heart failure mortality.[40] ARBs can be used as alternatives to ACE inhibitors in patients intolerant to ACE inhibitor, or in combination with ACE inhibitors.[41] Further analysis suggested the add-on ARB therapy to ACE inhibitors only has beneficial effects in heart failure patients who were not receiving a β-blocker.[42,43] Long-acting dihydropyridine calcium channel blockers have neutral effect on mortality in patients with heart failure, but they are useful for blood pressure control in those patients who are refractory to other agents.[44]

In contrast to systolic heart failure, very limited data are available on the treatment of diastolic heart failure. Again, aggressive blood pressure reduction with multiple agents to achieve regression of LVH is recommended. Calcium channel blockers may theoretically have several beneficial effects in patients with diastolic heart failure by their blood pressure and heart rate lowering effects and lusitropic properties. Previous studies have suggested that verapamil increases exercise capacity in patients with hypertension and diastolic heart failure.[45] However, recent studies suggested that candesartan was more effective than verapamil in improving symptoms and exercise capacity in those patients.[46] Indeed, the CHARM study suggested that treatment with ARBs reduced heart failure hospitalization in patients with heart failure and preserved the ejection fraction.[47]

Atrial fibrillation

Regarding treatment of atrial fibrillation, successful restoration and maintenance of sinus rhythm are conceptually expected to improve quality of life, reduce the incidence of strokes, heart failure and mortality, and avoid the use life-long anticoagulation. However, recent randomized trials have failed to show any superiority for a rhythm control strategy, primarily pharmacologic rate control plus anticoagulation strategy in terms of quality of life, stroke, or mortality.[48-51] These studies highlighted the low clinical efficacy of current antiarrhythmic agents to maintain sinus rhythm. This probably contributes to the stroke risk associated with rhythm control, especially in a high-risk hypertensive population. Therefore, in patients with hypertension and atrial fibrillation, unless contraindicated, oral anticoagulant with warfarin should be the mainstay of preventive therapy for stroke, irrespective of whether rate or rhythm control strategy is used. In high-risk patients with atrial fibrillation, including those with hypertension; age more than 65 years; prior history of stroke or transient ischemic attack, heart failure, diabetes, valvular heart diseases, and impaired left ventricular systolic function, oral anticoagulant reduces the risk of ischemic stroke by 68% and lowers mortality by 33%.[52] However, one of the major drawbacks of warfarin is the potential of increasing risk of hemorrhagic events. Therefore, the risks and benefits of warfarin therapy must be assessed for every individual patient. Compared with warfarin, aspirin is less effective in preventing stroke (22% risk reduction).[52] In hypertensive patients, aspirin can only be recommended for patients who refuse or cannot safely take warfarin.

In patients who need ventricular rate control, either β-blocker and/or rate-limiting calcium channel blockers (diltiazem or verapamil) are suitable initial choices of therapy in patients with hypertension (Table 62–2). In patients with impaired left ventricular or LVH, the use of class I and III antiarrhythmic agents is associated with an increase risk of proarrhythmia. In the latest American College of Cardiology (ACC)/American Heart Association (AHA)/European Society of Cardiology (ESC) guidelines for the management of atrial fibrillation, only amiodarone is recommended for rhythm control in patients with hypertension and LVH.[52]

The effect of specific classes of antihypertensive agents on the prevention of atrial fibrillation remains unclear. Recent studies suggest that blockade of the renin-angiotensin-aldosterone system with ACE inhibitors or ARBs may reduce the recurrence of atrial fibrillation, independent of blood pressure–lowering effect.[53,54] However, a meta-analysis failed to shown a significant reduction in atrial fibrillations with ACE inhibitors or ARBs.[55] The impact of ACE inhibitors or ARB in patients with atrial fibrillation is currently a focus of several major clinical trials, including the Atrial Fibrillation Clopidogrel Trial with Irbesartan for Prevention of Vascular Events (ACTIVE) and Ongoing Telmisartan Alone and in Combination with Ramipril Global Endpoint Trial/Telmisartan Randomized Assessment in ACE Intolerant Subjects with Cardiovascular Disease (ONTARGET/TRANSCEND).

Coronary heart disease

In patients with symptomatic coronary heart disease, the aims of treatment should include control of blood pressure, antiplatelet therapy with aspirin and/or clopidogrel, as well as reduction or cessation of other coronary artery risk factors, such as smoking, obesity, control of diabetes, and hyperlipidemia, relieving symptoms of angina, and preventing myocardial infarction. β-blockers, which reduce blood pressure, angina symptoms, and risk of myocardial infarction, should be considered as the first drug of choice

	JNC-7	ESH/ESC	BHS IV
COMPILING INDICATIONS OF VARIOUS ANTIHYPERTENSIVE DRUGS FROM THREE GUIDELINES FOR CONCOMITANT CARDIAC DISEASES			
Diuretic	**Thiazide-type** Heart failure	**Thiazide-type** Heart failure **Loop diuretic** Heart failure	**Thiazide-type** Heart failure
Beta-blockers	Heart failure Post myocardial infarction	Heart failure Post myocardial infarction Tachyarrhythmia	Heart failure Post myocardial infarction Angina pectoris
ACE inhibitors	Heart failure Post myocardial infarction	Heart failure Post myocardial infarction	Heart failure Post myocardial infarction Coronary artery diseases
ARB	Heart failure	Left ventricular hypertrophy	ACE intolerance in patients with heart failure and post myocardial infarction Left ventricular hypertrophy
Calcium channel blocker		Angina pectoris Supraventricular tachycardia	**Rate limiting** Angina pectoris

BHS IV, British Hypertension Society, IV revision; ESH/ESC, European Society of Hypertension/European Society of Cardiology; JNC-7, Joint National Committee on Prevention, Detection, Evaluation, and Treatment of High Blood Pressure, seventh report.

Table 62–2. Compelling Indications of Various Antihypertensive Drugs from Three Guidelines for Concomitant Cardiac Diseases

in hypertensive patients with symptomatic coronary heart disease (Table 62–2). Furthermore, in patients with coexisting heart failure due to myocardial infarction and/or hypertension, β-blockers (especially carvedilol or metoprolol) may be also used as part of heart failure therapy. In patients with adverse effects or contraindication to β-blockers, persistent angina symptoms or uncontrolled blood pressure, nondihydropyridine calcium channel blockers (diltiazem or verapmail) or long-acting dihydropyridine calcium channel blockers are appropriate alternative or add-on therapy for angina and hypertension. The use of short-acting dihydropyridine calcium channel blockers may increase the risk of adverse cardiac events and should be avoided. Furthermore, in hypertensive patients, aggressive lipid-lowering therapy with statins is effective for primary and secondary prevention of cardiovascular events.[55,56]

PROGNOSIS

Limited current systematic data are available on the long-term prognosis of hypertensive patients with each of these concomitant cardiac diseases. As discussed above, effective treatment of blood pressure can reduce the risk of heart failure and coronary heart disease, and probably also atrial fibrillation. In hypertensive patients who develop these concomitant cardiac diseases, the long-term risk of cardiovascular morbidity and mortality remains higher.

In patients who develop complications related to hypertension or poorly controlled blood pressure despite treatment, the potential of nonadherence to medications should be considered. Although uncontrolled blood pressure worsens the outcome in those patients, whether aggressive antihypertensive therapy below the current recommended guideline can improve their prognosis merits further investigation.

SUMMARY

With a growing aging population and advances in medical treatments, the number of hypertensive patients with concomitant cardiac diseases will be greatly increased. Despite all the major efforts and guidelines on the treatment of hypertension, a significant proportion of hypertensive patients are either not treated or have suboptimal blood pressure. The treatment of hypertension in patients with concomitant cardiac diseases often will require multiple pharmacologic agents for compelling indications as well as to achieve acceptable blood pressure control. Although different antihypertensive agents may have different advantages in different cardiac diseases, adequate blood pressure control continues to be primary goal of therapy. Future studies are needed to address the optimal blood pressure target and drug treatment regimen in different patient populations with concomitant cardiac diseases.

REFERENCES

1. Chobanian AV, Bakris GE, Black ER, et al. The seventh report of the Joint National Committee on Prevention, Detection, Evaluation, and Treatment of High Blood Pressure. The JNC 7 Report. *JAMA* 2003;289:2560–72.
2. Williams B, Poulter NR, Brown MJ, et al. British Hypertension Society guidelines for hypertension management 2004 (BHS-IV): summary. *BMJ* 2004;328:634–40.
3. Whitworth JA, World Health Organization, International Society of Hypertension Writing Group. 2003 World Health Organization (WHO)/International Society of Hypertension (ISH) statement on management of hypertension. *J Hypertens* 2003;21:1983–92.
4. European Society of Hypertension–European Society of Cardiology Guidelines Committee. 2003 European Society of Hypertension–European Society of Cardiology guidelines for the management of arterial hypertension. *J Hypertens* 2003;21:1011–53.
5. Hyman DJ, Pavlik VN. Characteristics of patients with uncontrolled hypertension in the United States. *N Engl J Med* 2001;345:479–86.
6. Healey JS, Connolly SJ. Atrial fibrillation: hypertension as a causative agent, risk factor for complications, and potential therapeutic target. *Am J Cardiol* 2003;91:9G–14G.
7. Gerdts E, Oikarinen L, Palmieri V, et al. Correlates of left atrial size in hypertensive patients with left

ventricular hypertrophythe Losartan Intervention for Endpoint Reduction in Hypertension (LIFE) Study. *Hypertension* 2002;39:739–43.
8. Kannel WB. Left ventricular hypertrophy as a risk factor: the Framingham experience. *J Hypertens Suppl* 1991;9:S3–8.
9. Van den Berg MP, Tuinenburg AE, Crijns HJ, et al. Heart failure and atrial fibrillation: current concepts and controversies. *Heart* 1997;77:309–13.
10. Lloyd-Jones DM, Larson MG, Leip EP, et al. Lifetime risk for developing congestive heart failure: the Framingham Heart Study. *Circulation* 2002;106:3068–72.
11. Flack JM, Neaton J, Grimm R Jr, et al. Blood pressure and mortality among men with prior myocardial infarction. Multiple Risk Factor Intervention Trial Research Group. *Circulation* 1995;92:2437–45.
12. Kostis JB, Davis BR, Cutler J, et al. Prevention of heart failure by antihypertensive drug treatment in older persons with isolated systolic hypertension. *JAMA* 1997;278:212–216.
13. MRC Working Party Medical Research Council. Trial of treatment in older adults: principal results. *BMJ* 1992;304:405–12.
14. Dahlof B, Lindholm LH, Hansson L, et al. Morbidity and mortality in the Swedish Trial in Old Patients with Hypertension (STOP-Hypertension). *Lancet* 1991;338:1281–5.

15. Staessen JA, R Fagard, L Thijs, et al. Randomised double-blind comparison of placebo and active treatment for older patients with isolated systolic hypertension (Syst-Eur). *Lancet* 1997;350:757–64.
16. Krum H, Gilbert RE. Demographics and concomitant disorders in heart failure. *Lancet* 2003;362:147–58.
17. Psaty BM, Manolio TA, Kuller LH, et al. Incidence of and risk factors for atrial fibrillation in older adults. *Circulation* 1997;96:2455–61.
18. Lloyd-Jones DM, Wang TJ, Leip EP, et al. Lifetime risk for development of atrial fibrillation: the Framingham Heart Study. *Circulation* 2004;110:1042–6.
19. Kannel WB, Abbott RD, Savage DD, McNamara PM. Epidemiologic features of chronic atrial fibrillation: the Framingham study. *N Engl J Med* 1982;306:1018–22.
20. Wolf PA, Dawber TR, Thomas HE Jr, Kannel WB. Epidemiologic assessment of chronic atrial fibrillation and risk of stroke: the Framingham study. *Neurology* 1978;28:973–7.
21. Stroke Prevention in Atrial Fibrillation Investigators. Predictors of thromboembolism in atrial fibrillation. II. Echocardiographic features of patients at risk. *Ann Intern Med* 1992;116:6–12.
22. Bhalla V, Isakson S, Bhalla MA, Lin JP, Clopton P, Gardetto N, et al. Diagnostic ability of B-type natriuretic peptide and impedance cardiography: testing to identify left ventricular dysfunction in

hypertensive patients. *Am J Hypertens* 2005;18:73S–81S.

23. Wei T, Zeng C, Chen L, Chen Q, Zhao R, Lu G, et al. Bedside tests of B-type natriuretic peptide in the diagnosis of left ventricular diastolic dysfunction in hypertensive patients. *Eur J Heart Fail* 2005;7:75–9.

24. Prisant LM. Hypertensive heart disease. *J Clin Hypertens* 2005;7:231–8.

25. Turnbull F and Blood Pressure Lowering Treatment Trialists' Collaboration. Effects of different blood-pressure–lowering regimens on major cardiovascular events results of prospectively-designed overviews of randomised trials. *Lancet* 2003;362: 1527–35.

26. Psaty BM, Lumley T, Furberg CD, et al. Health outcomes associated with various antihypertensive therapies used as first-line agents. A network meta-analysis. *JAMA* 2003;289:2534–44.

27. Yusuf S, Sleight P, Pogue J, et al. Effects of an angiotensin-converting-enzyme inhibitor, ramipril, on cardiovascular events in high-risk patients. The Heart Outcomes Prevention Evaluation Study Investigators. *N Engl J Med* 2000;342:145–53.

28. The ALLHAT Officers and Coordinators for the ALLHAT Collaborative Research Group. Major outcomes in high-risk hypertensive patients randomized to angiotensin-converting enzyme inhibitor or calcium channel blocker vs. diuretic. The Antihypertensive and Lipid-Lowering Treatment to Prevent Heart Attack Trial (ALLHAT). *JAMA* 2002;288:2981–97.

29. Julius S, Kjeldsen SE, Weber M, et al. Outcomes in hypertensive patients at high cardiovascular risk treated with regimens based on valsartan or amlodipine the VALUE randomized trial. *Lancet* 2004;363:2022–31.

30. Weber MA, Julius S, Kjeldsen SE, et al. Blood pressure dependent and independent effects of antihypertensive treatment on clinical events in the VALUE Trial. *Lancet* 2004;363:2032–9.

31. Dahlöf B, Devereux RB, Kjeldsen SE, et al. Cardiovascular morbidity and mortality in the Losartan Intervention for Endpoint reduction in hypertension study (LIFE): a randomised trial against atenolol. *Lancet* 2002;359:995–1003.

32. Dahlof B, Sever PS, Poulter NR, et al. Prevention of cardiovascular events with an antihypertensive regimen of amlodipine adding perindopril as required versus atenolol adding bendroflumethiazide as required, in the Anglo-Scandinavian Cardiac Outcomes Trial-Blood Pressure Lowering Arm (ASCOT-BPLA): a multicentre randomised controlled trial. *Lancet* 2005;366:895–906.

33. Poulter NR, Wedel H, Dahlof B, et al. Role of blood pressure and other variables in the differential cardiovascular event rates noted in the Anglo-Scandinavian Cardiac Outcomes Trial-Blood Pressure Lowering Arm (ASCOT-BPLA). *Lancet* 2005;366:907–13.

34. Hansson L, Zanchetti A, Carruthers SG, et al. Effects of intensive blood-pressure lowering and low-dose aspirin in patients with Hypertension: principal results of the Hypertension Optimal Treatment (HOT) randomised trial. HOT Study Group. *Lancet* 1998;351:1755–62.

35. Boutitie F, Gueyffier F, Pocock S, et al. J-shaped relationship between blood pressure and mortality in hypertensive patients: new insights from a meta-analysis of individual-patient data. *Ann Intern Med* 2002;136:438–48.

36. Gottdiener JS, Reda DJ, Williams DW, et al. Effect of single-drug therapy on reduction of left atrial size in mild to moderate hypertension: comparison of six antihypertensive agents. *Circulation* 1998;98:140–8.

37. Garg R, Yusuf S. Overview of randomized trials of angiotensin-converting enzyme inhibitors on mortality and morbidity in patients with heart failure. Collaborative Group on ACE Inhibitor Trials. *JAMA* 1995;273:1450–6.

38. Doughty RN, Rodgers A, Sharpe N, MacMahon S. Effects of beta-blocker therapy on mortality in patients with heart failure. A systematic overview of randomized controlled trials. *Eur Heart J* 1997;18:560–5.

39. McMurray J, Cohen-Solal A, Dietz R, et al. Practical recommendations for the use of ACE inhibitors, beta-blockers, aldosterone antagonists and angiotensin receptor blockers in heart failure: putting guidelines into practice. *Eur J Heart Fail* 2005;7:710–21.

40. Pitt B. Aldosterone blockade in patients with systolic left ventricular dysfunction. *Circulation* 2003;108:1790–4.

41. Pfeffer MA, Swedberg K, Granger CB, et al. Effects of candesartan on mortality and morbidity in patients with chronic heart failure: the CHARM-Overall programme. *Lancet* 2003;362: 759–66.

42. Cohn JN, Tognoni G. Valsartan Heart Failure Trial Investigators. A randomized trial of the angiotensin-receptor blocker valsartan in chronic heart failure. *N Engl J Med* 2001;345:1667–75.

43. McMurray JJ, Ostergren J, Swedberg K, et al. Effects of candesartan in patients with chronic heart failure and reduced left-ventricular systolic function taking angiotensin-converting-enzyme inhibitors: the CHARM-Added trial. *Lancet* 2003;362:767–71.

44. Packer M, O'Connor CM, Ghali JK, et al. Effect of amlodipine on morbidity and mortality in severe chronic heart failure. Prospective Randomized Amlodipine Survival Evaluation Study Group. *N Engl J Med* 1996;335:1107–14.

45. Setaro JF, Zaret BL, Schulman DS, Black HR, Soufer R. Usefulness of verapamil for congestive heart failure associated with abnormal left ventricular diastolic filling and normal left ventricular systolic performance. *Am J Cardiol* 1990;66:981–6.

46. Little WC, Wesley-Farrington DJ, Hoyle J, Brucks S, Robertson S, Kitzman DW, et al. Effect of candesartan and verapamil on exercise tolerance in diastolic dysfunction. *J Cardiovasc Pharmacol* 2004;43:288–93.

47. Yusuf S, Pfeffer MA, Swedberg K, et al. Effects of candesartan in patients with chronic heart failure and preserved left-ventricular ejection fraction: the CHARM-Preserved Trial. *Lancet* 2003; 362:777–81.

48. Wyse DG, Waldo AL, DiMarco JP, et al. A comparison of rate control and rhythm control in patients with atrial fibrillation. *N Engl J Med* 2002;347: 1825–33.

49. Van Gelder IC, Hagens VE, Bosker HA, et al. A comparison of rate control and rhythm control in patients with recurrent persistent atrial fibrillation. *N Engl J Med* 2002;347:1834–40.

50. Carlsson J, Miketic S, Windeler J, et al. Randomized trial of rate-control versus rhythm-control in persistent atrial fibrillation: the Strategies of Treatment of Atrial Fibrillation (STAF) study. *J Am Coll Cardiol* 2003;41:1690–6.

51. Hohnloser SH, Kuck KH, Lilienthal J. Rhythm or rate control in atrial fibrillation-Pharmacological Intervention in Atrial Fibrillation (PIAF): a randomised trial. *Lancet* 2000;356:1789–94.

52. Fuster V, Ryden LE, Asinger RW, et al. ACC/AHA/ESC guidelines for the management of patients with atrial fibrillation: executive summary. A report of the American College of Cardiology/ American Heart Association Task Force on Practice Guidelines and the European Society of Cardiology Committee for Practice Guidelines and Policy Conferences (Committee to Develop Guidelines for the Management of Patients with Atrial Fibrillation): developed in Collaboration with the North American Society of Pacing and Electrophysiology. *J Am Coll Cardiol* 2001;38:1231–66.

53. Madrid AH, Bueno MG, Rebollo JMG, et al. Use of irbesartan to maintain sinus rhythm in patients with long-lasting persistent atrial fibrillation. *Circulation* 2002;106:331–336.

54. Wachtell K, Lehto M, Gerdts E, et al. Angiotensin II receptor blockade reduces new-onset atrial fibrillation and subsequent stroke compared to atenolol the Losartan Intervention for End Point Reduction in Hypertension (LIFE) study. *J Am Coll Cardiol* 2005; 45:712–719.

55. Healey JS, Baranchuk A, Crystal E, et al. Prevention of atrial fibrillation with angiotensin-converting enzyme inhibitors and angiotensin receptor blockers: a meta-analysis. *J Am Coll Cardiol* 2005;45:1832–9.

56. Sever PS, Dahlof B, Poulter NR, et al. Prevention of coronary and stroke events in hypertensive patients who have average or lower-than-average cholesterol concentrations, in the Anglo-Scandinavian Cardiac Outcomes Trial—Lipid Lowering Arm (ASCOT-LLA): a multicentre randomised controlled trial. *Lancet* 2003;361: 1149–58.

57. Graham I. What impact will current trial data have on future guideline recommendations? *Am J Med* 2005; 118:42–7.

Chapter

63

Hypertensive Urgencies and Emergencies

Ehud Grossman and Franz H. Messerli

Definition

- A hypertensive crisis is defined as a severe elevation in blood pressure (BP), such as a diastolic BP above 120 to 130 mmHg, and is classified as either an emergency or urgency.

Clinical Implications

- Hypertensive emergencies are relatively rare and are said to be present only when BP elevation confers an immediate threat to the integrity of the cardiovascular system.

- In a hypertensive emergency, immediate reduction in BP is required to avoid further end-organ damage, generally by intravenous therapy in an intensive care setting, to lower the mean arterial pressure by 25% over the initial 2 to 4 hours with the most specific antihypertensive regimen. Fenoldopam, labetalol, nicardipine, and sodium nitroprusside are the most popular agents for treatment of hypertensive emergencies.

- Hypertensive urgencies are common and are said to be present when severe elevation in BP is not associated with end-organ injury.

- There is no scientific evidence that acute BP lowering is beneficial in hypertensive urgency. The appropriate approach is to lower BP gradually over 12 to 24 hours with oral antihypertensive agents. Any drug that lowers BP precipitously should be avoided.

Hypertensive crisis is defined as a severe elevation in blood pressure (BP), such as a diastolic BP above 120 to 130 mmHg; it can be subclassified as either emergent or urgent.[1,2] Hypertensive emergency is relatively rare and defined as such only when there is an immediate threat to the integrity of the cardiovascular system (Box 63–1). Patients with a hypertensive emergency require an immediate reduction in BP to avoid serious end-organ damage, generally by means of intravenous therapy in an intensive care setting.[2]

Unlike patients with a hypertensive emergency, patients with severe elevation in BP who have no evidence of progressive end-organ injury are classified as having an urgent hypertensive crisis and require only a gradual reduction in BP over a period of 12 to 24 hours.[2]

It has been estimated that approximately 1% of patients with hypertension will develop a hypertensive crisis at some point during their lives.[3] The incidence of hyper-

tensive crisis has increased over the past four decades. Hospital admissions for hypertensive emergency in the United States more than tripled between 1983 and 1990 from 23,000 to 73,000 per year.[3] According to one study, the prevalence of hypertensive crisis in an emergency room in 1 year is 3% of total patients, but 27% of all medical urgency emergencies.[4] Before it was possible to treat accelerated malignant hypertension, survival was 20% and 1%, for 1 and 5 years, respectively. During the last two decades survival improved, with a 10-year survival rate of 67% and mean survival of 18 years being reported.[5] Therapy has dramatically reduced immediate deaths from hypertensive encephalopathy, acute renal failure, hemorrhagic strokes, and congestive heart failure.

ETIOLOGY AND PATHOGENESIS

Hypertensive emergency can develop *de novo* or can complicate underlying essential or secondary hypertension.[3] Renal parenchymal diseases accounts for up to 80% of all secondary causes, with chronic pyelonephritis and glomerulonephritis being the most common diagnoses. The factors that lead to the severe and rapid BP elevation in patients with hypertensive emergency are poorly under-

---

Box 63–1

Definition of a Hypertensive Emergency

Moderate to severe elevation of arterial pressure associated with:

1. Malignant hypertension[a]
2. Intracranial hemorrhage
3. Atherothrombotic cerebral infarction
4. Acute congestive heart failure
5. Acute coronary insufficiency
6. Acute renal insufficiency
7. Acute aortic dissection
8. Adrenergic crisis (pheochromocytoma crisis, clonidine withdrawal, food and drug interactions with monoamine oxidase inhibitors, amphetamine overdose)
9. Eclampsia

[a]Malignant or accelerated hypertension is a syndrome characterized by elevated blood pressure accompanied by encephalopathy or nephropathy or by papilledema and/or microangiopathic hemolytic anemia.

stood. The rapidity of onset suggests a triggering factor superimposed on preexisting hypertension. The release of humoral vasoconstrictor substances from the stressed vessel wall is thought to be responsible for the initiation and perpetuation of the hypertensive emergency. Mild to moderate increase in BP does not affect target-organ perfusion because of the autoregulatory mechanisms. However, severe BP elevation above the autoregulatory threshold leads to transmission of the pressure to small distal vessels, causing endothelial injury. The endothelial dysfunction leads to increased vascular wall permeability, cell proliferation, and activation of the coagulation cascade and platelets, resulting ultimately in fibrinoid necrosis of small blood vessels, release of vasoconstrictor substances, and tissue ischemia. The initial vascular damage leads to a vicious cycle of further vascular injury, tissue ischemia, and release of more vasoconstrictor substances. Renal ischemia causes activation of the renin angiotension system that plays a central role in the initiation and perpetuation of the vascular injury characteristic to hypertensive emergency. In addition to activation of the renin–angiotensin system, vasopressin, endothelin, and catecholamines are postulated to play important roles in the pathogenesis of hypertensive emergencies.[6]

EVALUATION OF PATIENTS WITH HYPERTENSIVE CRISIS

Early triage is critical in an effort to ensure the most appropriate therapy for each patient.[7] A brief but thorough history should address duration as well as severity of hypertension, all current medications, including prescription and nonprescription drugs, and the use of recreational drugs. Direct questioning regarding the level of compliance with current antihypertensive medications may establish inadequacy of therapy. Information regarding neurologic, cardiovascular, and/or renal symptoms and specific manifestations, such as headache, seizures, chest pain, dyspnea, and edema is important for the correct diagnosis. A history of other comorbid conditions and prior cardiovascular or renal disease is critical for the initial evaluation.

Physical assessment should start with BP measurement in both arms, with an appropriate size cuff. A careful cardiovascular examination as well as a thorough neurological examination, including mental status, should be conducted. A careful funduscopic examination should be performed to detect hemorrhages, exudates, and/or papilledema.

Initial laboratory evaluation should include urinalysis with sediment examination, a stat chemistry profile, and an electrocardiogram. Laboratory results together with a complete history and thorough physical examination should enable a clinical assessment of the degree of target-organ involvement and should facilitate the selection of an appropriate antihypertensive agent for initial treatment.

Proteinuria, red blood cells, and/or cellular casts in the urine are suggestive of renal parenchymal disease. Electrolyte abnormalities and evidence of renal dysfunction may suggest secondary hypertension. The electrocardiogram should identify evidence of coronary ischemia and left ventricular hypertrophy, and pulse deficits should raise

the question of aortic dissection. A computed tomographic (CT) scan of the head should be considered when the clinical examination suggests cerebrovascular ischemia or hemorrhage, or in the comatose patient. The initial evaluation should help to decide whether to treat the patient with hypertensive crisis as emergency or urgency. The decision to treat as an emergency should prompt immediate admission to an intensive care unit for intravenous treatment and continuous BP monitoring.

GENERAL GUIDELINES FOR TREATMENT

The initial goal of the antihypertensive therapy is *not* to rapidly normalize BP but rather to prevent damage to target organs by gradually decreasing mean arterial pressure, while minimizing the risk of hypoperfusion.[8] Before discussing drug therapy for patients with hypertensive crisis it is important to emphasize that outcome data attesting to benefits of acutely lowering BP are not available. Thus most interventions currently used to treat hypertensive crisis have never been vigorously scrutinized. Much of the therapy, therefore, is entirely empirical and based on an attempt to best match pathophysiologic findings with pharmacologic properties of antihypertensive agents.

Several pharmacologic agents are available in the management of hypertensive crisis.[2] Those agents can be divided by mechanism of action and route of administration (parenteral vs. oral or sublingual) (Table 63–1).

Drug selection should be based on the severity of the crisis and on the specific hypertensive case. Emergency situations should aggressively treated typically using intravenous medication in units with monitoring facilities.[9]

PARENTERAL AGENTS

Several parenteral agents are available for the treatment of hypertensive emergencies (Table 63–2).

Sodium nitroprusside

Sodium nitroprusside is a short-acting direct vasodilator, requiring a constant intravenous infusion that can decrease BP in all patients irrespective of hypertension severity. The efficacy of sodium nitroprusside was compared with fenoldopam[10,11] with diazoxide and hydralazine[12] and with urapidil[13,14] in hypertensive crises, and was found to be effective in almost 100% of the cases.

The drug is light sensitive and should be shielded from light to prevent degradation. Sodium nitroprusside dilates both arteriolar resistance and venous capacitance vessels, thereby decreasing peripheral resistance without causing an increase in venous return.[2] The drug does not have any direct negative inotropic or chronotropic effects on the heart. By reducing the preload and afterload, sodium nitroprusside improves left ventricular function in patients with congestive heart failure and low cardiac output, and reduces myocardial oxygen demand in patients with ischemic heart disease.

The advantages of sodium nitroprusside in controlling hypertensive crisis in cardiac patients have been studied

DRUGS FOR TREATMENT OF HYPERTENSIVE CRISIS		
Drug	Mechanism of Action	Route of Administration
Sodium nitroprusside	Vasodilator	IV
Diazoxide	Vasodilator	IV
Hydralazine	Vasodilator	IV, IM
Nitroglycerin	Vasodilator	IV, SL
Nifedipine	CCB	PO
Nicardipine	CCB	IV, PO
Nimodipine	CCB	IV
Trimethaphan camsylate	Ganglionic blocker	IV
Phentolamine	α blocker	IV
Urapidil	α blocker with central serotonin-agonist activity	IV
Esmolol	β blocker	IV
Labetalol	α+β blocker	IV, PO
Captopril	ACE inhibitor	PO
Enalaprilat	ACE inhibitor	IV
Fenoldopam	Dopamine agonist	IV
Clonidine	α-2 agonist	PO
Furosemide	Loop diuretics	IV, PO
CCB, calcium channel blocker; IV, intravenous; IM, intramuscular; SL, sublingual; PO, oral.		

Table 63–1. Drugs for Treatment of Hypertensive Crisis

extensively. Recently, Khot et al.[15] reported their experience with nitroprusside in 25 normotensive patients with severe aortic stenosis and left ventricular dysfunction. Nitroprusside increased cardiac index that was associated with a significant increase in stroke volume and a significant fall in the systemic vascular resistance and pulmonary capillary wedge pressure. Nitroprusside was also well tolerated and improved renal function.

Several studies assessed the efficacy and safety of nitroprusside in ischemic heart disease. Kaplan and Jones[16] compared the effects of sodium nitroprusside and intravenous nitroglycerin in 20 patients during elective coronary artery surgery. Both regimens were effective in reducing intraoperative BP. However, nitroglycerin improved electrocardiographic ST segment depression in 8 of 10 patients, whereas sodium nitroprusside made the ST segment depression more pronounced in 3 of 10 patients. Decreased coronary perfusion pressure and intracoronary steal syndrome may be involved in the worsening of ischemia seen in patients receiving sodium nitroprusside. Flaherty et al.[17] found that sodium nitroprusside increased intrapulmonary shunting whereas nitroglycerin decreased it, thus making nitroglycerin more useful for managing patients with large intrapulmonary shunt or pulmonary hypertension.

Fremes et al.[18] found that nitroglycerin caused a greater reduction in myocardial oxygen demand and consumption than sodium nitroprusside in hypertensive patients after elective coronary bypass surgery. Therefore, if perioperative myocardial ischemia in the setting of postoperative hypertension is suspected, nitroglycerin may be a better antihypertensive agent.

In spite of the fact that sodium nitroprusside can increase intracranial pressure,[2] the fall in systemic pressure seems to block the rise in cerebral blood flow. It is therefore still recommended for management of some patients with encephalopathy and cerebrovascular accidents.[19] Despite its effectiveness as antihypertensive agent, sodium nitroprusside has not been used widely in pregnancy because of negative outcomes in animal experiments.[2]

Interaction of sodium nitroprusside with sulfhydryl groups in erythrocytes and tissues generates cyanide ions that are converted to thiocyanate by rhodanese in the liver, and then excreted by the kidney. However, with prolonged administration of sodium nitroprusside, or in patients with hepatic impairment, or renal insufficiency, free cyanide may accumulate, and interfere with aerobic metabolism, resulting in metabolic acidosis. Cyanide also interferes with the vasodilator action of sodium nitroprusside and may eventually lead to tachyphylaxis. Therefore, thiocyanate levels should be monitored periodically and maintained below 10 mg/100 mL in patients with hepatic impairment, renal insufficiency and in those receiving high dosages of sodium nitroprusside (3 µg/kg/min) or a prolonged infusion (>24–48 hours). It should be noted that the development of thiocyanate accumulation can not be predicted and even a dose that is considered to be safe may be toxic.[2] Thiocyanate toxicity includes fatigue, nausea, headache, disorientation, psychotic behavior, skin rashes, anorexia, convulsions, unexplained cardiopulmonary arrest, coma, diffuse encephalopathy, and even death.[2] When cyanide toxicity is diagnosed, it can be treated by the administration of amyl nitrate, sodium nitrate, and sulphydryl compound

PARENTERAL AGENTS FOR TREATMENT OF HYPERTENSIVE EMERGENCIES				
Drug	Dosage	Onset of Action	Duration of Action	Adverse Effects
Sodium nitroprusside	0.25–10 μg/kg/min	Immediate	1–2 minutes after infusion stopped	Nausea, vomiting, hypotension, muscle twitching, thiocyanate and cyanide toxicity mainly in patients with azotemia
Nitroglycerin	5-100 μg/min	1–5 minutes	5–10 minutes	Headache, nausea, tachycardia, vomiting, tolerance with prolonged use, methemoglobinemia
Labetalol hydrochloride	20–80 mg every 10–15 minutes, or 0.5–2 mg/min	5–10 minutes	3–6 hours	Vomiting, nausea, scalp tingling, bronchospasm, bradycardia, heart block, orthostatic hypotension
Fenoldopam mesylate	0.1–0.3 μg/kg/min	<5 minutes	30–60 minutes	Tachycardia, headache, nausea, flushing
Nicardipine hydrochloride	5-15 mg/h	5-10 minutes	15-90 minutes	Tachycardia, headache, flushing, local phlebitis
Esmolol hydrochloride	250–500 μg/kg/min IV bolus, then 50–100 μg/kg/min by infusion; may repeat bolus after 5 minutes or increase infusion to 300 μg/minute	1-2 minutes	10-30 minutes	Hypotension, nausea, asthma, first-degree heart block, heart failure
Urapidil	12.5–25 mg bolus followed by infusion of 5–40 mg/h	3–5 minutes	4–6 hours	Hypotension, headache, dizziness
Enalaprilat	0.625–5 mg every 6 hours	15 –30 minutes	6–12 hours	Hypotension, renal failure
Diazoxide	75–150 mg every 5 minutes, or 10–30 mg/min for 15–30 minutes	1–5 minutes	4–12 hours	Increased cardiac output and heart rate, precipitate ischemia, sodium retention, hyperglycemia, postural hypotension
Hydralazine	10–20 mg IV, or 10–50 mg IM; repeat every 4–6 hours	10–30 minutes	1–6 hours	Increased cardiac output and heart rate, headache, angina
Trimethaphan	1–15 mg/min	1–10 minutes	3–10 minutes after infusion stopped	Hypotension, tachyphylaxis, orthostatic effect, sympathetic blockade, respiratory arrest
Phentolamine	5–10 mg bolus	1–2 minutes	10–30 minutes	Tachycardia, flushing, headache, angina

Table 63–2. Parenteral Agents for Treatment of Hypertensive Emergencies

such as sodium thiosulphate. Thiosulphate can be used to prevent thiocyanate toxicity. It has also been demonstrated that hydroxocobalamin is safe and effective in preventing and treating cyanide toxicity associated with the use of nitroprusside.[3] In case of failure to respond to such therapy, hyperbaric oxygen therapy, hemodialysis, or charcoal hemoperfusion may prove beneficial; however, there is limited experience with this modes of therapy.[2] Considering the potential for severe toxicity with nitroprusside, this drug should only be used when other intravenous antihypertensive agents are not available and then only in specific clinical circumstances and in patients with normal renal and hepatic function. The duration of treatment

should be as short as possible and the infusion rate should not exceed 2 μg/kg per minute.

Nitroglycerin

Nitroglycerin is an antianginal as well as antihypertensive agent that dilates peripheral capacitance and resistance vessels. At higher doses nitroglycerin dilates arteriolar smooth muscle, thereby reducing peripheral resistance and afterload. It causes hypotension and reflex tachycardia, which are exacerbated by the volume depletion characteristic of hypertensive emergencies. Nitroglycerin reduces BP by reducing preload and cardiac output, which are undesirable effects in patients with compromised cerebral and renal perfusion. By diminishing preload, nitroglycerin decreases left ventricular end diastolic volume and pressure and myocardial wall tension, thus reducing myocardial oxygen consumption. These changes favor redistribution of coronary blood flow to the subendocardium, which is more vulnerable to ischemia. Nitroglycerin may dilate epicardial coronary vessels and their collaterals, and increase blood supply to ischemic regions. Continuous intravenous nitroglycerin is effective in decreasing the incidence of myocardial ischemia in patients with coronary artery disease undergoing cardiac and noncardiac surgery. Nitroglycerin is a better vasodilator of coronary conductance arteries than sodium nitroprusside and for that reason is preferred in the management of hypertensive crisis associated with acute coronary insufficiency.[19] Intravenous nitroglycerin infusion also has been used in controlling hypertensive crisis during pregnancy. Snyder et al.[20] reported the successful use of intravenous nitroglycerin in controlling hypertension during anesthesia for cesarean section, without neonatal depression or hypotension. The usual initial dose is 5 to 100 µg/min and can be titrated upward to a desired therapeutic endpoint. Doses as high as 200 to 300 µg/min may be required to achieve an adequate response. Onset of action is almost immediate with a very short duration of action of approximately 5 to 10 minutes.[2] Prolonged use of nitroglycerin is not associated with toxicity, but tolerance to its hemodynamic effects has been reported.[2] The main adverse effects are headache and tachycardia. The drug can also be used sublingually in selected patients.

Labetalol

Labetalol produces selective antagonism at the postsynaptic α-adrenoreceptors and nonselective antagonism at the β-adrenoreceptors. Labetalol reduces the systemic vascular resistance without reducing total peripheral blood flow. In addition, the cerebral, renal, and coronary blood flows are maintained. The drug can be given by repeated bolus of 20 to 80 mg every 10 to 15 minutes or by a continuous infusion of 0.5 to 2 mg/min. The average effective total dose is 200 mg. Labetalol is metabolized by the liver to form an inactive glucuronide conjugate. The hypotensive effect of labetalol begins within 5 to 10 minutes after its intravenous administration, reaching a peak at 5 to 15 minutes after administration and lasting for about 3 to 6 hours. The response rate in patients with hypertensive crisis is 80% to 93%.[2] The drug was found to be effective and safe in patients with myocardial infarction, in patients with acute postoperative hypertension after aortocoronary bypass surgery or surgery requiring general anesthesia, in neurovascular surgical patients, children with hypertensive crises, and hypertensive crisis complicating pregnancy.[2] The drug is contraindicated in patients with acute left ventricular failure, second- or third-degree atrioventricular block, and chronic obstructive pulmonary disease. Caution is needed to avoid postural hypotension if patients are allowed out of bed. Nausea, itching, tingling of the skin, and beta-blockade side effects may be noted. Transition to oral therapy with the same drug is not difficult.

Fenoldopam

Fenoldopam is a selective postsynaptic dopaminergic (DA_1) receptor agonist with weak α_2 antagonistic properties. Fenoldopam is a natriuretic agent that has potent vasodilator activity affecting primarily the renal vasculature.[21] Fenoldopam is rapidly and extensively metabolized by conjugation in the liver, without the participation of cytochrome P450 enzymes. The onset of action is within 5 minutes with the maximal response being achieved by 15 minutes. The duration of action is between 30 to 60 minutes with the pressure gradually returning to pretreatment values without rebound upon termination of the drug. Several clinical trials showed the effectiveness of intravenous fenoldopam in the treatment of severe hypertension and hypertensive crisis. At a dose of 0.2 to 0.5 µg/kg/min, fenoldopam decreases BP to desired levels within 5 to 40 minutes. Hemodynamically the drug induces a decrease in total peripheral resistance and in pulmonary vascular resistance with a slight elevation in heart rate. In another open, controlled, randomized, parallel trial, intravenous fenoldopam was compared to sodium nitroprusside in 18 patients with severe hypertension and mild renal failure.[11] Both antihypertensive agents successfully controlled BP in all patients. The rate of side effects was similar in both groups of patients. However, in two patients treated with sodium nitroprusside toxic levels of thiocyanate were detected. Thus fenoldopam may be superior to sodium nitroprusside for the control of hypertensive crisis in patients with decreased renal function.

In another comparative study, the electrocardiographic changes were recorded in 21 patients with hypertensive emergencies treated with either fenoldopam or sodium nitroprusside.[10] Both drugs reduced BP significantly in all patients. New T-wave inversion occurred in two patients treated with fenoldopam, and in four patients treated with sodium nitroprusside. Side effects included headache, flushing, tachycardia, and dizziness. Overall, tachycardia has occasionally been noted, and a dose-related increase in intraocular pressure has been observed in normotensive and hypertensive patients. It seems that fenoldopam is comparable to sodium nitroprusside, and can be the drug of choice in severely hypertensive patients with impaired renal function.

Nicardipine

Nicardipine is a dihydropyridine calcium antagonist with high vascular selectivity that can be administered intravenously.[22] The onset of action of intravenous nicardipine is between 5 and 10 minutes with duration of action of 15 to 90 minutes. It is an effective antihypertensive agent that decreases afterload by reducing total peripheral resistance without reducing cardiac output. Nicardipine improves left ventricular ejection fraction and pumping activity, both in normal and failing hearts.[2] The drug dilates more selectively the cerebral and coronary arteries than the remainder of the arterial tree, without changing heart rate. It may preserve tissue perfusion, and therefore may be advantageous in patients with ischemic disorders, such as coronary, cerebrovascular, and peripheral vascular disease. The drug is given as a continuous infusion at a starting dose of 5 mg/hr followed by increments of 2.5 mg/hr every 5 minutes until either reaching a maximal dose of 30 mg/hr or achieving the desired reduction in BP. Nicardipine has been used for the treatment of postoperative hypertension. In a double-blind study, intravenous nicardipine was compared with placebo in 123 patients with BP over 213/126 mmHg.[23] Of 73 patients who were treated with nicardipine, 67 patients achieved the therapeutic goal. Several side effects were reported; 30 patients had headache, 7 patients had hypotension, and 7 patients experienced nausea. Halpern et al.[24] and David et al.[25] found that nicardipine was as effective as sodium nitroprusside in patients with severe postoperative hypertension. Patients receiving intravenous nicardipine can then be easily switched to oral medication.

Esmolol

Esmolol is an ultra–short-acting β_1-selective adrenergic blocker. The onset of action of this agent is within 60 to 120 seconds and the duration of action is extremely short, about 10 to 30 minutes, because of its rapid metabolism by a specific plasma esterase. This characteristic provides a significant advantage because it is possible to titrate esmolol easily to the desired effect.[2] The drug can be administered either as a bolus injection or as a continuous intravenous infusion. The recommended loading dose is a bolus of 250 to 500 µg/kg/min followed by an infusion of 50 to 100 µg/kg/min. Esmolol is frequently combined with direct vasodilators to provide a more desirable hemodynamic profile. The negative chronotropic effect produced by esmolol may be beneficial in patients with ischemic heart disease. Esmolol has been used successfully with sodium nitroprusside in a few cases of hypertensive crises.[2]

Urapidil

Urapidil is a selective post-synaptic α_1 adrenoreceptor antagonist with strong vasodilating properties. The fact that it also antagonizes the pre-synaptic $5HT_1A$ (hydroxytryptamine) receptors explains the lack of reflex tachycardia in response to peripheral vasodilatation. Urapidil has a rapid onset of action, with a response rate of 81% to 100% in hypertensive emergencies.[26] Urapidil is given as an intravenous bolus at a dose of 12.5 to 25 mg followed by a continuous infusion at a rate of 5 to 40 mg/hr. It has no effect on coronary sinus blood flow, myocardial oxygen consumption, and myocardial lactate extraction, and it does not increase intracranial pressure. Adverse effects occur in 2% of all patients, and include hypotension, headache, and dizziness. Urapidil is safe and efficient in intraoperative hypertensive crises. In one study, the drug was given to 42 patients with intraoperative hypertensive crises. A significant reduction in BP was observed within 10 minutes in 81% of the patients.[27] In two studies the safety and efficacy of urapidil were compared with sodium nitroprusside. Response to treatment was similar in both treatment groups. However, BP re-elevation during the follow-up period was more common with sodium nitroprusside. Moreover, major side effects were more common in patients treated with sodium nitroprusside.[2] Since urapidil is equally effective compared to sodium nitroprusside with fewer adverse effects, urapidil is a reasonable alternative to sodium nitroprusside in the treatment of hypertensive emergency, especially in intraoperative hypertensive crises.

Enalaprilat

Enalaprilat is the only available angiotensin-converting enzyme (ACE) inhibitor that can be administered intravenously. Enalaprilat lowers BP within 15 to 30 minutes, but the BP response in hypertensive emergencies is unpredictable, in part because of variable degrees of plasma volume expansion. The initial recommended dose for enalaprilat is 0.625 to 1.25 mg administered over 5 minutes. The maximal single dose should not exceed 5 mg for patients receiving diuretics and 1.25 mg for patients with renal impairment.[2] The initial dose can be repeated after 1 hour if clinical response is inadequate. The total daily dose should not exceed 20 mg. In patients with severe renal insufficiency, the dose should be decreased because the compound is excreted primarily by the kidney.

Enalaprilat is more effective in patients with high-renin forms of hypertension, and may induce a dramatic fall in BP in patients who are volume depleted by previous dietary sodium restriction or diuretic use.[2] African Americans seem to respond poorly to enalaprilat, possibly because of their low renin levels. Because enalaprilat may induce severe hypotension in volume-depleted patients, it should be used with caution in patients who are at risk for cerebral hypotensive episode. In patients with hypertensive emergency, the response rate is about 65% and it is not dependent on the initial dose.[2] Thus a low dose of 0.625 mg may be adequate for initial treatment of hypertensive crisis.[28] In one study, enalaprilat was compared with intravenous urapidil and sublingual nifedipine in the management of hypertensive crisis. Only 70% of the patients in the enalaprilat group achieved goal BP (<180/95 mmHg within 45 minutes after start of treatment) versus 96% and 71% in the urapidil and nifedipine groups, respectively.[29]

The most common adverse effect is hypotension. The risk for hypotension increases in patients with evidence of renal hypertension, volume-depleted patients, and patients with prior use of diuretics. Enalaprilat is contraindicated in patients with evidence of bilateral renal artery stenosis or in patients with unilateral stenosis of a single kidney.[30] Thus enalaprilat is particularly useful in hypertensive emergencies associated with congestive heart failure or high renin levels, and can be easily replaced by oral enalapril for long-term maintenance therapy.

Diazoxide

Diazoxide is a direct rapid-acting vasodilator that decreases total peripheral resistance with a reflex increase in heart rate and cardiac output. The compensatory increase in cardiac output and heart rate can be blocked by concomitant beta blocker therapy. Since it does not cross the blood brain barrier, diazoxide has no direct effects on cerebral circulation, but of course cerebral blood flow will fall if systemic pressure is reduced below the lower limit of autoregulation. In the past, diazoxide was initially given as a rapid bolus of 300 mg. However, the standard rapid intravenous bolus administration may cause profound hypotension with subsequent myocardial ischemia and cerebrovascular insufficiency. The safer course is to give the drug either by smaller bolus doses of 75 to 150 mg intravenously, every 5 to 10 minutes or by a slow infusion of 10 to 30 mg/min for 15 to 30 minutes. These methods are equally effective and are associated with fewer adverse effects. The side effects of diazoxide include fluid retention, nausea, flushing, dizziness, and hyperglycemia. When using diazoxide, one must be aware of significant adverse effects such as postural hypotension, maternal and fetal hyperglycemia, and cessation of gestational labor that results from relaxation of the uterine smooth muscle. Diazoxide is contraindicated in patients with severe angina, acute myocardial infarction, dissecting aneurysm, and congestive heart failure. Because of potential side effects and the availability of new antihypertensive agents, the use of diazoxide in hypertensive emergencies decreased remarkably.[2]

Hydralazine

Hydralazine is a direct arteriolar vasodilator, with little effect on venous capacitance vessels, that produces a rapid BP decrease with diastolic pressure reduced more than systolic.[31] Its administration results in activation of baroreceptor reflexes leading to increased heart rate, myocardial contractility, and cardiac output, and augmented renal blood flow. Hydralazine can be given intravenously or intramuscularly in an initial dose of 10 to 50 mg. The drug should not be diluted with solutions containing dextrose or other sugars, because of its ability to form potentially toxic hydrazones.[31] The drug reduces systemic vascular resistance and BP in severe hypertension of pregnancy without a significant change in uteroplacental blood flow.[2]

Although hydralazine easily crosses the placenta, its relative safety and efficacy combined with extensive clinical experience have made it the most widely used antihypertensive agent in pregnancy-induced hypertension.[31] The major drawbacks of hydralazine are its side effects that include reflex tachycardia, salt and water retention, intense flushing, headache, nausea, vomiting, myocardial ischemia, and increased intracranial pressure. Therefore, the use of intravenous hydralazine is limited to patients with preeclampsia or eclampsia.[2]

Trimethaphan camsylate

Trimethaphan camsylate is a ganglionic blocker agent that inhibits both sympathetic and parasympathetic autonomic activity. It has a rapid onset and brief duration of action, and must be administered by continuous intravenous infusion with constant monitoring of BP. The usual starting dose is 0.5 to 1 mg/min. The dose is then titrated to achieve the desired BP level up to a maximum 15 mg/min. It is important to titrate the drug carefully, and to elevate the head of the patient's bed during the infusion to avoid severe postural hypotension. Trimethaphan camsylate is particularly useful in aortic dissection because it can be titrated carefully to permit smooth control of BP and because it decreases cardiac output and left ventricular ejection rate.

Tachyphylaxis develops frequently after 24 to 48 hours because of intravascular volume expansion, and this may be attenuated by the use of diuretics. Adverse effects include blurred vision, exacerbation of glaucoma, dry mouth, respiratory depression, nausea, constipation, fetal meconium ileus, paralytic ileus, impairment of renal blood flow with azotemia, and urinary retention. Because of the frequency and severity of side effects associated with this drug and the availability of more effective agents, it is now used only in patients with life-threatening disorders such as dissecting aortic aneurysm.[2,8]

Phentolamine

Phentolamine is a parenteral nonspecific α-adrenergic blocking agent with rapid onset and short-lasting hypotensive effect. It is given intravenously in boluses of 5 to 10 mg as necessary. Adverse effects include tachycardia, vomiting, and headache. In patients with coronary artery disease, phentolamine may induce angina pectoris or myocardial infarction. It is specifically useful in treatment of catecholamine-mediated hypertensive crises.[30] However, it is not consistently effective in other types of hypertensive emergencies.

OTHER AGENTS

Nimodipine

Nimodipine is a potent cerebral vasodilator that has been approved for use in relieving the vasospasm accompanying subarachnoid hemorrhage. Nimodipine has improved the outcome of patients with aneurysmal subarachnoid hemorrhage.[32,33] Its beneficial effect in aneurysmal subarachnoid hemorrhage seems to be unrelated to its hypotensive effect or to its cerebral vasodilator properties, and is perhaps related to preserving functioning neurons by preventing calcium influx to the ischemic cells. The drug is not recommended in hypertensive emergencies.[2]

Diuretics

In addition to an antihypertensive agent, a potent diuretic, usually furosemide, is given intravenously. The use of diuretics is somewhat controversial since most patients with hypertensive crisis are characterized by a contracted plasma volume. However, even if not given initially, a diuretic will likely be needed after other antihypertensives are used, since reactive renal sodium retention usually accompanies a fall in pressure and may blunt the efficacy of nondiuretic agents. Of note, if the patient is volume depleted, additional diuresis could be harmful.[2]

TREATMENT OF SPECIFIC HYPERTENSIVE EMERGENCIES

There is a multiplicity of disorders or diseases accompanying elevated BP that constitute a hypertensive crisis,

PREFERRED AGENTS FOR SPECIFIC HYPERTENSIVE EMERGENCY		
Emergency Condition	Preferred Agent	Comments
Hypertensive encephalopathy	Fenoldopam, labetalol, nicardipine or urapidil	Avoid methyldopa and diazoxide.
Cerebrovascular accident	Sodium nitroprusside, labetalol, urapidil, esmolol, nicardipine, nimodipine	Benefit from acute lowering of BP is uncertain.
Dissecting aortic aneurysm	Labetalol, or combination of nicardipine or fenoldopam or sodium nitroprusside with a β-blocker (metoprolol or esmolol), or trimethaphan	Titrate BP to the lowest possible level. Avoid hydralazine, diazoxide.
Acute left ventricular failure	Fenoldopam, or sodium nitroprusside with nitroglycerin, enalaprilat, urapidil, furosemide, morphine	Avoid labetalol, esmolol, diazoxide, hydralazine.
Coronary insufficiency	Nitroglycerin, labetalol, esmolol, nicardipine	BP should be reduced gradually. Avoid hydralazine, diazoxide.
Perioperative hypertension	Sodium nitroprusside, nitroglycerin, labetalol, urapidil, esmolol, nicardipine	Nitroglycerine is preferred in managing postcoronary bypass hypertension.
Eclampsia	Hydralazine, labetalol, urapidil, calcium antagonists	Avoid diuretics, trimethaphan, sodium nitroprusside, ACE inhibitor.
Catecholamine excess	Phentolamine, labetalol	Avoid diuretics, sodium nitroprusside.
Renal insufficiency	Fenoldopam, nicardipine, labetalol	Avoid β-blockers, sodium nitroprusside
BP, blood pressure.		

Table 63–3. Preferred Agents for Specific Hypertensive Emergency

and there is broad spectrum of pharmacologic agents that may be selected for treatment of these cases. Some agents that are useful for one hypertensive emergency may actually be contraindicated for another.[34] The recommended therapeutic approaches for specific conditions are summarized in Table 63–3.

Hypertensive encephalopathy

When mean arterial pressure reaches a critical level (around 180 mmHg), the previously constricted vessels are unable to withstand the pressure, counterregulation fails, and generalized vasodilatation ensues. Such a breakthrough of cerebral blood flow (CBF) leads to hyperperfusing the brain under high pressure, and results in cerebral edema and the clinical syndrome of hypertensive encephalopathy.[2] It is possible that many patients labeled as having "hypertensive encephalopathy" essentially had cerebrovascular events or intra-cranial space-occupying lesions, as brain imaging was less advanced in the past when this diagnosis was commonly made.

This scenario occurs at a much higher BP in patients with chronic hypertension than in previously normotensive persons. If untreated, the clinical picture progressively worsens, culminating in coma and death. Hypertensive encephalopathy is often indistinguishable from other acute neurologic complications of hypertension, such as cerebral infarction, subarachnoidal bleeding, or intracerebral hemorrhage. The only definite criterion to confirm diagnosis of hypertensive encephalopathy is a prompt improvement in the patient's condition in response to antihypertensive therapy.[35] First-choice drugs for this condition include intravenous fenoldopam, labetalol, nicardipine, or urapidil.

Cerebrovascular accidents
Intracerebral hemorrhage

As a result of intracerebral hemorrhage, intracerebral pressure rises and higher intra-arterial pressure is required to perfuse the brain adequately. In this condition, hypertension may be a result of increased intracerebral pressure and may resolve spontaneously within 48 hours.[35] Rapid reduction in BP may indeed prevent further bleeding, but at the risk of cerebral hypoperfusion.[1] One study compared the morbidity and mortality outcomes of patients with intracerebral hemorrhage according to their initial BP and the control of BP during the first 2 to 6 hours of presentation.[36] An improved outcome was observed in those who had an initial mean arterial pressure lower than 145 mmHg and in those who had their mean arterial pressure controlled below 125 mmHg. This retrospective study may suggest that markedly elevated BP may adversely affect the prognosis in hypertensive patients with intracerebral hemorrhage. Nevertheless, there is no consensus with regard to the advisability of reducing BP in these patients.[19] In any event the reduction should not exceed 20% of pretreatment BP level.[37] If BP is extremely elevated (diastolic pressure greater than 140 mmHg) and lasts more than 20 minutes, intravenous treatment is recommended.[38] The first drugs of choice for this condition include intravenous sodium nitroprusside, labetalol urapidil, esmolol, or nicardipine.[2] In one study, it was reported that nimodipine has improved the outcome of patients with aneurysmal subarachnoid hemorrhage.[33]

Acute ischemic stroke

Cerebral infarction causes impairment in autoregulation of CBF; thus elevated BP will accentuate perfusion through the damage tissue, leading to edema and compression of normal brain tissue. This provides evidence for carefully reducing BP in hypertensive patients with stroke. Conversely, because of local vasoconstriction, high arterial BP is required to perfuse jeopardized brain tissue around the infarct area. This provides evidence against reducing BP in acute ischemic stroke. Moreover, chronic hypertension and cerebral vascular disease move the autoregulation curve of CBF to the right so that a decrease in CBF occurs at a higher BP levels than in normal individuals. Therefore, cerebral hypoperfusion may appear at levels of BP that are still above the upper limit of normal. Patients with acute ischemic stroke demonstrate elevated BP levels on admission to the hospital. However, a spontaneous decrease in BP usually observed within the first 4 days after the event.[39] Moreover, no beneficial effect has been demonstrated by acute lowering of BP in patients with acute ischemic stroke. To the contrary, it has been shown that in patients with multiple stenosis of cerebral arteries, elevation of BP may improve the neurologic condition.

No antihypertensive treatment is recommended if BP is less than 180/105 mmHg. If BP is higher than 230/120 mmHg and persists more than 20 minutes, intravenous treatment is recommended. The target BP should be 160 to 170/95 to 100 mmHg for previously normotensive patients and 180 to 185/105 to 110 mmHg for previously hypertensive patients. The benefits to be derived from acutely lowering BP in patients with acute stroke of any kind remain conjectural and unsupported by good clinical or experimental studies. Sodium nitroprusside, labetalol, urapidil, esmolol, and nicardipine are the agents of choice whenever BP is to be reduced for patients with acute ischemic stroke. Results with nimodipine in this condition are equivocal so far.

Acute aortic dissection

Most untreated patients with acute aortic dissection die within 1 year, and most of the deaths occur within 2 weeks. Once diagnosis is suspected, attempts should be made to decrease the shear stress to the aortic wall with suitable agents. BP should be reduced within 15 to 30 minutes to the lowest tolerated level that preserves adequate organ perfusion. It has to be kept in mind that the force and velocity of ventricular contractions and pulsatile flow determine shear stress on the aortic wall. Drugs such as diazoxide or hydralazine that reflexively stimulate sympathetic activity and increase the shear stress on the aortic wall are contraindicated. Initial treatment should consist of labetalol or a combination of intravenous nicardipine or fenoldopam or sodium nitroprusside with intravenous β-blocking agent, most commonly metoprolol or esmolol. Used alone, sodium nitroprusside increases the velocity of ventricular contraction so that simultaneous β-blockade is obligatory. Trimethaphan camsylate, a ganglionic blocker, is also an alternative treatment.[2,30]

Acute left ventricular failure

Severe hypertension may precipitate acute left ventricular failure. Prompt reduction of BP decreases the work load of the failing myocardium and improves cardiac function.[35]

Immediate decrease of afterload with balanced vasodilating agent such as fenoldopam or sodium nitroprusside in combination with nitroglycerine is indicated in this circumstance.[2] Nitroglycerin alone is a reasonable alternative that has less afterload reducing capability than sodium nitroprusside, but may increase myocardial blood flow to ischemic areas in patients with acute myocardial ischemia. As urapidil has no influence on heart rate and myocardial oxygen consumption, it is a potential alternative to sodium nitroprusside and nitroglycerin if BP is insufficiently reduced. Concomitant therapy with oxygen, diuretics, or opioids may enhance efficacy of antihypertensive agents. Although the ACE inhibitors may be useful in this situation, there is a paucity of clinical experience concerning the therapeutic response to ACE inhibition in patients with acute left ventricular failure.[2] Drugs causing reflex tachycardia (diazoxide, hydralazine) or decreasing myocardial contractility (labetalol) should be avoided in this setting.[2]

Ischemic heart disease

Reduction of systemic BP by intravenous nitroglycerin reduces cardiac work, wall tension, and oxygen demand, and therefore has became the drug of choice for this crisis.[2] Intravenous nitroglycerine shortly after the onset of myocardial infarction may limit infarct size and improve ventricular ejection fraction.[40] Intravenous vasodilators, mainly sodium nitroprusside and nitroglycerin, have been tested in 11 trials involving 2170 patients with acute myocardial infarction and have reduced mortality by 43%. Cautious treatment of hypertension in patients with acute myocardial infarction is likely to be beneficial. Conversely, unnecessary reduction in BP could compromise an already unstable situation,[35] and therefore BP should be reduced gradually until symptoms subside or until the diastolic BP is approximately 100 mmHg.[2] Rapid reduction of BP with any drug may cause electrocardiographic changes.[10]

Initial treatment of patients with angina pectoris and severe hypertension includes sublingual nitroglycerin and morphine, followed by intravenous nitroglycerin if treatment is not successful. Nifedipine should not be used in this crisis, as it causes reflex tachycardia, increases myocardial oxygen demand, and may aggravate myocardial ischemia.[41]

Perioperative hypertension

Most of the time, perioperative hypertension is not an emergency in the usual sense, but parenteral agents frequently have to be used to control BP because patients are unable to receive medications orally. Severe hypertension may occur in some patients in the postoperative period, especially after open heart and carotid artery surgery. The etiology of this severe hypertension is mulifactorial, and includes withdrawal of antihypertensive drugs, pain, volume overload, and sympathetic activation.[35] In this setting, even moderate hypertension may jeopardize the integrity of the fresh vascular suture lines. Therapy should be individualized, and in some situations immediate lowering of the BP is warranted.[35] Hypotension is to be avoided in patients who have fresh vascular suture lines because of the danger of thrombosis.[19] Sodium nitroprusside is usually the agent of choice, provided that the patient is in an intensive care environment. Nitroglycerine administered intravenously may be the drug of choice for managing postcoronary bypass hypertension.[2] Labetalol, urapidil, esmolol, and nicardipine can also be used.

Eclampsia

Preeclampsia occurring in pregnancy is the syndrome of hypertension edema and proteinuria. Some of these patients may progress to eclampsia, which is associated with seizures and end-organ damage (cerebral hemorrhage, renal failure, microangiopathic hemolytic anemia).[42] The important part of safe treatment is to control hypertension, while keeping in mind the risk that reducing BP may further impair placental blood flow.

Hydralazine administered intravenously has been the drug of choice in recent years when diastolic BP is over 110 mmHg or when eclampsia supervenes; it is effective and does not decrease placental blood flow. Labetalol or calcium antagonists are possible alternative therapeutic approaches if hydralazine is ineffective.[42] Diuretics, trimethaphan camsylate, sodium nitroprusside, and ACE inhibitors should be avoided. If convulsions are imminent or occur, magnesium sulfate should be administered parenterally.

Excessive circulating catecholamines

Catecholamine-induced crises are characterized by a sudden increase in predominantly α-adrenergic tone. Plasma catecholamine levels are elevated in pheochromocytoma, rebound hypertension following clonidine withdrawal, hypertension associated with ingestion of sympathomimetics (cocaine hydrochloride, amphetamines, phencyclidine hydrochloride, lysergic acid diethylamide, and diet pills), and drug interaction of monoamine oxidase inhibitors with tyramine-rich food (certain beers, cheese, wine, chicken liver).[43] When this condition is suspected, the α-adrenergic–blocking drug, phentolamine, should be given. An alternative to phentolamine would be labetalol or sodium nitroprusside with β-blockers. A β-blocking drug may be needed if the patient has concomitant tachycardia or ventricular ectopy. Administration of β-blocking agent should always be preceded by α-blockade to prevent unopposed α-mediated peripheral vasoconstriction.[2]

Renal insufficiency

Deterioration of renal function in the face of elevated BP is considered a hypertensive emergency and requires lowering the BP. Therapy should reduce systemic vascular resistance without compromising the renal blood flow or glomerular filtration.[2] Fenoldopam, nicardipine, and labetalol are effective and well tolerated in these patients, and therefore should be used as the drugs of choice. Sodium nitroprusside is effective in these patients, but because of the high risk of thiocyanate toxicity it should not be used. β-blockers reduce the renal plasma flow and the glomerular filtration rate, and should therefore be used with caution if at all in these patients.

ORAL AGENTS FOR HYPERTENSIVE URGENCIES

During the last 20 years, the treatment focus for hypertensive urgencies has moved toward the use of oral agents. The ideal oral drug to treat hypertensive crisis should be one that has a rapid and smooth onset of action, few adverse effects, does not cause excessive hypotension, is convenient to monitor, and can be easily converted to a maintenance therapy.[44] The use of oral agents should be limited to hypertensive urgency as clearly recommended in the seventh report of the Joint National Committee on Prevention, Detection, Evaluation, and Treatment of High Blood Pressure (JNC 7).[9]

Captopril

Captopril, an ACE inhibitor was initially studied for treatment of hypertensive crisis in a few small uncontrolled studies using a dose of 25 mg sublingually.[45,46] Sublingual captopril is well tolerated and effective in reducing BP, the onset of action occurs within 5 to 10 minutes, and reaches a maximum within 30 minutes and lasts for at least 2 hours. Following oral administration of captopril on an empty stomach, maximal BP reduction is observed within 30 to 90 minutes.[2] Orally dissolved captopril seems to be more effective than captopril in standard oral administration. In one study,[47] sublingual administration of captopril reduced BP after 60 minutes from 196/112 to 154/90 mmHg with a response rate of 84%, whereas oral captopril reduced BP from 197/110 to only 182/99 mmHg with a response rate of 57%.

Patients with renal artery stenosis may suffer sudden severe deterioration of renal function. Undesirable effects are a rash and precipitous fall in BP in patients with suspected high renin levels.[2] In general, comparative trials have observed fewer side effects with captopril than with nifedipine administration. Most studies concluded that captopril should be considered as a first-line therapy in the acute management of hypertensive crisis.[2] However, as previously noted no outcome data are available that attest to benefits of captopril in this clinical situation.

Nifedipine

Nifedipine is a dihydropyridine calcium antagonist that lowers BP by peripheral vasodilatation with only mild negative inotropic and chronotropic effects. The advantages of nifedipine use are rapid onset of action and lack of central nervous system depression. Nifedipine is the most extensively studied agent for rapid control of BP, and until 1996 was used for acute BP lowering in hospitalized patients. After sublingual administration, the onset of action is within 1 to 5 minutes with a maximal effect at 20 to 30 minutes. The buccal absorption of nifedipine is minimal, and faster absorption and higher maximum concentrations were observed following the bite and swallow method when compared with other methods of dosing. The duration of action of a single dose of nifedipine is about 3 to 5 hours.[2] The most common adverse effect associated with nifedipine is reflex tachycardia secondary to pronounced vasodilatation. Some patients may experience symptoms of hypotension and flushing. Despite some reports on its efficacy and safety, sublingual nifedipine was not approved by the U.S. Food and Drug Administration for use in hypertensive emergency because of lack of scientific validation of advantageous use in this situation.

Nifedipine also has been associated with some severe adverse affects, including retinal ischemia, cerebral vascular accident, and myocardial ischemia and infarction.[41] Rapid uncontrolled pressure reduction may be harmful because it precipitates acute ischemic stroke or myocardial infarction. This has been emphasized with regard to short-acting nifedipine.[41] Therefore, the use of nifedipine capsules for hypertensive crisis should be abandoned. Oral nifedipine, however, may be used in hypertensive urgencies.

Nicardipine

Nicardipine is a second-generation dihydroperidine calcium antagonist that unlike nifedipine causes little, if any, increase in heart rate.[41] Nicardipine produces slower, and more prolonged decrease in BP than nifedipine, and therefore appears to be better tolerated. In a multicenter, randomized, double-blind, parallel placebo-controlled trial, 53 patients with hypertensive urgency were assigned to receive orally either 30 mg of nicardipine or placebo. Diastolic pressure decreased by 22.2 ±11.7 (SD) mmHg in the nicardipine group and only by 8.5 ±10.9 (SD) mmHg in the placebo group ($p<0.0001$). Adequate BP response was observed in 65% of the 26 patients treated with 30 mg of nicardipine and only in 22% of the 27 patients given the placebo ($p=0.002$). Of the 21 patients given the placebo who did not have an adequate BP response, 16 (76%) had adequate BP reduction after one open-label dose of 30 mg of nicardipine. Adverse events were reported in three patients given nicardipine and four patients given the placebo. Asymptomatic hypotension was noted in three patients, two in the nicardipine group, and one in the placebo group; one patient treated with nicardipine reported anxiety, headache, tachycardia, and chest pain.[48] During a 1-week follow-up, minor, well-tolerated adverse events were reported in the nicardipine group. Compared to nifedipine, it seems that oral nicardipine is safer and as effective a drug for the initial treatment of urgent hypertension.

Clonidine

Clonidine is a central-acting α_2-adrenergic receptor agonist that reduces BP by decreasing cerebral sympathetic outflow. Its action begins 30 to 60 minutes after administration, and its maximal effect is achieved within 1 to 4 hours and lasts for 6 to 8 hours.[2] A well-accepted method of clonidine administration in hypertensive crisis is by an oral loading regimen of an initial dose of 0.1 to 0.2 mg that may be repeated as needed. However, doses higher than 0.4 mg have little additional benefit in nonresponders.[2] Most studies report an average response rate of approximately 80%.[2] The drug should not be used in patients with altered mental status, because of its

common adverse effect of drowsiness.[2] In addition, clonidine can cause a significant decrease in CBF. One case of death from a progressive cerebral infarct following the administration of a cumulative clonidine dose of 0.4 mg was reported. Other complications associated with clonidine include dry mouth, occasional dizziness, and development of hypertensive crisis upon abrupt discontinuation of therapy. Due to its unpleasant side effects and its pharmacokinetics, the popularity of this drug is declining.

Labetalol

Labetalol is a unique antihypertensive agent that competitively inhibits both alpha- and beta-adrenergic receptors.[2] The alpha-blocking properties dominate in the treatment of hypertensive crisis. Labetalol reduces systemic vascular resistance and BP without inducing reflex tachycardia or change in cardiac output. Gonzalez et al.[49] conducted a dose–response study with labetalol in 36 patients. The maximal BP-lowering effect was seen at 2 hours, and BP control was maintained for 4 hours. An oral dose of 200 mg of labetalol was the most appropriate to maximize efficacy and tolerability. However, several other investigators used doses as high as 500 to 1200 mg to achieve BP control.[50] The initial dose should be 200 mg followed by hourly 200-mg doses to a maximal dose of 1200 mg. The response rate in patients with hypertensive urgency is 80% to 94%.[2] Because of its pharmacology, labetalol should not be used in patients with chronic obstructive lung disease, congestive heart failure, atrioventricular block, or bradycardia. Adverse effects include hypotension, dizziness, headache, nausea, vomiting, and flushing.

Other oral agents

The efficacy of other oral agents including methyldopa, phenoxybenzamine, losartan, valsartan, and direct-acting vasodilators, such as minoxidil and hydralazine, in treating hypertensive urgency has not been well studied. These drugs therefore have little if any role in the treatment of this condition.

TREATMENT OF HYPERTENSIVE URGENCIES

The most commonly seen hypertensive urgency is malignant-phase hypertension (MHT), which still occurs in the Third World and in clinical practices with a large migrant population.[51,52] MHT is usually defined clinically as a raised BP in association with bilateral retinal linear or flame-shaped hemorrhages and/or cotton-wool exudates and/or hard exudates, with or without papilledema. Malignant hypertension may be accompanied by other organ damage such as heart failure, kidney failure, and hypertensive encephalopathy. MHT affects under 1% of people with essential hypertension, but could occur in any form of hypertension. Afro-Caribbean patients tend to do badly, possibly because of their higher BPs and greater renal impairment at presentation, and not their ethnicity *per se*.

In uncomplicated MHT, the target-organ damage, which is retinopathy, occurs over days or weeks rather than minutes, and hence may be classed as a hypertensive "urgency" for managing blood pressure. In the setting of coexisting hypertensive encephalopathy or aortic dissection, the management would be the same as for a "hypertensive emergency."

The optimal approach in patients with a hypertensive urgency is to lower the BP gradually over 24 to 48 hours. This therapeutic approach requires a close follow-up of the patient in the first days after the acute event. When the cause of transient BP elevations is easily identified, such as pain or acute anxiety (as in panic disorders), the appropriate therapy is analgesic or anxiolytic medication. We have recently shown that antianxiety treatment with diazepam is as effective as sublingual captopril in patients with excessive hypertension.[53] When the cause of BP elevation is unknown, various oral antihypertensive agents are available. There are some reports attesting to the safety of intravenous drugs such as labetalol or urapidil in this setting, but this mode of treatment is not recommended. In the absence of any data comparing long-term outcome with the various agents, the choice of therapy should be based on efficacy and safety data.

The efficacy of the various oral antihypertensive agents seems to be similar, and it ranges in controlled trials between 96% to 98% for nifedipine, 79% to 100% for clonidine, 90% to 95% for captopril, 68% to 94% for labetalol, 65% to 91% for nicardipine, and 85% for nitroglycerine.[2] Acute lowering of BP may compromise cardiac and cerebral blood flow, especially in the elderly, and therefore may be associated with serious side effects. We have published a review of serious adverse effects following oral or sublingual administration of nifedipine capsule in hypertensive emergencies and pseudoemergencies.[41] Given the potential seriousness of adverse events, and the lack of any clinical documentation attesting to a benefit of rapid BP lowering, nifedipine capsules and any drug that lowers BP acutely to unpredictable levels should be avoided in hypertensive crisis. Of note oral agents should be used only in hypertensive urgency, and not emergency, and in this condition a slower reduction of BP over a period of hours to several days is more appropriate.

One should be careful not to be too aggressive in lowering BP, and to use the right agent for the right condition. When considering the appropriate agent, the mechanism of action and the profile of adverse effects should be taken into consideration. Nifedipine and to lesser degree captopril tend to increase heart rate and clonidine and labetalol tend to decrease it. This is particularly important in patients with ischemic heart disease. Other limitations are the use of labetalol in patients with bronchospasm and bradycardia and second and third degree heart blocks. Clonidine should be avoided if mental acuity is desired. Captopril should not be used in patients with bilateral renal artery stenosis or unilateral renal artery stenosis of a solitary kidney. All agents should be used carefully in volume-depleted patients.

TREATMENT OF SPECIFIC POPULATIONS

Hypertension in childhood

Hypertensive emergencies are rare events during childhood. Most children with hypertensive crisis have an underlying secondary cause of hypertension that is usually renal or renovascular in origin.[6] Extremely high BP may be seen in infants with autosomal recessive polycystic kidney disease. Extrarenal causes such as pheochromocytoma and neuroblastoma are less frequent. As in adults, the absolute BP values cannot be used as the only determinant of whether a child is experiencing a hypertensive emergency. In one study, as many as 24% of children presenting to the emergency room with hypertension required emergency management.[12] Of this group, 57 patients were treated with intravenous hydralazine or diazoxide to reduce BP within the first 12 to 24 hours. This management was associated with irreversible neurologic deficits in 4 out of the 57 patients. In a second subgroup of 53 patients, BP was reduced more gradually over 96 hours with either intravenous labetalol or sodium nitroprusside. In this subgroup no neurologic impairments were observed. Unfortunately, as in adults, a precise determination of what is safe for BP reduction has not been established. Intravenous treatment is often preferable due to greater ease in titrating BP.

In the absence of specific contraindications, a continuous infusion of nicardipine or sodium nitroprusside is preferable. Intravenous labetalol as a bolus injection followed by continuous infusion also may be used. Oral agents should be reserved for circumstances in which symptoms of end-organ toxicity are mild or absent.[54] Children have a more active renin-angiotensin system than adults, and a higher incidence of renal artery stenosis as a cause of severe hypertension. Therefore, the use of an ACE inhibitor should be withheld as long as the underlying cause for the hypertension is unknown.

Hypertension in the elderly

In general, older persons have a lower blood volume, lower plasma renin activity, and increased peripheral vascular resistance that affect the pharmacokinetics of some antihypertensive agents.[2] With age the decrease in glomerular filtration rate and blunted baroreceptor reflexes increase the risk of overdose and orthostatic hypotension. If supine hypertension is treated too vigorously, older patients may experience presyncope or actual syncope. The increase in systolic BP associated with age is actually atherosclerotic-related decrease in aortic distensability. In this setting, small changes in stroke volume can result in greater changes in systolic BP. Rapid reduction of BP is especially dangerous in elderly patients, and can cause transient ischemic attacks, strokes, angina, myocardial infarction, and syncope; therefore, low doses of antihypertensive agents should be used.

SUMMARY

Hypertensive crisis is defined as a severe elevation in BP, such as a diastolic BP above 120 to 130 mmHg, and can be subclassified into either emergency or urgency (Figure 63–1). Hypertensive emergencies are relatively rare, and are said to be present only when BP elevation confers an immediate treat to the integrity of the cardiovascular system. In this setting immediate reduction in BP is required, generally by intravenous therapy in an intensive care unit. Unlike emergencies, urgency is said to be present when severe elevation in BP is not associated with end-organ injury. Outcome data attesting to benefits of acutely lowering BP in this condition are not available.

Clearly, patients with hypertensive crises are not good candidates for prospective randomized trials. Therefore, the accepted approach for patients with hypertensive urgency is to lower the BP more gradually over 24 to 48 hours with oral antihypertensive agents. In many patients, panic or anxiety may be the precipitating factor for the BP elevation, and therefore anti-anxiety treatment may be initiated. If anxiety is not the cause, or an anti-anxiety agent does not lower the BP, then oral antihypertensive agent should be started. Any drug that lowers BP precipitously should be avoided. The efficacy of nifedipine, captopril, clonidine, labetalol, nicardipine, and nitroglycerin seems to be similar. Choice of the appropriate agent should be based on the underlying pathophysiologic and clinical findings, mechanism of action, and the potential adverse effects.

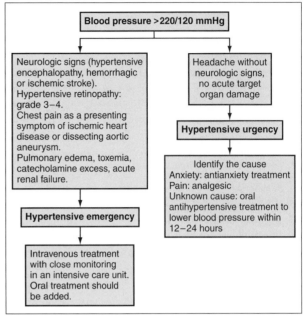

Figure 63–1. Therapeutic approach to hypertensive crisis.

REFERENCES

1. Calhoun DA, Oparil S. Treatment of hypertensive crisis. *N Engl J Med* 1990;323:1177–83.
2. Grossman E, Ironi AN, Messerli FH. Comparative tolerability profile of hypertensive crisis treatments. *Drug Safety* 1998;19:99–122.
3. Varon J, Marik PE. Clinical review: the management of hypertensive crises. *Crit Care* 2003;7:374–84.
4. Zampaglione B, Pascale C, Marchisio M, Cavallo-Perin P. Hypertensive urgencies and emergencies. Prevalence and clinical presentation. *Hypertension* 1996;27:144–7.
5. Kaplan NM. Management of hypertensive emergencies. *Lancet* 1994;344:1335–8.
6. Patel HP, Mitsnefes M. Advances in the pathogenesis and management of hypertensive crisis. *Curr Opin Pediatr* 2005;17:210–4.
7. Vidt DG. Emergency room management of hypertensive urgencies and emergencies. *J Clin Hypertens (Greenwich)* 2001;3:158–64.
8. Varon J, Marik PE. The diagnosis and management of hypertensive crises. *Chest* 2000;118:214–27.
9. Chobanian AV, Bakris GL, Black HR, Cushman WC, Green LA, Izzo JL Jr, et al. Seventh report of the Joint National Committee on Prevention, Detection, Evaluation, and Treatment of High Blood Pressure. *Hypertension* 2003;42:1206–52.
10. Gretler DD, Elliott WJ, Moscucci M, Childers RW, Murphy MB. Electrocardiographic changes during acute treatment of hypertensive

emergencies with sodium nitroprusside or fenoldopam. *Arch Intern Med* 1992; 152:2445–8.
11. Reisin E, Huth MM, Nguyen BP, Weed SG, Gonzalez FM. Intravenous fenoldopam versus sodium nitroprusside in patients with severe hypertension. *Hypertension* 1990;15:I59–62.
12. Deal JE, Barratt TM, Dillon MJ. Management of hypertensive emergencies. *Arch Dis Child* 1992; 67:1089–92.
13. Hirschl MM, Binder M, Bur A, Herkner H, Mullner M, Woisetschlager C, et al. Safety and efficacy of urapidil and sodium nitroprusside in the treatment of hypertensive emergencies. *Intensive Care Med* 1997;23:885–8.
14. van der Stroom JG, van Wezel HB, Vergroesen I, Kal JE, Koolen JJ, Dijkhuis JP, et al. Comparison of the effects of urapidil and sodium nitroprusside on haemodynamic state, myocardial metabolism and function in patients during coronary artery surgery. *Br J Anaesth* 1996;76:645–51.
15. Khot UN, Novaro GM, Popovic ZB, Mills RM, Thomas JD, Tuzcu EM, Hammer D, et al. Nitroprusside in critically ill patients with left ventricular dysfunction and aortic stenosis. *N Engl J Med* 2003;348:1756–63.
16. Kaplan JA, Jones EL. Vasodilator therapy during coronary artery surgery. Comparison of nitroglycerin and nitroprusside. *J Thorac Cardiovasc Surg* 1979;77:301–9.
17. Flaherty JT, Magee PA, Gardner TL, Potter A, MacAllister NP. Comparison of

intravenous nitroglycerin and sodium nitroprusside for treatment of acute hypertension developing after coronary artery bypass surgery. *Circulation* 1982; 65:1072–7.
18. Fremes SE, Weisel RD, Mickle DA, Teasdale SJ, Aylmer AP, Christakis GT, et al. A comparison of nitroglycerin and nitroprusside: I. Treatment of postoperative hypertension. *Ann Thorac Surg* 1985;39:53–60.
19. Gifford RW Jr. Management of hypertensive crises. *JAMA* 1991; 266:829–35.
20. Snyder SW, Wheeler AS, James FM 3rd. The use of nitroglycerin to control severe hypertension of pregnancy during cesarean section. *Anesthesiology* 1979; 51:563–4.
21. Tuncel M, Ram VC. Hypertensive emergencies: etiology and management. *Am J Cardiovasc Drugs* 2003;3:21–31.
22. Clifton GG, Cook ME, Bienvenu GS, Wallin JD. Intravenous nicardipine in severe systemic hypertension. *Am J Cardiol* 1989;64:16H–8H.
23. Wallin JD, Fletcher E, Ram CV, Cook ME, Cheung DG, MacCarthy EP, et al. Intravenous nicardipine for the treatment of severe hypertension. A double-blind, placebo-controlled multicenter trial. *Arch Intern Med* 1989; 149:2662–9.
24. Halpern NA, Goldberg M, Neely C, Sladen RN, Goldberg JS, Floyd J, et al. Postoperative hypertension: a multicenter, prospective, randomized comparison between intravenous

nicardipine and sodium nitroprusside. *Crit Care Med* 1992;20:1637–43.

25. David D, Dubois C, Loria Y. Comparison of nicardipine and sodium nitroprusside in the treatment of paroxysmal hypertension following aortocoronary bypass surgery. *J Cardiothorac Vasc Anesth* 1991;5:357–61.

26. Langtry HD, Mammen GJ, Sorkin EM. Urapidil. A review of its pharmacodynamic and pharmacokinetic properties, and therapeutic potential in the treatment of hypertension. *Drugs* 1989;38:900–40.

27. Fontana F, Allaria B, Brunetti B, Arienta R, Favaro M, Trivellato A, et al. Cardiac and circulatory response to the intravenous administration of urapidil during general anaesthesia. *Drugs Exp Clin Res* 1990;16:315–8.

28. Hirschl MM, Binder M, Bur A, Herkner H, Brunner M, Mullner M, et al. Clinical evaluation of different doses of intravenous enalaprilat in patients with hypertensive crises. *Arch Intern Med* 1995;155:2217–23.

29. Hirschl MM, Seidler D, Mullner M, Kurkciyan I, Herkner H, Bur A, et al. Efficacy of different antihypertensive drugs in the emergency department. *J Hum Hypertens* 1996;10(Suppl 3):S143–6.

30. Hirschl MM. Guidelines for the drug treatment of hypertensive crises. *Drugs* 1995;50:991–1000.

31. Abdelwahab W, Frishman W, Landau A. Management of hypertensive urgencies and emergencies. *J Clin Pharmacol* 1995;35:747–62.

32. Tettenborn D, Dycka J. Prevention and treatment of delayed ischemic dysfunction in patients with aneurysmal subarachnoid hemorrhage. *Stroke* 1990; 21:IV85–9.

33. Wong MC, Haley EC Jr. Calcium antagonists: stroke therapy coming of age. *Stroke* 1990;21:494–501.

34. Frohlich ED. American College of Chest Physicians' Consensus Panel on Hypertensive Emergencies. *Chest* 1990; 98:785–6.

35. Ram CV. Immediate management of severe hypertension. *Cardiol Clin* 1995; 13:579–91.

36. Dandapani BK, Suzuki S, Kelley RE, Reyes-Iglesias Y, Duncan RC. Relation between blood pressure and outcome in intracerebral hemorrhage. *Stroke* 1995;26:21–4.

37. Lavin P. Management of hypertension in patients with acute stroke. *Arch Intern Med* 1986;146:66–8.

38. Brott T, Reed RL. Intensive care for acute stroke in the community hospital setting. The first 24 hours. *Stroke* 1989; 20:694–7.

39. Britton M, Carlsson A, de Faire U. Blood pressure course in patients with acute stroke and matched controls. *Stroke* 1986;17:861–4.

40. Lau J, Antman EM, Jimenez-Silva J, Kupelnick B, Mosteller F, Chalmers TC. Cumulative meta-analysis of therapeutic trials for myocardial infarction. *N Engl J Med* 1992;327:248–54.

41. Grossman E, Messerli FH, Grodzicki T, Kowey P. Should a moratorium be placed on sublingual nifedipine capsules given for hypertensive emergencies and pseudoemergencies? *JAMA* 1996;276: 1328–31 (see comments).

42. Report of the National High Blood Pressure Education Program Working Group on High Blood Pressure in Pregnancy. *Am J Obstet Gynecol* 2000; 183:S1–22.

43. Grossman E, Messerli FH. High blood pressure. A side effect of drugs, poisons, and food. *Arch Intern Med* 1995; 155:450–60.

44. Gales MA. Oral antihypertensives for hypertensive urgencies. *Ann Pharmacother* 1994;28:352–8.

45. Case DB, Atlas SA, Sullivan PA, Laragh JH. Acute and chronic treatment of severe and malignant hypertension with the oral angiotensin-converting enzyme inhibitor captopril. *Circulation* 1981;64:765–71.

46. Tschollar W, Belz GG. Sublingual captopril in hypertensive crisis. *Lancet* 1985;2:34–5.

47. Di Veroli C, Pastorelli R. Acute captopril treatment in elderly hypertensive patients: a controlled study. *J Hypertens Suppl* 1988;6:S95–6.

48. Habib GB, Dunbar LM, Rodrigues R, Neale AC, Friday KJ. Evaluation of the efficacy and safety of oral nicardipine in treatment of urgent hypertension: a multicenter, randomized, double-blind, parallel, placebo-controlled clinical trial. *Am Heart J* 1995;129:917–23.

49. Gonzalez ER, Peterson MA, Racht EM, Ornato JP, Due DL. Dose-response evaluation of oral labetalol in patients presenting to the emergency department with accelerated hypertension. *Ann Emerg Med* 1991; 20:333–8.

50. Atkin SH, Jaker MA, Beaty P, Quadrel MA, Cuffie C, Soto-Greene ML. Oral labetalol versus oral clonidine in the emergency treatment of severe hypertension. *Am J Med Sci* 1992; 303:9–15.

51. Lip GYH, Beevers M, Beevers DG. Complications and survival of 315 patients with malignant-phase hypertension. *J Hypertens* 1995; 13:915–24.

52. Lip GYH, Beevers M, Beevers DG. The failure of malignant hypertension to decline: a survey of 24 years' experience. *J Hypertens* 1994;12: 1297–305.

53. Grossman E, Nadler M, Sharabi Y, Thaler M, Shachar A, Shamiss A. Antianxiety treatment in patients with excessive hypertension. *Am J Hypertens* 2005;18:1174–7.

54. Groshong T. Hypertensive crisis in children. *Pediatr Ann* 1996;25:368–71, 375–6.

Chapter

64 Renovascular Hypertension

Graham W. Lipkin, Puchimada Uthappa, and Jason Moore

Definition

- Renovascular hypertension (RVH) is a syndrome of arterial hypertension caused by reduced renal perfusion pressure secondary to a vascular lesion of the main renal artery or one of its branches.

- Atheromatous renovascular disease (ARVD) and fibromuscular dysplasia account for around 90% and 10% of renovascular hypertension, respectively.

- A significant renal artery stenosis is identified by a greater than 70% luminal area narrowing or 20-mmHg translesional pressure gradient. Lesser degrees of stenosis are unlikely to be causes of hypertension or chronic kidney disease.

Key Findings

- ARVD may present with RVH, ischemic nephropathy, flash pulmonary edema, and acute uremia following introduction of converting enzyme inhibitors or angiotensin receptor–blocking agents, or may be asymptomatic.

- ARVD, which is associated with widespread atheromatous disease, is progressive and portends a very high cardiovascular mortality.

- Magnetic resonance angiography (gadolinium contrasted) or computed tomographic angiography (in patients with normal renal function) are the investigations of choice for ARVD.

Clinical Implications

- In selected patients, percutaneous transluminal renal artery angioplasty (PTRA) is the treatment of choice for RVH caused by fibromuscular dysplasia. The use of stenting may successfully and durably correct ARVD, and may stabilize or improve chronic kidney disease and renovascular hypertension, as well as "flash" pulmonary edema secondary to ARVD.

- Controlled trials of PTRA (without stent) in RVH have shown little benefit in the control of blood pressure. Large multicenter randomized controlled trials of percutaneous renal artery endovascular stent insertion in patients with RVH and chronic kidney disease secondary to ARVD are underway.

Renovascular hypertension (RVH) is a syndrome of arterial hypertension caused by reduced renal perfusion pressure secondary to a vascular lesion of the main renal artery or one of its branches. RVH is the most common cause of secondary, potentially remediable hypertension (1% to 5%), and is usually caused by atheromatous renovascular disease (ARVD) (>90%) or fibromuscular dysplasia (FMD). Less common causes include arteritis (Takayasu's aortitis, giant cell arteritis and classical polyarteritis nodosa) thrombosis, embolism, dissection of the renal artery, neurofibromatosis and prior radiotherapy.[1] Where the lesion(s) subtend the entire renal mass, impaired renal function (ischemic nephropathy) may result. In patients aged over 50 years with chronic kidney disease, ARVD may contribute to renal damage in 14% to 25% of patients.[2] Correction of ARVD should ideally lead to the cure of hypertension and/or normalization of renal function. However, coexisting processes such as essential hypertension or renal parenchymal disease (such as diabetic, hypertensive, or atheroembolic nephropathy) frequently limit complete recovery in this patient group.[3]

It must be stressed that the finding of renovascular disease (RVD) in a patient with hypertension and/or impaired renal function does not necessarily indicate a causal relationship (see Figure 64–1). The prevalence of ARVD in a postmortem study was 5%, 18%, and 42% in those aged less than 64, 65 to 74, and 75 and older, respectively.[4] "Incidental" ARVD is not uncommon and has been increasingly identified. The functional significance of renal artery stenosis should be explored when considering intervention.

Since the 1980s, major advances have occurred in the understanding of pathophysiology, diagnosis (particularly noninvasive contrast magnetic resonance angiography (MRA) and computed tomography angiography (CTA), medical and interventional treatment (percutaneous transluminal renal artery angioplasty [PTRA] plus endoluminal stent insertion) of RVH. As medical treatment of hypertension has improved, the focus of intervention has shifted from blood pressure control to the preservation of renal function in patients with ischemic nephropathy due to significant renal artery stenosis. Nevertheless, the evidence base in this field is severely limited, and many key questions surrounding patient investigation and patient selection for revascularization await the outcome of ongoing prospective randomized trials.

This chapter focuses on practical clinical approaches to the identification, investigation, and treatment of RVH in native kidneys in adults. The 2006 American College of Cardiology/American Heart Association recommendations have been summarized in boxes after each section so as to inform best current practice.[1]

ANATOMY AND PATHOLOGY

Fibromuscular dysplasia

Fibromuscular dysplasia (FMD) accounts for less than 10% of cases of renal artery stenosis and encompasses an important group of non-atherosclerotic, non-inflammatory vascular diseases pathologically sub-classified by the arterial layer in which the lesion predominates.[5] The most frequent dysplastic pathology is medial fibroplasia, characterized by alternating aneurismal (intimal and medial thinning with loss of the internal elastic lamina) and stenotic (medial thickening and fibrosis) arterial segments. This leads to the classical "string of beads" appearance seen in angiography. In contrast to atheromatous disease, medial fibroplasia usually affects the mid and/or distal main renal artery (60% of cases) and less commonly intrarenal segmental branches (<10%). Bilateral renal artery involvement and involvement of extrarenal vascular beds, typically the extracranial carotid circulation, is seen in around one-third of cases. In the latter case, there is an association with intracranial aneurysm formation. Renal artery aneurysms may develop as the predominant clinical feature. Aneurysms larger than 2 cm are at risk of rupture, particularly in pregnancy. Intimal fibroplasia is identified as focal concentric stenoses at angiography. The differential diagnosis is of an arteritic process.[5]

The pathogenesis of FMD remains obscure, but mural ischemia, due to functional defects in the vasa vasorum during development, has been postulated. FMD of renal arteries is more common in younger women (second to fifth decade) and in those who smoke. A genetic component is suggested by the finding of FMD in increased frequency in first-degree family members and in people who carry certain angiotensin converting enzyme (ACE) gene polymorphisms.

Atherosclerotic renovascular disease

Atheromatous renovascular disease is the most common cause of renal artery stenosis. It can be considered primarily as a disease of the abdominal aorta, in which atheromatous plaques encroach on the ostia of the renal arteries. As such, over 80% of ARVD is ostial, and bilateral disease is found in 50% of cases.[6] At angiography, ostial disease is defined as a stenosis of up to 1 cm from the aortic lumen, which reflects massive aortic wall thickening often seen in this setting. Widespread atheroma of other arterial territories is common, particularly in peripheral vascular disease.

Atheromatous renovascular disease is commonly associated with reduced glomerular filtration rate (GFR) related to parenchymal renal damage that may be unrelated to the stenosis.[7] Typically, hypertensive nephropathy, atheroembolic damage, and diabetic glomerulonephropathy (where relevant) coexist. In the setting of critical narrowing, ischemic nephropathy or focal renal infarction can be superimposed. Unlike coronary artery stenosis, ARVD is usually characterized by slowly progressive stenoses. As such renal structure may be maintained by the development of collateral blood supply arising most commonly from adrenal and lumbar arteries even in the setting of renal artery occlusion. This should be considered in defining clinical management.[8]

Pathophysiology

It is important to emphasize that the finding of renal artery stenosis in a patient with hypertension and/or renal impairment may be incidental rather than causal, and therefore relief of stenosis may not be beneficial. Understanding the pathophysiology is essential to appropriate clinical management of this condition.

Animal models

Much of our understanding of the pathophysiologic mechanisms of renovascular hypertension stem from the seminal studies performed by Goldblatt of experimental renal artery clipping (stenosis) in dogs. The histology showed that there was a pattern of changes in the kidney with imposed narrowing including marked interstitial fibrosis and B- and T-cell infiltrate.

The two-kidney, one-clip (2K1C) model corresponds to unilateral renal artery stenosis. Renal hypoperfusion acutely activates the renin-angiotensin-aldosterone system resulting in angiotensin II–dependent hypertension. The mechanisms include vasoconstriction, sodium retention, aldosterone release, and augmentation of sympathetic nerve activation. This elevation of blood pressure (BP) results in a pressure natriuresis from the contralateral nonstenotic kidney preventing volume overload; however, systemic vasoconstriction persists. Although hypertension is sustained, plasma renin activity declines and raised BP may be subsequently maintained by alternative mechanisms such as enhanced oxidative stress, raised endothelin, and vasoconstrictor prostaglandin production together with vascular remodeling.[9] In this model, GFR is preserved by angiotensin II–dependent constriction of postglomerular arterioles maintaining intraglomerular pressure. This may explain the loss of GFR in patients with renal artery stenosis to the entire functioning renal mass treated with ACE inhibitors or ARB drugs. The central role of angiotensin II is confirmed by observations that "knockout" mice deficient in ATII receptors or normal animals pre-treated with converting enzyme inhibitors do not become hypertensive despite unilateral renal artery clipping.

The one-kidney, one-clip (1K-1C) model more closely corresponds to tight bilateral renal artery stenosis or unilateral renal artery stenosis to a sole functioning kidney. Initially raised BP is secondary to activation of the renin-angiotensin-aldosterone system. With time, volume overload secondary to progressive sodium retention develops and tends to lead to reduction in plasma renin activity. This sodium-dependent model of hypertension can be converted to an angiotensin-dependent model by restricting salt intake or by administering diuretics.

Clinical studies

In the clinical setting of bilateral renal artery stenosis or unilateral renal artery stenosis to a single functioning kidney, ACE inhibitors or angiotensin-receptor blocking (ARB) drugs may induce acute renal failure by reducing BP and by relieving angiotensin II–dependent postglomerular vasoconstriction and, as a consequence reducing glomerular filtration. Acute uremia following these agents is an increasingly common presentation of renal artery stenosis.

Failure to tolerate ACE-inhibitor/ARB drugs represents an increasing indication for renal revascularization. The clinical situation is more complex than in experimental studies. It is now clear that most but not all patients with bilateral RVD do indeed tolerate cautiously monitored ACE-inhibitor/ARB drugs.[10] Left ventricular hypertrophy, endothelial dysfunction, and renal interstitial fibrosis are striking features of renal artery stenosis and ischemic nephropathy. They appear to be in excess of that expected for BP and renal function when compared with essential hypertensive controls.[11,12] Aldosterone released by angiotensin II is now recognized to participate in regulation of tissue fibrosis and left ventricular hypertrophy. It may be an important mediator of these effects in patients with RVH, suggesting a further important role for drugs that block the renin-angiotensin-aldosterone system.

What degree of renal artery stenosis is significant in humans?

Understanding the degree of arterial stenosis at which the kidney suffers ischemia is critical to interpretation of clinical data (Figure 64–1). In healthy people, the kidneys account for 0.5% of body weight, receive 20% of cardiac output, and less than 10% of oxygen delivery is required for metabolic purposes of the kidney. Furthermore, autoregulation maintains renal blood flow and glomerular filtration over a wide range of arterial perfusion pressure. It is therefore not surprising that substantial renal artery luminal stenosis is required before renal ischemia ensues. Difficulties in interpretation of clinical studies are further compounded by known interobserver variability in assessing the degree of renal artery stenosis at angiography, the current "gold standard." In addition, there is inconsistent reporting of stenosis in clinical studies. Maximal luminal diameter or luminal area narrowing are reported interchangeably (two-dimensional assessment only). In experimental studies, luminal area narrowing of more than 75% is required to significantly reduce renal blood flow. Renal blood flow, GFR, and perfusion pressure rapidly diminish with greater narrowing.[13] Clinical studies demonstrate a clinically significant transstenotic peak pressure gradient to be greater than 20 mmHg (mean >10 mmHg). This corresponds to area stenosis of more than 75%, that is, greater than 50% reduction in renal artery diameter if the lesion is concentric.[14] Renal blood flow reduction is thus a late phenomenon in progressive renal artery stenosis, and is manifested only by severe stenosis. This issue complicates interpretation of much of the clinical intervention literature. Studies that include patients with only 50% to 70% of renal artery diameter narrowing have probably incorporated patients without "significant" disease.[15]

The clinical situation is much more complex and heterogeneous, and the relevance of animal models is unclear. There is significant species variability in response to renal ischemia; the Goldblatt model is induced acutely in contrast to the slowly progressive clinical situation in ARVD, which allows collateral circulation to develop. In humans, there is frequent pre-existing essential hypertension and renal parenchymal damage due to small-vessel hypertensive damage, cholesterol emboli, and coexistent diabetic renal disease (Figure 64–2). Wright et al.[7,16] demonstrated that in a group of patients with ARVD, there was no correlation between renal artery anatomy and baseline renal function or functional outcome following intervention. The same applies to studies comparing individual renal function and the severity of ARVD. Severe renal artery stenosis can lead to worsening renal interstitial fibrosis distal to a stenosis, but the mechanisms are incompletely understood.

CLINICAL PRESENTATION AND NATURAL HISTORY

Fibromuscular dysplasia

Fibromuscular dysplasia typically presents with hypertension in young women in the second to fifth decade of

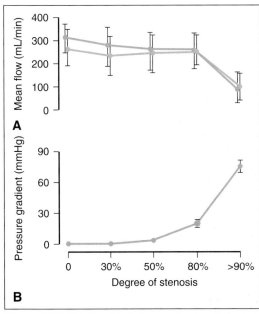

Figure 64–1. Relationship between degree of renal artery stenosis and renal blood flow in a canine model of renovascular disease. (Redrawn from Schoenberg SOM, et al. *J Am Soc Nephrol* 2000;11:2190–198.)

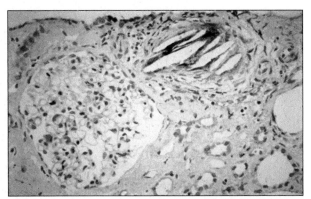

Figure 64–2. Severe chronic parenchymal renal disease due to athero-embolism in a patient with moderate renal artery stenosis.

life. Screening of a population with resistant hypertension identified the cause to be FMD in 16% of cases (Figure 64–3). However, evidence from screening of kidney donors indicates that "incidental" asymptomatic FMD may be relatively common, being detected in 3% to 6% of normotensive individuals.[17] The differential diagnosis includes atheromatous disease, arteritic processes, and rarely, connective tissue disorders Marfan's and Ehlers-Danlos syndrome. It is not usually difficult to distinguish FMD from atherosclerotic disease clinically. Patients with symptomatic FMD are usually younger and have no other evidence of atherosclerotic disease. At angiography FMD affects the middle/distal renal artery rather than the renal artery origin. In contrast ARVD is almost invariably associated with aortic atheroma.[2] Arteritic diseases such as Takayasu's aortitis and giant cell arteritis are typically associated with systemic symptoms and elevated acute phase markers. The natural history of FMD is variable and not necessarily benign. Progression of angiographic disease (new lesions, increasing stenosis or aneurysm dilatation) occurs in over a third of cases and loss of renal mass (>0.5 cm bipolar length) may be seen in two-thirds of cases, although renal artery occlusion and progressive renal failure are rare unless severe hypertension causes contralateral renal damage.[18,19]

Atheromatous renovascular disease

Atheromatous renovascular disease is relatively common but frequently asymptomatic and incidental to coexisting hypertension or chronic kidney disease[9] (Figure 64–4). Hansen et al.[20] studied the prevalence of ARVD using renal

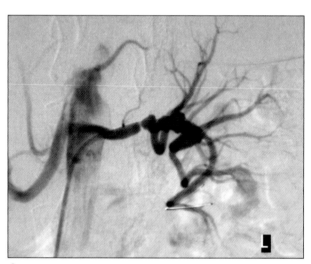

A

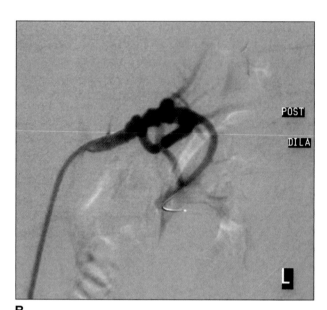

B

Figure 64–3. Catheter renal angiogram of 31-year-old female with severe hypertension due to fibromuscular dysplasia (medial fibroplasia). Left renal artery stenosis in setting of alternating stenosis and dilatation (**A**). Following successful left renal artery balloon angioplasty (**B**). Large right renal artery aneurysm that was managed surgically (**C**).

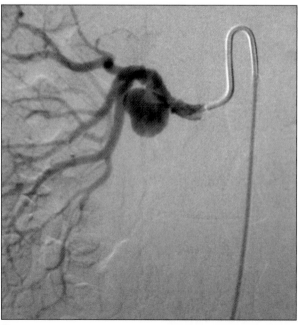

C

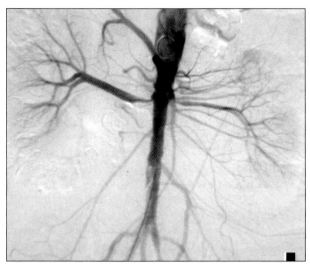

A

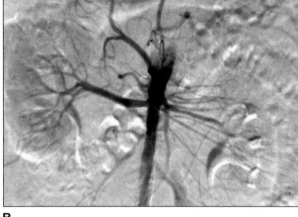

B

Figure 64–4. Catheter renal angiograms of a 55-year-old female with rapid worsening of hypertension on background of longstanding stable essential hypertension and mild chronic kidney disease. She suffered acute renal failure following introduction of converting enzyme inhibitor. Bilateral severe ostial atheromatous renal artery stenoses (**A**). Following successful bilateral percutaneous renal artery stent insertion. (**B**), renal function improved and antihypertensive drug therapy reduced. Twelve months later, serum creatinine and blood pressure rose. Repeat catheter angiography showing instent restenosis which was successfully treated with instent angioplasty (**C**).

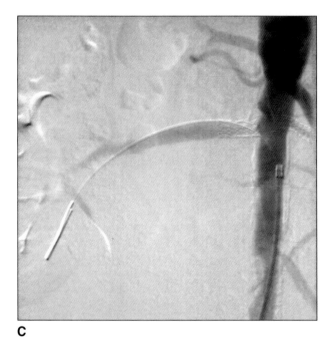

C

artery duplex ultrasound in individuals aged over 65. Of 834 participants, the overall prevalence of significant ARVD (>60%) was 6.8%. It was more frequent in men (9.1%) than women (5.5%). Contrary to previous studies, the prevalence was equal in black and white subjects.

The typical patient with ARVD is older (aged over 55), often with a long-standing history of essential hypertension, features of the metabolic syndrome or type II diabetes mellitus, and a background of ischemic heart disease, peripheral vascular, and cerebrovascular disease. The patient frequently has associated mild chronic kidney disease (as assessed by estimated creatinine clearance), and it is not unusual for the patient to have already undergone revascularization in another arterial territory. The prevalence of ARVD seems to be increasing as mortality from asso-

ciated coronary artery and cerebrovascular disease is diminishing.[9] Patients are living longer to be identified with more widespread manifestations of atheroma. It is also increasingly common to identify the lesion as the accuracy of screening tests has improved (MRI, CTA, and catheter aortography performed at the time of other indications such as peripheral vascular disease).

Clinically significant atheromatous renal artery stenosis (>75% stenosis or 20-mmHg translesional pressure drop) may present with one of the following clinical syndromes:
1. Renovascular hypertension
2. Ischemic nephropathy (chronic renal failure)
3. Acute renal failure following introduction of ACE inhibitor/ARB drugs
4. Resistant fluid retention/"flash" pulmonary edema

Box 64–1

Clinical Clues to Diagnosis of Renal Artery Stenosis: Recommendations of American College of Cardiology/American Heart Association, 2006

Class I

The performance of diagnostic studies to identify clinically significant renal artery stenosis is indicated in patients with:

- The onset of hypertension before age 30 years (*Level of evidence: B*)

- The onset of severe hypertension (as defined in *The Seventh Report of the Joint National Committee on Prevention, Detection, Evaluation, and Treatment of High Blood Pressure*, known as the JNC-7 report) after age 55 years (*Level of evidence: B*)

- The following characteristics: (a) accelerated hypertension, (b) resistant hypertension (defined as the failure to achieve goal blood pressure in patients who are adhering to full doses of an appropriate three-drug regimen that includes a diuretic), or (c) malignant hypertension (*Level of evidence: C*)

- New azotemia or worsening renal function after administration of an ACE inhibitor or an angiotensin-receptor blocking agent (*Level of evidence: B*)

- An unexplained atrophic kidney or a discrepancy in size between the two kidneys of greater than 1.5 cm (*Level of evidence: B*)

- Sudden unexplained pulmonary edema (especially in azotemic patients) (*Level of evidence: B*)

Renovascular hypertension

In patients with hypertension who are seen in specialist hypertension centers, renovascular hypertension is the underlying etiology in 0.5% to 4%.[1] Faced with a hypertensive patient, what features predict RVH?

Clinical markers for atheromatous renovascular hypertension

Kalra et al.[21] recently examined a 5% sample of the Medicare population (>1 million subjects included). The incidence of a new diagnosis of renovascular hypertension was 3.7 per hundred patient years in those older than 67. As compared with the general population, the diagnosis of RVH was associated with increased relative risk (RR) of existing chronic kidney disease (RR=2.5), essential hypertension (RR=2.4), peripheral vascular disease (RR=2.0), and ischemic heart disease (RR=1.7). The key clinical challenge is to distinguish hypertensive patients, or those with hypertension in association with chronic kidney disease, who have incidental ARVD, from those where the renal artery narrowing is etiological. A subsequent diagnosis for disease in other vascular territories was also high. The incidence quoted per thousand patient-years was 304 for ischemic heart disease, 259 for peripheral vascular disease, 195 for congestive cardiac failure, 176 for cerebrovascular

disease, 29 for dialysis requirement, and 116 for subsequent patient death. The risk in each of these cases is three- to five-fold that of the general population.

Screening in patients undergoing catheter angiography for other indications highlights the association of ARVD with widespread atheromatous disease. Renal arterial disease was present in 30% of patients undergoing screening renal artery angiography at the time of cardiac catheterization. Lesions likely to be hemodynamically significant have been reported in 11% to 18% of this patient group. Likewise in patients undergoing catheter angiography for investigation of aorto-iliac or peripheral vascular disease, several reports indicate a prevalence of significant ARVD of between 22% and 49%.[1]

Krijnen et al.[22] reviewed the patient population who were screened for the Dutch Renal Artery Stenosis Intervention Cooperative (DRASTIC) study. These authors sought to identify factors that were predictive of renovascular hypertension as opposed to essential hypertension. In multivariable analysis, the following factors favored RVH over those with essential hypertension: increasing age (odds ratio [OR]=1.8), atherosclerotic vascular disease (OR=1.8), recent-onset hypertension (OR=1.9), smoking history (OR=1.6), abdominal bruit (OR=5.4), and impaired renal function (OR=1.4 per 10 µmol/L increase). The clinical prediction appeared to be as sensitive and specific for ARVD as was the use of screening by captopril scintigraphy.

Renovascular hypertension and ischemic nephropathy

Detailed discussion of the management of ischemic chronic kidney disease is beyond the scope of this review. Nevertheless, it is important to recognize that chronic kidney disease is common in those patients with RVH due to ARVD. In patients over 50, ARVD is felt to be etiologic in 14% to 22% of patients with chronic kidney disease. One in eight patients entering dialysis programs has underlying severe ARVD.

Association with left ventricular hypertrophy

In a recent case–control series, Wright et al.[11] examined ambulatory BP and cardiac structure in patients with ARVD. Ninety-five percent of these patients had abnormal cardiac structure or function. As compared with matched patients with essential hypertension, those with ARVD have much greater left ventricular hypertrophy (79% vs. 46%). Those with bilateral renovascular disease had much greater LVH than those with unilateral disease. The cause of this excess LVH is unclear, but ambulatory BP monitoring identified the ARVD group to have less nocturnal fall in BP, and therefore the hypertensive load in the group with ARVD may be greater. In addition, activation of the renin angiotensin system is well known to be associated with left ventricular re-modeling and growth. This excess LVH may explain in part some of the increased mortality in this patient group.

Mortality in patients with renovascular hypertension secondary to atheromatous renovascular disease

As ARVD is associated with widespread atherosclerotic disease, it is not altogether unsurprising that the mortality rate in this population is particularly high. In a series of nearly 4000 patients undergoing screening at the time of cardiac catheterization, the 4-year survival rates for patients with and without ARVD was 57% and 89%, respectively. The mortality risk in this group is proportionate to the severity of renal artery narrowing. Four-year survival rates for individuals with ARVD of 50%, 75%, and 95% stenosis were 70%, 68%, and 48%, respectively. In those patients with bilateral ARVD, the 4-year survival was reportedly 47% as compared with 59% for those with unilateral disease. The severity of chronic kidney disease in those with renovascular hypertension due to atheroma also correlated with patient mortality. Three-year survival in this patient group with a creatinine of <1.4 mg/dL was 92%; for those with creatinine levels 1.5 to 1.9, it was 74%; and those with creatinine >2.0, it was only 51%.[23] Patients with RVH who progressed to end-stage renal failure had particularly high mortality rates. Mean life expectancy of individuals older than 65 with ARVD requiring dialysis was found to be only 2.7 years.[24] This compares with mean survival for patients with end-stage renal disease (ESRD) on dialysis secondary to malignant-phase hypertension and autosomal dominant polycystic kidney disease of around 6 and 11 years, respectively.

Natural history of atheromatous renovascular disease

The natural history of ARVD is one of progression. Early reports relied on retrospective analyses of serial angiograms performed in patients with either RVH or presumed ischemic nephropathy. Progression of renal artery stenosis occurred in 44% of 85 patients over a mean follow-up of 52 months and in 53% of 48 renal arteries over 7 years. High-grade stenosis (>75%) led to occlusion in 16% and 9%, respectively.[25,26] These studies probably overestimated the degree of progression, as the decision to repeat angiography is likely to have been influenced by clinical deterioration. The Dutch DRASTIC study group prospectively repeated angiography in patients with RVH due to ARVD at 1 year. Progression of stenosis or subsequent occlusion occurred in 20% and 9% of patients, respectively.[27] Similarly, Caps et al.,[28] using prospective Doppler ultrasound assessment of ARVD, demonstrated progression to be 35% at 3 years, and 51% at 5 years. Only 3% of arteries progressed to occlusion. Factors that were significantly associated with the risk of renal artery disease progression during follow-up: systolic BP of 160 mmHg or higher, diabetes mellitus, and high-grade (>60% stenosis) disease in either the ipsilateral or contralateral renal artery.

There are relatively little clinical data on the natural history of BP and renal function in patients with RVH due to ARVD. Baboolal et al.[29] reported the natural history of a retrospective series of 51 hypertensive patients with severe bilateral ARVD. The rate of loss of renal function overall was 4 mL/min/annum (range 1 to 8). The mortality rate was 45% at 5 years, reducing the final number reaching ESRD to 12%. Those with more advanced uremia and rapid progression were more likely to require dialysis. It is possible that the current rate of progression of chronic kidney disease in this group may be slower than histori-

cally reported. Aggressive lipid and BP control, particularly the more widespread use ACE inhibition, may be relevant. This has significance in defining the best clinical management and in the power calculations underlying ongoing clinical trials in this area.

DIAGNOSTIC TECHNIQUES FOR DETECTION OF RENAL ARTERY STENOSIS

The ideal test for renovascular hypertension should be safe, noninvasive, and provide good anatomic detail of the stenosis in the main renal artery, accessory renal arteries, or branches, with a high degree of sensitivity and specificity. It should have the potential to demonstrate surrounding anatomic structures including details of the renal parenchyma, aorta, and adrenal glands. Most importantly, the test should demonstrate the functional significance of the renal artery stenosis, as well as predict the BP and renal functional response to revascularization (Box 64–2).

Numerous studies in the 1970s and 1980s examined markers of activation of the renin angiotensin system (RAAS) whether at rest or stimulated. These included selective renal vein renin measurements or plasma renin activity measured before or after the administration of captopril, an ACE inhibitor. Standardization of sodium balance and drug therapy were critical, and the diagnostic accuracy against catheter angiography was poor. The tests have largely been abandoned in current clinical practice.

Captopril scintigraphy

Captopril renography detects the angiotensin-II dependence of glomerular filtration rate employing dynamic MAG-3 renography performed before and after administration of a single dose of captopril. In a positive test, there is a delay in the uptake, reduced peak uptake, prolonged parenchymal transit, and slow excretion of tracer. The reported accuracy of captopril renography in identifying patients with renovascular disease has been variable with reported sensitivity around 85% (range 45% to 94%) and speci-

---

Box 64–2

Diagnostic Methods for Renal Artery Stenosis: Recommendations of American College of Cardiology/American Heart Association, 2006

Class I

The following are recommended as a screening test to establish a diagnosis of renal artery stenosis:

1. Duplex ultrasonography (*Level of evidence: B*)
2. Computed tomographic angiography (in individuals with normal renal function) (*Level of evidence: B*)
3. Magnetic resonance angiography (*Level of evidence: B*)
4. When the clinical index of suspicion is high and the results of noninvasive tests are inconclusive, catheter angiography (*Level of evidence: B*)

ficity of around 93% (range 81% to 100%).[1] When compared with catheter angiography in the clinical setting, the sensitivity and specificity was only 74% and 59%, respectively.[30] Furthermore, the predictive accuracy is greatly restricted in those patients with bilateral renal artery stenosis, stenosis to a single functioning kidney and in those with impaired renal function. Therefore, the use of captopril renography as a diagnostic test is limited, although it may have a useful role in predicting the BP benefit of revascularization where the functional significance is uncertain in patients with normal renal function.

Duplex (Doppler with B-mode) ultrasound

In experienced centers duplex ultrasound has a sensitivity of 84% to 98% and a specificity of 62% to 99% when compared with catheter angiography for detecting significant renal artery stenosis. Both direct interrogation of the main renal artery and the downstream intrarenal arteries has been examined. Direct peak systolic velocity higher than 180 to 200 cm/s and renal to aortic ratio greater than 3.5 have been correlated with a stenosis of over 60%. An end diastolic velocity of more than 150 cm/s predicts renal artery stenosis higher than 80%. Measurements of intrarenal Doppler signals to arrive at indirect indices, such as resistive index (RI), are frequently combined. The use of contrast enhancement of ultrasound was explored in a large study with a crossover-randomized design. Visualization of the renal arteries was improved, but the sensitivity and specificity for the diagnosis of renal artery stenosis was not improved.[1]

In experienced hands, duplex Doppler ultrasound is an excellent technique to assess re-stenosis in renal arteries previously revascularized by metal stents (a major limitation of MRA in which the metal stent causes significant artifact). Intrarenal RI may also be of value in predicting the clinical outcome of revascularization by PTRA.

The limitations of duplex Doppler are that it is time consuming, very operator dependent, and is technically unsuccessful in 20% of patients due to overlying bowel gas or obesity. The technique also frequently fails to identify accessory arteries.

In the last decade, CT angiography (CTA) and contrast-enhanced (gadolinium) MR angiography (MRA) has become the accepted standard for noninvasive imaging of renal arteries. A meta-analysis showed the superiority of both of these techniques over both captopril renography and ultrasonography.[31]

Computed tomographic angiography

CTA has a sensitivity and specificity for detecting significant renal artery stenosis of 59% to 96%, and 82% to 98%, respectively (Figure 64–5). The technology is rapidly advancing. The method is based on rapid volume acquisition capabilities of scans timed after intravenous contrast bolus. Thirty-two and 64 row and flat-panel scanners are in development. With more recent scanners, sensitivity and specificity in excess of 90% against catheter angiography have been reported. In addition, CTA has the advantage over MRA of being able to detect re-stenosis within previously stented renal arteries. Nevertheless, the main

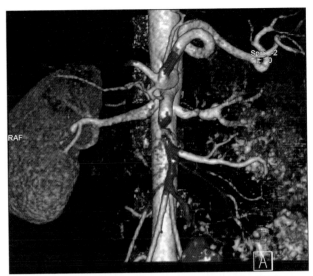

Figure 64–5. Computed tomography angiography (CTA) three-dimensional reconstruction of a patient demonstrating nonostial, left renal artery stenosis.

limitation of CTA in those patients with impaired renal function (in particular, those suffering from diabetes) is the risk of contrast nephropathy (100- to 150-mL contrast is typically employed). As technology improves, the required iodinated contrast dose may be reduced.

Gadolinium-enhanced magnetic resonance angiography

The sensitivity and specificity of MRA for the detection of renal artery stenosis are around 90% to 100% and 76% to 94%, respectively[31] (Figure 64–6). MRA has the major advantage that the contrast agent gadolinium is nonnephrotoxic in doses currently used. This facilitates its safe use in patients with impaired renal function. Three-dimensional image reconstructions greatly aid diagnosis and the planning of treatment for renal artery stenosis. In addition, newer technologies and improvements in acquisition speed and scanning technique continue to evolve. Contrast flow velocity and assessment of single-kidney GFR show early promise in investigating the functional significance of renal artery stenosis.

Some patients are unable to tolerate the claustrophobia induced by the more closed scanner designs. MRA may be less effective in the assessment of patients with FMD or with branch renal artery stenoses. Its other limitation is inability to re-image renal arteries that have previously undergone insertion of a stent (signal dropout artifact).

In due course, cross-sectional imaging may become the "gold standard" in assessment of the degree of luminal area narrowing, and replace catheter angiography, which is limited to two-dimensional assessment.

Selective renal artery catheter–contrast angiography

At present, selective renal artery catheter–contrast angiography remains the gold standard for the diagnosis of renal artery stenosis, which enables simultaneous percutaneous treatment of stenoses. It has now largely become

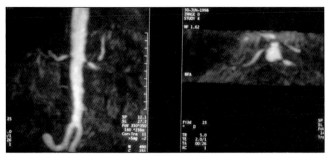

Figure 64–6. Gadolinium contrasted magnetic resonance angiography in a patient with severe hypertension and progressive chronic kidney disease demonstrating bilateral ostial renal artery stenosis (AP and coronal views).

a second-line investigation method used to guide percutaneous treatment after confirmation of the diagnosis by noninvasive screening tests. This is because of the higher risk of serious adverse outcomes in patients with impaired renal function and/or more advanced aortic and peripheral vascular atherosclerotic disease.

The risk of contrast-induced acute renal impairment in patients undergoing catheter renal angiography with chronic kidney disease is around 10% to 20%, and is even higher in individuals with concomitant diabetes, reaching between 20% and 50%.[32] Contrast-induced allergic reactions and atheromatous renal and lower extremity embolization, as well as groin hematoma, bleeding, and pseudo-aneurysm are also well described. Another disadvantage of this technique includes significant interobserver error in assessing the degree of stenosis. The incidence of complications is greater for the axillary or brachial approaches as compared with the femoral artery approach, even with the use of smaller size-4 French-gauge catheters. Major complications occur in 0.5% to 2% of patients with a mortality risk of 0.02% to 0.05%. The risk of iodinated contrast nephropathy can be reduced by minimizing contrast dose and by prehydration with intravenous normal saline to establish a good urine output prior to and 6 hours following the angiogram. N-acetyl-cysteine given before the examination and after for 48 hours appears beneficial as shown in meta-analyses, although the results are not uniform. Recently the use of iso-osmolar contrast as compared with low osmolality–contrast media has been shown to be associated with a lower risk of contrast nephropathy. Furthermore, other studies have shown a beneficial effect of prehydration with intravenous sodium bicarbonate. Intravenous aminophyline may also be protective.[33]

Alternative radiographic contrast media

Renal angiography employing carbon dioxide as a non-nephrotoxic contrast agent has been successfully used in patients undergoing renal arterial intervention studies.[34] Employing carbon dioxide as a contrast avoids nephrotoxicity but requires special equipment and is not widely available. Gadolinium (MRI contrast agent) is widely believed to be less nephrotoxic than iodinated contrast media. It is more expensive than other methods, and recent noncontrolled data suggest that it may not be without some risk of nephrotoxicity.[35] Gadolinium has recently been linked

to a severe condition of nephrogenic systemic fibrosis in patients with advanced renal failure, although this preliminary finding requires further confirmation.

Diagnosis/Imaging of fibromuscular dysplasia

At present spiral CT angiography and gadolinium-enhanced MRA cannot be relied on to adequately screen for FMD of the renal arteries. The current resolution of these techniques does not permit detailed review of branch renal artery lesions. In selected patients with a high clinical risk of FMD in whom intervention would be considered, it is advised to proceed directly to catheter angiography. In experienced centers, duplex sonography may have a role, as may captopril renography. Imaging technology is rapidly advancing, and as resolution improves these recommendations should be reviewed.[1]

CLINICAL MANAGEMENT AND PROGNOSIS

Fibromuscular dysplasia

Fibromuscular dysplasia is the second most common cause of RVH, and is an important potentially remediable condition. The underlying renal parenchyma is usually normal in the absence of hypertensive damage. Patients with FMD rarely suffer renal failure, and those with hypertension will respond to antihypertensive therapy or where indicated, to balloon angioplasty typically without the need for renal artery stent insertion.[2]

In patients with FMD, percutaneous revascularization should be considered with (1) recent onset hypertension where relief of stenosis may achieve "cure" of raised BP, (2) resistant hypertension or that associated with multiple drug side effects, and (3) development of loss of renal mass/function related to ischemic nephropathy.[5] The latter indicates the need for close follow-up of BP, renal function, and ultrasound-determined renal size and renal artery Doppler in this population.

There are no randomized trials comparing medical treatment alone against revascularization in patients with FMD. The outcome of 11 series of PTRA performed for treatment of hypertension in 455 patients is shown in Table 64–1.[5,36] The initial technical success rate of angioplasty is around 90% with stenosis rates at 2 years less than 10%. In this setting, renal artery stenting is reserved for "bailouts" (>50% residual stenosis after angioplasty or for complications). Cure (normotension without antihypertensive treatment) is achieved in around one-third of cases and a similar proportion showing improved BP control. Covered renal artery stents can be deployed where appropriate to exclude coexisting renal artery aneurisms from the circulation or, in rare cases, renal artery perforation or dissection. Surgery is reserved for cases not amenable to angioplasty/covered stenting, comprising a complex branch of arterial vessel disease requiring *ex vivo* reconstruction or aneurysm repair.[37] In experienced hands, the results are excellent.

REVIEW OF TRIALS OF PERCUTANEOUS RENAL ARTERY ANGIOPLASTY IN FIBROMUSCULAR DYSPLASIA (11 SERIES, 1983–2005)					
n	Technical Success (%)	Effect on Blood Pressure			Follow-up (Months)
		Cure (%)	Improved (%)	No Effect (%)	
455	87–100	22–59	22–63	7–30	12–96

Table 64-1. Review of Trials of Percutaneous Renal Artery Angioplasty in Fibromuscular Dysplasia (11 Series, 1983–2005)

Atherosclerotic renovascular disease
Medical therapy

Individuals with atherosclerotic disease and vascular disease should be treated according to recommendations in the Seventh report of the Joint national Committee on Prevention, Detection, Evaluation and Treatment of High Blood Pressure.[37a] ARVD is associated with high cardiovascular mortality, and as such, aggressive cardiovascular protection measures should be offered to suitable patients including smoking cessation, cholesterol control with statin therapy, and antiplatelet treatment. Multiple studies demonstrate that calcium-channel blockers, thiazide diuretics, and beta blockers appear effective in BP reduction in patients with ARVD.[2] Widespread use of angiotensin-converting enzyme (ACE) inhibitors or angiotensin-receptor blocking (ARB) agents has impacted on both the diagnosis and indications for invasive treatment of ARVD (Box 64–3).

Converting enzyme inhibitors or angiotensin-receptor blockers in renovascular hypertension

Prior to the availability of ACE inhibitors or AR blockers, BP control could only be achieved in less than 50% of patients with RVH secondary to ARVD who were referred to specialist centers. With the use of ACE inhibitors as well as the availability of new classes of antihypertensive agents in this population, 82% to 96% of patients achieve satisfactory BP control.[38]

Patients suffering from vascular disease or impaired left ventricular dysfunction (both of which are common in this patient population) treated with ACE/ARBs reduces mortality, compared to other antihypertensive drug classes.[10] Furthermore, ACE inhibitors/ARB drugs, compared to other antihypertensive agents, reduce the rate of progression of both diabetic and nondiabetic chronic kidney disease.[38] However, in patients with ARVD subtending the whole renal mass, there is a risk of acute uremia following treatment with these drugs. This occurs because glomerular filtration is preserved by angiotensin II–mediated post-glomerular vasoconstriction in these patients.

How much of a risk does this represent? Large clinical trials in populations at high risk of ARVD (congestive cardiac failure, ischemic heart disease) demonstrate a low rate of functional renal decline after ACE inhibition. Patient withdrawal as a result of acute renal failure or hyperkalemia from these trials is rare at 2% to 6%.[39] It should be recognized that a 20% rise in ACE inhibitor–induced creatinine may occur even in patients who do not suffer RVH. Hollenberg et al.[38] treated 136 patients with captopril, who were known to have ARVD in the entire renal mass. Only 6% developed a decline in renal function over 4 weeks, which was reversible on stopping treatment. In a randomized double-blind trial of enalapril versus a non–ACE inhibitor regime in patients with RVH, 20% in the ACE group developed a rise in creatinine.[40] Preliminary evidence suggests that these drugs may reduce mortality in the renovascular population. It appears that most patients with RVH can be safely treated with ACE inhibitors. Nevertheless, these drugs must be introduced with great caution in patients know to suffer, or be at high risk for ARVD. Caution must be taken to ensure that patients are not over-diuresed, and renal function must be checked 1 week prior to and 4 weeks after starting these agents or after drug dose escalation.

Increasingly, failure to tolerate ACE inhibition as a consequence of acute decline in renal function has become an important indication for investigation for ARVD. In suitable patients, an inability to tolerate ACE inhibitors due to acute uremia represents an important indication for intervention.[10,38]

Box 64–3

Medical Treatment of Renal Artery Stenosis: Recommendations of American College of Cardiology/American Heart Association, 2006

Class I

The following are effective medications for treatment of hypertension associated with unilateral renal artery stenosis:

- Angiotensin-converting enzyme inhibitors *(Level of evidence: A)*
- Angiotensin receptor blockers *(Level of evidence: B)*
- Calcium-channel blockers *(Level of evidence: A)*
- Beta-blockers *(Level of evidence: A)*

Revascularization for renovascular hypertension due to significant atheromatous disease

Procedural success and complication rate for angioplasty alone versus angioplasty and stent insertion

Over 75% of ARVD is ostial in origin (within 1 cm of the aortic lumen), and relates predominantly to aortic atheroma encroaching on the renal artery ostia. As such, balloon angioplasty alone is associated with a high immediate recoil rate and high likelihood of late re-stenosis. A single small randomized study (*n*=85) compared renal artery stent insertion with angioplasty for ostial renal artery stenosis associated with "critical" ARVD. Primary success rate (<50% residual stenosis) of angioplasty was 57% compared with 88% for stent (difference between groups was 31%, 95% confidence interval [CI]=12–50). At 6 months, the primary patency rate was 29% (12 patients) for PTRA, and 75% (30 patients) for PTRA plus stent (46%, CI=24–68). Restenosis after a successful primary procedure occurred in 48% of patients for PTRA and 14% for PTRA and stent (34%, CI=11–58).[41] Leertouwer et al.[42] performed a meta-analysis of published studies comprising 644 patients. Renal artery stent placement proved highly successful, with an initial adequate patency rate of 98% and a restenosis rate at 6- to -29 month–follow-up of 17%, compared to rates of 77% and 26%, respectively, for angioplasty alone. The "cure rate" for hypertension was higher (20% vs. 10%), but renal functional improvement was lower (30% vs. 38%) in those treated with stent placement versus angioplasty alone. The latter is unexplained, but may reflect increased athero-emboli associated with stent placement. Renal angioplasty alone has a better procedural outcome in truncal disease, which is similar to the outcome in primary stenting (Boxes 64–4 and 64–5).

PTRA is not a benign procedure in this frail population group. Major complication rates are the same for both procedures at around 10%. These complications include renal failure (5%), segmental renal infarction (1%) perinephric hematoma (1%), renal artery thrombosis/occlusion (0.7%), and groin hematoma (5%). Patient mortality was around 1% (CI=0–2).

Randomized controlled trials of percutaneous transluminal angioplasty plus medical therapy versus medical therapy alone in patients with atheromatous renovascular disease

The evidence base on which to guide therapy is limited to three somewhat flawed, small randomized trials of PTRA versus medical treatment in patients with RVH and ARVD[27,43,44] (see Table 64–2).

In the DRASTIC study, 106 patients with unilateral or bilateral ARVD of greater than 50%-diameter luminal narrowing were randomly allocated to PTRA (almost all angioplasty alone) or medical therapy with a follow-up of 12 months. Blood pressure did not differ between groups, although the defined daily dose (DDD) of antihypertensive drugs was reduced by one agent in the intervention group. Renal function was significantly better at 3 months in the angioplasty group, but no difference was found at 1 year. There are several shortcomings of this study. Forty-four

---

Box 64–4

Indications for Revascularization: Recommendations of American College of Cardiology/American Heart Association, 2006

Asymptomatic Stenosis

1. Percutaneous revascularization may be considered for treatment of an asymptomatic bilateral or solitary viable kidney with a hemodynamically significant renal artery stenosis. *(Level of evidence: C)*
2. The usefulness of percutaneous revascularization of an asymptomatic unilateral hemodynamically significant renal artery stenosis in a viable kidney is not well established and is presently clinically unproven. *(Level of evidence: C)*

Hypertension

1. Percutaneous revascularization is reasonable for patients with hemodynamically significant renal artery stenosis and accelerated hypertension, resistant hypertension, malignant hypertension, hypertension with an unexplained unilateral small kidney, and hypertension with intolerance to medication. *(Level of evidence: B)*

Preservation of Renal Function

1. Percutaneous revascularization is reasonable for patients with renal artery stenosis and progressive chronic kidney disease with bilateral renal artery stenosis or a renal artery stenosis to a solitary functioning kidney. *(Level of evidence: B)*
2. Percutaneous revascularization may be considered for patients with renal artery stenosis and chronic renal insufficiency with unilateral renal artery stenosis. *(Level of evidence: C)*

Impact of Renal Artery Stenosis on Congestive Heart Failure and Unstable Angina

1. Percutaneous revascularization is indicated for patients with hemodynamically significant renal artery stenosis and recurrent, unexplained congestive heart failure, or sudden, unexplained pulmonary edema. *(Level of evidence: B)*
2. Percutaneous revascularization is reasonable for patients with hemodynamically significant renal artery stenosis and unstable angina. *(Level of evidence: B)*

Box 64–5

Catheter-Based Interventions: Recommendations of American College of Cardiology/American Heart Association, 2006

1. Renal stent placement is indicated for ostial atherosclerotic renal artery stenosis lesions that meet the clinical criteria for intervention. *(Level of evidence: B)*
2. Balloon angioplasty with bailout stent placement if necessary is recommended for fibromuscular dysplasia lesions. *(Level of evidence: B)*

percent of patients initially allocated to drug treatment crossed over during the trial and received PTRA due to presumed failure of medical treatment. As expected, renal artery patency achieved with angioplasty alone was poor at the end of the study with post-PTRA restenosis occurring in 48% of patients. Some patients with stenosis of around 50% were unlikely to have hemodynamically significant renal artery disease. The UK, Scottish and Newcastle Renal Artery Stenosis Collaborative Group (SNRASCG) randomized 44 of 135 eligible patients with presumed RVH and unilateral or bilateral ARVD of at least

50% to angioplasty (without stent) or medical treatment alone. After a follow-up of 3 to 54 months, systolic BP was lower in the PTRA group. The benefit was confined to those with bilateral disease and no patient was cured. The same provisos apply to the significance of stenosis and long-term success of PTRA. The French EMMA group randomized 40 patients with RVH in the setting of hemodynamically significant ARVD. After 6 months BP and renal function were the same in both groups although the DDD in the PTRA group was lower. A quarter of patients crossed over from the medical to PTRA for resistant hypertension.

Systematic review of randomized trials

A systematic Cochrane Library review of balloon angioplasty versus medical therapy for hypertensive patients with renal artery obstruction has recently been published. Meta-analysis of the above three randomized controlled trials included a total of 210 patients.[45] Those treated with balloon angioplasty required less antihypertensive drugs and were more likely to have patent renal arteries at 12 months (OR=4.2, CI=1.8–9.8). Cardiovascular and renovascular complications were also significantly less in the intervention group (OR=0.32, CI=0.15–0.7. There was no impact on renal function. A second meta-analysis that examined changes from baseline did in fact suggest that a small improvement in BP occurred; however, the improvement was of borderline significance with wide

RANDOMIZED CONTROLLED TRIALS OF PTA PLUS MEDICAL THERAPY VS. MEDICAL THERAPY ALONE IN PATIENTS WITH ATHEROMATOUS RENAL ARTERY STENOSIS							
	PTA vs. Control (*n*)	Follow-up (Months)	Bilateral vs. Unilateral Stenosis	BP Outcome	Impact on Renal Function	Crossover (%) (Medical to PTA)	Comments
van Jaarsveld et al.[27]	50 vs. 56	12	Unilateral and bilateral	NS	Improved at 3 months, no change at 12 months	22 (44)	Reduced BP Rx (DDD fell 1.1) Re-stenosis in 48% Stent in 2 patients
Plouin et al.[44]	23 vs. 26	6	Unilateral (severe, >60%–75%)	NS (24-hour ambulatory blood pressure)	NS	7 (27) Refractory hypertension	Reduced BP Rx (0.78 DDD) 26% complication rate (4% major)
Webster et al.[43]	13 vs. 14	3–54	Unilateral (>50% stenosis)	NS	NS	0	BP fell during run-in period (pre-intervention)
	16 vs. 12	3–54	Bilateral (>50%)	152/83 vs. 171/91 (*p*<0.005)	NS	0	28% complication rate (arterial access site bleeding/ hematoma)

BP, blood pressure; DDD, defined daily doses of antihypertensives; NS, not significant; PTA, percutaneous transluminal angioplasty.

Table 64-2. Randomized Controlled Trials of PTA Plus Medical Therapy vs. Medical Therapy Alone in Patients with Atheromatous Renal Artery Stenosis

confidence intervals (*p*=0.06)(Figure 64–7).[46] Large randomized controlled studies in this area are required to define the true benefit and ideal patient selection for intervention.

Role of distal atheroembolic protection device at time of percutaneous transluminal renal artery angioplasty/stent

Manipulation of a guide wire and subsequent deployment of the angioplasty balloon and stent is associated with distal athero-emboli (mainly of cholesterol crystals) in coronary or carotid circulation. These emboli can adversely affect tissue microcirculation. Controlled trial evidence indicates that the deployment of distal protection devices at the time of angioplasty and/or stent in those areas captures cholesterol crystals and can lead to improved outcomes.[47] Clinical results following successful percutaneous renal artery revascularization in ARVD are variable. Stabilization or improvement of hypertension or renal impairment may result in some patients, while deterioration occurs in others. By extrapolation it is plausible that renal athero-emboli during PTRA may limit benefits in this setting. Indeed, recent preliminary evidence confirms generation of athero-emboli following PTRA, the magnitude of which can be limited by one distal protection device.[48] Technical improvement is required to adapt this treatment to the specific requirements for renal artery use. Importantly, the randomized CORAL study (Cardiovascular Outcomes with Renal Atherosclerotic Lesions) will examine whether these devices lead to better clinical outcomes when compared to renal stent placement alone.

Surgical management of atheromatous renovascular disease

The requirement for surgical intervention to accomplish renal revascularization in ARVD has diminished considerably since the late 1990s. The technical success and long-term durability of percutaneous renal artery stenting has largely replaced the previous main indication for surgery, namely ostial ARVD.[49] Traditionally, aorto-renal bypass employing saphenous vein conduits were used for single–renal artery bypass while trans-aortic renal endarterectomy was employed in the case of multiple renal arteries, often in combination with aortic reconstruction. Subsequently, extra-anatomic bypass procedures employing disease-free splenic or hepatic arteries have become more popular.[38] Reported surgical perioperative mortality rates are 2% to 6% as compared with around 1% for percutaneous intervention. In a highly comorbid patient group with generalized arteriopathy, complication rates following aorto-renal surgery are also significant, including periprocedure myocardial infarction (2% to 9% vs. 0% to 3%, respectively) and cholesterol embolization syndrome. The reported risks of surgical renal artery revascularization failure at 5 years ranges from 6% to 18% in experienced hands.[9] More recently, extra-anatomic bypass (splenic artery on the left and hepatic artery on the right) have gained acceptance. This approach avoids the need for surgery on a severely diseased aorta as well as the need for aortic cross-clamping in a group of patients with frequently compromised left ventricular function. Extra-anatomic bypass is associated with a lower mortality rate (2.9%) compared to aorto-renal bypass[37] (see Box 64–6).

A defined role for surgery remains in patients with ARVD requiring revascularization. Vascular surgical reconstruction is indicated for patients with a clinical indication for intervention who at the same time require aortic reconstruction, e.g., in the treatment of aortic aneurysm or severe aorto-iliac occlusive disease.[49] Combined surgery has increased mortality and morbidity rates as compared with aortic or renal artery surgery alone. Associated coronary and cerebrovascular diseases are common. Careful screening and, where possible, correction of critical disease

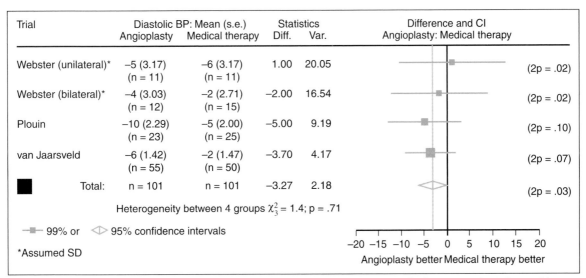

Figure 64–7. Meta-analysis of randomized controlled trials of angioplasty versus medical treatment in patients with renovascular hypertension due to atheromatous renal artery stenosis. Effect on diastolic blood pressure. (Redrawn from Ives N J, et al. *Nephrol Dial Transplant,* 2003. 18:298–304 with permission from Oxford University Press.)

in these areas in advance of aorto-iliac surgery, may improve outcome or enable focused surgical selection; this issue remains controversial.[50] Surgery may also be indicated when there are stenoses in multiple small renal arteries or early primary branching of the main renal artery. Bilateral renal artery occlusion causing acute renal failure where the renal parenchyma is preserved by collateral blood supply remains a strong indication for surgical treatment.[51]

Comparison of surgery versus percutaneous transluminal renal artery angioplasty for revascularization

Weibull et al.[52] performed the only randomized study comparing PTRA (without stenting) with surgical revascularization in 58 patients with unilateral renovascular disease. The primary patency rate at 2 years was 75% and 96% in the PTRA and surgical groups, respectively. The impact on BP or renal function was not significantly different, although 17% of the patients treated with PTRA underwent subsequent surgical intervention. Major morbidity was reported in 34% of surgically treated patients as compared with 17% of those receiving angioplasty. It is difficult to generalize these results to current clinical practice. The primary patency rate quoted is much higher than in other series after angioplasty alone—the patients studied had unilateral disease only and were all non-diabetic. As such, the patients were not typical of current practice and represented a relatively low-risk group. A clinical trial comparing renal artery revascularization by PTRA or surgery is now unlikely to be performed as the indications for the two procedures fall into different categories.

Predictors of intervention outcome in atheromatous renovascular disease

Both surgical renal revascularization and percutaneous renal artery stenting in selected patients durably correct renal arterial stenosis and improve BP control, and/or stabilize or improve renal function in selected patients with hemodynamically relevant renal artery stenosis. The clinical challenge is to identify individual patients who are likely to respond and then select them for intervention thereby sparing the remainder from the interventional risks. In surgical series, favorable response of BP and renal function to revascularization could be predicted by (1) serum creatinine <3 mg/dL, (2) preserved renal structure as defined by intraoperative histology, and (3) rapidly declining preoperative renal function.[53] In patients undergoing PTRA, rapidly declining pre-intervention renal function was also predictive of a beneficial result. Radermacher et al.[54,55] reported that a Doppler ultrasound–derived variable, intrarenal resistive index (RI) greater than 0.8, was a marker of poor outcome after PTRA. A higher RI is associated with more extensive renal parenchymal disease. Nevertheless, this study has been criticized due to its retrospective nature and use of angioplasty without stenting. Furthermore, these data have been challenged recently by a prospective uncontrolled study of renal stent placement in 241 patients by Zeller et al.[56] Normal renal parenchymal thickness, high baseline BP, and female sex independently predicted a favorable fall in BP. Another multivariable logistic regression analysis demonstrated that bilateral ARVD and mean arterial pressure higher than 110 mmHg to predict a beneficial BP response to renal artery stenting in patients with RVH.[57] The evidence base is limited at present.

Revascularization in special situations
Flash pulmonary edema

Pickering et al.[58] first described a syndrome of recurrent life-threatening pulmonary edema in patients with renal impairment who exhibit tight arterial stenosis to their whole renal mass (bilateral or unilateral to single functioning kidney). This was "cured" by surgical or percutaneous revascularization. Flash pulmonary edema is largely a diagnosis of exclusion, which is usually made after exclusion of other more common causes of pulmonary edema such as left ventricular systolic impairment or reversible myocardial ischemia. Alterations in circulatory homeostasis in these patients can provoke exacerbations of coronary ischemia and/or congestive cardiac failure (which frequently coexists,[59] due to peripheral vasoconstriction, direct effects of angiotensin II on the myocardium and/or volume overload).[1] Relief of renal artery stenosis may reduce angiotensin levels, increase GFR, enable natriuresis, and permit introduction of ACE inhibition. Furthermore, acute decline in renal function following introduction of a converting enzyme inhibitor in a patient with bilateral renal artery stenosis may limit optimal medical therapy of patients with impaired left ventricular systolic function, thereby predisposing them to decompensation and heart failure.

ONGOING RANDOMIZED CONTROLLED STUDIES OF PERCUTANEOUS TRANSLUMINAL RENAL ARTERY ANGIOPLASTY/STENTING FOR ATHEROMATOUS RENAL ARTERY STENOSIS						
Study (Recruitment Start/Projected End)	Target *n*	Stenosis (Site)	Renal Artery Intervention	Comparator Group	Primary Endpoint	Minimum Follow-up (Years)
ASTRAL (2000/07)	750	>50% (any)	Angioplasty ± stent	Medical (center specific)	Rate of chronic kidney disease progression	1
STAR (2000/06)[61]	140	>50% (ostial)	Stent	Medical (defined)	20% fall in CrCl	1
NITER (2003/07)[62]	100	>70% (ostial)	Stent	Medical (defined)	Death/dialysis or >20% fall glomerular filtration rate	3
CORAL (2005/07)[63]	1060	>60% (or >20 mmHg pressure drop)	Stent	Medical (defined)	Death/dialysis or major adverse cardiovascular events	2

Table 64-3. Ongoing Randomized Controlled Studies of Percutaneous Transluminal Renal Artery Angioplasty/Stenting for Atheromatous Renal Artery Stenosis

Stable congestive cardiac failure and angina

Preliminary evidence suggests that percutaneous renal revascularization in selected patients with ARVD and ischemic heart disease may lead to improved severity of angina (Canadian Cardiovascular Society Angina score) and/or symptomatic heart failure.[60] In these studies, the benefits were sustained over 8 months. Patients underwent percutaneous stenting of both coronary and renal artery stenoses or of renal artery stenosis alone. Those who underwent renal artery stenting alone seemed to gain the same cardiac benefits as those patients who underwent both procedures. It must be stressed that these results require confirmation by ongoing prospective randomized studies.

The ongoing ASTRAL (Angioplasty and Stent for Renal Artery Lesions) Trial (United Kingdom) and its heart and heart failure substudies, as well as the CORAL study, will hopefully answer these important questions.

SUMMARY

Many questions regarding the natural history, pathophysiology, and medical and surgical treatment of patients with renovascular hypertension remain unanswered. Despite this being a relatively common condition, the field is dogged by the lack of robust evidence on which to guide management. It is clear from existing evidence that we have extremely good diagnostic tools to identify the disease as well as percutaneous intervention that durably restores renal artery patency, albeit at some risk. Fortunately, ongoing randomized controlled trials should help resolve at least some of the pertinent issues (Table 64–3).

Inclusion criteria for ASTRAL (>700 patients recruited, target 750) allow a wide range of stenosis severity. This study recruits predominantly from UK and Australasia. This will enable subsequent broad predefined subgroup analysis. Researchers have already recruited three times the number of patients included in all previous randomized studies in this area. Two substudies look at the impact of PTRA on cardiac structure/function in those patients with preserved and impaired systolic function.

The North American CORAL study addresses whether medical therapy and stent placement for hemodynamically significant ARVD in patients with refractory systolic hypertension reduce the incidence of adverse cardiovascular and renal endpoints compared with medical therapy alone. The intervention subgroup also explores the important question of whether the deployment of a distal atheroembolic protection device at the time of stent placement improves outcomes compared with a stent alone.

REFERENCES

1. Hirsch AT, et al. ACC/AHA 2005 practice guidelines for the management of patients with peripheral arterial disease (lower extremity, renal, mesenteric, and abdominal aortic). *Circulation* 2006;113:463–654.
2. Safian RD, Textor SC. Renal-artery stenosis. *N Engl J Med* 2001;344:431–42.
3. Wright JR, et al. Clinicopathological correlation in biopsy-proven atherosclerotic nephropathy: implications for renal functional outcome in atherosclerotic renovascular disease. *Nephrol Dial Transplant* 2001;16:765–70.
4. Schwartz CJ, White TA. Stenosis of renal artery: an unselected necropsy study. *BMJ* 1964;5422:1415–21.
5. Slovut DP, Olin JW. Fibromuscular dysplasia. *N Engl J Med* 2004;350(18):1862–71.
6. Garovic V, Textor SC. Renovascular hypertension: current concepts. *Semin Nephrol* 2005;25:261–71.
7. Scoble JE, Cook GJ. Individual kidney function in atherosclerotic nephropathy. *Nephrol Dial Transplant* 1998;13:842–44.
8. Tuttle KR. Renal parenchymal injury as a determinant of clinical consequences in atherosclerotic renal artery stenosis. *Am J Kidney Dis* 2002;39:1321–22.
9. Garovic VD, Textor SC. Renovascular hypertension and ischemic nephropathy. *Circulation* 2005;112:1362–74.
10. Main J. Atherosclerotic renal artery stenosis, ACE inhibitors, and avoiding cardiovascular death. *Heart* 2005;91:548–52.

11. Wright, JR, et al. Left ventricular morphology and function in patients with atherosclerotic renovascular disease. *J Am Soc Nephrol* 2005;16:2746–53.

12. Higashi Y, et al. Endothelial function and oxidative stress in renovascular hypertension. *N Engl J Med* 2002;346(25):1954–62.

13. Schoenberg SO, et al. Correlation of hemodynamic impact and morphologic degree of renal artery stenosis in a canine model. *J Am Soc Nephrol* 2000;11:2190–98.

14. Gross CM, et al. Determination of renal arterial stenosis severity: comparison of pressure gradient and vessel diameter. *Radiology* 2001;220:751–56.

15. Zoccali CF, Mallamaci F, Finocchiaro P. Atherosclerotic renal artery stenosis: epidemiology, cardiovascular outcomes, and clinical prediction rules. *J Am Soc Nephrol* 2002;13(Suppl 3):S179–83.

16. Wright JR, et al. A prospective study of the determinants of renal functional outcome and mortality in atherosclerotic renovascular disease. *Am J Kidney Dis* 2002;39:1153–61.

17. Neymark E, et al. Arteriographic detection of renovascular disease in potential renal donors: incidence and effect on donor surgery. *Radiology* 2000;214:755–60.

18. Connolly JO, Woolfson RG. Renovascular hypertension: diagnosis and management. *BJU Int* 2005;96:715–20.

19. Mounier-Vehier C, et al. Parenchymal consequences of fibromuscular dysplasia renal artery stenosis. *Am J Kidney Dis* 2002;40:1138–45.

20. Hansen KJ, et al. Prevalence of renovascular disease in the elderly: a population-based study. *J Vasc Surg* 2002;36:443–51.

21. Kalra PA, et al. Atherosclerotic renovascular disease in United States patients aged 67 years or older: risk factors, revascularization, and prognosis. *Kidney Int* 2005;68:293–301.

22. Krijnen P, et al. Which patients with hypertension and atherosclerotic renal artery stenosis benefit from immediate intervention? *J Hum Hypertens* 2004;18:91–96.

23. Dorros G, et al. Four-year follow-up of Palmaz-Schatz stent revascularization as treatment for atherosclerotic renal artery stenosis. *Circulation* 1998;98:642–47.

24. Neggers SJ, van der Meulen J. Prediction rule for renal artery stenosis. *Ann Intern Med* 1999;131:228.

25. Tollefson DF, Ernst CG. Natural history of atherosclerotic renal artery stenosis associated with aortic disease. *J Vasc Surg* 1991;14:327–31.

26. Schreiber Jr MJ, Pohl MA, Novick AC. Preserving renal function by revascularization. *Annu Rev Med* 1990;41:423–29.

27. van Jaarsveld BC, et al. The effect of balloon angioplasty on hypertension in atherosclerotic renal-artery stenosis. Dutch Renal Artery Stenosis Intervention Cooperative Study Group. *N Engl J Med* 2000;342:1007–14.

28. Caps MT, et al. Prospective study of atherosclerotic disease progression in

the renal artery. *Circulation* 1998;98:2866–72.

29. Baboolal K, Evans C, Moore RH. Incidence of end-stage renal disease in medically treated patients with severe bilateral atherosclerotic renovascular disease. *Am J Kidney Dis* 1998;31:971–77.

30. Huot SJ, et al. Utility of captopril renal scans for detecting renal artery stenosis. *Arch Intern Med* 2002;162:1981–84.

31. Vasbinder GB, et al. Diagnostic tests for renal artery stenosis in patients suspected of having renovascular hypertension: a meta-analysis. *Ann Intern Med* 2001;135:401–11.

32. Parfrey PS, et al. Contrast material-induced renal failure in patients with diabetes mellitus, renal insufficiency, or both. A prospective controlled study. *N Engl J Med* 1989;320:143–49.

33. Barrett BJ, Parfrey PS. Clinical practice. Preventing nephropathy induced by contrast medium. *N Engl J Med* 2006;354:379–86.

34. Caridi JG, Stavropoulos SW, Hawkins Jr IF. Carbon dioxide digital subtraction angiography for renal artery stent placement. *J Vasc Interv Radiol* 1999;10:635–40.

35. Chiesa R, et al. Endovascular stenting for the nutcracker phenomenon. *J Endovasc Ther* 2001;8:652–55.

36. Alhadad A, et al. Revascularisation of renal artery stenosis caused by fibromuscular dysplasia: effects on blood pressure during 7-year follow-up are influenced by duration of hypertension and branch artery stenosis. *J Hum Hypertens* 2005;19:761–67.

37. Novick AC. Surgical revascularization for renal artery disease: current status. *BJU Int* 2005;95(Suppl 2):75–77.

37a. Chobanian AV, Bakris GL, Black HR, et al. The Seventh Report of the Joint National Committee on Prevention, Detection, Evaluation, and Treatment of High Blood Pressure: the JNC 7 report. *JAMA* 2003;289:2560–72.

38. Textor SC. Ischemic nephropathy: where are we now? *J Am Soc Nephrol* 2004;15:1974–82.

39. Schoolwerth AC, et al. Renal considerations in angiotensin converting enzyme inhibitor therapy: a statement for healthcare professionals from the Council on the Kidney in Cardiovascular Disease and the Council for High Blood Pressure Research of the American Heart Association. *Circulation* 2001;104:1985–91.

40. Franklin SS, Smith RD. Comparison of effects of enalapril plus hydrochlorothiazide versus standard triple therapy on renal function in renovascular hypertension. *Am J Med* 1985;79:14–23.

41. van de Ven PJ, et al. Arterial stenting and balloon angioplasty in ostial atherosclerotic renovascular disease: a randomised trial. *Lancet* 1999;353:282–86.

42. Leertouwer TC, et al. Stent placement for renal arterial stenosis: where do we stand? A meta-analysis. *Radiology* 2000;216:78–85.

43. Webster J, et al. Randomised comparison of percutaneous angioplasty vs continued medical therapy for hypertensive patients with atheromatous renal artery stenosis.

Scottish and Newcastle Renal Artery Stenosis Collaborative Group. *J Hum Hypertens* 1998;12:329–35.

44. Plouin PF, et al. Blood pressure outcome of angioplasty in atherosclerotic renal artery stenosis: a randomized trial. Essai Multicentrique Medicaments vs Angioplastie (EMMA) Study Group. *Hypertension* 1998;31:823–29.

45. Nordmann AJ, Logan AG. Balloon angioplasty versus medical therapy for hypertensive patients with renal artery obstruction. *Cochrane Database Syst Rev* 2003:CD002944.

46. Ives NJ, et al. Continuing uncertainty about the value of percutaneous revascularization in atherosclerotic renovascular disease: a meta-analysis of randomized trials. *Nephrol Dial Transplant* 2003;18:298–304.

47. Scoble JE. Do protection devices have a role in renal angioplasty and stent placement? *Nephrol Dial Transplant* 2003;18:1700–703.

48. Hagspiel KD, Stone JR, Leung DA. Renal angioplasty and stent placement with distal protection: preliminary experience with the FilterWire EX. *J Vasc Interv Radiol* 2005;16:125–31.

49. Hirsch AT, et al. ACC/AHA 2005 guidelines for the management of patients with peripheral arterial disease (lower extremity, renal, mesenteric, and abdominal aortic): executive summary. *J Am Coll Cardiol* 2006;47:1239–312.

50. McFalls EO, et al. Coronary-artery revascularization before elective major vascular surgery. *N Engl J Med* 2004;351:2795–804.

51. Kaylor WM, et al. Reversal of end stage renal failure with surgical revascularization in patients with atherosclerotic renal artery occlusion. *J Urol* 1989;141:486–88.

52. Weibull H, et al. Percutaneous transluminal renal angioplasty versus surgical reconstruction of atherosclerotic renal artery stenosis: a prospective randomized study. *J Vasc Surg* 1993;18:841–50; discussion 850–52.

53. Greco BA, Breyer JA. Atherosclerotic ischemic renal disease. *Am J Kidney Dis* 1997;29:167–87.

54. Radermacher J, et al. Use of Doppler ultrasonography to predict the outcome of therapy for renal-artery stenosis. *N Engl J Med* 2001;344:410–17.

55. Muray S, et al. Rapid decline in renal function reflects reversibility and predicts the outcome after angioplasty in renal artery stenosis. *Am J Kidney Dis* 2002;39:60–66.

56. Zeller T, et al. Predictors of improved renal function after percutaneous stent-supported angioplasty of severe atherosclerotic ostial renal artery stenosis. *Circulation* 2003;108:2244–249.

57. Rocha-Singh KJ, et al. Clinical predictors of improved long-term blood pressure control after successful stenting of hypertensive patients with obstructive renal artery atherosclerosis. *Catheter Cardiovasc Interv* 1999;47:167–72.

58. Pickering TG, et al. Recurrent pulmonary oedema in hypertension due to bilateral renal artery stenosis: treatment by angioplasty or surgical revascularisation. *Lancet* 1988;2:551–52.

59. MacDowall P, et al. Risk of morbidity from renovascular disease in elderly patients with congestive cardiac failure. *Lancet* 1998;352:13–16.

60. Khosla S, et al. Effects of renal artery stent implantation in patients with renovascular hypertension presenting with unstable angina or congestive heart failure. *Am J Cardiol* 1997;80:363–66.

61. Bax L, et al. The benefit of stent placement and blood pressure and lipid-lowering for the prevention of progression of renal dysfunction caused by atherosclerotic ostial stenosis of the renal artery. The STAR study: rationale and study design. *J Nephrol* 2003;16:807–12.

62. Scarpioni R, et al. Atherosclerotic renovascular disease: medical therapy versus medical therapy plus renal artery stenting in preventing renal failure progression: the rationale and study design of a prospective, multicenter and randomized trial (NITER). *J Nephrol* 2005;18:423–28.

63. Murphy TP, et al. The Cardiovascular Outcomes with Renal Atherosclerotic Lesions (CORAL) study: rationale and methods. *J Vasc Interv Radiol* 2005;16:1295–300.

Chapter

65 Proteinuria

Chris Isles

Definition

- Microalbuminuria and proteinuria are common in hypertensive diseases. They predict progressive renal failure and also amplify the risk of vascular disease. The heavier the proteinuria the greater the risk of progressive renal failure, whereas even microalbuminuria can amplify the risk of vascular disease.

- 24 hour urine collections are no longer recommended for quantification of urine albumin or protein. Microalbuminuria can be detected by the albumin:creatinine ratio and proteinuria by the protein:creatinine ratio, on untimed specimens of urine.

- Microalbuminuria is defined as an albumin:creatinine ratio between around 3 and 30 mg/mmol creatinine, and proteinuria by a protein:creatinine ratio > 45 mg/mmol creatinine.

Clinical Implications

- Control of blood pressure and renin angiotensin system blockade can reduce both microalbuminuria and proteinuria, which in turn may lead to a reduction in the risk of vascular disease and in the rate of progression of renal disease.

- The target of blood pressure for patients with microalbuminuria and proteinuria is <130/80 mmHg, though this is not always possible to achieve even with several antihypertensive drugs taken in combination.

- ACE inhibitors and/or angiotensin receptor blockers have both antihypertensive and antiproteinuric properties. They are indicated for diabetics with microalbuminuria and for non diabetics with protein:creatinine ratio exceeding 50 mg/mmol.

- The antiproteinuric effect of these drugs is related to the intensity of renin angiotensin system blockade and may be increased when ACE inhibitors and angiotensin receptor blockers are given in combination.

- Adverse effects of renin angiotensin system blockade include hyperkalaemia and worsening renal function, which is more likely to occur in patients with vascular disease.

- Statins may also have antiproteinuric effects although evidence to date suggests that these are less than those of drugs that block the renin angiotensin system.

Hypertension may lead to renal failure and renal disease commonly causes hypertension. Elevated blood pressure is an independent risk factor for chronic kidney disease (CKD)[1] and may also be the main reason why renal function declines with age.[2,3] Renal dysfunction is common among patients with diabetes or vascular disease, many of whom are significantly hypertensive. The pathogenesis of the renal failure in this setting is likely to include contributions from large vessel renal disease (i.e., atherosclerotic renal vascular disease), small vessel renal disease (so called hypertensive nephrosclerosis) and cholesterol embolism.

Proteinuria, the hallmark of glomerular disease, is also common in the hypertensive renal diseases, and greater in patients with hypertensive renal diseases who have impaired renal function. For example, glomerular filtration rate (GFR) and proteinuria in the 1094 African Americans with hypertensive renal disease who participated in the AASK trial, ranged from 20 to 65 mL/min/1.73 m^2 and 20 to 2023 mg/24 h, respectively. Approximately two-thirds had microalbuminuria and one-third proteinuria, although none had nephrotic-range proteinuria (>3 g/24 h). Proteinuria greater than 1 g/24 h was seen almost exclusively in patients with GFR less than 40 mL/min.[4]

Proteinuria, when present in hypertensive renal diseases, may accelerate the decline of renal function[4,5] and also amplify the risk of vascular disease.[6,7] For these reasons, a working knowledge of the measurement, implications, and management of proteinuria in patients with hypertension is likely to be helpful to today's clinicians.

MEASUREMENT OF PROTEINURIA

The literature on measurement on proteinuria is not a particularly easy read. This is partly because measurements may be of urinary albumin or urinary total protein, and because of the different units of measurement used in the United States and United Kingdom. Against this background, normal urine protein excretion is less than 150 mg/24 h. This comprises up to 30 mg of albumin, the remainder consisting of low-molecular-weight proteins freely filtered by the glomerulus and Tamm-Horsfall proteins and β_2-microglobulin that are secreted by the tubules. The relation between albumin and total protein excretion is nonlinear, such that albumin typically represents 50% of total urinary protein at 300 mg/L and 70% at 1 g/L.[8] Tests for proteinuria range from the semiquantitative urinalysis strip to measurement of albumin:creatinine and protein:creatinine ratios on spot urine samples, and finally to quantitative assay for all forms of protein in a 24-hour urine collection.

Urinalysis for proteinuria is recommended as part of the initial assessment of patients with hypertension by the

British Hypertension Society,[9] Scottish Intercollegiate Guidelines Network,[10] and National Institute for Clinical Excellence,[11] because persistent proteinuria may indicate underlying CKD, and is also associated with an increased risk of cardiovascular disease (CVD). The simple dipstick urinalysis strip is a useful initial test for proteinuria provided the following four limitations are recognized. First, the test strip is more sensitive to albumin than to globulin and may not detect Bence Jones protein (BJP). Consequently, a negative urinalysis does not exclude significant urinary protein loss in the setting of myeloma. Second, dipstick proteinuria measures albumin concentration in excreted urine volume, not the rate of albumin excretion, and is therefore highly influenced by the concentration or dilution of the urine sample. Third, it is insufficiently sensitive to detect microalbuminuria (MA). Fourth, it is at best semiquantitative. As a general rule, 2+ proteinuria equates to a protein output of around 1 g/24 h, but for all urinalysis showing 1+ proteinuria or more, a quantitative assessment is recommended.

The gold standard for quantitative assessment, with some qualification, remains the laboratory analysis of a 24-hour urine collection, which detects both albumin and globulins. The qualification is that 24-hour urines are notoriously difficult to collect as many patients fail to understand that the collection begins by discarding the first specimen on the first day and is completed by including the first specimen in the second day. Some idea of the completeness of a 24-hour urine collection can be gained by measuring urine creatinine. Twenty-four-hour urine collections in which the ratio of measured creatinine (MC) to estimated creatinine (EC) is between 0.75 and 1.25 are likely to be accurate, where EC excretion is given by the following formula[12]:

EC g/24 h = (140 minus age) × lean weight (kg) × 0.2 (× 0.85 if female)

Guidelines in the United States and United Kingdom suggest untimed "spot" urine samples should be used in preference to 24-hour urine collections to detect and monitor proteinuria, either by albumin:creatinine ratio or protein:creatinine ratio.[13,14] Although a first-morning urine specimen has been recommended[13,14] it is by no means clear that spot urines at other times of day are any less satisfactory. Three of eight studies in the National Kidney Foundation's DOQI report[13] evaluating urine protein:creatinine ratio concluded that a daytime sample was a better predictor of 24-hour urine protein than a first void. Two of the eight studies tested a daytime sample only, two reported little difference between first void and subsequent random urines, and one found that a first void was more accurate.[13] Surprisingly, only one of these eight studies attempted to confirm the accuracy of the 24-hour urine protein (gold standard) by simultaneous measurement of urine creatinine, which may account for at least some of the deviations from the line of unity reported in these studies.[13] The most recent contribution to the debate on timing of the spot urine sample has concluded that random urine samples through the day are all satisfactory substitutes for 24-hour proteinuria.[15]

The normal range for albumin:creatinine ratio in the United Kingdom is given as less than 2.5 mg/mmol in men and less than 3.5 mg/mmol in women, reflecting the fact that women generally excrete less creatinine in their urine than men.[16] MA, which is used primarily to identify people with diabetes who are at risk of developing nephropathy, and which is defined as an albumin excretion rate (AER) of 30 to 300 mg/24 h, can be inferred when the albumin:creatinine ratio is higher than 2.5 mg/mmol in men or higher than 3.5 mg/mmol in women and less than 30 mg/mmol in both sexes. For completeness, the American Diabetes Association expresses albumin:creatinine ratio as milligrams per gram. The Association's normal range is less than 30 for both men and women.[17] MA is defined as albumin:creatinine ratio of 30–300 (which corresponds rather conveniently with a urinary albumin excretion rate of 30–300 mg/24 h). Clinical proteinuria is suggested either by an albumin:creatinine ratio higher than 30 mg/mmol (United Kingdom) or 300 mg/g (United States), and is more appropriately assessed by the protein:creatinine ratio.[12] Table 65–1 presents thresholds for microalbuminuria and proteinuria by albumin and total urine protein excretion.

The normal range for total protein:creatinine ratio is less than 15 mg/mmol. MA is suggested by a protein:creatinine ratio of 15 to 44 mg/mmol, but is more appropriately assessed by the albumin:creatinine ratio (above). Protein:creatinine ratio >45 mg/mmol represents clinical proteinuria and is approximately equivalent to an AER >300 mg/24 h or to a total urinary protein excretion of 0.45 g/24 h.[14] For completeness, the Americans express protein:creatinine ratio in grams per gram. To convert mmol of creatinine to grams of creatinine, divide by 8.84 or approximate (as is commonly done) by accepting that 10 mmol of creatinine is roughly equivalent to 1 g of creatinine.

A more precise estimate of urinary protein excretion can be obtained by calculating estimated protein output in grams per 24 hours using the formula given below. It is clear from this formula that estimated protein output will be the same as protein:creatinine ratio when the estimated creatinine excretion is 1 g/24 h, which it is for a 70-year-old man weighing 70 kg (see formula for estimated creatinine excretion). Estimated protein output therefore adds value to protein:creatinine ratio in very light or very heavy subjects whose estimated creatinine excretion is either much less or much greater than 1 g/24 h.[18]

EPO g/24 h = protein/creatinine ratio × estimated creatinine excretion

RISKS OF PROTEINURIA

Renal risk of proteinuria

Much of the work on the pathophysiology of proteinuria and its relation to renal function comes from studies of diabetes in which the development of nephropathy typi-

THRESHOLDS FOR MICROALBUMINURIA AND PROTEINURIA BY ALBUMIN AND TOTAL URINE PROTEIN EXCRETION			
Albumin:Creatinine Ratio (ACR)	Albumin Excretion Rate (AER)	Protein:Creatinine Ratio (PCR)	Protein Excretion Rate (PER)
Normal			
<2.5 mg/mmol men	<30 mg/24 hours	<15 mg/mmol	<0.15 g/24 hours
<3.5 mg/mmol women			
<30 mg/g (U.S.)			
Microalbuminuria			
2.5–30 mg/mmol men	30–300 mg/24 hours	15–45 mg/mmol	0.15–0.45 g/24 hours
3.5–30 mg/mmol women			
30–300 mg/g (U.S.)		But better assessed by ACR or AER	
Proteinuria			
> 30 mg/mmol	> 300 mg/24 hours	> 45 mg/mmol	>0.45 g/24 hours
> 300 mg/g (U.S.)		But better assessed by PCR or PER	

Table 65–1. Thresholds for Microalbuminuria and Proteinuria by Albumin and Total Urine Protein Excretion

cally follows a biphasic pattern, which is characterized by MA and hyperfiltration initially before progressing to overt proteinuria with a fall in glomerular filtration.[19] A similar biphasic response has recently been shown in nondiabetic subjects,[20] although the rate of progression to clinical proteinuria is lower than in people with diabetes. New proteinuria (more than 300 mg/24 h) in the HOPE Study was recorded in 20% of diabetics with microalbuminuria but in only 5% nondiabetics with microalbuminuria.[21] It was not possible to judge whether this heralded future renal failure in nondiabetics, as there were very few cases of progressive failure during the 4 to 6 years of follow-up.[21] Microalbuminuria has also been shown to predict a small fall in creatinine clearance during 7 years of follow-up in patients with essential hypertension, although no data were presented in this study to show whether this was associated with progression from microalbuminuria to overt proteinuria.[22]

By contrast, overt proteinuria predicts renal outcome both in CKD[5,23] and in population studies.[24,25] The heavier the proteinuria the greater the risk (Figures 65–1 and 65–2). Relative risk of developing ESRD during 17 years of follow-up in a community-based program of 106,117 Japanese adults was 2.95 for men and 2.66 for women with ++ proteinuria (approximately 1 g/L). Similar findings have been reported from a population cohort of 8592 Dutch adults in whom urinary albumin excretion independently predicted the risk of developing a GFR of less than 60 mL/min.[25] Absolute risk of developing ESRD in these population studies was of course lower than that in the studies of CKD, because nearly all subjects in the population studies had normal renal function at the time of screening.[24,25]

Cardiovascular risk of proteinuria

Microalbuminuria is also an independent risk factor for cardiovascular disease, in which setting it amplifies risk in patients who have vascular disease or are at high risk of developing vascular disease. The best example of this is the Heart Outcomes Prevention Evaluation (HOPE) study where the presence of microalbuminuria was associated with substantially increased cardiovascular events in subjects with diabetes and also in those with pre-existing CHD, after adjusting for a number of competing risk factors including serum creatinine[6] (Figure 65–3). Microalbuminuria has been shown to carry similar relative risks for cardiovascular events in general population studies,[26–30] albeit with lower absolute risk than reported in HOPE.

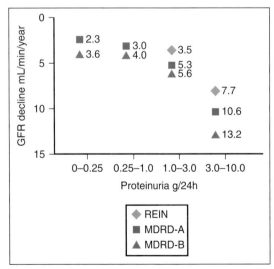

Figure 65–1. Relation between decline of GFR in milliliters per minute per year and proteinuria in grams per 24 hours in three studies. Baseline GFR was 38 to 46 mL/min in the Ramipril Efficacy in Nephropathy (REIN) study, 25 to 55 mL/min in the Modification of Diet in Renal Disease (MDRD-A) study, and 13 to 24 mL/min in the MDRD-B study. The data shown are for the usual care groups.

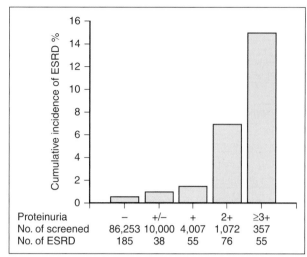

Figure 65–2. Cumulative incidence of end-stage renal disease by baseline proteinuria during 17 years of follow-up in a community-based program of 106,177 Japanese adults. (Data from Iseki K, Ikemiya Y, Iseki C, Takishita S. *Kidney Int* 2003;63:1468–74.)

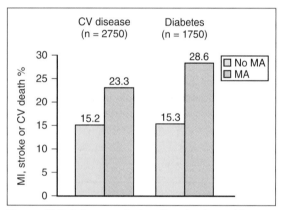

Figure 65–3. Influence of microalbuminuria on risk of MI, stroke or cardiovascular death in 4500 subjects in the HOPE placebo group who were followed for 4.5 years. Microalbuminuria was detected in 33% of those with diabetes and 15% of those with cardiovascular disease at baseline. (Data from Gerstein HC, Mann JF, Yi Q, et al. *JAMA* 2001;286:421–26.)

Several possible explanations for the association between microalbuminuria and cardiovascular risk have been proposed. It is unlikely that MA *per se* is the cause of the observed increase in risk. It is also unlikely simply to reflect the known higher prevalence of cardiovascular risk factors in MA, because MA continues to predict adverse outcomes after adjusting for the presence of these risk factors. It may, however, denote generalized endothelial dysfunction or abnormalities of coagulation and fibrinolysis, may be a marker of inflammation or may reflect a greater degree of end-organ damage in microalbuminuric subjects (reviewed by Sarnak et al.[31]).

BENEFITS OF TREATMENT

Blood pressure control

Most patients with proteinuric renal disease and raised serum creatinine have a clinical course characterized by relentless progression toward ESRD and dialysis. Control of hypertension is the single most effective intervention for those with proteinuria.[32] Progression to ESRD is reduced when proteinuria is decreased with larger reductions in proteinuria leading to lower rates of decline in GFR.[33] The much quoted MDRD study supports a target blood pressure as low as 125/75 mmHg when patients pass more than 1 g of protein per day,[5] although in other studies the benefits of such aggressive blood pressure control are not quite as convincing.[34,35]

The guideline writers currently favor a target blood pressure of below 130/80 mmHg for patients with CKD, the definition of which includes subjects with proteinuria alone.[36,37] They further recommend initiating treatment with an angiotensin converting enzyme (ACE) inhibitor or angiotensin receptor blocker (ARB), while recognizing that in order to achieve a blood pressure goal of less than 130/80 combination therapy will usually be required; also that co-prescription of lipid-lowering and antiplatelet therapy should be considered to reduce cardiovascular risk.[36,37] An integrated therapeutic intervention that includes antihypertensive drug therapy, statins, and aspirin has been tested with impressive benefits in patients with type 2 diabetes.[38]

Can blood pressure be lowered too far in hypertensive patient with proteinuric renal disease? A meta-analysis of 11 randomized controlled trials of ACE inhibitor therapy in 1860 nondiabetic patients suggests that it can. For patients with protein excretion higher than 1 g/day, optimum systolic blood pressure (SBP) was 110 to 129 mmHg. Reduction of SBP to less than 110 mmHg involving use of an ACE inhibitor led to worse renal outcomes in patients with pre-existing renal disease. For reasons that are not entirely clear, this J-shaped relationship between risk of progression of kidney disease and SBP was a feature of patients with significant proteinuria only, and was not observed in those with protein excretion of less than 1 g/day.[39]

Renin angiotensin system blockade

Notwithstanding the observations of Jafar et al.,[39] ACE inhibitors and ARBs have antiproteinuric properties that make them drugs of first choice in proteinuric patients.[40,41] A systematic review of 43 trials comprising 7545 patients showed that these two classes of drug had equivalent effects on renal outcomes.[42] Moreover, a recent study comparing the ACE inhibitor enalapril with the ARB telmisartan in type 2 diabetes and early nephropathy patients showed no significant differences between the effects of these two agents on a number of renal endpoints including change in glomerular filtration rate, serum creatinine level, urinary albumin excretion, and blood pressure.[43]

For patients with diabetes, the renal benefits of these drugs appear to extend across the whole range of proteinuria from MA to nephrotic range,[44–46] while for those with nondiabetic renal disease the threshold for benefit may be higher.[23,47,48] In a meta-analysis of 11 randomized trials of ACE inhibition in nondiabetic renal disease, patients with greater urine protein excretion at baseline benefited more from ACE inhibitor therapy, although the data were inconclusive as to whether benefit extended to those with baseline urine protein excretion of less than 0.5 g/24 h (protein:creatinine <50 mg/mmol)[41] (Figure 65–4).

The benefits of renin:angiotensin system (RAS) blockade appear to be directly proportional to the degree of RAS inhibition. Thus, low-dose ramipril had no effect on cardiovascular and renal outcomes of patients with type 2 diabetes and microalbuminuria,[49] whereas extreme doses of candesartan were more effective than conventional doses.[50] Remission of nephrotic range proteinuria by ACE inhibition to a level less than 1 g/24 h occurred only in 15% to 20% of patients with type 1 diabetes who were enrolled in an early study involving the short-acting ACE inhibitor captopril.[51] Incomplete inhibition of the RAS by ACE inhibitors and the fact that around 20% of treated patients still reach the combined endpoints of doubling serum creatinine or ERSD in randomized trials, has led to the hypothesis that better outcomes might be achieved by dual blockade of the RAS. This has since been tested in type 2 diabetes with microalbuminuria,[52] type 1 diabetes with established nephropathy,[53] and in nondiabetics with heavy proteinuria and either normal renal function[54] or established renal failure.[55,56] All have reported positive results.

The findings of Nakao et al.[56] are particularly relevant to current practice. Combination treatment with trandolapril and losartan was compared with trandolapril alone and losartan alone in 263 patients with nondiabetic renal disease whose baseline creatinine and protein output were 267 μmol/L and 2.5 g/24 h, respectively. During an average 2.9 years follow-up, only 11% of the combination

group reached the combined primary endpoint of time to doubling serum creatinine or ESRD, compared to 23% in each of the other two treatment groups. Urinary protein excretion decreased significantly in all three groups, but to a significantly greater extent in patients receiving trandolapril and losartan. In subgroup analyses, benefits could be shown for patients with baseline proteinuria higher than 1 g/24 h, but less convincingly at lower rates of urinary protein excretion (Figure 65–5).

The clinical importance of the Nakao study is that the patients treated are precisely those for whom most clinicians would avoid dual RAS blockade for fear of provoking hyperkalemia or aggravating their renal failure. What it proves is that the kidney may benefit even in advanced renal failure provided that patients are selected carefully enough and monitored closely thereafter. An initial rise in serum creatinine is a normal hemodynamic response to blockade of RAS in patients with CKD, but is not a reason to withhold or suspend treatment unless the increase is greater than 30% above baseline or hyperkalemia develops.[57] A particular concern is the risk of life-threatening hyperkalemia and/or acute renal failure requiring dialysis when a patient taking an ACE inhibitor or ARB becomes dehydrated. This occurs not uncommonly during intercurrent illnesses characterized by blood volume depletion, and diarrhea and vomiting.[58,59] Other circumstances in which renal function may be seriously compromised during RAS blockade include unsuspected bilateral renovascular disease[60] and co-prescription of a nonsteroidal anti-inflammatory drug.[61]

The possibility that the benefits of RAS blockade could be enhanced by drugs that lower blood pressure by other means has also been explored. The addition of felodipine to ramipril in patients with nondiabetic nephropathies gave no additional renoprotection despite further blood

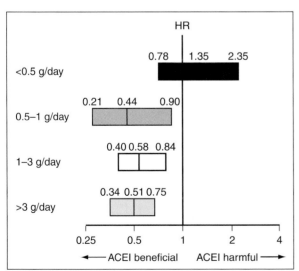

Figure 65–4. Meta-analysis of 11 randomized trials of ACE inhibition in nondiabetic renal disease showing hazard ratios for ACE inhibition on a composite endpoint of doubling serum creatinine or end-stage renal disease at various levels of baseline urinary protein excretion (Data from Jafar TH, Schmit CH, Landa M, et al. *Ann Intern Med* 2001;135:73–87.)

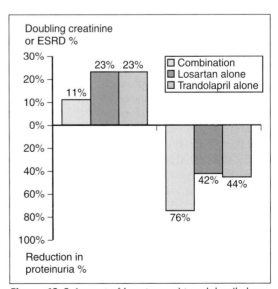

Figure 65–5. Impact of losartan and trandolapril alone and together on proteinuria and the composite renal endpoint of doubling serum creatinine or end-stage renal disease in 263 patients with nondiabetic renal disease. (Data from Nakao N, Yoshimura A, Morita H, Takada M, Kayano T, Ideura T. *Lancet* 2003;361:117–24.)

pressure reductions of 5/0 mmHg[62] and 4/3 mmHg.[63] Another recently published study in patients with type 2 diabetes and hypertension with normoalbuminuria, showed that the renoprotective effect of the ACE inhibitor trandolapril was not enhanced by the addition of the non–dihydropyridine calcium channel blocker, verapamil.[64]

Statins

HMG-CoA reductase inhibitors or statins are now firmly established as the lipid-lowering treatment of choice in both primary and secondary prevention settings of coronary and vascular events. Patients in the statin trials who had moderate renal impairment (estimated GFR at 30 to 60 mL/min) had higher rates of vascular disease than those with eGFR higher than 60 mL/min, and also benefited from statins.[65] The role of statins in patients with more advanced CKD is less secure. An observational study of the U.S. Renal Data System information suggested that statin use was independently associated with lower all cause (relative risk [RR] 0.68, 95% confidence interval [CI] 0.54–0.87) and cardiovascular mortality (RR 0.64, 95% CI 0.45–0.91),[66] but a randomized comparison of atorvastatin and placebo in dialysis patients with type 2 diabetes showed no such benefits.[67] The ALERT (Assessment of Lescol in Renal Transplantation) study of fluvastatin in renal transplant patients showed a reduction in a secondary endpoint of fatal coronary heart (CHD) and nonfatal myocardial infarction, but not in cardiovascular or total mortality.[68] Against this background, the results of AURORA (A study to evaluate the Use of Rosuvastatin in subjects On Regular haemodialysis: an Assessment of survival and cardiovascular events) are awaited with interest.[69]

The suggestion that statins might be good for the kidney as well as the heart is relatively new. Hyperlipidemia is thought to contribute to the progression of renal disease, either by a toxic effect on mesangial cells or by promoting intrarenal atherosclerosis.[70] Evidence is beginning to emerge that statins may have both antiproteinuric effects and benefits for renal function, although the mechanisms of benefit are as yet uncertain. A meta-analysis of 13 small randomized trials up to 1999 showed a slower rate of decline in GFR and a trend toward lower urinary protein excretion.[71] Athyros et al.,[72] in an analysis of the GREACE (Greek Atorvastatin and Coronary Heart Disease Evaluation) study reported that atorvastatin not only prevented decline but also improved renal function in patients who had established vascular disease and normal serum creatinine (less than 115 µmol/L) initially. Curiously, the authors did not provide details of urinary protein output in this analysis.

The most convincing evidence of renal benefit comes from a comparison of atorvastatin and placebo in 56 patients with CKD whose baseline proteinuria and creatinine clearance were 2.2 g/24 h and 50 mL/min, respectively. During 1 year of treatment, patients who received atorvastatin experienced less proteinuria and a slower rate of GFR decline[73] (Figure 65–6). The benefits shown in this study were in addition to those of treatment with ACEIs and ARBs. Similar findings have been reported by others,[74,75] although it has not been possible to show renal benefits for statins in patients with lesser degrees of proteinuria. In a randomized comparison of fosinopril and pravastatin in 864 mostly nondiabetic subjects with microalbuminuria and normal serum creatinine, fosinopril reduced urinary albumin excretion but pravastatin did not.[76]

SUMMARY

The detection of protein in the urine of a patient with hypertension has major implications for both doctor and patient. The limitations of the dipstick test are now widely recognized. Urine collection for 24 hours is no longer recommended as a means of quantifying proteinuria. Instead, the albumin:creatinine ratio is firmly established as the method of choice for detecting and quantifying microalbuminuria, as is the protein:creatinine ratio for patients with overt proteinuria. Estimated protein output, derived by multiplying the protein:creatinine ratio by the estimated creatinine excretion, is the most accurate of measures based on a spot urine sample. On the rare occasions that a 24-hour urine collection is required, its accuracy can be determined by the ratio of measured to expected creatinine excretion with values lying between 0.75 and 1.25 suggesting that the collection is likely to be complete.

Proteinuria predicts subsequent loss of renal function. Relative risk is similar in the general population and in those with CKD, although absolute risks are much higher in patients with CKD, particularly in those with heavier proteinuria. Proteinuria also predicts cardiovascular disease, but in contrast to the renal risks of proteinuria, cardiovascular risk can be increased by microalbuminuria.

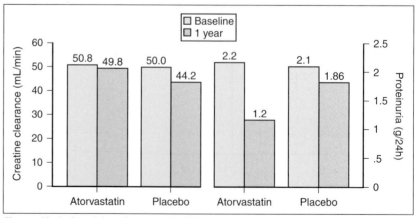

Figure 65–6. Creatinine clearance (milliliters per minute) and proteinuria (grams per 24 hours) in 56 patients with chronic kidney disease randomized to atorvastatin at 10 to 40 mg daily or placebo and followed for 1 year. Baseline creatinine clearance was 50.4 mL/min and baseline proteinuria 2.2 g/24 h. (Data from Bianchi S, Bigazzi R, Caiazza A, Campese VM. *Am J Kidney Dis* 2003;41:565–70.)

These observations may mean there are two types of proteinuria: "renal proteinuria," in which the magnitude of the renal risk is directly related to the level of the proteinuria, and "cardiovascular proteinuria" (usually microalbuminuria), which probably arises as a result of endothelial dysfunction. Cardiovascular proteinuria does not generally lead to progressive renal failure, although it does indicate associated increase in risk of vascular events, particularly in patients who already have vascular disease.

Treatment options for proteinuria include blood pressure control to less than 130/80 mmHg and possibly to less than 125/75 mmHg if proteinuria exceeds 1 g/

24 h. ACE inhibitors and ARBs have additional anti-proteinuric properties with trial evidence of benefit for diabetics with microalbuminuria and nondiabetics with proteinuric nephropathy exceeding 0.5 g/24 h (50 mg of protein/mmol creatinine). Dual blockade of the renin:angiotensin system is associated with greater renal benefit than by ACE inhibitor or ARB alone. The use of statins in patients with proteinuria remains controversial. The antiproteinuric effect of statins is not only less than the ability of this class of drugs to reduce vascular events but it is also likely to be less than the antiproteinuric effects of RAS blockade.

REFERENCES

1. Hsu CY, McCulloch CE, Darbinian J, Go AS, Uribarren C. Elevated blood pressure and risk of end stage renal disease in subjects without baseline kidney disease. *Arch Intern Med* 2005; 165:923–28.
2. Klag MJ, Whelton PK, Randall BL, et al. Blood pressure and end stage renal disease in men. *N Engl J Med* 1996; 334:13–18.
3. Haroun MK, Jaar BG, Hoffman SC, Comstock GW, Klag MJ, Coresh J. Risk factors for chronic kidney disease: a prospective study of 23,534 men and women in Washington County, Maryland. *J Am Soc Nephrol* 2003; 14:2934–41.
4. Lea J, Greene T, Hebert L, et al. The relationship between magnitude of proteinuria reduction and risk of end stage renal disease. Results of the African American Study of Kidney Disease and Hypertension. *Arch Intern Med* 2005;165:247–53.
5. Peterson JC, Adler S, Burkart JM, et al. Blood pressure control, proteinuria and the progression of renal disease: the Modification of Diet in Renal Disease Study. *Ann Intern Med* 1995;123:754–62.
6. Gerstein HC, Mann JF, Yi Q, et al. Albuminuria and risk of cardiovascular events, death and heart failure in diabetic and nondiabetic subjects. *JAMA* 2001;286:421–26.
7. Leoncini G, Sacchi G, Viazzi F, et al. Microalbuminuria identifies overall cardiovascular risk in essential hypertension: an artificial neural network-based approach. *J Hypertens* 2002;20:1315–21.
8. Newman DJ, Thakkar H, Medcalf EA, Gray MR, Price CP. Use of urine albumin measurement as a replacement for total protein. *Clin Nephrol* 1995;43:104–109.
9. Williams B, Poulter NR, Brown MJ, et al. Guidelines for management of hypertension: report of the Fourth Working Party of the British Hypertension Society, 2004. *J Hum Hypertens* 2004; 18:139–85.
10. Scottish Intercollegiate Guidelines Network. *Hypertension in Older People. A National Clinical Guideline, 2001;* Royal College of Physicians, London.
11. National Institute for Clinical Excellence. *Hypertension: management of hypertension in adults in primary care,*

2006: www.nice.org.uk/guidance/CG34 (accessed January 2007).
12. Wilmer WA, Rovin BH, Herbert CJ, Rao SV, Kumor K, Herbert LA. Management of glomerular proteinuria: a commentary. *J Am Soc Nephrol* 2003; 14:3217–32.
13. National Kidney Foundation/Kidney Disease Outcomes Quality Initiative. NKF K/DOQI clinical practice guidelines for chronic kidney disease. Guideline 5: assessment of proteinuria. *Am J Kidney Dis* 2002;39:S93–201 (available at www.kidney.org/professionals/kdoqi/gui delines).
14. Joint Specialty Committee for Renal Disease, Royal College of Physicians of London, and The Renal Association. *Chronic Kidney Disease in Adults: UK Guidelines for Identification, Management and Referral.* London: Royal College of Physicians of London, 2005.
15. Gaspari F, Perico N, Remuzzi G. Timed urine collections are not needed to measure urine protein excretion in clinical practice. *Am J Kidney Dis* 2006;47:1–7.
16. Scottish Intercollegiate Guidelines Network (SIGN). *Management of Diabetes.* SIGN publication 55. Edinburgh: SIGN, November 2001 (also available at www.sign.ac.uk).
17. American Diabetes Association. Clinical Practice Recommendations 2001. *Diabetes Care* 2001;24:S1–133 (see S69–72).
18. Ginsberg JM, Chang BS, Matarese RA, Garella S. Use of single voided urine samples to estimate quantitative proteinuria. *N Engl J Med* 1983; 309:1543–46.
19. Viberti GC, Hill RD, Jarret RJ, Argyropoulos A, Mahmud U, Keen H. Microalbuminuria as a predictor of clinical nephropathy in insulin dependent diabetes mellitus. *Lancet* 1982;1:1430–32.
20. Pinto-Sietsma S-J, Janssen WMT, Hillege HL, Navis G, De Zeeuw D, De Jong PE. Urinary albumin excretion is associated with renal function abnormalities in a nondiabetic population. *J Am Soc Nephrol* 2000; 11:1882–88.
21. Mann JFE, Gerstein HC, Yi Q-L, et al. Development of renal disease in people at high cardiovascular risk: results of the HOPE randomised study. *J Am Soc Nephrol* 2003;14:641–47.

22. Bigazzi R, Bianchi S, Baldari D, Campese VM. Microalbuminuria predicts cardiovascular events and renal insufficiency in patients with essential hypertension. *J Hypertens* 1998;16:1325–33.
23. Ruggenenti P, Perna A, Mosconi L, et al. Proteinuria predicts end stage renal failure in nondiabetic chronic nephropathies. *Kidney Int* 1997; 52(Suppl 63):S54–57.
24. Iseki K, Ikemiya Y, Iseki C, Takishita S. Proteinuria and the risk of developing end stage renal disease. *Kidney Int* 2003;63:1468–74.
25. Verhave JC, Gansevoort RT, Hillege HL, Bakker SJL, De Zeeuw D, De Jong PE, et al. An elevated urinary albumin excretion predicts de novo development of renal function impairment in the general population. *Kidney Int* 2004; 66(Supp 92):S18–21.
26. Kannel WB, Stampfer MJ, Castelli WP, Verter J. The prognostic significance of proteinuria: the Framlingham Study. *Am Heart J* 1984;108:1347–52.
27. Wagener DK, Harris T, Madans JH. Proteinuria as a biomarker: risk of subsequent morbidity and mortality. *Environ Res* 1994;66:160–72.
28. Miettinen H, Haffner SM, Lehto S, et al. Proteinuria predicts stroke and other atherosclerotic vascular disease in nondiabetic and non–insulin-dependent diabetic subjects. *Stroke* 1996;27:2033–39.
29. Hillege HL, Fidler V, Diercks GFH, et al. Urinary albumin excretion predicts cardiovascular and noncardiovascular mortality in general population. *Circulation* 2002;106:1777–82.
30. Muntner P, He J, Hamm L, Loria C, Whelton PK. Renal insufficiency and subsequent death resulting from cardiovascular disease in the United States. *J Am Soc Nephrol* 2002;13:745–53.
31. Sarnak MJ, Levey AS, Schoolwerth AC, Coresh J, Culleton B, Lee Hamm L, et al. Kidney disease as a risk factor for the development of cardiovascular disease. A statement from the American Heart Association Councils on kidney in cardiovascular disease, high blood pressure research, clinical cardiology, and epidemiology and prevention. *Circulation* 2003;108:2154–69.
32. Ruggenenti P, Schiepatti A, Remuzzi G. Progression, remission, regression of chronic renal diseases. *Lancet* 2001; 357:1601–608.

33. Rossing P, Hommel E, Smidt UM, Parving H-H. Reduction in albuminuria predicts beneficial effect on diminishing the progession of human diabetic nephropathy during antihypertensive treatment. *Diabetologia* 1994;37:511–6.

34. Schrier RW, Estacio RO, Esler A, Mehler P. Effects of aggressive blood pressure control in normotensive type 2 diabetic patients on albuminuria, retinopathy and stroke. *Kidney Int* 2002;61:1086–97.

35. Wright JT, Bakris G, Greene T, et al. Effects of blood pressure lowering and antihypertensive drug class on progression of hypertensive kidney disease. Results from the AASK Trial. *JAMA* 2002;288:2421–31.

36. Guidelines Committee. 2003 European Society of Hypertension—European Society of Cardiology Guidelines for the management of arterial hypertension. *J Hypertens* 2003;21:1011–53.

37. Chobanian AV, Bakris GL, Black HR, et al. The seventh report of the Joint National Committee on Prevention, Detection, Evaluation and Treatment of High Blood Pressure: the JNC7 Report. *JAMA* 2003;289:2560–72.

38. Gaede P, Vedel P, Larsen N, Jensen GV, Parving HH, Pedersin O. Multifactorial intervention and cardiovascular disease in patients with type 2 diabetes. *N Engl J Med* 2003;348:383–93.

39. Jafar TH, Stark PC, Schmid CH, et al. Progression of chronic kidney disease: the role of blood pressure control, proteinuria and angiotensin converting enzyme inhibition—a patient level meta analysis. *Ann Intern Med* 2003;139: 244–52.

40. Kshirsagar AV, Joy MS, Hogan SL, et al. Effect of ACE inhibitors in diabetic and nondiabetic chronic renal disease: a systematic overview of randomised placebo controlled trials *Am J Kidney Dis* 2000;35:695–707.

41. Jafar TH, Schmit CH, Landa M, et al. Angiotensin converting enzyme inhibitors and progression of nondiabetic renal disease; a meta analysis of patient level data. *Ann Intern Med* 2001;135:73–87.

42. Strippoli GFM, Craig M, Deeks JJ, Schena FP, Craig JC. Effects of angiotensin converting enzyme inhibitors and angiotensin 2 receptor antagonists on mortality and renal outcomes in diabetic nephropathy: systematic review. *BMJ* 2004;329: 818–31.

43. Barnett AH, Bain SC, Bowter B, et al. Angiotensin receptor blockade versus converting enzyme inhibition in type 2 diabetes and nephropathy. *N Engl J Med* 2004;351:1952–61.

44. Parving HH, Lehnert H, Brochner-Mortensen J, Gomis R, Andersen S, Arner P. The effect of irbesartan on the development of diabetic nephropathy in patients with type 2 diabetes. *N Engl J Med* 2001;345:870–78.

45. Lewis EJ, Hunsicker LG, Clarke WR, et al. Renoprotective effect of the angiotensin-receptor antagonist irbesartan in patients with nephropathy due to type 2 diabetes. *N Engl J Med* 2001;345:851–60.

46. Brenner BM, Cooper ME, De Zeeuw D, et al. The effects of losartan on renal and cardiovascular outcomes in patients with type 2 diabetes and nephropathy. *N Engl J Med* 2001;345:861–69.

47. Ruggenenti P, Perna A, Gherardi G, et al. Renal function and requirement for dialysis in chronic nephropathy patients on long-term ramipril: REIN follow-up trial. *Lancet* 1998;352:1252–56.

48. Ruggenenti P, Perna A, Gherardi G, et al. Renoprotective properties of ACE inhibition in nondiabetic nephropathies with non-nephrotic proteinuria. *Lancet* 1999;354:359–66.

49. Marre M, Lievre M, Chatellier G, et al. on behalf of the DIABHYCAR Study Investigators. Effects of low dose ramipril on cardiovascular and renal outcomes in patients with type 2 diabetes and raised excretion of urinary albumin: randomised, double blind, placebo controlled trial (the DIABHYCAR Study). *BMJ* 2004;328:495–99.

50. Weinberg AJ, Zappe DH, Ashton M, Weinberg MS. Safety and tolerability of high dose angiotensin receptor blocker therapy in patients with chronic kidney disease. *Am J Nephrol* 2004;24:340–45.

51. Hebert LA, Bain RP, Verme D, et al. Remission of nephrotic range proteinuria in type 1 diabetes. *Kidney Int* 1994; 46:1688–93.

52. Mogensen CE, Neldam S, Tikkanen I, et al. Randomised controlled trial of dual blockade of renin-angiotensin system in patients with hypertension, microalbuminuria and non-insulin dependent diabetes: the Candesartan and Lisinopril Microalbuminuria (CALM) study. *BMJ* 2000;321:1440–44.

53. Jacobsen P, Anderson S, Rossing K, Jensen BR, Parving H-H. Dual blockade of the renin angiotensin system versus maximum recommended dose of ACE inhibition in diabetic nephropathy. *Kidney Int* 2003;63:1874–80.

54. Laverman GD, Navis G, Henning RH, de Jong PE, de Zeeuw D. Dual renin angiotensin system blockade at optimal doses for proteinuria. *Kidney Int* 2002; 62:1020–25.

55. Campbell R, Sangalli F, Perticucci E, et al. Effects of combined ACE inhibitor and angiotensin II antagonist treatment in human chronic nephropathy. *Kidney Int* 2003;63:1094–103.

56. Nakao N, Yoshimura A, Morita H, Takada M, Kayano T, Ideura T. Combination treatment of angiotensin 2 receptor blocker and angiotensin converting enzyme inhibitor in nondiabetic renal disease (COOPERATE): a randomised controlled trial. *Lancet* 2003;361:117–24.

57. Bakris GL, Weir MR. Angiotensin converting enzyme inhibitor associated elevation in serum creatinine. *Arch Intern Med* 2000;160:685–93.

58. Stirling C, Houston J, Robertson S, et al. Diarrhoea, vomiting and ACE inhibitors—an important cause of acute renal failure. *J Hum Hypertens* 2003; 17:419–23.

59. McGuigan J, Robertson S, Isles C. Life threatening hyperkalaemia with diarrhoea during ACE inhibition. *Emerg Med J* 2005;22:154–55.

60. Brammah A, Robertson S, Tait G, Isles C. Bilateral renovascular disease causing cardiorenal failure. *BMJ* 2003; 326:489–91.

61. Gambaro G, Perazella MA. Adverse renal effects of anti-inflammatory agents: evaluation of selective and nonselective cyclooxygenase inhibitors. *J Intern Med* 2003;253:643–52.

62. Herlitz H, Harris K, Risler T, et al. The effects of an ACE inhibitor and a calcium antagonist on the progression of renal disease: the NEPHROS study. *Nephrol Dial Transplant* 2001;16: 2158–65.

63. Ruggenenti P, Perna A, Loriga G, et al. Blood pressure control for renoprotection in patients with non-diabetic chronic renal disease (REIN-2): multicentre randomised controlled trial. *Lancet* 2005;365:939–46.

64. Ruggenenti P, Fassi A, Ilieva AP, et al. Preventing microalbuminuria in type 2 diabetes. *N Engl J Med* 2004;351: 1941–51.

65. Tonelli M, Isles C, Curhan GC, et al. Effect of pravastatin on cardiovascular events in people with chronic kidney disease. *Circulation* 2004;110:1557–63.

66. Seliger SL, Weiss NS, Gillen DL, et al. HMG-CoA reductase inhibitors are associated with reduced mortality in end stage renal disease patients. *Kidney Int* 2002;61:297–304.

67. Wanner C, Krane V, Marz W, et al. Atorvastatin in patients with type 2 diabetes mellitus undergoing haemodialysis. *N Engl J Med* 2005;353:238–48.

68. Holdaas H, Fellstrom B, Jardine AG, et al. Effects of fluvastatin on cardiac outcomes in renal transplant recipients. *Lancet* 2003;361:2024–31.

69. Fellstrom BC, Holdaas H, Jardine AG. Why do we need a statin trial in haemodialysis patients? *Kidney Int* 2003;63(Suppl 84):S204–206.

70. Mason JC. The statins—therapeutic diversity in renal disease. *Curr Opin Nephrol Hypertens* 2005;14:17–24.

71. Fried LF, Orchard TJ, Kasiske LB. Effect of lipid reduction on the progression of renal disease: a meta-analysis. *Kidney Int* 2001;59:260–69.

72. Athyros VG, Mikhailidis DP, Papageorgiou AA, et al. The effect of statins versus untreated dyslipidaemia on renal function in patients with coronary heart disease. A sub group analysis of the Greek Atorvastatin and Coronary Heart Disease Evaluation (GREACE) study. *J Clin Pathol* 2004;57:728–34.

73. Bianchi S, Bigazzi R, Caiazza A, Campese VM. A controlled prospective study of the effects of atorvastatin on proteinuria and progression of kidney disease. *Am J Kidney Dis* 2003;41:565–70.

74. Lee T-M, Su S-F, Tsai C-H. Effect of pravastatin on proteinuria in patients with well controlled hypertension. *Hypertension* 2002;40:67–73.

75. Tonelli M, Moye L, Sacks FM, Cole T, Curhan G, et al. Effects of pravastatin on loss of renal function in people with moderate chronic renal insufficiency and cardiovascular disease. *J Am Soc Nephrol* 2003;14:1605–13.

76. Asselbergs FW, Diercks GFH, Hillege HL, et al. Effects of fosinopril and pravastatin on cardiovascular events in subjects with microalbuminuria. *Circulation* 2004;110:2809–16.

Chapter

66

Renin-Secreting Tumors and Other Renin-Secreting States

Michel Azizi, Pierre-François Plouin, and Laurence Amar

Key Findings

- Juxtaglomerular cell (JGC) tumors (JGCT) are very rare renin-secreting tumors originating from the JG apparatus.

- JGCT diagnosis remains difficult, but JGCT should be suspected in young patients with severe hypertension and secondary hyperaldosteronism associated with the secretion of large amounts of renin, after the elimination of other much more frequent causes of secondary hyperaldosteronism.

- The tumor is localized by thin-slice computerized tomography (CT) scan showing a small isodense or hypodense tumor with no enhancement or slight enhancement on contrast and an isosignal intensity on magnetic resonance image (MRI). Renal arteriography is required to rule out other causes of renin-dependent hypertension especially a stenosis affecting the distal renal artery or intrarenal arterial branches, usually caused by fibromuscular dysplasia. It shows a small avascular radiolucent area at the external contour of the kidney.

- Microscopic study of the tumor reveals the presence of specialized vascular smooth muscle cells showing endocrine differentiation and containing secretory cytoplasmic granules. These cells are very similar to those of normal renin-producing cells, and are strongly immunohistochemically labeled by renin and prorenin antibodies, confirming the diagnosis of JGCT. They are frequently associated with histamine-secreting mast cells.

- Conservative surgery with elective tumor resection is the preferred procedure.

PRIMARY RENINISM DUE TO TUMOR OF JUXTAGLOMERULAR APPARATUS

Renin may be produced by tumors of renal or extrarenal origin. This rare but severe form of secondary hypertension is usually referred to as primary reninism.[1] While very rare, this condition is of significance, as it may be confused with hyperaldosteronism and should attract specific management. Primary reninism is different from secondary reninism, which is caused by sodium depletion or by an abnormality of the extrarenal arteries or of the intrarenal arteries or arterioles, or other causes of excessive renin secretion by the kidney.

Juxtaglomerular cell (JGC) tumors (JGCT) are renin-secreting tumors that originate in the JG apparatus (Figure 66–1). The apparent prevalence (approximately 70 cases reported worldwide in the last review by Martin et al.[2]) and incidence (eight cases of renin-secreting JGCT among 30,000 hypertensive patients treated at a single hypertension clinic in Paris over a 15-year period[3]) of this disease are very low, possibly due to underestimation of its frequency. Indeed, it remains difficult to diagnose primary reninism due to a JGCT because (1) there are no specific clinical symptoms or laboratory results associated with these tumors, and (2) these tumors remain difficult to visualize and to localize, and neither hyperaldosteronism nor hyperreninemia is routinely defined in the vast majority of hypertensive patients worldwide.

ANATOMY AND PATHOLOGY

JGCT are usually small, well-circumscribed encapsulated cortical renal masses of less than 4 cm in diameter.[2,4] Larger JGCT, up to 8 or 9 cm in diameter, have been reported.[2,5] Large tumors must be differentiated histologically from papillary renal cell carcinomas, because these cancers may be associated with hypertension and may include either tumoral or non-tumoral renin containing-cells (see below). The distinction between JGCT and papillary renal cell carcinomas is based on various histological characteristics and is generally straightforward.

The cut surface of the JGCT is yellow to tan/gray with areas of hemorrhage.[2,4] The cell of origin of the JGCT is a modified smooth muscle cell from the vascular component of the JG apparatus. Light and electron microscopy studies reveal the presence of specialized vascular smooth muscle cells showing endocrine differentiation. JG cells are polygonal cells containing secretory cytoplamic granules, myofilaments, and attachment bodies[6] (see Martin et al.[2] for review). The ultrastructure of renin-secreting tumor cells is very similar to that of normal renin-producing cells, with the presence of secretory paracrystallin protogranules and round amorphous dense mature granules containing both prorenin and renin[7,8] (Figure 66–2). These cells are strongly labeled with antibodies against renin and prorenin, confirming the diagnosis of JGCT (Figures 66–3 and 66–4). *In situ* hybridization, gives a signal with tumor cells, including those not stained by the renin antibody.[9] Microscopy also shows that renin-secreting tumor cells are closely associated with capillaries and blood vessels and may occasionally show entrapped renal tubules. Histamine-secreting mast cells are frequent, accounting for up to 25% of all cells,[6,10] even though no mast cells are found in the normal or pathologic JG apparatus. This suggests that JGCT may

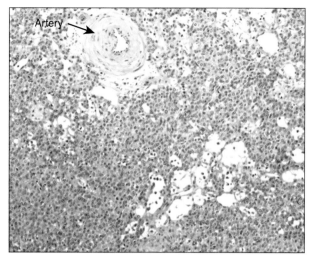

Figure 66–1. The juxtaglomerular cell tumor is characterized by a homogeneous proliferation of regular round cells without any atypia or marked proliferation. Note a thickened wall artery within the tumor reflecting highly activated local renin-angiotensin system. Hematoxylin-eosin. Original magnification ×10. (Courtesy of Patrick Bruveval, Hôpital Européen Georges Pompidou, Paris, France.)

release a factor attracting and favoring the growth of mast cells.

PATHOPHYSIOLOGY: AUTONOMY OF RENIN SECRETION

Human active renin is a 340–amino acid, aspartyl protease with a molecular weight of 40,000 Daltons and two N-glycosylation sites. It is secreted by the renal JG epithelioid cells, and synthesized in these cells as prorenin, which is activated by cleavage of an N-terminal 43-amino acid prosegment. Prorenin is also secreted into the blood. Total plasma renin concentration therefore corresponds to the concentration of both prorenin and active renin.

Active renin and prorenin originating from a JGCT or other tumor (see below) are the same molecules as physiologic renin and prorenin originating from normal kidneys, except for their secretion in excess, in an unregulated fashion.

In patients with JGCT, the renin response to various interventions known to inhibit or to stimulate renin is variable. Renin release from the JGCT usually responds to changes in posture and sodium intake, but this is not always so. Upright posture increases plasma renin activity (PRA) and/or plasma active renin concentration in about 70% of cases, whereas beta-blocker administration inhibits renin release, suggesting that beta-receptors may be present in these tumors.[4]

The demonstration that renin secretion by the tumor is autonomous is based on the inhibition of angiotensin II (Ang II) generation by angiotensin-converting enzyme (ACE) inhibitors or the blockade of angiotensin type 1 (AT1) receptors by Ang II receptor antagonists. Blockade of the renin-angiotensin system (RAS) consistently decreases

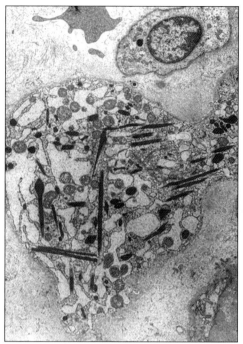

Figure 66–2. A tumor cell contains many renin granules exhibiting either an immature pattern with paracristallin shape or a mature pattern with a round shape and a homogeneous matrix. Original magnification ×2500. (Courtesy of Patrick Bruveval, Hôpital Européen Georges Pompidou, Paris, France.)

blood pressure (BP), demonstrating a direct role of Ang II in the maintenance of hypertension. In the absence of a renovascular disease or severe sodium depletion, a major decrease in BP in response to RAS blockade should lead to a search for renin-secreting JGCT. However, BP response to ACE inhibitors/AT1 receptor antagonists is

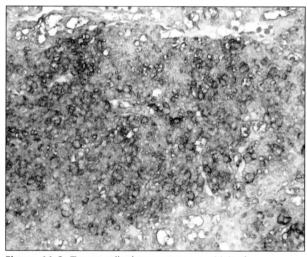

Figure 66–3. Tumor cells show a strong positivity for immunohistochemistry with renin antibody. Original magnification ×20. (Courtesy of Patrick Bruveval, Hôpital Européen Georges Pompidou, Paris, France.)

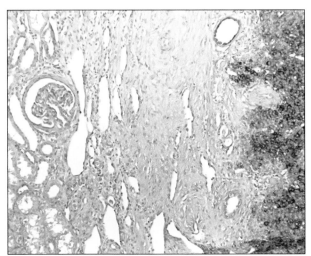

Figure 66–4. The tumor is clearly separated from the adjacent nontumoral kidney tissue in which it is developed. Note that renin production is abolished in the adjacent glomerulus due to the huge local renin production by the tumor cells. Renin immunohistochemistry. Original magnification ×10. (Courtesy of Patrick Bruveval, Hôpital Européen Georges Pompidou, Paris, France.)

not specific for JGCT, and may be observed in all cases of hypertension associated with RAS activation. Interestingly, blockade of the RAS frequently fails to increase circulating renin concentration, indicating that tumor renin secretion is autonomous. This autonomy may result from an absence of AT1 receptor expression in the tumors, leading to inactivation of the angiotensin-II negative feedback loop on renin secretion.[11]

CLINICAL PRESENTATION

Robertson et al.[12] provided the first description of a case of primary reninism in 1967, and the first histologic description of a JGCT was provided by Kihara et al.[13] JGCT generally occur in young male or female patients in their mid-20s, with a female/male ratio of approximately 1.9:1.[2,14] However, these tumors have also been reported in children[14] and older adults,[5] and due to their rarity the age-stratified prevalence is not adequately defined.

There are no specific features of hypertension due to a renin-secreting tumor. Indeed, the patient may present hypertension for several years before the discovery of the JGCT. One case of normotensive JGCT has been reported,[15] but in all other cases, hypertension has been severe, accelerated, or malignant with presence of thirst and polyuria.[1] Severe target-organ damage (e.g., alteration of optic fundi and left ventricular hypertrophy, proteinuria) and early complications (cerebrovascular accidents) may also be present. Hypertension may be resistant to conventional antihypertensive treatments, although this resistance is neither specific nor constant. As would be predicted, and unlike primary hyperaldosteronism, these tumors respond well to treatments blocking the RAS either by ACE inhibitors or AT1 receptor antagonists.

DIAGNOSTIC TECHNIQUES

Biological and hormonal parameters

The principal routine laboratory finding in almost all cases is severe hypokalemia at less than 3.0 mmol/L (occasionally as low as 1.9 mmol/L) due to secondary hyperaldosteronism associated with excess renin,[1,2,4,6,14] but normal serum K^+ values have been reported in some cases.[14] Mild hyponatremia may occur, due to the interaction of multiple factors.[4] Renal function is generally not impaired, although proteinuria is common[14] and/or plasma active renin concentration (PRA) is usually extremely high (more than five times the upper limit of the normal range), resulting in concomitantly high plasma Ang II and aldosterone concentrations. However, PRA levels may be only moderately high in some cases. There is no correlation between the tumor size and PRA.[16] Prorenin (inactive form of renin) determinations by trypsin activation or direct radioimmunoassay may facilitate diagnosis, because some tumors may release more prorenin due to abnormal processing or storage in tumor cells.[17]

The diagnosis of a renin-secreting tumor should therefore be considered in young patients with severe hypertension and secondary hyperaldosteronism associated with the secretion of large amounts of renin, after elimination of the most frequent diagnoses associated with these nonspecific clinical and biological conditions.

Tumor localization

JGCT localization takes place after the elimination of other much more frequent causes of severe hypertension with marked hyperreninism and hyperaldosteronism. The precise localization of the JGCT is a prerequisite for conservative surgery, limiting the extent of the surgical excision. Several methods may be used to localize the tumor.

Contrast-enhanced computerized tomography scans or magnetic resonance imaging

Thin-slice CT scan and MRI are the most reliable methods of tumor localization, and should be systematically performed whenever a renin-secreting JGCT is suspected, especially in patients with highly renin-dependent hypertension, a normal renal arteriogram, and two kidneys of similar size on renal ultrasound scans.

Noncontrast CT scan typically shows a small isodense or hypodense tumor at the external contour of the kidney, with no enhancement or slight enhancement after contrast injection[4,6] (Figure 66–5). On MRI, the tumor displays isosignal intensity with the adjacent normal renal parenchyma in both T1- and T2-weighted images (Figure 66–6). Its visibility can be enhanced by using pre- and post-contrast fat-saturated T1-weighted images and pre- and post-contrast fat-saturated SPRG (spoiled gradient recalled acquisition in steady state) images.[18]

Renal ultrasound

Renal ultrasound cannot be recommended as a screening test for JGCT diagnosis, because of its low sensitivity and specificity for such tumors. Most JGCT are hyper-

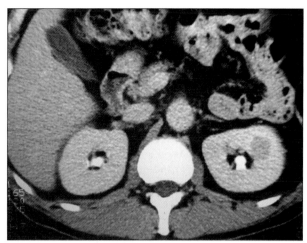

Figure 66–5. Computed tomography scan of a juxtaglomerular cell tumor in the left kidney.

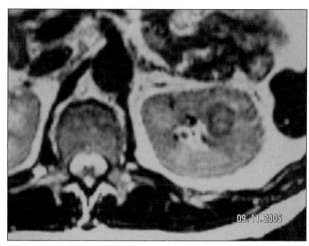

Figure 66–6. Magnetic resonance image of a juxtaglomerular cell tumor in the left kidney.

echogenic, but some may be isoechogenic or hypo-echogenic.[19]

Selective renal arteriography

Renal arteriography is required to rule out other causes of renin-dependent hypertension, especially a stenosis affecting the distal renal artery or intrarenal arterial branches that is usually caused by fibromuscular dysplasia. JGCT can be visualized on selective renal arteriograms with right and left anterior oblique views, as a small characteristic avascular radioluscent area at the external contour of the kidney. This image is highly suggestive of JGCT in the context of hypertension with reninism and hyperaldosteronism. However, it should be borne in mind that renal arteriography gives false negatives in as many as 60% of cases.[14] Renal arteriography alone is therefore not sufficient for formal exclusion of the diagnosis of JGCT. This invasive procedure is complemented by CT scans or MRI. Finally, renal arteriography can also be used for precise analysis of the renal vasculature before conservative surgery.

Selective and segmental renin measurements in renal veins

Although this procedure is performed in most cases, a clear increase in PRA in a renal vein or one of its branches is not always observed.[6,14] Negative lateralization of renal vein renin secretion was reported in 50% of the cases described by McVicar et al.[14] In most cases, renin concentration is only slightly high on the affected side, probably because the tumor is frequently located at the surface of the kidney and most of the venous blood from the tumor is collected by the pericapsular veins rather than draining into the main renal vein. Selective catheterization of the branches of the renal vein is commonly used and may occasionally help localization of the tumor, but it is increasingly recognized that this technique may also give misleading results. Modern diagnosis usually involves CT or MRI scanning combined with angiography.

PREOPERATIVE AND SURGICAL MANAGEMENT

Hypertension induced by renin-secreting JGCT is the best example of purely renin-dependent hypertension because hypertension should theoretically be cured by surgical removal of the tumor. If left undiagnosed and untreated, primary reninism can be lethal[20] or lead to severe complications due to severe hypertension.

Preoperative treatment aims to control hypertension control, with correction of hypovolemia in cases of malignant hyponatremic-hypertensive syndrome, and correction of hypokalemia. BP can be controlled by ACE inhibitors or AT1 receptor antagonists in association with other drugs, such as calcium channel blockers.[14] RAS blockers also decrease the intensity of secondary hyperaldosteronism, thereby correcting hypokalemia. Spironolactone and amiloride can also be used to lower blood pressure and correct the hypokalemia.

Conservative surgery with elective tumor resection is the preferred procedure because JGCT are small (2–3 cm) and superficial and can be easily dissected from the adjacent kidney tissue.[3] Careful palpation of the surface of the kidney usually reveals the presence of a superficial tumor, but perioperative ultrasound scans can also facilitate localization of the tumor.[3] Larger tumors may require more extensive surgery, such as partial nephrectomy, after perioperative elimination of the histological diagnosis of renal carcinoma. It is difficult to obtain enough appropriate tissue for JGCT diagnosis and it is therefore important to make the best possible use of the excised tumor for molecular and cell culture studies.[4,6,21]

PROGNOSIS

JGCT are technically benign in almost all cases although the consequences of uncontrolled hypertension and proteinuria clearly are not. Only one case of a very large (15 cm) malignant JGCT with pulmonary metastases has been reported.[22] Following JGCT removal, both PRA and

BP rapidly decrease to normal levels. Some patients may have persistent mild hypertension, which is readily controlled by current antihypertensive treatments[3] and may be caused by hypertension-induced vascular and/or kidney alterations.

HYPERENINEMIA AND SECONDARY HYPERALDOSTERONISM ASSOCIATED WITH RENAL TUMORS OTHER THAN THOSE OF JUXTAGLOMERULAR APPARATUS

Hypertension associated with reninism and secondary hyperaldosteronism are occasionally observed in patients with renal tumors other than JGCT. Almost 60% of cases of Wilms' tumor (nephroblastoma) in childhood are accompanied by hypertension.[23] These malignant tumors predominantly secrete prorenin, which is considered a tumor biomarker.[24] These tumors may secrete renin in infrequent cases, but hypertension may also be due to secondary reninism if the tumor compresses the kidney or the renal arteries.[23]

In some rare cases of renal cell carcinomas, hypertension associated with high levels of renin secretion has been noted.[25,26] Some of these carcinomas contain cells displaying positive staining for renin. These cases should be distinguished from cases of renin secretion occurring as a result of the compression of renal vessels by an expanding mass that synthesizes renin itself.

PRIMARY RENINISM ASSOCIATED WITH EXTRARENAL RENIN-SECRETING TUMORS

Excessive renin production may also occur in various other types of extra-renal tumor, but these tumors remain very rare in adults and are exceptional in children.[4] Several cases of ectopic renin-secreting cancers have been reported: lung cancers,[27] cancers originating from the uterogenital tract, ovarian and paraovarian tumors, adrenal carcinomas, oat cell carcinoma, epithelial liver hamartoma, orbital hemangiopericytoma, pancreatic cancer, angiolymphoid hyperplasia with eosinophilia, and other tumors (see reviews in Anderson et al.[28] and Balu et al.[29]). All these cases presented severe hypertension with hypokalemia, with a higher frequency in women than in men. Interestingly, patients with extrarenal renin-secreting tumors present higher concentrations of prorenin, the inactive precursor of renin, than do patients suffering from renal tumors, with extremely high plasma levels of prorenin and normal-to-high plasma active renin concentrations.[17,29,30] This may be due to (1) activation of the renin gene during cell multiplication, resulting in the synthesis of a large amount of prorenin, and (2) inefficient or incomplete processing of prorenin to generate active renin due to the absence of processing enzymes and specialized organelles in the neoplastic cells.[21] As for JGCT, complete surgical removal of the tumor usually cures the hypertension, but the final prognosis depends on the nature and the aggressiveness of the primary tumor.

It remains likely that the prevalence of extrarenal renin-secreting cancers is underestimated. The development of hypertension and hypokalemia during the course of a malignant disease should systematically lead to consideration of this diagnosis and to the determination of plasma prorenin and active renin concentrations.

OTHER RENIN-ANGIOTENSIN–DEPENDENT FORMS OF HYPERTENSION

Essential hypertension

About one-sixth of patients with benign essential hypertension have high renin levels.[31] Renin levels are also high in most patients with malignant hypertension. Renin concentration is very high in hyponatremic hypertensive syndrome, leading to hyperangiotensinemia with thirst, polyuria, and hyponatremia, and secondary aldosteronism with kaliuresis and systemic hypokalemia.[32] Malignant hypertension may be primary or, as in 45% of cases, the consequence of an underlying renal or adrenal disease.

Renal artery stenosis

Renal ischemia associated with renal artery stenosis is the most frequent condition occurring with renin-angiotensin–dependent hypertension and has been considered in detail elsewhere. Uni- or bilateral renal artery stenoses may cause renovascular hypertension, a form of hypertension that is reversible on nephrectomy or renal revascularization. About two thirds of stenoses are due to atherosclerosis, usually in patients over the age of 50. One-third are due to fibromuscular dysplasia, mostly in young female patients. This diagnosis should be considered in patients with recent, progressive, severe and/or resistant hypertension, in young hypertensive women (fibromuscular dysplasia), in patients with angina or arteritis (atherosclerosis), or in hypertensive patients with ACE inhibitor–induced increases in plasma creatinine concentration. The gold standard procedure for diagnosing renal artery stenosis is catheter angiography. For screening purposes, this invasive procedure can be replaced by CT angiography, magnetic resonance angiography, or duplex Doppler ultrasound. These techniques have estimated the frequency of renal artery stenosis at 1% in unselected patients with hypertension, and 10% to 30% in drug-resistant hypertensive patients.[33]

Other conditions with renal ischemia

A few conditions with chronic or acute intrarenal ischemia may also induce renin-dependent hypertension. These conditions include systemic diseases such as polyarteritis nodosa associated with widespread microaneurysms on renal angiogram and scleroderma in which BP and renal outcomes are greatly improved by ACE inhibitors, and segmental renal infarction.[34] Segmental renal infarction may result from renal embolism, renal artery thrombosis or dissection, or *in situ* thrombosis in cases of coagulation disorders. It usually presents as an abrupt onset of lumbar pain and hematuria followed by acute malignant hypertension, polyuria, hypokalemia, hyponatremia, and extremely high renin concentrations. The condition may revert spontaneously to normotension because the ischemic renal tissue, which releases large amounts of renin, causing renin-angiotensin–dependent hypertension, may subsequently progress to a silent renal scar. Diagnosis is made either by CT angiography or magnetic resonance angiography.

A renin-dependent form of hypertension was recently described in two young patients with a nonstenotic elongated aberrant renal artery associated with a marked decrease in flow to the renal tissue, and thus with renal tissue ischemia.[35] Hypertension was cured by partial nephrectomy in one case.

Renal tumors and cysts

Some large non–renin-secreting cysts and tumors may present as renin-dependent hypertension, the mechanism of RAS stimulation being renal artery compression. In selected cases with lateralized renal vein renin ratio, cyst drainage or tumor resection may improve or cure hypertension.[36] Activation of the RAS also occurs in hypertensive patients with polycystic kidney disease, presumably because stretching of the intrarenal vessels around cysts causes areas of intrarenal ischemia.[37]

Unilateral nonvascular small kidneys

Pyelonephritic scarring associated with urinary tract infection and bladder-ureter reflux can cause childhood hypertension and progressive degradation of renal function. PRA is often high and RAS activation has been implicated as a cause of hypertension.[38] High renin concentrations may also occur in cases of renal hypoplasia. In cases with a very small unilateral kidney and a lateralized renal vein renin ratio, unilateral nephrectomy may improve hypertension.

Non–renin-secreting extrarenal tumors

Pheochromocytoma is a catecholamine-secreting neoplasm of adrenal or extra-adrenal chromaffin tissue. Patients with pheochromocytoma usually have sustained or paroxysmal hypertension with headache, palpitations and excessive sweating. Diagnosis is based on the determination of plasma catecholamine levels or urinary excretion of catecholamine metabolites. The tumor is located by CT scan and metaiodobenzyl guanidine scintigraphy. The high BP levels associated with pheochromocytoma are caused by high plasma catecholamine levels both directly, through the stimulation of vascular adrenergic receptors, and indirectly, through RAS activation mediated by the adrenergic stimulation of JG cells and renal vasoconstriction.[39] Consequently, ACE inhibition may be used to control BP before surgery. In some very rare cases, pheochromocytoma may be associated with a renal artery stenosis (due to direct or indirect compression of the renal artery, or intense renal artery vasoconstriction

due to high levels of circulating cathecholamines, or to the presence of an atherosclerotic disease), which may itself stimulate renin release.[40] Finally, malignant hypertension with RAS activation has been reported in patients with pheochomocytoma.[40]

HYPERRENINEMIA WITH NORMAL BLOOD PRESSURE LEVELS

In most conditions with normal BP levels, hyperreninemia is a homeostatic response to reduced renal perfusion pressure or plasma flow. Conditions in which this is the case include dehydration, hemorrhage, adrenal insufficiency,[41] cardiac failure, and reduced plasma volume due to hypoproteinemia in patients with nephrotic syndrome or kidney failure and liver cirrhosis. Two genetic disorders are also associated with hyperreninemia and normal BP. Bartter's syndrome, or inherited hypokalemic metabolic alkalosis, is an autosomal recessive disorder characterized by salt wasting, insensitivity to the vasoconstrictive effects of Ang II, and consequently high renin levels with normal BP, hyperaldosteronism, and hypokalemia. Gitelman's syndrome resembles Bartter's syndrome, but patients also display hypomagnesemia and hypocalciuria. Recent advances in the field of molecular genetics have demonstrated that these diseases are caused by genetically different abnormalities resulting from mutations in genes encoding renal electrolyte transporters and channels.[42,43]

DRUG-INDUCED HYPERRENINEMIA

Independent of BP status, many drugs, especially those used to treat cardiovascular conditions, interfere with the RAS.[44] Diuretics, direct vasodilators (such as dihydralazine, minoxidil, phentolamine, prazosin, fenoldopam), ACE inhibitors, and AT1 receptor antagonists activate renin release and synthesis via different mechanisms (sodium depletion, reflex activation of the sympathetic system, and interruption of the Ang II–renin negative feedback loop, respectively). Hypokalemia, due in part to activation of the RAS, is also a hallmark of diuretic and laxative abuse. Nonselective β-agonists, such as isoproterenol and selective β2 agonists can also stimulate renin release.[44]

SUMMARY

Juxtaglomerular cell tumors are very rare renin-secreting tumors originating from the juxtaglomerular apparatus, and are benign in the vast majority of cases. Their diagnosis remains difficult, but these tumors should be suspected in young patients with severe hypertension and secondary hyperaldosteronism associated with secretion of large amounts of renin, after the elimination of other much more frequent causes of secondary hyperaldosteronism. Conservative surgery with elective tumor resection is the preferred procedure.

REFERENCES

1. Conn JW, Cohen EL, Lucas CP, et al. Primary reninism. Hypertension, hyperreninemia, and secondary aldosteronism due to renin-producing juxtaglomerular cell tumors. *Arch Intern Med* 1972;130(5):682.

2. Martin SA, Mynderse LA, Lager DJ, Cheville JC. Juxtaglomerular cell tumor: a clinicopathologic study of four cases and review of the literature. *Am J Clin Pathol* 2001;116(6):854.

3. Haab F, Duclos JM, Guyenne T, et al. Renin secreting tumors: diagnosis, conservative surgical approach and long-term results. *J Urol* 1995;153(6):1781.

4. Lindop GBM, Leckie BJ, Mimran A. Renin-secreting tumors. In: Robertson JIS, Nicholls MG, eds. *The Renin-Angiotensin System*. London: Gower Medical Publishing, 1993:54.1.

5. Kuroda N, Moriki T, Komatsu F, et al. Adult-onset giant juxtaglomerular cell tumor of the kidney. *Pathol Int* 2000;50(3):249.

6. Corvol P, Pinet F, Galen FX, et al. Seven lessons from seven renin secreting tumors. *Kidney Int Suppl* 1988;25:S38.

7. Camilleri JP, Hinglais N, Bruneval P, et al. Renin storage and cell differentiation in juxtaglomerular cell tumors: an immunohistochemical and ultrastructural study of three cases. *Hum Pathol* 1984;15(11):1069.

8. Lindop GB, Stewart JA, Downie TT. The immunocytochemical demonstration of renin in a juxtaglomerular cell tumour by light and electron microscopy. *Histopathology* 1983;7(3):421.

9. Bruneval P, Fournier JG, Soubrier F, et al. Detection and localization of renin messenger RNA in human pathologic tissues using in situ hybridization. *Am J Pathol* 1988;131(2):320.

10. Phillips G, Mukherjee TM. A juxtaglomerular cell tumour: light and electron microscopic studies of a renin-secreting kidney tumour containing both juxtaglomerular cells and mast cells. *Pathology* 1972;4(3):193.

11. Tanabe A, Naruse M, Naruse K, et al. Angiotensin II type 1 receptor expression in two cases of juxtaglomerular cell tumor: correlation to negative feedback of renin secretion by angiotensin II. *Horm Metab Res* 1999;31(7):429.

12. Robertson PW, Klidjian A, Harding LK, et al. Hypertension due to a renin-secreting renal tumour. *Am J Med* 1967;43(6):963.

13. Kihara I, Kitamura S, Hoshino T, et al. A hitherto unreported vascular tumor of the kidney: a proposal of "juxtaglomerular cell tumor." *Acta Pathol Jpn* 1968;18(2):197.

14. McVicar M, Carman C, Chandra M, et al. Hypertension secondary to renin-secreting juxtaglomerular cell tumor: case report and review of 38 cases. *Pediatr Nephrol* 1993;7(4):404.

15. Hayami S, Sasagawa I, Suzuki H, et al. Juxtaglomerular cell tumor without hypertension. *Scand J Urol Nephrol* 1998;32(3):231.

16. Brown JJ, Fraser R, Lever AF, et al. Hypertension and secondary hyperaldosteronism associated with a renin-secreting renal juxtaglomerular-cell tumour. *Lancet* 1973;2(7840):1228.

17. Baruch D, Corvol P, Alhenc-Gelas F, et al. Diagnosis and treatment of renin-secreting tumors. Report of three cases. *Hypertension* 1984;6(5):760.

18. Wang JH, Sheu MH, Lee RC. MR findings of renin-secreting tumor: a case report. *Abdom Imaging* 1998;23(5):533.

19. Raynaud A, Chatellier G, Baruch D, et al. Radiologic features of renin-producing tumors. A report of two cases. *Ann Radiol (Paris)* 1985;28(6):439.

20. Gherardi GJ, Arya S, Hickler RB. Juxtaglomerular body tumor: a rare occult but curable cause of lethal hypertension. *Hum Pathol* 1974;5(2):236.

21. Corvol P, Pinet F, Plouin PF, et al. Renin-secreting tumors. *Endocrinol Metab Clin North Am* 1994;23(2):255.

22. Duan X, Bruneval P, Hammadeh R, et al. Metastatic juxtaglomerular cell tumor in a 52-year-old man. *Am J Surg Pathol* 2004;28(8):1098.

23. Sukarochana K, Tolentino W, Kiesewetter WB. Wilms' tumor and hypertension. *J Pediatr Surg* 1972;7(5):573.

24. Carachi R, Lindop GB, Leckie BJ. Inactive renin: a tumor marker in nephroblastoma. *J Pediatr Surg* 1987;22(3):278.

25. Hollifield JW, Page DL, Smith C, et al. Renin-secreting clear cell carcinoma of the kidney. *Arch Intern Med* 1975;135(6):859.

26. Lindop GB, Leckie B, Winearls CG. Malignant hypertension due to a renin-secreting renal cell carcinoma—an ultrastructural and immunocytochemical study. *Histopathology* 1986;10(10):1077.

27. Soubrier F, Skinner SL, Miyazaki M, et al. Activation of renin in an anaplastic pulmonary adenocarcinoma. *Clin Sci (Lond)* 1981;61 Suppl 7:299s.

28. Anderson PW, Macaulay L, Do YS, et al. Extrarenal renin-secreting tumors: insights into hypertension and ovarian renin production. *Medicine (Baltimore)* 1989;68(5):257.

29. Balu L, Gasc JM, Boccon-Gibod L, et al. Arterial hypertension and ovarian tumour in a girl: what is the link? *Nephrol Dial Transplant* 2005;20(1):231.

30. Soubrier F, Devaux C, Galen FX, et al. Biochemical and immunological characterization of ectopic tumoral renin. *J Clin Endocrinol Metab* 1982;54(1):139.

31. Alderman MH, Madhavan S, Ooi WL, et al. Association of the renin-sodium profile with the risk of myocardial infarction in patients with hypertension. *N Engl J Med* 1991;324:1098.

32. Agarwal M, Lynn KL, Richards AM, Nicholls MG. Hyponatremic-hypertensive syndrome with renal ischemia: an underrecognized disorder. *Hypertension* 1999;33(4):1020.

33. Derkx FH, Schalekamp MA. Renal artery stenosis and hypertension. *Lancet* 1994;344(8917):237.

34. Elkik F, Corvol P, Idatte JM, Menard J. Renal segmental infarction: a cause of reversible malignant hypertension. *J Hypertens* 1984;2(2):149.

35. Kem DC, Lyons DF, Wenzl J, et al. Renin-dependent hypertension caused by nonfocal stenotic aberrant renal arteries: proof of a new syndrome. *Hypertension* 2005;46(2):380.

36. Luscher TF, Wanner C, Hauri D, et al. Curable renal parenchymatous hypertension: current diagnosis and management. *Cardiology* 1985;72(Suppl. 1):33.

37. Gabow PA. Autosomal dominant polycystic kidney disease. *N Engl J Med* 1993;329(5):332.

38. Goonasekera CD, Shah V, Wade AM, et al. 15-year follow-up of renin and blood pressure in reflux nephropathy. *Lancet* 1996;347(9002):640.

39. Plouin PF, Chatellier G, Rougeot MA, et al. Plasma renin activity in phaeochromocytoma: effects of beta-blockade and converting enzyme inhibition. *J Hypertens* 1988;6(7):579.

40. Robertson JIS. Pheochromocytoma and the renin system. In: Robertson JIS, Nicholls MG, eds. *The Renin-Angiotensin System*. London: Gower Medical Publishing, 1993:67–1.

41. Stockigt JR. The renin-angiotensin system in adrenal insufficiency. In: Robertson JIS, Nicholls MG, eds. *The Renin-Angiotensin System*. London: Gower Medical Publishing, 1993:68.1.

42. Lifton RP, Gharavi AG, Geller DS. Molecular mechanisms of human hypertension. *Cell* 2001;104(4):545.

43. Shaer AJ. Inherited primary renal tubular hypokalemic alkalosis: a review of Gitelman and Bartter syndromes. *Am J Med Sci* 2001;322(6):316.

44. Doig JK, Lees KR, Reid JL. The effects of drugs on the renin-angiotensin system in man. In: Robertson JIS, Nicholls MG, eds. *The Renin-Angiotensin System*. London: Gower Medical Publishing, 1993:80.1.

Chapter

67

Primary Hyperaldosteronism and Other Forms of Mineralocorticoid Hypertension

Hari Krishnan Parthasarathy and Thomas M. MacDonald

Key Findings

- Adrenal hypertension is the leading cause of secondary hypertension.
- Mineralocorticoid hypertension comprises a group of potentially curable syndromes.
- The genetic basis of several forms of mineralocorticoid hypertension has renewed interest in the role of steroid hormones in the control of blood pressure.
- Primary aldosteronism is the leading cause of mineralocorticoid excess.
- Unprovoked hypokalemia associated with hypertension strongly suggests mineralocorticoid hypertension.
- The use of the aldosterone:renin ratio as a screening test for aldosteronism has improved the rate of detection of the condition among hypertensives.
- Mineralocorticoid excess state can also be produced by an excess of other adrenal steroids apart from aldosterone, including deoxycorticosterone and cortisol.
- Rare inherited syndromes of mineralocorticoid excess include glucocorticoid-remediable aldosteronism, the syndrome of apparent mineralocorticoid excess, congenital adrenal hyperplasia, and Liddle syndrome.

Hypertension is the third most important cause of avoidable death worldwide and the second most important in developed countries.[1] In most cases, no underlying cause for a patient's raised blood pressure is apparent, and these cases are traditionally describe as "essential hypertension." Secondary causes of hypertension are uncommon; however, their importance is underlined by the fact that their recognition may in some cases lead to normalization of blood pressure. Importantly, several of these are associated with life-threatening complications and others are familial, stressing the need for careful family screening. It is, therefore, necessary to have a high index of suspicion to ensure that important rare endocrine causes of hypertension are not missed. In recent years, the genetic basis of several forms of mineralocorticoid hypertension has been elucidated, and this research has renewed interest in the role of steroid hormones in the control of blood pressure.

Mineralocorticoid hypertension comprises a fascinating group of potentially curable syndromes that lead to secondary hypertension (Box 67–1). Primary aldosteronism, which is comprised of various subsets, is the major syndrome in this group. Other rare but inherited syndromes

of mineralocorticoid excess include glucocorticoid-remediable aldosteronism (GRA), the syndrome of apparent mineralocorticoid excess (SAME), congenital adrenal hyperplasia (CAH), and Liddle syndrome.

PRIMARY ALDOSTERONISM

Primary aldosteronism is the leading cause of mineralocorticoid excess. It is characterized by autonomous hypersecretion of aldosterone from the adrenal cortex. It is either due to an adrenal adenoma or bilateral adrenal hyperplasia in more than 95% of cases. Adrenal carcinoma can be a rare cause of primary aldosteronism. Jerome Conn first characterized this syndrome in 1955.[2]

Much of the debate in the prevalence of primary aldosteronism is due to differences in the criteria used for defining the condition. Conn's syndrome of primary aldosteronism, which has been considered by many as a rare entity, was due to an aldosterone-producing adenoma (APA) that, if removed, may in many cases offer a potential cure for hypertension.[2] Therefore in earlier definitions, the syndrome was identified by the excessive autonomous secretion of aldosterone, leading to mineralocorticoid hypertension. This in turn is characterized by suppression of renin, expansion of body sodium content, expansion of plasma volume, and a tendency to hypokalemia. Using these criteria, the prevalence of aldosteronism was considered less than 1% in an unselected hypertensive population.[3,4] However, not all adrenal glands in subjects with primary aldosteronism contain an APA. Some specimens are hyperplastic with varying degrees of nodularity. The term idiopathic hyperaldosteronism (IHA) was coined to describe this condition. The spectrum of primary aldosteronism includes APA and IHA, which are clinically indistinguishable from each other (biochemically they can be distinguished as IHA responds to AII—aldosterone is stimulated—but APA does not), although patients with APA may present with more severe hypertension and hypokalemia. However, the more recent introduction of a raised aldosterone-renin ratio (ARR) to define the condition has led to the emergence of primary aldosteronism as an important cause of secondary hypertension in about 5% to 15% of so-called essential hypertensives.[5-9] There is an ongoing debate about whether this group of patients has true aldosteronism as first described by Conn. Moreover, in the majority of patients identified by a raised ARR, the real reason for the abnormality is the low level of renin rather than raised

Box 67–1

Causes of Mineralocorticoid Excess

Elevated Aldosterone

I. Primary Aldosteronism

Major Subtypes

- Aldosterone-producing adenoma (APA): usual, angiotensin unresponsive
- Idiopathic hyperaldosteronism (IHA) or bilateral adrenal hyperplasia (BAH): angiotensin responsive

Rare Subtypes

- Angiotensin II–responsive adenoma: atypical
- Primary adrenal hyperplasia (PAH): morphologically like IHA, physiologically like APA
- Glucocorticoid-remediable hyperaldosteronism (GRA) or familial hyperaldosteronism type I (FH-I) (AD)
- Familial hyperaldosteronism type II (FH-II): probably heterogeneous
- Aldosterone-producing adrenal carcinoma
- Aldosterone-producing ovarian carcinoma

Suppressed or Normal Aldosterone

II. Secondary Aldosteronism

Deoxy Corticosterone (DOC) Excess

- DOC-secreting adrenocortical carcinoma/adenoma
- Congenital adrenal hyperplasia ($\uparrow$ACTH)
  11β-Hydroxylase deficiency syndrome (AR)
  17α-Hydroxylase deficiency syndrome (AR)
- Primary cortisol resistance (AR/AD)

Cortisol Excess

- Deficiency of 11β-hydroxysteroid dehydrogenase (HSD)
- The syndrome of apparent mineralocorticoid excess (SAME)
  Inherited deficiency of HSD (AR)
  Ingested glycyrrhetinic acid (licorice and carbenoxolone) and $\downarrow$ HSD
  Other causes of cortisol excess exceeding the capacity of HSD: Cushing syndrome, exogenous steroids, neoplasms
  Primary cortisol resistance (AR/AD)
- Defects in amiloride sensitive sodium channels (ASSC)
  Liddle syndrome (mutations in β and γ subunits) (AD)

AD, autosomal dominant; AR, autosomal recessive.

---

aldosterone. In many patients, the level of aldosterone is within the normal range. It is uncertain how they differ from previously identified types of aldosteronism, and whether this phenomenon is synonymous with primary aldosteronism, as defined by earlier criteria.[10]

Anatomy and pathology

Aldosterone-producing adenoma

About two-thirds of patients with classic aldosteronism (hypertension, hypokalemia, low renin) have a unilateral solitary benign adenoma. This condition is more common among women and the most common age group is 30 to 40 years. The tumor is usually unilateral, less than 3 cm in diameter, encapsulated, well circumscribed, and solitary. It is usually solid with a golden-yellow to yellow-brown cut surface with no evidence of hemorrhage or necrosis. Histologically, in most adenomas the tumor cells resemble zona fasciculata cells more than glomerulosa cells due to numerous lipid-laden clear cells; however, occasionally these may appear pigmented due to lipofuscin or neuromelanin ("black adenoma").[11] The adjacent adrenal cortex is nonatrophic (i.e., normal or hypertrophied, which is contrary to expectations), or may even demonstrate focal or diffuse hyperplasia. The presence of intracytoplasmic lipid is fairly specific for adrenal cortical adenomas, and this helps to differentiate these from other adrenal pathologies such as metastasis, hemorrhage, and other primary adrenal neoplasms.

An adrenal nodule in an individual with confirmed primary aldosteronism can be an APA, an incidental finding, or a macronodule of hyperplasia in an individual with bilateral adrenal hyperplasia (BAH).[12,13] A nonsecretory adrenal mass can be incidentally discovered in 2% to 10% of all adults during imaging investigations of the abdomen.

Bilateral adrenal hyperplasia

Bilateral adrenal hyperplasia represents one-third of cases of classical primary aldosteronism. Some also use the term idiopathic hyperaldosteronism (IHA); the terms are often used interchangeably. It may be that the latter term is best reserved for those who have milder biochemical abnormalities and do not present with hypokalemia but who often do have adrenal hyperplasia. With the recent improved screening using aldosterone-renin ratio (ARR), BAH and IHA have been reported to constitute the most common forms of PA compared to APA.[14] Adrenal hyperplasia is characterized by a non-neoplastic increase in adrenal cells. It can be diffuse (most common) or nodular. The nodular variety can be micro- or macro-nodular. The nodular variety of hyperplasia can often be misdiagnosed as APA. Similarly, hyperplasia adjacent to bilateral APAs can be misdiagnosed as BAH. Clinical correlation with dynamic adrenal testing usually helps to differentiate between these conditions.

Unilateral adrenal hyperplasia

Cases of unilateral hyperplasia leading to primary aldosteronism (<1%) have been reported.[15]

Adrenal carcinoma

Aldosterone-producing adrenal carcinomas are rare.[16] Usually there is a global hypersecretion of all other adrenal hormones. Carcinoma is readily suspected by very high levels of aldosterone and its precursor steroids with loss of circadian rhythm. Hypokalemia is often profound. The tumors are usually large (200 g, 20 cm), and unencapsulated with a variegated cut surface due to hemorrhage, cysts, and necrosis. They often have soft, friable intratumoral nodules and often invade major veins.

Chemotherapeutic agents such as ketoconazole, aminoglutethemide, and mitotane are useful palliatively, but these are rarely curative. The prognosis is very poor (life expectancy of less than 6 months).[17]

Extra-adrenal tumors producing aldosterone

Aldosterone-producing tumors have been reported in the kidney and ovary.[18,19]

PATHOPHYSIOLOGY

Adrenal corticosteroids are classified as mineralocorticoids or glucocorticoids. Both types of hormone are secreted from the adrenal cortex—glucocorticoids (in large amounts) from the zona fasciculata, and mineralocorticoids (in small amounts) from the zona glomerulosa. Aldosterone secretion is under control of the renin–angiotensin system (Figure 67–1).

However, aldosterone secretion is also determined by several other factors, notably serum potassium and adreno-cortico-trophic hormone (ACTH) as well as other hormones (Figure 67–2). Certain drugs can also modify its secretion.

Aldosterone was first discovered by Simpson and colleagues in 1953. Aldosterone is a steroid hormone produced by the adrenal cortex. It may also be synthesized locally in the heart, blood vessels, and brain, implying a paracrine function,[20,21] although this is a contentious issue. Aldosterone has been conventionally associated with the control of fluid and electrolyte balance in epithelial tissues, and mainly in the kidney and distal colon. The best-known renal target sites for aldosterone are the cortical and outer medullary collecting tubules.[22–24] At the cortical collecting tubule, the principal role of mineralocorticoids is to enhance Na^+ reabsorption and K^+ secretion, while in the outer medullary collecting tubules,

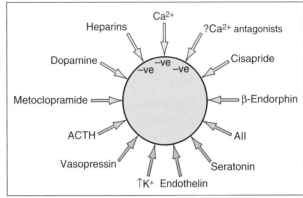

Figure 67–2. Factors regulating aldosterone secretion. ACTH – adrenocorticotrophic hormone.

aldosterone stimulates H^+ secretion. There are three types of cells in these segments: principal cells, intercalated A cells, and intercalated B cells. Principal cells reabsorb Na^+ through apical sodium channels and basolateral Na^+-K^+ ATPase. H^+ is excreted by intercalated B cells that have H^+-ATPase in the luminal membrane.[25] Aldosterone seems to have similar effects on Na^+ and K^+ transport in the colon.[26] The other epithelial targets for aldosterone are sweat glands, bile cannalicula, and endolymphatic sac of the ear.[27,28] The role of aldosterone in these target organs is unclear.

In addition to its classical epithelial effects, aldosterone has a variety of nonepithelial effects, including induction of inflammatory processes, collagen formation, fibrosis, and necrosis[29,30] (Figure 67–3). Interest in these effects has recently resurfaced; the effects had been noted as early as in the 1940s, even prior to the actual discovery of the aldosterone molecule by Selye.[31] In 1946, Selye reported on "a state of chronic stress" that developed in rats administered deoxycorticosterone acetate, an intermediate in the biosynthetic pathway of aldosterone with mineralocorticoid activity. This state resulted in an "adaptation syndrome," leading to formation of perivascular granulomas visible in the coronary, renal, and systemic vasculature.

Mineralocorticoid receptors

Apart from renal sites, mineralocorticoid receptors have been detected in the colon, ureter, bladder, salivary glands, brain, heart, and arterial system.[32–37] The mineralocorticoid receptor has been shown to be equally receptive to both mineralocorticoids and to glucocorticoids.[38] Relatively small amounts of aldosterone are able to bind to the mineralocorticoid receptor in preference to much higher concentrations of glucocorticoids (mainly cortisol). This selectivity is achieved through the expression of the enzyme 11β-hydroxysteroid dehydrogenase, which converts cortisol to cortisone (which does not bind to the receptor), but allows

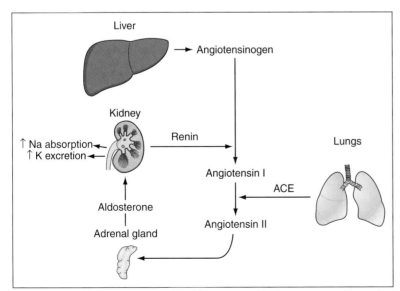

Figure 67–1. The renin–angiotensin–aldosterone axis. The common triggers for renin secretion are hypotension and hyponatremia.

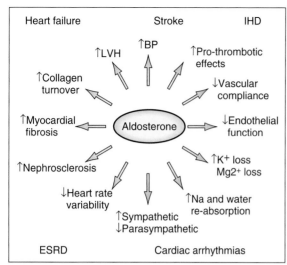

Figure 67–3. Deleterious effects of aldosterone. BP, blood pressure; ESRD, end-stage renal disease; IHD, ischemic heart disease; LVH, left ventricular hypertrophy.

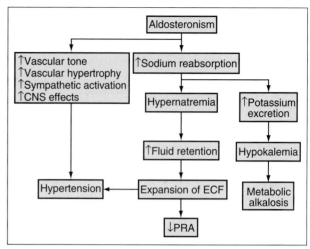

Figure 67–4. Pathophysiology of aldosteronism. ECF, extracellular fluid; PRA, plasma renin activity.

aldosterone to occupy the mineralocorticoid receptor.[39,40] Inhibition of this enzyme has the result that cortisol, usually classified as a glucocorticoid, acts as a potent mineralocorticoid.

Mineralocorticoid-based hypertension refers to hypertension caused by increased sodium and water retention by the kidney, and by expansion of the extracellular fluid compartment, which suppresses endogenous plasma renin activity.[41] There is also renal potassium loss leading to hypokalemia. Hypokalemia leads to metabolic alkalosis (Figure 67–4). Unlike most cases of secondary aldosteronism, edema is not a feature of primary aldosteronism, probably because of "escape" from progressive sodium retention due to increases in renal perfusion pressure and a secondary atrial natriuretic factor.[42] Nevertheless, in the short term, intravascular volume is reset at a higher volume, which leads to increased cardiac output and increased blood pressure. In the chronic state, hypervolemia cannot be consistently shown and other mechanisms including increase of vascular tone, vascular hypertrophy, activation of the sympathetic nervous system, and central effects of mineralocorticoids could potentially contribute to the hypertension.[43–45]

Hypokalemia

The presence of spontaneous or easily provoked hypokalemia ($K < 3.5$ mEq/L) in a patient with hypertension should provoke strong suspicion of primary aldosteronism. The classic case of primary aldosteronism presents with hypokalemia in association with metabolic alkalosis and low plasma renin activity. Of note, Conn first suggested that hypokalemia was a late manifestation of aldosteronism, and that many hypertensive patients may never reach this stage of the disease.[3,46]

Many authors have nonetheless considered primary aldosteronism a rare cause of hypertension among patients with normal serum potassium concentrations.[47–49] In recent years, evidence in support of Conn's belief has increased.[50] For example, Gordon and colleagues[5] studied 199 normokalemic hypertensives and postulated a 10% incidence of aldosteronism in their clinic population. There have been numerous similar reports worldwide.[14,51]

Hypokalemia leads to various clinical manifestations discussed in the following section. Other associated biochemical findings are suppressed plasma renin activity, hypernatremia, and hypomagnesemia.

CLINICAL PRESENTATIONS

Primary aldosteronism is commonly seen in the 30- to 50-year age group, and is more common in females. The clinical features of hyperaldosteronism are often nonspecific and variable.[52] However, a majority of cases are associated with hypertension. The phenotype depends largely on the underlying cause and the severity of the aldosterone excess. The classic symptoms of primary aldosteronism can be divided into cardiovascular, neuromuscular, and renal (Box 67–2). In the majority of cases, however, only subtle clues of hyperaldosteronism exist, such as the presence of refractory hypertension.

Primary aldosteronism is a significant cause of resistant hypertension in both black and white subjects.[53] Importantly, these patients tend to suffer from more severe hypertension.[54,55] Primary aldosteronism has been associated with malignant hypertension. However, in contrast to other causes of accelerated phase or "malignant" hypertension (who usually have high renin levels), the malignant phase of primary aldosteronism is associated with low renin levels.[56]

Hypokalemia rarely leads to weakness, flaccid paralysis, paraesthesia, and tetany.[57] Even more rare are secondary myositis and rhabdomyolysis. Magnesium loss might partly contribute to some of these symptoms. Nephrogenic diabetes insipidus, caused by reversible hypokalemic tubular damage and renal tubule antidiuretic hormone resistance due to the hypokalemia, can cause nocturia, polyuria, and polydipsia. In severe cases of hypokalemia, cardiac arrhythmias occur and can be life threatening.

Box 67–2

Clinical Manifestations of Primary Aldosteronism

Neuromuscular
- Paresthesia
- Tetany
- Flaccid paralysis
- Weakness

Cardiovascular
- Hypertension
- Left ventricular hypertrophy
- CCF
- Arrhythmias
- Retinopathy
- Headaches
- Renal
- Nephrogenic diabetes insipidus (polyuria, polydypsia, nocturia)

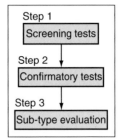

Figure 67–5. Three steps in the evaluation of primary aldosteronism.

Patients with primary aldosteronism have a tendency to impaired glucose tolerance resulting from the inhibitory effect of hypokalemia on insulin action and secretion.[58] However, diabetes mellitus is rare.

DIAGNOSTIC TECHNIQUES

Clinical signs and symptoms of primary aldosteronism are nonspecific. Hence, diagnostic techniques form a vital part in the initial screening, confirmation, and subtype evaluation of primary aldosteronism (Figure 67–5).

Screening tests
Serum potassium

Unprovoked hypokalemia associated with hypertension strongly suggests mineralocorticoid hypertension (Table 67–1). Hypokalemia provoked by diuretic use resistant

to replacement should also raise a high index of suspicion. However, normokalemic hyperaldosteronism has been widely reported[5,14,59,60] (Table 67–2). Therefore, hypokalemia is not a prerequisite for the diagnosis of hyperaldosteronism.

Other conditions requiring further screening tests for hyperaldosteronism are resistant hypertension, presence of an adrenal mass with hypertension, and evaluation of further causes for secondary hypertension.[61]

Aldosterone:renin ratio

Use of the ARR as a screening test for aldosteronism has improved the rate of detection of the condition among hypertensive patients (Figure 67–6). It has also enabled clinicians to overcome the shortcomings of using hypokalemia as a screening tool.

Units of measurement

Plasma aldosterone can be expressed in ng/dL (USA) and pmol/L SI units (in Europe, the conversion factor is 27.7). Plasma renin activity (PRA) is usually expressed as ng/mL Ang I/hr. However, a few investigators have used renin mass. Renin mass includes both active renin (contributing to PRA) and inactive renin. The relationship between renin mass and PRA is complex. The higher the renin mass, the greater the percentage of the renin that is active. For clarity, we will refer only to PRA. Most investigators consider the ARR level raised if it is higher than 25 when

STUDIES OF NORMOKALEMIC PRIMARY HYPERALDOSTERONISM					
Study	Number of Patients	Type of Patients	Incidence of Aldosteronism (%)	Normokalemia (%)	Confirmatory Tests
Gordon et al.[5]	199	Hypertension clinic	10	100	Salt loading, FST, ± adrenal vein sampling
Lim et al.[53]	465	Hypertension clinic	9.2	95	Salt loading, FST
Benchetrit et al.[61]	20	Low–renin resistant hypertensives	100	100	Salt loading
Bernini et al.[62]	125	Adrenal incidentaloma	4	100	Saline infusion, captopril test, ± adrenal vein sampling ± surgery
FST, finger skin temperature.					

Table 67–1. Studies of Normokalemic Primary Hyperaldosteronism

SCREENING TESTS FOR PRIMARY ALDOSTERONISM (OTHER THAN HYPOKALEMIA)			
Test	Procedure	Result	Comments
Serum potassium		Hypokalemia	Low sensitivity
Aldosterone:renin ratio	Plasma renin and aldosterone	Raised ratio	Ratio affected in low-renin hypertension and a variety of other factors
Captopril test	Sitting, plasma aldosterone before and 2 hours after oral captopril	Plasma aldosterone Unsuppressed in primary aldosteronism Suppressed in essential hypertension	Improves the specificity of aldosterone:renin ratio

Table 67–2. Screening Tests for Primary Aldosteronism (Other than Hypokalemia)

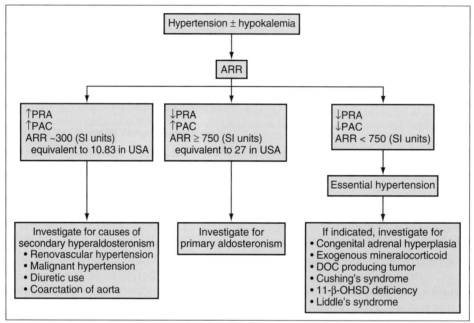

Figure 67–6. Using the ARR in hypertension. The ARR is the ratio between the PAC and PRA. (The PAC is expressed as pmol/L (SI units); in the United States the PAC is expressed as ng/dL. PRA is usually expressed as ng/mL/h.) ARR, aldosterone:renin ratio; PAC, plasma aldosterone concentration; PRA, plasma renin activity. (Modified from Young WF Jr. *Ann N Y Acad Sci* 2002;970:61–76, Blackwell Scientific.)

plasma aldosterone is expressed as ng/dL or greater than 750 when expressed as pmol/L.

Historical perspective on aldosterone:renin ratio

After the work of Hiramatsu and colleagues[62] in 1981, ARR began to be used more often in clinical practice. These researchers measured serum sodium and potassium levels, PRA (ng/mL/hr), plasma aldosterone (pg/mL) concentration, and ARR in 348 patients with hypertension. Nine patients with substantially elevated ARR levels were selected and hospitalized for further study. All nine patients then underwent scintigraphy with labeled cholesterol, venography, and surgical excision, and all had proven APA or Conn's syndrome. The serum concentration of potassium was subnormal in only three of the nine patients with APA. In patients with APA, administration of diuretics and salt restriction significantly

elevated PRA. However, even with diurnal and day-to-day variation of plasma aldosterone concentrations, it was found that the ARR was always elevated inappropriately to more than 400 ng/dL (equivalent to 1108 when plasma aldosterone is expressed in pmol/L). In contrast, after administration of diuretics, both the PRA and aldosterone levels increased significantly in patients with essential hypertension, but the ARR was always less than 200 (equivalent to 554 when plasma aldosterone is expressed in pmols/L). Hiramatsu and colleagues suggested that an ARR higher than 400 was a useful screening tool for the prediction of APA among hypertensive patients.

In spite of concerns over the sensitivity, specificity, and validity of the ARR,[63] it is widely accepted as a useful screening tool in aldosteronism.[14] A high ARR can be caused by a very low PRA and a normal aldosterone. Setting a lower limit for aldosterone (for example, 415 pmol/L) increases the specificity of the test. This is explained below. Use of high aldosterone levels along with raised ARR increases the specificity of ARR. The need for plasma aldosterone to be above normal, along with suppressed renin is seen by many as an important distinction between aldosteronism and low-renin hypertension. This is because very low renin concentrations will always result in a high ARR, as it is similar to dividing by zero. For this reason, many investigators also impose other criteria such as a minimum plasma level of aldosterone, and do not rely on just the calculated ratio alone. It should also be noted that plasma renin activity can be low in older and black people apart from those patients with "low-renin" hypertension,[64,65] and several hormonal and other factors can alter renin levels (Figure 67–7).

Moreover, the sensitivity and specificity of ARR depend on the cut-off values used. Most investigators would consider further evaluation for aldosteronism if the level of ARR is ≥25 when plasma aldosterone is expressed as ng/dL (or ≥750 when expressed as pmol/L) along with a raised plasma aldosterone concentration (PAC) of 15 ng/dL or more (equivalent to 415 in pmol/L).

Various factors that can cause false-positive or false-negative ARRs are summarized in Table 67–3. In particular, many antihypertensive medications can affect the ARR, and therefore measurements should be undertaken if possible after stopping them for a duration that varies depending on the drug. Patients should be off spironolactone therapy for at least 6 weeks before evaluation of ARR. Beta-blockers should be stopped for at least a week because they suppress renin. However, there is some evidence to suggest that calcium channel blockers have no significant effect on the ARR while angiotensin-converting enzyme (ACE) inhibitors and ARBs probably enhance the diagnostic value of a high ARR because these drugs will serve to raise renin and reduce aldosterone via their action or the renin–angiotensin–aldosterone

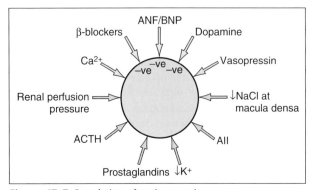

Figure 67–7. Regulation of renin secretion.
ANF – Atrial natriuretic factor.
BNP – Brain natriuretic peptide.
ACTH – Adrencorticotropic hormone.

system.[66,67] This latter action is the basis of the captopril suppression test.

Captopril suppression test

Acute administration of an ACE inhibitor such as captopril blocks angiotensin II synthesis, and hence decreases aldosterone secretion. The post-captopril ARR has been used to improve the specificity of diagnosing primary aldosteronism.

In 1983, Lyons and colleagues[68] measured plasma aldosterone concentrations 2 hours after the administration of 25 mg of captopril in 9 normotensive subjects, 10 patients with essential hypertension, and 12 patients with primary aldosteronism on an unrestricted diet. The study showed that ARR was suppressed in essential hypertensives and normotensives but was not suppressed in primary aldosteronism. The presence of an ARR above 35 before and after 50 mg of captopril had been demonstrated to increase both the sensitivity and specificity of ARR.[69]

CAUSES OF FALSE-POSITIVE AND FALSE-NEGATIVE ALDOSTERONE:RENIN RATIO	
Causes	Mechanisms
False-Positive Ratios	
β-blockers	↓ PRA
Very high-salt diet	↓ PRA
Renal impairment	Na retention, ↓ PRA
Nonsteroidal anti-inflammatory drugs	Na retention, ↓ PRA
Low-renin hypertension	↓ PRA
False-Negative Ratios	
Spironolactone	↑ PRA, ↑ Aldosterone (by feedback)
Angiotension-converting enzyme inhibitors/angiotensin receptor blockers	↑ PRA, ↓ Aldosterone
Calcium channel blockers	↓ Aldosterone
Diuretics other than spironolactone	Volume depletion, ↑ PRA
Hypokalemia	↓ Aldosterone
PRA, plasma renin activity.	

Table 67–3. Causes of False-Positive and False-Negative Aldosterone:Renin Ratio

Confirmatory tests

The basic principle of confirmatory tests for primary aldosteronism (Table 67–4) is to demonstrate that the secretion of aldosterone is autonomous and nonsuppressible with expansion of extracellular fluid volume. Thus sodium loading with or without fludrocortisone plus potassium supplementation to correct or prevent hypokalemia is the basis of most definitive tests; in a positive test, aldosterone is not suppressed by such maneuvers.

Subtype determination

Both hormonal studies and radiologic evaluation help to determine the underlying pathology for aldosteronism.

Hormonal studies

Posture test

The posture test has traditionally been used in subtype evaluation of aldosteronism. The physiologic basis is that on upright posture plasma aldosterone increases if the renin angiotensin aldosterone system (RAAS) is intact as in essential hypertension, normal subjects, and in IHA. However, in APA, where the RAAS is suppressed, posture does not stimulate aldosterone production and levels may actually decline. The circulating aldosterone levels in patients with APA show a diurnal variation due to sensitivity to ACTH, and are relatively unaffected by changes in angiotensin II levels. In contrast, IHA is characterized by increased sensitivity to a small change in angiotensin II that occurs when standing. Samples of PRA and plasma aldosterone are collected along with cortisol levels after overnight recumbency and 2 to 4 hours of upright posture. A significant decline in plasma aldosterone levels on upright posture (>30%) is supportive of APA. A corresponding fall in cortisol is usually seen, which reflects the fall in ACTH levels. The predictive value of posture test in distinguishing APA from IHA is around 80% to 90%.

However, this study is not fully discriminative of the subtypes; for instance, studies have shown that some patients with APA are sensitive to angiotensin II, and some patients with IHA are responsive to ACTH and show diurnal variation in aldosterone secretion. Moreover, the posture test does not help in the lateralization of an adenoma.

Blood levels of 18-OH-corticosterone are usually greater than 100 ng/dL in APA, whereas patients with IHA have lower levels.[70] A posture-induced decrease in aldosterone levels is also seen in glucocorticoid-remediable hypertension (GRA) because aldosterone is solely regulated by ACTH in this variant of aldosteronism.

However, with the advent of high-resolution imaging techniques and centers proficient in adrenal vein sampling (AVS), these hormonal studies are less often used.

Radiologic investigations

An adrenal CT scan is useful in differentiating adenomas from adrenal hyperplasias.[71] However, due to the spectrum of adrenal pathologies[72] seen in primary aldosteronism, misdiagnosis can occur.[73] Adenomas can often be associated with adjacent adrenal hyperplasia. On the other hand, hyperplasia of the adrenal gland is often nodular. Consequently, dynamic and hormonal testing should always be used in conjunction with imaging techniques for subtype evaluation.

Adrenal magnetic resonance imaging has been shown to be more sensitive and has improved diagnostic accuracy compared to the CT scan.[74] Dexamethasone-suppressed selenium-75-Nor-cholesterol adrenal scintigraphy has been found to be useful in the presence of equivocal AVS results in ruling out aldosterone-producing adenomas.[75]

Adrenal vein sampling

Adrenal vein catheterization was introduced about four decades ago for identification of the etiology of primary aldosteronism.[76] It forms the gold standard test to distin-

CONFIRMATORY TESTS FOR PRIMARY ALDOSTERONISM (DYNAMIC STUDIES)			
Test	Procedure	Result	Comments
Saline infusion	2 L of normal saline over 4-hour period	Plasma aldosterone unsuppressed	Contraindicated in severe hypertension, CCF, MI, stroke Does not differentiate adenoma and hyperplasia
Oral salt loading	110 mEq of sodium/day for 3 to 5 days	Urinary aldosterone 1. Partially suppressed (hyperplasia) 2. Unsuppressed (adenoma) 3. Total suppression (essential hypertension)	"Gold standard test" Differentiates adenoma, hyperplasia, and essential hypertension
Response to DOC or fludrocortisone	DOC or 9α-fludrocortisone for 2 to 3 days	Urinary aldosterone unsuppressed	Mineralocorticoid suppression tests provide little additional benefit over salt loading

Note: The basic principle of confirmatory tests for primary aldosteronism is to demonstrate that the secretion of aldosterone is autonomous and nonsuppressible to expansion of extracellular fluid volume.
CCF, congestive heart failure; DOC deoxycortisone; EH, essential hypertension; MI, myocardial infarction.

Table 67–4. Confirmatory Tests for Primary Aldosteronism (Dynamic Studies)

guish unilateral from bilateral disease. The success of adrenal vein catheterization depends on the operator's expertise. Bilateral adrenal venous sampling can be a challenging procedure. This is particularly true with catheterization of the right adrenal vein, because of its short limb and various anomalies.[77] Catheterization of the left adrenal vein, on the other hand, is usually simpler because of its longer trunk and uncommon anomalies. Adrenal veins are usually catheterized via the femoral approach using a Seldinger technique. Creating artificial gradients is avoided by keeping the patients supine before the AVS procedure. The time elapsing between catheterization of both adrenal veins should be kept to minimum. Blood should be drained by gravity or by gentle negative pressure when necessary. Samples of adrenal venous and infrarenal, inferior vena cava blood are collected for measurement of plasma aldosterone and cortisol. The selectivity of AVS on both sides is assessed with the ratio between cortisol levels in the right and left adrenal veins and the inferior vena cava plasma. In view of the risks of this invasive procedure, which include extravasation, adrenal vein thrombosis, and adrenal infarction, some authors advise that it should be used only if there is discordance among dynamic, hormonal, and imaging studies.[70] Young[61] recommends using AVS for subtype evaluation in confirmed aldosteronism in the presence of a unilateral hypodense nodule of more than 1 cm in patients aged over 40 years, if associated with features of a high probability of APA, including severe hypertension, profound hypokalemia (<3.0 mEq/L), higher plasma (>25 ng/dL), and urinary (>30 µg/day) levels of aldosterone. Young further recommends unilateral adrenalectomy if solitary unilateral macroadenoma of more than 1 cm is present along with confirmed aldosteronism in a younger patient (<40 years). AVS is advised in cases of confirmed features of aldosteronism and a high probability of APA, where the CT scan reveals any of the following features: minimal, unilateral, adrenal limb thickening; unilateral microadenoma (≤1 cm); or bilateral macroadenomas. AVS in these instances helps in detecting the source. However, in some centers, AVS is routinely used in all patients with confirmed primary aldosteronism.[78] Our own practice has been to use AVS only where we are considering surgical therapy. This is usually confined to younger, low operative risk subjects in whom the diagnosis of APA is unclear. We also like to see blood pressure and biochemical abnormalities normalize with spironolactone, as this is the group most likely to attain a "cure" with surgery. Therefore, older and high-risk subjects are usually treated medically, and we would only consider AVS exceptionally in such subjects.

MANAGEMENT

The management of primary aldosteronism (PA) depends on the etiology. The aim is to correct the hypertension and hypokalemia associated with aldosterone excess and to reduce associated morbidity and mortality. In APA and in some cases of adrenal hyperplasia, surgery is a good treatment choice, and in some patients this may be curative. In IHA and GRA and in subjects at high operative risk, medical management is indicated.

Surgical management

Cure rates (which might be defined as blood pressure <140/90 without medication, 6 months postsurgery) for APA and PAH postunilateral adrenalectomy range from 35% to 60%.[61,79,80] However, nearly all patients (~95%) show improved blood pressure control if treated in addition with medications when necessary. Resolution of hypertension usually takes from 1 to 6 months. All patients should have hypokalemia corrected and hypertension controlled prior to surgery. The preoperative blood pressure response to spironolactone often predicts the blood pressure response to surgery in APA. Laparoscopic adrenalectomy, although technically more demanding than open adrenalectomy, has been shown to decrease the hospital stay and late incisional complications.[81] In patients with APA who are reluctant to undergo surgery, super-selective, adrenal arterial embolization using high-concentration ethanol have been shown to be an option.[82]

Medical treatment

Medical treatment is the therapy of choice in IHA and for subjects at high operative risk from surgery. It is also indicated before and in addition to surgical treatment of APA for control of hypertension and hypokalemia and also when surgery is not possible. Hypertension in IHA or PAH responds poorly to bilateral adrenalectomy, although potassium wasting is corrected.

Nonpharmacologic factors contributing to a successful medical therapy are dietary sodium restriction (<100 mEq/day), weight loss, alcohol restriction, and aerobic exercise where relevant. It is instructive to remember that a very low sodium diet can correct all biochemical and hemodynamic abnormalities seen in Conn's syndrome and that prior to the advent of mineralocorticoid antagonists, this was the mainstay of treatment.

Spironolactone has traditionally been the main stay in medical therapy. The range of doses used varies from 12.5 mg/day in milder cases to as much as 500 mg/day. Spironolactone is highly effective in the control of hypertension and hypokalemia. However, spironolactone has numerous metabolic, endocrine, gastrointestinal, hepatic, and renal side effects (Table 67–5). Spironolactone lacks specificity for mineralocorticoid receptors and binds to both progesterone and androgen receptors leading to various endocrine side effects. Gynecomastia can often be troublesome. However, in low doses (no more than 25 mg per day) spironolactone is tolerated well. A mistake often made is to up-titrate the dose too quickly, given that it can take up to 3 months for the full pharmacodynamic effects to be seen.

Eplerenone, a selective aldosterone receptor antagonist, is a derivative of spironolactone and has been shown to have a lower incidence of androgenic and progestogenic side effects. However, it is also a less-potent mineralocorticoid antagonist than spironolactone. Eplerenone selectively binds to mineralocorticoid receptors relative to

ADVERSE EFFECTS OF SPIRONOLACTONE	
System	**Side Effects**
Digestive	Gastric bleeding
	Ulceration
	Gastritis
	Diarrhea
	Cramping
	Nausea
	Vomiting
Metabolic/endocrine	Hyperkalemia
	Hyponatremia
	Gynecomastia
	Impotence
	Dysmenorrhea
	Amenorrhea
	Postmenopausal bleeding
	Deepening of voice
	Hirsutism
	Decreased libido
	Carcinoma of breast (reported but cause–effect not proved)
Hematologic	Agranulocytosis
Hypersensitivity	Fever
	Urticaria
	Rash
	Anaphylaxis
	Vasculitis
Nervous system/psychiatric	Mental confusion
	Ataxia
	Headache
	Drowsiness
	Lethargy
Hepatobiliary	Mixed cholestatic/hepatocellular toxicity; one reported fatality
Renal	Renal dysfunction/failure

Table 67–5. Adverse Effects of Spironolactone

its binding to glucocorticoid, progesterone, and androgen receptors. The efficacy and safety of eplerenone in hypertension have been assessed in numerous clinical trials, whether as monotherapy or concomitantly with other antihypertensive medications. Eplerenone was approved by the Food and Drug Administration in 2002 for the treatment of hypertension.[83] Weinberger and colleagues[84] randomized 417 patients with mild to moderate hypertension to eplerenone (in different doses), spironolactone, or placebo. The mean changes in both office systolic blood pressure (SBP) and diastolic blood pressure (DBP) and 24-hour ambulatory blood pressures were significantly greater for all doses of eplerenone compared to placebo. Furthermore, a dose–response effect was observed with eplerenone. On a molecular weight basis, however, eplerenone was only 50% to 75% as potent as spironolactone. There were no antiandrogenic or progestational side effects seen with eplerenone. However, at present there are no published data on its efficacy in aldosteronism; we are aware though of at least one unpublished study where subjects with aldosteronism were random-

ized to spironolactone or eplerenone. The antihypertensive effect of spironolactone was greater in this trial.

In some countries, a metabolite of spironolactone, potassium canrenoate, is available for oral administration. Its adverse effect profile is similar to spironolactone. However, some say that it has fewer endocrine side effects.[85] In animals, there have been reports of carcinogenicity. In 2-year studies in the rat, oral administration of potassium canrenoate was associated with myelocytic leukemia and hepatic, thyroid, testicular, and mammary tumors.[86]

Amiloride and triamterene may be used as alternatives in those intolerant to spironolactone or eplerenone.[87–89] These drugs have a direct effect on the renal tubule to impair sodium reabsorption in exchange for potassium and hydrogen.

Nifedipine has been tried in aldosteronism, and has been shown to decrease aldosterone secretion from APA.[90,91] It seems to have both acute and chronic antihypertensive effects in aldosteronism.[92] There are a few studies reported in literature to the effect that other calcium channel blockers including verapamil and diltiazem might be useful in treating primary aldosteronism.[93]

OTHER SUBTYPES OF ALDOSTERONISM

Glucocorticoid-remediable aldosteronism

Glucocorticoid-remediable aldosteronism is also known as familial hyperaldosteronism type 1 (FH-1) or glucocorticoid-suppressible hyperaldosteronism (GSH). It is a rare inherited form of primary aldosteronism that was first described clinically by Sutherland and colleagues in 1966.[94] It is characterized by classic features of primary aldosteronism, but is completely reversible by exogenous glucocorticoid (hence, the name of glucocorticoid suppressible/remediable aldosteronism). The hormonal basis of GRA was first postulated by Ulick and colleagues.[95] They first identified increased levels of hybrid steroids including 18-oxo-cortisol and 18-hydroxy-cortisol,[96] and later postulated that the disorder might be due to defective acquisition of the aldosterone synthase enzymatic activity (methyl oxidase activity) by zona fasciculata.[95]

Genetic basis

It was Lifton and colleagues who elucidated the genetic basis of GRA[97] (Figure 67–8). They identified a hybrid or chimeric gene arising from unequal crossing-over and fusing of regulatory sequences of steroid 11 beta-hydroxylase (CYP11β1) to coding sequences of aldosterone synthase (CYP11β2) genes by studying 12 kindreds with GRA.[98] This hybrid gene is regulated by ACTH (because the regulatory portion of CYP11β1 is ACTH sensitive) and produces aldosterone (due to the coding portion of CYP11β2, which is now without its usual regulatory portion sensitive to angiotensin II). This leads to aldosterone production that is then regulated by ACTH instead of angiotensin II.

Clinical features

GRA is an autosomal dominant disorder. The phenotype is extremely variable.[99–101] Patients can present with mild

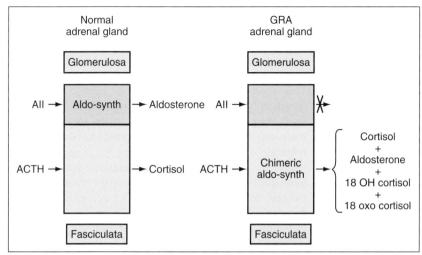

Figure 67–8. The genetic basis of glucocorticoid-remediable aldosteronism.

hypertension and normal biochemistry, and can be clinically indistinguishable from patients with essential hypertension, but it can also present with fatal hypertensive stroke in men aged 20 to 40 years.[102] The disorder commonly begins during childhood.[103] Women who have GRA with chronic hypertension seem to be at increased risk for exacerbation of hypertension during pregnancy.[104] The most affected have normal potassium levels. Neither the differences in gene cross-over points nor plasma steroid levels seem to correlate with degrees of hypertension.[105]

Jamieson and colleagues[105] observed that patients inheriting GRA from their mothers have higher blood pressure and plasma aldosterone concentration compared to those who inherited the syndrome from their fathers. Hence they postulated permanent programming of mineralocorticoid-dependent, blood-pressure regulatory mechanisms due to chronic intrauterine exposure to PA.[105] Dulhy and colleagues[106] observed reciprocal correlation of blood pressure with urinary kallikrein excretion, and postulated possible interaction of gene mutation with other blood-pressure regulatory mechanisms.

Diagnosis

Glucocorticoid-remediable aldosteronism can masquerade as essential hypertension because most affected subjects are normokalemic and their blood pressures can range from mildly to severely elevated.[99] Many patients are refractory to usual antihypertensive agents but may become hypokalemic if potassium-wasting diuretics (e.g., bendrofluazide at 2.5 mg) are administered.[107] GRA should be considered in a patient with hypertension of early onset or a history of early-onset hypertension in first-degree relatives, if there is a significant family history of early hemorrhagic stroke, precipitation of hypokalemia when treated with potassium-wasting diuretics, and the refractoriness of the blood pressure to standard treatments.[102,107] A screening policy targeted at these individuals has been shown to be effective.[108]

Patients with GRA have raised ARR (>30). PRA will be suppressed unless mineralocorticoid antagonists have been used as therapeutic agents. Therefore, nonsuppressed PRA levels in the absence of such therapies makes diagnosis of GRA unlikely. However, the presence of a suppressed PRA level is nonspecific. Aldosterone blood levels or urinary aldosterone excretion rates are usually normal or mildly elevated, but the levels may be inappropriate for the intake of sodium because production is solely regulated by ACTH.[109]

The disorder is characterized by increased excretion of 18-oxo-cortisol and 18-hydroxy-cortisol in urine, and these provide a sensitive and highly specific test to confirm diagnosis of GRA.[96,109] However, their measurement necessitates 24-hour collection and the assay is not widely available. Dexamethasone suppression testing (DST) is also used to differentiate this disorder from other causes of primary aldosteronism. A fall in aldosterone to nearly undetectable levels after low-dose DST (0.5 mg of dexamethasone orally every 6 hours over 2 to 4 days) in GRA is expected, and reflects the sole control of aldosterone by ACTH in this disorder.[109] PA is measured before and after oral dexamethasone administration to determine the extent to which aldosterone is suppressed by the glucocorticoid. A post-DST aldosterone level of less than 4 ng/dL has been shown to demonstrate high sensitivity and specificity.[110] A definitive diagnosis can only be reached by identification of the CYP11B1/ CYP11B2 chimeric gene in genomic DNA using either Southern blotting[98] or the long PCR technique.[111,112]

Therapy
Glucocorticoid suppression

Dexamethasone suppression does not always result in normalization of blood pressure in GRA. This might be due to various causes, such as the duration of hypertension, end-organ injury, concomitant essential hypertension, and autonomous production of aldosterone in patients with longstanding GRA.[109] Great care should be taken due to side effects associated with excessive doses of suppressive glucocorticoids, especially in children. Iatrogenic Cushing's syndrome and impaired linear growth in children have resulted from such overdosing.[103] The smallest effective doses of shorter-acting agents such as prednisone or hydrocortisone are used. Target blood pressure in children should be guided by age-specific blood pressure percentiles, and linear growth should be monitored to detect any slowing as a result of overtreatment. The therapeutic goal should be normotension, and not normalization of biochemical markers such as urinary 18-oxosteroid or serum aldosterone levels, because these remain elevated in the majority of patients who normalize blood pressure. Titrating therapy to normalize laboratory values could unnecessarily increase the risk of Cushingoid side effects.[107]

Antihypertensive medications

Mineralocorticoid antagonists, including spironolactone, amiloride, and triamterene, can be used as second-line agents to treat hypertension in GRA. Dihydropyridine calcium channel blockers have also been used in GRA.[109]

Familial hyperaldosteronism type 2

Gordon and colleagues[113] have described another familial variety of hyperaldosteronism (familial hyperaldosteronism type 2), which has been described as more common than FH-1. FH-2 does not involve inheritance of the hybrid gene and is not glucocorticoid-remediable; it was first described in 1991.[114,115] About 32 Australian families (80 patients) with FH-2 have been identified thus far.[113] Nine of the 32 families have demonstrated vertical transmission of phenotype between successive generations, consistent with autosomal dominant inheritance. The mode of inheritance in the remaining families remains unknown. FH-2 has been linked to the chromosome 7p22 region in some families. However, the syndrome is thought to be genetically heterogenous.[113] The clinical, biochemical, and morphologic characteristics of patients with FH-2 are similar to those with classic primary aldosteronism.

CONDITIONS OF MINERALOCORTICOID EXCESS WITH SUPPRESSED OR NORMAL ALDOSTERONE

A mineralocorticoid excess state can also be produced by adrenal steroids other than aldosterone. These are due to either excess deoxy corticosterone (DOC) or cortisol. Other conditions of mineralocorticoid excess with normal or suppressed aldosterone are defects in the amiloride-sensitive sodium channels (Liddle syndrome) or defective mineralocorticoid receptors.

Deoxycorticosterone excess

Excessive DOC can lead to a mineralocorticoid excess state and hypertension. DOC excess can arise from adrenal tumors or congenital adrenal hyperplasia.

DOC-secreting tumors

Adrenal tumors producing excess DOC vary from benign adrenocortical adenomas to metastatic adrenocortical carcinomas.[116] DOC-producing adrenal tumors are very rare. They can present with hypertension and hypokalemia.[117]

Congenital adrenal hyperplasia

The syndromes of congenital adrenal hyperplasia (CAH) associated with mineralocorticoid excess are 17α-hydroxylase and 11β-hydroxylase deficiencies.

17α-hydroxylase deficiency

17α-hydroxylase deficiency is a rare variety of CAH. Patients with 17α-hydroxylase deficiency have alterations in their CYP17 gene that encodes the P450C17 enzyme. This enzyme plays a central role in steroidogenesis, and is essential for the production of cortisol and sex steroids (Figure 67–9).

The block in the production of cortisol and sex steroids stimulates ACTH via a feedback mechanism that in turn stimulates excess production of DOC and corticosterone. This leads to hypertension and hypokalemia and surprisingly low levels of aldosterone. It is believed to result from the feedback inhibition of the suppressed renin–angiotensin system in the presence of excess salt retention due to excess DOC. Deficiency in sex hormones leads to incomplete masculinization and pseudo-hermaphroditism in males and primary amenorrhea in women. Most affected 46XY males are phenotypically females. The characteristic steroid profile is marked elevation of deoxycorticosterone and corticosterone, slightly elevated pregnenolone and progesterone, and decreased aldosterone and cortisol. Treatment with glucocorticoid replacement corrects hypertension and hypokalemia.

11β-hydroxylase deficiency

11β-hydroxylase deficiency presents as hypertension, hypokalemia, and virilization in infants.[118] This deficiency results from mutations in the CYP11B1 gene.[119] 11β-hydroxylase deficiency leads to cortisol, corticosterone, and aldosterone production blocks. Activation of ACTH by feedback leads to stimulation of excess androgens. Excess DOC leads to signs of mineralocorticoid excess in the form of hypertension and hypokalemia. The typical steroid profile includes elevated 11-deoxycorticosterone and 11-deoxycortisol. Plasma androstenedione and testosterone are also elevated. PRA and aldosterone are suppressed. Recommended treatment consists of glucocorticoid replacement, which relieves hypertension and hypokalemia and helps normal development of the child.

CORTISOL EXCESS

Syndrome of apparent mineralocorticoid excess

The mineralocorticoid receptor (MR) is nonselective in vitro, and cannot distinguish between the glucocorticoid cortisol and its natural ligand, aldosterone. 11β-hydroxysteroid dehydrogenase type 2 (11β-HSD2) plays a crucial role in converting hormonally active cortisol to inactive cortisone, thereby conferring specificity on the mineralocorticoid receptor (MR).[120] Two isoforms of human 11β-HSD have been described, but it is the NAD-dependent type 2 isoform (11β-HSD2) that is expressed in the mineralocorticoid target tissues, kidney, and colon. Mutations in the gene encoding 11β-HSD2 account for an autosomal recessive inherited form of hypertension, the syndrome of "apparent mineralocorticoid excess" (AME), in which cortisol induces hypertension and hypokalemia with suppression of plasma renin and aldosterone concentrations.[121,122] It is caused by defective 11β-HSD2, allowing cortisol, which has higher (100 to 1000 times) circulating levels than aldosterone, to bind to the MR and to act as a potent mineralocorticoid.

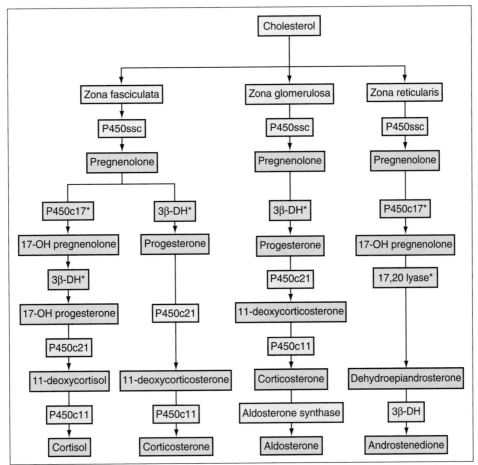

Figure 67–9. The pathways of steroid biosynthesis and the effect of spironolactone. P450ssc, P450-linked side–chain cleaving enzyme; P450c17, 17α-hydroxylase; 3β-DH, 3β-dehydrogenase; P450c21, 21β-hydroxylase; P450c11, 11β-hydroxylase. 17,20 lyase is the same as 17,20 desmolase in the testis. Asterisks represent enzymes inhibited by spironolactone. (Adapted from King MW. On steroid hormones, May 2006. Available at: *http://web.indstate.edu/thcme/mwking/steroid-hormones.html.*)

Clinical features

The syndrome is salt sensitive and autosomal recessive inherited form of hypertension. SAME shows a close correlation between disease phenotype and genotype.[123] The *in vitro* enzymatic activity conferred by each mutation is strongly correlated with the ratio of cortisone to cortisol metabolites in the urine, with age of diagnosis, and with birth weight, suggesting that the biochemical and clinical phenotype of AME is largely determined by genotype. Patients with mutations resulting in little or no 11β-HSD2 activity present in early life with a severe phenotype. On the other hand, patients presenting in late adolescence or early adulthood with mild forms of AME (also referred to as AME type 2) have been found to harbor mutations that result in a partially functional 11β-HSD2 protein with attenuated activity.[124]

This syndrome usually manifests in childhood with hypertension, hypokalemia, and low PRA. Other clinical features include moderate intrauterine growth retardation and postnatal failure to thrive. Complications of severe hypokalemia include nephrocalcinosis, rhabdomyolysis, and nephrogenic diabetes insipidus. Complications of

hypertension include cerebrovascular accidents and death during infancy or adolescence.

Diagnosis

An elevated ratio of cortisol to cortisone metabolites in the urine (tetrahydrocortisol plus allo tetrahydrocortisol to tetrahydrocortisone ([THF + aTHF]/THE]) is considered diagnostic.

Treatment

A low-salt diet, potassium supplementation, and spironoactone have been the mainstay in treating SAME.[125] Therapy with spironolactone results in growth, weight gain, and blood pressure control. Triamterene inhibits the tubular sodium channel and has also been successfully used. Amiloride has similar effects, and is also effective therapy for AME. The dihydropyridine calcium-channel blocker, nifedipine, has been useful for hypertension in SAME. Angiotensin-converting enzyme inhibitors have been shown to enhance renal 11-HSD activity, and might be useful in patients with partial enzyme defects.[126]

Ingested glycyrrhetinic acid causing deficiency of 11β-hydroxysteroid dehydrogenase

Both licorice and carbenoxolone contain glycyrrhetinic acid. Excess consumption of licorice has been well known to produce hypokalemia and hypertension. Active components of licorice are glycyrrhetinic acid and glycyrrhizic acid. Carbenoxolone is a hemisuccinate derivative of glycyrrhetinic acid, which is used in the treatment of acid peptic disease. Carbenoxolone produces sodium retention, hypokalemia, and hypertension. A mechanism similar to SAME explains the mineralocorticoid excess state seen following the ingestion of these compounds containing glycyrrhetinic acid. Glycyrrhetinic acid is a potent inhibitor of 11β-HSD.[127,128]

The syndrome of primary cortisol resistance

The syndrome of primary cortisol resistance (SPCR) is a rare familial cause of cortisol and DOC excess due to a defect in the glucocorticoid receptor.[129] SPCR may be the outcome of mutations of the glucocorticoid receptor or the reduced number of receptors.[130,131] ACTH is stimulated via feedback mechanisms, and there is overproduction of cortisol, mineralocorticoids, and androgens. In its severe form, hypertension and hypokalemic alkalosis are present, owing to increased secretion of the sodium-retaining mineralocorticoids. In subjects with a less-severe resistance to cortisol, there are no clinical abnormalities and the disease is revealed only by detailed examination of several parameters of cortisol metabolism. Excess androgens in women can result in acne, hirsutism, menstrual irregularities, anovulation, and infertility. In men, it may lead to infertility, and in children, to precocious puberty.[132]

Other causes of cortisol excess

The most common causes of cortisol excess leading to hypertension (due to its mineralocorticoid activity), including Cushing syndrome and exogenous steroids, are dealt with in Chapter 69.

Liddle syndrome (Pseudohyperaldosteronism)

The amiloride-sensitive epithelial sodium channel (ENaC) is expressed in the distal part of the renal tubule where it constitutes the rate-limiting step of Na^+ reabsorption, under the control of aldosterone. ENaC is composed of three subunits—alpha, beta, and gamma. Activating mutations of the C terminus of beta or gamma subunits of ENaC lead to a rare form of autosomal dominant hypertension described by Liddle in 1963, and is characterized by increased Na^+ and water reabsorption which stimulates primary aldosteronism.[133] There could be a variety of mutations affecting the ENaC, the genes of which are located on chromosome 16p13-p12.[134–136] Liddle's syndrome is an autosomal dominant form of salt-sensitive hypertension. The classic description of Liddle's syndrome includes early severe hypertension with hypokalemia, metabolic alkalosis, and suppressed PRA and aldosterone (hence the term "pseudohyperaldosteronism"). These abnormalities are not reversed by spironolactone. This syndrome has also been reported as sporadic cases due to *de novo* mutations without a family history.[137]

Gain of function receptor mutations

Rarely, mutations can occur in the mineralocorticoid receptors[138] that result in gain of mineralocorticoid function.[138] Those subjects present with early onset hypertension that is often made worse by pregnancy. They have a suppressed PRA and aldosterone.

SUMMARY

Mineralocorticoid excess remains the leading cause of secondary hypertension. Mineralocorticoid hypertension comprises a group of potentially curable syndromes and a high index of suspicion is needed. Unprovoked hypokalemia associated with hypertension strongly suggests mineralocorticoid hypertension. The genetic basis of several rare forms of mineralocorticoid hypertension has provided insight into the pathophysiology of hypertension. Clearly there is more to discover about mineralocorticoid hypertension and further research is needed.

REFERENCES

1. Ezzati M, Lopez AD, Rodgers A, Vander Hoorn S, Murray CJ. Selected major risk factors and global and regional burden of disease. *Lancet* 2002;360:1347–60.
2. Conn JW. Presidential address. I. Painting background. II. Primary aldosteronism, a new clinical syndrome. *J Lab Clin Med* 1955;45:3–17.
3. Conn JW. Normokalemic primary aldosteronism: a detectable cause of curable "essential hypertension." *JAMA* 1965;193:200–6.
4. Tucker RM, Labarthe DR. Frequency of surgical treatment for hypertension in adults at the Mayo Clinic from 1973 through 1975. *Mayo Clin Proc* 1977; 52:549–5.

5. Gordon RD, Stowasser M, Tunny TJ, Klemm SA, Rutherford JC. High incidence of primary aldosteronism in 199 patients referred with hypertension. *Clin Exp Pharmacol Physiol* 1994;21:315–8.
6. Lim PO, Dow E, Brennan G, Jung RT, MacDonald TM. High prevalence of primary aldosteronism in the Tayside hypertension clinic population. *J Hum Hypertens* 2000;14:311–5.
7. Loh KC, Koay ES, Khaw MC, Emmanuel SC, Young WF Jr. Prevalence of primary aldosteronism among Asian hypertensive patients in Singapore. *J Clin Endocrinol Metab* 2000;85:2854–9.
8. Mosso L, Fardella C, Montero J, Rojas P, Sanchez O, Rojas V, et al.

[High prevalence of undiagnosed primary hyperaldosteronism among patients with essential hypertension]. *Rev Med Chil* 1999;127:800–6.
9. Nishikawa T, Omura M. Clinical characteristics of primary aldosteronism: its prevalence and comparative studies on various causes of primary aldosteronism in Yokohama Rosai Hospital. *Biomed Pharmacother* 2000; 54(Suppl 1):83s–85s.
10. Connell JM, Fraser R, MacKenzie S, Davies E. Is altered adrenal steroid biosynthesis a key intermediate phenotype in hypertension? *Hypertension* 2003;41:993–9.
11. Erem C, Hacihasanoglu A, Cinel A, Cobanoglu U, Ersoz HO, Ahmetoglu A,

et al. Adrenal black adenoma associated with Cushing's syndrome. *Endocrine* 2004;25:253–7.

12. Barzon L, Sonino N, Fallo F, Palu G, Boscaro M. Prevalence and natural history of adrenal incidentalomas. *Eur J Endocrinol* 2003;149:273–85.

13. Magill SB, Raff H, Shaker JL, Brickner RC, Knechtges TE, Kehoe ME, et al. Comparison of adrenal vein sampling and computed tomography in the differentiation of primary aldosteronism. *J Clin Endocrinol Metab* 2001;86: 1066–71.

14. Mulatero P, Stowasser M, Loh KC, Fardella CE, Gordon RD, Mosso L, et al. Increased diagnosis of primary aldosteronism, including surgically correctable forms, in centers from five continents. *J Clin Endocrinol Metab* 2004;89:1045–50.

15. Mansoor GA, Malchoff CD, Arici MH, Karimeddini MK, Whalen GF. Unilateral adrenal hyperplasia causing primary aldosteronism: limitations of I-131 norcholesterol scanning. *Am J Hypertens* 2002;15:459–64.

16. Seccia TM, Fassina A, Nussdorfer GG, Pessina AC, Rossi GP. Aldosterone-producing adrenocortical carcinoma: an unusual cause of Conn's syndrome with an ominous clinical course. *Endocr Relat Cancer* 2005;12:149–59.

17. Biglieri EG, Kater CE, Mantero F. *Hypertension: Pathophysiology, Diagnosis and Management.* 2nd ed. New York: Raven Press, 1995.

18. Abdelhamid S, Muller-Lobeck H, Pahl S, Remberger K, Bonhof JA, Walb D, et al. Prevalence of adrenal and extra-adrenal Conn syndrome in hypertensive patients. *Arch Intern Med* 1996;156: 1190–5.

19. Kulkarni JN, Mistry RC, Kamat MR, Chinoy R, Lotlikar RG. Autonomous aldosterone-secreting ovarian tumor. *Gynecol Oncol* 1990;37:284–9.

20. Takeda Y, Miyamori I, Yoneda T, Iki K, Hatakeyama H, Blair IA, et al. Production of aldosterone in isolated rat blood vessels. *Hypertension* 1995; 25:170–3.

21. Takeda Y, Yoneda T, Demura M, Miyamori I, Mabuchi H. Cardiac aldosterone production in genetically hypertensive rats. *Hypertension* 2000; 36:495–500.

22. Gross JB, Imai M, Kokko JP. A functional comparison of the cortical collecting tubule and the distal convoluted tubule. *J Clin Invest* 1975;55:1284–94.

23. Stone DK, Seldin DW, Kokko JP, Jacobson HR. Mineralocorticoid modulation of rabbit medullary collecting duct acidification. A sodium-independent effect. *J Clin Invest* 1983; 72:77–83.

24. Schwartz GJ, Burg MB. Mineralocorticoid effects on cation transport by cortical collecting tubules in vitro. *Am J Physiol* 1978;235:F576–85.

25. Endou H, Hosoyamada M. *Diuretics: Potassium-Retaining Diuretics, Aldosterone Antagonists.* 2nd ed. London: Springer, 1995.

26. Binder HJ, McGlone F, Sandle GI. Effects of corticosteroid hormones on the electrophysiology of rat distal colon: implications for Na+ and K+ transport. *J Physiol* 1989;410:425–41.

27. Omland E, Mathisen O. Mechanism of ursodeoxycholic acid- and canrenoate-induced biliary bicarbonate secretion and the effect on glucose- and amino acid-induced cholestasis. *Scand J Gastroenterol* 1991;26:513–22.

28. Mori N, Yura K, Uozumi N, Sakai S. Effect of aldosterone antagonist on the DC potential in the endolymphatic sac. *Ann Otol Rhinol Laryngol* 1991; 100:72–5.

29. Schachter M. Aldosterone antagonism: new ideas, new drugs. *Br J Cardiol* 2002;9:533–7.

30. Struthers AD. Aldosterone: cardiovascular assault. *Am Heart J* 2002;144:S2–7.

31. Selye H. The general adaptation syndrome and the diseases of adaptation. *Clin Endocrinol J Clin Endocrinol* 1946;6:117–230.

32. Lombes M, Farman N, Oblin ME, Baulieu EE, Bonvalet JP, Erlanger BF, et al. Immunohistochemical localization of renal mineralocorticoid receptor by using an anti-idiotypic antibody that is an internal image of aldosterone. *Proc Natl Acad Sci U S A* 1990;87:1086–8.

33. Grillo C, Vallee S, McEwen BS, De Nicola AF. Properties and distribution of binding sites for the mineralocorticoid receptor antagonist [3H]ZK 91587 in brain. *J Steroid Biochem* 1990;35:11–5.

34. Young M, Fullerton M, Dilley R, Funder J. Mineralocorticoids, hypertension, and cardiac fibrosis. *J Clin Invest* 1994;93:2578–83.

35. Lombes M, Oblin ME, Gasc JM, Baulieu EE, Farman N, Bonvalet JP. Immunohistochemical and biochemical evidence for a cardiovascular mineralocorticoid receptor. *Circ Res* 1992;71:503–10.

36. Meyer WJ 3rd, Nichols NR. Mineralocorticoid binding in cultured smooth muscle cells and fibroblasts from rat aorta. *J Steroid Biochem* 1981; 14:1157–68.

37. Pearce P, Funder JW. High-affinity aldosterone binding sites (type I receptors) in rat heart. *Clin Exp Pharmacol Physiol* 1987;14:859–66.

38. Arriza JL, Weinberger C, Cerelli G, Glaser TM, Handelin BL, Housman DE, et al. Cloning of human mineralocorticoid receptor complementary DNA: structural and functional kinship with the glucocorticoid receptor. *Science* 1987;237:268–75.

39. Walker BR. Defective enzyme-mediated receptor protection: novel mechanisms in the pathophysiology of hypertension. *Clin Sci Clin Sci (Lond)* 1993;85:257–63.

40. Funder JW, Pearce PT, Smith R, Smith AI. Mineralocorticoid action: target tissue specificity is enzyme, not receptor, mediated. *Science* 1988;242:583–5.

41. Ferriss JB, Beevers DG, Brown JJ, Davies DL, Fraser R, Lever AF, et al. Clinical, biochemical and pathological features of low-renin ("primary") hyperaldosteronism. *Am Heart J* 1978;95:375–88.

42. Gonzalez-Campoy JM, Romero JC, Knox FG. Escape from the sodium-retaining effects of mineralocorticoids: role of ANF and intrarenal hormone systems. *Kidney Int* 1989;35:767–77.

43. Gomez-Sanchez EP, Zhou M, Gomez-Sanchez CE. Mineralocorticoids, salt and high blood pressure. *Steroids* 1996;61:184–8.

44. Walker BR, Connacher AA, Webb DJ, Edwards CR. Glucocorticoids and blood pressure: a role for the cortisol/cortisone shuttle in the control of vascular tone in man. *Clin Sci Clin Sci (Lond)* 1992;83:171–8.

45. Ullian ME, Hazen-Martin DJ, Walsh LG, Davda RK, Egan BM. Carbenoxolone damages endothelium and enhances vasoconstrictor action in aortic rings. *Hypertension* 1996;27:1346–52.

46. Conn JW. Plasma renin activity in primary aldosteronism. *JAMA* 1964;190:222–5.

47. Kaplan NM. Commentary on the incidence of primary aldosteronism. *Arch Intern Med* 1969;123:152–4.

48. Kaplan NM. Cautions over the current epidemic of primary aldosteronism. *Lancet* 2001;357:953–4.

49. Fishman LM, Kuchel O, Liddle GW, et al. Incidence of primary aldosteronism: uncomplicated "essential" hypertension. *JAMA* 1968; 205:85–90.

50. Bravo EL, Tarazi RC, Dustan HP, Fouad FM, Textor SC, Gifford RW, et al. The changing clinical spectrum of primary aldosteronism. *Am J Med* 1983;74:641–51.

51. Lim PO, Dow E, Brennan G, Jung RT, MacDonald TM. High prevalence of primary aldosteronism in the Tayside hypertension clinic population. *J Hum Hypertens* 2000;14:311–5.

52. Drury PL, Besser GM. Adrenal cortex. In: Hall R, Besser M, eds. *Fundamentals of Clinical Endocrinology.* 4th ed. London: Churchill Livingstone, 1989.

53. Calhoun DA, Nishizaka MK, Zaman MA, Thakkar RB, Weissmann P. Hyperaldosteronism among black and white subjects with resistant hypertension. *Hypertension* 2002; 40:892–6.

54. Mosso L, Carvajal C, Gonzalez A, Barraza A, Avila F, Montero J, et al. Primary aldosteronism and hypertensive disease. *Hypertension* 2003;42:161–5.

55. Strauch B, Zelinka T, Hampf M, Bernhardt R, Widimsky J Jr. Prevalence of primary hyperaldosteronism in moderate to severe hypertension in the Central Europe region. *J Hum Hypertens* 2003;17:349–52.

56. Zarifis J, Lip GY, Leatherdale B, Beevers G. Malignant hypertension in association with primary aldosteronism. *Blood Press* 1996;5:250–4.

57. Ma JT, Wang C, Lam KS, Yeung RT, Chan FL, Boey J, et al. Fifty cases of primary hyperaldosteronism in Hong Kong Chinese with a high frequency of periodic paralysis. Evaluation of techniques for tumour localisation. *Q J Med* 1986;61:1021–37.

58. Corry DB, Tuck ML. The effect of aldosterone on glucose metabolism. *Curr Hypertens Rep* 2003;5:106–9.

59. Benchetrit S, Bernheim J, Podjarny E. Normokalemic hyperaldosteronism in patients with resistant hypertension. *Isr Med Assoc J* 2002;4:17–20.

60. Bernini G, Moretti A, Argenio G, Salvetti A. Primary aldosteronism in normokalemic patients with adrenal incidentalomas. *Eur J Endocrinol* 2002; 146:523–9.

61. Young WF Jr. Primary aldosteronism: management issues. *Ann N Y Acad Sci* 2002;970:61–76.

62. Hiramatsu K, Yamada T, Yukimura Y, Komiya I, Ichikawa K, Ishihara M, et al. A screening test to identify aldosterone-producing adenoma by measuring plasma renin activity. Results in hypertensive patients. *Arch Intern Med* 1981;141:1589–93.

63. Montori VM, Young WF Jr. Use of plasma aldosterone concentration-to-plasma renin activity ratio as a screening test for primary aldosteronism. A systematic review of the literature. *Endocrinol Metab Clin North Am* 2002;31:619–32, xi.

64. Kaplan NM. Caution about the overdiagnosis of primary aldosteronism. *Mayo Clin Proc* 2001;76:875–6.

65. Fray JC, Russo SM. Mechanism for low renin in blacks: studies in hypophysectomised rat model. *J Hum Hypertens* 1990;4:160–2.

66. Seifarth C, Trenkel S, Schobel H, Hahn EG, Hensen J. Influence of antihypertensive medication on aldosterone and renin concentration in the differential diagnosis of essential hypertension and primary aldosteronism. *Clin Endocrinol (Oxf)* 2002;57:457–65.

67. Gallay BJ, Ahmad S, Xu L, Toivola B, Davidson RC. Screening for primary aldosteronism without discontinuing hypertensive medications: plasma aldosterone-renin ratio. *Am J Kidney Dis* 2001;37:699–705.

68. Lyons DF, Kem DC, Brown RD, Hanson CS, Carollo ML. Single dose captopril as a diagnostic test for primary aldosteronism. *J Clin Endocrinol Metab* 1983;57:892–6.

69. Rossi E, Regolisti G, Negro A, Sani C, Davoli S, Perazzoli F. High prevalence of primary aldosteronism using postcaptopril plasma aldosterone to renin ratio as a screening test among Italian hypertensives. *Am J Hypertens* 2002;15:896–902.

70. Litchfield WR, Dluhy RG. Primary aldosteronism. *Endocrinol Metab Clin North Am* 1995;24:593–612.

71. White EA, Schambelan M, Rost CR, Biglieri EG, Moss AA, Korobkin M. Use of computed tomography in diagnosing the cause of primary aldosteronism. *N Engl J Med* 1980; 303:1503–7.

72. Lim PO, Struthers AD, MacDonald TM. The neurohormonal natural history of essential hypertension: towards primary or tertiary aldosteronism? *J Hypertens* 2002;20:11–5.

73. Young WF Jr, Klee GG. Primary aldosteronism. Diagnostic evaluation. *Endocrinol Metab Clin North Am* 1988; 17:367–95.

74. Rossi GP, Chiesura-Corona M, Tregnaghi A, Zanin L, Perale R, Soattin S, et al. Imaging of aldosterone-secreting adenomas: a prospective comparison of computed tomography and magnetic resonance imaging in 27 patients with suspected primary aldosteronism. *J Hum Hypertens* 1993;7:357–63.

75. Rossi G, Chiesura-Corona M, Gregianin M. Diagnosis and treatment of primary hyperaldosteronism. *Ann Intern Med* 1995;123:73–4.

76. Mitty HA, Nicolis GL, Gabrilove JL. Adrenal venography: clinical-roentgeno-graphic correlation in 80 patients. *Am J Roentgenol Radium Ther Nucl Med* 1973;119:564–75.

77. Stack SP, Rosch J, Cook DM, Sheppard BC, Keller FS. Anomalous left adrenal venous drainage directly into the inferior vena cava. *J Vasc Interv Radiol* 2001;12:385–7.

78. Gordon RD, Stowasser M, Rutherford JC. Primary aldosteronism: are we diagnosing and operating on too few patients? *World J Surg* 2001;25:941–7.

79. Blumenfeld JD, Sealey JE, Schlussel Y, Vaughan ED Jr, Sos TA, Atlas SA, et al. Diagnosis and treatment of primary hyperaldosteronism. *Ann Intern Med* 1994;121:877–85.

80. Jeck T, Weisser B, Mengden T, Erdmenger L, Grune S, Vetter W. Primary aldosteronism: difference in clinical presentation and long-term follow-up between adenoma and bilateral hyperplasia of the adrenal glands. *Clin Invest* 1994;72:979–84.

81. Thompson GB, Grant CS, van Heerden JA, Schlinkert RT, Young WF Jr, Farley DR, et al. Laparoscopic versus open posterior adrenalectomy: a case–control study of 100 patients. *Surgery* 1997;122:1132–6.

82. Hokotate H, Inoue H, Baba Y, Tsuchimochi S, Nakajo M. Aldosteronomas: experience with superselective adrenal arterial embolization in 33 cases. *Radiology* 2003;227:401–6.

83. Food and Drug Administration. Inspra description, 2003. Available at: *http://www.fda.gov.*

84. Weinberger MH, Roniker B, Krause SL, Weiss RJ. Eplerenone, a selective aldosterone blocker, in mild-to-moderate hypertension. *Am J Hypertens* 2002;15:709–16.

85. Traina M, Vizzini GB. [Controlled study of the effect of long-term administration of canrenoate potassium in cirrhotic ascites]. *Minerva Med* 1986;77:87–91.

86. Pfizer Inc. Aldactone: full US prescribing information. Available at: *www.pfizer.com.*

87. Griffing GT, Cole AG, Aurecchia SA, Sindler BH, Komanicky P, Melby JC. Amiloride in primary hyperaldosteronism. *Clin Pharmacol Ther* 1982;31:56–61.

88. Stowasser M, Gordon RD, Gunasekera TG, Cowley DC, Ward G, Archibald C, et al. High rate of detection of primary aldosteronism, including surgically treatable forms, after 'non-selective' screening of hypertensive patients. *J Hypertens* 2003;21:2149–57.

89. Mantero F, Opocher G, Rocco S, Carpene G, Armanini D. Long-term treatment of mineralocorticoid excess syndromes. *Steroids* 1995;60:81–6.

90. Nadler JL, Hsueh W, Horton R. Therapeutic effect of calcium channel blockade in primary aldosteronism. *J Clin Endocrinol Metab* 1985;60:896–9.

91. Yokoyama T, Shimamoto K, Iimura O. [Mechanism of inhibition of aldosterone secretion by a Ca2+ channel blocker in patients with essential hypertension and patients with primary aldosteronism]. *Nippon Naibunpi Gakkai Zasshi* 1995; 71:1059–74.

92. Carpene G, Rocco S, Opocher G, Mantero F. Acute and chronic effect of nifedipine in primary aldosteronism. *Clin Exp Hypertens A* 1989;11:1263–72.

93. Opocher G, Rocco S, Murgia A, Mantero F. Effect of verapamil on aldosterone secretion in primary aldosteronism. *J Endocrinol Invest* 1987;10:491–4.

94. Sutherland DJ, Ruse JL, Laidlaw JC. Hypertension, increased aldosterone secretion and low plasma renin activity relieved by dexamethasone. *CAMJ* 1966;95:1109–19.

95. Ulick S, Chan CK, Gill JR Jr, Gutkin M, Letcher L, Mantero F, et al. Defective fasciculata zone function as the mechanism of glucocorticoid-remediable aldosteronism. *J Clin Endocrinol Metab* 1990;71:1151–7.

96. Ulick S, Chu MD. Hypersecretion of a new corticosteroid, 18-hydroxycortisol in two types of adrenocortical hypertension. *Clin Exp Hypertens A* 1982;4:1771–7.

97. Lifton RP, Dluhy RG, Powers M, Rich GM, Gutkin M, Fallo F, et al. Hereditary hypertension caused by chimaeric gene duplications and ectopic expression of aldosterone synthase. *Nat Genet* 1992;2:66–74.

98. Lifton RP, Dluhy RG, Powers M, Rich GM, Cook S, Ulick S, et al. A chimaeric 11 beta-hydroxylase/aldosterone synthase gene causes glucocorticoid-remediable aldosteronism and human hypertension. *Nature* 1992;355:262–5.

99. Rich GM, Ulick S, Cook S, Wang JZ, Lifton RP, Dluhy RG. Glucocorticoid-remediable aldosteronism in a large kindred: clinical spectrum and diagnosis using a characteristic biochemical phenotype. *Ann Intern Med* 1992;116:813–20.

100. Stowasser M, Bachmann AW, Jonsson JR, Tunny TJ, Klemm SA, Gordon RD. Clinical, biochemical and genetic approaches to the detection of familial hyperaldosteronism type I. *J Hypertens* 1995;13:1610–3.

101. Gates LJ, MacConnachie AA, Lifton RP, Haites NE, Benjamin N. Variation of phenotype in patients with glucocorticoid remediable aldosteronism. *J Med Genet* 1996; 33:25–8.

102. Litchfield WR, Anderson BF, Weiss RJ, Lifton RP, Dluhy RG. Intracranial aneurysm and hemorrhagic stroke in glucocorticoid-remediable aldosteronism. *Hypertension* 1998; 31:445–50.

103. Dluhy RG, Anderson B, Harlin B, Ingelfinger J, Lifton R. Glucocorticoid-remediable aldosteronism is associated with severe hypertension in early childhood. *J Pediatr* 2001;138:715–20.

104. Wyckoff JA, Seely EW, Hurwitz S, Anderson BF, Lifton RP, Dluhy RG. Glucocorticoid-remediable aldosteronism and pregnancy. *Hypertension* 2000;35:668–72.

105. Jamieson A, Slutsker L, Inglis GC, Fraser R, White PC, Connell JM. Glucocorticoid-suppressible hyperaldosteronism: effects of crossover site and parental origin of chimaeric gene on phenotypic expression. *Clin SciClin Sci (Lond)* 1995;88:563–70.

106. Dluhy RG, Lifton RP. Glucocorticoid-remediable aldosteronism (GRA): diagnosis, variability of phenotype and regulation of potassium homeostasis. *Steroids* 1995;60:48–51.

107. McMahon GT, Dluhy RG. Glucocorticoid-remediable aldosteronism. *Cardiol Rev* 2004;12:44–8.

108. Gates LJ, Benjamin N, Haites NE, MacConnachie AA, McLay JS. Is random screening of value in detecting glucocorticoid-remediable aldosteronism within a hypertensive population? *J Hum Hypertens* 2001;15:173–6.

109. Dluhy RG, Lifton RP. Glucocorticoid-remediable aldosteronism. *J Clin Endocrinol Metab* 1999;84:4341–4.

110. Litchfield WR, New MI, Coolidge C, Lifton RP, Dluhy RG. Evaluation of the dexamethasone suppression test for the diagnosis of glucocorticoid-remediable aldosteronism. *J Clin Endocrinol Metab* 1997;82:3570–3.

111. Jonsson JR, Klemm SA, Tunny TJ, Stowasser M, Gordon RD. A new genetic test for familial hyperaldosteronism type I aids in the detection of curable hypertension. *Biochem Biophys Res Commun* 1995;207:565–71.

112. MacConnachie AA, Kelly KF, McNamara A, Loughlin S, Gates LJ, Inglis GC, et al. Rapid diagnosis and identification of cross-over sites in patients with glucocorticoid remediable aldosteronism. *J Clin Endocrinol Metab* 1998;83:4328–31.

113. So A, Duffy DL, Gordon RD, Jeske YW, Lin-Su K, New MI, et al. Familial hyperaldosteronism type II is linked to the chromosome 7p22 region but also shows predicted heterogeneity. *J Hypertens* 2005;23:1477–84.

114. Gordon RD, Stowasser M, Tunny TJ, Klemm SA, Finn WL, Krek AL. Clinical and pathological diversity of primary aldosteronism, including a new familial variety. *Clin Exp Pharmacol Physiol* 1991;18:283–6.

115. Stowasser M, Gordon RD, Tunny TJ, Klemm SA, Finn WL, Krek AL. Primary aldosteronism: implications of a new familial variety. *J Hypertens Suppl* 1991;9:S264–5.

116. Irony I, Biglieri EG, Perloff D, Rubinoff H. Pathophysiology of deoxycorticosterone-secreting adrenal tumors. *J Clin Endocrinol Metab* 1987;65:836–40.

117. Wada N, Kubo M, Kijima H, Yamane Y, Nishikawa T, Sasano H, et al. A case of deoxycorticosterone-producing adrenal adenoma. *Endocr J* 1995;42:637–42.

118. Rosler A, Leiberman E, Cohen T. High frequency of congenital adrenal hyperplasia (classic 11 beta-hydroxylase deficiency) among Jews from Morocco. *Am J Med Genet* 1992;42:827–34.

119. Krone N, Riepe FG, Gotze D, Korsch E, Rister M, Commentz J, et al. Congenital adrenal hyperplasia due to 11-hydroxylase deficiency: functional characterization of two novel point mutations and a three-base pair deletion in the CYP11B1 gene. *J Clin Endocrinol Metab* 2005;90:3724–30.

120. Stewart PM. 11 beta-Hydroxysteroid dehydrogenase: implications for clinical medicine. *Clin Endocrinol (Oxf)* 1996;44:493–9.

121. New MI, Stoner E, DiMartino-Nardi J. Apparent mineralocorticoid excess causing hypertension and hypokalemia in children. *Clin Exp Hypertens A* 1986;8:751–72.

122. Wilson RC, Nimkarn S, New MI. Apparent mineralocorticoid excess. *Trends Endocrinol Metab* 2001;12:104–11.

123. White PC, Agarwal AK, Nunez BS, Giacchetti G, Mantero F, Stewart PM. Genotype–phenotype correlations of mutations and polymorphisms in HSD11B2, the gene encoding the kidney isozyme of 11beta-hydroxysteroid dehydrogenase. *Endocr Res* 2000;26:771–80.

124. Li A, Tedde R, Krozowski ZS, Pala A, Li KX, Shackleton CH, et al. Molecular basis for hypertension in the "type II variant" of apparent mineralocorticoid excess. *Am J Hum Genet* 1998;63:370–9.

125. White PC, Mune T, Agarwal AK. 11 beta-Hydroxysteroid dehydrogenase and the syndrome of apparent mineralocorticoid excess. *Endocr Rev* 1997;18:135–56.

126. Riddle MC, McDaniel PA. Renal 11 beta-hydroxysteroid dehydrogenase activity is enhanced by ramipril and captopril. *J Clin Endocrinol Metab* 1994;78:830–4.

127. Stewart PM, Wallace AM, Valentino R, Burt D, Shackleton CH, Edwards CR. Mineralocorticoid activity of liquorice: 11-beta-hydroxysteroid dehydrogenase deficiency comes of age. *Lancet* 1987;2:821–4.

128. MacKenzie MA, Hoefnagels WH, Jansen RW, Benraad TJ, Kloppenborg PW. The influence of glycyrrhetinic acid on plasma cortisol and cortisone in healthy young volunteers. *J Clin Endocrinol Metab* 1990;70:1637–43.

129. Chrousos GP, Vingerhoeds A, Brandon D, Eil C, Pugeat M, DeVroede M, et al. Primary cortisol resistance in man. A glucocorticoid receptor-mediated disease. *J Clin Invest* 1982;69:1261–9.

130. Iida S, Gomi M, Moriwaki K, Itoh Y, Hirobe K, Matsuzawa Y, et al. Primary cortisol resistance accompanied by a reduction in glucocorticoid receptors in two members of the same family. *J Clin Endocrinol Metab* 1985;60:967–71.

131. Malchoff DM, Brufsky A, Reardon G, McDermott P, Javier EC, Bergh CH, et al. A mutation of the glucocorticoid receptor in primary cortisol resistance. *J Clin Invest* 1993;91:1918–25.

132. Chrousos GP, Detera-Wadleigh SD, Karl M. Syndromes of glucocorticoid resistance. *Ann Intern Med* 1993;119:1113–24.

133. Liddle GW, Bledsoe T, Coppage WS Jr. A familial renal disorder simulating primary aldosteronism but with negligible aldosterone secretion. *Trans Assoc Am Physicians* 1963;76:199–213.

134. Shimkets RA, Warnock DG, Bositis CM, Nelson-Williams C, Hansson JH, Schambelan M, et al. Liddle's syndrome: heritable human hypertension caused by mutations in the beta subunit of the epithelial sodium channel. *Cell* 1994;79:407–14.

135. Bubien JK, Ismailov, II, Berdiev BK, Cornwell T, Lifton RP, Fuller CM, et al. Liddle's disease: abnormal regulation of amiloride-sensitive Na+ channels by beta-subunit mutation. *Am J Physiol* 1996;270:C208–13.

136. Auberson M, Hoffmann-Pochon N, Vandewalle A, Kellenberger S, Schild L. Epithelial Na+ channel mutants causing Liddle's syndrome retain ability to respond to aldosterone and vasopressin. *Am J Physiol Renal Physiol* 2003;285:F459–71.

137. Yamashita Y, Koga M, Takeda Y, Enomoto N, Uchida S, Hashimoto K, et al. Two sporadic cases of Liddle's syndrome caused by de novo ENaC mutations. *Am J Kidney Dis* 2001;37:499–504.

138. Geller DS. A mineralocorticoid receptor mutation causing human hyptertension. *Curr Opin Nephrol Hypertens* 2001;10:661–65.

Chapter

68 Glucocorticoid Hypertension

Steven Miller and John M. C. Connell

Definitions

- Glucocorticoid hypertension occurs in florid form in Cushing's syndrome.
- Cushing's syndrome can result from pharmacologic excess of glucocorticoid, a pituitary ACTH-secreting adenoma, adrenal adenoma or carcinoma, or ectopic secretion of ACTH.

Key Findings

- Excess glucocorticoid action leads to additional cardiovascular and metabolic risk factors including central obesity, glucose intolerance, and dyslipidemia.
- In the ectopic ACTH syndrome, the hypertension is characterized by activation of the mineralocorticoid receptor by cortisol, leading to hyporeninemic hypokalemia
- The mechanisms underlying glucocorticoid hypertension include sodium retention, central sympathetic activation and altered vascular endothelial function
- Patients with glucocorticoid hypertension do not have consistent abnormalities of the RAAS or sympathetic nervous system
- Patients with the metabolic syndrome share several features of Cushing's syndrome
- Recent evidence suggests that altered local regulation of glucocorticoid metabolism by the 11α-HSD1 enzyme results in increased receptor activation in omental fat and liver in patients with metabolic syndrome

Clinical Implications

- Hypertension in patients with gross glucocorticoid excess can be resistant to antihypertensive agents; no one specific class of drug is best
- Novel agents to inhibit local cortisol regeneration by 11α-HSD 1 may offer alternative strategies to manage features of glucocorticoid excess in the metabolic syndrome

tension. In this chapter the role of glucocorticoids in the genesis of high blood pressure will be considered in detail.

The importance of glucocorticoid production to cardiovascular health is illustrated by the circumstance of lack of cortisol production in patients with either primary or secondary adrenal failure. In these circumstances glucocorticoid deficiency results in a syndrome characterized by hypotension and a significant risk of premature death. In contrast, gross cortisol excess, in the form of Cushing's syndrome, if unrecognized can result in severe hypertension, and associated metabolic dysfunction, including hyperglycemia, dyslipidemia and a prothrombotic tendency. Indeed, in a careful reanalysis of the presenting features of Cushing's syndrome, Ross et al.[1] suggested that high blood pressure was an important and frequent accompaniment of this syndrome and helped distinguish it from "simple obesity." Thus, hypertension is a common accompaniment of glucocorticoid excess and that glucocorticoid-mediated hypertension is associated with several other cardiovascular risk factors

The morbidity associated with cortisol excess[2] is substantial, and the risk of death is largely accounted for by excess cardiovascular events, illustrating the importance of glucocorticoid action and regulation of vascular function. In this chapter we will address the mechanisms that underlie glucocorticoid hypertension, the clinical presentations that are characterized by glucocorticoid excess and the way in which steroid hormones may contribute to the wider occurrence of atherosclerosis and vascular occlusive disease in the population.

REGULATION OF CORTISOL PRODUCTION AND ACTION

Cortisol is produced in the zona fasiculata of the adrenal cortex in a series of biosynthetic reactions from the precursor cholesterol.[3] These steps involve sequential hydroxylation reactions catalyzed by P450 enzymes that are encoded by distinct and separate genes (Figure 68–1). The key steps in cortisol production include the initial transport of cholesterol from the cell cytoplasm to within the mitochondrion by the steroid acute regulatory (STAR) protein. The initial step in cortisol synthesis involves cleavage of the side chain of cholesterol and production of the hormone pregnenolone. Subsequent steps include hydroxylations at the 17 and 21 positions, and the final hydroxylation at the 11 position. This last step, catalyzed by the enzyme 11α-hydroxylase, is a key and rate-limiting

Steroid hormones produced by the adrenal cortex are essential to health and homeostasis. The two principal adrenal steroids in man are cortisol, which is primarily a glucocorticoid, and aldosterone, which is classified as a mineralocorticoid. This distinction has become blurred in recent years, but still forms a useful means of identifying the key actions of the two hormones. When produced in excess, cortisol and aldosterone produce significant and contrasting syndromes, both of which include hyper-

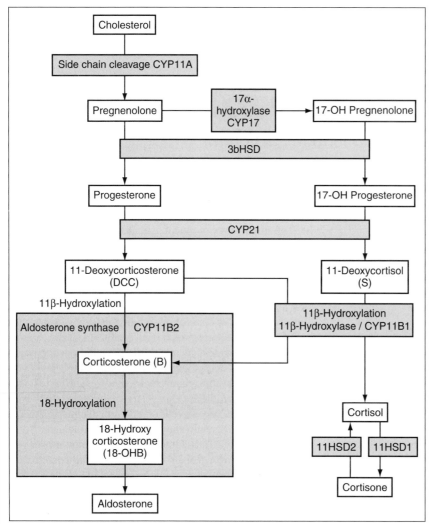

Figure 68–1. Schematic representation of adrenocorticoid synthesis and metabolism. Intermediate corticosteroid metabolites are in white, enzymes in grey. (3bHSD, 3β-hydroxysteroid dehydrogenase; CYP21, 21-hydroxylase; 11HSD1/11HSD2, 11a-hydroxylase. (Adapted from Connell JM, Fraser R, MacKenzie S, Davies E. *Hypertension* 2003;41:993–999.)

subjects with pathologic syndromes of cortisol excess, this diurnal variation is lost. The complex feedback system described ensures that cortisol levels are regulated, normally within a well-defined range in day-to-day circumstances.[5]

The mineralocorticoid hormone, aldosterone, is produced by zona glomerulosa cells of the adrenal cortex. It is regulated, principally, by angiotensin-II and potassium,[6] and has an important role in the control of sodium and potassium homeostasis by regulating the absorption and secretion, respectively, of these ions in the cortical-collecting duct of the kidney. The actions of aldosterone and the regulation of the hormone and its role in blood pressure will not be considered in detail here but are fully reviewed in Chapter 67.[7]

Steroid hormones exert their main effects through interaction with specific receptors that are located in the cell cytoplasm. On binding of ligand, these receptors translocate to the nucleus where they bind to particular receptor recognition sequences on the promoter regions of specific genes, leading to activation or repression of gene expression.[8,9] Glucocorticoid receptors form part of a superfamily of nuclear hormone receptors that also includes the mineralocorticoid receptor, estrogen receptor, vitamin D receptor, and others. Glucocorticoid receptors are widely distributed in tissues leading to pleiotrophic actions on human physiology. Activation of the glucocorticoid receptor has effects on metabolic function, immune modulation, and growth and development.[10]

In addition to binding to the glucocorticoid receptor, cortisol binds with high affinity, *in vitro*, to the mineralocorticoid receptor that has, as its natural ligand, aldosterone.[11] Indeed, the affinity of this receptor for cortisol is at least equivalent to that of aldosterone. However, in normal circumstances this receptor is protected from binding by cortisol by the action of the enzyme 11α-hydroxy steroid dehydrogenase type 11 (HSD2). This enzyme acts as a dehydrogenase to convert cortisol to its inactive metabolite, cortisone, which does not have significant affinity for the glucocorticoid or mineralocorticoid receptor.[12] This enzyme is found in close proximity to the mineralocorticoid receptor (within the same cell) in the majority of tissues where the receptor has a key mineralocorticoid action (such as the distal renal tubule). In this circumstance, cortisol is unable to access the receptor, allowing aldosterone to act as the key activating ligand (see below).[13]

step within the pathway; the enzyme 11-hydroxylase is encoded by the gene CYP11B1. Expression of the genes involved in cortisol production and of the STAR protein is regulated by the pituitary hormone ACTH.[4] Thus, ACTH deficiency leads to loss of expression of these key steroid hydroxylase genes and limits the ability of the adrenal gland to produce cortisol. In contrast, chronic ACTH excess leads to increased expression of these genes and, in addition, hyperplasia of adrenal cortical tissue. This, over time, leads to an increased capacity for production of cortisol from the adrenal glands.

Cortisol production by the adrenal cortex is controlled by the pituitary hormone ACTH. In turn, ACTH secretion is controlled through a negative feedback mechanism; in addition, pituitary ACTH production is regulated by input from the hypothalamus via corticotrophin-releasing hormone. ACTH (and cortisol) responds acutely to stress (hypoglycemia). There is a pronounced diurnal variation in ACTH (and thus of cortisol) so that levels are highest in the early morning and lowest in the late evening. In

Altered glucocorticoid receptor function has been investigated as a possible explanation for some of the glucocorticoid-mediated effects that might contribute to essential hypertension. Thus, studies have suggested that increased sensitivity of the receptor to glucocorticoids might change vascular reactivity by demonstrating, for example, increased skin blanching in response to application of topical glucocorticoid.[14] In other investigations, variation in the gene encoding the glucocorticoid receptor has been linked to the risk of inheriting hypertension. In an early study, Harrap et al.[15] reported a restriction fragment–length polymorphism of the glucocorticoid receptor gene that was associated with an increased risk of developing high blood pressure in later life in a normotensive population. However, this has not been subsequently confirmed, although other studies have demonstrated the same variation is associated with a risk of morbid obesity.[16,17] Thus, it is unlikely that major variation in glucocorticoid receptor sensitivity is a key factor that underlies the risk of developing glucocorticoid hypertension in patients with cortisol excess.

Glucocorticoid receptor activation is clearly central to the effects of glucocorticoid to alter blood pressure and regulate cardiovascular physiology. For example, in the kidney, activation of the glucocorticoid receptor will increase proximal sodium tubular reabsorption and, in addition, change the sensitivity of the renal tubule to the actions of vasopressin. Together, these actions will contribute to the effects of glucocorticoid on sodium and water homeostasis. Glucocorticoid receptors are also expressed in human vascular smooth muscle cells within blood vessels, and their activation will lead to a change in cell growth, and potentiation of response to a range of pressor hormones.[18] Effects on the central nervous system will alter stress response and sympathetic outflow, the effects of which on the heart lead to a change in cardiac output. Specific effects of glucocorticoids on the endothelium regulate production of endothelial nitric oxide; glucocorticoid administration can be shown to reduce nitric oxide synthase (iNOS) expression, along with availability of its cofactor (tetra-hydro biopterin) and substrate (L-arginine).[19] Taken together these actions will lead to altered circulating volume, cardiac output, and vascular responsiveness. It is easy to understand, therefore, how glucocorticoids can have an acute and chronic effect on blood pressure homeostasis.

Aldosterone binding to the mineralocorticoid receptor leads to a distinct set of events that include increased activity of the epithelial sodium transporter in the cortical-collecting duct of the kidney, resulting in net sodium reabsorption at that site. In addition, activation of this receptor has effects on other tissues that lead to increased cardiac collagen synthesis, altered vascular endothelial function, altered baroreceptor sensitivity, and an increase in central sympathetic outflow.[20–22] As indicated above, cortisol normally does not activate this mineralocorticoid receptor in peripheral tissues. However, in situations of severe cortisol excess (e.g., in patients with the ectopic ACTH syndrome), grossly excessive levels of cortisol overwhelm the capacity of the enzyme HSD2, allowing cortisol to access and activate mineralocorticoid receptor.[23] In these circumstances, cortisol action results in classic mineralocorticoid effects that include increased sodium reabsorption and potassium loss. The clinical presentation of this is discussed above. It has been proposed that the capacity of this enzyme (11a-HSD2) might be reduced in some subgroups of patients with essential hypertension. Thus, it may be that polymorphic variation at this locus leads to altered sodium sensitivity, although definitive studies that prove this to be the case are lacking.

METABOLISM OF GLUCOCORTICOIDS AND CARDIOVASCULAR DYSFUNCTION

Cortisol is metabolized to the inactive hormone, cortisone, as described above by the enzyme 11HSD2. This enzyme is located in classic mineralocorticoid target tissues such as the kidney. The reverse reaction (predominantly a reductase) by which cortisone is converted to cortisol is catalyzed by the enzyme 11-hydroxylase steroid dehydrogenase type 1. This enzyme is present in a number of key glucocorticoid target tissues, including adipose and liver. By this means there is local regulation of cortisol generation close to the site of action. Thus, cortisol availability to the glucocorticoid receptor can be increased (by 11HSD type 1) or decreased (by 11HSD type 2). Cortisol metabolism is also carried out by reduction of the "A" ring of the molecule by 5a-reductase, which generates tetrahydro cortisol. This alters bioavailability of the hormone. Thus, the net ability of cortisol to activate glucocorticoid receptors is determined not only by production rate within the adrenal cortex, but also by local generation and inactivation by the enzyme systems discussed above.[3] This leads to a complex circumstance in normal physiology; the way in which local glucocorticoid action may be modulated in a subtle manner in central obesity and essential hypertension remains a subject of considerable debate. Nevertheless, syndromes of gross cortisol excess accounted for by increased production in the adrenal cortex provide clear examples of how glucocorticoid excess can lead to profoundly abnormal cardiovascular homeostasis.

Syndromes and experiments in which activity of these enzymes is either increased or decreased illustrate the way in which local regulation of cortisol availability can be important. Thus, patients who have lost the function of the enzyme 11HSD2 (which inactivates cortisol) have a syndrome characterized by increased cortisol availability to the mineralocorticoid receptor.[24] This is characterized by severe hypertension with low renin and hypokalemia. In contrast, where the enzyme 11HSD1 is deficient, an unusual syndrome develops in which patients have a relative inability to regenerate cortisol from cortisone.[25] This leads to a net increase in ACTH drive to the adrenal; consequently, cortisol levels in the circulation are not significantly abnormal. However, in this circumstance adrenal androgen production is increased; thus affected individuals can present with a syndrome resembling that of the polycystic ovary syndrome.[25] However, blood pressure levels in this circumstance are not reported to be consistently elevated.

In animal models in which 11HSD1 is knocked out, there is clear evidence of reduced glucocorticoid action in the liver, and improved insulin sensitivity and resistance to the development of obesity.[26,27] In the converse circumstance, where the enzyme is specifically overexpressed in adipose tissue, regeneration of active glucocorticoid is enhanced. This produces a syndrome characterized by obesity, metabolic dysregulation, and hypertension.[28] This presentation has a remarkable similarity to the human metabolic syndrome, and it is tempting to speculate (see below) that local increased availability of cortisol within visceral fat and liver is a key contributor to metabolic dysfunction and risk of hypertension and diabetes. In contrast to animal data from knockout mice, there may be a paradox that blood pressure is not elevated in human 11HSD1 deficiency.

In summary, the regulation of cortisol production is complex and reflects both endocrine diurnal variation, classic negative feedback regulation, and local autocrine and paracrine mechanisms that lead to the ability to closely regulate the excess of glucocorticoids to the glucocorticoid and mineralocorticoid receptors. This complexity, coupled with the multiple sites of action and tissue-specific and varied effects of glucocorticoid, makes the understanding of glucocorticoid hypertension difficult. The experiments discussed above where specific enzyme systems are disrupted confirm, however, the key importance of glucocorticoid action in regulating cardiovascular function. In addition, the complex normal physiology of cortisol metabolism described identifies several mechanisms by which cortisol availability may be locally regulated and glucocorticoid action increased. How this contributes to obesity or hypertension within the general population remains the subject of considerable debate. Nevertheless, syndromes of gross cortisol excess, which are accounted for by increased production of the hormone by the adrenal cortex, provide clear examples of how glucocorticoid excess can lead to hypertension and altered metabolic homeostasis.

HOW DO GLUCOCORTICOIDS RAISE BLOOD PRESSURE?

The way in which glucocorticoid excess leads to hypertension has been the subject of a large number of studies in animal models and humans over the years. However, despite this intense effort, a full understanding of glucocorticoid hypertension remains elusive. There is no doubt that patients with gross cortisol excess have severe hypertension that is often resistant to therapy. These patients also have central obesity, dyslipidemia (mainly hypertriglyceridemia), and glucose intolerance, and have many features in common with the metabolic syndrome,[29,30] although this is less so, if the new IDF definition of metabolic syndrome is used. Many of the actions of glucocorticoids that lead to these changes are easy to appreciate; activation of glucocorticoid receptors will, clearly, favor central weight gain. Increased hepatic glycogenolysis and increased fat deposition within the liver, resistance to the action of the hormone insulin, and disturbed lipid

metabolism leading to increased levels of LDL cholesterol, are also consequences of glucocorticoid excess. However, the way in which glucocorticoids specifically raise blood pressure is less evident.

Some of the effects of glucocorticoids on blood pressure may be very long-standing. For example, evidence suggests that early life exposure to glucocorticoids determines long-term cardiovascular function. Animals exposed to high doses of glucocorticoid *in utero* have an increased lifetime risk of developing glucose intolerance and high blood pressure.[31,32] In human studies, it has been shown that there is an association between low birth weight and subsequent long-term regulation of the hypothalamic/pituitary/adrenal axis.[33] Thus, normotensive adults with low birth weight (who subsequently have a risk of becoming hypertensive in later life) have higher morning cortisol levels than subjects with normal birth weight.[34] The way in which this relationship develops and its importance in long-term development of hypertension remain unclear, but serve to illustrate the possible importance of glucocorticoids in the long-term regulation of cardiovascular function.

In addition to these very long-term "programming" mechanisms, several shorter-term mechanisms that may allow glucocorticoids to regulate cardiovascular function have been studied.

Sodium status and volume

The ability of cortisol to activate the mineralocorticoid receptor in circumstances of severe excess of the hormone has been discussed above. In such patients there is sodium retention, expansion of plasma volume and of total body exchangeable sodium (as reflected by suppression of renin), and potassium wasting. However, the majority of patients with glucocorticoid excess have normal levels of renin and do not have substantial expansion of body sodium content. Thus, although short-term administration of hydrocortisone to normal humans does lead to profound antinatriuresis, chronic cortisol excess appears not always to be associated with substantial volume expansion. Sodium restriction does not prevent the development of glucocorticoid-mediated hypertension in experimental circumstances.[35] Furthermore, administration of a mineralocorticoid receptor antagonist such as spironolactone does not prevent glucocorticoid-induced hypertension in human subjects or in animal models.[36]

A rise in cardiac output (by administration)

Short-term administration of glucocorticoids can increase cardiac output. However, in experimental circumstances prevention of this rise in cardiac output (by the administration of beta-blockers) does not inhibit development of glucocorticoid hypertension, and a rise in cardiac output as a consequence of acute glucocorticoid administration is unlikely to be a primary pathogenic mechanism.

Central sympathetic activation

Steroid hormones have profound effects on central nervous system (CNS) function, so that administration of glucocorticoid leads to a rise in sympathetic activation.

For example, local administration of corticosterone within the ventricular system of the brain raises blood pressure acutely.[37] However, this is likely to be a consequence of direct mineralocorticoid receptor activation within the brain, and the influence of circulating glucocorticoids on the CNS in relation to blood pressure regulation is less well understood.

Pressor responsiveness

Administration of hydrocortisone to human subjects increases pressor responsiveness to agents such as phenylephrine.[18] The mechanism of this remains unclear; in the long term this may reflect a change in vascular geometry so that responsiveness to any pressor agent is increased. However, in the short term it is likely that there is a change in α-receptor sensitivity or density in vascular smooth muscle cells. In addition, however, there is evidence that glucocorticoid receptor activation leads to a decrease in availability of endothelial nitric oxide.[38] Effects in relation to this appear to be specific. Thus, in animal studies the effects of glucocorticoid on NO availability are uncertain, whereas in human studies it seems clear that nitric oxide availability (as assessed by blood flow response to acetylcholine) is impaired in subjects given an acute short-term course of glucocorticoid.

In summary, there are a variety of potential mechanisms by which cortisol excess can raise blood pressure. Many of these can be shown to be present under short-term experimental circumstances when pharmacologic doses of glucocorticoids are administered. Thus, Brotman et al.[39] recently studied the effects of short-term dexamethasone administration in normal subjects, and showed a rise in blood pressure that was associated with a fall in heart rate and a change in a number of inflammatory markers. However, how this translates into long-term alteration on blood pressure regulation remains unclear. Evidence suggests that multiple pathways are involved in development of glucocorticoid hypertension. The one that dominates may in part be determined by the absolute level of glucocorticoid. Thus, in subjects with very marked overproduction of cortisol (as in the ectopic ACTH syndrome), the effect of cortisol on sodium and water metabolism may predominate, leading to a volume-dependent form of hypertension. In more subtle cortisol excess, long-term effects of glucocorticoid on vascular geometry and endothelial nitric oxide synthesis may become the dominant way in which blood pressure elevation is maintained.

CLINICAL PRESENTATIONS OF GLUCOCORTICOID-MEDIATED HYPERTENSION

Exogenous glucocorticoid excess

The commonest circumstance in which glucocorticoids cause hypertension relates to pharmacologic use in the treatment of patients with inflammatory and other disorders. Hypertension and altered vascular risk are important causes of morbidity and mortality in these patients. For example, in a survey of a large population within the Tayside Region (Scotland) of patients given a range of glucocorticoids, Wei et al.[40] reported a marked excess of cardiovascular disease. A confounding factor in this study was, of course, the notion that patients prescribed glucocorticoids may have had increased cardiovascular risk due to underlying disorders (such as inflammatory arthritis), and the absolute impact of glucocorticoid prescription on hypertension and cardiovascular risk remains to be determined. Nevertheless, even when data in this study were corrected for other known confounding factors, vascular excess risk remained, and it seems likely that glucocorticoid prescription is associated with a potentially independent long-term effect to increase cardiovascular event rate in addition to an impact on blood pressure.

Endogenous glucocorticoid excess
Cushing's disease

Cushing's disease remains the most common cause of endogenous cortisol excess. The disorder, due to increased ACTH secretion from the anterior pituitary, results in a syndrome characterized by overproduction of cortisol. Patients with untreated Cushing's disease have markedly increased 5-year mortality from cardiovascular disease, which is accounted for by hypertension, glucose intolerance, and dyslipidemia.[2,41] Effective treatment of ACTH excess cures the condition. However, it is noteworthy that excess cardiovascular morbidity and mortality remain in patients following successful treatment of Cushing's disease,[42] suggesting that glucocorticoid excess may confer increased long-term risk that is not relieved by normalizing cortisol levels.

Ectopic ACTH syndrome

The ectopic ACTH syndrome results in very severe cortisol excess. This can develop in patients with bronchial carcinoma, but is also seen in a variety of other circumstances, including bronchial carcinoid tumors. In the circumstance of gross cortisol hypersecretion, the capacity of the 11HSD2 enzyme to metabolize cortisol to cortisone is overwhelmed, allowing the hormone access to the mineralocorticoid receptor. Patients occasionally develop severe hypertension, associated with suppression of renin and hypokalemia. In this condition, the mechanism of hypertension is clearly due to mineralocorticoid receptor activation. However, this is a rare and unusual circumstance that does not reflect the general cardiovascular state of patients with less severe aspects of glucocorticoid excess.

Adrenal tumors

Adrenal tumors that release cortisol are most frequently benign. In patients with unilateral adrenal adenomas, hypertension and metabolic dysfunction resulting from cortisol excess is common. In such patients with marked excess of cortisol, the diagnosis is straightforward. However, it has become clear in recent years that a number of patients present with adrenal adenomas that produce cortisol at a much lower level; in many instances, circulating plasma cortisol is not increased in comparison with normal subjects. Such adrenal "incidentalomas" were thought not to have any significant clinical syndrome associated with them. However, it is now clear that in a number of patients, cortisol production by the tumor does contribute to cardiovascular morbidity.[43] In particular, low-grade cortisol excess from apparent adrenal incidentalomas is associated with an increased risk of high blood pressure and other cardiovascular disturbance including glucose intolerance and hypercholesterolemia. For this reason it is important that careful studies are made of cortisol production and its suppressability in all patients with apparent nonfunctioning adrenal adenomas.

Although the majority of such adrenal tumors are benign, adrenal lesions that are malignant can also be associated with increased cortisol production. In this circumstance, mortality from the underlying adrenal lesion is high, and the response to chemotherapy and radiotherapy is disappointing.

While the majority of patients with unilateral cortisol-producing tumors show no evidence of excess production of other steroid hormones that might contribute to cardiovascular dysfunction, patients with adrenal carcinomas may present with a range of excess hormone production, including secretion of precursor hormones (such as deoxycorticosterone) that can have important mineralocorticoid actions. In addition, a small number of patients can present with increased production of both cortisol and aldosterone. In this circumstance, hypertension may occur as a result of both increased mineralocorticoid and glucocorticoid effects.

CONTRIBUTION OF GLUCOCORTICOIDS TO METABOLIC SYNDROME

The above instances illustrate how major pathophysiologic glucocorticoid excess presents with the clinical features of Cushing's syndrome. However, it has been observed that patients with the metabolic syndrome have several clinical features that resemble Cushing's syndrome, although cortisol levels are not significantly elevated in this circumstance. Thus, patients with the metabolic syndrome have central obesity, glucose intolerance, dislipidemia, and hypertension.[44] In recent years, studies have focused on the notion that glucocorticoid excess might contribute to some of these manifestations. Additionally, there have been suggestions in the past that ACTH-dependent cortisol overproduction might contribute to the development of essential hypertension. For example, in the late 1980s, Whitworth et al.[45] demonstrated that dexamethasone treatment caused blood pressure to fall in patients with hypertension, and argued that this evidence of high blood pressure was a consequence of adrenal-derived steroids under the influence of ACTH. This concept has not been studied in detail by other investigators, although there is no clear evidence that there is a general overproduction of glucocorticoid in hypertensive patients.

The notion that the metabolic syndrome might represent a subtle form of increased glucocorticoid action has, however, been investigated.[46,47] There is evidence of a small increase in cortisol metabolite excretion in subjects with obesity, although this is very much less than would

normally be found in patients with classic Cushing's syndrome.[48] Plasma cortisol levels, in contrast, are slightly lower than would be expected. These data have been interpreted as showing evidence of increased cortisol metabolic clearance (with a corresponding small increase in secretion rate) in obese patients. Cortisol is metabolized by several routes that are discussed above. Studies suggest that there is, in obesity, an increase in "A" ring reduction of cortisol that might account for the altered metabolic clearance noted.[49] The biological significance of this remains uncertain.

In addition to evidence of increased cortisol clearance, other studies have suggested that the activity of 11HSD1 is increased in the metabolic syndrome. Again, the significance of this remains unclear. Studies by Walker et al.[50] suggest that the expression of the enzyme in adipose tissue (particularly subcutaneous fat) is increased in obesity, while other studies[51] have suggested that this is not the case in visceral adipose tissue, although visceral obesity is more commonly associated with most features of the metabolic syndrome, including hypertension. Nevertheless, it has been suggested that an increase in generation of cortisol from cortisone within omental fat results in enhanced cortisol delivery to the liver in obese patients. This would be expected to lead to a range of changes, including altered hepatic fat metabolism and, possibly, an increase in hepatic cytokine production. In turn, this might lead to a change in peripheral glucose disposal. In other circumstances increased secretion of cytokines (including IL6 and TNFα) from the liver has been shown to cause insulin resistance at the level of skeletal muscle and adipose tissue.[52] If these data can be extrapolated to effects of increased local availability of cortisol, it is possible that altered regulation of cortisol metabolism within omental fat results in a change in whole body regulation of glucose disposal that favors the development of insulin resistance and, in some subjects, progression to diabetes mellitus. This notion is supported by studies in which the adipose HSD1 enzyme expression has been increased using a tissue-specific enhancer. In mice with this overexpression, central obesity develops as does hypertension and glucose intolerance.[53] In mice, in contrast, where the corresponding gene is knocked out in the liver, there is evidence of a resistance to obesity during high fat feeding.[27] Thus, it is possible that a local increase is cortisol delivery to the liver may set in process mechanisms that give rise to generalized insulin resistance with hypertension. The mechanism for the rise in blood pressure in this circumstance remains to be fully determined. However, there is an association between generalized insulin resistance and hypertension and some other circumstances[54] that may, in part, represent reduced vascular endothelial nitric oxide production,[55] although a cause-and-effect relationship between insulin resistance and hypertension remains unclear. However, in this circumstance, it is possible that the altered production of hepatic cytokines leads to a direct cytokine-mediated impairment of endothelial nitric oxide availability that alters, in the long term, blood vessel contractility and structure.

THERAPEUTIC ASPECTS

The uncertainty regarding the exact mechanisms for glucocorticoid-mediated hypertension means that specific treatment targeted to key pathways is unlikely to be successful. For example, although use of a mineralo-corticoid receptor antagonist is of benefit in patients with aldosterone excess, this is unlikely to prove beneficial unless patients have cortisol excess to the extent that there is increased activation of the mineralocorticoid receptor (as in the ectopic ACTH syndrome). This is a rare circumstance. In other patients, the response to anti-hypertensive therapy can be variable. Patients often require a combination of treatment, and blood pressure can prove resistant. It is clear that the most important consideration is early action to normalize cortisol production. As noted above, however, there is evidence that significant cardiovascular morbidity remains in patients following successful treatment of Cushing's disease.

The implications of the role of cortisol regeneration in patients with the metabolic syndrome has led to thera-peutic consideration of development of inhibitors of the HSD1 enzyme that might reduce cortisone to cortisol metabolism within omental fat. Such drugs might, in theory, prove valuable in treatment of the metabolic syndrome. It is less certain how effective they would be in patients with gross glucocorticoid excess presenting as part of Cushing's syndrome.

SUMMARY

Patients with glucocorticoid excess suffer substantial cardiovascular morbidity and have increased mortality. Evidence from specific syndromes and from population studies of patients taking exogenous glucocorticoids indi-cate that there is, indeed, significant risk of hypertension in patients with glucocorticoid excess. The underlying mechanisms that give rise to this remain unclear; several potential pathways that may raise blood pressure have been implicated. At present it seems likely that gluco-corticoids raise blood pressure through a range of different mechanisms that will include central activation of sympa-thetic outflow, alteration of vascular endothelial function (through change of availability of nitric oxide) and, poten-tially, increased activation of the mineralocorticoid recep-tor in specific circumstances. It is important to recognize that hypertension in this patient group is part of a cardio-vascular syndrome that also includes glucose intolerance and dislipidemia. Thus, treatment of patients with gluco-corticoid excess needs to focus not only on blood pressure–lowering but also on other aspects of metabolic management including treatment of hypercholesterolemia, and specific glucose-lowering strategies.

REFERENCES

1. Ross EJ, Marshall-Jones P, Friedman M. Cushing's syndrome: diagnostic criteria. *Q J Med* 1966;35:149–92.
2. Etxabe J, Vazquez JA. Morbidity and mortality in Cushing's disease: an epidemiological approach. *Clin Endocrinol (Oxf)* 1994;40:479–84.
3. Arlt W, Stewart PM. Adrenal corticosteroid biosynthesis, metabolism, and action. *Endocrinol MetabEndocrinol Metab Clin North Am* 2005;34:293–313.
4. Liu J, Heikkila P, Kahri AI, Voutilainen R. Expression of the steroidogenic acute regulatory protein mRNA in adrenal tumors and cultured adrenal cells. *J Endocrinol* 1996;150:43–50.
5. Jacobson L. Hypothalamic-pituitary-adrenocortical axis regulation. *Endocrinol MetabEndocrinol Metab Clin North Am* 2005;34:271–92.
6. Jamieson A, Fraser R. Developments in the molecular biology of corticosteroid synthesis and action: implications for an understanding of essential hypertension. *J Hypertens* 1994;12:503–509.
7. Connell JM, Davies E. The new biology of aldosterone. *J Endocrinol* 2005;186:1–20.
8. Evans RM. The steroid and thyroid hormone receptor superfamily. *Science* 198813;240:889–95.
9. Aranda A, Pascual A. Nuclear hormone receptors and gene expression. *Physiol Rev* 2001;81:1269–304.
10. Rashid S, Lewis GF. The mechanisms of differential glucocorticoid and mineralocorticoid action in the brain

and peripheral tissues. *Clin Biochem* 2005;38:401–409.
11. Sheppard K, Funder JW. Mineralocorticoid specificity of renal type I receptors: in vivo binding studies. *Am J Physiol* 1987;252(2 Pt 1):E224–9.
12. Walker BR, Best R. Clinical investigation of 11 beta-hydroxysteroid dehydrogenase. *Endocr Res* 1995;21:379–87.
13. Krozowski Z, Li KX, Koyama K, Smith RE, Obeyesekere VR, Stein-Oakley A, et al. The type I and type II 11beta-hydroxysteroid dehydrogenase enzymes. *J Steroid Biochem Mol Biol* 1999;69:391–401.
14. Marks R, Barlow JW, Funder JW. Steroid-induced vasoconstriction: glucocorticoid antagonist studies. *J Clin Endocrinol Metab* 1982;54:1075–77.
15. Watt GC, Harrap SB, Foy CJ, Holton DW, Edwards HV, Davidson HR, et al. Abnormalities of glucocorticoid metabolism and the renin-angiotensin system: a four-corners approach to the identification of genetic determinants of blood pressure. *J Hypertens* 1992;10:473–82.
16. Lin RC, Wang WY, Morris BJ. Association and linkage analyses of glucocorticoid receptor gene markers in essential hypertension. *Hypertension* 1999;34:1186–92.
17. Weaver JU, Hitman GA, Kopelman PG. An association between a Bc1I restriction fragment length polymorphism of the

glucocorticoid receptor locus and hyperinsulinaemia in obese women. *J Mol Endocrinol* 1992;9:295–300.
18. Yang S, Zhang L. Glucocorticoids and vascular reactivity. *Curr Vasc Pharmacol* 2004;2:1–12.
19. Whitworth JA, Schyvens CG, Zhang Y, Andrews MC, Mangos GJ, Kelly JJ. The nitric oxide system in glucocorticoid-induced hypertension. *J Hypertens* 2002;20:1035–43.
20. Schiffrin EL, Franks DJ, Gutkowska J. Effect of aldosterone on vascular angiotensin II receptors in the rat. *Can J Physiol Pharmacol* 1985;63:1522–27.
21. Jazayeri A, Meyer WJ 3rd. Mineralocorticoid-induced increase in beta-adrenergic receptors of cultured rat arterial smooth muscle cells. *J Steroid Biochem* 1989;33:987–91.
22. Taddei S, Virdis A, Mattei P, Salvetti A. Vasodilation to acetylcholine in primary and secondary forms of human hypertension. *Hypertension* 1993;21(6 Pt 2):929–33.
23. Stewart PM. Cortisol as a mineralocorticoid in human disease. *J Steroid Biochem Mol Biol* 1999;69:403–408.
24. Monder C, Shackleton CH, Bradlow HL, New MI, Stoner E, Iohan F, et al. The syndrome of apparent mineralocorticoid excess: its association with 11 beta-dehydrogenase and 5 beta-reductase deficiency and some consequences for corticosteroid metabolism. *J Clin Endocrinol Metab* 1986;63:550–57.

25. Jamieson A, Wallace AM, Andrew R, Nunez BS, Walker BR, Fraser R, et al. Apparent cortisone reductase deficiency: a functional defect in 11beta-hydroxysteroid dehydrogenase type 1. *J Clin Endocrinol Metab* 1999; 84:3570–74.

26. Walker BR. Steroid metabolism in metabolic syndrome X. *Best Pract Res Clin Endocrinol Metab* 2001;15:111–22.

27. Kotelevtsev Y, Holmes MC, Burchell A, Houston PM, Schmoll D, Jamieson P, et al. 11beta-hydroxysteroid dehydrogenase type 1 knockout mice show attenuated glucocorticoid-inducible responses and resist hyperglycemia on obesity or stress. *Proc Natl Acad Sci U S A* 199723;94:14924–29.

28. Paterson JM, Morton NM, Fievet C, Kenyon CJ, Holmes MC, Staels B, et al. Metabolic syndrome without obesity: Hepatic overexpression of 11beta-hydroxysteroid dehydrogenase type 1 in transgenic mice. *Proc Natl Acad Sci U S A* 2004 4;101:7088–93 (Epub April 26, 2004).

29. Peeke PM, Chrousos GP. Hypercortisolism and obesity. *Ann N Y Acad Sci* 199529;771:665–76.

30. Friedman TC, Mastorakos G, Newman TD, Mullen NM, Horton EG, Costello R, et al. Carbohydrate and lipid metabolism in endogenous hypercortisolism: shared features with metabolic syndrome X and NIDDM. *Endocr J* 1996;43:645–55.

31. Levitt NS, Lindsay RS, Holmes MC, Seckl JR. Dexamethasone in the last week of pregnancy attenuates hippocampal glucocorticoid receptor gene expression and elevates blood pressure in the adult offspring in the rat. *Neuroendocrinology* 1996;64:412–18.

32. Barker DJ. In utero programming of cardiovascular disease. *Theriogenology.* 2000 15;53:555–74.

33. Clark PM. Programming of the hypothalamo-pituitary-adrenal axis and the fetal origins of adult disease hypothesis. *Eur J Pediatr* 1998; 157(Suppl 1):S7–10.

34. Economides DL, Nicolaides KH, Linton EA, Perry LA, Chard T. Plasma cortisol and adrenocorticotropin in appropriate and small for gestational age fetuses. *Fetal Ther* 1988;3:158–64.

35. Tonolo G, Fraser R, Connell JM, Kenyon CJ. Chronic low-dose infusions of dexamethasone in rats: effects on blood pressure, body weight and plasma atrial natriuretic peptide. *J Hypertens* 1988;6:25–31.

36. Li M, Wen C, Fraser T, Whitworth JA. Adrenocorticotrophin-induced hypertension: effects of mineralocorticoid and glucocorticoid receptor antagonism *J Hypertens* 1999;17:419–26.

37. Gomez-Sanchez EP, Venkataraman MT, Thwaites D, Fort C. ICV infusion of corticosterone antagonizes ICV-aldosterone hypertension. *Am J Physiol* 1990;258(4 Pt 1):E649–53.

38. Radomski MW, Palmer RM, Moncada S. Glucocorticoids inhibit the expression of an inducible, but not the constitutive, nitric oxide synthase in vascular endothelial cells. *Proc Natl Acad Sci U S A* 1990;87(24):10043–47.

39. Brotman DJ, Girod JP, Posch A, Jani JT, Patel JV, Gupta M, et al. Effects of short-term glucocorticoids on hemostatic factors in healthy volunteers. *Thromb Res* 2005 (Epub, Jul 7).

40. Wei L, MacDonald TM, Walker BR. Taking glucocorticoids by prescription is associated with subsequent cardiovascular disease. *Ann Intern Med* 2004 16;141:764–70.

41. Sacerdote A, Weiss K, Tran T, Rokeya Noor B, McFarlane SI. Hypertension in patients with Cushing's disease: pathophysiology, diagnosis, and management. *Curr Hypertens Rep* 2005;7:212–18.

42. Lindholm J, Juul S, Jorgensen JO, Astrup J, Bjerre P, Feldt-Rasmussen U, et al. Incidence and late prognosis of Cushing's syndrome: a population-based study. *J Clin Endocrinol Metab* 2001;86:117–23.

43. Terzolo M, Bovio S, Pia A, Conton PA, Reimondo G, Dall'Asta C, et al. Midnight serum cortisol as a marker of increased cardiovascular risk in patients with a clinically inapparent adrenal adenoma. *Eur J Endocrinol* 2005;153: 307–15.

44. Eckel RH, Grundy SM, Zimmet PZ. The metabolic syndrome. *Lancet* 2005; 365:1415–28.

45. Whitworth JA, Gordon D, McLachlan-Troup N, Scoggins BA, Moulds RW.

Dexamethasone suppression in essential hypertension: effects on cortisol and blood pressure. *Clin Exp Hypertens A* 1989;11:323–35.

46. Bahr V, Pfeiffer AF, Diederich S. The metabolic syndrome X and peripheral cortisol synthesis. *Exp Clin EndocrinolExp Clin Endocrinol Diabetes* 2002;110:313–18.

47. Stewart PM. Tissue-specific Cushing's syndrome uncovers a new target in treating the metabolic syndrome—11beta-hydroxysteroid dehydrogenase type 1. *Clin Med* 2005;5:142–46.

48. Galvao-Teles A, Graves L, Burke CW, Fotherby K, Fraser R. Free cortisol in obesity; effect of fasting. *Acta Endocrinol (Copenh)* 1976;81:321–29.

49. Rask E, Walker BR, Soderberg S, Livingstone DE, Eliasson M, Johnson O, Andrew R, Olsson T. Tissue specific changes in cortisol metabolism in obese women: increased adipose II beta-hydroxysteroid dehydrogenase Type I activity. *J Clin End Metab* 2002;87:3330–3336.

50. Andrew R, Phillips DI, Walker BR. Obesity and gender influence cortisol secretion and metabolism in man. *J Clin Endocrinol Metab* 1998;83:1806–809.

51. Rask E, Olsson T, Soderberg S, Andrew R, Livingstone DE, Johnson O, et al. Tissue-specific dysregulation of cortisol metabolism in human obesity. *J Clin Endocrinol Metab* 2001;86:1418–21.

52. Tomlinson JW, Sinha B, Bujalska I, Hewison M, Stewart PM. Expression of 11beta-hydroxysteroid dehydrogenase type 1 in adipose tissue is not increased in human obesity. *J Clin Endocrinol Metab* 2002;87:5630–35.

53. Kobayashi K. Adipokines: therapeutic targets for metabolic syndrome. *Curr Drug Targets* 2005;6:525–29.

54. Tomlinson JW, Stewart PM. The functional consequences of 11beta-hydroxysteroid dehydrogenase expression in adipose tissue. *Horm Metab Res* 2002;34: 746–51.

55. Sharma AM, Chetty VT. Obesity, hypertension and insulin resistance. *Acta Diabetol* 2005;42(Suppl 1):S3–S8.

56. Sowers JR. Insulin resistance and hypertension. *Am J Physiol Heart Circ Physiol* 2004;286:H1597–602.

Chapter

69

Cushing's Syndrome and Human Glucocorticoid Hypertension

Fernando Elijovich and Cheryl L. Laffer

Definition

- Cushing's syndrome is a cluster of clinical features produced by exaggerated action of glucocorticosteroids that are either stimulated by hypothalamo-pituitary or ectopic ACTH, hypersecreted by diseased adrenal glands, or given as therapeutic agents.

Clinical Implications

- Major manifestations include truncal obesity, hypertension, insulin resistance, overt diabetes, and dyslipidemia. These features, resembling the "metabolic syndrome," are associated with a large increase in cardiovascular morbidity and mortality.

- Stigmata of Cushing's syndrome may be absent; a high index of suspicion is required to establish the diagnosis when only isolated features are present (e.g., hypertension).

- Despite advances in definitive pituitary and adrenal surgeries, pharmacologic management to suppress synthesis or block the action of glucocorticoids may be required for severe disease, recurrences, or incurable etiology.

Cushing's syndrome has been considered an infrequent endocrinopathy (incidence 0.24 cases/100,000/year and prevalence of 1 to 4/100,000 in the general population,[1] or 5 cases/1000 hypertensive subjects in a referral tertiary care health center[2]), but nonetheless deserving of prompt identification and treatment because of its poor prognosis. Employing the World Health Organization–International Society of Hypertension classification, more than 80% of patients with Cushing's syndrome fall within high cardiovascular risk categories, and duration of disease is a major risk predictor, emphasizing the need for early recognition and therapy. Total and cardiovascular[1] mortalities are four- and five-fold higher than in the general population, respectively. In a study of 151,000 Scottish individuals without pre-existing cardiovascular disease (with 470,000 person-years follow-up), 46% of patients on chronic glucocorticoid therapy had 6.90 and 2.56/1000 person-year increases in absolute and relative covariate-adjusted risks for a cardiovascular event, respectively.[3]

Increasing use of computerized tomography and magnetic resonance imaging of the abdomen over the last two decades made it apparent that 5% of subjects have unsuspected, incidentally discovered adrenal masses.

Investigation of these "incidentalomas" showed that 5% to 20% of them are functional, secreting adrenal steroids autonomously and often producing clinically inapparent hypercortisolism with associated hypertension. Combined prevalence of clinical and subclinical forms of Cushing's syndrome is about 79/100,000. This is much higher than previously suspected, and suggests that undetected hypercortisolism may cause or contribute to blood pressure elevation in 150,000 to 600,000 subjects in the United States who carry a diagnosis of "essential" hypertension. Therefore, clinicians must seek subtle signs of Cushing's syndrome in all hypertensive patients and proceed with cost-effective screening if they are present. It has been argued that concomitant obesity, nonfamilial diabetes in both sexes and hirsutism in females, as well as otherwise unexplained menstrual irregularities, should prompt screening for hypercortisolism in hypertensive subjects.

In this chapter we will review the clinical features, diagnostic approach, and therapeutic options for the diverse forms of Cushing's syndrome. Also, we will discuss the complex and not fully understood mechanisms of hypertension and its treatment in states of glucocorticoid excess.

CLINICAL PRESENTATION

Clinical features

A list of common and uncommon features of Cushing's syndrome is shown in Table 69–1. Frequencies represent a compilation from many literature sources.

Hypertension

Hypertension is present in 70% to 80% of pituitary and adrenal Cushing's syndrome,[4] but less commonly (~20%) in chronic exogenous glucocorticoid therapy. It can be severe and refractory to therapy, and is usually salt resistant. Blood pressure correlates with age in Cushing's syndrome and fails to be normalized by successful therapy of hypercortisolism in about 30% of patients, suggesting that glucocorticoid hypertension may often be concomitant with or superimposed on essential hypertension.[4]

Circadian rhythm of blood pressure

Out of several forms of secondary hypertension in which the normal circadian rhythm of blood pressure is attenuated, abolished, or reversed, Cushing's syndrome is the one in which this abnormality (lack of nocturnal blood

FREQUENCY OF SYMPTOMS AND SIGNS OF CUSHING'S SYNDROME			
Frequency Organ System	>70%	40% to 69%	<40%
Cardiovascular	Hypertension		
Metabolic	Glucose intolerance		Overt diabetes
General		Muscle weakness	Headaches
Adipose Tissue	Obesity Moon facies	Truncal obesity "Buffalo hump"	
Cutaneous	Skin thinning Facial plethora Hirsutism	Purple striae Ecchymoses Acne	Female balding
Bone	Osteopenia	Osteoporosis Back pain	Fractures
Other	Menstrual abnormalities Decreased libido Impotence	Neuropsychiatric symptoms	Recurrent infections Poor wound healing Renal lithiasis
Note: Based on composite data from several publications.			

Table 69–1. Frequency of Symptoms and Signs of Cushing's Syndrome

pressure "dip") is most consistently observed, even in subjects without hypertension. The circadian rhythm of heart rate is preserved, indicating that the hypothalamo-pituitary-adrenal axis exerts specific control of blood pressure (not heart rate) variability. Nocturnal dipping is always absent in Cushing's syndrome of long duration, suggesting an interaction between hypertension itself and hypercortisolism in determining loss of the circadian rhythm of blood pressure. Glucocorticoid treatment of collagen vascular disorders or renal disease reduces nocturnal dipping as much as endogenous Cushing's syndrome, whereas this is not so in dexamethasone-induced hypertension in the rat,[5] indicating that the effect is species-specific. Nocturnal dipping is more commonly normalized by surgical cure of adrenal than of pituitary Cushing's,[6] and is restored to normal by cyproheptadine (inhibition of ACTH release[7]), suggesting that the effect of glucocorticoids on blood pressure variability is exerted in the central nervous system.

Lack of nocturnal dipping of blood pressure is a known risk factor for exaggerated hypertensive target-organ damage, and antihypertensive drugs of several families do not correct it in patients with Cushing's syndrome. Therefore, the need to quickly address definitive therapy of Cushing's syndrome cannot be overemphasized.

Obesity

Weight gain of Cushing's syndrome results in characteristic redistribution of subcutaneous fat leading to truncal obesity, moon facies, and supraclavicular and dorsal cervical ("buffalo hump") fat pads (see Figure 69–1). However, none of these features is specific for the obesity of glucocorticoid excess. Weight gain and growth retardation are prominent features of pediatric Cushing's syndrome, in which hypertension is not as prevalent as in adults (~50%).

Dermatologic features

Purple striae (Figure 69–1), dermal thinning, and easy bruising are common clinical signs, useful to alert the clinician regarding the possibility of hypercortisolism in patients who are being evaluated for obesity or hypertension. In contrast, hirsutism is more likely to be associated with primary obesity in hypertensive women.

Metabolic abnormalities

Diabetes mellitus type 2 and hyperlipidemia are present in approximately 40% of patients, but glucose intolerance is much more prevalent (~90%). These metabolic abnormalities are specific to the glucocorticoid excess because they regress after surgical therapy, improve with pharmacologic inhibition of glucocorticoid synthesis, are also produced by exogenous glucocorticoids, and can be reduced when the latter are given on alternate days. Metabolic factors account for the fact that cardiovascular damage of Cushing's syndrome can be observed in the absence of hypertension.[4]

Neuropsychiatric manifestations

Depression and cognitive impairment of Cushing's syndrome are associated with reduced brain volume and diminished cerebral glucose metabolism (measured with PET 18-fluorodeoxyglucose scanning[8]), which are somewhat reversible with therapy. In children, neuropsychiatric manifestations are frequent but subtle, often overlooked as behavioral problems.

Other

Severe osteoporosis in the young (even when an isolated manifestation), unexplained recurrent infections, myopathy (proximal muscle weakness), erectile dysfunction, and gynecomastia should prompt the search for subtle clinical stigmata of hypercortisolism. Nephrolithiasis, owing to

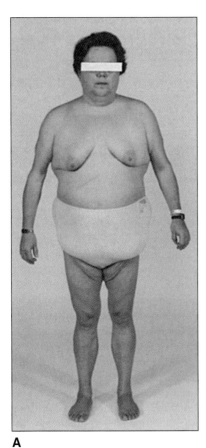

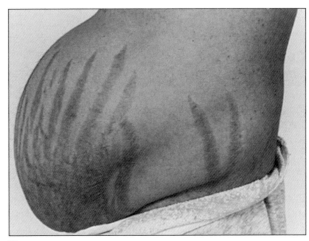

B
Figure 69–1. A: The left panel shows a patient with typical features of Cushing's syndrome including moon facies, supraclavicular fat pads and truncal obesity. **B:** On the right, characteristic wide purple striae are seen on the abdomen. (From *Endocrinology Online*, 5th ed. Philadelphia. Elsevier, 2006.)

A

a combination of hypercalciuria, hyperuricosuria, hyper-cystinuria, hyperoxaluria, and diminished citrate excretion, occurs in 20% to 25% of Cushing's patients.

Complications and damage of target organs
Neuro-ophthalmologic complications and stroke

Rare neurologic complications include paralysis of oculomotor cranial nerves due to compression by large pituitary adenomas, and spinal epidural lipomatosis, an abnormal growth of epidural fat that produces compressive thoracolumbar myelopathy and radiculopathy. Epidural lipomatosis is more common in Cushing's syndrome caused by ectopic ACTH secretion and glucocorticoid therapy. It is often missed when symptoms are nonspecific, but can be easily detected by magnetic resonance imaging (MRI). Successful surgical decompression has been achieved in severe cases but a conservative approach is indicated if it is milder.[9]

Ischemic and hemorrhagic strokes occur in Cushing's syndrome, which are not unexpected in severe hypertension. Funduscopic changes may reflect hypertensive retinopathy or the effect of a large neighboring pituitary tumor. Glaucoma and exophthalmos are common with exogenous glucocorticoid therapy but rare in endogenous Cushing's syndrome. Proximal muscle weakness may be due to hypokalemia or to underlying malignancy in ectopic Cushing's syndrome.

Left ventricular hypertrophy

Left ventricular hypertrophy (LVH) was not more prominent in Cushing's syndrome than in essential hypertension, and less in these two groups than in primary hyperaldosteronism in one study.[10] In contrast, others found severe LVH by electrocardiographic criteria and asymmetric LV septal hypertrophy (up to 32 mm) by echocardiogram in all patients. The latter was more prevalent in Cushing's syndrome than in essential hypertension or primary aldosteronism, suggesting a contribution of cortisol to LVH independent of blood pressure.[11] This is consistent with an observed relationship between LV mass and urine free cortisol in essential hypertension but not normal subjects.[12] However, echocardiographic relative wall thickness did not correlate with urine cortisol in another study of Cushing's syndrome.[13] Regardless of their mechanisms, LVH and asymmetric septal hypertrophy normalized with successful surgical therapy in both studies.

Vascular complications

Delayed scar tissue formation by glucocorticoids may explain the increased risk for rupture of the LV free wall after myocardial infarction in patients on chronic therapy with these agents. A similar mechanism may account for the reported aortic and large conduit artery aneurysms and dissections in patients with Cushing's syndrome, although these are not more frequent than expected in an illness characterized by atherosclerotic vascular disease.

Cushing's syndrome in pregnancy

Pregnancy in women with Cushing's syndrome is uncommon because glucocorticoids inhibit gonadotrophin-releasing hormone and stimulate androgens, resulting in ovulatory disturbance, amenorrhea, oligomenorrhea, infertility, and abortions. As opposed to the predominance of pituitary Cushing's in nonpregnant subjects, the cause in pregnant women is usually adrenal. Diagnosis is often delayed, assuming instead pre-eclampsia or gestational diabetes, to the point that adrenal adenomas have been accidentally discovered during Cesarean sections. Maternal (hypertension, diabetes, congestive heart failure, delayed wound healing, HELLP syndrome) and fetal (growth retardation, death in utero, prematurity) morbidities and mortalities are increased. Although normal births occur, the consensus is to intervene to reduce the risk of fetal loss. Multiple forms of therapy (pituitary and adrenal surgery, pharmacologic suppression of cortisol synthesis, and pituitary radiation) have been employed, with variable success.

Associated clinical conditions

Patients with Cushing's syndrome may present with the manifestations of the underlying illness responsible for ectopic secretion of ACTH (discussed later) or with those of associated conditions unrelated to the hypercortisolism. Some of them are authentic associations, whereas others are coincidental. Among the former are adrenal myelolipomas (benign tumors containing scattered islands of erythroblasts, myeloid and lymphocytic cells), sometimes found next to or combined with adrenal adenomas; and atrial myxomas that may or may not be part of Carney's syndrome. Concomitant pituitary corticotroph and lactotroph adenomas with hyperprolactinemia, and somatotroph adenomas with acromegaly have been reported.

Difficulties in clinical diagnosis

High blood pressure, weight gain, and glucose intolerance are most commonly produced by essential hypertension, primary obesity, and insulin resistance, three prevalent diseases that many times occur in combination (e.g., the metabolic syndrome). It is therefore very easy to overlook the diagnosis of Cushing's syndrome, which has a similar phenotype. This is particularly so when obesity is not clearly truncal or cutaneous stigmata are absent. Moreover, Cushing's syndrome may present with isolated features, be paucisymptomatic in the elderly, or subclinical in incidentalomas. The mean delay, from the retrospective assessment of the onset of symptoms to diagnosis, is about 3 years, with a range extending up to 8 years.[14] However, improvement of laboratory and imaging techniques has increased physicians' awareness. Referrals of subjects who will have confirmed Cushing's syndrome in a specialized center have tripled since the late 1980s.[15]

CAUSES OF CUSHING'S SYNDROME: ANATOMY, PATHOLOGY, AND DIFFERENTIAL FEATURES

ACTH-dependent and ACTH-independent Cushing's syndrome

Figure 69–2 provides a schematic representation of the causes of Cushing's syndrome. The top panel represents the normal stimulation of pituitary ACTH release by hypothalamic corticotrophic releasing hormone (CRH), leading to normal cortisol secretion by the zona fasciculata of the adrenal cortex. The three orange lines depict the inhibitory feedback loops that fine-tune the system (ACTH on CRH and cortisol on both CRH and ACTH). Exaggerated release of ACTH by a pituitary adenoma (second panel) is designated as Cushing's disease (after its description by Harvey Cushing in 1919). There is feedback inhibition of CRH by ACTH (with a few exceptions to be discussed later), while that of ACTH by cortisol is diminished or absent. Adrenal adenomas, carcinomas, or hyperplasia produce ACTH-independent, autonomous secretion of cortisol (third panel). The latter inhibits both hypothalamic CRH and pituitary ACTH. The fourth and fifth panels depict ectopic production of ACTH or CRH (the former much more common) by a malignant tumor. Ectopic CRH stimulates pituitary ACTH, hence adrenal cortisol, with inhibition of hypothalamic CRH, whereas ectopic ACTH stimulates production of cortisol by the adrenal cortex, with feedback inhibition of CRH and pituitary ACTH. Finally, when Cushing's syndrome is secondary to exogenous administration of synthetic glucocorticoids (the most common cause now, due to use of high-dose steroids in oncology and immunology), the whole endogenous axis is inhibited, as shown in the bottom panel.

In the following sections we will describe the anatomy and differential clinical characteristics of the entities that produce ACTH-dependent and ACTH-independent Cushing's syndrome.

Pituitary adenomas

Ten to 15% of all pituitary adenomas secrete ACTH. They are the most common cause of endogenous hypercortisolism (70%), four to five times more frequent in women than men, and also the most common cause in the elderly, in whom increased prevalence of cancer does not lead to excess ectopic Cushing's syndrome. Only in pregnancy is adrenal Cushing's more common than Cushing's disease.

Most ACTH-producing tumors are single microadenomas (85%), the size of which is often below the limit of detection for current imaging modalities. Corticotrophs of ACTH-secreting adenomas are monoclonal, consistent with proliferation of a founder cell that developed a spontaneous somatic mutation. This is in contrast to the polyclonal corticotrophs stimulated by CRH of ectopic sources. Microscopically (Figure 69–3), ACTH adenomas show basophilic (rarely chromophobic) cells, strong PAS and lead-hematoxylin positivity, and a prominent Golgi

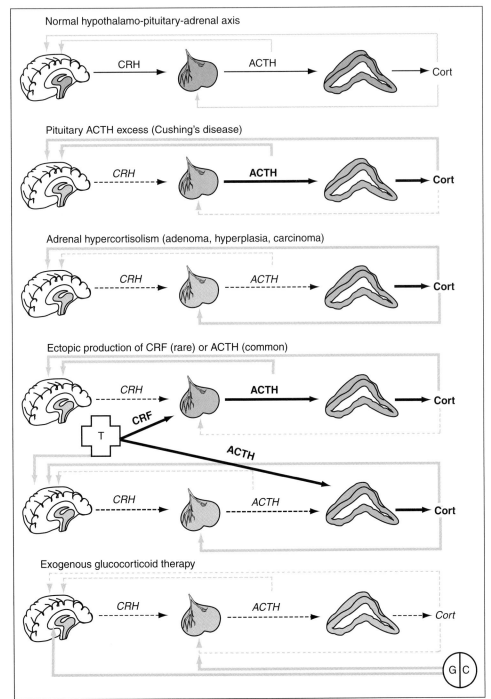

Figure 69–2. Schematic representation of the normal hypothalamo-pituitary-adrenal axis (*top panel*) and its alteration by the diverse causes of endogenous and exogenous glucocorticoid excess in humans. For description of each panel, see text. Normal function is depicted by blue organs, hyperfunction by green, and hypofunction by orange. Thick black lines and arrows and bolded letters signify excess stimulation, whereas thick orange lines indicate excess inhibition. Dashed thin black lines and *lightface italicized* letters indicate loss of normal stimulation. Dashed thin orange lines show loss of normal inhibition. ACTH, adrenocorticotropin; Cort, cortisol; CRH, corticotropin-releasing hormone; GC, tablet of therapeutic synthetic glucocorticoid; T, CRH- or ACTH-producing tumor.

apparatus harboring secretory granules that stain with immunoperoxidase (ACTH or other pro-opiomelanocortin–derived peptides). Large adenomas greater than 3 cm are seen only in 1% to 2% of cases, may invade surrounding tissues (60%), and have impaired secretory exocytosis

with lower ACTH levels and lesser prevalence of hypertension. Other causes of clinically inapparent Cushing's disease have been reported, including coincidental coexistence of mutations of adrenal 21-hydroxylase or dysfunction of 11-β-hydroxy-steroid dehydrogenase type

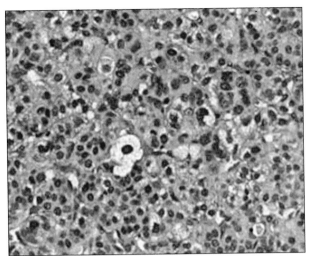

Figure 69–3. Photomicrograph of the histologic aspect of a pituitary adenoma. The monomorphic aspect of these cells, which usually stain positive with PAS, is accounted for by their monoclonal origin; see text. (From Kumar V, Abbas AK, Nelson F, eds. *Robbins and Cotran Pathologic Basis of Disease*, 7th ed. Philadelpha: Elsevier Saunders, 2005.)

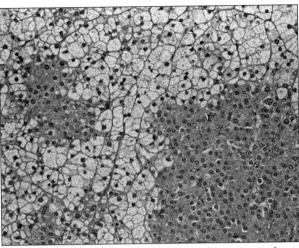

Figure 69–4. Photomicrograph of the histologic aspect of an adrenal adenoma. The specimen contains a mixture of the two classical cell types observed in this entity: clear, lipid-containing (lightly stained on the picture), and compact, lipid-poor (darker stained) cells. (From Korobkin M, Giordano TJ, Brodeur FJ, et al. *Radiology* 1996;200:743–7.)

1 (11bHSD1), reducing adrenal synthesis of cortisol or its tissue generation from cortisone, respectively.

As opposed to acromegaly, Cushing's disease is rarely due to multiple pituitary adenomas. When present, they may all secrete ACTH or be a combination of ACTH and prolactin- or growth-hormone–secreting tumors. Corticotrophs can also cluster into hyperplastic nodules, not adenomas, suggesting that hypothalamic stimulation by CRH may be the cause of hypercortisolism in these rare cases.

Extra-pituitary corticotroph adenomas are many times located in the cavernous sinus. They are often undetectable by imaging techniques and only found at autopsy. In one reported case, Cushing's disease was produced by leptomeningeal masses representing intracranial dissemination of a pituitary adenoma that was nonfunctional when resected years earlier.[16]

Adrenal adenomas

These benign tumors are responsible for 10% to 20% of all cases of endogenous Cushing's syndrome. The typical adrenal adenoma is a well-delimited yellowish-brown tumor that histologically resembles the normal gland (cords of clear and compact cells) (Figure 69–4), and rarely exceeds 25 to 35 g. Unusual variants include multiple adenomas in one or both adrenal glands, extra-adrenal location in the urinary tract, and so-called "black adenomas," which are larger, have higher than usual attenuation in a CT scan, and lack reduction of signal intensity in T1-MRI. They consist of polygonal cells with brown granules containing lipofuscin-like pigment and many lysosomes by electron microscopy. While traditional adenomas usually present with overt Cushing's syndrome, "black adenomas" may present only with hypertension.[17]

Analogous to carcinomas, cortisol-producing adenomas may have concomitant secretion of aldosterone, or lack of suppression of aldosterone by paradoxical hyperplasia of the zona glomerulosa, in which case they present with significant hypokalemia. They may also produce testosterone and other androgens, presenting with virilization and masked Cushing's syndrome.

Adrenal carcinoma

Adrenal carcinomas are the cause of ~5% of cases of Cushing's syndrome. They are large tumors, occasionally palpable, with all the macroscopic (necrosis, hemorrhage, capsular invasion, neovascularization) and microscopic (pleomorphic nuclei and prominent mitoses) pathologic characteristics of malignancy.

In addition to cortisol, adrenal carcinomas commonly secrete steroids with mineralocorticoid activity, such as combinations of 11-deoxycorticosterone, 11-deoxycortisol, and 17-α-hydroxyprogesterone, suggesting defective 11-β hydroxylation, isolated deoxycorticosterone, or aldosterone. Severe hypertension and hypokalemia may suggest primary hyperaldosteronism, but cortisol secretion is not suppressible. Androgenic steroids may also be secreted and produce clinical virilization. The steroid profiles of individual patients may be very different, but they remain constant during the course of the disease in each subject.

Adrenal hyperplasia

All forms of adrenal hyperplasia account for about 2% of endogenous Cushing's syndrome.

Micronodular hyperplasia

Several forms of adrenal hyperplasia can produce ACTH-independent secretion of cortisol with Cushing's syndrome. In the primary micronodular form, micronodules of clear cells, arranged in cords or acini, sometimes macroscopic, coexist with surrounding areas of diffuse hyperplasia. In children, the disease may not be easily identified because the adrenal glands are not enlarged. Another variant without much enlargement of the adrenals is primary pigmented nodular adrenocortical hyperplasia (PPNAD), which is characterized by eosinophilic cells with dark lipofuscin pigment and areas of atrophy.

It has been argued that micronodular hyperplasia may be a form of "tertiary" Cushing's syndrome, in which the hyperplastic adrenals acquired secretory autonomy after a period of ACTH stimulation, and also that it may represent hypersensitivity of the adrenal gland to normal ACTH levels.

Primary pigmented nodular adrenocortical hyperplasia can be secondary to mutations of the type-1 alpha-regulatory subunit of cAMP-dependent protein kinase A,[18] and can also be a component of Carney's syndrome (visceral and cutaneous myxomata, pituitary and testicular tumors, and spotty skin pigmentation).[19] When not a part of this syndrome, PPNAD commonly presents with hypertension or severe osteopenia.

Macronodular hyperplasia

This rare form, also known as ACTH-independent massive bilateral adrenal disease (AIMBAD), derives its name from the fact that adrenal glands may reach weights up to 200 g with nodules up to 5 cm in diameter. The cortical macronodules have clear cells whereas the rest of the gland has disorganization of its structure.

A characteristic feature is that adrenocortical cells have abnormal expression of receptors for non-ACTH substances; hence, their agonists stimulate cortisol secretion. Examples include angiotensin II stimulation that can be prevented with the AT1 receptor blocker candesartan,[20] vasopressin stimulation via V1a and V1b receptors,[21] and catecholamine stimulation prevented by propranolol in a case with adrenal binding sites with the properties of β-1 and β-2 adrenoceptors.[22] Familial and nonfamilial forms of abnormal cortisol responsiveness to gastric inhibitory polypeptide (GIP), documented *in vitro* with tissue from resected adenomas, are characterized by food-induced Cushing's syndrome that can be suppressed by octreotide, indicating that cells from the macronodules may have heterotopic receptors for GIP.[23]

Patients with macronodular hyperplasia are older, with longer duration of disease and higher prevalence of hypertension than those with the micronodular form. There is frequent hypoandrogenism due to atrophy of the zona reticularis and occasional hypersecretion of DOC and 18-OH-DOC with significant hypokalemia. Lack of Nelson's syndrome after bilateral adrenalectomy attests to ACTH independence. Treatment has included simultaneous bilateral laparoscopic adrenalectomy, although unilateral surgery (to avoid lifelong hormone replacement) and ketoconazole have also been used.

Unilateral nodular hyperplasia

This is an extremely rare condition first described in 1980. Patients present with severe hypertension and classic biochemical features of Cushing's syndrome with imaging suggesting a unilateral adenoma but with gross, histologic, and electron microscopy findings of nodular hyperplasia in one gland and suppression (lack of response to ACTH) in the contralateral one.[24] Suppression of cortisol by high-dose dexamethasone may lead to the mistaken diagnosis of Cushing's disease. The nodules contain a mix of clear and compact cells that exhibit immunoreactivity for several enzymes involved in synthesis of steroids, and large mitochondria by electron microscopy, indicating exaggerated steroidogenesis.

Incidentalomas and Cushing's syndrome

Incidentalomas are found in approximately 4% to 5% of the nearly half a million imaging studies of the abdomen carried out yearly in the United States for reasons other than adrenal disease. When the term was coined, the prevailing view was that these adrenal nodules were nonfunctioning and benign. Increased use of computed tomography (CT) scanning and MRI and accumulation of larger series of patients made it apparent that this interpretation was erroneous.

Low prevalence of adrenal carcinomas (0.25/1000 in the population and 3.2% in large series of incidentalomas[25]) does not justify systematic exclusion workup.[26] CT-diagnosed adrenal cysts, myelolipomas, homogeneous masses with low attenuation, and nodules without change of size in 6 months may be considered benign.[26] Tumors greater than 6 cm are usually taken to surgery, whereas those less than 4 cm are managed conservatively, although size criteria are not extremely accurate. Percutaneous needle biopsy has been used, but it is not devoid of risk.

All patients with incidentalomas must have measurement of plasma or urine catecholamine metabolites. Although pheochromocytomas are at most 3.4% of all incidentalomas,[25] they may be silent (no hypertension) but fatal during anesthesia or surgery, when unsuspected and unprepared with alpha-blockers.

Excluding these two potentially fatal conditions, 80% to 90% of incidentalomas are nonfunctional.[25] Patients with hypertension must have measurements of serum potassium and aldosterone:renin ratio to exclude rare cases (0.9%[25]) of unsuspected primary hyperaldosteronism that may have presented via accidental discovery of an adrenal nodule.

The remaining 5% to 20% incidentalomas have autonomous or excessive cortisol secretion that may be completely silent. This has led to the recommendation that all patients must undergo a 1-mg dexamethasone suppression test[26] for diagnosis and also to prevent postoperative adrenal crises. Subclinical Cushing's syndrome is not actually that "silent." The prevalences of hypertension, diabetes, obesity, and abnormal lipids in all incidentalomas exceed those in the general population, whereas in those with confirmed hypercortisolism, hypertension and diabetes may be present in 90% and 40%, respectively, not different from their prevalence in overt Cushing's syndrome.[27] Metabolic risk factors such as increased fasting glucose and insulin, total cholesterol, triglycerides, fibrinogen, insulin-resistance index, and waist to hip ratio, as well as organ damage such as atherosclerotic plaques and increased carotid intima-media thickness are also more frequent in cortisol-producing than in nonfunctioning incidentalomas. The causal relationship between the cortisol-producing adrenal incidentalomas and these clinical manifestations has been repeatedly confirmed by improvement of hypertension and metabolic abnormalities after surgical resection.[28]

Biochemical screening for hypercortisolism in adrenal incidentalomas is somewhat different from overall testing for Cushing's syndrome. The early suggestion that reduced DHEA levels was a specific finding has not been confirmed.[25] In addition to dexamethasone suppression, midnight serum cortisol values greater than 5.4 µg/dL, suppressed responses to CRH, and excess uptake of iodomethylnorcholesterol are useful to identify functioning nodules. In contrast, urine free cortisol is not reliable because it is not elevated until Cushing's syndrome is fully established.

Normal results of screening have been observed in patients who nonetheless had tumors with immunoreactive evidence for increased steroidogenesis,[29] which may explain why some nodules deemed nonfunctional and managed conservatively develop hypercortisolism on follow-up. Although this may happen up to 10 years after initial diagnosis, the general consensus is that after 4 years without evidence for steroid secretion, no further follow-up is warranted.[26]

Management of malignant or functioning incidentalomas with clinical repercussion (pheochromocytomas or Cushing's syndrome) is surgical, preferably with laparoscopy. In contrast, it remains controversial whether surgery is required for functioning nodules with negligible clinical repercussion, or with minimal clinical manifestations and high risk (e.g., patients older than 75 years).

Ectopic Cushing's syndrome

Ectopic Cushing's syndrome is a nonpituitary, nonadrenal hypercortisolism caused by ACTH secreted from malignant or neuroendocrine cells. It is responsible for 6% to 15% of all causes of endogenous Cushing's syndrome. Table 69–2 shows the tumors that produce it, grouped by organ system and relative frequencies (compiled from several series in the literature). The cause of ectopic ACTH production may be the loss of normal downregulated transcription of the pro-opiomelanocortin gene by malignant cells.[30] However, there are other causes such as secretion of CRH by pheochromocytomas, ganglioneuroblastomas, prostate carcinoma, bronchial carcinoids, and medullary thyroid carcinomas; local release of IL-6 by pheochromocytomas with stimulation of neighboring adrenal cortex; concomitant ACTH and CRH secretion by prostate carcinomas; concomitant production of catecholamines and cortisol by rare mixed adrenal corticomedullary adenomas; and ectopic production of cortisol by rare forms of ovarian cancer. Co-secretion of ACTH with insulin, gastrin, and glucagon (pancreatic islet cell carcinomas), PTH (small cell lung cancer), catecholamines (neuroendocrine tumors), calcitonin (thyroid medullary carcinoma) and endothelin, neuropeptide Y and ghrelin (carcinoids[31]) has been described but is usually clinically silent, except for the symptoms of a pheochromocytoma. ACTH immunoreactivity can be demonstrated in neuroendocrine and malignant cells, whereas some tumors (e.g., carcinoids) express a multiplicity of heterotopic receptors, including those for ghrelin, growth hormone secretagogue, vasopressin V3, CRH, and somatostatin. They may be linked to ACTH secretion, as demonstrated

TUMORS THAT PRODUCE ECTOPIC CUSHING'S SYNDROME			
Frequency Organ System	>20%	5-19%	<5%
Lung	Small cell cancer Bronchial carcinoid		Adenocarcinoma Squamous cancer
Thymus	Carcinoid		Epithelial cancer
Pancreas		Islet cell tumors	Cystadenoma
Neuroendocrine		Pheochromocytoma Medullary thyroid cancer	Paraganglioma Neuroblastoma Medulloblastoma
Urogenital			Wilm's tumor Hypernephroma Prostate cancer Ovarian cancer Ovarian carcinoid Sertoli cell tumor Cervical cancer
Gastrointestinal			Colon cancer Gastric cancer Esophageal cancer Ileal cancer Appendicular cancer

Note: Composite data from several publications.

Table 69–2. Tumors That Produce Ectopic Cushing's Syndrome

by the stimulatory effect of hexarelin, a growth hormone secretagogue,[31] and their presence can be exploited for localization purposes (e.g., somatostatin receptor scintigraphy).[32]

The course of ectopic Cushing's syndrome differs from that of ACTH-dependent pituitary disease in several aspects. First, its development is rapid, over the course of a few months, consistent with the pace of progression of malignant disease. Second, Cushing's stigmata may be absent because some (e.g., redistribution of adipose tissue) require a long time to be established. Third, levels of ACTH are higher than those in Cushing's disease and produce significant cutaneous and mucosal pigmentation. A similar situation is present in rare cases of pituitary carcinomas, which although not actually ectopic, have marked hyperpigmentation due to very high ACTH levels.[33] Fourth, severe hypercortisolism leads to hypokalemia (up to 57%[34]) with muscle weakness, probably explained by saturation of 11bHSD2, which allows activation of mineralocorticoid receptors by cortisol.[34] Fifth, hypertension is common (78%) and severe, requiring three or more drugs in almost half of the subjects.[34] Finally, there may be local (primary organ or metastasis) or systemic (anorexia, weight loss) symptoms of malignancy, as well as neuropsychiatric manifestations and rare forms with cyclical course.[31]

Mistaken diagnoses of pituitary Cushing's have been made when the cause of ectopic Cushing's evolves slowly, ACTH is suppressed by high-dose dexamethasone, and the source is not readily apparent (e.g., carcinoids). Also, when the initial finding is adrenal hyperplasia (secondary to ACTH stimulation), the diagnosis of ectopic Cushing's may not be suspected until after demonstration of ACTH dependency of the hypercortisolism.

Although treatment of ectopic Cushing's syndrome is that of the primary tumor, drugs that inhibit synthesis or actions of glucocorticoids may be required either temporarily for symptomatic management or permanently when the causative cancer is incurable.

DIAGNOSTIC TESTING

Laboratory tests
Screening

Screening for Cushing's syndrome is conducted with tests that assess hypersecretion of cortisol, autonomy of its secretion, and loss of its diurnal variation. No test is perfect, the choice depends on the clinical situation, and interpretation of results may be complex. It has been stated that, "Clinicians who have never missed the diagnosis of Cushing's syndrome or have never been fooled by attempting to establish its cause should refer their patients with suspected hypercortisolism to someone who has."[35]

Secretion of cortisol in bursts leads to overlapping morning serum levels in normal individuals and patients with Cushing's syndrome, precluding their use for screening. Assessment of diurnal variation of cortisol is cumbersome and expensive, requiring hospitalization. Moreover,

diurnal variation is found in 30% of Cushing's patients and is absent in 20% of normal subjects. Midnight serum cortisol is a better discriminator (only 3% to 4% of Cushing's patients have normal levels), as is midnight salivary cortisol, which is highly correlated with serum cortisol and avoids hospitalization.

Overnight 1-mg dexamethasone suppression (serum cortisol 8 to 9 hours later less than 5 μg/dL in normal subjects and more than 10 μg/dL in Cushing's syndrome) is the most commonly used screening test. In populations with low prior probability (e.g., obese hypertensive subjects or all incidentalomas), the test is useful to exclude Cushing's syndrome. In contrast, when prior probability is high (i.e., overt clinical features), normal cortisol suppression does not exclude it because it can occur in a few subjects with mild hypercortisolism,[35] or with low clearance (i.e., high plasma levels) of dexamethasone, which misleadingly suppresses cortisol. Furthermore, "falsely positive" lack of cortisol suppression is observed in clinical situations designated as "Pseudocushing's." They include 30% to 40% of obese subjects (increased metabolic clearance rate for cortisol and urine free cortisol), 50% of patients with major depression (cortisol hypersecretion), and many chronic alcohol abusers (hypercortisolism attributed to the stress of repeated alcohol intoxication). Drugs that accelerate liver metabolism of dexamethasone, and the mere stress of hospitalization also produce falsely positive results.

Urine free cortisol excretion above the maximum normal (~100 μg/day) may be enough to support the diagnosis in patients with clinically obvious Cushing's syndrome. A level greater than 300 μg/day is required when clinical findings are equivocal, and repeated collections may be needed. Sensitivity of urine free cortisol as a screening test is very high, but there are documented false negatives owing to renal insufficiency or mild hypercortisolism.[35]

Cushing's syndrome versus Pseudocushing's

Confirmation by a 2-day, low-dose (0.5 mg × 4 doses per day) dexamethasone suppression test used to be the norm after a positive screening, but is now reserved for patients without definitive clinical features in whom free urine cortisol is between 100 and 300 μg/day. The normal response is a serum cortisol less than 5 μg/dL and urine free cortisol lower than 20 μg/day. Because patients with Pseudocushing's may have false-positive results, a combination of the low-dose dexamethasone suppression test, followed by CRH stimulation is currently considered the best discriminator. Lesser suppression of cortisol by dexamethasone in Cushing's syndrome leads to exaggerated response to ensuing CRH, whereas the latter is blunted in Pseudocushing's patients.[35]

ACTH-dependent versus ACTH-independent hypercortisolism

Once hypercortisolism is confirmed, determining whether it is ACTH-dependent or -independent has been simplified by the development of highly sensitive and specific immunoradiometric ACTH assays. Values less than 5 pg/mL indicate adrenal origin of Cushing's syndrome, a range from high normal to 200 pg/mL is characteristic of pituitary Cushing's, while those more than 200 pg/mL are usually (but not always) observed in patients with ectopic ACTH-producing tumors. Few (~5%) cases of pituitary Cushing's may have levels less than 10 pg/mL on presentation, but they will exceed this value after a bolus injection of CRH, whereas this response will be absent in adrenal Cushing's. Lack of suppression of cortisol by either 8 mg overnight or 2-day high-dose dexamethasone was also used to establish diagnosis of adrenal Cushing's, but it has been rarely needed for this purpose since the advent of accurate ACTH assays.

Once adrenal hypercortisolism is confirmed, the next diagnostic steps are straightforward and include adrenal imaging to define the cause, and a search for unusual steroids if malignancy is suspected.

Pituitary versus ectopic Cushing's syndrome

In contrast, ACTH-dependent Cushing's syndrome requires further work up because 20% to 25% of patients with ectopic Cushing's will have ACTH levels in the 100 to 200 pg/mL range, that is, overlapping those of subjects with pituitary disease. Differential diagnosis cannot rely on imaging techniques because 30% to 50% of pituitary adenomas and one-third of bronchial carcinoids are below the detection size for pituitary MRI or chest CT. Furthermore, detecting an incidental pituitary tumor may be misleading in a patient who has ectopic Cushing's syndrome. High-dose dexamethasone (50% suppression of cortisol in pituitary Cushing's), although used, is not completely reliable because 10% to 30% of ectopic Cushing's patients may show a positive response, particularly those with bronchial carcinoids. Alternative tests include assessment of the ACTH responses to CRH and metyrapone (11-β-hydroxylase inhibitor), which will be larger in pituitary than in ectopic Cushing's syndrome.

Inferior petrosal sinus sampling, a somewhat invasive test, is required in patients without an apparent tumor and equivocal ACTH levels. A petrosal sinus versus peripheral vein ACTH gradient of 2:1 or higher baseline, or 3:1 or higher after CRH stimulation establishes the diagnosis of pituitary Cushing's. An additional benefit of this test is that it provides the surgeon with information about the location of the pituitary adenoma, on the basis of lateralization of petrosal sinus ACTH values.

Radiology
Pituitary imaging

Detection of pituitary microadenomas (<1 cm) by MRI has improved with use of gadolinium contrast and rapid sequential imaging. The latter identifies 70% of microadenomas with a resolution of 5 mm. A positive MRI (such as those shown in Figure 69–5) allows for adenomectomy in more than 80% of cases, whereas in the absence of an MRI finding, the surgeon identifies an adenoma in only half.[36] Doppler techniques and ACTH sampling from peripituitary veins have been employed intraoperatively to locate an adenoma, with variable results. Techniques that are still experimental include neurotransmitter-receptor ligand imaging by SPECT, using 123-I-IBZM for dopamine D2, or 111-In-DTPA-octreotide for somatostatin receptors.[37] In a few cases, the pituitary adenoma had uptake of 18-F-fluorodeoxyglucose by PET scanning.[38]

Adrenal imaging

Arteriography and adrenal venous sampling for Cushing's syndrome are of historical interest. Contrast dye and purposeful injection of toxic substances led to remission

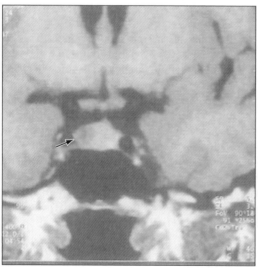
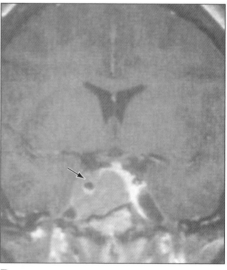

A   **B**

Figure 69–5. MRI films showing pituitary micro- and macro-adenomas (**A** and **B**, respectively), causing Cushing's disease. Tumors (arrows) appear hypodense, and the magnitude of displacement of the pituitary stalk is proportional to their size. While microadenomas are usually cured by surgery, macroadenomas that extend outside the sella turcica usually recur. (From Larsen PR, ed. *Williams Textbook of Endocrinology*, 10th ed. Philadelphia: Saunders, 2003.)

of disease in a few cases (sometimes with adrenal insufficiency), by necrosis of the adenoma. As opposed to its usefulness in primary hyperaldosteronism, adrenal venous sampling in Cushing's syndrome yielded overlapping results between different adrenal causes.

CT scan and MRI of the adrenal are now part of the routine evaluation and detect adrenal tumors with a resolution of 1 cm (see left panel of Figure 69–6). Presence of fat within a nodule suggests adenoma while necrosis, hemorrhage, and calcification are clues suggesting carcinoma. Although CT/MRI are not as accurate for imaging of adrenal hyperplasia, they may suggest primary pigmented nodular hyperplasia when normal-sized adrenals contain very small nodules with normal internodal tissue, and ACTH-independent macronodular hyperplasia when there is extreme enlargement of the glands and nodules greater than 2 to 3 cm (Figure 69–6, right panel). MRI performs slightly better than CT for differentiation between adenomas and malignancies, owing to better tissue characterization and multiplanar visualization of blood vessels.[39] Ultrasonography has also been used successfully to locate and identify adrenal masses, but is very operator dependent.

The uptake of 6-β-(131-I)-iodomethyl-19-norcholesterol by cortisol-hypersecreting adrenal tissue correlates with the magnitude of the hyperfunction. Adrenal scintigraphies with this isotope and with selenium-75-6-seleno-methyl-cholesterol are better than CT/MRI for detection of bilateral adrenocortical hyperplasia,[40] for differentiating it from unilateral adenomas or carcinomas, and for recognition of functioning lesions located far from the adrenal glands.

Recent reports have described utility of 18-F-fluorodeoxyglucose PET scanning for differentiation between malignant and nonmalignant adrenal masses.[41]

Others have described uptake in adrenal hyperplasia. Positron emission tomography (PET) scanning with the 11-β-hydroxylase tracer (11)-C-metomidate distinguishes cortical from noncortical adrenal masses and Conn's syndrome from Cushing's adenomas. The latter distinction is due to preserved expression of 11-β-hydroxylase in the gland contralateral to the Conn's adenoma, versus its suppression in Cushing's syndrome. Further studies are needed to assess the clinical utility of this imaging modality.

Imaging of ectopic, ACTH-secreting tumors

The choice of radiologic technique to detect ACTH-secreting malignancies or neuroendocrine tumors depends on the organ of origin. In the absence of clues, the search should begin at the chest (x-rays and CT scan) because ~50% of these tumors are intrathoracic. Pancreatic tumors and pheochromocytoma may have to be investigated with abdominal CT, MRI, or scintigraphy. Thyroid nuclear scanning may also be required.

When ectopic Cushing's syndrome has been diagnosed by extremely high ACTH levels or by inferior petrosal sinus sampling but the tumor is not found, multiple selective venous catheterization and sampling throughout the body may be required to locate the source of ACTH secretion, particularly in slowly growing carcinoids that may not become radiologically detectable for years.

Alternative methods to identify carcinoid tumors include the use of radiolabeled octreotide-like compounds, which may be taken up when the tumor expresses somatostatin receptors, and more recently whole-body PET scanning with (11)-C-5-hydroxytryptophan, an isotope that is taken up by neuroendocrine cells, and may become the technique of choice for imaging of these tumors.[42]

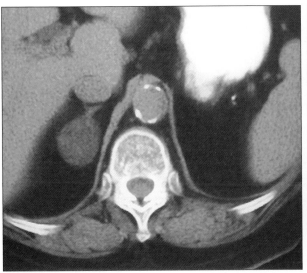
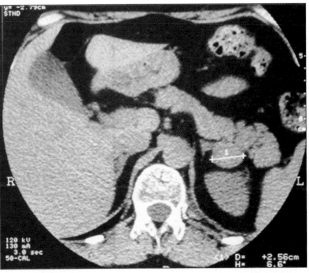

A **B**

Figure 69–6. Classic examples of cortisol-secreting adrenal disorders. The *left* CT scan depicts a lipid-rich adenoma with obvious low attenuation. The *right* panel shows a large nodule (bars for size assessment) in a patient with enlarged adrenal glands due to nodular hyperplasia. (**A**, from Dunnick NR, Korobkin M. *Am J Roentgenol* 2002;179:559–68; **B**, From *Endocrinology Online*, 5th ed. Philadelphia: Elsevier, 2006.)

If a radiologic technique identifies a tumor, but its causative role is equivocal, percutaneous needle biopsy and detection of pro-opiomelanocortin secretory granules or mRNA in the tissue will provide the confirmation required to carry out a surgical excision.

PATHOPHYSIOLOGY OF HUMAN GLUCOCORTICOID HYPERTENSION

The basic biochemistry and physiology of steroidogenesis are extensively reviewed in Chapter 68. In this section, we will review the pathophysiologic mechanisms that are pertinent for the understanding of human glucocorticoid-induced hypertension.

The mechanisms of blood pressure elevation by glucocorticoids are not well known, but our understanding has been enhanced by the realization that in addition to glucocorticoid secretion rates and plasma levels, tissue levels and access to tissue receptors are major determinants of glucocorticoid action. In this regard, a major regulator is the 11-β-hydroxysteroid dehydrogenase (11bHSD) "shuttle," composed of two enzymes that are distant congeners with conserved domains but different tissue distributions and actions. The type 2 isoform (11bHSD2), a dehydrogenase that converts cortisol into cortisone, is expressed in tissues in which the actions of aldosterone are physiologically important (e.g., kidney, gut epithelium, and regions of the central nervous system) and in vascular smooth muscle. Its main function is to "protect" against activation of the mineralocorticoid receptor by cortisol, which circulates in much higher concentrations compared to aldosterone, but binds with equal affinity to its receptor. Intracellular topology of 11bHSD2 (endoplasmic reticulum, facing the cytoplasm)[43] is consistent with its function as a regulator of mineralocorticoid receptor binding, a unique example of receptor specificity not due to protein structure, but to the actions of a neighboring enzyme. Failure of this "protection" (e.g., loss of function mutations of 11bHSD2 in the familial syndrome of apparent mineralocorticoid excess or inhibition of its action by licorice or carbenoxolone) leads to a clinical picture indistinguishable from that of primary hyperaldosteronism, in which the "mineralocorticoid" is cortisol.

The type 1 isoform (11bHSD1) is ubiquitous and can function bidirectionally, converting cortisol to cortisone as a dehydrogenase or cortisone to cortisol as a reductase. The latter function is more common, and is important for local tissue generation of cortisol in organs that regulate lipid and carbohydrate metabolism, such as liver hepatocytes and visceral fat adipocytes. Intracellular topology of 11bHSD1 (endoplasmic reticulum, facing the lumen)[43] is consistent with its function as a pre-receptor amplifier of glucocorticoid signals.

Glucocorticoids and long-term regulation of blood pressure ("programming")

Animal studies have demonstrated that materno-fetal malnutrition with low birth weight leads to exaggerated rates of hypertension in the adult offspring, an effect that is mimicked by administration of glucocorticoids during very defined, species-specific time windows in pregnancy.

Both malnutrition during pregnancy and glucocorticoid excess decrease the ability of placental 11bHSD2 to protect the placental glucocorticoid receptor and the fetus from abnormal exposure to maternal glucocorticoids. Malnutrition inhibits expression of placental 11bHSD2, whereas glucocorticoid excess saturates its catalytic activity. Inhibition of 11bHSD2 with carbenoxolone also enhances hypertension in the offspring, and its effects can be prevented by adrenalectomy, confirming the roles of the enzyme and glucocorticoids, respectively. Furthermore, offspring hypertension cannot be produced with other interventions that reduce birth weight, such as placental embolization. Finally, in rats and humans, normal levels of placental 11bHSD2 are highly variable and correlate with weight of neonates.

The mechanisms by which fetal glucocorticoid excess leads to adult hypertension are controversial. It has been suggested that even without fetal growth retardation, there is altered nephrogenesis with lower nephron numbers, tubular disruption and glomerulointerstitial fibrosis in the adult offspring, and that glomerulosclerosis is more important than reduction of nephron number. In contrast, data by others suggest that glucocorticoid-induced low birth weight is more important than effects on 11bHSD for development of hypertension, and that the latter is not clearly related to fetal renal abnormalities. Alternative explanations include altered expression of angiotensinogen and angiotensin receptors in the kidney and central nervous system of the offspring (although the circulating renin-angiotensin system is unaffected), vascular hypersensitivity to vasoconstrictors, increased expression of vascular smooth muscle contractile proteins, and controversial results on decreased expression of nitric oxide synthase.

Programming of metabolic abnormalities such as insulin resistance, and reduced insulin content of pancreatic beta cells by glucocorticoids may contribute to diabetes and the hypertension of the metabolic syndrome. These effects are gender specific and can be blocked by concomitant stimulation of 11bHSD by leptin, indicating regulation of the effects of fetal exposure to glucocorticoids by this peptide.[44]

In humans, glucocorticoid programming may act via a permanently imprinted change in the adult pattern of expression of the glucocorticoid receptor via actions on its promoter,[45] although this effect is not present in other species. Regardless of its mechanism, low birth weight in humans is associated with higher blood pressure, glucose intolerance and higher rates of diabetes in childhood and adulthood, and also with higher plasma cortisol levels throughout adult life. Even when given prenatally, that is, late in pregnancy, glucocorticoids lead to higher systolic and diastolic blood pressures as early as age 14.[46]

Glucocorticoids, essential hypertension, and the metabolic syndrome

Studies in rodent models for essential hypertension or the metabolic syndrome suggest that there may be a role for glucocorticoids in these conditions in humans. The hypertension of SHR, a rat strain with increased expression of vascular endothelial glucocorticoid receptors,[47] is prevented by adrenalectomy and restored by glucocorticoids, not mineralocorticoids. In obese SHR, adrenalectomy prevents the hypertension and also the development of metabolic abnormalities and renal damage. Corticosterone increases blood pressure in lean Zucker rats, whereas mifepristone (glucocorticoid receptor antagonist) reduces it in obese rats of the strain, by effects unrelated to hyperinsulinemia or renin.

11bHSD2 mRNA and activity are reduced in DahlSS rats, a model for salt-sensitive essential hypertension, in which there is urinary excretion of inhibitors of 11bHSD2. This suggests that salt sensitivity of blood pressure may be mediated by glucocorticoid activation of mineralocorticoid receptors. Adipose tissue overexpression of 11bHSD1 in transgenic mice leads to abnormalities indistinguishable from those of the human metabolic syndrome, including insulin resistance, dyslipidemia, and salt-sensitive hypertension,[48] the latter associated with activation of the renin-angiotensin system and abnormalities of the renal distal tubular epithelium. Therefore, glucocorticoid effects on both isoforms of the 11bHSD shuttle may participate in salt-sensitive hypertension.

In humans with the metabolic syndrome, 11bHSD1 is overexpressed in adipocytes.[49] Transcriptional inhibition of this enzyme by PPAR-alpha agonists in the liver[50] and PPAR-gamma agonists[51] in adipose tissue may explain the improvement of metabolic abnormalities and modest antihypertensive effect of these agents. Consistent with this, metabolic abnormalities and early severe hypertension are present in rare patients with loss-of-function mutations of PPAR-gamma.[52] Also, a myocardial deficit of 11bHSD2, where this isoform is coexpressed with the mineralocorticoid receptor, may contribute to LV hypertrophy in essential hypertension, as suggested by the positive relationship between cortisol:cortisone ratios and LV mass in these patients.[53]

Hypercortisolism (urine free cortisol:creatinine ratios greater than two standard deviations above those of normal subjects) may also play a role in 20% of essential hypertensive patients, who are usually salt sensitive with low PRA and serum aldosterone. This is supported by negative correlations between urine cortisol and both PRA and aldosterone in unselected hypertensive patients, suggesting that subtle hypercortisolism may play a role in the pathogenesis of low-renin essential hypertension.[54] Finally, increased affinity of glucocorticoid receptors for cortisol has been demonstrated with a dermal vasoconstriction assay in patients with essential hypertension and the metabolic syndrome.

Mineralocorticoid mechanisms in hypertension of glucocorticoid-excess states

Mineralocorticoid and glucocorticoid mechanisms are very different but the former may participate in diseases primarily characterized by glucocorticoid excess. Severe hypokalemia, metabolic alkalosis, or therapeutic responses

to spironolactone, which are not common in pure glucocorticoid hypertension, may become prominent clinical features if there is excess mineralocorticoid activity. The steroid responsible for the latter may actually be cortisol itself, when the catalytic capacity of 11bHSD2 (close to saturation at the physiologic range) is surpassed by very high cortisol levels, or when the activity of the enzyme is impaired.

Familial glucocorticoid resistance due to mutations in the ligand-binding domain of the glucocorticoid receptor,[55] is an example of the former situation. It leads to feedback stimulation of the hypothalamo-pituitary-adrenal axis and exaggerated secretion of cortisol. However, manifestations of glucocorticoid excess are absent because of the receptor abnormality. Symptoms relate to hypermineralocorticism produced by saturation of 11bHSD2 by high levels of cortisol and hyperandrogenism owing to ACTH stimulation of the adrenal gland.

Examples of impaired activity of 11bHSD2 include the syndrome of apparent mineralocorticoid excess (loss-of-function mutations of 11bHSD2), and inhibition of this enzyme by use of licorice or by therapy with carbenoxolone. These entities are best regarded as differential diagnoses of primary hyperaldosteronism, since the abnormality is entirely linked to aberrant activation of the mineralocorticoid receptor. In ectopic Cushing's syndrome, high levels of ACTH and cortisol are responsible for both the glucocorticoid and mineralocorticoid clinical features, via saturation of 11bHSD2, which is worsened by diminished A-ring reduction and turnover of cortisol. A negative correlation between cortisol:cortisone ratios and serum potassium proves that this mechanism is responsible for the hypokalemia of ectopic Cushing's syndrome.

It has been argued that the same mechanism plays a role, albeit of much lesser magnitude, in all forms of endogenous Cushing's disease because ACTH-stimulated cortisol:cortisone ratios in these patients are higher than in normal subjects. Whatever the mechanism for this subtle deficiency of 11bHSD2 activity, it is independent of ACTH, because it is observed in both Cushing's disease and adrenal Cushing's syndrome.

Mineralocorticoids such as aldosterone and 18-oxo steroids are usually not hypersecreted in pituitary Cushing's disease. However, there have been isolated reports of hypersecretion of desoxycorticosterone and of 18-oxo-cortisol with increased 18-oxo:cortisol and 18-oxo:aldosterone ratios, compared to normal subjects. The reason for the former is not clear. The latter may reflect increased cortisol supply to adrenal 18-hydroxylase.

In adrenal Cushing's syndrome, a whole host of different mineralocorticoids can be secreted, including 16-β-hydroxydehydroepiandrosterone, 19-nor-desoxycorticosterone, deoxycorticosterone, aldosterone, and combinations. In all cases but that of aldosterone, the secretion of this steroid is suppressed. Plasma renin activity is sometimes not inhibited, probably due to concomitant stimulation of liver angiotensinogen by cortisol.

Effects of glucocorticoids on ion pumps and transporters

Glucocorticoids affect the function of many cation transporters. Effects on vascular smooth muscle transport may modify vascular reactivity to vasoconstrictors. Those on renal transport of sodium may determine changes in systemic hemodynamics via changes in salt balance. We will review the relevance of these actions for changes in salt balance and hemodynamics in human glucocorticoid hypertension. A scheme of the major actions of gluco- corticoids on transporters throughout the nephron is provided in Figure 69–7.

Renal tubular Na⁺/H⁺ exchanger

Glucocorticoids increase the rate of Na^+-dependent H^+ efflux in acid-loaded proximal tubular cells and that of Na^+ entry in normal-pH, sodium-depleted isolated renal cells. Concomitant stimulation of the basolateral $Na^+/CO3H^-$ transporter (NCB-1) contributes to the overall increase in proximal tubular bicarbonate reabsorption by glucocorticoids. Kinetic studies indicate that the effect on Na^+/H^+ exchange is mediated by increased number of exchangers (Vmax) without change in affinity (Km). Of the four known isoforms (NHE-1 to -4), glucocorticoids stimulate the apical, amiloride-resistant NHE-3 (as opposed to aldosterone effects on NHE-2). Stimulation of basolateral amiloride-sensitive NHE-1 is controversial. Acute transport effects occur before increases in NHE-3 mRNA, indicating enhanced trafficking to the apical mem- brane,[56] or enhanced translational efficiency of NHE-3 mRNA. Increased trafficking is mediated by glucocorticoid- stimulated transcription of serum and glucocorticoid induced kinase-1 (SGK1), which after interaction with the regulatory protein NHERF2 phosphorylates a conserved Ser663 of NHE-3.[57,58] Mutations of this site and use of a "dead" kinase abolish NHE-3 trafficking. Chronic stimu- lation of NHE-3 by glucocorticoids is due to enhanced transcription, mediated by an interaction between bound glucocorticoid receptors and cis-acting elements of the NHE-3 gene. Neither turnover rate of NHE-3 mRNA nor endocytic retrieval of the transporter from the membrane[56] is affected by glucocorticoids.

In whole animals, natriuresis may occur despite fourfold stimulation of cortical NHE-3 mRNA by glucocorticoids, as if systemic factors (e.g., renal hemodynamics) may be more important in determining overall sodium excretion. Also, ACTH inhibits NHE-3 expression, suggesting that Na^+/H^+ exchange of Cushing's disease may be the net

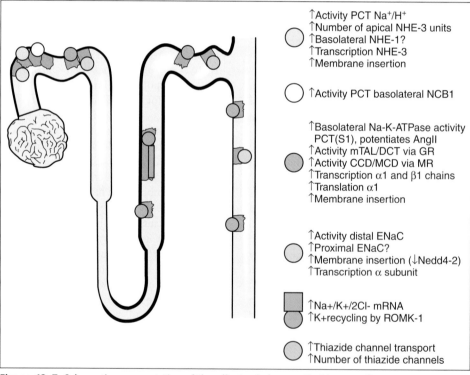

Figure 69–7. Schematic representation of the effects of glucocorticoids on sodium transporters throughout the nephron. The transporters are color coded and their location in the basolateral or apical membrane is depicted. The major actions of glucocorticoids are described on the right. A detailed description of these effects appears in the text. CCD and MCD, cortical and medullary collecting ducts; DCT, distal convoluted tubule; ENaC, epithelial sodium channel; GR, glucocorticoid receptor; MR, mineralocorticoid receptor; mTAL, medullary thick ascending limb of Henle; Na+/K+/2Cl-, the mTAL cotransporter; NCB1, sodium bicarbonate transporter; Nedd4-2, a protein involved in ubiquitination steps for removal of ENaC from the membrane; NHE-1 and -3 designate isoforms of the proximal Na+/H+ exchanger; PCT and PCT(S1), proximal convoluted tubule and its S1 segment; ROM-K1, mTAL cellular potassium channel that recycles K+ to the lumen.

result of opposing effects of cortisol and ACTH. In normotensive humans, dexamethasone inhibits Na^+/H^+ exchange activity in lymphocytes, via activation of glucocorticoid receptors, whereas in patients with Cushing's disease and adrenal Cushing's syndrome, Na^+/H^+ activity is spontaneously increased in mononuclear leukocytes. Therefore, the role of Na^+/H^+ exchange in human glucocorticoid hypertension remains to be settled.

Renal tubular Na-K-ATPase

Glucocorticoids and mineralocorticoids stimulate the function of renal Na-K-ATPase—the major basolateral sodium transporter across all segments of the nephron—in isolated tubules and cultured tubular cells, that is, independent of hemodynamic effects or renal sodium load.

Transcriptional mechanisms had been suspected because specific receptor antagonists prevent hydrocortisone activation of Na-K-ATPase. They were confirmed by demonstration of an interaction between bound nuclear glucocorticoid receptors and specific oligonucleotide sequences in the genes for the two human subunit isoforms (alpha-1 and beta-1) that constitute the renal heterodimeric Na^+ pump. A combined mineralocorticoid and glucocorticoid receptor responsive element in these sequences has been confirmed by their ability to confer mineralocorticoid and glucocorticoid activation to heterologous promoters.

Nontranscriptional mechanisms had also been suspected because glucocorticoid-stimulated Na-K-ATPase activity does not correlate with abundance of mRNA subunits and is inhibited by blockers of protein synthesis. It is now known that glucocorticoids increase translation efficiency of rat mRNA for alpha (not beta) subunit isoforms, without intervention of the glucocorticoid receptor. In contrast, there is no effect of glucocorticoids on mRNA stability. Finally, concomitant with increased biosynthesis, glucocorticoids augment insertion of functional pumps in the basolateral membrane, independent of the presence of active Na^+ transport. Experiments in xenopus oocytes suggest that SGKs may be involved in this step, as they are in the trafficking of NHE-3.[59]

Nephron-segment specificity for the stimulatory actions of mineralocorticoids and glucocorticoids on Na-K-ATPase has been shown in experiments with separate steroid replacement of adrenalectomized animals. Glucocorticoids stimulate activity of this enzyme in the S1 convoluted segment of the proximal tubule but not in the straight, S2, and S3 segments. Stimulatory effects of dexamethasone at the medullary thick ascending limb and the distal convoluted tubule are not blocked by spironolactone, whereas those on cortical and medullary collecting ducts are, as if in the latter segments dexamethasone activates the mineralocorticoid receptor.

In humans, erythrocyte 86-rubidium uptake, a measure of Na-K-ATPase activity, is increased by ACTH and synthetic glucocorticoids. The latter also increase synthesis of alpha subunit mRNA (alpha-2) and total pump pool size in skeletal muscle.[60] In patients with Cushing's syndrome, Na-K-ATPase activity of erythrocyte ghosts is spontaneously increased, and greater than those in essential hypertension, renal disease, and primary hyperaldosteronism.

In contrast to its inhibitory effect on NHE-3, ACTH increases ouabain-sensitive Na^+ transport, similar to glucocorticoids.[61] Despite this, and despite the potent stimulatory effect of synthetic or endogenous glucocorticoids on renal Na-K-ATPase, the baseline net proximal tubular reabsorption of Na^+ is not much increased by glucocorticoid excess. The effect of glucocorticoids may be much more important in potentiating the action of other substances that increase proximal tubular Na^+ reabsorption, such as angiotensin II,[62] thus exerting an indirect effect on blood pressure regulation by this mechanism.

Loop of Henle, distal nephron, and the epithelial sodium channel

There are very few studies about effects of glucocorticoids on the Na-K-2Cl cotransporter of the medullary thick ascending limb of the loop of Henle. Dexamethasone increases its mRNA and protein contents in the rat, in a glucocorticoid receptor–dependent manner and concomitant with increased cotransport activity. This action may be more important for acid-base balance ($NH4^+$ cotransport) than for net sodium reabsorption. Glucocorticoids also simulate activity of ROMK1, the K^+ channel that recycles luminal K^+ to the cells of the thick ascending limb, via the same interaction between SGK1 and NHERF2 that participates in stimulation of NHE-3.[57] Recycling of K^+ by ROMK1 is indispensable for the functioning of Na-K-2Cl. Therefore, stimulation of the latter by glucocorticoids may be due to the ROMK1 effect. Direct stimulation of Na-K-2Cl transport by dexamethasone has been shown in trabecular meshwork cells of the eye, an effect that may be linked to ophthalmologic complications of glucocorticoid therapy, such as glaucoma.

An additional effect of glucocorticoids in the distal nephron is to increase binding of (3H)-metolazone, that is, to increase the density of thiazide channels. This may contribute to enhanced sodium reabsorption in the distal convoluted tubule.

The most important distal Na^+ transporter is the epithelial sodium channel (ENaC), an amiloride-sensitive, heterotrimeric (alpha, beta, and gamma subunits) protein that is the major effector of aldosterone action in the kidney but is also expressed in many other epithelia. Activated glucocorticoid receptors augment transcription of the human alpha subunit chain by interacting with a glucocorticoid-responsive element in the 5′-flanking region of the gene.[63] In addition, transcriptional stimulation of SGK1 by glucocorticoids interferes with a ubiquitin ligase (Nedd4-2) that removes channels from the mouse collecting duct membranes for proteasome processing.[64] Hence, glucocorticoids also increase channel activity by increasing their number in the membrane.

In intestinal and airway/alveolar epithelia,[65] glucocorticoid-induced ENaC transport is associated with transcription of its inducible beta and gamma subunits, while the alpha chain is constitutively activated and less subject to regulation. ENaC is also regulated by glucocorticoids in ocular ciliary and semicircular canal duct epithelia, which may be important to explain some of their therapeutic actions.

In the kidney, glucocorticoid stimulation of ENaC is associated with increased transcription of the alpha subunit[63,66] and post-translational mechanisms related to transcriptional stimulation of SGK1.[67] Most studies of transport activity have been conducted in tissues or cells representing the distal nephron, but there is also evidence for glucocorticoid-stimulation of a proximal tubular ENaC. As opposed to the studies on airway epithelium, conducted with human cells, there is no clear evidence that effects of glucocorticoids on renal ENaC play a role in the hypertension of Cushing's syndrome.

Glucocorticoids and transport abnormalities in vascular smooth muscle

Dexamethasone increases Ca^{2+} influx in isolated vascular smooth muscle cells and in aortic rings of rabbits made hypertensive by its *in vivo* administration. *In vitro* effects occur in minutes, are blocked by glucocorticoid but not mineralocorticoid receptor antagonists, and also by nifedipine. Binding experiments indicate that increased Ca^{2+} influx is mediated by the increased number of high-affinity, dihydropyridine-sensitive, membrane calcium channels. In contrast, Ca^{2+} efflux is halved by dexamethasone and aldosterone in aortic myocytes, the action of the former being 100-fold more potent. The effect is due to transcriptional inhibition of the Na^+/Ca^{2+} exchanger, with 90% reduction of its mRNA.

Dexamethasone doubles 22-Na^+ incorporation into vascular smooth muscle cells, an action that is blocked by the competitive glucocorticoid receptor antagonist RU 486 and requires protein synthesis, suggesting a genomic mechanism. Transport may be via the Na^+/H^+ exchanger because hydrocortisone doubles the rate of recovery of smooth muscle intracellular pH following acidification, with increased Vmax (but no change in Km) for this exchanger. Smooth muscle synthesis of mRNA and protein is involved, as proved by blockade of the effect with actinomycin D and cycloheximide. Vascular smooth muscle Na-K-ATPase activity is also increased by glucocorticoids *in vitro*, that is, independent of blood pressure. The effect may be mediated by glucocorticoid-stimulated synthesis of mRNA and protein for alpha- and beta-subunit isoforms, as shown in skeletal muscle, where glucocorticoids increase tritiated ouabain binding.

In summary, exaggerated intracellular Ca^{2+} stores, via both increased Ca^{2+} influx and decreased Ca^{2+} efflux, and alterations in vascular smooth muscle Na^+ transport, may account for vascular hyperresponsiveness to vasoconstrictor stimuli in Cushing's syndrome, an issue that will be discussed further below.

Effects of ACTH and glucocorticoids on salt and water metabolism, plasma volume, and systemic and regional hemodynamics

Despite almost uniform stimulation of sodium reabsorption by nephron transporters, the effects of ACTH and glucocorticoids on salt balance in the whole animal are not straightforward. The synthetic glucocorticoids increase natriuresis and contract plasma volume in animals and humans, an effect that has been exploited for the therapy of refractory edematous states (Figure 69–8, left). Natriuresis can be blocked by glucocorticoid but not mineralocorticoid receptor antagonists, and is associated with activation of the renal dopamine system and renal vasodilation.[68] Increases in single nephron plasma flow and glomerular filtration rate in methylprednisolone-hypertensive rats are pronounced enough to accelerate the progression of proteinuria and glomerular sclerosis in models of partial renal ablation.[69]

ACTH increases water and salt intake in most species, including humans.[70] The mechanism does not involve the brain renin-angiotensin system. A mix of glucocorticoids and mineralocorticoids is required to reproduce the effect of ACTH, which is usually associated with hypernatremia.[70,71] Hence, ACTH-induced mineralocorticoid activity seems to play a role.

Effects of ACTH on renal sodium handling are species dependent. Increased salt intake may contribute to ACTH-induced natriuresis despite stimulation of nephron sodium transporters. However, this does not explain why ACTH natriuresis is only observed in rats, rabbits, and dogs.[71] The reason is the different magnitude of pressure natriuresis among species (Figure 69–8, right). In ACTH-hypertensive dogs, servo-controlling renal arterial pressure to keep it in the normal range leads to reversal of sodium losses and unmasking of ACTH-induced salt and water retention.[72] Pressure natriuresis is such an important determinant of the renal action of ACTH that this peptide does not produce hypertension in the dog, unless salt excretion is impaired by other means.[71]

In contrast, ACTH produces sodium retention in sheep and humans.[70] In sheep, the effect is transient, whereas in humans it is sustained and reproduced by cortisol (albeit of lesser magnitude). Therefore, normotensive and hypertensive subjects develop plasma and extracellular fluid volume expansion,[73] and have increased total exchangeable sodium when given ACTH. These changes trigger release of atrial natriuretic peptide and inhibition of plasma renin activity, even during salt depletion. Moreover, plasma volume expansion is exaggerated by glucocorticoid-induced fluid shifts from the intra- to the extra-cellular compartment,[74] owing to increased Na-K-ATPase activity. However, plasma volume is increased in some[75] but not all patients[76] with Cushing's syndrome, perhaps due to differences in the severity of blood pressure elevation and consequent pressure natriuresis.

The hemodynamic pattern of glucocorticoid hypertension is similar in all species, consisting of increased cardiac output and normal total peripheral resistance. High cardiac output is initially caused by faster heart rate, but later by increased stroke volume. It precedes elevation of blood pressure, indicating transient compensatory vasodilation. When total peripheral resistance returns to normal, hypertension develops. Loss of the initial compensatory vasodilation can be prevented by pretreating ACTH-hypertensive sheep with either nisoldipine or minoxidil, indicating that recovery of vascular tone is not calcium dependent. If cardiac output is reduced to normal by atenolol or dietary potassium supplementation, blood

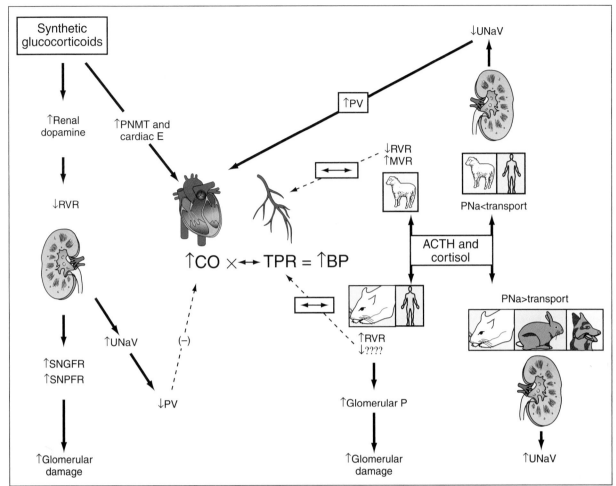

Figure 69–8. The figure illustrates differences in renal sodium handling, renal hemodynamics, and plasma volume produced by synthetic versus endogenous glucocorticoids and ACTH. The actions of the latter on the kidney are species specific, depending on the gain of the pressure–natriuresis mechanism (PNa). Despite these differences, the systemic hemodynamic pattern of the hypertension is common to all situations (high CO, and normal TPR). Question marks represent an unknown vascular bed that must sustain vasodilation to offset renal vasoconstriction in rat and humans, for maintenance of normal TPR. For a detailed explanation of these mechanisms, see text. BP, blood pressure; CO, cardiac output; E, epinephrine; MVR, mesenteric vascular resistance; P, capillary pressure; PNMT, phenylethanolamine N-methyltransferase; PV, plasma volume; RVR, renal vascular resistance; SNGFR, single nephron glomerular filtration rate; SNPFR, single nephron plasma flow rate; TPR, total peripheral resistance; UNaV, natriuresis.

pressure remains elevated. This indicates a shift to the hemodynamic pattern of normal cardiac output with high total peripheral resistance, suggesting resetting of blood pressure control to higher values. These observations explain why the hemodynamics of human glucocorticoid hypertension may vary from a pattern of increased cardiac output with normal total peripheral resistance[73] to exactly the opposite,[77] or a combined increase in cardiac output and vasoconstriction.[75]

Although total peripheral resistance is normal, regional hemodynamic changes vary among species (Figure 69–8, right). In sheep, ACTH and combinations of steroids are renal and skeletal muscle vasodilators. Total peripheral resistance is unaltered because mesenteric vasoconstriction offsets these changes, contributing to the establishment of high cardiac output hypertension. In contrast, ACTH and cortisol are renal vasoconstrictors in rats and humans. In rats, cortisol participates in the physiologic

renal vasoconstrictor response to salt-depletion. Their renal vasoconstrictor response to ACTH is prevented by L-arginine and reversed by ramipril, indicating participation of the nitric oxide and renin-angiotensin systems. Reduction of cardiac output by atenolol and decreased total peripheral resistance by minoxidil do not fully restore blood pressure to normal, whereas normalization of renal (but not total) peripheral resistance by ramipril corrects the hypertension. This observation supports a major role for renal vasoconstriction in glucocorticoid-induced hypertension in rats. Increased renal vascular resistance and reduced renal blood flow also occur in normal humans given ACTH or cortisol, even if the renal vasculature is preconstricted by salt depletion. Changes are more prominent in postglomerular vessels, with elevated glomerular filtration rate and filtration fraction. The vascular bed that offsets renal vasoconstriction and maintains normal total peripheral resistance in humans or rats is not known.

It can be concluded that ACTH and all glucocorticoids have the potential for the production of progressive glomerular dysfunction, either via glomerular hyperfiltration when they are renal vasodilators, or via glomerular hypertension when they are predominantly vasoconstrictors of the postglomerular vasculature.

Effects of glucocorticoids on vasoactive systems

A major reason by which the mechanisms of glucocorticoid-induced blood pressure elevation is not fully understood, is that the actions of these agents on vasoactive systems differ if studied in cells, tissues, whole animals, or humans. We will review the findings that are relevant for understanding of human glucocorticoid hypertension. Because of their complexity, an extensive but focused summary is provided in Table 69–3.

Renin-angiotensin system

Glucocorticoids increase synthesis of angiotensinogen. The effect is transcriptional, with increased mRNA in liver and other tissues,[78] can be inhibited by actinomycin D, and is mimicked by estrogens, but not by mineralocorticoids. Conversely, adrenalectomy reduces angiotensinogen mRNA and this can be prevented with a glucocorticoid receptor agonist.

In methylprednisolone-hypertensive rats, increased angiotensinogen leads to higher plasma renin concentration and activity, which account for blood pressure response to the angiotensin receptor blocker saralasin.[79] Once salt depleted, activation of the renin-angiotensin system is no longer different from that of normal salt-depleted rats and the blood pressure response to captopril is diminished. Because there is no change in circulating or tissue angiotensin-converting enzyme,[80] the data suggests a defect in non–angiotensin-mediated effects of the converting enzyme inhibitor during salt depletion. Lesions of the AV3V region prevent or improve blood pressure elevation and abolish the responses to saralasin and captopril,[81] indicating a role for the central nervous system in the control of the renin-dependent component of the hypertension of this model.

Other prohypertensive effects of the renin-angiotensin system include ACTH downregulation of the vasodilatory angiotensin AT2 receptor in arteries of sheep, dexamethasone-induction of angiotensin-converting enzyme in vascular smooth muscle cells, and increased AT1 receptor number in vessels of SHR given a glucocorticoid agonist, but their role in glucocorticoid hypertension is not known.

In humans, glucocorticoid-induced synthesis of angiotensinogen is associated with protein heterogeneity that may affect the kinetics of the renin-substrate reaction.[82] Increased angiotensin II in Cushing's syndrome, which correlates with serum cortisol, may be the result of this effect, because plasma renin activity is usually normal (although its response to salt depletion may be exaggerated). In the few cases in which plasma renin is suppressed, there is usually concomitant excess mineralocorticoid activity. The antihypertensive effect of saralasin has been used as a test of renin-dependency of the hypertension of Cushing's syndrome and was found to be significant in some but not all patients.

Arginine vasopressin

Dexamethasone doubles the density of arginine vasopressin (AVP) V1a receptors in vascular smooth muscle cells by increasing stability of its mRNA.[83] However, a vasopressor role for AVP in states of glucocorticoid excess is unlikely because these steroids actually blunt osmotic and nonosmotic release of AVP, inhibiting its mRNA expression in the parvocellular paraventricular nucleus. Methylprednisolone-induced hypertension is of the same magnitude in Brattleboro as in Wistar rats. Also, a nonpeptide V1a receptor antagonist fails to reduce blood pressure in rats with ACTH hypertension.[84] Both observations confirm lack of a vasoconstrictor role for AVP in glucocorticoid hypertension.

Stimulation of ACTH release by vasopressin is exerted via V1b (also called V3) receptors in corticotrophs. These receptors are overexpressed in ACTH-secreting pituitary adenomas and bronchial carcinoids.[85] Although it is not clear how much AVP contributes to secretion of ACTH by these tumors, there is great interest in the recent development of oxindole compounds that are specific blockers for V1b receptors.[86] Direct stimulation of cortisol by AVP occurs in cases of ACTH-independent macronodular adrenal hyperplasia with "illicit" expression of V1a receptors. It is now known that these receptors are expressed in normal adrenal cortex and overexpressed in compact cells of adrenal adenomas and less commonly carcinomas.[85] Therefore, V1a receptor antagonists could attenuate hypercortisolism in these patients, as they do in macronodular adrenal hyperplasia.[87]

Endothelin system

Glucocorticoids increase the pre-pro-endothelin-1 gene transcription rate in rat vessels and vascular smooth muscle cells, acting on their receptors. Release of endothelin-1 from vascular smooth muscle, not endothelium, is enhanced. Moreover, in the kidney, they downregulate expression of the natriuretic ETb receptor. Although these are prohypertensive actions, glucocorticoids also decrease ETa receptor mRNA and binding sites in vascular smooth muscle cells of normal rats and SHR.

In humans, the evidence is predominantly against a role for endothelin-1 in glucocorticoid hypertension. Increased production of this peptide by human endothelial cells exposed to glycyrrhizic acid (an inhibitor of 11bHSD2) is most likely a mineralocorticoid effect of the corticosterone employed in these experiments.[88] In contrast, dexamethasone decreases release of endothelin-1 by human monocytes, baseline and cytokine-stimulated pre-pro-endothelin-1 mRNA expression in a pulmonary epithelial cell line, and the number of ETa receptors in endothelium derived from human brain microvessels.

Consistent with the information above, ETa receptor blockers prevent hypertension in glycyrrhizic acid-induced,[88] but not ACTH hypertension in the rat. There are no data on these receptor blockers in glucocorticoid hypertension in humans.

SUMMARY OF ACTIONS OF GLUCOCORTICOIDS ON VASOACTIVE SYSTEMS

Vasoactive System	Gene and Cell Effects	Actions in experimental animals	Role in experimental hypertension	Findings in humans	Findings in Cushing's Syndrome	Relevance for therapy
RAS	↑ Transcription of AGTN gene	↑ AGTN, PRC and PRA, in MP-HTN rat	Captopril ↓ BP in MP-HTN rat	AGTN protein heterogeneity	Nl PRA, ↑ AGTN, ↑ AngII	ACE-inhibitors and losartan ↓ BP
	↑ IP3 by AngII in VSM	↑↓ Vascular sensitivity to AngII infusion				
	↑ VSMC/adrenal V1a receptors by ↑ mRNA stability		No ↓ MP-HTN in DI rat			V1b blockers for ↓ ACTH release?
AVP	↑ V1b pituitary receptors		No ↓ ACTH-HTN with V1 antagonist			
	↓ AVP release					
	↓ Hypothalamic AVP mRNA					
	↑IP3 by AVP in VSM					
ET	↑ Transcription PP-ET gene, ↑ ET1 release, ↓ ETa receptor in VSMC	No ↑ vascular sensitivity to ET1 in sheep ACTH-HTN	ETa blocker ↓ BP in licorice but not ACTH-HTN rats	Endothelial cells + licorice = ↑ ET1		Effect of ET antagonists?
	↓ ETb kidney receptor			Monocytes + dexa = ↓ET1		
	↓ Vascular sensitivity to ET1 in vitro					
PG	↓ COX-2 mRNA, ↓mRNA stability	↓ Renal but not VSM PGI2 in dexa-HTN rat and dog	No ↑ BP by indomethacin but ↓ BP by PGI2 in dexa-HTN dogs			
		↓ PGE2 in renal cells and urine but not in tissue of MP-HTN rat				
ANP	↑ Atrial synthesis and content	↑ Plasma levels and cGMP-action in ADX	↓ Plasma level in rat-dog HTN	↑ Function in Addison's	↑ Plasma levels (higher in GC therapy)	Effect of ANP analogs?
		↓ CGRP and cGMP in normal rat	↑ action in sheep HTN	↑ Plasma level but ↑ NEP in normal humans		
NO	↓ eNOS/iNOS expression	↓ Plasma NO2:NO3	No GC-HTN in eNOS knockout mice	↓ Transcription eNOS gene and ↓ mRNA stability in endothelial cells	↓ Urine NO2:NO3, but no ↑ with L-Arg	Effect of NO donors?
	↓ L-arginine availability	↓ Response to ACh	↓ BP by L-Arg in rat ACTH-HTN but not dexa-HTN	↓ NO2:NO3 and Ach responses but no ↓ BP with L-Arg in F-HTN		
	↓ THB4 synthesis					

SECONDARY HYPERTENSION : Cushing's Syndrome and Human Glucocorticoid Hypertension

Table continued

SUMMARY OF ACTIONS OF GLUCOCORTICOIDS ON VASOACTIVE SYSTEMS—CONT'D

Vasoactive System	Gene and Cell Effects	Actions in experimental animals	Role in experimental hypertension	Findings in humans	Findings in Cushing's Syndrome	Relevance for therapy
OXS	↑ XO in kidney cells	Allopurinol ↓ XO in rat dexa-HTN but not iso-prostanes in ACTH-HTN	Allopurinol ↓ BP in rat dexa-HTN but not ACTH-HTN	Endothelial cells: ↑ XO, NADPH and H2O2, OO-NO-	↑ FVR, responsive to vitC in GC therapy	Effect of antioxidants?
	↑↓ Effects on tissue antioxidant enzymes	Tempol does not ↓ isoprostanes in either	Tempol ↓ BP in both rat dexa- and ACTH-HTN	VSMC: ↓ ROS generation	↑ XO in RA	
					↑ Isoprostanes with topical but ↓ with inhaled GCs	
VEGF	GC ↓ mRNA and protein by ↑ mRNA turnover			↑ Plasma levels in EH correlate with TOD	↑ Expression in adrenal tumors	Prevention of TOD with anti VEGF mAbs?
	ACTH ↑ expression in adrenal cells				↑ Plasma levels in adrenal and pituitary Cushing's > than in EH	Future receptor antagonists?
SNS	↓ DBH and TH transcription, and ↑ cardiac PNMT	↑ Plasma NE + E and cardiac E	↓ BP by αCH3Tyr in rat dexa-HTN	↑ Plasma NE + E by ACTH	↓ Plasma NE + E, and responses to glucagon	Variable antihypertensive effect of antiadrenergic agents
		↑↓ BP effects on CNS	No ↓ BP with clonidine or renal denervation in sheep ACTH-HTN	Trimethaphan does not prevent ↑ BP by F	Normal NE:E adrenal vein ratio and E clearance	
		↓ Baroreflexes			Negative correlation plasma NE/UFC	
					↑ Response to NE but not PE	
					↑ Responses to AngII	

αCH3Tyr, alphamethyltyrosine; ACE, angiotensin-converting enzyme; ACTH, adrenocorticotropin; ADX, adrenalectomized; AGTN, angiotensinogen; AngII, angiotensin II; ANP, atrial natriuretic peptide; AVP, arginine vasopressin; BP, blood pressure; CGRP, calcitonin gene-related peptide; CNS, central nervous system; COX-2, cyclooxygenase isoform 2; DBH, dopamine-beta-hydroxylase; dexa, dexamethasone; DI, diabetes insipidus; E, epinephrine; EH, essential hypertension; eNOS and iNOS, endothelial and inducible nitric oxide synthases; ET, endothelin; ETa and ETb, endothelin receptor types; F, cortisol; FVR, forearm vascular resistance; GC, glucocorticoids; H2O2, hydrogen peroxide; HTN, hypertension; IP3, inositol-3-phosphate; L-Arg, l-arginine; MP, methylprednisolone; NADPH, nicotine adenine phosphate oxidase; NE, norepinephrine; NEP, neutral endopeptidases; NO, nitric oxide species; NO2:NO3, nitrite:nitrate ratio; OO-NO-, peroxynitrite; OXS, oxidative stress systems; PE, phenylephrine; PG, prostaglandins; PGE2, prostaglandin E2; PGI2, prostacyclin; PNMT, phenylethanolamine N-methyltransferase; PP-ET, pre-proendothelin; PRA, plasma renin activity; PRC, plasma renin concentration; RA, rheumatoid arthritis; RAS, renin-angiotensin system; ROS, reactive oxygen species; SNS, sympathetic nervous system; THB4, tetrahydrobiopterin; TH, tyrosine hydroxylase; TOD, target-organ damage; UFC, urine free cortisol; V1a and V1b, vasopressin receptor types; VEGF, vascular endothelial growth factor; VSM, vascular smooth muscle; VSMC, VSM cells; XO, xanthine oxidase.

Table 69–3. Summary of Actions of Glucocorticoids on Vasoactive Systems

Prostaglandins and the kallikrein-kinin system

Glucocorticoids tonically inhibit expression of COX-2 by destabilizing its mRNA,[89] but it is not clear whether decreased availability of vasodilatory natriuretic prostaglandins participates in glucocorticoid hypertension. Renal prostacyclin is markedly inhibited by dexamethasone in rats and dogs, but glucocorticoids do not affect baseline levels of prostacyclin in vascular smooth muscle. These agents blunt the effect of some, but not all stimuli for prostacyclin synthesis in vascular smooth muscle, suggesting that their action is mediated by phospholipase A2, not inhibition of COX.

Glucocorticoids inhibit synthesis of PGE2 in renomedullary interstitial, tubular, and mesangial cells, but are paradoxically unable to normalize increased renal PGE2 produced by adrenalectomy, and increase its content in normal renal papillae. Urine excretion of PGE2 is unaltered in methylprednisolone-induced hypertension in rats but decreased in dexamethasone-treated dogs. In the latter, infusion of prostacyclin reduces blood pressure, whereas indomethacin does not worsen the hypertension, suggesting that inhibition of endogenous prostaglandins plays a major role. In contrast, infusion of prostacyclin does not improve ACTH hypertension in sheep, despite the fact that these animals have increased vascular sensitivity to prostaglandins—a compensatory, albeit ineffectual, mechanism to the hypertension.

Analogous results have been described for the kallikrein-kinin system. Glucocorticoids inhibit the action of bradykinin on its B1 receptor in isolated blood vessels, and decrease kallikrein excretion in Dahl rats and dogs. In the latter, infusion of bradykinin reduces blood pressure, whereas a bradykinin receptor antagonist does not worsen the hypertension, suggesting that inhibition of renal kallikrein by glucocorticoids plays a role in blood pressure elevation. However, the antihypertensive effect of trandolapril in human Cushing's disease is associated with paradoxical further reduction of urine kallikrein excretion.[90]

Therefore, it is not clearly established that a deficiency in the action of these two vasodilatory natriuretic systems plays a major role in glucocorticoid hypertension.

Natriuretic peptides and ouabain

Replacement of glucocorticoids in adrenalectomized animals stimulates atrial synthesis, increases plasma levels, and restores impaired function (increased diuresis, natriuresis, and urinary cyclic GMP) of atrial natriuretic peptide (ANP) in response to water or salt loading. Glucocorticoid activation of ANP could be considered the positive limb of a feedback loop, because ANP inhibits adrenal production of glucocorticoids, not only aldosterone. In Addison's disease dexamethasone also restores impaired diuretic and natriuretic responses to infusion of human ANP.

However, in the absence of adrenal insufficiency, dexamethasone inhibits CGRP[91] (a physiologic stimulus for ANP release), blunts the stimulation of cyclic GMP by ANP in vascular smooth muscle of normal rats by acting on glucocorticoid receptors, and upregulates neutral endopeptidases that degrade ANP in vascular smooth muscle of normal humans in a dose-dependent, protein synthesis–dependent manner. The latter two effects may counter the actions of ANP, even if plasma levels in humans are increased by glucocorticoids as reported by others.[92] Therefore, inhibition of the action of natriuretic peptides might be a pathogenetic mechanism in glucocorticoid hypertension.

Plasma ANP is decreased in glucocorticoid-induced hypertension in the rat and dog, but its hemodynamic actions are enhanced in ACTH-induced hypertension in sheep, perhaps because of concomitant plasma volume expansion. In human Cushing's disease,[93] and more so in patients on chronic high-dose prednisone therapy,[93] plasma levels of ANP are markedly elevated, but infusions of the peptide produce half the expected urine cyclic GMP response, with consequent decreases in diuresis and natriuresis.[94] Infusion of nesiritide could provide more information on the role of atrial natriuretic peptides in the hypertension of Cushing's syndrome, but this has not been explored to date.

Endogenous ouabain-like compounds are increased in systemic and adrenal vein plasma of patients with Cushing's syndrome, although lack of change with adrenalectomy suggests an extra-adrenal origin. In a patient with ectopic Cushing's syndrome and a 40-fold elevation in the levels of a compound indistinguishable from authentic ouabain (by chromatography and binding properties), there was a direct correlation of its plasma concentration with the magnitude of blood pressure elevation during the course of the disease and therapy.[95] This suggests a compensatory response to plasma volume expansion that contributed to vasoconstriction via inhibition of vascular smooth muscle Na-K-ATPase.

Nitric oxide and erythropoietin

Glucocorticoids downregulate eNOS in many organs,[96] prevent expression of iNOS in response to endotoxin or cytokines (explaining their therapeutic effect in septic shock), decrease L-arginine availability in endothelial cells by downregulating amino acid transporters and impairing regeneration from citrulline, and reduce synthesis of tetrahydrobiopterin, a necessary cofactor for the action of eNOS, by inhibiting the enzyme GTP-cyclohydrolase.[97] These actions on the nitric oxide system account for decreased plasma nitrite:nitrate ratios, attenuation of relaxation responses to acetylcholine, equipotent hypertensive effects of dexamethasone and eNOS inhibitors, and lack of development of glucocorticoid hypertension in eNOS knockout mice.[96,98]

In ACTH and corticosterone hypertension of the rat, reduced kidney expression of iNOS and eNOS leads to increased renal vascular resistance and hypertension that can be prevented or ameliorated by L-arginine, lipopolysaccharide stimulation, or the NO donor isosorbide,[99] but not by tetrahydrobiopterin. The inhibitor N-nitro L-arginine blocks the beneficial effect of L-arginine. These data indicate a deficit in nitric oxide generation, not diminished L-arginine availability in these models. In contrast, in dexamethasone-induced hypertension in the rat, L-arginine does not improve blood pressure, despite increasing plasma nitrite:nitrate ratio, suggesting differences in the participation of the NOS system in ACTH versus synthetic steroid hypertension.

In human endothelial cells, activated glucocorticoid receptors inhibit eNOS by decreasing binding of the transcription factor GATA to the eNOS gene promoter and by impairing mRNA stability, both leading to diminished eNOS mRNA and protein.[98] Consistent with this, cortisol-induced hypertension in normal humans is associated with reduced plasma nitrite:nitrate concentration (without changes in arginine cellular uptake, plasma levels, or stimulation of endogenous eNOS inhibitors), and with impaired forearm vasodilator responses to acetylcholine, indistinguishable from those to NOS antagonists. However, L-arginine does not prevent cortisol-induced reduction of nitrite:nitrate ratios or blood pressure elevation,[100] indicating that there may be additional defects that preclude the normal actions of nitric oxide.

It has been speculated that erythropoietin may be responsible because cortisol increases its levels in humans,[101] and the vascular actions of erythropoietin are mediated by resistance to the actions of NO. However, data on ACTH hypertension in the rat do not support this speculation; in this model ACTH reduces erythropoietin levels, and the concentration of the renal hormone is inversely related to the magnitude of blood pressure elevation.[102]

There is only one report about the nitric oxide system in a patient with Cushing's syndrome. Urinary excretions of nitrate and nitrite were reduced and could not be corrected by L-arginine.[103] Therefore, the hypertension of the naturally occurring disease may have mechanisms similar to that of normal volunteers given cortisol.

Oxidative stress

Increased generation of oxygen radicals may impair nitric oxide vasodilatation by scavenging of nitric oxide and formation of peroxynitrite. Glucocorticoids activate xanthine oxidase in renal cell preparations but decrease its serum levels in patients with rheumatoid arthritis.[104] Allopurinol, an inhibitor of xanthine oxidase, reduces blood pressure and muscle levels of this enzyme in dexamethasone hypertensive rats,[105] but does not affect blood pressure or plasma isoprostanes in ACTH hypertension, in which the source of superoxide is NADPH oxidase.[106]

Actions of glucocorticoids on antioxidant enzymes are complex because they are tissue dependent. Renal tissue catalase, superoxide dismutase, glutathione peroxidase, and glutathione S-transferase are increased by glucocorticoids in rats, conferring protection against oxidative glomerular damage. In the heart *in vivo*, effects on antioxidant enzymes are opposite.[107] Effects on skeletal muscle superoxide dismutase and lymphoid tissue catalase depend on the organ studied. Moreover, in the same experiment in the liver, glucocorticoids concomitantly increase and decrease the contents of various antioxidant enzymes.[108] The superoxide dismutase mimetic tempol is able to prevent or ameliorate blood pressure in

dexamethasone and ACTH hypertension in rats, despite the various enzymes involved in generating oxygen radicals.[109,110] However, improvement of hypertension is not associated with reduction of isoprostane concentrations, making it unclear whether the antihypertensive effect of tempol is due to reduced oxidative stress.

The issue is not less complex in humans. Glucocorticoids increase hydrogen peroxide and peroxynitrite by stimulation of both NADPH and xanthine oxidase in human endothelial cells,[111] but they decrease generation of superoxide anion in response to several stimuli in vascular smooth muscle, an action mediated by decreased expression of p22 phox, a major subunit of NADPH oxidase.[112] The pro-oxidative endothelial effect seems to predominate, as assessed by decreased forearm dilatory responses to hyperemia (reversible with vitamin C) in patients treated with glucocorticoids.[111] Finally, there is evidence for both anti- and pro-oxidant effects in humans receiving chronic glucocorticoid therapy. For example, markers of oxidative stress are increased in patients receiving fluocinonide cream for the treatment of psoriasis,[113] whereas plasma isoprostanes and erythrocyte catalase decrease in those using glucocorticoid inhalers for the treatment of asthma.[114] Exploring a role for oxidative stress in human glucocorticoid hypertension in direct fashion will have to wait for the development of specific and effective antioxidant agents for human use, an achievement that has been elusive to date.

Vascular endothelial growth factor

Vascular endothelial growth factor (VEGF), a cytokine best known for its angiogenic and endothelial mitogenic effects, is also a powerful activator of the nitric oxide system in vascular tissues. VEGF stimulates nitric oxide release by human endothelial cells and rabbit vessels and relaxes dog coronary arteries by a mechanism enhanced by L-arginine and attenuated or abolished by inhibitors of nitric oxide synthase. Exaggerated VEGF-induced aortic relaxation in SHR is consistent with a deficient nitric oxide system in this rat strain. In whole animals, the beneficial coronary vasodilation produced by VEGF is nonetheless accompanied by severe hypotension associated with decreased cardiac output and total peripheral resistance, both of which are prevented by nitric oxide synthase inhibitors.[115]

Glucocorticoids dose dependently inhibit VEGF expression (mRNA and protein) by a nontranscriptional increase in VEGF mRNA turnover.[116] In nonvascular tissues, this effect decreases VEGF-induced vascular permeability, probably accounting for the beneficial effects of glucocorticoids in inflammatory cutaneous disorders,[116] asthma, diabetic retinopathy, and the edema that accompanies several types of brain tumors.

It is thus conceivable that glucocorticoid hypertension involves a deficit in VEGF-dependent vasodilation. Paradoxically, however, plasma VEGF levels are increased in essential hypertensive patients, and more so in those with hypertension due to Cushing's syndrome.[117] VEGF is expressed in normal adrenal fasciculata and glomerulosa cells and participates in terminal differentiation of the endothelium into the fenestrated phenotype that is characteristic of endocrine glands.[118] ACTH, in an action that is opposite to that of glucocorticoids, stimulates adrenal cell VEGF expression,[119] thus modulating the tight balance between steroid-secreting cells and their capillary vessels. Because VEGF is overexpressed in adrenal tumor cells,[120] this could be the source for increased levels of the peptide in Cushing's syndrome. However, VEGF plasma levels are equally increased in ACTH-dependent and -independent human hypercortisolism, which does not support this interpretation.[117] In adrenal carcinomas, the phenotype consists of overexpression of VEGF despite very low capillary density.[121] Therefore, it is conceivable that increased VEGF in hypertension (whether essential or in Cushing's syndrome) is a compensatory response to rarefaction of the microvasculature. Regardless of the mechanism of its increased plasma levels, VEGF may participate in target-organ damage of Cushing's syndrome via remodeling of atherosclerotic plaques. This is supported by observations in a large number of essential hypertensive patients, in whom VEGF correlated with cardiovascular risk factors and could be decreased by their successful therapy.[122]

Glucocorticoids and the autonomic nervous system

Glucocorticoids stimulate all major enzymes of the catecholamine biosynthetic pathway. Effects on adrenal medullary tyrosine hydroxylase include increased enzyme mRNA and activity, with augmented tissue and plasma concentrations of norepinephrine and epinephrine. The effect is transcriptional, via a glucocorticoid receptor responsive element in the tyrosine hydroxylase gene,[123] and functionally significant, as demonstrated by prevention of dexamethasone-induced hypertension by alpha-methyl-p-tyrosine.[124] Analogously, transcriptional stimulation of dopamine beta-hydroxylase mRNA by dexamethasone has been demonstrated in isolated cells. Stimulatory effects on cardiac phenylethanolamine N-methyltransferase (PNMT)—the enzyme that converts norepinephrine into epinephrine in adrenal and non-adrenal tissues—with consequent increased myocardial epinephrine, may explain increases in cardiac output despite plasma volume contraction in dexamethasone hypertension and play a role in hemodynamic responses to stress.[125]

In contrast, modulatory effects of glucocorticoids on central nervous system control of the circulation are varied. For example, pressor responses elicited by corticosterone in the rostral ventrolateral medulla are glucocorticoid receptor dependent, whereas those produced by dexamethasone in the nucleus tractus solitarius are not.[126] Moreover, dexamethasone is depressor when given into the cerebral ventricles.[127] Clonidine fails to inhibit ACTH hypertension in sheep as if brainstem alpha-2–mediated sympathetic inhibition were impaired in this model, which is consistent with previously demonstrated alpha-2 adrenoceptor hyperactivity in glucocorticoid hypertension. Blunting of baroreflexes in rats and sheep could contribute to glucocorticoid-induced hypertension. However, renal denervation does not prevent ACTH hyper-

tension in sheep, making it doubtful that abnormalities in baroreflex control of heart rate or renal sympathetic nerves play a major role.

In normal humans, ACTH increases norepinephrine and epinephrine concentration in the adrenal vein, as if there were a role for the pituitary hormone in regulation of adrenal medullary function. However, hemodynamic responses to mental stress are not altered by dexamethasone, suggesting that glucocorticoids may not be major regulators of overall autonomic function in response to usual stimuli.[128] In Cushing's syndrome, epinephrine: norepinephrine ratios in adrenal vein blood (a marker of PNMT activity) and the metabolic clearance rate of epinephrine are normal, while plasma catecholamines and their response to glucagon are diminished, suggesting that the adrenal medulla does not play a role in the hypertension. Also, neuropeptide Y levels are not different from those in controls, indicating that the direct vasoconstrictor effect of this peptide and its ability to enhance vascular responses to norepinephrine are not involved in the hypertension of Cushing's disease. Finally, there are two major observations against a significant participation of the autonomic nervous system in the hypertension of Cushing's disease: the ganglionic blocker trimethaphan does not prevent cortisol-induced hypertension in normal volunteers;[129] and in Cushing's syndrome, there is a negative correlation between plasma norepinephrine levels and urine free cortisol excretion.[130]

Glucocorticoids and vascular reactivity

Vascular smooth muscle glucocorticoid receptors mediate the transport actions discussed in a previous section and have also been implicated in vascular hypersensitivity to constrictor agents. For example, generation of inositol-triphosphate by angiotensin II and AVP in vascular smooth muscle cells is enhanced by dexamethasone, and prevented by glucocorticoid receptor blockers.

Whether there is vascular hyperreactivity in organ preparations or whole animals with glucocorticoid excess is less clear. Hypersensitivity to the constrictor action of endothelin-1 in sheep arteries[88] does not result in an endothelin pressor effect in ACTH hypertension. Increased pressor action of norepinephrine may be a mineralocorticoid effect of glucocorticoids, as suggested by experiments in 11bHSD2 knockout mice or humans given licorice or carbenoxolone. In methylprednisolone-induced hypertension in the rat, responses to exogenous angiotensin II depend on salt balance, that is, not on the steroid.[79,80]

Results are equally controversial in humans. Forearm vascular resistance after glucocorticoids may be increased[4] or unchanged.[131] The cold pressor test (a measure of adrenergic responsiveness) is not modified by dexamethasone,[132] whereas cutaneous vasoconstriction after topical cortisol or beclomethasone is increased in essential hypertensive patients.[133] In patients with Cushing's syndrome, hyperresponsiveness to exogenous norepinephrine infusion[134] and normal responses to phenylephrine[135] have both been reported. Angiotensin II infusions are equipressor in patients with Cushing's syndrome with normal plasma renin and in subjects with Conn's syndrome and renin suppression. This implies hyperreactivity in the former, since responses to exogenous angiotensin II should be inversely related to the prevailing level of activation of the endogenous renin-angiotensin system.[136] Finally, methylprednisolone improves myocardial function in experimental heart failure by increasing beta-adrenergic receptor density, without effect on isoproterenol-stimulated adenylyl cyclase activity,[137] whereas in patients with Cushing's syndrome, enhanced hemodynamic responses to isoproterenol are unrelated to adrenoceptor numbers and remain unexplained.[138]

TREATMENT OF CUSHING'S SYNDROME AND GLUCOCORTICOID HYPERTENSION

Pharmacologic therapy
Treatment of hypercortisolism

The primary treatment of Cushing's syndrome, discussed in the next section, is surgical. Therefore, medical therapy is reserved for incurable malignant disease, recurrences after transsphenoidal pituitary surgery, high surgical-risk patients, and transient management of severe hypertension or other manifestations of hypercortisolism to decrease surgical risk.

Hypercortisolism can be improved by blocking adrenal steroid synthesis, regulating release of ACTH by the pituitary gland, or targeting expression of aberrant receptors in tumors. Residual uncontrolled hypertension may require use of conventional antihypertensive agents.

Metyrapone and op'DDD, older inhibitors of steroid synthesis, are not much used any longer, although the former may still have a role in the management of ACTH-independent macronodular adrenal hyperplasia of the elderly.[139]

Aminoglutethimide is an anticonvulsant that blocks CYP450 hydroxylation steps in the conversion of cholesterol to pregnenolone, with consequent inhibition of cortisol, aldosterone, and androgens. It has been used in all forms of hypercortisolism but is more effective in adrenal (including carcinoma) and ectopic Cushing's syndrome. In pituitary Cushing's disease, it produces further stimulation of ACTH, which overcomes its inhibitory action. Its use may be combined with metyrapone.

Ketoconazole, an antifungal imidazole, diminishes cortisol secretion and action via decreased synthesis of cholesterol, inhibition of 11-β-hydroxylase, and partial blockade of the glucocorticoid receptor. After a few weeks of therapy, its effects are sustained in Cushing's disease. Its major drawback is the potential for liver toxicity, which requires periodic monitoring of laboratory tests. It may lead to adrenal insufficiency, requiring dose adjustments.

Mitotane inhibits steroid synthesis via actions on mitochondrial hydroxylases but also induces microsomal hydroxylases that alter the metabolism of 17-OH compounds. In addition, its metabolites are toxic to mitochondria, producing cell necrosis of the zonae reticularis and fasciculata. There is relative sparing of the glomerulosa, which explains the lack of need for mineralocorticoid

replacement even when cortisol secretion becomes subnormal. Finally, mitotane inhibits ACTH production, preventing its secretion in response to cortisol suppression. It is effective, combined with pituitary radiation, after failure of transsphenoidal surgery or when patients cannot undergo surgery. The necrotizing effect of mitotane makes it useful for the treatment of adrenal carcinoma. It is currently given as adjuvant therapy immediately after the surgery for the primary tumor[140] because it is unclear that it prolongs survival once metastases have occurred.

Mifepristone (RU-486), a specific antagonist of glucocorticoid receptors, is a substituted 19-norsteroid that improves the clinical manifestations of Cushing's syndrome, usually without changing ACTH or cortisol levels. However, ACTH of pituitary tumors may occasionally overcome the receptor blockade. It is approved in the United States as an antiprogestin agent to induce abortion. Experience in the treatment of Cushing's syndrome is limited, but it seems to be efficacious and devoid of major side effects.

Agents used to modulate release of ACTH in pituitary Cushing's disease include serotonin antagonists (cyproheptadine, ketanserin, and ritanserin), dopamine agonists (bromocriptine and cabergoline), the GABA agonist valproic acid, and somatostatin analogs of the octreotide family. In ACTH-independent adrenal macronodular hyperplasia, transient inhibition of cortisol secretion has been achieved with blockade of aberrant receptors for gastric inhibitory polypeptide (octreotide), catecholamines (propranolol), dopamine (cabergoline), LH (leuprolide), AVP (OPC-21268), and angiotensin II (candesartan). Finally, there is experimental evidence that retinoic acid[141] and the PPAR-gamma agonist rosiglitazone[142] inhibit ACTH secretion and have antiproliferative effects in cultured corticotrophs, but a role for these agents in the treatment of human disease is yet to be determined.

Antihypertensive agents

No systematic comparison of antihypertensive agents has been conducted in patients with Cushing's syndrome, probably because the focus is on the treatment of the primary disease. There are isolated reports on their use before surgery or for management of severe hypertension. Initially, central sympatholytic agents (e.g., clonidine) and beta-blockers were recommended. The latter were thought to have central nervous system actions because they reduced blood pressure in glucocorticoid hypertensive rats with excised renal medullae.[143] Use of diuretics was discouraged owing to their potential to increase the cardiovascular manifestations of adrenal insufficiency after correction of the hypercortisolism. More recently, it was shown that diuretics, calcium channel blockers, and angiotensin-converting enzyme inhibitors were equally effective in glucocorticoid hypertension. Failure to normalize blood pressure is usually due to unremitting hypercortisolism, not to the choice of antihypertensive agents, and can be overcome by pretreatment with or addition of ketoconazole.

Efficacy of the angiotensin-converting enzyme inhibitors captopril, benazepril,[144] and trandolapril,[90] and the angiotensin receptor blocker losartan is consistent with increased synthesis of angiotensinogen in animals and humans with glucocorticoid hypertension and with responses to captopril in methylprednisolone-induced hypertension in the rat.[80] In essential hypertension, the blood pressure effect of these agents correlates with their ability to decrease 11-oxycorticosteroids.[144] Hence, the latter effect may also participate in glucocorticoid hypertension. Plasma renin activity predicts the effect of blockade of the renin-angiotensin system in Cushing's syndrome. In the few cases in which mineralocorticoid activity is prominent and plasma renin suppressed, angiotensin-converting enzyme inhibitors will not be as effective.[145]

Our review of pathophysiologic mechanisms in the hypertension of glucocorticoid excess predicts beneficial effects for agents that have not yet been tested in the hypertension of Cushing's syndrome or exogenous glucocorticoid excess. For example, tetrahydrobiopterin, L-arginine, and vitamin C supplementation are simple nutritional interventions that may improve nitric oxide synthase activity, endothelium-dependent relaxation, and blood pressure. Also, taking into consideration that activation of the endothelin system by glucocorticoids is more likely a mineralocorticoid effect, there is a rationale for the use of spironolactone and eplerenone, even in the absence of clinical evidence for excess mineralocorticoid activity. Effects of mineralocorticoid receptor blockers could be enhanced by their combined use with the ET(a) receptor blockers bosentan or darusentan,[88] a possibility that has not yet been tested.

Pituitary surgery

Adrenalectomy was used indiscriminately to eradicate excess cortisol before there was clear understanding of the multiple causes of Cushing's syndrome. It was complicated, when the origin was pituitary, by Nelson's syndrome (i.e., de-repression of ACTH secretion with tumor growth and hyperpigmentation). Currently, detection of the different causes of Cushing's syndrome with biochemical and imaging tests, and development of microsurgical techniques allow for cause-specific therapies.

The treatment of choice for Cushing's disease is transsphenoidal pituitary surgery,[36] usually preceded by a few weeks of medical treatment to decrease surgical risk. Adenomectomy is preferred, when the tumor is located by MRI or found by the surgeon. Hemihypophysectomy is carried out when the tumor is not located, but there was lateralization of ACTH secretion by inferior petrosal sinus sampling. Total hypophysectomy may be required otherwise, but is only conducted with the patient's full understanding of the problems of lifelong multihormone replacement. When fertility is an issue, adrenalectomy and medical therapy are better treatment choices. Successful adenomectomy is currently achieved in 80% to 90% of cases, the mortality rate is negligible (~1-2%), but complications (pituitary insufficiency, diabetes insipidus, and cerebrospinal fluid leaks) may occur in 10% to 30% of procedures. The success rate is lower in macroadenomas that extend to the dura.

Abnormal corticotroph remnants may be inhibited for prolonged periods, but are the cause of late recurrences. Lack of postoperative hypocortisolism with need for replacement is a predictor of delayed recurrence.[146] Over a decade, success rates drop to ~50%. If a recurrence occurs early, diagnostic error needs to be considered. For example, failure to suppress ACTH after surgery may indicate an undiagnosed cause of CRH hypersecretion. Overall, when Cushing's disease persists after surgery, re-exploration, radiation, and adrenalectomy are possible alternatives.

Immediate postoperative glucocorticoid replacement is tapered rapidly, relying on cortisol measurements. Pseudotumor cerebrii[147] may occur if replacement is insufficient. Testing for recovery of the pituitary-adrenal axis is usually begun after 6 to 12 months. If the need for chronic replacement is established, patients must receive instructions regarding titration of dosage in case of illness or stress. Evidence for other hormone deficiencies must also be sought out.

Pituitary radiation

High-voltage cobalt 60, the most common form of pituitary radiation, is used when surgery is not possible or has failed. The response rate is about 50%, with preservation of pituitary and adrenal function and no need for glucocorticoid replacement. Recurrences are rare, but medical therapy is required because it takes months for the effect of radiation to be established. A rare but severe delayed complication is radiation necrosis of the brain.

More powerful forms of radiation (proton beam, radioactive needle implant) are more effective but commonly lead to panhypopituitarism. The gamma knife (stereotactic radiosurgery) has been used for visible remnant adenomas and also in the primary therapy of Cushing's disease.

Adrenalectomy in pituitary Cushing's disease

Despite the major improvement in complication rates with laparoscopic, compared to open, adrenalectomy, bilateral adrenalectomy in Cushing's disease should be reserved for special circumstances, because it may lead to Nelson's syndrome and its complications, including local tumor invasion and a rare malignant course. Adrenalectomy is preferred over radiation to preserve fertility, but radiation may nonetheless be required if there are early skin or radiologic changes suggestive of Nelson's syndrome. Glucocorticoid and mineralocorticoid replacement will be required lifelong.

Surgical management of adrenal Cushing's syndrome

Laparoscopic adenomectomy or unilateral adrenalectomy is the current treatment of choice for benign adrenal adenomas. Success rates approach 100%, even in large tumors,[148] although there have been recurrences in cases with bilateral adenomas or ectopic adrenal tissue. Patients require long-term (minimum of 6 months) glucocorticoid replacement until the normal function of the hypothalamo-pituitary-adrenal axis is restored, due to preexisting chronic suppression of the contralateral gland.

Bilateral adrenalectomy is the treatment for micro- and macro-nodular forms of adrenal hyperplasia, usually with good results. Choice of laparoscopy versus open adrenalectomy in the macronodular form depends on the size of the glands. Lifelong glucocorticoid and mineralocorticoid replacements are required.

Optimal management of adrenal carcinoma is controversial and prognosis is poor (<40% survival at 5 years), particularly when the primary tumor is large. Aggressive debulking surgery, including that of multiple metastases, does not improve outcomes significantly. Palliative radiation therapy and chemotherapy are not very useful. Use of mitotane has been discussed in the section on medical therapy, with dramatic responses in some cases, but controversial results in metastatic disease, for which survival is usually less than 1 year. Tumor embolization has been employed to produce necrosis of inoperable masses.

Treatment of ectopic Cushing's syndrome

Extensive review of the oncologic approach to the multiple diverse tumors producing ACTH (or rarely CRH) is beyond the scope of this chapter. It is of note, however, that nonmetastatic carcinoid tumors are those with the highest likelihood of cure by combined surgery and radiotherapy, provided that they can be located by radiologic means.

Medical therapy for nonresectable cancers in ectopic Cushing's syndrome has variable success, because blockade of synthesis of glucocorticoids and that of glucocorticoid receptors may be overcome by persistent ACTH hypersecretion, particularly when plasma levels are very high. In such situations, and also in patients who cannot tolerate the side effects of cortisol-suppressing therapy, bilateral adrenalectomy may be considered to control hypercortisolism. Obviously, the appropriateness of this surgery must be considered within the framework of expected survival; for instance, it may be indicated for slowly evolving carcinoids but not for rapidly growing cancers.

PROGNOSIS

Remission of hypertension and other clinical manifestations after successful treatment of hypercortisolism

Cure and recurrence rates for all forms of Cushing's syndrome have been discussed in the previous section. However, successful correction of hypercortisolism does not necessarily lead to complete resolution of clinical manifestations. Hypertension persists in 25% of patients with cured pituitary Cushing's disease[146] and in 10% to 30% of those with cured adrenal Cushing's syndrome,[149,150] although medication requirements may decrease in some. One possible explanation, derived from the fact that these percentages are similar to the prevalence of essential hypertension in the general population, is that these patients had, while the Cushing's disease or syndrome was active, a combination of essential and glucocorticoid-induced hypertension.

However, many findings suggest that residual hypertension (historically called meta-glucocorticoid hypertension) may be caused by nonreversible, glucocorticoid-induced organ damage. For example, in children, hypertension of Cushing's syndrome resolves in almost all subjects 1 year after surgery. In adults, the predictors of lack of cure for hypertension (age,[151] and duration or severity of glucocorticoid hypertension) are all determinants of target-organ damage. Finally, the rate at which blood pressure returns to normal after cure of Cushing's syndrome correlates negatively with the magnitude of renal damage assessed by biopsy.[149]

Obesity (55%), menstrual abnormalities (41%), and diabetes (22%) may also persist after successful treatment of hypercortisolism, whereas hirsutism, neuropsychiatric manifestations, and myopathy are more likely to disappear.[150] Vascular damage established during Cushing's syndrome and lack of complete reversibility of hypertension and metabolic features probably account for the residual incidence of cardiovascular and cerebrovascular disease during long-term follow-up of subjects with cured hypercortisolism.[151]

Overall long-term prognosis

A recent study has shown that despite the cure of Cushing's disease, there may be long-term effects on quality of life, particularly if there is residual hypopituitarism with glucocorticoid dependency and requirements for other hormone replacements. Women and older patients are most commonly affected and nonspecific symptoms, such as fatigue, prevail.[152]

Life expectancy of patients with Cushing's disease and benign adrenal Cushing's syndrome has sustained dramatic improvement due to the advances in therapy. Hence, in the early 1950s, 5-year mortality rates were about 50%. In contrast, a recent European epidemiologic study demonstrated that successful transsphenoidal surgery restores mortality to levels indistinguishable from those in the general population.[153] Although these results may appear inconsistent with the evidence for residual hypertension and metabolic abnormalities described above, it may simply mean that their impact is no longer different from that of similar prevalence rates for these disorders in the general population.

SUMMARY

Cushing's disease and syndrome, although endocrinopathies, are also cardiovascular diseases in terms of their major clinical manifestations and prognosis. Hypertension and the abnormalities in lipid and carbohydrate metabolism are the major determinants of morbidity and mortality. The mechanisms underlying the hypertension of glucocorticoid excess are varied, depending on the nature of the steroid (synthetic vs. endogenous), and the species studied. In humans, the renin-angiotensin system, exaggerated oxidative stress, and abnormalities in nitric oxide play a role in vasoconstriction. Arginine vasopressin regulation of ACTH and cortisol secretion by pituitary and adrenal adenomas may be amenable to therapy with V1b blockers in development. The VEGF response to microvascular rarefaction may also be a therapeutic target for prevention of target-organ damage.

In contrast, some traditionally mentioned pathogenic mechanisms, such as abnormalities in the sympathetic nervous system, vascular hyperreactivity to vasoconstrictors, and deficient vasodilatory systems (e.g., ANP and prostaglandins), are of more questionable relevance and no clear therapeutic usefulness.

Studies on the pathophysiologic mechanisms of glucocorticoid hypertension have also revealed possible roles for glucocorticoids in the pathogenesis of essential hypertension. Moreover, a role has been established for the tissue 11bHSD shuttle in the pathogenesis of the metabolic syndrome, which provided impetus for further research on relationships among glucocorticoids, PPAR alpha and gamma nuclear receptors, and their therapeutic manipulation. Finally, knowledge about the role of prenatal glucocorticoids in the determination of long-term, adult arterial pressure will certainly have an impact on the management of obstetric maternal and fetal disorders.

These nonendocrine results of research on the hypertension of human glucocorticoid excess may turn out to be the most important, since progress in the reliable cure of Cushing's disease and syndrome continues, owing to improvements in biochemical diagnosis, imaging techniques, and microsurgery.

REFERENCES

1. Etxabe J, Vazquez JA. Morbidity and mortality in Cushing's disease: an epidemiological approach. *Clin Endocrinol* 1994;40:479–84.

2. Anderson GH Jr, Blakeman N, Streeten DH. The effect of age on prevalence of secondary forms of hypertension in 4429 consecutively referred patients. *J Hypertens* 1994; 12:609–15.

3. Wei L, MacDonald TM, Walker BR. Taking glucocorticoids by prescription is associated with subsequent cardiovascular disease. *Ann Intern Med* 2004;141:764–70.

4. Mantero F, Boscaro M. Glucocorticoid-dependent hypertension. *J Steroid Biochem Mol Biol* 1992;43:409–13.

5. Kim CY, Imai Y, Itoi K, et al. Analysis of circadian variation of blood pressure and heart rate in dexamethasone-induced hypertensive rats. *Clin Exp Hypertens* 1996;18:65–76.

6. Zacharieva S, Orbetzova M, Stoynev A, et al. Circadian blood pressure profile in patients with Cushing's syndrome before and after treatment. *J Endocrinol Invest* 2004;27:924–30.

7. Prattichizzo FA. Arterial hypertension in Cushing's disease: the 24-hour pressure profile without and during treatment with beta-blockers or cyproheptadine. *G Ital Cardiol* 1994; 24:533–8.

8. Brunetti A, Fulham MJ, Aloj L, et al. Decreased brain glucose utilization in patients with Cushing's disease. *J Nucl Med* 1998;39:786–90.

9. Bodelier AG, Groeneveld W, van der Linden AN, Haak HR. Symptomatic epidural lipomatosis in ectopic Cushing's syndrome. *Eur J Endocrinol* 2004;151:765–9.

10. Tanabe A, Naruse M, Naruse K, et al. Left ventricular hypertrophy is more prominent in patients with primary aldosteronism than in patients with other types of secondary hypertension. *Hypertens Res* 1997;20:85–90.

11. Sugihara N, Shimizu M, Kita Y, et al. Cardiac characteristics and postoperative courses in Cushing's syndrome. *Am J Cardiol* 1992; 69:1475–80.

12. Duprez D, De Buyzere M, Paelinck M, et al. Relationship between left ventricular mass index and 24-h urinary free cortisol and cortisone in essential arterial hypertension. *J Hypertens* 1999;17:1583–8.

13. Fallo F, Budano S, Sonino N, et al. Left ventricular structural characteristics in Cushing's syndrome. *J Hum Hypertens* 1994;8:509–13.

14. Fekete Z, Landin-Wilhelmsen K, Jakobsson KE, Petruson B. Follow-up of Cushing syndrome in western Sweden. More than one treatment method needed for cure, hormonal deficiencies common. *Lakartidningen* 2002;99:4635–9.

15. Cavagnini F, Pecori Giraldi F. Epidemiology and follow-up of Cushing's disease. *Ann Endocrinol (Paris)* 2001;62:168–72.

16. Giordana MT, Cavalla P, Allegranza A, Pollo B. Intracranial dissemination of pituitary adenoma. Case report and review of the literature. *Ital J Neurol Sci* 1994;15:195–200.

17. Fujita R, Yamashiro Y, Igarashi T, et al. A case of adrenal black adenoma associated with Cushing's syndrome. *Acta Urol Jpn* 1988;34:2155–9.

18. Lacroix A, Bourdeau I. Bilateral adrenal Cushing's syndrome: macronodular adrenal hyperplasia and primary pigmented nodular adrenocortical disease. *Endocrinol Metab Clin North Am* 2005;34:441–58.

19. Hsin SC, Hsieh MC, Hwang SJ, et al. Carney complex, a familial Cushing's syndrome due to primary pigmented nodular adrenocortical disease: a case report. *Kaohsiung J Med Sci* 2002; 18:627–31.

20. Nakamura Y, Son Y, Kohno Y, et al. Case of adrenocorticotropic hormone-independent macronodular adrenal hyperplasia with possible adrenal hypersensitivity to angiotensin II. *Endocrine* 2001;15:57–61.

21. Miyamura N, Taguchi T, Murata Y, et al. Inherited adrenocorticotropin-independent macronodular adrenal hyperplasia with abnormal cortisol secretion by vasopressin and catecholamines: detection of the aberrant hormone receptors on adrenal gland. *Endocrine* 2002; 19:319–26.

22. Lacroix A, Tremblay J, Russeau G, et al. Propranolol therapy for ectopic (beta)-adrenergic receptors in adrenal Cushing's syndrome. *N Engl J Med* 1997;337:1429–34.

23. Lacroix A, Bolte E, Tremblay J, et al. Gastric inhibitory polypeptide-dependent cortisol hypersecretion—a new cause of Cushing's syndrome. *N Engl J Med* 1992;327:974–81.

24. Josse RG, Bear R, Kovacs K, Higgins HP. Cushing's syndrome due to unilateral nodular adrenal hyperplasia: a new pathophysiological entity? *Acta Endocrinol (Copenh)* 1980;93:495–504.

25. Mantero F, Masini AM, Opocher G, et al. Adrenal incidentaloma: an overview of hormonal data from the National Italian Study Group. *Horm Res* 1997;47:284–9.

26. National Institutes of Health. NIH state-of-the-science statement on management of the clinically inapparent adrenal mass ("incidentaloma"). *NIH Consens State Sci Statements* 2002;19:1–25.

27. Rossi R, Tauchmanova L, Luciano A, et al. Subclinical Cushing's syndrome in patients with adrenal incidentaloma: clinical and biochemical features. *J Clin Endocrinol Metab* 2000;85:1440–8.

28. Bernini G, Moretti A, Iacconi P, et al. Anthropometric, haemodynamic, humoral and hormonal evaluation in patients with incidental adrenocortical adenomas before and after surgery. *Eur J Endocrinol* 2003;148:213–9.

29. Midorikawa S, Sanada H, Hashimoto S, et al. Analysis of cortisol secretion in hormonally inactive adrenocortical incidentalomas: study of in vitro steroid secretion and immunohistochemical localization of steroidogenic enzymes. *Endocr J* 2001;48:167–74.

30. White A, Clark AJ, Stewart MF. The synthesis of ACTH and related peptides by tumors. *Baillières Clin Endocrinol Metab* 1990;4:1–27.

31. Arnaldi G, Mancini T, Kola B, et al. Cyclical Cushing's syndrome in a patient with a bronchial neuroendocrine

tumor (typical carcinoid) expressing ghrelin and growth hormone secretagogue receptors. *J Clin Endocrinol Metab* 2003;88:5834–40.

32. Beuschlein F, Hammer GD. Ectopic pro-opiomelanocortin syndrome. *Endocrinol Metab Clin North Am* 2002;31:191–234.

33. Fachnie JD, Zafar MS, Mellinger RC, et al. Pituitary carcinoma mimics the ectopic adrenocorticotropin syndrome. *J Clin Endocrinol Metab* 1980;50:1062–5.

34. Torpy DJ, Mullen N, Ilias I, Nieman LK. Association of hypertension and hypokalemia with Cushing's syndrome caused by ectopic ACTH secretion: a series of 58 cases. *Ann N Y Acad Sci* 2002;970:134–44.

35. Findling JW, Raff H. Diagnosis and differential diagnosis of Cushing's syndrome. *Endocrinol Metab Clin North Am* 2001;30:729–47.

36. Salenave S, Gatta B, Pecheur S, et al. Pituitary magnetic resonance imaging findings do not influence surgical outcome in adrenocorticotropin-secreting microadenomas. *J Clin Endocrinol Metab* 2004;89:3371–6.

37. De Herder WW, Lamberts SW. Imaging of pituitary tumours. *Baillières Clin Endocrinol Metab* 1995;9:367–89.

38. Komori T, Martin WH, Graber AL, Delbeke D. Serendipitous detection of Cushing's disease by FDG positron emission tomography and a review of the literature. *Clin Nucl Med* 2002; 27:176–8.

39. Galanski M, Peters PE. Computerized tomography and nuclear magnetic resonance tomography in adrenal gland diseases. *Bildgebung* 1987–89; 56:147–55.

40. Gross MD, Shapiro B. Scintigraphic studies in adrenal hypertension. *Semin Nucl Med* 1989;19:122–43.

41. Zettinig G, Mitterhauser M, Wadsak W, et al. Positron emission tomography imaging of adrenal masses: (18)F-fluorodeoxyglucose and the 11beta-hydroxylase tracer (11)C-metomidate. *Eur J Nucl Med Mol Imaging* 2004;31: 1224–30.

42. Orlefors H, Sundin A, Garske U, et al. Whole-body (11)C-5-hydroxytryptophan positron emission tomography as a universal imaging technique for neuroendocrine tumors: comparison with somatostatin receptor scintigraphy and computed tomography. *J Clin Endocrinol Metab* 2005;90:3392–400.

43. Frey FJ, Odermatt A, Frey BM. Glucocorticoid-mediated mineralocorticoid receptor activation and hypertension. *Curr Opin Nephrol Hypertens* 2004;13:451–8.

44. Stocker CJ, Arch JR, Cawthorne MA. Fetal origins of insulin resistance and obesity. *Proc Nutr Soc* 2005;64: 143–51.

45. Seckl JR, Meaney MJ. Glucocorticoid programming. *Ann N Y Acad Sci* 2004; 1032:63–84.

46. Doyle LW, Ford GW, Davis NM, Callanan C. Antenatal corticosteroid therapy and blood pressure at 14 years of age in preterm children. *Clin Sci* 2000;98:137–42.

47. DeLano FA, Schmid-Schonbein GW. Enhancement of glucocorticoid and mineralocorticoid receptor density

in the microcirculation of the spontaneously hypertensive rat. *Microcirculation* 2004;11:69–78.

48. Seckl JR, Morton NM, Chapman KE, Walker BR. Glucocorticoids and 11beta-hydroxysteroid dehydrogenase in adipose tissue. *Recent Prog Horm Res* 2004;59:359–93.

49. Engeli S, Bohnke J, Feldpausch M, et al. Regulation of 11beta-HSD genes in human adipose tissue: influence of central obesity and weight loss. *Obes Res* 2004;12:9–17.

50. Hermanowski-Vosatka A, Gerhold D, Mundt SS, et al. PPARalpha agonists reduce 11betahydroxysteroid dehydrogenase type 1 in the liver. *Biochem Biophys Res Commun* 2000; 279:330–6.

51. Berger J, Tanen M, Elbrecht A, et al. Peroxisome proliferator-activated receptor-ligands inhibit adipocyte 11-hydroxysteroid dehydrogenase type 1 expression and activity. *J Biol Chem* 2001;276:12629–35.

52. Barroso I, Gurnell M, Crowley VE, et al. Dominant negative mutations in human PPARgamma associated with severe insulin resistance, diabetes mellitus and hypertension. *Nature* 1999;402:880–3.

53. Glorioso N, Filigheddu F, Parpaglia PP, et al. 11beta-Hydroxysteroid dehydrogenase type 2 activity is associated with left ventricular mass in essential hypertension. *Eur Heart J* 2005;26:498–504.

54. Krall P, Mosso L, Carvajal C, et al. Free urinary cortisol is elevated in patients with low-renin essential hypertension. *Rev Med Chil* 2004;132:1053–9.

55. Kino T, Vottero A, Charmandari E, Chrousos GP. Familial/sporadic glucocorticoid resistance syndrome and hypertension. *Ann N Y Acad Sci* 2002;970:101–11.

56. Bobulescu IA, Dwarakanath V, Zou L, et al. Glucocorticoids acutely increase cell surface Na+/H+ exchanger–3 (NHE3) by activation of NHE3 exocytosis. *Am J Physiol* 2005;289: F685–91.

57. Yun CC. Concerted roles of SGK1 and the Na+/H+ exchanger regulatory factor 2 (NHERF2) in regulation of NHE3. *Cell Physiol Biochem* 2003;13: 29–40.

58. Wang D, Sun H, Lang F, Yun CC. Activation of NHE3 by dexamethasone requires phosphorylation of NHE3 at Ser663 by SGK1. *Am J Physiol* 2005; 289:C802–10.

59. Henke G, Setiawan I, Bohmer C, Lang F. Activation of Na+/K+-ATPase by the serum and glucocorticoid-dependent kinase isoforms. *Kidney Blood Press Res* 2002;25:370–4.

60. Rhee MS, Perianayagam A, Chen P, et al. Dexamethasone treatment causes resistance to insulin-stimulated cellular potassium uptake in the rat. *Am J Physiol* 2004;287:C1229–37.

61. Khan I, Cheng B. Selective suppression of renal Na+/H+ exchanger isoform-3 by prolonged stimulation of rats with adrenocorticotropic hormone. *Endocrine* 2001;16:189–94.

62. Brem AS. Insights into glucocorticoid-associated hypertension. *Am J Kidney Dis* 2001;37:1–10.

63. Sayegh R, Auerbach SD, Li X, et al. Glucocorticoid induction of epithelial sodium channel expression in lung and renal epithelia occurs via trans-activation of a hormone response element in the 5'-flanking region of the human epithelial sodium channel alpha subunit gene. *J Biol Chem* 1999; 274:12431–7.

64. Itani OA, Stokes JB, Thomas CP. Nedd4-2 isoforms differentially associate with ENaC and regulate its activity. *Am J Physiol* 2005;289: F334–46.

65. Ramminger SJ, Richard K, Inglis SK, et al. A regulated apical Na(+) conductance in dexamethasone-treated H441 airway epithelial cells. *Am J Physiol* 2004;287:L411–9.

66. Schulz-Baldes A, Berger S, Grahammer F, et al. Induction of the epithelial Na+ channel via glucocorticoids in mineralocorticoid receptor knockout mice. *Pflugers Arch* 2001;443:297–305.

67. Itani OA, Liu KZ, Cornish KL, et al. Glucocorticoids stimulate human sgk1 gene expression by activation of a GRE in its 5'-flanking region. *Am J Physiol* 2002;283:E971–9.

68. Aguirre JA, Ibarra FR, Barontini M, et al. Effect of glucocorticoids on renal dopamine production. *Eur J Pharmacol* 1999;370:271–8.

69. Garcia DL, Rennke HG, Brenner BM, Anderson S. Chronic glucocorticoid therapy amplifies glomerular injury in rats with renal ablation. *J Clin Invest* 1987;80:867–74.

70. Whitworth JA, Saines D, Thatcher R, et al. Blood pressure, renal and metabolic effects of ACTH in normotensive man. *Clin Sci* 1981; 61:269s–72s.

71. Lohmeier TE, Carroll RG. Chronic potentiation of vasoconstrictor hypertension by adrenocorticotropic hormone. *Hypertension* 1982;4:138–48.

72. Woods LL, Mizelle HL, Hall JE. Control of sodium excretion in NE-ACTH hypertension: role of pressure natriuresis. *Am J Physiol* 1988;255:R894–900.

73. Whitworth JA, Saines D, Andrews J, et al. Haemodynamic response to ACTH administration in essential hypertension. *Clin Exp Pharmacol Physiol* 1981;8:553–6.

74. Levitt MF, Bader ME. Effect of cortisone and ACTH on fluid and electrolyte distribution in man. *Am J Med* 1951; 11:715–23.

75. Agrest A, Finkielman S, Elijovich F. Hemodynamics of arterial hypertension in Cushing's syndrome. *Medicina (B Aires)* 1974;34:457–62.

76. Hifumi S, Morise T, Honjo A, et al. Total blood volume in essential and secondary hypertension. *Folia Endocrinol Jpn* 1982;58:790–5.

77. Komissarenko IV, Slavnov VN, Cheban AK, et al. Pathogenesis of the arterial hypertensive syndrome in Itsenko-Cushing disease. *Probl Endokrinol (Mosk)* 1982;28:28–31.

78. Kunapuli SP, Benedict CR, Kumar A. Tissue specific hormonal regulation of the rat angiotensinogen gene expression. *Arch Biochem Biophys* 1987;254:642–6.

79. Krakoff LR, Selvadurai R, Sutter E. Effect of methylprednisolone upon arterial pressure and the renin angiotensin system in the rat. *Am J Physiol* 1975;228:613–7.

80. Elijovich F, Krakoff LR. Effect of converting enzyme inhibition on glucocorticoid hypertension in the rat. *Am J Physiol* 1980;238:H844–8.

81. Marson O, Ribeiro AB, Tufik S, et al. Role of the anteroventral third ventricle region and the renin angiotensin system in methylprednisolone hypertension. *Hypertension* 1981; 3:II-142–6.

82. Eggena P, Hidaka H, Barrett JD, Sambhi MP. Multiple forms of human plasma renin substrate. *J Clin Invest* 1978;62:367–72.

83. Murasawa S, Matsubara H, Kizima K, et al. Glucocorticoids regulate V1a vasopressin receptor expression by increasing mRNA stability in vascular smooth muscle cells. *Hypertension* 1995;26:665–9.

84. Fraser TB, Turner SW, Wen C, et al. Vasopressin V1a receptor antagonism does not reverse adrenocorticotrophin-induced hypertension in the rat. *Clin Exp Pharmacol Physiol* 2000; 27:866–70.

85. Arnaldi G, de Keyzer Y, Gasc JM, et al. Vasopressin receptors modulate the pharmacological phenotypes of Cushing's syndrome. *Endocr Res* 1998; 24:807–16.

86. Serradeil-Le Gal C, Wagnon J, Valette G, et al. Nonpeptide vasopressin receptor antagonists: development of selective and orally active V1a, V2 and V1b receptor ligands. *Prog Brain Res* 2002; 139:197–210.

87. Daidoh H, Morita H, Hanafusa J, et al. In vivo and in vitro effects of AVP and V1a receptor antagonist on Cushing's syndrome due to ACTH-independent bilateral macronodular adrenocortical hyperplasia. *Clin Endocrinol* 1998; 49:403–9.

88. Ruschitzka F, Quaschning T, Noll G, et al. Endothelin 1 type a receptor antagonism prevents vascular dysfunction and hypertension induced by 11beta-hydroxysteroid dehydrogenase inhibition: role of nitric oxide. *Circulation* 2001;103:3129–35.

89. Ristimaki A, Narko K, Hla T. Down-regulation of cytokine-induced cyclo-oxygenase-2 transcript isoforms by dexamethasone: evidence for post-transcriptional regulation. *Biochem J* 1996;318:325–31.

90. Zacharieva S, Torbova S, Orbetzova M, et al. Trandolapril in Cushing's disease: short-term trandolapril treatment in patients with Cushing's disease and essential hypertension. *Methods Find Exp Clin Pharmacol* 1998;20:433–8.

91. Watson RE, Supowit SC, Zhao H, et al. Role of sensory nervous system vasoactive peptides in hypertension. *Braz J Med Biol Res* 2002;35:1033–45.

92. Weidmann P, Matter DR, Matter EE, et al. Glucocorticoid and mineralocorticoid stimulation of atrial natriuretic peptide release in man. *J Clin Endocrinol Metab* 1988;66:1233–9.

93. Soszynski P, Slowinska-Srzednicka J, Kasperlik-Zaluska A, Zgliczynski S. Endogenous natriuretic factors: atrial natriuretic hormone and digitalis-like substance in Cushing's syndrome. *J Endocrinol* 1991;129:453–8.

94. Sala C, Ambrosi B, Morganti A. Blunted vascular and renal effects of exogenous atrial natriuretic peptide in patients with Cushing's disease. *J Clin Endocrinol Metab* 2001;86:1957–61.

95. Goto A, Yamada K, Hazama H, et al. Ouabainlike compound in hypertension associated with ectopic corticotropin syndrome. *Hypertension* 1996;28:421–5.

96. Wallerath T, Godecke A, Molojavyi A, et al. Dexamethasone lacks effect on blood pressure in mice with a disrupted endothelial NO synthase gene. *Nitric Oxide* 2004;10:36–41.

97. Mitchell BM, Dorrance AM, Webb RC. GTP cyclohydrolase 1 downregulation contributes to glucocorticoid hypertension in rats. *Hypertension* 2003;41:669–74.

98. Wallerath T, Witte K, Schafer SC, et al. Down-regulation of the expression of endothelial NO synthase is likely to contribute to glucocorticoid-mediated hypertension. *Proc Natl Acad Sci U S A* 1999;96:13357–62.

99. Andrews MC, Schyvens CG, Zhang Y, et al. Nitric oxide donation lowers blood pressure in adrenocorticotrophic hormone-induced hypertensive rats. *Clin Exp Hypertens* 2004;26:499–509.

100. Kelly JJ, Williamson P, Martin A, Whitworth JA. Effects of oral L-arginine on plasma nitrate and blood pressure in cortisol treated humans. *J Hypertens* 2001;19:263–8.

101. Kelly JJ, Martin A, Whitworth JA. Role of erythropoietin in cortisol-induced hypertension. *J Hum Hypertens* 2000; 14:195–8.

102. Zhang Y, Andrews MC, Schyvens CG, et al. Adrenocorticotropic hormone, blood pressure, and serum erythropoietin concentrations in the rat. *Am J Hypertens* 2004;17:457–61.

103. Saruta T. Mechanism of glucocorticoid-induced hypertension. *Hypertens Res* 1996;19:1–8.

104. Miesel R, Zuber M. Elevated levels of xanthine oxidase in serum of patients with inflammatory and autoimmune rheumatic diseases. *Inflammation* 1993;17:551–61.

105. Wallwork CJ, Parks DA, Schmid-Schonbein GW. Xanthine oxidase activity in the dexamethasone-induced hypertensive rat. *Microvasc Res* 2003;66:30–7.

106. Zhang Y, Chan MM, Andrews MC, et al. Apocynin but not allopurinol prevents and reverses adrenocorticotropic hormone-induced hypertension in the rat. *Am J Hypertens* 2005;18:910–6.

107. Valen G, Kawakami T, Tahepold P, et al. Pretreatment with methylprednisolone protects the isolated rat heart against ischaemic and oxidative damage. *Free Radic Res* 2000;33:31–43.

108. McIntosh L, Hong K, Sapolsky R. Glucocorticoids may alter antioxidant enzyme capacity in the brain: baseline studies. *Brain Res* 1998;791:209–14.

109. Zhang Y, Jang R, Mori TA, et al. The anti-oxidant tempol reverses and partially prevents adrenocorticotrophic hormone-induced hypertension in the rat. *J Hypertens* 2003;21:1513–8.

110. Zhang Y, Croft KD, Mori TA, et al. The antioxidant tempol prevents and partially reverses dexamethasone-induced hypertension in the rat. *Am J Hypertens* 2004;17:260–5.

111. Iuchi T, Akaike M, Mitsui T, et al. Glucocorticoid excess induces superoxide production in vascular endothelial cells and elicits vascular endothelial dysfunction. *Circ Res* 2003;92:81–7.

112. Marumo T, Schini-Kerth VB, Brandes RP, Busse R. Glucocorticoids inhibit superoxide anion production and p22 phox mRNA expression in human aortic smooth muscle cells. *Hypertension* 1998;32:1083–8.

113. Gavan N, Popa R, Orasan R, Maibach H. Effect of percutaneous absorption of fluocinolone acetonide on the activity of superoxide dismutase and total antioxidant status in patients with psoriasis. *Skin Pharmacol* 1997; 10:178–82.

114. Dworski R, Murray JJ, Roberts LJ 2nd, et al. Allergen-induced synthesis of F(2)-isoprostanes in atopic asthmatics. Evidence for oxidant stress. *Am J Respir Crit Care Med* 1999;160:1947–51.

115. Horowitz JR, Rivard A, van der Zee R, et al. Vascular endothelial growth factor/vascular permeability factor produces nitric oxide-dependent hypotension. Evidence for a maintenance role in quiescent adult endothelium. *Arterioscler Thromb Vasc Biol* 1997;17:2793–800.

116. Gille J, Reisinger K, Westphal-Varghese B, Kaufmann R. Decreased mRNA stability as a mechanism of glucocorticoid-mediated inhibition of vascular endothelial growth factor gene expression by cultured keratinocytes. *J Invest Dermatol* 2001;117:1581–7.

117. Zacharieva S, Atanassova I, Orbetzova M, et al. Vascular endothelial growth factor (VEGF), prostaglandin E2 (PGE2) and active renin in hypertension of adrenal origin. *J Endocrinol Invest* 2004;27:742–6.

118. Gaillard I, Keramidas M, Liakos P, et al. ACTH-regulated expression of vascular endothelial growth factor in the adult bovine adrenal cortex: a possible role in the maintenance of the microvasculature. *J Cell Physiol* 2000; 185:226–34.

119. Thomas M, Keramidas M, Monchaux E, Feige JJ. Role of adrenocorticotropic hormone in the development and maintenance of the adrenal cortical vasculature. *Microsc Res Tech* 2003; 61:247–51.

120. Katoh R. Angiogenesis in endocrine glands: special reference to the expression of vascular endothelial growth factor. *Microsc Res Tech* 2003;60:181–5.

121. Bernini GP, Moretti A, Bonadio AG, et al. Angiogenesis in human normal and pathologic adrenal cortex. *J Clin Endocrinol Metab* 2002;87:4961–5.

122. Felmeden DC, Spencer CG, Belgore FM, et al. Endothelial damage and angiogenesis in hypertensive patients: relationship to cardiovascular risk factors and risk factor management. *Am J Hypertens* 2003;16:11–20.

123. Hagerty T, Fernandez E, Lynch K, et al. Interaction of a glucocorticoid-responsive element with regulatory sequences in the promoter region of the mouse tyrosine hydroxylase gene. *J Neurochem* 2001;78:1379–88.

124. Kumai T, Asoh K, Tateishi T, et al. Involvement of tyrosine hydroxylase up regulation in dexamethasone-induced hypertension of rats. *Life Sci* 2000;67:1993–9.

125. Krizanova O, Micutkova L, Jelokova J, et al. Existence of cardiac PNMT mRNA in adult rats: elevation by stress in a glucocorticoid-dependent manner. *Am J Physiol* 2001;281:H1372–9.

126. Wang LL, Ou CC, Chan JY. Receptor-independent activation of GABAergic neurotransmission and receptor-dependent nontranscriptional activation of phosphatidylinositol 3-kinase/protein kinase Akt pathway in short-term cardiovascular actions of dexamethasone at the nucleus tractus solitarii of the rat. *Mol Pharmacol* 2005;67:489–98.

127. Nakamoto H, Suzuki H, Kageyama Y, et al. Central nervous system mediates an antihypertensive property of glucocorticoid hypertension in dogs. *J Hypertens* 1995;13:1169–79.

128. Seematter G, Battilana P, Tappy L. Effects of dexamethasone on the metabolic responses to mental stress in humans. *Clin Physiol Funct Imaging* 2002;22:139–44.

129. Williamson PM, Tam SH, Kelly JJ, Whitworth JA. Ganglion blockade does not prevent cortisol-induced hypertension in man. *Clin Exp Pharmacol Physiol* 2005;32:294–6.

130. Cameron OG, Starkman MN, Schteingart DE. The effect of elevated systemic cortisol levels on plasma catecholamines in Cushing's syndrome patients with and without depressed mood. *J Psychiatr Res* 1995;29:347–60.

131. van Uum SH, Hermus AR, Sweep CG, et al. Short-term cortisol infusion in the brachial artery, with and without inhibiting 11 beta-hydroxysteroid dehydrogenase, does not alter forearm vascular resistance in normotensive and hypertensive subjects. *Eur J Clin Invest* 2002;32:874–81.

132. Scherrer U, Vollenweider P, Randin D, et al. Suppression of insulin-induced sympathetic activation and vasodilation by dexamethasone in humans. *Circulation* 1993;88:388–94.

133. Walker BR, Best R, Shackleton CH, et al. Increased vasoconstrictor sensitivity to glucocorticoids in essential hypertension. *Hypertension* 1996;27:190–6.

134. Heaney AP, Hunter SJ, Sheridan B, Brew Atkinson A. Increased pressor response to noradrenaline in pituitary dependent Cushing's syndrome. *Clin Endocrinol* 1999;51:293–9.

135. McKnight JA, Rooney DP, Whitehead H, Atkinson AB. Blood pressure responses to phenylephrine infusions in subjects with Cushing's syndrome. *J Hum Hypertens* 1995;9:855–8.

136. Yasuda G, Shionoiri H, Umemura S, et al. Exaggerated blood pressure response to angiotensin II in patients with Cushing's syndrome due to adrenocortical adenoma. *Eur J Endocrinol* 1994;131:582–8.

137. Nishimura H, Yoshikawa T, Kobayashi N, et al. Effects of methylprednisolone on hemodynamics and beta-adrenergic receptor signaling in rabbits with acute left ventricular failure. *Heart Vessels* 1997;12:84–91.

138. Ritchie CM, Sheridan B, Fraser R, et al. Studies on the pathogenesis of hypertension in Cushing's disease and acromegaly. *Q J Med* 1990;76:855–67.

139. Omori N, Nomura K, Omori K, et al. Rational, effective metyrapone treatment of ACTH-independent bilateral macronodular adrenocortical hyperplasia (AIMAH). *Endocr J* 2001;48:665–9.

140. Schteingart DE, Motazedi A, Noonan RA, et al. Treatment of adrenal carcinomas. *Arch Surg* 1982;117:1142–6.

141. Paez-Pereda M, Kovalovsky D, Hopfner U, et al. Retinoic acid prevents experimental Cushing syndrome. *J Clin Invest* 2001;108:1123–31.

142. Heaney AP, Fernando M, Melmed S. PPAR-gamma receptor ligands: novel therapy for pituitary adenomas. *J Clin Invest* 2003;111:1381–8.

143. Burris J, Waeber B, Nussberger J, Brunner HR. Blood pressure and heart rate response to central beta-blockade in conscious rats with glucocorticoid-induced hypertension. *J Cardiovasc Pharmacol* 1985;7:121–4.

144. Olbinskaya LI, Golubev SA, Bolshakova TD. Influence of benazepril and captopril on blood pressure, glucocorticoids and progesterone in essential hypertensives. *J Hum Hypertens* 1993;7:603–6.

145. Greminger P, Vetter W, Groth H, et al. Captopril in Cushing's syndrome. *Klin Wochenschr* 1984;62:855–8.

146. Ludecke DK, Niedworok G. Results of microsurgery in Cushing's disease and effect on hypertension. *Cardiology* 1985;72:91–4.

147. Parfitt VJ, Dearlove JC, Savage D, et al. Benign intracranial hypertension after pituitary surgery for Cushing's disease. *Postgrad Med J* 1994;70:115–7.

148. Kuriansky J, Saenz A, Astudillo E, et al. Laparoscopic adrenalectomy in the elderly. *J Laparoendosc Adv Surg Tech A* 1999;9:317–20.

149. Aso Y, Kinoshita K. Postoperative improvement of hypertension in primary aldosteronism and Cushing's syndrome. *Urol Int* 1975;30:386–95.

150. Ross EJ, Linch DC. The clinical response to treatment in adult Cushing's syndrome following remission of hypercortisolaemia. *Postgrad Med J* 1985;61:205–11.

151. Sapienza P, Cavallaro A. Persistent hypertension after removal of adrenal tumours. *Eur J Surg* 1999;165:187–92.

152. van Aken MO, Pereira AM, Biermasz NR, et al. Quality of life in patients after long-term biochemical cure of Cushing's disease. *J Clin Endocrinol Metab* 2005;90:3279–86.

153. Lindholm J, Juul S, Jorgensen JO, et al. Incidence and late prognosis of Cushing's syndrome: a population-based study. *J Clin Endocrinol Metab* 2001;86:117–23.

Chapter

70

Oral Contraceptives, Hormone Replacement Therapy, and Hypertension

Talma Rosenthal and Suzanne Oparil

Key Findings

- Oral contraceptives provide the most reliable and convenient means of contraception and are safe for use in younger, healthy, normotensive women.

- Oral contraceptives are associated with increases in blood pressure that are usually minor and resolve quickly with cessation of use.

- High-risk women, including those with uncontrolled hypertension, established cardiovascular or thromboembolic disease, breast cancer, or smoking, should not use combined estrogen–progestin oral contraceptives.

- To minimize risks while preserving benefits, guidelines specify that combined oral contraceptives should contain low doses of estrogen (<35 or <50 μg of ethinyl estradiol) and the "lowest progestin dose." Progestin-only contraceptives, delivered by oral, intramuscular, or intrauterine routes, provide safe alternatives to combined oral contraceptives for high-risk women.

- Medical management of oral contraceptive users with hypertension should include frequent monitoring of blood pressure and aggressive cardiovascular risk factor reduction, including smoking cessation.

- Estrogens, particularly 17β-estradiol, have anti-inflammatory, vasoprotective, and favorable hemodynamic effects when administered to healthy women in the early postmenopausal years. These benefits are not seen in older postmenopausal women for reasons that are not clearly understood.

- Menopausal hormones generally do not increase blood pressure but do increase risk of stroke, thromboembolic disease, and coronary heart disease events in older postmenopausal women.

Clinical Implications

- Menopausal hormones are not recommended for the prevention or treatment of cardiovascular disease in postmenopausal women.

- Combined estrogen–progestin menopausal hormones are indicated only for treatment of vasomotor symptoms and symptoms of vulvovaginal atrophy associated with menopause and for prevention of postmenopausal osteoporosis.

- Menopausal hormones should be administered in the lowest doses and for the shortest time period needed to achieve the desired clinical effect.

The introduction of the oral contraceptives (OCs) in the 1960s was met almost immediately with reports of severe hypertension in some users,[1,2] and suspicions that OCs might evoke stroke.[3,4] These reports led to a series of observational studies that found higher blood pressures among OC users than nonusers, although differences in cohort size and dosages and types of OCs resulted in variations in the magnitude of blood pressure differences between the two groups.[4–13] The average difference in systolic and diastolic blood pressure between OC users and nonusers in these studies was, respectively, 5 to 7 mmHg and 1 to 3 mmHg for white American women. Blood pressure usually returned to pretreatment levels within 3 to 6 months when OC use was discontinued. The Nurses' Health Study found that current users of OCs had a statistically significant increased risk of hypertension compared with never users that resolved quickly with cessation of OC use.[13]

Most of the studies conducted in the 1960s and 1970s on the cardiovascular effects of the OCs used formulations containing 80 or 100 μg estrogen, vastly different from the 30 to 35 μg estrogen in today's agents.[14] In addition, these earlier formulations contained high doses (>50 μg, often 100 μg) of ethinyl estradiol (EE), a synthetic estradiol that is activated in the liver, and was subsequently found to have deleterious side effects. One of the ways that OCs were made safer was reducing hormone content.[15] The amount of EE in the "low-dose formulations" was reduced to 35 μg in the 1970s and to as low as 15 μg in some formulations today.[16] Seibert et al.[17] were unable to substantiate harmful cardiovascular effects of OCs containing less than 35 μg EE.

OCs have been reported in numerous studies to increase the risk of stroke.[3,6,14] The original studies were carried out when OCs contained higher doses of estrogen (80 to 150 μg) and progesterone. When doses were reduced to 30 to 50 μg of estrogen, the results of studies varied, with some finding increased risk for stroke and others not.[14] For example, the European arm of a WHO (World Health Organization) study found that women older than 35 years who used OCs containing less than 50 μg of estrogen did not have a higher risk for ischemic stroke than nonusers.[17]

Recommendations of the American College of Obstetrics and Gynecology (ACOG) and the WHO for use of combined estrogen–progestin OCs in women with characteristics that might increase the risk of adverse effects are summarized in Table 70–1.[18–20] A variety of concomitant conditions, including uncontrolled hypertension, smoking, established cardiovascular disease (CVD), breast cancer, and thromboembolic disease, are considered absolute contraindications to OC use due to unacceptable health risk. Medical management of OC users with hypertension should include frequent monitoring of blood pressure and aggressive CVD risk factor modification, including smoking cessation.

In contrast to OCs, menopausal hormones (hormone replacement therapy [HRT]) have not been shown to increase blood pressure in either normotensive or hypertensive postmenopausal women.[21–26] These differences in blood pressure effect may be related to the dosage and molecular forms of estrogen used in menopausal HRT and in OC. Estrogens in HRT are usually natural estrogens, while estrogens in OC are usually synthetic.[5,27] The estrogenic component of HRT, particularly 17β-estradiol, has been shown in some studies to lower both systolic and diastolic blood pressure, particularly nighttime blood pressure, in healthy normotensive, prehypertensive, and hypertensive postmenopausal women when administered in the first few years following cessation of menses.[22,27,28] Further, both oral and transdermal estradiol have been shown to attenuate the age-related rise in blood pressure.[29]

In older postmenopausal women, the effect of HRT on blood pressure appears to be minimal, but HRT regimens, particularly those that contain progestins, increase the risk of stroke, thromboembolic disease, and coronary heart disease events in this population.[30,31] Accordingly, HRT is not recommended for the prevention of CVD in post-

RECOMMENDATIONS OF THE AMERICAN COLLEGE OF OBSTETRICS AND GYNECOLOGY AND WORLD HEALTH ORGANIZATION FOR USE OF COMBINED ESTROGEN–PROGESTIN ORAL CONTRACEPTIVES IN WOMEN WITH CHARACTERISTICS THAT MIGHT INCREASE RISK OF ADVERSE EFFECTS		
Condition	**Risk Status**	**Comment**
Age		
Menarche to <40 years	No Restriction	
>40 years	Benefit>Risk	
Smoking		
Age <35 years	Benefit>Risk	OCP users who smoked were at increased risk of CVD, especially MI, compared with those who did not smoke. The risk of MI increased with increasing number of cigarettes smoked per day.
Age >35 years		
<15 cigarettes/day	Risk>Benefit	
>15 cigarettes/day	Risk Unacceptable	
Obesity: >30 kg/m² body mass index	Benefit>Risk	Obese women who used OCPs were at increased risk of VTE compared with nonusers. The absolute risk of VTE remained small. Data are limited regarding the impact of obesity on COC effectiveness.
Multiple risk factors for CVD (older age, smoking, diabetes, and hypertension)	Risk>Benefit: May be Unacceptable	When a woman has multiple major risk factors, any of which alone would substantially increase the risk of CVD, use of COCs may increase her risk to an unacceptable level.
Hypertension		
History of hypertension, current BP unknown	Risk>Benefit	Women who did not have a BP check before COC use had increased risk of acute MI and stroke.
Adequately controlled hypertension	Risk>Benefit	Women adequately treated for hypertension are at reduced risk of acute MI and stroke as compared with untreated women. COC users with adequately controlled and monitored hypertension should be at reduced risk of acute MI and stroke compared with untreated hypertensive COC users.
Elevated BP levels Systolic 140–159 or diastolic 90–99	Risk>Benefit	Among women with hypertension, COC users were at increased risk of stroke, acute MI, and peripheral arterial disease compared with nonusers.
Systolic >160 or diastolic >100	Risk Unacceptable	
Vascular disease	Risk Unacceptable	
History of high BP during pregnancy (currently normotensive)	Benefit>Risk	Women who had history of high BP in pregnancy, who also used COCs, had an increased risk of MI and VTE, compared with COC users who did not have a history of high BP during pregnancy. The absolute risks of acute MI and VTE in this population are small.

RECOMMENDATIONS OF THE AMERICAN COLLEGE OF OBSTETRICS AND GYNECOLOGY AND WORLD HEALTH ORGANIZATION FOR USE OF COMBINED ESTROGEN–PROGESTIN ORAL CONTRACEPTIVES IN WOMEN WITH CHARACTERISTICS THAT MIGHT INCREASE RISK OF ADVERSE EFFECTS—cont'd

Condition	Risk Status	Comment
DVT/PE		
History of or current DVT/PE	Risk Unacceptable	
Family history of DVT/PE (first-degree relatives)	Benefit>Risk	
Major surgery		
With prolonged immobilization	Risk Unacceptable	
Without prolonged immobilization	Benefit>Risk	
Minor surgery without immobilization	No Restriction	
Known thrombogenic mutations (e.g., factor V Leiden; prothrombin mutation; protein S, protein C, and antithrombin deficiencies)	Risk Unacceptable	Routine screening not appropriate because of the rarity of these conditions and high cost of screening. Among women with thrombogenic mutations, COC users had a 2- to 20-fold higher risk of thrombosis than nonusers.
Ischemic heart disease	Risk Unacceptable	
Stroke	Risk Unacceptable	
Hyperlipidemias		Routine screening inappropriate due to rarity of conditions and high cost. Base assessment on type, severity, and presence of other cardiovascular risk factors.
Headaches		
Nonmigrainous	No Restriction	Classification depends on accurate diagnosis of severe headaches that are migrainous and those that are not. Any new headaches or marked changes in headaches should be evaluated. Classification is for women without other risk factors for stroke. Stroke risk increases with age, hypertension, and smoking.
Migraine without aura		Women who also had aura had a higher stroke risk than those without aura. COC users had a two- to four-fold increased risk of stroke versus nonusers.
Age <35	Benefit>Risk	
Age >35	Risk>Benefit	
With aura, at any age	Risk Unacceptable	
Diabetes		
History of gestational disease	No Restriction	Patient should be assessed according to severity of condition.
Nonvascular disease		
Noninsulin dependent	Benefit>Risk	
Insulin dependent	Benefit> Risk	
Nephropathy/retinopathy/neuropathy	Risk>Benefit/Risk Unacceptable	
Other vascular disease or diabetes of >20 years duration	Risk>Benefit/Risk Unacceptable	Patient should be assessed according to severity of condition.

COC, combination oral contraceptive; CVD, cardiovascular disease; DVT, deep venous thrombosis; MI, myocardial infarct; OCP, oral contraceptive; PE, pulmonary embolism.

From World Health Organization. In: *Improving Access to Quality Care in Family Planning: Medical Eligibility Criteria for Contraceptive Use.* 3rd ed. Geneva: World Health Organization, 2004.

Table 70–1. Recommendations of the American College of Obstetrics and Gynecology and World Health Organization for Use of Combined Estrogen–Progestin Oral Contraceptives in Women with Characteristics that Might Increase Risk of Adverse Effects

menopausal women.[32] Combined (estrogen plus progestin) HRT is indicated only for the treatment of vasomotor symptoms and symptoms of vulvovaginal atrophy associated with the menopause and for prevention of postmenopausal osteoporosis. Most guidelines suggest that HRT be administered in the lowest doses and for the shortest time period needed to achieve the desired clinical effect.[32]

In this chapter we review the mechanisms by which estrogens and progestins alter blood pressure, and the important clinical studies of the effects of OCs and HRT on blood pressure and related target-organ damage.

MECHANISMS

Estrogens

Estrogens reduce blood pressure, and thereby CVD risk, by multiple mechanisms, including modulation of nitric oxide (NO)-mediated vascular responses,[33–36] inhibition of sympathetic nervous system activity and vasoconstrictor responses to sympathetic stimulation,[37,38] suppression of the renin–angiotensin system,[39,40] inhibition of plasminogen-activator inhibitor type-1 (PAI-1) and endothelin,[41] and enhanced production of natriuretic peptides[42] and prostacyclin[43] (Figure 70–1).

NO-Mediated vascular responses

Estrogen acts on the endothelium to increase the production of the vasodilators NO and prostacyclin[35,36] (Figure 70–1). Physiologic levels of estradiol potentiate endothelium-dependent, flow-mediated vasodilation in postmenopausal women, in part by modifying the synthesis/release/bioactivity of the powerful vasodilator NO.[33] It has been suggested that gender differences in vascular tone may be accounted for by the increased NO release from the endothelium in women compared to men. This gender difference tends to disappear in menopause when the circulating level of estrogen falls. Circulating levels of NO metabolites in postmenopausal women are generally less than 25 µmol/L, most likely because of estrogen deficiency, and treatment with oral or transdermal unopposed estrogen or tibolone has been shown, at least in the short term, to increase NO metabolites in these women.[44] Whether these endothelium-mediated effects on NO synthesis/release can be sustained over many years of menopausal hormone treatment is unknown.

Estrogen increases circulating NO/NO metabolite levels by a variety of mechanisms. It stimulates expression and activation of endothelial nitric oxide synthase (eNOS) via both genomic and nongenomic mechanisms, enhances Ca^{2+} dependent NO release from endothelial cells, and modulates generation of reactive oxygen species and reduces oxidative stress by inhibiting NADPH oxidase. Thus, the effects of estrogen on the NO pathway are related to its antioxidant effects, which increase the bioavailability of NO.[45] These antioxidant/NO potentiating effects of estrogen inhibit the adhesion of activated monocytes to the endothelium, the initiating phase of atherosclerosis, thus protecting the vasculature against plaque formation via a mechanism that is independent of blood pressure.[46]

Sympathoinhibition

Estrogen supplementation in healthy perimenopausal women attenuates the pressor, glucocorticoid, and catecholamine responses to stress, suggesting that it inhibits sympathetic outflow from the central nervous system.[37] These effects may explain part of the apparently beneficial actions of estrogen on the acute symptoms of menopause and on long-term cardiovascular risk. Presynaptic modulation of norepinephrine release is another major way in which estrogen is thought to reduce the sympathetic response.[38] Further, estrogen therapy has been shown to improve baroreceptor sensitivity, thus lowering blood pressure and rate pressure product at rest and during physiologic challenge.[47] Perimenopausal women given estrogen supplementation show both an attenuated vasoconstrictor response to norepinephrine and diminished total body norepinephrine spillover, a measure of reduced sympathetic neural activity.[48] Estrogen blunts the vasoconstrictor response to norepinephrine and other sympathetic mediators by inhibiting Ca^{2+} entry into vascular smooth muscle cells, thus lowering intracellular free Ca^{2+} and attenuating the ability of the muscle to contract[49] (Figure 70–1). Thus, by mediating endothelium-dependent vasodilation and modulating sympathetically mediated vasoconstriction, estrogen may play an important role in regulating vascular tone and compliance and therefore blood pressure in women.[50] Mode of delivery seems to play a role here, since muscle sympathetic nerve activity and blood pressure in postmenopausal women are decreased by chronic transdermal estrogens but not oral estrogens.[51,52] These differential effects of oral vs. transdermal estrogen treatment have been attributed to induction of insulin-like growth factor-1 (IGF-1) deficiency and increased adiposity/reduced lean body mass by oral estrogens.[51,53–55] Sympathetic overactivity related to IGF-1 deficiency and/or increased adiposity opposes the direct inhibitory effect of estrogen on sympathetic nerve discharge, which is unopposed during transdermal estrogen treatment.

Aortic stiffness

Central arterial stiffness and wave reflections increase with advancing age and elevate systolic and pulse pressure.[56] Pulse wave analysis of 333 apparently healthy women in the Framingham Heart Study offspring cohort revealed a marked age-related increase in aortic stiffness, assessed by carotid-femoral pulse wave velocity. Augmentation of arterial stiffness with increasing age is more prominent in women than in men,[57] and appears to be further accelerated by occurrence of menopause.[58] A cross-sectional study of 3149 Japanese women undergoing annual health screening examination revealed that the relationship between age and the brachial-ankle pulse wave velocity, an index of central arterial stiffness, has the form of a quadratic curve with a slope that steepens after menopause.[59] Limitations of this study include its cross-sectional design, reliance on self-report for definition of menopausal status, and the

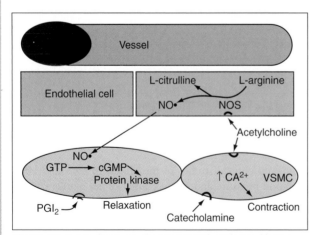

Figure 70–1. Mechanisms of estrogen-induced vasodilation. Estrogen relaxes vascular smooth muscle by increasing PGI2 and NO levels; decreases vasoconstriction by acting as a calcium antagonist. (Redrawn with modification from *Heart Lung* 2001;30:401–426.)

lack of precision of brachial-ankle pulse wave velocity in assessing central arterial stiffness. Nevertheless, because of the large number of women examined, this study provides important evidence that menopause, and probably estrogen deficiency, has unfavorable effects on central arterial stiffness. To test the hypothesis that loss of hormonal modulation contributes to the rapid increase in arterial stiffness seen in the perimenopausal period, the effects of HRT and selective estrogen receptor modulators on arterial stiffness and blood pressure in perimenopausal women have been examined.[60–63] HRT decreased pulse wave velocity and increased arterial compliance without major effects on blood pressure in these studies, indicating that ovarian hormones have favorable effects on central arterial stiffness that are independent of blood pressure. While the responsible cellular/molecular mechanisms have not been defined precisely, it is thought that impaired endothelial function and increased NO bioavailability play a major role.

Suppression of renin-angiotensin-aldosterone system

Estrogen modulates expression of several components of the renin-angiotensin-aldosterone cascade, including renin, angiotensinogen, angiotensin-converting enzyme (ACE), and the angiotensin AT_1 receptor[39,40] (Figure 70–2). Renin levels are lower in women than in men, and in postmenopausal women receiving estrogen therapy than in those not receiving estrogen.[39,64] Both endogenous estrogen and estrogen replacement therapy are associated with reduced plasma renin and prorenin concentrations, serum ACE activity and tissue ACE and AT_1 receptor expression in women and experimental animals.[39,64–69] Additionally, estrogen induces production of the heptapeptide Ang 1-7, a potent vasodilator and inhibitor of smooth muscle cell growth,[68] and inhibits angiotensin-induced aldosterone secretion in ovariectomized animals.[70] This effect appears to be mediated by a posttranscriptional mechanism by which estradiol interferes with ribosomal efficiency for AT_1 receptor translation.[71] In contrast, estrogen stimulates synthesis of angiotensinogen in liver and isolated hepatocytes, probably by binding to an estrogen response element in the angiotensinogen gene promoter.[72,73] This pro-hypertensive effect of estrogen on the initial step of the cascade opposes its inhibitory actions on downstream components. Thus, estrogen has a dichotomous effect on the renin-angiotensin-aldosterone system, whereby it increases the initial substrate (angiotensinogen) but inhibits the generation and biological action of the active hormones (angiotensin II and aldosterone), thus tending to reduce blood pressure and related target organ damage.

Renal effects

Postmenopausal women are more salt sensitive than premenopausal women, and salt sensitivity correlates inversely with levels of circulating ovarian hormones in the former group.[74,75] Further, a strong sodium–blood pressure association that is independent of age has been identified in postmenopausal women, suggesting that postmenopausal salt sensitivity is related to hormonal changes rather than aging.[76] Estrogen protects against salt-induced increases in blood pressure, at least in part by increasing the sensitivity of the pressure–natriuresis relationship and augmenting renal excretion of sodium.[77] In young normotensive women, the pressure–natriuresis relationship is steep during all phases of the menstrual cycle and during oral contraceptive use, indicating insensitivity to salt. However, the pressure–natriuresis curve is shifted to the right in menopausal women, indicating that BP becomes salt-sensitive after the menopause (Figure 70–3).

To test directly the hypothesis that loss of ovarian hormones increases the salt sensitivity of blood pressure, blood pressure responses to intravenous saline and furosemide challenge were examined in healthy normotensive women immediately prior to and 4 months after surgical menopause.[78] The prevalence of salt sensitivity, defined as a decrease of more than 10 mmHg in systolic blood pressure between salt loading and salt depletion, doubled after surgical menopause, and nearly 40% of salt-resistant

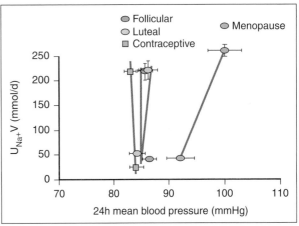

Figure 70–3. Pressure–natriuresis relationship in normotensive women during the normal menstrual cycle, during use of oral contraceptives and after menopause. All women received randomly a diet low in sodium (40 mmol Na⁺/day) and high in sodium (250 mmol Na⁺/day) for 1 week. Blood pressure was measured over 24 hours using ambulatory blood pressure monitoring. (Redrawn from *Am J Hypertens* 2004;17:994–1001.)

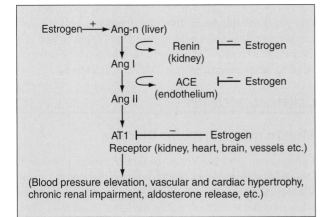

Figure 70–2. The influence of estrogen on the cascade leading to angiotensin II formation and subsequent receptor activation. (Redrawn from *Cardiovasc Res* 2002;53:672–77.)

women developed salt sensitivity without an associated increase in blood pressure during this period (Figure 70–4). Consistent with observations from epidemiologic studies that hypertension may not develop until 5 to 10 years after menopause, the investigators concluded that loss of ovarian hormones may unmask a population of women who, with aging, are at high risk for development of hypertension and CVD.

Progestins

The progestins generally antagonize the effects of estrogen on vascular tone. Native progesterone has minimal effects on endothelium-dependent and endothelium-independent relaxation of arteries *in vivo* and *in vitro*, but co-administration of progesterone with estrogen blunts both modes of vasodilator response to the latter hormone.[79,80] The synthetic progestin medroxyprogesterone acetate (MPA) is a more potent antagonist of estrogen than native progesterone. In ovariectomized monkeys, MPA but not progesterone reduced or completely abolished endothelium-dependent vasorelaxation in response to administration of conjugated equine estrogen in doses comparable to those administered to humans.[81] Likewise, in ovariectomized monkeys subjected to coronary vasospasm induced by direct stimulation, progesterone plus estradiol protected, while MPA plus estradiol failed, to protect against vasospasm.[82]

Progesterone and MPA have differential effects on human umbilical vein endothelial cells *in vitro*: progesterone stimulates eNOS activity, does not alter stimulatory effects of estradiol on eNOS, and augments estradiol-induced ERK 1/2 phosphorylation and Akt phosphorylation, while MPA does not alter eNOS activity, blunts estradiol-induced increases in eNOS activity, and reduces estradiol-dependent ERK 1/2 phosphorylation.[83] Thus, progesterone and MPA are not equivalent, since they have distinct biological effects on vasoactive mediators and intracellular signaling pathways, as well as differential effects on the actions of estradiol.

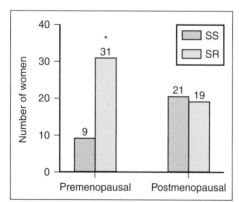

Figure 70–4. Number of study participants with salt sensitivity (SS) and salt resistance (SR) just before (premenopausal) and 4 months after hysterectomy and ovariectomy (postmenopausal). *Significant increase in number of women with SS after surgical menopause (p=0.01). (Redrawn from *Hypertension* 2006;47:1168–74.)

Vascular remodeling

Native progesterone has a dose-dependent inhibitory effect on DNA synthesis and proliferation in rat aortic smooth muscle cells *in vitro*.[84] Progesterone appears to be vasoprotective, while MPA produces unfavorable effects on the vascular injury response by antagonizing the modulatory effects of estrogen on vascular remodeling in response to various stresses, including mechanical injury. In the setting of vascular injury, exogenous native progesterone, administered alone and with estradiol, has variable effects on neointima formation and does not alter the actions of co-administered estrogen. This may be related to variable partial conversion of progesterone to estrogen *in vivo*. In contrast, MPA has no independent biological effect, but blunts the antiproliferative and anti-inflammatory effects of estradiol in the balloon-injured carotid artery of the ovariectomized rat.[85–87] MPA increases neointima formation in injured arteries of intact female rats and abolishes the anti-inflammatory and vasoprotective (inhibition of neointima formation) effects of estradiol in ovariectomized animals. The latter effect of MPA may be mediated by its demonstrated interference with nuclear factor-κB suppression by estrogen.[83]

Renin-angiotensin-aldosterone system

Progesterone may stimulate components of the renin-angiotensin-aldosterone system and may be a competitive inhibitor of mineralocorticoid receptors.[88,89] In women undergoing ovarian stimulation for *in vitro* fertilization, there is a positive relationship between progesterone levels and plasma renin activity during and after ovulation and throughout pregnancy.[88] Progesterone increases plasma renin activity and aldosterone levels in Sprague-Dawley rats and increases baseline and angiotensin II–stimulated aldosterone production in isolated zona glomerulosa cells.[90] Thus, progesterone has complex and directionally opposite effects on components of the renin-angiotensin-aldosterone system that regulate both blood pressure and target organ damage.

Renal effects

Progesterone produces natriuresis in humans.[91,92] This natriuretic effect results from mineralocorticoid-independent direct action on the distal nephron: progesterone increases Ca^{2+} reabsorption and Na^+ excretion in the distal but not the proximal tubule of the rabbit kidney, and progesterone receptors are found in the distal nephron but not the proximal tubules.[93] Whether these effects can be extrapolated to other progestins (e.g., MPA) is unknown.

CLINICAL STUDIES

Menopausal hormone therapy

Endogenous estradiol tends to lower blood pressure.[94] Observational studies of blood pressure through the menstrual cycle have demonstrated that blood pressure is lower when estradiol levels peak during the luteal phase than when they are at their nadir during the follicular phase.[95–97] The rise in blood pressure seen later in life in women has been related to menopause, in addition to aging *per se*, and been attributed to estrogen withdrawal, overproduction of pituitary hormones, weight gain, or a combination of these and other yet undefined neurohumoral influences.[5,98] The menopause is associated with a significant increase in blood pressure in cross-sectional studies.[99] Further, a prospective study of blood pressure in premenopausal, perimenopausal, and postmenopausal women demonstrated an age-dependent 4- to 5-mmHg increase in systolic blood pressure and a tripling in risk of developing hypertension in postmenopausal women over a 5-year follow-up period[100] (Figure 70–5).

Studies of the effects of HRT on blood pressure have reported somewhat inconsistent findings, including blood pressure–neutral,[23,101] blood pressure–lowering,[27–29,102–107] and blood pressure–elevating effects,[108–111] likely due to differences in patient populations studied and in hormone preparations administered, as well as to methodologic differences in blood pressure measurement. In the Postmenopausal Estrogen/Progestin Interventions (PEPI) trial, which enrolled 875 healthy normotensive early postmenopausal women, assignment to conjugated equine estrogen (CEE) (0.625 mg/day) plus or minus three progestin regimens did not impact systolic or diastolic blood pressure when compared with placebo controls.[23] Systolic blood pressure increased in all three treatment groups over the 3-year follow-up period, but there were no differences between treatments. Similarly, the Lipid Research Clinics Program follow-up study found no differences in systolic or diastolic blood pressures between HRT users and nonusers, although the latter had significantly higher body weight.[101]

In contrast, the Baltimore Longitudinal Study on Aging found that HRT has favorable effects on blood pressure in postmenopausal women.[29] This observational study followed 226 normotensive, postmenopausal women for an average of 5.7 years, 75 using both estrogen and progestin, and 149 using neither. There was a smaller increase in systolic blood pressure over time in women taking HRT than those not taking HRT, and the difference was greater at older ages (Figure 70–6). Diastolic blood pressure was not affected by HRT in this study. Similarly, the Framingham Heart Study reported that the average systolic blood pressure of HRT users was 139.4 mmHg (standard error [SE]=22.4 mmHg), compared with 142.1 mmHg (SE=23.4 mmHg) in nonusers.[102] The Rancho Bernardo study also reported HRT users had systolic and diastolic blood pressures that

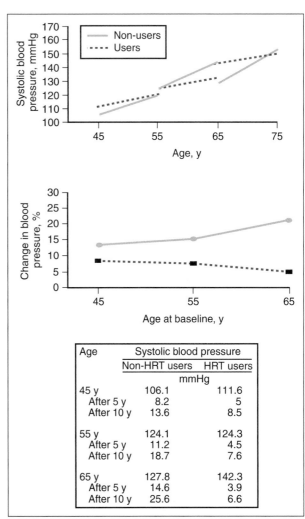

Age	Systolic blood pressure	
	Non-HRT users	HRT users
	mmHg	
45 y	106.1	111.6
After 5 y	8.2	5
After 10 y	13.6	8.5
55 y	124.1	124.3
After 5 y	11.2	4.5
After 10 y	18.7	7.6
65 y	127.8	142.3
After 5 y	14.6	3.9
After 10 y	25.6	6.6

Figure 70–6. Results of a mixed-effects model predicting average changes in systolic blood pressure over time at different ages at first visit. The table below the graph shows the predicted average systolic blood pressure at first visit and the predicted average increase at different follow-up points (**top**). Predicted average increase in systolic blood pressure in hormone replacement therapy users (*dotted line*) and nonusers (*solid line*) over a mean follow-up of 10 years. Average predicted changes in systolic blood pressure are expressed as percentages to take into account the difference in starting systolic blood pressure at first visit in different age groups. The final model of the mixed-effects linear regression has been used to construct the figure (**bottom**). (Redrawn from *Ann Intern Med* 2001;135:229–38.)

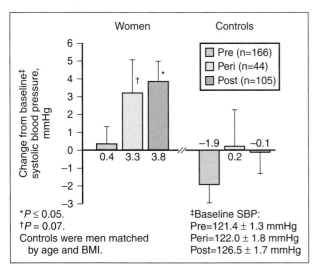

Figure 70–5. The cross-sectional association between the conventionally measured blood pressure and age. The relationship with age was studied cross-sectionally in 166 premenopausal (systolic blood pressure [SBP]=121.4±1.3 mmHg), 44 perimenopausal (SBP=122.0±1.8 mmHg), and 105 postmenopausal (126.5±1.7 mmHg) women and male controls. Values are regression slopes expressed in mmHg per 10 years (standard error), adjusted for body mass index and antihypertensive treatment. *p≤0.05 slopes; †p=0.07. (Reprinted by permission from Macmillan Publishers Ltd: from *J Hum Hypertens* 1997;11:507–14.)

were 2 to 4 mmHg lower than those of nonusers.[103] A follow-up study on a subset of these women[104] showed that those on combined estrogen/progestin had systolic blood pressures 5 mmHg lower than women on estrogen alone, and 7 mmHg lower than women who had never used hormones ($p<0.01$).

A review of papers published since 1960 and listed in MEDLINE found that risk of developing hypertension during HRT was very low.[25] Indeed, blood pressure was often even lowered with HRT treatment: these authors' study of 1397 hypertensive postmenopausal women showed that various transdermal HRT regimens lowered blood pressure by an average of 7 (systolic)/9 (diastolic) mmHg. Remarkably, only 30 patients (0.22%) developed increased blood pressure. A recent study carried out in 161 postmenopausal women with hypertension showed that systolic blood pressure remained unaffected and diastolic blood pressure was reduced during HRT administration.[26] This was an extension of an earlier cohort of 75 hypertensive menopausal women, where the introduction of HRT did not adversely affect mean blood pressure, despite a small increase in mean weight.[112] However, few high-risk participants were enrolled in the study, and the authors cautioned that blood pressure should be monitored regularly in hypertensive postmenopausal women receiving HRT.

The Women's Health Initiative (WHI) collected data on risk factors for CVD, including blood pressure, from 98,705 women aged 50 to 79 years, the largest multiethnic, best-characterized cohort of postmenopausal women ever studied.[108] WHI found that current hormone use was associated with a 25% greater likelihood of having hypertension compared to past use or no prior use. The estrogen-plus-progestin clinical trial component of WHI, a placebo-controlled trial of HRT (CEE 0.625 mg/day plus MPA 2.5 mg/day) in 16,608 postmenopausal women, found a small (~1 mmHg) increase in systolic blood pressure in the active treatment group compared to the placebo control group.[109,110] Importantly, the trial found significant increases in risk of CVD, including coronary heart disease, stroke, and venous thromboemboli, as well as increased risk of invasive breast cancer in the HRT group. Following publication of the WHI results, consensus panels recommended against use of HRT for chronic disease prevention in postmenopausal women, and promotion and prescribing of HRT fell drastically. Prescriptions for the fixed dose combination of CEE plus MPA declined by 66%, and those for unopposed CEE fell by 33%[113–115] (Figure 70–7). Transdermal hormone preparations were less affected, and transvaginal and low-dose preparations gained in usage.

The Estrogen Replacement Trial (ERT) in the WHI randomized 5310 postmenopausal women who had undergone hysterectomy to CEE (0.625 mg/day) and an equal number to placebo.[111] In the CEE group, there was a 1.1-mmHg increase from baseline in systolic blood pressure at 1 year that persisted throughout the 6.8 years of follow-up and was not seen in the placebo group. There was no difference in diastolic blood pressure between treatment groups. In contrast, administration of transdermal estradiol in physiologic doses to healthy postmenopausal women has been shown to lower nocturnal systolic, diastolic, and mean blood pressure when compared to placebo in studies that employed ambulatory blood pressure monitoring.[105–107] The selective benefits of transdermal estradiol over oral conjugated estrogen on blood pressure may relate to delivery

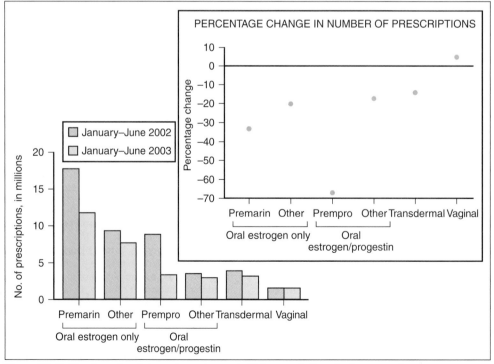

Figure 70–7. Number of and percentage change in U.S. prescriptions for hormone therapy, January–June 2002 to January–June 2003 by formulation. (Redrawn from *JAMA* 2004;291:47–53.)

of lower, more sustained levels of circulating estrogen without a potentially proinflammatory first-pass effect in the liver.[116]

A mechanistic study that compared 6 months of treatment with transdermal estradiol (0.05 mg/day) plus oral MPA (2.5 mg/day) to oral CEE (0.625 mg/day) plus the same progestin dose in healthy postmenopausal smokers, demonstrated more consistent and pronounced reductions in blood pressure, total peripheral resistance, and circulating norepinephrine levels, and increases in endothelium-dependent vasodilation and vascular β-adrenoreceptor responsiveness in the transdermal estradiol group[117] (Figure 70–8). These relationships held during both resting and stress conditions. Importantly, serum estrogen (estradiol and esterone) concentrations were lower and

more reflective of premenopausal values during transdermal estrogen treatment compared to CEE.

Whether the improvements in endothelial function and other determinants of vascular integrity observed in this short-term study translate to vasoprotection and prevention of atherosclerosis with transdermal estradiol is being tested in the ongoing Kronos Early Estrogen Prevention Study (KEEPS).[118] KEEPS is evaluating the effectiveness of CEE (0.45 mg/day) or transdermal estradiol (50 μg/week) in combination with cyclic oral micronized progesterone and placebo in preventing the progression of vascular disease, as assessed by ultrasound measurement of carotid intimal-medial thickness and electron beam tomographic measurement of coronary artery calcification in women aged 42 to 56 years who are within 36 months of their final menstrual period. The placebo-controlled Early versus Late Intervention Trial with Estradiol (ELITE) is testing whether oral 17β-estradiol (1 mg/day) can slow the progression of vascular disease assessed by surrogate endpoints in postmenopausal women.[119] ELITE is randomizing women according to their number of years since menopause (<6 vs. ≥10) to receive either oral 17β-estradiol (1 mg/day) or placebo; women with a uterus also receive vaginal progesterone gel (or placebo gel) for the last 10 days of each month. Carotid artery thickness by ultrasound is the primary endpoint of the trial. Surrogate endpoints for vascular disease will be measured in both trials in lieu of morbid and mortal CVD events, which are rare in the perimenopausal age group.

Remarkably, and in contrast to the other outcome trials of menopausal hormone therapy, the ERT component of the WHI showed no significant effect of unopposed CEE on coronary heart disease risk.[111] There was even a statistically significant time trend in coronary heart disease occurrence that suggested a modest benefit with long-term use. Possible explanations for the discrepancy in effects of the two hormone regimens (CEE plus MPA vs. unopposed CEE) that were tested in WHI include the deleterious effects of the progestin MPA, which has been shown in preclinical studies to negate the anti-inflammatory and vasoprotective effects of 17β-estradiol in the setting of acute vascular injury,[85–87] as well as differences in study populations (with or without hysterectomy) and baseline risk factors, duration of intervention, and follow-up, and play of chance.[113,120]

Another surprising finding of the ERT component of the WHI is that CEE appears to have more favorable effects in younger than older women.[111] Estimated hazard ratios for CEE for several outcomes, including coronary heart disease, were lower for women in their fifties than for older women (Figure 70–9). Although the differences in hazard ratios across age groups were not statistically significant, the results are consistent with the concept, supported by both human and animal studies, that aging and prolonged hormone deprivation may attenuate the hemodynamic, anti-inflammatory, neurohormonal, and vasoprotective effects of estrogen.[121–124] For example, HRT has been shown to alter hemodynamics (blood pressure, heart rate, cardiac output, systemic vascular resistance, and plasma norepinephrine levels) under resting and behavioral stress conditions in women who were within 5 years after menopause but not in

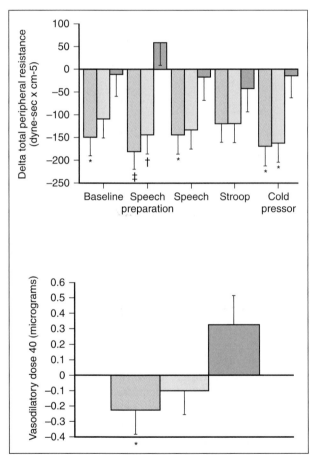

Figure 70–8. Change from pretreatment levels (post-treatment–pretreatment) in total peripheral resistance during baseline rest and stressors in women randomly assigned to transdermal estrogen (*n*=34, *p*<0.05), oral conjugated equine estrogen (*n*=33), or placebo (*n*=21). Orange bar=transdermal (*n*=31); green bar=oral (*n*=30); blue bar=placebo (*n*=21). *p*<0.05, *p*<0.01, *p*<0.001 versus placebo (**top**). Change from pretreatment levels (post-treatment–pretreatment) in the dose of isoproterenol required to decrease vascular resistance by 40% in women randomly assigned to transdermal estrogen (n=29), oral conjugated equine estrogen (n=29), or placebo (n=21). Orange bar=transdermal (n=29); green bar=oral (n=29); blue bar=placebo (n=21). *p*<0.05 versus placebo (**bottom**). (Redrawn from *Obstet Gynecol* 2004;103:169–80.)

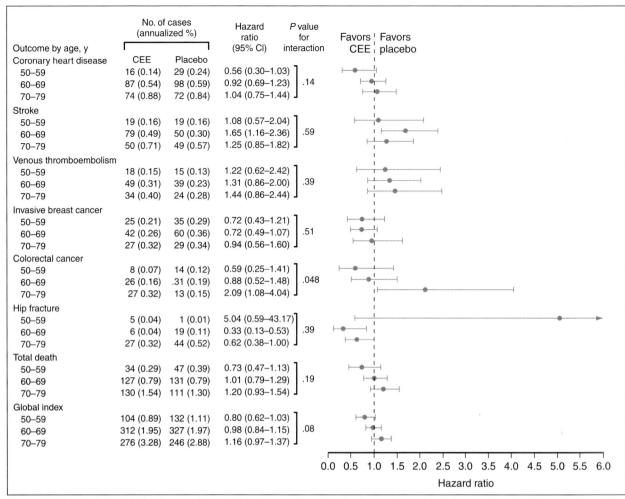

Figure 70–9. Selected clinical outcomes by participant age and randomization assignment. Data are plotted as hazard ratios with error bars showing 95% confidence intervals. CEE, conjugated equine estrogen; CI, confidence interval. (Redrawn with permission from *JAMA* 2004;291:1701–12.)

those more than 5 years postmenopausal[121] (Figure 70–10). HRT was associated with a major reduction (–8.5 mmHg) in blood pressure in women at less than 5 years post-menopause, but had no depressor effect in those who were five or more years postmenopausal. Systemic vascular resistance and plasma norepinephrine also trended downward in response to HRT only in women who were less than 5 years postmenopausal.

The positive studies of HRT and ERT on blood pressure and vascular function discussed previously were carried out in healthy women in the early years postmenopause; the studies that showed harmful or neutral effects of HRT or estrogen on CVD outcomes were carried out in older women (average age ≥60 years) who were many years postmenopause.[109–111] The KEEPS and ELITE studies are testing the hypothesis that HRT initiated at the time of menopause will delay the onset of subclinical CVD, ultimately providing cardiovascular benefit to women.

The selective estrogen receptor modulators (SERMs) are agents that bind to estrogen receptors and produce estrogen-agonist effects in some tissues and estrogen-antagonist effects in others. Raloxifene, the most widely used SERM,

has favorable effects on markers of cardiovascular risk, including LDL cholesterol and fibrinogen, and therefore its effects on coronary outcomes have been tested in women with or at increased risk for coronary heart disease.[124] The Raloxifene Use for Heart Disease (RUTH) trial tested the effects of raloxifene 60 mg/d compared to placebo on coronary events (death from coronary causes, myocardial infarction, or hospitalization for an acute coronary syndrome) and invasive breast cancer in 10,101 postmenopausal women (mean age 67.5 years) with coronary heart disease or multiple CVD risk factors over a median 5.6 years of follow-up. Raloxifene treatment had no significant effect on the risk of primary coronary events, all-cause mortality, or total stroke, but was associated with increases in fatal stroke and venous thromboembolism. The authors did not comment on blood pressure. Their main conclusion was that the benefits of raloxifene in reducing risks of invasive breast cancer and vertebral fracture, demonstrated in RUTH, should be weighed against the increased risks of venous thromboembolism and fatal stroke. There is no evidence that raloxifene or any other SERM has a role in blood pressure management or CVD prevention.

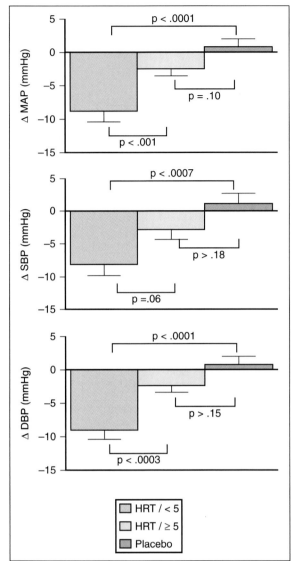

Figure 70–10. Change (Δ) in MAP, SBP, and DBP after 6 months of treatment in the three study groups (HRT-treated/postmenopausal <5 years; HRT-treated/postmenopausal ≥5 years; placebo). Δ values are averaged across rest and task periods (cold pressor, active and passive speech, paper and computerized Stroop). The HRT/<5 group showed significantly greater decreases in MAP and DBP compared with the HRT/≥5 group, which did not differ significantly from placebo. DBP, diastolic blood pressure; HRT, hormone replacement therapy; MAP, mean arterial pressure; SBP, systolic blood pressure. (Redrawn from *Am J Obstet Gynecol* 2004;190:1052–58.)

Recommendation

Pending the availability of data supporting the benefits of initiating HRT and/or ERT in the perimenopausal period in preventing CVD, caution is advised. Menopausal hormone treatment is not recommended for the prevention or treatment of CVD, and if administered for other indications, such as relief of hot flashes and vaginal dryness, use of the lowest effective dose for the shortest period of time needed to relieve menopausal symptoms is recommended. Unopposed estrogen treatment is recommended for women who have undergone hysterectomy; combined estrogen

plus low-dose progestin treatment is required for women with intact uteri to prevent unwanted uterine bleeding and endometrial carcinoma.

In relation to HRT use and BP management, we would suggest the following approach:

1. All clinicians should measure blood pressure before starting HRT.
2. In a normotensive postmenopausal woman, blood pressure should be measured annually following the start of HRT. One exception may be the use of Premarin, where a follow-up blood pressure measurement should be made at 3 months, due to a possible rare idiosyncratic rise in blood pressure.[125]
3. In hypertensive menopausal women, blood pressure should at least be measured initially and thereafter at 6-month intervals, although if blood pressure is labile or difficult to control, three-month measurements should be done.
4. If a hypertensive woman on HRT demonstrates a rise in blood pressure, careful monitoring or observation and perhaps alteration or increase of antihypertensive treatment should be given.

Oral contraceptives
Combined estrogen–progestin oral contraceptives

Since the doses of estrogen and the types of progestin in combined oral contraceptive (COC) preparations have changed over time, published reports of the effects of COCs on blood pressure have been inconsistent and sometimes conflicting. However, the largest and most carefully conducted studies have concluded that use of COCs generally produces modest blood pressure elevation, with development of hypertension in a subgroup of women, and improvement of blood pressure upon withdrawal in most. Further, increases in blood pressure are major contributors to the adverse effects of COCs on the vasculature and to the increased prevalence of CVD, particularly stroke, among COC users.[126]

A cross-sectional survey (Health Survey for England) of a sociodemographically representative sample of 3545 premenopausal English women, 892 of whom were current users of OCs (815 COCs and 77 progestin-only contraceptives [POCs]), revealed that mean blood pressures adjusted for age were significantly higher among COC users (125/70 mmHg) than among nonusers (123/68 mmHg, $p<0.001$)[127] (Figure 70–11). Interestingly, blood pressures tended to be lower among POC users than among nonusers, although the numbers were small and the difference statistically nonsignificant. Blood pressure differences between users and nonusers tended to increase with age such that there was a 4-mmHg excess in systolic blood pressure in OC users aged 35 years and older, a number compatible with increased CVD risk at the population level. The results were not altered by adjustment for body mass index (lower among OC users), alcohol intake (higher among OC users), physical activity, and antihypertensive treatment.

The Health Survey for England did not collect detailed information about the formulations and durations of current and past OC use, making it impossible to assess the impact of estrogen dose on blood pressure. However, a contem-

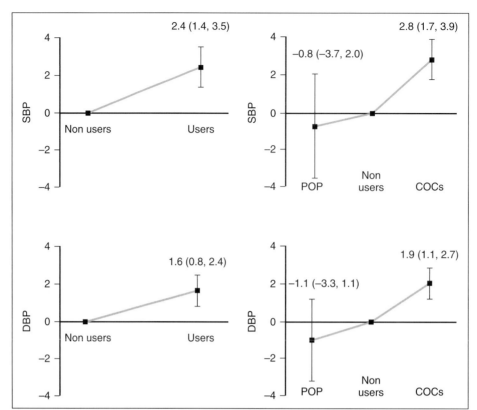

Figure 70–11. Differences in blood pressure (mmHg) between oral contraceptive users and nonusers, adjusted for age, body mass index, smoking, alcohol consumption, physical activity and treatment for hypertension. Confidence interval in parentheses. COCs, combined oral contraceptives; DBP, diastolic blood pressure; POP, progestogen-only pills; SBP, systolic blood pressure. (Redrawn from *J Hypertens* 1997;15:1063–68.)

poraneous study of OC use in the United Kingdom showed that more than 90% of users of COCs used products containing less than 35 μg of estrogen,[128] suggesting that the blood pressure effects observed in the Health Survey for England related mainly to low-dose estrogen contraceptives. The authors concluded that even low-dose COCs constitute a health risk, and recommend that women have their blood pressures checked before they receive COCs and that their blood pressures be monitored on a regular basis during COC use. For women with preexisting hypertension, POCs were recommended.

The Nurses' Health Study II (NHS II), a prospective cohort study of 68,297 premenopausal women free of CVD, documented the magnitude of the problem of OC-induced hypertension in the United States. The multivariate risk for the development of hypertension among current users of OCs compared with never-users was 1.8 (confidence interval [CI] 1.5–2.3).[13] Absolute risk was small, however (only 41.5 cases of hypertension per 10,000 person-years could be attributed to OC use), and risk decreased quickly with cessation of OC use (past users had only a slightly increased [relative risk 1.2, CI=1.0–1.4] risk compared with never-users).

Importantly, however, there is evidence that prolonged use of OCs and continuation of OC treatment in women with established hypertension lead to increased prevalence and severity of hypertension and progressive difficulty in

blood pressure control.[13,129] In a prospective cross-sectional study of 171 women who were referred to a specialized hypertension clinic, of whom 66 were current users of OCs, 26 were users of other contraceptive methods, and 79 were nonusers of contraception, OC use was associated with increased diastolic blood pressure and poor blood pressure control, independent of age, body mass index, and antihypertensive drug treatment. Diastolic blood pressure was significantly higher in OC users (100±16 mmHg) than in those using other contraceptive methods (93±15 mmHg) and in nonusers (93±14 mmHg). Systolic blood pressure was also higher in OC users, although the difference was not statistically significant. Blood pressure control (<140/90 mmHg) was achieved in only 17% of OC users, versus 35% of users of alternate methods and 32% of nonusers (*p*=0.046 for trend), and a higher proportion of OC users had stage 2 or 3 hypertension according to JNC VI (Joint National Committee on Prevention, Detection, Evaluation, and Treatment of High Blood Pressure, 6th report) criteria. These differences in blood pressure control could not be related to a lower intensity of antihypertensive treatment for OC users. Finally, there was a significant positive association between duration of OC use, adjusted for age, and levels of both systolic and diastolic blood pressure, supporting the findings of the Nurses' Health Study II, in which the cohort using OC for more than 6 years had an increased risk of developing hypertension (Hazard ratio 2.1, CI=1.6–27).[13] In this cross-sectional study, information about formulation of the OC used was available from 60% of participants: 62% of these used low-dose (≤30 μg estrogen) and 38%, high-dose (≥50 μg estrogen) OCs. Use of POCs was not reported. This study lends further support to the recommendation that POCs or alternative contraceptive methods be used rather than COCs in women with established hypertension.

COC use has been associated with increases in blood pressure, plasma renin activity, and aldosterone excretion, and these elevated blood pressure and hormone levels have been shown to normalize within weeks of COC withdrawal. In the absence of appropriate control data from COC users who did not develop hypertension, these findings suggest, but do not prove, that the hypertension-promoting effects of COCs are related to activation of the renin-angiotensin-aldosterone system and attendant alterations in intrarenal hemodynamics and salt and water handling.[130] Alternative mechanisms that have been adduced to explain the pressure effects of COCs include increases in sympathetic nervous system activity[131] and insulin resistance,[132] and alterations in hemodynamics[133] and adrenal cortical function.[134] Definitive evidence supporting these putative mechanisms is lacking, and mechanistic research in the area is hampered by the low prevalence of oral contraceptive-induced hypertension, the difficulty of carrying out controlled experiments in human subjects, and the unavailability of suitable animal models.

Progestin-only oral contraceptives

The finding of the Health Survey for England that POCs do not increase blood pressure confirmed the observations of previous investigators.[135,136] Further, it has been shown that the type and dose of progestin included in COCs can influence the effect of the estrogenic component on blood pressure.[137,138] A review of published literature (PUBMED and Cochrane database), which included three prospective controlled trials and one cross-sectional survey published in the period 1970–1994,[127,135,136,139] revealed no significant association of high blood pressure with use of POCs ("minipills") for up to 2 to 3 years of follow-up.[140] This neutral effect on blood pressure was seen with some POCs even among women who had developed blood pressure elevations while taking COCs.[136,141] Further, the second-generation progestin norgestrel has been reported to reduce blood pressure in women with a history of hypertension, resulting in a recommendation that it be used in women with a history of blood pressure elevation with COC or long-acting progestin use, as well as women with preexisting hypertension.[136,139,140] Importantly, there is no randomized controlled trial designed to examine the effect of POCs on blood pressure. Thus, the highest level of evidence on this important issue is lacking.

It is important to note that various progestins have differential effects on blood pressure and other CVD risk factors. For example, norethisterone, a first-generation progestin that was developed in the 1960s, has been shown to elevate blood pressure in women with a history of COC-induced hypertension[136] and levonorgestrel (Norplant) implants have been reported to elevate blood pressure and increase the risk of developing borderline hypertension (now referred

to as prehypertension).[142–144] The third-generation progestins, including desogestrel, gestodene, and norgestimate, which came into use in Europe in the 1980s and in the United States in the 1990s, were developed to minimize the androgenic side effects of the earlier progestins, including acne, insulin resistance, sodium retention, and adverse effects on blood pressure and lipoproteins. They contain reduced doses and different types of progestins from earlier preparations.[145]

Drospirenone, a novel fourth-generation progestin, contains a 17a-spironolactone group that confers a mineralocorticoid antagonist effect similar to that described for progesterone.[146–149] Drospirenone is eight times as potent a mineralocorticoid receptor antagonist as spironolactone, has antiandrogenic effects, and resembles natural progesterone more closely than conventional synthetic progestins.[148,149] Thus, a 3-mg drospirenone dose is equivalent to 25 mg of spironolactone, the usual antihypertensive dose of the latter agent. Compared to placebo, drospirenone in a dose of 2 mg/day has been shown to effect a natriuresis and weight loss in normal menstruating young women.[146] A combination of 3 mg of drospirenone plus 30 μg EE, currently available as an oral contraceptive, reduces blood pressure and body weight and effects a negative sodium balance when compared to COC preparations containing 30 μg EE plus 150 μg levonorgestrel, a synthetic progestin that has no mineralocorticoid receptor antagonist activity.[150] Thus, drospirenone effectively counteracts the sodium-retaining and aldosterone-stimulating effects of EE, suggesting that it may be useful as an antihypertensive agent.[149,150]

The combination of drospirenone plus 17β-estradiol has been shown in randomized placebo-controlled trials to be effective in lowering blood pressure in hypertensive postmenopausal women.[151–154] The 3 mg of drospirenone plus 1 mg of 17β-estradiol combination reduced blood pressure by ~9/5 mmHg in postmenopausal women with stage 1 hypertension who were being treated with an angiotensin-converting enzyme inhibitor or an angiotensin receptor blocker for hypertension.[151,152] Further, in a larger (213 participants) 12-week placebo-controlled study in post-menopausal women with stage 1 hypertension, treatment with 3 mg of drospirenone plus 1 mg of 17β-estradiol reduced clinic blood pressure by 14/8 mmHg compared to 7/3 mmHg for the placebo (p<0.0001).[153] In a subgroup of 43 women subjected to ambulatory blood pressure monitoring, 24-hour blood pressure fell by 9/4 mmHg (vs. 2/2 mmHg with placebo, p=0.002/0.07). Potassium homeostasis was evaluated in this study because mineralocorticoid receptor blockade has been associated with significant increases in serum potassium.[150,155] No significant changes from baseline in potassium levels or in the incidence of hyperkalemia were noted with drospirenone treatment.

Most recently, a rigorous dose-ranging study of the drospirenone–17β-estradiol combination compared to estradiol alone and placebo has been carried out in 750 postmenopausal women with stage 1 to stage 2 hypertension using both ambulatory and clinic blood pressure monitoring.[154] Significant dose-dependent decreases in systolic and diastolic blood pressure in clinic and on 24-hour ambulatory recording were seen with the 2- and 3-mg doses of drospirenone plus 17β-estradiol; the 1-mg dose, estradiol alone, and placebo were ineffective (Figure 70–12). The treatment-induced blood pressure reductions persisted throughout the 24-hour dosing period and were similar in magnitude to those previously reported for the selective mineralocorticoid receptor antagonist eplerenone. There were no significant changes from baseline in potassium in any treatment group. Given the proven efficacy of the drospirenone–estradiol combination in treatment of vasomotor symptoms associated with menopause and prevention of endometrial bleeding/hyperplasia,[156] it appears to have advantages in the treatment of hypertensive postmenopausal women. A caveat in this regard is the possibility of precipi-

tating hyperkalemia, particularly in those with renal insufficiency and on concomitant angiotensin-converting enzyme inhibitor and/or angiotensin receptor blocker treatment. Longer-term safety studies will likely be needed to clarify this issue.[149]

Recommendation

COCs have a favorable risk–benefit ratio for healthy women who are free of CVD and major CVD risk factors, including hypertension.[18] Both the WHO and ACOG recommend use of COCs containing low doses of estrogen (<35 μg EE by WHO; <50 μg EE combined with the "lowest progestin

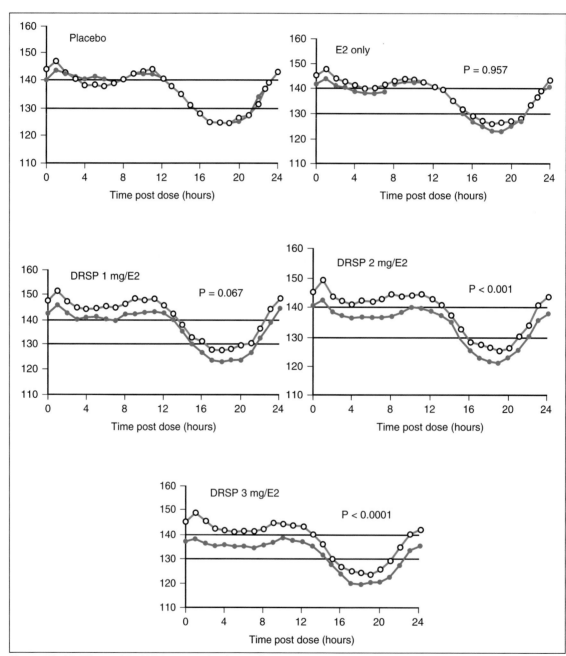

Figure 70–12. Effects of DRSP/E2 versus placebo on the coprimary endpoint of ambulatory systolic blood pressure over 24 hours at baseline and after 8 weeks of double-blind therapy that included placebo, E2 alone, 1-mg DRSP/E2, 2-mg DRSP/E2, and 3-mg DRSP/E2. Baseline period is the o—o , and treatment period is the ●—● . (Redrawn from *Hypertension* 2006;48:246–53.)

dose" by ACOG) for these women.[18,19,20,157] Progestin-only methods, including POCs, depot medroxyprogesterone acetate (MPA), and intrauterine devices are recommended as safer than COCs for women with established CVD, at high risk for CVD, migraine headaches with focal neurologic signs, or history of thromboembolic disease.[19] Table 70–2 summarizes current WHO recommendations with comments on the evidence base for them.[20] ACOG recommendations are similar.[19]

CONCLUSIONS AND PERSPECTIVES

Ovarian hormones play an important role in women's health, providing the most reliable and convenient means of contraception and of relieving menopausal symptoms. Hormone therapy also has other benefits, including the regulation of menstrual irregularities and relief of dysmenorrhea in menstruating women, and prevention of vulvovaginal atrophy and osteoporosis/fractures in postmenopausal women. Further, natural estrogens, principally 17β-estradiol and natural progesterone (but not synthetic progestins), have biological effects that protect the vasculature from oxidative and inflammatory injury and prevent cardiovascular disease. These functions have been adduced by some to account for the 10- to 15-year delay in presentation of clinical cardiovascular disease and events in women compared to men.

Despite these impressive benefits, hormone therapy, both in the form of oral contraceptives and menopausal hormone treatment, poses substantial risks, particularly for women with preexisting cardiovascular disease or multiple cardiovascular risk factors. Principal among these conditions are history of ischemic heart disease, cerebrovascular, peripheral arterial and renal disease, deep-vein thrombosis/pulmonary embolism, hypertension, smoking, diabetes, and older age.

To minimize the risks of oral contraceptives, while at the same time preserving their benefits for the majority of younger, lower-risk women, guidelines specify that combined oral contraceptives should contain low doses of estrogen (<35 or <50 µg of ethinyl estradiol) and the "lowest progestin dose" (Table 70–1).[19,20] Recommendations for use of combined oral contraceptives are then stratified according to the risk status of the woman. For example, ACOG guidelines comment that for healthy nonsmoking women, it is appropriate to continue use of combined oral contraceptives until age 50 to 55 years, after weighing the risks and benefits.[19] Risk of venous thromboembolic disease and atherosclerotic cardiovascular disease with combined oral contraceptive use increases rapidly after age 35 to 40, particularly in the presence of multiple cardiovascular risk factors, and is unacceptable for some, such as smokers over age 35 years and those with stage 2 hypertension (blood pressure >160 mmHg systolic or >100 mmHg diastolic) (Table 70–1). Progestin-only oral contraceptives, depot MPA injections, or the levonogestrel intrauterine system provide safe alternatives to combined oral contraceptives for these high-risk women.

Despite evidence from observational studies that estrogen treatment is associated with reduced risk of coronary heart disease in postmenopausal women, menopausal hormone therapy has lost favor in recent years because of reports of increased stroke and coronary heart disease risk in randomized controlled trials. Guidelines recommend that menopausal hormone therapy not be used for the prevention of cardiovascular disease and, if used for the treatment of menopausal symptoms, that it be administered in the lowest doses and for the shortest time period needed to achieve the desired clinical effect.[32] However, estrogens, particularly 17β-estradiol, have been shown to have anti-inflammatory, vasoprotective, and favorable hemodynamic effects when administered to healthy women in the early postmenopausal years. Clinical trials are testing whether regimens of estrogen with or without natural progesterone are vasoprotective and effective in preventing atherosclerosis when administered to women within a few years postmenopause.[118,119] The combination of drospirenone, a progestin with mineralocorticoid receptor antagonist effects plus 17β-estradiol has been shown to lower blood pressure, and is being evaluated as menopausal hormone therapy in hypertensive women.[146,154]

REFERENCES

1. Laragh JH, Sealey JE, Ledingham JGG, Newton MA. Oral contraceptives—renin, aldosterone and high blood pressure. *JAMA* 1967;201:918–22.
2. Woods JW. Oral contraceptives and hypertension. *Lancet* 1967;2:653–54.
3. Lorentz IT. Parietal lesion and Enavid. *BMJ* 1962;2:1191.
4. Crane MG, Harris JJ, Winsor W 3rd. Hypertension, oral contraceptive agents, and conjugated estrogens. *Ann Intern Med* 1971;74:13–21.
5. Morley Kotchen J, Kotchen TA. Impact of female hormones on blood pressure: review of potential mechanisms and clinical studies. *Curr Hypertens Rep* 2003;5:505–12.
6. Stern MP, Brown BW, Haskell WL, et al. Cardiovascular risk and use of estrogens or estrogen–progestagen combinations. *JAMA* 1976;235:811–15.

7. Fisch JR, Frank J. Oral contraceptive and blood pressure. *JAMA* 1977;237:2499–503.
8. Royal College of general practitioners' oral contraception study. Effect on hypertension and benign breast disease of progestogen component in combined oral contraceptives. *Lancet* 1977;8012:624–26.
9. Ostrander LD, Lamphiear DE, Block WD, et al. Oral contraceptives and physiological variables. *JAMA* 1980;244:677–79.
10. Godsland IF, Crook D, Devenport M, Wynn V. Relationship between blood pressure, oral contraceptive use and metabolic risk markers for cardiovascular disease. *Contraception* 1995;52:143–49.
11. Sherif K. The effects of hormone replacement therapy and oral

contraceptive pills on blood pressure. *Prog Cardiovasc Nurs* 2000;15:21–23.
12. Murayama N, Matsunaga A, Tangbanluekal L, et al. Effects of oral contraceptive use on body mass index and blood pressure among female villagers in north-east Thailand. *J Biosoc Sci* 2003;35:243–61.
13. Chasan-Taber L, Willett WC, Manson JE, et al. Prospective study of oral contraceptives and hypertension among women in the United States. *Circulation* 1996;94:483–89.
14. Siritho S, Thrift AG, McNeil JJ, et al. Melbourne Risk Factor Study (MERFS) Group. Risk of ischemic stroke among users of the oral contraceptive pill: the Melbourne Risk Factor Study (MERFS) Group. *Stroke* 2003;34:1575–80

15. Tanis BC, Rosendaal FR. Venous and arterial thrombosis during oral contraceptive use: risks and risk factors. *Semin Vasc Med* 2003;3:69–83.

16. Allais G, De Lorenzo C, Mana O, Benedetto C. Oral contraceptives in women with migraine: balancing risks and benefits. *Neurol Sci* 2004;25:S211–14.

17. Seibert C, Barbouche E, Fagan J, et al. Prescribing oral contraceptives for women older than 35 years of age. *Ann Intern Med* 2003;138:54–64.

18. Pettiti DB. Combination estrogen-progestin oral contraceptives. *N Engl J Med* 2003;349:1443–50.

19. American College of Obstetricians and Gynecologists Practice Bulletin. Use of hormonal contraception in women with coexisting medical conditions: clinical management guidelines for obstetrician-gynecologists. *Obstet Gynecol* 2006;107:1453–72.

20. World Health Organization. Low dose combined oral contraceptives. In: *Improving Access to Quality Care in Family Planning: Medical Eligibility Criteria for Contraceptive Use.* 3rd ed. Geneva: World Health Organization, 2004.

21. Wren BG, Routledge DA. Blood pressure changes: oestrogens in climacteric women. *Med J Aust* 1981;2:528–31.

22. Lutola H. Blood pressure and hemodynamics in postmenopausal women during estradiol-17 beta substitution. *Am Clin Res* 1983;15(Suppl 38):1–121.

23. The Writing Group for the PEPI Trial. Effects of estrogen or estrogen/progestin regimens on heart disease risk factors in postmenopausal women: the Postmenopausal Estrogen/Progestin Interventions (PEPI) trial. *JAMA* 1995;273:199–208.

24. Cushman M, Meilahn EN, Psaty BM, et al. Hormone replacement therapy, inflammation, and hemostasis in elderly women. *Arterioscler Thromb Vasc Biol* 1999;19:893–99.

25. Mueck AO, Seeger H. Effect of hormone therapy on BP in normotensive and hypertensive postmenopausal women. *Maturitas* 2004;49:189–203.

26. Karalis I, Beevers G, Beevers M, Lip G. Hormone replacement therapy and arterial blood pressure in postmenopausal women with hypertension. *Blood Press* 2005;14:38–44.

27. Cagnacci A, Rovati L, Zanni A, et al. Physiological doses of estradiol decrease nocturnal blood pressure in normotensive postmenopausal women. *Am J Physiol* 1999;276:H1355–60.

28. Seely EW, Walsh BW, Gerhard MD, Williams GH. Estradiol with or without progesterone and ambulatory blood pressure in postmenopausal women. *Hypertension* 1999;33:1190–94.

29. Scuteri A., Bos AJG, Brant LJ, et al. Hormone replacement therapy and longitudinal changes in blood pressure in postmenopausal women. *Ann Intern Med* 2001;135:229–38.

30. Writing Group for the Women's Health Initiative. Risk and benefits of estrogen plus progestin in health postmenopausal women: principal results from the Women's Health Initiative randomized controlled trial. *JAMA* 2002;288:321–33.

31. The Women's Health Intitiative Steering Committee. Effects of conjugated equine estrogen in postmenopausal women with hysterectomy: the Women's Health Initiative Randomized Controlled Trial. *JAMA* 2004;291:1701–12.

32. Mosca L, Appel LJ, Benjamin EJ, et al. Evidence-based guidelines for cardiovascular disease prevention in women. *J Am Coll Cardiol* 2004;43:900–21.

33. Orshal JM, Khalil RA. Gender, sex hormones, and vascular tone. *Am J Physiol Regul Integr Comp Physiol* 2004;286:R233–49.

34. Edwards DP. Regulation of signal transduction pathways by estrogen and progesterone. *Annu Rev Physiol* 2005;67:335–76.

35. Schwerz DA, Penckofer S. Sex differences and the effects of sex hormones on hemostasis and vascular reactivity. *Heart Lung* 2001;30:401–26.

36. Halligan SC, Lerman A. Hormone replacement therapy and coronary endothelial function in postmenopausal women. *Mayo Clin Proc* 2005;80:824–28.

37. Komesaroff PA, Esler MD, Sudhir K. Estrogen supplementation attenuates glucocorticoid and catecholamine responses to mental stress in perimenopausal women. *J Clin Endocrinol Metab* 1999;84:606–10.

38. Sofowora GG, Singh I, He HB, et al. Effect of acute transdermal estrogen administration on basal, mental stress and cold pressor-induced sympathetic responses in postmenopausal women. *Clin Auton Res* 2005;15:193–99.

39. Schunkert H, Danser AH, Hense HW, et al. Effects of estrogen replacement therapy on the renin-angiotensin system in postmenopausal women. *Circulation* 1997;95:39–45.

40. Fischer M, Baessler A, Schunkert H. Renin angiotensin system and gender differences in cardiovascular system. *Cardiovasc Res* 2002;53:672–77.

41. Wilcox J, Hatch I, Gentzshein E, et al. Endothelin levels decrease after oral and nonoral estrogen in postmenopausal women with increased cardiovascular risk factors. *Fertil Steril* 1997;67:273–77.

42. Karjalainen AH, Ruskoaho H, Vuolteenaho, et al. Effects of estrogen replacement therapy on natriuretic peptides and blood pressure. *Maturitas* 2004;47:201–208.

43. Geary GG, Krause DN, Duckles SP. Estrogen reduces mouse cerebral artery tone through endothelial NOS- and cyclooxygenase-dependent mechanisms. *Am J Physiol Heart Circ Physiol* 2000;279:H511–19.

44. Kesim MD, Aydin Y, Erden M, Atis A. Nitric oxide in postmenopausal women taking three different HRT regimens. *Maturitas* 2005;50:52–57.

45. Gerhard M, Walsh BW, Tawakol A, et al. Estradiol therapy combined with progesterone and endothelium-dependent vasodilation in postmenopausal women. *Circulation* 1998;98:1158–63.

46. Mori M, Tsukahara F, Yoshioka T, et al. Suppression by 17-estradiol of monocyte adhesion to vascular endothelial cells is mediated by estrogen receptors. *Life Sci* 2004;75:599–609.

47. De Meersman RE, Zion AS, Giardina EGV, et al. Estrogen replacement, vascular distensibility, and blood pressures in postmenopausal women. *Am J Physiol* 1998;274:H1539–44.

48. Sudhir K, Elser MD, Jennings GL, Komesaroff PA. Estrogen supplementation decreases norepinephrine-induced vasoconstriction and total body norepinephrine spillover in perimenopausal women. *Hypertension* 1997;30:1538–43.

49. Crews JK, Khalil RA. Gender-specific inhibition of Ca^{2+} entry mechanisms of arterial vasoconstriction by sex hormones. *Clin Exp Pharmacol Physiol* 1999;26:707–15.

50. Sung BH, Ching M, Izzo JL Jr, et al. Estrogen improves abnormal norepinephrine-induced vasoconstriction in postmenopausal women. *J Hypertens* 1999;17:523–28.

51. Vongpatanasin W, Tuncel M, Mansour Y, et al. Transdermal estrogen replacement therapy decreases sympathetic activity in postmenopausal women. *Circulation* 2001;103:2903–2908.

52. Weitz G, Elam M, Born J, et al. Postmenopausal estrogen administration suppresses muscle sympathetic nerve activity. *Clin Endocrinol Metab* 2001;86:344–48.

53. O'Sullivan AJ, Crampton LJ, Freund J, et al. The route of estrogen replacement confers divergent effects on substrate oxidation and body composition in postmenopausal women. *J Clin Invest* 1998;102:1035–40.

54. Duanmu Z, Iapanowski K, Dunbar JC. Insulin-like growth factor-I decreases sympathetic nerve activity: the effect is modulated by glycemic status. *Proc Soc Exp Biol Med* 1997;216:93–97.

55. Scherrer U, Randin D, Tappy L, et al. Body fat and sympathetic nerve activity in healthy subjects. *Circulation* 1994;89:240–63.

56. Mitchell GF, Parise H, Benjamin EJ, et al. Changes in arterial stiffness and wave reflection with advancing age in healthy men and women: the Framingham Heart Study. *Hypertension* 2004;43:1239–45.

57. Tomiyama H, Yamashina A, Arai T, et al. Influences of age and gender on results of noninvasive brachial-ankle pulse wave velocity measurement—a survey of 12517 subjects. *Atherosclerosis* 2003;166:303–309.

58. London GM, Guerin AP, Pannier B, et al. Influences of sex on arterial hemodynamics and blood pressure: role of body height. *Hypertension* 1995;26:514–19.

59. Zaydun G, Tomiyama H, Hashimoto H, et al. Menopause is an independent factor augmenting the age-related increase in arterial stiffness in the early postmenopausal phase. *Atherosclerosis* 2006;184:137–42.

60. Rajkumar C, Kingwell BA, Cameron JD, et al. Hormonal therapy increases arterial compliance in postmenopausal women. *J Am Coll Cardiol* 1997;30:350–56.

61. McGrath BP, Liang YL, Teede H, et al. Age-related deterioration in arterial structure and function in postmenopausal women: impact of hormone replacement therapy. *Arterioscler Thromb Vasc Biol* 1988;18:1149–56.

62. Kawecka K, Czarnecka D, Olszanecka A, et al. The effect of hormone replacement therapy on arterial blood pressure and vascular compliance in postmenopausal women with arterial hypertension. *J Hum Hypertens* 2002;16:509–16.

63. Soares da Costa L, Amorin de Oliviera M, Siquiera Martins Rubim V, et al. Effects of hormone replacement therapy or raloxifene on ambulatory blood pressure and arterial stiffness in treated hypertensive postmenopausal women. *Am J Cardiol* 2004;94:1453–56.

64. Danser AH, Derkx FH, Schalekamp MA, et al. Determinants of interindividual variation of renin and prorenin concentrations: evidence for a sexual dimorphism of (pro)renin levels in humans. *J Hypertens* 1998;16:853–62.

65. Proudler AJ, Ahmed AL, Crook D, et al. Hormone replacement therapy and serum angiotensin-converting enzyme activity in postmenopausal women. *Lancet* 1995;346:89–90.

66. Brosnihan KB, Weddle D, Anthony MS, et al. Effects of chronic hormone replacement on the renin-angiotensin system in cynomolgus monkeys. *J Hypertens* 1997;15:719–26.

67. Dean SA, Tan J, O'Brien, Leenen FH. 17β-estradiol downregulates tissue angiotensin-converting enzyme and ANG II type 1 receptor in female rats. *Am J Regul Integr Comp Physiol* 2005;288:R759–66.

68. Brosnihan KB, Li P, Ganten D, Ferrario CM. Estrogen protects transgenic hypertensive rats by shifting the vasoconstrictor-vasodilator balance of RAS. *Am J Integr Comp Physiol* 1997;273:R1908–15.

69. Nickenig G, Baumer AT, Crohe C, et al. Estrogen modulates AT₁ receptor gene expression *in vitro* and *in vivo*. *Circulation* 1998;97:2197–201.

70. Roesch DM, Tian Y, Zheng W, et al. Estradiol attenuates angiotensin-induced aldosterone secretion in ovariectomized rats. *Endocrinology* 2000;141:4629–36.

71. Wu Z, Maric C, Roesch DM, et al. Estrogen regulates adrenal angiotensin AT₁ receptors by modulating AT₁ receptor translation. *Endocrinology* 2003;144:3251–61.

72. Klett C, Ganten D, Hellman W, et al. Regulation of angiotensinogen synthesis and secretion by steroid hormones. *Endocrinology* 2002;130:3660–68.

73. Feldmer M, Laking M, Takahashi S, et al. Glucocorticoid- and estrogen-responsive elements in the 5'-flanking region of the rat angiotensinogen gene. *J Hypertens* 1991;9:1005–12.

74. Myers J, Morgan T. The effect of sodium intake on the blood pressure related to age and sex. *Clin Exp Hypertens A* 1983;5:99–118.

75. Tominaga T, Suzuki M, Ogata Y, et al. The role of sex hormones and sodium intake in postmenopausal hypertension. *J Hum Hypertens* 1991;5:495–500.

76. Yamori Y, Liu L, Ikeda K, et al. Different associations of blood pressure with 24-hr urinary sodium excretion among pre- and post-menopausal women. WHO Cardiovascular Diseases and Alimentary Comparison (WHO-CARDIAC) Study. *J Hypertens* 2001;19:535–38.

77. Pechere-Bertschi A, Burnier M. Female sex hormones, salt, and blood pressure regulation. *Am J Hypertens* 2004;17:994–1001.

78. Schulman IH, Aranda P, Raij L, et al. Surgical menopause increases salt sensitivity of blood pressure. *Hypertension* 2006;47:1168–74.

79. Miller VM, Vanhoutte PM. Progesterone and modulation of endothelium-dependent responses in canine coronary arteries. *Am J Physiol* 1991;261:R1022–27.

80. Jiang CW, Sarrel PM, Lindsay DC, Poole-Wilson PA, Collins P. Progesterone induces endothelium-independent relaxation of rabbit coronary artery *in vitro*. *Eur J Pharmacol* 1992;211:163–67.

81. Williams JK, Honore EK, Washburn SA, Clarkson TB. Effects of hormone replacement therapy on reactivity of atherosclerotic coronary arteries in cynomolgous monkeys. *J Am Coll Cardiol* 1994;24:1757–61.

82. Miyagawa K, Rosch J, Stanczyk F, Hermsmeyer K. Medroxyprogesterone interferes with ovarian steroid protection against coronary vasospasm. *Nat Med* 1997;3:324–27.

83. Simoncini T, Mannella P, Fornari L, et al. Differential signal transduction of progesterone and medroxyprogesterone acetate in human endothelial cells. *Endocrinology* 2004;145:5745–56.

84. Lee WS, Harder JA, Yoshizumi M, et al. Progesterone inhibits arterial smooth muscle cell proliferation. *Nat Med* 1997;3:1005–1008.

85. Oparil S, Levine RL, Chen SJ, et al. Sexually dimorphic response of the balloon injured rat carotid artery to hormone treatment. *Circulation* 1997;95:1301–1307.

86. Xing D, Miller AP, Novak L, et al. Estradiol and progestins differentially modulate leukocyte infiltration after vascular injury. *Circulation* 2004;109:234–41.

87. Levine RL, Chen SJ, Durand J, et al. Medroxyprogesterone attenuates estrogen-mediated inhibition of neointima formation after balloon injury of the rat carotid artery. *Circulation* 1996;94:2221–27.

88. Sealey JE, Itskovitz-Eldor J, Rubattu S, et al. Estradiol- and progesterone-related increases in the renin-aldosterone system: Studies during ovarian stimulation and early pregnancy. *J Clin Endocrinol Metab* 1994;79:258–64.

89. Myles K, Funder JW. Progesterone binding to mineralocorticoid receptors: *in vitro* and vivo studies. *Am J Physiol* 1996;270:E601–607.

90. Braley LM, Menachery AI, Yao T, et al. Effect of progesterone on aldosterone secretion in rats. *Endocrinology* 1996;137:4773–78.

91. Landau RL, Bergenstal DM, Lugibihl K, Kascht ME. The metabolic effects of progesterone in man. *J Clin Endocrinol* 1955;15:1194–215.

92. Oparil S, Ehrlich EN, Lindheimer MD. Effect of progesterone on renal sodium handling in man: Relation to aldosterone excretion and plasma renin activity. *Clin Sci Mol Med* 1975;49:139–47.

93. Brunette MG, Leclerc M. Renal action of progesterone: effect on calcium reabsorption. *Mol Cell Endocrinol* 2002;194:183–90.

94. Dubey RK, Oparil S, Imthurn B, Jackson EK. Sex hormones and hypertension. *Cardiovasc Res* 2002;53:688–708.

95. Dunne FP, Barry DG, Ferriss JB, et al. Changes in blood pressure during the normal menstrual cycle. *Clin Sci* 1991;81:1991;515–18.

96. Karpanou EA, Vyssoulis GP, Georgoudi DG, et al. Ambulatory blood pressure changes in the menstrual cycle of hypertensive women: Significance of plasma renin activity values. *Am J Hypertens* 1993;6:654–59.

97. Chapman AB, Zamudio S, Woodmansee W, et al. Systemic and renal hemodynamic changes in the luteal phase of the menstrual cycle mimic early pregnancy. *Am J Physiol* 1997;273:F777–82.

98. Miller AP, Bittner VB, Oparil S. *Hypertension*. In: *Women and Heart Disease*. 2nd ed. Wenger N, Collins P, eds. London: Taylor and Francis, 2005:441–53.

99. Staessen JA, Celis H, Fagard R. The epidemiology of the association between hypertension and menopause. *J Hum Hypertens* 1998;12:587–92.

100. Staessen JA, Ginocchio G, Thijs L, Fagard R. Conventional and ambulatory blood pressure and menopause in a prospective population study. *J Hum Hypertens* 1997;11:507–14.

101. Bush TL, Barrett-Connor E, Cowan LD, et al. Cardiovascular mortality and noncontraceptive use of estrogen in women: results of the Lipid Research Clinics' program follow-up study. *Circulation* 1987;75:1102–109.

102. Kannel WB, Hjortland MC, McNamara PM, Gordon T. Menopause and risk of cardiovascular disease: the Framingham study. *Ann Intern Med* 1976;85:447–52.

103. Barrett-Connor E, Brown WV, Turner J, et al. Heart disease risk factors and hormone use in postmenopausal women. *JAMA* 1979;241:2167–69.

104. Barrett-Connor E, Wingard DI, Criqui MH. Postmonopausal estrogen use and heart disease risk factors in the 1980s. Rancho Bernardo, Calif., revisited. *JAMA* 1989;14:2095–100.

105. Mercuro G, Zoncu S, Pilia I, et al. Effects of acute administration of transdermal estrogen on postmenopausal women with systemic hypertension. *Am J Cardiol* 1997;80:652–55.

106. Mercuro G, Zoncu S, Piano D, et al. Estradiol-17β reduces blood pressure and restore the normal amplitude of the circadian blood pressure rhythm in postmenopausal hypertension. *Am J Hypertens* 1998;11:909–13.

107. Butkevich A, Abraham C, Phillips RA. Hormone replacement therapy and 24-hour blood pressure profile of postmenopausal women. *Am J Hypertens* 2000;13:1039–41.

108. Wassertheil-Smoller S, Psaty B, Greenland P, et al. Association between cardiovascular outcomes and antihypertensive drug treatment in older women. *JAMA* 2004;292:2849–59.

109. Writing Group for the Women's Health Initiative Investigators. Risks and benefits of estrogen plus progestin in healthy postmenopausal women: principal results from the Women's Health Intitiative randomized controlled trial. *JAMA* 2002;288:321–33.

110. Manson JE, Hsai J, Johnson KC, et al. Estrogen plus progestin and the risk of coronary artery disease. The Women's Health Initiative: a randomized trial. *N Engl J Med* 2003;349:523–34.

111. Anderson GL, Limacher M, Assaf AR, et al. Effects of conjugated equine estrogen in postmenopausal women with hysterectomy: the Women's Health Initiative randomized controlled trial. *JAMA* 2004;291:701–12.

112. Lip GYH, Beevers M, Churchill D, Beevers DG. Hormone replacement therapy and blood pressure in hypertensive women. *J Hum Hypertens* 1994;8:491–94.

113. Oparil S. Women's health: hormone replacement therapy. In: Brunner H, ed. *The Year in Hypertension: 2005.* Oxford: Clinical Publishing, 2006:197–234.

114. Hersh AL, Stefanick ML, Stafford RS. National use of postmenopausal hormone therapy: annual trends and response to recent evidence. *JAMA* 2004;291:47–53.

115. Majumdar SR, Almasi EA, Stafford RS. Promotion and prescribing of hormone replacement therapy after report of harm after the Women's Health Initiative. *JAMA* 2004;292:1983–88.

116. Miller AP, Chen YF, Xing D, et al. Hormone replacement therapy and inflammation: interactions in cardiovascular disease. *Hypertension.* 2003;42:657–63.

117. Girdler SS, Hinderliter AL, Wells EC, et al. Transdermal versus oral estrogen therapy in postmenopausal smokers: hemodynamic and endothelial effects. *Obstet Gynecol* 2004;103:169–80.

118. Harman SM, Brinton EA, Cedars M, et al. KEEPS: the Kronos Early Estrogen Prevention Study. *Climacteric* 2005;8:3–12.

119. Early versus Late Intervention Trial with Estradiol (ELITE). Home page. Available at: www.usc.edu/schools/medicine/ research/centers_programs/aru.elite.html.

120. Stefanick ML, Cochrane BB, Hsia J, et al. The Women's Health Initiative post-menopausal hormone trials: overview and baseline characteristics of participants. *Ann Epidemiol* 2003;13:S78–86.

121. Brownley KA, Hinderliter AL, West SG, et al. Cardiovascular effects of 6 months of hormone replacement therapy versus placebo: differences associated with years since menopause. *Am J Obstet Gynecol* 2004;190:1052–58.

122. Miller AP, Xing D, Feng W, Fintel M, Chen YF, Oparil S. Aged rats lose vasoprotective and anti-inflammatory actions of estrogen in injured arteries. *Menopause* 2006; December 28 E.pub ahead of print.

123. Phillips LS, Langer RD. Postmenopausal hormone therapy: critical reappraisal and a unified hypothesis. *Fertil Steril* 2005;83:558–66.

124. Barrett-Connor E, Mosca L, Collins P, et al. Effects of raloxifene on cardiovascular events and breast cancer in postmenopausal women. *N Engl J Med* 2006;355:125–37.

125. Crane MG, Harris JJ, Winsor W. Hypertension, oral contraceptive agents and conjugated estrogens. *Ann Intern Med* 1971;74:13–21.

126. Prentice RL. On the ability of blood pressure effects to explain the relation between oral contraceptives and cardiovascular disease. *Am J Epidemiol* 1988;127:213–19.

127. Dong W, Colhoun HM, Poulter NR. Blood pressure in women using oral contraceptives: results from the Health Survey for England 1994. *J Hypertens* 1997;15:1063–68.

128. World Health Organization Collaborative Study of Cardiovascular Disease and Steroid Hormone Contraception. A multinational case–control study of cardiovascular disease and steroid hormone contraceptives: description and validation of methods. *J Clin Epidemiol* 1995;48:1513–47.

129. Lubianca JN, Faccin CS, Fuchs FD. Oral contraceptives: a risk factor for uncontrolled blood pressure among hypertensive women. *Contraception* 2003;67:19–24.

130. Hollenberg NK, Williams GF, Burger B, et al. Renal blood flow and its response to angiotensin II. An interaction between oral contraceptive agents, sodium intake and the renin-angiotensin system in healthy young women. *Clin Res* 1976;38:35–40.

131. Rockson SG, Stone RA, Gunnells JC, et al. Plasma dopamine β-hydroxylase activity in oral contraceptive hypertension. *Circulation* 1975;51:916–23.

132. Godsland IF, Crook D. Update on the metabolic effects of steroidal contraceptives and their relationship to cardiovascular disease risk. *Am J Obstet Gynecol* 1994;170:1528–36.

133. Walters WAW, Lim YL. Haemodynamic changes in women taking oral contraceptives. *J Obstet Gynaecol Br Commonw* 1970;77:1007–12.

134. Burke CW. Biologically active cortisol in plasma of oestrogen-treated adrenal subjects. *BMJ* 1969;2:798–800.

135. Hall WD, Douglas MB, Blumenstein B, Hatcher RA. Blood pressure and oral progestational agents. A prospective study of 199 black women. *Am J Obstet Gynecol* 1980;136:344–48.

136. Wilson ESB, Cruikshank J, McMaster M, Weir RJ. A prospective controlled study of the effect on blood pressure of contraceptive preparations containing different types and dosages of progestagen. *Br J Obstet Gynaecol* 1984;91:1254–60.

137. Royal College of General Practitioners. *Oral Contraceptives and Health.* New York: Pittman, 1974:34–42.

138. Khaw KT, Peart WS. Blood pressure and contraceptive use. *BMJ* 1985;285:403–407.

139. Spellacy WN, Birk SA. The effect of intrauterine devices, oral contraceptives, estrogens, and progestogens and blood pressure. *Am J Obstet Gynecol* 1972;112:912–19.

140. Hussain SF. Progestogen-only pills and high blood pressure: is there an association? A literature review. *Contraception* 2004;69:89–97.

141. Weir RJ, Briggs E, Mack A, et al. Blood pressure in women taking oral contraceptives. *BMJ* 1974;1:533–35.

142. Meirik O, Farley TM, Sivin I. Safety and efficacy of levonorgestrel implant, intrauterine device, and sterilization. *Obstet Gynecol* 2001;97:539–47.

143. Croxatto HB, Urbancsek J, Massai R, et al. A multicentre efficacy and safety study of the single contraceptive implant Implanon. Implanon Study Group. *Hum Reprod* 1999;14:976–81.

144. Sivin I. Risks and benefits, advantages and disadvantages of levonorgestrel-releasing contraceptive implants. *Drug Saf* 2003;26:303–35.

145. Sitruk-Ware R. Pharmacological profile of progestins. *Maturitas* 2004;47:277–83.

146. Oelkers W, Berger V, Bolik A, Bahr V, Hazard B, Beier S, et al. Dihydrospirorenone—a new progestogen with antimineralocorticoid activity: effects on ovulation, electrolyte excretion and the renin-aldosterone system in normal women. *J Clin Endocrinol Metab* 1991;73:837–42.

147. Elger W, Beier S, Pollow K, et al. Conception and pharmacodynamic profile of drospirenone. *Steroids* 2003;68:891–905.

148. Oelkers W. Drospirenone, a progestogen with antimineralocorticoid properties: a short review. *Mol Cell Endocrinol* 2004;217:255–61.

149. Sica DA. Drospirenone: an antihypertensive in waiting. *Hypertension* 2006;48:205–206.

150. Oelkers W, Foidart JM, Dombrovicz N, et al. Effects of a new oral contraceptive containing an antimineralocorticoid progestogen, drospirenone, on the renin-aldosterone system, body weight, blood pressure, glucose tolerance, and lipid metabolism. *J Clin Endocrinol Metab* 1995;80:1816–21.

151. Preston RA, Alonso A, Panzitta D, et al. Additive effect of drospirenone/ 17β-estradiol in hypertensive postmenopausal women receiving enalapril. *Am J Hypertens* 2002;15:816–22.

152. Preston RA, White WB, Pitt B, et al. Effects of drospirenone/17β-estradiol on blood pressure and potassium balance in hypertensive postmenopausal women. *Am J Hypertens* 2005;18:797–804.

153. White WB, Pitt B, Preston RA, Hanes V. Antihypertensive effects of drospirenone with 17β-estradiol, a novel hormonal treatment in postmenopausal women with stage 1 hypertension. *Circulation* 2005;112:1979–84.

154. White WB, Hanes V, Chauhan V, Pitt B. Effects of a new hormone therapy, drospirenone and 17β-estradiol, in postmenopausal women with hypertension. *Hypertension* 2006;48:246–53.

155. Rosendorff C. Progestin and potassium. *Am J Hypertens* 2005;18:741–43.

156. Archer DF, Thorneycroft IH, Foegh M, et al. Long-term safety of drospirenone-estradiol for hormone therapy: a randomized, double-blind, multicenter trial. *Menopause* 2005;12:716–27.

Chapter

71 Drug-Induced Hypertension

Ehud Grossman and Franz H. Messerli

Key Findings

- A variety of therapeutic agents and chemical substances can induce transient or sustained hypertension, exacerbate well-controlled hypertension, or antagonize the effects of antihypertensive therapy.

- Careful evaluation of a patient's drug regimen and exposure to chemicals may identify chemically induced hypertension.

- Diagnosis of drug-induced hypertension may obviate the need for unnecessary, costly, and potentially dangerous evaluations, and prevent the need for lifelong antihypertensive therapy.

- When drug- or chemical-induced hypertension is identified, discontinuation of the causative agent should be recommended.

- When it is not possible to avoid chemical agents that cause hypertension, institution of appropriate antihypertensive treatment is indicated.

Most patients with hypertension have essential hypertension or well-known forms of secondary hypertension such as renal disease or renal artery stenosis or common endocrine diseases (hyperaldosteronism or pheochromocytoma). Physicians are less aware of rare and unusual forms of hypertension such as drug-induced hypertension. To secure a more complete diagnosis, an accurate and detailed medical history should include specific inquiries concerning foods, poisons, and medications that patients do not consider to be drugs, and therefore frequently omit from their history. Identification of the intake of these substances is important because their elimination can obviate the need for unnecessary, costly, and potentially dangerous evaluations, treatments, or both.[1,2]

Hypertension related to drugs and other substances represents an important modifiable and often unnoticed source of secondary hypertension (Table 71–1). This chapter reviews therapeutic agents or chemical substances that may elevate blood pressure (BP) by different mechanisms of action.

STEROIDS

Hypertension occurs in about 20% of patients treated with high doses of synthetic corticosteroids. Oral cortisol increases BP in a dose-dependent fashion. At a dose of 80 to 200 mg/day, the peak increases in systolic pressure is of the order of 15 mmHg. Increased BP is usually apparent within 24 hours.[2] Glucocorticoid-induced hypertension is more common in elderly patients, and in patients with a positive family history of essential hypertension. Hemodynamically, ACTH and adrenocortical steroids increase BP through increasing cardiac output, with little change in peripheral resistance.[1] The mechanism of glucocorticoid-induced hypertension remains uncertain and it seems to be multifactorial. The mechanisms of action of the various steroids are related to their glucocorticoid or mineralocorticoid effects, which include retention of salt and water (mineralocorticoid effect), redistribution of body fluid with increase in plasma volume and cardiac output (glucocorticoid effect), increased peripheral vascular responsiveness to vasoactive agents (mineralocorticoid and glucocorticoid effects), and activation of the central and peripheral nervous systems.[1] Of note, mineralocorticoid activity is not essential for steroids to induce an increase in BP. It has been shown that using synthetic steroids with glucocorticoid activity and little or no mineralocorticoid activity produced no effects on body weight, urinary sodium excretion, plasma volume and hematocrit, but increased BP significantly.[3] Glucocorticoids modify multiple intracellular and extracellular biochemical processes but have limited direct effects on BP. In the proximal tubule, glucocorticoids do not induce a change in sodium transport directly but serve to enhance the activity of many existing pathways and transporters. Conversely, the distal tubule and collecting duct are responsive to glucocorticoids. Glucocorticoids are able to bind to mineralocorticoid receptors (MRs) and glucocorticoid receptors (GRs) and stimulate sodium reabsorption. Protein binding of the glucocorticoids in serum and the metabolic activity of local 11 β-hydroxysteroid dehydrogenase (11β-HSD) limit access of these steroids to both MRs and GRs. Inhibition of 11β-HSD with licorice or abnormality of this enzyme may enhance access of steroids to both MRs and GRs thereby causing BP elevation.[4] Recent evidence suggests that the nitric oxide system also plays a key role in the hypertension produced by glucocorticoids. Glucocorticoid actions at various sites in the nitric oxide synthase (NOS) pathway may result in elevated BP. These include: alterations in L-arginine availability or transport, NOS2 and NOS3 downregulation, reduced cofactor bioavailability, NOS uncoupling, a concomitant elevation in reactive oxygen species and removal of nitric oxide (NO) from the vascular environment, alterations in whole body antioxidant status, and erythropoietin-induced resistance to NO.[5] Inhaled corticosteroids during

LIST OF MEDICATIONS THAT MAY INCREASE BLOOD PRESSURE

Ingredient	Clinical Use Steroids	Notes
Glucocorticoid	Replacement therapy, rheumatic disease, collagen disease, dermatologic disease, allergic state, ophthalmic disease, inflammatory bowel disease, respiratory disease, hematologic and neoplastic disease, nephropathies	Dose-dependent, sustained increase mainly in systolic BP
Mineralocorticoid		Dose-dependent, sustained increase in BP characterized by hypokalemia, metabolic alkalosis, and suppressed plasma renin activity and aldosterone levels
Licorice	Flavoring and sweetening agent	
Carbenoxolone	Ulcer medication	
9-alpha fluoroprednisolone	Skin ointments, antihemorrhoid cream	
9-alpha fluorocortisol	Ophthalmic drops, and nasal sprays	
Ketoconazole	Antimycotic	
	Sex Hormones	
Estrogen	Contraception, replacement therapy	Mild, sustained BP elevation, more common in premenopausal women. Severe hypertension has been reported.
Progesterone	Prostate cancer	
Androgens	Anabolic effect	
Danazol (semisynthetic androgen)	Endometriosis, hereditary angioedema	Mild dose-dependent, sustained increase in systolic BP
	Anesthetics, Narcotics	
Ketamine hydrochloride	Anesthetic agent	Transient severe increase in BP has been reported
Fentanyl citrate	Narcotic analgesic and anesthetic agent	
Scopolamine	Preanesthetic medication, motion sickness	
Naloxone hydrochloride	Opioid overdose	Transient BP elevation
	Drugs Affecting Sympathetic Nervous System	
Phenylephrine hydrochloride	Upper respiratory decongestant, ophthalmic drops	Dose-dependent, sustained increase in BP
Dipivalyl adrenaline hydrochloride	Ophthalmic drops	Severe HT has been reported
Epinephrine (with β blocker)	Local anesthetic, anaphylactic reaction bronchodilatation, decongestant antihemorrhoidal treatment	
Phenylpropanolamine	Anorectic, upper respiratory decongestant	
Pseudoephedrine hydrochloride	Upper respiratory decongestant	
Tetrahydrozoline hydrochloride	Ophthalmic vasoconstrictor drops	
Naphazoline hydrochloride	Ophthalmic vasoconstrictor and nasal decongestant drops	
Oxymetazoline hydrochloride	Upper respiratory decongestant drops	
Caffeine	Analgesia, vascular headache, beverages	Acute transient increase in BP
Herbal products	Complementary and alternative medicine	Mainly relate to dietary supplements that contain ephedra alkaloids
Cocaine	Local anesthetics	Transient severe increase in BP especially when used with β-blockers
	Antiemetic Agents	
Metoclopramide	Antiemetic	Transient increase in BP in association with cancer
Alizapride	Antiemetic	
Prochlorperazine	Antiemetic	

Ingredient	Clinical Use Steroids	Notes
LIST OF MEDICATIONS THAT MAY INCREASE BLOOD PRESSURE—cont'd		
Other Agents		
Yohimbine hydrochloride	Impotence	Acute, dose-dependent increase in BP
Sibutramine	Weight loss	
Clozapine	Antipsychotic agent	
Glucagon	Prevent bowel spasm	Only in patients with pheochromocytoma
Physostigmine	Reverse anticholinergic syndrome	
Ritodrine hydrochloride	Inhibition of preterm labor	Hypertensive crisis has been reported
Antidepressant Agents		
MAOIs	Antidepressive agents	Mainly with sympathomimetic amines and with certain foods containing tyramine
Selegiline	Used mainly for Parkinson's disease	
Tricyclic antidepressants	Antidepressive agent	More common in patients with panic disorders
Buspirone	Anxiolytic agent	Mild dose-dependent increase in BP
Fluoxetine	Antidepressive agents	In combination with selegiline
Thioridazine hydrochloride	Psychotic and depressive disorders	Massive overdose may cause severe HT
Carbamazepine	Bipolar depression and seizures	
Lithium	Manic depressive illness	Acute intoxication can cause severe HT
Immunosuppressive Agents		
Cyclosporine A	Immunosuppressive agent, prophylaxis of organ rejection, autoimmune disease, dermatologic disorders	Dose-dependent mild to moderate increase in BP. Severe HT has been reported
Tacrolimus	Prophylaxis of organ rejection	Produces less hypertension than cyclosporine A
Rapamycin	Prophylaxis of organ rejection	Produces little BP increase
Antineoplastic Agents		
Alkylating agents	Antineoplastic agent	
Paclitaxel	Antineoplastic agent	
Cis-diamminedichloroplatinium	Antineoplastic agent	Only during intra-arterial administration
Recombinant human erythropoietin	Anemia of renal failure	Dose-related, mild increase in BP. Hypertensive crisis with encephalopathy has been reported
Alcohol	Beverage	Dose-dependent, sustained increase in BP
Disulfiram	Management of alcoholism	Slight increase in BP. Severe HT may occur in alcoholic-induced liver disease
NSAIDs	Rheumatic disease	Mild dose-dependent increase in BP
Heavy Metals		
Lead	Industry	
Cadmium	Industry	The association between cadmium exposure and hypertension is equivocal
Arsenic	Industry	
Bromocriptine mesylate	Suppression of lactation, and prolactin inhibition in prolactinoma	Severe HT with stroke has been reported following the use for suppression of lactation
Venoms	Sting of scorpion	
Amphotericin B	Fungal infections	
Protease inhibitor	Anti-HIV treatment	

BP, blood pressure; HT, hypertension.

Table 71–1. List of Medications That May Increase Blood Pressure

pregnancy do not increase the risk of pregnancy-induced hypertension or preeclampsia.[6]

Cessation of steroid therapy usually leads to normalization of BP. However, there is one report that reduction in steroid therapy in nine patients with steroid-requiring asthma was associated with a rise in BP. In these patients, BP elevations were resistant to diuretic therapy, but responded rapidly to angiotensin-converting enzyme inhibitor.[1]

Certain exogenous compounds such as 9-alpha fluoro-prednisolone and 9-alpha fluorocortisol have mineralo-corticoid activity. Other compounds such as licorice and carbenoxolone have mineralocorticoid-like activity by inhibition of the 11 beta-HSD enzyme. Excess consumption of these compounds may produce arterial hypertension characterized by increased exchangeable sodium and blood volume, hypokalemia with metabolic alkalosis, and suppressed plasma renin and aldosterone levels.[1] Prolonged use of high-dose ketoconazole may alter enzymatic degradation of steroids leading to mineralocorticoid-related hypertension.[1] Skin ointments, antihemorrhoidal preparations, ophthalmic drops, and nasal sprays may contain substances with mineralocorticoid activity (9-alpha-fluoroprednisolone) and sympathetic amines. Their excessive use may even cause severe arterial hypertension.[1] Discontinuation of these substances is recommended to lower BP. However, when steroid treatment is mandatory, a diuretic is the drug of choice, since volume overload is the main mechanism by which steroids raise BP; careful monitoring of potassium is necessary.

SEX HORMONES

Oral contraceptives induce hypertension in approximately 5% of users of high-dose pills that contain at least 50 μg of estrogen and 1 to 4 mg of progestin.[2] There is a two- to three-fold increased risk of hypertension in women taking oral contraceptives compared with age-matched controls using alternative methods of contraception.[2] This risk seems to correlate with the estrogen and progesterone dose, but even the newer generations of oral contraceptive drugs with lower doses of estrogen tend to increase the risk of hypertension.[2] The increased pressure is usually minimal; however, severe hypertensive episodes, including malignant hypertension, have been reported. Women with a history of high BP during pregnancy, those with a family history of hypertension, cigarette smokers, obese, black, or diabetic women, and those with renal diseases may respond with a greater increase in BP.[1] The risk of hypertension decreased quickly with cessation of oral contraceptives, and past users appeared to have only a slightly increased risk. Several mechanisms have been postulated to be involved in BP increase associated with oral contraceptive drugs, including activation of the renin-angiotensin-aldosterone system; the latter is activated by estrogens via amplified synthesis of angiotensinogen in the liver, thus resulting in increased intracellular volume and cardiac output, and as a consequence, hypertension.[2] The oral contraceptive effect probably relates to the exogenous administration of high levels of estrogens and/or progesterones in women who already have "physiologically normal"

levels of these hormones, while in postmenopausal women, natural hormone levels are low, and (low-dose) hormone replacement therapy (HRT) merely restores the hormone levels to physiologic levels. The pressor effects of estrogens in oral contraceptives and in HRT are therefore likely to be different.[2]

Postmenopausal estrogen replacement therapy (ERT) has minimal effect on arterial pressure in normotensive women, and rare cases of estrogen-induced hypertension represent an idiosyncratic reaction to ERT.[2] Recently the use of ERT was associated with increased cardiovascular morbidity and mortality, and therefore it is not routinely recommended.[7–10] Cessation of oral contraceptives is recommended when hypertension has developed.

Men receiving estrogen for the treatment of prostate cancer may also exhibit an increase in BP.[1] Danazol, a semisynthetic androgen that is used in the treatment of endometriosis and hereditary angioedema, was reported to induce hypertension due to fluid retention.[1]

ANESTHETICS AND NARCOTICS

Ketamine hydrochloride, widely used as an anesthetic in children, has been reported to severely increase arterial pressure.[1] A case of hypertension and pulmonary edema triggered by ketamine in a pregnant woman with a history of cocaine abuse has also been reported.[1] The mechanism by which ketamine hydrochloride increases BP is not completely understood. In one study,[1] clonidine—which suppresses sympathetic activity—was found to be effective in reducing the hypertensive response to ketamine.

High-dose fentanyl used as an anesthetic agent in valvular and coronary heart surgery may increase BP.[1] A case is reported in which hypertensive crisis occurred in a patient anesthetized with high-dose fentanyl-diazepam-oxygen.[1]

Scopolamine, a belladonna alkaloid, has a central anticholinergic activity. A case is reported in which 0.1 mg of scopolamine intravenously administered during surgery induced marked hypertension in a patient with type 4 hereditary sensory and autonomic neuropathy.[1] The simultaneous use of vasoconstrictors (felypressin) with topical cocaine can result in severe hypertension.[1] Hypertensive responses to naloxone (opiate antagonist), especially during attempted reversal of narcotic-induced anesthesia in hypertensive patients, have also been reported. Naloxone seems to acutely reverse the antihypertensive effects of clonidine, and can thereby cause an acute hypertensive emergency.[1] Naloxone also partially ameliorates the hypotension associated with various forms of shock. Endogenous opioids appear to regulate BP in some hypertensive patients, and antagonizing their effect may increase BP.[2]

DRUGS AFFECTING THE SYMPATHETIC NERVOUS SYSTEM

Agents that directly activate the sympathetic nervous system

Phenylephrine, a sympathomimetic agent with a potent vasoconstrictor activity, has been reported to severely increase arterial pressure following its administration in an ophthalmic solution.[1] The most important factor in the development of hypertension from topically applied phenylephrine is the total dose administered; it appears that infants, because of their immature degradation pathways, are more susceptible than adults.[1] Recently pulmonary edema was described in a child who developed severe hypertension after the inadvertent administration of a large dose of topical nasal phenylephrine, followed by the beta-adrenergic antagonist esmolol.[11] Dipivalyl adrenaline, an adrenaline prodrug used topically in the management of chronic simple glaucoma, can also increase BP in treated hypertensive patients.[1]

The concomitant use of sympathomimetic agents and β-blockers can severely increase arterial pressure because of unopposed α-adrenergic vasoconstriction. Severe hypertensive crises were reported in a hypertensive patient treated with propranolol after subcutaneous epinephrine injection for anaphylactic reaction; after administering a local anesthetic containing epinephrine to a patient previously treated with propranolol, and after administration of levonordefrin during dental treatment to a patient receiving propranolol.[1] In diabetic hypertensive patients treated with both insulin and propranolol, hypoglycemic episodes may be accompanied by severe hypertension due to excessive vasoconstriction mediated by α-receptors and rising epinephrine levels.[1] If β-antagonists must be used in insulin-dependent diabetic patients, $β_1$-selective antagonists appear to be the better choice. If hypertensive episodes occur, arterial pressure can be reduced by α-receptor antagonists.[1] In a prospective study, hypoglycemia was induced by insulin injection in diabetic patients who were previously treated with a placebo, atenolol, or propranolol.[1] Arterial pressure increased significantly in the group treated with propranolol, strengthening the concept that the β-receptor selectivity of these agents determines the change in arterial pressure.

Over-the-counter drugs

Most nonprescription anorectics contain combinations of an antihistamine and an adrenergic agonist (usually phenylpropanolamine [PPA], ephedrine, pseudoephedrine, or caffeine). All act by potentiating presynaptic norepinephrine release and by directly activating adrenergic receptors. Known toxic effects of these substances include hypertension, tachycardia, ventricular ectopy, agitation, psychosis, and seizure.[1] Alpha-adrenergic intoxication induced by nasal decongestant and cough medications containing massive doses of oxymetazoline hydrochloride, phenylephrine hydrochloride, and ephedrine hydrochloride has been reported to result in severe hypertension, cardiomegaly, and congestive heart failure in a 34-year-old man.[1] Severe hypertensive crisis was reported in a young man after ingestion of seven Trinalin tablets (120 mg of pseudoephedrine and 1 mg of azatadine sulfate per tablet). Labetalol given intravenously was very effective treatment.[1] PPA is the active ingredient in most diet aids and many decongestant agents, and is also used as a substitute for amphetamine. In a recent meta-analysis, Salerno et al.[12] showed that PPA caused a small, but significant increase in systolic BP.

The effect was more pronounced with shorter-term administration, higher doses of medication, and immediate-release formulations. Excessive doses may result in severe hypertension and, in rare instances, hypertensive encephalopathy, intracerebral hemorrhage, and death.[1] Of note, PPA was recently withdrawn from the market in the United States and is therefore no longer available.

Agents that indirectly activate the sympathetic nervous system
Caffeine

Caffeine can acutely and transiently increase BP by increasing peripheral resistance.[1] The reaction to caffeine is more pronounced in males, in those with a positive family history, and in African-American subjects.[1,2,13] Several investigators showed by using ambulatory BP monitoring that caffeine may increase BP levels.[13,14] Caffeine may cause persistent BP effects in persons who are regular consumers, even when daily intake is at moderately high levels.[15] In a recent meta-analysis, Noordzij et al.[16] found that regular caffeine intake increases BP; however, when ingested through coffee, the BP effect of caffeine is small. In one case report, intravenous caffeine, used to increase the length of seizure during electroconvulsive therapy, caused hypertension and tachycardia.[1] The effect of caffeine on the cardiovascular system is not homogenous. In a recent study, Sudano et al.[17] showed that in nonhabitual coffee drinkers, coffee enhanced the cardiovascular response to mental stress with an additional increase in systolic BP, whereas in habitual drinkers, the response is blunted.[17] It seems that strategies for encouraging reduced dietary levels of caffeine should be considered.[18] Of note, concomitant medications, such as monoamine oxidase inhibitors (MAOIs), antihypertensive drugs, oral contraceptives, and nonsteroidal anti-inflammatory drugs seem to increase the risk of hypertension.[1]

Herbal products

Herbal products that are popular have the potential to increase BP and to interfere with antihypertensive treatment.[19–28] The evidence is anecdotal, and therefore it is impossible to estimate the true incidence of these adverse effects. Several reports showed that dietary supplements that contain ephedra alkaloids can increase BP.[22,26] Some herbs can have a significant influence on concurrently administered drugs.[28] Hypertension was reported after coadministration of ginkgo and a diuretic thiazide.[25]

Cocaine

Cocaine intoxication and abuse is characterized by adrenergic overactivity associated with increased BP. Cocaine use is associated with acute but not chronic hypertension. Severe hypertension has been reported to occur in subjects treated with propranolol, because of unopposed peripheral α-stimulation.[1] Hypertensive encephalopathy secondary to cocaine abuse was reported in a 40-year-old woman who was treated successfully with nitroprusside and captopril.[1] Cocaine ingestion during pregnancy increases the risk of early placental abruption and BP elevation that are less responsive to conventional therapy than pregnancy-induced hypertension.[1]

Antiemetic agents

Antiemetic agents such as metoclopramide, alizapride, and prochlorperazine, have been reported to increase BP transiently.[1] Metoclopramide—an antiemetic agent classified as an antagonist of central and peripheral dopamine receptors—has been reported to increase BP transiently in patients treated with cisplatin.[1] The exact mechanism responsible for the rise in BP is unclear. Two other antiemetics, alizapride and prochlorperazine, were found to have a similar effect on BP.[1]

Yohimbine hydrochloride

Yohimbine hydrochloride—an α_2-adrenoceptor antagonist that is approved for treatment of erectile dysfunction—may increase BP.[1,2,29] In normal volunteers and in patients with panic disorders, oral administration at doses used clinically may slightly increase BP.[1] However, in hypertensive patients oral yohimbine was reported to induce a significant increase in mean arterial pressure.[29] The magnitude of the pressor response was related to baseline norepinephrine levels and to the yohimbine-induced increment in plasma norepinephrine levels.[29] Thus yohimbine increases BP by stimulation of the sympathetic nervous outflow, and the drug should be administered with caution to patients with evidence for increased basal sympathetic outflow or those undergoing concurrent treatment with tricyclic antidepressants or other drugs that interfere with neuronal uptake or metabolism of norepinephrine.

Sibutramine

Sibutramine, a novel serotonin and noradrenaline reuptake inhibitor, is an antiobesity drug. It reduces food intake by enhancing the physiologic response of postingestive satiety and increases energy expenditure. By activating the sympathetic nervous system, the drug may increase heart rate and BP.[30–33] In obese hypertensive patients, the BP reduction achieved by weight loss may negate the potential BP increase related to the drug.[34,35] In a recent combined analysis of two placebo-controlled trials, sibutramine treatment did not elicit a critical increase in BP even in hypertensive patients.[36] Nevertheless, obese patients being treated with sibutramine should be monitored periodically for changes in BP.

Clozapine

Clozapine is an antipsychotic agent that is used for schizophrenic symptoms in patients refractory to classical antipsychotics. This drug may raise BP by sympathetic activation.[1] Several case reports of pseudopheochromocytoma syndrome associated with clozapine have been described.[1,37] Sympathetic overactivity and BP were normalized upon treatment discontinuation. It is not clear whether long-term use of clozapine may induce hypertension. Lund et al.[38] did not find an increased risk to develop hypertension, whereas Henderson et al.[39] showed increased rates of hypertension in patients treated with clozapine.

Nonspecific agents

Glucagon may produce a catecholamine-mediated rise in BP in patients with pheochromocytoma.[40] Blocking the α-adrenoceptors by either intravenous phentholamin or oral agents such as phenoxybenazamine or doxazosin may prevent catastrophic cardiovascular events.

Administration of physostigmine, a centrally acting cholinergic agent, to patients with Alzheimer's disease was accompanied by a rise in BP, probably due to direct sympathetic activation.[1] A hypertensive crisis was reported in a pregnant woman who was treated with ritodrine hydrochloride for inhibition of preterm labor. This was related to its inherent pharmacology as a beta-mimetic drug.[1]

ANTIDEPRESSANT AGENTS

Monoamine oxidase inhibitors (MAOIs) exert their effects by delaying the metabolism of sympathomimetic amines and 5-hydroxytryptophan, and by increasing the store of norepinephrine in postganglionic sympathetic neurons. MAOIs are used to treat psychiatric patients with depression. Hypertensive crisis, the most serious toxic effect of these agents, has been reported more frequently when MAOIs were taken concomitantly with exogenous sympathomimetic amines.[1]

Certain foods containing tyramine, such as cheese (Parmiggiano), beer, wine (Chianti), snails, chicken liver, yeast, coffee, citrus fruits, avocados, canned figs, broad beans, chocolate, and bananas, may interact with MAOIs to cause hypertensive crisis. A patient treated with isoniazid who ate Swiss cheese had recurrent episodes of severe hypertension.[1] There are some reports of MAOIs that cause severe hypertensive reaction even without use of concomitant medications.[1] Among the various MAOIs, tranylcypromine is the most hazardous because of its stimulant action, whereas moclobemide and brofaromine are the least likely to induce hypertensive reaction.[1] Selegiline, a type-B MAOI mainly used for Parkinson's disease, may also increase BP.[41] A case of hypertensive crisis was reported when selegiline was coadministered with other anti-Parkinson's agents or dopamine.[42,43]

Tricyclic antidepressants block the reuptake of the neurotransmitters in the synapse in the central nervous system. There are some reports that these agents increase BP, mainly in patients with panic disorders.[1]

Buspirone, a serotonin receptor type 1 α-agonist, has also been reported to increase BP.[1] It is speculated that buspirone increases BP by its metabolite 1-2 pyrimidinyl piperazine, which is an α_2-adrenoceptor antagonist, and therefore should not be used concomitantly with an MAOI. A small but sustained and dose-dependent increase in arterial pressure seems to occur with other serotonin agonists as well. Venlafaxine has a dose-dependent effect on BP that is clinically significant at high dosages.[2] Episodes of severe hypertension were described in patients treated with other antidepressant agents such as fluoxetine, fluoxetine plus selegiline, and thioridazine.[1]

Carbamazepine used for bipolar depression and seizures may also induce hypertension.[44] In rare cases, lithium intoxication has been accompanied by severe hypertension. The exact mechanism for this phenomenon is not known.[1]

IMMUNOSUPPRESSIVE AGENTS

Cyclosporine A (CyA) is a potent, orally active immuno-suppressive drug used in human organ transplantation and in autoimmune diseases, such as psoriasis, primary biliary cirrhosis, rheumatoid arthritis, type 1 diabetes mellitus, myasthenia gravis, and uveitis. The major side effects of cyclosporine are nephrotoxicity and arterial hypertension.

The incidence of cyclosporine associated hypertension (CAH) varies with the patient population under evaluation. The greatest experience to date has been with patients undergoing organ transplantation with kidney recipients representing the largest single group.[1] In 212 cyclosporine-treated renal transplant recipients, the prevalence of arterial hypertension was as high as 81.6% at 1 year after transplantation.[1] The presence of hypertension before transplantation, a plasma creatinine level higher than 2 mg/dL at 1 year, and a maintenance therapy with corticosteroids were positively associated with CAH. In a large cohort of 1267 kidney transplant patients who received an immunosuppressive regimen based on CyA, usually in association with azathioprine and steroids, the rate of hypertension was 32.7% at 1 year of transplantation.[45]

For patients undergoing bone marrow transplantation, the evidence of an excess incidence of hypertension due to cyclosporine appears to be more compelling. In recipients of bone marrow transplants, a 57% incidence of hypertension was reported in cyclosporine-treated patients, compared with a 4% incidence in methotrexate-treated patients.[1] The frequency of CAH in cardiac transplant recipients is approaching 100%, and virtually all patients develop hypertension soon after transplantation, independent of renal impairment and irrespective of conventional risk factors associated with CAH.[1]

In liver transplant recipients, CAH is also frequent and occurred in more than 70% of the patients.[1] In liver transplant recipients with cyclosporine-related hypertension, conversion to a low dose of cyclosporine and azathioprine lowered the BP.[1] Using cyclosporine A microemulsion (CyA-ME) with C2 rather than C0 monitoring reduced the risk of developing hypertension to 42%, a rate that is similar to the rate with tacrolimus.[46] Substitution of CyA with mycophenolate mofetil may improve BP control.[47]

CAH is also common in patients with autoimmune disease treated with cyclosporine. In one study, 11% of 321 patients with autoimmune disease treated with cyclosporine for up to 2 years developed new-onset hypertension.[1] Among 16 normotensive patients with idiopathic autoimmune uveitis who were treated with cyclosporine orally at an initial dosage of 5 mg/kg of body weight per day for at least 2 years, 81% developed hypertension.[1] Some investigators studied the effects of cyclosporine on BP after short- and long-term treatment for dermatologic disorders.[1,48] In 21 psoriatic patients, cyclosporine at 14 mg/kg per day increased systolic BP by 10% and diastolic BP by 16% after 4 weeks of treatment.[1] There was a significant correlation between cyclosporine trough levels and diastolic BP. During a long-term follow-up, patients with psoriasis who were treated with cyclosporine exhibited a dose-related increase in the mean diastolic BP, and 5 out of 10 patients who were treated with cyclosporine at more than 3 mg/kg per day became hypertensive.[1]

Several potential mechanisms may contribute to the development of CAH. These include the nephrotoxic effects *per se*, and renal vasoconstriction, which has been documented in both animals and humans.[1,49] The nephrotoxic effects can be mediated by one or more of several mechanisms, including stimulation of the renal sympathetic nervous system, imbalance in the production of renal vasoconstrictor eicosanoids and/or failure of vasodilatory prostaglandin synthesis, alteration of the renin-angiotensin-aldosterone system, and a direct vasoconstriction effect mediated by either stimulation of endothelin synthesis or interference with the production of endothelial-derived relaxation factor.[1] However, elevation of BP can also be observed without clinically detectable renal abnormalities. Thus nonrenal factors need to be considered in the pathogenesis of CAH.

Cyclosporine can cause direct vasoconstriction[2] and thereby increase BP. The role of the sympathetic nervous system in cyclosporine-induced vasoconstriction was suggested by some investigators.[1] Scherrer et al.[50] found a 2.7-fold higher rate of sympathetic-nerve firing in heart-transplant recipients receiving cyclosporine than those not receiving cyclosporine.

Increases in thromboxane production can also contribute to the vasoconstrictor effects of cyclosporine.[2]

The renin-angiotensin-aldosterone system has also been extensively investigated. Animal experiments indicated that cyclosporine stimulates plasma renin activity. However, subsequent studies in humans have consistently shown a suppressed renin-angiotensin system, extracellular volume expansion, and a sodium-avid state in transplant recipients with CAH.[2] Increased production of endothelin and reduced release of endothelial-derived relaxing factor may also contribute to the vasoconstrictive effects of cyclosporine.[2] Cyclosporine also causes increased vascular sensitivity to humoral and neurogenic stimuli.[2] Interference with intracellular calcium homeostasis could produce hypertension by direct action on resistance vessels.[2]

The occurrence of CAH is unrelated to age, sex, or race.[2] While most patients present with mild to moderate asymptomatic BP elevation, others may rapidly develop severe hypertension and encephalopathy. CAH is characterized by a disturbed circadian rhythm with the absence or reversal of the normal nocturnal fall in BP.[49] BP usually falls after the withdrawal or substitution of cyclosporine immunosuppression but may not remit completely. Furthermore, it is often not possible to discontinue therapy. Calcium antagonists have been used successfully to lower BP, but they can increase cyclosporine blood levels.[51] Multidrug therapy is usually necessary to control CAH.

Tacrolimus, another immunosuppressive agent that inhibits calcineurin, may also induce hypertension. However, it produces less hypertension than cyclosporin A, and therefore conversion to tacrolimus may be considered in patients with CAH.[52,53]

Rapamycin, a novel immunosuppressive agent, that does not inhibit calcineurin, produces little nephrotoxicity and hypertension.[54]

ANTINEOPLASTIC AGENTS

Several alkylating agents can increase BP. In one series, 15 of 18 patients treated with multiple alkylating agents following autologous bone marrow transplantation developed hypertension.[1] The hypertension was unrelated to plasma renin activity, aldosterone, and catecholamines, but was related to digoxin-like immunoreactive factor. Hypertensive reactions associated with paclitaxel treatment has been reported.[2]

Cis-diamminedichloroplatinium (CDDP) is an organic platinum compound with an antineoplastic effect. It has been demonstrated in four of five patients that intra-arterial administration of CDDP produces sustained systemic hypertension. This complication has not been observed in patients receiving the drug by the intravenous route. The etiology of the hypertension remains obscure.[2]

RECOMBINANT HUMAN ERYTHROPOIETIN

Recombinant human erythropoietin (r-HuEPO) is effective in correcting the anemia of patients with end-stage renal failure, and patients with malignancies. r-HuEPO can lead to an increase in BP that appears to be dose related. Systemic hypertension has been reported to develop, or to worsen, in 20% to 30% of patients treated with r-HuEPO worldwide.[55] The greatest increases in BP affect daytime systolic and nighttime diastolic BP.[1,2] Hypertension may develop in some patients as early as 2 weeks and in others as late as 4 months after the start of r-HuEPO treatment.[1,2] Hypertension has not proved to be a serious general problem in the r-HuEPO treated patient; however, few cases of hypertensive crisis with encephalopathy have been reported.[1,2]

Several risk factors for the development, or worsening, of hypertension after r-HuEPO therapy, have been identified. They include the presence of pre-existing hypertension, rapid increase in hematocrit, a low baseline hematocrit before r-HuEPO administration, high doses and intravenous route of administration, the presence of native kidneys, a genetic predisposition to hypertension, and possibly a younger age.[1,2,56] There are several potential mechanisms by which r-HuEPO therapy may increase BP in hemodialysis patients. They include increased blood viscosity, the loss of hypoxic vasodilation, the activation of neurohumoral systems (catecholamines, the renin-angiotensin system), and especially a direct vascular effect. This last mechanism is supported by several data sets, and many factors may be involved in its pathogenesis (increased cell calcium uptake, imbalance in local vasoactive agents, with increased synthesis of ET-1, mitogenic effect, and a platelet-dependent mechanism).[57–62] Hemodynamically, r-HuEPO increases BP by a marked increase in peripheral resistance associated with only a mild decrease in cardiac output.[1] By optimizing dialysis treatment, paying close attention to volume regulation, giving r-HuEPO subcutaneously and in a fashion to increase hematocrit gradually, the occurrence of hypertension can be minimized.[56]

The hypertension associated with r-HuEPO has not generally been too difficult to control. The BP can usually be controlled with a combination of fluid removal with dialysis and conventional antihypertensive therapy. If these measures are unsuccessful, the dose of r-HuEPO should be lowered or therapy should be held for several weeks. Phlebotomy of 500 mL of blood may rapidly lower BP in refractory patients.

ALCOHOL

Excessive alcohol use has clearly been shown to raise BP and can also increase resistance to antihypertensive therapy. Small doses of ethanol slightly increase heart rate, cardiac output, and BP. The exact mechanisms mediating the acute effects are not yet clear; however, acute increases in plasma epinephrine and norepinephrine levels have been reported, reflecting an increase in sympathetic nervous activity.[1] Increased plasma renin levels in heavy drinkers, and increased plasma cortisol levels have been reported. In heavy drinkers, withdrawal from alcohol as well as drinking were found to increase BP, probably because of a hyperadrenergic state.[1]

Apart from the acute effects of alcohol, an increased prevalence of hypertension has been shown in heavy drinkers.[1,2] In the Australian Risk Factor Prevalence Study, 7% of the prevalence of hypertension was attributed to alcohol consumption, whereas in the Kaiser-Permanente Study, the rate for men was 11%.[1] It was found that the greater the quantity of alcohol consumption, the higher the prevalence of hypertension.

The BP effects of alcohol are independent of obesity, salt intake, cigarette smoking, and potassium intake, and there is a dose–response relationship for the hypertensive effects of alcohol. In a prospective cohort study of 3900 Japanese men, Yoshita et al.[63] found that annual systolic BP increase was greater in those who consumed 300 g/week or more of alcohol than nondrinkers. Baseline diastolic BP was associated with alcohol consumption and was significantly higher in drinkers consuming 200 g/week or more than nondrinkers. Therefore moderation of alcohol intake is recommended as an initial therapy for mild hypertension. A reasonable approach is to limit daily alcohol consumption to less than 200 g/week.

Disulfiram

Disulfiram is commonly used as a pharmacologic adjunct in the treatment of alcoholism. Administration of 500 mg per day of disulfiram for 2 to 3 weeks has been reported to increase BP slightly. A low dose of 125 mg per day of this agent may also increase BP. It seems that changes in peripheral or central noradrenergic activity are responsible for the increase in arterial pressure.

NONSTEROIDAL ANTI-INFLAMMATORY DRUGS

Nonsteroidal anti-inflammatory drugs (NSAIDs) can induce an increase in BP and interfere with antihypertensive treatment, nullifying its effect.[1] Two meta-analyses have demonstrated that, after pooling data drawn from published reports of randomized trials of younger adults, NSAID use produces a clinically significant increment in mean BP of 5 mmHg.[1] Elderly patients, those with pre-existing hypertension, salt-sensitive patients, patients with renal failure and patients with renovascular hypertension are at a higher risk to develop severe hypertension when treated with NSAIDs.[64–68] The mechanisms whereby NSAIDs raise BP are not fully understood. Inhibiting the synthesis of prostaglandins (PGs) from arachidonic acid via the two isoforms of cyclooxygenase (COX), COX-1 and COX-2, is probably the main mechanism of action.[1] Interference with both the control of vascular resistance and the regulation of extracellular volume homeostasis has been suggested, but several other putative mechanisms such as moderation of adrenergic activity or resetting of the baroreceptor response may also be involved.[1] NSAIDs may interact with some antihypertensive agents such as diuretics, beta-blockers, and ACE inhibitors, and do not interact with calcium antagonists and central-acting drugs (actions of these drugs are apparently unrelated to production of PGs).[1] NSAIDs vary considerably in their effect on BP.[69] Armstrong and Malone[69] found in a recent study that among the various NSAIDs, indomethacin, naproxen, and piroxicam were associated with the greatest increase in BP. They also showed that among the selective NSAIDs, rofecoxib is more likely than celecoxib to raise systolic BP.[69] In a recent meta-analysis, Aw et al.[70] showed that selective COX-2 inhibitors increase BP more than the nonselective agents. However, there is evidence that patients receiving celecoxib experience less increase in BP compared with those receiving rofecoxib. A recent study by Sowers et al.[71] showed that at equally effective doses for osteoarthritis management, treatment with rofecoxib but not celecoxib or naproxen induced a significant increase in 24-hour systolic BP. Low-dose aspirin has no effect on BP control in hypertensive patients. It is wise to balance the risk of an increase in BP against the expected benefit of treatment with an NSAID. In patients who take NSAIDs, calcium antagonists would appear to be a preferred choice to other antihypertensive agents.[72]

HEAVY METALS

Epidemiologic studies confirmed the high incidence of hypertension among patients exposed to lead.[73–76] Even at low levels of exposure (40 μg/dL), blood lead level was positively associated with both systolic and diastolic BP and risks of hypertension among women aged 40 to 59 years. The relationship between blood lead level and hypertension was most pronounced in postmenopausal women.[77] History of lead exposure influences hypertension and elevated BP during pregnancy.[78] Lead exposure affects the renin angiotensin system, and induces sympathetic hyperreactivity by acting on central and peripheral sympathetic junctions.[1] These results provide support for continued efforts to reduce lead levels in the general population, especially in women.

A retrospective study of 311 male workers in an alkaline battery factory indicated a possible relationship between exposure to cadmium oxide and the development of hypertension.[1] Several other studies also showed an association between cadmium exposure and hypertension.[79,80] However,

other epidemiologic studies have failed to show such a relationship.[1,81] In a recent study, environmental exposure to cadmium was not associated with higher conventional BP or 24-hour ambulatory BP measurements, or with increased risk for hypertension.[82]

Some studies suggest that arsenic exposure also may induce hypertension in humans.[83,84]

OTHER AGENTS

Bromocriptine

Bromocriptine mesylate is commonly used for prolactin inhibition and suppression of puerperal lactation. Although bromocriptine often has a hypotensive effect, severe hypertension with subsequent stroke has been reported in the postpartum period.[1] Patients with pregnancy-induced hypertension are at increased risk to develop hypertension. The suppression of lactation is no longer a Food and Drug Administration–approved use for bromocriptine.

Scorpions and black widow spiders

Venoms of scorpions (especially the South American species) and spiders (particularly the black widow spider, *Latrodectus mactans*) commonly produce a clinical picture of profuse perspiration, lacrimation, vomiting, convulsion, and cardiovascular collapse. However, occasionally hypertension and bradycardia occur. Hypertension is mediated by a massive discharge of catecholamines into the circulation produced by the venom, and therefore β- or α-blockade is effective in this condition.[1]

Amphotericin B

Amphotericin B (AmB) is the mainstay of therapy for serious fungal infections. A few cases of severe hypertension associated with the use of AmB deoxycholate have been reported in the literature, and one case report of hypertension associated with a lipid-containing preparation of the medication have been described.[1]

Anti-HIV treatment

One case report of severe hypertension and renal atrophy associated with the protease inhibitor indinavir has been described.[85] Hypertensive crisis secondary to phenylpropanolamine interacting with triple-drug therapy for HIV prophylaxis has also been reported.[86] In addition, potential drug interactions exist between antiretroviral medications, particularly the protease inhibitors and antihypertensive medications.

SUMMARY

A variety of therapeutic agents and chemical substances can increase blood pressure and even induce hypertension. These agents increase arterial pressure by either causing sodium retention and volume expansion or activate directly or indirectly the sympathetic nervous system. Some agents act directly on arteriolar smooth muscle.

For a few agents the mechanism is mixed or unknown. In general, these pressure increases are small and transient:

however, severe hypertension involving encephalopathy, stroke and irreversible renal failure have been reported. Careful evaluation of a patient's drug regimen may obviate the need for unnecessary, costly, and potentially dangerous evaluations and prevent the need for lifelong antihypertensive therapy.

Using these agents should be avoided in hypertensive patients and in subjects with pre-hypertension. When it is not possible to avoid chemical agents that cause hypertension, institution of appropriate antihypertensive treatment is indicated.

REFERENCES

1. Grossman E, Messerli FH. High blood pressure. A side effect of drugs, poisons, and food. *Arch Intern Med* 1995;155(5):450–60.
2. Grossman E, Messerli FH. Management of drug-induced and iatrogenic hypertension. In: Izzo JL Jr, Black HR, eds. *Hypertension Primer*. 3rd ed. Dallas: Lippincott Williams & Wilkins, 2003:516–9.
3. Sinclair AM, Isles CG, Brown I, Cameron H, Murray GD, Robertson JW. Secondary hypertension in a blood pressure clinic. *Arch Intern Med* 1987; 147(7):1289–93.
4. Brem AS. Insights into glucocorticoid-associated hypertension. *Am J Kidney Dis* 2001;37(1):1–10.
5. Whitworth JA, Schyvens CG, Zhang Y, Andrews MC, Mangos GJ, Kelly JJ. The nitric oxide system in glucocorticoid-induced hypertension. *J Hypertens* 2002;20(6):1035–43.
6. Martel MJ, Rey E, Beauchesne MF, Perreault S, Lefebvre G, Forget A, et al. Use of inhaled corticosteroids during pregnancy and risk of pregnancy induced hypertension: nested case-control study. *BMJ* 2005;330(7485):230.
7. Cushman M, Kuller LH, Prentice R, Rodabough RJ, Psaty BM, Stafford RS, et al. Estrogen plus progestin and risk of venous thrombosis. *JAMA* 2004; 292(13):1573–80.
8. Rossouw JE, Anderson GL, Prentice RL, LaCroix AZ, Kooperberg C, Stefanick ML, et al. Risks and benefits of estrogen plus progestin in healthy postmenopausal women: principal results From the Women's Health Initiative randomized controlled trial. *JAMA* 2002;288(3):321–33.
9. Wassertheil-Smoller S, Hendrix SL, Limacher M, Heiss G, Kooperberg C, Baird A, et al. Effect of estrogen plus progestin on stroke in postmenopausal women: the Women's Health Initiative: a randomized trial. *JAMA* 2003; 289(20):2673–84.
10. Lokkegaard E, Jovanovic Z, Heitmann BL, Keiding N, Ottesen B, Hundrup YA, et al. Increased risk of stroke in hypertensive women using hormone therapy: analyses based on the Danish Nurse Study. *Arch Neurol* 2003;60(10):1379–84.
11. Son JS, Lee SK. Pulmonary edema following phenylephrine intranasal spray administration during the induction of general anesthesia in a child. *Yonsei Med J* 2005;46(2):305–8.
12. Salerno SM, Jackson JL, Berbano EP. The impact of oral phenylpropanolamine on blood pressure: a meta-analysis and review of the literature. *J Hum Hypertens* 2005;19(8):643–52.
13. Savoca MR, MacKey ML, Evans CD, Wilson M, Ludwig DA, Harshfield GA. Association of ambulatory blood pressure

and dietary caffeine in adolescents. *Am J Hypertens* 2005;18(1):116–20.
14. Lane JD, Pieper CF, Phillips-Bute BG, Bryant JE, Kuhn CM. Caffeine affects cardiovascular and neuroendocrine activation at work and home. *Psychosom Med* 2002;64(4):595–603.
15. Lovallo WR, Wilson MF, Vincent AS, Sung BH, McKey BS, Whitsett TL. Blood pressure response to caffeine shows incomplete tolerance after short-term regular consumption. *Hypertension* 2004;43(4):760–5.
16. Noordzij M, Uiterwaal CS, Arends LR, Kok FJ, Grobbee DE, Geleijnse JM. Blood pressure response to chronic intake of coffee and caffeine: a meta-analysis of randomized controlled trials. *J Hypertens* 2005;23(5):921–8.
17. Sudano I, Spieker L, Binggeli C, Ruschitzka F, Luscher TF, Noll G, et al. Coffee blunts mental stress-induced blood pressure increase in habitual but not in nonhabitual coffee drinkers. *Hypertension* 2005;46(3):521–6.
18. James JE. Critical review of dietary caffeine and blood pressure: a relationship that should be taken more seriously. *Psychosom Med* 2004;66(1):63–71.
19. Zahn KA, Li RL, Purssell RA. Cardiovascular toxicity after ingestion of "herbal ecstacy." *J Emerg Med* 1999; 17(2):289–91.
20. Yates KM, O'Connor A, Horsley CA. "Herbal Ecstasy": a case series of adverse reactions. *N Z Med J* 2000;113(1114): 315–7.
21. Ruck B, Shih RD, Marcus SM. Hypertensive crisis from herbal treatment of impotence. *Am J Emerg Med* 1999;17(3):317–8.
22. Richard CL, Jurgens TM. Effects of natural health products on blood pressure. *Ann Pharmacother* 2005; 39(4):712–20.
23. Pharand C, Ackman ML, Jackevicius CA, Paradiso-Hardy FL, Pearson GJ. Use of OTC and herbal products in patients with cardiovascular disease. *Ann Pharmacother* 2003;37(6):899–904.
24. Kuczkowski KM. Herbal ecstasy: cardiovascular complications of khat chewing in pregnancy. *Acta Anaesthesiol Belg* 2005;56(1):19–21.
25. Izzo AA, Di Carlo G, Borrelli F, Ernst E. Cardiovascular pharmacotherapy and herbal medicines: the risk of drug interaction. *Int J Cardiol* 2005;98(1):1–14.
26. Haller CA, Benowitz NL. Adverse cardiovascular and central nervous system events associated with dietary supplements containing ephedra alkaloids. *N Engl J Med* 2000;343(25):1833–8.
27. Ernst E. Cardiovascular adverse effects of herbal medicines: a systematic review of the recent literature. *Can J Cardiol* 2003;19(7):818–27.

28. Awang DV, Fugh-Berman A. Herbal interactions with cardiovascular drugs. *J Cardiovasc Nurs* 2002;16(4):64–70.
29. Grossman E, Rosenthal T, Peleg E, Holmes C, Goldstein DS. Oral yohimbine increases blood pressure and sympathetic nervous outflow in hypertensive patients. *J Cardiovasc Pharmacol* 1993;22(1):22–6.
30. Kim SH, Lee YM, Jee SH, Nam CM. Effect of sibutramine on weight loss and blood pressure: a meta-analysis of controlled trials. *Obes Res* 2003; 11(9):1116–23.
31. McMahon FG, Fujioka K, Singh BN, Mendel CM, Rowe E, Rolston K, et al. Efficacy and safety of sibutramine in obese white and African American patients with hypertension: a 1-year, double-blind, placebo-controlled, multicenter trial. *Arch Intern Med* 2000;160(14):2185–91.
32. McMahon FG, Weinstein SP, Rowe E, Ernst KR, Johnson F, Fujioka K. Sibutramine is safe and effective for weight loss in obese patients whose hypertension is well controlled with angiotensin-converting enzyme inhibitors. *J Hum Hypertens* 2002;16(1):5–11.
33. Sramek JJ, Leibowitz MT, Weinstein SP, Rowe ED, Mendel CM, Levy B, et al. Efficacy and safety of sibutramine for weight loss in obese patients with hypertension well controlled by beta-adrenergic blocking agents: a placebo-controlled, double-blind, randomised trial. *J Hum Hypertens* 2002;16(1):13–9.
34. Gokcel A, Karakose H, Ertorer EM, Tanaci N, Tutuncu NB, Guvener N. Effects of sibutramine in obese female subjects with type 2 diabetes and poor blood glucose control. *Diabetes Care* 2001;24(11):1957–60.
35. Hazenberg BP. Randomized, double-blind, placebo-controlled, multicenter study of sibutramine in obese hypertensive patients. *Cardiology* 2000;94(3):152–8.
36. Jordan J, Scholze J, Matiba B, Wirth A, Hauner H, Sharma AM. Influence of Sibutramine on blood pressure: evidence from placebo-controlled trials. *Int J Obes Relat Metab Disord* 2005;29(3):509–16.
37. Krentz AJ, Mikhail S, Cantrell P, Hill GM. Drug points: pseudophaeochromocytoma syndrome associated with clozapine. *BMJ* 2001;322(7296):1213.
38. Lund BC, Perry PJ, Brooks JM, Arndt S. Clozapine use in patients with schizophrenia and the risk of diabetes, hyperlipidemia, and hypertension: a claims-based approach. *Arch Gen Psychiatry* 2001;58(12):1172–6.
39. Henderson DC, Daley TB, Kunkel L, Rodrigues-Scott M, Koul P, Hayden D. Clozapine and hypertension: a chart

review of 82 patients. *J Clin Psychiatry* 2004;65(5):686–9.

40. Grossman E, Goldstein DS, Hoffman A, Keiser HR. Glucagon and clonidine testing in the diagnosis of pheochromocytoma. *Hypertension* 1991;17(6 Pt 1):733–41.

41. Selegiline: a second look. Six years later: too risky in Parkinson's disease. *Prescrire Int* 2002;11(60):108–11.

42. Ito D, Amano T, Sato H, Fukuuchi Y. Paroxysmal hypertensive crises induced by selegiline in a patient with Parkinson's disease. *J Neurol* 2001;248(6):533–4.

43. Rose LM, Ohlinger MJ, Mauro VF. A hypertensive reaction induced by concurrent use of selegiline and dopamine. *Ann Pharmacother* 2000;34(9):1020–4.

44. Jette N, Veregin T, Guberman A. Carbamazepine- induced hypertension. *Neurology* 2002;59(2):275–6.

45. Snanoudj R, Kriaa F, Arzouk N, Beaudreuil S, Hiesse C, Durrbach A, et al. Single-center experience with cyclosporine therapy for kidney transplantation: analysis of a twenty-year period in 1200 patients. *Transpl Proc* 2004;36(Suppl 2):83S–88S.

46. Levy G, Villamil F, Samuel D, Sanjuan F, Grazi GL, Wu Y, et al. Results of LIS2T, a multicenter, randomized study comparing cyclosporine microemulsion with C2 monitoring and tacrolimus with C0 monitoring in de novo liver transplantation. *Transplantation* 2004; 77(11):1632–8.

47. Moreno JM, Rubio E, Gomez A, Lopez-Monclus J, Herreros A, Revilla J, et al. Effectiveness and safety of mycophenolate mofetil as monotherapy in liver transplantation. *Transpl Proc* 2003;35(5):1874–6.

48. Markham T, Watson A, Rogers S. Adverse effects with long-term cyclosporin for severe psoriasis. *Clin Exp Dermatol* 2002;27(2):111–4.

49. Cifkova R, Hallen H. Cyclosporin-induced hypertension. *J Hypertens* 2001;19(12):2283–5.

50. Scherrer U, Vissing SF, Morgan BJ, Rollins JA, Tindall RS, Ring S, et al. Cyclosporine-induced sympathetic activation and hypertension after heart transplantation. *N Engl J Med* 1990;323(11):693–9.

51. Rodicio JL. Calcium antagonists and renal protection from cyclosporine nephrotoxicity: long-term trial in renal transplantation patients. *J Cardiovasc Pharmacol* 2000;35(Suppl 1):S7–11.

52. Jardine AG. Assessing the relative risk of cardiovascular disease among renal transplant patients receiving tacrolimus or cyclosporine. *Transpl Int* 2005;18(4):379–84.

53. Dikow R, Degenhard M, Kraus T, Sauer P, Schemmer P, Uhl W, et al. Blood pressure profile and treatment quality in liver allograft recipients-benefit of tacrolimus versus cyclosporine. *Transpl Proc* 2004; 36(5):1512–5.

54. Morales JM, Andres A, Rengel M, Rodicio JL. Influence of cyclosporin, tacrolimus and rapamycin on renal function and arterial hypertension after renal transplantation. *Nephrol Dial Transplant* 2001;16(Suppl 1):121–4.

55. Smith KJ, Bleyer AJ, Little WC, Sane DC. The cardiovascular effects of erythropoietin. *Cardiovasc Res* 2003;59(3):538–48.

56. Luft FC. Erythropoietin and arterial hypertension. *Clin Nephrol* 2000; 53(Suppl 1):S61–4.

57. Miyashita K, Tojo A, Kimura K, Goto A, Omata M, Nishiyama K, et al. Blood pressure response to erythropoietin injection in hemodialysis and predialysis patients. *Hypertens Res* 2004;27(2):79–84.

58. Rodrigue ME, Moreau C, Lariviere R, Lebel M. Relationship between eicosanoids and endothelin-1 in the pathogenesis of erythropoietin-induced hypertension in uremic rats. *J Cardiovasc Pharmacol* 2003; 41(3):388–95.

59. Shimada N, Saka S, Sekizuka K, Tanaka A, Takahashi Y, Nakamura T, et al. Increased endothelin: nitric oxide ratio is associated with erythropoietin-induced hypertension in hemodialysis patients. *Ren Fail* 2003;25(4):569–78.

60. Stefanidis I, Mertens PR, Wurth P, Bach R, Makropoulos W, Mann H, et al. Influence of recombinant human erythropoietin therapy on plasma endothelin-1 levels during hemodialysis. *Int J Artif Organs* 2001;24(6):367–73.

61. Ksiazek A, Zaluska WT, Ksiazek P. Effect of recombinant human erythropoietin on adrenergic activity in normotensive hemodialysis patients. *Clin Nephrol* 2001;56(2):104–10.

62. Vaziri ND. Vascular effects of erythropoietin and anemia correction. *Semin Nephrol* 2000;20(4):356–63.

63. Yoshita K, Miura K, Morikawa Y, Ishizaki M, Kido T, Naruse Y, et al. Relationship of alcohol consumption to 7-year blood pressure change in Japanese men. *J Hypertens* 2005;23(8):1485–1490.

64. de Leeuw PW. Nonsteroidal anti-inflammatory drugs and hypertension. The risks in perspective. *Drugs* 1996; 51(2):179–87.

65. Johnson AG. NSAIDs and increased blood pressure. What is the clinical significance? *Drug Safety* 1997; 17(5):277–89.

66. Whelton A. Nephrotoxicity of nonsteroidal anti-inflammatory drugs: physiologic foundations and clinical implications. *Am J Med* 1999;106(5B): 13S–24S.

67. Johnson AG. NSAIDs and blood pressure. Clinical importance for older patients. *Drugs Aging* 1998;12(1):17–27.

68. Ruoff GE. The impact of nonsteroidal anti-inflammatory drugs on hypertension: alternative analgesics for patients at risk. *Clin Ther* 1998;20(3):376–87, discussion 375.

69. Armstrong EP, Malone DC. The impact of nonsteroidal anti-inflammatory drugs on blood pressure, with an emphasis on newer agents. *Clin Ther* 2003;25(1):1–18.

70. Aw TJ, Haas SJ, Liew D, Krum H. Meta-analysis of cyclooxygenase-2 inhibitors and their effects on blood pressure. *Arch Intern Med* 2005;165(5):490–6.

71. Sowers JR, White WB, Pitt B, Whelton A, Simon LS, Winer N, et al. The effects of cyclooxygenase-2 inhibitors and nonsteroidal anti-inflammatory therapy on 24-hour blood pressure in patients with hypertension, osteoarthritis, and type 2 diabetes mellitus. *Arch Intern Med* 2005;165(2):161–8.

72. Polonia J. Interaction of antihypertensive drugs with anti-inflammatory drugs. *Cardiology* 1997;88(Suppl 3):47–51.

73. Glenn BS, Stewart WF, Links JM, Todd AC, Schwartz BS. The longitudinal association of lead with blood pressure. *Epidemiology* 2003;14(1):30–6.

74. Nomiyama K, Nomiyama H, Liu SJ, Tao YX, Nomiyama J, Omae K. Lead induced increase of blood pressure in female lead workers. *Occup Environ Med* 2002;59(11):734–8.

75. Telisman S, Pizent A, Jurasovic J, Cvitkovic P. Lead effect on blood pressure in moderately lead-exposed male workers. *Am J Ind Med* 2004;45(5):446–54.

76. Vupputuri S, He J, Muntner P, Bazzano LA, Whelton PK, Batuman V. Blood lead level is associated with elevated blood pressure in blacks. *Hypertension* 2003; 41(3):463–8.

77. Nash D, Magder L, Lustberg M, Sherwin RW, Rubin RJ, Kaufmann RB, et al. Blood lead, blood pressure, and hypertension in perimenopausal and postmenopausal women. *JAMA* 2003;289(12):1523–32.

78. Rothenberg SJ, Kondrashov V, Manalo M, Jiang J, Cuellar R, Garcia M, et al. Increases in hypertension and blood pressure during pregnancy with increased bone lead levels. *Am J Epidemiol* 2002;156(12):1079–87.

79. Satarug S, Nishijo M, Ujjin P, Vanavanitkun Y, Moore MR. Cadmium-induced nephropathy in the development of high blood pressure. *Toxicol Lett* 2005;157(1):57–68.

80. Kosanovic M, Jokanovic M, Jevremovic M, Dobric S, Bokonjic D. Maternal and fetal cadmium and selenium status in normotensive and hypertensive pregnancy. *Biol Trace Elem Res* 2002;89(2):97–103.

81. Sirivarasai J, Kaojarern S, Wananukul W, Deechakwan W, Srisomerarn P. Non-occupational lead and cadmium exposure and blood pressure in Thai men. *Asia Pac J Public Health* 2004;16(2):133–7.

82. Staessen JA, Kuznetsova T, Roels HA, Emelianov D, Fagard R. Exposure to cadmium and conventional and ambulatory blood pressures in a prospective population study. Public Health and Environmental Exposure to Cadmium Study Group. *Am J Hypertens* 2000;13(2):146–56.

83. Rahman M, Tondel M, Ahmad SA, Chowdhury IA, Faruquee MH, Axelson O. Hypertension and arsenic exposure in Bangladesh. *Hypertension* 1999;33(1):74–8.

84. Chen CJ, Hsueh YM, Lai MS, Shyu MP, Chen SY, Wu MM, et al. Increased prevalence of hypertension and long-term arsenic exposure. *Hypertension* 1995;25(1):53–60.

85. Cattelan AM, Trevenzoli M, Naso A, Meneghetti F, Cadrobbi P. Severe hypertension and renal atrophy associated with indinavir. *Clin Infect Dis* 2000;30(3):619–21.

86. Khurana V, de la Fuente M, Bradley TP. Hypertensive crisis secondary to phenylpropanolamine interacting with triple-drug therapy for HIV prophylaxis. *Am J Med* 1999;106(1):118–9.

Chapter 72

Catecholamines, Pheochromocytoma, and Hypertension: Genomic Insights

Fangwen Rao, Ryan Friese, Gen Wen, Lian Zhang, Yuqing Chen, Madhusudan Das, Kuixing Zhang, Bruce A. Hamilton, Nicholas J. Schork, Laurent Taupenot, Sushil K. Mahata, Michael G. Ziegler, and Daniel T. O'Connor

Key Findings

- Knowledge of catecholamine biosynthesis, vesicular storage, exocytotic release, and metabolism is crucial to the effective diagnosis and management of patients with pheochromocytoma.

- Discovery of naturally occurring common genetic variation in the catecholamine-storage vesicle protein chromogranin A opened the way to understanding interindividual differences in the storage and release process.

- Common genetic variation at the locus encoding the rate-limiting enzyme in catecholamine biosynthesis, tyrosine hydroxylase, seems to have pleiotropic effects on catecholamine production, stress physiology, and genetic risk of developing hypertension.

- Elucidation of the chromosomal positions of loci encoding the components of the sympathetic neuroeffector junction should assist in further studies of how allelic variation at such loci influences the development of hypertension.

The catecholamines (norepinephrine, epinephrine, and dopamine) are both neurotransmitters and circulating hormones.[1] Catecholamines possess a catechol (3,4-dihydroxyphenyl) modification of the aromatic phenyl ring. Norepinephrine is released from terminals of postganglionic axons of the sympathetic nervous system, as well as central nervous system noradrenergic axons. Adrenal medullary chromaffin cells store both epinephrine and norepinephrine in secretory vesicles.

Chromaffin cells arise embryologically from neuroectoderm. Adrenal precursor cells differentiate first in response to cortisol, and ultimately into sympathetic neurons in response to nerve growth factor. Such cells also migrate to form paraganglia, collections of chromaffin cells beside the aorta. The largest periaortic cluster, often found near the inferior mesenteric artery, is the organ of Zuckerkandl. Both chromaffin cells and postganglionic sympathetic axons are part of the effector limb of the sympathetic branch of the autonomic nervous system and are innervated by thoracolumbar preganglionic axons emerging from the spinal cord.

Catecholamines are released from the adrenal medulla into the circulation through the adrenal vein. Norepinephrine from sympathetic neurons is released presynaptically, acting as a cell-to-cell neurotransmitter. Circulating plasma norepinephrine influences blood pressure and heart rate under extreme circumstances of sympathetic activation. Relatively selective adrenal catecholamine release occurs during syncope and insulin-evoked hypoglycemia, while dynamic exercise selectively stimulates sympathetic neuronal norepinephrine release.

CATECHOLAMINE BIOSYNTHESIS AND METABOLISM

Catecholamine biosynthesis starts with phenylalanine, which is converted to tyrosine by phenylalanine hydroxylase. Tyrosine is hydroxylated to dihydroxyphenylalanine (DOPA) by tyrosine hydroxylase, the rate-limiting enzymatic step in catecholamine biosynthesis. DOPA decarboxylase then converts DOPA to dopamine, which is carried by the vesicular monoamine transporter from the cytosol into the catecholamine storage vesicle, where dopamine β-hydroxylase converts it to norepinephrine. In sympathetic axons and in ~15% to 20% of chromaffin cells, norepinephrine is the final catecholamine product. In ~80% to 85% of chromaffin cells, a further enzymatic step occurs: phenylethanolamine-N-methyltransferase, a cytosolic enzyme, catalyzes the N-methylation of norepinephrine to epinephrine.

Catecholamines in noradrenergic axons and chromaffin cells are sequestered in membrane-limited organelles called catecholamine storage vesicles (or chromaffin granules in chromaffin cells). Chromaffin granule cores contain not only catecholamines but also soluble proteins such as dopamine β-hydroxylase and chromogranin A (Figure 72–1).

The process of catecholamine discharge from chromaffin cells and sympathetic axons is "exocytosis," wherein all soluble components of the granule are co-released and ultimately make their way to the circulation.

Neuronal uptake (or "reuptake") is the major route of catecholamine removal from synaptic clefts and plasma

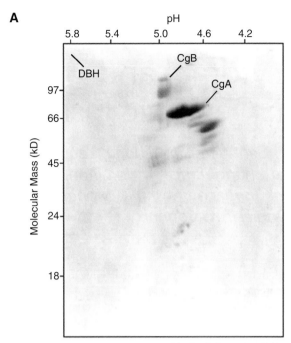

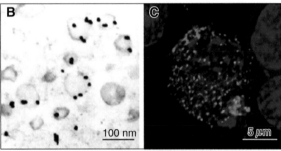

Figure 72–1. Localization of chromogranins within dense-core secretory granules of sympathoadrenal chromaffin cells. **A,** Resolution of bovine chromaffin-vesicle, soluble core proteins by two-dimensional SDS-PAGE gel electrophoresis, followed by Coomassie blue staining of separated proteins. **B,** Immunogold electron microscopy of bovine chromaffin cells. The electron-dense spherical or oblong structures are dense core secretory chromaffin granules. The 8- to 12-nm diameter black particles are immunogold labeling of CgA with rabbit antibovine CgA, indicating the presence of CgA in several secretory granules. **C,** Subcellular distribution of a human CgA-EGFP (enhanced green fluorescent protein) chimeric photoprotein in living sympathoadrenal PC12 cells. CgA-EGFP expressing PC12 cells are examined by three-dimensional (3D) deconvolution microscopy. Nuclei were visualized with (blue) Hoechst 33342 dye. Optical sections along the z axis were acquired with increments of 200 nm using 100× oil immersion objectives to generate 3D views of the photoprotein distribution. CgA-EGFP displays a bright, punctate/vesicular fluorescence signal, especially within the subplasmalemmal region, indicating storage of the chimera in chromaffin secretory granules. CgA, chromogranin A; CgB, chromogranin B; DBH, dopamine β-hydroxylase. (Åsa Thureson-Klein prepared the electron micrograph of immuno-localization of CgA in chromaffin granules of the bovine adrenal medulla. From Taupenot L, Harper KL, O'Connor DT. *N Engl J Med* 2003;348:1134–49.)

(Figure 72–2). Characteristics of this process are its location at the presynaptic axonal membrane, high affinity, stereoselectivity, saturability, dependence on extracellular sodium, and specific pharmacologic inhibition by agents such as tricyclic antidepressants (e.g., desipramine) and cocaine. Non-neuronal uptake may be mediated by the organic cation transporter (OCT) family, especially OCT3. After neuronal uptake, cytosolic catecholamines can be either retransported into storage vesicles or deaminated by the enzyme monoamine oxidase (MAO) to yield the unstable intermediate dihydroxyphenylglycolaldehyde, which is then metabolized to dihydroxyphenylglycol (DHPG) (Figure 72–2).[2] The enzyme catechol O-methyltransferase (COMT), which acts on both catecholamines and DHPG, is present mainly in the cytosol of liver and kidney cells, and also in chromaffin cells. COMT adds a methyl group to one of the hydroxyl oxygens on the catecholamines' dihydroxyphenyl rings to yield either metanephrine (i.e., methoxyepinephrine from epinephrine), normetanephrine (i.e., methoxynorepinephrine from norepinephrine), or methoxytyramine (from dopamine). The metanephrines can then be deaminated by MAO to yield vanillylmandelic acid (VMA), whereas deamination of methoxytyramine by MAO yields homovanillic acid. DHPG is also a substrate for COMT in the formation of MHPG. In the liver, alcohol dehydrogenase oxidizes MHPG to VMA. Thus complete enzymatic degradation of catecholamines to VMA (from epinephrine or norepinephrine) or homovanillic acid (from dopamine) involves the sequential action of two enzymes (MAO and COMT), either of which may initiate the process, followed by an alcohol dehydrogenase step in the liver. In the blood stream, catecholamines have a very short half-life, ~1 to 2 minutes. They are cleared from the circulation largely by neuronal uptake, but in addition are subject to direct renal excretion or sulfoconjugation of a ring hydroxyl group by SULT1A3 in the gastrointestinal tract.

CATECHOLAMINE ACTION

Catecholamine (adrenergic) G protein–coupled receptors are specific for particular ligands (agonists and antagonists) and thereby classified as subtypes of the α (α_1a,b,c, α_2a,b,c) and β (beta$_{1,2,3}$) classes. The hemodynamic effects of circulating norepinephrine require extreme concentrations. Whereas plasma norepinephrine may vary normally over a range of 200 to 1000 pg/mL during physiologic stimulation of sympathetic neuronal activity, far higher concentrations of infused norepinephrine (in excess of 1000 to 2000 pg/mL) are required to substantially affect the blood pressure or heart rate. At β-receptors, norepinephrine is a strong agonist at β_1 (cardiac inotropic and chronotropic) sites, although a relatively weak agonist at β_2 (vascular, vasodilatory) sites. At α-receptors, norepinephrine is an effective agonist at both α_1 (vascular, vasoconstrictive) and α_2 (neuronal and vascular) sites. Infused norepinephrine acutely raises both systolic and diastolic

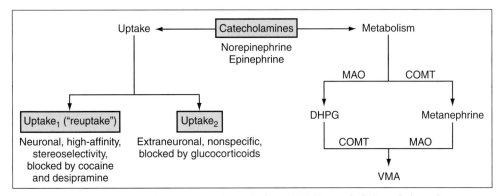

Figure 72–2. Catecholamine disposition and metabolism. COMT, catechol-*O*-methyltransferase; DHPG, dihydroxyphenylglycol; MAO, monoamine oxidase; VMA, vanillylmandelic acid. (From O'Connor DT. In: Bennett JC, Plum F, eds. *Cecil Textbook of Medicine.* 22nd ed. Philadelphia: WB Saunders, 2004:1419–24.)

blood pressure by actions on both β_1- and α-adrenergic receptors, with vasoconstriction accompanied by reflex bradycardia. The hemodynamic effects of circulating epinephrine (50 to 500 pg/mL) differ from those of norepinephrine. At β-receptors, epinephrine is an agonist at both the β_1- and β_2-sites. It is also a more potent agonist than norepinephrine at both the α_1- and α_2-sites. During acute infusion, it increases systolic blood pressure, heart rate, and cardiac output, with a fall in diastolic blood pressure and systemic resistance, the latter effects resulting from actions at β_2-adrenergic receptors.

With chronically elevated circulating catecholamines, the hemodynamic profile may change substantially, in part as a consequence of desensitization of catecholamine target organs resulting from adaptive changes in both receptor and postreceptor responses.

PHEOCHROMOCYTOMA

Introduction and location

Pheochromocytoma is a chromaffin cell neoplasm causing symptoms and signs of episodic catecholamine release, including paroxysmal hypertension.[1] The tumor is an unusual cause of hypertension and accounts for at most ~0.1% to 0.2% of cases of high blood pressure. In population-based cancer studies, its frequency was about two cases per million population. The diagnosis of pheochromocytoma is typically made in young to middle-aged adults, most commonly in the fourth or fifth decade of life; about 10% of diagnoses are made in children (usually male). Autopsy series indicate that the incidence of pheochromocytoma increases progressively with age. In adults, no gender difference is seen in the incidence of pheochromocytoma.

About 90% of pheochromocytomas exist as solitary, unilateral, encapsulated adrenal medullary tumors. About 10% are bilateral, more commonly seen in several members of a family, ~40% to 70% of whose members may

have bilateral tumors. The tumors are vascular, and large ones often contain internal hemorrhagic or cystic areas. Reported sizes have ranged from less than 1 g to several kilograms; the average is about 40 g. About 10% of tumors are extra-adrenal (paragangliomas), and 90% of these are intra-abdominal, most commonly arising from chromaffin cells near the aortic bifurcation in the organ of Zuckerkandl or near the kidney. Other sites include the paravertebral sympathetic ganglia, the urinary bladder, other autonomic ganglia (celiac, superior, or inferior mesenteric), the thorax (including the posterior mediastinum, the heart, and para-cardiac regions), and the neck (in sympathetic ganglia, the carotid body, cranial nerves, or the glomus jugulare). Bilateral and extra-adrenal tumors are more common in children. Histologically, oval groups of cells, in clusters or "nests," stain for chromogranin A; a less frequently used stain identifies neuron-specific enolase. Fewer than 10% of the tumors are malignant; malignancy occurs more frequently in extra-adrenal tumors and is diagnosed by local invasion or distant metastases, but cannot be judged reliably from the histologic appearance. Local invasion commonly involves adjacent vascular structures such as the inferior vena cava. Distant metastatic sites include bone, lung, lymph nodes, and liver. Bilateral adrenal medullary hyperplasia has been reported in gene carriers from kindreds with multiple endocrine neoplasia (MEN) type 2. This hyperplasia may be a precursor of pheochromocytoma.

The "rule of 10s" is useful to recall approximate frequencies of pheochromocytoma that vary from the usual: ~10% bilateral, ~10% extra-adrenal, ~10% malignant, ~10% familial, ~10% pediatric, and ~10% without blood pressure elevation.

Etiology, heredity, and familial forms

Familial pheochromocytomas constitute up to 10% of the total and are more frequently bilateral, although less commonly malignant. A careful family history is essential, and relatives of patients with the familial syndromes should be screened for pheochromocytoma; biochemical screening is often not sufficient, and imaging studies are also recommended in this high-risk group.

Von Hippel-Lindau syndrome (VHLS) is an autosomal dominant disorder resulting from germline mutations at the VHL tumor suppressor locus on chromosome 3p25-p26. Its manifestations include pheochromocytoma (in about 14% of gene carriers), retinal angioma, cerebellar hemangioblastoma, renal cysts and carcinoma, pancreatic cysts, and epididymal cystadenoma.[3,4] Accordingly, all patients with pheochromocytoma deserve careful funduscopic examination. Pheochromocytoma occurs in type 2 VHLS, in which missense mutations (especially Arg238Trp or Arg238Gln) lie in a region of the VHL gene product that binds transcriptional elongation factors. Pheochromocytomas do not occur in type 1 VHLS, which is caused by deletion or premature termination (nonsense) VHL mutations.

MEN type 2A and type 2B (Sipple's syndrome) are autosomal dominant disorders arising from germline mutations on chromosome 10q11.2 in the RET proto-oncogene, which encodes a neurotrophin co-receptor tyrosine kinase. The features of MEN type 2A include pheochromocytoma (in about 40% of gene carriers), medullary thyroid carcinoma, and primary hyperparathyroidism (adenoma or hyperplasia). Because of this syndrome, it is wise to screen all pheochromocytoma patients for medullary thyroid carcinoma with serum calcitonin. MEN type 2B features include pheochromocytoma, medullary thyroid carcinoma, multiple mucosal neuromas (of the lips, tongue, buccal mucosa, eyelids, conjunctivae, corneas, and gastrointestinal tract), and a marfanoid body habitus (but without lens or aortic abnormalities). RET mutations in MEN 2A affect one of five Cys residues in the juxtamembrane extracellular domain, perhaps resulting in intermolecular disulfide formation and consequent constitutive activation of the kinase. The most common RET mutation in MEN 2B, Met981Thr, seems to alter the substrate specificity of the kinase.

The clinical presentation of pheochromocytoma may differ in MEN 2 versus VHLS: MEN 2 patients may be more symptomatic, have a higher incidence of hypertension, and higher plasma metanephrines, but lower plasma catecholamines than VHLS patients. Pheochromocytomas in VHLS patients exhibit a more noradrenergic phenotype characterized by selective increases in urinary and plasma normetanephrine and sometimes norepinephrine, whereas tumors in MEN 2 patients exhibit an adrenergic phenotype, characterized by additional and consistent increases in plasma and urinary metanephrine, sometimes associated with increases in epinephrine.

Hereditary neurofibromatosis (von Recklinghausen's disease), an autosomal dominant disorder resulting from mutations at the NF1 (neurofibromin) locus on chromosome 17q11.2, is manifested as neurofibromas and café au lait spots; about 1% of patients with neurofibromatosis have pheochromocytoma. Inactivating germline mutations at the SDHB (succinate dehydrogenase small subunit D) locus on chromosome 11q23 may also cause susceptibility to familial pheochromocytoma, as well as familial paragan-

glioma. Familial pheochromocytoma may also occur in isolation; whether such families represent disease processes etiologically distinct from von Hippel-Lindau syndrome or MEN is not clear.

In the 90% to 95% of pheochromocytomas that are sporadic, the cause of the neoplastic process remains obscure, although loss of heterozygosity on chromosomes 1p, 3p, 17p, and 22q suggests somatic cell deletion mutation of one autosomal allele at as-yet-uncharacterized tumor suppressor loci.

Because pheochromocytoma can be a curable form of hypertension, the diagnosis is important to consider in each new case of hypertension. However, because hypertension is so commonly encountered in clinical practice (>20% to 25% of the adult population) and pheochromocytoma is so distinctly unusual (<0.1% to 0.2% of patients with hypertension), laboratory evaluation should be selective, guided by the degree of clinical suspicion, and based on practical criteria outlined below (Box 72–1).

Clinical manifestations: symptoms and signs

Paroxysmal symptoms (such as the triad of episodic palpitations, diaphoresis, and headache) are the classic features of pheochromocytoma. These paroxysmal "attacks" characteristically begin abruptly, may last for minutes to hours, and subside gradually, with a frequency varying from many times daily to one or more per week (most commonly) or even every few months. Less common symptoms include apprehension or anxiety, tremulousness, pain in the chest or abdomen, weakness, or weight loss. In some series, more than 90% of patients have experienced paroxysmal symptoms of one or more of the classic triad. Autopsy series indicate that as many as 50% to 75% of pheochromocytomas may be undiagnosed during life, thus suggesting that many pheochromocytomas do not give rise to these classic symptomatic features. Patients older than 60 years with pheochromocytoma are especially likely to report minor or no symptoms.

Other features in the history may suggest pheochromocytoma. Affected patients may report an increase in blood pressure after receiving certain antihypertensive drugs, especially β-adrenergic antagonists and guanethidine, or they may experience a remarkable fall in blood pressure after receiving alpha$_1$-adrenergic antagonists such as prazosin. Hypertension in such patients is relatively refractory to medical management. A history of extreme blood pressure lability during intubation, surgery, or induction of general anesthesia also suggests possible pheochromocytoma. A family history of pheochromocytoma, von Hippel-Lindau syndrome, or MEN 2 should prompt an evaluation for pheochromocytoma. Paroxysmal symptoms on micturition or bladder distention, or painless gross hematuria may suggest pheochromocytoma of the bladder; the diagnosis is confirmed by cystoscopy.

Hypertension (usually severe and refractory to antihypertensive medications) is the cardinal sign of pheochromocytoma, although it is nonspecific and may be insensitive. In about half of patients, hypertension is sustained, with intermittent blood pressure surges in half or more

Box 72–1

Practical Diagnostic Approach to Pheochromocytoma

Clinical Clues or "Tipoffs"

- History
  Paroxysmal symptoms (classic triad is headache, diaphoresis, palpitations)
  History of extraordinarily labile or refractory hypertension
  Family history of pheochromocytoma, von Hippel-Lindau syndrome, or multiple endocrine neoplasia (MEN)
  Incidental adrenal abnormality on abdominal imaging test (rarely)
- Physical examination
  Labile, refractory hypertension
  Orthostatic hypotension
  von Hippel-Lindau syndrome, or multiple endocrine neoplasia–associated findings (retinal angiomas, thyroid enlargement, mucosal neuromas)

Biochemical Confirmation (only after clue or tipoff; begin with urinary tests)

- Urinary catecholamines and metabolites (24-hour sample or 2-hour sample after a paroxysm; metanephrines, the initial screening test)
- Plasma catecholamines (if urinary values are equivocal; take care to obtain a basal, resting sample)
- Clonidine suppression test (if plasma catecholamines are in the equivocal 1000 to 2000 pg/mL range)
- Plasma chromogranin A (storage vesicle protein released with catecholamines; also elevated by renal failure)

Anatomic Localization (only after biochemical confirmation)

- By morphology (most sensitive, less specific)
  Computed tomography (the imaging test most frequently obtained)
  Magnetic resonance imaging (may have advantages for extra-adrenal tumors)
- By function (most specific, less sensitive)
  Radiolabeled [131I]–MIBG scanning (accumulates in functioning chromaffin tissue)

From O'Connor DT. In: Bennett JC, Plum F, eds. *Cecil Textbook of Medicine.* 22nd ed. Philadelphia: WB Saunders, 2004:1419–24.

---

cytoma in hypertensives should be selective and focused on subjects who display some relevant clue to pheochromocytoma on history, physical examination, or screening laboratory evaluation. If interpretation of urinary measurements is not clear-cut, evaluation should proceed to plasma measurements, which require more careful sampling technique. The number and diversity of biochemical tests obtained should parallel the clinical index of suspicion. If suspicion is low, a single screening test may suffice, usually 24-hour urinary metanephrine excretion. If suspicion is high, multiple tests, including urine and plasma, are in order. Because anatomic or imaging studies may detect nonspecific adrenal abnormalities in up to 2% of the population, such studies should not be undertaken unless biochemical tests are positive.

Routine/Screening tests

Results of routine screening tests obtained for other purposes (such as general health maintenance) may provide tip-offs. Hyperglycemia is common, and about half of patients with pheochromocytoma manifest carbohydrate intolerance; frank diabetes requiring insulin is unusual. Lactic acidosis occurs rarely, even without shock. Serum lactate dehydrogenase activity may be elevated from adrenal isoenzyme 3.[5] Rarely, pheochromocytoma may be an incidental finding on computed tomography (CT) or magnetic resonance imaging (MRI) of the abdomen undertaken for other indications.

Urine biochemical tests

Widely available tests measure urinary free (unconjugated) catecholamines and catecholamine metabolites: the metanephrines and vanillylmandelic acid (VMA).[6] A 24-hour urine sample is collected, and creatinine is measured in the same sample as an index of adequacy and completeness of collection. Of the available urinary tests, increased fractionated metanephrines (separately measured normetanephrine and metanephrine) have the highest diagnostic sensitivity for pheochromocytoma. Normal test results for urinary fractionated metanephrines are therefore useful for excluding pheochromocytoma. Inadequate specificity makes it difficult to reliably confirm pheochromocytoma from an increased test result. Testing of urinary VMA is less sensitive than testing of metanephrines. Urinary excretion of metanephrines and VMA remains normal until the very end stage of renal disease, so elevated levels validly diagnose pheochromocytoma.

False-positive assay results have been greatly minimized in recent years with the introduction of more specific assay methods based on separation of catecholamines and metabolites in urine by high-pressure liquid chromatography. False-positive increases in free catecholamines may result from exogenous sources, such as catecholamines (which may be administered surreptitiously), alpha-methyldopa (but VMA excretion is characteristically normal), L-DOPA, labetalol, sympathomimetic amines (which release endogenous catecholamines from their stores), and fluorescent drugs such as tetracycline. Misleading elevations of endogenous catecholamines may occur as a consequence of the sympathoadrenal responses

---

of these; in about 40%, hypertension is paroxysmal, with relatively normal blood pressure between surges. Hypertensive surges may be precipitated by abdominal manipulation, but generally no antecedent is noted. The heart rate is usually elevated during blood pressure surges but may decline as a result of physiologic reflex bradycardia. Orthostatic hypotension is variably observed. As many as 15% to 20% of patients may have cholesterol gallstones.

Laboratory diagnosis

Because hypertension is common and pheochromocytoma so rare, further biochemical evaluation for pheochromo-

to shock, hypoglycemia, physical exertion, increased intracranial pressure, or withdrawal of central alpha$_2$-agonists such as clonidine. False-positive metanephrine elevations may result from excessive catecholamines (exogenous or endogenous) or the use of tricyclic antidepressants, MAO inhibitors, or propranolol (which interferes with the spectrophotometric assay). False-positive elevations in VMA may occur after ingesting carbidopa (a peripheral DOPA decarboxylase inhibitor) or MAO inhibitors.

Blood biochemical tests

Biochemical tests on blood samples offer the advantage of patient convenience but the disadvantage that even minor physical or mental stress can result in false-positive elevations. Plasma catecholamines are best sampled from a supine, resting patient in whom an indwelling antecubital venous cannula has been in place for at least 15 minutes. Plasma assay methods generally provide reliable results with the usual normal resting norepinephrine value being 200 to 400 pg/mL and the normal resting epinephrine value being 20 to 60 pg/mL. Most patients with pheochromocytoma have markedly elevated (>2000 pg/mL) resting plasma catecholamine (norepinephrine plus epinephrine) values; plasma concentrations elevated beyond this point strongly suggest pheochromocytoma. The upper limit of normal (norepinephrine plus epinephrine) is less than 1000 pg/mL. Values between 1000 and 2000 pg/mL are equivocal and may represent either pheochromocytoma or sympathoadrenal activation by physical or mental stress. In these subjects the clonidine suppression test discussed below is of particular value.

False-positive plasma catecholamine elevations may result from the same factors that produce false-positive urinary elevations but are a more severe problem because measurements are made at only one point. These factors include physical stress, such as trauma, surgery, upright posture, acute venipuncture, hypoglycemia, hypovolemia, hypotension, cold, and sodium depletion, or mental stress such as anxiety or pain. Drugs that increase plasma catecholamines include sympathomimetic amines, which release catecholamines from their stores; cocaine, which blocks catecholamine reuptake; and abrupt clonidine withdrawal. Illnesses known to elevate plasma catecholamines include both acute (e.g., myocardial infarction, diabetic ketoacidosis, or sepsis) and chronic conditions (e.g., congestive heart failure, anemia, respiratory failure, or hypothyroidism). Factors that diminish plasma catecholamines include drugs (clonidine, reserpine, and α-methylparatyrosine), autonomic neuropathy, and congenital deficiency of dopamine β-hydroxylase activity.

As with urine biochemical tests, plasma catecholamine sampling during a paroxysmal attack of hypertension is of value. A finding of normal plasma catecholamines when blood pressure is elevated is quite a useful negative result. Because only extreme elevations of plasma norepinephrine perturb blood pressure, the finding of normal plasma catecholamines while blood pressure is elevated argues strongly against pheochromocytoma as the cause.

Plasma metanephrine measurements are also highly sensitive and specific for diagnosis of pheochromocytoma,[2] although the measurements are not as widely available as plasma catecholamines. Other components of the catecholamine storage vesicle core are released into the blood stream by pheochromocytomas. The plasma concentration of chromogranin A is elevated in patients with pheochromocytoma, with a diagnostic sensitivity of 83% and specificity of 96%.[6] It is not substantially elevated by acute venipuncture, nor is it affected by drugs used in treatment or diagnosis of pheochromocytoma. Because chromogranin A is released by a variety of neuroendocrine secretory vesicles, its plasma concentration is also elevated in other neuroendocrine neoplasia.[7] Chromogranin A values are also elevated in renal insufficiency because of retained immunoreactive fragments of the protein.[8]

Pharmacologic tests for pheochromocytoma are generally not necessary because the diagnosis can usually be confirmed by urine and plasma biochemical measurements at rest or during spontaneous blood pressure surges. The clonidine suppression test is of value if plasma catecholamine elevations in a patient with suspected pheochromocytoma are equivocal (i.e., from 1000 to 2000 pg/mL). The rationale for the test is that pheochromocytoma chromaffin cells, unlike normal adrenal medullary chromaffin cells, are not innervated; hence catecholamine release from pheochromocytoma chromaffin cells is autonomous and not susceptible to manipulation by drugs that decrease efferent sympathetic outflow, such as the central α$_2$-agonist clonidine. Blood is obtained for plasma catecholamines before and 3 hours after a single oral dose of 0.3 mg clonidine. In a subject without pheochromocytoma, plasma norepinephrine should fall to less than 500 pg/mL after clonidine. A positive test (failure of catecholamines to decline after clonidine) is sensitive but may not be entirely specific for pheochromocytoma. Although catecholamine levels do not fall after clonidine administration in pheochromocytoma, the blood pressure fall is comparable to that seen in essential hypertensives. To prevent inordinate falls in blood pressure during the test, prior volume depletion should be avoided; the test is most safely done in subjects whose diastolic blood pressure before clonidine is 100 mmHg or higher. Because beta-blockers such as propranolol diminish circulating norepinephrine clearance (and hence plasma norepinephrine responses to clonidine), their use should be discontinued 48 hours before and during the test. The test remains valid during alpha-blockade.

Catecholamine provocative tests (such as the glucagon or tyramine tests) are used in only a few centers because of the potential hazard posed by inordinate catecholamine release.

Anatomical localization

Tumor localization allows for planning the proper surgical route. Ninety-five percent of pheochromocytomas are in the abdomen, and the great majority of these can be visualized by one of three modalities: CT, MRI, or [^{131}I]-metaiodobenzylguanidine (MIBG) scintigraphy. CT and MRI are highly sensitive, although nonspecific because they visualize any mass lesion, not just pheochromocytomas.

[^{131}I]-MIBG, a radiolabeled analogue of guanethidine, is transported into chromaffin cells by the reuptake cell membrane catecholamine carrier. Because it accumulates in chromaffin cells, an MIBG abnormality is extraordinarily specific (about 98%) for pheochromocytoma, although somewhat less sensitive (85% to 90%) than CT or MRI. [^{123}I]-MIBG is also used extensively outside the United States. MIBG imaging is especially useful for metastatic, recurrent, or extra-adrenal tumors. Abdominal ultrasonography is a safe imaging tool but is less sensitive than CT or MRI. Plain abdominal radiography, intravenous urography (pyelography), air insufflation retroperitoneal pneumography, arteriography, and venography are no longer done to localize pheochromocytoma. Indeed, arteriography or venography of the tumor may trigger hypertensive crises.

Differential diagnosis

Because many conditions can mimic the diagnostic features of pheochromocytoma, as many as 90% of patients who have some feature of the tumor turn out not to have one after diagnostic testing. Examples include certain drugs, such as surreptitiously self-administered epinephrine or isoproterenol. Abrupt withdrawal from clonidine can provoke a sympathoadrenal discharge with "rebound" blood pressure elevation. Subjects treated with MAO inhibitors for depression may have hypertensive crises if they inadvertently ingest foods rich in tyramine.

Disease states causing or simulating catecholamine excess and hypertension include thyrotoxicosis; acute intracranial disturbances such as subarachnoid hemorrhage or posterior fossa masses; hypertensive crisis of paraplegia, which can be initiated by visceral manipulation or bladder distention; and hypoglycemia, especially in the presence of beta-blockade. Damage to carotid sinus baroreceptors by surgery or tumor may result in baroreflex failure, with episodic blood pressure and plasma catecholamine surges; clonidine is the drug of choice.[9] Episodic surges in plasma dopamine have been described in some patients with episodic blood pressure elevation but without pheochromocytoma; the mechanism has not been established.[10] Some patients with symptomatic blood pressure surges have underlying unrecognized emotional trauma, which may respond to psychotherapy.

Pathophysiology and complications

Although circulating catecholamine excess is the ultimate cause of hypertension in pheochromocytoma, the correlation of blood pressure with plasma catecholamines is modest. Desensitization to catecholamine effects may contribute to underdiagnosis of the tumor in the elderly. In addition to catecholamines, pheochromocytomas also release a number of potentially vasoactive substances that may modify blood pressure. Hemodynamic studies suggest that elevations in systemic vascular resistance rather than cardiac output account for the blood pressure rise.

Acute norepinephrine infusion leads to plasma volume contraction, and a past mainstay of pheochromocytoma management has been an effort to re-expand plasma volume, either spontaneously after therapeutic α-blockade or with preoperative saline infusion. However, recent careful measurements of plasma volume indicate that on average it is not as contracted as once believed. Orthostatic hypotension is variably observed in pheochromocytoma. It cannot be clearly attributed to plasma volume contraction and probably reflects catecholamine desensitization, the effects of vasodilator peptides and catecholamines and dysautonomia.

The major catecholamine secreted by most pheochromocytomas is norepinephrine. Small intra-adrenal tumors (especially early in the course of MEN type 2) may secrete predominantly epinephrine. Pure epinephrine secretion by pheochromocytomas is rare.

Cardiomyopathy (myocarditis) occurs in a minority of patients with pheochromocytoma, presumably as a consequence of catecholamine excess. This process is generally reversible after tumor removal, and congestive heart failure responds to preoperative α-adrenergic blockade. In most patients, however, the degree of myocardial left ventricular hypertrophy on cardiac ultrasonography is no different from that seen in essential hypertension.

MANAGEMENT

Preoperative preparation and drug treatment

After diagnosis of pheochromocytoma, the patient is prepared for surgery with adrenergic blockade for a period of 1 to 4 weeks. During α-blockade, any catecholamine-induced plasma volume contraction is allowed to correct itself. α-blockade is usually accomplished with oral phenoxybenzamine, an irreversible, noncompetitive antagonist that acts predominantly (although not exclusively) at α_1-receptors. The drug is begun at 5 mg twice daily, and the dose is adjusted gradually upward by increments of 10 mg every 1 to 4 days to a maximum of 50 to 100 mg twice daily. The usual dose range required is 30 to 80 mg/day. Treatment goals are to normalize blood pressure (<160/<90 mmHg), prevent paroxysmal hypertension, and abolish tachyarrhythmias (ventricular extrasystoles, less than one to five per minute) without inducing intolerable orthostatic hypotension (i.e., orthostatic falls of >85/>45 mmHg). Side effects of an adequate phenoxybenzamine dosage include orthostatic hypotension, tachycardia, nasal congestion, dry mouth, diplopia, and ejaculatory dysfunction. In patients intolerant of phenoxybenzamine, one can use the α_1-selective antagonists doxazosin (at 2 to 8 mg orally once daily) or prazosin (at 0.5 to 16 mg/day, orally two to four times daily). Some authorities advocate the initial use of the newer, more selective alpha$_1$-selective antagonists (e.g., doxazosin) in preference to phenoxybenzamine, since phenoxybenzamine's alkylation of α-receptors may cause prolonged α-blockade contributing to postoperative hypotension, and its minor action on presynaptic α_2-receptors may contribute to increased sympathetic neuronal norepinephrine release, causing undesirable chronotropic and inotropic effects in the heart.

If blood pressure or tachyarrhythmias, including sinus tachycardia, are not fully controlled by α-blockade, beta-blockade is instituted with oral propranolol, 10 to 40 mg four times daily. Beta-blockade must not be undertaken before α-blockade has been instituted; after blockade of vasodilatory vascular beta$_2$-adrenergic receptors, catecholamines' continued access to vasoconstrictive α$_1$-receptors, may induce unopposed vasoconstriction and exacerbation of hypertension. Beta-blockade may be especially useful for predominantly epinephrine-secreting tumors. The more β$_1$-selective antagonists atenolol (50–100 mg/day) or metoprolol (50–200 mg/day), or the combined alpha/beta-antagonist labetalol (100–400 mg/day), are alternatives to propranolol, and are preferable in the view of some authorities. In subjects with contraindications to beta-blockade, lidocaine, or amiodarone can be used for tachyarrhythmias.

If combined management with α- plus β-adrenergic antagonists is not fully effective (especially in patients with widespread, unresectable malignant pheochromocytoma), the tyrosine hydroxylase inhibitor α-methylparatyrosine is added at an oral dose of 0.25 to 1.0 g four times daily. Its use may be complicated by sedation, fatigue, anxiety, diarrhea, or extrapyramidal reactions.

For acute management of severe hypertensive crises, intravenous nitroprusside is effective. Intravenous nonselective α$_1$/α$_2$-blockade with phentolamine (1 to 2 mg bolus, then by further incremental doses or continuous infusion) is also useful. If a pressor response is accompanied by tachycardia, the combined α- and β-adrenergic antagonist labetalol (intravenous 5-mg incremental doses) may also be useful. Calcium channel blockade with sublingual nifedipine (10 mg broken under the tongue) has also been used.

Opiates (narcotic analgesics), narcotic antagonists (such as naloxone), histamine, adrenocorticotropic hormone, saralasin, glucagon, or indirect sympathomimetic amines (such as phenylpropanolamine or tyramine) should be avoided. All of these agents may provoke hypertensive surges by releasing catecholamines from the tumor. Drugs that block catecholamine reuptake, such as tricyclic antidepressants (e.g., desipramine), cocaine, or guanethidine, may worsen hypertension. Beta-adrenergic antagonists, by blocking vasodilatory vascular β$_2$-receptors, may cause unopposed α-mediated vasoconstriction by circulating catecholamines and thereby result in severe hypertension, unless α-blockade is first instituted beforehand. Dopaminergic antagonists (such as metoclopramide or sulpiride) may result in hypertension, and should be avoided.

Operative and perioperative management

Autopsy series indicate that even clinically unsuspected cases of pheochromocytoma can be lethal. At least 90% of pheochromocytomas are benign, and surgical resection provides a cure, although up to 25% of patients may retain some lesser degree of hypertension. Residual tumor may be diagnosed by urinary catecholamine measurement 1 to 2 weeks postoperatively. The operative mortality of pheochromocytoma resection should not exceed 2% to 3%. Patients should be followed for at least 10 years postoperatively, because of the small (~5%) risk of late tumor recurrence. Perioperative complications were more frequent in patients with higher blood pressures, higher catecholamine/metabolite excretion, recurrent/multiple surgical excisions, or prolonged anesthesia. In malignant pheochromocytoma, the individual course is highly vari-

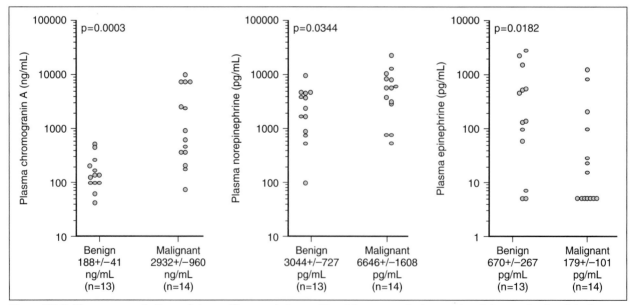

Figure 72–3. Plasma concentrations of chromaffin granule transmitters (chromogranin A, norepinephrine, and epinephrine) in subjects with pheochromocytoma (*n*=27 patients) stratified by tumor behavior, benign (*n*=13) versus malignant (*n*=14). Individual values are shown from samples obtained prior to treatment. Normal ranges: chromogranin A, 48.0 (SE) ±3.0 ng/mL; norepinephrine 200 ±7.8 pg/mL; epinephrine 18.0 ±1.5 pg/mL. The lower limit of detection for plasma epinephrine is 5 pg/mL. To convert chromogranin A from ng/mL to µg/L, multiply by 1.0. To convert epinephrine from pg/mL to pmol/L, multiply by 5.458. To convert norepinephrine from pg/mL to nmol/L, multiply by 0.005911. (From Rao F, Keiser HR, O'Connor DT. *Hypertension* 2000;36:1045–52.)

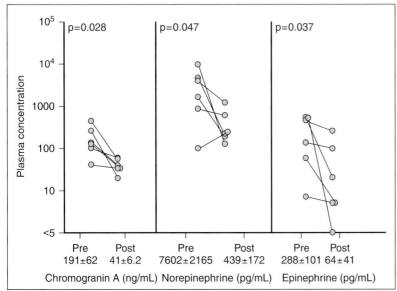

Figure 72–4. Response of chromaffin granule transmitter concentrations to successful surgical resection of benign adrenal pheochromocytoma (*n*=6 patients). Postoperative nadir values were analyzed (samples obtained at 4.1 ±2.0, [range 0.7–13.5] months after resection). Normal ranges: chromogranin A, 48.0 ±3.0 ng/mL; norepinephrine 200 ±7.8 pg/mL; epinephrine 18.0 ±1.5 pg/mL. Paired comparisons were made by the nonparametric Wilcoxon signed rank test. To convert chromogranin A from ng/mL to μg/L, multiply by 1.0. To convert epinephrine from pg/mL to pmol/L, multiply by 5.458. To convert norepinephrine from pg/mL to nmol/L, multiply by 0.005911. (From Rao F, Keiser HR, O'Connor DT. *Hypertension* 2000;36:1045–52.)

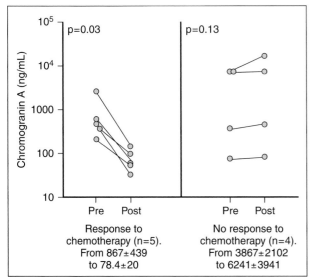

Figure 72–5. Changes in chromaffin granule transmitter (chromogranin A) concentrations in plasma after intravenous combination chemotherapy for malignant pheochromocytoma, stratified by response to chemotherapy: *n*=5 patients with response to chemotherapy versus *n*=4 patients with no response to chemotherapy. Postchemotherapy nadir values were analyzed (in the four nonresponders, samples obtained at 6.6 ±1.1 [range 4–9] months after initiation of treatment; in the five responders, samples obtained at 13.2 ±2.5 [range 6.5–22] months after initiation of treatment). Normal range: chromogranin A, 48.0 ±3.0 ng/mL. (From Rao F, Keiser HR, O'Connor DT. *Hypertension* 2000;36:1045–52.)

able, but long-term 50% survival is less than 5 years.

Several surgical approaches are feasible, depending on the particular characteristics of the pheochromocytoma; the experience of the surgeon is crucial. Laparoscopic adrenalectomy is increasingly used and may result in faster postoperative recovery. The entire adrenal gland harboring a pheochromocytoma is usually excised, but during excision of bilateral pheochromocytomas, a section of cortex from one adrenal gland may be left in place, to prevent steroid dependency. Anesthetic management is guided by selection of agents that do not cause catecholamine release or potentiate its dysrhythmic effects.[11] Intravenous glucose replacement (5% dextrose in water or saline) should be given to prevent hypoglycemia, a frequent occurrence after tumor removal. Times at which hypertensive surges are likely to occur include anesthetic induction, intubation, tumor palpation, and ligation of tumor veins. If intraoperative hypotension occurs, the initial treatment should be saline infusion to expand intravascular volume. Norepinephrine infusion is appropriate only after plasma volume expansion to euvolemia.

For intraoperative blood pressure surges, intravenous nitroprusside is often used. Alternatively, α-blockade can be accomplished with intravenous phentolamine (an α_1- and α_2-antagonist), starting with a 1- to 2-mg dose and proceeding to infusion. The calcium channel antagonist nicardipine has also been used.

In the postoperative period, the following problems occur with some frequency:

1. *Hypotension.* Most commonly, hypotension results from hypovolemia and responds to saline infusion; several liters may be required, often with the guidance of central pressure measurements. After volume repletion, norepinephrine can be infused if needed.

2. *Hypertension.* Plasma catecholamine levels may remain elevated for several days even after complete pheochromocytoma resection. Even 2 weeks postoperatively, up to one-fourth of patients still have hypertension. At this time the differential diagnosis includes residual unresected tumor, essential hypertension, or hypertension secondary to renal damage caused by prior hypertension. A urine collection for catecholamines, obtained at least 1 to 2 weeks after tumor resection, may clarify matters.

3. *Hypoglycemia.* After correction of catecholamine excess, insulin release may be increased and end-organ responsiveness to insulin augmented, resulting in hypoglycemia. Hypoglycemia may masquerade as refractory hypotension. Infusion of glucose (5% dextrose in water or saline) during the intraoperative and immediate postoperative period is useful.

Malignant pheochromocytoma

Although most pheochromocytomas are well-encapsulated, localized growths, approximately 5% to 10% are malignant. Malignancy is diagnosed by the biologic behavior of the tumor in the form of adjacent tissue invasion or distant metastatic spread. Extra-adrenal tumors are more likely to metastasize than are primary adrenal ones. Catecholamine biosynthesis tends to be especially deranged in malignant tumors, with secretion of substantial amounts of DOPA and dopamine (metabolized to homovanillic acid, which can be detected in the urine). Increased plasma DOPA in pheochromocytoma suggests malignancy. Extreme elevations in plasma norepinephrine or chromogranin A may suggest malignant pheochromocytoma; serial chromogranin A measurements can then be used to gauge tumor response to treatment.[12]

In patients with malignant pheochromocytoma, α- and β-adrenergic blockade with phenoxybenzamine and propranolol remains the mainstay of management of the symptoms and signs of catecholamine excess. If catecholamine effects are not controlled, the tyrosine hydroxylase inhibitor α-methylparatyrosine can be effective at 0.25 to 1.0 g four times daily.

Metastases tend to be slow-growing, and the natural history of malignant pheochromocytoma is variable; the 5-year survival rate is less than 50%. Common sites of metastasis are the retroperitoneum, skeleton (bone), lymph nodes, and liver. Periodic surgical debulking may help control symptoms. The response to chemotherapy has generally been disappointing, but the combination of vincristine, cyclophosphamide, and dacarbazine shows promise in many patients. Skeletal metastases show some response to irradiation, although the neoplasm is not particularly susceptible to radiation therapy. High-dose (~500 mCi cumulative dose) repeated radiation therapy with intravenous [131I]-MIBG remains experimental but is of value in some patients.

CHROMOGRANIN A IN PHEOCHROMOCYTOMA: DIAGNOSIS, TREATMENT, AND PROGNOSIS

Neurons and neuroendocrine cells contain membrane-delimited pools of peptide hormones, biogenic amines, and neurotransmitters with a characteristic electron-dense appearance on transmission electron microscopy (Figure 72–2). These vesicles, which are present throughout the neuroendocrine system and in a variety of neurons, store and release chromogranins and secretogranins (also known as "granins"), a unique group of acidic, soluble secretory

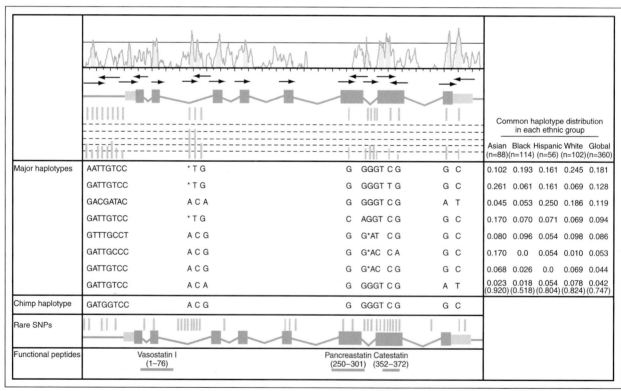

Figure 72–6. Resequencing strategy for the human chromogranin A gene, and identified variants. Conserved noncoding sequences between mouse and human chromogranin A were visualized with VISTA. Location of common (*upper*) and rare (*lower*) single nucleotide polymorphisms (SNPs) relative to exons and conserved noncoding sequences is indicated by position. *Red rods* represent nonsynonymous SNPs, and *black rods* represent synonymous SNPs. Nucleotides in red color in chimpanzee haplotype indicates the minor allele in the human sequence. Computationally reconstructed haplotypes are indicated along with their relative frequencies in ethnogeographic groups within our sample population. Nucleotide deletions in haplotype sequences are indicated by asterisk (*). (From Wen G, Mahata SK, Cadman PE, Mahata M, Ghosh S, Mahapatra NR, et al. *Am J Hum Genet* 2004;74:197–207.)

proteins.[7] The three "classic" granins are chromogranin A (CgA), which was first isolated from chromaffin cells of the adrenal medulla; chromogranin B, initially characterized in a rat pheochromocytoma cell line; and secretogranin II (sometimes called chromogranin C), which was originally described in the anterior pituitary. Because of their ubiquitous distribution in neuroendocrine and nervous-system tissues and their co-secretion with resident peptide hormones and biogenic amines, granins are valuable indicators of sympathoadrenal activity and clinically useful markers of secretion from normal and neoplastic neuroendocrine cells. Indeed, numerous studies have documented the clinical value of detecting granins in tissues and measuring circulating levels of granins, particularly chromogranin A. In addition to providing information about the neuroendocrine character of various neoplasms, measurement of chromogranin A has yielded insights into the pathogenesis of essential hypertension.

Several circulating granins are sensitive biomarkers for pheochromocytoma. Elevation of plasma CgA is used diagnostically in suspected pheochromocytoma, and in familial syndromes such as von Hippel-Lindau syndrome,[3,4] multiple endocrine neoplasia (MEN) type 2 (MEN2), and neurofibromatosis. In sporadic pheochromocytoma, elevation of plasma CgA concentration was 83% sensitive and 96% specific for the diagnosis, and CgA concentration correlated with tumor mass.[6] Drugs commonly used to diagnose or treat pheochromocytoma, such as phentolamine, tyramine, clonidine, and metoprolol, do not significantly alter serum CgA levels. Furthermore, unlike plasma epinephrine and norepinephrine, plasma CgA levels can distinguish between malignant and benign pheochromocytoma. In one study, CgA levels of 188 ±40.5 (SE) ng/mL signified benign disease while much higher levels of (2932 ±960 ng/mL) suggested malignancy.[12] Serum CgA may not provide adequate diagnostic

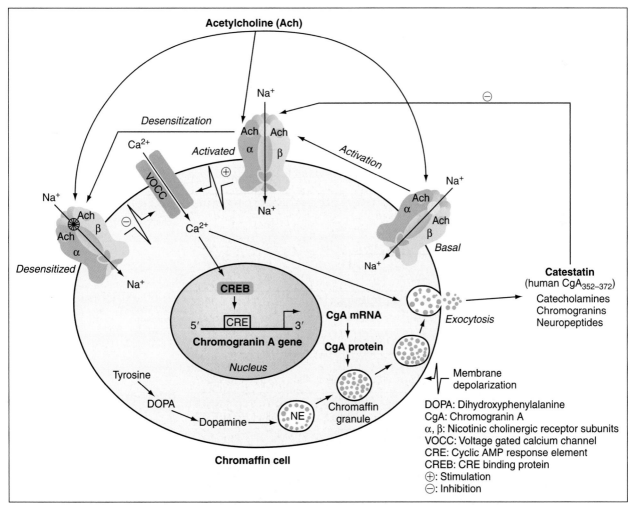

Figure 72–7. Autocrine negative feedback regulation of nicotinic cholinergic processes by catestatin variants. The diagram illustrates nicotinic cholinergic receptor activation in chromaffin cells by the endogenous agonist, acetylcholine (Ach), with subsequent mobilization of signal transduction (initially ligand-gated extracellular Na⁺ entry); then Ca²⁺ entry through voltage-operated calcium channels. Farther downstream, activation of secretion and transcription ("stimulus transcription coupling") is also illustrated. Agonist stimulation of nicotinic receptor activation (opening of the cation pore formed by the alpha and beta subunits), followed by receptor desensitization (closing of the cation pore) is depicted. Finally, the actions of catestatin, co-released by exocytosis with catecholamines, are shown on several nicotinic cholinergic processes: receptor activation, initial cationic signaling, subsequent signaling to secretion and transcription, and finally receptor desensitization. (From Mahata SK, Wen G, Mahapatra N, Mahata N, Hamilton BA, O'Connor DT. *Mol Pharmacol* 2004;66:1180–91.)

specificity for pheochromocytoma in patients with impaired renal function.[8,13,14] However, this limitation can be overcome by evaluating renal function in the patient,[8,13,14] and combining measurement of CgA with plasma catecholamines, which may provide lower diagnostic sensitivity, but improved specificity and positive predictive value.[14] In factitious pheochromocytoma, normal plasma CgA may be a valuable clue to the diagnosis.[15] Measurements of CgB and SgII may also be of diagnostic value in patients with suspected pheochromocytoma. Indeed, plasma CgB was elevated in 81% of patients,[16] and an increase of four- to five-fold for plasma secretoneurin was observed.[17]

Rao et al.[12] studied plasma concentrations of chromaffin granule transmitters (chromogranin A, norepinephrine, and epinephrine) in patients with pheochromocytoma ($n=27$), both benign ($n=13$) and malignant ($n=14$). Patients with benign pheochromocytoma were studied before and after surgical removal ($n=6$), while patients with malignant pheochromocytoma were evaluated before and after chemotherapy cycles of cyclophosphamide/dacarbazine/vincristine (nonrandomized trial in $n=9$).

In the diagnosis of pheochromocytoma (benign or malignant), Rao et al.[12] found a progressive rise ($p<0.0001$) in plasma chromogranin A, from control subjects (48.0 ± 3.0 SE ng/mL) to benign pheochromocytoma (188 ± 40.5 SE ng/mL) to malignant pheochromocytoma (2932 ± 960 SE ng/mL). Parallel changes were seen for plasma norepinephrine ($p<0.0001$). When stepwise linear regression was allowed to select the model, the independent variable best predicting the distinction of pheochromocytoma versus control was norepinephrine (multiple $R=0.417$, $R^2=0.174$, adjusted $R^2=0.149$, $T=2.67$, $F=7.14$, $p=0.011$).

Both plasma chromogranin A ($p=0.0003$) and norepinephrine ($p=0.0344$) were higher in malignant than benign pheochromocytoma (Figure 72–3), although plasma epinephrine was actually lower ($p=0.0182$) in malignant tumors. In a stepwise multivariate analysis, plasma chromogranin A elevation proved to be the most significant difference between benign and malignant tumors (adjusted $R^2=0.202$, $F=7.56$, $p=0.011$).

In the treatment of pheochromocytoma, Rao et al.[12] found that after surgical excision of benign pheochromocytomas, chromogranin A ($p=0.028$), norepinephrine ($p=0.047$), and epinephrine ($p=0.037$) all fell to values near normal (Figure 72–4). During chemotherapy of malignant pheochromocytoma ($n=9$) (Figure 72–5), plasma chromogranin A ($p=0.047$) and norepinephrine ($p=0.02$) fell, but not epinephrine. After chemotherapy, five clinical "responders" showed declines in chromogranin A (by ~91%, $p=0.03$) and norepinephrine (also by ~91%, $p=0.03$) but not epinephrine ($p=0.31$). By contrast,

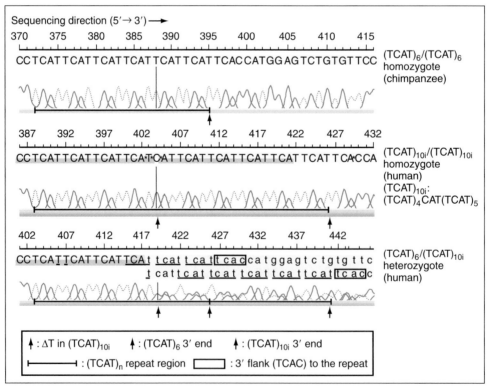

Figure 72–8. Determination of tyrosine hydroxylase (TCAT)$_n$ genotype by resequencing a 475-bp amplicon in tyrosine hydroxylase intron A from human genomic DNA. The ABI-3100 sequence trace data display window from PolyPhred is shown, along with the direction of sense-strand sequencing (5'◊3'). Results are shown for a (TCAT)$_6$/(TCAT)$_6$ homozygote, a (TCAT)$_{10i}$/(TCAT)$_{10i}$ heterozygote, and a (TCAT)$_6$/(TCAT)$_{10i}$ homozygote. (TCAT)$_{10i}$: (TCAT)$_4$CAT(TCAT)$_5$. Sequencing from the opposite (antisense) direction confirmed each genotype. (From Zhang L, Rao F, Wessel J, Kennedy BP, Rana BK, Taupenot L, et al. *Physiol Genomics* 2004;19:277–91. Used with permission.)

four "nonresponders" showed no significant decline in any of the transmitters (all $p=0.13$).

Rao et al.[12] concluded that plasma chromogranin A is an effective tool in the diagnosis of pheochromocytoma, and markedly elevated chromogranin A may point to malignant pheochromocytoma. During chemotherapy of malignant pheochromocytoma, chromogranin A can be used to gauge tumor response and relapse.

CATECHOLAMINE STORAGE AND RELEASE: COMMON HUMAN GENETIC VARIATION IN CHROMOGRANIN A

Chromogranin A (CgA) expression and activity have been proposed as "intermediate phenotypes" in human essential hypertension.[18] Family studies have shown substantial heritability of hypertension, yet the specific genes leading to chronic, pathologic increases in blood pressure remain poorly understood. Genetic analyses of complex traits such as hypertension are complemented by the use of intermediate phenotypes—simpler, often monogenic traits with earlier penetrance than the ultimate disease phenotype.[19] The CgA locus likely controls intermediate phenotypes that contribute to hypertension.[18] CgA is overexpressed in chromaffin cells of genetic (SHR, spontaneously hypertensive rat)[19,20] and acquired (renovas-

cular)[21] rodent models of human essential hypertension, and twin studies have shown significant heritability of circulating CgA in humans.[22] Furthermore, circulating levels of the CgA catestatin fragment, which inhibits nicotinic receptor-induced secretion of catecholamines,[23] are decreased in hypertensive patients as well as in normotensive patients at genetic risk (i.e., one or both parents have hypertension) of developing the disease.[18]

Wen et al.[24] studied the effect of sequence variation within the CgA gene to identify genetic variants that might quantitatively and/or qualitatively alter the protein and its bioactive peptide products. The investigators resequenced all eight exons and adjacent intronic regions, ~1.2 kilobases of the 5' promoter region, and two highly conserved intronic regions from 180 ethnically diverse human subjects living in urban southern California (San Diego). Wen et al.[24] identified 53 single nucleotide polymorphisms (SNPs) and 2 single-base insertion/deletions in the resequenced regions (Figure 72–6). Seventeen of the polymorphisms occurred in the coding region of the gene, while 11 of the 17 encoded amino acid substitutions. Three of these nonsynonymous coding SNPs—Gly364Ser, Pro370Leu, and Arg374Gln—were relatively uncommon (minor allele frequency 0.3% to 3.1%) variants of the catestatin region, where they appear the ability of the peptide to inhibit catecholamine secretion.

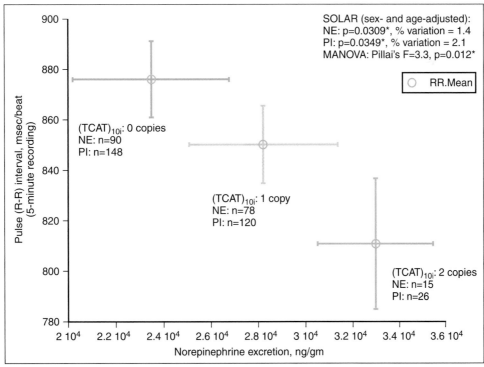

Figure 72–9. Tyrosine hydroxylase polymorphism: pleiotropy and phenotypic clusters. $(TCAT)_{10i}$ joint predictions of biochemical (renal norepinephrine excretion) and physiologic (pulse interval) phenotypes in twins. Clusters are displayed as mean value plus or minus one standard error of the mean for each trait, by generalized estimator equations. Joint prediction of two traits by one genotype was tested by multivariate analysis of variance (MANOVA), wherein the model contains one independent variable (genotype) and two dependent variables (biochemical and physiological). MANOVA: Pillai's trace F=3.30, $p=0.012$; Wilks' lambda F=3.38, $p=0.011$. Hotelling's trace F=3.46, $p=0.009$; Roy's largest root F=7.054, $p=0.001$. (From Zhang L, Rao F, Wessel J, Kennedy BP, Rana BK, Taupenot L, et al. *Physiol Genomics* 2004;19:277–91. Used with permission.)

The functional significance of individual SNPs on the expression of CgA and its peptide products was examined. One-way analysis of variance with Bonferroni correction for multiple comparisons identified three SNPs in the promoter region that were significantly associated with plasma CgA concentrations. These three SNPs were in absolute linkage disequilibrium with each other, thus indicating possible haplotype-specific effects. The authors tested the functional significance of inferred promoter haplotypes by placing the haplotypes upstream of a luciferase reporter and assaying expression in PC12 rat chromaffin cells. The promoter SNPs resolved into 6 relatively common haplotypes, each differing in the ability to promote transcription and regulate gene expression.

To determine the functional significance of amino acid substitution SNPs occurring in the catestatin peptide, the authors synthesized wild-type and variant synthetic peptides and assayed their potency for inhibition of nicotinic cholinergic-stimulated catecholamine release from PC12 chromaffin cells.[25] The two SNPs resulted in greater than 10-fold differences in the ability of catestatin to inhibit catecholamine release. Figure 72–7 summarizes the role of the catecholamine release-inhibitory peptide catestatin in sympathochromaffin function.

Thus genetic variation within the chromogranin A locus can quantitatively and qualitatively affect the protein and its bioactive peptide products, further supporting the role of CgA as an important contributor to and intermediate phenotype for hypertension.

CATECHOLAMINE BIOSYNTHESIS: COMMON FUNCTIONAL HUMAN GENETIC VARIATION IN RATE-LIMITING ENZYME TYROSINE HYDROXYLASE

Tyrosine hydroxylase (TH) is the rate-limiting enzyme in catecholamine biosynthesis.[26] Zhang et al.[27] employed the classic twin study design to probe the influence of tyrosine hydroxylase polymorphisms on autonomic traits. Previous studies have shown associations between the microsatellite tetranucleotide repeat $(TCAT)_n$ polymorphism within intron A of the human tyrosine hydroxylase gene, hypertension,[28] and blood pressure regulation. Zhang et al.[27] investigated the relationship between biochemical (catecholamine) and physiologic autonomic phenotypes, heritability estimates, and $(TCAT)_n$ genotypes within the twin population. The twin study consisted of 103 monozygotic (MZ) and 45 dizygotic (DZ) twin pairs of European ancestry (white) from urban southern California (San Diego). Thirty subjects were hypertensive while the remaining individuals were normotensive.

Biochemical and physiologic autonomic phenotypes measured included plasma and urinary catecholamines (norepinephrine and epinephrine), basal blood pressure, pulse interval (R-R interval or heart period, in milliseconds per beat), and blood pressure and pulse interval responses to cold stress (i.e., the "cold pressor test": immersion of one hand in ice water). Heritability for each of the autonomic phenotypes was determined and each subject was genotyped for the $(TCAT)_n$ microsatellite. Sequencing

revealed six alleles of the $(TCAT)_n$ microsatellite repeat, differing in number of consecutive TCAT repeats: $(TCAT)_6$, $(TCAT)_7$, $(TCAT)_8$, $(TCAT)_9$, $(TCAT)_{10}$, and the imperfect repeat $(TCAT)_4CAT(TCAT)_5$, also known as $(TCAT)_{10i}$. The two most common alleles observed were $(TCAT)_6$ and $(TCAT)_{10i}$ (Figure 72–8).

Biochemical phenotypes showed substantial heritability (h^2): plasma norepinephrine (NE) $h^2=55.3 \pm 8.0\%$, $p<0.0001$; plasma epinephrine (EPI) $h^2=61.4 \pm 9.8\%$, $p=0.0460$; urinary NE $h^2=32.5 \pm 9.6\%$, $p=0.001$; urinary EPI $h^2=47.1 \pm 8.8\%$, $p<0.0001$. Basal heart rate and basal blood pressure also showed significant heritability, with heart rate ($h^2=61 \pm 6\%$, $p<0.0001$) showing substantially more heritability than either systolic blood pressure (SBP) ($h^2=26\pm8\%$, $p=0.0016$) or diastolic blood pressure (DBP) ($h^2=18 \pm9\%$, $p=0.0359$). Cold stress–induced changes in heart rate (delta HR $h^2=36 \pm8\%$, $p<0.0001$) and blood pressure (delta SBP $h^2=23 \pm9\%$, $p=0.0098$; delta DBP $h^2=32 \pm8\%$) were also heritable. As positive controls, the heritability of weight ($h^2=87 \pm2\%$, $p<0.0001$) and height ($h^2=93 \pm1\%$, $p<0.0001$) were computed to verify the reliability of the heritability estimates.

Significant correlations between biochemical and physiologic traits with mechanistic implications for autonomic control of blood pressure were reported: (1) a positive correlation between renal NE excretion and resting SBP

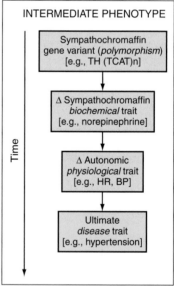

Figure 72–10. Tyrosine hydroxylase $(TCAT)_n$ polymorphism and "intermediate phenotypes" in the autonomic system. In the "intermediate phenotype" schema,[36] biochemical traits are postulated to be determined earlier and more proximately by genotype than are physiologic traits. Δ, change; BP, blood pressure; HR, heart rate; TH, tyrosine hydroxylase. (From Zhang L, Rao F, Wessel J, Kennedy BP, Rana BK, Taupenot L, et al. *Physiol Genomics* 2004; 19:277–91. Used with permission.)

(Pearson R=0.48, R^2=0.23, n=111, $p<10^{-7}$), and (2) a positive correlation between renal NE excretion and SBP increase in response to cold stress (R=0.30, R^2=0.09, n=112, p=0.001).

Zhang et al.[27] used a variance components method to determine the effect of variation of individual $(TCAT)_n$ microsatellite alleles on autonomic trait heritability. To maximize statistical power, the variance components analysis focused only on the most common alleles: $(TCAT)_6$ and $(TCAT)_{10i}$. An increase in $(TCAT)_6$ copy number (from 0 to 1 to 2 alleles) was associated with increased basal pulse interval (p=0.007), as well as basal (p=0.0003) and post–cold-stress (p=0.0001) heart rate. In contrast, an increase in $(TCAT)_{10i}$ copy number was associated with decreased pulse interval (p=0.0349), increased plasma epinephrine (p=0.0133), and increased renal NE excretion (p=0.0309). The $(TCAT)_6$ and $(TCAT)_{10i}$ alleles exerted directionally opposite effects on pulse interval.

The $(TCAT)_6/(TCAT)_6$ homozygous, $(TCAT)_6/(TCAT)_{10i}$ heterozygous, and $(TCAT)_{10i}/(TCAT)_{10i}$ homozygous diploid genotypes also exerted effects on autonomic phenotypes, specifically basal and post-stress heart rate. Within the diploid genotypes, the $(TCAT)_6$ allele exerted a dose-dependent direct effect on basal pulse interval and inverse effect on pre- and post-stress heart rate. Conversely, the $(TCAT)_{10i}$ allele displayed a dose-dependent inverse effect on basal pulse interval, and a direct effect on pre- and post-stress heart rate. Finally, Zhang et al.[27] suggested that the $(TCAT)_n$ polymorphisms of tyrosine hydroxylase exhibit pleiotropy (i.e., one gene influences multiple phenotypes), since $(TCAT)_{10i}$ allele copy number predicted both pulse interval (inverse relationship) and renal norepinephrine excretion (direct relationship) in a dose-dependent fashion (multivariate analysis of variance: Pillai F=3.30, p=0.012) (Figure 72–9).

TCAT allele frequencies also differed in subjects stratified by genetic risk of hypertension. Thus the catecholamine and stress physiologic traits may represent "intermediate phenotypes" in the pathway whereby common human genetic variation influences ultimate disease traits, such as hypertension (Figure 72–10).

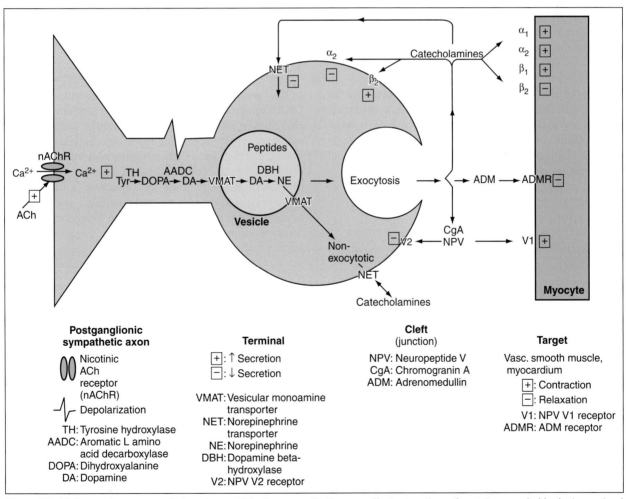

Figure 72–11. Pre- and post-synaptic locations, within the sympathetic neuroeffector junction, of proteins encoded by loci examined. The schematic neuron is illustrative of the functions of an efferent postganglionic sympathetic axon, innervating such cardiovascular targets as vascular smooth myocytes or cardiac myocytes. Note that the biosynthesis and vesicular uptake of catecholamines (although not soluble peptides) can take place throughout the neuron, even in the terminus. By contrast, vesicular soluble peptides (e.g., chromogranin A and neuropeptide Y) can only enter the vesicle as it buds off the Golgi apparatus in the cell soma. (From Chitbangonsyn SW, Mahboubi P, Walker D, Rana BK, Diggle KL, Timberlake DS, et al. *J Hum Hypertens* 2003;17:319–24.)

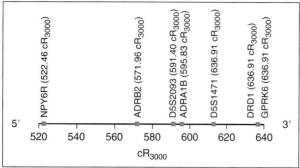

Figure 72–12. Chromosomal clusters of adrenergic candidate loci observed during radiation hybrid (RH) mapping: human chromosome 5q. The map units are cR3000, where one cR3000 corresponds to ~270 kbp. Chromosome 5q cluster in a region linked to systolic blood pressure. The microsatellite marker linked to systolic blood pressure variation in sibling pairs is D5S1471, while the microsatellite associated with systolic blood pressure variation is D5S2093. A neuroeffector candidate locus newly mapped by the RH technique to chromosome 5q is ADRA1B. Other locus positions are already in the public domain (www.ncbi.nlm.nih.gov/genome/guide/human). ADRA1B, alpha$_1$-adrenergic receptor; ADRB2, β$_2$-adrenergic receptor; DRD1, dopamine receptor isoform 1; GPRK6, G protein–coupled, receptor kinase isoform 6; NPY6R, neuropeptide Y receptor isoform 6 (pseudogene). (From Chitbangonsyn SW, Mahboubi P, Walker D, Rana BK, Diggle KL, Timberlake DS, et al. *J Hum Hypertens* 2003;17:319–24.)

Zhang et al.[27] thus presented compelling evidence for the role of allelic variation at the tyrosine hydroxylase locus in regulation of biochemical and physiologic autonomic phenotypes, with mechanistic implications for regulation of blood pressure and, ultimately, the development of hypertension.

SYMPATHETIC NEUROEFFECTOR JUNCTION GENOMICS

Allelic variation at multiple genetic loci may contribute to hypertension. Since autonomic or sympathetic dysfunction may play an early, pathogenic, heritable role in hypertension, we evaluated candidate loci likely to contribute to such dysfunction, including the components of the sympathetic neuroeffector junction (Figure 72–11): catecholamine biosynthetic enzymes, catecholamine transporters, neuropeptides, and adrenergic receptors.[29] Since chromosomal locations and physical map positions of many of these loci had not yet been identified, we used the GeneBridge4 human/hamster radiation (somatic cell) hybrid library panel (resolution ~1 to ~1.5 Mb), along with specifically designed oligonucleotide primers and PCR (200–400 bp products) to position these loci in the human genome. Primers were designed from sequences outside the coding regions (3'-flanking or intronic segments) to avoid cross-species (hamster) amplification. Chromosomal positions were assigned in cR (centi-Ray) units (~270 kbp/cR3000 for GeneBridge 4). A total of 13 loci were newly assigned chromosomal positions; of particular interest was a cluster of adrenergic candidate loci on chromosome 5q (including ADRB2, ADRA1A, DRD1, GPRK6, and the NPY6R pseudogene), a region harboring linkage peaks for blood pressure (Figure 72–12). Such physical map positions will enable more precise selection of polymorphic microsatellite and single nucleotide polymorphism markers at these loci, to aid in linkage and association studies of autonomic-sympathetic dysfunction in human hypertension.

SUMMARY

In the "postgenomic era," information on interindividual DNA sequence variation will become more readily available, and applicable to complex human traits such as systemic hypertension and other catecholaminergic disorders. Careful human phenotyping may be essential to understanding the consequences of genetic variants in the catecholaminergic pathway for autonomic function. Such study designs as the classical twin method[27] present many advantages for the elucidation of the hereditary basis of common human phenotypic variation. Coupling of such human study designs with increasingly powerful and rapid advances in genome technology[29] may ultimately provide a comprehensive picture of the role of the genome in determination of sympathochromaffin activity.

REFERENCES

1. O'Connor DT. Adrenal medulla, catecholamines and pheochromocytoma. In: Goldman L, Ausiello D, eds. *Cecil Textbook of Medicine*. 22nd ed. Philadelphia: WB Saunders, 2004:1419–24.
2. Eisenhofer G, Huynh T-T, Hiroi M, Pacak K. Understanding catecholamine metabolism as a guide to the biochemical diagnosis of pheochromocytoma. *Rev Endocr Metab Disord* 2001;2:297–311.
3. Hsiao RJ, Neumann HP, Parmer RJ, et al. Chromogranin A in familial pheochromocytoma: diagnostic screening value, prediction of tumor mass, and post-resection kinetics indicating two-compartment distribution. *Am J Med* 1990;88:607–13.
4. Neumann HP, Berger DP, Sigmund G, et al. Pheochromocytomas, multiple endocrine neoplasia type 2, and von Hippel-Lindau disease. *N Engl J Med* 1993;329:1531–8.
5. O'Connor DT, Gochman N. Lactic dehydrogenase activity in human pheochromocytoma. *JAMA* 1983;249:383–385.
6. Hsiao RJ, Parmer RJ, Takiyyuddin MA, O'Connor DT. Chromogranin A storage and secretion: sensitivity and specificity for the diagnosis of pheochromocytoma. *Medicine (Baltimore)* 1991;70:33–45.
7. Taupenot L, Harper KL, O'Connor DT. The chromogranin-secretogranin family. *N Engl J Med* 2003;348:1134–49.
8. Hsiao RJ, Mezger MS, O'Connor DT. Chromogranin A in uremia: progressive retention of immunoreactive fragments. *Kidney Int* 1990;37:955–64.
9. Robertson D, Hollister AS, Biaggioni I, et al. The diagnosis and treatment of baroreflex failure. *N Engl J Med* 1993(Nov 11);329(20):1449–55.
10. Kuchel O. Peripheral dopamine in hypertension and associated conditions. *J Hum Hypertens* 1999;9:605–15.
11. Prys-Roberts C. Phaeochromocytoma: recent progress in its management. *Br J Anaesth* 2000;85:44–57.

12. Rao F, Keiser HR, O'Connor DT. Malignant pheochromocytoma: chromaffin granule transmitters and response to treatment. *Hypertension* 2000;36:1045–1052.

13. O'Connor DT, Pandlan MR, Carlton E, et al. Rapid radioimmunoassay of circulating chromogranin A: in vitro stability, exploration of the neuroendocrine character of neoplasia, and assessment of the effects of organ failure. *Clin Chem* 1989;35:1631–7.

14. Canale MP, Bravo EL. Diagnostic specificity of serum chromogranin-A for pheochromocytoma in patients with renal dysfunction. *J Clin Endocrinol Metab* 1994;78:1139–44.

15. Kailasam MT, Parmer RJ, Stone RA, et al. Factitious pheochromocytoma: novel mimickry by Valsalva manuever and clues to diagnosis. *Am J Hypertens* 1995; 8:651–5.

16. Stridsberg M, Husebye ES. Chromogranin A and chromogranin B are sensitive circulating markers for phaeochromocytoma. *Eur J Endocrinol* 1997;136:67–73.

17. Ischia R, Gasser RW, Fischer-Colbrie R, et al. Levels and molecular properties of secretoneurin-immunoreactivity in the serum and urine of control and neuroendocrine tumor patients. *J Clin Endocrinol Metab* 2000;85:355–60.

18. O'Connor DT, Kailasam MT, Kennedy BP, et al. Early decline in the catecholamine release-inhibitory peptide catestatin in humans at genetic risk of hypertension. *J Hypertens* 2002;20(7):1335–45.

19. O'Connor DT, Takiyyuddin MA, Printz MP, et al. Catecholamine storage vesicle protein expression in genetic hypertension. *Blood Press* 1999;8(5–6): 285–95.

20. Schober M, Howe PR, Sperk G, et al. An increased pool of secretory hormones and peptides in adrenal medulla of stroke-prone spontaneously hypertensive rats. *Hypertension* 1989; 13(5):469–74.

21. Takiyyuddin MA, De Nicola L, Gabbai FB, et al. Catecholamine secretory vesicles. Augmented chromogranins and amines in secondary hypertension. *Hypertension* 1993;21(5):674–9.

22. Takiyyuddin MA, Parmer RJ, Kailasam MT, et al. Chromogranin A in human hypertension. Influence of heredity. *Hypertension* 1995;26(1):213–20.

23. Mahata SK, Mahata M, Wakade AR, O'Connor DT. Primary structure and function of the catecholamine release inhibitory peptide catestatin (chromogranin A(344–364)): identification of amino acid residues crucial for activity. *Mol Endocrinol* 2000;14(10):1525–35.

24. Wen G, Mahata SK, Cadman PE, et al. Both rare and common polymorphisms contribute functional variation at CHGA, a regulator of catecholamine physiology. *Am J Hum Genet* 2004;74:197–207.

25. Sushil K. Mahata SK, Wen G, et al. The catecholamine release-inhibitory "catestatin" fragment of chromogranin A: naturally occurring human variants with different potencies to affect chromaffin cell secretory responses. *Mol Pharmacol* 2004;66:1180–91.

26. Flatmark T. Catecholamine biosynthesis and physiological regulation in neuroendocrine cells. *Acta Physiol Scand* 2000;168:1–17.

27. Zhang L, Rao F, Wessel J, et al. Functional allelic heterogeneity and pleiotropy of a repeat polymorphism in the tyrosine hydroxylase locus: prediction of catecholamine secretion and cardiovascular response to stress in twins. *Physiol Genomics* 2004; 19:277–291.

28. Sharma P, Hingorani A, Jia H, et al. Positive association of tyrosine hydroxylase microsatellite marker to essential hypertension. *Hypertension* 1998;32(4):676–82.

29. Chitbangonsyn SW, Mahboubi P, Walker D, et al. Physical mapping of autonomic/sympathetic candidate genetic loci for hypertension in the human genome: a somatic cell radiation hybrid library approach. *J Hum Hypertens* 2003;17:319–24.

Chapter

73

Nonadrenal Endocrine Hypertension

J. Enrique Silva

Key Findings

- Thyroid dysfunction, hyperparathyroidism, and acromegaly are frequently associated with changes in systemic arterial blood pressure or overt hypertension.

- Thyroid hormone increases cardiac contractility and reduces systemic vascular resistance, which leads to increased cardiac output and pulse pressure. Hyperthyroidism is associated with increases in pulmonary arterial pressure, while there is little effect on mean systemic blood pressure.

- Hypothyroidism is frequently associated with increased mean blood pressure and reduced amplitude of pulse pressure.

- Primary hyperparathyroidism is frequently associated with increases in blood pressure. Elevated serum calcium, changes in intracellular calcium, increased 1,25-di-OH vitamin D, and the so-called parathyroid hypertensive factor are likely contributors.

- Given acutely, parathyroid hormone reduces blood pressure, but chronically leads to functional abnormalities, and with time, to vascular remodeling.

- Hypertension is frequently found in acromegaly, and cardiovascular disease is the main cause of mortality in these patients.

- Because of the progression from functional abnormalities to tissue remodeling, particularly in primary hyperparathyroidism and acromegaly, these conditions should be diagnosed early and treated promptly.

Systemic arterial hypertension is a central manifestation of endocrine diseases involving hypersecretion of the adrenal cortex, adrenal medulla, or extra-adrenal chromaffin tissues. These conditions are discussed in other chapters in Section 3 of this volume. However, hormones from other glands have important hemodynamic effects or may affect vascular biology; hence, diseases disrupting their hormones frequently have an impact on hemodynamics and blood pressure (BP). Among these conditions, thyroid dysfunction, hyperparathyroidism, and acromegaly are frequently associated with changes in systemic arterial BP or overt hypertension.

HYPERTENSION AND THYROID DYSFUNCTION

The biological effects of thyroidal secretion, called thyroid hormone (TH) here (calcitonin is not included in this

discussion), are for the most part mediated by triiodothyronine (T_3), although the major product of thyroidal secretion is thyroxine (T_4). T_3 is about 10 times more active than T_4 and more than 80% of T_3 is produced outside the thyroid in humans from 5'deiodination of T_4.[1] The effects of TH are largely the result of modifying the transcription of specific genes by T_3, which is mediated by nuclear TH receptors (TRs). These are ligand-activated transcription factors that, upon binding T_3 (or T_4, or a suitable analog), will recruit to the regulatory elements of those genes other transcription factors that will ultimately modify their transcription by RNA polymerase II (see Bassett et al.[2] for review). TRs are the product of two genes, TRα and TRβ, which generate various products by alternate splicing or from the use of diverse promoters. Only TRα1, TRβ1, TRβ2, and TRβ3 are *bona fide* receptors in that they can both bind TH and mediate effects of TH on the transcription of specific genes.[2] TRs are ubiquitously distributed, indicating that most tissues are, or can be, directly affected by TH. Given the ubiquitous presence of TRs, TH can affect tissues directly as well as indirectly, that is, as a consequence of its effects in other tissues or as part of homeostatic responses to effects in the body. Thus, TH increases oxygen consumption in all tissues (except the brain, spleen, and testes[3]), resulting in augmented oxygen demands and more heat production, thereby creating the need to increase cardiac output and heat dissipation.

Thyroid hormone effects on cardiovascular system and hemodynamics

The cardiovascular effects of TH are quite prominent and dramatic, and have been recognized by clinicians since the early descriptions of thyrotoxicosis by Parry et al. in the 19th century (see Kahaly and Dillmann[4] and references). It has long been known that myocardial contractility is increased by TH continuously from the hypothyroid to hyperthyroid state.[5] Such effect is the result of the modified expression of several genes. Among others, TH stimulates the expression of myosin heavy-chain alpha (MHCα), while it inhibits the expression of MHCβ, and also stimulates the expression of sarco-endoplasmic reticulum, calcium-dependent ATPase 2 (SERCA2). These changes largely account for the increased velocity and force of contraction and accelerated relaxation seen in response to TH. Thus, MHCα is catalytically more efficient than MHCβ, which explains faster contraction, whereas the increase in SERCA2 explains a greater release of sarcoplasmic calcium during systole, increasing the force of contraction and a faster reuptake during diastole that accelerates relaxation.[4] These effects may be enhanced by a concomitant decrease in the expression of phospholamban and increase in ryanodine channels, causing less inhibition of SERCA2 and increased calcium flux into the cytosol during systole, respectively. TH also has a direct chronotropic effect, as well as increasing the rates of depolarization and repolarization, and shortening the duration of the action potential in the sinoatrial node. These effects are mediated by T_3-dependent acceleration of the ion currents in the sinoatrial node and the conduction system, and result from increases in Na+ pump density and enhancement of Na+ and K+ permeability, as well as stimulation of the ID L-type Ca channels, which also serve important pacemaker functions.[6]

All of these effects are believed to result from the direct action of T_3 on the expression of specific genes, which are independent from effects on sympathetic activity and responsiveness (discussed below). TRs are present in the heart[7] and in blood vessels.[8,9] Both TRα and TRβ are expressed in the heart, with TRα1 being the predominant receptor.[10] Mice with deletion of this receptor have lower heart rates, yet the rate responds normally to adrenergic stimulation,[11,12] whereas the role of TRβ is less well characterized but evidenced by the fact that mice devoid of both receptor isoforms have an even lower heart rate than the TRα-deficient model.[13] However compelling the evidence that TH directly affect genes concerned with heart contractility, TH response elements (TREs) have been so far identified and characterized only in the MHCα and β genes and the SERCA2 gene (reviewed by Kahaly and Dillmann[4]).

In addition to its direct effects on the heart, TH affects myocardial function via increasing its responsiveness to adrenergic stimulation. The density of β-adrenergic receptors (β-AR) in the heart is increased in the hyperthyroid state,[14] which is known now to reflect an increase in $β_1$-AR gene transcription mediated by a TRE.[15] However, it is very likely that the increased $β_1$-AR receptor density is not the main factor in the enhanced responsiveness. Indeed, TH also stimulates the adrenergic pathways at post-receptor levels, increasing Gs protein and reducing Gi α and β,[16] enhancing the cAMP responses to a much higher level than expected from about double of the $β_1$-AR number.

Altogether, the direct effects of TH on the myocardium and the TH-mediated increase in responsiveness to catecholamines converge to increase cardiac output and circulatory velocity. The more rapid and energetic contraction causes the systolic BP to increase faster and to higher levels. In addition, TH markedly reduces systemic vascular resistance (SVR) and increases blood volume.[17] SVR is three to four times lower in the hyperthyroid than in the hypothyroid state, with intermediate values in the euthyroid condition, and together with the expanded blood volume, the reduced SVR importantly contributes to the augmented cardiac output of hyperthyroid states. The reduced SVR also causes a rapid reduction in intra-arterial pressure after the systolic peak and this is usually associated with reduced diastolic BP. Typically, hyperthyroid patients have modestly elevated systolic pressure (140 to 150 mmHg)

with reduced diastolic pressure (50 to 70 mmHg), and greater amplitude of pulse pressure even at high heart rates.

It is not entirely clear how TH causes a reduction in SVR. A major factor could be enhanced responsiveness of vascular smooth muscle to $β_2$-AR–mediated effects of catecholamines. This is supported by the marked increase in SVR caused by propranolol, a nonselective $β_1$-$β_2$–AR blocker,[18] compared with the modest effect of the selective $β_1$-AR agent, bisoprolol.[19] In addition, T_3 can directly relax vascular smooth muscle in vitro,[20] although the physiologic significance of this mechanism is to be demonstrated. Yet another possible contributing mechanism is augmented production of nitric oxide,[21] but again, the significance of this finding in human physiology and disease has not been established.

Clinically, the hyperdynamic state of thyrotoxicosis is characterized, subjectively, by palpitations, felt as forceful, rapid "pounding" on the chest, and objectively, by tachycardia, hyperdynamic precordium, increased pulse pressure, and usually modestly elevated systolic pressure with normal or modestly reduced diastolic BP, and normal or modestly increased mean arterial blood pressure. The skin is warm and well perfused, with rapid capillary filling. In otherwise normal individuals, the thyrotoxic hyperdynamic state is usually of no consequence. The judicious use of β-AR blockers ameliorates the clinical translation of this state and is objectively associated with a significant reduction of heart rate and less so of systolic BP, while diastolic blood pressure may increase modestly and pulse amplitude is reduced. Except in individuals with pre-existing hypertension, in whom BP may become harder to control, arterial hypertension is generally not a clinical problem in hyperthyroid patients. Systolic BP rarely surpasses 150 mmHg, and generally can be reduced, along with the hyperdynamic circulation, by modest doses of β-AR blocking agents. No additional treatment is necessary. In patients with pre-existing hypertension, this may worsen, which is caused by the hyperdynamic state and the reduced effectiveness of antihypertensive drugs owing to stimulation by TH of drug clearance, angiotensinogen-converting enzyme and sympathetic activity. However, it is rarely necessary to adjust the treatment, sufficing to give, or increase the dose of, β-AR antagonists and treat rapidly the thyrotoxic state (Figure 73–1A).

Pulmonary hypertension has been reported in hyperthyroidism with increasing frequency[22-24] (Figure 73–1B). It seems to be more frequent in women than in men. It is likely that the pulmonary vascular bed is less compliant than the systemic arterial bed, and cannot accommodate the increased cardiac output as the systemic bed does. Indeed, experimental hyperthyroidism is associated with greater right than left ventricular hypertrophy.[25] The frequency of pulmonary hypertension is likely underestimated, and will be better appreciated as more Doppler studies are done. In one study, 9 of 17 untreated patients with Graves disease had elevated pulmonary arterial pressure, with an average or mean of 29 mmHg,[22] whereas another study found 41% of patients with systolic pulmonary pressures higher than 35 mmHg.[23] The thyrotoxic

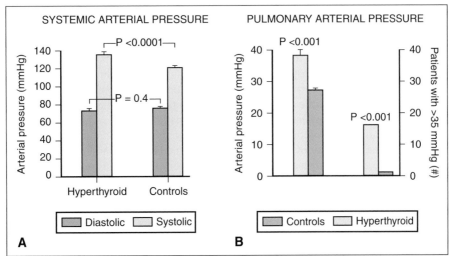

Figure 73–1. Changes in systemic and pulmonary arterial pressures in patients with thyrotoxicosis. Values are means (± standard error of the mean) of 39 cases and 39 matched euthyroid controls. **A,** Systolic and diastolic systemic blood pressures. In this study, diastolic blood pressure was not significantly reduced in the hyperthyroid patients. **B,** Systolic pulmonary hypertension in the same cohort of patients. The right axis shows the number of cases with systolic blood pressures greater than 35 mmHg, which included 16 in the hyperthyroid group and only 1 among the controls. (Data from Merce J, Ferras S, Oltra C, Sanz E, Vendrell J, Simon I, et al. *Am J Med* 2005;118:126–31.)

pulmonary hypertension is reversible with treatment, especially since it is related to the thyroid status, specifically the thyrotoxic state[22–24]; however, its clinical impact is to be defined. It is expected that patients with pre-existing secondary or primary pulmonary hypertension have a significant worsening of their condition if they become thyrotoxic, possibly with development of overt right-sided congestive heart failure, requiring aggressive treatment of the hyperthyroid state.

Effects of hypothyroidism on sympathetic activity, vascular physiology, and blood pressure

The hemodynamic effects of hypothyroidism are essentially the opposite of those described for hyperthyroidism. Myocardial contraction is slower and less energetic, and diastolic relaxation is delayed. Cardiac output is reduced and SVR is increased as much as 70%.[4,17] Clinical findings include bradycardia and reduced skin perfusion and pulse amplitude. Frequently, hypothyroidism is considered a cause of hypertension, but the reported prevalence of hypertension among hypothyroid patients is highly variable.[26–29] Nonetheless, the majority of longitudinal studies of patients with chronic hypothyroidism show modest increases in systolic and, more consistently, in diastolic BP that disappear upon treatment with T_4 (see Fletcher and Weetman[26]). Hypothyroid patients sometimes have unequivocal hypertension that reverts with correction of the hypothyroid status.[28,30,31] Interestingly, among nearly 700 patients with newly diagnosed hypertension, 3.6% had previously unrecognized hypothyroidism.[28]

The mechanisms leading to hypertension in hypothyroidism are probably multiple. The increase in SVR plays

a central role, and whether it leads to frank hypertension may depend on the magnitude of the increase and the participation of other factors and mechanisms. Increased SVR is caused by the lack of TH both locally at the blood vessel level, and indirectly by the enhancing effect on sympathetic activity due to hormone absence. In addition, the lack of TH could conceivably result in changes in the concentration or activity of other factors regulating the tone and lumen of resistance vessels. Chronic hypothyroidism is associated with increased circulating levels of norepinephrine.[32–34] Furthermore, sympathetic activity in muscle is increased,[35] and its vascular bed is a major determinant of SVR. Enhanced sympathetic stimulation, however, is not the only factor. The number and proportion of β-AR and α-AR in the vasculature seem also to play a significant role. The number of β_2-AR, which are involved in vasodilatation in important vascular beds, such as muscle, is reduced, whereas that of α1-AR is increased.[36] Interestingly, the pressor response to exogenous norepinephrine is reduced in muscle,[37] which is possibly due to desensitization caused by the tonic increase in sympathetic activity. The presence of TRs in vascular smooth muscle cells[20] is an indication that these cells have at least the potential to respond directly to TH. Little is known, however, as to what genes are affected by TH. It has been recently found that T_3 reduces the expression of type-1 angiotensin II receptors in vascular muscle cells[38] at the transcriptional and post-transcriptional level. T_3 also induces relaxation of vascular smooth muscle cells *in vitro*, which is believed to be a nongenomic effect of TH.[20] Additional evidence indicating a direct effect of TH in blood vessels is the presence in vascular smooth muscle cells of type-2 T_4 5'deiodinase (D2), which catalyzes the conversion of T_4 into the 10-fold more active T_3.[39,40]

The experimental observations mentioned here suggest that vascular tone and BP are more sensitive to TH than one would anticipate from past observations in individuals with overt, long-term hypothyroidism. Indeed, relationships between BP and TH homeostasis are demonstrable even in euthyroid individuals as well as in short-term hypothyroidism. Thus, in hypertensive individuals, the serum-free T_4 index and TSH are lower and higher, respectively, than in appropriately matched controls.[41] Moreover, serum FT_4I is inversely correlated to the sensitivity of BP to salt, and both TSH and FT_4I are directly and inversely related, respectively, to renal vascular resistance.[41] In a study of short-term hypothyroidism, normotensive subjects with stage 1 of differentiated thyroid cancer maintained on L-T_4 were studied 6 weeks after withdrawal of the hormone (in preparation for whole-body scanning with ^{131}I) and then 2 months after resuming treatment. There was a modest but significant increase of both systolic and diastolic pressures during the hypothyroid phase. This was associated with a nearly twofold increase of norepinephrine and epinephrine, and the daytime diastolic BP was inversely related to the T_3 levels during the replacement with L-T_4.[42]

Altogether, these studies suggest that vascular tone is highly dependent on TH via direct as well as indirect effects such as increased sympathetic tone. Such influences are reversible but, if prolonged and severe, they may lead to irreversible remodeling of the vasculature. Such conceptualization is supported by more recent and detailed studies. One such study reports increased SVR and aortic stiffness in patients with hypothyroidism, which were significantly greater in those who were also hypertensive.[30] In about 50% of the hypothyroid patients with hypertension, the treatment with LT$_4$ was associated with a normalization of BP and a significant reduction of SVR and aortic stiffness, whereas these latter changes did not occur or were less pronounced in the other half with persistent hypertension after euthyroidism was achieved.[30] When all patients were pooled, the reduction in systolic BP was significantly correlated to the reduction in aortic stiffness (r=0.83, $p<0.001$).[30] Reasons for the normalization of BP with LT$_4$ treatment in only half of the hypothyroid patients are not clear, but certainly the difference was not due to the degree of hypothyroidism because there were no differences in TSH, FT$_4$, or FT$_3$ between responders and nonresponders. The nonresponsive group had greater SVR and aortic stiffness, suggesting a more pronounced change in vasculature, but whether this was related to duration of the hypothyroidism or the presence of other factors is not readily evident.[30]

Systemic arterial hypertension is rarely a clinical challenge in hypothyroidism. Besides, with the availability of inexpensive and accurate TSH assays, severe, protracted hypothyroidism is currently less frequently seen. From a practical point of view, hypothyroidism should be considered in a patient with newly diagnosed hypertension, whereas hypothyroid patients with hypertension, particularly if moderate, should not be rushed into extensive investigation or treatment without correcting the hypothyroidism.

HYPERTENSION IN PRIMARY HYPERPARATHYROIDISM

Numerous studies show that systemic arterial hypertension is more frequent in patients with primary hyperparathyroidism (PHP) than in the appropriately matched general population.[43–46] A number of vascular abnormalities have been reported in patients with PHP, some of which may play a pathogenic role while others may be consequence of vascular stress. PHP patients have endothelial dysfunction as revealed by impaired flow-mediated dilation of medium-size arteries,[47] which is reversible after successful parathyroidectomy.[48] However, the mechanical properties of the arteries such as isobaric distensibility, pulse wave velocity, and intima media thickness, were not altered by recent-onset PHP, nor were they modified by parathyroidectomy in patients with PHP without hypertension or kidney involvement or any other known vascular risk factor such as diabetes or hypercholesterolemia.[49]

More recently, a study showed increased arterial stiffness in mild PHP.[50] The authors used the augmentation index (AI) as a measure of stiffness. The AI basically represents the increase in systolic pressure due to the reflection of the initial pressure wave caused by the ventricular ejection, the timing and magnitude of which are functions of artery compliance. When corrected by all confounding variables, PHP was a stronger predictor of elevated AI than age, gender, smoking, hypertension, hyperlipidemia, or diabetes, and AI correlated significantly with the levels of PTH and inversely with radius mineral density, used in the study as a cumulative effect of PTH.[50] The discrepancy between these two reports[49,50] is probably explained by age and length of the disease, as in the latter[50] patients were significantly older and had been hyperparathyroid for longer time periods than in the aforementioned study.[49] Altogether, these results suggest that PHP is associated with functional abnormalities of blood vessels that lead to hypertension, but vascular remodeling takes time and probably requires the contribution of other factors. Compensatory mechanisms may be one such factor and a source of variability in the timing and magnitude of the elevation of blood pressure in PHP. For example, patients with PHP have higher levels of adrenomedullin, a vasodilator, and while mean levels are higher among those that are hypertensive, not all hypertensive patients with PHP have high adrenomedullin.[51]

The mechanisms leading to vascular changes and hypertension in PHP have been only partially identified and are not yet well characterized. Acute injections of parathyroid hormone (PTH) itself cause hypotension in a dose-dependent manner in several species, but most prominently in dogs.[52] PTH-related peptide (PTHrP), acting on the same receptors, also has a clear vasodilating effect.[53] Furthermore, these hormones cause substantial reduction of intracellular calcium in vascular smooth muscle,[54,55] although in some instances a transient increase has been reported.[56] PTH receptors have been identified in endothelial cells.[57,58] Another potential mechanism mediating an acute vasodilating response is a reduction of endothelin-1, because this is sensitive to inhibition by PTHrP acting presumably via the PTH receptor.[59]

How then to explain the higher frequency of hypertension in patients with PHP? As mentioned above, in spite of the acute vasodilating effects of PTH, there is an impaired dilation response to increase flow that is reversible with parathyroidectomy.[47,48] There are several possible mechanisms to explain the hypertension and impaired dilation responses. One is obviously hypercalcemia, whether general or limited to a vascular territory (i.e., forearm), has been associated with impaired endothelial vasodilatory function, and when systemic, with a significant increase in blood pressure.[60] It has been found that intracellular calcium is increased in platelets of patients with PHP, in proportion to the increase in serum Ca and PTH. Interestingly, platelet Ca is increased and more than in PHP in patients with essential hypertension, which lends support to the use of platelets as surrogates for vascular smooth muscle. In PHP, platelet Ca normalized promptly following parathyroidectomy.[61] Another interesting factor is that hypercalcemic states, PHP included, are associated with increased levels of norepinephrine and, most importantly, increased pressor response to exogenous norepinephrine.[62]

In addition to the effects of PTH on blood vessels, several lines of evidence point to effects on myocardial contractility. One study showed no effect of acutely injected PTH on myocardial contractility, but in patients with PHP there were changes suggesting increased heart sympathetic activity such as shortening of the relaxation and loss of circadian variation of heart rate.[63] Two other studies showed increased ejection fraction (EF) and cardiac output in patients with PHP that were at least partially reversible with parathyroidectomy.[64,65] Finally, other investigations have shown left ventricular hypertrophy, above and beyond the expected from the hypertension.[66,67] Thus, it appears that increased cardiac output, which is, at least in part, adrenergically mediated, could contribute to the hypertension seen in patients with PHP.

Finally, parathyroid hypertensive factor (PHF) is also a contributing factor. PHF was discovered in the circulation of spontaneously hypertensive rats (SHR). Injected into normotensive rats, PHF causes a delayed (60 to 90 min) increase in arterial BP (see Pang et al.[68] for a review). Subsequent studies in animals and then in isolated parathyroid cells or tissues showed that the source of this factor was the parathyroid glands.[69,70] The chemical structure has not yet been completely defined, but is believed to be a peptide linked to a phospholipid.[69,71,72] About 30% to 40% of patients with hypertension have elevated PHF, most notably those exhibiting a low-renin, salt-sensitive form of hypertension, in whom PHF correlates well with BP.[73] The PHF mechanism of action was shown to rely mainly on the opening of L-type calcium channels in vascular smooth muscle cells with an increase in intracellular Ca^{2+} and possibly sensitization to norepinephrine and perhaps other hypertensive factors.[74] It is possible that PHF is responsible for the hypertension in a substantial portion of patients with PHP. In 9 of 10 of these patients with hypertension, PHF was elevated and its elevation predicted a BP reduction following parathyroidectomy.[75]

It is also very interesting that circulating Ca^{2+} regulates PHF, and its secretion can be reduced by substances acting on the parathyroid calcium sensor receptor,[76] whereas 1,25-di-OH vitamin D3 stimulates its secretion, and more in SHR than in their normotensive cognates.[77] These are interesting observations that have the potential to explain clinical observations such as the beneficial effect of calcium supplementation in the management of hypertension.[78] Elevation of PTH in hyperparathyroidism might contribute to hypertension via increasing the synthesis of 1,25-di-OH vitamin D3 by the kidney, which will in turn increase the secretion of PHF.

Although several studies have reported BP normalization in significant fractions of the PHP cohorts studied,[44–46] others have failed to document a significant reduction in BP following successful surgical treatment of the PHP.[79–81] It is likely that discrepancies derive from differences in the populations studied and in the endpoints of the studies. In two of these studies, the hypertensive patients had more severe disease with greater kidney damage[80,81] than the normotensive patients, suggesting that they had moved into a phase of irreversibility due to end-organ damage. The third study compared blood pressure longtime after the surgery (15 years) with that existing prior to parathyroidectomy in a cohort with a mean age of 58, and during this period many patients became hypertensive, regardless of treatment and calcium status.[79] In general, these three studies[79–81] aimed at assessing the long-term cardiovascular risk of not surgically treating the primary hyperparathyroidism. However, in another large cohort study in Denmark that compared patients surgically treated with those kept under observation, the authors observed no difference in the prevalence of hypertension, but mortality during the follow-up occurred in 31% of surgically treated patients compared to 37% of conservatively treated patients (Figure 73–2).[82] There are limits to this study. First, the overall frequency of hypertension in both groups was very low, 4% to 5%, but more important was the bias that

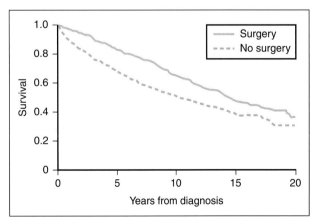

Figure 73–2. Kaplan-Meier plot of survival in surgically and conservatively treated patients with primary hyperparathyroidism. Death during follow-up occurred in 591 (31%) surgically treated patients and 474 (37%) conservatively treated patients. (Redrawn from Vestergaard P, Mosekilde L. *BMJ* 2003;327:530–34.)

patients undergoing surgery are generally those with more severe hyperparathyroidism and more end-organ damage.

From a practical viewpoint, it is reasonable to accept the potential of PHP to cause hypertension or enhance essential or secondary pre-existing hypertension. If PHP is not prolonged, and there is no evidence of arterial and kidney damage, parathyroidectomy is likely to result in reduction of BP or in making pre-existing hypertension more manageable.

HYPERTENSION IN ACROMEGALY

Hypertension is frequently found in at least one-third of patients with acromegaly.[83,84] In a recent study, systolic BP descended from 132 to 121 mmHg in 15 of 30 patients considered "cured" after treatment of acromegaly ($p<0.003$), whereas in the same patients diastolic BP decreased from 88 to 80 mmHg ($p=0.09$).[85] In another study, mean arterial BP was significantly higher in patients with acromegaly, and failed to decrease overnight as it did in normotensive controls.[86] Together with insulin resistance, dyslipidemia, and probably direct effects of growth hormone (GH) and insulin-like growth factor I (IGF-I) on the heart, hypertension contributes to increased mortality due to cardiovascular events in patients with acromegaly. The rate of cardiovascular events in patients with acromegaly is three to four times that of the appropriately matched general population, and ranks as the major cause of death in patients with this disease.[83] As in the case of hyperparathyroidism, discussed previously, the mechanisms leading to hypertension in acromegaly have not been totally defined, and they seem to be multiple and of variable importance depending on individual backgrounds, severity, and duration of the disease.

Of the multiple abnormalities observed in the heart of patients with acromegaly,[83,87] increased cardiac output and stroke volume[84,87] may be early contributing factors to the increase in systolic BP. Globally, vascular peripheral resistance is reduced,[84] which may explain why diastolic BP is not as elevated as systolic pressure. On the other hand, diastolic dysfunction is common (particularly during exercise) in acromegalic patients,[85,87] and is associated with a progressive reduction in EF.[88] Diastolic dysfunction is the result of the trophic effects of GH and IGF-I on cardiomyocytes as well as increased interstitial collagen accumulation, all of which leads to myocardial stiffness.[89] As the heart starts to fail, it ceases to play any role in the hypertension, which is now maintained by changes in the arteries and kidney. Heart failure in acromegaly is due to a combination of muscle hypertrophy and stiffness (note that acromegaly *per se* is not usually associated with dilated cardiomyopathy).

There are acute and long-term systemic and vascular effects of acromegaly that are likely to contribute significantly to the hypertension observed in these patients. Most important among these are fluid and sodium retention, endothelial dysfunction, and arterial remodeling. More speculative and perhaps less important are the roles of insulin resistance and the sympathetic nervous system.

That GH promotes fluid and sodium retention, as it has been shown in individuals with deficiency and excess of this hormone, as well as in adults treated with GH.[90] The consensus is that this effect is ultimately mediated by IGF-I, as this can nicely mimic these effects of GH.[91,92] Probably central to the fluid retaining effect is the stimulation of the renin-angiotensin-aldosterone system (RAAS), because its blockade cancels the volume expansion induced by GH or IGF-I.[93] The injection of GH to normal volunteers is associated with fluid and sodium retention concomitantly with an increase in renin and a seven-fold increase in circulating aldosterone, without changes in plasma osmolality or antidiuretic hormone concentration.[94] An important factor in the activation of RAAS is the potential inhibition of atrial natriuretic factor (ANF) by GH-IGF-I, derepressing RAAS.[92] The importance of these mechanisms in maintaining hypertension in the long term remains unclear, because population studies do not show a clear correlation of hypertension with levels of renin, aldosterone, or responses of the RAAS to standard challenges.[95] It is reasonable to think that somehow elevated GH can ultimately increase the responsiveness of target cells to angiotensin or aldosterone, or both.

Even though studies on endothelial function in acromegaly are scarce and at times difficult to reconcile, the notion that endothelial dysfunction occurs in this condition is widely accepted.[83] In spite of reduced global vascular peripheral resistance, Chanson et al.[84] found decreased brachial artery blood flow with significantly higher forearm vascular resistance in acromegalic patients compared with matched controls. Since other studies have demonstrated increased renal blood flow, glomerular hyperfiltration,[96] and increased functional liver plasma flow,[97] it is well accepted that the chronic excess of GH differentially affects various vascular beds, causing heterogeneity in the distribution of cardiac output in acromegaly.[98] Defective artery dilation in response to increased blood flow is considered a marker of endothelial dysfunction, and may explain the failure of the brachial arterial territory to accommodate increased flow pressure. Recently, Maison et al.[99] reported impaired endothelium-dependent vasodilatation in acromegalic patients together with exaggerated sympathetic-mediated vasoconstrictor response. Flow-mediated dilatation of the brachial artery was significantly lower in acromegalic patients than in healthy and risk-factor–matched controls (by 64% and 47%, respectively).[100] The contributions of insulin resistance of acromegaly and of high levels of GH or IGF-I to endothelial dysfunction are unclear.

In addition to functional abnormalities, several investigators have reported arterial remodeling with increased intima media thickness (IMT), and narrowing of the arterial lumens together with hypertrophic remodeling of small arteries.[85,101,102] These changes probably require a long time to take effect, and to some extent they may regress with treatment.[102] It is most interesting that such changes are also seen in transgenic mice overexpressing bovine GH.[103] These mice have higher BP than wild-type genotype controls, and their blood vessels show increased IMT and other changes seen in patients with acromegaly. Notably, BP in these mice is not salt-sensitive and the arteries do not respond to manipulations of vasomotor tone such as norepinephrine, sodium nitroprusside, and acetylcholine. Since these mice have been chronically exposed to GH (i.e., congenitally), such results support the notion that chronic exposure to GH causes blood vessel remodeling, making the hypertension difficult or impossible to control. In addition, IGF-I elevation in acromegaly seemingly stimulates vascular growth factors, such as angiogenin and endostatin, the concentrations of which correlates with IGF-I levels.[104]

These observations together suggest that, as occurs in hyperparathyroidism, functional abnormalities lead somehow to arteriolar remodeling, which in turn makes hypertension irreversible or less responsive to successful treatment of the acromegaly. Only longitudinal studies could confirm this hypothesis (difficult to implement because of ethical considerations). But even if this sequence remains hypothetical, the studies mentioned here provide support to the idea of promptly correcting the high GH/IGF-I levels to reduce the risk of morbidity and mortality due to cardiovascular events.

tissue, hypertension is not a central manifestation of most endocrine diseases. Thyroid dysfunction, primary hyperparathyroidism, and acromegaly are frequently associated with significant hemodynamic changes and increases in arterial BP. These are, of course, of more clinical significance in previously hypertensive individuals. In spite of the dramatic effects of thyrotoxicosis on the heart and vasculature, hypertension is rarely of clinical significance. Hypothyroidism may more frequently associate with hypertension and its correction, particularly when severe, is followed by a reduction in arterial pressure. Primary hyperparathyroidism and acromegaly are frequently associated with elevations of BP, and cardiovascular disease is the leading cause of death in protracted acromegaly. In both conditions, factors leading to elevation in BP are multiple. Likewise, in both conditions abnormalities are initially functional and reversible, but with time lead to vascular remodeling and irreversibility, adding support to the tendency of diagnosing and treating these conditions early and radically, that is, eliminating the source of the hormonal excess.

SUMMARY

Except for endocrine diseases associated with hypersecretion of the adrenal cortex, adrenal medulla, or chromaffin

REFERENCES

1. Bianco AC, Salvatore D, Gereben B, Berry MJ, Larsen PR. Biochemistry, cellular and molecular biology, and physiological roles of the iodothyronine selenodeiodinases. *Endocr Rev* 2002;23:38–89.
2. Bassett JH, Harvey CB, Williams GR. Mechanisms of thyroid hormone receptor-specific nuclear and extra nuclear actions. *Mol Cell Endocrinol* 2003;213:1–11.
3. Barker SB, Klitgaard HM. Metabolism of tissues excised from thyroxine-injected rats. *J Physiol (Lond)* 1952;170:81–86.
4. Kahaly GJ, Dillmann WH. Thyroid hormone action in the heart. *Endocr Rev* 2005;26:704–708.
5. Buccino RA, Spann JF Jr, Pool PE, Sonneblick EH, Braunwald E. Influence of the thyroid state on the intrinsic contractile properties and energy stores of the myocardium. *J Clin Invest* 1967;46:1669–82.
6. Dillmann WH. Cellular action of thyroid hormone on the heart. *Thyroid* 2002;12:447–52.
7. Oppenheimer JH, Schwartz HL, Surks MI. Tissue differences in the concentration of triiodothyronine nuclear binding sites in the rat liver, kidney, pituitary, heart, brain, spleen and testes. *Endocrinology* 1974;95:897–903.
8. Dietrich JB, Kuchler-Bopp S, Boutillier S, Ittel ME, Reeber A, Zaepfel M, et al. Expression of thyroid hormone receptors alpha and beta–1 messenger RNAs in human endothelial cells. The T3

hormone stimulates the synthesis of the messenger RNA of the intercellular adhesion molecule–1. *Cell Mol Biol* 1997;43:1205–12.
9. Hu RM, Wu LM, Frank HJ, Pedram A, Levin ER. Insulin stimulates thyroid hormone receptor alpha gene expression in cultured bovine aortic endothelial cells. *Mol Cell Endocrinol* 1994;103:65–71.
10. Trost SU, Swanson E, Gloss B, Wang-Iverson DB, Zhang H, Volodarsky T, et al. The thyroid hormone receptor-beta-selective agonist GC–1 differentially affects plasma lipids and cardiac activity. *Endocrinology* 2000;141:3057–64.
11. Marrif H, Schifman A, Stepanyan Z, Gillis MA, Calderone A, Weiss RE, et al. Temperature homeostasis in transgenic mice lacking thyroid hormone receptor alpha gene products. *Endocrinology* 2005;146:2872–84.
12. Johansson C, Gothe S, Forrest D, Vennstrom B, Thoren P. Cardiovascular phenotype and temperature control in mice lacking thyroid hormone receptor-β or both α1 and β. *Am J Physiol* 1999;276:H2006–12.
13. Forrest D, Vennstrom B. Functions of thyroid hormone receptors in mice. *Thyroid* 2000;10:41–52.
14. Williams LT, Lefkowitz RJ, Watanabe AM, Hathaway DR, Besch HR Jr. Thyroid hormone regulation of beta-adrenergic receptor number. *J Biol Chem* 1977;252:2787–89.
15. Bahouth SW, Cui X, Beauchamp MJ, Park EA. Thyroid hormone induces

beta1-adrenergic receptor gene transcription through a direct repeat separated by five nucleotides. *J Mol Cell Cardiol* 1997;29:3223–37.
16. Silva JE. Thermogenesis and the sympathoadrenal system in thyrotoxicosis. In: Braverman LE, Utiger RD, eds. *Werner and Ingbar's The Thyroid: A Fundamental and Clinical Text.* 9th ed. Philadelphia: Lippincott-Williams & Wilkins, 2005:607–20.
17. Klein I, Ojamaa K. Thyroid hormone and the cardiovascular system. *N Engl J Med* 2001;344:501–509.
18. Kahaly GJ, Wagner S, Nieswandt J, Mohr-Kahaly S, Ryan TJ. Stress echocardiography in hyperthyroidism. *J Clin Endocrinol Metab* 1999;84:2308–13.
19. Palmieri EA, Fazio S, Palmieri V, Lombardi G, Biondi B. Myocardial contractility and total arterial stiffness in patients with overt hyperthyroidism: acute effects of beta1-adrenergic blockade. *Eur J Endocrinol* 2004;150:757–62.
20. Ojamaa K, Klemperer JD, Klein I. Acute effects of thyroid hormone on vascular smooth muscle. *Thyroid* 1996;6:505–12.
21. Quesada A, Sainz J, Wangensteen R, Rodriguez-Gomez I, Vargas F, Osuna A. Nitric oxide synthase activity in hyperthyroid and hypothyroid rats. *Eur J Endocrinol* 2002;147:117–22.
22. Marvisi M, Brianti M, Marani G, Del Borello R, Bortesi ML, Guariglia A. Hyperthyroidism and pulmonary hypertension. *Respir Med* 2002;96:215–20.

23. Merce J, Ferras S, Oltra C, Sanz E, Vendrell J, Simon I, et al. Cardiovascular abnormalities in hyperthyroidism: a prospective Doppler echocardiographic study. *Am J Med* 2005;118:126–31.

24. Soroush-Yari A, Burstein S, Hoo GW, Santiago SM. Pulmonary hypertension in men with thyrotoxicosis. *Respiration* 2005;72:90–94.

25. Hu LW, Benvenuti LA, Liberti EA, Carneiro-Ramos MS, Barreto-Chaves ML. Thyroxine-induced cardiac hypertrophy: influence of adrenergic nervous system versus renin-angiotensin system on myocyte remodeling. *Am J Physiol Regul Integr Comp Physiol* 2003;285:R1473–80.

26. Fletcher AK, Weetman AP. Hypertension and hypothyroidism. *J Hum Hypertens* 1998;12:79–82 [review].

27. Streeten DH, Anderson GH Jr, Wagner S. Effect of age on response of secondary hypertension to specific treatment. *Am J Hypertens* 1990;3:360–65.

28. Streeten DH, Anderson GH Jr, Howland T, Chiang R, Smulyan H. Effects of thyroid function on blood pressure. Recognition of hypothyroid hypertension. *Hypertension* 1988;11:78–83.

29. Anderson GH Jr, Blakeman N, Streeten DH. The effect of age on prevalence of secondary forms of hypertension in 4429 consecutively referred patients. *J Hypertens* 1994;12:609–15.

30. Dernellis J, Panaretou M. Effects of thyroid replacement therapy on arterial blood pressure in patients with hypertension and hypothyroidism. *Am Heart J* 2002;143:718–24.

31. Bing RF, Briggs RS, Burden AC, Russell GI, Swales JD, Thurston H. Reversible hypertension and hypothyroidism. *Clin Endocrinol (Oxf)* 1980;13:339–42.

32. Coulombe P, Dussault JH. Catecholamine metabolism in thyroid disease. II. Norepinephrine secretion rate in hyperthyroidism and hypothyroidism. *J Clin Endocrinol Metab* 1977;44:1185–89.

33. Christensen NJ. Increased levels of plasma noradrenaline in hypothyroidism. *J Clin Endocrinol Metab* 1972;35:359.

34. Polikar R, Kennedy B, Ziegler M, O'Connor DT, Smith J, Nicod P. Plasma norepinephrine kinetics, dopamine-beta-hydroxylase, and chromogranin-A, in hypothyroid patients before and following replacement therapy. *J Clin Endocrinol Metab* 1990;70:277–81.

35. Fagius J, Westermark K, Karlsson A. Baroreflex-governed sympathetic outflow to muscle vasculature is increased in hypothyroidism. *Clin Endocrinol (Oxf)* 1990;33:177–85.

36. Bilezikian JP, Loeb JN. The influence of hyperthyroidism and hyperthyroidism on α- and β-adrenergic receptor systems and adrenergic responsiveness. *Endocr Rev* 1983;4:378–88.

37. Bramnert M, Hallengren B, Lecerof H, Werner R, Manhem P. Decreased blood pressure response to infused noradrenaline in normotensive as compared to hypertensive patients with primary hypothyroidism. *Clin Endocrinol (Oxf)* 1994;40:317–21.

38. Fukuyama K, Ichiki T, Takeda K, Tokunou T, Iino N, Masuda S, et al. Downregulation of vascular angiotensin II type 1 receptor by thyroid hormone. *Hypertension* 2003;41:598–603.

39. Yasuzawa-Amano S, Toyoda N, Maeda A, Kosaki A, Mori Y, Iwasaka T, et al. Expression and regulation of type 2 iodothyronine deiodinase in rat aorta media. *Endocrinology* 2004;145:5638–45.

40. Mizuma H, Murakami M, Mori M. Thyroid hormone activation in human vascular smooth muscle cells: expression of type II iodothyronine deiodinase. *Circ Res* 2001;88:313–18.

41. Gumieniak O, Perlstein TS, Hopkins PN, Brown NJ, Murphey LJ, Jeunemaitre X, et al. Thyroid function and blood pressure homeostasis in euthyroid subjects. *J Clin Endocrinol Metab* 2004;89:3455–61.

42. Fommei E, Iervasi G. The role of thyroid hormone in blood pressure homeostasis: evidence from short-term hypothyroidism in humans. *J Clin Endocrinol Metab* 2002;87:1996–2000.

43. Heath H III, Hodgson SF, Kennedy MA. Primary hyperparathyroidism. Incidence, morbidity, and potential economic impact in a community. *N Engl J Med* 1980;302:189–93.

44. Broulik PD, Horky K, Pacovsky V. Blood pressure in patients with primary hyperparathyroidism before and after parathyroidectomy. *Exp Clin Endocrinol* 1985;86:346–52.

45. Ringe JD. Reversible hypertension in primary hyperparathyroidism—pre- and post-operative blood pressure in 75 cases. *Klin Wochenschr* 1984;62:465–69.

46. Diamond TW, Botha JR, Wing J, Meyers AM, Kalk WJ. Parathyroid hypertension. A reversible disorder. *Arch Intern Med* 1986;146:1709–12.

47. Kosch M, Hausberg M, Vormbrock K, Kisters K, Rahn KH, Barenbrock M. Studies on flow-mediated vasodilation and intima-media thickness of the brachial artery in patients with primary hyperparathyroidism. *Am J Hypertens* 2000;13:759–64.

48. Kosch M, Hausberg M, Vormbrock K, Kisters K, Gabriels G, Rahn KH, et al. Impaired flow-mediated vasodilation of the brachial artery in patients with primary hyperparathyroidism improves after parathyroidectomy. *Cardiovasc Res* 2000;47:813–18.

49. Kosch M, Hausberg M, Barenbrock M, Posadzy-Malaczynska A, Kisters K, Rahn KH. Arterial distensibility and pulse wave velocity in patients with primary hyperparathyroidism before and after parathyroidectomy. *Clin Nephrol* 2001;55:303–308.

50. Rubin MR, Maurer MS, McMahon DJ, Bilezikian JP, Silverberg SJ. Arterial stiffness in mild primary hyperparathyroidism. *J Clin Endocrinol Metab* 2005;90:3326–30.

51. Letizia C, Caliumi C, Delfini E, Celi M, Subioli S, Diacinti D, Minisola S, D'erasmo E, Mazzuoli GF. Adrenomedullin concentrations are elevated in plasma of patients with primary hyperparathyroidism. *Metab Clin Exp* 2003;52:159–62.

52. Pang PK, Tenner TE Jr, Yee JA, Yang M, Janssen HF. Hypotensive action of parathyroid hormone preparations on rats and dogs. *Proc Natl Acad Sci U S A* 1980;77:675–78.

53. Massfelder T, Helwig JJ, Stewart AF. Parathyroid hormone-related protein as a cardiovascular regulatory peptide. *Endocrinology* 1996;137:3151–53.

54. Ishikawa M, Ouchi Y, Han SZ, Akishita M, Kozaki K, Toba K, et al. Parathyroid hormone-related protein reduces cytosolic free Ca2+ level and tension in rat aortic smooth muscle. *Eur Eur J Pharmacol* 1994;269:311–17.

55. Shan J, Wu X, Pang PK. Human parathyroid hormone fragment(1–34) and human [Ala25,26,27]parathyroid hormone fragment(1–34): their vascular and intracellular calcium regulating action in vascular smooth muscle cells. *J Pharmacol Exp Ther* 1994;268:19–24.

56. Kawashima H. Parathyroid hormone causes a transient rise in intracellular ionized calcium in vascular smooth muscle cells. *Biochem Biophys Res Commun* 1990;166:709–14.

57. Isales CM, Sumpio B, Bollag RJ, Zhong Q, Ding KH, Du W, et al. Functional parathyroid hormone receptors are present in an umbilical vein endothelial cell line. *Am J Physiol Endocrinol Metab* 2000;279:E654–62.

58. Jiang B, Morimoto S, Yang J, Niinoabu T, Fukuo K, Ogihara T. Expression of parathyroid hormone/parathyroid hormone-related protein receptor in vascular endothelial cells. *J Cardiovasc Pharmacol* 1998;31(Suppl 1):S142–44.

59. Jiang B, Morimoto S, Fukuo K, Hirotani A, Tamatani M, Nakahashi T, et al. Parathyroid hormone-related protein inhibits indothelin–1 production. *Hypertension* 1996;27:360–63.

60. Nilsson IL, Rastad J, Johansson K, Lind L. Endothelial vasodilatory function and blood pressure response to local and systemic hypercalcemia. *Surgery* 2001;130:986–90.

61. Fardella C and Rodriguez-Portales JA. Intracellular calcium and blood pressure: comparison between primary hyperparathyroidism and essential hypertension. *J Endocrinol Invest* 1995;18:827–32.

62. Vlachakis ND, Frederics R, Valasquez M, Alexander N, Singer F, Maronde RF. Sympathetic system function and vascular reactivity in hypercalcemic patients. *Hypertension* 1982;4:452–58.

63. Barletta G, De Feo ML, Del BR, Lazzeri C, Vecchiarino S, La VG, et al. Cardiovascular effects of parathyroid hormone: a study in healthy subjects and normotensive patients with mild primary hyperparathyroidism. *J Clin Endocrinol Metab* 2000;85:1815–21.

64. Otto AC, Nel MG, Van Staden JA, Dunn M, Van AA, Nel R. Enhanced myocardial contractility associated with hypercalcaemia of hyperparathyroidism—a case study in six patients. *Cardiovasc J S Afr* 2003;14:141–43.

65. Georgiannos SN, Jenkins BJ, Goode AW. Cardiac output in asymptomatic primary hyperparathyroidism: a stigma of early cardiovascular dysfunction? *Int Surg* 1996;81:171–73.

66. Almqvist EG, Bondeson AG, Bondeson L, Nissborg A, Smedgard P, Svensson SE. Cardiac dysfunction in mild primary hyperparathyroidism assessed

by radionuclide angiography and echocardiography before and after parathyroidectomy. *Surgery* 2002;132:1126–32.

67. Piovesan A, Molineri N, Casasso F, Emmolo I, Ugliengo G, Cesario F, et al. Left ventricular hypertrophy in primary hyperparathyroidism. Effects of successful parathyroidectomy. *Clin Endocrinol (Oxf)* 1999;50:321–28.

68. Pang PK, Benishin CG, Shan J, Lewanczuk RZ. PHF: the new parathyroid hypertensive factor. *Blood Press* 1994;3:148–55.

69. Benishin CG, Labedz T, Guo DD, Lewanczuk RZ, Pang PK. Identification and purification of parathyroid hypertensive factor from organ culture of parathyroid glands from spontaneously hypertensive rats. *Am J Hypertens* 1993;6:134–40.

70. Benishin CG, Lewanczuk RZ, Pang PK. Purification of parathyroid hypertensive factor from plasma of spontaneously hypertensive rats. *Proc Natl Acad Sci U S A* 1991;88:6372–76.

71. Benishin CG, Lewanczuk RZ, Shan J, Pang PK. Purification and structural characterization of parathyroid hypertensive factor. *J Cardiovasc Pharmacol* 1994;23(Suppl 2):S9–13.

72. Chang E, Hamet P, Tremblay J. Biochemical characteristics of a calmodulin-phosphodiesterase activator increased in spontaneously hypertensive mice and rats. *J Cardiovasc Pharmacol* 1994;23(Suppl 2):S42–49.

73. Lewanczuk RZ, Resnick LM, Ho MS, Benishin CG, Shan J, Pang PK. Clinical aspects of parathyroid hypertensive factor. *J Hypertens* 1994;12(Suppl):S11–16.

74. Shan J, Benishin CG, Lewanczuk RZ, Pang PK. Mechanism of the vascular action of parathyroid hypertensive factor. *J Cardiovasc Pharmacol* 1994;23(Suppl 2):S1–S8.

75. Lewanczuk RZ, Pang PK. Expression of parathyroid hypertensive factor in hypertensive primary hyperparathyroid patients. *Blood Press* 1993;2:22–27.

76. Rybczynska A, Boblewski K, Lehmann A, Orlewska C, Foks H, Drewnowska K, et al. Calcimimetic NPS R-568 induces hypotensive effect in spontaneously hypertensive rats. *Am J Hypertens* 2005;18:364–71.

77. Sutherland SK, Nemere I, Benishin CG. Regulation of parathyroid hypertensive factor secretion by vitamin D(3) analogs in parathyroid cells derived from spontaneously hypertensive rats. *J Cell Biochem* 2005;96:97–108.

78. Kawano Y, Yoshimi H, Matsuoka H, Takishita S, Omae T. Calcium supplementation in patients with essential hypertension: assessment by office, home and ambulatory blood pressure. *J Hypertens* 1998;16:1693–99.

79. Lind L, Jacobsson S, Palmer M, Lithell H, Wengle B, Ljunghall S. Cardiovascular risk factors in primary hyperparathyroidism: a 15-year

follow-up of operated and unoperated cases. *J Intern Med* 1991;230:29–35.

80. Rapado A. Arterial hypertension and primary hyperparathyroidism. Incidence and follow-up after parathyroidectomy. *Am J Nephrol* 1986;6(Suppl 1):49–50.

81. Sancho JJ, Rouco J, Riera-Vidal R, Sitges-Serra A. Long-term effects of parathyroidectomy for primary hyperparathyroidism on arterial hypertension. *World J Surg* 1992;16:732–35.

82. Vestergaard P, Mosekilde L. Cohort study on effects of parathyroid surgery on multiple outcomes in primary hyperparathyroidism. *BMJ* 2003;327:530–34.

83. Clayton RN. Cardiovascular function in acromegaly. *Endocr Rev* 2003;24:272–77.

84. Chanson P, Megnien JL, del PM, Coirault C, Merli I, Houdouin L, et al. Decreased regional blood flow in patients with acromegaly. *Clin Endocrinol (Oxf)* 1998;49:725–31.

85. Colao A, Spiezia S, Cerbone G, Pivonello R, Marzullo P, Ferone D, et al. Increased arterial intima-media thickness by B-M mode echodoppler ultrasonography in acromegaly. *Clin Endocrinol (Oxf)* 2001;54:515–24.

86. Terzolo M, Matrella C, Boccuzzi A, Luceri S, Borriero M, Reimondo G, et al. Twenty-four hour profile of blood pressure in patients with acromegaly. Correlation with demographic, clinical and hormonal features. *J Endocrinol Invest* 1999;22:48–54.

87. Vitale G, Pivonello R, Lombardi G, Colao A. Cardiac abnormalities in acromegaly. Pathophysiology and implications for management. *Treat Endocrinol* 2004;3:309–18.

88. Colao A, Cuocolo A, Marzullo P, Nicolai E, Ferone D, Della Morte AM, et al. Impact of patient's age and disease duration on cardiac performance in acromegaly: a radionuclide angiography study. *J Clin Endocrinol Metab* 1999;84:1518–23.

89. Ciulla MM, Epaminonda P, Paliotti R, Barelli MV, Ronchi C, Cappiello V, et al. Evaluation of cardiac structure by echoreflectivity analysis in acromegaly: effects of treatment. *Eur J Endocrinol* 2004;151:179–86.

90. Moller J. Effects of growth hormone on fluid homeostasis. Clinical and experimental aspects. *Growth Horm IGF Res* 2003;13:55–74.

91. Cittadini A, Stromer H, Katz SE, Clark R, Moses AC, Morgan JP, et al. Differential cardiac effects of growth hormone and insulin-like growth factor-1 in the rat. A combined in vivo and in vitro evaluation. *Circulation* 1996;93:800–809.

92. Moller J, Jorgensen JO, Moller N, Hansen KW, Pedersen EB, Christiansen JS. Expansion of extracellular volume and suppression of atrial natriuretic peptide after growth hormone

administration in normal man. *J Clin Endocrinol Metab* 1991;72:768–72.

93. Moller J, Moller N, Frandsen E, Wolthers T, Jorgensen JO, Christiansen JS. Blockade of the renin-angiotensin-aldosterone system prevents growth hormone–induced fluid retention in humans. *Am J Physiol* 1997;272:E803–808.

94. Ho KY, Weissberger AJ. The antinatriuretic action of biosynthetic human growth hormone in man involves activation of the renin-angiotensin system. *Metab Clin Exp* 1990;39:133–37.

95. Kraatz C, Benker G, Weber F, Ludecke D, Hirche H, Reinwein D. Acromegaly and hypertension: prevalence and relationship to the renin-angiotensin-aldosterone system. *Klin Wochenschr* 1990;68:583–87.

96. Dullaart RP, Meijer S, Marbach P, Sluiter WJ. Effect of a somatostatin analogue, octreotide, on renal haemodynamics and albuminuria in acromegalic patients. *Eur J Clin Invest* 1992;22:494–502.

97. Avagnina P, Martini M, Terzolo M, Sansoe G, Peretti P, Tinivella M, et al. Assessment of functional liver mass and plasma flow in acromegaly before and after long-term treatment with octreotide. *Metab Clin Exp* 1996;45:109–13.

98. Evans LM, Davies JS. Heterogeneous haemodynamics in acromegaly: evidence of endothelial dysfunction? *Clin Endocrinol (Oxf)* 1998;49:711–12.

99. Maison P, Demolis P, Young J, Schaison G, Giudicelli JF, Chanson P. Vascular reactivity in acromegalic patients: preliminary evidence for regional endothelial dysfunction and increased sympathetic vasoconstriction. *Clin Endocrinol (Oxf)* 2000;53:445–51.

100. Brevetti G, Marzullo P, Silvestro A, Pivonello R, Oliva G, di Somma C, et al. Early vascular alterations in acromegaly. *J Clin Endocrinol Metab* 2002;87:3174–79.

101. Rizzoni D, Porteri E, Giustina A, De CC, Sleiman I, Boari GE, et al. Acromegalic patients show the presence of hypertrophic remodeling of subcutaneous small resistance arteries. *Hypertension* 2004;43:561–65.

102. Smith JC, Lane H, Davies N, Evans LM, Cockcroft J, Scanlon MF, et al. The effects of depot long-acting somatostatin analog on central aortic pressure and arterial stiffness in acromegaly. *J Clin Endocrinol Metab* 2003;88:2556–61.

103. Bohlooly Y, Carlson L, Olsson B, Gustafsson H, Andersson IJ, Tornell J, et al. Vascular function and blood pressure in GH transgenic mice. *Endocrinology* 2001;142:3317–23.

104. Silha JV, Krsek M, Hana V, Marek J, Weiss V, Jezkova J, et al. The effects of growth hormone status on circulating levels of vascular growth factors. *Clin Endocrinol (Oxf)* 2005;63:79–86.

Chapter

74 Coarctation of the Aorta

Richard A. Krasuski and Fetnat Fouad-Tarazi

Definition

- Coarctation of the aorta (CoA) is an important cause of secondary hypertension with the potential to serve as a model for the understanding of essential hypertension.

- CoA is a very common defect, accounting for ~8% of all congenital heart defects. Approximately 50% to 85% of patients with CoA also have a bicuspid aortic valve.

Clinical Implications

- Symptomatic patients with a peak gradient over 30 mmHg on invasive measurement or a similar gradient in asymptomatic patients with upper extremity hypertension that becomes severe with exercise or is associated with left ventricular hypertrophy should have intervention.

- Other evolving indications for treatment include the presence of concurrent aortic aneurysms and symptomatic aneurysms of the circle of Willis. Young women who wish to bear children are also at risk.

- Surgery has remained the mainstay approach to native CoA, although percutaneous intervention is an alternative.

- Despite intervention, hypertension is more prevalent in these patients, developing at a far younger age than would normally be expected.

Coarctation of the aorta (CoA) is an important cause of secondary hypertension with the potential to serve as a model for the understanding of essential hypertension. This chapter reviews the prevalence, pathophysiology, presenting features, invasive and noninvasive assessment, treatment and long-term clinical outcome of this congenital anomaly.

DEFINITION AND PREVALENCE

Coarctation of the aorta (CoA) refers to a narrowing in the descending aorta (Figure 74–1), typically in the location of the takeoff of the left subclavian artery and the ligamentum arteriosum (ductus arteriosus). Anatomically it can occur just before the ductus, at the ductus, or just after the ductus. In its rarest form, CoA can involve the abdominal segment of the aorta (<2% of all cases).[1] Adults with a previously undiagnosed CoA will almost always have postductal lesions. The lesion itself is either a localized narrowing or a hypoplastic segment of the aorta, with the former lesion being much more common.

CoA is a very common defect, accounting for an estimated 8% of all congenital heart defects.[2] Although distributed fairly evenly between genders among infants, older patients have a male predominance. Approximately 50% to 85% of patients with CoA also have a bicuspid aortic valve.[3] If there are no other anatomic abnormalities (with the exception of the biscupid valve), the lesion is referred to as a "simple coarctation."[4] If accompanied by other cardiac anomalies it is referred to as a "complex coarctation."

Patients with complex CoA typically are diagnosed early in childhood, while simple CoA may not be recognized until adulthood. It is estimated that CoA may account for up to 0.2% of all adults with hypertension, and is therefore a lesion with which hypertension specialists should become familiar.[5]

ANATOMY AND DEVELOPMENT

There are two main hypotheses that have been proposed to explain CoA formation.[1] In the hemodynamic theory, there is an abnormal angle between the ductus arteriosus and the aorta leading to abnormal blood flow and subsequently reduced growth of the descending aorta. By the time the ductus closes, this segment of aorta is hypoplastic and results in partial obstruction. Supporting this theory is the high incidence of CoA in congenital heart disease patients with decreased aortic flow *in utero*, and the absence of CoA in patients with right heart obstructive disease. The "ectopic ductal tissue" hypothesis proposes that tissue from the ductus arteriosus abnormally extends into the descending aorta, and this ectopic ductal tissue then constricts during ductal closure. While compelling, the latter theory does not easily explain the common occurrence of hypoplasia of the aortic arch and isthmus seen with CoA.

In addition to bicuspid aortic valves, other pathologic abnormalities have been described in patients with both simple and complex CoA. This includes the above mentioned hypoplasia of the transverse aortic arch (region between the left common carotid artery and left subclavian artery) and aortic isthmus (region between the left subclavian artery and ductus arteriosus).[6] Dilatation of descending aorta just beyond the CoA, often referred to as "poststenotic dilatation," is typically present as well.[7] There may also be an inherent structural weakness of the ascending aorta in a so-called "cystic medial necrosis" pattern, usually seen in patients with concurrent bicuspid aortic valve. This abnormality appears to

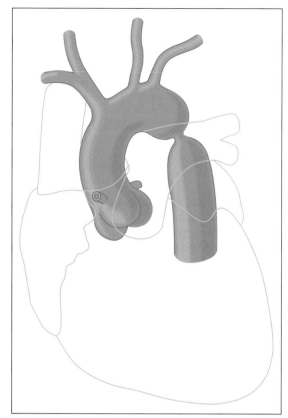

Figure 74–1. Coarctation of the aorta.

increase the risk of aortic dissection.[8] Similarly, the presence of Berry aneurysms in the cerebral circulation (found in up to 10% of patients with CoA) appears to increase the risk of intracranial hemorrhage.[9,10]

PATHOPHYSIOLOGY AND PRESENTATION

Presentation during infancy is most common among patients with complex CoA. Heart failure resulting from significant hemodynamic compromise can necessitate early repair. For simple CoA, the lesion is most often discovered during childhood or early adolescence by the recognition of otherwise unexplained hypertension or by the presence of a loud systolic murmur. The most common presentation in adults is the fortuitous discovery during secondary work-up for systemic hypertension.[11] Although early theories focused solely on the role of mechanical obstruction of aorta as the source of blood pressure elevation, a better understanding of the humoral pathways of blood pressure regulation has provided a stronger explanation for hypertension in CoA. Renal hypoperfusion secondary to the CoA generally leads to a state of activation of the renin-angiotensin-aldosterone system and subsequent increased production of angiotensin and aldosterone. Plasma renin and aldosterone levels typically return to nearly normal levels after arterial pressure increases and renal perfusion is restored toward normal. Activation of the central sympathetic nervous system has also been suggested to play an additional role in the development of hypertension.

In most children and adults with significant CoA, there is upper extremity hypertension and the development of collateral vessels around the coarctation to the lower extremity. These collateral channels often create a continuous murmur heard over the back, and involvement of the intercostal arteries leads to the familiar rib notching seen on chest radiography (Figure 74–2). Lower extremity hypoperfusion can also lead to symptoms of leg fatigue during exercise in up to half of patients.[12]

PHYSICAL EXAMINATION

The examination of a patient with suspected CoA requires careful diligence on the part of the practitioner, as the physical findings can be subtle and often overlooked. In addition to upper extremity hypertension, the fundoscopic examination will generally show the classic retinopathic changes of long-standing hypertension including pulsatile, U-shaped, corkscrew arterioles.[13] An essential aspect of the examination in patients with suspected CoA is careful palpation of pulses in all four extremities as well as the simultaneous palpation of the femoral and brachial pulses. A significant delay or decrement in the femoral pulse should lead one to suspect CoA, particularly in the absence of known peripheral vascular disease. Blood pressures can be taken in the arm and leg, and a decrement of 20 mmHg or greater in the systolic blood pressure in the legs is suggestive of CoA. Of note, diastolic blood pressure generally does not differ. Simultaneous palpation of the brachial pulses is also helpful, particularly to differentiate a pre-ductal coarctation where the left pulse will be diminished and possibly delayed from the right pulse.

DIAGNOSTIC WORK-UP

The electrocardiogram of the patient with CoA often demonstrates the voltage abnormalities of left ventricular

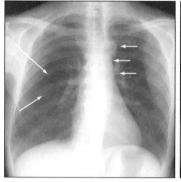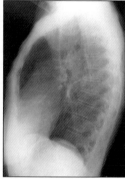

Figure 74–2. Chest x-ray of coarctation. A chest x-ray that demonstrates the classic findings in an adult patient with unrepaired coarctation of the aorta. *Short arrows* point out the "number 3" sign resulting from the focal narrowing. Rib notching (*long arrows*) is seen on the inferior portion of the posterior ribs (third to ninth) and results from pressure erosion caused by dilated intercostal arteries that serve as collateral blood flow between the internal mammary arteries and the descending aorta. (Photo courtesy of Richard White, MD.)

hypertrophy, while the presence of prominent, coved ST segment depressions and deeply inverted T waves are more suggestive of concurrent bicuspid aortic valve.[1] The chest x-ray in CoA can range from essentially normal to pathognomonic. The most classic finding is the presence of rib notching that signifies the presence of collateral flow through dilated posterior intercostal arteries (Figure 74–2). This finding is very important, because it helps to differentiate CoA from pseudocoarctation (Figure 74–3). The latter lesion is an unusual anomaly associated with buckling or kinking of the aorta in the region of the ligamentum arteriosum.[1] This is often related to long-standing hypertension and is associated with elongation, tortuosity, and dilatation of the descending aorta. Although this lesion is by no means benign, it is called "pseudo" because of the lack of true obstruction to flow (no evident gradient).

Echocardiography with a focus on the descending aorta is an excellent noninvasive manner in which to make the clinical diagnosis of CoA in patients with suspicious clinical findings.[14] A resting peak systolic velocity of 3.2 or more meters per second or a diastolic velocity of 1.0 or more meters per second suggests a significant coarctation. Echocardiography also allows interrogation of the aortic valve and the assessment of the ascending aortic root.

Magnetic resonance imaging has now become the choice imaging modality preoperatively to size the aorta and the coarctation region (Figure 74–4) and postoperatively to follow patients.[15,16] In the event of a contraindication (pacemaker or severe claustrophobia) or lack of availability, computer tomography is a reasonable alterative.

INDICATIONS FOR INTERVENTION

Symptomatic patients with a peak gradient over 30 mmHg on invasive measurement or a similar gradient in asymptomatic patients with upper extremity hypertension that becomes severe with exercise or is associated with left ventricular hypertrophy should be considered for intervention. Other evolving indications for treatment include

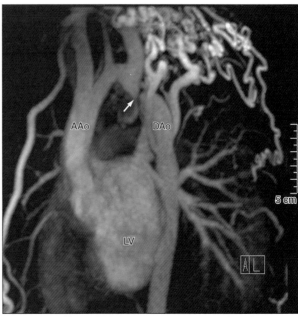

Figure 74–4. Magnetic resonance image of a patient with unrepaired coarctation of the aorta. Magnetic resonance angiogram of the heart and great vessels in a patient with unrepaired coarctation of the aorta. There are prominent collateral vessels which drain into the descending aorta below the coarcted segment (*arrow*) and maintain lower extremity perfusion. AAo, ascending aorta; DAo, descending aorta; LV, left ventricle. (Photo courtesy of Janine Arruda, MD.)

the presence of concurrent aortic aneurysms and symptomatic aneurysms of the circle of Willis. Young women who wish to bear children are also at risk, as placental flow may be inadequate should they become pregnant.[17]

THERAPEUTIC MODALITIES

Surgery

Surgery has remained the mainstay approach to native CoA since its first description in 1945.[18] Several different techniques have been developed over time with the most notable options being resection and end-to-end anastomosis, prosthetic patch aortoplasty, interposition (tube bypass) grafting, and subclavian to aortic bypass (Figure 74–5). The procedural choice is often dictated by the unique anatomy of the coarctation, including the need for significant mobilization of the aorta and the presence of extensive collateral vessels. Resection with end-to-end anastomosis remains the most popular surgical option, and has the advantage of limiting the use of prosthetic material. This may reduce the degree of inflammation at the anastomosis site, and therefore reduces the risk of recoarctation. In one large series, the risk of re-operation in extended follow-up was the lowest (<2%) using this technique.[19]

Several large surgical series describing CoA repair have been published with a large range of perioperative and long-term morbidity and mortality reported.[20] Complications during the procedure are most common with the

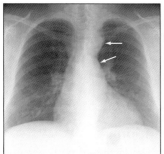
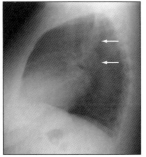

Figure 74–3. Chest x-ray of pseudocoarctation. A chest x-ray that demonstrates the classic findings of unrepaired pseudocoarctation of the aorta. The arrows mark the "double-left aortic arch sign," which can appear very similar to the "number 3" sign of coarctation. Because there is no physiologic obstruction, there is an absence of collateral vessel development and subsequent rib notching. (Photo courtesy of Richard White, MD.)

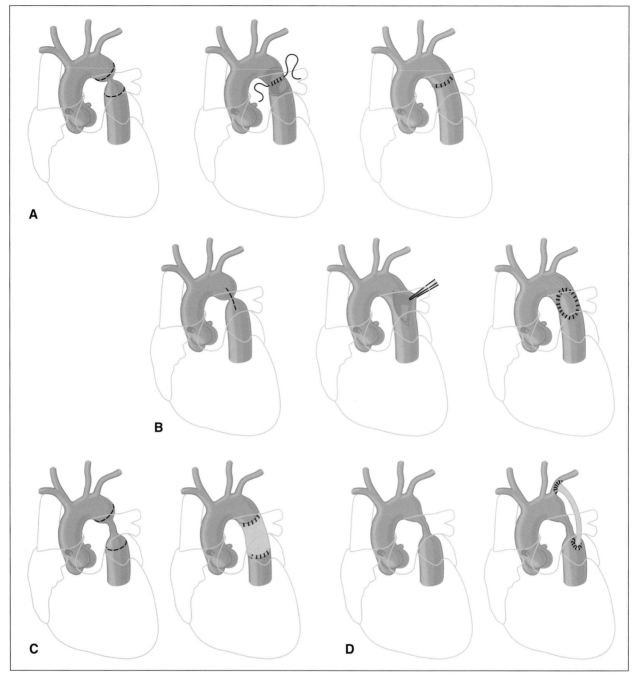

Figure 74–5. Surgical approaches to coarctation repair. The most commonly used techniques to repair aortic coarctation over the years include resection and end-to-end anastomosis (**A**), prosthetic patch aortoplasty (**B**), tube interposition bypass grafting (**C**), and subclavian to aortic bypass (**D**).

repair of complex coarctation, while operative mortality may be less than 1% for simple coarctation.[4] Unique perioperative complications include chylothorax, damage to the recurrent laryngeal or phrenic nerves, ischemic bowel, parenchymal lung injury, and spinal chord ischemia and paraplegia.[19] There is a long-term risk of pseudoaneurysm formation, particularly in patients receiving a patch aortoplasty, as well as a risk for recoarctation.[21] Patients also remain at a substantially higher risk of developing hypertension (see below) despite proper repair, but are even more likely to be hypertensive if residual coarctation is present.[22] The optimal timing for repair appears to be in

the range of 2 to 5 years where the risk of long-term complications appears to be the lowest.[4]

Percutaneous intervention

Recently some success has been achieved with percutaneous intervention in young patients with native coarctation.[23] Older patients, however, should still be considered for surgery if they are viable candidates. Percutaneous angioplasty has been performed since 1982,[24] and the availability of stents has recently led to improved outcomes, to the extent that percutaneous intervention is now considered the procedure of choice in patients with recoarctation following surgery.[25] Stents are particularly effective in preventing complications from recoil of the aorta following angioplasty. The size of the stent should never be larger than the native aorta. Intravascular ultrasound has been very useful in ensuring that there is adequate apposition of the stent against the aortic wall.

Several large series of angioplasty/stent patients suggest success rates of 65% to 100% with a complication rate of ~10%. Problems to watch for include recoarctation and aneurysm formation at the site of intervention, blood pressure problems including hypo- and hypertension, and paraplegia. Endocarditis prophylaxis remains important, even if the residual gradient is minimal (Figure 74–6). Postcoarctation aneurysm formation occurred commonly when angioplasty alone was used to treat native coarctation, but appears to be less of a concern with the wider use of stents.[25]

LONG-TERM CLINICAL OUTCOMES

The natural history of CoA prior to the modern era of surgical and percutaneous repair was unfortunately quite poor with one large series showing a mortality rate of 25% by age 20, 50% by age 32, 75% by age 46, and 92% by age 60.[26] Although surgical and percutaneous interventions have greatly mitigated this risk, epidemiologic studies still suggest that premature morbidity and mortality remain common in this patient population. In fact, two long-term studies found the mean age of death to be under 40.[27,28] Later problems after coarctation may be due to recoarctation or aneurysm formation at the anastomotic site.[15] Or they may be secondary to associated lesions such as Berry aneurysms of the brain or a bicuspid aortic valve. In at least 5% of patients, re-operation for the aortic valve will be necessary at some point in the future. Also associated with the bicuspid valve is a strong

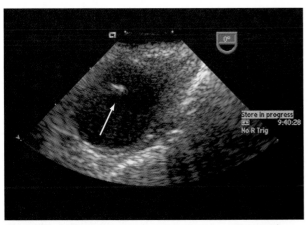

Figure 74–6. The presence of endarteritis in a patient with prior percutaneous balloon angioplasty. A transesophageal echocardiographic view of a linear strand (*arrow*) emanating from the aortic wall just distal to the site of prior percutaneous intervention to a coarcted segment of the descending aorta. This patient had blood cultures positive for *Staphylococcus aureus* and the lesion was later confirmed to be a vegetation. He was successfully treated with surgery and prolonged intravenous antibiotics.

predilection for aortic dilatation and the potential for aortic dissection. Finally, there is evidence that hypertension is substantially more prevalent in these patients, developing at a far younger age than would normally be expected. Hypertension is likely an important mediator of the accelerated atherogenesis reported in patients with CoA. Of late deaths in CoA, up to one-third are related to acute myocardial infarction, so the importance of cardiovascular risk reduction in these patients should not be overlooked.

HYPERTENSION IN THE COARCTATION PATIENT

Probably the best recognized complication resulting from CoA is hypertension. It is thought to directly contribute to the poor prognosis associated with unrepaired coarctation by increasing the risk of myocardial infarction, intracranial hemorrhage, aortic dissection, and congestive heart failure. In one early series, 25% of unrepaired patients died before age 20, 50% before age 32, 75% before age 46, and 90% before age 58. It was previously hoped that relieving the obstruction would cure the hypertension and return normal life expectancy. Although advancements in both surgical and percutaneous repairs have greatly impacted on the morbidity and mortality of this disorder, the longevity of patients with CoA still appears significantly reduced compared to patients without CoA.

The hypertension in patients with CoA prior to repair is unique, as it affects only the upper extremities. Thus, vascular beds above the CoA are subjected to hypertensive changes while vascular beds below the CoA are generally normotensive or even occasionally hypotensive. Several mechanisms have been proposed to explain the genesis of hypertension in CoA patients.[29] The first is that the stenosis leads to high mechanical resistance to cardiac output that subsequently increases pressure. The second is increased activation of the renin-angiotensin-aldosterone system through underperfusion of the kidneys, the so-called "Goldblatt phenomenon." Finally, the neural hypothesis proposes that baroreceptors in the aorta above the obstruction are reset to facilitate blood flow to the lower parts of the body. It is quite likely that all three mechanisms work in concert in CoA patients to increase blood pressure.

After coarctation repair, blood pressure returns to normal in the upper extremity in the majority of patients, particularly in the young. The development of systemic hypertension following CoA repair should prompt a thorough evaluation to exclude restenosis at the site of surgical or percutaneous repair. In such case, re-intervention may be warranted, which can relieve obstruction and lead to a reduction in upper extremity blood pressure.

The incidence of so called "late hypertension" in repaired CoA patients still far exceeds the incidence of essential hypertension in the general population, suggesting that long-standing perturbations of normal homeostatic mechanisms are present in CoA patients. Previous studies have used fairly conservative definitions for hypertension (including systolic blood pressure higher than 160 and diastolic blood pressure higher than 90 or 95 mmHg) and have been limited by relatively short follow-up periods, and therefore underestimate the true prevalence of hypertension in patients with repaired CoA. In general, the older the patient is at the time of repair, the greater the likelihood of developing long-standing hypertension. One short-duration follow-up series (median 7.5 years) showed that in the absence of recoarctation, no patients operated on prior to age 4 weeks developed hypertension, while over a quarter of patients operated on after 1 year of age developed hypertension.[30] The optimal timing of repair, however, has been greatly debated over the years, and it now appears that performing surgery at age 5 to 6 years (prior to entering primary school) best limits the risk of restenosis and improves long-term clinical outcome.[4]

While surgery is most effective in the younger patient, it is important to recognize that repair of the adult with CoA can still result in a significant systolic blood pressure reduction and reduce the need for antihypertensive therapy[31,32]; similar results may also be seen with percutaneous interventions. The hypertension that eventually develops despite coarctation repair is almost indistinguishable from essential hypertension, and has led to the study of coarctation patients and animal models of coarctation to gain greater insight into essential hypertension. The primary mechanism is believed to be increased activity of the renin-angiotensin-aldosterone system and volume retention. At the heart of this may be the presence of a small residual gradient at the site of coarctation repair. In a study of 73 patients with repaired coarctation with residual gradients of less than 20 mmHg, the ratio between the diameter of the aorta at the repair site to the diameter at the diaphragmatic aorta was among the strongest independent predictors of elevated ambulatory blood pressure and carotid intimal-medial thickness.[22] Subtle gradients may become particularly more pronounced during exercise when the cardiac output increases significantly.[33,34]

Another mechanism likely to be involved is a reduction in cardiopulmonary baroreceptor sensitivity. The proximal thoracic aorta in CoA has been shown to be stiffer[35] and more fibrotic,[36] which may result in less stretch and activation in response to elevated blood pressure.[37] Such a diminished response remains present more than 10 years after corrective surgery.[38]

Aside from affecting the baroreflex, a stiff, fibrotic ascending aorta may be part of a generalized defect in arterial elasticity and/or reactivity that may result in abnormal vascular function and subsequently hypertension.[29] Several studies have demonstrated abnormal vascular reactivity to various interventions including intra-arterial norepinephrine,[39] reactive hyperemia,[40] and nitrates.[41] It remains unknown, however, whether these vascular abnormalities are a cause or merely a consequence of hypertension.

MEDICAL THERAPY FOR LATE HYPERTENSION

It is generally accepted that antihypertensive therapy should be initiated for any coarctation patient with a resting blood pressure higher than 140/90 mmHg, once the presence of a significant gradient has been properly excluded. Similar to essential hypertension target organ damage such as left ventricular hypertrophy is readily found in hypertensive patients with CoA,[42,43] and therapy may help to prevent these complications. As in patients with essential hypertension, therapy should be initiated and lower goals targeted in the presence of high-risk features such as diabetes and renal insufficiency. Although inhibitors of the renin-angiotensin system are often mentioned as the preferred therapeutic agents for patients with CoA,[44] no long-term efficacy studies exist to confirm the benefits of this strategy.

Up to a third of repaired CoA patients are normotensive at rest but develop a profound hypertensive response to exercise.[45–47] Although there are studies suggesting that normal individuals with a hypertensive response to exercise have a higher risk of developing hypertension or experiencing a cardiovascular event,[48–50] no such evidence exists for CoA patients, and treatment for such patients can therefore not be recommended at this time.[51]

SUMMARY

Coarctation of the aorta is an important cause of secondary hypertension. It is estimated that coarctation accounts for approximately 0.2% of all adults with hypertension. Patients with complex coarctation typically are diagnosed early in childhood, while simple coarctation may not be recognized until adulthood. Coarctation may be associated with other anatomic changes such as bicuspid aortic valve, hypoplasia of the transverse aortic arch and aortic isthmus, poststenotic dilatation of the descending aorta, and cystic medial necrosis of the ascending aorta. The clinical diagnosis of coarctation is suggested by the presence of hypertension in the upper extremities with significantly lower blood pressure in the lower extremities, by the presence of collateral channels manifested as rib notching on the chest x-ray, and by EKG evidence of left ventricular hypertrophy. Echocardiography is an excellent noninvasive tool for diagnosing coarctation of the aorta in patients with suspicious clinical findings. Magnetic resonance imaging has now become the choice imaging modality preoperatively to size the aorta and the coarctation lesion, and is very useful in postoperative follow-up. In the event of a contraindication to MRI or lack of availability, computer tomography scanning is a reasonable alternative.

Interventional therapy for coarctation of the aorta is indicated in the presence of a peak gradient over 30 mmHg, a significant hypertensive response to exercise testing or with concurrent aortic aneurysm or symptomatic aneurysm of the circle of Willis. Surgery remains the mainstay in the treatment of native coarctation of the aorta, although some success has recently been achieved with percutaneous intervention in younger patients. Percutaneous intervention appears particularly effective in the treatment of recoarctation. Postinterventional "late hypertension" is well recognized, and suggests long-standing perturbations of normal homeostatic mechanisms in coarctation patients. Re-coarctation or aneurysm formation at the anastomotic site may also occur. Consequently, follow-up after surgical treatment is a necessity. Medical therapy is indicated for "late hypertension." Overall, the hypertension in coarctation and "late hypertension" carries at least the same cardiovascular risk as hypertension in the general population, including accelerated atherogenesis, and increased risk of myocardial infarction and stroke. Consequently, the importance of cardiovascular risk reduction in these patients should not be overlooked.

REFERENCES

1. Perloff JG. Coarctation of the aorta. In: *Clinical Recognition of Congenital Heart Disease.* 5th ed. Philadelphia: Saunders, 2003:403–29.

2. Hoffman JI, Kaplan S. The incidence of congenital heart disease. *J Am Coll Cardiol* 2002;39:1890–900.

3. Therrien J, Webb G. Clinical update on adults with congenital heart disease. *Lancet* 2003;362:1305–13.

4. Webb G. Treatment of coarctation and late complications in the adult. *Cardiovasc SurgSemin Thorac Cardiovasc Surg* 2005;17:139–42.

5. Prisant LM, Mawulawde K, Kapoor D, Joe C. Coarctation of the aorta: a secondary cause of hypertension. *J Clin Hypertens (Greenwich)* 2004; 6:347–50, 352.

6. Rao PS. Coarctation of the aorta. *Curr Cardiol Rep* 2005;7:425–34.

7. Edwards JE. Aneurysms of the thoracic aorta complicating coarctation. *Circulation* 1973;48:195–201.

8. Oliver JM, Gallego P, Gonzalez A, Aroca A, Bret M, Mesa JM. Risk factors for aortic complications in adults with coarctation of the aorta. *J Am Coll Cardiol* 2004;44:1641–47.

9. Connolly HM, Huston J 3rd, Brown RD Jr, Warnes CA, Ammash NM, Tajik AJ. Intracranial aneurysms in patients with coarctation of the aorta: a prospective magnetic resonance angiography study of 100 patients.*Mayo Clin Proc* 2003; 78:1491–99.

10. Hodes HL, Steinfeld L, Blumenthal S. Congenital cerebral aneurysms and coarctation of the aorta. *Arch Pediatr* 1959;76:28–43.

11. Kaemmerer H. Aortic coarctation and interrupted aortic arch. In: Gatzoulis MA, Webb GD, Daubeney PEF, eds. *Diagnosis and Managment of Adult Congenital Heart Disease.* New York: Churchill Livingstone, 2003:253–64.

12. Glancy DL, Morrow AG, Simon AL, Roberts WC. Juxtaductal aortic coarctation. Analysis of 84 patients studied hemodynamically, angiographically, and morphologically after age 1 year. *Am J Cardiol* 1983; 51:537–51.

13. Johns KJ, Johns JA, Feman SS. Retinal vascular abnormalities in patients with coarctation of the aorta. *Arch Ophthalmol* 1991;109:1266–68.

14. Weyman AE, Caldwell RL, Hurwitz RA, Girod DA, Dillon JC, Feigenbaum H, et al. Cross-sectional echocardiographic detection of aortic obstruction. 2. Coarctation of the Aorta. *Circulation* 1978;57:498–502.

15. Celermajer DS, Greaves K. Survivors of coarctation repair: fixed but not cured. *Heart* 2002;88:113–14.

16. Marx GR. "Repaired" aortic coarctation in adults: not a "simple" congenital heart defect. *J Am Coll Cardiol* 2000; 35:1003–1006.

17. Kupferminc MJ, Lessing JB, Jaffa A, Vidne BA, Peyser MR. Fetomaternal blood flow measurements and management of combined coarctation and aneurysm of the thoracic aorta in pregnancy. *Acta Obstet Gynecol Scand* 1993;72:398–402.

18. Crafoord C, Nylin G. Congenital coarctation of the aorta and its surgical treatment. *Cardiovasc SurgJ Thorac Cardiovasc Surg* 1945;14:347–61.

19. Corno AF, Botta U, Hurni M, Payot M, Sekarski N, Tozzi P, et al. Surgery for aortic coarctation: a 30 years experience. *Eur J Cardiothorac Surg* 2001;20:1202–206.

20. Rothman A. Coarctation of the aorta: an update. *Curr Probl Pediatr* 1998; 28:33–60.

21. Vriend JW, Mulder BJ. Late complications in patients after repair of aortic coarctation: implications for management. *Int J Cardiol* 2005; 101:399–406.

22. Vriend JW, Zwinderman AH, de Groot E, Kastelein JJ, Bouma BJ, Mulder BJ. Predictive value of mild, residual descending aortic narrowing for blood pressure and vascular damage in patients after repair of aortic coarctation. *Eur Heart J* 2005;26:84–90.

23. Fawzy ME, Awad M, Hassan W, Al Kadhi Y, Shoukri M, Fadley F. Long-term outcome (up to 15 years) of balloon angioplasty of discrete native coarctation of the aorta in adolescents and adults. *J Am Coll Cardiol* 2004; 43:1062–67.

24. Singer MI, Rowen M, Dorsey TJ. Transluminal aortic balloon angioplasty for coarctation of the aorta in the newborn. *Am Heart J* 1982;103:131–32.

25. Piechaud JF. Stent implantation for coarctation in adults. *J Interv Cardiol* 2003;16:413–18.

26. Campbell M. Natural history of coarctation of the aorta. *Br Heart J* 1970;32:633–40.

27. Cohen M, Fuster V, Steele PM, Driscoll D, McGoon DC. Coarctation of the aorta. Long-term follow-up and prediction of outcome after surgical correction. *Circulation* 1989;80:840–5.

28. Presbitero P, Demarie D, Villani M, Perinetto EA, Riva G, Orzan F, et al. Long term results (15–30 years) of surgical repair of aortic coarctation. *Br Heart J* 1987;57:462–67.

29. de Divitiis M, Rubba P, Calabro R. Arterial hypertension and cardiovascular prognosis after successful repair of aortic coarctation: a clinical model for the study of vascular function. *Nutr Metab Cardiovasc Dis* 2005;15:382–94.

30. Seirafi PA, Warner KG, Geggel RL, Payne DD, Cleveland RJ. Repair of coarctation of the aorta during infancy minimizes the risk of late hypertension. *Ann Thorac Surg* 1998;66:1378–82.

31. Ozkokeli M, Gunduz H, Sensoz Y, Ates M, Gunay R, Tayyareci G, et al. Blood pressure changes after aortic coarctation surgery performed in adulthood. *J Card Surg* 2005; 20:319–21.

32. Ozyazicioglu A, Ates A, Yekeler I, Balci AY, Bozkurt E. Repair of coarctation of the aorta in adults and hypertension. *Cardiovasc Surg* 2003;11:353–57.

33. Freed MD, Rocchini A, Rosenthal A, Nadas AS, Castaneda AR. Exercise-induced hypertension after surgical repair of coarctation of the aorta. *Am J Cardiol* 1979;43:253–58.

34. James FW, Kaplan S. Systolic hypertension during submaximal exercise after correction of coarctation of aorta. *Circulation* 1974;50(Suppl 2):II27–34.

35. Sehested J, Baandrup U, Mikkelsen E. Different reactivity and structure of the prestenotic and poststenotic aorta in human coarctation. Implications for baroreceptor function. *Circulation* 1982;65:1060–65.

36. Niwa K, Perloff JK, Bhuta SM, Laks H, Drinkwater DC, Child JS, et al. Structural abnormalities of great arterial walls in congenital heart disease: light and electron microscopic analyses. *Circulation* 2001;103:393–400.

37. Beekman RH, Katz BP, Moorehead-Steffens C, Rocchini AP. Altered baroreceptor function in children with systolic hypertension after coarctation repair. *Am J Cardiol* 1983;52:112–17.

38. Johnson D, Perrault H, Vobecky SJ, Trudeau F, Delvin E, Fournier A, et al. Resetting of the cardiopulmonary baroreflex 10 years after surgical repair of coarctation of the aorta. *Heart* 2001; 85:318–25.

39. Gidding SS, Rocchini AP, Moorehead C, Schork MA, Rosenthal A. Increased forearm vascular reactivity in patients with hypertension after repair of coarctation. *Circulation* 1985;71:495–99.

40. Gardiner HM, Celermajer DS, Sorensen KE, Georgakopoulos D, Robinson J, Thomas O, et al. Arterial reactivity is significantly impaired in normotensive young adults after successful repair of aortic coarctation in childhood. *Circulation* 1994; 89:1745–50.

41. de Divitiis M, Pilla C, Kattenhorn M, Zadinello M, Donald A, Leeson P, et al. Vascular dysfunction after repair of coarctation of the aorta: impact of early surgery. *Circulation* 2001;104(Suppl): I165–70.

42. de Divitiis M, Pilla C, Kattenhorn M, Donald A, Zadinello M, Wallace S, et al. Ambulatory blood pressure,

left ventricular mass, and conduit artery function late after successful repair of coarctation of the aorta. *J Am Coll Cardiol* 2003;41:2259–65.

43. Krogmann ON, Rammos S, Jakob M, Corin WJ, Hess OM, Bourgeois M. Left ventricular diastolic dysfunction late after coarctation repair in childhood: influence of left ventricular hypertrophy. *J Am Coll Cardiol* 1993; 21:1454–60.

44. Swan L, Ashrafian H, Gatzoulis MA. Repair of coarctation: a higher goal? *Lancet* 2002;359:977–78.

45. Markel H, Rocchini AP, Beekman RH, Martin J, Palmisano J, Moorehead C, et al. Exercise-induced hypertension after repair of coarctation of the aorta: arm versus leg exercise. *J Am Coll Cardiol* 1986;8:165–71.

46. Pelech AN, Kartodihardjo W, Balfe JA, Balfe JW, Olley PM, Leenen FH. Exercise in children before and after coarctectomy: hemodynamic, echocardiographic, and biochemical assessment. *Am Heart J* 1986; 112:1263–70.

47. Sigurdardottir LY, Helgason H. Exercise-induced hypertension after corrective surgery for coarctation of the aorta. *Pediatr Cardiol* 1996;17:301–307.

48. Allison TG, Cordeiro MA, Miller TD, Daida H, Squires RW, Gau GT. Prognostic significance of exercise-induced systemic hypertension in healthy subjects. *Am J Cardiol* 1999;83:371–75.

49. Sharabi Y, Ben-Cnaan R, Hanin A, Martonovitch G, Grossman E. The significance of hypertensive response to exercise as a predictor of hypertension and cardiovascular disease. *J Hum Hypertens* 2001;15:353–56.

50. Singh JP, Larson MG, Manolio TA, O'Donnell CJ, Lauer M, Evans JC, et al. Blood pressure response during treadmill testing as a risk factor for new-onset hypertension. The Framingham Heart Study. *Circulation* 1999;99:1831–36.

51. Swan L, Goyal S, Hsia C, Hechter S, Webb G, Gatzoulis MA. Exercise systolic blood pressures are of questionable value in the assessment of the adult with a previous coarctation repair. *Heart* 2003;89:189–92.

Chapter

75 Hypertension Due to Central Nervous System Dysfunction

J. David Spence

Definition and Key Features

- Conditions affecting the central nervous system that may cause severe paroxysmal hypertension include stroke and brainstem lesions, carotid endarterectomy, general anesthesia, epilepsy, electroconvulsive therapy, and quadriplegia.
- The principal differential diagnosis is pheochromocytoma.

Therapy

- Management of hypertension in acute stroke must avoid sudden hypotension, which may aggravate ischemia. Labetalol is effective.
- In the management of hypertension in quadriplegic patients, it is important to avoid bladder distension. A beta-adrenergic antagonist in combination with a competitive alpha-blocker is effective.
- During electroconvulsive therapy ganglionic blockade may be achieved with trimethaphan camsylate.
- Epilepsy-related hypertension may be managed with administration of trimethaphan or phenoxybenzamine.

Short-term blood pressure is regulated by the autonomic nervous system (see Chapters 17 and 18). This reflex regulation of blood pressure from beat to beat depends on several key structures: the anterior hypothalamus and brainstem nuclei including the nucleus of the tractus solitarius, baroreceptors in the carotid artery, aorta and heart, stretch receptors in the bowel, bladder, ureters and kidneys, and the intermediolateral cell column, which represents in a sense the "lower motor neurons" of the autonomic system (Figure 75-1).

When these structures are damaged, or their function is disrupted by lesions or events in the central nervous system, severe hypertension can result. Failure of the peripheral autonomic nerves, as in diabetes or amyloidosis (including amyloidosis secondary to "benign" monoclonal gammopathy), causes severe postural hypotension because reflex control of blood pressure is lost. Although hypertension secondary to dysfunction of the central nervous system is uncommon, the syndromes are instructive. Effective management of such events requires an understanding of the mechanisms. For those reasons, this chapter will discuss several examples of hypertension due to disorders of the central nervous system.

ANATOMY AND PATHOLOGY

The hypothalamus has been called the head ganglion of the autonomic nervous system. It has extensive connections with the limbic system, and with the brainstem, so that in addition to influencing the body through pituitary secretions, the hypothalamus is involved in blood pressure regulation via central nervous system control. Nuclei in the brainstem receive inputs from baroreceptors in the heart, aorta, and carotid arteries via the hypoglossal (IXth cranial) nerve. The nucleus of the tractus solitarius, present bilaterally in the lower medial medulla (Figure 75-2), is involved in integrating blood pressure as sensed by the baroreceptors, and sends inputs down the spinal cord to the intermediolateral column (Figure 75-3). These inputs may be inhibitory or excitatory. From the intermediolateral cell column impulses go via cholinergic fibers to sympathetic ganglia, where a multiplier effect occurs: for every one preganglionic fiber approximately 100 postganglionic adrenergic fibers travel to structures including peripheral veins and arteries. Excitatory impulses from the brainstem result in vasoconstriction, whereas inhibitory impulses result in vasodilation. Thus within seconds an elevation of blood pressure is sensed by the baroreceptors, integrated in the brainstem, and vasodilation results from downward inhibitory traffic; a reciprocal sequence results from a drop in blood pressure. This mechanism can be thought of as reflex control of blood pressure through a reflex loop that has its afferent limb in the baroreceptors, integration in the brainstem, descending traffic to the spinal cord, and its efferent limb in preganglionic nerves.

PATHOPHYSIOLOGY

Central nervous system regulation of blood pressure can become disordered at several levels: the hypothalamus, brainstem, baroreceptors, and spinal cord.

Lesions of the hypothalamus may cause severe hypertension either as the result of damage such as infarction, or may be paroxysmally be activated leading to severe hypertension in the setting of epilepsy.

Lesions of the brainstem, including infarction, tumor and compression by vascular loops, may lead to severe hypertension because baroreceptor reflex integration is disturbed by damage to the nucleus of the solitary tract.

Disruption of baroreceptor nerves during carotid endarterectomy or neck dissection for cancer disrupts reflex control of blood pressure by eliminating the afferent limb of the reflex.

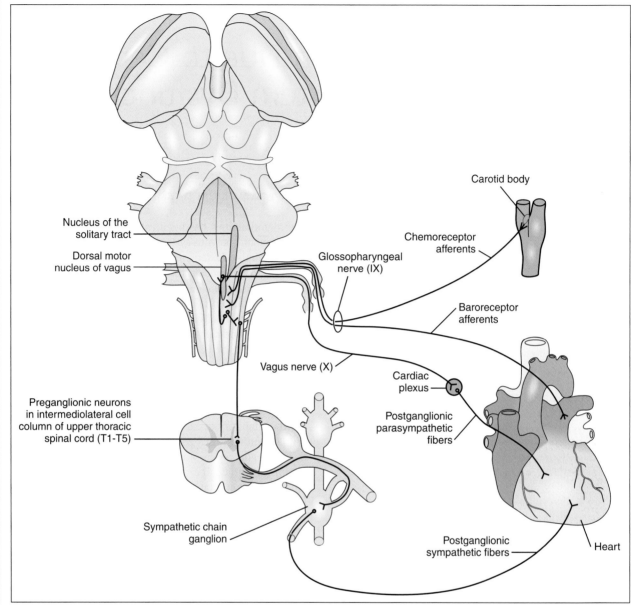

Figure 75–1. Reflex integration of blood pressure. Afferents from baroreceptors in the heart, aorta, and carotid artery ascend via the glossopharyngeal (IXth cranial) nerve to the nucleus of the solitary tract. Descending inputs go via the vagus to the heart and down to the intermediolateral cell column of the spinal cord (T_1-T_5). (Redrawn from Purves D, Augustine GJ, Fitzpatrick D, et al. *Neuroscience.* 2nd ed. Sunderland, MA: Sinauer Associates, Inc., 2001, Figure 21.7.)

In quadriplegic patients, damage to the cervical cord interrupts the connections between the brainstem and the intermediolateral cell column (which is located in the thoracic cord). Distension of viscera including the ureter, kidneys, bladder, or bowel causes afferent traffic to the spinal cord, which leads to reflex activation of sympathetic nerves in the intermediolateral cell column and a rise in blood pressure that can no longer be corrected by the brainstem in response to baroreceptor input. The result is severe hypertension with bradycardia, because the vagus is intact.

In patients under deep general anesthesia the reflex control of blood pressure may be impaired, with the potential for severe hypertension related to visceral distension or traction. In patients who undergo carotid endarterectomy or neck dissection for cancer, the baroreceptor nerves may be damaged, so that the afferent loop of the reflex is lost.

CLINICAL PRESENTATIONS

Several cases are presented below to illustrate the various presentations of hypertension attributable to central nervous system dysfunction.

Hypertension as consequence of stroke and brainstem lesions

In 1974, Mazey[1] described a syndrome resembling pheochromocytoma following a stroke. Two years later, the author

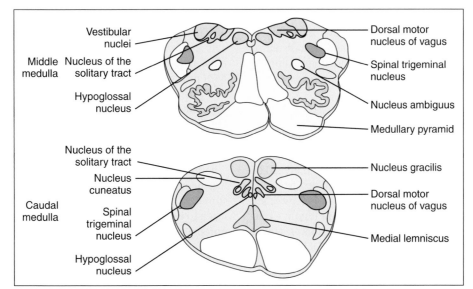

Figure 75–2. The dorsal motor nucleus of the vagus, and the nucleus of the solitary tract, in the lower medulla. (Redrawn from Purves D, Augustine GJ, Fitzpatrick D, et al. *Neuroscience.* 2nd ed. Sunderland, MA: Sinauer Associates, Inc., 2001.)

admitted a 36-year-old woman with no previous history of hypertension, who presented with a brainstem infarction and severe labile hypertension, ranging from 200/100 to 230/130, with a heart rate of 70 to 80 per minute. She was shaky and sweaty, raising the possibility of pheochromocytoma. Most of her findings were consistent with lateral

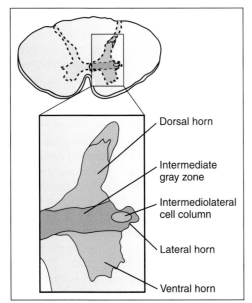

Figure 75–3. Intermediolateral cell column. In the thoracic cord (T_1–T_5), the intermediolateral cell column represents the equivalent of the "lower motor neurons" of the sympathetic nervous system. Their axons terminate on the sympathetic ganglia. (Redrawn from Purves D, Augustine GJ, Fitzpatrick D, et al. *Neuroscience.* 2nd ed. Sunderland, MA: Sinauer Associates, Inc., 2001, Figure 21.2.)

medullary syndrome, but she had some pontine involvement, and some features of medial medullary syndrome. Her cerebral angiogram showed bilateral lesions at the C1-2 level typical of chiropractic injury, and upon questioning she reported that she had undergone chiropractic manipulation with rotation of the neck the day before her stroke. Plasma catecholamines were initially moderately elevated, with a plasma norepinephrine that was three times the upper limit of normal for the author's laboratory. She was managed initially with phenoxybenzamine and propranolol, but over the course of 3 weeks her blood pressure settled down and these medications were gradually stopped. She made a good recovery from her brainstem infarction.

Such patients present a "chicken-and-egg" problem; often it is assumed that the hypertension caused the stroke, rather than the reverse. It seems that in this case the severe hypertension was due to interruption of baroreceptor reflexes by damage to the nucleus of the tractus solitarius (NTS); this problem is more common with brainstem infarctions than with carotid territory ischemia, but Nathan and Reis[2,3] showed that severe hypertension with 100-fold elevations of plasma renin and elevated catecholamines could be produced in rats with lesions of either the NTS or of the anterior hypothalamus. Thus a large infarction with carotid occlusion affecting the hypothalamus might also present in this way. Reis and Doba[4] also presented a case of hypertension secondary to a mass lesion of the brainstem. Tumors of the fourth ventricle can also cause hypertension, presumably by irritating or compressing structures in the floor of the ventricle, and basilar artery aneurysm has been described with a syndrome resembling pheochromocytoma.[5]

Jannetta[6] showed that several paroxysmal cranial nerve syndromes such as tic doloureux, hemifacial spasm, vertigo, and glossopharyngeal neuralgia may be due to pulsatile compression of the involved cranial nerves by vascular loops, and that surgical decompression is an effective treatment in many such cases. Similarly, Levy et al.[7] have proposed that paroxysmal hypertension, and even sustained hypertension, may be due to medullary compression by vascular loops, and relieved by surgical decompression.

Cushing reflex

A 32-year-old auto mechanic presented to the emergency room after a witnessed generalized tonic-clonic seizure. He was comatose, with right hemiplegia, bilateral papilledema, and a blood pressure of 236/130 mmHg. The house staff admitted him with a diagnosis of hypertensive encephalopathy, but his examination the next morning was more consistent with a left hemisphere lesion. Computerized tomography showed a large brain tumor, with a 2-cm midline shift. On biopsy, the lesion was a high-grade glioma. He died several weeks later. It seems likely that his markedly elevated blood pressure was due to a Cushing reflex, with elevation of blood pressure secondary to raised intracranial pressure.

Hypertension in patients with quadriplegia

A 23-year-old quadriplegic man presented to the neurosurgery service with a C5–6 lesion sustained a month earlier by diving into a quarry and striking his head on a rock. He was being taught to empty his bladder with a tap maneuver, and during this session he became very pale and diaphoretic, and developed a severe headache. His blood pressure was 230/130 mmHg, and he was developing acute pulmonary edema. With catheterization and emptying of the bladder, the entire syndrome abated immediately.

Several years later I was consulted about a similar event with severe hypertension and an intracerebral hemorrhage triggered by bladder distension in a young man with quadriplegia. Such patients with quadriplegia and severe hypertension during bladder distension had high plasma catecholamines during bladder distension in the course of a cystometrogram, and the elevation of plasma catecholamines during bladder distension could be blunted by treatment with phenoxybenzamine. This syndrome has been described by several authors.[8–10] Severe paroxysms of hypertension have also been described in quadriplegia during lithotripsy.[11]

Hypertension during general anesthesia

During surgery for treatment of a cerebral aneurysm, hypotension often is induced to reduce the risk of catastrophic hemorrhage in the event of rupture of the aneurysm during clipping. I report here one case where, despite efforts to achieve hypotension with trimethaphan camsylate, the patient's blood pressure did not fall, and she was not producing urine despite having been given 500 mL of mannitol to slacken her brain. It was found that her urinary catheter was kinked, and once the kink was removed, her blood pressure decreased dramatically. It appears that the general anesthetic had interfered with reflex control of blood pressure, so that the stimulus from bladder distension had caused hypertension. Reflex

activation of blood pressure by bladder distension, and termination of that activation by bladder emptying probably account also for micturition syncope and the hypotension sometimes seen after catheterization of old men with prostatic obstruction.

A related phenomenon is the severe hypertension that sometimes occurs after removal of a pheochromocytoma. During the surgery, the general anesthetic inactivates the autonomic system; but in the recovery room when the patient begins to shiver and experience piloerection, severe hypertension may develop even though the tumor has been successfully removed, because catecholamine stored in the sympathetic nerve boutons requires about a week to be exhausted. (Approximately 80% of discharged norepinephrine is taken back up into the bouton after discharge, so it is recycled and takes some time to be depleted.) It is therefore advisable to leave a phentolamine infusion hanging for some time after removal of a pheochromocytoma in case it is needed. (A missed pheochromocytoma in the case of multiple pheochromocytomas is another possible cause of this phenomenon. It is for that reason that abdominal exploration during removal of a pheochromocytoma is advocated, rather than posterior removal of the single recognized pheochromocytoma.)

Hypertension in patients undergoing carotid endarterectomy

A 67-year-old woman underwent right carotid endarterectomy because of severe symptomatic stenosis. A left carotid endarterectomy had been performed 3 years earlier because of symptomatic severe stenosis. Preoperatively she was mildly hypertensive, with pressures around 150/90, and was being treated with propranolol. Immediately postoperatively, she became extremely hypertensive, with a blood pressure of 250/150 mmHg, with shaking, diaphoresis, and pallor that raised the possibility of pheochromocytoma. She was treated with phentolamine and phenoxybenzamine; indeed over the next 2 days she exhausted the entire supply of phenoxybenzamine in the city, and an emergency supply had to be flown in. Her plasma catecholamines were elevated to around four times the upper limit of normal, but extensive investigation including computerized tomography and nuclear medicine scanning with metaiodobenzylguanidine ruled out pheochromocytoma. Her blood pressure stabilized over the course of a month. Rebound hypertension from propranolol withdrawal was a consideration, but a virtually identical experience several years later with a patient who underwent bilateral neck dissection with cancer suggests that interruption of baroreceptor reflexes by the neck dissection was a more likely cause.

This problem is distinctly unusual and no case was reported among the 1108 patients randomized to endarterectomy in the North American Carotid Endarterectomy trial.[12] However, it has been suggested that the problem is more common than is recognized.[13,14] There does not appear to be a long-term effect of carotid endarterectomy on blood pressure.[15]

A more common problem is moderate hypertension following endarterectomy, with a syndrome resembling unilateral hypertensive encephalopathy. This syndrome of cerebral hyperperfusion[16] appears to be due to hypertension (possibly related to the neck dissection[17,18]) with sudden increased perfusion pressure after a severe stenosis is alleviated. Breakthrough of cerebral autoregulation in this circumstance probably results from high pressure entering a circulatory bed that was previously under low pressure, with the consequent loss of hypertensive remodeling of the resistance vessels.

Hypertension in epilepsy

Rarely, epilepsy may present with a syndrome resembling pheochromocytoma.[19] Seizures originating in the diencephalon,[19] hypothalamus,[20] or temporal lobe[21] can elevate blood pressure and plasma catecholamines, presumably by activating hypothalamic, limbic, and insular structures relating to autonomic function. In addition to elevation of plasma norepinephrine, hypothalamic seizures have been shown to elevate levels of prolactin and adrenocorticotropic hormone.[20]

Hypertension in patients undergoing electroconvulsive therapy

Some patients have severe hypertension, in the range of 250/150 mmHg, immediately after electroconvulsive (ECT) therapy. Extensive investigation ruled out pheochromocytoma in both cases. It is suspected that this syndrome, which may be more common with bilateral than with unilateral ECT, is pathophysiologically similar to the severe hypertension that may occur with epilepsy.

DIAGNOSTIC TECHNIQUES

In these conditions the diagnosis is made by recognizing and understanding the pathophysiology as described in this chapter, and by exclusion of pheochromocytoma and other causes that may be contributing. For example, in addition to cervical spinal cord transection, obstruction to outflow of urine by a kinked catheter or by prostatic disease may be the immediate cause of the hypertension; catheterization, or suprapubic drainage may be needed in emergency circumstances with severe hypertension and pulmonary edema.

The principal differential diagnosis is that of pheochromocytoma, and the association of bladder distension with paroxysms of hypertension, diaphoresis, and pallor will raise the specter of a pheochromocytoma related to the bladder. A second competing problem of the chicken-and-egg variety is that seizures may complicate severe hypertension from other causes, so that it may be thought that the epilepsy was the cause of the hypertension, rather than the result of the hypertension. This has been described with renovascular hypertension[22] and pheochromocytoma.[23] In my experience, it is much more common for the seizures to be secondary to the hypertension, rather than the epilepsy being the cause of the hypertension.

The differentiation of pheochromocytoma from quadriplegic hypertensive crises requires careful and thoughtful investigation.[10,24] Plasma catecholamines will be elevated to several times above the lab reference range in many of these cases, but seldom are extremes of catecholamine elevation seen as with pheochromocytoma. A 24-hour urine collection for metanephrine will be more abnormal in pheochromocytoma, and in most of these circumstances such as pseudopheochromocytoma following stroke, the syndrome settles down over several weeks. In the meantime if blood pressure is very difficult to control, it may be necessary to go on to imaging studies, including computed tomography, MRI, or nuclear medicine imaging with metaiodobenzylguanidine, which can identify pheochromocytomas anywhere from the bladder to the base of the skull.

MANAGEMENT

Management of hypertension in acute stroke

In the past, many experts recommended that the elevation of blood pressure during acute stroke should remain untreated, since abrupt lowering of blood pressure to levels that are too low may exacerbate brain ischemia. However, that recommendation is too simplistic, as sometimes the blood pressure must be treated.[25] For example, in a patient whose stroke is caused by aortic dissection that occludes a carotid artery and at the same time occludes a renal artery, the severe hypertension from the renal artery occlusion must be treated. Similarly, a patient with severe hypertension who is in pulmonary edema with a recent myocardial infarction that has caused an embolic stroke must have the hypertension treated on account of the pulmonary edema and myocardial ischemia. Recently the Acute Candesartan Cilexitil in Stroke Survivors (ACCESS) trial[26] showed that treatment with candesartan in acute stroke was associated with improved outcomes; however, to conclude that the improvement was due to blood pressure reduction is problematic; benefits may have been related to protective effects of angiotensin receptor blockade.[27]

The real issue is not whether to treat hypertension in acute stroke; it is how to treat it. The principal concern is to avoid sudden hypotension that may aggravate ischemia; for this reason sublingual nifedipine should never be used in acute stroke.[28] Intravenous drugs such as labetolol are probably best for this purpose, but before initiating treatment with a beta blocker it is important to draw blood for plasma renin and aldosterone, so that the underlying cause of the severe hypertension can be identified and treated specifically after the crisis has resolved.[29,30]

This topic is discussed in detail in Chapter 48 and is also touched on in Chapter 71.

Management of hypertension in quadriplegic patients

Attention to avoidance of bladder distension is part of management, but I have found that phenoxybenzamine was successful in a number of cases. Unfortunately this drug (a noncompetitive blocker of alpha receptors, and therefore better suited to paroxysmal hypertension such as with pheochromocytoma) is increasingly difficult to obtain, so it may be more practical to use beta-adrenergic antagonists in combination with the less satisfactory competitive alpha-blocker such as doxazosin (which is longer acting than terazosin or prazosin). Phentolamine infusion may be used in short-term settings in hospital. Stimulation with transcutaneous electrical nerve stimulation has been described as a treatment for paroxysmal hypertension during colonic distension in quadriplegic rats,[31] so this may offer an alternative in some cases. Clonidine has been used to treat this condition,[32] but because of my experience with severe rebound hypertension from clonidine withdrawal, I avoid using this drug.

Electroconvulsive therapy

A good approach to the management of severe hypertension during electroconvulsive therapy was described by Petrides et al.[33] using intravenous trimethaphan camsylate (Arfonad). They found that a bolus of 15 mg was more effective than lower doses. This treatment is physiologically sound, as it represents ganglionic blockade. It is also practical, as anesthetists are commonly involved in the care of patients during electroconvulsive therapy, which is a brief scheduled event. Nicardipine and labetolol in combination have been used to treat this problem,[34,35] but because these drugs are competitive antagonists, they are less logical, and in my view less likely to be effective than ganglionic blockade.

Epilepsy

By analogy with hypertension during electroconvulsive therapy, it seems likely that trimethaphan may also be useful therapy during hypertensive emergencies caused by diencephalic epilepsy; however, for preventing hypertension during seizures that occur outside the hospital setting, phenoxybenzamine would be the most effective therapy if available.

Here an explanation is in order for the need for a noncompetitive alpha receptor antagonist. Paroxysmal hypertension due to discharge of catecholamines from sympathetic nerve boutons is best treated with phenoxybenzamine because it is a noncompetitive antagonist. It binds covalently to alpha receptors, so that when a norepinephrine molecule arrives the receptor is already occupied (Figure 75–4). Because the paroxysm releases such a flood of catecholamines, it is not possible to treat this effectively with competitive alpha-blockers: in order to have enough antagonist on board to deal with the paroxysm when it happens, the blood pressure while standing would be so low between paroxysms that the patient would not be able to walk around. This principle applies equally to the management of pheochromocytoma and to that of disorders of reflex control of blood pressure in which severe hypertension results from paroxysmal sympathetic discharge.

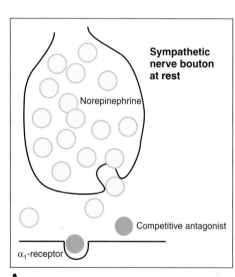

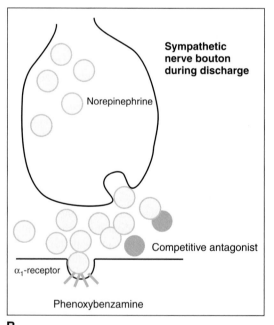

A **B**

Figure 75–4. Noncompetitive α-receptor antagonism with phenoxybenzamine. Norepinephrine (white circles) is released from a sympathetic nerve bouton, stimulating the postsynaptic α₁-receptor. Competitive antagonists such as phentolamine or doxazosin (*purple circles*) block the stimulation by competing for the receptor. This is successful at reasonable doses of antagonist while the sympathetic nerves are quiescent (*left above*), but when a paroxysmal discharge floods the synaptic space with excess norepinephrine (*right above*), the effect of the competitive antagonist is overcome by norepinephrine's competition for the receptor. Phenoxybenzamine (*purple bars*) binds covalently to the receptor, so that no matter how much norepinephrine is present in the synaptic space, the receptor cannot respond. This principle is the reason that phenoxybenzamine is the preferred α-blocker for severe paroxysmal hypertension due to adrenergic agonism, such as in pheochromocytoma, or in hypertension due to central nervous system disorders that cause loss of reflex control of blood pressure.

PROGNOSIS

The prognosis of hypertension secondary to lesions of the central nervous system depends on how high the pressure goes, how well and how quickly it is controlled, and in part on the premorbid state of the vasculature. Patients who previously had low blood pressure will be at greater risk from a sudden severe rise in pressure because they will not have adaptive hypertrophy of their resistance vessels, and they will therefore be more likely to sustain a brain hemorrhage or hypertensive encephalopathy. In the longer term, the severe hypertension due to loss of reflex blood pressure control generally abates over several weeks with acute lesions such as stroke or carotid dissection. Surgical removal of the brainstem compression generally resolves the problem within days. The prognosis in epileptic cases depends on control of the epilepsy, and in this regard it is worth considering surgical treatment of the epilepsy if there is an accessible lesion, as surgical treatment of epilepsy is much more effective than medical therapy in resistant cases.[36,37] Hypertension during electroconvulsive therapy can usually be managed, and because it occurs during a planned procedure, the management is usually successful.

The principal exception is the syndrome of hypertension during bladder distension due to cervical cord transaction, which may continue for years.

SUMMARY

Lesions of the central nervous system can cause acute severe hypertension due to loss of reflex control of blood pressure. The principal differential diagnosis is pheochromocytoma. When bladder distension is the trigger for the hypertensive crisis, emptying the bladder will usually solve the immediate crisis, but longer-term management will usually be required to prevent recurrence. For severe hypertension due to electroconvulsive therapy, because it is a brief scheduled event, the ganglionic blocker trimethaphan camsylate is a practical therapy. However, for most of these conditions more long-term therapy is required, and phenoxybenzamine, because it binds covalently to alpha-receptors, is the treatment of choice.

It is therefore a problem, not only for the management of pheochromocytoma but also for the management of reflex disorders of blood pressure regulation such as the conditions described in this chapter, that phenoxybenzamine is now so difficult to obtain. It is hoped that regulatory authorities and the pharmaceutical industry will address it. Development of an alternative noncompetitive antagonist might be an alternative to making phenoxybenzamine more readily available, but the market is so small that such a product should probably be regarded as an orphan drug.

REFERENCES

1. Mazey RM, Kotchen TA, Ernst CB. A syndrome resembling pheochromocytoma following a stroke. Report of a case. *JAMA* 1974; 230:575–7.
2. Nathan MA, Reis DJ. Chronic labile hypertension produced by lesions of the nucleus tractus solitarii in the cat. *Circ Res* 1977;40:72–81.
3. Nathan MA, Reis DJ. Fulminating arterial hypertension with pulmonary edema from release of adrenomedullary catecholamines after lesions of the anterior hypothalamus in the rat. *Circ Res* 1975;37:226–35.
4. Reis DJ, Doba N. Hypertension as a localizing sign of mass lesions of brainstem. *N Engl J Med* 1972;287: 1355–6.
5. Emanuele MA, Dorsch TR, Scarff TB, Lawrence AM. Basilar artery aneurysm simulating pheochromocytoma. *Neurology* 1981;31:1560–1.
6. Jannetta PJ. Outcome after microvascular decompression for typical trigeminal neuralgia, hemifacial spasm, tinnitus, disabling positional vertigo, and glossopharyngeal neuralgia (honored guest lecture). *Clin Neurosurg* 1997;44:331–83.
7. Levy EI, Scarrow AM, Jannetta PJ. Microvascular decompression in the treatment of hypertension: review and update. *Surg Neurol* 2001;55:2–10.
8. Chua KS, Kong KH, Tan ES. Paroxysmal hypertension in a C4 spinal cord injury—a case report. *Ann Acad Med Singapore* 1995;24:470–2.

9. Naftchi NE, Demeny M, Lowman EW, Tuckman J. Hypertensive crises in quadriplegic patients. Changes in cardiac output, blood volume, serum dopamine-beta-hydroxylase activity, and arterial prostaglandin PGE2. *Circulation* 1978;57:336–41.
10. Mathias CJ, Christensen NJ, Corbett JL, Frankel HL, Spalding JM. Plasma catecholamines during paroxysmal neurogenic hypertension in quadriplegic man. *Circ Res* 1976; 39:204–8.
11. Chen L, Castro AD. Autonomic hyperreflexia during extracorporeal shock-wave lithotripsy (ESWL) in quadriplegic patients. *Can J Anaesth* 1989;36:604–5.
12. Barnett HJ, Taylor DW, Eliasziw M, et al. Benefit of carotid endarterectomy in patients with symptomatic moderate or severe stenosis. North American Symptomatic Carotid Endarterectomy Trial Collaborators. *N Engl J Med* 1998; 339:1415–25.
13. De Toma G, Nicolanti V, Plocco M, et al. Baroreflex failure syndrome after bilateral excision of carotid body tumors: an underestimated problem. *J Vasc Surg* 2000;31:806–10.
14. Timmers HJ, Wieling W, Karemaker JM, Lenders JW. Baroreflex failure: a neglected type of secondary hypertension. *Neth J Med* 2004;62:151–5.
15. Eliasziw M, Spence JD, Barnett HJ. Carotid endarterectomy does not affect long-term blood pressure: observations from the NASCET. North American

Symptomatic Carotid Endarterectomy Trial. *Cerebrovasc Dis* 1998;8:20–4.
16. Streifler JY, Israel D, Melamed E. The hyperperfusion syndrome: an under-recognized complication of carotid endarterectomy. *Isr Med Assoc J* 2004;6:54–6.
17. Timmers HJ, Buskens FG, Wieling W, Karemaker JM, Lenders JW. Long-term effects of unilateral carotid endarterectomy on arterial baroreflex function. *Clin Auton Res* 2004;14:72–9.
18. Timmers HJ, Wieling W, Karemaker JM, Lenders JW. Cardiovascular responses to stress after carotid baroreceptor denervation in humans. *Ann N Y Acad Sci* 2004;1018:515–9.
19. Charoenlarp K, Buranakitjaroen P, Gulprasutdilog S, Prayoonwiwat N, Jaroonvesama N. Diencephalic epilepsy resembling pheochromocytoma: a first reported case in Thailand. *J Med Assoc Thai* 1995;78:332–6.
20. Cerullo A, Tinuper P, Provini F, et al. Autonomic and hormonal ictal changes in gelastic seizures from hypothalamic hamartomas. *Electroencephalogr Clin Neurophysiol* 1998;107:317–22.
21. Brown RW, McLeod WR. Sympathetic stimulation with temporal lobe epilepsy. *Med J Aust* 1973;2:274–6.
22. Chen TY, Huang LT, Liang CD, Ko SF, Fang CY. Renal artery stenosis presenting with status epilepticus: a report of one case. *Acad Emerg Med* 2002;9:1445–7.
23. Leiba A, Bar-Dayan Y, Leker RR, Apter S, Grossman E. Seizures as a presenting symptom of phaeochromocytoma in

a young soldier. *J Hum Hypertens* 2003;17:73–5.

24. Manger WM, Davis SW, Chu DS. Autonomic hyperreflexia and its differentiation from pheochromocytoma. *Arch Phys Med Rehabil* 1979;60:159–61.

25. Spence JD, Del Maestro RF. Hypertension in acute ischemic strokes. *Treat. Arch Neurol* 1985;42:1000–2.

26. Schrader J, Luders S, Kulschewski A, et al. The ACCESS Study: evaluation of acute candesartan cilexetil therapy in stroke survivors. *Stroke* 2003;34:1699–703.

27. Spence JD. Hypertension and stroke. *Can J Neurol Sci* 2002;29:113–4.

28. Spence JD, Paulson OB, Strandgaard S. Hypertension and stroke. In: Messerli FH, ed. *The ABCs of Antihypertensive Therapy*. 2nd ed. New York: Lippincott Williams & Wilkins, 2000:279–96.

29. Spence JD. The current epidemic of primary aldosteronism: causes and consequences. *J Hypertens* 2004; 22:2038–9.

30. Spence JD. Physiologic tailoring of therapy for resistant hypertension: 20 years' experience with stimulated renin profiling. *Am J Hypertens* 1999;12:1077–83.

31. Collins HL, DiCarlo SE. TENS attenuates response to colon distension in paraplegic and quadriplegic rats. *Am J Physiol Heart Circ Physiol* 2002;283:H1734–9.

32. Mathias CJ, Reid JL, Wing LM, Frankel HL, Christensen NJ. Antihypertensive effects of clonidine in tetraplegic subjects devoid of central sympathetic control. *Clin Sci (Lond)* 1979;57(Suppl 5):425s–8s.

33. Petrides G, Maneksha F, Zervas I, Carasiti I, Francis A. Trimethaphan (Arfonad) control of hypertension and tachycardia during electroconvulsive therapy: a double-blind study. *J Clin Anesth* 1996;8:104–9.

34. Avramov MN, Stool LA, White PF, Husain MM. Effects of nicardipine and labetalol on the acute hemodynamic response to electroconvulsive therapy. *J Clin Anesth* 1998;10:394–400.

35. Zhang Y, White PF, Thornton L, Perdue L, Downing M. The use of nicardipine for electroconvulsive therapy: a dose-ranging study. *Anesth Analg* 2005;100:378–81.

36. Wiebe S. Effectiveness and safety of epilepsy surgery: what is the evidence? *CNS Spectr* 2004;9:120–32.

37. Wiebe S, Blume WT, Girvin JP, Eliasziw M. A randomized, controlled trial of surgery for temporal-lobe epilepsy. *N Engl J Med* 2001;345:311–8.

Chapter

76 Sleep Apnea and Hypertension

Peter Y. Hahn and Virend K. Somers

Key Findings

- Obstructive sleep apnea (OSA) is a common disorder affecting 5% to 25% percent of men and women worldwide.

- OSA is characterized by repetitive partial or total collapse of the pharyngeal airway resulting in arousals and sleep fragmentation.

- Risk factors for OSA include age, male sex, obesity, and retrognathia.

- OSA is diagnosed using polysomnography and is defined by a respiratory disturbance index (RDI) of more than five per hour.

- OSA patients are at increased risk of developing cardiovascular diseases, including hypertension (HTN).

- Disordered sympathetic activation, endothelial dysfunction, inflammation, and insulin resistance may play a role in the development of HTN in OSA.

- Positive airway pressure (PAP) treats OSA by acting as a pneumatic splint, thereby preventing the pharyngeal airway from collapse.

- PAP reduces both nocturnal and daytime blood pressure in OSA patients with HTN.

Obstructive sleep apnea (OSA) is a common disorder affecting 5% to 25% of men and women worldwide.[1] The prevalence of OSA has been reported to be equivalent to that of diabetes. Patients with OSA have a high prevalence of cardiovascular disease, including hypertension, ischemic heart disease, heart failure, and stroke. Epidemiologic studies show that OSA is an important risk factor for the development of systemic hypertension.[2,3] There appears to be direct linear relationship between incidence of hypertension and the severity of OSA.[3] The seventh report by the Joint National Committee on the Detection, Prevention, Evaluation and Treatment of High Blood Pressure (JNC-7) lists OSA as first on the list of causes of secondary hypertension.[4] Although the mechanisms linking OSA and hypertension remain incompletely understood, disordered sympathetic activation, endothelial dysfunction, and inflammation are thought to play important roles. To date, several studies have demonstrated that treatment of OSA has beneficial effects on the treatment and control of systemic hypertension.[5,6] OSA patients already on anti-hypertensive treatment appear to derive particular benefit, suggesting that OSA as a cause of resistant hypertension. Recognizing and diagnosing sleep apnea in patients with hypertension is important considering the potential effective treatments currently available for OSA.

ANATOMY AND PATHOLOGY

The human upper airway is a compliant structure that is susceptible to collapse during inspiration. Obesity is an important risk factor for OSA. Obesity can result in increased fat deposition around the neck resulting in an increased positive pressure outside the airway thereby predisposing to collapse. Any reduction in cross-sectional area of the pharynx and in particular reduced lateral dimensions of the pharynx increases the risk of upper airway collapse. Concordantly, large tonsils, long prominent soft palate, macroglossia, or posterior displacement of the mandible (retrognathia) have all been shown to increase the risk of OSA (Figure 76–1).

Although anatomic predisposition is important, decreased pharyngeal dilator muscle function during sleep also plays an equally important role in the development of upper airway collapse characteristic of obstructive sleep apnea. During the awake state, neuromuscular input to the pharyngeal dilator muscles (e.g., glossopharyngeal) actively keeps the airway patent. Neuromuscular input to the pharyngeal muscles consists of a complex interplay of innervation of over 20 different upper airway muscles (Figure 76–2). This complex system consists of an underlying tonic activation and intermittent phasic activation of the muscles. The phasic activation is a reflex mechanism counteracting the pulses of increased negative intrathoracic pressure generated during inspiration. Both phasic and tonic activation are increased during wakefulness in patients with OSA compared to controls. This is thought to be due to the increased activity required to keep the anatomically compromised airway open. With sleep onset, however, neuromuscular input to the dilator muscles is decreased. The loss of this input puts the airway at increased risk of collapse in individuals with anatomic predisposition leading to obstructive breathing events (Figure 76–3).

PATHOPHYSIOLOGY

Normal sleep is characterized by a state of cardiovascular "relaxation." Blood pressure, both systolic and diastolic, decrease with sleep onset (stages 1 and 2) and with deepening levels of NREM sleep (stages 3 and 4). Heart rate and cardiac output also decrease during NREM sleep. These changes

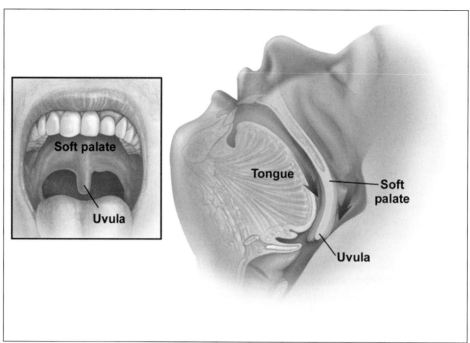

Figure 76–1. Prominent soft palate and uvula.

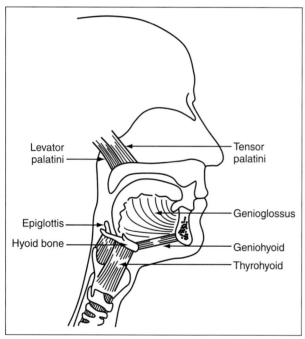

Figure 76–2. Schematic representation of muscles important in the maintenance of upper airway patency.

are likely due to the reduction in sympathetic nervous activity and the progressive rise in parasympathetic activity. During REM sleep, there is increased variability in blood pressure and heart rate with levels approaching those of relaxed wakefulness. Sympathetic nervous activity has been found to be increased during REM sleep, which likely accounts for these findings. Obstructive sleep apnea, however, results in acute hemodynamic effects that disrupt cardiovascular relaxation during sleep.

During obstructive apneas, hypoxemia and hypercapnia stimulate peripheral and central chemoreceptors leading to an increase in sympathetic activity.[7] A progressive rise in sympathetic activity is noted during apneas followed by a peak with arousal and resumption of breathing. Increased SNA results in increased peripheral vascular resistance. Concordantly, blood pressure increases progressively during the apnea and also peaks with arousal (Figure 76–4). Although heart rate and cardiac output decrease during obstructive apneas, both increase dramatically with arousal and resumption of breathing. This increase in cardiac output in the face of continuing severe peripheral vasoconstriction contributes to the large increase in blood pressure observed with arousals.

While much is known regarding the acute hemodynamic effects of OSA, the mechanisms underlying the association of OSA and systemic hypertension remain incompletely understood. Disordered sympathetic activity, however, may play an important role in the development of hypertension in these patients. Patients with OSA have evidence of a heightened sympathetic drive that is present even during wakefulness. This heightened sympathetic drive in patients with OSA is associated with faster heart rates, decreased heart rate variability, and increased blood pressure variability.[8] Previous studies have demonstrated that individuals with decreased heart rate variability are at increased risk of developing future hypertension, while increased blood pressure variability results in target-organ damage.[9]

Abnormal relaxation of the endothelium is thought to represent a nascent form of atherosclerosis and may lead to the development of hypertension and other cardiovascular disorders. Studies have demonstrated that OSA is an independent risk factor for the development of endothelial dysfunction. Patients with OSA who are free of overt cardiovascular or vascular disease have been shown to have

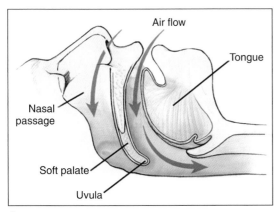

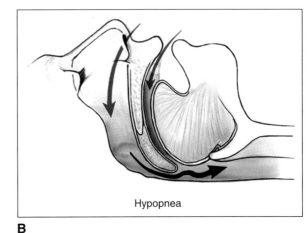

Hypopnea

A

B

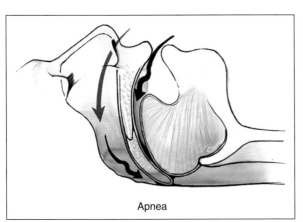

Apnea

C

Figure 76–3. Schematic representation of a patent upper airway. Obstructed breathing manifesting as a hypopnea and apnea are illustrated.

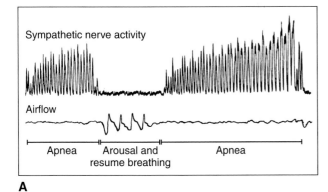

A

B

Figure 76–4. Sympathetic nerve activity rises progressively during an apnea followed by a decrease after arousal and resumption of breathing. Blood pressure gradually rises during the apnea and peaks with arousal.

impaired resistance vessel endothelial function.[2,10] Whether conduit vessel (brachial artery) endothelial function is also impaired is controversial. Disordered sympathetic nervous activity (SNA) may play a role in the development of endothelial dysfunction in patients with OSA, as may inflammation, disordered coagulation, and metabolic dysfunction.

The adhesion of leukocytes to the endothelium can result in impaired endothelial function by interfering with endothelial cell–derived, nitric oxide–dependent vasodilation. Several studies have shown that adhesion molecule expression (ICAMs, VCAMs) is increased in OSA, which suggests that the endothelium is "primed" for leukocyte binding.[11] Furthermore, monocytes isolated from patients with OSA have been shown to have increased expression of adhesion molecules and to have increased *in vitro* binding to cultured endothelial cells. Several studies have also found decreased levels of NO breakdown products in OSA further suggesting impaired synthesis. Levels of inflammatory markers C-reactive protein (CRP) and serum amyloid A (SAA) as well as various cytokines (TNF-a, IL-6,

IL-8) are elevated in patients with OSA also suggesting a state of heightened inflammatory response.[12,13] CRP may directly damage the endothelium, as may reactive oxygen species (ROS), which have also been shown to be increased in patients with OSA.[14] ROS, which can be produced during hypoxia-reoxygenation episodes, may also stimulate leukocyte production of cytokines and upregulation of adhesion molecules on the endothelium.

Other hormonal factors may play a role in the development of hypertension in OSA. Endothelin-1, a potent vasoconstrictor, may be elevated in patients with OSA,[15] and may play a role in the development of hypertension. Dysregulation of leptin, an adipocyte-derived hormone that suppresses appetite and promotes satiety, may also be involved. Leptin is elevated in obese patients, but even further elevated in patients with OSA, suggesting a state of leptin insensitivity. Administration of leptin in an animal model resulted in increases in blood pressure.[16] VEGF, an angiogenesis factor important for normal blood vessel growth is also elevated in OSA, which suggests activation of a protective response to endothelial dysfunction. It remains unclear, however, whether it is the repetitive apneas, arousals, or hypoxemia that is the primary mechanism responsible for these findings.

There is also accumulating evidence linking OSA with glucose intolerance and insulin resistance. Patients with OSA have increased levels of fasting blood glucose, insulin, and glycosylated hemoglobin.[17,18] Furthermore, the severity of OSA appears to correlate with the degree of insulin resistance. The risk of overt diabetes may be increased in patients with severe OSA. The mechanisms underlying this relationship are unclear, but likely are associated with sympathetic activation and sleep deprivation. Glucose intolerance and other metabolic disturbances in OSA may potentially play a role in the development of hypertension in these patients.

CLINICAL PRESENTATIONS

The predominant risk factor for OSA is obesity (body mass index [BMI] >25), and specifically the android pattern of obesity with fat deposition in the neck and trunk.[19] Male sex, increasing age, African-American race, and family history of OSA have also been shown to be risk factors. Postmenopausal status in women is also a risk factor thought to be due to the loss of the protective effects of female hormones.[20] Some studies suggest that hormone replacement therapy (HRT) decreases the prevalence of OSA in postmenopausal women.[21] Although less well defined, smoking and a history of chronic nasal congestion are also considered to be risk factors for OSA.

Patients with OSA may present with both nocturnal symptoms and daytime complaints (Box 76–1). Common nocturnal symptoms include snoring, witnessed apneic pauses, awakenings with choking/gasping or dyspnea, and snort-arousals. Restless sleep, nocturia, and diaphoresis are also common complaints. Most patients with OSA do not complain about difficulty falling asleep. However, studies have suggested that sleep-onset insomnia is not an uncommon complaint. Bruxism, or teeth grinding, has also been

---

Box 76–1

Nocturnal and Daytime Symptoms of Obstructive Sleep Apnea

Daytime Symptoms

Sleepiness
Morning dry mouth
Morning headache
Poor concentration
Cognitive dysfunction
Personality changes
Mood disturbance
Erectile dysfunction
Lower extremity edema

Nocturnal Symptoms

Snoring
Snorts, gasping, choking spells
Restless sleep
Frequent arousals
Nocturia
Diaphoresis
Insomnia
Bruxism
Palpitations

---

shown to be a frequently cited complaint. Patients often will present to the physician primarily due to bed partner complaints or concerns regarding these symptoms.

Common daytime symptoms of OSA include excessive daytime sleepiness (EDS), tiredness and fatigue, cognitive difficulties, and changes in mood. Excessive daytime sleepiness is a common presenting symptom of patients with OSA and can be present with any severity level of OSA. EDS, however, does not correlate directly with OSA severity as measured by the apnea-hypopnea index (AHI), and patients with severe OSA may have no daytime complaints of sleepiness. Sleepiness is often mild and may present predominantly during inactive situations such as during reading, watching TV, while riding as a passenger in a car, and while sitting quietly after lunch. Patients with more severe sleepiness, however, may fall asleep during active situations such as eating, during conversations, and while driving. A commonly used clinical tool to measure the degree of self-reported sleepiness is the Epworth Sleepiness Scale. Many patients, however, complain more of tiredness, fatigue, and lack of energy as opposed to daytime sleepiness.

It is important to note that studies have shown that men and women often have very different clinical presentations. Women report less snoring and witnessed apneas and more daytime fatigue, morning headaches, and complaints of mood disturbance.[22] One study found that women were twice as likely as men to be treated for depression before their OSA diagnosis was established.

On physical examination, increased neck size, retroposition of the mandible or maxilla, large soft palate, and lateral narrowing of the pharyngeal walls have all been shown to be good predictors of OSA.[23] Increased neck circumference (>40 cm) in particular has been shown to be a better predictor of OSA than BMI.[24] Reduced mandibular body length can be manifested by retrognathia (small chin) or overjet (upper teeth resting anteriorly to lower teeth). The relationship between OSA and retroposition of the maxilla is most striking in young patients with craniofacial abnormalities such as Down's syndrome. Obesity itself is associated with increased fat deposition in the tongue, soft palate, uvula, and parapharyngeal fat pads, all of which can compromise upper airway space. Lateral narrowing of the pharyngeal walls may be an important anatomic predictor of OSA.

DIAGNOSTIC TECHNIQUES

Obstructive sleep apnea is diagnosed using overnight polysomnography. Polysomnography (PSG) consists of continuous measurement of nasal pressure, oxygen saturation, electroencephalogram, electro-oculogram, chin and lower extremity electromyography, electrocardiogram, and chest and abdomen plethysmography (Figure 76–5). PSG is performed in the setting of a sleep laboratory and the patient is monitored continuously via video by certified sleep technicians. Important indices determined during PSG include the overall AHI, AHI according to sleep stage and position, and the arousal index (AI). An apnea is defined as the absence of airflow for 10 seconds in the setting of continued respiratory effort (Figure 76–6). A hypopnea is considered to be a decrease in airflow greater than 50% for 10 seconds associated with a 4% drop in saturation and arousal (Figure 76–7). Although there is no universally accepted definition of a respiratory effort–related arousal (RERA) or "snort arousals," they are generally accepted to consist of a transient decrease in air flow followed by an

arousal and normalization of airflow. Crescendo snoring prior to the arousal and mild desaturation of less than 4% after is commonly observed. Simply put, RERAs describe events that do not meet definitions for apneas or hypopneas.

Obstructive sleep apnea has been defined as an AHI of more than five per hour. OSA can be purely positional with obstructive events only occurring during supine sleep. OSA occurring only during REM sleep is also not uncommonly observed. The obstructive sleep apnea syndrome (OSAS) is OSA associated with symptoms of excessive daytime sleepiness, mood disturbance, or impaired cognition. Upper airway resistance syndrome (UARS) was described in 1998 and has been considered to represent a mild form of OSA, where RERAs result in sleep disruption and symptoms of excessive daytime sleepiness.[25] The recently published International Classification of Sleep Disorders-2 (ICSD2), however, defines OSA as more than five respiratory events (apneas, hypopneas, or RERAs) per hour with symptoms, or more than 15 without symptoms. The new ICSD incorporates UARS as part of OSA, given the essentially identical underlying pathophysiology. Generally accepted is the concept that OSA lies on a spectrum that includes severe OSA with cor pulmonale on one end of the spectrum and simple snoring on the other.

MANAGEMENT

Several treatment options exist for OSA, including positional therapy, weight loss, continuous positive airway pressure (CPAP), oral appliances, and surgery. A subset of patients has position-dependent OSA. Positional therapy utilizing tennis balls sewn into the back of a nightshirt is often effective in the treatment of these patients. Weight

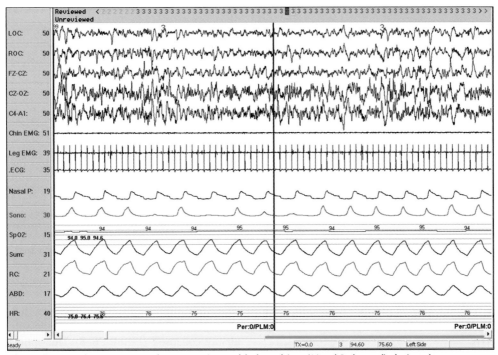

Figure 76–5. Polysomnogram demonstrating stable breathing (*Nasal P* channel) during slow wave sleep. Note the snoring (*Sono* channel).

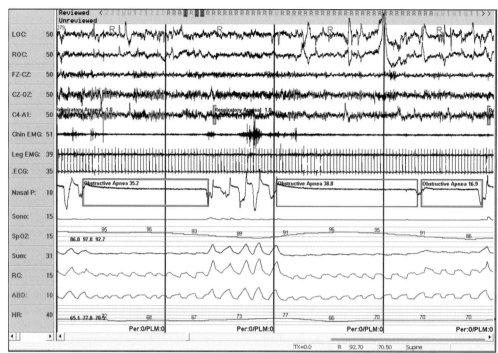

Figure 76–6. Obstructive apneas are demonstrated with absence of flow (*Nasal P* channel) despite continued respiratory efforts (*RC* and *ABD* channels). Note thoracoabdominal paradox (*arrows*) during the apnea, which resolves with resumption of breathing.

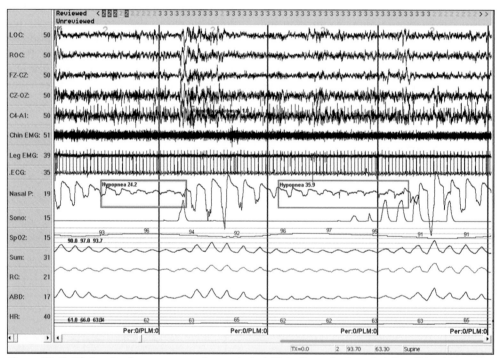

Figure 76–7. Obstructive hypopneas are demonstrated. Note the reduction of airflow (*Nasal P* channel) during the hypopnea followed by arousal and resumption of breathing. Note the decreased saturation following the hypopneas (*SpO2* channel).

loss should be recommended in most OSA patients. Loss of 10% of body weight results in an approximately 20% reduction in AHI.[26]

The primary treatment for obstructive sleep apnea is positive airway pressure in the form of nasal CPAP. CPAP effectively provides a constant pressure to the pharyngeal airway, and thereby acts as pneumatic splint preventing airway collapse[27] (Figure 76–8). The optimal pressure of CPAP is largely a function of sleep stage and position, with the highest pressures usually being required during supine

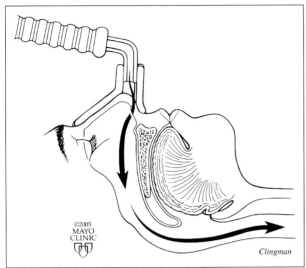

Figure 76–8. CPAP provides positive pressure to the pharyngeal airway thereby preventing collapse.

REM sleep. Pressures between 5 and 15 cm H_2O are commonly used. The optimal CPAP for any given patient is determined during polysomnography. A split-night protocol using both a diagnostic study and CPAP titration over the course of one night is increasingly being used. Although autotitrating CPAP (auto-APA) devices are available, they are not currently recommended for use in determining optimal CPAP pressure in the unattended home setting.

Numerous studies have demonstrated the beneficial effects of CPAP on the daytime and nocturnal symptoms of OSA. However, compliance with CPAP can be a problem in some patients. Depending on the type of surveillance used (e.g., surreptitious) and definition of compliance, overall CPAP compliance is reported to be between 50% and 80%. Rhinorrhea, nasal congestion, headache, and claustrophobic symptoms are common complaints. The degree of sleepiness prior to treatment appears to predict favorable compliance. Interestingly, higher CPAP pressure levels are not associated with decreased compliance. A heated humidifier as part of the CPAP unit and close follow-up 1 month post-CPAP initiation may increase compliance. Compliance is certainly an important issue given that only 46% of patients in one study were reported to use CPAP at least 4 hours for 70% of nights. It is generally accepted that at least 4 hours of usage is required for adequate treatment of daytime symptoms. Despite hope that auto-CPAP or bi-level PAP (bi-PAP) might be better tolerated due to lower mean pressure, studies suggest these may not lead to increased compliance. Other treatments for OSA include oral appliances and surgery. Oral appliances reposition the mandible in a forward position during sleep thereby, increasing upper airway space, and have been shown to be effective in patients with mild to moderate OSA. This therapy is contraindicated in patients with temporal mandibular joint problems or edentulous patients. Current surgical options include uvulopalapharyngoplasty (UPPP) and maxillomandibular advancement (MMA). Gastric bypass procedures can also result in indirect treatment of OSA through their effects on weight loss. The most commonly performed surgical procedure for OSA, UPPP, is unfortunately effective in only about 50% of cases, with effectiveness being measured as at least a 50% decrease in AHI.[28] Many patients will require further treatment of OSA, including CPAP. Patients with milder OSA and those with more pronounced retropalatal obstruction (as opposed to retroglossal) may have more benefit. MMA usually consists of forward advancement of the mandible and maxilla utilizing titanium plates. MMA can be very effective for OSA, with studies documenting approximately a 90% to 95% success rate. Patients with retrognathia may derive particular benefit. Tracheostomy, which allows complete bypass of the collapsible upper airway, was the routine treatment for OSA before the era of CPAP. Although highly effective, it is currently uncommonly used except in severe cases unresponsive to other therapy modalities.

PROGNOSIS

Several studies have demonstrated beneficial effects of CPAP on blood pressure. There has been general agreement on the beneficial effects of CPAP on nocturnal blood pressure. Early studies demonstrated that CPAP restores the normal nocturnal dip in blood pressure (BP) in patients with OSA.[7] The effects on daytime blood pressure, however, have been more controversial, perhaps because early studies were small and observational. Recently, however, several randomized controlled studies have been reported using subtherapeutic or "sham" CPAP.[5,29] Becker et al.[6] reported the largest decrease in blood pressure with CPAP. In a study using noninvasive continuous BP monitoring, OSA patients treated with therapeutic CPAP for 9 weeks had a 10-mmHg decline in daytime systolic and diastolic BP. Patients in this study had at least moderate to severe OSA with a mean AHI of 63, which fell to 3 with CPAP. Interestingly, the subtherapeutic CPAP group did not have a significant change in daytime BP despite having a noticeable reduction in AHI from 65 to 33. Another study by Peperell et al.[5] also showed reduction in daytime BP, albeit a smaller one, in OSA patients treated with CPAP versus sham CPAP. There was an overall reduction in mean BP of 3.4 mmHg. Although they used the oxygen desaturation index (ODI) as opposed to AHI, there appeared to be a greater reduction in daytime mean BP in patients with severe OSA (ODI >33) and patients on antihypertensive medications. CPAP may also have beneficial effects on complications of systemic hypertension including congestive heart failure, atrial fibrillation, and ischemic heart disease.[30–32]

The mechanisms by which CPAP decreases nocturnal and daytime blood pressure are likely multiple. By eliminating obstructive breathing (apneas, hypopneas, RERAs), repetitive arousals, and the resulting large swings in intrathoracic pressure, CPAP has obvious beneficial acute physiologic effects on the heart. Disordered sympathetic activity and endothelial function appear to be normalized.[33] CPAP has also been shown to result in decreased inflammatory markers, cytokines, and endothelin-1, as well as improving glucose metabolism in patients with OSA.[34]

SUMMARY

Obstructive sleep apnea is a common condition. It is characterized by recurrent partial or total collapse of the upper airway, resulting in intermittent hypoxia and hypercapnia, sleep fragmentation, and daytime sequelae. There is compelling evidence that OSA may be an important risk factor for the development of cardiovascular disease, especially systemic hypertension. Even mild OSA appears to place individuals at a higher risk of developing systemic hypertension. Although the exact mechanisms for this association are incompletely understood, increased sympathetic activity, endothelial dysfunction, inflammation, and disordered metabolism may play important roles. Effective treatments for OSA include positional therapy and weight loss, CPAP, oral appliances, and surgery. Recent studies suggest that CPAP therapy for OSA results in a decrease in both nighttime and daytime blood pressure. Patients already using antihypertensive medications may derive particular benefit, suggesting that OSA may be a cause of resistant hypertension.

REFERENCES

1. Young T, Palta M, Dempsey J, Skatrud J, Weber S, Badr S. The occurrence of sleep-disordered breathing among middle-aged adults. *N Engl J Med* 1993;328(17):1230–5.
2. Nieto FJ, Young TB, Lind BK, et al. Association of sleep-disordered breathing, sleep apnea, and hypertension in a large community-based study. Sleep Heart Health Study. *JAMA* 2000;283(14):1829–36.
3. Peppard PE, Young T, Palta M, Skatrud J. Prospective study of the association between sleep-disordered breathing and hypertension. *N Engl J Med* 2000;342(19):1378–84.
4. Chobanian AV, Bakris GL, Black HR, et al. The Seventh Report of the Joint National Committee on Prevention, Detection, Evaluation, and Treatment of High Blood Pressure: the JNC 7 report. *JAMA* 2003;289(19):2560–72.
5. Pepperell JC, Ramdassingh-Dow S, Crosthwaite N, et al. Ambulatory blood pressure after therapeutic and subtherapeutic nasal continuous positive airway pressure for obstructive sleep apnoea: a randomised parallel trial. *Lancet* 2002;359(9302):204–10.
6. Becker HF, Jerrentrup A, Ploch T, et al. Effect of nasal continuous positive airway pressure treatment on blood pressure in patients with obstructive sleep apnea. *Circulation* 2003;107(1):68–73.
7. Somers VK, Dyken ME, Clary MP, Abboud FM. Sympathetic neural mechanisms in obstructive sleep apnea. *J Clin Invest* 1995;96(4):1897–904.
8. Narkiewicz K, Montano N, Cogliati C, van de Borne PJ, Dyken ME, Somers VK. Altered cardiovascular variability in obstructive sleep apnea. *Circulation* 1998;98(11):1071–7.
9. Singh JP, Larson MG, Tsuji H, Evans JC, O'Donnell CJ, Levy D. Reduced heart rate variability and new-onset hypertension: insights into pathogenesis of hypertension: the Framingham Heart Study. *Hypertension* 1998;32(2):293–7.
10. Kato M, Roberts-Thomson P, Phillips BG, et al. Impairment of endothelium-dependent vasodilation of resistance vessels in patients with obstructive sleep apnea. *Circulation* 2000;102(21):2607–10.
11. Ohga E, Nagase T, Tomita T, et al. Increased levels of circulating ICAM-1, VCAM-1, and L-selectin in obstructive sleep apnea syndrome. *J Appl Physiol* 1999;87(1):10–4.

12. Shamsuzzaman AS, Winnicki M, Lanfranchi P, et al. Elevated C-reactive protein in patients with obstructive sleep apnea. *Circulation* 2002;105(21):2462–4.
13. Vgontzas AN, Papanicolaou DA, Bixler EO, Kales A, Tyson K, Chrousos GP. Elevation of plasma cytokines in disorders of excessive daytime sleepiness: role of sleep disturbance and obesity. *J Clin Endocrinol Metab* 1997;82(5):1313–6.
14. Schulz R, Mahmoudi S, Hattar K, et al. Enhanced release of superoxide from polymorphonuclear neutrophils in obstructive sleep apnea. Impact of continuous positive airway pressure therapy. *Am J Respir Crit Care Med* 2000;162(2 Pt 1):566–70.
15. Saarelainen S, Seppala E, Laasonen K, Hasan J. Circulating endothelin-1 in obstructive sleep apnea. *Endothelium* 1997;5(2):115–8.
16. Shek EW, Brands MW, Hall JE. Chronic leptin infusion increases arterial pressure. *Hypertension* 1998;31(1 Pt 2):409–14.
17. Punjabi NM, Ahmed MM, Polotsky VY, Beamer BA, O'Donnell CP. Sleep-disordered breathing, glucose intolerance, and insulin resistance. *Respir Physiol Neurobiol* 2003;136(2–3):167–78.
18. Punjabi NM, Sorkin JD, Katzel LI, Goldberg AP, Schwartz AR, Smith PL. Sleep-disordered breathing and insulin resistance in middle-aged and overweight men. *Am J Respir Crit Care Med* 2002;165(5):677–82.
19. Young T, Peppard PE, Gottlieb DJ. Epidemiology of obstructive sleep apnea: a population health perspective. *Am J Respir Crit Care Med* 2002;165(9):1217–39.
20. Redline S, Kump K, Tishler P, Browner I, Ferrette V. Gender differences in sleep-disordered breathing in a community-based sample. *Am J Respir Crit Care Med* 1994;149:722–6.
21. Shahar E, Redline S, Young T, et al. Hormone-replacement therapy and sleep-disordered breathing. *Am J Respir Crit Care Med* 2003;16:16.
22. Chervin R. Sleepiness, fatigue, tiredness, and lack of energy in obstructive sleep apnea. *Chest* 2000;118:372–9.
23. Kushida CA, Efron B, Guilleminault C. A predictive morphometric model for the obstructive sleep apnea syndrome. *Ann Intern Med* 1997;127(8 Pt 1):581–7.
24. Davies RJ, Stradling JR. The relationship between neck circumference,

radiographic pharyngeal anatomy, and the obstructive sleep apnoea syndrome. *Eur Respir J* 1990;3(5):509–14.
25. Suzuki M, Otsuka K, Guilleminault C. Long-term nasal continuous positive airway pressure administration can normalize hypertension in obstructive sleep apnea patients. *Sleep* 1993;16(6):545–9.
26. Smith PL, Gold AR, Meyers DA, Haponik EF, Bleecker ER. Weight loss in mildly to moderately obese patients with obstructive sleep apnea. *Ann Intern Med* 1985;103(6 Pt 1):850–5.
27. Sullivan CE, Issa FG, Berthon-Jones M, Eves L. Reversal of obstructive sleep apnoea by continuous positive airway pressure applied through the nares. *Lancet* 1981;1(8225):862–5.
28. Larsson LH, Carlsson-Nordlander B, Svanborg E. Four-year follow-up after uvulopalatopharyngoplasty in 50 unselected patients with obstructive sleep apnea syndrome. *Laryngoscope* 1994;104(11 Pt 1):1362–8.
29. Faccenda JF, Mackay TW, Boon NA, Douglas NJ. Randomized placebo-controlled trial of continuous positive airway pressure on blood pressure in the sleep apnea-hypopnea syndrome. *Am J Respir Crit Care Med* 2001;163(2):344–8.
30. Kaneko Y, Floras JS, Usui K, et al. Cardiovascular effects of contineous positive airway pressure in patients with heart failure and obstructive sleep apnea. *N Engl J Med* 2003;348:1233–41.
31. Kanagala R, Murali NS, Friedman PA, et al. Obstructive sleep apnea and the recurrence of atrial fibrillation. *Circulation* 2003;107(20):2589–94.
32. Peled N, Abinader EG, Pillar G, Sharif D, Lavie P. Nocturnal ischemic events in patients with obstructive sleep apnea syndrome and ischemic heart disease: effects of continuous positive air pressure treatment. *J Am Coll Cardiol* 1999;34(6):1744–9.
33. Hedner J, Darpo B, Ejnell H, Carlson J, Caidahl K. Reduction in sympathetic activity after long-term CPAP treatment in sleep apnoea: cardiovascular implications. *Eur Respir J* 1995;8(2):222–9.
34. Saarelainen S, Hasan J, Siitonen S, Seppala E. Effect of nasal CPAP treatment on plasma volume, aldosterone and 24-h blood pressure in obstructive sleep apnea. *J Sleep Res* 1996;5(3):181–5.

PHARMACOLOGIC AND NONPHARMACOLOGIC INTERVENTIONS AND TREATMENT GUIDELINES

Section 4

Daniel W. Jones and Chim C. Lang

Chapter

77 Diuretics

John F. Setaro and Marvin Moser

Key Findings

- Most hypertension patients will require a diuretic in some form to achieve adequate blood pressure (BP) regulation and a reduction in cardiovascular (CV) events.

- Low-dose diuretics may be given in combination with beta blockers, angiotensin-converting enzyme inhibitors, angiotensin receptor blockers, calcium channel blockers, or other drugs with excellent BP-reducing effects.

- Black and elderly patients, who are characteristically more sensitive to sodium, exhibit a greater response to diuretics than younger or white individuals.

- Despite questions concerning the metabolic effects of thiazide diuretics, newer trials and guidelines have reaffirmed their safety and effectiveness in initial management of high BP and as an element of combination therapy in more complex cases.

- Diuretic-associated hypokalemia is dose related and can be minimized by using combination agents such as spironolactone/thiazide or an angiotensin-converting enzyme inhibitor or angiotensin-2 receptor-blocker with thiazide.

- Contemporary strict BP treatment goals will require that diuretics continue to play a major role in hypertension therapy.

INTRODUCTION

Diuretics, in particular thiazide compounds, were the earliest forms of practical and well-tolerated antihypertensive drugs introduced in the modern therapeutic era. Numerous large randomized clinical trials have demonstrated the value of these agents in reducing morbidity and mortality in the hypertensive patient. Despite questions raised concerning the metabolic effects of thiazide diuretics, newer trials and guidelines have reaffirmed their primacy in the safe and effective initial management of high BP and as an element of combination therapy in more complex or difficult cases. Contemporary strict BP treatment goals will require that diuretics continue to play a major role in hypertension therapy.

HISTORICAL BACKGROUND

Thiazide diuretics were introduced initially in 1957 and were quickly accepted as therapy for hypertension because they were effective, inexpensive, and well tolerated and

because they could be used once daily in contrast to existing agents.[1] Large randomized clinical trials in hypertensive patients subsequently proved their effectiveness in reducing morbidity and mortality. This chapter surveys the physiology and pharmacology of diuretics, examines early trial evidence, assesses the metabolic implications of diuretic use, and discusses recent trials and management guidelines that confirm the key role of diuretics in hypertensive patients.

PHYSIOLOGY AND PHARMACOLOGY OF DIURETIC COMPOUNDS

There are four classes of diuretics. *Thiazide-type diuretics* (including hydrochlorothiazide, chlorthalidone, bendroflumethiazide, methyclothiazide, and metolazone) inhibit the reabsorption of sodium in the early distal renal tubule (Figure 77–1).[2] These are most effective in patients who have normal serum creatinine values (< 1.5 mg/dl), although metolazone may also be effective despite some renal impairment. *Indoline derivatives* (including indapamide) may also interfere with calcium influx into vascular smooth muscle cells.[3] *Loop diuretics* (furosemide, bumetanide, torsemide, and ethacrynic acid) are compounds that act more rapidly in the proximal region, inhibiting sodium reabsorption in the loop of Henle. These are ideally suited for patients with evidence of renal impairment.

Potassium-sparing diuretics (amiloride, triamterene, spironolactone, and eplerenone) are active in the distal tubule and inhibit the exchange of sodium for potassium. Amiloride and triamterene inhibit potassium secretion directly and thus can help maintain potassium homeostasis. Both of these agents are weak diuretics, however, and are most effective in combination with hydrochlorothiazide. Spironolactone and eplerenone inhibit aldosterone by competitive or direct blockade of the aldosterone receptor, respectively. Both are potassium-sparing as well as antihypertensive agents. Eplerenone may be particularly useful in male patients because as a direct inhibitor it is free of anti-androgenic effects (mastodynia, gynecomastia, sexual dysfunction) in contrast to spironolactone.

Initially, when diuretics are given plasma volume decreases—lowering cardiac output and arterial BP. Later, volume rises toward normal and cardiac output normalizes. However, BP remains low, with reduced peripheral vascular resistance.[4] This effect is attributable to direct arterial relaxation via alterations in ion flux across vascular smooth muscle cells, which likely occurs as an autoregulatory

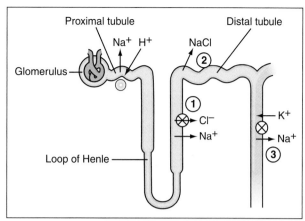

Figure 77–1. Diuretics: sites of action. (1) Loop agents, (2) thiazide diuretics, and (3) potassium-sparing diuretics. (Redrawn from Moser M. *Clinical Management of Hypertension, Seventh Edition*. Caddo, OK: Professional Communications 2004, with permission.)

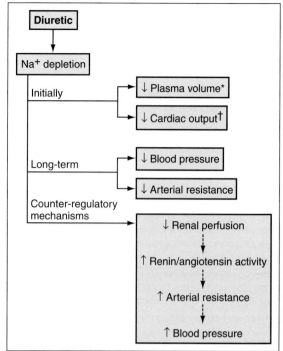

Figure 77–2. Physiology of diuretic action. Plasma volume and cardiac output decrease (a,b), returning to normal after several weeks, with long-term reduction in vascular resistance and blood pressure. Although consequent stimulation of the renin-angiotensin system does not lead to a rise in blood pressure, this counter-regulatory mechanism can be addressed to attain further improvements in blood pressure control by adding an angiotensin-converting enzyme inhibitor, angiotensin receptor blocker, or beta blocker. (Redrawn from Moser M. *Clinical Management of Hypertension, Seventh Edition*. Caddo, OK: Professional Communications 2004, with permission.)

response to reduced BP (Figure 77–2).[5] High dosages were used in the past, such as 50 to 200 mg of hydrochlorothiazide, although it is now recognized that 12.5 to 25 mg are effective doses in most patients. The Systolic Hypertension in the Elderly Program (SHEP) employed low-dose chlorthalidone (12.5 mg) to attain goal BP values in nearly half of the subjects.[6]

Low-dose hydrochlorothiazide (12.5 mg) reduces BP in up to two-thirds of diuretic-responsive patients, with an additional 15% responding to 25 mg. Up to 90% may respond to 50 mg daily, but above this dosage side effects may become troublesome. Diuretics lower BP by 10-15/5–10 mmHg compared to a placebo effect, with a greater effect on systolic BP. This is of importance in the treatment of older patients who have isolated systolic hypertension.[6] Black and elderly patients, who are characteristically more sensitive to sodium, exhibit a greater response to diuretics than younger or white individuals.[7]

Low-dose diuretics may be given in combination with beta blockers, angiotensin-converting enzyme inhibitors, angiotensin receptor blockers, calcium channel blockers, or other drugs with excellent BP-reducing effects (Figure 77–2). Such combinations may permit a return to normotensive BP levels in 80% of patients.[8] The reduction in plasma volume with a diuretic stimulates the renin angiotensin aldosterone system. Consequently, additional BP lowering occurs when agents such as beta blockers, angiotensin-converting enzyme inhibitors, or angiotensin receptor blockers that inhibit the system are added to a diuretic.

EARLY EVIDENCE FROM RANDOMIZED CLINICAL TRIALS

Diuretics and beta blockers were used in the majority of randomized trials conducted before 1995, with the optional addition of vasodilators or centrally acting agents when initial therapies were insufficient to achieve BP targets. A pooled analysis of 17 placebo-controlled trials revealed that subjects treated with these medications experienced a 52% lower incidence of congestive heart failure, 38% reduction in stroke morbidity and mortality, 35% less left ventricular hypertrophy, 21% less vascular mortality, and a 16% lower incidence of coronary events.[9] Active therapy also prevented progression to more severe stages of hypertension.[9] Another meta-analysis of 18 trials of antihypertensive therapy confirmed stroke reduction with active therapy, with a lesser beneficial effect on coronary heart disease events.[10]

Studies that used diuretics as part of a treatment regimen included the Veterans Administration Study, which reported significant stroke reduction in subjects who had severe and moderately severe hypertension—with a beneficial trend in regard to coronary outcomes.[11] The Hypertension Detection and Follow-up Program (HDFP), where diuretics were administered as first-step therapy in subjects with less severe hypertension, demonstrated a 45% reduction in stroke mortality and a 20% reduction in coronary event mortality in the more intensively treated subjects.[12]

The SHEP, using diuretics (and beta blockers, if necessary), reported a 54% reduction in heart failure, 30% reduction in myocardial infarctions, 37% reduction in stroke, and 25% fewer transient ischemic neurologic attacks.[6] Based on these findings, as well as on data from more recent trials, all of the Joint National Committee (JNC) Reports on the Detection, Evaluation, and Treatment of High Blood Pressure (from the first in 1977 and including the 2003 JNC 7 Report) have recommended diuretics as one of the preferred agents for the initiation of antihypertensive therapy in most patients.[13,14]

METABOLIC ISSUES IN DIURETIC USE

Diuretic compounds are generally well tolerated, and two large prospective controlled series reported only a 3% withdrawal rate for adverse effects in subjects randomized to diuretic therapy.[15,16] However, questions have been raised by the observation that BP-lowering therapy in large clinical trials has significantly reduced pressure-related complications (stroke, congestive heart failure, renal impairment, and left ventricular hypertrophy). Although there were improvements in coronary heart disease outcomes (angina, fatal and nonfatal myocardial infarction),[6,12] these were somewhat less than predicted by epidemiologic data. Some investigators believe that metabolic changes from diuretics may account for this shortfall. Several explanations have been advanced to account for this phenomenon.

First, atherosclerotic coronary heart disease is a long-term multifactorial process whose outcome may not be affected by short-term manipulation of a single risk factor such as high BP. It is possible that the short duration of the diuretic-based treatment trials compared to the longer duration of epidemiologic follow-up explains an apparent shortfall in coronary heart disease benefit. For instance, a 12/4–5 mmHg reduction in BP predicts a decrease of approximately 20 to 25% in coronary heart disease events over 10+ years.

In the three- to five-year clinical trials, a decrease in BP of this magnitude led to only 16% fewer coronary events. Newer studies, however, indicate that longer-term BP reduction improves coronary event rates to a greater degree than that seen in shorter-term trials. In the ALLHAT (Anti-hypertensive and Lipid-Lowering Treatment to Prevent Heart Attack Trial) study, for example—which compared a diuretic, angiotensin-converting enzyme inhibitor, and calcium channel blocker—thiazide diuretics reduced coronary events to the same extent as competing agents.[17]

The metabolic side effects of thiazide diuretics (electrolyte, lipid, and glucose changes) were originally advanced as reasons for the less than dramatic reduction of CHD events in the early studies The claim was that these may negate some of the advantages of BP lowering. These questions have been addressed elsewhere.[9,18] Specific components of the "metabolic debate" are reviewed in material following. In general, the results of recent trials such as ALLHAT have negated these speculations.

Electrolytes

Diuretic-associated hypokalemia is dose related. Up to one-third of patients show a decrease in serum potassium, ranging from 0.5 to 0.8 mEq/L when given high doses of hydrochlorothiazide (50 to 100 mg daily). The use of an intermediate dose of 25 mg hydrochlorothiazide results in a decrease in potassium of 0.3 to 0.4 mEq/L, with minimal effects seen at 12.5 or 6.25 mg daily. Potassium-sparing diuretics may be advisable in patients who are especially sensitive to hypokalemia—particularly in older individuals, those taking digitalis preparations, or diabetic patients whose insulin utilization may be affected by hypokalemia.

Hypokalemia can also be minimized by using combination agents such as spironolactone/thiazide or an angiotensin-converting enzyme inhibitor or angiotensin-2 receptor blocker with thiazide. The potassium-conserving tendencies of the former medications serve to offset potassium loss caused by the latter. However, diuretic-induced hypokalemia with presently recommended doses is not infrequently of clinical significance.

One report argued that thiazide-related hypokalemia could provoke increased ventricular ectopy, including ventricular tachycardia and sudden death.[19] In the Multiple Risk Factor Intervention Trial (MRFIT), subjects with abnormal electrocardiograms in the special care higher-dose diuretic group had a higher coronary heart disease mortality compared to usual care patients who received lower doses of diuretics. This finding, however, was likely a statistical anomaly.[20,21] Retrospective non-randomized case-control studies questioned the increased incidence of sudden death in diuretic-treated patients, yet comparative groups were not adequately matched in these series.[22,23]

Anecdotal reports of hypokalemia in cardiac arrest victims who had received thiazide diuretics aroused some concern. However, 24- and 48-hour Holter monitoring studies with prospective controlled trials of high-dose thiazide-treated subjects showed no significant increase in simple or complex ventricular ectopy—whether in the presence or absence of left ventricular hypertrophy despite the presence of some hypokalemia.[6,16,24] The use of diuretics results in regression of left ventricular hypertrophy, itself an independent risk factor for ventricular rhythm disturbances.[25] Finally (and perhaps most importantly), recent large studies employing diuretics compared to placebo, angiotensin-converting enzyme inhibitors, or calcium channel blockers failed to report any increase in sudden cardiac death in groups receiving diuretics.[6,18,26] Thus, hypokalemia is less of an issue with low doses of diuretics—especially when these agents are used with other medications in attempts to lower BP to attain present BP goals.[27–30]

Lipid changes

Over the course of the first year of treatment, thiazide diuretics may increase total and low-density lipoprotein cholesterol by 5 to 7%, without changes in high-density lipoprotein cholesterol concentration. Two small studies suggested that thiazide agents increase serum lipid concentrations significantly,[30–32] whereas large long-term clinical trials using diuretics show no change or even a decline in total cholesterol in diuretic-assigned cohorts.[33] Trials that demonstrated no lipid effects include the Medical Research Council Study (MRC), the Medical Research

Council Study in the Elderly (MRC-Elderly), the Metoprolol Atherosclerosis Prevention in Hypertension Study (MAPHY), and the Heart Attack Primary Prevention in Hypertension Study (HAPPHY).[34–37]

Other series report improved lipid levels the diuretic treatment study arms. For example, a decrease in total cholesterol was noted in subjects in the HDFP of 232 to 223 mg/dl in the active diuretic treatment (special care) group,[38] and similar results have been noted in other diuretic-assigned subjects in multiple large prospective studies. These investigations include the Multiple Risk factor Intervention Trial (MRFIT), the European Working Party on High Blood Pressure in the Elderly Study (EWPHE), the Treatment of Mild Hypertension Study (TOMHS), the Verapamil in Hypertension Atherosclerosis Study (VHAS), and ALLHAT.

The data in ALLHAT are confounded by the significant number of subjects who were taking statin agents at the trial's conclusion.[16,18,20,39,40] Despite slightly higher mean cholesterol levels in the diuretic compared to the lisinopril or amlodipine arms at the conclusion of ALLHAT, coronary heart disease rates were similar among study groups.[18] In SHEP and HDFP, CV morbidity and mortality were decreased with the use of diuretics, regardless of baseline lipid values.[6,38] Based on these findings, it would appear that thiazide diuretics can be used safely irrespective of the lipid status of an individual.

Glucose and insulin metabolism

Although thiazide diuretics may adversely affect insulin sensitivity and glucose utilization, unfavorable clinical outcomes with these medications have not been reported in large prospective trials. Significant vascular risks arise from insulin resistance and abnormal glucose tolerance in an increasingly obese and diabetic population. Yet in large studies employing thiazide diuretics only minimal changes in fasting glucose are observed, and newly incident diabetes (NOD) is increased by only 0.6% more than placebo.[6,34,36,38,39,41]

Given that typical older hypertensive patients may have been minimally insulin resistant upon study entry, a higher rate of diuretic-induced progression to overt diabetes would be expected if indeed diuretics caused diabetes. Although hypertensive individuals show a greater tendency toward development of diabetes than normotensive patients, people who have received diuretics have not required antidiabetic medication any more frequently than those given other antihypertensive compounds.[42]

Comparative data in new onset of diabetes

The ALLHAT investigators noted a small increase in serum glucose and an absolute increase of 3.5% in new-onset diabetes in the thiazide- compared to lisinopril-treated patients (11.6 versus 8.1%), yet there was a similar frequency of CV events in the diuretic therapy group in this five-year study.[18] Diabetic subjects in ALLHAT who received diuretics had coronary heart disease outcomes equal to diabetic subjects who received lisinopril or amlodipine, and experienced fewer strokes or episodes of heart failure compared with lisinopril.

Heart failure was less frequent in diabetic or non-diabetic thiazide-treated patients compared with the amlodipine cohort.[18] In the Controlled Onset Verapamil Investigation of Cardiovascular End Points (CONVINCE) trial, diabetic individuals had equal CV outcomes whether they were assigned to verapamil, diuretic, or beta blocker.[43] Potential metabolic changes associated with diuretic use are summarized in Table 77–1. Of some interest is the theory that hypokalemia itself may mediate the development of diabetes, given the tendency of drugs that raise potassium levels to have the lowest rates of new-onset diabetes (angiotensin-converting enzyme inhibitors and angiotensin receptor blockers).[44]

THIAZIDE DIURETICS: POTENTIAL METABOLIC ALTERATIONS	
Metabolic Change	Comments
Hypokalemia	Can be minimized by using lower dosages. Avoid if possible, especially in diabetics and patients taking digitalis. Replace as appropriate.
Hyperlipidemia	Short term: total cholesterol and low-density lipoproteins increased 5 to 7% (effect may be less with lower dosages). No effect on high-density lipoproteins. Long term: few measurable effects. Same degree of reduction in cardiovascular events in subjects with hyperlipidemia or normal cholesterol levels.
Increased insulin	Insulin resistance increased, but only small average rise in blood glucose levels in long-term resistance trials in diuretic-treated versus placebo subjects. Some difference in new-onset diabetes when compared with other medications. Overall cardiovascular mortality reduced to same or greater extent in diabetics versus non-diabetics.
Hyperuricemia	Gout in fewer than 3% of patients. If diuretic is essential, allopurinol can be used.
Hypercalcemia	May be advantageous in treatment of osteoporosis and prevention of fractures.

Table 77–1 Thiazide Diuretics: Potential Metabolic Alterations

Another perspective on this question arises from the observation that in most studies diabetic patients receiving diuretics experienced fewer adverse CV outcomes than non-diabetics on diuretics, reflecting the safety and usefulness of diuretics in diabetic hypertensive persons.[45] The SHEP trial results illustrate this point (Figure 77–3).[6] The importance of BP reduction using effective and well-tolerated agents was again confirmed in the United Kingdom Prospective Diabetes Study Group (UKPDS) trial, in which tighter versus less strict BP control (a difference of –10/–5 mmHg) led to better outcomes with respect to both macrovascular and microvascular events. There was no difference in outcomes between angiotensin-converting enzyme inhibitor versus diuretic/beta-blocker combination groups.[46]

In diabetic patients, angiotensin receptor blockers can delay or reverse the progression of nephropathy and prevent the occurrence of end-stage renal disease. They are thus indicated for this patient group.[47–49] To attain the new BP goal of 130/80 mmHg in diabetic patients (JNC 7 2003), thiazide diuretics may have to be added to a multi-drug program—particularly because diabetic patients tend to be sodium sensitive with consequent volume expansion.[14,50] Overall, most large hypertension trials conducted in the last several decades have employed thiazide diuretics as a component of a multi-drug regimen.

The prospect of preventing diabetes in at-risk patients has stimulated interest with the publication of at least three trials that report the prevention of new-onset type 2 diabetes by using inhibitors of the renin-angiotensin-aldosterone system. Agents studied include captopril in the Captopril Prevention Project (CAPP), ramipril in the Heart Outcomes Prevention Evaluation study (HOPE), and losartan in the Losartan Intervention for Endpoint reduction in hypertension study (LIFE).[51–53] In a significant number of subjects in these and most of the trials, diuretic therapy was necessary to reach BP goals.

Although the mechanism by which diabetes is possibly prevented by inhibitors of the renin angiotensin system is unclear, it has been proposed that these agents defend potassium balance.[44] For example, in the Valsartan Antihypertensive Long-term Use Evaluation (VALUE) trial the incidence of new-onset diabetes was 3.3% less in the group treated with the angiotensin receptor blocker valsartan compared with the calcium channel blocker amlodipine.[54] An equal number of subjects in both arms received thiazide diuretics as well, with hypokalemia more common in the amlodipine group.

The fewer cases of NOD in the Valsartan group are presumably based on this drug's tendency to elevate potassium, which has been theorized to play a role in diabetes prevention.[44,54] It is therefore reasonable to initiate therapy using a combination of a diuretic and an angiotensin-converting enzyme inhibitor or diuretic and angiotensin receptor blocker in hypertensive patients who are obese, have a family history of diabetes, or have personal criteria for the diagnosis of metabolic syndrome. This is especially true in patients with stage 2 hypertension.

RECENT STUDIES AND PRESENT RECOMMENDATIONS

Recent studies have underscored the role of diuretics as initial therapy for patients who have high BP.[14] For other patients (including those with resistant hypertension, diabetes, or renal impairment), diuretics should form the essential core of a multi-drug regimen.[14,27,50,55]

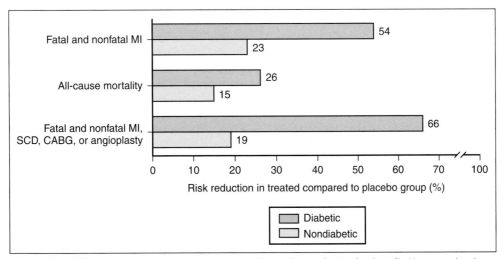

Figure 77–3. Effect of treatment in reducing morbidity and mortality in the Systolic Hypertension in the Elderly Program (SHEP) study using low-dose thiazide diuretic (with beta blocker added as needed) versus placebo. CABG, coronary artery bypass surgery; MI, myocardial infarction; SCD, sudden cardiac death. Open bars: diabetic cohort receiving active treatment (n = 283) versus placebo (n = 300). Filled bars: non-diabetic cohort receiving active treatment (n = 2080) versus placebo (n = 2069). (Redrawn from Moser M. *Clinical Management of Hypertension, Seventh Edition.* Caddo, OK: Professional Communications 2004, with permission.)

Role of aldosterone inhibitors

Recently, published data have led to a renewed appreciation for the role of aldosterone-inhibiting diuretics in hypertension management—especially when hypertension is drug resistant.[56] In resistant hypertension patients, it has been reported that there is a relatively high prevalence of primary aldosteronism[57] and that there may be an overlap between essential hypertension and subtle forms of hyperaldosteronism. This typically occurs in the form of bilateral adrenal hyperplasia rather than discrete adenoma. If essential hypertension and mild aldosteronism were part of a continuum, it would explain the excellent reponse to spironolactone across a broad spectrum of hypertension patients.

Obesity may be a factor that amplifies the hypertensive and vascular risks of aldosterone.[58] A published analysis from the Framingham Heart Study shows that initially normotensive individuals who have higher baseline serum aldosterone concentrations are more likely to develop hypertension later in contrast to those with lower baseline concentrations.[59] In one study, when the mineralocorticoid receptor inhibitor spironolactone was added to the multi-drug programs of resistant hypertension patients (which included other diuretics and inhibitors of the renin-angiotensin system) mean BP over six months decreased 25/12 mmHg.[60] This suggests that minrealocorticoid receptor-inhibiting diuretics can play an important role in managing difficult-to-treat hypertensive patients, and raises the prospect that dual diuretic programs may be safe and effective.

Hypertension trials employing diuretics

In several recent controlled prospective trials, the principal role of diuretics has been validated. In diabetic hypertensive patients, a combined regimen of beta blockers and diuretics with tight BP control produced favorable CV outcomes over a nine-year study (UKPDS).[46] In the CONVINCE trial, a calcium channel blocker verapamil was not proved superior to either a beta blocker or a thiazide diuretic in preventing unfavorable CV events.[43] In the PROGRESS (Perindopril Protection Against Recurrent Stroke Study) investigation, the angiotensin-converting enzyme inhibitor perindopril required the addition of the diuretic indapamide before significant benefit could be observed in regard to reduction of stroke and transient ischemic neurologic attacks in hypertensive patients who had previously suffered a CVA.[61]

In the INCLUSIVE (Irbesartan/HCTZ Blood Pressure Reductions in Diverse Patient Populations) study, 77% of patients achieved a systolic BP goal and 83% achieved a diastolic BP goal when given a combination of hydrochlorothiazide and an angiotensin receptor blocker.[8] The MIDAS (Multicentre Isradapine Diuretic Atherosclerosis Study) evaluated a short-acting dihydropyridine calcium channel blocker and a diuretic and reported fewer CV events in the diuretic group.[62] In the VHAS, long-acting verapamil possessed no advantage in preventing CV events over diuretic therapy.[40]

The INSIGHT (International Nifedipine GITS Study: Intervention as a Goal in Hypertension Treatment) investigation assessed long-acting nifedipine compared to a diuretic in combination with a potassium-sparing component, showing no difference between the two groups in overall CV outcomes.[63] The NORDIL trial comparing diltiazem to a beta-blocker/diuretic reported no overall event difference.[26] The Swedish Trial in Old Patients with Hypertension-2 (STOP-2) reported no difference in outcomes among older hypertension patients treated with diuretics, calcium channel blockers, or angiotensin-converting enzyme inhibitors.[64] In each instance, diuretic compounds were equivalent to or better than newer, more expensive agents.

ALLHAT

ALLHAT analyzed 33,000 high-risk hypertensive patients over a five-year period.[18] The trial sought to determine outcome differences among patients randomized to a diuretic (low-dose chlorthalidone), a calcium channel blocker (amlodipine), or an angiotensin-converting enzyme inhibitor (lisinopril). An earlier alpha-adrenergic blocker arm of the study (doxazosin) was terminated when investigators reported a significant excess in congestive heart failure events in the doxazosin group compared to the diuretic group.

To reach goal BP in ALLHAT, beta blockers, reserpine, clonidine, and hydralazine were permitted as second- or third-step agents. Study participants represented a high-risk group for adverse hypertensive CV outcomes: average age was 67 years, 35% were black, and 36% were diabetic.[18] Results showed fewest overall CV events in the diuretic-assigned patients, but there was no difference among the groups in the primary outcome of fatal or non-fatal coronary events. Compared with lisinopril-treated patients, patients on diuretics had fewer strokes and heart failure events (particularly in blacks). Compared with amlodipine-treated patients, the diuretic group had fewer severe heart failure events causing death or hospitalization.

Some differences among treatment groups may reflect overall BP differences. Systolic BP was 0.8 mmHg higher in the amlodipine compared to chlorthalidone groups, a significant difference in a trial with very large numbers of participants. The ALLHAT authors reported a 4-mmHg lower average systolic BP in blacks and a 3-mmHg lower average in subjects older than 65 years of age treated with chlorthalidone compared to the angiotensin-converting enzyme inhibitor. Previous clinical and investigative experience affirms that elderly and black individuals respond better to diuretic agents. If other compounds are used, they probably should be used with diuretics to lower BP more effectively Such a combination, however, was not permitted by the ALLHAT protocol—perhaps accounting for the lesser effectiveness of therapy in the non-diuretic-treated patients.[65]

In a similar fashion, the inability to use diuretics as initial therapy may have biased the results of the ASCOT (Anglo-Scandinavian Cardiac Outcomes Trial–Blood Pressure Lowering Arm) trial.[66] In this study, subjects received a calcium channel blocker (amlodipine) or a beta blocker (atenolol) as initial therapy. As a second drug, an angiotensin-converting enzyme inhibitor (perindopril) could be added to amlodipine, and a thiazide diuretic (bendroflumethiazide) could be added to atenolol.

Overall CV outcomes were more favorable in the amlodipine/perindopril group compared to the atenolol/bendroflumethiazide group, a finding perhaps linked to the 2.7/1.9-mmHg BP difference favoring amlodipine/perindopril at the study conclusion.[66] The primary outcome of CHD events, however, was similar in the two groups. This study was conducted in predominantly older Caucasian males. The findings therefore may not apply to a non-European, younger, or female population. Moreover, it is interesting to speculate whether results may have been different if diuretics had been given first (with beta blockers added later) in light of the overall excellent record of using diuretics in this age group.

Recommendations

As previously mentioned, the equivalent primary outcome results and the more favorable secondary CV endpoint results for the diuretic-treated group in ALLHAT contradict arguments that the possible metabolic changes as a result of diuretics detract from their protective potential.[67] More than half of the ALLHAT study participants were not fully controlled on monotherapy, multi-drug treatment being required. Based on ALLHAT and many other trials, JNC 7 continued to advocate diuretics as first-step therapy in most cases—acknowledging that many (if not a majority of) patients will need a multi-drug program.[14]

Compelling reasons for starting with other agents (such as angiotensin-converting enzyme inhibitors or angiotensin receptor blockers) include heart failure, diabetes, diabetic nephropathy, or a desire to prevent diabetes in individuals at risk. Additional studies have confirmed the protective role of inhibitors of the renin-angiotensin system. In the Australian National Blood Pressure-2 trial, there was a marginally significant benefit in CV event reduction favoring a program based on an angiotensin-converting enzyme compared to a diuretic-based program[68] (but only in men). Less than two-thirds of subjects continued the study drug throughout the protocol, and the demographics of the study were different from those of ALLHAT (more Caucasians, few blacks)—factors that may limit the application of these findings to other populations.

SUMMARY AND PERSPECTIVES

Most hypertension patients will require a diuretic in some form to achieve adequate BP regulation and a reduction in CV events. These agents have been widely used for nearly five decades, with an unequaled record of safety and effectiveness across diverse populations. Current recommendations favor initiating therapy with diuretics. Perhaps more important than the question of how one begins therapy is the question of how one ends it. For most hypertension patients, this will consist of a multi-drug program including diuretics to attain BP targets that duplicate benefits observed in clinical trials.

REFERENCES

1. Moser M, Macaulay AI. Chlorothiazide as an adjunct in the treatment of essential hypertension. *Am J Card* 1959;3:214.
2. Moser M. *Clinical Management of Hypertension, Seventh Edition.* Caddo, OK:Professional Communications 2004.
3. Zempel G, Ditlevsen J, Hoch M, et al. Effects of indapamide on Ca+2 entry into vascular smooth muscle cells. *Nephron* 1997;76:460–65.
4. Tarazi RC, Dustan HP, Frolich ED. Long term thiazide therapy in essential hypertension: Evidence for persistent alteration in plasma volume and renin activity. *Circulation* 1970;41:709–17.
5. Colas B, Collin T, Safraou F, et al. Direct vascular actions of methyclothiazide in remodeled mesenteric arteries from hypertensive patients. *Am J Hypertens* 2001;14:989–94.
6. SHEP Cooperative Research Group. Prevention of stroke by antihypertensive drug treatment in older persons with isolated systolic hypertension: Final results of the Systolic Hypertension in the Elderly Program (SHEP). *JAMA* 1991;265:3255–64.
7. Weinberger, MH. Salt sensitivity of blood pressure in humans. *Hypertension* 1996;27(2):481–90.
8. Neutel JM, Saunders E, Bakris GL, et al., on behalf of the INCLUSIVE Investigators. The efficacy and safety of low- and high- dose fixed combinations of irbesaartan/hydrochlorothiazide in patients with uncontrolled systolic blood pressure on monotherapy: The INCLUSIVE Trial. *J Clin Hypertens* 2005;7:578–86.
9. Moser M, Hebert P. Prevention of disease progression, left ventricular hypertrophy, and congestive heart failure in the hypertension treatment trials. *J Am Coll Cardiol* 1996;27:1214–18.
10. Psaty BM, Smith NL, Siscovick DS, et al. Health outcomes associated with antihypertensive therapies used as first line agents. *JAMA* 1997;277:739–45.
11. Veterans Cooperative Study Group on Antihypertensive Agents. Effects of treatment on morbidity in hypertension: Results in patients with diastolic blood pressures averaging 115 through 129 mm Hg. *JAMA* 1967; 202:1028–34.
12. Hypertension Detection and Followup Cooperative group (HDFP). Five-year findings of the Hypertension Detection and Follow-up Program. I. Reduction in mortality of persons with high blood pressure, including mild hypertension. *JAMA* 1979;242:2562–71.
13. Moser M, Guyther JR, Finnerty F, et al. The First Report of the Joint National Committee on Detection, Evaluation, and Treatment of High Blood Pressure (JNC I). *JAMA* 1977;237:255.
14. JNC 7. The Seventh Report of the Joint National Committee on Prevention, Detection, Evaluation, and Treatment of High Blood Pressure (JNC 7). *Hypertension.* 2003;42:1206–52.
15. Materson BJ, Reda DJ, Cushman WC, et al. Single-drug therapy for hypertension in men: A comparison of six antihypertensive agents with placebo. The Department of Veterans Affairs Cooperative Study Group on Antihypertensive Agents. *N Engl J Med* 1993;328:914–21.
16. Neaton, JD, Grimm RH, Prineas RJ, et al. Treatment of Mild Hypertension Study (TOMHS): Final results. Treatment of Mild Hypertension Study Group. *JAMA* 1993;270:713–24.
17. ALLHAT Officers and Coordinators for the ALLHAT Collaborative Research Group. Major outcomes in high-risk hypertensive patients randomized to angiotensin-converting enzyme inhibitor or calcium channel blocker vs. diuretic: The Anti-hypertensive and Lipid-Lowering Treatment to Prevent Heart Attack Trial (ALLHAT). *JAMA* 2002; 288:2981–97.
18. Hebert PR, Moser M, Mayer J, Glynn RJ, Hennekens CH. Recent evidence on drug therapy of mild to moderate hypertension and decreased risk of coronary heart disease. *Arch Intern Med* 1993;153:578–81.

19. Holland OB, Nixon JV, Kuhnert I. Diuretic-induced ventricular ectopic activity. *Am J Med* 1981;770:762–68.

20. Multiple Risk Factor Intervention Trial Research Group (MRFIT). Mortality rates after 10.5 years for participants in the Multiple Risk Factor Intervention Trial. *JAMA* 1990;263:1795–1801.

21. Papademetriou V. Diuretics, hypokalemia, and cardiac arrhythmia: A 20-year controversy. *J Clin Hypertens* 2006; 8:86–92.

22. Siscovick DS, Raghunathan TE, Psaty BM, et al. Diuretic therapy for hypertension and the risk of primary cardiac arrest. *N Engl J Med* 1994; 330:1852–57.

23. Hoes AW, Grobbee DE, Hubsen J, et al. Diuretics, beta-blockers, and the risk of sudden cardiac death in hypertension patients. *Ann Intern Med* 1995;123: 481–87.

24. Papademetriou V, Burris JF, Notargiacomo A, Fletcher RD, Freis ED. Thiazide therapy is not a cause of arrhythmia in patients with systemic hypertension. *Arch Intern Med* 1988;148:1272–76.

25. Moser M, Setaro JF. Antihypertensive drug therapy and regression of left ventricular hypertrophy: A review with a focus on diuretics. *Eur Heart J* 1991; 12:1034–39.

26. Hansson L, Hedner T, Lund-Johansen P, et al., for the NORDIL Study Group. Randomised trial of effects of calcium antagonists compared with diuretics and beta-blockers on cardiovascular morbidity and mortality in hypertension: The Nordic Diltiazem Study. *Lancet* 2000;356:359–65.

27. Setaro JF, Black HR. Refractory hypertension. *N Engl J Med* 1992; 327:543–47.

28. Taler SJ, Textor SC, Augustine JE. Resistant hypertension: Comparing hemodynamic management to specialist care. *Hypertension* 2002; 39:982–88.

29. Garg JP, Elliott WJ, Folker A, Izhar M, Black HR. Resistant hypertension revisited: A comparison of two university-based cohorts. *Am J Hypertens* 2005;18:619–26.

30. Calhoun DA. Resistant or difficult-to-treat hypertension. *J Clin Hypertens* 2006;8:181–86.

31. Middeke M, Weisweiler P, Schwandt P, et al. Serum lipoprotein during antihypertensive therapy with beta-blockers and diuretics: A controlled long term comparative trial. *Clin Cardiol* 1987;10:94–8.

32. Lind L, Pollare T, Berne C. Long-term metabolic effects of antihypertensive drugs. *Am Heart J* 1994;128:1177–83.

33. Moser M. Current hypertension management: Separating fact from fiction. *Cleve Clin J Med* 1993; 60:27–37.

34. MRC Working Party. Medical Research Council trial of treatment of mild hypertension: Principal results. *Br Med J* 1985;291:97–104.

35. MRC Working Party. Medical Research Council trial of treatment of hypertension in older adults: Principal results. *Br Med J* 1992;304:405–12.

36. Wilhelmsen L, Berglund G, Elmfeldt D, et al. Beta-blockers versus diuretics in hypertensive men: Main results from the HAPPHY trial. *J Hypertens* 1987; 5:561–72.

37. Wikstrand J, Warnold I, Olsson G, et al. Primary prevention with metoprolol in patients with hypertension: Mortality results from the MAPHY Study. *JAMA* 1988;259:1976–82.

38. Williams R, Schneider KA, Borhani NO, et al. The relationship between diuretics and serum cholesterol in Hypertension Detection and Follow-up Program participants. *Am J Prev Med* 1986; 2:248–55.

39. Amery A, Birkenhager W, Brixko P, et al. Mortality and morbidity results from the European Working Party on High Blood Pressure in the Elderly Trial. *Lancet* 1985;1:1349–54.

40. Rosei EA, Dal Palu C, Leonetti G, Magnani B, Pessina A, Zanchetti A. Clinical results of the verapamil in hypertension and atherosclerosis study. VHAS Investigators. *J Hypertens* 1997; 15:1337.

41. Dahlof B, Lundholm L, Hanson L, et al. Morbidity and mortality in the Swedish Trial of Older Patients with Hypertension (STOP-Hypertension). *Lancet* 1991;338: 1281–85.

42. Gurwitz JH, Bohn RL, Glynn RJ, Monane M, Mogun H, Avorn J. Antihypertensive drug therapy and the initiation of treatment for diabetes mellitus. *Ann Intern Med* 1993;118:273–78.

43. Black HR, Elliott WJ, Grandits G, et al., for the CONVINCE Research Group. Principal results of the Controlled Onset Verapamil Investigation of Cardiovascular Endpoints (CONVINCE) Trial. *JAMA* 2003;289:2073–82.

44. Carter BL, Basile J. Development of diabetes with thiazide diuretics: The potassium issue. *J Clin Hypertension* 2005;7:638–40.

45. Curb JD, Pressel SL, Cutler JA, et al. Effect of diuretic-based antihypertensive treatment on cardiovascular disease risk in older diabetic patients with isolated systolic hypertension. *JAMA* 1996; 276:1886–92.

46. United Kingdom Prospective Diabetes Study Group. Tight blood pressure control and risk of macrovascular and microvascular complications in Type 2 diabetes: (UKPDS). *Br Med J* 1998; 317:703–13.

47. Brenner BM, Cooper ME, DeZeeuw D, Keane WF, Mitch WE, Parving HH, et al. Effects of losartan on renal and cardiovascular outcomes in patients with type 2 diabetes and nephropathy. *N Engl J Med* 2001;345:861–69.

48. Lewis EJ, Hunsicker LG, Clarke WR, et al. Renoprotective effect of the angiotensin receptor antagonist irbesartan in patients with nephropathy due to Type 2 diabetes. *N Engl J Med* 2001;345:851–60.

49. Parving HH, Lehnert H, Brochner-Mortensen J, Gomis R, Andersen S, Arner P, et al., for the Irbesartan in Patients with Type 2 Diabetes and Microalbuminuria Study Group. The effect of irbesartan on the development of diabetic nephropathy in patients with Type 2 diabetes. *N Engl J Med* 2001;345:870–78.

50. Bakris GL. A practical approach to achieving recommended blood pressure goals in diabetic patients. *Arch Intern Med* 2001;161:2661–67.

51. Hansson L, Lindholm LH, Niskanen L, et al. Effect of angiotensin converting enzyme inhibition compared with conventional therapy on cardiovascular morbidity and mortality in hypertension: The Captopril Prevention Project (CAPP) randomized trial. *Lancet* 1999;353: 611–16.

52. Heart Outcomes Prevention Evaluation (HOPE) Study Investigators. Effects of an angiotensin converting enzyme inhibitor, ramipril, on cardiovascular events in high risk patients. *N Engl J Med* 2000;342:145–53.

53. Dahlof B, Devereux RB, Kjeldsen SE, et al., for the LIFE Study Group. Cardiovascular morbidity and mortality in the Losartan Intervention for Endpoint reduction in hypertension study (LIFE): A randomized trial against atenolol. *Lancet* 2002;359:995–1003.

54. Julius S, Kjeldsen SE, Meber M, for the VALUE Trial Group. Outcomes in hypertensive patients at high cardiovascular risk treated with regimens based on valsartan or amlodipine: The VALUE randomized trial. *Lancet* 2004;363:2022–31.

55. Yakovlevitch M, Black HR. Resistant hypertension in a tertiary care clinic. *Arch Intern Med* 1991;151:1786–92.

56. Nishizaka MK, Calhoun DA. Use of aldosterone antagonists in resistant hypertension. *J Clin Hypertens* 2004;6:458–60.

57. Calhoun DA, Nishizaka MK, Zaman A, et al. High prevalence of primary aldosteronism among black and white subjects with resistant hypertension. *Hypertension* 2002;40:892–96.

58. Goodfriend TL. Aldosterone: A hormone of cardiovascular adapation and maladaptation. *J Clin Hypertens* 2006; 8:133–39.

59. Vasan RS, Evans JC, Larson MG, et al. Serum aldosterone and the incidence of hypertension in nonhypertensive persons. *N Engl J Med* 2004;351:33–41.

60. Nishizaka MK, Zaman MA, Calhoun DA. Efficacy of low-dose spironolactone in subjects with resistant hypertension. *Am J Hypertens* 2003;16:925–30.

61. PROGRESS Collaborative Group. Randomised trial of a perindopril-based blood pressure lowering regimen among 6105 individuals with previous stroke or transient ischaemic attack. *Lancet* 2001;358:1033–41.

62. Borhani NO, Mercuri M, Borhani PA, et al. Final outcome results of the Multicentre Isradipine Diuretic Atherosclerosis Study (MIDAS): A randomized controlled trial. *JAMA* 1996;276:785–91.

63. Brown MJ, Palmer CR, Cataigne A, et al., for the INSIGHT Study Group. Morbidity and mortality in patients randomized to double blind treatment with a long acting calcium channel blocker or diuretic in the International Nifedipine GITS Study: Intervention as a Goal in Hypertension Treatment (INSIGHT). *Lancet* 2000;356:366–72.

64. Hansson L, Lindholm LH, Ekbom T, et al. Randomised trial of old and new antihypertensive drugs in elderly patients: Cardiovascular mortality and morbidity in the Swedish Trial of Old Patients with Hypertension-2 Study (STOP-2). *Lancet* 1999;354:1751–56.

65. Singer GM, Setaro JF. The ALLHAT Study: Implications for the management of resistant hypertension. *J Clin Hypertens* 2005;7:31–2.

66. Dahlof B, Sever PS, Poulter NR, et al., for the ASCOT investigators. Prevention of cardiovascular events with an antihypertensive regimen of amlodipine adding perindopril as required versus atenolol adding bendroflumethiazide as required, in the Anglo-Scandinavian Cardiac Outcomes Trial-Blood Pressure Lowering Arm (ASCOT-BLA): A multicenter randomized controlled trial. *Lancet* 2005;366:895–906.

67. Moser M. Results of the ALLHAT Trial: Is the debate about initial antihypertensive drug therapy over? *J Clin Hypertens* 2003;5:5–8.

68. Wing LMH, Reifel CM, Ryan P, et al. A comparison of outcomes with angiotensin converting enzyme inhibitors and diuretics for hypertension in the elderly. Australian National Blood Pressure Study 2. *N Eng J Med* 2003;348:583–92.

Chapter

78

Beta Blockers in Hypertension

Gurusher S. Panjrath and Franz H. Messerli

Key Findings

- Beta blockers (β-blockers) are used widely as antihypertensive agents.
- Evidence regarding primary prevention of cardiovascular morbidity and mortality is lacking.
- Multiple randomized controlled trials (RCTs) have shown β-blockers to be blood-pressure-lowering drugs.
- β-blockers should *only* be used in combination with other drug classes for controlling hypertension.
- Selection of β-blocker should be done based on patient profile and other co-morbid conditions.
- β-blockers are indicated in patients with chronic heart failure (CHF), arrhythmias (e.g., atrial fibrillation), or post myocardial infarction (MI).
- Until further evidence is available, β-blockers are not suitable as first-line agents for uncomplicated hypertension.

INTRODUCTION

Since the first description of the use of propanolol in 1964 in the treatment of hypertension,[1] β-blockers have become a popular choice for controlling hypertension. β-blockers have traditionally played a widespread role in hypertension therapy and are recommended as first-line agents along with other classes of antihypertensive drugs per the *Seventh Report of the Joint National Committee on Prevention, Detection, Evaluation, and Treatment of High Blood Pressure* (JNC VII) guidelines.[2,3] Other cardiovascular disorders (such as angina pectoris, post-MI, and arrhythmias) are also indications for β-blockers.

MECHANISM OF ACTION

β-blockers are competitive antagonists and are classified based on their selectivity for β1 or β2 receptors. Further characterization is based on the presence of partial β-agonist activity [otherwise known as intrinsic sympathomimetic activity (ISA)], on lipid solubility, and on combined alpha- and beta-blocking activity. The common characteristic required for their role in lowering blood pressure is β-receptor antagonism.

The beta receptor and selectivity

The β-adrenoreceptor is a polypeptide with a molecular weight of 67,000. Catecholamines (agonists) and β-blockers (antagonist) serve as first messengers on the β-receptor, which is present on the surface of target cells. Catecholamines form a complex with the receptor that usually activates adenyl cyclase (via the Gs protein), resulting in formation of intracellular cyclic adenosine monophosphate (cyclic AMP).[4] Subsequently, metabolic or physiologic events are stimulated or inhibited by cyclic AMP. Whereas some of the cyclic AMP is metabolized by phosphodiesterase (PDE), some activates protein kinase via dissociation of 'R' and catalytic subunits. Phosphorylation of catalytic subunits results in the final effects.

Beta-adrenoreceptors vary in their distribution (Table 78–1) among organ systems.[5] An significant inter-species and inter-individual variance exists in their distribution.[6,7] β1-adrenoreceptors are predominantly found in cardiac and adipose tissues, whereas β2-adrenoreceptors are present in tissues such as bronchi and vasculature.[8] The β1-receptor mediates renin release and the effects of catecholamines and sympathetic activity on the cardiac tissue. Effect of β-blockers on either receptor depends on receptor selectivity and drug concentration. Selectivity is lost with increasing doses of the drug.

At lower concentrations of drug action is preferential to specific receptors. For example, low plasma concentrations of a selective β_2 agonist will favorably bind β_2 receptors. As plasma concentrations of the β_2 agonist increase, binding becomes less selective.

Blood pressure lowering

The mechanism of blood pressure lowering by β-blockers may be multifactorial. Four possible modes are described in the following material (Figure 78–1). The first possibility is diminished sympathetic outflow mediated by effects on the central nervous system (CNS). Hydrophilic agents such as practolol and sotalol do not decrease peripheral sympathetic activity while lowering blood pressure.[8] Thus, although the effects on the CNS may contribute to the mechanism of blood pressure lowering for certain drugs it may be difficult to use this to explain the efficacy of β-blockers (which lack the capacity to cross the blood/brain barrier).

The second possibility is that diminished cardiac output may contribute to lowering blood pressure. There is a drop in cardiac output in response to β-blockers, accompanied by increased peripheral resistance.[9] Continued therapy results in a decrease in peripheral resistance (although above pre-treatment levels) and thus may not alone explain the mechanism of blood pressure lowering.[10]

DISTRIBUTION OF α- AND β-RECEPTORS AND MEDIATED EFFECTS		
Receptor Subtype	**Organ System**	**Effect**
α	Blood vessel	↑ Constriction
	Uterus	↑ Contraction
	Pancreas	↓ Insulin secretion
β1	Heart	↑ Heart rate
	Kidneys	↑ Contractility
	Adipose tissue	↑ Conduction
	Parathyroid glands	↑ Excitation
		↑ Automaticity
		↑ Renin secretion
		↑ Lipolysis
		↑ Secretion
β2	Heart	↑ Heart rate
	Blood vessels	↑ Contractility
	Skeletal muscle	↑ Conduction
	Liver	↑ Excitation
	Lungs	↑ Automaticity
	Pancreas	↑ Vasodilation
	Uterus	↑ Vasodilation
	Urinary bladder	↑ Glycogenolysis
	Gastrointestinal	↑ Contractility
	Gall bladder and ducts	↑ Potassium uptake
	Nerve terminals	↑ Glycogenolysis
	Thyroid	↑ Bronchodilation
	Parathyroid glands	↑ Insulin and glucagon secretion
		↑ Relaxation
		↑ Adrenaline release
		↑ T4-T3 conversion
		↑ Secretion

Table 78–1. Distribution of α- and β-receptors and Mediated Effects

A third possibility is inhibition of renin secretion from the kidneys and a subsequent decrease in plasma angiotensin II.[11] Although studies have shown a correlation between reduction in blood pressure with β-blocker use and decreased plasma renin levels,[12] this may not fully explain the action of all members of this class.[13] Plasma renin levels were found to increase with β-blockers in combination with an ISA such as pindolol, with blood pressure reduction achieved.[10] Furthermore, techniques such as concomitant diuretic use or upright posture helped overcome the inhibitory effect of β-blockers on renin release while maintaining blood pressure control.

A fourth possibility is the uptake and accumulation of adrenaline in sympathetic nerve terminals and their stimulation of pre-synaptic β2 receptor release of noradrenaline and elevation of blood pressure.[14] Inhibitory effects upon stimulation of pre-synaptic β2 adrenergic receptors by adrenaline have also been suggested to explain the reduction in arterial pressure.[10] Nonselective blockers (e.g., propranolol) inhibit noradrenaline, whereas β1 selective agents (e.g., atenolol) do not inhibit β2 receptors but are still good blood-pressure-lowering agents.[15] In addition, β2 selective agents are not blood-pressure-lowering agents *per se* (undermining the importance of this mechanism).[16]

Structure/Activity relationships

Most β-blocking agents vary widely in their chemical structure but contain a common aminopropanol moiety linked to an aromatic system.[17] They are commonly prepared as racemic mixtures and consist of pairs of optical isomers.[18–20] Most of the β-blocking effect, which is useful in treating hypertension, is attributed to the negative levorotatory (l) stereoisomer. The dextrorotatory (d) form may not have many clinical benefits other than in d-sotalol and nebivolol, where it has antiarrhythmic and vasodilatory properties.[21,22] Membrane-stabilizing activity is a function of both forms (d and l).

PHARMACOKINETICS OF BETA BLOCKERS

Wide variances exist in the pharmacokinetics of this class of drugs (Tables 78–2 and 78–3). Despite similarities in their chemical structures, a number of differences arise in their pharmacokinetics (which are attributed to variations in aromatic ring).[19] Drugs in this class can be divided into arylethanolamines (e.g., sotalol) and aryloxypropanololamines (e.g., propanolol, atenolol, and pindolol). β-blocking drugs can be further characterized on the basis of absorption in the gut, lipid solubility, first-pass metabolism,

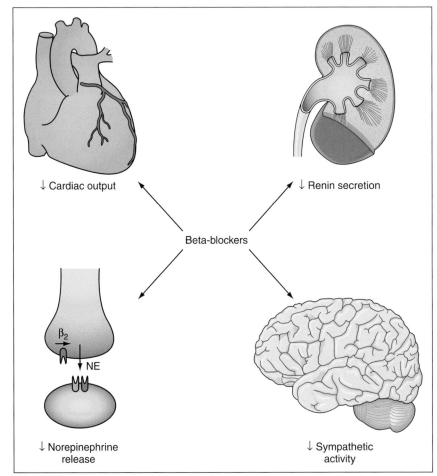

Figure 78–1. Mechanism of action for blood pressure lowering by β-blockers. Several modes of action have been proposed for the blood-pressure-lowering effect. The four most probable modes are depicted in this figure. No single mechanism can explain the effect for all agents in this class of drug.

low and variable oral bioavailability because they are metabolized in the wall of the gastrointestinal tract and in the liver. Lipid-soluble drugs show unpredictable absorption levels in patients receiving drugs that alter metabolism and hepatic blood flow. They also show unpredictable absorption levels under other low-flow conditions, with decreased hepatic circulation in the elderly and in patients with congestive heart failure and liver cirrhosis.[25,26]

In contrast, hydrophilic agents have relatively poorer absorption from the gut, are excreted from the kidneys relatively unchanged, and have poor transport across the blood/brain barrier. These drugs tend to have a longer half-life, which is further increased under conditions of reduced glomerular filtration rate (renal insufficiency and in the elderly).[27] These drugs show minimal interaction with other liver-metabolized drugs.

Relationships among dose, plasma concentration, and clinical effect

Lipid-soluble drugs of predominantly hepatic metabolism have wide variations in plasma concentrations.[28,29] In contrast, drugs with renal clearance have lower variations in plasma levels because they are excreted essentially unchanged. No clear relationship exists between β-blocker plasma concentrations and their clinical effects.[30] Wide variability exists among patients in regard to the relationship between plasma concentration and effect achieved.[28] A number of explanations have been offered in regard to this variation. One explanation posits that differences in sympathetic tone result in, for example, a higher concentration of drugs being required by individuals with increased sympathetic tone.

Body fat distribution (especially in regard to lipid-soluble drugs) and flat dose-response curves are among the other mechanisms suggested. A flat dose-response curve may result in minor changes in clinical effects despite variations in plasma concentrations. In addition, plasma concentrations of pharmacologically active metabolites of certain drugs (such as propranolol and acebutolol) that may not be detectable on standard plasma assays have been suggested as causes of this discordance.

Intrinsic sympathetic activity

Certain β-blockers possess partial agonist properties.[31] ISA caused by a beta-adrenoceptor-blocking drug results in a number of different pharmacologic properties. Most profound are the central hemodynamic effects. β-blockers

blood/brain barrier crossing ability, concentration within cardiac tissue, biotransformation, and renal clearance.

Absorption from the gut among this class of drugs remains fairly constant, with few exceptions.[23] Bioavailability of these drugs is variable. Whereas some of them are metabolized in the liver and thus have a shorter half-life, others are largely excreted by the kidneys unchanged and thus have a longer average half-life.

Absorption

Generally, β-blockers are absorbed from the gastrointestinal tract via passive diffusion. The majority of the β-blockers are well absorbed in the small intestine. Exceptions (e.g., nadolol and atenolol) are not well absorbed from the gut.[24] Rates of absorption ranges vary from 30% for nadolol to more than 90% for the majority of the other agents in this class. Where absorption tends to be rapid for the short-acting lipid-soluble drugs, water-soluble drugs take longer. Other factors that interfere with absorption of drugs in the gastric tract include gastric emptying time and the presence of food.

Lipid solubility

Absorption of lipid-soluble drugs from the gastrointestinal tract is rapid and complete. These drugs have a relatively

PHARMACOKINETICS OF BETA-BLOCKING DRUGS							
Drug	Half-life (h)	Absorption (%)	Bioavailability (%)	Protein Binding (%)	Lipid Solubility	Clearance *Liver/Kidney*	
Acebutolol	7–13	>90	20–60	25	Low	++++	+
Atenolol	6–9	50	45–50	<5	Low	+	++++
Betaxolol	14–22	>90	=80	50	Low	+++++	——
Bisoprolol	6–9	=90	90	=33	Low	++	++
Bucindolol	3–4	=90	=30	95	Moderate	++++	+
Carteolol	6	=90	=90	23–30	Low	——	+++++
Carvedilol	7	>90	=30	98	Moderate	++++	+
Celiprolol	5–6	H30	30–75	22–24	Low	++	+++
Esmolol[a]	9 min	——	——	55	Low	——	——
Labetalol	6	>90	=33	=50	Moderate	+++++	——
Metoprolol	3–4	>90	50	12	Moderate	+++++	——
Nadolol	12–24	H30	30–40	=30	Low	——	+++++
Nebivolol	22	>90	12–96	98	NA	+++++	——
Oxprenolol	1–4	H90	19–74	80	Moderate	+++++	——
Penbutolol	1–3	>90	=100	80–98	High	++++	+
Pindolol	3–4	>90	90	57	Moderate	+++	++
Propranolol	2–5	>90	30–70	93	High	+++++	——
Sotalol	7–18	70–90	75–90	0	Low	+	++++
Timolol	4–5	>90	50–75	=10	Moderate	++++	+

a. Esmolol is metabolized by erythrocyte esterases.

Table 78–2. Pharmacokinetics of Beta-blocking Drugs

PHARMACODYNAMIC PROPERTIES OF BETA-BLOCKING AGENTS				
Agent	Selectivity	ISA	MSA	Additional Properties
Acebutolol	$\beta1$	+	+	—
Atenolol	$\beta1$	—	—	—
Betaxolol	$\beta1$	—	—	—
Bisoprolol	$\beta1$	—	—	—
Bucindolol	$\beta1, \beta2$	—	—	—
Carteolol	$\beta1, \beta2$	+	—	—
Carvedilol	$\beta1, \beta2, \alpha1$	—	+ +	Anti-oxidative
Celiprolol	$\beta1, \alpha2$	+	—	—
Esmolol	$\beta1$	—	—	—
Labetalol	$\beta1, \beta2, \alpha1$	+	—	—
Metoprolol	$\beta1$	—	—	—
Nadolol	$\beta1, \beta2$	—	—	—
Nebivolol	$\beta1$	+	—	NO release
Oxprenolol	$\beta1, \beta2$	+	+	—
Penbutolol	$\beta1, \beta2$	+	—	—
Pindolol	$\beta1, \beta2$	+	—	—
Propranolol	$\beta1, \beta2$	—	+ +	—
Sotalol	$\beta1, \beta2$	—	—	—
Timolol	$\beta1, \beta2$	—	—	—

Abbreviations: ISA, intrinsic sympathetic activity; MSA, membrane-stabilizing activity.

Table 78–3. Pharmacodynamic Properties of Beta-blocking Agents

with a significant degree of ISA interact with both binding and activation sites on the beta receptor. Although these drugs attach avidly to the binding sites, they tend to have low affinity for the activation site. The overall effect depends on the sympathetic state. Conditions with low sympathetic tone (e.g., during rest/sleep) are associated with a sufficient degree of ISA and a resultant decreased reduction in heart rate and cardiac output. If the drug possesses β2 ISA, stimulation of β2 vasodilator receptors may result in less of a decrease in peripheral blood flow.

In contrast, during conditions of high sympathetic tone (e.g., exercise)—and if full dosages of the drugs are used—β-blockade predominates and a β-blocking drug with ISA produces less of an increase in heart rate. In asthmatic subjects, the modest β-stimulant action on bronchial smooth muscle is not important, as these patients are potentially sensitive to any receptor blockade. Down-regulation of β-receptors by β-blocking drugs with ISA prevents post-beta-blocking drug hypersensitivity upon withdrawal of the agent. In contrast, β-blockade with drugs without ISA results in up-regulation of β-receptors. Upon discontinuing the drug, rebound phenomena resulting from uninhibited stimulation by catecholamines characterized by palpitations and anxiety are seen.[32] Patients with ischemic disease are at risk of cardiovascular events (including myocrdial infarction and death) following abrupt β-blocker withdrawal.

Membrane-stabilizing activity

Membrane-stabilizing activity refers to the ability of certain drugs to exert a quinidine-like effect by reducing the rate of rise of intra-cardiac action potential or by reducing local anesthetic activity. β-blockers interact with sodium channels to produce this effect, although such actions appear to occur only at doses much higher than those required to produce effective β-blockade. Not all β-blockers possess this characteristic. Certain β-blockers (such as metoprolol and pindolol) have weak effects, whereas drugs such as atenolol have none. Membrane-stabilizing activity does not contribute to the lowering of blood pressure.

DRUG INTERACTIONS

Interactions with other drugs can be understood using an example of propanolol, which traditionally represents this class.[33] The bioavailability of propanolol (a liver-metabolized drug) is decreased by agents (e.g., alcohol, phenytoin, rifampin, Phenobarbital, and smoking) that induce hepatic biotransformation enzymes. These agents decrease the plasma concentration and half-lives of lipophilic β-blockers. In contrast, drugs (e.g., cimetidine, hydralazine, and so on) that inhibit hepatic enzymes can increase lipophilic β-blocker bioavailability.[34] Concomitant use of antiarrythmic drugs and calcium antagonists may cause sinus nodes or conduction anomalies.

Nonsteroidal anti-inflammatory drugs (NSAIDs) may have an antagonistic effect on the antihypertensive effect of β-blockers.[35] Elderly blacks are at the greatest risk. The mechanism of the hypertensive effects of NSAIDs seems primarily related to their ability to block the cyclo-oxygenase pathway of arachidonic acid metabolism, with a resultant decrease in prostaglandin formation. Co-administration of clonidine and β-blocker can result in elevated blood pressure,[36] and stopping clonidine in the presence of propranolol has been shown to result in cerebral hemorrhage.[37]

ADVERSE EFFECTS

The adverse effects of β-blockers are usually due to blockade of $β_2$-receptor-mediated functions such as bronchodilation, vasodilation, and mobilization of glucose and free fatty acids. β-blockers can result in a wide range of side effects, depending on the dose and population (Box 78–1). Usage should be determined based on risk/benefit comparison in a particular clinical scenario. Although it is necessary to observe caution regarding side effects, it is important to remember the utility of β-blockers in patients with peripheral vascular disease, coronary artery disease, and diabetes (especially post-MI or involving CHF).

Cardiovascular

By virtue of their chronotropic effects, β-blockers reduce heart rate, reduce the firing rate of ectopic pacemakers, decrease conduction, and increase the refractory time of the AV node (resulting in bradycardia and atrioventricular (AV) block). These effects are predominantly observed in patients with sinus nodes or conduction abnormalities. Caution should be exercised when prescribing other negative chronotropes such as diltiazem, verapamil, or digoxin. β-blockers may worsen symptoms of peripheral vascular disease by producing cold extremities and Raynaud's phenomenon. β-blockers with vasodilatory effects result, and β1-selective agents may produce lesser effects on peripheral vasculature.

As mentioned previously, β-blockade with a nonselective blocker results in up-regulation of β-receptors. Suddenly

---

Box 78–1

Adverse Effects Related to Beta-blocker Use

General: Arthralgias, asthenia, fatigue, diaphoresis, edema, myalgia, pharyngitis, urinary retention
CNS: Depression, dizziness, hallucinations, headache, insomnia, nightmares, paresthesias
Eye: Lacrimation, ocular irritation, xerosis
Cardiovascular: Orthostatic hypotension, peripheral vasoconstriction, peripheral edema, QT prolongation, sinus bradycardia, syncope, torsade de pointes, ventricular tachycardia, angina, AV block, cardiac arrest
Respiratory: Bronchospasm, wheezing, dyspnea
Gastrointestinal: Jaundice, diarrhea, dyspepsia, hepatic necrosis, nausea, vomiting, constipation, flatulence, hypoglycemia, elevated liver function tests
Sexual: Ejaculation dysfunction, impotence, libido decrease, orgasmic dysfunction in women
Skin: Skin hyperpigmentation, alopecia, exfoliative dermatitis, pruritis
Metabolic: Weight gain, increased cholesterol and triglycerides, increased insulin resistance

discontinuing the drug exposes the up-regulated receptors to uninhibited catecholamines, resulting in symptoms such as hypertension, arrhythmias, anxiety, and increased risk of myocardial ischemia in susceptible patients.[38,39]

Metabolic

Nonselective β-blockers in insulin-dependent diabetes mellitus may mask warning symptoms of hypoglycemia, including tremor and tachycardia. Other symptoms (such as sweating) persist. Selective β-blockers are preferable in insulin-dependent diabetics.[40] Data on the effects of β-blockers on serum lipoproteins is conflicting. β-blockers have been shown to increase triglyceride levels and decrease high-density lipoprotein (HDL) levels.[41–43]

β-blockers with ISA have a smaller effect on serum lipoproteins compared to those lacking it. A review of 474 studies demonstrated that increase in triglyceride levels and effect on HDL was diminished with cardio-selective agents.[44] β-blocker use is often associated with an increase in body weight.[45] Thus, its use in uncomplicated obese hypertensives is further affected by unwanted weight gain.

Pulmonary

Use of β-blockers in patients with asthma or significant reactive airway disease can lead to increased airway resistance and even to life-threatening bronchospasm. Although the threat of worsening airway disease exists, certain patients with chronic obstructive pulmonary disease may benefit from β-blockade.[46] Chronic obstructive pulmonary disease in the absence of any significant reactive component is not a contraindication to the use of β-blockers.

Sexual dysfunction

Certain patients may experience worsening impotence or loss of libido. Higher rates of impotence were seen in a propanolol group compared to placebo in the MRC mild hypertension study.[47,48] Ejaculation dysfunction is another side effect associated with β-blocker use.

Central effects

As mentioned previously, central effects are more common with lipophilic agents compared to hydrophilic agents.[49] Central effects include fatigue, headache, sleep disturbance, insomnia, vivid dreams, nightmares, and depression.

CLINICAL USE AND INDICATIONS

Hypertension

β-adrenoreceptor-blocking drugs are recommended, along with thiazides, as one of the first-line drugs in initial treatment of hypertension. Although all of these first-line agents have a near equal ability to lower blood pressure in large clinical studies, their efficacy may differ depending on demographic groups and other co-morbid conditions. When considering the initial class of drug, age, race, metabolic side effects, cardiovascular disease, and concomitant disease states should be taken into account. Guidelines recommend blood pressure reduction to levels based on risk profile. A greater reduction should be achieved in high-risk patients.

While maintaining adequate blood pressure control, it is quintessential that the antihypertensive agent should reduce cardiovascular morbidity and mortality. β-blockers as a class have failed to show any role in primary prevention in uncomplicated hypertension. Hence, they should not be recommended as first-line agents in uncomplicated hypertension.

Based on recent trial evidence, β-blockers were removed as first-, second-, and third-line agents by the guidelines of the British Hypertension Society. However, not all agree with this position. In 2003, the *Seventh Report of the Joint National Committee on Prevention, Detection, Evaluation, and Treatment of High Blood Pressure* (JNC 7) still considered β-blockers as appropriate drugs for primary prevention in uncomplicated hypertension. We may select a β-blocker for hypertensive patients who are symptomatic from excessive sympathetic activity, although there is no outcome evidence in this regard.

β-blockers that have traditionally been recommended for the initial treatment of hypertension include propranolol, metoprolol, and atenolol. All β-blocker are similar in efficacy to control blood pressure regardless of whether they are cardio-selective (β1-specific) or nonselective (β1 and β2), possess ISA, or are lipid/water soluble. However, they differ in their metabolic effects and ability to reduce cardiovascular morbidity and mortality, especially in hypertensives without risk factors.[50] Box 78–2 compares the differential effect of newer and traditional agents on the hemodynamic profile of patients.

Beta blockers and ethnic differences

Ethnic differences exist in responses to β-blockers in patient populations.[51] The reason for this difference is not clear, but results suggest differences in hepatic metabolism may be an important contributory factor. For example, propanolol is least responsive in blacks.[52] In contrast, Chinese patients have been shown to be more sensitive to beta-blockade effect in comparison to white patients.[53]

β-blockers also tend to be less effective as monotherapy in black/Afro-Caribbean populations, possibly due to the low renin state in this ethnic group (especially in older subjects).

Box 78–2

Unfavorable Hemodynamic and Metabolic Effects of Beta Blockers

- Decrease in cardiac output and heart rate; increase in vascular resistance
- Low efficacy in reducing LV hypertrophy
- Reduced renal blood flow and glomerular infiltrate rate
- Minimal effect on arterial stiffness
- Increased risk of new-onset diabetes, triglycerides
- Decrease in high-density lipoproteins
- Decrease in exercise tolerance

This can largely be overcome by co-administration of a diuretic.

Beta blockers in chronic heart failure

Recent clinical trials have demonstrated the beneficial effects of β-blocker therapy on survival in CHF due to systole dysfunction. Based on data from these trials, β-blocker therapy has become part of standard therapy for patients with CHF, in addition to angiotensin-converting enzyme inhibitors and diuretics. Whether clinical effects of certain β-blockers are the result of properties such as antioxidant effects or of enhanced nitric oxide production is not certain. β-blockers (particularly those with vasodilatory properties) have beneficial hemodynamic, metabolic, and renal responses. These drugs have been effective in the reduction of long-term cardiovascular morbidity and mortality in patients with CHF and in survivors of acute MI.

In a recently reported COMET (Carvedilol or Metoprolol European Trial) report,[54] effects of carvedilol and metoprolol were compared in patients with CHF due to left ventricular (LV) systolic dysfunction. Patients with ejection fractions (EF) <35% (N = 1,151) were randomized to equivalent β-blocking doses of either drug. Carvedilol treatment was associated with a significant 17% greater reduction in all-cause mortality ($P = 0.0017$) and a 20% greater reduction in cardiovascular mortality ($P = 0.0004$) compared to metoprolol therapy.

Beta blockers in post myocardial infarction patients

The use of β-blockers in post-MI has been shown to reduce cardiovascular mortality. Noteworthy trials demonstrating the role of beta blockade in MI are the β-blocker Heart Attack Trial (BHAT)[55], the Norwegian Multicenter Study of Timolol after Myocardial Infarction,[56] and the Carvedilol Post-Infarct Survival Control in LV Dysfunction (CAPRICORN) trial.[57]

The BHAT compared the incidence of coronary incidence defined as recurrent nonfatal definite reinfarction plus fatal coronary heart disease in 3,837 patients receiving propanolol or placebo. Patients were followed up for an average of 25 months and the trial was terminated early on evidence of clear differences in reduction of coronary incidence in the propranolol group. An incidence of 10% was observed in the propranolol group compared with 13% in the placebo group, which was a reduction of 23%. The incidence of definite nonfatal reinfarction was lower (by 15.6%), and that of definite or probable nonfatal reinfarction was also lower (by 14.7%).[55,58]

Similarly, timolol was compared to placebo in the Norwegian timolol study in 1,884 patients followed for 12 to 33 months. One hundred fifty-two patients in the placebo group and 98 in the timolol group died. The life-table cumulative probability of total death was 21.9% in the placebo group and 13.3% in the timolol group, corresponding to a relative reduction of 39.4% ($P = 0.0003$). One hundred thirty-one nonfatal reinfarctions were confirmed in the placebo group and 90 were confirmed in the timolol group, including events among withdrawn patients. The life-table probability rate of reinfarction was

16.4% in the placebo and 11.8% in the timolol group ($P = 0.001$). It was concluded that chronic treatment with timolol in survivors of acute MI who can tolerate beta-adrenergic blockade is effective in reducing both total mortality and reinfarction over 33 months.[56]

The CAPRICORN trial compared the effect of carvedilol and placebo on cardiovascular end points in 1,959 survivors of acute MI with reduced EFs. Carvedilol-treated patients experienced a significant 23% greater reduction in all-cause mortality ($P = 0.031$), a 25% greater reduction in cardiovascular death ($P = 0.024$), and a 41% greater reduction in nonfatal recurrent MI ($P = 0.014$) compared with placebo-treated patients. Another trial comparing carvedilol and atenolol in MI survivors with normal EF found carvedilol to significantly lower a composite score of cardiovascular events better than atenolol.[53]

Blacks, patients 80 years old or older, and those with a LV EF below 20%, serum creatinine concentration greater than 1.4 mg per deciliter, or diabetes mellitus had a lower percentage of reduction in mortality. However, given the higher mortality rates in these subgroups the absolute reduction in mortality was similar to or greater than that among patients with no specific risk factors. After MI, patients with conditions often considered contraindications to beta-blockade (such as pulmonary disease and older age) and those with nontransmural infarction benefit from β-blocker therapy.[59] Controlled trials in patients who are post-MI with normal or close to normal LV function are needed to assess use of β-blockers in this subgroup.[60]

Beta blockers in acute coronary syndromes

Role of β-blockers in acute settings have been primarily based on results from two major trials conducted in the 1980s: metoprolol in acute myocardial infarction (MIAMI)[61,62] and first international study of infarct survival (ISIS-1).[63] Results from ISIS-1 show non-significant reduction of early in-hospital events described as nonfatal cardiac arrests and reinfarctions with the use of atenolol compared to placebo. Subsequent necropsy of patients with complications in the ISIS-1 study failed to reveal any considerable role of mechanisms such as limitation of infarct size or prevention of reinfarction or cardiac arrest.

The extent of thrombolytic use in these studies is also not clear. In the absence of data pertaining to concomitant use of thrombolytics in these patients, added benefits of β-blockers in acute events is still debatable. The recently reported Clopidogrel and Metoprolol in Myocardial Infarction Trial (COMMIT/CCS-2)[64] showed that early use of β-blockers in acute MI was associated with increased risk of cardiogenic shock. Results from this study of more than 45,000 patients suggest avoiding intravenous use of β-blocker and use of β-blockers in general within 12 hours of acute MI.

Beta blockers in diabetes mellitus

As previously mentioned, β-blockers were relatively contraindicated in diabetes until recently. Nonselective β-blockers can prevent normalization of blood sugar after an episode of hypoglycemia in patients on insulin. This is accompanied by a rise in blood pressure and reflex brady-cardia. The risk of developing diabetes is high in nondiabetic hypertensives on treatment with β-blocking agents.[65–68] Similarly, the efficacy of β-blockers in reducing cardiovascular and all-cause mortality in diabetics is not impressive. The Losartan Intervention for Endpoint Reduction in Hypertension (LIFE) trial[69] showed that atenolol was less effective than the angiotensin receptor blocker (losartan) in reducing cardiovascular events and all-cause mortality in mainly elderly hypertensives with diabetes.

The United Kingdom Prospective (UKPDS) study showed a non-significant difference between β-blockers (atenolol) and ACE inhibitors (captopril) in type 2 diabetics with hypertension in preventing all primary macrovascular and microvascular endpoints.[70] Captopril and atenolol were equally effective in reducing the risk of macrovascular endpoints. Similar proportions of patients in the two groups showed deterioration in retinopathy by two grades after nine years (31% in the captopril group and 37% in the atenolol group) and developed clinical-grade albuminuria at 300 mg/L (5 and 9%, respectively). Data from this trial showed that young, middle aged diabetics witnessed the most reduction in cardiovascular endpoints. This difference in outcomes was attributed to β-blockade in a relatively higher sympathetic state in the younger age group, and to subsequent stimulation of normally functioning beta-1 receptors.[71] β-blockers utilized in the type 2 diabetic patients resulted in an even greater decrease in cardiac events than in the nondiabetic patients.

Recent evidence shows that benefits of β-blocker reign over the risks in high-risk patients, such as patients post-MI.[72] The COMET showed that use of carvedilol resulted in a decrease in new onset of diabetes in patients with heart failure.[54] The Glycemic Effects in Diabetes Mellitus: Carvedilol-Metoprolol Comparison in Hypertensives (GEMINI) trial[73] compared carvedilol and metoprolol (third- and second-generation β-blockers, respectively) in patients with hypertension and type 2 diabetes. Both treatment groups had similar blood pressure lowering. Mean HbA1c increased with metoprolol (0.15% [0.04%]; $P < .001$) but not carvedilol (0.02% [0.04%]; $P = 0.65$). Insulin sensitivity improved with carvedilol (–9.1%; $P = 0.004$) but not metoprolol (–2.0%; $P = 0.48$). Progression to microalbuminuria was less frequent with carvedilol than with metoprolol (6.4 versus 10.3%; odds ratio, 0.60; 95% CI, 0.36 to 0.97; $P = 0.04$). More participants withdrew due to worsening glycemic control in the metoprolol group.

Unfortunately, traditional β-blockers are associated with the worsening of insulin resistance, deterioration of glycemic control, peripheral vasoconstriction, potentially worsening peripheral vascular disease, and more frequent and severe hypoglycemia. The newer β-blockers have unique properties, including alpha1-blockade, and they lower insulin resistance, improve glycemic control, and vasodilate resistance arterioles.

Beta blockers in the elderly and those with left ventricular hypertrophy

The JNC 7 guidelines made the recommendation that systolic blood pressure be the primary target for the diagnosis and care of older persons with hypertension.[3] Multiple studies have provided evidence that increased large artery thickening and stiffness[74] and endothelial dysfunction in healthy elderly persons, which were earlier considered to be part of normal aging process, along with the resulting increase in systolic and pulse pressure may be related to a greater risk of manifestation of hypertension, to atherosclerosis, and to other associated cardiovascular events.[75]

Hypertension, especially in the elderly, is marked by reduced cardiac output and increased peripheral vascular resistance.[76,77] In addition, there is a decrease in renal blood flow and glomerular filtration rate and an increase in proteinuria.[78–83] Unlike the other classes of antihypertensive agents that reduce blood pressure by lowering peripheral vascular resistance while preserving cardiac output, traditional β-blockers lower blood pressure by reducing cardiac output through their negative inotropic effect and induce a compensatory increase in vascular tone mediated through a_1 vascular receptors (Box 78–2). In addition, nonselective β-blockers can also promote vasoconstriction by blocking vasodilatory $β_2$ vascular receptors.[84]

Long-term β-blocker therapy produces homeostatic regulatory adjustments that can improve cardiac output but still be depressed compared to original state. These adjustments may decrease vascular resistance to some degree, but cardiac output will remain distinctly elevated (often above pre-treatment levels).[85,86] Traditional β-blockers further decrease renal blood flow and glomerular filtration rate and have no effect on proteinuria.[81,82,87,88] Similarly, older agents have no effect on arterial stiffness or hypertrophy.[89,90] Cardioselective β-blockers with low lipid solubility have a preferable side-effect profile in older persons.

β-blockers that are lipophilic cross the blood/brain barrier, possibly causing more sedation, depression, and sexual dysfunction in older patients.[22] Particularly in older patients, β-blockers as a class can cause bradycardia, conduction abnormalities, and development of heart failure if started too aggressively in patients with preexisting LV dysfunction.[6,22,23] β-blockers should be tapered before discontinuation to minimize the risk of reflex tachycardia.

A meta-analysis of 10 placebo-controlled hypertension trials of more than 16,000 elderly patients (= 60 years) found that although traditional β-blockers significantly lowered blood pressure they were ineffective in preventing coronary heart disease (defined as fatal or nonfatal MI and sudden cardiac death, cardiovascular mortality, and all-cause mortality).[91] In addition, a meta-analysis of 80 double-blind randomized controlled trials with 3,767 hypertensive patients found that β-blockers were the least effective in reducing LV mass compared with ARBs, calcium channel antagonists (CCAs), and ACE inhibitors despite similar blood pressure reduction among these antihypertensive drug classes ($P = 0.004$).[92]

The lesser effectiveness of β-blockers, compared with angiotensin II receptor antagonists, on LV mass reduction is in accordance with the results of one of the largest trials on antihypertensive treatment in patients with LV hypertrophy [the Losartan Intervention for Endpoint Reduction in Hypertension (LIFE) study]. In that study, losartan was more effective in reducing electrocardiographically determined LV hypertrophy than was atenolol. The beneficial effects on LV hypertrophy were partly responsible for the better cardiovascular outcome in patients treated with losartan.

A randomized study with 42 elderly patients with hypertension concluded that the β-blocker atenolol failed to reduce LV mass compared to the CCA verapamil after six months of treatment despite comparable blood pressure lowering.[93] In a randomized double-blind study of 19 untreated hypertensive patients treated with the ARB losartan or atenolol treatment, atenolol-treated patients failed to demonstrate a reduction in LV mass despite comparable blood pressure reduction in both groups.[94] In addition, a meta-analysis of 80 double-blind randomized controlled trials with 3,767 hypertensive patients found that β-blockers were the least effective in reducing LV mass compared with ARBs, CCAs, and ACE inhibitors despite similar blood pressure reduction among these antihypertensive drug classes ($P = 0.004$).[92]

A randomized study with 42 elderly patients with hypertension concluded that atenolol failed to reduce LV mass compared to verapamil after six months of treatment despite comparable blood pressure lowering.[93] In a randomized double-blind study of 19 untreated hypertensive patients treated with losartan or atenolol treatment, atenolol-treated patients failed to demonstrate a reduction in LV mass despite comparable blood pressure reduction in both groups.[94]

The poor efficacy of β-blockers in the elderly may be attributed to unfavorable effects on the hemodynamics in the vasculature and end organs and to metabolism. Table 78–4 summarizes the effect of traditional β-blockers on the hemodynamic profile. Newer agents with peripheral vasodilating properties have a more favorable profile. Based on results from trials and inherent properties of β-blockers that result in a less than favorable effect, β-blocking drugs are not suitable as first-line agents in the elderly without other co-morbid conditions such as CHF or MI.[95]

Beta blockers and cardiac arrhythmias

Hypertensive patients are prone to both supraventricular and ventricular arrhythmias. The most common sustained cardiac rhythm disorder is atrial fibrillation, and the β-

blockers have a role for rate control in permanent AF.[96] In paroxysmal AF, β-blockers may also be useful for the suppression of paroxysms and maintenance of sinus rhythm, as well as the facilitation of cardioversion in persistent AF.

BETA BLOCKERS AND PRIMARY PREVENTION

Hypertension is a well-recognized risk factor for the development of serious cardiovascular disease. Multiple prospective observational studies have documented a strong, continuous, graded, and independent association between blood pressure and mortality risk due to stroke, coronary artery disease (CAD), or other vascular causes.[97] Hypertension also doubles the risk of developing congestive heart failure, which is augmented by the presence of CAD.[98,99] Hypertension also similarly increases the risk of developing end-stage renal disease.[100]

Using a variety of antihypertensive agents to lower elevated blood pressure to <140/90 mmHg has consistently decreased cardiovascular events. Systematic overviews of multiple trials show that reducing diastolic blood pressure by as little as 7.5 mmHg results in 46% and 29% relative risk reductions in stroke and CAD, respectively.[101] Even reducing systolic blood pressure by as little as 2 mmHg can lower the risk of stroke by 10% and CAD mortality by 7%.[97] The largest single randomized controlled blood pressure trial, the Antihypertensive and Lipid-Lowering Treatment to Prevent Heart Attack Trial (ALLHAT),[102] reported that lowering blood pressure with a diuretic, an ACE inhibitor, or a CCA significantly improved cardiovascular endpoints. Unfortunately, however, β-blockers were not directly studied in this landmark trial.

In a recent review of clinical hypertension trials, although β-blockers significantly lowered blood pressure there was no convincing evidence to support their effectiveness in reducing cardiovascular morbidity and mortality, including fatal and nonfatal stroke and MI. A meta-analysis of 10 placebo-controlled hypertension trials of more than 16,000 elderly patients (> 60 years) similarly found that although traditional β-blockers significantly lowered blood pressure they were ineffective in preventing coronary heart disease, defined as fatal or nonfatal MI and sudden cardiac death,

COMPARISON OF TRADITIONAL AND NEWER BETA-BLOCKING AGENTS[a]

Function	Ideal Drug	Traditional Beta Blockers	Carvedilol
Mean arterial blood pressure	Decrease	Decrease	Decrease
Total peripheral resistance	Decrease	Increase	Decrease
Cardiac output	None	Decrease	None
Heart rate	None/decrease	Decrease	None/decrease
Activation of sympathetic nervous system	Decrease	Decrease	Decrease
Renin-angiotensin-aldosterone system	Decrease	Decrease	Decrease
Lipid metabolism	None/positive	Negative	None
Glucose metabolism	None/positive	Negative	None
a. Newer agents have a more beneficial metabolic and hemodynamic profile.			

Table 78–4. Comparison of Traditional and Newer Beta-blocking Agents[a]

cardiovascular mortality, and all-cause mortality.[91] Another recent meta-analysis showed that although atenolol reduced blood pressure greater than placebo and comparably to other antihypertensive agents there was no difference in mortality or MI compared to placebo and there was an increased risk of mortality and stroke compared with other antihypertensives. However, the risk of stroke with atenolol was lower compared to placebo.[103]

NEWER AGENTS

Nonselective β-blockers (such as propranolol, and the β_1-selective blockers atenolol and metoprolol) have traditionally played a role in the treatment of hypertension. β-blockers successfully lower elevated blood pressure but are less effective in reducing the risk of morbidity and mortality associated with hypertension-related cardiovascular diseases (including stroke and CAD) compared with other antihypertensive agents such as diuretics, ACE inhibitors, and CCAs. The mechanisms by which traditional β-blockers lower blood pressure differ significantly from those of other antihypertensive agents. β-blockers lower cardiac output and induce a compensatory increase in peripheral vascular resistance. This reflex increase in a_1-adrenergic activity may in turn lead to metabolic consequences that can promote CAD, decrease insulin sensitivity and glucose utilization, increase triglyceride levels, and decrease HDL cholesterol levels.

The availability of vasodilating β-blockers represents a significant change from the hemodynamic, renal, and metabolic responses associated with traditional β-blocker therapy (Table 78–4). Newer agents with a combined alpha and beta effect maintain cardiac output, have a lower effect on heart rate, and decrease blood pressure by decreasing systemic vascular resistance.[50] These newer agents thus have a more preferential hemodynamic profile. Carvedilol increases plasma flow to the kidneys as opposed to the decreased glomerular filtration rate seen with traditional β-blockers. These properties are an advantage, especially in the elderly (in whom the cardiac output is low and systemic vascular resistance elevated).

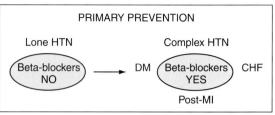

Figure 78–2. Algorithm for β-blocker use. Beta-blocking agents should not be used for management of hypertension in patients with no other co-morbid conditions. In patients with hypertension and congestive heart failure, post-MI, or diabetes, beta-blocking agents should be a first-line agent.

The beneficial effect of carvedilol on systemic resistance is similar to ACE inhibitors and calcium channel blockers. Carvedilol was found superior to traditional β-blockers on many levels in addition to its hemodynamic properties. One aspect is the lower rate of new-onset diabetes compared to traditional β-blockers, owing to its effect on increase of glucose utilization, in turn decreasing circulating insulin levels and hence improving insulin sensitivity. Carvedilol seems to have fewer metabolic adverse effects than traditional β-blockers. Furthermore, carvedilol has a beneficial effect on lipid profile or a neutral effect on atherogenicity. This may be of particular importance in younger patients, who will be exposed to these drugs for a longer duration.

FUTURE POSSIBILITIES

β-blockers have been popular antihypertensive agents in clinical practice. However, the efficacy of β-blockers has been poorly documented. Guidelines relating to β-blocker use need to be readdressed (Figure 78–2). Further outcome trials on the role of newer β-blockers in the primary prevention of cardiovascular events and mortality in uncomplicated hypertension and the elderly are warranted.

REFERENCES

1. Prichard BN, Gillam PM. Use of propranolol (inderal) in treatment of hypertension. *Br Med J* 1964;5411:725–27.
2. Chobanian AV, Bakris GL, Black HR, et al. The Seventh Report of the Joint National Committee on Prevention, Detection, Evaluation, and Treatment of High Blood Pressure: The JNC 7 report. *JAMA* 2003;289(19):2560–72.
3. Chobanian AV, Bakris GL, Black HR, et al. Seventh Report of the Joint National Committee on Prevention, Detection, Evaluation, and Treatment of High Blood Pressure. *Hypertension* 2003;42(6):1206–52.
4. Lefkowitz RJ, Caron MG, Stiles GL. Mechanisms of membrane-receptor regulation: Biochemical, physiological, and clinical insights derived from studies

of the adrenergic receptors. *N Engl J Med* 1984;310(24):1570–79.
5. Lands AM, Arnold A, McAuliff JP, et al. Differentiation of receptor systems activated by sympathomimetic amines. *Nature* 1967;214(88):597–98.
6. Minneman KP, Hedberg A, Molinoff PB. Comparison of beta adrenergic receptor subtypes in mammalian tissues. *J Pharmacol Exp Ther* 1979;211(3):502–08.
7. Hedberg A, Minneman KP, Molinoff PB. Differential distribution of beta-1 and beta-2 adrenergic receptors in cat and guinea-pig heart. *J Pharmacol Exp Ther* 1980;212(3):503–08.
8. Cruickshank JM. *Beta Blockers in Clinical Practice, Second Edition.* Edinburgh: Churchill-Livingstone 1994:1–1204.

9. Colfer HT, Cottier C, Sanchez R, Julius S. Role of cardiac factors in the initial hypotensive action by beta-adrenoreceptor blocking agents. *Hypertension* 1984;6(2/1):145–51.
10. Man In't Veld AJ, Schalekamp MA. Effects of 10 different beta-adrenoceptor antagonists on hemodynamics, plasma renin activity, and plasma norepinephrine in hypertension: The key role of vascular resistance changes in relation to partial agonist activity. *J Cardiovasc Pharmacol* 1983;5(1):S30–45.
11. Buhler FR, Laragh JH, Baer L, et al. Propranolol inhibition of renin secretion: A specific approach to diagnosis and treatment of renin-dependent hypertensive diseases. *N Engl J Med* 1972;287(24):1209–14.

12. Castenfors J, Johnsson H, Oro L. Effect of alprenolol on blood pressure and plasma renin activity in hypertensive patients. *Acta Med Scand* 1973;193(3):189–95.

13. Hansson L. Beta-adrenergic blockade in essential hypertension: Effects of propranolol on hemodynamic parameters and plasma renin activity. *Acta Med Scand Suppl* 1973;550:1–40.

14. Richards AM, Nicholls MG, Espiner EA, et al. Diurnal patterns of blood pressure, heart rate and vasoactive hormones in normal man. *Clin Exp Hypertens A* 1986;8(2):153–66.

15. Vincent HH, Man In't Veld AJ, Boomsma F, et al. Elevated plasma noradrenaline in response to beta-adrenoceptor stimulation in man. *Br J Clin Pharmacol* 1982;13(5):717–21.

16. Dahlof B, Andren L, Svensson A, Hansson L. Antihypertensive mechanism of beta-adrenoceptor antagonism: The role of beta 2-blockade. *J Hypertens Suppl* 1983;1(2):112–15.

17. Fitzgerald DG. Beta-adrenoceptor antagonism. In: van Zwieten PA (ed.), *Pharmacology of antihypertensive drugs.* Amsterdam: Elsevier 1984:249–306 (*Handbook of hypertension,* Vol. 3.)

18. Conolly ME, Kersting F, Dollery CT. The clinical pharmacology of beta-adrenoceptor-blocking drugs. *Prog Cardiovasc Dis* 1976;19(3):203–34.

19. Frishman W. Clinical pharmacology of the new beta-adrenergic blocking drugs. Part 1: Pharmacodynamic and pharmacokinetic properties. *Am Heart J* 1979;97(5):663–70.

20. Koch-Weser J, Frishman WH. Beta-adrenoceptor antagonists: New drugs and new indications. *N Engl J Med* 1981;305(9):500–06.

21. Singh BN, Deedwania P, Nademanee K, et al. Sotalol: A review of its pharmacodynamic and pharmacokinetic properties, and therapeutic use. *Drugs* 1987;34(3):311–49.

22. McNeely W, Goa KL. Nebivolol in the management of essential hypertension: A review. *Drugs* 1999;57(4):633–51.

23. Opie LH SE, Frishman WH, et al. Beta blocking agents. In LH Opie, WH Frishman, et al. (eds.), *Drugs for the Heart, Fourth Edition.* Philadelphia: W. B. Saunders 1995:1–30.

24. McDevitt DG. Comparison of pharmacokinetic properties of beta-adrenoceptor blocking drugs. *Eur Heart J* 1987;8(M):9–14.

25. Cruickshank JM. The clinical importance of cardioselectivity and lipophilicity in beta blockers. *Am Heart J* 1980;100(2):160–78.

26. McDevitt DG. Pharmacological characteristics of beta blockers and their role in clinical practice. *J Cardiovasc Pharmacol* 1986;8(6):S5–11.

27. Borchard U. Pharmacokinetics of beta-adrenoceptor blocking agents: Clinical significance of hepatic and/or renal clearance. *Clin Physiol Biochem* 1990;8(2):28–34.

28. Johnsson G, Regardh CG. Clinical pharmacokinetics of beta-adrenoreceptor blocking drugs. *Clin Pharmacokinet* 1976;1(4):233–63.

29. Shand DG. Pharmacokinetic properties of the beta-adrenergic receptor blocking drugs. *Drugs* 1974;7(1):39–47.

30. Galletti F, Fasano ML, Ferrara LA, et al. Obesity and beta blockers: Influence of body fat on their kinetics and cardiovascular effects. *J Clin Pharmacol* 1989;29(3):212–16.

31. Prichard BN. Pharmacologic aspects of intrinsic sympathomimetic activity in beta-blocking drugs. *Am J Cardiol* 1987;59(13):13F–17F.

32. Hart GR, Anderson RJ. Withdrawal syndromes and the cessation of antihypertensive therapy. *Arch Intern Med* 1981;141(9):1125–27.

33. Routledge PA, Shand DG. Clinical pharmacokinetics of propranolol. *Clin Pharmacokinet* 1979;4(2):73–90.

34. Mutschler E, Spahn H, Kirch W. The interaction between H2-receptor antagonists and beta-adrenoceptor blockers. *Br J Clin Pharmacol* 1984;17(1):51S-57S.

35. Beckmann ML, Gerber JG, Byyny RL, et al. Propranolol increases prostacyclin synthesis in patients with essential hypertension. *Hypertension* 1988;12(6):582–88.

36. Warren SE, Ebert E, Swerdlin AH, et al. Clonidine and propranolol paradoxical hypertension. *Arch Intern Med* 1979;139(2):253.

37. Vernon C, Sakula A. Fatal rebound hypertension after abrupt withdrawal of clonidine and propranolol. *Br J Clin Pract* 1979;33(4):112,121.

38. Houston MC, Hodge R. Beta-adrenergic blocker withdrawal syndromes in hypertension and other cardiovascular diseases. *Am Heart J* 1988;116(2/1):515–23.

39. Psaty BM, Koepsell TD, Wagner EH, et al. The relative risk of incident coronary heart disease associated with recently stopping the use of beta blockers. *JAMA* 1990;263(12):1653–57.

40. Cruickshank JM. Beta blockers continue to surprise us. *Eur Heart J* 2000;21(5):354–64.

41. Weidmann P, Ferrier C, Saxenhofer H, et al. Serum lipoproteins during treatment with antihypertensive drugs. *Drugs* 1988;35(6):118–34.

42. Grimm RH Jr. Antihypertensive therapy: Taking lipids into consideration. *Am Heart J* 1991;122(3/2):910–18.

43. Roberts WC. Recent studies on the effects of beta blockers on blood lipid levels. *Am Heart J* 1989;117(3):709–14.

44. Kasiske BL, Ma JZ, Kalil RS, Louis TA. Effects of antihypertensive therapy on serum lipids. *Ann Intern Med* 1995;122(2):133–41.

45. Sharma AM, Pischon T, Hardt S, et al. Hypothesis: Beta-adrenergic receptor blockers and weight gain: A systematic analysis. *Hypertension* 2001;37(2):250–54.

46. Chen J, Radford MJ, Wang Y, et al. Effectiveness of beta blocker therapy after acute myocardial infarction in elderly patients with chronic obstructive pulmonary disease or asthma. *J Am Coll Cardiol* 2001;37(7):1950–56.

47. Medical Research Council Working Party on Mild to Moderate Hypertension. Adverse reactions to bendrofluazide and propranolol for the treatment of mild hypertension. 1981;2(8246):539–43.

48. Messerli FH, Grossman E. Beta blocker therapy and depression. *JAMA* 2002;288(15):1845–46.

49. Salem SA, McDevitt DG. Central effects of beta-adrenoceptor antagonists. *Clin Pharmacol Ther* 1983;33(1):52–57.

50. Messerli FH, Grossman E. beta blockers in hypertension: Is carvedilol different? *Am J Cardiol* 2004;93(9A):7B-12B.

51. Charney B, Meyer BR, Frishman WH, et al. Gender, race, and genetic issues in cardiovascular pharmacotherapeutics. In WH Frishman (ed.), *Cardiovascular Pharmacotherapeutics.* New York: McGraw Hill 1997:1347–61.

52. Johnson JA, Burlew BS, Stiles RN. Racial differences in beta-adrenoceptor-mediated responsiveness. *J Cardiovasc Pharmacol* 1995;25(1):90–96.

53. Zhou HH, Koshakji RP, Silberstein DJ, et al. Altered sensitivity to and clearance of propranolol in men of Chinese descent as compared with American whites. *N Engl J Med* 1989;320(9):565–70.

54. Poole-Wilson PA, Swedberg K, Cleland JG, et al. Comparison of carvedilol and metoprolol on clinical outcomes in patients with chronic heart failure in the Carvedilol or Metoprolol European Trial (COMET) randomised controlled trial. *Lancet* 2003;362(9377):7–13.

55. The beta blocker heart attack trial: Beta blocker Heart Attack Study Group. *JAMA* 1981;246(18):2073–74.

56. Pedersen TR. The Norwegian Multicenter Study of Timolol after Myocardial Infarction. *Circulation* 1983;67(6/2):I49–53.

57. Dargie HJ. Effect of carvedilol on outcome after myocardial infarction in patients with left-ventricular dysfunction: The CAPRICORN randomised trial. *Lancet* 2001;357(9266):1385–90.

58. A randomized trial of propranolol in patients with acute myocardial infarction. II. Morbidity results. *JAMA* 1983;250(20):2814–19.

59. Gottlieb SS, McCarter RJ, Vogel RA. Effect of beta-blockade on mortality among high-risk and low-risk patients after myocardial infarction. *N Engl J Med* 1998;339(8):489–97.

60. Mickley H, Eiskjaer H, Botker HE. Is an additional post-myocardial infarction beta blocker trial required in the era of early revascularization? *Eur Heart J* 2004;25(1):96–97.

61. Metoprolol in acute myocardial infarction: Mortality. The MIAMI Trial Research Group. *Am J Cardiol* 1985;56(14):15G-22G.

62. Metoprolol in acute myocardial infarction (MIAMI): A randomised placebo-controlled international trial. The MIAMI Trial Research Group. *Eur Heart J* 1985;6(3):199–226.

63. Randomised trial of intravenous atenolol among 16 027 cases of suspected acute myocardial infarction: ISIS-1. First International Study of Infarct Survival Collaborative Group. *Lancet* 1986;2(8498):57–66.

64. Chen ZM, Pan HC, Chen YP, et al. Early intravenous then oral metoprolol in 45,852 patients with acute myocardial infarction: Randomised placebo-controlled trial. *Lancet* 2005;366(9497):1622–32.

65. Skarfors ET, Lithell HO, Selinus I, Aberg H. Do antihypertensive drugs precipitate diabetes in predisposed men? *BMJ* 1989;298(6681):1147–52.

66. Bengtsson C, Blohme G, Lapidus L, et al. Diabetes incidence in users and non-users of antihypertensive drugs in relation to serum insulin, glucose tolerance and degree of adiposity: A 12-year prospective population study of women in Gothenburg, Sweden. *J Intern Med* 1992;231(6):583–88.

67. Pollare T, Lithell H, Selinus I, Berne C. Sensitivity to insulin during treatment with atenolol and metoprolol: A randomised, double blind study of effects on carbohydrate and lipoprotein metabolism in hypertensive patients. *BMJ* 1989;298(6681):1152–57.

68. Lithell H, Pollare T, Vessby B. Metabolic effects of pindolol and propranolol in a double-blind cross-over study in hypertensive patients. *Blood Press* 1992;1(2):92–101.

69. Dahlof B, Devereux RB, Kjeldsen SE, et al. Cardiovascular morbidity and mortality in the Losartan Intervention for Endpoint reduction in hypertension study (LIFE): A randomised trial against atenolol. *Lancet* 2002;359(9311):995–1003.

70. UK Prospective Diabetes Study Group. Efficacy of atenolol and captopril in reducing risk of macrovascular and microvascular complications in type 2 diabetes: UKPDS 39. *BMJ* 1998;317(7160):713–20.

71. Cruickshank JM. Beta blockers and diabetes: The bad guys come good. *Cardiovasc Drugs Ther* 2002;16(5):457–70.

72. Kjekshus J, Gilpin E, Cali G, et al. Diabetic patients and beta blockers after acute myocardial infarction. *Eur Heart J* 1990;11(1):43–50.

73. Bakris GL, Fonseca V, Katholi RE, et al. Metabolic effects of carvedilol vs metoprolol in patients with type 2 diabetes mellitus and hypertension: A randomized controlled trial. *JAMA* 2004;292(18):2227–36.

74. Folkow B. Physiological aspects of primary hypertension. *Physiol Rev* 1982;62(2):347–504.

75. Lakatta EG, Levy D. Arterial and cardiac aging: major shareholders in cardiovascular disease enterprises. Part I: Aging arteries: a "setup" for vascular disease. *Circulation* 2003;107(1):139–46.

76. Messerli FH, Sundgaard-Riise K, Ventura HO, et al. Essential hypertension in the elderly: Haemodynamics, intravascular volume, plasma renin activity, and circulating catecholamine levels. *Lancet* 1983;2(8357):983–86.

77. Lund-Johansen P, Ormvik P. Hemodynamic patterns of untreated hypertensive disease. In JH BB Laragh (ed.), *Hypertension: Pathophysiology, Diagnosis, and Management,*

Second Edition. New York: Raven Press 1995:323–42.

78. Hollenberg NK, Epstein M, Basch RI, Merrill JP. "No man's land" of the renal vasculature: An arteriographic and hemodynamic assessment of the interlobar and arcuate arteries in essential and accelerated hypertension. *Am J Med* 1969;47(6):845–54.

79. London GM, Safar ME, Sassard JE, et al. Renal and systemic hemodynamics in sustained essential hypertension. *Hypertension* 1984;6(5):743–54.

80. Schmieder RE, Schachinger H, Messerli FH. Accelerated decline in renal perfusion with aging in essential hypertension. *Hypertension* 1994;23(3):351–57.

81. Maki DD, Ma JZ, Louis TA, Kasiske BL. Long-term effects of antihypertensive agents on proteinuria and renal function. *Arch Intern Med* 1995;155(10):1073–80.

82. Kasiske BL, Kalil RS, Ma JZ, et al. Effect of antihypertensive therapy on the kidney in patients with diabetes: A meta-regression analysis. *Ann Intern Med* 1993;118(2):129–38.

83. Mogensen CE. Microalbuminuria predicts clinical proteinuria and early mortality in maturity-onset diabetes. *N Engl J Med* 1984;310(6):356–60.

84. Weber K, Bohmeke T, van der Does R, Taylor SH. Comparison of the hemodynamic effects of metoprolol and carvedilol in hypertensive patients. *Cardiovasc Drugs Ther* 1996;10(2):113–17.

85. Man In't Veld AJ, Van den Meiracker AH, Schalekamp MA. Do beta blockers really increase peripheral vascular resistance? Review of the literature and new observations under basal conditions. *Am J Hypertens* 1988;1(1):91–96.

86. Lund-Johansen P. Hemodynamic consequences of long-term beta blocker therapy: A 5-year follow-up study of atenolol. *J Cardiovasc Pharmacol* 1979;1(5):487–95.

87. Bauer JH. Diabetic nephropathy: Can it be prevented? Are there renal protective antihypertensive drugs of choice? *South Med J* 1994;87(10):1043–53.

88. Bauer JH, Brooks CS. The long-term effect of propranolol therapy on renal function. *Am J Med* 1979;66(3):405–10.

89. Schiffrin EL, Deng LY, Larochelle P. Progressive improvement in the structure of resistance arteries of hypertensive patients after 2 years of treatment with an angiotensin I-converting enzyme inhibitor: Comparison with effects of a beta blocker. *Am J Hypertens* 1995;8(3):229–36.

90. Schiffrin EL, Deng LY, Larochelle P. Effects of a beta blocker or a converting enzyme inhibitor on resistance arteries in essential hypertension. *Hypertension* 1994;23(1):83–91.

91. Messerli FH, Grossman E, Goldbourt U. Are beta blockers efficacious as

first-line therapy for hypertension in the elderly? A systematic review. *JAMA* 1998;279(23):1903–07.

92. Klingbeil AU, Schneider M, Martus P, et al. A meta-analysis of the effects of treatment on left ventricular mass in essential hypertension. *Am J Med* 2003;115(1):41–46.

93. Schulman SP, Weiss JL, Becker LC, et al. The effects of antihypertensive therapy on left ventricular mass in elderly patients. *N Engl J Med* 1990;322(19):1350–56.

94. Schiffrin EL, Park JB, Intengan HD, Touyz RM. Correction of arterial structure and endothelial dysfunction in human essential hypertension by the angiotensin receptor antagonist losartan. *Circulation* 2000;101(14):1653–59.

95. Grossman E, Messerli FH. Why beta blockers are not cardioprotective in elderly patients with hypertension. *Curr Cardiol Rep* 2002;4(6):468–73.

96. Lip GYH, Tello-Montoliu A. Management of atrial fibrillation. *Heart* 2006;92:1177–82.

97. Lewington S, Clarke R, Qizilbash N, et al. Age-specific relevance of usual blood pressure to vascular mortality: A meta-analysis of individual data for one million adults in 61 prospective studies. *Lancet* 2002;360(9349):1903–13.

98. Haider AW, Larson MG, Franklin SS, Levy D. Systolic blood pressure, diastolic blood pressure, and pulse pressure as predictors of risk for congestive heart failure in the Framingham Heart Study. *Ann Intern Med* 2003;138(1):10–16.

99. Vasan RS, Levy D. The role of hypertension in the pathogenesis of heart failure: A clinical mechanistic overview. *Arch Intern Med* 1996;156(16):1789–96.

100. Klag MJ, Whelton PK, Randall BL, et al. End-stage renal disease in African-American and white men: 16-year MRFIT findings. *JAMA* 1997;277(16):1293–98.

101. MacMahon S, Peto R, Cutler J, et al. Blood pressure, stroke, and coronary heart disease. Part 1: Prolonged differences in blood pressure: Prospective observational studies corrected for the regression dilution bias. *Lancet* 1990;335(8692):765–74.

102. ALLHAT Officers and Coordinators for the ALLHAT Collaborative Research Group. Major outcomes in high-risk hypertensive patients randomized to angiotensin-converting enzyme inhibitor or calcium channel blocker vs diuretic: The Antihypertensive and Lipid-Lowering Treatment to Prevent Heart Attack Trial (ALLHAT). *JAMA* 2002;288(23):2981–97.

103. Carlberg B, Samuelsson O, Lindholm LH. Atenolol in hypertension: is it a wise choice? *Lancet* 2004;364(9446):1684–89.

Chapter

79 Calcium Antagonists

Stefano Taddei, Lorenzo Ghiadoni, Agostino Virdis, and Antonio Salvetti

Key Findings

- Non-dihydropyridine calcium antagonists are less potent vasodilators, but also show chronotropic, dromotropic, and inotropic effect.
- Calcium antagonists have potent antioxidant effects that are relevant to the restoration of endothelial function.
- Calcium antagonists lower blood pressure in primary and secondary hypertension and in special populations, including elderly and black individuals.
- Calcium antagonists effectively reduce left ventricular mass and prevent atherosclerosis, as well as reduce the occurrence of stroke.

INTRODUCTION

After the pioneering observation by Fleckenstein in 1967 that reduction of calcium movement into cardiac myocytes determined a negative inotropic effect, calcium antagonist drugs were developed for the treatment of several disorders (mainly of the cardiovascular apparatus) —including high blood pressure, angina pectoris, supraventricular tacharrhythmia, Raynoud's phenomenon, hypertrophic cardiomyopathy, pulmonary hypertension, migraine, and esophageal spasm. However, despite this large variety of clinical indications treatment of hypertension remains the main indication for the utilization of this drug class throughout the world because calcium antagonists represent one of the cornerstones for the therapy of this disease.

The term *calcium antagonist* was coined by Fleckenstein to convey the fact that these agents produced *in vitro* effects similar to those exerted by specific antagonists. Later, the International Union of Basic and Clinical Pharmacology proposed the term *calcium channel blocker* (CCB). Finally, in addition to this more common term these drugs are also designated as *calcium entry blockers*, *calcium blockers*, *calcium channel antagonists*, and *calcium channel inhibitors*. All of these terms have the same meaning.

Recent years have seen the emergence of the need for stricter blood pressure control in the general population. Utilization of this drug class in cardiovascular medicine has thus gained new relevance. This is due to the undisputed efficacy of these compounds in reducing blood pressure values independently of the characteristics of the patients (age, race, sodium repletion, pathogenesis of hypertension), their notable flexibility for use in combination therapy, and the extensive availability of clinical intervention trials demonstrating the effectiveness of this drug class on target organ damage and cardiovascular events (including a high safety profile).

MECHANISMS OF ACTION

Calcium in its ionized form (Ca^{2+}) is generally considered the ubiquitous second messenger, and Ca channels regulate the entry of Ca^{2+} into the cytoplasm. Thus, cells utilize Ca from two different sources: Ca^{2+} entering from the outside or Ca^{2+} released from internal stores. Ca^{2+} enters the cell through a variety of plasmalemmal ion channels such as voltage-operated channels, receptor-operated channels, store-operated channels, and non-selective channels. Voltage-operated channels have been divided into at least three subtypes based on their conductance and voltage sensitivity. The channels best characterized are the L (long-lasting), T (transient), and N (neuronal) subtypes. The main effect of calcium antagonists is blockade of calcium entry into cells by acting on the L subtype and changing the opening mode for these channels to a preponderance of short-lived rather than long-acting channels and switching them to long-lived closed state.[1,2]

From the clinical point of view, calcium antagonists are divided into different classes according to their chemical structure. The three main classes are (1) phenylalkylamines (prototype is verapamil), (2) benzothiazepines (prototype is diltiazem), and (3) dihydropyridines (prototype is nifedipine). Less specific agents are categorized as diphenylpiperazines (cinnarizine, flunarizine) and diarylaminopropylamines (bepridil).

It must be stressed that each of the calcium antagonists of cardiovascular interest (namely, verapamil, diltiazem, nifedipine, and all other dihydropyridines) has a completely different molecular structure, and as a consequence different receptor sites on Ca channels (although receptors for verapamil and diltiazem have some overlapping sites). This concept is important in explaining the various hemodynamic properties of these compounds.

After the first generation of calcium antagonists, characterized by rapid onset of action and very short half-life, second- and third-generation drugs were developed with compounds characterized by a longer duration of action attributable to pharmacokinetic properties or extended-release mechanisms (Box 79–1). Second- and third-generation drugs are therefore associated with slower onset and longer duration of action, with lower reflex sympathetic nervous system activation and fewer side effects.[3]

The cardiovascular activity of the three classes of calcium antagonists shows important differences: verapamil has more significant effects on cardiac performance (determining a negative chronotropic, dromotropic, and inotropic effect), while causing modest vasodilation; dihydropyridines are potent and almost pure vasodilators (with some slight difference between nifedipine and the other dihydropyridines); and diltiazem has intermediate effects between verapamil and dihydropyridines. Among the various dihydropyridines, nifedipine shows a modest negative inotropic effect that has no clinical relevance in patients with preserved left ventricular function (such as the majority of patients with essential hypertension). Newer dihydropyridines are characterized by more pronounced vascular selectivity caused by an increased lipophilicity.[2]

The pharmacokinetics of calcium antagonists are characterized by nearly complete absorption after oral administration, associated with marked reduction in bioavailability because of first-pass hepatic metabolism. The effect of the prototypes is evident within 30 to 60 minutes after the oral dose, but it is obviously delayed with the extended-release formulation or longer-acting agents (Box 79–1). These agents are all bound to plasma proteins to a significant extent (70 to 90%), and their elimination half-lives vary widely, ranging from 1.3 to 64 hours. During repeated oral administration, bioavailability and half-life may increase because of saturation of hepatic metabolism. In patients with hepatic cirrhosis, the bioavailability and half-life of calcium antagonists may be increased and dosage should be decreased accordingly. On the other hand, no dose adjustment is required in patients with renal failure.

The main mechanism through which calcium antagonists lower blood pressure values is the reduction in peripheral vascular resistances (Figure 79–1). This effect is the consequence of several properties of this drug class. Basically, through the reduction in cytosolic free calcium concentrations calcium antagonists are potent vasodilators, an effect mainly observed at the level of resistance arteries. In addition, these drugs can interfere with several vasocon-strictors acting through intracellular calcium mobilization, including alpha-adrenergic agonists (norepinephrine, phenylephrine) or angiotensin II. Finally, calcium antagonists also induce mild natriuresis, thereby averting volume retention, a negative effect usually common to direct vasodilators (Figure 79–1). Compared to dihydropyridines, verapamil and diltiazem prove to be less potent as vasodilating agents, although their negative chronotropic, dromotropic, and inotropic effects can contribute to antihypertensive activity (Figure 79–1).[4]

The clinical efficacy of calcium antagonists as single agents is well documented not only in patients with mild to moderate or severe essential hypertension but in special populations, including patients with primary aldosteronism or pheochromocytoma, hypertensive emergency, cyclosporine-induced hypertension, and hypertension (in elderly and black patients). It is worth noting that nifedipine is considered the first-choice drug in pregnancy-induced hypertension.[5]

Calcium antagonists can be effectively combined with all other antihypertensive drug classes, apart from diuretics. Although the association between calcium antagonists and diuretics has been employed in intervention clinical trials, it has no mechanistic rationale because (as previously stated) calcium antagonists themselves have a natriuretic activity and several studies have documented that these two drug classes show no antihypertensive additive effect. The only exception concerns patients with renal failure, who often require both calcium antagonists and loop diuretics to obtain adequate blood pressure control.[5]

Another limitation to therapy with calcium antagonists is the combination of verapamil or diltiazem with beta blockers because of prolongation of atrioventricular conduction time as well as an additive negative inotropic effect.[1] In contrast, the combination of dihydropyridines

---

Box 79–1

Classification of Calcium Antagonists

- *First generation:* verapamil, diltiazem, nifedipine, felodipine, isradipine nicardipine, nitrendipine
- *Second generation:* verapamil SR, diltiazem CD, nifedipine XL, nifedipine GITS, felodipine ER, isradipine CR
- *Third generation:*
  - Long plasma half-life: amlodipine
  - Long receptor half-life: barnedipine, lercanidipine, lacidipine, manidipine

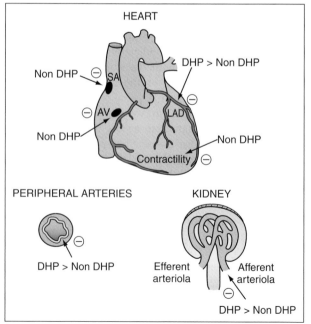

Figure 79–1. Mechanisms of action of calcium antagonists (DHP, dihydropyridines).

and beta blocker is an ideal and effective combination in the treatment of essential hypertension.

Metabolic effects are considered of primary relevance in the treatment of hypertensive patients because of the need to reduce the global cardiovascular risk. Calcium antagonists show a neutral effect on lipid and glucose profile. However, prospective randomized trials have clearly documented that treatment using this drug class is associated with a reduced incidence of new cases of diabetes mellitus compared to diuretic and beta-blocker-based treatment.

ANTIATHEROSCLEROTIC EFFECT

One of the relevant characteristics of calcium antagonists that could be clinically important in the prevention of cardiovascular disease is the antiatherosclerotic effect. Some aspects of the pathogenesis of atherosclerosis depend on calcium-regulated cell processes such as chemotaxis, cell migration and adhesion, proliferation, lipid uptake, and endothelial necrosis. In experimental models, most of these processes are inhibited by calcium chelating agents and calcium antagonists.[6] In addition, a large body of evidence indicates that an early event in the atherosclerotic disease process is endothelial dysfunction, which promotes a constellation of processes that contribute to plaque development (including vasoconstriction, thrombosis, inflammation, oxidation, and proliferation). In the healthy endothelium, nitric oxide (NO) protects the vessel wall not only by inducing vasodilation but through various anti-inflammatory benefits (including scavenging of superoxide, inhibition of platelet aggregation, reduced hyperadhesiveness of leukocytes, and interference with platelet aggregation). Essential hypertension is causally associated with endothelial dysfunction, which results in reduced NO availability because of the production of oxidative stress.

These alterations lead to increased vessel wall permeability to atherogenic lipids and inflammatory cells such as monocytes and T lymphocytes. Consequently, it is believed that the cascade of events leading to the formation of atherosclerotic plaques includes the penetration of damaged vessel walls by monocytes/macrophages and their development into cholesterol-rich foam cells (mediated by oxidized low density lipoprotein (LDL)) and the proliferation of vascular smooth muscle cells followed by their migration toward the vascular lumen. This view is increasingly supported by mounting evidence demonstrating the association of endothelial dysfunction with carotid and coronary atherosclerosis, both in patients with essential hypertension and those with atherosclerotic disease. Finally, the presence of endothelial dysfunction has been associated with the occurrence of cardiovascular events in several longitudinal studies, especially in patients with coronary atherosclerosis.

Calcium antagonists are powerful compounds that interfere with the cascade of events leading to the development of atherosclerosis. Such effects are mediated not only by the interaction with intracellular calcium but by the strong antioxidant activity that characterizes this drug class. A positive effect of calcium antagonists (mainly of

the dihydropyridine type) on endothelial function in different vascular beds has been documented in essential hypertension and coronary artery disease. Thus, one-year treatment with nifedipine gastro-intestinal therapeutic system (GITS) (but not the β-blocker atenolol) improved relaxation to acetylcholine in gluteal subcutaneous resistance-size small arteries of essential hypertensive patients.[7]

This beneficial effect of calcium antagonists on endothelial function was confirmed in the coronary vascular bed by the demonstration that intracoronary infusion of two different calcium antagonists, the dihydropyridine nicardipine and the benzothiazepine-like diltiazem, improved endothelium-dependent dynamic exercise-induced vasomotion in stenotic epicardial vessels of normotensive subjects and in normal and stenotic epicardial vessels of essential hypertensive patients.[8] In addition, the ENCORE study[9] showed that treatment with nifedipine GITS resulted in a significantly greater improvement of response to acetylcholine as compared to the placebo group in epicardial arteries of patients with coronary artery disease. Finally, several positive studies are also available in the forearm microcirculation of essential hypertensive patients.[10]

In particular, extensive evidence indicates that different dihydropyridine calcium antagonists (including lacidipine,[11,12] nifedipine GITS,[13] isradipine,[14] and lercanidipine[15]) significantly increase the forearm vasodilation to acetylcholine or bradykinin. The potential mechanism by which calcium antagonists could exert their beneficial activity on endothelial dysfunction is very likely to be an antioxidant activity.[16] This hypothesis is reinforced by evidence that calcium antagonists can restore NO availability and decrease oxidative stress in essential hypertensive patients (Figure 79–2).[12,13,15]

As discussed later in the chapter, this specific effect of calcium antagonists on endothelial dysfunction could account for the well-documented effect of preventing atherosclerosis in the coronary and carotid arteries exerted by these compounds. It is also conceivable that the restoration of endothelial dysfunction might play a role in long-term reduction of cardiovascular events.

INDICATIONS

Calcium antagonists are first-choice drugs for the treatment of essential hypertension. As stated previously, they can be used in all essential hypertensive patients. However, to better understand the specific beneficial effects that can derive from this drug class it is necessary to examine the available clinical evidence on target organ damage and clinical events (Box 79–2).

EFFECTS OF CALCIUM ANTAGONISTS ON TARGET ORGAN DAMAGE

Left ventricular hypertrophy (LVH)

Although several studies have assessed the effects of various antihypertensive drugs on LVH by echocardiographic determination of left ventricular mass (LVM), only

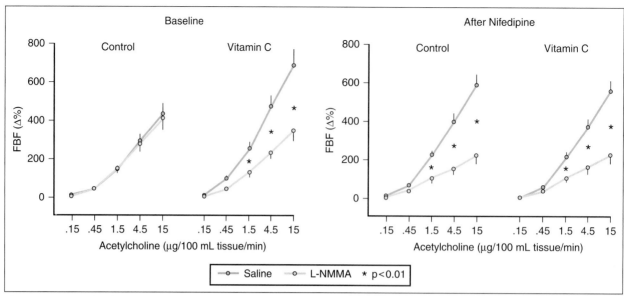

Figure 79–2. Graphs show a study performed in essential hypertensive patients documenting that calcium antagonists can restore endothelial function by improving NO availability through an antioxidant effect. At baseline, in essential hypertensive patients vasodilation (measured by strain-gauge venous plethysmography) induced by intrabrachial infusion of acetylcholine is resistant to L-NMMA, indicating the presence of impaired NO availability. When the agonist is repeated in presence of the intrabrachial infusion of vitamin C (an antioxidant), the vasodilation to acetylcholine is increased and the ability of L-NMMA to inhibit the relaxing effect of the endothelial agonist is restored, demonstrating the presence of oxidative stress-induced impairment in NO availability. After three months of nifedipine GITS administration, the response to acetylcholine is increased compared to baseline (whereas L-NMMA clearly blunts the vasodilation induced by the agonist). It is worth noting that after nifedipine treatment the facilitating effect of vitamin C is prevented. Thus, calcium antagonists can restore NO-dependent relaxation by an antioxidant mechanism. (Modified from Taddei S, Virdis A, Ghiadoni L, et al. Restoration of nitric oxide availability after calcium antagonist treatment in essential hypertension. *Hypertension* 2001;37:943.)

a few studies have followed sufficiently strict criteria to provide reliable information.[5] Consequently, meta-analyses cannot provide indisputable evidence. However, as reviewed elsewhere[17] angiotension converting enzyme (ACE) inhibitors and calcium antagonists seem to be more efficient than other antihypertensive drugs in reducing LVM. A more recent meta-analysis of 80 trials, also including patients treated with angiotensin II receptor blockers (ARB), indicated that ARBs, ACE inhibitors, and calcium antagonists similarly reduce LVM by approximately 10 to 13%. This effect was marginally greater than that of diuretics (–8%) and significantly greater than that of β-blockers (–6%).[18]

It is relevant to specifically quote three studies[19–21], performed with the application of strict methodological criteria to evaluate the effect of antihypertensive drugs on LVM changes. The ELVERA trial, a study in elderly newly diagnosed hypertensive patients, showed that monotherapy with nifedipine or lisinopril while similarly reducing clinic blood pressure caused a similar and significant decrease in LVM at one-year and even more at two-year follow-up.[19]

The PRESERVE trial, a randomised, double-blind study in essential hypertensive patients with LVH, demonstrated that amlodipine- and enalapril-based treatment (in combination with hydrochlorothiazide and atenolol) similarly reduced clinic blood pressure and LVM at one-year follow-up.[20] Finally, in a large group of essential hypertensive patients participating in the ELSA study lacidipine- and atenolol-based treatments significantly and similarly

reduced clinic and ambulatory blood pressure and the LVM index at one- and four-year follow-up (Figure 79–3).[21]

Interestingly, in this study changes in LVM were significantly associated with mean 24-hour systolic blood pressure changes. A similar correlation, although less consistent, was found with clinic blood pressure in the ELVERA[19] and PRESERVE studies.[20] It can be concluded from these studies that in hypertensive patients treatments with dihydropyridine calcium antagonists, ACE inhibitors, and β-blockers are equally effective in reducing LVM when blood pressure values are similarly lowered. Such a finding supports the primary role of hemodynamic load lowering to achieve LVM reduction.

Atherosclerosis of carotid arteries

Several randomized trials have compared the long-term effects of calcium antagonists on carotid intima-media thickness (IMT). In the PREVENT study,[22] performed in patients with angiographic evidence of coronary artery disease, amlodipine significantly reduced the progression of mean maximal (M-max) IMT in three-year follow-up compared to placebo.

The MIDAS study[23] compared the effect of isradipine and hydrochlorothiazide on the rate of change of IMT in hypertensive patients and indicated that the rate of progression of M-max IMT did not significantly differ between the two treatment groups over three years. However, six months after randomization M-max increased significantly more in the diuretic group (a difference that

Box 79–2

Clinical Trials Cited

- AASK: African American Study of Kidney disease and hypertension
- ACTION: A Coronary disease Trial Investigating Outcome with Nifedipine GITS
- ALLHAT: Antihypertensive and Lipid-lowering treatment to prevent Heart Attack Trial
- ASCOT-BPLA: Anglo-Scandinavian Cardiac Outcomes Trial, Blood Pressure Lowering Arm
- BENEDICT: Bergamo Nephrologic Diabetes Complication Trial
- CAMELOT: Comparison of AMlodipine versus Enalapril to Limit Occurrences of Thrombosis
- CONVINCE: Controlled Onset Verapamil Investigation of Cardiovascular End Points
- ELSA: European Lacidipine Study on Atherosclerosis
- ELVERA: Effects of amlodipine and lisinopril on Left VEntricular mass and diastolic function (E/A RAtio)
- ENCORE: Evaluation of Nifedipine and Cerivastatin ON Recovery of coronary Endothelial function
- ESPIRAL: Efecto del tratamiento antihipertensivo Sobre la Progresion de la Insuficiencia RenAL en pacientes no diabeticos
- IDNT: Irbesartan Diabetic Nephropathy Trial
- INSIGHT: Intervention as a Goal in Hypertension Treatment
- INTACT: International Nifedipine Trial on Antiatherosclerotic Therapy
- INVEST: International Verapamil-Trandolapril Study
- MARVAL: MicroAlbuminuria Reduction Valsartan
- NORDIL: NORdic DILtiazem
- MIDAS: Multicenter Isradipine Diuretic Atherosclerosis Study
- MOSES: MOrbidity and mortality after Stroke, Eprosartan compared with nitrendipine for Secondary prevention
- NICS-EH: National Intervention Cooperative Study in Elderly Hypertensive
- PRESERVE: Prospective Randomized Enalapril Study Evaluating Regression of Ventricular Enlargement
- PREVENT: Prospective Randomized Evaluation of the Vascular Effects of Norvasc Trial
- RENAAL: Reduction of Endpoints in NIDDM (non-insulin-dependent diabetes mellitus) with the Angiotensin II Antagonist Losartan
- SYST-EUR: SYSTolic hypertension in EURope
- Valsartan Antihypertensive Long-term Use Evaluation
- Verapamil in Hypertension and Atherosclerosis Study

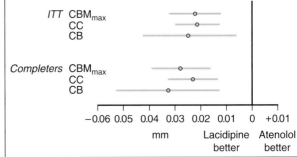

Figure 79–3. Estimated treatment effect of lacidipine versus atenolol on mean maximum intima media thickness (IMT) of the four far walls in the distal common carotids and carotid bifurcations bilaterally (CBMmax), common carotid (CC), and carotid bifurcation (CB) IMT changes using repeated measurements model analysis. Mean changes over the treatment period (approximately four years; circles) and their 95% confidence intervals are illustrated by the bars. Values to the left of the 0 line indicate less progression with lacidipine. The intention-to-treat population consisted of all patients randomized to double-blind medication who had the baseline ultrasound scan and at least one follow-up scan, including scans performed after withdrawal (mean follow-up 3.75 years). The completer population was made up of patients who actually completed the four years of the study under randomized medication. (Modified from Agabiti-Rosei E, Trimarco B, Muiesan ML, et al. Cardiac structural and functional changes during long-term antihypertensive treatment with lacidipine and atenolol in the European Lacidipine Study on Atherosclerosis (ELSA). *J Hypertens* 2005;23:1091.)

Moreover, this significant difference was detectable in diseased segments, indicating that the calcium antagonist is more efficient than the diuretic in slowing down the progression of carotid lesions.

The VHAS[24] trial, which compared the effect of verapamil slow-release and chlorthalidone on IMT changes in hypertensive patients, indicated that at four-year follow-up the rate of change in carotid artery IMT (although tending to be smaller in the verapamil group) did not significantly differ compared to the chlorthalidone group. However, because in carotid arteries with M-max > 1.2 mm the rate of IMT progression during long-term treatment was dependent on baseline value, the slope of the regression rate of M-max changes related to initial M-max was significantly steeper in the verapamil compared to the chlorthalidone group. This finding indicated a greater effectiveness of the calcium antagonist in inducing a structural regression in the carotid wall, despite a blood pressure reduction similar to that observed with the diuretic.

In a subgroup of the INSIGHT study, common carotid artery IMT progressed significantly in patients treated with Co-Amilozide but not in those on nifedipine GITS for a follow-up ranging from two to four years.[25] Finally, the ELSA study (the largest available randomized double-blind long-term study) compared the effect of lacidipine and atenolol (associated with hydrochlorothiazide in about 35% of patients) on IMT and plaque of common carotid artery and carotid bifurcation of essential hypertensive

persisted over the entire three-year duration of the study). As a consequence, at the end of the study the average difference in M-max IMT change from baseline was significantly lower in the isradipine group despite a greater reduction in systolic blood pressure in the diuretic group.

patients during four-year follow-up.[26] Treatment with lacidipine significantly reduced the four-year progression of IMT compared to atenolol treatment.

Moreover, patients with plaque progression were significantly less common (and patients with plaque regression significantly more common) in the lacidipine group. It is worth noting that although clinic blood pressure was similarly reduced by both treatments 24-hour ambulatory blood pressure was greatly reduced in the atenolol group. Therefore, this study was able to show a greater effect of lacidipine not only in slowing the progression of IMT but in plaque progression and regression (despite a smaller ambulatory blood pressure reduction). Such a finding supports the antiatherosclerotic action of lacidipine independently of its antihypertensive action. In conclusion, overall data from the previously described studies show uniform evidence of the beneficial action of calcium antagonists on atherosclerotic carotid lesions, with a superiority of these drugs over diuretic and β-blocker therapy.

Atherosclerosis of coronary arteries

Placebo-controlled studies, in which coronary atherosclerosis was assessed by coronary angiography, have given contrasting results. The INTACT study showed that nifedipine reduced the incidence of new lesions by 28% in a follow-up of one year,[27] and the Montreal study indicated that nicardipine reduced the progression of minimal lesions in patients with 5 to 7.5% stenosis in at least four coronary artery segments at two-year follow-up.[28] By contrast, in the PREVENT study treatment with amlodipine had no effect on angiographic progression of coronary atherosclerosis.[22]

However, in a substudy of CAMELOT[29] (a double-blind randomized trial comparing amlodipine or enalapril with placebo in patients with angiographically documented coronary artery disease) the progression of arteriosclerosis was evaluated by intravascular ultrasound at baseline and after 24 months. The results showed a trend toward a lesser progression of atheroma volume in the amlodipine group versus placebo, with significantly less progression in the subgroup with systolic blood pressure greater than the mean. In the coronary calcification substudy of the INISIGHT trial,[30] total calcium score (measured by double-helical computed tomography) was significantly lower in the nifedipine-GITS-treated group than in the Co-Amilozide recipients during the first and third years (a finding that suggests that nifedipine GITS can slow the progression of coronary calcification). Thus, available data indicate that treatment with calcium antagonists exerts a modest or no effect on coronary atherosclerosis.

Finally, with regard to the REGRESS trial (a randomized placebo-controlled study aimed at evaluating the effect of two-year treatment with the statin pravastatin on progression/regression of angiographically documented atherosclerosis of patients with normal to moderately raised serum cholesterol), revision of the results indicated that the addition of various dihydropyridine and non-dihydropyridine calcium antagonists had a synergistic effect with pravastatin in retarding the progression of coronary atherosclerosis.[31]

Renal protection

Dihydropyridine calcium antagonists, and probably to a lesser extent non-dihydropyridine calcium antagonists, induce renal vasodilation and increase glomerular filtration rate (GFR) by relaxing the afferent arteriole. However, in hypertensive patients with preserved renal function this effect can impair renal autoregulation with no effect on (or even increase of) intra-glomerular pressure. In addition, calcium antagonists do not improve glomerular membrane permeability and selectivity, and thus lack any direct effect on proteinuria (as shown by drugs blocking the renin-angiotensin system). Therefore, the capacity of calcium antagonists to protect the kidney in hypertensive patients and in patients with diabetic and nondiabetic nephropathy may depend on the mere capacity of these drugs to reduce systemic blood pressure.[32,33]

This possibility is clearly demonstrated by several controlled clinical studies that indicate that blood pressure reduction induced by calcium antagonists is a major mechanism leading to renal protection. A post hoc analysis of the SYST-EUR trial in older patients with isolated systolic hypertension indicates that blood pressure lowering with nitrendipine significantly reduced the risk of proteinuria (especially in diabetic patients) and the risk of mild renal dysfunction, with a slight but significant decrease in serum creatinine concentrations in patients with proteinuria at entry.[34] In addition, it is worth noting that after a mean follow-up of five years very strict and similar blood pressure control by enalapril or nitrendipine attained a similar degree of renal protection.[35,36]

Post hoc analysis from the ALLHAT study indicates that in high-risk hypertensive patients with reduced GFR but with well-controlled blood pressure values (about 135 to 75 mmHg) the risk of end-stage renal disease (ESRD) (or = 50% GFR reduction) was similar in the total study population and diabetic subgroup independent of the treatment (chlorthalidone, amlodipine, or lisinopril).[37] However, the data on renal outcome from ALLHAT, which apparently contradict available evidence indicating the specific ability of drugs blocking the RAS to protect the kidney beyond blood pressure reduction,[38] should be cautiously evaluated due to the several limitations of this study—such as selection bias (patients with nephropathies treated with ACE inhibitors not enrolled), lack of acknowledgement of the underlying kidney disease, no data on proteinuria, and the great prevalence of cardiovascular events (which could have masked renal outcomes).[37]

Moreover, these results contrast with other studies comparing calcium antagonists with diuretics in hypertensive patients. The INSIGHT trial showed that in spite of similar blood pressure control both the rate of decline in creatinine clearance and the occurrence of renal insufficiency were significantly lower in patients treated with nifedipine GITS compared to those receiving the diuretic combination hydrochlorothiazide and amiloride.[39] These data suggest that antihypertensive treatment based on a long-acting dihydropyridine calcium antagonist may offer better renoprotection than therapy based on diuretics.

This hypothesis is further supported by the results of SYST-EUR, which indicated that serum creatinine did not change in patients on nitrendipine monotherapy but increased in patients treated with hydrochlorothiazide.[34] It is also supported by the NICS-EH study, which reported that abnormally elevated serum urea nitrogen was observed less frequently in patients treated with sustained-release nicardipine compared to those receiving a thiazide diuretic.[40] Finally, available evidence indicates that calcium antagonists can improve renal function in cyclosporine-treated patients.[41,42]

Diabetic nephropathy

Primary prevention of the occurrence of incipient nephropathy does not seem to occur with calcium antagonists. The BENEDICT study demonstrated that verapamil does not prevent or delay the occurrence of microalbuminuria and does not enhance the beneficial effect of the ACE inhibitor trandolapril on prevention of diabetic nephropathy in type 2 diabetic patients with hypertension.[43]

With regard to the progression of incipient to overt nephropathy, although calcium antagonists have no effect in type 1 diabetic patients with incipient nephropathy[32] results in type 2 diabetics are more controversial. Available evidence indicates that dihydropyridine calcium antagonists, in reducing blood pressure, can reduce the urinary albumin excretion (UAE) rate[32] and prevent the progression to overt nephropathy. It is worth noting that if blood pressure is strictly controlled[35,36] or greatly reduced[44] this effect is basically the same as that observed with ACE inhibitors.

However, in type 2 diabetic patients when blood pressure is reduced but not perfectly controlled (as in the MARVAL study) valsartan (an AT-1 receptor antagonist) significantly reduced the UAE rate whereas amlodipine had no significant effect. In addition, valsartan induced regression to normoalbuminuria in a significantly greater proportion of patients than the calcium antagonist. This study therefore reinforces the view that blockade of the renin-angiotensin system adds a specific beneficial effect to blood pressure control as a means of reducing the UAE rate and thereby slowing down the progression to overt nephropathy and increasing regression to normoalbuminuria in type 2 diabetic patients with microalbuminuria.[45,46]

As far as the prevention of progression to overt nephropathy is concerned, several studies performed in a small number of type 1 and type 2 diabetic patients with overt nephropathy indicated that calcium antagonists decrease or do not change either proteinuria or GFR in a relatively short-term follow-up.[32] A four-year prospective study in a small number of hypertensive type 1 diabetic patients with overt nephropathy indicated that nisoldipine and lisinopril, although similarly reducing blood pressure, had a similar effect on the rate of decline in GFR (although only lisinopril significantly reduced proteinuria).[47] Moreover, a 4.5-year follow-up open study in a small number of hypertensive African Americans with type 2 diabetes indicated that verapamil sustained release significantly reduced the rate of decline in creatinine clearance and of creatinemia doubling compared to atenolol.[48]

However, the IDNT study comparing irbesartan with amlodipine and placebo in a large number of hyper-

tensive type 2 diabetic patients indicated that given similar blood pressure reduction the AT-1 receptor antagonist was superior to the dihydropyridine calcium antagonist in reducing the doubling of serum creatinine and marginally the occurrence of ESRD. In addition, these endpoints did not differ between the amlodipine and placebo groups.[49]

These results suggest that calcium antagonists do not exert a specific renal protective action beyond blood pressure reduction in hypertensive type 2 diabetic patients with overt nephropathy. However, as shown by the results of the RENAAL study dihydropyridine calcium antagonists are decisive in providing adequate blood pressure reduction without reducing the efficacy of the AT-1 receptor antagonist losartan on hard renal endpoints (including ESRD).[50] Thus, calcium antagonists can be effective and safely used in combination therapy, which is very often needed to control blood pressure in diabetic patients with nephropathy.

The results appear to be similar in patients with non-diabetic nephropathy. The AASK study,[51] performed in African Americans with hypertensive renal disease, showed that ramipril was superior to amlodipine (despite a similar blood pressure control) in determining a significant reduction of GFR decline (the primary endpoint) as well as the rate of secondary endpoints, including GFR decline >50% or by 25 mL/min per 1.73 m^2 and ESRD. In addition, proteinuria increased in the amlodipine group but declined in the ramipril group during the first six months of treatment and thereafter tended to rise in both groups, although with a significantly greater increase in the amlodipine group. However, the superiority of the ACE inhibitor was detectable only in patients with baseline proteinuria, without a significant difference in non-proteinuric patients.[51]

Moreover, in the same study the rate of decline in GFR was slower for amlodipine than metoprolol in non-proteinuric patients, but faster for amlodipine than metoprolol in proteinuric patients. Finally, only in patients with proteinuria was the risk for ESRD or death significantly lower in the metoprolol group compared to the amlodipine group.[52] Taken together, these results indicate that treatment with an ACE inhibitor, and to a lesser extent with a β-blocker, is superior to treatment with a dihydropyridine calcium antagonist in slowing the progression of proteinuria in hypertensive patients with nephroangiosclerosis. However, in non-proteinuric patients the calcium antagonist seems to have the same efficacy as the other two treatments.

Two other studies have confirmed the superiority of an ACE inhibitor compared to a dihydropyridine calcium antagonist in hypertensive patients with mild proteinuria and nondiabetic nephropathies. In a randomized double-blind study, at one-year follow-up enalapril (which greatly reduced blood pressure) significantly reduced proteinuria, whereas the latter was unmodified by manidipine (the rate and slope of creatinine clearance was similar with both treatments).[53] In addition, the ESPIRAL study demonstrated that fosinopril greatly reduced blood pressure values compared to nifedipine GITS, and significantly improved renal survival as evaluated by time to serum creatinine doubling or dialysis while reducing proteinuria (which was unchanged by the calcium antagonist).[54] Finally, another controlled study in hypertensive patients with primary glomerulonephritis and heavy proteinuria demonstrated that only trandolapril, in monotherapy or even better if combined with verapamil, significantly reduced proteinuria (which was unchanged by verapamil and atenolol treatment).[55]

It is therefore possible to conclude from the available information that hypertensive patients with diabetic or nondiabetic nephropathy, especially with microalbuminuria or proteinuria, should receive a compound blocking the renin-angiotensin system as a first-line therapy.[56] However, calcium antagonists must be considered part of a combination therapy that will be required in most patients to reach target blood pressure control.

EFFECTS OF CALCIUM ANTAGONISTS ON CLINICAL EVENTS

Placebo-controlled studies indicate that calcium-antagonist-based therapy reduces major cardiovascular events and cardiovascular death, as well as the total rate of stroke and all cardiac endpoints in elderly hypertensive patients.[3] As shown in Table 79–1, results from meta-analyses of placebo-controlled trials indicate that conventional therapy based on diuretics and β-blockers,[57] ACE inhibitors,[58] and calcium antagonists[58] similarly reduced cardiovascular outcomes. Furthermore, a recent meta-analysis of placebo-controlled trials in diabetic patients indicates that calcium antagonists reduce the risk of stroke by 53%, coronary artery disease by 40%, major cardiovascular events by 28%, cardiovascular deaths by 46%, and total mortality by 17%.[59]

The benefit achieved in these placebo-controlled studies was related to the degree of blood pressure reduction.[57,58] In addition, greater risk reductions were produced by regimens targeted to reach lower blood pressure goals.[58] Taken together, these results indicate that blood pressure lowering is the major component of the benefit of antihypertensive drug treatment, including that with calcium antagonists.[5,60] However, the results of these meta-analyses indicate that calcium antagonists do not reduce (or even tend to increase) the risk of heart failure, whose incidence was independent of blood pressure reduction.[58,59] However, the lack of protective action of calcium antagonists on heart failure (despite blood pressure reduction) is apparently contradicted by the results of the ACTION trial, which aimed to investigate the effect of long-acting nifedipine GITS in patients with stable angina receiving antianginal drugs (including β-blockers in about 80% of patients).[61]

This study showed that at 4.9-year follow-up nifedipine GITS, although reducing blood pressure by 5/3 mmHg, did not change fatal and nonfatal coronary events and total mortality but achieved a significant 29% reduction in new overt heart failure (a component of primary combined endpoint) as well as an 18% reduction in coronary angiography and a 21% reduction in coronary bypass surgery (two secondary endpoints).[61] Moreover, a predefined subgroup analysis of hypertensive patients (baseline blood pressure values ≥140/90 mmHg) indicated that nifedipine GITS significantly reduced new overt heart failure by 38%, any stroke or transient ischemic attacks (TIA) by 28%, and debilitating stroke by 33%—without affecting the rate of all-cause death, cardiovascular death, and myocardial infarction.[62]

Therefore, in agreement with the results of other placebo-controlled studies in patients with stable coronary artery disease[22,29,63,64] long-acting dihydropyridine calcium antagonists appear to be safe, do not increase the risk of hard coronary outcomes, and offer the additional advantage of reducing angina-related events such as hospitalization for unstable angina[22,29] and revascularization procedures.[22,29,63,64] Although the direct effect of calcium antagonists on heart failure (tested in placebo-controlled trials) is still an open question,[58] results from studies designed to provide drug class comparison indicate that calcium antagonists provide less protection from heart failure compared to conventional therapy or ACE inhibitors.[58]

On the question of the clinical efficacy of calcium antagonists compared to other drug classes, seven large long-term controlled clinical trials based on cardiovascular outcomes allow a comparison of calcium antagonists

PERCENT RISK REDUCTION IN CARDIOVASCULAR EVENTS INDUCED BY ACTIVE TREATMENT WITH CONVENTIONAL THERAPY ACE INHIBITORS AND CALCIUM ANTAGONISTS VERSUS PLACEBO			
Outcome	Conventional Therapy[a,57]	ACE Inhibitors[58]	Calcium Antagonists[58]
Stroke	−38	−28	−38
Coronary heart disease	−16	−20	−22
Heart failure	Not assessed	−18	+21[b]
Major cardiovascular events	Not assessed	−22	−18
Cardiovascular deaths	−21	−20	−22
Total mortality	−12	−12	−11[b]
a. Conventional therapy is based principally on diuretics and beta blockers. b. Not significant.			

Table 79–1. Percent Risk Reduction in Cardiovascular Events Induced by Active Treatment with Conventional Therapy ACE Inhibitors and Calcium Antagonists Versus Placebo

versus conventional therapy,[65-68] ACE inhibitors,[65,69,70] and ARB.[71] Data obtained so far show no difference in primary endpoints between calcium antagonists and other drug classes (Table 79–2). However, a differential effect of calcium antagonists compared to the other drug classes can be observed on different cardiovascular outcomes.

A recent prospectively designed meta-analysis, and therefore not biased by *a posteriori* selection of trials, including nine studies comparing calcium antagonists with conventional therapy and six studies comparing calcium antagonists with ACE inhibitors showed that the risk of major cardiovascular events and cardiovascular and total mortality was similar when calcium-antagonist-treated groups were compared to those on conventional therapy or ACE inhibitors.[58] Moreover, another randomized controlled study (INVEST, not included in the meta-analysis) compared outcomes in older hypertensive patients with coronary artery disease treated with a verapamil- or atenolol-based strategy (both treatments being mainly associated with an ACE inhibitor and a thiazide diuretic).

The results of this study showed that the rate of cardiovascular and total mortality did not differ between the two treated groups.[70] Finally, the VALUE trial (a randomized double-blind study performed in hypertensive patients at high cardiovascular risk) was designed to test the hypothesis that with the same blood pressure control an ARB (valsartan) would reduce cardiac mortality and morbidity more than a dihydropyridine calcium antagonist (amlodipine). The results at a 4.2-year follow-up showed that although blood pressure was greatly reduced in the amlodipine arm cardiovascular and total mortality did not differ between the treated groups.[71]

Overall, these data indicate that Ca-antagonist-based treatment exerts an effect on cardiovascular and total mortality similar to that exerted by treatments based on conventional therapy, ACE inhibitors, and ARBs. The data on coronary artery disease (CAD) events are even more interesting, considering the past controversy on the possible adverse effect of calcium antagonists on this outcome.[72]

The result from the previously quoted meta-analysis[58] indicates that the risk of coronary artery disease events in calcium-antagonist-treated patients did not differ from that of patients receiving conventional therapy or ACE inhibitors, a finding in agreement with the more recent INVEST[70] study (not included in the meta-analysis). Moreover, a post hoc analysis from the ALLHAT study showed that given similar blood pressure control the primary outcome of fatal CAD and nonfatal myocardial infarction did not differ between amlodipine and lisinopril in essential hypertensive patients with CAD at baseline.

However, a very recent meta-analysis—including 14 placebo-controlled studies (six with calcium antagonists and eight with ACE inhibitors) and 18 studies comparing conventional therapy versus calcium antagonists (13 studies) or ACE inhibitors (5 studies) and modeling the risk of coronary artery disease on group difference in achieved systolic blood pressure—indicated that (1) the risk of coronary artery disease was not significantly different between regimens based on calcium antagonists and conventional therapy, (2) the risk of coronary artery disease decreased by 15% per 10 mmHg reduction in systolic blood pressure, and (3) independently of blood pressure difference ACE inhibitors were superior to calcium antagonists in the prevention of coronary artery disease.[73]

In the VALUE trial, the risk of myocardial infarction was significantly greater in the valsartan-treated patients compared to those receiving amlodipine.[71] This difference was partially but not fully explained by differences in blood pressure control.[74]

CONTROLLED CLINICAL TRIALS OF CARDIOVASCULAR OUTCOMES COMPARING CALCIUM ANTAGONISTS WITH OTHER DRUG CLASSES IN HYPERTENSIVE PATIENTS			
Study	Drugs	Primary Endpoint	Relative Risk (95% CI)
STOP-2[65]	Felodipine, isradipine vs D/βB	Fatal stroke, MI, and other CV deaths	0.97 (0.80–1.17)
STOP-2[65]	Enalapril, lisinopril, vs D/βB	Fatal stroke, MI, and other CV deaths	1.01 (0.84–1.22)
NORDIL[66]	Diltiazem vs D/βB	Fatal stroke, MI, and other CV deaths	1.00 (0.87–1.15)
CONVINCE[68]	Verapamil vs atenolol/HCTZ	First occurrence of stroke and MI, CV mortality	1.02 (0.88–1.18)
INVEST[70]	Verapamil vs atenolol	CHD morbidity and mortality	1.02 (0.92–1.15)
INSIGHT[67]	Nifedipine vs HCTZ/amiloride	CV mortality, MI, HF, stroke	1.10 (0.91–1.34)
ALLHAT[69]	Chlorthalidone vs amlodipine	CHD morbidity and mortality	0.99 (0.91–1.08)
ALLHAT[69]	Lisinopril vs amlodipine	CHD morbidity and mortality	1.01 (0.91–1.11)
VALUE[71]	Valsartan vs amlodipine	CHD morbidity and mortality	1.04 (0.94–1.15)
Abbreviations: CI, confidence intervals; MI, myocardial infarction; CV, cardiovascular; CHD, coronary heart disease; HF, heart failure; D, diuretics; βB, beta-blockers; HCTZ, hydrochlorothiazide; and ACE-I, angiotensin-converting enzyme.			

Table 79–2. Controlled Clinical Trials of Cardiovascular Outcomes Comparing Calcium Antagonists with Other Drug Classes in Hypertensive Patients

Finally, the MOSES study was a randomized open trial in a relatively small number of hypertensive patients with a history of documented cerebrovascular disease. The study compared an ARB (eprosartan) with nitrendipine, which showed at four-year follow-up that cardiovascular events (mainly including acute coronary syndrome and heart failure) were significantly lower in the eprosartan compared to the nitrendipine arm.[75] It can therefore be concluded that long-acting calcium antagonists are as effective as other drug treatments for prevention of coronary artery disease in hypertensive patients, a finding that strongly contradicts the hypothesis of a possible negative effect of these drugs on coronary artery disease events. However, the possibility exists that beyond blood pressure reduction treatment with ACE inhibitors is superior to that with calcium antagonists in preventing coronary artery disease events.

With regard to the prevention of cerebrovascular disease, meta-analyses indicate a marginally lower risk of stroke in calcium-antagonist-treated patients compared to those receiving conventional therapy[58,76] and ACE inhibitors.[58] A more recent meta-analysis, including 13 studies comparing calcium antagonists with other antihypertensive treatments, showed a 10% significant reduction in the risk of stroke in patients treated with calcium antagonists. This beneficial effect was unrelated to the degree of systolic blood pressure reduction.[77] The superiority of calcium antagonists compared to conventional therapy and ACE inhibitors in reduction of the risk of stroke is further confirmed by the previously quoted meta-analysis.[73]

In the VALUE trial, the risk of fatal and nonfatal stroke was marginally lower in the amlodipine than in the valsartan group[71]—a difference that can be explained by differences in blood pressure control.[74] However, in the MOSES study given the same blood pressure reduction total cerebrovascular events (including recurrent events, but not first cerebrovascular events) were significantly lower in the eprosartan compared to the nitrendipine arm.[75] One may therefore conclude that calcium antagonists seem to be more effective compared to conventional therapy and ACE inhibitors in stroke prevention, whereas comparative data with AT-1 receptor antagonists are too scanty to draw definitive conclusions.

Decisive demonstration of the effectiveness of calcium-antagonist-based treatment derives from the ASCOT-BPLA trial, which compared amlodipine-based treatment (plus perindopril in about 50% of patients) with atenolol-based treatment (plus bendroflumethiazide in about 55% of patients) in hypertensive patients with moderately high cardiovascular risk.[78] This study, which was stopped prematurely after 5.5 years of median follow-up owing to a significant difference in mortality in the two treatment arms, showed that amlodipine-based treatment [although not significantly reducing (10%) the primary endpoint of nonfatal myocardial infarction plus fatal coronary artery disease] significantly decreased secondary endpoints, including nonfatal myocardial infarction (excluding silent myocardial infarction) plus fatal coronary artery disease (–13%), total coronary events (–13%), total cardiovascular events and procedures (–16%), all-cause mortality (–11%), and cardiovascular mortality (–24%) and fatal and nonfatal stroke (–23%). It also decreased tertiary endpoints, such as unstable angina (–32%), peripheral arterial disease (–35%), development of diabetes (–30%), and renal impairment (–15%).

Therefore, the ASCOT-BPLA study shows the superiority of an antihypertensive regimen based on a dihydropyridine calcium antagonist (with the combination of an ACE inhibitor when necessary) compared to a beta-blocker-based treatment with the eventual addition of a thiazide diuretic for the prevention of most cardiovascular events associated with hypertension.[78] It is worth noting that the beneficial effect of the calcium antagonist is partially but not fully explained by the different effect not only on blood pressure but on other cardiovascular risk factors, including high density lipoprotein (HDL) cholesterol, triglycerides, glucose, potassium, and body weight.[79]

COMPLICATIONS

Calcium antagonists are generally well-tolerated compounds. Among possible side effects caused by this drug class, the most common manifestations are related to vasodilation (observed particularly with the dihydropyridines). These main side effects include headache, flushing, and reflex tachycardia.[4] They are usually benign, appear with the first dosing, and spontaneously disappear in a few days. From a clinical point of view, a more troublesome adverse effect of dihydropyridine calcium antagonists is ankle edema.

Usually, this side effect appears after several weeks of treatment and is specifically related to arteriolar vasodilation. It is dose dependent, and available evidence suggests that it is less evident with newer calcium antagonists (including lacidipine, lercanidipine, and possibly barnedipine). Although ankle edema is not dangerous for the patient, it can determine some discomfort or cause esthetic problems. If the patient tolerates this side effect, treatment can be continued. However, another possibility is to add an ACE inhibitor or an AT-1 receptor antagonist (which can reduce the severity of ankle edema). It is also important to note that given the mechanistic cause of the ankle edema the association of diuretic treatment is totally ineffective. Finally, although diltiazem treatment sometimes induces ankle edema (although with a lesser incidence compared with dihydropyridine calcium antagonists) such an effect is only very rarely observed with verapamil.

Non-dihydropyridine calcium antagonists may have side effects related to the specific cardiac mechanism of action.[1] Verapamil and diltiazem can lead to bradycardia, atrioveutricular block, and worsening of congestive heart failure. It is therefore important to assess heart rate and P-R interval on EKG before administering one of these compounds. In addition, if the patient has clinical symptoms that could be related to heart failure it is crucial to evaluate left ventricular function by echocardiography. As well as these expected side effects, verapamil treatment can also induce constipation, which is usually not seen with diltiazem or dihydopyridines. However, this characteristic of verapamil can be useful when treating patients with chronic diarrhea.

CHAPTER
79

PHARMACOLOGIC TREATMENT : Calcium Antagonists

Another side effect specifically related to calcium antagonist treatment is gingival hypertrophy. This effect is not frequent, but it occurs both with dihydripyridines and non-dihydropyridines. It is reversible by withdrawal of treatment. Other less common side effects may include digital dysesthesia, nausea, and occasionally minor elevation of the liver function test.

A special comment is needed concerning massive utilization of sublingual nifedipine in hypertensive emergencies. This treatment is extremely dangerous because the rapid and powerful vasodilating effect can frequently cause cerebrovascular or coronary ischemia, and in any case there is little or no absorption of the drug from the buccal mucosa. Because in most cases the urgent reduction of blood pressure values is overestimated the utilization of sublingual nifedipine should be avoided in common clinical practice and reserved as a procedure for selected and monitored patients in emergency care units.

Finally, it is necessary to consider some harmful drug interactions. Earlier, attention was drawn to the dangerous combination between verapamil or diltiazem and beta blockers, which can sum their effects of heart rate, A-V conduction, and left ventricular contractility. In addition, verapamil (and sometimes other calcium antagonists) can cause an increase in plasma digoxin concentrations, although toxicity from the cardiac glycoside rarely develops.

In conclusion, calcium antagonists are well-tolerated compounds with very few side effects. It is also important to observe that although some of the side effects may cause discomfort for the patients none of these effects is life-threatening, and the physician has the possibility of adjusting the treatment without serious and/or permanent damage to patients.

SUMMARY

Calcium antagonists are very effective antihypertensive drugs. These compounds can be divided into dihydropyridine and non-dihydropyridine calcium antagonists. Dihydropyridines are pure vasodilators, whereas non-dihydropyridines (verapamil and diltiazem) are associated with a lesser ability to vasodilate (with a chronotropic,

dromotropic, and inotropic effect). However, all calcium antagonists induce a significant dose-dependent reduction in blood pressure values (with few and non-life-threatening side effects). The main adverse reaction caused by these compounds is ankle edema, which although discomforting is not dangerous to patients.

Usually, no specific indication exists for the utilization of calcium antagonists because these compounds are effective in any form of hypertension—including secondary hypertension, sodium repleted hypertension, black and elderly patients, and pregnancy-induced hypertension (although in this case the evidence is limited to nifedipine). Dihydropyridine calcium antagonists are effective as combination therapy with all the other antihypertensive drug classes, with the exclusion of diuretics (except in patients with heart failure). In contrast, non-dihydropyridine calcium antagonists cannot be associated with beta blockers, to avoid the sum of the cardiac effects.

The clinical relevance of these compounds is supported by the evidence that calcium antagonists are as effective as ACE inhibitors and AT-1 receptor antagonists in reversing left ventricular hypertrophy. In addition, they show antiatherosclerotic properties, probably related to their antioxidant properties and the consequent restoration of endothelial function. Evidence from clinical trials indicates that these compounds are effective in reducing the occurrence of stroke and myocardial infarction, whereas discordant results are available on the prevention of heart failure. Calcium antagonists have no specific effects in protecting renal function, as observed with drugs blocking the renin angiotensin system, but they can be useful in treating patients with diabetic and nondiabetic nephropathy because of their ability to lower blood pressure values.

In the future it will be necessary to investigate whether some specific characteristic of calcium antagonists, including their antiatherosclerotic activity, might be clinically relevant. However, only results from large numbers of patients and especially a more prolonged period of observation will give further information on the possible clinical implications of calcium antagonist treatment.

REFERENCES

1. Robertson RM, Robertson D. Drugs used for the treatment of myocardial ischemia. In Hardman JG, Goodman Gilman A, Limbird LE (eds), Goodman and Gilman's *The Parmacological Basis of Therapeutics, Ninth Edition.* New York: McGraw-Hill 1996:759–769.
2. Opie LH. *Clinical Use of Calcium Channel Antagonist Drugs.* Boston: Kluver Academic Publishers 1990:1.
3. Grossman E, Messerli FH. Calcium antagonists. *Prog Cardiovasc Dis* 2004; 47:34.
4. Oates JA. Antihypertensive agents and drug therapy of hypertension. In Hardman JG, Goodman Gilman A, Limbird LE (eds), Goodman & Gilman's *The Parmacological Basis of Therapeutics,*

Ninth Edition. New York: McGraw-Hill 1996:780–808.
5. European Society of Hypertension-European Society of Cardiology. Guidelines for the management of arterial hypertension. *J Hypertens* 2003;21:1011.
6. Henry PD. Atherogenesis, calcium and calcium antagonists. *Am J Cardiol* 1990;66:31–61.
7. Schiffrin EL, Deng LY. Structure and function of resistance arteries of hypertensive patients treated with a beta-blocker or a calcium channel antagonist. *J Hypertens* 1996;14:1247.
8. Frielingsdorf J, Seiler C, Kaufmann P, et al. Normalization of abnormal coronary vasomotion by calcium

antagonists in patients with hypertension. *Circulation* 1996;93:1380.
9. Effect of nifedipine and cerivastatin on coronary endothelial function in patients with coronary artery disease: The ENCORE I study (Evaluation of Nifedipine and Cerivastatin on Recovery of Coronary Endothelial Function). *Circulation* 2003;107:422.
10. Taddei S, Virdis A, Ghiadoni L, et al. Effects of antihypertensive drugs on endothelial dysfunction: Clinical implications. *Drugs* 2002;62:265.
11. Taddei S, Virdis A, Ghiadoni L, et al. Lacidipine restores endothelium-dependent vasodilation in essential hypertensive patients. *Hypertension* 1997;30:1606.

12. Taddei S, Virdis A, Ghiadoni L, et al. Effect of calcium antagonist or beta blockade treatment on nitric oxide-dependent vasodilation and oxidative stress in essential hypertensive patients. J Hypertens 2001;19:1379.

13. Taddei S, Virdis A, Ghiadoni L, et al. Restoration of nitric oxide availability after calcium antagonist treatment in essential hypertension. Hypertension 2001;37:943.

14. Perticone F, Ceravolo R, Maio R, et al. Calcium antagonist isradipine improves abnormal endothelium-dependent vasodilation in never treated hypertensive patients. Cardiovasc Res 1999;41:299.

15. Taddei S, Virdis A, Ghiadoni L, et al. Calcium antagonist treatment by lercanidipine prevents hyperpolarization in essential hypertension. Hypertension 2003;41:950.

16. Lupo E, Locher R, Weisser B, Vetter W. In vitro antioxidant activity of calcium antagonists against LDL oxidation compared with alpha-tocopherol. Biochem Biophys Res Commun 1994;203:1803.

17. Kozakova M, Buralli S, Palombo C, Salvetti A. Surrogate end-points of antihypertensive treatment: Left ventricular hypertrophy and structural alteration of carotid arteries. Heart Drug 2001;1:89.

18. Klingbeil AU, Schneider M, Martus P, et al. A meta-analysis of the effects of treatment on left ventricular mass in essential hypertension. Am J Med 2003;115:41.

19. Terpstra WF, May JF, Smit AJ, et al. Long-term effects of amlodipine and lisinopril on left ventricular mass and diastolic function in elderly, previously untreated hypertensive patients: The ELVERA trial. J Hypertens 2001;19:303.

20. Devereux RB, Palmieri V, Sharpe N, et al. Effects of once-daily angiotensin-converting enzyme inhibition and calcium channel blockade-based antihypertensive treatment regimens on left ventricular hypertrophy and diastolic filling in hypertension: The prospective randomized enalapril study evaluating regression of ventricular enlargement (preserve) trial. Circulation 2001;104:1248.

21. Agabiti-Rosei E, Trimarco B, Muiesan ML, et al. Cardiac structural and functional changes during long-term antihypertensive treatment with lacidipine and atenolol in the European Lacidipine Study on Atherosclerosis (ELSA). J Hypertens 2005;23:1091.

22. Pitt B, Byington RP, Furberg CD, et al. Effect of amlodipine on the progression of atherosclerosis and the occurrence of clinical events. Circulation 2000; 102:1503.

23. Borhani NO, Mercuri M, Borhani PA, et al. Final outcome results of the Multicenter Isradipine Diuretic Atherosclerosis Study (MIDAS): A randomized controlled trial. JAMA 1996;276:785.

24. Zanchetti A, Rosei EA, Dal Palu C, et al. The Verapamil in Hypertension and Atherosclerosis Study (VHAS): Results of long-term randomized treatment with either verapamil or chlorthalidone on carotid intima-media thickness. J Hypertens 1998;16:1667.

25. Simon A, Gariepy J, Moyse D, Levenson J. Differential effects of nifedipine and co-amilozide on the progression of early carotid wall changes. Circulation 2001;103:2949.

26. Zanchetti A, Bond MG, Hennig M, et al. Calcium antagonist lacidipine slows down progression of asymptomatic carotid atherosclerosis: Principal results of the European Lacidipine Study on Atherosclerosis (ELSA), a randomized, double-blind, long-term trial. Circulation 2002;106:2422.

27. Lichtlen PR, Hugenholtz PG, Rafflenbeul W, et al. Retardation of angiographic progression of coronary artery disease by nifedipine: Results of the International Nifedipine trial on Antiatherosclerotic Therapy (INTACT). Lancet 1990;335:1109.

28. Waters D, Lesperance J, Francetich M, et al. A controlled clinical trial to assess the effect of a calcium channel blocker on the progression of coronary atherosclerosis. Circulation 1990; 82:1940.

29. Nissen SE, Tuzcu EM, Libby P, et al. Effect of antihypertensive agents on cardiovascular events in patients with coronary disease and normal blood pressure: The CAMELOT study, a randomized controlled trial. JAMA 2004;292:2217.

30. Motro M, Shemesh J. Calcium channel blocker nifedipine slows down progression of coronary calcification in hypertensive patients compared with diuretics. Hypertension 2001;37:1410.

31. Jukema JW, Zwinderman AH, van Boven AJ, et al. Evidence for a synergistic effect of calcium channel blockers with lipid-lowering therapy in retarding progression of coronary atherosclerosis in symptomatic patients with normal to moderately raised cholesterol levels: The REGRESS Study Group. Arterioscler Thromb Vasc Biol 1996;16:425.

32. Salvetti A, Mattei P, Sudano I. Renal protection and antihypertensive drugs: Current status. Drugs 1999;57:665.

33. Segura J, Garcia-Donaire JA, Ruilope LM. Calcium channel blockers and renal protection: Insights from the latest clinical trials. J Am Soc Nephrol 2005; 16:S64.

34. Voyaki SM, Staessen JA, Thijs L, et al. Follow-up of renal function in treated and untreated older patients with isolated systolic hypertension: Systolic Hypertension in Europe (Syst-Eur) Trial Investigators. J Hypertens 2001;19:511.

35. Estacio RO, Jeffers BW, Gifford N, Schrier RW. Effect of blood pressure control on diabetic microvascular complications in patients with hypertension and type 2 diabetes. Diabetes Care 2000;23:B54.

36. Schrier RW, Estacio RO, Esler A, Mehler P. Effects of aggressive blood pressure control in normotensive type 2 diabetic patients on albuminuria, retinopathy and strokes. Kidney Int 2002;61:1086.

37. Rahman M, Pressel S, Davis BR, et al. Renal outcomes in high-risk hypertensive patients treated with an angiotensin-converting enzyme inhibitor or a calcium channel blocker vs a diuretic: A report from the Antihypertensive and Lipid-Lowering Treatment to Prevent Heart Attack Trial (ALLHAT). Arch Intern Med 2005; 165:936.

38. Remuzzi G, Ruggenenti P, Perico N. Chronic renal diseases: Renoprotective benefits of renin-angiotensin system inhibition. Ann Intern Med 2002; 136:604.

39. de Leeuw PW, Ruilope LM, Palmer CR, et al. Clinical significance of renal function in hypertensive patients at high risk: Results from the INSIGHT trial. Arch Intern Med 2004;164:2459.

40. Randomized double-blind comparison of a calcium antagonist and a diuretic in elderly hypertensives: National Intervention Cooperative Study in Elderly Hypertensives Study Group. Hypertension 1999;34:1129.

41. Rodicio JL, Morales JM, Ruilope LM. Lipophilic dihydropyridines provide renal protection from cyclosporin toxicity. J Hypertens Suppl 1993; 11:S21.

42. Rahn KH, Barenbrock M, Fritschka E, et al. Effect of nitrendipine on renal function in renal-transplant patients treated with cyclosporin: A randomised trial. Lancet 1999;354:1415.

43. Ruggenenti P, Fassi A, Ilieva AP, et al. Preventing microalbuminuria in type 2 diabetes. N Engl J Med 2004;351:1941.

44. Baba S. Nifedipine and enalapril equally reduce the progression of nephropathy in hypertensive type 2 diabetics. Diabetes Res Clin Pract 2001;54:191.

45. Parving HH, Lehnert H, Brochner-Mortensen J, et al. The effect of irbesartan on the development of diabetic nephropathy in patients with type 2 diabetes. N Engl J Med 2001; 345:870.

46. Opie LH, Parving HH. Diabetic nephropathy: Can renoprotection be extrapolated to cardiovascular protection? Circulation 2002;106:643.

47. Tarnow L, Rossing P, Jensen C, et al. Long-term renoprotective effect of nisoldipine and lisinopril in type 1 diabetic patients with diabetic nephropathy. Diabetes Care 2000; 23:1725.

48. Bakris GL, Mangrum A, Copley JB, et al. Effect of calcium channel or beta-blockade on the progression of diabetic nephropathy in African Americans. Hypertension 1997;29:744.

49. Lewis EJ, Hunsicker LG, Clarke WR, et al. Renoprotective effect of the angiotensin-receptor antagonist irbesartan in patients with nephropathy due to type 2 diabetes. N Engl J Med 2001;345:851.

50. Bakris GL, Weir MR, Shanifar S, et al. Effects of blood pressure level on progression of diabetic nephropathy: Results from the RENAAL study. Arch Intern Med 2003;163:1555.

51. Agodoa LY, Appel L, Bakris GL, et al. Effect of ramipril vs amlodipine on renal outcomes in hypertensive nephrosclerosis: A randomized controlled trial. JAMA 2001;285:2719.

52. Wright JT Jr., Bakris G, Greene T, et al. Effect of blood pressure lowering and antihypertensive drug class on progression of hypertensive kidney disease: Results from the AASK trial. JAMA 2002;288:2421.

53. Del Vecchio L, Pozzi M, Salvetti A, et al. Efficacy and tolerability of manidipine in the treatment of hypertension in

patients with non-diabetic chronic kidney disease without glomerular disease: Prospective, randomized, double-blind study of parallel groups in comparison with enalapril. *J Nephrol* 2004;17:261.

54. Marin R, Ruilope LM, et al. A random comparison of fosinopril and nifedipine GITS in patients with primary renal disease. *J Hypertens* 2001;19:1871.

55. Dissociation between blood pressure reduction and fall in proteinuria in primary renal disease: A randomized double-blind trial. *J Hypertens* 2002; 20:729.

56. Jafar TH, Stark PC, Schmid CH, et al. Progression of chronic kidney disease: The role of blood pressure control, proteinuria, and angiotensin-converting enzyme inhibition (a patient-level meta-analysis). *Ann Intern Med* 2003;139:244.

57. Collins R, MacMahon S. Blood pressure, antihypertensive drug treatment and the risks of stroke and of coronary heart disease. *Br Med Bull* 1994;50:272.

58. Turnbull F. Effects of different blood-pressure-lowering regimens on major cardiovascular events: Results of prospectively-designed overviews of randomised trials. *Lancet* 2003;362: 1527.

59. Turnbull F, Neal B, Algert C, et al. Effects of different blood pressure-lowering regimens on major cardiovascular events in individuals with and without diabetes mellitus: Results of prospectively designed overviews of randomized trials. *Arch Intern Med* 2005;165:1410.

60. Chobanian AV, Bakris GL, Black HR, et al. The Seventh Report of the Joint National Committee on Prevention, Detection, Evaluation, and Treatment of High Blood Pressure: The JNC 7 report. *JAMA* 2003;289:2560.

61. Poole-Wilson PA, Lubsen J, Kirwan BA, et al. Effect of long-acting nifedipine on mortality and cardiovascular morbidity in patients with stable angina requiring treatment (ACTION trial): Randomised controlled trial. *Lancet* 2004;364:849.

62. Lubsen J, Wagener G, Kirwan BA, et al. Effect of long-acting nifedipine on mortality and cardiovascular morbidity in patients with symptomatic stable angina and hypertension: The ACTION trial. *J Hypertens* 2005;23:641.

63. Jorgensen B, Simonsen S, Endresen K, et al. Restenosis and clinical outcome in patients treated with amlodipine after angioplasty: Results from the Coronary AngioPlasty Amlodipine REStenosis Study (CAPARES). *J Am Coll Cardiol* 2000;35:592.

64. Dens JA, Desmet WJ, Coussement P, et al. Long term effects of nisoldipine on the progression of coronary atherosclerosis and the occurrence of clinical events: The NICOLE study. *Heart* 2003;89:887.

65. Hansson L, Lindholm LH, Ekbom T, et al. Randomised trial of old and new antihypertensive drugs in elderly patients: Cardiovascular mortality and morbidity the Swedish Trial in Old Patients with Hypertension-2 study. *Lancet* 1999;354:1751.

66. Hansson L, Hedner T, Lund-Johansen P, et al. Randomised trial of effects of calcium antagonists compared with diuretics and beta-blockers on cardiovascular morbidity and mortality in hypertension: The Nordic Diltiazem (NORDIL) study. *Lancet* 2000;356:359.

67. Brown MJ, Palmer CR, Castaigne A, et al. Morbidity and mortality in patients randomised to double-blind treatment with a long-acting calcium-channel blocker or diuretic in the International Nifedipine GITS study: Intervention as a Goal in Hypertension Treatment (INSIGHT). *Lancet* 2000; 356:366.

68. Black HR, Elliott WJ, Grandits G, et al. Principal results of the Controlled Onset Verapamil Investigation of Cardiovascular End Points (CONVINCE) trial. *JAMA* 2003;289:2073.

69. Major outcomes in high-risk hypertensive patients randomized to angiotensin-converting enzyme inhibitor or calcium channel blocker vs diuretic: The Antihypertensive and Lipid-Lowering Treatment to Prevent Heart Attack Trial (ALLHAT). *JAMA* 2002;288:2981.

70. Pepine CJ, Handberg EM, Cooper-DeHoff RM, et al. A calcium antagonist vs a non-calcium antagonist hypertension treatment strategy for patients with coronary artery disease: The International Verapamil-Trandolapril Study (INVEST), a randomized controlled trial. *JAMA* 2003;290:2805.

71. Julius S, Kjeldsen SE, Weber M, et al. Outcomes in hypertensive patients at high cardiovascular risk treated with regimens based on valsartan or amlodipine: The VALUE randomised trial. *Lancet* 2004;363:2022.

72. Effects of calcium antagonists on the risks of coronary heart disease, cancer and bleeding: Ad Hoc Subcommittee of the Liaison Committee of the World Health Organisation and the International Society of Hypertension. *J Hypertens* 1997;15:105.

73. Verdecchia P, Reboldi G, Angeli F, et al. Angiotensin-Converting Enzyme Inhibitors and Calcium Channel Blockers for Coronary Heart Disease and Stroke Prevention. *Hypertension* 2005;11:11.

74. Weber MA, Julius S, Kjeldsen SE, et al. Blood pressure dependent and independent effects of antihypertensive treatment on clinical events in the VALUE Trial. *Lancet* 2004;363:2049.

75. Schrader J, Luders S, Kulschewski A, et al. Morbidity and Mortality After Stroke, Eprosartan Compared with Nitrendipine for Secondary Prevention: Principal results of a prospective randomized controlled study (MOSES). *Stroke* 2005;36:1218.

76. Staessen JA, Wang JG, Thijs L. Cardiovascular prevention and blood pressure reduction: A quantitative overview updated until 1 March 2003. *J Hypertens* 2003;21:1055.

77. Angeli F, Verdecchia P, Reboldi GP, et al. Calcium channel blockade to prevent stroke in hypertension: A meta-analysis of 13 studies with 103,793 subjects. *Am J Hypertens* 2004;17:817.

78. Dahlöf B, Sever PS, Poulter NR, et al. Prevention of cardiovascular events with an antihypertensive regimen of amlodipine adding perindopril as required versus atenolol adding bendroflumethiazide as required, in the Anglo-Scandinavian Cardiac Outcomes Trial-Blood Pressure Lowering Arm (ASCOT-BPLA): A multicentre randomised controlled trial. *Lancet* 2005;366:895.

79. Poulter NR, Wedel H, Dahlöf B, et al. Role of blood pressure and other variables in the differential cardiovascular event rates noted in the Anglo-Scandinavian Cardiac Outcomes Trial-Blood Pressure Lowering Arm (ASCOT-BPLA). *Lancet* 2005;366:907.

Chapter

80 Angiotensin-Converting Enzyme Inhibitors

Alan H. Gradman and Darren Traub

Key Findings

- Angiotensin-converting enzyme inhibitors (ACE inhibitors) inhibit the conversion of the inactive decapeptide angiotensin I to the active vasopressor angiotensin II. ACE inhibitors also prevent the breakdown of bradykinin, a potent endothelium-dependent vasodilator.

- Although the 12 currently available ACE inhibitors differ in their pharmacokinetics and pharmacodynamics, all ACE inhibitors are capable of producing a clinically effective blood pressure (BP) response when dosed appropriately.

- ACE inhibitors effectively reduce BP and cardiovascular endpoints in unselected patients with hypertension.

- Currently, ACE inhibitors are the only drug class recommended for all of the "compelling indications" in the recent JNC-7 hypertension guidelines.

- Experimental models and clinical trials have shown that ACE inhibitors effectively reduce target organ pathology, including regression of left ventricular hypertrophy and fibrosis, reversal of vascular hypertrophy, reduction of proteinuria, and the development of end-stage renal disease.

- ACE inhibitors are recognized as preferred treatment for patients with hypertension complicated by heart failure; coronary artery disease or history of myocardial infarction (MI); diabetes; or chronic kidney disease. It is also used for recurrent stroke prevention (JNC-7).

- The maximum BP response to ACE inhibitors is achieved in approximately four to six weeks.

- By activating the renin-angiotensin system, low-dose diuretics combined with ACE inhibitors produce additive BP reduction and improve responder rates to ACE inhibition.

- In patients with renal insufficiency, an initial rise in serum creatinine (SCr) of up to 30% above baseline levels can be expected with initiation of ACE inhibitor therapy. This elevation of SCr usually stabilizes within two to three weeks and represents a hemodynamic (not a toxic) effect.

- ACE inhibitors are well tolerated by a broad population of hypertensive patients. The most common side effect is a persistent nonproductive cough, reported in 0.5 to 20% of patients.

INTRODUCTION

The first ACE inhibitor, teprotide, was derived from the venom of the Brazilian arrowhead viper (*Bothrops jararaca*).[1] When it became available for clinical testing in 1973, the role of the renin-angiotensin system (RAS) as an endocrine system involved in the regulation of BP and volume status had been established for almost a century.[2] Activation of the RAS induced by experimental renal artery stenosis had been shown to produce marked hypertension, and it was originally postulated that inhibiting the RAS would be beneficial primarily in treating renovascular hypertension. The wider therapeutic potential of inhibiting ACE became apparent following the observation that teprotide effectively lowered BP in patients with essential hypertension.

Almost 25 years after their introduction, the role of ACE inhibitors in cardiovascular medicine continues to expand as new beneficial effects are discovered, tested in animal models, and evaluated in clinical trials. ACE inhibitors have been shown to reduce BP and cardiovascular endpoints in unselected patients with hypertension. They are among the most effective category of antihypertensive drugs. In the recent JNC-7 report, ACE inhibitors are the only drug class recommended for all of the six categories of "compelling indications" for which directed drug therapy is advised.[3]

ACE inhibitors have been shown to improve symptoms and survival in patients with heart failure, decrease proteinuria and the progression of both diabetic and non-diabetic renal disease, reduce myocardial infarction (MI) and post-infarction ventricular remodeling in patients with coronary artery disease, decrease the incidence of new-onset diabetes, reduce the progression of diabetic retinopathy, and in conjunction with diuretics attenuate the risk of stroke and transient ischemic attacks in patients with symptomatic cerebrovascular disease. Importantly, these achievements are obtained with a favorable side effect profile that allows ACE inhibitors to be well tolerated by the vast majority of treatment-eligible patients.[4–12]

The importance of angiotensin II in the pathogenesis of atherosclerosis, left ventricular hypertrophy, vascular/ventricular remodeling, and glomerulosclerosis has placed the RAS and drugs that block its effects at the center of investigation of virtually all aspects of hypertensive disease and its complications.[13] Evidence that the RAS plays a critical role in the development of the structural precursors of cardiovascular complications in the hypertensive population has led to interest in the ability of ACE inhibitors to produce therapeutic benefits beyond those achieved through BP reduction alone.

It is now generally accepted that the effectiveness of ACE inhibitors in slowing the progression of renal disease is due to a combination of antihypertensive and organ-specific effects. Likewise, their ability to confer protection against the occurrence of MI in high-risk populations is apparently due to direct effects on the vasculature in addition to BP reduction. Further delineation of the direct organ protective effects of ACE inhibitors remains an area of active investigation.[13]

MECHANISM OF ACTION

ACE inhibitors competitively inhibit ACE, thus preventing the conversion of the inactive decapeptide angiotensin I to the active octapeptide vasopressor angiotensin II. ACE inhibitors also prevent the breakdown of the endothelium-dependent vasodilator bradykinin (Figure 80–1).

Pharmacodynamics
Humoral effects

ACE inhibitors inhibit the conversion of the inactive decapeptide angiotensin I to the active octapeptide angiotensin II. Following ACE inhibitor administration, the pressor response to intravenous infusion of angiotensin I (but not angiotensin II) is blocked. Short-term administration of ACE inhibitors causes a reduction in plasma and tissue angiotensin II levels. Plasma aldosterone levels are also reduced.[14–16] These changes, along with increases in circulating bradykinin, account for the immediate hemodynamic effects of ACE inhibitors.[17]

Over a period of days to a few weeks, loss of negative feedback inhibition by angiotensin II results in an increase in plasma renin activity (PRA) and circulating levels of angiotensin I, the ACE substrate. Driven by increased substrate availability and elaboration via non-ACE enzymatic pathways such as chymase, angiotensin II reaccumulates in the plasma during chronic dosing. Circulating levels of angiotensin II and aldosterone often return to pre-therapeutic levels, particularly at trough drug concentrations.[14,16,18,19] Despite this phenomenon of "ACE escape," BP reduction and other favorable hemodynamic alterations are maintained with chronic therapy, indicating that suppression of circulating angiotensin II does not fully explain the antihypertensive effect of ACE inhibitors.[14–16,19]

Role of bradykinin

ACE, also referred to as kininase II, is the principal enzyme responsible for the metabolism of bradykinin (a potent endothelium-dependent vasodilator). Bradykinin induces vasodilation by stimulating production of nitric oxide, the arachidonic acid metabolites prostacyclin (PGI-2) and PGE-2, and endothelium-derived hyperpolarizing factor. The brief duration of action and rapid degradation of bradykinin (plasma half-life of 15 to 30 seconds) has made it difficult to investigate its role in ACE inhibitor therapy.[14,20–22] Development of bradykinin receptor antagonists has helped clarify the important contribution of bradykinin to the acute and chronic actions of ACE inhibitors.[14] In normotensive and hypertensive salt-depleted subjects, addition of the selective BK$_2$ receptor antagonist icitabant (HOE 140) significantly reduced the acute hypotensive effect of captopril.[17]

Small studies in heart failure patients demonstrate blunting of the vasodilatory effects of chronic ACE inhibition following infusion of bradykinin receptor antagonists.[20,22] In dog models of heart failure induced by right ventricular pacing, animals receiving a bradykinin receptor antagonist in conjunction with enalapril developed increased cardiac fibrosis (types I and III collagen deposition) and increased left ventricular filling pressures compared to dogs receiving enalapril alone.[23] Animal models also suggest that bradykinin has anti-fibrotic effects in the renal interstitium.[24] Increased bradykinin levels may contribute to the anti-thrombotic properties of ACE inhibitors by increasing endothelial tPA release.[25,26] Bradykinin is thought to be responsible for ACE-inhibitor-induced cough and for the infrequent but clinically serious adverse reaction of angioedema.[27]

Hemodynamic effects

The acute hemodynamic effects of ACE inhibitors are the result of inhibition of angiotensin II formation and prevention of bradykinin degradation.[14,17,28] Vasoconstriction is reduced in both small and large arteries, with resultant decline in systemic vascular resistance. Venous capacitance is increased through venodilation.[28,29] In contrast to direct-acting vasodilators, ACE inhibitors do not provoke reflex tachycardia or increases in cardiac contractility. Baroreceptor function and cardiovascular reflexes are maintained, and responses to postural changes and exercise are virtually unimpaired. Vasodilation (without a compensatory increase in cardiac output) leads to a reduction in systolic, diastolic, and mean arterial BP.[28,30]

The magnitude of the initial BP reduction correlates positively with pre-treatment PRA and angiotensin II levels. Patients with a highly activated renin-angiotensin system caused by salt and water depletion or other conditions demonstrate an exaggerated acute hypotensive response to ACE inhibitors.[14,28,31] With chronic administration, BP continues to decline for a period of four to six weeks. In contrast to the acute effects, BP reduction with chronic administration is independent of pretreatment PRA.[14,16,28,32,33]

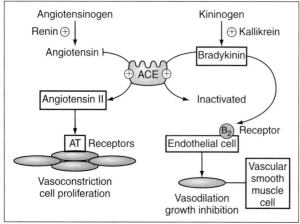

Figure 80–1. Mode of action of ACE inhibition.

Structure activity relationships

ACE inhibitors are structurally heterogeneous molecules, of which 12 chemical entities are currently available in the United States and/or the European Union (EU). All ACE inhibitors reduce ACE activity by competitive inhibition, achieved by binding to the zinc ion on the active site of the ACE molecule. The agents can be divided into three classes according to the functional group that serves as the ligand for ACE: sulfhydryl-, carboxyl-, and phosphinyl-containing groups. Captopril, the first available ACE inhibitor, and zofenopril are the only approved agents with a sulfhydryl group serving as a ligand for the ACE molecule. Fosinopril is the only agent with a phosphinyl group. All other ACE inhibitors use a carboxyl group to bind to ACE.

The potency of an ACE inhibitor is determined by the zinc ligand as well as the number and chemical structure of auxillary binding sites, which further enhance the ACE/drug interaction. Although the strength of binding between the sulfhydryl group and the zinc ion is greater than that for the carboxyl group, enalapril and other carboxyl analogues are actually more potent than captopril because of their additional binding sites. Differences in potency, however, are of little clinical relevance. A similar degree of ACE inhibition can be achieved by adjusting drug dosage.[34–37] Captopril's sulfhydryl moiety appears to be responsible for the side effects of dysgeusia and maculopapular skin rash seen with this agent.[38]

Pharmacokinetics

ACE inhibitors differ in their absorption, bioavailability, time to onset of action, duration of action, lipophilicity, and mode of elimination (see Table 80–1). The lipophilicity of an ACE inhibitor may influence the degree of tissue penetration and distribution.[16,34,35] With the exception of captopril and lisinopril, all ACE inhibitors are administered as ester-containing pro-drugs. In general, these pro-drugs have greater oral bioavailability compared to their active metabolites. They remain biologically inactive until hydrolyzed in the liver or the gastrointestinal mucosa by first-pass metabolism into their active diacid form. The active form is designated by the suffix at (e.g., enalaprilat).

Patients with severe hepatic dysfunction may not be able to adequately activate the pro-drug or may have a significant delay in activation. This problem has not been reported in patients with stable modest liver dysfunction. Although neither captopril nor lisinopril require hepatic activation, only lisinopril has almost exclusive renal elimination and may provide the most predictable pharmacokinetics in cirrhotic patients.[34,35]

Differences in bioavailability exist among ACE inhibitors. This has limited clinical significance if appropriate doses of an agent are used. Captopril and moexipril have potential drug/food interactions. A 50% decrease in the rate, but not necessarily the extent, of absorption may occur with either agent. These drugs should be administered one hour before meals.[35]

All ACE inhibitors are capable of producing clinically relevant BP reduction. The dose-response curve for ACE inhibitors is relatively steep at lower doses and flattens considerably as the plateau is approached. There is no convincing evidence for greater maximum BP-reducing potency of one ACE inhibitor versus another provided each drug is administered at a dose that reaches the plateau of the dose-response curve.[16,34,39]

The duration of clinically significant BP reduction differs among ACE inhibitors. Results of 24-hour BP monitoring studies indicate that fosinopril, lisinopril, perindopril, ramipril, and trandolapril can be administered once daily. Captopril, enalapril, benazepril, quinapril, and moexipril often require twice-daily dosing to achieve sustained BP reduction over a 24-hour period.[34,35,40] At higher doses, further up-titrating the dose of an ACE inhibitor will produce little incremental effect in peak BP reduction but may favorably extend the duration of BP response. By taking advantage of this dose-response relationship, shorter-acting drugs such as enalapril or benazepril can be used as once-a-day medications provided high-enough doses are given.[39,32]

Most ACE inhibitors have dual routes of elimination via the renal and hepatobiliary systems. ACE inhibitors are predominantly excreted as active compounds. The molecular size and lipophilicity of an ACE inhibitor influence the route of elimination. Larger molecular size and higher lipophilicity increase biliary excretion. When one route of elimination is compromised, accumulation of active drug may occur. Fosinopril is the only ACE inhibitor in which there is a compensatory increase in hepatobiliary elimination in the setting of renal insufficiency. Thus, total body clearance of fosinopril does not appreciably differ with any degree of renal insufficiency, permitting the use of the usual dosage in patients with any degree of renal impairment. All other ACE inhibitors require an initial dosage reduction, usually by one-half, when administered to patients with moderate to severe renal insufficiency. Plasma clearance of trandolapril is reduced in patients with either renal or hepatic insufficiency, requiring a lower starting dose.[33,35]

Organ-specific effects of ACE inhibitors
Renal

The effects of ACE inhibitors on renal hemodynamics are a consequence of blocking angiotensin II formation. Experimental evidence indicates that a significant contribution to the renal effects is accounted for by local ACE inhibition in the renal parenchyma.[41] ACE inhibitors reduce mesangial cell contractility, thereby increasing glomerular capillary area.[42] Renal vascular resistance is decreased and renal blood flow increases in many patients. ACE inhibitors dilate postglomerular efferent arterioles to a greater degree than the preglomerular afferent arterioles.

This discrepancy in vasodilation results in a net reduction in glomerular capillary hydrostatic pressure. As a consequence, GFR remains the same or falls despite the overall increase in renal plasma flow. The reduction in glomerular filtration rate (GFR) may lead to an increase in serum creatinine concentration, usually less than 10 to 20%. This reflects the renal hemodynamic effects of ACE

PHARMACOKINETICS OF ACE INHIBITORS

Drug	Labeled Indications				Duration of Action (h)	Serum Half-life (h)	Dosing for Hypertension	Elimination
	Hypertension	Heart Failure/ LV Dysfunction	Diabetic Nephropathy	Risk Prevention*				
Sulfhydryl-containing Captopril	√	√, √[1]	√		6 – 10[3]	<2	25–50 mg bid – tid	renal
Zofenopril	√	√			24	5–6	7.5–30 mg in 1–2 doses	renal + hepatic
Carboxyl-containing Benazepril	√				24[3]	11	10–40 mg in 1–2 doses	primarily renal
Cilazepril	√	√			24	9	2.5–10 mg once daily	renal
Enalapril	√	√, √[2]			12–24[3]	11	5– 40 mg in 1–2 doses	renal
Lisinopril	√	√			24	11–12	10–40 mg once daily	renal
Moexipril	√				24	2–9	7.5–30 mg in 1–2 doses	hepatic > renal
Perindopril	√			√	24	3–10	2–8 mg once daily	renal
Quinapril	√	√			24	2	10–80 mg in 1–2 doses	renal
Ramipril	√	√[1]		√	24	13–17	2.5–20 mg in 1–2 doses	renal > hepatic
Trandolapril	√	√[1]			24	10	1–4 mg once daily	renal > hepatic
Phosphinyl-containing Fosinopril	√	√			24	12	10–80 mg once daily	renal = hepatic[4]

* = Reduce risk of MI, stroke, and death from cardiovascular causes.
1 = Post-myocardial infarction.
2 = Asymptomatic LV dysfunction.
3 = Dose related.
4 = Compensatory hepatobiliary excretion in the setting of renal insufficiency.

Table 80–1. Pharmacokinetics of ACE Inhibitors and labeled indications

inhibition (not renal toxicity). ACE inhibitors promote natriuresis by decreasing proximal tubular and collecting-duct Na+ reabsorption and by blocking activation of adrenal AT_1 receptors by angiotensin II. The resulting reduction in aldosterone release leads to decreased sodium reabsorption and potassium excretion in the collecting ducts.[43]

Reduction of intraglomerular hypertension is of paramount importance to the renal protective action of ACE inhibitors. Elevated intraglomerular pressure caused by hyperfiltrating states such as diabetes or a reduction in nephron mass impairs the size-selective function of the glomerular permeability barrier and causes protein ultrafiltration. The excessive protein traffic activates tubular epithelium, leading to elaboration of inflammatory and pro-fibrotic cytokines. The net effect is fibroblast proliferation, increased synthesis, and decreased breakdown of extracellular matrix proteins in the mesangium and interstitium (leading to glomerulosclerosis and interstitial fibrosis).[5]

Control of systemic hypertension does not necessarily translate into reduction of intraglomerular hypertension. Animal models of two-thirds nephrectomy have demonstrated that control of systemic BP with vasodilators and a diuretic, both of which elevate plasma renin levels, leads to angiotensin-II-mediated efferent arteriolar vasoconstriction and continued intraglomerular hypertension. When ACE inhibitors were administered at doses producing an equivalent reduction in systemic BP, glomerular capillary pressure returned to near-normal values. In this model, ACE inhibition prevented proteinuria and the development of glomerulosclerosis. Triple antihypertensive therapy without ACE inhibition led to proteinuria and glomerulosclerosis similar to untreated controls.[44] Animal models and human studies have demonstrated that the renal protection afforded by ACE inhibitors is associated with a reduction in the expression of both plasminogen activator inhibitor (PAI-1) and the growth factor TGF-β.[45–47]

Left ventricular hypertrophy and fibrosis

In spontaneously hypertensive (SHR) rats, early administration of ACE inhibitors to young animals who do not yet exhibit hypertension prevents the development of left ventricular hypertrophy (LVH). ACE inhibitors produce LVH regression in older animals with established hypertension (a result not seen when similar degrees of BP reduction are induced by direct-acting vasodilators such as hydralazine or with diuretics). Rats with LVH produced by abdominal aortic banding exhibit a decrease in left ventricular mass when treated with ramipril at doses too low to reduce BP, indicating a direct myocardial effect.[48] Reduction of interstitial collagen content and restructuring of the myocardial extracellular matrix with ACE inhibition contributes to LVH mass regression, improves diastolic dysfunction, and reduces the tendency to arrhythmogenesis.[49]

In humans, reduction of left ventricular mass has been documented after eight weeks of ACE inhibitor therapy.[50] Early meta-analyses suggested that for equal reductions in BP ACE inhibitors had a greater effect on LVH regression.[51,52] More recent meta-analyses and head-to-head comparisons with dihydropiridine calcium antagonists suggest that ACE inhibitors, angiotensin receptor blockers (ARBs), and calcium channel blockers exert similar effects.[53] A recent meta-analysis of 80 trials and 3,767 patients found that when adjusted for the decrease in diastolic BP and treatment duration ARBs (13%) produced the greatest reduction in left ventricular mass index, followed closely by calcium antagonists (11%) and ACE inhibitors (10%). There was no statistical difference among these three drug classes. All three classes were superior to beta blockers and diuretics.[53]

The LVH associated with hypertension consists of perivascular and myocardial fibrosis, medial thickening of intramyocardial coronary arteries, and myocyte hypertrophy. In one elegant study, the effect of ACE inhibition on myocardial fibrosis in hypertensive patients was studied directly. Thirty-five patients with hypertension and normal coronary angiograms received either lisinopril (n = 18) or hydrochlorothiazide (n = 17) for a six-month period. Left ventricular biopsies were performed at baseline and at the end of the treatment period. Myocardial fibrosis, measured by left ventricular collagen volume fraction and hydroxyproline concentration, decreased significantly with lisinopril compared to hydrochlorothiazide (HCTZ) (which showed no change to a small increase in both parameters). Diastolic function as determined by echocardiography improved with lisinopril but not with HCTZ.[54]

Vascular hypertrophy

Remodeling of small resistance arteries represents one of the earliest manifestations of target organ damage and is characterized by an increase in the media thickness to lumen ratio. Animal models and human studies document the ability of ACE inhibitors to prevent or reverse vascular hypertrophy, remodeling, and fibrosis. In SHR, initiation of perindopril from age 4 to 24 weeks results in a dose-dependent reduction of BP and media-to-lumen ratio of small resistance arteries leading to an increase in lumen diameter. Interestingly, BP in treated animals remained below controls even at 36 weeks (12 weeks after cessation of the ACE inhibitor).

This study and others performed in young SHR indicate that at least in this animal model of genetically determined hypertension short-term administration of ACE inhibitors at a critical period of growth can have lasting effects on cardiovascular structure and the development of hypertension.[55,56] ACE inhibitor administration in older SHR induces regression of both vascular and cardiac hypertrophy. Administration of the direct-acting vasodilator hydralazine and beta blockers, however, does not produce equivalent hypertrophy regression when given at doses that produce comparable BP reduction.[32]

In humans, investigators have utilized subcutaneous gluteal specimens to study the effects of various antihypertensive agents on the structure and function of resistance vessels. In one study, previously untreated males with essential hypertension were treated with cilazapril versus atenolol for a two-year period. BP reduction was similar for both groups throughout the study. Gluteal biopsies were obtained after one and two years of treatment. After one year, the media-to-lumen ratio of the cilazapril-treated group was significantly reduced (whereas that of atenolol-treated patients remained unchanged). At year 2 of therapy, the media-to-lumen ratio of the cilazapril-treated group demonstrated continued regression and was statistically no different from arteries derived from normotensive control subjects. Cilazapril was also found to improve endothelial dysfunction. At baseline, patients with hypertension demonstrated reduced vasodilation in response to acetylcholine infusion. After two years of treatment, the response to acetylcholine was similar in cilazapril-treated patients and normotensive controls.[57–59]

Improving vascular compliance is emerging as an important therapeutic objective in the management of hypertension.[60,61] Antihypertensive therapy can reduce aortic stiffness passively by reducing mean arterial BP. Animal models and in vitro study of human smooth muscle cells also suggest that chronic ACE inhibitor therapy may generate pharmacologic remodeling of the arterial wall, leading to BP-independent reduction in large arterial stiffness. When human aortic smooth muscle cells were incubated with ramiprilat for 10 weeks, staining for collagen was reduced by >50%, whereas staining for elastin and fibrillin-1 increased by more than three- and fourfold, respectively. The elastin/collagen ratio increased sevenfold.[62] In older SHR, treatment with perindopril decreased aortic stiffness by reducing BP and caused regression of medial hypertrophy and a decrease in the collagen content of the aortic wall.[63]

Based on studies of arterial wave reflections, ACE inhibitors appear to be quite effective in reducing larger-artery stiffness in humans. In a study of 2,187 patients with essential hypertension, treatment with perindopril reduced pulse pressure and pulse wave velocity after two months of therapy. Continued improvement in these parameters was noted after six months of treatment.[64] In patients with peripheral arterial disease, six months of treatment with ramipril significantly increased arterial compliance and reduced pulse wave velocity and augmentation index.[62] As the structure and composition of the larger arteries cannot be directly assessed in humans, it is difficult to demonstrate conclusively that favorable hemodynamic alterations are the result of structural remodeling and changes in arterial composition.

Atherosclerosis

Atherosclerosis is the anatomical substrate for the majority of cardiovascular endpoints in hypertensive patients. It is a complex multifactorial process that begins with endothelial dysfunction and involves vascular inflammation, lipid accumulation, and smooth muscle cell growth and migration. Angiotensin II and ACE are intimately involved in every stage of atherosclerotic lesion development and in the events that lead to vascular complications.[65,66] A significant body of evidence indicates that ACE inhibitors exert salutary effects on the complications of atherosclerosis. Whether these effects are in

part independent of BP reduction is a subject of continuing controversy.

ACE inhibitors improve endothelial vasodilator function and appear to do so better than other available classes of antihypertensive agents. By blocking angiotensin-II-induced reactive oxygen species (ROS) formation, ACE inhibitors prevent nitric oxide (NO) degradation and increase NO release. In healthy volunteers, quinaprilat enhanced radial artery diameter during reactive hyperemia. Vasodilation was abolished by the bradykinin receptor antagonist HOE 140, suggesting that this effect is bradykinin mediated.[21] Several studies comparing ACE inhibitors to other commonly used antihypertensive drugs have been performed. In a prospective study of 168 hypertensive patients comparing the ACE inhibitor perindopril to other antihypertensive treatments (including beta blockers, calcium channel blockers, and an angiotensin receptor blocker), perindopril alone improved vasodilation during reactive hyperemia.[67] In a similar trial of 296 hypertensive patients performed in Japan comparing the effects of various antihypertensive drug classes, ACE-inhibitor-treated patients had significantly greater vasodilatation following forearm occlusion compared to patients taking calcium channel blockers, beta blockers, and thiazide diuretics.[68]

The Trial on Reversing Endothelial Dysfunction (TREND) study demonstrated that chronic administration of an ACE inhibitor can improve abnormal endothelial function in atherosclerotic coronary arteries. Patients with coronary artery disease who demonstrated reduced vasodilator or a vasoconstrictor response to intracoronary acetylcholine infusion were randomized to receive quinapril or placebo for a six-month period. A target arterial segment at the site of a noncritical (<40%) stenosis was studied at baseline and again at the end of the blinded treatment period. Whereas the placebo group demonstrated no change in vascular response to acetylcholine infusion, the target arteries of quinapril-treated patients showed a marked (statistically significant) improvement in endothelial-mediated dilatation. A significant number of quinapril-treated patients had complete resolution of abnormal vasoconstriction seen at baseline.[69]

ACE inhibitors retard the development of atherosclerotic lesions in multiple animal models of hyperlipidemia, including the rabbit, hamster, mini-pig, cynomolgus monkey, and apolipoprotein E-deficient mice.[70] Without correcting hyperlipidemia, delapril (in a dose-dependent fashion) inhibited the development of atherosclerosis (expressed as aortic area covered by lesions) in cholesterol-fed rabbits.[71] Captopril reduced aortic atherosclerosis in the normotensive Watanabe hyperlipidemic rabbit model and in the cynomolgus monkey.[70,72] In apo E-deficient mice, fosinopril given at a dose insufficient to produce a hypotensive effect reduced atherosclerotic lesion size and increased the resistance of LDL to oxidation.[70,73] This property of ACE inhibitors is independent of bradykinin.[74]

Human studies on prevention and regression of atherosclerosis with ACE inhibitors have yielded inconsistent results. Two large studies have been performed to assess the ability of ACE inhibitors to inhibit carotid atherosclerosis and two studies have evaluated coronary atherosclerosis. In the Prevention of Atherosclerosis with Ramipril-2 (PART-2) study, patients with a history of cardiovascular events were assigned to ramipril or placebo. After four years of follow-up, neither carotid artery wall thickness nor carotid plaque burden differed between the two groups.[75] Ramipril reduced progression of carotid atherosclerosis by 0.008 mm/year compared to placebo in the Study to Evaluate Carotid Ultrasound Changes in Patients Treated with Ramipril and Vitamin E (SECURE), a sub-study of the Heart Outcomes Prevention Evaluation (HOPE) study. Several studies have failed to demonstrate any effect of ACE inhibitors on the progression of coronary artery disease.[76] Therapy with ACE inhibitors has also been unsuccessful in preventing restenosis following coronary angioplasty or stent placement.[77]

CLINICAL INDICATIONS

Hypertension

All available ACE inhibitors are approved for the treatment of hypertension. Based on outcome data, the *Seventh Report of the Joint National Committee on the Prevention, Detection, Evaluation and Treatment of High Blood Pressure* (JNC-7), the World Health Organization/International Society of Hypertension, and the European Society of Hypertension/European Society of Cardiology recognize ACE inhibitors as an option for first-line therapy in patients with essential hypertension. ACE inhibitors are recognized as preferred treatment for patients with hypertension complicated by heart failure, coronary artery disease (CAD) or history of MI, diabetes, or chronic kidney disease (as well as for recurrent stroke prevention).[3]

The magnitude of BP reduction seen after ACE inhibitor administration depends on a number of factors, including the degree of elevation in baseline BP, intravascular volume status, and demographic characteristics of the population studied. White subjects have the most consistent response to ACE inhibitors. Sodium restriction, which activates the RAS, increases the magnitude of BP reduction after ACE inhibitor administration. For these reasons, the reported response rate (usually defined as diastolic BP reduction of ≥ 10 mmHg or BP normalization) to ACE inhibitor monotherapy is quite variable (ranging from 20 to 70%).[78]

There is no convincing evidence for greater hemodynamic efficacy of one ACE inhibitor compared to another, provided that each drug is titrated to its effective dose. ACE inhibitors generally reduce BP within several hours of oral administration. The maximum response to an administered dose is achieved after approximately four to six weeks. Patients with a highly activated RAS and very high PRA, as occurs in renal artery stenosis, may show an immediate and profound hypotensive response to ACE inhibitors. There is little relationship, however, between pretreatment PRA and the magnitude of long-term BP reduction.[14,16,32]

Concomitant aspirin administration (ASA) does not seem to affect the BP response to ACE inhibitors. BP was not altered when ASA 81 or 325 mg was administered to patients receiving chronic stable dosing with enalapril. Subgroup analysis from the Hypertension Optimal Treatment (HOT) trial revealed no interaction between low-dose (75 mg daily) ASA with the BP-lowering effect of antihypertensive agents, including combinations that included ACE inhibitors.[79–81]

Demographic subgroups
African Americans

Although individual responses vary, BP reduction and responder rates after ACE inhibitor administration are less in African Americans compared to Caucasians. The magnitude of mean diastolic BP reduction in most studies is approximately one-half to two-thirds that seen in white patients. This has been attributed to the tendency of African Americans toward low-renin, volume-expanded, salt-sensitive hypertension.[14,82] The abolition of racial differences in response to ACE inhibitors when diuretics are coadministered lends credence to this theory. However, there may be inherent mechanistic differences mediating BP response in whites and African Americans. In a study using trandolapril, white and black hypertensive patients were given 1-mg, 2-mg, or 4-mg doses of this agent.

A 1-mg dose of trandolapril resulted in a 6.1-mmHg mean decrease in baseline sitting diastolic pressure for whites. Black patients required 4 mg of trandolapril to achieve the same BP response. Despite the robust differences in BP response, a similar reduction in serum ACE activity was achieved for each dose of trandolapril in both populations. There were also no racial differences in the trandolaprilat concentrations required to achieve a given level of serum ACE inhibition.[83] In general, African Americans require a higher dose of ACE inhibitor to achieve therapeutic BP reductions. However, the maximum response cannot be equalized regardless of dose. Despite these differences in BP response, in black patients with renal disease, diabetes, and heart failure ACE inhibitors appear to produce endpoint reductions comparable to those of whites (indicating a dissociation between hemodynamic and tissue protective effects).[84,85]

The elderly

More than two-thirds of patients over age 65 have hypertension and are candidates for antihypertensive drug therapy. With aging, there is progressive loss of distensibility of the aorta and large conduit arteries. Diastolic BP remains the same or decreases, whereas systolic BP rises.[58] Low PRA is seen in the elderly, but unlike African Americans it is the result of age-related changes in the RAS axis and not a consequence of volume expansion. Although this might theoretically render elderly individuals less responsive to ACE inhibitors, BP reduction and responder rates are equivalent in studies comparing younger and older individuals.[86–88]

ACE inhibitors are generally well tolerated in older patients. These agents do not interfere with (and may even improve) baroreceptor sensitivity in elderly hypertensive individuals. With the exception of occasional first-dose hypotension, orthostatic hypotension is quite rare and occurs less often than with diuretics and most other vasodilating agents. Cerebral blood flow is well maintained and improvement has been documented in the BP range in which effective cerebral autoregulation is maintained. Cognitive function is unaffected by ACE inhibitors. When prescribing ACE inhibitors to the elderly, age-related decline in renal function must be taken into account. Drug elimination may be slower. Dosage and dosing intervals often need to be adjusted. First-dose hypotension can be avoided by starting elderly patients at lower doses and gradually increasing the dose over days to weeks.[86–88]

Rational use of ACE inhibitors in combination

It is estimated that approximately 75% of patients with hypertension require two or more drugs to achieve the BP goals specified in JNC-7. Devising effective drug combinations is therefore an essential element of antihypertensive therapy. The goal is to combine drugs with complimentary pharmacologic mechanisms of action in order to produce additive BP reduction. For ACE inhibitors, diuretics and calcium channel blockers constitute the preferred combination partners.[89,90]

The combination of an ACE inhibitor and a low-dose thiazide diuretic constitutes one of the most successful approaches to contemporary combination therapy. From an evolutionary perspective, the primary purpose of the RAS is to protect the organism from salt and water depletion. Because the pharmacologic action of diuretics is to increase urinary sodium excretion and reduce intravascular volume, their administration results in renin release and increased angiotensin II production. Coadministration of an ACE inhibitor blocks this activation and leads to additive BP reduction. In addition, the hypokalemia associated with diuretic therapy is often blunted or abolished by ACE inhibitors (which tend to promote potassium retention by reducing the availability of aldosterone).[90]

Dihydropyridine calcium channel blockers are also effective in combination with ACE inhibitors. When combined with ACE inhibitors, additive BP reduction is achieved. Addition of an ACE inhibitor has the added benefit of partially neutralizing the lower extremity edema, which is the most frequent dose-limiting side effect of calcium channel blockers. The edema seen with these agents is not the result of sodium retention but is due to a selective reduction in arteriolar resistance and an increase in capillary hydrostatic pressure. ACE inhibitors, by lowering post-capillary resistance, decrease the pressure gradient and the stimulus to fluid extravasation. In a study of 707 patients randomized to receive enalapril, felodipine, and their combination, the incidence of edema was reduced from 10.8% with felodipine monotherapy to only 4.1% in patients receiving the combination.[29,90]

In patients requiring three antihypertensive agents, the combination of an ACE inhibitor, diuretic, and calcium channel blocker offers an excellent combination of complementary pharmacology, additivity of BP reduction, and proven effectiveness in achieving endpoint protection.

ENDPOINT TRIALS

The Captopril Prevention Project (CAPPP) compared the effects of ACE inhibition to conventional therapy (beta blockers and/or diuretics) on cardiovascular morbidity and mortality in 10,985 hypertensive patients.[91] Captopril was prescribed in a dose of up to 100 mg/day given once or twice daily. At a mean follow-up of 6.1 years, there was no difference in the primary endpoint (a composite of MI, stroke, and cardiovascular death). There was a trend in favor of lower cardiovascular mortality in the captopril arm (relative risk 0.77). The rate of MI was similar, but stroke was more common with captopril (relative risk 1.25, $p = 0.004$). The incidence of newly diagnosed diabetes was significantly lower with captopril therapy (relative risk 0.79, $p = 0.007$), a finding replicated in later trials with ACE inhibitors.

The dosing regimen for captopril in CAPPP was unconventional. Captopril has a known duration of action of 6 to 10 hours. Nonetheless, 48% of captopril-treated patients received the drug once daily (raising the possibility that 24-hour BP control was inadequate). Target diastolic BP was more rapidly achieved with conventional treatment, and both systolic and diastolic BPs were on average 2 mmHg higher in the captopril arm throughout the trial. Stroke is an endpoint that is exquisitely sensitive to BP and the 2-mmHg difference could account for up to a 15% difference in the cerebrovascular accident (CVA) event rate.

In the smaller diabetic arm, equal BP reduction was obtained throughout the trial. The rate of CVA was the same among diabetics in both arms and the combined primary endpoint was significantly lower with captopril treatment (relative risk 0.59, $p = 0.019$). The CAPPP trial showed that even with slightly less BP control ACE inhibitor therapy was at least equivalent to conventional beta blocker and diuretic therapy in preventing cardiovascular complications.

The Antihypertensive and Lipid-Lowering Treatment to Prevent Heart Attack Trial (ALLHAT) is the largest hypertension trial conducted to date.[92] It involved 42,416 patients over age 55 with hypertension and at least one additional coronary heart disease (CHD) risk factor. The study compared chlorthalidone, amlodipine, lisinopril, and doxazosin as first-line therapy. The doxazosin arm was terminated early due to an increased event rate compared to chlorthalidone. At a mean follow-up of 4.9 years, there was no difference among the three remaining treatment groups in the primary endpoint of fatal CHD or nonfatal MI. The occurrence of new-onset heart failure and stroke was higher in the lisinopril arm.

Some have interpreted ALLHAT as showing an advantage of diuretic-based therapy compared to ACE inhibitors. However, as in CAPPP on-treatment BPs were higher in the ACE inhibitor group throughout the trial (2 mmHg), with the difference being greatest in the first two years of therapy (4 mmHg). The increased stroke rate with lisinopril was entirely driven by the 35% of the population who were African American (relative risk 1.40). In this subgroup, BP remained an average of 4 mmHg higher with lisinopril compared to chlorthalidone throughout the trial.

In ALLHAT, combination of the ACE inhibitor with its two preferred combination partners (diuretics and calcium channel blockers) was not permitted. Atenolol, clonidine, and hydralazine were the designated step 2 drugs, and most patients received atenolol as add-on therapy. Because ACE inhibitors and beta blockers when combined do not produce additive BP reduction, this artificial treatment regimen may well account for the higher BPs observed in the lisinopril arm. In ALLHAT, as in CAPPP, the ACE inhibitor achieved equality with regard to the primary endpoint despite a disadvantage in terms of BP control.

The Second Australian National Blood Pressure Study (ANBP2) compared outcomes with an ACE inhibitor (enalapril recommended) or a diuretic-based regimen (hydrochlorothiazide recommended) in a relatively healthy hypertensive population.[93] BP reductions were similar throughout the five-year study duration. There was a statistically significant 11% lower incidence for the primary endpoint of all cardiovascular events or death from any cause favoring the ACE-inhibitor-based regimen. The difference in outcomes was driven mainly by a reduction in MI in the ACE inhibitor group. There was no difference in stroke rate.

In the Second Swedish Trial in Old Patients with Hypertension (STOP-2), 6,614 elderly patients (ages 70 to 84) with a systolic BP >180 and/or diastolic BP >105 were randomly assigned to one of three treatment groups: conventional therapy with beta blockers and/or diuretics, the ACE inhibitor enalapril or lisinopril, or the calcium antagonist felodipine or isradipine.[94] Similar BP control was obtained throughout the trial. At 4.5 years follow-up, the combined endpoint of fatal stroke, fatal MI, and other fatal cardiovascular disease was the same in the three groups. There were significantly fewer MIs and episodes of congestive heart failure in patients treated with ACE inhibitors compared to those receiving calcium channel blockers.

Taken together, the major outcome trials indicate that ACE inhibitors are excellent first-line agents in hypertensive patients of any age. A meta-analysis performed by the Blood Pressure Lowering Treatment Trialists' Collaboration concluded that there is no reliable evidence of a difference between ACE-inhibitor-based regimens and conventional beta-blocker/diuretic-based regimens for preventing major cardiovascular events. There was also no reliable evidence of a difference between ACE-inhibitor-based regimens and calcium-antagonist-based regimens (with the exception of a lower incidence of heart failure with ACE inhibitor therapy).[95]

Renal protection

Therapeutic goals in the treatment of patients with hypertension and kidney disease are to normalize BP, reduce proteinuria, and slow or arrest the deterioration in renal function. Effective BP control *per se* delays the progression of renal dysfunction. JNC-7 recommends a BP goal of <130/80 mmHg for patients with chronic kidney disease defined by either a GFR <60 mL/min per 1.73 m² or the presence of albuminuria >300 mg/day, regardless of GFR. Compelling evidence that reduction in protein excretion by at least 30% below baseline is associated with a marked decrease in renal disease progression has led the National Kidney Foundation to recommend that therapies used to treat BP also target proteinuria reduction.

In patients with renal disease, specifically those with proteinuria, blockade of the renin-angiotensin system affords end-organ protection clearly superior to that obtained with other classes of antihypertensive agents. This appears to be the case in normotensive as well as hypertensive individuals, and the treatment effect is greater than can be accounted for on the basis of BP reduction alone. The renal protection afforded by ACE inhibitors is intricately linked to producing a decline in protein excretion. This applies to both diabetic and non-diabetic kidney disease.

In patients with diabetic nephropathy, ACE inhibitors have been more extensively studied in patients with type I diabetes. The benefits of ACE inhibition can be demonstrated early in the course of the disease. Administration of captopril to normotensive type I diabetics with microalbuminuria significantly reduced both the albumin excretion rate and the fraction of patients who progressed to clinical proteinuria, the hallmark of the rapidly progressive phase of diabetic nephropathy.[96] In a landmark study, 409 type I diabetics with urinary protein excretion >500 mg/day and serum creatinine concentration <2.5 mg/dL were randomized to receive captopril 25 mg three times daily or placebo.[97,98] After a median follow-up of three years, captopril reduced the risk of doubling of serum creatinine by 48% and the combined endpoint of death, dialysis, and transplantation by 50% (Figure 80–2).

The data for renal protection with ACE inhibitors in type II diabetes are somewhat less robust, but are consistent with the view that ACE inhibitors provide renal protection in this population and are approximately equivalent in their efficacy to ARBs. In normotensive and

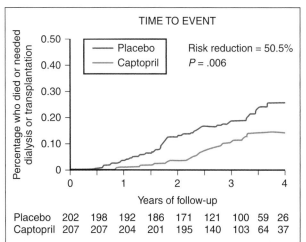

Figure 80–2. Captopril in diabetic nephropathy: end-stage renal disease (ESRD) or death. In patients with renal disease, specifically those with proteinuria, ACE inhibitors afford end-organ protection clearly superior to that obtained with other classes of antihypertensive agents. (Redrawn from Lewis EJ, Hunsicker LG, Bain RP, Rohde RD. The effect of angiotensin-converting-enzyme inhibition on diabetic nephropathy: The Collaborative Study Group. *N Engl J Med* 1993;329:1456–62.)

hypertensive type II diabetics, enalapril has been shown to reduce the progression from microalbuminuria to proteinuria and to protect against decline in GFR.[99,100] In the recently published Diabetics Exposed to Telmisartan and Enalapril (DETAIL) study, enalapril 20 mg/day was compared to the ARB telmisartan (at a dose of 80 mg/day) in 250 patients with early diabetic nephropathy and a serum creatinine level <1.6. After five years of treatment, GFR declined by 17.9 mL/min per 1.73 m² in the telmisartan group and 14.9 mL/min per 1.73 m² in enalapril-treated patients. This trend in favor of the ACE inhibitor was not statistically significant.[101]

In hypertensive patients with type II diabetes, the progression from normal urinary albumin excretion to microalbuminuria can be delayed by treatment with an ACE inhibitor. This protective effect was demonstrated in the Bergamo Nephrologic Diabetes Complications (BENEDICT) trial. Treatment with the ACE inhibitor trandolapril or the combination of trandolapril plus verapamil delayed the onset of microalbuminuria compared to placebo or verapamil treatment alone. The results of this study further support the value of treating hypertensive type II diabetics with an ACE inhibitor.[102]

A number of well-conducted studies have confirmed that ACE inhibitors also confer renal protection in patients with non-diabetic nephropathy. In the Ramipril Efficacy in Nephropathy (REIN) study, patients were classified into two groups based on degree of proteinuria (stratum 1, of 1 to 3 g/24 h, and stratum 2 of >3 g/24 h) and randomized to receive ramipril or placebo. BPs in the two arms were almost identical throughout the study. Urinary protein excretion decreased significantly at one month in the ramipril group and remained lower than baseline throughout the study period. After 16 months, the study was prematurely terminated in stratum 2 patients (baseline protein excretion of >3 g/day) because of a highly significant reduction in the rate of GFR decline (0.53 versus 0.88 mL/min per month ramipril versus placebo). Risk reduction was correlated with the percentage decrease from baseline in urinary protein excretion.[103]

Analysis of stratum 1 patients (1 to 3 g/24 h protein excretion) revealed that ramipril significantly benefited those with a basal GFR of less than 45 mL/min and proteinuria of at least 1.5 g/day. Patients with the most severe renal dysfunction (basal GFR of 10 to 30 mL/min per 1.73 m²) experienced a 22% reduction in decline in GFR and a 33% reduction in progression to end-stage renal disease (ESRD) without increased risk of major adverse events. These findings are important because many physicians are reluctant to start ACE inhibitors in patients with more severe renal dysfunction. Such patients may actually derive the greatest benefit from ACE inhibition.[104]

Although ACE inhibitors are less effective as BP-reducing agents in African Americans, renal protective effects are preserved. In the African American Study of Kidney Disease and Hypertension (AASK) trial, ramipril was more effective than amlodipine or metoprolol in slowing the progression of hypertensive nephrosclerosis.[85]

A significant decrease in proteinuria was seen with ramipril, whereas patients treated with amlodipine had an increase in proteinuria. In concordance with previous trials, the treatment effect was greater in the patient subgroup with baseline proteinuria UP/Cr >0.22 (approximately 300 mg/day).

A meta-analysis of 1,860 patients with non-diabetic renal disease concluded that ACE inhibitors reduce the risk for doubling of serum creatinine or progression to end-stage renal disease by 30% compared to other antihypertensive regimens. Patients with greater baseline urinary protein excretion benefit the most from ACE inhibitor therapy. The data were inconclusive for patients with baseline urinary excretion less than 0.5 g/day.[105,106]

Combining an ACE inhibitor with an ARB has theoretical advantages for renal protection. There is emerging evidence that in some patient populations this combination provides superior reduction in proteinuria and renal protection than either agent alone. In the combination treatment of angiotensin-II receptor blocker and angiotensin-converting-enzyme inhibitor in non-diabetic renal disease (COOPERATE) trial, 263 Japanese patients with non-diabetic nephropathy were randomized to receive trandolapril, losartan, or their combination. The dose of trandolapril was selected as that dose beyond which further proteinuria reduction could not be achieved. The combination therapy group demonstrated further reduction in proteinuria and improvement in renal survival despite equality of on-treatment BPs in the three treatment groups.[107]

When initiating ACE inhibitor therapy in patients with decreased renal function, a few caveats should be kept in mind. There may be an initial elevation in serum creatinine level of up to 30% from baseline. This usually occurs within the first two weeks of therapy, stabilizes within two to four weeks, and is often transient. When a more significant elevation in serum creatinine occurs, an explanation should be sought. Common causes include renal artery stenosis, volume depletion from concomitant diuretic use, and the use of non-steroidal anti-inflammatory drugs (NSAIDs). Review of trial data indicates that acute limited increases in serum creatinine of up to 30% correlate with slower rates of long-term decline in renal function. Careful monitoring of electrolytes upon initiation or up-titration of ACE inhibitors is recommended for patients with more severe renal dysfunction.[43,108]

Cardiac protection

In the context of antihypertensive therapy, cardiac protection refers to the ability of a drug to protect the heart from (1) MI, (2) progressive deterioration in ventricular function after MI or other processes initiating ventricular dysfunction, and (3) mortality related to cardiac events. With regard to cardiac protection, JNC-7 delineates three categories of "compelling indications" (i.e., subgroups of patients in whom certain drug classes are preferred). These include those with heart failure due to systolic dysfunction or prior/recent MI and patients at high risk for clinical coronary events. ACE inhibitors are designated as a preferred therapy in each of these patient groups.

The Survival and Ventricular Enlargement (SAVE) trial was the first study to show cardiac protection by ACE inhibitors in patients with recent MI[109] (Figure 80–3). It was undertaken after animal models showed that ACE inhibitors could reduce ventricular dysfunction and improve survival following experimental MI. The study randomized 2,231 patients with LVEF <40% and no overt signs of heart failure to treatment with captopril or placebo. After an average 3.5 years, the captopril group demonstrated a reduction in all-cause mortality (19%) and the number of patients developing clinical heart failure. An unexpected finding was a 25% reduction in the risk of recurrent MI.

The post-MI trials validated the results of SAVE. The Acute Infarction Ramipril Efficacy (AIRE) trial included 2,006 patients with clinically overt heart failure symptoms after MI randomized to receive ramipril at a dose of 5 mg bid.[110] Follow-up averaged 15 months. The primary endpoint of all-cause mortality was 27% lower in the ramipril arm. The secondary endpoint of progression to severe heart failure, re-infarction, or stroke was reduced by 19%. The reduction in MI was statistically significant. In the Trandolapril Cardiac Evaluation (TRACE) study, post-MI patients with left ventricular dysfunction after MI were studied.[111] Mortality and progression to severe heart failure were reduced in patients randomized to trandolapril. A non-significant reduction in MI risk was observed. The six-year follow-up of TRACE patients documented that median life expectancy was prolonged by 15.3 months in trandolapril-treated patients.[112]

SAVE, AIRE, and TRACE firmly established ACE inhibitors as first-line therapy for patients with asymptomatic left ventricular dysfunction following acute MI. A meta-analysis of the three trials revealed a reduction in mortality from 29.1% in placebo to 23.4% with ACE inhibitor treatment, at an average follow-up of 2.6 years.[113] It was estimated that to avoid one death about 15 patients required therapy for 2.5 years. Cumulative reduction in the development of chronic heart failure was also observed. The reduction in re-infarction apparent in these trials laid the groundwork for evaluating the vascular protective effect of ACE inhibitors in broader high-risk populations with normal left ventricular function.[113]

The HOPE trial evaluated whether ramipril at a dose of 10 mg daily could reduce the composite endpoint of MI, stroke, or death from cardiovascular causes in a population at high risk for cardiovascular events.[114] More than 9,000 patients, age 55 years or older, with a history of known vascular disease or diabetes plus at least one other cardiovascular risk factor were randomized to ramipril 10 mg/day or placebo. Patients were excluded if they had heart failure or were known to have an ejection fraction below 40%. The mean BP at entry was 139/79 mmHg in both groups.

The study was not designed as a hypertension trial, and patients with hypertension required ongoing BP treatment in order to be eligible for participation. The BP of patients in the ramipril arm was reduced by a mean of 3/2 mmHg compared to placebo. The primary composite endpoint of MI, stroke, or cardiovascular mortality was 22% lower in the ramipril group. Each of the components of the composite endpoint was reduced with ramipril: cardiovascular death by 26%, MI by 20%, and stroke by 32%. The benefits were consistent across all subgroups of patients, including diabetics with no previously documented vascular disease.

It has been debated whether the cardiovascular protection afforded by ramipril was the result of BP reduction or was in part related to non-BP related effects. It is clear that endpoint reduction exceeded what would be predicted by the relatively small difference in mean BP between the placebo and treatment groups. However, subsequent analysis of 38 patients with peripheral arterial disease in whom ambulatory BP monitoring was performed revealed a larger difference in 24-hour BP (10/4 mmHg), mainly caused by a pronounced BP lowering effect at night (17/8 mmHg). It is difficult, however, to derive far-reaching conclusions from such a small subgroup.[115] Regardless of the BP effect, the overall trial result validated the cardiovascular protective effects of ACE inhibitor therapy in a population not previously thought to require either antihypertensive therapy or to be candidates for ACE inhibition.

Further evidence for cardiac protection by ACE inhibitors came from the European Trial on Reduction of Cardiac Events with Perindopril in Stable Coronary Artery Disease (the EUROPA study).[116] In EUROPA, 13,655 patients with stable coronary artery

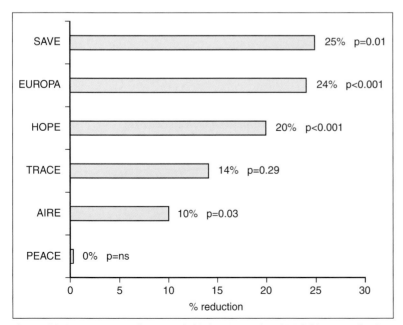

Figure 80–3. Prevention of myocardial infarction with ACE inhibitors. Reduction in the incidence of myocardial infarction compared to placebo in studies of patients who are post-MI and/or at high-risk for cardiovascular events.

disease and without clinical evidence of heart failure were randomized to perindopril 8 mg/day or placebo. The baseline BP was 137/82 in both groups. After randomization, BP in the perindopril group was reduced by an average of 5/2 mmHg compared to placebo. Perindopril treatment was associated with a significant reduction in the primary endpoint of cardiovascular mortality, non-fatal MI, and resuscitated cardiac arrest (relative risk reduction 20%). The risk of MI was reduced by 24%. In a post hoc analysis of the EUROPA data, no relationship was noted between either baseline BP or BP reduction during blinded treatment and endpoint reduction.

The results of the Prevention of Events with Angiotensin Converting Enzyme Inhibition (PEACE) trial, comparing trandolapril with placebo in a population with stable coronary artery disease, are at variance with HOPE and EUROPA.[117] There was no reduction in the incidence of the primary endpoint of death from cardiovascular causes, MI, or coronary revascularization. This negative result may be due to the fact that the study was statistically underpowered, to the relatively low dose of trandolapril utilized, to the low adherence to treatment noted in the study, or to the fact that the population studied exhibited a very low cardiovascular mortality in the placebo group (0.8%/year). Meta-analysis of data from HOPE, EUROPA, and PEACE combined demonstrate an overall reduction in mortality.[118]

Reduction in diabetes

ACE inhibitors (and ARBs) consistently reduce the risk of diabetes development compared to placebo or other antihypertensive agents (Table 80–2). The first study to report a decrease in the incidence of new-onset diabetes with ACE inhibition was the CAPPP study, which compared captopril to beta blocker and diuretic therapy in patients with diastolic hypertension.[91] The incidence of new onset diabetes mellitus (DM) was 21% lower in captopril-treated patients. In the HOPE study, a 34% relative risk reduction for development of new-onset diabetes with ramipril was noted. A small sub-study of the

HOPE trial found that fasting glucose increased more with placebo than with ramipril.[114,119–121]

In ALLHAT, the incidence of new-onset DM was highest in the chlorthalidone group (11.6%) and lowest in the lisinopril-treated patients, lisinopril versus chlorthalidone 30% risk reduction (8.1%). The incidence in the amlodipine (9.8%) arm was intermediate.[92] In ANBP-2, there was a 31% lower incidence of new-onset diabetes with enalapril compared to hydrochlorothiazide.[93]

Cerebrovascular disease

The Perindopril Protection Against Recurrent Stroke Study (PROGRESS) randomized 6,105 patients with a history of a stroke or transient ischemic attack (TIA) within five years to receive perindopril ± indapamide or placebo irrespective of BP. Administration of indapamide was at the discretion of the investigator. There were no BP criteria mandating combination therapy.[9] Fifty percent of patients were already receiving antihypertensive therapy. BP at baseline averaged 147/86 mmHg in both treatment arms and was reduced by a mean of 9/4 mmHg in the active therapy compared to the placebo group. The results demonstrated a highly significant 28% risk reduction for stroke after four years of follow-up. Normotensive patients as well as hypertensives experienced significant stroke risk reduction.[122]

Post hoc analysis indicated that patients receiving perindopril monotherpy showed no benefit, whereas patients receiving both drugs showed a 43% risk reduction for stroke. It is noteworthy that PROGRESS was designed as a combination therapy trial and was not powered to detect statistical differences between the monotherapy and combination arms. Because of its unusual study design, the PROGRESS data are subject to several interpretations: (1) that BP reduction *per se* regardless of baseline BP is valuable in reducing recurrent cerebrovascular events, (2) that ACE inhibition improves prognosis in this patient population, and (3) that a diuretic or a diuretic in combination with an ACE inhibitor improves prognosis. Recognizing these uncertainties,

ACE INHIBITORS: ROLE IN THE PREVENTION OF DIABETES			
Trial	**Population**	**Intervention**	**Diabetes**
HOPE	High-risk CVD	Ramipril vs. placebo	↓34%
CAPPP	HTN	Captopril vs. beta blockers/ diuretics	↓21%
SOLVD sub-study	Heart failure	Enalapril vs. placebo	↓21%
ANBP-2	HTN	Enalapril vs. HCTZ	↓31%
ALLHAT	High-risk HTN	Lisinopril vs. chlorthalidone	↓30%
ALLHAT	High-risk HTN	Lisinopril vs. amlodipine	↓17%

ACE inhibitors consistently reduce the incidence of new-onset diabetes compared to placebo or other antihypertensive agents. The mechanism for the apparent improvement in glucose tolerance with ACE inhibition remains to be delineated. Data from Yusuf S, et al. *JAMA* 2001; 286:1882–85; Hansson L, et al. *Lancet* 1999;353;611–16; Vermes E, et al. *Circulation* 2003; 107:1291–96; Wing LMH, et al. *N Engl J Med* 2003;348:583–92; and ALLHAT. *JAMA* 2002; 288:2981–97.

Table 80–2. ACE Inhibitors: Role in the Prevention of Diabetes

JNC-7 recommends the combination of an ACE inhibitor and a diuretic for secondary prevention in patients who have sustained a stroke or transient ischemic attack.[3,122]

ADVERSE EVENTS AND COMPLICATIONS

ACE inhibitors are well tolerated in most patients. They do not cause excessive fatigue or other central nervous system symptoms. As with all classes of antihypertensive medications, symptomatic hypotension can occur. This is more likely to happen in patients who are sodium or volume depleted and in whom the RAS is activated, making BP more angiotensin dependent. Hypotension can be minimized by starting with a low dose of ACE inhibitor and gradually titrating upward or by withholding diuretic therapy for a few days prior to starting ACE inhibitors. Patients who become hypotensive after receiving ACE inhibitors while volume depleted will often tolerate them without difficulty in a volume-repleted state.[123]

Hyperkalemia resulting from the anti-aldosterone effect of ACE inhibitors is a recognized side effect of therapy. In patients with normal renal function, a small and clinically insignificant rise in serum potassium routinely occurs. Hyperkalemia (defined as serum potassium >5.1) occurred in 11% of patients who had received prescriptions for ACE inhibitors in an outpatient Veterans Affairs medical center. The strongest predictor of hyperkalemia was a serum creatinine level >1.6 mg/dL.[124] Patients with baseline low aldosterone levels (as occurs in diabetics and the elderly) are predisposed to developing hyperkalemia. Concomitant use of NSAIDs, potassium supplements, and potassium-sparing diuretics also increase the risk for hyperkalemia.

Alternatively, use of thiazide and loop diuretics can prevent hyperkalemia. When prescribing an ACE inhibitor to a patient with risk factors for hyperkalemia, it is advisable to start at a low dose and check serum potassium concentrations one week after drug initiation and after any increase in dose.[125]

When renal function declines with chronic ACE inhibitor therapy, an explanation should be sought. Common reasons include hypoperfusion secondary to reduced cardiac output, volume depletion from excessive diuretic use, the presence of renal artery stenosis or the use of NSAIDs. In these settings, ACE inhibitors interfere with the kidney's compensatory mechanism for maintaining GFR. The ACE inhibitor should be temporarily discontinued while precipitating factors are corrected. Once renal function has stabilized, therapy can be resumed in some patients.[43,108]

The most common side effect of ACE inhibitors and the most frequent reason for drug discontinuation in clinical trials is a persistent nonproductive cough reported in 0.5 to 20% of patients.[126] The etiology of the cough is incompletely understood. It likely results from the accumulation of substances normally metabolized by ACE, including bradykinin and tachykinins (such as substance P). Increased synthesis of NO in the pulmonary epithelium and enhanced production of prostaglandins may

be contributory factors.[127] The cough is reported more frequently by women than by men. An increased prevalence of ACE-inhibitor-associated cough has been reported in Asian populations, with rates up to 53%.[128]

The cough is generally characterized as troublesome or annoying, rather than disabling, and does not result in pulmonary dysfunction. It usually begins within one week of starting therapy. In some cases it may have a delayed onset of up to six months. Once the drug is stopped, the cough usually disappears within one to seven days. However, it can take as long as four weeks to subside. Upon re-challenge with the same or another ACE inhibitor the cough will almost always recur. The cough appears to be dose independent, but its frequency may be reduced with a decrease in dosage. Failure of a clinician to consider ACE inhibitor therapy as a possible etiology for cough can lead to unnecessary evaluations and treatment. A simple four- to seven-day trial of drug withdrawal is an easy way of making the diagnosis. If the cough is mild and tolerable, the ACE inhibitor can be continued. Alternatively, substitution with an AT_1 receptor blocker is well tolerated.[126–129]

Angioneurotic edema is a rare but potentially fatal side effect of ACE inhibitors requiring immediate medical attention. Clinical manifestations include well-demarcated non-pitting edema of the tongue, lips, eyelids, or other parts of the face. Edema of the mucous membranes of the mouth, throat, and nose may also occur. Edema of the gastrointestinal tract has also been reported. Dysphagia can be a presenting symptom. Involvement of the upper respiratory tract can result in life-threatening airway compromise.[126–130] The incidence of angioedema associated with ACE inhibitor use is approximately 0.1 to 1.2%. In the Omapatrilat Cardiovascular Treatment vs. Enalapril (OCTAVE) trial, angioedema occurred in 86 of 12,557 (0.68%) patients treated with enalapril. The occurrence of angioedema does not appear to be influenced by dosage, age, or gender. African Americans are predisposed to ACE-inhibitor-associated angioedema with relative risks of 3 to 4.5 times that of white patients.[130,131]

The pathogenesis of angioedema is thought to be the same as that of ACE inhibitor-induced cough; namely, increased activity of bradykinin. Interestingly, cough and angioneurotic edema generally occur independently. The risk of angioedema is greatest within the first eight weeks of initiating therapy and declines thereafter. It can, however, occur within a few hours or be delayed for up to five years. In a retrospective analysis of 82 patients with documented angioedema while using ACE inhibitors, the risk of a recurrent episode was 10 times higher if ACE inhibitor therapy was reinstituted. The mean time between recurrent episodes was 11 months (range 0.6 to 34 months). The variable temporal relationship between ACE inhibitor administration and the occurrence of angioedema may contribute to a failure to recognize the association and discontinuation of the drug. Patients who develop angioedema while taking ACE inhibitors should not be re-challenged with any agent of this class.[126–131]

A few idiosyncratic side effects appear to be unique to captopril, including a maculopapular skin rash, taste disturbances, membranous glomerulopathy, and leukopenia. Leukopenia is particularly rare and occurs more frequently in patients with collagen vascular disease. These undesirable effects were much more common when captopril was used in excessively high doses (600 to 1,200 mg/day) and are rarely encountered with current dosing regimens.[38] Finally, ACE inhibitors are embryopathic. Use in the second and third trimester of pregnancy can cause renal dysgenesis, oligohydramnios, pulmonary hypoplasia, and neonatal death. All ACE inhibitors carry an FDA "black box" warning against use during the second and third trimesters of pregnancy.[123,132]

CONCLUSIONS

ACE inhibitors are among the most commonly prescribed and well-studied class of antihypertensive agents. They are effective in lowering BP in all patient populations, although the magnitude of the BP response is decreased in individuals of African descent. Despite the lack of long-term suppression in plasma angiotensin II levels, they maintain their BP-lowering effect without the development of tolerance. Their tolerability profile is generally benign and common side effects are limited to nonproductive cough and to increases in serum creatinine and potassium in susceptible individuals, primarily those with volume depletion, renal insufficiency, or heart failure. Importantly, ACE inhibitors do not interfere with cognitive function or cardiovascular reflexes.

Large-scale clinical trials have found ACE inhibitors to be as effective or more effective compared to other antihypertensive drug classes in reducing the long-term cardiovascular complications of hypertension. The totality of evidence supports the concept that ACE inhibitors are competitive but offer no particular endpoint advantage compared to low-dose diuretics and calcium channel blockers when broad hypertensive populations are studied. A consistent advantage of ACE inhibitors relates to the relative reduction in the incidence of new-onset diabetes compared to populations treated with other antihypertensive agents (excluding ARBs).

In patients with established end-organ disease, ACE inhibitors often constitute preferred antihypertensive therapy. This is particularly true in patients with renal disease and proteinuria regardless of etiology. It is also true in patients with left ventricular systolic dysfunction with or without heart failure. In these patients, ACE inhibitors attenuate long-term deterioration in ventricular function and improve both symptoms and survival. ACE inhibitors also decrease the incidence of MI in this population and in other patients with established coronary heart disease. In these selected patient populations with end-organ disease, the beneficial effects of ACE inhibitors are to some extent independent of BP reduction and appear to be related to organ-specific effects reflecting the critical role of the RAS in the development of the pathologic substratum for cardiovascular events.

REFERENCES

1. Cushman DW, Ondetti MA. History of the design of captopril and related inhibitors of angiotensin converting enzyme. *Hypertension* 1991; 17:589–92.

2. Basso N, Terragno NA. History about the discovery of the renin-angiotensin system. *Hypertension* 2001;38:1246–49.

3. Chobanian AV, Bakris GL, Black HR, et al. The seventh report of the joint national committee on prevention, detection, evaluation, and treatment of high blood pressure: The JNC 7. *JAMA* 2003;289:2560–72.

4. Flather M, Yusuf S, Kober L, et al. Long-term ACE-inhibitor therapy in patients with heart failure or left-ventricular dysfunction: A systematic review of data from individual patients. *Lancet* 2000;355:1575–81.

5. Yu, HT. Progression of chronic renal failure. *Arch Intern Med* 2003;163: 1417–29.

6. Givertz MM. Manipulation of the renin-angiotensin system. *Circulation* 2001;104:e14–18.

7. Pfeffer MA, Lama GA, Vaughan DE, et al. Effect of captopril on progressive ventricular dilatation after anterior myocardial infarction. *N Engl J Med* 1988;319:80–86.

8. Khalil ME, Basher AW, Brown EF, Alhaddad IA. A remarkable medical story: Benefits of angiotensin-converting enzyme inhibitors in cardiac patients. *J Am Coll Cardiol* 2001;37:1757–64.

9. Jandeleit-Dahm KAM, Tikellis C, Reid CM, et al. Why blockade of the renin-angiotensin system reduces the incidence of new-onset diabetes. *J Hypertens* 2005;23:463–73.

10. Chaturvedi N, Sjolie A, Stephenson JM, et al. Effect of lisinopril on progression of retinopathy in normotensive people with type 1 diabetes. *Lancet* 1998;351:28–31.

11. Progress Collaborative Group. Randomised trial of a perindopril-based blood-pressure-lowering regimen among 6,105 individuals with previous stroke or transient ischaemic attack. *Lancet* 2001;358:1033–41.

12. Anderson C. Blood pressure-lowering for secondary prevention of stroke: ACE inhibition is the key. *Stroke* 2004; 34:1333–36.

13. Dzau VJ, Bernstein K, Celermajer D, et al. The relevance of tissue angiotensin-converting enzyme: Manifestations in mechanistic and endpoint data. *Am J Cardiol* 2001;88(suppl):1L-20L.

14. Brown NJ, Vaughan DE. Angiotensin-converting enzyme inhibitors. *Circulation* 1998;97:1411–20.

15. Oates JA, Wood AJJ. Converting-enzyme inhibitors in the treatment of hypertension. *N Engl J Med* 1988; 319:1517–25.

16. Salvetti A. Newer ACE inhibitors-A look at the future. *Drugs* 1990;6:800–28.

17. Gainer JV, Morrow JD, Loveland A, et al. Effect of bradykinin-receptor blockade on the response to angiotensin-converting enzyme inhibitors in normotensive and hypertensive subjects. *N Engl J Med* 1998;339:1285–92.

18. Forclaz A, Maillard M, Nussberger J, et al. Angiotensin II receptor blockade: Is there truly a benefit of adding an ACE inhibitor? *Hypertension* 2003;41:31–36.

19. Azizi M, Menard J. Combined blockade of the renin-angiotensin system with angiotensin-converting enzyme inhibitors and angiotensin II type I receptor antagonists. *Circulation* 2004;109:2492–99.

20. Cruden NLM, Witherow FN, Webb DJ et al. Bradykinin contributes to the systemic hemodynamic effects of chronic angiotensin-converting enzyme inhibition in patients with heart failure. *Arterioscler Thromb Vasc Biol* 2004;24:1043–48.

21. Hornig, B, Kohler C, Drexler H. Role of bradykinin in mediating vascular effects of angiotensin-converting enzyme inhibitors in humans. *Circulation* 1997;95:1115–18.

22. Witherow FN, Helmy A, Webb DJ, et al. Bradykinin contributes to the vasodilator effects of chronic angiotensin-converting enzyme inhibition in patients with heart failure. *Circulation* 2001;104:2177–81.

23. Fujii M, Atsuyuki W, Tsutamoto T, et al. Bradykinin improves left ventricular diastolic function under long-term angiotensin-converting enzyme inhibition in heart failure. *Hypertension* 2002;39:952–57.

24. Schanstra JP, Neau E, Drogoz P, et al. In vivo bradykinin B2 receptor activation reduces renal fibrosis. *J Clin Invest* 2002;110:371–79.

25. Pretorius M, Rosenbaum D, Vaughan DE, Brown NJ. Angiotensin-converting enzyme inhibition increases human vascular tissue-type plasminogen activator release through endogenous bradykinin. *Circulation* 2003;107:579–85.

26. Murphy L, Vaughan D, Brown N. Contribution of bradykinin to the cardioprotective effects of ACE inhibitors. *Eur Heart J Supplements* 2003;5(A):A37–41.

27. Dykewicz MS. Cough and angioedema from angiotensin-converting enzyme inhibitors: New insight into mechanisms and management. *Curr Opin Allergy Clin Immunol* 2004;4:267–70.

28. Rotmensch HH, Vlasses PH, Ferguson RK. Angiotensin converting enzyme inhibitors. *Med Clin N Amer* 1988;72:399–425.

29. Gradman AH, Cutler NR, Davis PJ, et al. Combined enalapril and felodipine extended release (ER) for systemic hypertension. *Am J Cardiol* 1997;79:431–35.

30. Jackson EK. Renin and angiotensin. In JG Hardman, LE Limbird (eds.). *Goodman and Gilman's The Pharmacological Basis of Therapeutics, Tenth Edition.* New York: McGraw-Hill, 2001:809–41.

31. Laragh JH, Sealy JE. Causal roles of plasma renin in hypertension, and in heart attack, heart failure, stroke and kidney failure, and the unique value of anti-renin system drugs in prevention and treatment. In HR Ulfendahl, M Aurell (eds.). *Renin-Angiotensin.* London: Portland Press 1998:273–302.

32. Sica DA. Pharmacotherapy review: Angiotensin-converting enzyme inhibitors. *J Clin Hypertens* 2005; 7:485–88.

33. Renin angiotensin system antagonists. *Drug Facts and Comparisons* 2005; 632–45.

34. Leonetti G, Cuspidi C. Choosing the right ace inhibitor. *Drugs* 1995; 4:516–35.

35. White, CM. Pharmacologic, pharmacokinetic, and therapeutic differences among ACE inhibitors. *Pharmacotherapy* 1998;18:588–99.

36. Ondetti MA. Structural relationships of angiotensin converting-enzyme inhibitors to pharmacologic activity. *Circulation* 1988;77(1):174–78.

37. Thind GS. Angiotensin converting enzyme inhibitors: Comparative structure, pharmacokinetics, and pharmacodynamics. *Cardiovasc Drugs and Therapy* 1990;4:199–206.

38. Raia JJ, Barone JA, Byerly WG, Lace CR. Angiotensin-converting enzyme inhibitors: A comparative review. *DICP Ann Pharmacother* 1990; 24:506–25.

39. Sica DA. Angiotensin-converting enzyme inhibitors. In *Hypertension Primer, Second Edition.* Baltimore: Lippincott Williams & Wilkins 1999:426–29.

40. Zannad F. Trandolapril. How does it differ from other angiotensin converting enzyme inhibitors? *Drugs* 1993;46(2):172–82.

41. Hollenberg NK, Fisher NDL. Renal circulation and blockade of the renin-angiotnesin system: Is angiotensin-converting enzyme the last word? *Hypertension* 1995;26:602–09.

42. Salvetti A. Angiotensin-converting enzyme inhibitors in the treatment of mild to moderate essential hypertension. *Am J Hypertens* 1989; 2:94S-99S.

43. Schoolwerth AC, Sica DA, Ballermann BJ, Wilcox CS. Renal considerations in angiotensin converting enzyme inhibitor therapy. *Circulation* 2001; 104:1985–91.

44. Anderson S, Rennke HG, Brenner BM. Therapeutic advantage of converting enzyme inhibitors in arresting progressive renal disease associated with systemic hypertension. *J Clin Invest* 1986;77:1993–2000.

45. Fogo AB. The Role of angiotensin II and plasminogen activator inihibitor-1 in progressive glomerulopathies. *AJKD* 2000;35:179–88.

46. Ma LJ, Nakamura S, Aldigier MR, et al. Regression of glomerulosclerosis with high-dose angiotensin inhibition is linked to decreased plasminogen activator inhibitor-1. *J Am Soc Nephrol* 2005;16:966–76.

47. Shin GT, Kim SJ, Ma KA, et al. ACE inhibitors attenuate expression of renal transforming growth factor-B1 in humans. *Am J Kidney Dis* 2000; 36:894–902.

48. Lonn EM, Yusuf S, Jha P, et al. Emerging role of angiotensin-converting enzyme inhibitors in cardiac and vascular protection. *Circulation* 1994;90:2056–69.

49. Pahor M, Bernabei R, Sgadari A, et al. Enalapril prevents cardiac fibrosis and arrhythmias in hypertensive rats. *Hypertension* 1991;18:148–57.

50. Sonnenblick EH. Perindopril treatment for congestive heart failure. *Am J Cardiol* 2001;88:19i-27i.

51. Dahlof B, Pennert K, Hansson L. Reversal of left ventricular hypertrophy in hypertensive patients: A meta-analysis of 109 treatment studies. *Am J Hypertens* 1992;5:95–110.

52. Cruickshank JM, Lewis J, Moore V, Dodd C. Reversibility of left ventricular hypertrophy by differing types of antihypertensive therapy. *J Hum Hypertens* 1992;6:85–90.

53. Klingbeil AU, Schneider M, Martus P et al. A meta-analysis of treatment on left ventricular mass in essential hypertension. *Am J Med* 2003;115:41–46.

54. Brilla CG, Funck RC, Rupp H. Lisinopril-mediated regression of myocardial fibrosis in patients with hypertensive heart disease. *Circulation* 2000;102:1388–93.

55. Thybo NK, Korsgaard N, Eriksen S, et al. Dose-dependent effects of perindopril on blood pressure and small-artery structure. *Hypertension* 1994;23:659–66.

56. Harrap SB, Van der Merwe WM, Griffin SA. Brief angiotensin converting enzyme inhibitor treatment in young spontaneously hypertensive rats reduces blood pressure long-term. *Hypertension* 1990;16:603–14.

57. Schiffrin EL, Deng LY, Larochelle P. Effects of a B-blocker or a converting enzyme inhibitor on resistance arteries in essential hypertension. *Hypertension* 1994;23:83–91.

58. Schiffrin EL, Deng LY, Larochelle P. Progressive improvement in the structure of resistance arteries of hypertensive patients after 2 years of treatment with an angiotensin I-converting enzyme inhibitor: Comparison with effects of a B-Blocker. *Am J Hypertens* 1995; 8:229–36.

59. Schiffrin EL, Deng LY. Comparison of effects of angiotensin I-converting enzyme inhibition and B-blockade for 2 years on function of small arteries from hypertensive patients. *Hypertension* 1995;25(2):699–703.

60. Laurent S, Boutouyrie P, Asmar R, et al. Aortic stiffness is an independent predictor of all-cause and cardiovascular mortality in hypertensive patients. *Hypertension* 2001;37:1236–41.

61. Guerin AP, Blacher J, Pannier B, et al. Impact of aortic stiffness attenuation on survival of patients in end-stage renal failure. *Circulation* 2001; 103:987–92.

62. Ahimastos AA, Natoli AK, Lawler A, et al. Ramipril reduces large-artery stiffness in peripheral arterial disease and promotes elastogenic remodeling in cell culture. *Hypertension* 2005; 45:1194–99

63. Levy BI, Michel JB, Salzmann JL, et al. Long-term effects of angiotensin-converting enzyme inhibition on the arterial wall of adult spontaneously hypertensive rats. *Am J Cardiol* 1993; 71:8E-16E.

64. R Asmar, Topouchian J, Pannier B, et al. Pulse wave velocity as endpoint in large-scale intervention trial: The Complior(R) study. *Journal of Hypertension* 2001;19:813–18.

65. Schieffer B, Schieffer E, Hilfiker-Kleiner D. Expression of angiotensin II and interleukin 6 in human coronary atherosclerotic plaques: Potential implications for inflammation and plaque instability. *Circulation* 2001; 101:1372–78.

66. Diet F, Pratt RE, Berry GJ, et al. Increased accumulation of tissue ACE in human atherosclerotic coronary artery disease. *Circulation* 1996; 94:2756–67.

67. Ghiadoni L, Magagna A, Versari D, et al. Different effect of antihypertensive drugs on conduit artery endothelial function. *Hypertension* 2003;41:1281–86.

68. Higashi Y, Sasaki S, Nakagawa K, et al. A comparison of angiotensin converting enzyme inhibitors, calcium antagonsits, beta-blockers and diuretic agents on reactive hyperemia in patients with essential hypertension: A multicenter study. *J Am Coll Cardiol* 2000;35:284–91.

69. Mancini GB, Henry GC, Macaya C, et al. Angiotensin-converting enzyme inhibition with quinapril improves endothelial vasomotor dysfunction in patients with coronary artery disease: The TREND (Trial on Reversing Endothelial Dysfunction) Study. *Circulation* 1996;94:258–65.

70. Brasier AR, Recinos A, Eledrisi MS. Vascular inflammation and the renin-angiotensin system. *Arterioscler Thromb Vasc Biol* 2002;22:1257–66.

71. Hernandez A, Barberi L, Ballerio G, et al. Delapril slows the progression of atherosclerosis and maintains endothelial function in cholesterol-fed rabbits. *Atherosclerosis* 1987;137: 71–76.

72. Hayek T, Attias J, Smith J, et al. Antiatherosclerotic and antioxidative effects of captopril in apolipoprotein E-deficient mice. *J Cardiovasc Pharmacol* 1998;31:540–44.

73. Hayek T, Attias J, Coleman R, et al. The angiotensin converting enzyme inhibitor, fosinopril, and the angiotensin II receptor antagonist, losartan, inhibit LDL oxidation and attenuate atherosclerosis independent of lowering blood pressure in apolipoprotein E deficient mice. *Cardiovasc Res* 1999;44:579–87.

74. Keidar S, Attias J, Coleman R, et al. Attenuation of atherosclerosis in apolipoprotein E-deficient mice by ramipril is dissociated from its antihypertensive effect and from potentiation on of bradykinin. *J Cardio Pharm* 2000;35:64–72.

75. MacMahon S, Sharpe S, Sharpe N, et al. Randomized, placebo-controlled trial of the angiotensin-converting enzyme inhibitor, ramipril, in patients with coronary or other occlusive arterial disease: PART-2 collaborative research group. Prevention of atherosclerosis with ramipril. *J Am Coll Cardiol* 3:438–43.

76. Lonn EM, Yusuf S, Dzavik V, et al. Effects of Ramipril and Vitamin E on Atherosclerosis: The study to evaluate carotid ultrasound changes in patients treated with ramipril and vitamin E. *Circulation* 2001;103:919–25.

77. Ribichini F, Wijns W, Ferrero V, et al. Effect of angiotensin-converting enzyme inhibition on restenosis after coronary stenting. *Am J Cardiol* 2003;91:154–58.

78. Materson BJ, Reda DJ, Cushman WC. Single drug therapy for hypertension in men: A comparison of six antihypertensive agents with placebo. *N Engl J Med* 1993;328:914–21.

79. Cleland JGF, John J, Houghton T. Does aspirin attenuate the effect of angiotensin-converting enzyme inhibitors in hypertension or heart failure. *Curr Opin Nephrol Hypertens* 2001;10:625–31.

80. Nawarskas JJ, Townsend RR, Cirigliano MD, et al. Effect of aspirin on blood pressure in hypertensive patients taking enalapril or losartan. *A J Hypertens* 1999;12:784–89.

81. Zanchetti A, Hansson L, Leonetti G. Low-dose aspirin does not interfere with the blood pressure lowering effect of antihypertensive therapy. *J Hypertens* 2002;20:1015–22.

82. Weinberger MH. Blood pressure and metabolic responses to hydrochlorothiazide, captopril, and the combination in black and white mild-to-moderate hypertensive patients. *J Cardiovasc Pharmaco* 1985;7:S52–55.

83. Weir MR, Gray JM, Paster R, et al. Differing mechanisms of action of angiotensin-converting enzyme inhibition in black and white hypertensive patients. *Hypertension* 1995;25:124–30.

84. Douglas JG, Bakris GL, Epstein M. Management of high blood pressure in African Americans. *Arch Intern Med* 2003;163:525–41.

85. Wright JT, Bakris G, Greene T, et al. Effect of blood pressure lowering and antihypertensive drug class on progression of hypertensive kidney disease: Results from the AASK trial. *JAMA* 2002;288:2421–31.

86. Ravid M, Ravid D. ACE inhibitors in elderly patients with hypertension. *Drugs and Aging* 1996;8:29–37.

87. Smith WM, Gomez HJ. The use of benazepril in hypertensive patients age 55 and over. *Clin Cardiol* 1991; 14(IV):IV79–82.

88. Hajjar I. Postural blood pressure changes and orthostatic hypotension in the elderly patient: impact of antihypertensive medications. *Drugs Aging* 2005;22:55–68.

89. Gradman AH. Managing high-risk patients with hypertension: Focus on the renin-angiotensin system. *J Clin Hypertens* 2004;6:501–08.

90. Gradman AH. Drug combinations. In [eds.] *Hypertension Primer, Second Edition.* Baltimore: Lippincott Williams & Wilkins 1999:408–11.

91. Hansson L, Lindholm LH, Niskanen L, et al. Effect of angiotensin-converting-enzyme inhibition compared with conventional therapy on cardiovascular morbidity and mortality in hypertension: The Captopril Prevention Project (CAPPP) randomised trial. *Lancet* 1999;353:611–16.

92. The ALLHAT Officers and Coordinators for the ALLHAT Collaborative Research Group. Major outcomes in high-risk hypertensive patients randomized to angiotensin-converting enzyme inhibitor or calcium channel blocker vs. diuretic: The antihypertensive and lipid-lowering treatment to prevent heart attack trial. *JAMA* 2002; 288:2981–97.

93. Wing LMH, Reid CM, Ryan, et al. Second Australian National Blood Pressure Study (ANBP2)-comparative outcome trial of ACE inhibitor-and diuretic-based treatment of hypertension in the elderly: Principal results. *N Engl J Med* 2003;348:583–92.

94. Hansson L, Lindholm LH, Ekbom T, et al. Randomised trial of old and new antihypertensive drugs in elderly patients: Cardiovascular mortality and morbidity the Swedish Trial in Old Patients with Hypertension-2 study. *Lancet* 1999;354:1751–56.

95. Blood Pressure Lowering Treatment Trialists' Collaboration. Effects of different blood-pressure-lowering regimens on major cardiovascular events: results of prospectively-designed overviews of randomized trials. *Lancet* 2003;362:1527–35.

96. Viberti G, Mogensen CE, Groop LC, Pauls JF. Effect of captopril on progression to clinical proteinuria in patients with insulin-dependent diabetes mellitus and microalbuminuria. European Microalbuminuria Captopril Study Group. *JAMA* 1994;271:275–79.

97. Lewis EJ, Hunsicker LG, Bain RP, Rohde RD. The effect of angiotensin-converting-enzyme inhibition on diabetic nephropathy. The Collaborative Study Group. *N Engl J Med* 1993;329:1456–62.

98. Bakris GL, Williams M, Dworkin L., et al. Preserving renal function in adults with hypertension and diabetes: A consensus approach. *Am J Kid Diseases* 2000;36:646–61.

99. Ravid M, Savin H, Jutrin I, et al. Long-term effect of ACE inhibition on development of nephropathy in diabetes mellitus type II. *Kidney Int Suppl* 1994;45:S161–64.

100. Lebovitz HE, Wiegmann TB, Cnaan A, et al. Renal protective effects of enalapril in hypertensive NIDDM: Rode of baseline proteinuria. *Kidney Int Suppl* 1994;45:S150–54.

101. Barnett AH, Bain SC, Bouter P, et al. Angiotensin-receptor blockade versus converting-enzyme inhibition in type 2 diabetes and nephropathy. *N Engl J Med* 2004;351:1952–61.

102. Ruggenenti P, Fassi A, Ilieva A, et al. and the Bergamo Nephrologic Diabetes Complications Trial (BENEDICT) Investigators. Preventing microalbuminuria in type 2 diabetes. *N Engl J Med* 2004;351:1941–51.

103. The GISEN Group (Gruppo Italiano di Studi Epidemiologici in Nefrologia). Randomised placebo-controlled trial of effect of ramipril on decline in glomerular filtration rate and risk of terminal renal failure in proteinuric, non-diabetic nephropathy. *Lancet* 1997;349:1857–63.

104. Ruggenenti P, Perna A, Gherardi G, et al. Renoprotective properties of ACE-inhibition in non-diabetic nephropathies with non-nephrotic proteinuria. *Lancet* 1999;354:359–64.

105. Jafar TH, Schmid CH, Landa M, et al. Angiotensin-converting enzyme inhibitors and progression of nondiabetic renal disease: A meta-analysis of patient-level data. *Ann Intern Med* 2001;135:73–87.

106. Jafar TH, Stark PC, Schmid CH, et al. Progression of chronic kidney disease: the role of blood pressure control, proteinuria, and angiotensin-converting enzyme inhibition: A patient-level meta-analysis. *Ann Intern Med* 2003;139:244–52.

107. Nakao N, Yoshimura A, Morita H, et al. Combination treatment of angiotensin-II receptor blocker and angiotensin-converting-enzyme inhibitor in non-diabetic renal disease (COOPERATE): A randomised controlled trial. *Lancet* 2003;361:117–24.

108. Bakris GL, Weir MR. Angiotensin-converting enzyme inhibitor-associated elevations in serum creatinine: Is this a cause for concern? *Arch Intern Med* 2000;160:685–93.

109. Pfeffer MA, Braunwald E, Moye LA, et al. Effect of captopril on mortality and morbidity in patients with left ventricular dysfunction after myocardial infarction: Results of the Survival and Ventricular Enlargement Trial. The SAVE investigators. *N Engl J Med* 1992;327:669–77.

110. Acute Infarction Ramipril Efficacy (AIRE) Study Investigators. Effect of ramipril on mortality and morbidity of survivors of acute myocardial infarction with clinical evidence of heart failure. *Lancet* 1993;342:821–28.

111. Kober L, Torp-Pedersen C, Carlsen JE, et al. The Trandolapril Cardiac Evaluation (TRACE) Study Group: A clinical trial of the angiotensin-converting-enzyme inhibitor trandolapril in patients with left ventricular dysfunction after myocardial infarction. *N Engl J Med* 1995;333:1670–76.

112. Torp-Pedersen C, Kober L, for the TRACE Study Group. Effect of ACE inhibitor trandolapril on life expectancy of patients with reduced left-ventricular function after acute myocardial infarction. *Lancet* 1999; 354:9–12.

113. Flather MD, Yusuf S, Kober L, et al. Long-term ACE-inhibitor therapy in patients with heart failure or left-ventricular dysfunction: A systematic overview of data from individual patients. *Lancet* 2000;355:1575–81.

114. Yusuf S, Sleight P, Pogue J, et al. Effects of an angiotensin-converting-enzyme inhibitor, ramipril, on cardiovascular events in high-risk patients. The Heart Outcomes Prevention Evaluation Study Investigators. *N Engl J Med* 2000; 342:145–53.

115. Svensson P, de Faire U, Sleight P, Yusuf S, Ostergren J. Comparative effects of ramipril on ambulatory and office blood pressures: A HOPE substudy. *Hypertension* 2001; 38:E28–32.

116. Fox KM. Efficacy of perindopril in reduction of cardiovascular events among patients with stable coronary artery disease: Randomised, double-blind, placebo-controlled, multicentre trial (the EUROPA study). *Lancet* 2003;362:782–88.

117. The PEACE Trial Investigators. Angiotensin-converting-enzyme inhibition in stable coronary artery disease. *N Engl J Med* 2004; 351:2058–68.

118. Yusuf, S, Pogue, J, Myers MG, McCullough C, Pfeffer MA, Domanski MJ, Braunwald E. ACE Inhibition in Stable Coronary Artery Disease. *N Engl J Med* 2005; 352:937–39

119. Yusuf S, Gerstein H, Hoogwerf B, et al, and the HOPE Study Investigators. Ramipril and the development of diabetes. *JAMA* 2001;286:1882–85.

120. Lim HS, MacFadyen RJ, Lip GYH. Diabetes Mellitus, the renin-angiotensin-aldosterone system, and the heart. *Arch Intern Med* 2004; 164:1737–44.

121. Gress TW, Nieto FJ, Shahar E, et al. Hypertension and antihypertensive therapy as a risk factor for type 2 diabetes mellitus. *NEJM* 2000; 342:905–912.

122. Randomised trial of a perindopril-based blood-pressure-lowering regimen among 6,105 individuals with previous stroke or transient ischaemic attack. *Lancet* 2001;358:1033–41.

123. Hussar DA. The angiotensin-converting enzyme inhibitors (ACEIs). *The Drug Advisor* 2002;1:1–8.

124. Reardon LC, Macpherson DS. Hyperkalemia in outpatients using angiotensin-converting enzyme inhibitors: How much should we worry? *Arch Intern Med* 1998; 158:26–32.

125. Palmer BF. Managing hyperkalemia caused by inhibitors of the renin-angiotensin-aldosterone system. *N Engl J Med* 2004;351:585–92.

126. Israili ZH, Hall DW. Cough and angioneurotic edema associated with angiotensin-converting enzyme inhibitor therapy. *Ann Int Med* 1992; 117:234–42.

127. Dykewicz MS. Cough and angioedema from angiotensin-converting enzyme inhibitors: New insight into mechanisms and management. *Curr Opin Allergy Clin Immunol* 2004;4:267–70.

128. Nishizawa A. Angiotensin-converting enzyme inhibitor induced cough among Asians. *Proceedings of UCLA Healthcare* 2000;4:35–38.

129. Pylypchuk GB. ACE inhibitor-versus angiotensin II blocker-induced cough and angioedema. *Ann Pharmacother* 1998;32:1060–66.

130. Brown NJ, Snowden M, Griffin MR. Recurrent angiotensin-converting enzyme inhibitor-associated angioedema. *JAMA* 1997;278:232–33.

131. Kostis JB, Kim HJ, James Rusnak J, et al. Incidence and characteristics of angioedema associated with enalapril. *Arch Intern Med* 2005;165:1637–42.

132. The Task Force on ACE-inhibitors of the European Society of Cardiology. Expert consensus document on angiotensin converting enzyme inhibitors in cardiovascular disease. *Eur Heart J* 2004;25:1454–70.

Chapter

81 Angiotensin II Receptor Blockers

Hans R. Brunner

Key Findings

- Renin via angiotensin II induces cardiovascular risk independent of blood pressure (BP).

- Blockade of the renin-angiotensin system reduces risk beyond BP reduction.

- Angiotensin-converting enzyme inhibitors (ACEIs) and angiotensin receptor antagonists (ARBs) act similarly and mainly by blocking the renin-angiotensin system.

- ARBs have an antihypertensive efficacy comparable to that of other classes of antihypertensive agents.

- In patients with congestive heart failure, ARBs alone or in addition to ACEIs improve cardiac function and reduce cardiac death.

- In patients with type 2 diabetic nephropathy ARBs have been shown to provide clear renal protection, but optimal BP control is imperative.

- In many trials, so far ARBs have been shown to reduce the risk of new-onset diabetes.

- So far ARBs are the only class of antihypertensive agents available that exhibit a side effect profile comparable to placebo. Consequently, high doses of ARBs can and should be administered to obtain maximal therapeutic benefit. Whether the combination of maximal doses of ACEIs and ARBs can exert additive effects remains doubtful.

There is a continuous and independent relationship between BP and risk of cardiovascular disease events, including myocardial infarction, heart failure, stroke, and renal disease.[1,2] Consequently, the primary goal in the treatment of hypertensive patients is to achieve the maximum reduction in the long-term total risk of cardiovascular and renal morbidity and mortality.[1,3] The importance of lowering BP in reducing the risk of cardiovascular events has been demonstrated in various controlled clinical trials.[4,5] In addition to the lowering of BP per se, successful realization of the primary goal of treatment also requires consideration and appropriate management of co-morbidities, such as diabetes or preexisting cardiovascular disease.[1,6]

The renin-angiotensin system (RAS) plays an important physiologic role in the preservation of hemodynamic stability and the pathogenesis of many cardiovascular disease states, including hypertension, heart failure, nephropathy, atherosclerosis, and myocardial infarction.[7,8] The RAS is present in the systemic circulation, as well as in a variety of tissue types, including brain, heart, blood

vessel, adrenal gland, and kidney tissue.[9,10] The maladaptive effects of the RAS are mediated by the actions of angiotensin II, which is the major RAS effector peptide.[7,8,11] As well as controlling cardiovascular homeostasis, angiotensin II contributes to cellular growth and replication, and is involved with inflammation and oxidative stress.[12–15] Consequently, RAS activity contributes to the pathophysiology of hypertension, renal disease, atherosclerosis, diabetes, and heart failure.[12] Inhibition of the RAS has been shown to play an important role in lowering BP and in reducing the risk of development or progression of the conditions associated with hypertension.

Angiotensin II receptor blockers (ARBs) are the newest class of approved antihypertensive agents. These imidazole derivatives were developed with a specific and unique purpose: to block angiotensin II receptor binding. This chapter provides an overview of ARBs, focusing on their efficacy and tolerability in reducing BP patients with hypertension. The chapter also examines the evidence from some key clinical trials relating to their efficacy in treating related conditions and co-morbidities.

The RAS and evolution of ARBs

Angiotensin II is central to many of the pathologic changes that occur in hypertension and cardiovascular disease, and thus agents that interrupt the RAS are prime candidates for reducing BP and preventing or ameliorating disease processes.[16] Pharmacologic inhibition of the RAS has indeed proven to be a successful therapeutic strategy, and has helped to define the contribution of the system to BP control and the pathogenesis of diseases such as hypertension, congestive heart failure, and chronic renal failure.[17] The first major breakthrough in this regard was development of the angiotensin-converting enzyme (ACE) inhibitors, which are now recognized as an important therapeutic class in the control of hypertension.[1,17] Clinical studies have also shown that ACE inhibitors are able to reduce morbidity and mortality in a wide range of patients, including those with ischemic heart disease, heart failure, diabetic nephropathy, and stroke.[1,18–24]

Angiotensin II, which is converted from angiotensin I by angiotensin-converting enzyme (ACE), is the major end product of the RAS cascade—a series of reactions that starts with the cleavage of angiotensinogen by renin (Figure 81–1). From the RAS cascade, it can be seen that ACE is not an ideal target for RAS blockade.[17] One reason is that ACE is not specific for angiotensin I, and this lack of specificity (leading to accumulation of kinins and other

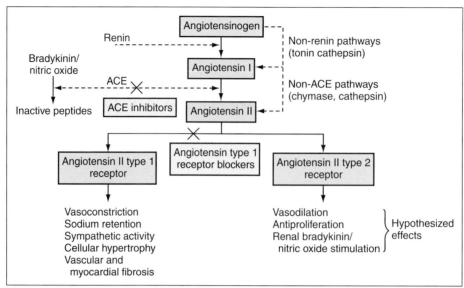

Figure 81–1. Schematic of the renin-angiotensin system and its inhibitors.

peptides) is the source of some of the most common side effects of ACE inhibitors, including cough and angio-oedema.[25,26] Another potential drawback is that non-ACE-dependent pathways exist for conversion of angiotensin I, which may contribute to incomplete or temporary suppression of angiotensin II production associated with ACE inhibitors.[17]

There is also the issue of the effects ACE inhibition may exert on the different types of angiotensin II receptor. At least four types of receptor for angiotensin II are known (AT1, AT2, AT3, and AT4).[27] The AT1 and AT2 subtypes are the most well characterized, but the role of the AT2 receptor remains to be fully defined. The physiologic effects of angiotensin II mediated by the AT1 receptor include vasoconstriction, stimulation of renal sodium reabsorption, increased collagen deposition, and cellular proliferation.[28] It has been proposed that the AT2 receptor antagonizes the vasoactive effects of the AT1 receptor, but experimental findings are inconsistent[29–31] and the function of the AT2 receptor remains controversial.[32] Thus, it is not clear whether inhibition of AT2 receptor function (as

would be expected with ACE inhibition) is clinically beneficial or detrimental.

In principle, blockade of the RAS at the rate-limiting step between renin and angiotensinogen would provide specific blockade of the system. However, the development of suitable candidate molecules for renin inhibition has been slow.[17] Such agents may soon become available,[33] and their introduction is awaited with interest. Blockade of the RAS at the level of the AT1 receptor (which would provide specific blockade, obviate angiotensin escape, and allow continued activation of the AT2 receptor) is an attractive option. Compared with ACE inhibition, it was hypothesized that inhibition of angiotensin II at the level of the AT1 receptor should result in at least equal antihypertensive efficacy with a reduced incidence of side effects.

Several orally active ARBs have now been successfully developed (Table 81–1). Losartan was the first orally active ARB available on the market (approved for use in 1995), and olmesartan is the most recent ARB to have been successfully launched for the treatment of hyper-

PHARMACOKINETICS AND RECOMMENDED DOSAGE OF CURRENTLY AVAILABLE ANGIOTENSIN RECEPTOR BLOCKERS FOR THE TREATMENT OF HYPERTENSION						
Drug Name	Bioavailability (%)	Terminal Half-life (h)	Protein Binding (%)	Conversion to Active Metabolite	Dosing	Starting/Maximum Recommended Dose (mg/day)
Losartan (Cozaar)	≈30	6–9	99.8	Yes	OD	50/100
Candesartan (Amias)	15	5–9	>99	Yes	OD	16/32
Irbesartan (Aprovel)	60–80	11–15	(90–92)*	No	OD	150/300
Valsartan (Diovan)	25	6–9	94–97	No	OD	80/320
Eprosartan (Teveten)	13	5–9	98	No	OD	600/800
Telmisartan (Micardis)	40–60	≈24	>99.5	No	OD	40/80
Olmesartan (Olmetec)	26	11–15	>99	Yes	OD	10/40
OD = once daily, * = probably higher.						

Table 81–1. Pharmacokinetics and Recommended Dosage of Currently Available Angiotensin Receptor Blockers for the Treatment of Hypertension

tension (approved for use in 2002). ARBs have the same mechanism of action, exhibiting high-affinity competitive AT1 receptor binding with almost no affinity for the AT2 receptor.[34] Structural differences between the ARBs contribute to variable degrees of "insurmountable" AT1 blockade. These range from classic competitive antagonism of the receptor with losartan to very slow dissociation from the receptor and almost complete insurmountable blockade with candesartan and olmesartan.[35,36] Surmountable antagonists are those that produce parallel rightward shifts of agonist dose-response curves *in vitro* with no alteration of the maximal response, whereas insurmountable antagonists also depress the maximal response. Insurmountable antagonism, which is due to slow dissociation of the antagonist from the receptor, should help to ensure sustained activity when concentrations of angiotensin II increase in response to an interrupted negative feedback loop—with no rebound effect upon ARB withdrawal.[34] Insurmountable blockade is, however, difficult to achieve at doses used clinically.[34]

ARBs also have different pharmacokinetic profiles.[34] The bioavailability of ARBs ranges from 13% for eprosartan to about 60% for irbesartan and telmisartan. The terminal half-lives of losartan, eprosartan, valsartan, and possibly candesartan are relatively short (<10 hours). Irbesartan and olmesartan have longer half-lives (11 to 15 hours), and telmisartan has the longest half-life of all

ARBs (approximately 24 hours). Once-daily oral dosing is claimed to be sufficient to provide effective antihypertensive treatment with all of the commercially available agents. Analyses of clinical studies comparing the efficacy of olmesartan with losartan, valsartan, and irbesartan appear to support this (Table 81–2).[37,38] Olmesartan produced the greatest decreases in BP, but BP levels were reduced from baseline during the last 2 and 4 hours of the dosing interval with all of the ARBs studied.[38] A recent analysis of a comparison between olmesartan and candesartan showed that both agents produced substantial reductions from baseline during the last 2 and 4 hours of the dosing interval, with olmesartan again providing better BP control over 24 hours.[39]

Blood-pressure-lowering efficacy and tolerability of ARBs

The hypothesis behind the rational pharmacologic development of ARBs has been confirmed: a number of clinical trials have now shown ARBs to be at least as effective as other classes of antihypertensive drugs (ACE inhibitors, β-blockers, calcium channel antagonists, and diuretics), with an excellent tolerability profile.[40]

Comparative efficacy

A comprehensive meta-analysis of 43 randomized placebo-controlled trials involving losartan, valsartan, irbesartan,

LEAST SQUARES MEAN REDUCTIONS FROM BASELINE IN SYSTOLIC BLOOD PRESSURE (SBP) AND DIASTOLIC BLOOD PRESSURE (DBP) AS ASSESSED BY AMBULATORY BP MONITORING AFTER 8 WEEKS OF TREATMENT WITH LOSARTAN (50 MG/DAY), VALSARTAN (80 MG/DAY), IRBESARTAN (150 MG/DAY), OR OLMESARTAN (20 MG/DAY) IN A RANDOMIZED DOUBLE-BLIND STUDY[37,38]				
Mean Reduction from Baseline (mmHg)	Losartan (n=134)	Valsartan (n=130)	Irbesartan (n=134)	Olmesartan (n=136)
24-hour:				
SBP	9.0**	8.1***	11.3	12.5
DBP	6.2**	5.6***	7.4	8.5
Daytime (0800–1959 h):				
SBP	10.9**	10.2***	13.8	14.7
DBP	7.2***	7.0***	8.8	10.2
Nighttime (2000–0759 h):				
SBP	7.3*	6.1***	8.8	10.3
DBP	5.2	4.2**	5.9	6.8
Last 2 hours of monitoring[a]:				
SBP	6.9*	5.1***	7.7	10.1
DBP	5.8	3.2***	5.4	7.1
Last 4 hours of monitoring[a]:				
SBP	7.1*	4.7***	7.4	9.8*
DBP	5.4	3.1***	4.9	6.8

[a]Includes the morning BP surge time period, beginning at approximately 0600 h.[106]
*p<0.05 versus olmesartan; **p<0.001 versus olmesartan; ***p<0.001 versus olmesartan.

Table 81–2. Least Squares Mean Reductions from Baseline in Systolic Blood Pressure (SBP) and Diastolic Blood Pressure (DBP) as Assessed by Ambulatory BP Monitoring After 8 Weeks of Treatment with Losartan (50 mg/day), Valsartan (80 mg/day), Irbesartan (150 mg/day), or Olmesartan (20 mg/day) in a Randomized Double-blind Study[37,38]

and candesartan suggested that agents within the ARB class of drugs have comparable antihypertensive efficacy.[41] However, studies that have directly compared the effects of ARBs are beginning to reveal some differences among agents.[37,38,42–44] These differences among ARBs seem to be mainly related to selected dose and duration of action of drug, with longer-acting ARBs such as irbesartan, telmisartan, and olmesartan providing more effective 24-hour control of BP than shorter-acting agents such as losartan and valsartan, particularly over the latter stages of the dosing interval.

In addition to assessing the efficacy of an antihypertensive agent over an entire dosing interval, 24-hour ambulatory BP monitoring (ABPM) values may provide a more accurate assessment of a patient's risk for cardiovascular events than cuff BP values.[45,46] Several head-to-head trials of ARBs have used ABPM as an indication of comparative antihypertensive efficacy. A 6-week double-blind randomized placebo-controlled study that involved more than 200 patients with mild to moderate essential hypertension compared the antihypertensive efficacy of telmisartan 40 or 80 mg/day with losartan 50 mg/day. Analysis of ABPM results revealed both doses of telmisartan to be significantly more effective than losartan in reducing mean 24-hour diastolic and systolic BP (DBP and SBP) (Figure 81–2).[44] Compared with losartan, telmisartan

80 mg produced significantly greater reductions in DBP and SBP during all monitored periods (day, night, and morning), whereas telmisartan 40 mg produced significantly greater reductions in DBP and SBP during the nighttime period and DBP during the morning period.

Olmesartan is another ARB with a longer half-life that has been assessed using ABPM. An 8-week double-blind randomized trial involving more than 500 patients with mild to moderate essential hypertension compared olmesartan (20 mg/day) with losartan (50 mg/day), valsartan (80 mg/day), and irbesartan (150 mg/day). The dosages of ARBs used in this study were the recommended starting doses for these agents at the time the study was carried out. The results of this comparison showed that reductions in mean 24-hour day, night, and morning DBP and SBP with olmesartan were generally significantly greater than those obtained with losartan and valsartan and equivalent to reductions obtained with irbesartan (Table 81–2).[37,38] A similar study comparing olmesartan (20 mg/day) with candesartan (8 mg/day) also showed significantly greater reductions in mean 24-hour day, night, and morning DBP and SBP with olmesartan.[43]

Tolerability

The adverse event profile of ARBs is similar to that of placebo.[47,48] Moreover, unlike other antihypertensive drug

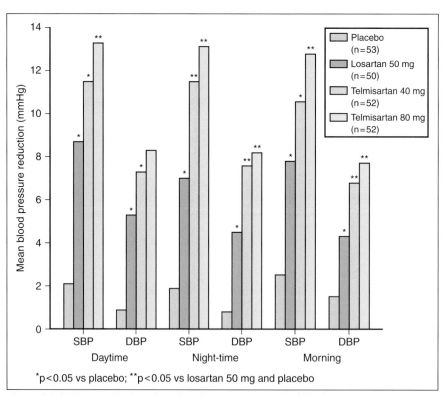

Figure 81–2. Mean reductions from baseline in mean systolic blood pressure (SBP) and diastolic blood pressure (DBP) for daytime (0600 to 2200 hours), nighttime (2201 to 0559 hours) and morning (0600 to 1159 hours) as measured by 24-hour ambulatory blood pressure monitoring after 6 weeks of therapy with telmisartan 40 or 80 mg/day, losartan 50 mg/day, or placebo in a randomized double-blind study. (Redrawn from Mallion J, Siche J, Lacourciere Y. ABPM comparison of the antihypertensive profiles of the selective angiotensin II receptor antagonists telmisartan and losartan in patients with mild-to-moderate hypertension. Reprinted by permission from Macmillan Publishers Ltd: *J Hum Hypertens* 1999;13(10):657–64, with permission.)

classes no clear class-specific adverse effects have been attributed to ARBs (Table 81–3).[48,49] The cough frequently encountered with ACE inhibitors is not an issue with ARBs, which makes them excellent alternatives for patients intolerant to ACE inhibitors.[50,51] Angio-oedema is another side effect of ACE inhibitors that seems to be related to the accumulation of bradykinin, although this may not be the only mechanism of action.[26] Some cases of angio-oedema have also been reported with losartan, but it is not clear that these cases are really linked to the drug.[17,48] The relative freedom of ARBs from adverse effects that limit compliance has contributed to enhanced patient adherence and low discontinuation rates associated with their use in clinical studies.[52–54] Patients also appear to be more likely to persist with long-term treatment when an ARB is prescribed as the initial agent.[54] ARBs also have no clinically important interactions with other agents commonly used in patients with hypertension,[48] indicating that they can be safely combined with other classes of antihypertensive agents.[55] The chronic nature of hypertension means that treatments are likely to be prescribed to patients for many years. In this regard, the excellent tolerability profile of ARBs is an important feature.

Dose and dosing intervals

ARBs have been shown to dose-dependently inhibit the pressor effects of exogenous angiotensin II.[34] However, dose recommendations for clinical use (Table 81–1) are based on antihypertensive efficacy, and ARBs are considered to have a rather flat BP dose-response curve.[40] Almost all ARBS have been shown to lower BP over 24 hours when given once per day in patients with mild to moderate hypertension.[40] However, although full blockade of angiotensin II around the clock is a clear therapeutic goal ARBs may not necessarily achieve this goal when administered according to prescribed doses as monotherapy.[56,57]

Blockade of the RAS for the duration of 24 hours can be achieved by combining relatively low ARB doses with an ACE inhibitor.[58] However, this strategy is limited by the side effects of ACE inhibition. It has also been shown that twice-daily administration of ARBs with a relatively short duration of action or an increase in dose for ARBs with longer durations of action can produce as much blockade of the RAS as adding an ACE inhibitor to currently recommended clinical doses.[59,60] Forclaz et al. demonstrated that when losartan 100 mg was given twice daily to normotensive subjects it produced a high degree of 24-hour RAS inhibition (77% blockade of SBP response to exogenous angiotensin I at trough). This was comparable to that achieved with losartan 100 mg once daily plus lisinopril 20 mg/day (76%), and approximately double the inhibition achieved with once-daily administration of losartan 100 mg (35%).[59] Possibly because of its longer half-life, a similar effect was not seen with twice-daily administration of telmisartan 80 mg.[59]

These results have been confirmed by the more recent findings of Hasler et al., who compared olmesartan with lisinopril in a similar context. They showed that olmesartan 20 mg/day produced a similar degree of 24-hour RAS inhibition to lisinopril 20 mg/day (58% of SBP response to angiotensin at trough for both). The combination of lisinopril 20 mg/day plus olmesartan 20 mg/day produced a higher degree of inhibition (80%), which was comparable to that produced by olmesartan 80 mg/day (76%).[60] Thus, in terms of blocking the vascular effects of angiotensin higher doses of longer-acting ARBs such as olmesartan are as effective as lower doses of the same compounds combined with an ACE inhibitor. Findings such as these provide a rationale for the use of higher doses of ARBs. Because ARBs do not exhibit any dose-dependent adverse effects, it is unlikely that there will be any safety concerns associated with increased dosing.[59,60]

ADVERSE EFFECT PROFILES OF ANTIHYPERTENSIVE DRUG CLASSES					
Adverse Effect	ARBs	ACE Inhibitors	Diuretics	β-blockers	CCBs
Headache	−	−	−	−	+
Flush	−	−	−	−	+[b]
Oedema	−	±[a]	−	−	+
Dyspnoea	−	−	−	+	−
Bradycardia/arrhythmia	−	−	−	+	+[c]
Fatigue	−	−	±	+	−
Cold extremities	−	−	−	+	−
Impotence	−	−	+	+	−
Gout	−	−	+	−	−
Cough	−	+	−	−	−
Orthostatic hypertension	−	−	+	−	−

+ indicates drug class-associated adverse effect; − indicates adverse effect not associated with drug class; ± indicates adverse effect may be associated with drug class. (Adapted from Mazzolai and Burnier.[48])
[a]Development of angio-oedema appears to involve accumulation of bradykinin, but it is not clear whether this is the unique mechanism[26]; [b]mainly with dihydropyridines; [c]occurring mainly with diltiazem and verapamil. ARBs = angiotensin II receptor blockers, ACE = angiotensin-converting enzyme, CCBs = calcium channel blockers.

Table 81–3. Adverse Effect Profiles of Antihypertensive Drug Classes

Outcome studies involving ARBs

The benefits of lowering BP are undisputed. However, because hypertension increases the risk of cardiovascular disease and other conditions a full range of outcomes are necessary to evaluate the efficacy of antihypertensive medication.[61] The best source of clinical evidence upon which physicians should base decisions about the treatment of patients is generally regarded as "hard endpoints" obtained from large randomized clinical trials with antihypertensive agents.[62] These include all-cause mortality, cardiovascular disease-specific mortality, and morbidity. Intervention trials are usually limited to a duration of =5 years, and thus it is often only when patients with high absolute cardiovascular risk are studied that differences in hard endpoint outcomes among antihypertensive drug classes are seen.[63] Consequently, many important outcome trials involving ARBs have been conducted in a range of patients at relatively high risk of morbidity and mortality from conditions such as cardiovascular disease and stroke (Table 81–4).

Studies in high-risk patients with hypertension

Various trials have been conducted with ARBs in hypertension, but there are three major cardiovascular outcome trials of ARBs in high-risk patients with hypertension that merit particular interest. These are the Losartan Intervention for Endpoint (LIFE) study,[64] the Study on Cognition and Prognosis in the Elderly (SCOPE),[65] and the Valsartan Antihypertensive Long-term Use Evaluation (VALUE) study.[55] Add-on treatment with diuretics and other antihypertensive drugs were permitted as required to lower BP to goal in all of these trials. Composite outcome endpoints, major cardiovascular outcome endpoints, and BP results from these three trials are outlined in Table 81–5.

LIFE

The LIFE study[64] provided some of the first evidence that ARBs may have possible cardiovascular protective effects beyond the powerful independent effects of lowering BP. In this large study, 9193 patients with primary hypertension and electrocardiographic evidence of left ventricular hypertrophy were randomly assigned to at least 4 years'

treatment with losartan or the β-blocker atenolol at equal doses (50 to 100 mg). The primary composite endpoint of cardiovascular mortality, stroke, and myocardial infarction was reached at a rate of 23.8 per 1000 patient-years of follow-up in the losartan group versus 27.9 with atenolol. This resulted in a significant 13% reduction of relative risk of the composite endpoint in the losartan-based treatment group compared to the atenolol-based regimen. The difference was due mainly to a highly significant 25% reduction in the relative risk of fatal or nonfatal stroke. Rates of myocardial infarction and cardiovascular mortality were not significantly different between the treatment groups. The losartan-based regimen produced substantial BP reductions that were similar to those obtained with the atenolol-based regimen. However, at the end of follow-up the reduction in sitting SBP was 1 mmHg greater with losartan than with atenolol.

Diabetes is a major independent indicator risk factor for cardiovascular disease, and patients with diabetes have at least a twofold higher risk of cardiovascular disease than nondiabetic individuals.[66] Diabetes is also closely associated with hypertension, and hypertension is approximately twice as common in patients with diabetes compared with nondiabetic patients.[67] Moreover, in patients who are already at high risk because of hypertension diabetes mellitus approximately doubles the risk of cardiovascular disease.[68] As expected, the incidences of cardiovascular morbidity and mortality in the subgroup of patients with diabetes who participated in the LIFE study were higher than in the overall population. The relative risk of the primary endpoint in the subgroup of patients with diabetes (n=1195) was significantly reduced by 24% with losartan versus atenolol ($p<0.05$), and the relative risk of death from cardiovascular disease was also significantly reduced (relative risk 0.63; $p<0.5$).[69] Adjustment for SBP had little effect on these results. Notably, in the lower-risk category of patients without vascular disease or diabetes the relative risk of the primary endpoint also significantly favored losartan (relative risk 0.82; $p<0.05$).

The overall LIFE trial results have led some to comment that a treatment strategy based on combining an ARB with a low dose of hydrochlorothiazide provides cardioprotection at least equal to that provided by β-blockers, greater protection from stroke (despite almost equal

KEY CLINICAL TRIALS INVOLVING ANGIOTENSIN II RECEPTOR BLOCKERS PER CLINICAL CONDITION			
High-risk Hypertension	Coronary Artery Disease/Myocardial Infarction	Diabetes Mellitus and/or Renal Disease	Congestive Heart Failure
LIFE[64]	VALIANT[87]	RENAAL[93]	ELITE I and II[84,85]
SCOPE[65]	OPTIMAAL[83]	IDNT[94]	Val-HeFT[81]
VALUE[71]		IRMA 2[92]	CHARM[100]
LIFE = Losartan Intervention for Endpoint Reduction in Hypertension, SCOPE = Study of Cognition and Prognosis in the Elderly, VALUE = Valsartan Antihypertensive Long-term Use Evaluation, VALIANT = VALsartan in Acute myocardial iNfarcTion, OPTIMAAL = Optimal Therapy in Myocardial Infarction with Angiotensin II Antagonist Losartan, RENAAL = Reduction of Endpoints in NIDDM with the Angiotensin II Antagonist Losartan, IDNT = Irbesartan Diabetic Nephropathy Trial, IRMA 2 = Irbesartan MicroAlbuminuria Type 2 Diabetes Mellitus, ELITE = Evaluation of Losartan in the Elderly, Val-HeFT = Valsartan in Heart Failure Trial, and Candesartan in Heart Failure-Assessment of Reduction in Mortality and Morbidity.			

Table 81–4. Key Clinical Trials Involving Angiotensin II Receptor Blockers per Clinical Condition

	LIFE		SCOPE		VALUE	
	Losartan	Atenolol	Candesartan	Placebo	Valsartan	Amlodipine
PRIMARY COMPOSITE AND COMPONENT CARDIOVASCULAR AND OUTCOME RESULTS FROM THE LOSARTAN INTERVENTION FOR ENDPOINT (LIFE) STUDY,[64] STUDY ON COGNITION AND PROGNOSIS IN THE ELDERLY (SCOPE),[65] AND THE VALSARTAN ANTIHYPERTENSIVE LONG-TERM USE EVALUATION (VALUE) STUDY[71]						
Primary composite outcome[a]:						
Rate/1000 patient-years	23.8	27.9	26.7	30.0	25.5	24.7
Relative risk for ARB vs. comparator (%)[b]	–13*		–11		+4	
Cardiac mortality:						
Rate/1000 patient-years	9.2	10.6	15.6	16.6	9.2	9.2
Relative risk for ARB vs comparator (%)[b]	–11		≈–5		+1	
Stroke[c]:						
Rate/1000 patient-years	10.8	14.5	7.4	10.3	10.0	8.7
Relative risk for ARB vs. comparator (%)[b]	–25**		–28*		+15	
Myocardial infarction[c]:						
Rate/1000 patient-years	9.2	8.7	5.9	5.2	11.4	9.6
Relative risk for ARB vs comparator (%)[b]	+7		≈+11		+19*	
Blood pressure reduction (mm Hg):						
SBP	30.2	29.1*	21.7	18.5**	15.2	17.3***
DBP	16.6	16.8	10.8	9.2**	8.2	9.9***

[a]LIFE composite endpoint = cardiovascular mortality, stroke and myocardial infarction; SCOPE composite endpoint = cardiovascular mortality, nonfatal stroke or nonfatal myocardial infarction; VALUE composite endpoint = sudden cardiac death, fatal or nonfatal myocardial infarction, death during or after percutaneous coronary intervention or coronary artery bypass graft, fatal heart failure, death associated with recent myocardial infarction on autopsy, heart failure requiring hospital management, or emergency procedures to prevent myocardial infarction. [b]In the LIFE study, relative risk was adjusted for degree of left ventricular hypertrophy and Framingham risk score at randomization. In the SCOPE study, adjustments were not specified. In the VALUE study, relative risk was adjusted for age, the presence of coronary heart disease, and the presence of left ventricular hypertrophy at baseline. [c] These outcomes refer to fatal or nonfatal events for the LIFE and VALUE studies, and to nonfatal events for the SCOPE study. *$p<0.05$; **$p''0.001$; ***$p<0.0001$.

Table 81–5. Primary Composite and Component Cardiovascular and Outcome Results from the Losartan Intervention for Endpoint (LIFE) Study,[64] Study on Cognition and Prognosis in the Elderly (SCOPE),[65] and the Valsartan Antihypertensive Long-term Use Evaluation (VALUE) Study[71]

BP control), and the benefit of fewer adverse effects.[63] There is, however, still room for improvement in terms of outcome. It has been hypothesized that because once-daily administration of losartan 100 mg cannot provide sustained high RAS blockade over 24 hours higher doses of losartan administered twice daily might enhance the differences in outcome between losartan and atenolol.[63] This again underlines the issue of dosing with ARBs and the need for clinical trials to assess the efficacy of using doses higher than those currently prescribed.

SCOPE

A significant ARB-associated reduction in the risk of stroke has been observed versus placebo in SCOPE, the first large-scale clinical trial to determine the effects of an ARB on cardiovascular outcomes in elderly patients.[65] A total of 4964 hypertensive elderly patients (mean age 76 years) were randomized to 3 to 5 years' treatment with candesartan 8 to 16 mg/day or placebo. However, it

should be noted that 84% of patients in the control group received active antihypertensive agents to control BP. A 10.9% risk reduction for candesartan versus placebo in the composite primary endpoint of major cardiovascular events (cardiovascular death, nonfatal myocardial infarction, and nonfatal stroke) was not statistically significant. The SCOPE researchers remarked that when compared with the control group the reductions in event rate seen in SCOPE were of similar magnitude to those observed in the losartan group versus atenolol in LIFE. As in the LIFE study, the effect of the ARB was driven by the reduction in stroke, with the risk of nonfatal stroke being significantly reduced by 28% in the candesartan treatment group. There were no significant differences between the treatment groups with regard to fatal, nonfatal, or total myocardial infarction; fatal stroke; cardiovascular mortality; or total mortality. A 3.2/1.6-mmHg greater reduction in BP was observed in favor of the candesartan group in the SCOPE study, which probably explains most of the reduction in nonfatal stroke observed with the ARB. Evidence from meta-regression analysis shows that even relatively small reductions in BP are important in terms of stroke reduction.[70]

VALUE

The aim of the VALUE study was to test the hypothesis that valsartan would be more effective than the calcium channel blocker amlodipine in preventing cardiac morbidity and mortality for the same degree of BP lowering.[71] In the VALUE study, 15,245 hypertensive patients at high cardiovascular risk were randomized to 4 to 6 years' treatment with antihypertensive regimens based on valsartan 80 to 160 mg/day or amlodipine 5 to 10 mg/day. There was no difference in the primary composite endpoint of cardiac morbidity and mortality between the two treatment groups. Stroke was less common in the amlodipine group, but the difference between the treatment groups did not reach statistical significance. Myocardial infarction was significantly more frequent in the valsartan group. Unfortunately for the interpretation of the trial results, patients treated with amlodipine-based therapy had significantly greater reductions in BP than patients treated with the valsartan-based regimen.

The differences in BP control in favor of amlodipine were sufficiently large to have major endpoint effects. These confounded the ability to test the primary hypothesis of VALUE, which was dependent on there being similar BP control between the two treatment groups.[72] One of the most interesting aspects of the VALUE data relates to the speed of onset of antihypertensive efficacy. After 1 month of treatment, BP control in the amlodipine group was substantially lower in the valsartan group (4.0/2.1 mmHg). This BP difference between the two groups had decreased to 2.1/1.6 mmHg by 6 months, and remained stable thereafter. For all endpoints, the highest odds ratios in favor of amlodipine were observed during the first 6 months of the trial (when BP differences between the treatment groups were greatest) (Figure 81–3). In the following months, when the difference in BP was relatively low, odds ratios were attenuated. In an attempt to overcome inequal-

ities in BP, serial median matching at 6 months was used to create 5006 valsartan-amlodipine patient pairs matched for SBP (mean 139.9 mmHg) and other variables. In this analysis, most outcomes (including the primary endpoint) were similar for the two regimens.[72]

During the latter stages of the VALUE trial, there was a persistent trend toward fewer admissions for heart failure in the valsartan group. However, the overall difference (which resulted in an 11% relative risk reduction) did not reach statistical significance.[71] In the post-hoc analysis of results, using serial median matching at 6 months the heart failure endpoint was significantly less likely with valsartan than with amlodipine ($p<0.05$).[72] The steady trend for a benefit of valsartan with regard to reduction of heart failure was consistent with the original VALUE study hypothesis and is also consistent with other research suggesting that a reduction in heart failure is seen with drugs that block the RAS.[70]

When data for both the valsartan and amlodipine treatment groups were pooled, immediate responders (patients who when switched from previous treatment to study drug had not increased in BP by 1 month, or those previously untreated who had an initial decrease in SBP of ≥10 mmHg) had significant advantages in relation to combined cardiac events, stroke, and all-cause death during the remainder of the study.[72] Such findings indicate that prompt control of BP, independent of drug type, was the main determinant of event rates in the VALUE study.

The results of the VALUE trial emphasize the importance of prompt BP lowering. Consequently, it has been recommended that instead of treatment initiation involving immediate rollover to a low dose of study drug (as occurred with valsartan in VALUE) more stringent initial control f BP should be an ethical requirement for clinical trials involving patients with hypertension.[72] It is, for example, important to adequately and rapidly titrate ARBs, and the addition of a low-dose thiazide diuretic at the first treatment step should be considered in high-risk hypertensive patients.[1,6] When the VALUE study was designed, the usual clinical dose range for valsartan was 80 to 160 mg/day. It has subsequently been shown that higher doses are

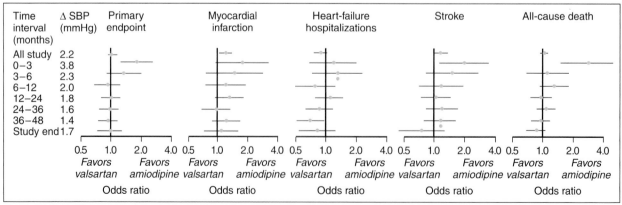

Figure 81–3. Differences in blood pressure between treatment groups, and odds ratios for the primary endpoint, secondary endpoints, and all-cause death during consecutive time periods in the VALUE study. Bars show 95% confidence intervals. (Redrawn from Julius S, Kjeldsen SE, Weber M, et al. Outcomes in hypertensive patients at high cardiovascular risk treated with regimens based on valsartan or amlodipine: The VALUE randomised trial. *Lancet* 2004;363(9426):2022–31, with permission from Elsevier.)

required for full angiotensin II blockade,[57] and a 160- to 320-mg/day dose range has now been approved. It should be noted that speed of onset of antihypertensive action is not an issue for ARBs, and that studies have shown substantial BP reduction with ARBs such as olmesartan and candesartan after a single week of treatment.[43]

Patients with isolated systolic hypertension

With increasing age, a gradual stiffening of the large arteries occurs, typically resulting in loss of elasticity and compliance and a consequent continuous elevation of SBP. Isolated systolic hypertension (ISH) is the most common form of hypertension in the elderly and a major risk factor for cardiovascular disease. Angiotensin II is believed to contribute to the development of endothelial dysfunction and vascular remodeling associated with hypertension, and it has been hypothesised that ARBs may be particularly useful in patients with ISH.[73]

The ISH substudy of LIFE involved 1326 patients with ISH (SBP between 160 and 200 mmHg and DBP <90 mmHg). This substudy demonstrated that compared to atenolol the adjusted relative risk of cardiovascular mortality was reduced by 46% with losartan ($p=0.01$), and the risk of stroke decreased by 40% ($p<0.05$).[74] BP was reduced by 28/9 mmHg in both arms of the study. These results are consistent with those reported in a subgroup analysis of outcome results in SCOPE patients with ISH (1518 patients had SBP >160 mmHg and DBP <90 mmHg) in which a reduction of 42% in the relative risk of stroke was observed for candesartan versus control.[75] BP reduction was slightly better with the candesartan-based regimen (2.0/1.2 mmHg advantage). It is possible that this small difference could account for part of the observed benefit with regard to stroke, but it was calculated that it should only account for a 15% difference between the treatment groups, suggesting that the beneficial effect of AT1 receptor blockade on stroke was not a result of BP reduction alone.[75]

Preventing new-onset diabetes mellitus

Several studies have suggested that blockade of the RAS may protect against the development of new-onset type 2 diabetes.[76] During the VALUE trial, the incidence of new-onset diabetes was significantly lower with valsartan-based than with amlodipine-based regimens (32 versus 41 cases per 1000 patient-years), resulting in a 23% relative risk reduction ($p<0.0001$).[71] There was a 25% risk reduction in the incidence of new-onset diabetes in the losartan treatment group relative to the atenolol treatment group during the LIFE trial ($p=0.001$).[64] During the SCOPE study, new-onset diabetes was reported in 4.3% of patients in the candesartan treatment group and 5.3% in the control group, but the difference did not reach statistical significance ($p=0.09$).[65] The SCOPE researchers commented that the lower rate of new-onset diabetes in the candesartan group versus the control group was similar in size to that observed in the LIFE study.

The VALUE results are particularly interesting because the calcium channel blocker comparison group is considered to be metabolically neutral, suggesting that AT1 receptor blockade had a positive effect on long-term glucose metabolism.[71] β-blockade, however, may decrease insulin sensitivity and increase the risk for the development of diabetes. Thus, a detrimental effect of atenolol may have contributed to the difference between losartan and atenolol with regard to new-onset diabetes in the LIFE study.[63,77,78] The SCOPE researchers also commented that a likely contribution to the reduced incidence of diabetes for patients receiving the ARB in their trial was that the use of diuretics and/or β-blockers reduced insulin sensitivity in the control group.[65]

It is well known that diabetes increases the cardiovascular consequences of hypertension. However, the duration of the VALUE trial was not long enough for cardiovascular complications of new-onset diabetes to emerge. Longer-term trials would be required to ascertain the true extent of benefits of ARBs on morbidity and mortality due to cardiovascular and renal disease in patients with hypertension.[79]

Patients with heart failure or acute myocardial infarction

The value of ACE inhibitors in reducing mortality rates and major nonfatal cardiovascular events in patients with chronic heart failure caused by left ventricular systolic dysfunction and in those with acute myocardial infarction is well established.[80] Evidence from clinical trials now suggests that when used at appropriate clinically effective doses ARB regimens lead to reductions in the risk of death and cardiovascular events in patients with heart failure and left ventricular systolic dysfunction or a high-risk acute myocardial infarction. The extent of these effects is comparable to that seen with ACE inhibitors, and additive benefits may be produced in patients with chronic heart failure when ARBs and ACE inhibitors are used in combination.[50,81–83]

Head-to-head comparisons of ARBs and ACE inhibitors

The 48-week Evaluation of Losartan in the Elderly (ELITE) study involved 722 ACE-inhibitor-naïve elderly patients with symptomatic heart failure. ELITE was designed to determine whether ARB blockade with losartan 50 mg once daily offered safety and efficacy advantages over ACE inhibition with captopril 50 mg three times daily.[84] As expected, losartan was generally better tolerated than captopril. However, unexpectedly a 46% risk reduction for all-cause mortality was seen with losartan compared to captopril ($p<0.05$). However, the ELITE II trial (n=3152), which was subsequently designed as a superiority trial to prospectively compare the two treatments on all-cause mortality, failed to find a significant difference between the treatment groups over a mean 1.5 years of follow-up (hazard ratio of 1.13 for total mortality in the losartan versus the captopril treatment group).[85] The once-daily 50-mg dose of losartan used in the ELITE trials was certainly too low to be optimally effective and provide reliable results. This led to the initiation of a heart failure outcome trial in which losartan 50 mg is being compared to 150 mg/day.[86]

In the Optimal Therapy in Myocardial Infarction with the Angiotensin II Antagonist Losartan (OPTIMAAL) trial,[83] 5477 patients with acute myocardial infarction and signs or symptoms of heart failure during the acute phase were randomized to the same losartan/captopril regimens used in the ELITE studies and followed for a mean 2.7 years. A nonsignificant difference in the primary total mortality outcome was seen in favor of captopril (relative risk 1.13, $p=0.07$), and non-inferiority of losartan could not be proved.

Subsequently, in the Valsartan in Acute Myocardial iNfarcTion (VALIANT) trial[87] valsartan 160 mg once daily was found to be as effective as captopril 50 mg twice daily in reducing the risk of major cardiovascular events in patients after acute myocardial infarction. In the VALIANT trial, 14,703 patients with acute myocardial infarction complicated by heart failure, left ventricular dysfunction, or both were randomized to one of three treatment arms: valsartan 160 mg bid, captopril 50 mg tid, or a combination of valsartan 80 mg bid + captopril 50 mg tid and followed for a median of 25 months. The risks of mortality from any cause and from cardio-vascular mortality were similar in the three treatment groups. In an imputed placebo analysis, valsartan was shown to preserve 99.6% of the mortality benefit of captopril. The rate of the secondary endpoint of death from cardiovascular causes, recurrent myocardial infarction, or hospitalization for heart failure was also similar in the three groups.

Combining an ARB and an ACE inhibitor

The Valsartan Heart Failure Trial (Val-HeFT)[81] and the Candesartan in Heart Failure: Assessment of Reduction in Mortality and Morbidity (CHARM)-Added trial[82] found that addition of an ARB to standard therapy involving ACE inhibitors provided additive clinical benefits in patients with chronic heart failure. This is in apparent contrast to the results of the VALIANT trial, which indicated no such benefits of combining an ARB with ACE inhibitor therapy in high-risk acute myocardial infarction patients.[87] However, it should be noted that the results of Val-HeFT were driven by the small subgroup (7%) of patients who did not receive an ACE inhibitor because of intolerance.

In the Val-HeFt trial, patients (n=5010) were random-ized to placebo or valsartan 160 mg twice daily, which were added to standard treatment (this included an ACE inhibitor in 93% of patients) and followed for a mean of 23 months. Although there was no reduction in mortality (relative risk 1.02), valsartan significantly reduced the risk of the composite co-primary endpoint (mortality, cardiac arrest with resuscitation, hospitalization for heart failure, or administration of inotropic or vasodilator drugs for =4 hours without hospitalization) by 13.2% ($p<0.01$). This was mainly driven by a 27.5% reduction in the risk of hospitalization for heart failure ($p<0.001$).

In CHARM-Added, patients taking an ACE inhibitor (n=2548) were randomized to either placebo or a target dose of candesartan 32 mg once daily and followed for a mean of 41 months. Candesartan significantly reduced the risk of the primary outcome (cardiovascular death or hospitalization for worsening heart failure) by 15%, and the risk of both primary endpoint components was also significantly reduced from 16 to 17% ($p<0.05$ for all outcomes). It has been suggested that the cardiovascular mortality benefit associated with the ARB in the CHARM-Added study may have been due to the fact that these patients had more advanced disease over a longer follow-up than patients in Val-HeFT.[86,88]

In CHARM, many patients with chronic heart failure remained symptomatic despite treatment with an ACE inhibitor. One consequence of this is that "ACE escape" could have occurred in such patients, resulting over time in increased levels of angiotensin II.[86] In contrast, only 14% of the VALIANT patients had previous chronic heart failure and many may have had relatively short-lived activation of the RAS, in which environment an ARB and ACE inhibitor were started simultaneously. In addition, different ARB inhibitor doses used in the VALIANT, CHARM-Added, and Val-HeFT trials may have affected outcomes, and this appears to be a much more likely explanation. In the VALIANT combination arm, the dose of valsartan was half that used in both the monotherapy arm and Val-HeFT study. Thus, it was unlikely that the relatively low dose of valsartan was equivalent to the dose of candesartan used in CHARM-Added.

An ARB as an alternative to an ACE inhibitor

The CHARM-Alternative trial[50] was the first randomized trial to evaluate an ARB in ACE inhibitor-intolerant patients with chronic heart failure. Patients (n=2028), most of whom were unable to take ACE inhibitors because of cough (72%), were randomized to placebo or a target dose of candesartan 32 mg once daily and followed for a median duration of 33.7 months. The risk of death from a cardiovascular cause or hospitalization for heart failure was significantly reduced by 23% with candesartan ($p<0.001$). The researchers noted that this result was similar in magnitude to reductions in these outcomes previously seen with ACE inhibitors in other trials. Risk reduction for the primary endpoint was mainly driven by a 32% relative risk reduction of hospital admission for heart failure ($p<0.0001$). Reduction in the risk of cardiovascular death in patients receiving valsartan (hazard ratio of 0.85) was not statistically significant, but did reach significance in a covariate-adjusted analysis (hazard ratio 0.80; $p<0.05$). Candesartan was almost as well tolerated as placebo in the CHARM-Alternative ACE-inhibitor intolerant group of patients.

Renal protection in patients with type 2 diabetes

In general, chronic renal disease can be a cause or conse-quence of hypertension. The majority of patients with chronic renal disease have hypertension, and without intervention this can result in a vicious cycle of worsening renal function and hypertension.[89,90] Diabetic renal disease is consequently closely linked with cardiovascular disease, and there are many similarities between renal and cardiovascular disease regarding the role of endothe-lial dysfunction and angiotensin-II-mediated cellular proliferation.[91]

Trials such as the Irbesartan MicroAlbuminuria Type 2 Diabetes Mellitus (IRMA 2),[92] Reduction of Endpoints in NIDDM with the Angiotensin II Antagonist Losartan (RENAAL),[93] and the Irbesartan Diabetic Nephropathy Trial (IDNT)[94] suggested that ARBs may have renoprotective effects that are independent of BP-lowering effects in patients with diabetes. Also worthy of mention is the more recent Angiotensin-Receptor Blockade Versus Converting-Enzyme Inhibition in Type 2 Diabetes and Nephropathy (DETAIL) study. This demonstrated that antihypertensive treatment based on the ARB telmisartan was equivalent to therapy based on the ACE inhibitor enalapril in providing renoprotection, as assessed by change in glomerular filtration rate in hypertensive patients with type 2 diabetes and early nephropathy.[95]

Patients with microalbuminuria

One of the earliest markers of nephropathy is microalbuminuria, a persistent increased urinary albumin excretion (UAE) rate of 20 to 200 µg/min or an albumin-to-creatinine ratio of 30/300 mg/g.[96] Microalbuminuria is more prevalent in diabetic and hypertensive populations,[97] and is a known risk factor for progression to further stages of nephropathy as well as for cardiovascular risk in patients with hypertension.[1,3] Clinical studies with ARBs have shown that they can reduce the rate of progression of diabetic nephropathy.

A total of 590 hypertensive patients with type 2 diabetes and persistent microalbuminuria were enrolled in the IRMA 2 trial, a randomized placebo-controlled 2-year trial of irbesartan at a dose of either 150 mg/day or 300 mg/day.[92] Over the course of the study, irbesartan reduced the rate of progression to clinical macroalbuminuria (a more advanced and clinically overt stage of nephropathy). After adjustment for the baseline level of microalbuminuria and the BP level achieved during the study, the relative risk of diabetic nephropathy was reduced by 44% for irbesartan 150 mg compared with placebo ($p=0.05$) and by 68% in the 300-mg group ($p<0.001$). This again highlights the importance of complete blockade of the RAS, independent of BP control.

The DETAIL study randomly assigned 250 patients with type 2 diabetes and early nephropathy (approximately 82% of whom had microalbuminuria) to receive telmisartan 80 mg/day or enalapril 20 mg/day.[95] After 5 years, the difference between the treatment groups in mean change in glomerular filtration was –3.0 ml/min/1.73m² (95% confidence interval –7.6 to 1.6 ml/min/1.73m²). The lower 95% confidence interval boundary of –7.6 ml/min/1.73m² was greater than –10 ml/min/1.73m, which was the predefined level for a clinically significant difference between the groups—indicating that telmisartan was not inferior to enalapril. The study authors commented that with respect to renoprotection the results of the DETAIL study were consistent with those of the IRMA 2 trial.

Patients with macroalbuninuria

ARBs delayed progression from macroalbuminuria toward end-stage renal disease in the IDNT and the RENAAL studies.[93,94] Both of these studies were designed to investigate the effects of ARBs on renal outcomes in patients with type 2 diabetes mellitus and overt nephropathy. In RENAAL, in addition to their standard antihypertensive therapy 1523 patients were randomized to receive losartan (50 to 100 mg/day) or placebo, and were followed up for a mean of 3.4 years. The IDNT study enrolled 1715 patients who were randomized to receive irbesartan 300 mg/day, amlodipine 10 mg/day, or placebo and followed for a mean 2.6 years. The primary outcome in both trials was a composite endpoint of a doubling of the baseline serum creatinine concentration, end-stage renal disease, or death. As shown in Table 81–6, risk of the primary endpoint was significantly reduced in both studies. A slowing of the rate of progression of nephropathy was reflected in a significant increase in the time to a doubling of the serum creatinine concentration, which is a measure that approximates a halving of the glomerular filtration rate. In the RENAAL study, losartan reduced the risk of end-stage renal disease by 28%. Patients treated with amlodipine in the IDNT trial had worse renal outcomes than those in the irbesartan group, although there was

RISK OF PRIMARY COMPOSITE AND COMPONENT ENDPOINTS IN THE REDUCTION OF ENDPOINTS IN NIDDM WITH THE ANGIOTENSIN II ANTAGONIST LOSARTAN (RENAAL) STUDY[93] AND THE IRBESARTAN DIABETIC NEPHROPATHY TRIAL (IDNT)[94]

| | Unadjusted Difference in Risk (%) | | |
| | IDNT | | RENAAL |
	Irbesartan vs. Placebo	Irbesartan vs. Amlodipine	Losartan vs. Placebo
Primary composite outcome[a]	–20*	–23**	–16*
Doubling of serum creatinine concentration	–33**	–37***	–25**
End-stage renal disease	–23	–23	–28**
Death	–8	+4	+2

[a]Doubling of the serum creatinine concentration, end-stage renal disease, or all-cause death.
*$p<0.05$; **$p<0.01$; ***$p<0.001$.

Table 81–6. Risk of Primary Composite and Component Endpoints in the Reduction of Endpoints in NIDDM with the Angiotensin II Antagonist Losartan (RENAAL) Study[93] and the Irbesartan Diabetic Nephropathy Trial (IDNT)[94]

equal control of BP in the two groups. Corrections for any disparities in BP control between the treatment groups did not reverse the renoprotective effects afforded by the ARBs in either study.

Patients with normoalbuminuria

Diabetic nephropathy develops slowly, and the early pathologic changes of extracellular matrix accumulation in the glomeruli and interstitium are clinically silent. Thus, nephropathy has already started by the time microalbuminuria is detected. Studies such as IRMA 2 and IDNT strongly suggest that interfering with the RAS has renoprotective benefits. However, the patients in those studies already had clinically detectable diabetic nephropathy. Thus, the question remains as to the extent of the benefit that might be possible with earlier inhibition of the RAS (i.e., in diabetic patients without any overt clinical signs nephropathy).

The Bergamo Nephrologic Diabetes Complications (BENEDICT) study recruited patients with diabetes and hypertension who were normoalbuminuric. This study showed that ACE inhibition was able to reduce the development of microalbuminuria compared to the calcium channel blockade.[98] However, the possible benefits of ARBs in diabetic patients without overt nephropathy are not yet known. This question is now being addressed by the Randomized Olmesartan and Diabetes Microalbuminuria Prevention (ROADMAP) study. This primary prevention study has been designed to determine whether olmesartan can prevent or delay the development of microalbuminuria in patients with type 2 diabetes and normoalbuminuria who are at risk of developing nephropathy due to the presence of at least one cardiovascular risk factor. In addition to assessing olmesartan's effects on microalbuminuria, the design and size of the ROADMAP study are such that it should allow assessment of whether such early intervention will translate into protection from cardiovascular and renal events and mortality.[99] Such studies would help provide conclusive answers about whether BP reduction alone is responsible for renal protection or whether inhibiting the RAS is also required for these benefits.

Recommendations regarding use of ARBs in clinical practice

Evidence suggests that specific drug classes may have benefits that may extend their BP-lowering effects and that may be particularly beneficial for certain groups of patients.[1,3] As mentioned previously, reducing the risk of cardiovascular disease should be the main aim of therapy (rather than simply reducing elevated BP). The choice of drugs for individual patients should be tailored to the patients' risk profile, including the presence or absence of target organ damage, clinical cardiovascular or renal disease, or diabetes.

Randomized clinical trials have demonstrated that ARBs have clinical benefits in a range of conditions that predispose patients to cardiovascular events, including left ventricular hypertrophy, isolated systolic hypertension, diabetes, micro- or macroalbuminuria, heart failure, and coronary artery disease.[64,69,74,81,83,87,92,94,100] The results of

these trials are reflected in both U.S. and European hypertension management guidelines, which list heart failure with left ventricular systolic dysfunction, diabetes, and kidney disease as conditions in which there is compelling clinical evidence favoring the use of ARBs.[1,3] A role for ARBs as alternatives to ACE inhibitors (especially in patients intolerant of ACE inhibitors, or as additions to ACE inhibitors in patients with heart failure) is recommended.[1,3] Here, of course, it should be remembered that when used at a sufficiently high dose or with a more frequent dosing interval ARBs can produce the same degree of RAS inhibition as the addition of an ARB to an ACE inhibitor (without the side effects of ACE inhibitors). As well as supporting the use of ARBs as effective alternative or additional therapies to ACE inhibitors in patients with chronic heart failure, recent chronic heart failure guidelines state that use of ARBs should be considered in ACE inhibitor-intolerant patients with acute myocardial infarction complicated by heart failure and/or left ventricular systolic dysfunction.[101]

In terms of renoprotection, ARBs are suggested as a logical first choice for inclusion in the antihypertensive regimens of patients with diabetes mellitus and hypertension.[1,3] Recent guidelines for the management of chronic kidney disease specifically recommend ARBs as preferred antihypertensive agents for patients with diabetic renal disease or nondiabetic renal disease with albuminuria.[102]

The future for ARBs

In addition to hypertension, ARBs have been approved for use (or are either registered or in pre-registration stages) for several other indications, including congestive heart failure, post-myocardial infarction, and diabetic nephropathy. In addition, ongoing and planned trials are likely to extend the indications for which ARBs are approved even further. Pharmaceutical companies and research institutions now register the clinical studies with which they are involved, and this provides insights into possible directions for agents in clinical development.

Searching Internet sites that list these trials (such as *http://clinicaltrials.gov/* and *http://www.controlledtrials.com/*) reveals that a considerable number of studies involving ARB have been completed, are in progress, or are being prepared. The diabetes-sparing potential of ARBs is being investigated in trials such as the ongoing Nateglinide and Valsartan in Impaired Glucose Tolerance Outcomes Research (NAVIGATOR) trial.[103] The effects of ARBs in patients with atherosclerosis are uncertain, but studies such as the Effect of Valsartan on Endothelial Function, Oxidative Stress, Carotid Atherosclerosis, and Endothelial Progenitor Cells (EFFERVESCENT) trial and the Multi-centre Olmesartan Atherosclerosis Regression Evaluation (MORE) trial are likely to change this. If successful, such studies may further increase the number of indications for which ARBs are approved.

Many patients with hypertension will require at least 2 antihypertensive medications to achieve BP goals, and treatment guidelines suggest that one of these should be a thiazide diuretic.[1,3] The antihypertensive efficacy of ARBs has been shown to be potentiated by the addition of a thiazide diuretic,[40] and several ARBs are now available or being launched as fixed combination treatments with hydrochlorothiazide. Significant cardiovascular benefits have been reported with calcium channel blockers (CCBs),[104] and studies of treatments combining these with ARBs are also ongoing or planned.

Multifactorial interventions that combine agents that target different aspects of cardiovascular risk may provide a means for more effective reduction of cardiovascular risk.[105] Thus, agents such as statins may come to play an important role in reducing cardiovascular risk in patients with hypertension, and combinations of ARBs with statins is a logical development. The future is likely to see more developments involving rational combinations of different

drug classes for use in high-risk patients. Such combinations are likely to be based on long-term reduction of risk of cardiovascular and other diseases, such as diabetes and nephropathy. As such, it is apparent that ARBs are uniquely placed in terms of their known and potential efficacy and excellent tolerability profile and are likely to play an increasingly central role in the management of hypertension and cardiovascular risk.

ACKNOWLEDGMENTS

I would like to thank Phil Jones and Joanne Dalton of Adis Communications, who provided editorial support during the writing of this chapter.

REFERENCES

1. Chobanian AV, Bakris GL, Black HR, Cushman WC, Green LA, Izzo JL Jr., et al. The Seventh Report of the Joint National Committee on Prevention, Detection, Evaluation, and Treatment of High Blood Pressure: The JNC 7 report. *JAMA* 2003;289(19):2560–72.

2. Lewington S, Clarke R, Qizilbash N, Peto R, and Collins R. Age-specific relevance of usual blood pressure to vascular mortality: a meta-analysis of individual data for one million adults in 61 prospective studies. *Lancet* 2002; 360(9349):1903–13.

3. 2003 European Society of Hypertension-European Society of Cardiology guidelines for the management of arterial hypertension. *J Hypertens* 2003;21(6):1011–53.

4. Hansson L, Zanchetti A, Carruthers SG, Dahlof B, Elmfeldt D, Julius S, et al. Effects of intensive blood-pressure lowering and low-dose aspirin in patients with hypertension: Principal results of the Hypertension Optimal Treatment (HOT) randomised trial. HOT Study Group. *Lancet* 1998; 351(9118):1755–62.

5. Neal B, MacMahon S, Chapman N. Effects of ACE inhibitors, calcium antagonists, and other blood-pressure-lowering drugs: Results of prospectively designed overviews of randomised trials. Blood Pressure Lowering Treatment Trialists' Collaboration. *Lancet* 2000;356(9246):1955–64.

6. European Society of Hypertension-European Society of Cardiology, 2003 European Society of Hypertension-European Society of Cardiology guidelines for the management of arterial hypertension. *J Hypertens* 2003;21(6):1011–53.

7. Brewster UC, Setaro JF, Perazella MA. The renin-angiotensin-aldosterone system: Cardiorenal effects and implications for renal and cardiovascular disease states. *Am J Med Sci* 2003; 326(1):15–24.

8. Jacoby DS, Rader DJ. Renin-angiotensin system and atherothrombotic disease: From genes to treatment. *Arch Intern Med* 2003;163(10):1155–64.

9. Carey RM, Siragy HM. Newly recognized components of the renin-angiotensin system: Potential roles in cardiovascular and renal regulation. *Endocr Rev* 2003;24(3):261–71.

10. Johnston CI, Volhard Lecture F.. Renin-angiotensin system: A dual tissue and hormonal system for cardiovascular control. *J Hypertens Suppl* 1992;10(7):S13–26.

11. Kim S, Iwao H. Molecular and cellular mechanisms of angiotensin II-mediated cardiovascular and renal diseases. *Pharmacol Rev* 2000;52(1):11–34.

12. Volpe M, Savoia C, De Paolis P, Ostrowska B, Tarasi D, Rubattu S. The renin-angiotensin system as a risk factor and therapeutic target for cardiovascular and renal disease. *J Am Soc Nephrol* 2002;13(Suppl 3):S173–78.

13. Nickenig G, Harrison DG. The AT(1)-type angiotensin receptor in oxidative stress and atherogenesis. Part I: Oxidative stress and atherogenesis. *Circulation* 2002;105(3):393–96.

14. Cheng ZJ, Vapaatalo H, Mervaala E. Angiotensin II and vascular inflammation. *Med Sci Monit* 2005; 11(6):RA194–205.

15. Dzau VJ. Theodore Cooper Lecture: Tissue angiotensin and pathobiology of vascular disease: a unifying hypothesis. *Hypertension* 2001; 37(4):1047–52.

16. Dzau V. The cardiovascular continuum and renin-angiotensin-aldosterone system blockade. *J Hypertens Suppl* 2005;23(1):S9–17.

17. Burnier M, Brunner HR. Angiotensin II receptor antagonists. *Lancet* 2000; 355(9204):637–45.

18. Effect of enalapril on mortality and the development of heart failure in asymptomatic patients with reduced left ventricular ejection fractions. The SOLVD Investigattors. *N Engl J Med* 1992;327(10):685–91.

19. Pfeffer MA, Braunwald E, Moye LA, Basta L, Brown EJ Jr., Cuddy TE, et al. Effect of captopril on mortality and morbidity in patients with left ventricular dysfunction after myocardial infarction: Results of the survival and ventricular enlargement trial. The SAVE Investigators. *N Engl J Med* 1992; 327(10):669–77.

20. Yusuf S, Sleight P, Pogue J, Bosch J, Davies R, Dagenais G. Effects of an angiotensin-converting-enzyme inhibitor, ramipril, on cardiovascular events in high-risk patients. The Heart Outcomes Prevention Evaluation Study Investigators. *N Engl J Med* 2000; 342(3):145–53.

21. Lewis EJ, Hunsicker LG, Bain RP, Rohde RD. The effect of angiotensin-converting-enzyme inhibition on diabetic nephropathy. The Collaborative Study Group. *N Engl J Med* 1993;329(20):1456–62.

22. Randomised trial of a perindopril-based blood-pressure-lowering regimen among 6,105 individuals with previous stroke or transient ischaemic attack. *Lancet* 2001;358(9287):1033–41.

23. Effects of enalapril on mortality in severe congestive heart failure. Results of the Cooperative North Scandinavian Enalapril Survival Study (CONSENSUS). The CONSENSUS Trial Study Group. *N Engl J Med* 1987; 316(23):1429–35.

24. Khalil ME, Basher AW, Brown EJ Jr., Alhaddad IA. A remarkable medical story: Benefits of angiotensin-converting enzyme inhibitors in cardiac patients. *J Am Coll Cardiol* 2001;37(7):1757–64.

25. Israili ZH, Hall WD. Cough and angioneurotic edema associated with angiotensin-converting enzyme inhibitor therapy: A review of the literature and pathophysiology. *Ann Intern Med* 1992;117(3):234–42.

26. Nussberger J, Cugno M, Amstutz C, Cicardi M, Pellacani A, Agostoni A. Plasma bradykinin in angio-oedema. *Lancet* 1998;351(9117):1693–97.

27. Wagenaar LJ, Voors AA, Buikema H, van Gilst WH. Angiotensin receptors in the cardiovascular system. *Can J Cardiol* 2002;18(12):1331–39.

28. Oliverio MI, Coffman TM. Angiotensin-II-receptors: New targets for antihypertensive therapy. *Clin Cardiol* 1997;20(1):3–6.

29. Munzenmaier DH, Greene AS. Opposing actions of angiotensin II on microvascular growth and arterial blood pressure. *Hypertension* 1996; 27(3 Pt 2):760–65.

30. Hein L, Barsh GS, Pratt RE, Dzau VJ, Kobilka BK. Behavioural and cardiovascular effects of disrupting the angiotensin II type-2 receptor in mice. *Nature* 1995;377(6551):744–47.

31. D'Amore A, Black MJ, Thomas WG. The angiotensin II type 2 receptor causes constitutive growth of cardiomyocytes and does not antagonize angiotensin II type 1 receptor-mediated hypertrophy. *Hypertension* 2005;46(6):1347–54.

32. Reudelhuber TL. The continuing saga of the AT2 receptor: A case of the good, the bad, and the innocuous. *Hypertension* 2005.;6(6):1261–62.

33. Gradman AH, Schmieder RE, Lins RL, Nussberger J, Chiang Y, Bedigian MP. Aliskiren, a novel orally effective renin inhibitor, provides dose-dependent antihypertensive efficacy and placebo-like tolerability in hypertensive patients. *Circulation* 2005;111(8):1012–18.

34. Burnier M, Maillard M. The comparative pharmacology of angiotensin II receptor antagonists. *Blood Press* 2001;10(S1):6–11.

35. Vanderheyden PM, Fierens FL, De Backer JP, Fraeyman N, Vauquelin G. Distinction between surmountable and insurmountable selective AT1 receptor antagonists by use of CHO-K1 cells expressing human angiotensin II AT1 receptors. *Br J Pharmacol* 1999;126(4):1057–65.

36. Mizuno M, Sada T, Ikeda M, Fukuda N, Miyamoto M, Yanagisawa H, et al. Pharmacology of CS-866, a novel nonpeptide angiotensin II receptor antagonist. *Eur J Pharmacol* 1995;285(2):181–88.

37. Oparil S, Williams D, Chrysant SG, Marbury TC, Neutel J. Comparative efficacy of olmesartan, losartan, valsartan, and irbesartan in the control of essential hypertension. *J Clin Hypertens (Greenwich)* 2001;3(5):283–91,318.

38. Smith DH, Dubiel R, Jones M. Use of 24-hour ambulatory blood pressure monitoring to assess antihypertensive efficacy: A comparison of olmesartan medoxomil, losartan potassium, valsartan, and irbesartan. *Am J Cardiovasc Drugs* 2005;5(1):41–50.

39. Brunner H, Arakawa K. Antihypertensive efficacy of olmesartan medoxomil and candesartan cilexetil in achieving 24-hour blood pressure reductions and ambulatory blood pressure goals. *Clin Drug Invest* 2005 (submitted).

40. Burnier M. Angiotensin II type 1 receptor blockers. *Circulation* 2001; 103(6):904–12.

41. Conlin PR, Spence JD, Williams B, Ribeiro AB, Saito I, Benedict C, et al. Angiotensin II antagonists for hypertension: are there differences in efficacy? *Am J Hypertens* 2000; 13(4 Pt 1):418–26.

42. Kassler-Taub K, Littlejohn T, Elliott W, Ruddy T, Adler E. Comparative efficacy of two angiotensin II receptor antagonists, irbesartan and losartan in mild-to-moderate hypertension. Irbesartan/Losartan Study Investigators. *Am J Hypertens* 1998;11(4 Pt 1):445–53.

43. Brunner HR, Stumpe KO, Januszewicz A. Antihypertensive efficacy of olmesartan medoxomil and candesartan cilexetil assessed by 24-hour ambulatory blood pressure monitoring in patients with essential hypertension. *Clin Drug Invest* 2003; 23(7):419–430.

44. Mallion J, Siche J, Lacourciere Y. ABPM comparison of the antihypertensive profiles of the selective angiotensin II receptor antagonists telmisartan and losartan in patients with mild-to-moderate hypertension. *J Hum Hypertens* 1999;13(10):657–64.

45. Clement DL, De Buyzere ML, De Bacquer DA, De Leeuw PW, Duprez DA, Fagard RH, et al. Prognostic value of ambulatory blood-pressure recordings in patients with treated hypertension. *N Engl J Med* 2003;348(24):2407–15.

46. Staessen JA, Thijs L, Fagard R, O'Brien ET, Clement D, de Leeuw PW, et al. Predicting cardiovascular risk using conventional vs ambulatory blood pressure in older patients with systolic hypertension. Systolic Hypertension in Europe Trial Investigators. *JAMA* 1999; 282(6):539–46.

47. Mancia G, Seravalle G, Grassi G. Tolerability and treatment compliance with angiotensin II receptor antagonists. *Am J Hypertens* 2003;16(12):1066–73.

48. Mazzolai L, Burnier M. Comparative safety and tolerability of angiotensin II receptor antagonists. *Drug Saf* 1999; 21(1):23–33.

49. McDonald MA, Simpson SH, Ezekowitz JA, Gyenes G, Tsuyuki RT. Angiotensin receptor blockers and risk of myocardial infarction: systematic review. *BMJ* 2005;331(7521):873.

50. Granger CB, McMurray JJ, Yusuf S, Held P, Michelson EL, Olofsson B, et al. Effects of candesartan in patients with chronic heart failure and reduced left-ventricular systolic function intolerant to angiotensin-converting-enzyme inhibitors: the CHARM-Alternative trial. *Lancet* 2003;362(9386):772–76.

51. Lacourciere Y, Lefebvre J. Modulation of the renin-angiotensin-aldosterone system and cough. *Can J Cardiol* 1995; 11(Suppl F):33F–39F.

52. Oparil S, Silfani TN, Walker JF. Role of angiotensin receptor blockers as monotherapy in reaching blood pressure goals. *Am J Hypertens* 2005; 18(2 Pt 1):287–94.

53. Bloom BS. Continuation of initial antihypertensive medication after 1 year of therapy. *Clin Ther* 1998; 20(4):671–81.

54. Gerth WC. Compliance and persistence with newer antihypertensive agents. *Curr Hypertens Rep* 2002; 4(6):424–33.

55. Volpe M, Tocci G, Pagannone E. Angiotensin II-receptor antagonist in the treatment of hypertension. *Curr Hypertens Rep* 2005;7(4):287–93.

56. Mazzolai L, Maillard M, Rossat J, Nussberger J, Brunner HR, Burnier M. Angiotensin II receptor blockade in normotensive subjects: A direct comparison of three AT1 receptor antagonists. *Hypertension* 1999; 33(3):850–55.

57. Maillard MP, Wurzner G, Nussberger J, Centeno C, Burnier M, Brunner HR Comparative angiotensin II receptor blockade in healthy volunteers: The importance of dosing. *Clin Pharmacol Ther* 2002;71(1):68–76.

58. Azizi M, Menard J. Combined blockade of the renin-angiotensin system with angiotensin-converting enzyme inhibitors and angiotensin II type 1 receptor antagonists. *Circulation* 2004;109(21):2492–99.

59. Forclaz A, Maillard M, Nussberger J, Brunner HR, Burnier M. Angiotensin II receptor blockade: Is there truly a benefit of adding an ACE inhibitor? *Hypertension* 2003;41(1):31–6.

60. Hasler C, Nussberger J, Maillard M, Forclaz A, Brunner HR, Burnier M. Sustained 24-hour blockade of the renin-angiotensin system: a high dose of a long-acting blocker is as effective as a lower dose combined with an angiotensin-converting enzyme inhibitor. *Clin Pharmacol Ther* 2005; 78(5):501–07.

61. Weber M. Guidelines for assessing outcomes of antihypertensive treatment. *Am J Cardiol* 1999; 84(2A):2K–4K.

62. Conlin P. Redifining efficacy of antihypertensive therapies beyond blood pressure reduction: The role of angiotensin II antagonists. *Int J Clin Pract* 2005;59(2):214–24.

63. Brunner HR, Gavras H. Angiotensin blockade for hypertension: A promise fulfilled. *Lancet* 2002;359(9311): 990–92.

64. Dahlof B, Devereux RB, Kjeldsen SE, Julius S, Beevers G, de Faire U, et al. Cardiovascular morbidity and mortality in the Losartan Intervention For Endpoint reduction in hypertension study (LIFE): A randomised trial against atenolol. *Lancet* 2002;359(9311): 995–1003.

65. Lithell H, Hansson L, Skoog I, Elmfeldt D, Hofman A, Olofsson B, et al. The Study on Cognition and Prognosis in the Elderly (SCOPE): Principal results of a randomized double-blind intervention trial. *J Hypertens* 2003;21(5):875–86.

66. Howard BV, Rodriguez BL, Bennett PH, Harris MI, Hamman R, Kuller LH, et al. Prevention Conference VI: Diabetes and Cardiovascular Disease. Writing Group I: Epidemiology. *Circulation* 2002;105(18):e132–37.

67. National High Blood Pressure Education Program Working Group, National High Blood Pressure Education Program Working Group report on hypertension in diabetes. *Hypertension* 1994;23(2): 145–58;discussion 159–60.

68. Zanchetti A, Ruilope LM. Antihypertensive treatment in patients with type-2 diabetes mellitus: What guidance from recent controlled randomized trials? *J Hypertens* 2002; 20(11):2099–2110.

69. Lindholm LH, Ibsen H, Dahlof B, Devereux RB, Beevers G, de Faire U, et al. Cardiovascular morbidity and mortality in patients with diabetes in the Losartan Intervention For Endpoint reduction in hypertension study (LIFE): A randomised trial against atenolol. *Lancet* 2002;359(9311):1004–10.

70. Staessen JA, Wang JG, Thijs L. Cardiovascular prevention and blood pressure reduction: A quantitative overview updated until 1 March 2003. *J Hypertens* 2003;21(6):1055–76.

71. Julius S, Kjeldsen SE, Weber M, Brunner HR, Ekman S, Hansson L, et al. Outcomes in hypertensive patients at high cardiovascular risk treated with regimens based on valsartan or amlodipine: The VALUE randomised trial. *Lancet* 2004; 363(9426):2022–31.

72. Weber MA, Julius S, Kjeldsen SE, Brunner HR, Ekman S, Hansson L, et al. Blood pressure dependent and independent effects of antihypertensive treatment on clinical events in the VALUE Trial. *Lancet* 2004;363(9426): 2049–51.

73. Volpe M. Treatment of systolic hypertension: Spotlight on recent studies with angiotensin II antagonists. *J Hum Hypertens* 2005;19(2):93–102.

74. Kjeldsen SE, Dahlof B, Devereux RB, Julius S, Aurup P, Edelman J, et al. Effects of losartan on cardiovascular morbidity and mortality in patients with isolated systolic hypertension and left ventricular hypertrophy: A Losartan Intervention for Endpoint Reduction (LIFE) substudy. *JAMA* 2002; 288(12):1491–98.

75. Papademetriou V, Farsang C, Elmfeldt D, Hofman A, Lithell H, Olofsson O, et al. Stroke prevention with the angiotensin II type 1-receptor blocker candesartan in elderly patients with isolated systolic hypertension: The Study on Cognition and Prognosis in the Elderly (SCOPE). *J Am Coll Cardiol* 2004;44(6):1175–80.

76. Jandeleit-Dahm KA, Tikellis C, Reid CM, Johnston CI, Cooper ME. Why blockade of the renin-angiotensin system reduces the incidence of new-onset diabetes. *J Hypertens* 2005; 23(3):463–73.

77. Gress TW, Nieto FJ, Shahar E, Wofford MR, Brancati FL. Hypertension and antihypertensive therapy as risk factors for type 2 diabetes mellitus. Atherosclerosis Risk in Communities Study. *N Engl J Med* 2000;342(13): 905–12.

78. Lindholm LH. Valsartan treatment of hypertension: Does VALUE add value? *Lancet* 2004;363(9426):2010–11.

79. Cheung BM, Cheung GT, Lauder IJ, Lau CP, Kumana CR. Meta-analysis of large outcome trials of angiotensin receptor blockers in hypertension. *J Hum Hypertens* 2005.

80. McMurray JJ, Pfeffer MA, Swedberg K, Dzau VJ. Which inhibitor of the renin-angiotensin system should be used in chronic heart failure and acute myocardial infarction? *Circulation* 2004;110(20):3281–88.

81. Cohn JN, Tognoni G. A randomized trial of the angiotensin-receptor blocker valsartan in chronic heart failure. *N Engl J Med* 2001;345(23): 1667–75.

82. McMurray JJ, Ostergren J, Swedberg K, Granger CB, Held P, Michelson EL, et al. Effects of candesartan in patients with chronic heart failure and reduced left-ventricular systolic function taking angiotensin-converting-enzyme inhibitors: The CHARM-Added trial. *Lancet* 2003;362(9386):767–71.

83. Dickstein K, Kjekshus J. Effects of losartan and captopril on mortality and morbidity in high-risk patients after acute myocardial infarction: The OPTIMAAL randomised trial. Optimal Trial in Myocardial Infarction with Angiotensin II Antagonist Losartan. *Lancet* 2002;360(9335): 752–60.

84. Pitt B, Segal R, Martinez FA, Meurers G, Cowley AJ, Thomas I, et al. Randomised trial of losartan versus captopril in patients over 65 with heart failure (Evaluation of Losartan in the Elderly Study, ELITE). *Lancet* 1997; 349(9054):747–52.

85. Pitt B, Poole-Wilson PA, Segal R, Martinez FA, Dickstein K, Camm AJ, et al. Effect of losartan compared with captopril on mortality in patients with symptomatic heart failure: Randomised trial, the Losartan Heart Failure Survival Study ELITE II. *Lancet* 2000;355(9215): 1582–87.

86. Swedberg K, McMurray JJ. Angiotensin receptor blockers and heart failure: Atill CHARMing after VALIANT? *Eur Heart J* 2004;25(5):357–58.

87. Pfeffer MA, McMurray JJ, Velazquez EJ, Rouleau JL, Kober L, Maggioni AP, et al. Valsartan, captopril, or both in myocardial infarction complicated by heart failure, left ventricular dysfunction, or both. *N Engl J Med* 2003;349(20):1893–1906.

88. Mielniczuk L, Stevenson LW. Angiotensin-converting enzyme inhibitors and angiotensin II type I receptor blockers in the management of congestive heart failure patients: What have we learned from recent clinical trials? *Curr Opin Cardiol* 2005; 20(4):250–55.

89. Mailloux LU. Hypertension in chronic renal failure and ESRD: Prevalence, pathophysiology, and outcomes. *Semin Nephrol* 2001;21(2):146–56.

90. Adler AI, Stevens RJ, Manley SE, Bilous RW, Cull CA, Holman RR. Development and progression of nephropathy in type 2 diabetes: The United Kingdom Prospective Diabetes Study (UKPDS 64). *Kidney Int* 2003;63(1):225–32.

91. Brewster UC, Perazella MA. The renin-angiotensin-aldosterone system and the kidney: Effects on kidney disease. *Am J Med* 2004;116(4):26372.

92. Parving HH, Lehnert H, Brochner-Mortensen J, Gomis R, Andersen S, Arner P. The effect of irbesartan on the development of diabetic nephropathy in patients with type 2 diabetes. *N Engl J Med* 2001;345(12):870–78.

93. Brenner BM, Cooper ME, de Zeeuw D, Keane WF, Mitch WE, Parving HH, et al. Effects of losartan on renal and cardiovascular outcomes in patients with type 2 diabetes and nephropathy. *N Engl J Med* 2001;345(12):861–69.

94. Lewis EJ, Hunsicker LG, Clarke WR, Berl T, Pohl MA, Lewis JB, et al. Renoprotective effect of the angiotensin-receptor antagonist irbesartan in patients with nephropathy due to type 2 diabetes. *N Engl J Med* 2001;345(12):851–60.

95. Barnett AH, Bain SC, Bouter P, Karlberg B, Madsbad S, Jervell J, et al. Angiotensin-receptor blockade versus converting-enzyme inhibition in type 2 diabetes and nephropathy. *N Engl J Med* 2004;351(19):1952–61.

96. National Kidney Foundation. K/DOQI Clinical Practice Guidelines for Chronic Kidney Disease: Evaluation, Classification, and Stratification. 2000 [cited 2005 December 12].

97. Diercks GF, van Boven AJ, Hillege JL, de Jong PE, Rouleau JL, van Gilst WH. The importance of microalbuminuria as a cardiovascular risk indicator: A review. *Can J Cardiol* 2002; 18(5):525–35.

98. Ruggenenti P, Fassi A, Ilieva AP, Bruno S, Iliev IP, Brusegan V, et al. Preventing microalbuminuria in type 2 diabetes. *N Engl J Med* 2004; 351(19):1941–51.

99. Haller H, Viberti G, Mimran A, Remuzzi G, Rabelink A, Ritz E, et al. Preventing Microalbuminuria in Patients with Diabetes: Rationale and Design of the Randomised Olmesartan and Diabetes Microalbuminuria Prevention (ROADMAP) Study. *J Hypertens* 2006 (in press).

100. Pfeffer MA, Swedberg K, Granger CB, Held P, McMurray JJ, Michelson EL, et al. Effects of candesartan on mortality and morbidity in patients with chronic heart failure: The CHARM-Overall programme. *Lancet* 2003;362(9386):759–66.

101. Swedberg K, Cleland J, Dargie H, Drexler H, Follath F, Komajda M, et al. Guidelines for the diagnosis and treatment of chronic heart failure: Executive summary (update 2005). The Task Force for the Diagnosis and Treatment of Chronic Heart Failure of the European Society of Cardiology. *Eur Heart J* 2005;26(11):1115–40.

102. K/DOQI clinical practice guidelines on hypertension and antihypertensive agents in chronic kidney disease. *Am J Kidney Dis* 2004;43(5 Suppl 1): S1–290.

103. Prisant LM. Preventing type II diabetes mellitus. *J Clin Pharmacol* 2004; 44(4):406–13.

104. Dahlof B, Sever PS, Poulter NR, Wedel H, Beevers DG, Caulfield M, et al. Prevention of cardiovascular events with an antihypertensive regimen of amlodipine adding perindopril as required versus atenolol adding bendroflumethiazide as required, in the Anglo-Scandinavian Cardiac Outcomes Trial-Blood Pressure Lowering Arm (ASCOT-BPLA): A multicentre randomised controlled trial. *Lancet* 2005;366(9489):895–906.

105. Williams B. Recent hypertension trials: implications and controversies. *J Am Coll Cardiol* 2005;45(6):813–27.

106. White WB. Cardiovascular risk and therapeutic intervention for the early morning surge in blood pressure and heart rate. *Blood Press Monit* 2001; 6(2):63–72.

Chapter

82 Alpha Adrenoreceptor Antagonists

Henry L. Elliott

Key Findings

- Selective alpha-1-adrenoreceptor antagonist drugs effectively block sympathetically mediated vasoconstrictor responses and thereby reduce peripheral vascular resistance (and blood pressure).

- There are no significant clinical contraindications to selective alpha-1-antagonist drugs. In fact, they have beneficial effects on glucose and lipid metabolism.

- Doxazosin is currently the preferred agent, particularly as an "add-on" treatment for all types of hypertension and as a combination partner with all classes of antihypertensive drug.

- Doxazosin (GITS formulation) has been shown to improve clinical outcomes when used in combination with other conventional antihypertensive drugs (see ASCOT results).

It is generally accepted that the sympathetic nervous system plays a role in the initiation and maintenance of the increased peripheral vascular resistance characteristic of established essential hypertension. Increases in arteriolar and venous tone, and hence blood pressure, are principally mediated by noradrenaline released from sympathetic nerve terminals and acting at alpha 1 adrenoceptors located post-junctionally in the blood vessel wall (Figure 82–1).[1] Essential hypertension reflects, at least in part, an enhanced alpha adrenergic vasoconstrictor influence on blood pressure regulation.

As with most receptor systems, further research has identified several alpha adrenoreceptor subtypes. For example, the alpha-1b subtype is found in the urinary tract and is targeted in the treatment of benign prostatic hyperplasia (BPH). However, the classical post-junctional alpha-1 adrenoreceptor remains the primary target for blocking sympathetically mediated vasoconstrictor mechanisms and thereby promoting a reduction in blood pressure. Because an alpha-1 adrenoreceptor antagonist drug reduces vascular smooth muscle tone and peripheral vascular resistance without interfering with myocardial contractility, it appears to fulfill the fundamental requirements for an effective antihypertensive agent.

CLINICAL PHARMACOLOGY

Mechanism of action

The particular advantage of selective alpha-1 antagonists (alpha-1 blockers), compared to nonselective alpha antago-

nist agents, is that they do not interfere with local feedback control mechanisms involving prejunctional alpha adrenoceptors within the neurovascular junction (Figure 82–1).[2] Thus, "spillover" of catecholamines into the systemic circulation (which occurs as a consequence of the blocked reuptake via pre-synaptic alpha-2 adrenoceptors) is significantly reduced. Accordingly, the risk of cardiac stimulation and reflex cardioacceleration during chronic treatment is reduced. Of the selective alpha-1 blockers developed for the treatment of hypertension, the prototype drug prazosin has largely been superseded by longer-acting quinazoline derivatives, particularly doxazosin (see Box 82–1). Other agents with selective alpha-1 blocking activity, such as tamsulosin and alfuzosin and the unrelated agent indoramin, now have little or no place in the routine management of hypertension but are retained for the use in the management of BPH.

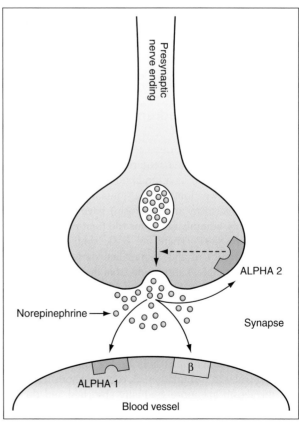

Figure 82–1. Depiction of the neuroeffector junction and the locations of pre- and post-junctional alpha adrenoceptors.

Box 82–1

Drugs with Alpha-1 Adrenoreceptor Antagonist Activity

Nonselective:
- Phenoxybenzamine
- Phentolamine

Selective:
- Quinazoline derivatives (prazosin, doxazosin, terazosin)
- Non-quinazolines: indoramin

Multiple actions:
- Carvedilol
- Labetalol

Nonselective alpha adrenoreceptor antagonists

Two nonselective agents—phentolamine (by parental administration) and the longer-acting agent phenoxybenzamine (by oral administration)—retain occasional clinical roles in specialist circumstances. These agents are used in the management of hypertension associated with the rare catecholamine-secreting tumor pheochromocytoma either as part of the perioperative management or as a constituent of the long-term antihypertensive drug treatment when surgical correction is not possible. These drugs may also have a role in the treatment of hypertensive crises associated with (for example) overdosage of sympathomimetic drugs, with autonomic dysreflexia, or as a consequence of the rebound hypertensive response that follows the abrupt withdrawal of centrally acting antihypertensive drugs such as clonidine.

Selective alpha-1 adrenoreceptor antagonists

Prazosin (the prototype quinazoline alpha-1 blocker) was a short-acting agent that required multiple daily dosing (unless administered as a modified release formulation), whereas the newer longer-acting quinazoline derivatives (including doxazosin and terazosin) have been licensed for once-daily administration for the treatment of hypertension (Box 82–1). There are basic similarities in the pharmacokinetics of the quinazoline derivatives, which have almost complete absorption from the gastrointestinal tract, bioavailability in the range of 40 to 70%, and hepatic metabolism as the principal route of elimination. Prazosin achieves its peak plasma concentrations within about 1 to 2 hours and has a relatively short half-life of about 4 to 6 hours. This translates to a short duration of action and the requirement for multiple daily dosing, unless used in a modified release formulation. In contrast, both terazosin and doxazosin are more gradually absorbed and do not achieve their peak plasma concentrations until 2 to 4 hours post-dose (with elimination half-lives in the range 8 to 16 hours). These characteristics lead to a more gradual onset

of action and a more sustained antihypertensive effect. For illustrative purposes, the clinical pharmacokinetic parameters of doxazosin and the prototype drug prazosin are compared in Table 82–1.

More recently, to further refine the pharmacokinetic characteristics and improve the therapeutic profile a once-daily GITS (Gastrointestinal Therapeutic System) formulation of doxazosin has been introduced.[3] In practical terms, and for the routine management of hypertensive patients, doxazosin is now the most important quinazoline derivative and the most widely studied.

Specific pharmacokinetic studies with doxazosin

Pharmacokinetic studies have been undertaken in elderly patients, and although there were some age-related differences in the disposition characteristics neither the bioavailability nor clearance of doxazosin was significantly altered and the overall conclusion was that age was unlikely to influence the disposition of doxazosin to any clinically significant extent.[4] In patients with varying degrees of renal impairment, there were no significant differences in half-life.[5] There is no evidence that the pharmacokinetics of doxazosin are either time or dose dependent, and for dosages between 1 and 16 mg the steady-state pharmacokinetics show proportional increases in plasma concentration and in area under the concentration time curve (AUC).[6]

Pharmacokinetic/pharmacodynamic relationships

The relationship between the response to doxazosin and either drug dose or plasma drug concentration has been investigated in several studies. For example, in a clinical study of antihypertensive efficacy a linear relationship was identified with a progressive increase in effect with oral doses of 2, 4, and 8 mg.[6] In a more detailed study, using integrated concentration-effect analysis (pharmacokinetic-pharmacodynamic modeling), linear relationships among dose, plasma drug concentration, and blood pressure response were identified in individual hypertensive subjects after single and multiple dosing.[7] The consistency of the response to doxazosin has also been investigated in the same individual after oral and intravenous administration.[8]

COMPARISON OF THE CLINICAL PHARMACOKINETICS OF DOXAZOSIN AND PRAZOSIN		
Parameters	Doxazosin	Prazosin
Bioavailability (%)	62–74	44–69
Volume of distribution (1/kg)	0.97–1.70	0.51–0.81
Clearance (ml/min/kg)	1–2	2–4
Elimination half-life (h):		
Single doses	9–16	2–4
Multiple doses	13–22	2–4

Table 82–1. Comparison of the Clinical Pharmacokinetics of Doxazosin and Prazosin

TOMHS: FINAL BP RESULTS, BP REDUCTIONS, CHANGE FROM BASELINE		
	Systolic	Diastolic
Chlorthalidone	14.6*	11.1* mmHg
Amlodipine	14.1*	12.2*
Acebutalol	13.9*	11.5*
Doxazosin	13.4*	11.2*
Enalapril	11.3	9.7
Placebo	8.6	8.6

*p<0.01 versus placebo. (From Neaton JD, Grimm JRH, Prineas RJ, et al. Treatment of mild hypertension study. Final results. *JAMA* 1993;270:713–24, with permission.)

Table 82–2. TOMHS: Final BP Results, BP Reductions, Change from Baseline

The results of these studies confirm the consistency and reproducibility of the concentration-effect relationship in individual hypertensive patients whereby an increase in dosage leads to an increase in blood pressure response. In addition, the relative magnitude of the chronic blood pressure response to doxazosin is well correlated with that of the acute response. The results of these studies also confirm that doxazosin, despite its close structural similarities to prazosin, is qualitatively different—with a gradual onset of action (even after intravenous administration) directly attributable to the parent drug and independent of an active metabolite.

CLINICAL INDICATIONS

Hypertension

Hypertension is the principal indication for treatment with a classical alpha-1 adrenoreceptor antagonist drug.

Antihypertensive efficacy

Early comparative clinical studies showed that the blood-pressure-lowering effects of various alpha-1 blockers were similar and generally shown to be equivalent to alternative classes of antihypertensive drug. A useful illustrative example was the Treatment of Mild Hypertension Study (TOMHS). TOMHS was a randomized placebo-controlled parallel group study in 902 patients with mild (borderline) hypertension who were treated for 4 years with representative agents from the major antihypertensive drug classes (including the alpha blocker doxazosin) with the dosage constrained to 2 mg once daily.[9] There were modest blood pressure reductions with all active treatments, and the principal blood pressure results are summarized in Table 82–2. Overall, the blood pressure reductions were similar with all active treatments in TOMHS and significantly greater than with placebo.

First-line treatment in essential hypertension (limited role)

There is little doubt that selective alpha blockers are clinically useful antihypertensive drugs. However, some recent doubts have been cast on the effectiveness of doxazosin as a first-line antihypertensive agent not only in terms of blood pressure reduction but in terms of risk reduction (particularly with respect to cardiac failure and stroke prevention). Thus, in the management of uncomplicated patients with essential hypertension alpha-1 adrenoreceptor antagonist drugs (including doxazosin) are no longer considered routine first-line agents. This is principally due to the general perception of a disappointing outcome result in ALLHAT (Antihypertensive and Lipid-Lowering Treatment to Prevent Heart Attack Trial).[10]

In ALLHAT, patients receiving doxazosin as their initial antihypertensive drug treatment were found to have poorer blood pressure control (by about 2 to 3 mmHg for systolic blood pressure; Figure 82–2) and higher incidences of heart failure and stroke relative to chlorthalidone-based treatment (Table 82–3). For this reason, doxazosin was prematurely withdrawn as a first-line treatment in ALLHAT. As a result, its role as a first-line option has been revised in most guidelines.

ALLHAT was the first prospective clinical outcome trial to incorporate and evaluate first-line treatment with an alpha-1 blocker (doxazosin), and the result is of major importance. It must be noted that there were no differences in the primary outcome measures of fatal CHD or nonfatal myocardial infarction. However, there were significant outcome differences because of higher rates for stroke and congestive heart failure and for angina and coronary revascularization procedures. Whether or not this is a simple and direct reflection of the small blood pressure difference in relatively high-risk patients remains unclear. The target blood pressure of less than 140/90 mmHg was achieved in 64% of the chlorthalidone group compared to 58% in the doxazosin group, and after 4 years of treatment the achieved blood pressures were respectively 135/76 and 137/76 mmHg.

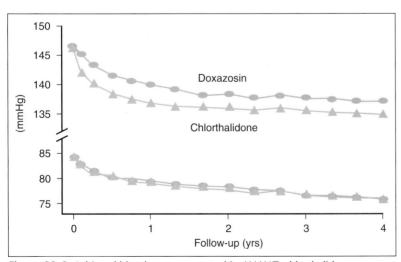

Figure 82–2. Achieved blood pressure control in ALLHAT: chlorthalidone versus doxazosin.

ALLHAT OUTCOMES PER 100 PATIENTS PER 4 YEARS		
	Chlorthalidone (n=15,268)	Doxzaosin (n=9067)
Primary endpoints:		
Nonfatal MI and fatal CHD	6.3	6.26 n.s
Secondary endpoints:		
Total mortality	9.08	9.62 n.s
CHD	11.97	13.06 (*p*<0.05)
STROKE	3.61	4.23 (*p*<0.04)
CVD (inc. CCF)	21.76	25.45 (*p*<0.001)
From The ALLHAT Collaborative Research Group: Major Cardiovascular Events in Hypertensive Patients Randomised to Doxazosin vs Chlorthalidone. *JAMA* 2000;283:1967–75.		

Table 82–3. ALLHAT Outcomes per 100 Patients per 4 Years

First-line treatment in special patient groups (examples)

Elderly hypertensive patients

The effectiveness of doxazosin in elderly patients, relative to young patients, has been reviewed in a survey involving 1486 patients of greater than 65 years of age.[11] In brief, the blood pressure reduction of 23/15 mmHg in those patients aged more than 65 years was directly comparable to the reduction of 21/14 mmHg in the younger group. Importantly, this study also provided substantial support for the good overall tolerability profile of doxazosin even though the elderly group reported more frequent episodes of dizziness (10.9 versus 5.1%). However, these authors concluded that this particular symptomatic complaint occurs more frequently in older patients in general and did not constitute a particular problem in relation to the doxazosin treatment.

Patients with hypertension and diabetes mellitus

The effectiveness of doxazosin has been compared with that of atenolol in a double-blind crossover comparative study involving 12 weeks of active treatment in hypertensive type I diabetic patients. Overall, there were modest reductions in blood pressure at 12/9 mmHg with doxazosin and 12/8 mmHg with atenolol.[12] However, only during the doxazosin phase was there any significant reduction in microalbuminuria. This potential benefit was not observed during the atenolol treatment phase. Several other clinical studies have confirmed the effectiveness of doxazosin in the management of hypertensive type II diabetic patients.

Patients with hypertension and renal disease

Alpha blockers are extensively metabolized, and there is no significant accumulation in patients with renal impairment. In addition, combination regimens are usually necessary in such patients and the alpha blockers can usefully be combined with all other types of agent.

Combination antihypertensive treatment (preferred/usual role)

Following the relative disappointment of ALLHAT, there has been a deliberate repositioning of doxazosin as a combination partner. Thus, unless there is a very particular reason for initiating antihypertensive treatment with doxazosin (in a man with mild hypertension and BPH, for example) improvement in blood pressure control through the addition of doxazosin has become the preferred role. Because the majority of hypertensive patients require two or more drugs to reach target (<140/90 mmHg), it is important to establish that this is a safe and effective strategy. As emphasized in several recent national and international guidelines, intensive treatment to provide "tight" or optimal blood pressure control frequently requires combinations of antihypertensive drugs, particularly in high-risk patients. This combination role might be a particularly useful and important component of the regimens used in patients with renal impairment, for example, or with metabolic problems (particularly disorders of lipid and glucose metabolism) because other agents would be relatively contraindicated in such conditions. The antihypertensive efficacy of this combination approach to treatment has been confirmed both in specific small-scale studies and in major clinical outcome studies.

Specific combination treatment studies

Usefully additive antihypertensive activity has been observed when doxazosin has been combined with representatives from other major antihypertensive drug classes. For example, the effectiveness of amlodipine alone (10 mg daily), doxazosin alone (4 mg daily), and the combination of these two drugs was investigated in patients with moderate to severe hypertension.[13] There were significant additive effects with the combination, particularly on standing blood pressure—whereby an additional reduction of 10/8 mmHg was achieved with the combination relative to amlodipine alone. There was no evidence of any significant reflex cardioacceleration or any increased likelihood of postural hypotension.

Also of interest was a small but well-designed study investigating the combination of enalapril and doxazosin in 9 hypertensive patients.[14] Standing blood pressure was reduced by 12/8 mmHg by doxazosin alone (4 mg daily) and by 9/6 mmHg with enalapril alone (20 mg daily). However, the combination of doxazosin and enalapril, with dosages constrained to respectively 1 mg and 5 mg daily, was associated with a significantly greater reduction of 23/20 mmHg (*p*<0.02). Indeed, the effectiveness of this combination might be particularly useful in the management of the diabetic hypertensive not only by virtue of the antihypertensive efficacy but because of the combination of positive metabolic effects and the potential for nephroprotection. Thus, doxazosin now appears to be established as a combination partner for all antihypertensive drug treatments when blood pressure control requires improvement.

Combination studies with doxazosin in routine patient care

The usefulness and effectiveness of doxazosin as a general "add-on" therapy was specifically studied in a double-blind placebo-controlled study of 70 hypertensive patients who were inadequately controlled on existing treatment.[15] Sitting and standing blood pressures were significantly reduced by (on average) 12.4/4.9 and 10.5/3.8 mmHg, respectively. Fatigue was the only symptomatic adverse effect, which was reported significantly more often in the doxazosin group (24 versus 3%). There were small but significant reductions in LDL and total cholesterol during doxazosin treatment by approximately 4.8 and 9.1%, respectively (placebo adjusted).

The GATES (Doxazosin GITS As Combination Therapy in Hypertensive Patients: An Efficacy and Safety) study was designed to clarify the role of doxazosin (GITS) as an add-on treatment. This was a randomized prospective placebo-controlled study designed to assess the responses to the addition of doxazosin GITS in 167 patients not adequately controlled with either one or two conventional antihypertensive drugs.[16] In brief, adding doxazosin GITS improved blood pressure control by an average of 9/8 mmHg such that 27% of previously uncontrolled patients achieved target. Because of adverse effects, there were some treatment withdrawals: 5 (5.6%) and 2 (2.3%) patients assigned doxazosin and placebo, respectively, were withdrawn because of perceived adverse drug reactions.

Doxazosin as a combination treatment in a clinical outcome trial (ASCOT)

The role of doxazosin GITS as an add-on treatment has been further assessed in ASCOT (Anglo-Scandinavian Cardiac Outcomes Trial).[17] The principal result in ASCOT was that antihypertensive treatment based on the combination of amlodipine and perindopril was significantly more effective than the combination of atenolol with bendroflumethiazide.[12] The treatment algorithm (flow diagram) is shown in Figure 82–3, with doxazosin as a suitable combination treatment following initial treatment with either thiazide/β-blocker or CCB/ACE inhibitor. The specific details of the impact of doxazosin are not yet published, but it is noted that 40% of the nondiabetic hypertensive patients and 68% of the diabetic patients in ASCOT had not achieved target blood pressure at the end of the trial despite an average of 2.2 antihypertensive drugs. In practice, therefore, there is a clear place for doxazosin as a "third" or "add-on" drug if blood pressure targets are to be achieved in 100% of patients.

Hypertension and related disorders

As with most antihypertensive drugs, claims have been made that alpha-1 antagonists possess nonhemodynamic pharmacologic properties that might lead to additional cardiovascular benefits. Beneficial metabolic effects on glucose and lipid metabolism have been most extensively studied as a specific additional property of alpha blockers. Although not considered an additional specific property of an alpha-1 blocker, regression of left ventricular (LV) hypertrophy is assessed for most types of antihypertensive drug because it is an important surrogate for improved cardiovascular outcomes in patients receiving antihypertensive drug treatment.

Metabolic effects

The small but potentially beneficial effects of alpha blockers on glucose and lipid metabolism have been consistently

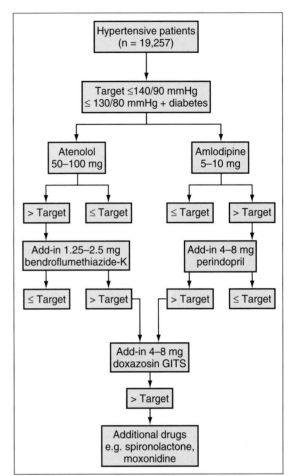

Figure 82–3. Treatment flow diagram in ASCOT.

identified. In fact, alpha-1 adrenoreceptor antagonist drugs are the only antihypertensive treatments consistently shown to have beneficial effects on plasma lipid profiles with modest reductions in total and LDL cholesterol and a small increase in HDL cholesterol. For example, in TOMHS doxazosin was associated with a significant increase in the total/HDL-cholesterol ratio by 2.6 compared to 1.2 with placebo ($p<0.001$), and compared to 1 to 2 with acebutolol, 1.5 with amlodipine, and 1.4 with chlorthalidone ($p<0.01$). This metabolic improvement is linked to the beneficial effect alpha blockers have on insulin responsiveness leading to increased peripheral glucose uptake. Thus, selective alpha blockers may be particularly well suited for the treatment of hypertensive patients with type II diabetes mellitus.[18,19] Of particular additional interest, and linked to the beneficial effect on insulin responsiveness, was an observation that doxazosin treatment in patients with CHD resulted in significant dose-dependent increases in t-PA concentration leading to a net increase in fibrinolytic potential.[20]

Regression of LV hypertrophy

Effective blood pressure reduction is the primary requirement for promoting the regression of LV hypertrophy, and whether or not different pharmacologic properties lead to a greater effectiveness remains to be clearly established in clinical studies. The results of a meta-analysis indicate that treatment based on alpha blockers is correspondingly as effective as treatment based on most types of antihypertensive drug[21] (Figure 82–4). This effect has also been demonstrated in a small study of 11 hypertensive patients over a 6-month treatment period.[22] However, in this study not only was there a significant reduction in LV mass index—from 128.5 to 114 g/m² (a reduction of 12%)—but left ventricular systolic and diastolic function were also shown to be improved.

Genitourinary effects

Alpha blockers (particularly those with effects on the alpha-1b receptor subtype) are well recognized to have effects on the genitourinary system. Accordingly, alpha blockers are used for the relief of obstructive urinary symptoms in males with benign prostatic hyperplasia/ hypertrophy (BPH). Unfortunately, this predictable pharmacologic effect may occasionally lead to urinary incontinence in females.

There is evidence also that male sexual dysfunction occurs less frequently with alpha blockers than with other types of antihypertensive agent. This was seen in TOMHS, where erectile dysfunction was reported in only 3% of patients receiving doxazosin compared to 17% of patients receiving chlorthalidone. There is no evidence that this effect can be used therapeutically, although it may occasionally prove helpful to change to doxazosin treatment when a hypertensive male is having erectile problems during treatment with a thiazide diuretic.

Congestive cardiac failure

The role of selective alpha-1 antagonist drugs in the management of congestive cardiac failure was studied in the 1980s. The results were disappointing, and this indication is of historical interest only.

COMPLICATIONS

Cardiovascular effects

Historically, the "first dose effect" with symptomatic orthostatic hypotension and possible syncope, accompanied by tachycardia and palpitations, is probably the most well-known adverse effect of alpha-blocking drugs. This well-recognized complication occurred upon treatment initiation but in general occurred only with short-acting and rapid-onset agents, particularly the prototype drug prazosin. In retrospect, these dramatic (and worrying) hypotensive reactions were attributable to the use of unnecessarily high starting doses—particularly in patients who were salt/volume depleted or receiving other antihypertensive treatment such as thiazide diuretics and beta blockers. The newer agents (including doxazosin), with a more gradual onset of effect and longer duration of action, administered in initially low dosages have minimized the risk of this dramatic early response. Unfortunately, although doxazosin continues to be associated to some extent with the "bad publicity" that surrounded prazosin it is of particular interest that the incidence of syncope with doxazosin in TOMHS was identical to that of the other drug groups[9] (Table 82–4).

Adverse effects on other systems

With respect to tolerability, there were overall similarities between doxazosin and chlorthalidone in ALLHAT. For example, the most common reasons offered by the patients for discontinuing medication during the 4 years of trial were symptomatic adverse effects (20% in the chlorthalidone group and 19% in the doxazosin group); an unspecified refusal in 30 and 29%, respectively; and because of abnormal laboratory values in 5 and 1%, respectively.

As with most antihypertensive drugs, nonspecific upper-gastrointestinal symptoms with nausea and abdominal discomfort have been reported. Similarly, drowsiness, fatigue, confusion, and malaise have occasionally been reported. Because of their (unwarranted) reputation for causing profound postural falls in blood pressure there have been concerns that alpha blockers might impair cerebral perfusion, particularly in elderly hypertensives. This has not been confirmed in clinical studies.

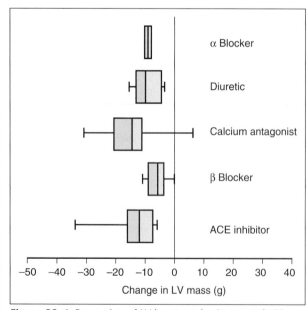

Figure 82–4. Regression of LV hypertrophy (meta-analysis). (Redrawn from Jennings GL, Wong J. Assessment of hypertensive organ damage. In: Hansson L, Birkenhager WH (eds.). *Handbook of Hypertension, Volume 18*. Amsterdam: Elsevier, 1997.)

TOMHS: SELECTED ADVERSE EFFECTS		
Drug Syncope	**Reported (%)**	**Impotence (%)**
Chlorthalidone	0	12
Acebutolol	1	8
Doxazosin	1	0
Enalapril	2	4
Amlodipine	1	3
Placebo	4	6

From Neaton JD, Grimm JRH, Prineas RJ, et al. Treatment of mild hypertension study: Final results. *JAMA* 1993;270:713–24, with permission.

Table 82–4. TOMHS: Selected Adverse Effects

SUMMARY

Alpha-1-adrenoreceptor antagonist drugs have the immediate attraction that there are no patient co-morbidities that constitute absolute contraindications to their use. Thus, alpha blockers can safely and appropriately be administered to hypertensive patients with concomitant disease states such as diabetes mellitus or obstructive airway disease or renal impairment. However, it is difficult to ignore the disappointing results of ALLHAT, which have been taken to suggest that doxazosin and other alpha-1 blockers should no longer be considered routine first-line agents but alternative or additional agents.

Overall, the recent evidence favoring intensive blood pressure control has clearly identified the requirement for combination drug treatments if lower blood pressure targets are to be attained. The role of doxazosin GITS as an effective add-on treatment has been established in GATES, for example, and the predicted results of ASCOT suggest that this additive antihypertensive effect translates to outcome benefits particularly in patients with high levels of absolute cardiovascular risk (for example, those with diabetes mellitus or with concomitant hypercholesterolemia). Because high-risk patients benefit most from intensive antihypertensive treatment, there are clear indications that a drug such as doxazosin (with its favorable metabolic profile) might be particularly useful as an add-on antihypertensive drug treatment. Overall, the tolerability profile of doxazosin has been shown to be similar (albeit not superior) to that of any of the competitor antihypertensive drug classes in TOMHS and ALLHAT (for example).

In summary, a selective alpha-1-adrenoreceptor antagonist drug (and particularly doxazosin) retains a useful and important role as a combination partner for all other types of antihypertensive drug. This role may be particularly important in patients at high cardiovascular risk because of hypertension that is proving difficult to control or because of concomitant metabolic problems such as obesity or type II diabetes mellitus.

REFERENCES

1. Reid JL. Alpha-adrenoceptors in hypertension. In: Kobinger W, Ahlquist RP (eds.) Alpha and beta adrenoceptors and the cardiovascular system. Amsterdam: Excerpta Medica. 1984:161–217.

2. Langer SZ, Cavero I, Massingham R. Recent developments in non-adrenergic neurotransmission and its relevance to the mechanism of action of certain antihypertensive agents. *Hypertension* 1980;2:372–82.

3. Chung M, Vashi V, Puente J, et al. Clinical pharmacokinetics of doxazosin in a controlled-release gastrointestinal therapeutic system (GITS) formulation. *Br J Clin Pharmacol* 1999;48:678–87.

4. Elliott HL, Meredith PA, Reid JL. Pharmacokinetic overview of doxazosin. *Am J Cardiol* 1987;59:786–818.

5. Bailey RR, Begg E, Carlson R, Sharman R. Single-dose pharmacokinetics of doxazosin in healthy volunteers and patients with renal insufficiency. *N Z Med J* 1985;98:248.

6. Cubeddu LX, Fuynmayor N, Caplan N, Ferry D. Clinical pharmacology of doxazosin in patients with essential hypertension. *Clin Pharmacol Ther* 1987;41:439–49.

7. Donnelly R, Elliott HL, Meredith PA, Reid JL. Concentration-effect relationships and individual responses to doxazosin in essential hypertension. *Br J Clin Pharmacol* 1989;28:517–26.

8. Meredith PA, Elliott HL, Kelman AW, et al. Concentration-effect relationships and individual responses to doxazosin in essential hypertension. *Br J Clin Pharmacol* 1989;28:517–26.

9. Neaton JD, Grimm JRH, Prineas RJ, et al. Treatment of mild hypertension study: Final results. *JAMA* 1993; 270:713–24.

10. The ALLHAT Collaborative Research Group: Major Cardiovascular Events in Hypertensive Patients Randomised to Doxazosin vs Chlorthalidone. *JAMA* 2000;283:1967–75.

11. Langdon CG, Packard RS. Doxazosin in hypertension: Results of a general practice study in 4809 patients. *Br J Clin Pract* 1994;46:1–6.

12. Winocour PH. Contrasting renal and metabolic effects of alpha-and beta-adrenergic blockade in mildly hypertensive type I (insulin-dependent) diabetic subjects. *Nutr Metab Cardiovasc Dis* 1995;5:217–24.

13. Brown MJ, Dickerson JEC. Alpha-blockade and calcium antagonism: An effective and well-tolerated combination for the treatment of resistant hypertension. *J Hypertens* 1995;13:701–07.

14. Brown MJ, Dickerson JEC. Synergism between alpha I blockade and angiotensin converting enzyme inhibition in essential hypertension. *J Hypertens* 1991;6:362–63.

15. Black HR, Sollins JS, Garofalo JL. The addition of doxazosin to the Therapeutic Regimen of Hypertensive Patients inadequately controlled with other antihypertensive medications: A randomised, placebo-controlled study. *Am J Hypertens* 2000;13:468–74.

16. Black H, Keck M, Meredith P, et al. An efficacy and safety study of doxazosin gastrointestinal therapeutic system as combination therapy in hypertensive patients. New York: American Society of Hypertension. 2004.

17. Dahloff B, Sever PS, Poulter NR, for the ASCOT investigators. Prevention of cardiovascular events with an antihypertensive regimen of amlodipine adding perindopril as required versus atenolol adding bendroflumethiazide as required, in the Anglo-Scandinavian Cardiac Outcomes Trial-Blood-Pressure Lowering Arm (ASCOT - BPLA): A multicentre randomised controlled trial. *Lancet* 2005;366:895–906 (in press).

18. Giorda C, Appendino M, Mason MG, et al. Alpha-I blocker doxazosin improves peripheral insulin sensitivity in diabetic hypertensive patients. *Metabolism* 1995;44:673–76.

19. Giordana M, et al. Effects of angiotensin-converting enzyme inhibitors, Ca^{2+} channel antagonists and alpha-adrenergic blockers on glucose and lipid metabolism in NIDDM patients with hypertension. *Diabetes* 1995;44:665–71.

20. Zehetgruber M, Christ G, Gabriel H, et al. Effect of antihypertensive treatment with doxazosin on insulin sensitivity and fibrinolytic parameters. *Thromb Haemost* 1998;79:378–82.

21. Jennings GL, Wong J. Assessment of hypertensive organ damage. In: Hansson L, Birkenhager WH (eds.). *Handbook of Hypertension, Volume 18.* Amsterdam: Elsevier Science, 1997.

22. Agabati-Rosei E, Miuiesan ML, Eizzoni D, et al. Reduction of left ventricular hypertrophy after long term antihypertensive treatment with doxazosin. *J Hum Hypertens* 1992;6:9–15.

Chapter

83

Centrally Acting Agents

Domenic A. Sica

Key Findings

- Centrally acting agents stimulate α_2-receptors and/or imadozoline receptors on adrenergic neurons located within the rostral ventrolateral medulla, thereby reducing sympathetic outflow. Centrally acting agents also stimulate peripheral α_2-receptors, which for the most part is of limited clinical significance.

- Central alpha-agonists have had a lengthy history of use—starting with α-methyldopa, which has seen its use decline because of annoying side effects.

- Patients requiring multi-drug therapy with otherwise resistant hypertension (such as diabetic and/or renal failure patients) are generally responsive to these drugs, as are patients with sympathetically driven forms of hypertension.

- Perioperative forms of hypertension respond well to clonidine. In addition, an anesthesia- and analgesia-sparing property of these drugs may offer a unique clinical benefit.

- Clonidine can be used adjunctively with other therapies in heart failure (HF), particularly when hypertension is present. Sustained-release moxonidine, however, is associated with early mortality and morbidity when used in the patient with HF.

- Escalating doses of drugs in this class often bring on salt and water retention, in which case a diuretic becomes useful adjunctive therapy.

- Drugs that reduce sympathetic neurotransmission have been some of the first compounds used in the treatment of hypertension. These agents are effective antihypertensives and establish a favorable hemodynamic profile in the course of reducing blood pressure (BP).

- The side-effect profile of compounds in this class is unpleasant and is a consideration that ultimately has some bearing on patient compliance.

INTRODUCTION

Although complex, and not understood in full detail, a relationship exists between the centrally modulated activated sympathetic nervous system (SNS) and hypertension. SNS activation is also an important element of HF pathophysiology and influences various developmental aspects of the metabolic syndrome. It has been estimated that from 15 to 30% of essential hypertension patients have a primary neurogenic stimulus as an etiology for their hypertension.[1]

One aspect of the SNS contribution to hypertension that has proven bothersome is how best to experimentally establish an activity/effect relationship. The idea that plasma concentrations of catecholamines [particularly norepinephrine (NE)] faithfully reflect what transpires at nerve endings or within the central nervous system (CNS) is one that has died hard. In that regard, the measurement of circulated NE reflects a delicate balance between afferent signals and catecholamine release, metabolism, uptake, and sensitivity of the adrenergic receptors. Thus, many experiments attempting to establish the SNS contribution to various aspects of the hypertensive state were predestined to failure based on interpretive considerations relating to plasma NE concentrations.[2]

Nonetheless, vascular resistance is inversely related to the fourth power of vascular diameter, and the arteriolar sympathetic tone has a considerable influence on peripheral resistance. Sympathetic stimulation also has important effects related to stimulation of renal sodium reabsorption and renal release of renin. As a result of these multiple effects, sympathetic stimulation also has important effects on BP.

In more general terms, sympathetic activation (as reflected by an increase in both heart rate and/or plasma catecholamine levels) is regarded as a determinant of hypertension development and thus a target with some considerable potential for drug treatment. However, centrally acting antihypertensive agents still prove effective even in the absence of apparent signs of SNS activation.[3,4] Of note, SNS activity need not be measurably abnormal but rather can perpetuate the hypertensive state if merely increased (albeit inappropriately so) relative to a patient's hemodynamic, volume, and neurohumoral circumstances. In addition, the SNS is adjoined to other regulatory pathways in a manner such that even a normal level of activity can unduly contribute to the prevailing BP. This is particularly the case when the interrelationship between the sympathetic and renin-angiotensin systems is considered.

MECHANISM OF ACTION

Molecular aspects of drug action and pharmacokinetics

For effect, α-methyldopa (the first drug in this class) requires local conversion within the brain to an active metabolite (α-methylnorepinephrine). The antihypertensive action of α-methyldopa was originally believed to be via tissue inhibition of dopa decarboxylase followed by a depletion of biogenic amines. However, this mechanism contributes minimally to its BP-lowering effect. Instead, α-methyldopa lowers BP by conversion to α-methylnorepinephrine—an active metabolite that displaces NE from the α-adrenergic receptor (e.g., the concept of a false neurotransmitter; Figure 83–1).[5]

The other agents in this class do not require metabolic conversion and are functionally active as their respective intact molecules. For their main pharmacodynamic effect to occur, compounds in this drug class must cross the blood/brain barrier to gain access to their effect compartment within the CNS. As such, there is an implicit time lag between plasma concentrations and antihypertensive effect. The pharmacokinetics of the various centrally acting agents are similar, with a few noteworthy exceptions (Tables 83–1 and 83–2). The onset of action varies among the compounds in this class, with clonidine showing activity within 15 to 30 minutes of intake.

These compounds typically have a large volume of distribution, which in part relates to compartmentalization in the CNS. The systemic half-life for compounds in this class is not necessarily representative of their pharmacodynamic half-life. This finding relates to receptor affinity and depot effects in deep-tissue compartments. Finally, moxonidine and rilmenidine are extensively renally cleared and call for their being carefully dose adjusted in the patient with renal failure.[6,7]

Pharmacodynamics

Centrally acting drugs stimulate central vasomotor adrenergic receptors (e.g., nucleus tractus solitarii), thereby inhibiting central sympathetic outflow to the heart and peripheral vasculature. These compounds stimulate α_2-receptors on adrenergic neurons found within the rostral ventrolateral medulla, a site that adjusts sympathetic outflow. Plasma catecholamine levels drop with centrally acting therapy, which may also relate to the stimulation of presynaptic α_2-receptors in peripheral locations.

Clonidine stimulates both α_2-receptors and imidazoline (I_1)-receptors as the basis for its peripheral sympathoinhibition. Guanfacine is considered a more selective alpha$_2$-receptor agonist than clonidine (Table 83–3). Unlike clonidine, guanfacine does not inhibit dopamine turnover. More selective I_1 receptor agonists, such as moxonidine and rilmelidine, activate I_1-receptors within the rostral ventrolateral medulla in the brain stem (with moxonidine having up to a 30-fold greater affinity for I_1 than alpha$_2$ receptors). In the course of I_1 receptor agonism, the firing rate of bulbospinal sympathoexcitatory neurons decreases, peripheral sympathoinhibition ensues, and BP is reduced. The antihypertensive activity of moxonidine and rilmenidine correlates most closely with its I_1-receptor binding (Figure 83–2).[8]

The physiologic effects of withdrawal of SNS tone include parallel and balanced falls in peripheral vascular resistance and systolic/diastolic BP. The reduction in peripheral resistance seen persists during long-term treatment. Despite the vasodilator action of drugs in this class, reflex tachycardia does not develop—and heart rate may be somewhat reduced in the course of treatment. Cardiac output and renal blood flow typically remain unchanged with drugs in this class.[9]

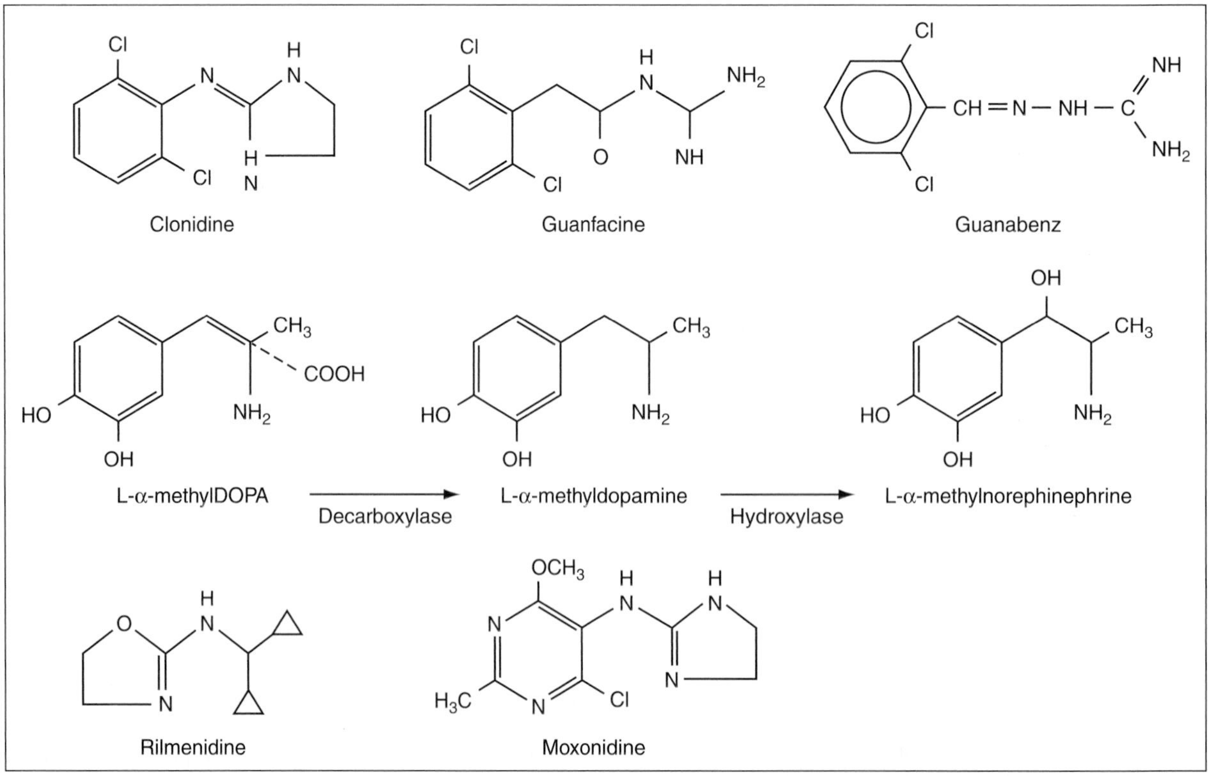

Figure 83–1. Chemical structures of various centrally acting antihypertensive agents.

PHARMACOKINETICS OF CENTRALLY ACTING COMPOUNDS					
Drug	Absorption (%)	Tmax (hrs.)	Protein Binding (%)	Volume of Distribution (L/kg)	Half-life (hrs.)
α-methyldopa	25	2.0	< 15	0.6	1.7
Clonidine	75–100	1.5–2.0	20–40	2.0	6–15
Guanabenz	75	2–5	90	7.4–13.4	6–14
Guanfacine	> 90	1.5–4.0	70	6.3	17
Moxonidine	80–90	0.5–3.0	5.8–7.9	3.0	2–3
Rilmenidine	100	1.7	10–11	315–325 L	8.5

Table 83–1. Pharmacokinetics of Centrally Acting Compounds

RENAL AND PREGNANCY CONSIDERATIONS WITH CENTRALLY ACTING COMPOUNDS				
Drug	Renal Elimination[a] (%)	Dialyzability	Dose Adjustment in Renal Failure	FDA Pregnancy Category
α-methyldopa	70	Yes	Yes	C
Clonidine	58	Yes, but limited	No	C
Guanabenz	< 5	No	No	C[b]
Guanfacine	50	Limited	No	B[c]
Moxonidine[d]	50–75	Not known	Yes	Not classified
Rilmenidine[d]	52–93	Yes	Yes	Not classified

a. Elimination of the intact molecule.

b. FDA category C: Either studies in animals have revealed adverse effects on the fetus (teratogenic or embryocidal or other) and there are no controlled studies in women or studies in women and animals are not available. Drugs should be given only if the potential benefit justifies the potential risk to the fetus.

c. FDA category B: Either animal reproduction studies have not demonstrated a fetal risk but there are no controlled studies in pregnant women or animal reproduction studies have shown an adverse effect (other than a decrease in fertility) that was not confirmed in controlled studies in women in the first trimester (and there is no evidence of a risk in later trimesters).

d. Not available in the United States and thus the basis for no FDA pregnancy categorization.

Table 83–2. Renal and Pregnancy Considerations with Centrally Acting Compounds

CENTRAL NERVOUS SYSTEM RECEPTORS AS TARGETS OF CENTRALLY ACTING ANTIHYPERTENSIVES	
Compound	Receptor
α-methyldopa	α₂
Guanfacine	α₂
Guanabenz	α₂
Clonidine	α₂ and I₁
Moxonidine	I₁ > α₂
Rilmenidine	I₁ > α₂

Table 83–3. Central Nervous System Receptors as Targets of Centrally Acting Antihypertensives

During exercise, these compounds reduce peripheral vascular resistance—suggesting that exercise-related changes in SNS activity are blocked. Centrally acting agents also reduce plasma renin activity (PRA), and with long-term treatment regress left ventricular hypertrophy.[10] Agents in this class tend to produce dose-dependent salt-and-water retention, and as a result their effectiveness may diminish over time. This pseudotolerance to a BP-lowering effect can be undone with diuretic therapy.

INDICATIONS/CONTRAINDICATIONS AND OBJECTIVES OF THERAPY

Indications

The antihypertensive efficacy of both central α₂-receptor and I₁-receptor agonists is well established, having been confirmed in large numbers of patients with essential hypertension. Clonidine, the standard in this class, has been shown in the Veterans Affairs Cooperative Study to be somewhat more effective in whites than in blacks (and is recognized as being more effective in older than in younger blacks).[3] Centrally acting compounds compare favorably with other first-line antihypertensive drug classes—such as diuretics, beta blockers, angiotensin-converting enzyme (ACE) inhibitors, and calcium-channel blockers (CCBs)—in effectiveness. These compounds are also useful adjunctive therapies related to most other antihypertensive medication classes, paticularly with vasodilators in that they can attenuate the pulse-rate change that occurs as these drugs reduce BP.

Centrally acting compounds are particularly useful for patients who have hypertension with associated anxiety, especially that marked by sympathetic overactivity. Drugs in this class are metabolically neutral and can be used safely in the diabetic patient. In addition, patients with

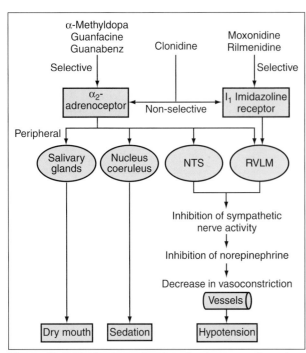

Figure 83–2. Mechanisms of action of various centrally acting antihypertensive agents. Dry mouth and sedation are side effects mediated by α_2-receptor but not I_1-receptor stimulation. (Adapted with permission from van Zwieten PA. The renaissance of centrally acting antihypertensive drugs. *J Hypertens* 1999;17:S15–21.)

chronic obstructive pulmonary disease safely tolerate these compounds. Clonidine is used in the perioperative setting in that it has the ability to control the sympathetically driven hypertension common to this setting and the ability to provide an anesthetic- and analgesic-sparing effect.[11]

Drug differentiation and mode of delivery considerations

All five drugs that comprise the centrally acting medication class similarly reduce BP if comparable doses are being used (Box 83–1). α-Methyldopa and clonidine are the only two drugs in this class available for intravenous administration. Clonidine is the only compound in the class that is available in a transdermal delivery system.[12] Onset of action and effect half-life are two of the main features that separate compounds in this class. Clonidine seems to have the quickest onset of action and the shortest duration of effect. The half-life of drugs in this class is widely variable and poorly correlates with the duration of medication effect.[6,7] As regards all compounds in this class, final dosing recommendations should be based on local prescribing information because there is a considerable geographic disparity in both usage and regulatory approval.

α-Methyldopa

From the early 1960s to the latter part of the 1970s, α-methyldopa was a popular drug for the treatment of hypertension. During that time it was found to be useful in all types and degrees of severity of hypertension.[5] Methyldopa is available in an intravenous formulation as an ester of the parent drug and has been used for hyper-

tensive emergencies. Treatment of hypertensive urgencies and emergencies with intravenous α-methyldopa has been supplanted by more effective drugs. With time and the availability of newer better tolerated antihypertensive medications, oral α-methyldopa also began to fall out of favor—although it still retains a niche status in the treatment of pregnancy-induced hypertension.[13] There is little evidence of adverse effects on fetal development with α-methyldopa. When used in doses ranging from 250 mg to 2.0 g per day it effectively reduces supine BP without causing orthostatic hypotension.

Clonidine

Oral clonidine has a rapid onset of action (30 to 60 minutes) and is of particular utility for managing hypertensive urgencies. However, it is relatively short acting and in managing hypertensive urgencies often requires frequent dosing.[14] A transdermal patch delivery system for clonidine provides a constant amount of drug for seven days, but it takes one to two days to attain peak effect and this effect lingers from 8 to 24 hours after the patch is removed.[15] Drug is best absorbed from the patch when it is placed on the chest or upper arm and not the lower torso.[16] Transdermal clonidine is very useful in the management of the labile hypertensive patient who requires multiple medications, the hospitalized patient who cannot take medications by mouth, and the patient prone to early morning surges in BP. At equivalent doses, transdermal clonidine is more likely than oral clonidine to precipitate salt and water retention.[12]

Guanabenz

Guanabenz is mechanistically similar to clonidine but is somewhat longer acting. It is less likely to cause rebound hypertension (Figure 83–3), fluid retention, and orthostatic hypotension. Therapy should generally begin with 4 mg twice daily, with increments up to a total daily dose of as much as 64 mg. The most noteworthy metabolic action of guanabenz is a reduction in total cholesterol levels in the order of 10 to 20%. The presumed mechanism for this may be related to inhibition of hepatic cholesterol production and triglyceride synthesis, as well as stimulation of fatty acid oxidation.[17]

Guanfacine

Guanfacine differs from the other members of this class in that its prolonged (24 hours) duration of action typically allows it to be dosed once daily.[18] Guanfacine appears to enter the brain more slowly and to maintain its antihypertensive effect longer than guanabenz. It is preferably dosed in the evening so that it can then blunt the early morning catecholamine surge. Evening dosing also allows any sedative effect to play out during sleep. As with other agents in this class, it works best when combined with a small dose of diuretic—which optimizes BP lowering. Guanfacine may be useful as an alternative to clonidine in patients developing intolerable sedation with the latter, and in patients recognized as being noncompliant with clonidine.[19] Finally, guanfacine has orphan drug status for the fragile-X syndrome, which is the most common inherited cause of mental retardation.

Box 83–1

Dosing Considerations with Centrally Acting Agents

Available Compounds

α-methyldopa, clonidine, guanfacine, guanabenz, moxonidine, rilmenidine

Dosing Considerations

α-Methyldopa

Oral α-methyldopa is initially given two to three times daily in a dose of 250 mg. Individual maintenance doses are in the range of 0.5 to 2.0 g/day in two to three divided doses.

Clonidine

Oral clonidine is best given two to three times daily. Starting doses are in the order of 0.1 mg two to three times daily, with dose increase up to as high as 0.6 mg two to three times daily. A small dose of clonidine (0.1 to 0.2 mg twice daily) augments the BP-lowering effect of most other agents and can be reliably used as add-on therapy. Clonidine is a short-acting compound, and thus patients with excessive sympathetic activity can have a short-lived response to it. If being given together with a beta blocker, rebound hypertension is more common when it is abruptly stopped and beta-blocker therapy is continued. In certain countries, transdermal clonidine is available. The transdermal system dose range allows for release of 0.1 to 0.3 mg per 24 hours. There is a one- to two-day delay in the onset of action after initial patch application with transdermal clonidine, making it inappropriate for the management of hypertensive emergencies. Conversely, removal of the transdermal delivery system for clonidine does not immediately eliminate drug effect. Clonidine can also be used intravenously for perioperative hypertension, with a dose of 0.15 mg given two to four times daily. These side effects can also occur at lower doses.

Guanfacine

The initial response to guanfacine is delayed compared to clonidine, but its longer duration of action allows it to be effectively dosed in a range of 1 to 3 mg given once or twice daily in a split dose. Withdrawal phenomena are significantly less pronounced than observed with clonidine, which may relate to its longer duration of action. Adverse effects increase significantly with doses in excess of 1 mg/day.

Guanabenz

Guanabenz is given by mouth as the acetate, but doses are usually expressed in terms of the base. Guanabenz acetate 5 mg is equivalent to about 4 mg of guanabenz. In hypertension, the usual dose is 4 mg twice daily initially; the daily dose may be increased by amounts of 4 to 8 mg every 1 to 2 weeks according to response. Doses of up to 32 mg twice daily have been used.

Moxonidine

0.2 mg once daily. As needed, the dose can be slowly increased to 0.4 or a maximum of 0.6 mg. The dose must be reduced to 0.2 to 0.4 mg/day in patients with moderate renal failure (GFR of 30-60 mL/min) and the drug should not be used at GFR values less than 30 mL/min.

Rilmenidine

1 mg once daily, if necessary to be increased to 2 mg in one oral dose. At GFR values < 15 mL/min it should be given in a dose of 1 mg every other day.

Overdose

Large doses can paradoxically increase blood pressure particularly with clonidine.

Moxonidine

Moxonidine reduces BP as effectively as most first-line antihypertensives when used as monotherapy and is an effective adjunctive therapy in combination with other antihypertensive agents.[6] Moxonidine does not reduce heart rate, as can occur with clonidine. The plasma half-life of moxonidine is only on the order of 2 to 3 hours. Thus, its much longer duration of action suggests CNS retention and tight binding to imidazoline I_1 receptors. Unlike other centrally acting agents, moxonidine undergoes extensive renal clearance and its dose has to be carefully adjusted according to the glomerular filtration rate (GFR).[20]

The United Kingdom licensed prescribing information states that in patients with moderate renal impairment (GFR 30 to 60 mL/min) single doses of moxonidine should not exceed 200 μg and the daily dose should not exceed 400 μg. Moxonidine should not be given in severe impairment (GFR < 30 mL/min). In addition, moxonidine should

not be used in severe forms of HF and only with considerable caution in patients with moderate HF.[21]

Rilmenidine

Numerous studies have demonstrated that oral rilmenidine 1 to 2 milligrams (mg) daily, alone or in combination with other antihypertensives, is well tolerated and effective in the treatment of mild to moderate hypertension.[7] An oral dosage of 1 mg daily appears to provide the optimum ratio of efficacy to tolerability (i.e., a lower incidence of adverse effects). Rilmenidine appears to enhance parasympathetic tone, which may account for the lack of effect on heart rate while producing a reduction in BP.[22]

Uses independent of blood pressure

Centrally acting agents (in particular, clonidine) have a number of alternative uses beyond BP reduction. As such, they can be used to good effect in disease states other

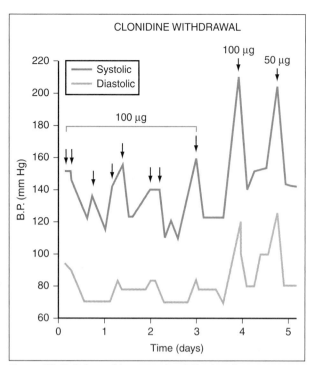

Figure 83–3. Rebound hypertension following the discontinuation of clonidine.

than hypertension. For example, clonidine may be used to provide migraine prophylaxis, to alleviate post-traumatic stress syndrome, to suppress postmenopausal flushing, to minimize alcohol and opioid withdrawal symptoms, and to manage open-angle glaucoma.

Clonidine is also useful in various diarrheal states, including that which occasionally accompanies the short-gut syndrome.[23] Clonidine has also been used in the perioperative period both as an adjuvant to general and/or regional anesthesia; to improve analgesia after systemic, spinal, or peripheral opioids; and to control postoperative sympathetic responses.[11] Of note, clonidine sympatholytic activity primarily affects tonic activity and less so the reactivity of the SNS, which is a valuable pharmacologic feature in the perioperative setting.

The sympathoinhibition that occurs with clonidine can provide a diuretic-enhancing effect in cirrhotic patients with ascites and is viewed as a secondary approach to counteract the sympathetic hyperactivity, which distinguishes HF.[24] In this regard, modest doses of clonidine significantly attenuate cardiac and renal sympathetic tone in HF, which may conceivably counter the salt and water retention that marks this disease state.[25] Oral clonidine also appears to control ventricular rate in new-onset atrial fibrillation, with an efficacy comparable to that of standard agents.[26] Finally, clonidine can be used for the diagnosis of pheochromocytoma. When 0.1 mg of clonidine is administered hourly for three doses, plasma NE levels fall in patients with essential hypertension but remain elevated in patients with a pheochromocytoma.[27]

Alternatives to therapy

If centrally acting agents are being used simply as add-on therapy in a multi-drug regimen, the issue of intolerance is resolved most simply by discontinuing the offending medication. In other instances (in which use of centrally acting agents are of a more crucial nature), drug classes such as beta blockers, combined alpha/beta blockers, and peripheral alpha blockers can be substituted. However, the occasional patient with a strong SNS component to their hypertension will develop paradoxical hypertension with beta-blocker therapy. Finally, in certain patients with a sympathetically driven form of hypertension behavioral modification strategies and/or anxiolytic therapy can be used. This approach can often keep the dose of a centrally acting agent in a tolerable range.

Cost effectiveness

Centrally acting agents can be quite cost-effective therapies in that these compounds are for the most part available generically. Thus, they minimally affect the incremental cost of hypertension management when multi-drug therapy is required to reach treatment goals. The considerably higher cost of transdermal clonidine has, however, proven a disincentive to its more widespread use despite its better tolerance.

COMPLICATIONS

Class side-effect considerations

As with any antihypertensive agent that inhibits SNS activity, most anticipated side effects (postural hypotension, weakness, sodium and water retention, gastrointestinal symptoms) may be related to the adrenolytic action or to the resultant override of parasympathetic function, or to both. Somnolence and dry mouth (40%) are the most common adverse drug reactions and are the major reason central sympatholytics are discontinued.[28,29] I_1-receptor stimulants appear to have a better tolerability profile, causing less dry mouth and drowsiness.[6,7]

Other CNS depressants (such as sedative-hypnotics, benzodiazepines, antihistamines and/or ethanol) may add to the sedative effects within this drug class. The dry mouth with centrally acting agents relates to a α_2-mediated drop-off in salivary flow rate and can be very annoying. If central-acting therapy is sufficiently long lived it can increase the likelihood of dental caries, periodontal disease, or oral candidiasis.[30]

Class-member-specific side-effect considerations
Methyldopa

The intestinal absorption of α-methyldopa, and therefore its therapeutic effect, is reduced by simultaneously ingested iron. Additional side effects characteristic of α-methyldopa include somnolence and depressive reactions, which may relate to a change in brain biogenic amines.[28,29] Hypersensitivity reactions, including hepatitis and Coombs-positive hemolytic anemia (due to the appearance of an antibody with specificity for red cell Rh determinants), have been observed with α-methyldopa. This occurs in 10 to 20% of patients receiving at least 1 g of α-methyldopa daily over several months.[31]

In general, α-methyldopa can be continued in the presence of a positive direct Coombs test alone. However, if anemia occurs therapy should be withdrawn. A drug-induced hepatitis (with fever, eosinophilia, and increased transaminase values) can occur with α-methyldopa. This appears to be a self-limited process that remits with drug discontinuation. α-Methyldopa may also produce a flu-like syndrome marked by high fever (drug-induced fever). α-Methyldopa and its metabolic products can interfere with some assays for catecholamines and can interfere with other therapeutic agents, such as levodopa, bromocriptine, and monoamine oxidase inhibitors.

Clonidine

Clonidine can suppress sinus and atrioventricular nodal function, with the result sometimes being significant brady-cardia. Patients with chronic kidney disease (CKD) and sinus node dysfunction are at risk of significant brady-cardia with clonidine.[32] In these patients, clonidine is best avoided. If clonidine is suddenly discontinued during treatment with high doses (usually > 1.0 mg, but some-times lower doses), rebound hypertension may occur secondarily to an excessive sympathetic discharge.[33] Rebound hypertension may be more prominent if beta-blocker therapy is ongoing at the time of clonidine discon-tinuation. Such a rebound phenomenon has not been seen with moxonidine and rilmenidine.[6,7]

Skin hypersensitivity to the transdermal clonidine occurs in 15 to 20% of patients. Skin reactions to transdermal clonidine can include subjective signs of pruritus and objective findings such as erythema, scaling, vesiculation, excoriation, and induration. Hyperpig-mentation, depigmentation, and pseudolymphoma can also occur.[12] Allergic dermatitis occurs more commonly in whites than in blacks, and more commonly in women than in men.

Potential causes of the allergic contact dermatitis could be active drug, adhesive, diffusion membrane, solvent, or enhancer. Most studies have indicated that skin reactions are related to the active drug itself and not to other factors.[12] Clonidine overdose produces paradoxical hypertension when the depressor effects of central α$_2$-adrenergic receptor stimulation are exceeded by the pressor effects of peripheral α$_2$-adrenergic receptor stimulation, resulting in a predominantly vasoconstrictor response.[34]

Guanfacine

Tricyclic antidepressants, such as imipramine and amitripty-line, reduce the antihypertensive action of guanfacine (and clonidine) in that they are antagonists of the same central α$_2$-receptors these compounds target.[35]

Guanabenz

The incidence of sedation in clinical trials is dose dependent and ranges from 20 to 50% with guanabenz. However, guanabenz-related sedation appears to diminish with time in patients receiving maintenance treatment. Guanabenz

has not been associated with weight gain and/or clinically apparent sodium retention.[36]

Moxonidine/Rilmenidine

Monoamine oxidase inhibitors should not be given together with these compounds. Both compounds have fewer side effects than is the case with clonidine and α-methyldopa, owing to a lesser affinity for α$_2$-receptors.[6,7]

CONTRAINDICATIONS

Epidural clonidine hydrochloride is not recommended for obstetrical, postpartum, or perioperative pain management. The risk of hemodynamic instability, especially hypoten-sion and bradycardia, from epidural clonidine hydrochloride may be unacceptable in these patients. All centrally acting agents are contraindicated in those with hypersensitivity to the compound. On a compound-specific basis, moxoni-dine is contraindicated in both advanced CKD and severe HF.[6] Although not specifically contraindicated, clonidine should be used cautiously in patients with sinoatrial and/or atrioventricular disease—particularly if the patient is already bradycardic.[32]

SIDE EFFECT MANAGEMENT

The side effects with centrally acting compounds can be most directly treated by discontinuing the compound to blame. However, there are sufficient patients for whom BP control is heavily dependent on therapy with centrally acting agents making medication discontinuation a less than desirable choice. In such cases, several therapy options exist. Medication can be split-dosed such that the same total daily dose is given but more frequently and at lower individual doses. This often lessens the sedating effect of these compounds, which is the most common reason for medication discontinuation and one that is drug concentration dependent.

In addition, nighttime dosing is an alternative—in which case the sedating effects of these medications can be exploited to facilitate sleeping. However, the decrease in salivary flow that accompanies these therapies (in particular, with clonidine) can be quite discomfiting and may promote caries development. If so, salivary substitutes can be considered. Another treatment option is to lower the total daily dose of a centrally acting agent and direct therapy to alternative drug classes that are less side-effect provoking. Within-class switches are sometimes of use. For example, a patient intolerant of either the sedating effects or the rebound hypertension with clonidine may be switched to a less sedating compound (such as guanfacine or even more so moxonidine or rilmenidine).[37] However, moxonidine and rilmenidine are not as widely available as guanfacine.

A final consideration is that a patient intolerant of oral clonidine can be converted to the transdermal form of clonidine, with which the side effects of sedation, fatigue, and/or dry mouth are considerably less. The transdermal delivery system can be particularly useful in reducing the risk of rebound hypertension.[12] Transdermal clonidine has a not insignificant number of patients in whom it causes a skin rash.[38] Treatment with hydrocortisone cream or over-the-counter antacids (magnesium-aluminum hydroxide suspension) has been used in an attempt to ameliorate skin reactions. Hydrocortisone cream (0.5%), whether applied under or around the edges of the patch, has occasionally been effective in preventing (or lessening) the contact dermatitis. However, this has been poorly studied other than for the observation that pretreatment of the skin with hydrocortisone increases clonidine absorption and thereby plasma levels.[36]

The variable response to hydrocortisone may reflect the relative weakness of this compound as a corticosteroid. Alternatively, an aerosolized spray of the more potent corticosteroid beclomethasone seems to favorably impact the skin sensitization seen with transdermal clonidine. The drying effect of the steroid spray does not affect the adhesion of the patch to the skin surface, which has been viewed as a drawback with hydrocortisone cream.[39,40]

SUMMARY

Centrally acting antihypertensive compounds remain an important tool in the management of hypertension. There are significant numbers of patients whose hypertension is linked to the SNS in such a way that these drugs remain primary first-line therapies. However, centrally acting antihypertensive compounds are used most regularly in an adjunctive role for general control of hypertension irrespective of its origin.

The prototype compounds in this class (α-methyldopa and clonidine) are used less regularly because of a fairly onerous side-effect profile. However, there are several choices within the centrally acting antihypertensive medication class that increase the chances of finding a well-tolerated compound. Centrally acting antihypertensive compounds are fairly diversified in their actions and not only reduce BP but favorably influence a number of non-hypertensive conditions linked to sympathetic activity

REFERENCES

1. Rahn KH, Barenbrock M, Hausberg M. The sympathetic nervous system in the pathogenesis of hypertension. *J Hypertens* Suppl 1999;17:S11–14.
2. Grassi G, Esler M. How to assess sympathetic activity in humans. *J Hypertens* 1999;17:719–34.
3. Materson BJ, Reda DJ, Cushman WC. Department of Veterans Affairs single-drug therapy of hypertension study: Revised figures and new data. Department of Veterans Affairs Cooperative Study Group on Antihypertensive Agents. *Am J Hypertens* 1995;8:189–92.
4. Materson BJ, Kessler WB, Alderman MH, et al. A multicenter, randomized, double-blind dose-response evaluation of step-2 guanfacine versus placebo in mild to moderate hypertension. *Am J Cardiol* 1986;57:32E–37E.
5. Frohlich ED. Methyldopa: Mechanisms and treatment 25 years later. *Arch Intern Med* 1980;140:954–59.
6. Fenton C, Keating G, Lyseng-Williamson, Katherine A. Moxonidine: A review of its use in essential hypertension. *Drugs* 2006;66:477–96.
7. Reid JL. Rilmenidine: A clinical overview. *Am J Hypertens* 2000;13:106S–111S.
8. van Zwieten PA. The renaissance of centrally acting antihypertensive drugs. *J Hypertens* Suppl 1999;17:S15–21.
9. Goldberg M, Gehr M. Effects of alpha$_2$ agonists on renal function in hypertensive humans. *J Cardiovasc Pharmacol* 1985;7(8):S34–S37.
10. Mohammed S, Fasola AF, Privitera PJ, et al. Effect of methyldopa on plasma renin activity in man. *Circ Res* 1969;25:543–48.
11. Doman T, Clarkson K, Rosenfeld BA, et al. Effects of clonidine on prolonged postoperative sympathetic response. *Crit Care Med* 1997;25:1147–52.
12. Sica DA, Grubbs R. Transdermal clonidine: Therapeutic considerations. *J Clin Hypertens (Greenwich)* 2005;7:558–62.

13. Chobanian AV, Bakris GL, Black HR, et al. Joint National Committee on Prevention, Detection, Evaluation, and Treatment of High Blood Pressure: Seventh report of the Joint National Committee on Prevention, Detection, Evaluation, and Treatment of High Blood Pressure. *Hypertension* 2003;42:1206–52.
14. Houston MC. Treatment of hypertensive emergencies and urgencies with oral clonidine loading and titration. *Arch Intern Med* 1986;146:586–89.
15. MacGregor TR, Matzek KM, Keirns JJ, et al. Pharmacokinetics of transdermally delivered clonidine. *Clin Pharmacol Ther* 1985;38:278–84.
16. Hopkins K, Aarons L, Rowland M. Absorption of clonidine from a transdermal therapeutic system when applied to different body sites. In MA Weber, CJ Mathias (eds.), *Mild Hypertension*. Darmstadt, Germany: Steinkopf Verlag 1984:143.
17. Capuzzi DM, Cevallos WH. Inhibition of hepatic cholesterol and triglyceride synthesis by guanabenz acetate. *J Cardiovasc Pharmacol* 1984;6(5):S847–52.
18. Oster JR, Epstein M. Use of centrally acting sympatholytic agents in the management of hypertension. *Arch Intern Med* 1991;151:1638–44.
19. Cornish LA. Guanfacine hydrochloride: A centrally acting antihypertensive agent. *Clin Pharm* 1988;7:187–97.
20. Kirch W, Hutt HJ, Planitz V. The influence of renal function on clinical pharmacokinetics of moxonidine. *Clin Pharmacokinet* 1988;15:245–53.
21. Cohn JN, Pfeffer MA, Rouleau J, et al. Adverse mortality effect of central sympathetic inhibition with sustained-release moxonidine in patients with heart failure (MOXCON). *Eur J Heart Fail* 2003;5:659–67.

22. Zannad F, Aliot E, Florentin J, et al. Hemodynamic and electrophysiologic effects of a new alpha 2-adrenoceptor agonist, rilmenidine, for systemic hypertension. *Am J Cardiol* 1988;61:67D–71D.
23. Buchman AL, Fryer J, Wallin A, et al. Clonidine reduces diarrhea and sodium loss in patients with proximal jejunostomy: A controlled study. *J Parenter Enteral Nutr* 2006;30:487–91.
24. Azevedo ER, Newton GE, Parker JD. Cardiac and systemic sympathetic activity in response to clonidine in human heart failure. *J Am Coll Cardiol* 1999;33:186–91.
25. Aggarwal A, Esler MD, Morris MJ, et al. Regional sympathetic effects of low-dose clonidine in heart failure. *Hypertension* 2003;41:553–57.
26. Simpson CS, Ghali WA, Sanfilippo AJ, et al. Clinical assessment of clonidine in the treatment of new-onset rapid atrial fibrillation: A prospective, randomized clinical trial. *Am Heart J* 2001;142:E3.
27. Bravo EL, Tarazi RC, Fouad FM, et al. Clonidine-suppression test: a useful aid in the diagnosis of pheochromocytoma. *N Engl J Med* 1981;305:623–26.
28. van Zwieten PA, Thoolen MJ, Timmermans PB. The hypotensive activity and side effects of methyldopa, clonidine, and guanfacine. *Hypertension* 1984;6:II28–33.
29. Webster J, Koch HF. Aspects of tolerability of centrally acting antihypertensive drugs. *J Cardiovasc Pharmacol* 1996;27:S49–54.
30. Watson GE, Pearson SK, Bowen WH. The effect of chronic clonidine administration on salivary glands and caries in the rat. *Caries Res* 2000;34:194–200.
31. Carstairs KC, Breckenridge A, Dollery CT, Worlledge SM. Incidence of a positive direct coombs test in patients on alpha-methyldopa. *Lancet* 1966;2:133–35.

32. Byrd BF III, Collins HW, Primm RK. Risk factors for severe bradycardia during oral clonidine therapy for hypertension. *Arch Intern Med* 1988;148:729–33.

33. Hansson L, Hunyor SN, Julius S, Hoobler SW. Blood pressure crisis following withdrawal of clonidine (Catapres, Catapresan), with special reference to arterial and urinary catecholamine levels, and suggestions for acute management. *Am Heart J* 1973;85:605–10.

34. Domino LE, Domino SE, Stockstill MS. Relationship between plasma concentrations of clonidine and mean arterial pressure during an accidental clonidine overdose. *Br J Clin Pharmacol* 1986;21:71–74.

35. Buckley M, Felly J. Antagonism of antihypertensive effects of guanfacine by tricyclic antidepressants [letter]. *Lancet* 1991;337:1173.

36. Braden G, Alvis R, Walker BR, Cox M. Effects of guanabenz on sodium and water homeostasis. *J Clin Hypertens* 1987;3:397–404.

37. Wilson MF, Haring O, Lewin A, et al. Comparison of guanfacine versus clonidine for efficacy, safety and occurrence of withdrawal syndrome in step-2 treatment of mild to moderate essential hypertension. *Am J Cardiol* 1986;57:43E–49E.

38. Ito MK, O'Connor DT. Skin pretreatment and the use of transdermal clonidine. *Am J Med* 1991;91:42S–49S.

39. Tom GR, Premer R. Hydrocortisone cream in clonidine patch dermatitis. *Ann Pharmacother* 1994;28:889–90.

40. McChesney JA. Preventing the contact dermatitis caused by a transdermal clonidine patch (letter). *West J Med* 1991;154:736.

Chapter
84 Vasodilators

Gordon T. McInnes

Key Findings

- Vasodilators reduce blood pressure primarily by actions on vascular smooth muscle.
- Vasodilators can be classified as adrenergic inhibitors (ganglion-blocking drugs and post-ganglionic adrenergic inhibitors) and direct-acting vascular smooth muscle relaxants (hydralazine/endralazine, minoxidil, diazoxide, sodium nitroprusside, and potassium channel agonists).
- Vasodilators are effective antihypertensive agents but are associated with severe side effects.
- Vasodilators now have a very restricted clinical role, mainly in hypertensive emergencies and in patients with severe hypertension refractory to other agents.

INTRODUCTION

Over the past three decades, antihypertensive drug therapy has made a tremendous impact on morbidity and mortality from cardiovascular disease. Because rigorous control of blood pressure is needed to maximally improve outcome and few patients achieve this with first-choice therapy, a wide selection of antihypertensive agents is desirable.

The lower blood pressure that occurs with most antihypertensive drugs is associated with decreased peripheral vascular resistance. In some cases, this effect is indirect as a result of actions upon neural or humoral control systems or through an autoregulatory response to lower blood pressure. Other drugs have direct actions upon vascular smooth muscle.

Among the most effective antihypertensive drugs are those that inhibit sympathetic activity. This may be achieved at practically any anatomic level of adrenergic function. The term *vasodilator* was originally reserved for direct-acting vascular smooth muscle relaxants. Individual vasodilators may act upon resistance vessels, large arteries, or venous capacitance vessels.

Differential actions at these sites play a major role in the hemodynamic profile of the drugs[1] (Table 84–1). A predominant action upon the resistance vessels causes an immediate fall in blood pressure, activation of baroreceptor reflexes, and increased cardiac output.[2] Orthostatic hypotension is not seen. By contrast, relaxation of the venous capacitance vessels causes a reduction of venous return to the heart and a fall in cardiac output associated with a fall in blood pressure.[3] Cardiovascular baroreceptors are again activated.

Changes in the patterns of the large arterial waveform resulting from large arterial relaxation and dilatation of resistance vessels may have important consequences for the development of atheroma. These changes may not be reflected in blood pressure measured conventionally in the brachial artery.[4] Therefore, it seems possible that different types of vasodilators may have differential consequences for cardiovascular morbidity, although there are no endpoint data to define a particularly favorable pattern.

There are other consequences of vasodilator therapy apart from activation of the sympathetic nervous system. Parasympathetic withdrawal contributes to the cardiac response.[5] Renin and aldosterone levels are usually increased, partly as a result of increased sympathetic activity and partly as a result of decreased renal arterial perfusion pressure.[6] Agents that have a predominant action upon resistance vessels produce edema by increased capillary hydrostatic pressure resulting in disturbance of the Starling equilibrium. This is not seen with venodilator drugs.

Every direct-acting smooth muscle vasodilator and most adrenergic inhibitors induce compensatory sodium and water retention and extracellular fluid volume expansion following reduction of arterial pressure.[7,8] To maintain persistent and steady contraction of fluid volume, concomitant diuretic therapy is needed. A thiazide is generally the best choice for patients with relatively normal renal function because duration of action is greater than that of a loop diuretic. The diuretic enhances antihypertensive action by maintaining constriction of the extracellular and intracellular compartments.

ROLE OF VASODILATORS IN HYPERTENSION

The heterogeneous action of vasodilators is reflected in the different indications for usage. Because of the availability of newer better-tolerated drugs, in most developed countries use is restricted to management of patients with severe hypertension not readily controlled with other agents, parenteral treatment of hypertensive emergencies, and control of hypertension in pregnancy.

Whereas use of vasodilators has decreased drastically in favor of newer agents with different mechanisms of action, these agents continue to be used widely around the world. This is undoubtedly related to the availability of generic formulations and lower cost.

CORRELATION OF RELATIVE ACTIVITY OF VASODILATOR DRUGS IN RESISTANCE AND CAPACITANCE VESSELS WITH CIRCULATORY EFFECTS			
	Arterioselective	Nonselective	Vesoselective
Cardiac output	↓↑	↑	↓ (upright)
Arterial pressure	↓	↓	↓ (greater upright)
Central venous pressure	No change	No change	↓
Pulmonary artery pressure	↑		↓

Table 84–1. Correlation of Relative Activity of Vasodilator Drugs in Resistance and Capacitance Vessels with Circulatory Effects

MECHANISM OF ACTION AND PHARMACOKINETICS

Adrenergic inhibitors

Central adrenergic efferent impulses pass through major cardiovascular centers in the hypothalamus, medulla, and other subcortical areas of the spinal cord to synapse with second neurons located in the sympathetic ganglia at the thoracolumbar level of the spinal column. These most distal neurons are stimulated at the ganglion level by the release of acetylcholine from the terminals of the central neurons, thereby propagating the peripheral outflow of adrenergic impulses. Neural impulses (passing distally via the adrenergic neurons) reach the heart or blood vessels, where norepinephrine is released from nerve terminals. Norepinephrine stimulates the effector organ (heart, venule, or arteriole) by attachment to specific binding sites, alpha- or beta-adrenergic receptors. Norepinephrine is metabolized within the nerve terminal by monoamine oxidase in the mitochondria.

Binding of norepinephrine at the effector receptor may result in several possible processes. Stimulation of the beta-adrenergic receptor will produce vasoconstriction of the arteriole and venule. Stimulation of the alpha-adrenergic receptor will promote peripheral vasodilatation and increase heart rate, myocardial contractility, and myocardial metabolism.

There are many loci at which antihypertensive agents may inhibit the adrenergic nerve stimulus, including efferent sensory pathways from the heart, vessels, and mechanoreceptors; centrally at the ganglion level; or at the nerve terminal. Certain antihypertensive agents may also inhibit norepinephrine biosynthesis or block its action at the adrenergic receptor.

Ganglion-blocking drugs

Ganglion blockers act by occupying receptor sites on the post-ganglionic axon to stabilize the membrane against acetylcholine stimulation. These drugs have no effect on pre-ganglionic acetylcholine release, cholinesterase activity, post-ganglionic neuronal catecholamine release, or vascular smooth muscle contractility.[9]

Adrenergic transmission to the heart and vessels is impaired, with the result that heart rate, myocardial contractility, and total peripheral resistance are reduced. The fall in arterial pressure and vascular resistance is not as great in the supine as in the upright position because the adrenergic venomotor effect is enhanced by the gravitational effect of pooling blood when the patient is upright. Examples include hexamethonium, pentolinium, mecamylamine, pempidine, chlorisondamine, and trimetaphan. The only widely used agent in this class, trimetaphan, is excreted by glomerular filtration and active secretion (30% is unchanged in urine).

Post-ganglionic adrenergic inhibitors

When acetylcholine stimulates the post-ganglionic axon at the ganglionic levels, the impulse is propagated and cumulates in the release of norepinephrine at the nerve terminal with stimulation of adrenergic receptors in the vascular smooth muscle membrane. The impulse can be interrupted pharmacologically by a variety of mechanisms, including depletion of neurohumoral stores at the nerve terminal, prevention of norepinephrine uptake by the nerve terminal, inhibition of catecholamine biosynthesis, and therapeutic introduction of false neurotransmitters that block the adrenergic receptors on vascular smooth muscle.

Rawolfia alkaloids

Reserpine and more than 20 related compounds deplete the myocardium, blood vessels, adrenergic nerve terminals, adrenal medulla, and brain of catecholamines and serotonin.[10] By depleting the nerve terminal of norepinephrine stores and inhibiting norepinephrine re-uptake, adrenergic transmission is altered so that vascular resistance falls. With prolonged treatment, the persistent arterial hypotension is associated with slight decreases in renal blood flow and glomerular filtration rate. This may be related to the reduction in cardiac output or a venodilator effect similar to that of ganglion-blocking drugs.[10] Reserpine has oral bioavailability of 30%. Plasma half-life is prolonged (one to two weeks). Plasma protein binding is 96%.

Adrenergic neuron-blocking agents

These agents interfere with adrenergic neurotransmission at the post-ganglionic nerve terminals. Like reserpine there is depletion of catecholamine stores in nerve terminals, blood vessels, and the myocardium, but unlike reserpine there is little effect on catecholamine stores in the adrenal glands or brain.

After ingestion, there is a transient pressor phase associated with increased heart rate and cardiac output related to catecholamine release. A prolonged period of cardiac, vascular, and nerve terminal catecholamine depletion follows, associated with progressive reduction in systemic arterial pressure (explained by reduction in vascular resistance). Hypotension is less marked in the supine posture or with agents that simultaneously contract or prevent reexpansion of plasma volume.[7,8]

Guanethidine has oral absorption of 50 to 60% despite undergoing quite extensive pre-systemic metabolism (30 to 40%). Plasma half-life is two to eight days, and protein binding is less than 10%. Metabolism is in the liver. Bethanidine has complete oral absorption and undergoes no significant pre-systemic metabolism. Plasma half-life is 8 to 15 hours. Plasma protein binding is less than 10%. Bethanidine is excreted unchanged in the urine.

Debrisoquine has oral absorption of less than 85%. There is no pre-systemic metabolism and half-life is 10 to 26 hours. Protein binding is 25%. Metabolism is subject to genetic polymorphism via the P450 isoenzyme P450 II DI. Some 92% of Caucasians are extensive metabolizers, and 8% have poor metabolizer phenotypes. Plasma concentrations are several-fold higher in poor metabolizers. Bretylium was withdrawn as an antihypertensive agent because of incomplete and variable absorption after oral administration, rapid occurrence of tolerance, and a high rate of side effects. This drug is unsuitable for long-term use.

Monoamine oxidase inhibitors

Examples include pargyline, transcylypramine, phenylzine, and iproniazid. Pargyline was introduced primarily as an antihypertensive agent. Only a relatively few hypertensive individuals were studied and results were not striking.

Veratrium alkaloids

These agents alter the responsiveness of vagal efferent nerve fibers in the coronary sinus, left ventricle, and carotid sinus so that any pressure will result in altered nerve traffic. The stimulus is interpreted in the medullary vasomotor center as reflecting a higher pressure than actually exists, as a result of an induced delay in the vagal repolarization process.

The altered input in the cerebral vasomotor centers results in a reflexive fall in blood pressure and heart rate. The latter response may be abolished by atropine. Because adrenergic function is not blocked but only reset at a different pressure level, the usual postural and adrenergic reflexive responses are not altered. The result is a significant fall in peripheral resistance with little change in cardiac output despite marked bradycardia. Cerebral and renal blood flow and glomerular filtration rate remain normal unless the hypotensive response is excessive.

Direct-acting vascular smooth muscle relaxants

Agents in this class act by decreasing arteriolar resistance. Mechanisms of action are variable, although the final common pathway is vascular smooth muscle relaxation (Figure 84–1).

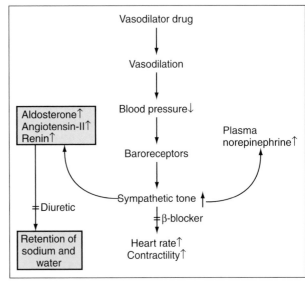

Figure 84–1. Reflex mechanisms triggered by vasodilation induced by vasodilator drugs.

Hydralazine

Hydralazine is a dilator of resistance vessels and has little action on venous beds.[11] After intravenous administration, hydralazine has slow onset of action of 15 to 20 minutes. Blood pressure fall is accompanied by baroreceptor-mediated sympathetic activation with tachycardia and sweating. After oral administration, onset of action is gradual and the duration of action is prolonged. The peak effect is seen 30 to 120 minutes after dosing. Higher doses do not increase the peak blood pressure reduction but prolong the duration of action.

The precise mode of action is unknown, but hydralazine causes activation of guanylate cyclase and accumulation of cyclic guanosine monophosphate (GMP).[12] By altering cellular calcium metabolism, hydralazine interferes with the movement of calcium that is responsible for initiating or maintaining the contractile state of vascular smooth muscle. Accumulation of cyclic GMP stimulates cyclic GMP-dependent protein kinase. This eventually leads to dephosphorylation of the light chain of myosin, which is thought to be involved in the contractile process in the phosphorylated form. Preferential dilation of arterioles (versus veins) minimizes postural hypotension, promotes increased cardiac output, and tends to lower diastolic more than systolic blood pressure. Blood flow increases in coronary, cerebral, and renal vascular beds.

In addition, a component of action is dependent on the presence of intact endothelium. Hydralazine may cause release of nitric oxide from the vascular endothelium. Hydralazine also stimulates the renin-angiotensin aldosterone (RAAS) system. This, together with a compensatory increase in heart rate and contractility, tends to counteract the antihypertensive effect.

Hydralazine is rapidly and completely (100%) absorbed from the gastrointestinal tract after oral administration.[11] The time to maximum serum concentration is one to two hours. Biotransformation commences in the gut wall and during first-pass through the liver (pre-systemic metabolism of 65 to 90%).[11] The liver is the major site of metabolism of hydralazine. Of the administered dose, 80% is excreted in the urine almost entirely as metabolites. The major metabolic pathways are N-acetylation and hydroxylation, with subsequent glucuronidation. Plasma half-life is two to four hours.[11] Plasma protein binding is 87%.

The acetylation pathway is subject to genetic polymorphism. Elimination is more rapid in "fast acetylators" than in "slow acetylators." "Slow acetylators" have almost twice the plasma concentration of "fast acetylators." This leads to greater antihypertensive effect and greater risk of side effects in "slow acetylators."

Endralazine

Endralazine is a vasodilator chemically similar to hydralazine. Acetylation is not a major route of metabolism and therefore response is not related to acetylator phenotype.[13]

Minoxidil

Treatment is associated with dilatation of resistance vessels.[14] There is little or no action on the venous bed. Minoxidil acts by activation of adenosine triphosphate (ATP)-sensitive potassium channels in arterial smooth muscle.[15] As a result, the smooth muscle membrane is hyperpolarized and calcium influx though voltage-gated calcium channels is inhibited. Cytosolic calcium concentration is reduced.

Oral absorption is 100%. Plasma half-life is 2.8 to 4.2 hours and plasma protein binding is negligible. Minoxidil is extensively metabolized in the liver. A sulphated metabolite is pharmacologically active and probably accounts for much of the activity of the parent drug.

Diazoxide

Diazoxide is a non-natriuretic thiazide congener that is an extremely potent vasodilator,[16] acting on resistance vessels and without effect on the venous bed.[17] The mode of action is opening of ATP-sensitive potassium channels in vascular smooth muscle cells.

Oral absorption is 85 to 95%. Plasma half-life is 28 hours. More than 90% of diazoxide is protein blood. Elimination is primarily by glomerular filtration. About 20% is metabolized in the liver to inactive metabolites.

Sodium nitroprusside

Sodium nitroprusside is administered as a slow intravenous infusion to produce rapidly reversible decrease in blood pressure.[18] The mode of action is to increase GMP within vascular smooth muscle activating vasorelaxation. This effect is probably mediated by non-enzymatic degradation of nitric oxide. The result is activation of vascular smooth muscle soluble guanylate cyclase with generation of cyclic adenosine monophosphate (AMP).[19]

Sodium nitroprusside is mainly excreted through the kidney. Clearance is extremely rapid. Half-life for blood pressure lowering is 32 to 40 seconds. The antihypertensive effect is potentiated in renal failure, although because a dose-titration regimen is employed adjustment of dose is unnecessary. The drug is metabolized non-enzymatically to cyanide, which reacts with thiosulphates to form thiocyanate (which is also excreted through the kidney).[20] The metabolic products of sodium nitroprusside are not active in the cardiovascular system.

Other potassium channel agonists

The recognition that minoxidil and diazoxide act through smooth muscle potassium channels increased interest in other agents with a similar mode of action and that may not give rise to the same serious side effects.[15,21] Hyperpolarization of the vascular smooth muscle membrane inhibits the opening of voltage-operated calcium channels and increases excretion of calcium by sodium-calcium exchange, inhibiting intracellular calcium release and increasing uptake of norepinephrine by the extraneuronal catecholamine transporter. In addition, potassium channel activators cause vasodilatation of small and large arteries but have little effect on the venous circulation.

Pinacidil has high oral absorption. Its half-life is 1.6 to 2.9 hours. Plasma protein binding is 40%. Metabolism and elimination is by biotransformation in the liver via cytochrome P-450, followed by renal elimination. Nicorandil has a nitrate moiety incorporated in the molecule. This significantly modifies the pharmacologic vasodilator profile.[22] Thus, nicorandil increases smooth muscle cyclic GMP.[23] Tachycardia is transient and cardiac output is not usually increased.

INDICATIONS/CONTRAINDICATIONS AND OBJECTIVES

Adrenergic inhibition
Ganglion-blocking drugs

Because interference with transmission of the autonomic impulse at the ganglia level impairs adrenergic and parasympathetic impulse transmission, the clinical use of ganglion blockers is associated with severe side effects and unwanted parasympathetic inhibition. With the advent of newer agents, ganglion blockers have become mostly of academic interest.

The exception is trimetaphan, which is still useful as an antihypertensive agent. Trimetaphan is delivered by slow intravenous infusion.[24] The starting dose is 0.5 to 2 mg/min and the adequate dose is usually 0.5 to 6 mg/min. Reduction of arterial pressure is immediate. Marked interindividual variability necessitates direct arterial blood pressure monitoring. When the infusion is discontinued, return of arterial pressure to pre-infusion levels is prompt. Thus, when administered in severe hypertension long-acting antihypertensive therapy must be initiated before discontinuing the infusion.

Trimetaphan can be used in hypertension with dissecting aortic aneurysm where the drug reduces velocity of ventricular ejection and hence sheering force. In controlling hypertension in acute aortic dissection, during surgery, and in arteriography, trimetaphan may be more manageable than agents with more prolonged action. Under these circumstances, ganglion blockade will not be associated with the secondary reflexive stimulation of the heart that is found with other vasodilators.

There are several contraindications to trimetaphan, including atheromatous vascular disease because of reduced blood supply, pyloric stenosis because of compromised gastric outflow via ganglionic blockade and in pregnancy because of the risk of paralytic or meconium ileus in the newborn. The duration of action of suxamethonum is prolonged by inhibition of pseudocholinesterase. The neuro-muscular blocking action of trimetaphan enhances non-depolarizing muscle relaxants.

Rawolfia alkaloids

Reserpine and similar alkaloids are efficacious in reducing arterial pressure when used with a diuretic.[25,26] Reserpine is generally added to the treatment regimen if response to a thiazide (or thiazide-like) diuretic is inadequate. Reserpine is also useful in treating hypertensive emergencies.[27] The maintenance dose of reserpine is up to 0.1 mg daily. Because reserpine has a long half-life, a loading dose is employed to obtain a reasonably rapid steady-state concentration.

Reserpine is contraindicated absolutely in depression and in those with a history of depression. The drug is also contraindicated in severe renal failure and is best avoided in peptic ulceration, ulcerative colitis, or asthma. Reserpine may cause complications in the neonate if used in pregnancy. These include nasal obstruction (anosmia), bradycardia, and hypothermia. Thus, reserpine is no longer a drug of choice in hypertensive emergencies in pregnancy. A reduced dose is recommended in the elderly.

Several drug interactions have been reported. There is enhanced peripheral vasodilatation and hypotension with alcohol. Enhanced falls in blood pressure are also seen with glyceryl trinitrate, L-dopa, fenfluramine, and phenothiazines. The pressor effects of phenylephrine and catecholamines are enhanced, whereas the effect of direct-acting amines (such as ephedrine) is diminished. There is excessive central nervous system excitation with monomine oxidase inhibitors. Reserpine lowers the convulsive threshold in epilepsy. The bradycardic effect of digoxin and the negative isotropic effects of antiarrhythmic agents, such as disopyramide and quinidine, are enhanced. There is increased myocardial depression with halothane and increased prolactin/breast enlargement with the oral contraceptive steroids.

Adrenergic neuron-blocking agents
Guanethidine

Because of prolonged action and because sympathetic inhibition is usually maximal at night, guanethidine needs to be administered only once daily. The starting dose of 10 mg is titrated to the required dose, which is usually 25 to 75 mg daily although up to 200 to 300 mg daily may be needed. Antihypertensive effect can be hastened by initiation with a loading dose.

Because fluid retention and expanded intravascular and extracellular fluid volumes are prominent, a diuretic is indicated, with the caveat that patients should be monitored carefully for hypokalemia and impaired renal excretory function. The phenomenon is due to fluid expansion because impairment of drug absorption over time seems unlikely. However, the common adverse effect of diarrhea may reduce absorption. Abrupt withdrawal is not associated with rebound hypertension because of the prolonged half-life. The mechanism of action leads to postural hypotension,

particularly after exercise or circumstances favoring vasodi-latation (such as heat, alcohol, or pyrexia). This is a particular risk in the elderly and when a diuretic is added.

When urgent reduction of blood pressure is indicated, guanethidine can be given parenterally (intramuscular or intravenous). A slow intravenous infusion or intramuscular injection avoids the initial pressor response due to cate-cholamine release. The maximum effect after intramuscular use is seen in one to two hours. Guanethidine is safe in pregnancy. Loss of blood pressure control may be due to drug interactions. Uptake into adrenergic nerve endings is reduced by concomitant tricyclic antidepressant therapy.

Bethanidine

The initial dose of 5 to 10 mg three times daily is titrated as necessary to a maximum dose of 200 mg daily. Bethanidine was widely used as third drug in combination with a thiazide and a beta blocker. The drug accumulates in renal failure, whereby antihypertensive effects may be enhanced.

Debrisoquine

The dose range is 20 to 400 mg daily, administered by twice- or thrice-daily dosing regimens. Debrisoquine is used with a beta blocker and diuretic to avoid fluid retention. Poor metabolizers respond to 10 mg twice daily, which is therefore the usual starting dose unless the metabolic phenotype is known. The starting dose is 40 mg twice daily in extensive metabolizers.

Adrenergic neuron-blocking agents are contraindicated in pheochromocytoma. Withdrawal of neurally released norepinephrine induces extreme sensitivity to circulating catecholamines. These drugs may exaggerate hypertension consequent on sudden release of catecholamines from the tumor.

Monoamine oxidase inhibitors

Monamine oxidase inhibitors may aggravate hypertension by inhibition of norepinephrine metabolism. Because monoamine oxidase is inhibited in the post-ganglionic nerve terminal, several weak pressor amines accumulate at this site. These substances are believed to act as false neurohumoral transmitters, tending to elevate blood pressure. Because of the potentially severe hypertensive crisis that may be associated with use, these drugs should be con-sidered primarily of academic interest in the treatment of hypertension.

Veratrium alkaloids

Clinical use has been severely restricted by side effects.

Direct-acting smooth muscle relaxants

With the fall in total peripheral resistance and arterial pressure, reflex stimulation of the heart occurs so that tachy-cardia and palpitation results frequently unless the cardiac reflex responses are offset by an adrenergic inhibitor (usually a beta blocker). These agents should not be administered to hypertensive patients with heart failure, myocardial infarction, angina, or aortic dissection because the reflexive cardiac effects will aggravate the underlying cardiac condition.

Hydralazine

Hydralazine entered the therapeutic armamentarium shortly after the ganglian-blocking agents and was one of the most effective drugs in the 1950s.[28] Usage declined rapidly in the 1960s but hydralazine returned to regular usage in stepped-care regimens of the late 1960s, in combination with a beta blocker and diuretic. Hydralazine has largely been replaced by other peripherally acting drugs and is now not widely used, although the drug remains effective and safe in specialist hands.

Hydralazine is usually administered three or four times daily, preferably starting with an individual dose of 12.5 to 25 mg. A lower dose (10 mg) may be used if there are side effects. The dose is then increased as necessary to a maximum of 200 to 300 mg daily. Slow acetylators show greater lowering of blood pressure.[11] The daily dose should not exceed 200 mg. High doses are more likely to be associated with development of anti-nuclear antibodies (ANA) and a lupus-like syndrome.[11] The acetylator phenotype can be determined readily by a simple urinary test of sulphonamide acetylation.[29] Periodic full blood count and ANA titers are recommended during chronic hydralazine therapy. Because hydralazine undergoes hepatic metabolism, dose adjustment is unnecessary in renal impairment.

Pretreatment with a beta blocker prevents sympathetic activation, reduces side effects, and potentiates the anti-hypertensive action.[30] Hydralazine is used with a beta blocker and diuretic to control moderate to severe hypertension. Where renal function is seriously impaired, a loop diuretic rather than a thiazide is needed to avoid edema. A multi-center trial[31] evaluated hydralazine, labetalol, methyldopa, prazosin, and placebo for value as a third drug when added to ongoing beta-blocker and diuretic treatment. Overall, hydralazine was the most generally suitable third drug.

Much of the early information demonstrating that anti-hypertensive therapy can diminish morbidity and mortality involved hydralazine-treated patients.[25,26,32,33] A combination of reserprine, hydrochlorothiazide, and hydralazine was used in the landmark Veterans Administration Cooporative Study Group Trials,[25] which demonstrated unequivocally the merits of antihypertensive therapy not only in severe but in moderate hypertension.

For urgent control of blood pressure, hydralazine can be given parenterally. Onset of action is in 15 minutes,[2] but the dose and frequency of administration required for blood pressure control are highly variable, the long duration of action makes dose titration difficult, and many patients do not respond adequately to any dose of hydralazine. Therefore, hydralazine is not an ideal drug for hypertensive emergencies. Sodium nitroprusside is more effective if continuous monitoring in an intensive therapy unit is available.

Although there have been no formal studies in pregnancy, and although the drug is teratogenic in some animals, hydralazine is widely used in pregnant women.[34] The main contraindication is coronary artery disease because increased cardiac output increases cardiac work and may provoke angina and myocardial ischemia or infarction. However, if hypertension is severe reduction in blood pressure and cardiac work will more than compensate. In mitral valve disease, hydralazine may increase pulmonary artery pressure and induce congestive heart failure. Endralazine lowers blood pressure over 24 hours with once-daily dosing.[35]

Minoxidil

Because of the severity of adverse effects, usage is limited to severe hypertension unresponsive to other treatments.[36] Minoxidil is usually administered twice daily with an initial dose of 2.5 to 5 mg. Once-daily dosing is sometimes employed. The maximum daily dose is usually 50 mg, although doses up to 100 mg have been used.

Pretreatment with a beta blocker limits sympathetic activation.[37] Sodium retention requires concomitant diuretic therapy in most. A loop diuretic is often necessary. Minoxidil is excreted into breast milk and therefore is best avoided in breast-feeding mothers. Safety in pregnancy has not been established.

Diazoxide

Oral diazoxide can be used in resistant hypertension as a twice-daily regimen, although the long half-life suggests that once-daily treatment may be sufficient. A graded sustained fall in blood pressure usually results. The initial dose is 50 to 100 mg twice daily, increasing as necessary to a total daily dose of 1 g.[38] The severity of side effects has rendered this usage largely obsolete.

Intravenous diazoxide is still occasionally used in the treatment of hypertensive emergencies. Diazoxide has been useful for the patient with hypertensive encephalopathy, and in those with severe, malignant, or accelerated hypertension (without heart failure) for whom rapid and immediate reduction in arterial pressure is mandatory. Blood pressure is lowered rapidly and consistently but rarely below normal. The first dose is usually effective and the action persists for several hours. The maximal daily dose is 150 mg. Higher doses previously used were associated with unacceptable hypotension and exacerbation of ischemic heart disease. For the same reason, rapid infusion is no longer recommended and the bolus should be administered over about 10 minutes.[39] Repeated doses can be administered every 5 to 15 minutes until target blood pressure is achieved. After each dose, the patient should remain recumbent and should be closely monitored for 30 minutes.

Diazoxide has been successful in severe hypertension in children. The usual effective dose is 5 mg/kg. Hypertensive crises induced by pheochromocytoma or due to monoamine oxidase inhibitor therapy should not be treated with diazoxide because blood pressure responds more specifically to alpha blockers. Safety in pregnancy has not been demonstrated conclusively.

Contraindications include subarachnoid hemorrhage, intracerebral hemorrhage, postoperative bleeding, functional hypoglycemia, and hypersensitivity to thiazides. In the case of dissection of aortic aneurysms, the increase in stroke volume and left ventricular ejection rate reflexively induced by diazoxide augment stresses in the aortic wall. The antidiuretic properties of diazoxide can lead to significant fluid retention which may precipitate congestive heart failure in patients with impaired cardiac reserve.

Sodium nitroprusside

Sodium nitroprusside is used for the short-term treatment of severely hypertensive patients at high risk, to normalize blood pressure before and during surgery for renal artery stenosis or pheochromocytoma, in hypotensive anesthesia, and in dissecting aortic aneurysm. Sodium nitroprusside is useful in hypertensive emergencies because of rapid onset of action, titratability, and rapid reversibility of excess blood pressure reduction.

The absence of tachycardia in most patients means that sodium nitroprusside is free of the cardiac symptoms produced by some other vasodilators. The drug is administered dissolved in 5% dextrose in water as an intravenous infusion using an infusion pump or drip regulator. The infusion should be protected from light using aluminum foil.

The drip rate is titrated against blood pressure. The average dose is 0.5 to 8.0 µg/kg/min. The rate should be increased slowly to prevent or reduce compensatory reactions (sharp rises in catecholamines and renin, tachycardia, and tachyphylaxis). The infusion should not be terminated abruptly to prevent excessive rebound in blood pressure. The starting dose is 0.3 to 1.0 µg/kg/min and is increased gradually until the desired blood pressure reduction is achieved, preferably while monitoring intra-arterial blood pressure. To avoid excessive levels of cyanide and to lessen the possibility of precipitous blood pressure reduction, the maximum recommended dose is 8 µg/kg/min. If this is insufficient, another approach should be tried.

Prolonged infusions are undesirable because of the risk of thiocyanate intoxication, but if continuous therapy over several days is required acid/base balance should be assessed by measurement of plasma bicarbonate, lactate, and the lactate/pyruvate ratio. This is a more sensitive measure of intoxication than plasma concentration of thiocyanate or cyanide under these conditions because toxicity is associated with the development of acidosis.

Sodium nitroprusside is contraindicated in severe liver impairment, Leber's optic atrophy, and tobacco amblyopia. Precaution is needed in disturbed cerebral blood flow because of the risk of too rapid lowering of blood pressure. Caution is also required in hypothyroidism because thiocyanate inhibits iodine uptake and binding by the thyroid. Care should be taken in renal failure because excretion of thiocyanate is decreased.

Other potassium channel agonists
Pinacidil

Greatest experience in hypertension is with this agent.[40] Pinacidil is usually administered as a sustained-release preparation. In doses ranging from 12.5 to 37.5 mg twice daily, pinacidil has a useful blood-pressure-lowering action. Dose-dependent edema offsets the antihypertensive effect. This can be overcome by concomitant diuretic. Pinacidil is contraindicated in congestive heart failure and should be used with caution in coronary or cerebrovascular disease and tachyarrhythmias because of the tendency to tachycardia.

Because pinacidil undergoes hepatic metabolism, dose reduction is advised in severe hepatic dysfunction and in the elderly because renal clearance of the metabolite is reduced. Nevertheless, pinacidil has been used with success

in renal hypertension. Intravenous pinacidil can be used in emergencies. Because of tachycardia, pinacidil has no advantage over other drugs.

Nicarandil

Intravenous use produces a fall in blood pressure, but oral treatment (20 to 40 mg daily) in normotensive subjects during exercise produces little effect on blood pressure.

Chromakalim

This agent has been much less extensively investigated, but chromakalim lowers blood pressure in both hypertensive and normotensive subjects following oral doses of 0.75 to 1.5 mg.[41]

COMPLICATIONS

Major complications are listed in Tables 84–2 through 84–5.

Adrenergic inhibitors
Ganglion-blocking drugs

As a result of reduction in vasomotor tone, treated patients will pool blood in dependent capacitance vessels. This effect explains the phenomenon of orthostatic hypotension that can be associated with syncope.[42] To enhance the antihypertensive effect in the supine posture, it is necessary to reduce intravascular (and extracellular) fluid volume and prevent the expansion of blood volume.[7,8] Prolonged therapy with trimetaphan for 48 to 72 hours is associated with refractory responses (tachyphylaxis).[43]

Reduction in cardiac output results in at least proportionate reduction of renal blood flow, sometimes associated with reduced creatinine clearance.[44] Because parasympathetic inhibition also results from ganglionic blockade, tonic activity leads to risk of paralytic ileus and acute urinary retention. Thus, abdominal pain with reduced bowel sounds, constipation, or reduced urinary output in a patient with aortic dissection may not reflect extension of the dissection into the mesenteric or renal arteries but instead may be a side effect of treatment. Other adverse drug reactions with trimetaphan include asthma attacks because of histamine release. Large doses may provoke muscle relaxation leading to cardiac arrest.

Rawolfia alkaloids

Parasympathetic activity remains unopposed, explaining many common side effects (including bradycardia, prolonged atrioventricular conduction, increased gastric acid excretion with possible secondary peptic ulceration, and frequency of bowel movements). These adverse effects may be counteracted by parasympathetic inhibitors.

Although arterial dilatation with increased blood flow has been considered greatest in the skin, other vascular beds are also involved. The frequent complaint of nasal mucosal congestion and suffiness is ameliorated by nasally administered vasoconstrictors.[45] However, prolonged use may result in chemical rhinitis.

As a result of depletion of brain catecholamines and serotonin, there may be behavioral alterations and subtle

ADVERSE REACTIONS DUE TO ADRENERGIC INHIBITORS: GANGLION BLOCKERS AND RAWOLFIA ALKALOIDS

Drug	Common Side Effects	Other Side Effects
Ganglion blockers	■ Orthostatic hypotension ■ Tachyphylaxis ■ Reduced creatinine clearance	■ Paralytic ileus ■ Urinary retention ■ Asthma ■ Respiratory arrest
Rawolfia alkaloids	■ Bradycardia ■ Prolonged AV conduction ■ Nasal stuffiness ■ Depression	■ Peptic ulceration ■ Diarrhea ■ Bronchospasm ■ Increased appetite ■ Fluid retention, weight gain ■ Loss of libido, impotence ■ Menstrual irregularities ■ Amenorrhea ■ Galactorrhea ■ Ocular palsies ■ Extrapyramidal symptoms

Table 84–2. Adverse Reactions Due to Adrenergic Inhibitors: Ganglion Blockers and Rawolfia Alkaloids

ADVERSE REACTIONS DUE TO ADRENERGIC INHIBITORS: ADRENERGIC NEURON-BLOCKING AGENTS, MONOAMINE OXIDASE INHIBITORS, AND VERATRIUM ALKALOIDS

Drug	Common Side Effects	Other Side Effects
Adrenergic neuron blockers	■ Orthostatic hypotension ■ Muscle weakness ■ Bradycardia ■ Diarrhea ■ Retrograde ejaculation ■ Fluid retention ■ Dizziness ■ Nasal stuffiness ■ Lethargy	■ Nausea and vomiting ■ Thrombocytopenia ■ Loss of scalp hair ■ Dry mouth ■ Blurred vision ■ Anorexia ■ Epigastric discomfort ■ Itch, rashes, and urticaria
Monoamine oxidase inhibitors	■ Euphoria ■ Insomnia ■ Acute psychosis ■ Severe hypertension with certain foods	■ Hepatocellular necrosis ■ Blood dyscrasias
Veratrium alkaloids	■ Nausea and vomiting ■ Excessive salivation ■ Diaphoresis ■ Blurred vision ■ Mental confusion	

Table 84–3. Adverse Reactions Due to Adrenergic Inhibitors: Adrenergic Neuron-blocking Agents, Monoamine Oxidase Inhibitors, and Veratrium Alkaloids

or overt depression (sometimes leading to suicide).[46] Less severe central complications include drowsiness and nightmares. Parkinsonism, dyskinesia, and dystonia can result from dopamine depletion in the basal ganglia. Congestive heart failure may be precipitated or worsened.

Adrenergic neuron-blocking drugs

Because of coincidental inhibition of venous tone,[45] venous return to the heart is reduced by peripheral pooling of blood in dependent areas of the body with upright posture. As a result, orthostatic hypertension is prominent.[47]

Associated with the resulting fall in cardiac output, there is a proportionate reduction in organ blood flow. Severe hypotension may aggravate angina and lead to myocardial infarction, cerebrovascular insufficiency with syncope, or even stroke. The renal and splanchnic territories may receive a smaller proportion of total cardiac output, but glomerular filtration rate and renal function appear to return to normal with time.[48] With reducing skeletal muscle blood flow and adrenergic innervation of skeletal muscle, weakness may result. This can be exacerbated by diuretic treatment.[49] Muscle weakness may be aggravated still further during and immediately after exercise.[50]

ADVERSE REACTIONS DUE TO DIRECT-ACTING VASCULAR SMOOTH MUSCLE RELAXANTS: HYDRALAZINE AND MINOXIDIL		
Drugs	**Common Side Effects**	**Other Side Effects**
Hydralalzine	■ Headache ■ Nasal stuffiness ■ Tachycardia ■ Palpitation ■ Flushing ■ Sweating ■ Peripheral neuropathy ■ Lupus reaction	■ Fluid retention, edema ■ Drug fever ■ Skin eruptions ■ Blood dyscrasias ■ Purpura
Minoxidil	■ ECG changes ■ Fluid retention, edema ■ Hirsutism ■ Flushing ■ Palpitation ■ Headache	■ Nasal stuffiness ■ Nausea ■ Breast tenderness ■ Skin reactions

Table 84–4. Adverse Reactions Due to Direct-acting Vascular Smooth Muscle Relaxants: Hydralazine and Minoxidil

ADVERSE REACTIONS DUE TO DIRECT-ACTING VASCULAR SMOOTH MUSCLE RELAXANTS: DIAZOXIDE, SODIUM NITROPRUSSIDE, AND OTHER POTASSIUM CHANNEL AGONISTS		
Drug	**Common Side Effects**	**Other Side Effects**
Diazoxide	■ Hyperglycemia ■ Tachycardia ■ Palpitation ■ Fluid retention, edema ■ Hypertrichosis ■ Headache	■ Chest pain ■ Extrapyrimidal reactions ■ Skin rashes ■ Hypotension ■ Acute pancreatitis ■ Fever ■ Lymphadenopathy ■ Gout ■ Blood dyscrasias/purpura ■ Nausea and vomiting ■ Abdominal pain, ileus, and diarrhea
Sodium nitroprusside	■ Hypothyroidism ■ Methemoglobinemia ■ Nausea and vomiting ■ Headache	■ Restlessness ■ Muscle twitching ■ Cyanide intoxication
Other potassium channel agonists	■ Headache ■ Dizziness ■ Palpitation ■ Tachycardia ■ Edema	■ Hypertrichosis ■ Nausea dyspepsia ■ Rashes ■ Increased ANA titers

Table 84–5. Adverse Reactions Due to Direct-acting Vascular Smooth Muscle Relaxants: Diazoxide, Sodium Nitroprusside, and Other Potassium Channel Agonists

Some side effects (orthostatic hypotension, excessive hypotension, bradycardia, increased gastric excretion) result from unopposed parasympathetic activity and impaired adrenergic function. Similarly, diarrhea, retrograde ejaculation, and fluid retention may be explained by reduced adrenergic transmission. Many of these side effects may be counteracted by reduction in dosage or the addition of a parasympatholytic agent or diuretic.

Because these agents act by entering the nerve terminal, any agent that prevents this will block the action. This is the means by which tricyclic antidepressants act,[51] and therefore these classes of drugs should not be prescribed concomitantly. Drugs that reduce efferent sympathetic output enhance postural hypotension and bradycardia. Examples include alpha blockers, beta blockers, and ganglion blockers. Cardiac glycosides may also enhance bradycardia.

Monoamine oxidase inhibitors

The major side effects are centrally mediated mental and emotional reactions, including euphoria, insomnia, and acute psychosis. More important is the severe hypertensive crisis following the ingestion of foods containing tyramine, such as aged cheeses, beer, sherry, Chianti, and herring.[52]

Veratrium alkaloids

Because of the narrow therapeutic index, the effective control of arterial pressure is not infrequently associated with side effects.

Direct-acting vascular smooth muscle relaxants

Side effects common to these agents include headache and nasal stuffiness attributable to local vasodilatation, fluid retention, and edema. The latter effects can result in pseudotolerance.

Hydralazine

Peripheral neuropathy is dose dependent and is rare at doses up to 200 mg daily.[53] This complication is more common in slow acetylators. Neuropathy is first manifest by paraesthesia, numbness, and tingling of the extremities. Pyridoxine deficiency is the likely cause and correction can be achieved by administration of pyridoxine.[11]

The lupus reaction gives rise to malaise, myalgia, and arthralgia/arthritis, and is associated with raised ANA titers.[54] Raised titers are often encountered in asymptomatic patients and are not a contraindication to continuation, although the lupus syndrome is. Hydralazine does not worsen idiopathic systemic lupus erythematosis.

There may be more severe signs of systemic illness such as weight loss, splenomegaly, and effusion in serous cavities. Rashes may also occur. If not diagnosed promptly, the degree of temporary disability may be severe. Renal and cerebral involvement is rare. The hydralazine lupus reaction usually occurs after six months of therapy at doses over 400 mg daily and is almost always seen in slow acetylators. Patients with HLA DR4 phenotype are particularly susceptible.[55] The syndrome resolves when the drug is withdrawn, although months or years may be required for complete clearing.[11] After withdrawal of hydralazine, positive tests for ANA may persist for years.

Although the lupus reaction is reduced substantially at daily doses of 200 mg or less, there is still a significant incidence. In one study,[56] the incidence was 6.7% over three years. No cases were seen at 50 mg daily, 5.4% with 100 mg daily, and 10.4% with 200 mg daily. The incidence was higher in women (11.6%) than in men (2.8%). In women taking 200 mg daily, the three-year incidence was 19.4%. Thus, the true incidence of lupus syndrome is unacceptably high.

Decrease in white cell count is more common in blacks. Mild gastrointestinal side effects sometimes occur but present no clinical problems at conventional doses. Endralazine is not associated with the lupus syndrome.

Minoxidil

Increase in cardiac work may account for electrocardiograph (ECG) changes, which are often observed during the first few days of therapy. ECG changes include ST depression and T-wave inversion[57] but are not associated with cardiac enzyme elevation. However, reflex tachycardia may provoke angina in those with ischemic heart disease. Pulmonary edema may be the consequence of increased cardiac output.

An uncommon cardiac adverse event is pericardial effusion, which is rarely associated with tamponade.[58] Deaths have been reported. Dependent edema and ascites are extremely common.

A very common side effect of minoxidil is hirsutism, which is particularly bothersome in women. Hypertrichosis mainly affects the forehead and face and is most apparent in dark-haired individuals. There is no pharmacologic treatment for excess hair growth, and the only remedy is removal of hair or discontinuation of the drug. After discontinuation, hair growth reverses in a few months.

Diazoxide

Diazoxide shares the adverse effects of minoxidil. In addition, diazoxide causes impairment of glucose tolerance in the majority of patients. Hyperglycemia is due to inhibition of insulin secretion. The effect is probably mediated by action upon pancreatic islet cell potassium channels and can be reversed by sulphanylurea drugs.[38] Diabetic betoacidosis and hyperosmolar non-ketonic coma are infrequent but can develop very rapidly. Conventional therapy with insulin and restoration of fluid and electrolyte balance is usually effective.

Increased hepatic enzymes, uremia, reduced creatinine clearance, reversible nephrotic syndrome, decreased urine output, hematuria, and albuminuria occur very occasionally. Thrombocytopenia with or without purpura may require discontinuation. Drug interactions include bleeding with anticoagulants and hypotension with beta blockers. Diuretics potentiate hyperuricemia by inhibition of tubular secretion of uric acid.

Sodium nitroprusside

Retrosternal discomfort, palpitation, dizziness, and abdominal discomfort can occur if blood pressure reduction is too rapid. Cyanide intoxication is rare unless the recommended dose is exceeded. Metabolic acidosis may be followed by hypoxia and tetanic spasms.

Other potassium channel agonists

When used as monotherapy, side effects of pinacidil are dose related. ECG T-wave changes have been reported in the initial phase of treatment.[40] Hypertrichosis is seen occasionally.[59]

SUMMARY

Vasodilators are highly effective antihypertensive agents that dominated the management of hypertension in the 1950s and 1960s. However, treatment with these agents is associated with an unacceptable level of adverse reactions. With the advent of newer and better-tolerated antihypertensive agents, their use has declined dramatically. Many vasodilators can now be considered only of historical interest.

In developed countries, vasodilators have a limited clinical role. Some direct-acting vascular smooth muscle relaxants continue to have utility in the management of hypertensive emergencies (notably sodium nitroprusside) and in severe hypertension refractory to other antihypertensive agents (notably minoxidil). In developing countries, however (where the cost of newer agents may be prohibitive), vasodilators continue to be prescribed more widely. The safe and effective long-term use of these drugs requires careful attention to adverse reactions with concomitant administration of beta blockers and diuretics to avoid the consequences of reflex cardiac stimulation and salt and water retention.

REFERENCES

1. Van Zwieten PA. Vasodilator drugs with direct action on smooth muscle. In PA Van Zweiten (ed). *Handbook of Hypertension, Volume III*. Amsterdam: Elsevier 1984:307–46.
2. Ablad B. A study of the mechanism of the haemodynamic effects of hydralazine in man. *Acta Pharmacol Toxicol* 1963;20(Suppl 1):1–53.
3. Christensson B, Nordenvelt I, Westling H, White T. Haemodynamic effects of nitroglycerine in normal subjects during supine and sitting exercise. *Br Heart J* 1969;31:80–82.
4. O'Rourke M. Vasodilatation and arterial compliance. Recent innovations on beta blockade: The role of vasodilatation. *RSM Round Table Series* 1990;17:94–104.
5. Man in t'Veld AJ, Wenting GJ, Boomsma F, Verhoeven RP, Schalekamp MADH. Sympathetic and parasympathetic components of reflex cardiostimulation during vasodilator treatment of hypertension. *Br J Clin Pharmacol* 1980;9:547–51.
6. Koch-Weser J. Vasodilator drugs in the treatment of hypertension. *Arch Intern Med* 1974;133:1017–27.
7. Dustan HP, Cumming GR, Corcoran AC, et al. A mechanism of chlorothiazide-enhanced effectiveness of antihypertensive ganglioplegic drugs. *Circulation* 1959;19:360–65.
8. Dustan HP, Tarazi RC, Bravo EL. Dependence of arterial pressure on intravascular volume in treated hypertensive patients. *N Engl J Med* 1972;286:861–66.
9. Patton WDM. Transmission and block in autonomic ganglia. *Pharmacol Rev* 1954;6:59–67.
10. Brest AN, Onesti G, Swartz C, et al. Mechanisms of antihypertensive drug therapy. *JAMA* 1970;211:480–84.
11. Koch-Weser J. Drug therapy: Hydralazine. *N Eng J Med* 1976;295:320–23.
12. Rapaport RM, Draznin MB, Muirad F. Endothelial-dependent vasodilator and nitrovasodilator-induced relaxation may be mediated through cyclic GMP formation and cyclic GMP-dependent protein phosphoylation. *Trans Assoc Am Phys* 1983;96:19–30.
13. Holmes DG, Bogers WA, Wideroe JE, Huunan-Seppola A, Wideroe B. Endralazine, a new peripheral vasodilator: Absence of effect of acetylators status on antihypertensive effect. *Lancet* 1983;1:670–71.
14. Bryan RK, Hoobler SW, Rosenzweig J, Weller JM, Purdy JM. Effect of minoxidil on blood pressure and haemodynamics in severe hypertension. *Am J Cardiol* 1977;39:796–801.

15. Andersson KE. Clinical pharmacology of potassium channel openers. *Pharmacol Toxicol* 1992;70:244–54.
16. Koch-Weser J. Diazoxide. *N Engl J Med* 1976;294:1271–73.
17. Standen NB, Quayle JM, Davies NW, Brayden JE, Huang Y, Nelson MT. Hyperpolarizing vasodilators activate ATP sensitive K^+ channels in arterial smooth muscle. *Science* 1989;245:177–80.
18. Cohn N, Burke P. Nitroprusside. *Ann Intern Med* 1979;91:752–57.
19. Schroder H, Noack E, Muller R. Evidence for a correlation between nitric oxide formation by cleavage of organic nitrates and activation of guanylate cyclase. *J Mol Cell Cardiol* 1985;17:931–34.
20. Verndier IR. Sodium nitroprusside: Theory and practice. *Postgrad Med J* 1974;50:576–81.
21. Richer C, Pratz J, Mulder P, Mondot S, Giudicelli JF, Cavero I. Cardiovascular and biological effects of K^+ channel openers A class of drugs with vasorelaxant and cardioprotective properties. *Life Sci* 1990;47:1693–1705.
22. Frampton J, Buckley MM, Filton A. Nicorandil: A review of its pharmacology and therapeutic effects in angina pectoris. *Drugs* 1992;44:625–55.
23. Kinoshita M, Sakai K. Pharmacology and therapeutic effects of nicorandil. *Cardiovasc Drug Ther* 1990;4:1075–88.
24. Bhatia S, Frohlich ED. A hemodynamic comparison of agents useful in hypertensive emergencies. *Am Heart J* 1973;85:367–73.
25. Veterans Administration Cooperative Study Group on Antihypertensive Agents: Effects of treatment on morbidity in hypertension. II. Results in patients with diastolic blood pressure averaging 90 through 114 mmHg. *JAMA* 1970;213:1143–52.
26. Veterans Administration Cooperative Study Group on Antihypertensive Agents. Effects of treatment on morbidity in hypertension. I. Results in patients with diastolic blood pressures averaging 115 through 129 mmHg. *JAMA* 1967;202:116–22.
27. Canary JJ, Schaaf M, Duffy BJ, et al. Effects of oral and intramuscular administration of reserpine in thyrotoxicosis. *N Engl J Med* 1957;257;435–42.
28. Freis ED, Rose JC, Higgins TF, Finnerty FA, Kelly RT. The hemodynamic effects of hypotensive drugs in man: 41 - hydrazinophthalazine. *Circulation* 1953;8:197–204.
29. Schroder H. Simplified method for determining acetylators phenotype. *BMJ* 1972;3:506–07.

30. Zacest R, Gilmore E, Koch-Weser J. Treatment of essential hypertension with combined vasodilatation and beta adrenergic blockade. *N Engl J Med* 1972;286:617–22.
31. McAraevey D, Ramsey LE, Latham L, et al. "Third drug" trial: Comparative study of antihypertensive agents added to treatment when blood pressure remains uncontrolled by beta-blocker plus thiazide diuretics. *BMJ* 1984;288:106–11.
32. Australian Therapeutic Trial in Mild Hypertension Management Committee. The Australian Therapeutic Trial in Mild Hypertension. *Lancet* 1980;i:1261–67.
33. Hypertension Detection and Follow-Up Program Co-operative Group: Five year findings of the Hypertension Detection and Follow-Up Program. 1. Reduction in mortality of persons with high blood pressure, including mild hypertension. *JAMA* 1979;242:2562–71.
34. Liedholm H, Melander A. Drug selection in the treatment of pregnancy hypertension. *Obstet Gynaecol* 1984;118:49–55.
35. McGourty JC, Silas JH, Pidgeon J. Comparison of once daily endralazine with placebo in the treatment of hypertension uncontrolled by a beta-blocker and diuretic. *Eur J Clin Pharmacol* 1985;29:401–03.
36. Swales JD, Bing RF, Heagerty AM, Pohl JF, Russell GI, Thurston H. Treatment of refractory hypertension. *Lancet* 1982;1:894–96.
37. Brunner HR, Jaeger P, Ferguson RK, Jequier E, Turini G, Gavras H. Need for beta blockade in hypertension reduced with long-term minoxidil. *BMJ* 1978;2:385–88.
38. Pohl JEF, Thurston H, Swales JD. Hypertension with renal impairment: Influence of intensive therapy. *QJ Med* 1974;43:569–81.
39. Garrett BN, Kaplan NM. Efficacy of slow infusion of diazoxide in the treatment of severe hypertension without organ hyperperfusion. *Am Heart J* 1982;103:390–94.
40. Friedel HA, Brogden RN. Pinacidil: A review of its pharmacodynamic and pharmacokinetic properties and therapeutical potential in the treatment of hypertension. *Drugs* 1990;39:929–67.
41. Donnelly R, Elliott HL, Meredith PA, Reid JL. Clinical studies with a potassium channel activator chromakalim in normotensive and hypertensive subjects. *J Cardiovasc Pharmacol* 1990;16:790–95.
42. Freis ED, Rose JC, Partenope EA, et al. The hemodynamic effects of hypotensive drugs in man. II. Hexamethonium. *J Clin Invest* 1953;32:1285–98.

43. Finnerty FA, Witkin L, Fazekas JF. Cerebral hemodynamics in acute hypotension. *J Clin Invest* 1954;33:933.

44. Ullmann TD, Menczel J. The effect of a ganglion blocking agent (hexamethonium) on renal function and on excretion of water and electrolytes in hypertension and in congestive heart failure. *Am Heart J* 1956;52:106–20.

45. Gaffney FE, Bryant WM, Braunwald E. Effect of reserpine and guanethidine on venous reflexes. *Circ Res* 1962;11:889–94.

46. Freis ED. Mental depression in hypertensive patients treated for long periods with large doses of reserpine. *N Engl J Med* 1954;251:1006–08.

47. Cohn JD, Liptak TE, Freis ED. Hemodynamic effect of guanethidine in man. *Circ Res* 1963;12:298–307.

48. Villareal H, Exaire JB, Rubio V, et al. Effects of guanethidine and bretylium tosylate on systemic and renal hemodynamics in essential hypertension. *Am J Cardiol* 1964;14:633–40.

49. Bowman WC, Notts MW. Actions of sympathomimetic amines and their antagonists on skeletal muscle. *Pharmacol Rev* 1969;21:27–72.

50. Khatri IM, Cohn HN. Mechanism of exercise hypotension after sympathetic blockade. *Am J Cardiol* 1970;25:329–38.

51. Mitchell JR, Cavenaugh JH, Arias L, et al. Guanethidine and related agents III Antagonism by drugs which inhibit the norepinephrine pump in man. *J Clin Invest* 1970;49:1596–1604.

52. Goldberg LI. Monoamine oxidase inhibitors: Adverse reactions and possible mechanisms. *JAMA* 1964;190:456–62.

53. Raskin NH, Fishman RA. Pyridoxine-deficiency neuropathy due to hydralazine. *N Engl J Med* 1965;273:1182–85.

54. Perry HM, Tan EM, Karmody S, Sakamoto A. Relation of acetyl transferase activity to anti-nuclear antibodies and toxic symptoms in hypertensive patients treated with hydralazine. *J Lab Clin Med* 1970;76:114–25.

55. Batchelor JR, Welsh KI, Tinoco RM, Dollery CT, Hughes GRV, Bernstein R, et al. Hydralazine-induced systemic lupus erythematosus: Influence of HLA DR and sex on susceptibility. *Lancet* 1980;1:1107–09.

56. Cameron HA, Ramsay LE. The lupus syndrome induced by hydralazine: A common complication of low dose treatment. *BMJ* 1984;289:408–09.

57. Hall D, Froer KL, Rudolph W. Serial electrocardiographic changes during long-term treatment of severe hypertension with minoxidil. *J Cardiovasc Pharmacol* 1980;2(2):S200–05.

58. Reichgott MJ. Minoxidil and pericardial effusion: An idiosyncratic reaction. *Clin Pharmacol Ther* 1981;30:64–70.

59. Goldberg MR. Clinical pharmacology of pinacidil: A prototype for drugs that affect potassium channels. *J Cardiovasc Pharmacol* 1988;12(2):S41–47.

Chapter

85

Novel Drug Treatments for Hypertension

Henry Krum and Jennifer Martin

Key Findings

- The treatment of hypertension is becoming more difficult because of the lower blood pressure (BP) targets set by evidence-based guideline recommendations.

- The renin-angiotensin-aldosterone system remains one of the key targets for therapeutic intervention in the treatment of systemic hypertension.

- Renin as an early and rate-limiting step in renin-angiotensin system activity is a particularly attractive therapeutic target.

- Newer renin inhibitors have been developed that overcome many of the limitations of older agents, particularly bioavailability.

- Aldosterone is an important independent hormone involved in the progression of a number of major cardiovascular disease states, including systemic hypertension.

- Selective aldosterone blockers (e.g., eplerenone) have been developed that do not possess the antiandrogenic and progestational adverse effects of earlier agents such as spironolactone.

- Aldosterone synthase inhibitors represent an alternative approach to blockade of the adverse actions of aldosterone on the cardiovascular system.

- Endothelin is another more recently described hormonal system that may be involved in the pathogenesis of essential hypertension.

- Endothelin receptor antagonists lower BP but will undoubtedly be reserved as third- or fourth-line agents for refractory disease because of side effects and teratogenicity.

- Rho-kinase is a recently described cell-signaling pathway that may be of relevance in the progression of hypertension.

- Blockade of the rho-kinase system should produce effects on BP complementary to blockade of other systems such as the renin-angiotensin-aldosterone pathway. Rho-kinase inhibitors have been developed and have been shown to exert vasodilator effects in hypertensive patients.

Treatment of essential hypertension has advanced considerably in the past few decades. We now have agents that are highly effective at lowering BP, are associated with minimal side effects, and are able to be given on a once-daily basis to aid adherence to therapy. The question therefore arises as to why we need new treatments in the management of this condition. There are several reasons for this. One of the most important is that target BP goals continually move lower, based on epidemiologic and intervention study data. This is particularly true of hypertension associated with co-morbid conditions such as diabetes mellitus. For this reason, monotherapy alone is usually not able to lower BP to these target levels in many patients. The use of multiple classes of agents within the individual patient has therefore become the norm. However, certain agents cannot be used together with (and/or interfere with) the BP-lowering efficacy of other agents. Therefore, the clinical need for new therapies as add-on treatments for refractory hypertension and to attack new targets still remains highly relevant. This chapter assesses the development of new therapies directed at new targets and new approaches to old targets in the management of essential hypertension.

RENIN INHIBITORS

Blockade of the renin-angiotensin-aldosterone system (RAAS) is an important therapeutic strategy not only for the treatment of hypertension but for the clinical benefits it provides beyond BP reduction, such as in the management of heart failure and progressive kidney disease. To date, interruption of this system has been effected at multiple steps that include enzyme inhibition (angiotensin-converting enzyme and renin) in addition to receptor blockade (angiotensin II type 1 receptor and aldosterone) (Figure 85–1).

Angiotensin II, a major effector molecule of this system, is produced via a two-step process in which angiotensinogen (synthesised primarily in the liver) is cleaved by the aspartic peptidase renin (produced in the juxtaglomerular cells of the kidney) to give rise to angiotensin I. This biologically inactive decapeptide is then converted to the active octapeptide angiotensin II by the di-peptidyl carboxypeptidase angiotensin-converting enzyme (ACE) or by a range of other proteases that include chymase.

Although highly effective, the therapeutic response achieved with both ACE inhibitors and angiotensin receptor blockers (ARBs) is limited by the reactive rise in renin (and thus angiotensin peptides) that occurs with both drug classes. Renin is not only the rate-limiting step in angiotensin II formation but shows remarkable substrate specificity for angiotensinogen, making it an attractive target for therapeutic inhibition. Furthermore, the recent identification of a renin receptor in the glomerular mesangium and in arterial subendothelium suggests the possibility of additional advantages of renin inhibition beyond those of ACE inhibitors

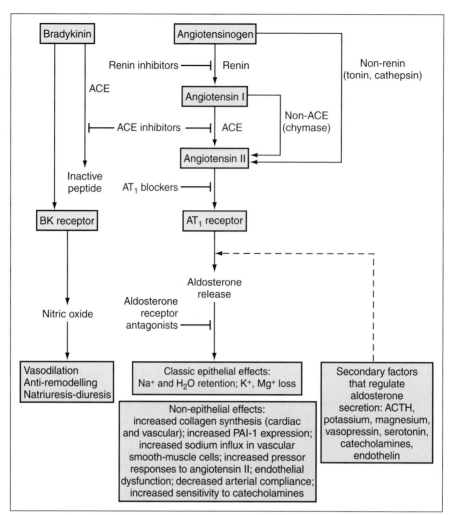

Figure 85–1. The renin-angiotensin-aldosterone system: a key regulator of blood pressure. Renin (a protease secreted into the circulation in response to various physiological stimuli) cleaves the protein angiotensinogen to produce the inactive decapeptide angiotensin I. Cleavage of angiotensin I by angiotensin-converting enzyme (ACE) produces the active octapeptide angiotensin II (as shown, ACE also inactivates bradykinin, and there are alternative routes for the generation of angiotensin II). Angiotensin II activates the angiotensin II type 1 (AT1) receptor, a member of the G-protein-coupled receptor superfamily. Many of these effects, such as vasoconstriction and stimulation of aldosterone synthesis and release (which leads to sodium retention), tend to elevate blood pressure. Angiotensin II also activates the AT2 receptor, the effects of which (Box 85–1) are less well understood but which could antagonize many of the effects of activation of the AT1 receptor. Various points shown in the renin-angiotensin-aldosterone cascade have been the targets for pharmacologic intervention, and inhibitors of ACE, angiotensin-receptor blockers, and aldosterone-receptor antagonists are in clinical use at present. ACTH, adrenocorticotropic hormone; BK receptor, bradykinin receptor. (From Zaman MA, Oparil S, Calhoun DA. Drugs targeting the renin-angiotensin-aldosterone system. *Nature Rev Drug Discovery* 2002;Vol 1 No. 8:1:621–36.)

and ARBs.[1] For instance, binding of renin to this receptor not only increases its catalytic efficiency in angiotensin I formation but converts the otherwise inert pro-renin into an active moiety. Moreover, the interaction between either renin or pro-renin with its receptor leads to activation of the potentially pathogenetic mitogen-activated protein kinase (MAPK) pathway in the absence of angiotensin peptide formation.[1]

Despite the attractiveness of renin inhibition and the success of early compounds in validating it as therapeutic target, further drug development had been marred by issues

of potency, bioavailability, duration of action, and costs of synthesis.[2] For instance, although potent, renin inhibitors such as remikiren and enalkiren showed poor oral biovavailability. Although this was improved somewhat with agents such as zankiren and terlakiren,[3] further development of renin inhibitors was halted in the mid 1990s—apparently for commercial reasons in the setting of angiotensin receptor blockers.[4]

More recently, programs to develop renin inhibitors have been reactivated. However, drug design for these new programs has been based on X-ray crystallography of renin's active site with computational modeling rather than on the structure of angiotensinogen—leading to the synthesis of a series of novel renin inhibitors with the hope of overcoming previous problems.[5] Of these, aliskiren (2(S),4(S),5(S),7(S)-N-(2-carbamoyl-2-methylpropyl)-5-amino-4-hydroxy-2,7-diisopropyl-8-[4-methoxy-3-(3-methoxypropoxy)phenyl]-octanamid hemifumarate, SPP100, Speedel/Novartis) is the most advanced of the new class of orally active, nonpeptide, low-molecular-weight renin inhibitors. It has several favorable attributes in its profile, including being highly potent (IC_{50} 0.6 nM) and specific for human renin with a plasma $T_{1/2}$ of approximately 24 hours.[5] In healthy volunteers, aliskiren (40 to 640 mg/day) orally was well tolerated, inducing a dose-dependent decrease in plasma renin activity and in angiotensin I and II concentrations.[6] In 226 patients with mild to moderate essential hypertension, aliskiren (37.5 to 300 mg/day) led to a dose-dependent reduction in ambulatory BP.[7] More recently, in a larger trial 652 hypertensive subjects were randomized to receive either the ARB irbesartan or aliskiren 150, 300, or 600 mg.[8] Over an 8-week study period, aliskiren 150 mg/day was as effective as irbesartan 150 mg/day in lowering BP (with similar safety and tolerability).

Based on these studies, it seems likely that renin inhibitors will provide improvements in cardiovascular and renal morbidity. Whether these agents are similar, inferior, or superior to ACE inhibitors and ARBs is at present unclear. Similarly, extensive clinical evaluation with hard endpoints will be required to ascertain whether the combination of renin inhibition with ACE inhibitors and/or ARBs in providing more complete blockade of the RAS also leads to further improvements in morbidity and mortality.

NOVEL ALDOSTERONE BLOCKERS

The hormone aldosterone has been a well-known target for therapeutic intervention for many decades. Aldosterone, as a hormone, was first described in 1954 when its steroid structure was discovered.[9] It was known to have potent actions on sodium retention and potassium excretion at the renal distal convoluted tubule, and to a lesser extent at other epithelial sites such as salivary glands and the gastrointestinal tract. These so-called epithelial effects are mediated via the binding of aldosterone to the mineralocorticoid (type I glucocorticoid receptor), interaction of the ligand-receptor complex with DNA, and eventual modulation of gene expression.[10]

Recent evidence suggests that aldosterone also exerts a variety of nonepithelial effects based on the discovery of mineralocorticoid receptors in multiple nonepithelial sites.[11] In contrast to interactions with nuclear receptors, nonepithelial effects of aldosterone appear to be mediated via a second messenger system that involves the activation of a sodium hydrogen anti-porter.[10] These nonepithelial receptors have been found to be present in heart[12] and vascular tissue,[13] the stimulation of which causes pathologic fibrosis and remodeling. There are also recently discovered nonepithelial actions of aldosterone on kidneys, including direct induction of glumerulosclerosis and proteinuria (which may occur independently of effects on BP).

As would be predicted by its sites of action, stimulation of mineralocorticoid receptors contributes not only directly to hypertension but to its complications. These include left ventricular hypertrophy and concomitant heart failure (via inhibition of necrosis), pathologic fibrosis, increased catecholamine release, and stimulation of cardiac arrhythmias.

Selective aldosterone receptor blockers

Spironolactone has been approved for many decades in the treatment of mineralocorticoid hypertension, ascites associated with portal hypertension and chronic heart failure. It has been widely used for the treatment of undifferentiated (essential) hypertension. However, this agent has been limited by its nonspecificity for mineralocorticoid receptors, including antiandrogenic and pro-estrogenic actions. For example, in the RALES trial 10% of male patients noted gynecomastia.[14]

On this basis, a more highly selective agent for the mineralocorticoid receptor was developed by replacing the 17-alpha-thoacetyl group with a carbomethoxy group.[15] This new agent (eplerenone) has been studied in a large program exploring the potential benefits of this agent as monotherapy and add-on therapy in patients with essential hypertension, both undifferentiated and in those with low-renin/high-aldosterone plasma levels.

To date, a number of double-blind randomized clinical trials have contributed to the database for the efficacy and safety of eplerenone in systemic hypertension. Key study program results are summarized below. An 8-week study randomized 417 patients with mild to moderate hypertension to eplerenone in different doses, spironolactone, or placebo.[16] The mean changes in systolic blood pressure (SBP) and diastolic blood pressure (DBP), both from baseline to final visit and based on 24-hour ambulatory BP monitoring, were significantly greater for all eplerenone groups than the placebo group. Furthermore, the antihypertensive effect of eplerenone increased in a dose-response fashion. Eplerenone (100 mg) reduced BP by 75% compared to spironolactone (100 mg) and displayed an adverse event profile similar to placebo. In particular, no antiandrogenic or progestational side effects were observed.

The effects of eplerenone on left ventricular hypertrophy and renal function associated with mild to moderate hypertension were assessed in a 9-month study of patients who received one of eplerenone (n=50), enalapril (n=54), or the combination (n=49).[17] Whereas BP effects were similar, mean reductions in left ventricular mass were 7.6%, 10.5%, and 14.1% in the three groups, respectively (p=0.007 eplerenone versus combination, p=0.107 enalapril versus combination). The equivalent figures for reductions in urinary albumin to creatinine ratio (UACR) were, respectively, 24.9%, 37.4%, and 52.6% (p=0.001 eplerenone versus combination, p=0.038 enalapril versus combination). More cough was experienced by patients assigned to the enalapril group than the eplerenone group (14.1% versus 3.1%, p=0.033).

To assess the renal effects of eplerenone, 257 hypertensive patients with type 2 diabetes mellitus and microalbuminuria were prescribed eplerenone (n=89), enalapril (n=83), or the combination (n=85) for 24 weeks.[18] Reductions in

UACR were 62%, 45%, and 74% for the three groups, respectively (p=0.015 eplerenone versus enalapril, p=0.018 combination versus eplerenone and p<0.001 combination versus enalapril) despite similar reductions in BP. Both drugs were well tolerated (with no reports of gynecomastia), but hyperkalemia occurred in 8, 2, and 8 subjects of the eplerenone, enalapril, and combination groups, respectively.

To examine if low-renin essential hypertension was more responsive to aldosterone receptor antagonism than antagonism of angiotensin II (due to greater salt sensitivity), a sample of patients with this condition received either eplerenone (n=86) or losartan (n=82) for 8 weeks, after which hydrochlorothiazide could have been added if necessary for another 8 weeks.[19] At week 8, mean change in SBP/DBP was significantly greater in the eplerenone group (–15.8/–9.3 mmHg versus –10.1/–6.7 mmHg, p=0.017/0.050). At week 16, mean change in SBP/DBP had evened out (–18.3/–10.8 mmHg versus –15.0/–9.8 mmHg), but fewer patients in the eplerenone group required dual therapy (32.5 versus 55.6%). Increases in renin activity were similar, but the increase in aldosterone levels was greater for the eplerenone group (week 8: +74.7% versus –18.7%, p<0.001; week 16: +89.8% versus –5.5%, p<0.001). The adverse effect profiles were similar.

An 8-week study assessed the coadministration of eplerenone with one of the following ACE inhibitors or ARBs among patients with mild to moderate hypertension: ACE inhibitor plus eplerenone (n=87), ACE inhibitor plus placebo (n=90), ARB plus eplerenone (n=83), or ARB plus placebo (n=81).[20] ARB plus eplerenone was significantly more effective than ARB alone in reducing BP (SBP/DBP: –16.0/–12.7 mmHg versus –9.2/–9.3 mmHg; p=0.001/p=0.004), whereas ACE inhibitor plus eplerenone seemed to be more effective than an ACE inhibitor alone in reducing SBP only (SBP/DBP: –13.4/–9.9 mmHg versus –7.5/–8.0 mmHg, p=0.002/p=0.134). Adverse events did not differ significantly across the treatment groups and were generally not severe.

These observations were further analyzed as group data, combining the ACE inhibitor and ARB groups.[21] Compared to placebo, SBP/DBP was reduced by 5.9/2.4 mmHg more in the eplerenone group (p<0.001 and p=0.006, respectively) additional to ACE inhibitor or ARB. In an ad hoc analysis, neither baseline values of plasma renin activity serum aldosterone (or the ratio) predicted BP response to treatment.[21]

In summary, the effect of eplerenone on BP and left ventricular mass appears similar to that of ACE inhibitors, but eplerenone may confer greater reno-protection and be associated with fewer adverse events. It also appears superior to ARBs for the treatment of patients with low-renin hypertension. If BP is uncontrolled by ACE inhibitor or ARB alone, the addition of eplerenone can be safely considered, and need not be dictated by plasma renin activity nor aldosterone levels. Among patients with diabetes mellitus, eplerenone combined with ACE inhibitor appears to more efficacious than either agent alone in regressing left ventricular mass and renal impairment, and these effects may occur independently of BP reduction.

The caveat is that the long-term efficacy and safety profile of eplerenone remains uncertain. With regard to safety, there is no data at present to suggest that eplerenone is less likely to cause clinically significant hyperkalemia than spironolactone. Nevertheless, these data suggest considerable promise for eplerenone in the management of systemic hypertension. Other than hypertension, eplerenone has been found to be a potential new treatment for chronic heart failure post-myocardial infarction in a major multinational randomized clinical trial, EPHESUS.[22]

Aldosterone synthase inhibitors

Another approach to blocking the effects of mineralocorticoid receptor activation is to inhibit the production of the endogenous ligand aldosterone. This can be achieved via several approaches to interference with the pathway of aldosterone synthesis. The last step in this pathway is conversion to mature aldosterone by the enzyme aldosterone synthase.

Interestingly, transgenic overexpression of aldo-synthase results primarily in marked coronary endothelium-dependent dilatation.[23] Selective aldo-synthase inhibitors have been developed and are currently undergoing preclinical evaluation. One advantage may be the absence of reflex activation of the renin-angiotensin system as occurs with specific aldosterone receptor blockers where there is upstream activation of renin and angiotensin II to overcome the blockade. On the other hand, there are often multiple pathways of generation of mature peptides and blocking aldo-synthase may not result in complete blockade of synthesis of mature aldosterone. This is analogous to similar observations with ACE inhibitors where other enzymes such as chymase may be operative in the conversion of angiotensin-I to angiotensin-II. Further study is required to determine the extent of the BP-lowering efficacy and safety of this approach to blocking aldosterone.

BLOCKADE OF THE ENDOTHELIN SYSTEM

Background

The endothelin family comprises three 21-amino-acid peptides (ET-1, ET-2, ET-3) with autocrine and paracrine actions.[24] Of these isoforms, ET-1 is by far the most vasoactive, mediating intense vasoconstriction upon exogenous infusion.

The 21-amino-acid endothelins are formed within endothelial (and other) cells from conversion of larger precursor peptides. Pre-pro endothelin (212 amino acids) is converted via specific endopeptidases to a 39-amino-acid peptide, pro- or "big" endothelin.[25] Big endothelin is in turn cleaved to the 21-amino-acid peptide via an endothelin-converting enzyme (ECE). ECE is a membrane-bound zinc-containing metalloprotease. A series of ECE isoforms has been described, with ECE-1 thought the major iso-enzyme involved in conversion of big-ET to ET-1 in the peripheral vasculature. Furthermore, other proteases (e.g., neutral endopeptidase) are also capable of this conversion.

Preformed 21-amino-acid endothelin is released in response to known endogenous stimuli such as low shear stress, thrombin, transforming growth factor-β, tumor necrosis factor-α, angiotensin II, and vasopressin,[26] Endothelin produced by vascular endothelial cells is released predominantly in an abluminal direction [i.e., away from the lumen of the peripheral blood vessel toward the vascular smooth muscle cell (VSMC)], upon which it mediates net vasoconstriction.

Endothelin mediates vasoconstriction via ET_A and ET_B receptors located on VSMCs. The ET_A receptor has greater affinity for ET-1 than other endothelin isoforms, whereas the ET_B receptor has similar affinity for all endothelin isoforms. Following binding of ET-1 to specific endothelin receptors, G-protein-dependent activation of phospliase C occurs, leading to the formation of inositol triphosphate and a rapid increase of intracellular calcium (mediating contraction).[27]

In addition to VSMC endothelin receptors, ET_B receptors are located on endothelial cells and mediate vasodilation upon agonist activation. These vasodilator responses largely occur due to activation of nitric oxide and to a lesser extent vasodilator prostaglandins (e.g., prostacyclin) located within the endothelial cell.[28]

ET-1 binds to these cell surface receptors, which are then internalized. The peptide is then degraded by various proteases, including neutral endopeptidase. There are some data to support the view that the ET_B receptor plays the key role in the removal of ET-1 from the circulation.[29]

The contribution of endothelin to increased vascular tone in patients with essential hypertension is somewhat controversial. In some studies, there was an enhanced vasodilator response to the administration of the ET_A receptor antagonist BQ-123 in hypertensive patients compared to normal subjects. Furthermore, blockade of ET_B receptor by BQ-788 resulted in a decrease in blood flow in normal subjects but an increase in hypertensive patients, suggesting that an impairment of ET_B-receptor-mediated vasodilation is consistent with endothelial dysfunctional in these patients. However, other studies have shown no difference in vasodilator responsiveness between normal and hypertensive subjects to ET receptor blockade.

Therapeutic blockade of the endothelin system in hypertension

There have been two major approaches to blockade of this system: (1) endothelin receptor antagonists that block (1) ET_A or both ET_A and ET_B receptor subtypes and (2) inhibition of the endothelin-converting enzyme, particularly the ECE_1 isoform.

Endothelin receptor blocking agents

There have been two major studies in human essential hypertension of endothelin receptor blockade. The study by Krum et al.[30] was a 4-week examination of endothelin blockade in patients with mild essential hypertension (n=293) conducted with bosentan (dual ET receptor blocker) at 4 doses: 100 mg once daily, 500 mg once daily, 1000 mg once daily, and 1000 mg twice daily. These doses were compared to placebo and enalapril 20 mg once daily as active comparator.

At doses of 500 m/day or higher, bosentan lowered trough BP by up to 5.7 mmHg, significantly greater than placebo and similar to the BP-lowering effects of enalapril (5.8 mmHg). On 24-hour BP monitoring, mean daytime BP levels were significantly reduced by bosentan at all doses. The BP-lowering effect of bosentan was diminished at 24 hours in all but the twice-daily dose regimen.

Pharmacologic blockade of the endothelin receptor was confirmed by increased levels of the agonist to the receptor, endothelin-1. The BP-lowering activity of bosentan was not associated with evidence of reflex activation of neurohormonal systems. Specifically, there was no activation of the renin-angiotensin system (as measured by plasma levels of renin and angiotensin II) or the sympathetic nervous system (as measured by plasma levels of noradrenaline). This latter observation provided neurochemical support for the observed lack of reflex increase in heart rate in response to endothelin blockade and supported endothelin being a facilitator of both renin-angiotensin and sympathetic nervous system activity.

The second study is the HEAT study of the ETA selective receptor antagonist darusentan in a similar essential hypertension population[31] (n=392). There were significant reductions in BP at all dose levels compared to placebo with the active treatment, without a reflex increase in heart rate.

Endothelin-converting enzyme inhibitors

Pharmacologic inhibition of the endothelin-converting enzyme has been able to be achieved for some years. The metalloprotease inhibitor phospharamidon inhibits ECE. However, this agent also inhibits cleavage of other metalloproteases and as such is unsuitable for mechanistic studies requiring selective blockade of the ECE enzyme. Other agents have been developed that nonselectively block ECE as well as other metalloproteases such as angiotensin-converting enzyme (ACE) and neutral endopepetidase (NEP). These NEP/ACE/ACE inhibitors (e.g., CGS 26303) may be of therapeutic potential in their own right. However, they do not permit assessment of the contribution of ECE to various diseases. More recently, highly selective ECE inhibitors have been developed and studied *in vitro* and in various animal models.[32]

SLV-306 has been developed as an NEP/ECE inhibitor and has been found to produce significant reductions in BP in undifferentiated essential hypertension patients.[33] This approach may offer advantages over NEP/ACE inhibition, which has been plagued by the side effect of excess angioneurotic edema. It is currently in late phase II trials for both hypertension and the indication of chronic heart failure.

Adverse effect profile of endothelin blockade in human hypertension

In the 4-week study of bosentan in hypertension[30] there was a small but dose-related increase in vasodilator-type side effects such as headache, flushing and leg edema. Similar vasodilator-type symptoms were observed with darusentan. Although these events were minor and not debilitating, they have to be viewed in the context of the asymptomatic nature of the disease and modern antihypertensive therapy where placebo-like tolerability has been achieved with agents such as angiotensin II receptor antagonists. Furthermore, ET receptor antagonists are first-trimester teratogens in animals. It may be for these reasons there has been considerable reluctance by the pharmaceutical industry to pursue endothelin receptor antagonism in the broad patient group of mild to moderate essential hypertension.

A further problem with bosentan has been elevated transaminases and bile acids in a small percentage of the population. This appears to be dose related in hypertension, and has been reported in patients with heart failure in the REACH-1[34] and ENABLE[35] studies. It is unclear whether this is a side effect specific for bosentan, found in mixed ET_A receptor antagonists only or in all ET receptor antagonists, be they ET_A selective or mixed.

Current place of endothelin receptor antagonists in hypertension

With the adverse effect profile as described, endothelin receptor antagonists are unlikely to become first-line monotherapy for the treatment of hypertension. However, there still remains a role for these agents as add-on therapy in patients with refractory hypertension, particularly where endothelin has been specifically implicated in the progression of disease.

Two areas that appear to fulfill these criteria are in low-renin cyclosporine-induced hypertension and in the African-American population. Moreover, the use of the agent bosentan is limited for this indication because of

a profound pharmacokinetic drug interaction resulting in large increases in bosentan plasma levels with cyclosporine coadministration.

A pathogenic role for ET has been proposed in hypertension associated with use of the immunosuppressant cyclosporine.[36] Post-transplantation hypertension and atherosclerosis are major and increasing complications in the post-transplantation patient. Increased ET receptor messenger RNA has been found in the mesenteric vasculature of cyclosporine-treated rats. ET peptide is increased in rat cardiac allograft coronary vasculopathy and bosentan therapy attenuates the vasculopathy. Cyclosporine-induced renal vasoconstriction is reduced by ET_A receptor antagonism with BQ-123, and bosentan blocks cyclosporine-induced hypertension in rats and marmosets.[37] Furthermore, increased ET peptide expression is observed in diseased coronary arteries post cardiac transplantation and in the neointima of the renal vasculature following kidney transplantation. However, clinical trials of ET blockade in this patient population have not yet been reported.

Hypertension in the African-American population has been associated with marked elevations in plasma ET concentrations.[38] Furthermore, these patients generally comprise a low-renin population where ET blockade has been demonstrated to be most effective in BP lowering in animal models of hypertension. Plasma levels of ET and BP can both be lowered by conventional therapies, but the hypothesis that the ET system is an appropriate target for specific blockade in this patient population has not been clinically tested.

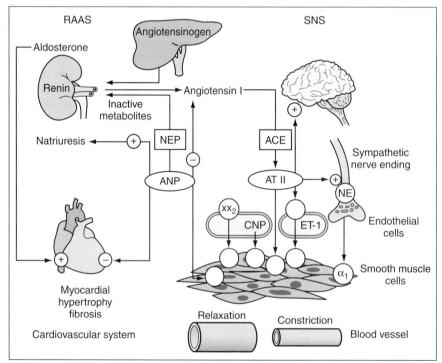

Figure 85–2. Cardiovascular regulation by sympathetic nervous system (SNS), RAAS, ANP, and local mediators. ET-1, endothelin; AT II, angiotensin II. (From Corti R, Burnett JC Jr, Rouleau JL, et al. Vasopeptidase inhibitors: A new therapeutic concept in cardiovascular disease? *Circulation* 2001;104:1856–62.)

Conclusions

There is now considerable evidence that endothelin plays a role in the pathogenesis and progression of essential hypertension, other forms of systemic hypertension, and many hypertension-related disorders. This conclusion is based on several observations in animals and man comprising measurement of plasma levels, expression of gene and peptide in arteries, and vascular responsiveness to endothelin blockade. Furthermore, endothelin appears to have a role in cardiovascular disease beyond merely being a vaso-constrictor peptide but also having additional effects as a mitogen and growth promoter.

The limited clinical studies of endothelin blockade in hypertension conducted thus far demonstrate the potential for these agents to lower BP without reflex activation of other neurohormonal systems. There may be particular advantages in targeting populations particularly where endothelin has been more directly pathogenically implicated (such as black hypertension and cyclosporine-induced hypertension). Furthermore, endothelin blockade may be a preferred agent in hypertensive patients with concomitant diseases where the peptide has been pathogenically implicated (and the antagonist therapy approved for treatment)—such as pulmonary arterial hypertension. However, widespread acceptance of endothelin receptor antagonists for the treatment of hypertension (even as ancillary agents) will not occur until drugs are developed without significant side effects at the doses used to achieve beneficial BP-lowering effects.

VASOPEPTIDASE INHIBITION

The humoral control of the cardiovascular system involves both vasoconstrictive and vasodilatory peptides, with the natriuretic peptides (ANP, BNP, CNP) providing endoge-

NATRIURETIC PEPTIDES HAVE CONTRASTING BIOLOGICAL EFFECTS TO ANG II		
Angiotensin II		Natriuretic Peptides
↑	Blood pressure	↓
↓	Renal sodium secretion	↑
↑	Aldosterone	↓
↓	Renin secretion	↓
↑	Sympathetic nerve activity	↓
↑	Cell proliferation	↓
↑	Hypertrophy	↓

Corti R, Burnett JC, Jr., Rouleau JL, Ruschitzka F, Luscher TF. Vasopeptidase inhibitors: a new therapeutic concept in cardiovascular disease? *Circulation.* 2001;104:1856-1862

Table 85–1. Natriuretic Peptides Have Contrasting Biological Effects to Ang II

nous antagonism to angiotensin II (Figure 85–2, Table 85–1). The natriuretic peptides are removed from the circulation primarily as a result of enzymatic degradation by neutral endopeptidase (NEP) and to a lesser extent through clearance by the natriuretic clearance receptor.[39] Moreover, in addition to the natriuretic peptides, NEP also catalyzes the degradation of the vasodilatory kinins and adrenomedullin. Thus, in theory inhibition of the renin-angiotensin-aldosterone system combined with potentiation of the natriuretic peptide/kinin should lead to improved cardiovascular hemodynamics and sodium/ water balance. Moreover, the structural similarities in the active sites of both NEP and ACE had made the simultaneous inhibition of these two enzymes an attractive target for drug development (Figure 85–3). Indeed, a number of such dual vaso-peptidase inhibitors (VPIs) entered pre-clinical and clinical development in the 1990s. These agents (which vary in their inhibitory activity for ACE and NEP) include omapatrilat, SA 7060, MDL 100240, MDL 10017, fasidotril, sampatrilat, alatriopril, CGS 30440, and S 21402.[40]

Of the dual vasopeptidase inhibitors, omapatrilat has been the most extensively studied in clinical trials. Initial studies with this compound showed it to be superior to ACE inhibitors as an anti-hypertensive agent[41] and in the treatment of heart failure.[42] Although the benefits beyond ACE inhibition were initially attributed to it, omapatrilat was shown to be a weak diuretic (with thiazides diuretic providing additional BP reduction).[43] These findings led to the conclusion that the efficacy of omapatrilat in hypertension and heart failure may be attributable to the potentiation of kinins. Despite the immense enthusiasm generated by initial studies, the larger definitive studies were not greeted with such enthusiasm.

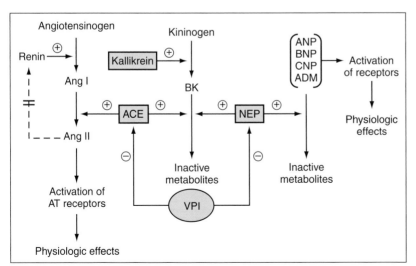

Figure 85–3. Major components of the renin-angiotensin, natriuretic peptide, and kinin-kallikrein systems. VPIs reduce the formation of angiotensin II (Ang II) and increase levels of natriuretic peptides by decreasing their degradation. These effects of VPIs are mediated by inhibiting ACE and NEP. ADM, adrenomedullin; ANP, atrial natriuretic peptide; BNP, brain natriuretic peptide; CNP, C-type natriuretic peptide. (From Gilbert RE, Kelly DJ, Atkins RC. Novel approaches to the treatment of progressive renal disease. *Curr Opin Pharmacol* 2001:1:183–89. With permission from Elsevier.)

For instance, in the omapatrilat cardiovascular treatment versus enalapril (OCTAVE) trial 25,302 hypertensive subjects were randomized to receive either omapatrilat 80 mg or enalapril 40 mg once daily. Omapatrilat reduced SBP 3.6 mmHg more than enalapril at week 8, with less use of adjunctive antihypertensive therapy needed to reach BP target. However, angioedema was much more frequent with omapatrilat than enalapril (2.17 versus 0.68%)—with two omapatrilat-treated subjects experiencing airway compromise.[44] Although the mechanisms underlying the development of angioedema with omapatrilat are incompletely understood, this adverse effect is viewed as pharmacodynamic rather than idiosyncratic (with rapid increases in bradykinin being contributory).[45]

In the Omapatrilat Versus Enalapril Randomized Trial of Utility in Reducing Events (OVERTURE) study, 5770 patients with New York Heart Association class II to IV heart failure were randomized to treatment with either enalapril 10 mg twice daily or omapatrilat 40 mg once daily for a mean of 15 months.[46] Although omapatrilat reduced the risk of death and hospitalization, it was not more effective than ACE inhibition alone in reducing the risk of a primary clinical event. Again, a trend to an increased likelihood of angioedema was noted (omapatrilat 0.8% and enalapril 0.5%).

Thus, despite the immense theoretical appeal of blocking both ACE and NEP the limited incremental benefit of this drug class along with the greater possibility of angioedema limit its potential utility. However, the fact that newer VPIs such as M100240 (Sanofi Aventis) are entering early-phase human trials[47] suggests that this class of drug may still have a future in the clinic.

V RHO-KINASE INHIBITORS

The pathophysiology of hypertension involves several processes, including abnormally increased activation of myosin-II-regulated calcium signaling, impaired nitric oxide production, and pathologic remodeling of the vascular wall. Rho-kinase, a serine-threonine kinase, is an important mediator of these pathways. Increased activity of the Rho-kinase-mediated pathway in vascular smooth muscle has been demonstrated to have a central role in the genesis of enhanced vasoconstriction in animal models of hypertension,[48,49] as well as in similar conditions with abnormal tonic smooth muscle contraction such as erectile dysfunction, vasospastic angina, pulmonary hypertension, and bronchodilation. Thus, inhibition of this pathway is theoretically appealing.

Rho-kinase pathway

An appreciation of the therapeutic potential of rho-kinase inhibitors is aided by an understanding of the mechanism of smooth muscle cell tone. Myosin II is the major molecular protein in smooth muscle cells, and its effects are controlled by electromechanical coupling (regulated by changes in cytoplasmic calcium contractility) and by phosphorylation/dephosphorylation of the myosin regulatory light chain (MLC). In fact, phosphorylation of MLC is one of the most important steps for vascular smooth muscle contraction and was traditionally believed to have been regulated by a simple Ca-calmodulin-dependent activation of myosin light chain kinase (MLCK) and myosin phosphatase (MLCP). Evidence for the involvement of the small GTPase RhoA in calcium sensitivity in smooth muscle has now been demonstrated.[50]

The exchange of GDP for GTP on RhoA and translocation of RhoA from the cytosol to the membrane are markers of RhoA activation. Activated RhoA binds to the rho-binding domain of rho-kinase, activating it. Rho-kinase is an important regulator of MLCP. When activated, it phosphorylates MLC via the myosin-binding subunit (MBS) of MLCP. Phosphorylation of MLC causes actin/myosin cross-bridge formation and muscle contraction. Relaxation is mediated by the dephosphorylation of MLC (Figure 85–4).

The endothelium has important roles to play in hypertension, one of the most important being the production of nitric oxide (NO). NO is an important mediator of smooth muscle function through its ability to induce vasodilation and to inhibit vasoconstriction.

RhoA has recently been found to have an important role in endothelial function. Interestingly, the role of RhoA in the endothelium arose from studies using HMG-CoA reductase inhibitors, which in addition to lowering LDL cholesterol decrease post-translational acylation of RhoA GTPase, increasing endothelial nitric oxide synthase (eNOS) expression and enhancing endothelial function. Thus, the importance of the RhoA/Rho-kinase pathway (by suppressing eNOS in endothelial cells and thus decreasing the synthesis of NO) in understanding endothelial dysfunction is now being recognized.

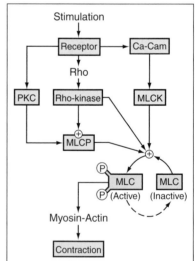

Figure 85–4. Effect of rho-kinase, PKC, and MLCK and MLCP in arterial smooth muscle. PKC, protein kinase C; MLC, myosin light chain; MLCK, myosin light chain kinase; MLCP, myosin light chain phosphatase. (From Kandabashi T, Shimokawa H, Miyata K, et al. Inhibition of myosin phosphatase by upregulated rho-kinase plays a key role for coronary artery spasm in a porcine model with interleukin-1b. *Circulation* 2000;101:1319–23.)

As well as its role in the regulation of actin-myosin contractility, rho-kinase plays an important role in the remodeling of the actin cytoskeleton via its role in adhesion, migration, proliferation, and cytokinesis of vascular smooth muscle cells. Rho-kinase is upregulated in a mouse model of myocardial infarction (MI)[51] and is known to be involved in the *in vivo* pathogenesis of vascular remodelling[52] and in cardiac hypertrophy.[53]

Mechanism of action of rho-kinase inhibitors

The rho-rhokinase pathway can be inhibited at several stages: at the receptor by antagonists to the activating agonist (such as antagonists to arachadonic acid or PKC); by hydrolysis of bound GTP to GDP (preventing activation of RhoA); by complexing of free RhoA, preventing activation of rho-kinase and inhibition of MLCP; and by direct inhibition of rho-kinase (Figure 85–5).

The three most specific inhibitors of rho-kinase to date are hydroxyfasudil, fasudil, and Y-27632. Hydroxy-fasudil is 1-(5 isoquinolinesulfonyl)-homopiperazine (HA-1077), fasudil is (S)-(+)-2-methyl-1-[(4-methyl-5-isoquinoline)sulfonyl]-homopiperazine (H-1152P), and Y-27632 (Welfide Corporation, Osaka, Japan) is a (+)-(R)-trans-4-(1-aminoethyl)-N-(4-pyridyl) cyclohexanecarboxamide dihydrochloride monohydrate.

The compounds differ in their ability to inhibit rho-kinase. In particular, H-1152P (fasudil) has a greater affinity for rho-kinase, as compared to HA-1077 (hydroxy-fasudil) and Y-27632 (Table 85–2). These rho-kinase inhibitors also

KI VALUES OF RHO-KINASE INHIBITORS FOR SER/THR PROTEIN KINASES			
	Ki (µM)	Rho-kinase	Inhibitor
Protein kinase	**H-1152P**	**HA-1077**	**Y-27632**
Rho-kinase	0.0016	0.33	0.14
PKA	0.63	1.0	25
PKC	9.27	9.3	26
MLCK	10.1	55	>250

Adapted from Sasaki Y, Suzuki M, Hidaka H. The novel and specific rho-kinase inhibitor (S)-(+)-2-methyl-1-[(4-methyl-5-isoquinoline)sulfonyl]-homopiperazine as a probing molecule for rho-kinase-involved pathway. *Pharmacology & Therapeutics* 2002;93:226 with permission from Elsevier.

Table 85–2. Ki Values of Rho-kinase Inhibitors for Ser/Thr Protein Kinases

have varying degrees of affinity for other serine-threonine kinases.

Pharmacodynamics of rho-kinase inhibitors

Activated rho-kinase phosphorylates the catalytic site of myosin light-chain phosphatase, causing smooth muscle contraction. In addition to inhibition of both *in vivo* and *in vitro* rho-kinase, the three currently available rho-kinase inhibitors inactivate the myosin-binding subunit of myosin light-chain phosphatase—preventing phosphorylation of MLC by rho-kinase in vascular smooth muscle cells.[54,55]

HA-1077, originally developed as an isoquinoline derivative of N-(2-guanidinoethyl)-5-isoquinolinesulfon-amide (a calcium channel antagonist), is a vasodilator of the cerebral and coronary vasculature that inhibits the vascular contraction induced by agonists such as norepinephrine, histamine, angiotensin II, and endothelin. Continuous infusion of HA-1077 results in a dose-dependent decrease in peripheral vascular resistance and increased cardiac output, without a significant change in the right atrial pressure. Although its initial effects were thought to be due to calcium channel inhibition, HA-1077 displays vasodilatation even when these channels are antagonized. HA-1077, like the other rho-kinase inhibitors, inhibits other protein kinases (such as protein kinase C) but has a lower Ki for rho-kinase. For example, the inhibitory effect of fasudil on rho-kinase is >100 times more potent than on protein kinase C and myosin light-chain kinase. The IC50 value of fasudil has been established as 1.9 mol/L when tested *in vitro*[56] and a comparable dose of intra-coronary fasudil (100 µg/kg) suppressed

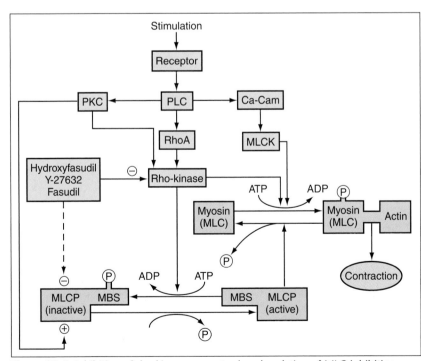

Figure 85–5. Inhibition of rho-kinase prevents phosphorylation of MLC-inhibiting contraction. PLC, phospholipase C; Ca, calcium; CaM, calmodulin; PKC, protein kinase C, MLCK, myosin light chain kinase; MLCP, myosin light chain phosphatase; MBS, myosin binding subunit. (From Kandabashi T, Shimokawa H, Miyata K, et al. Inhibition of myosin phosphatase by upregulated rho-kinase plays a key role for coronary artery spasm in a porcine model with interleukin-1b. *Circulation* 2000;101:1319–23.)

coronary artery spasm in an *in vivo* porcine model[57] (300 μg/min for 15 minutes suppressed coronary artery spasm in humans).[49]

The effects of Y-27632 have similarly been assessed using a number of cardiovascular models. In the halothane anesthetized canine model,[58] an intravenous dose of 0.01 mg/kg of Y-27632 significantly decreased the total peripheral vascular resistance and increased the cardiac output. Moreover, a 10 times higher dose of Y-27632 (0.1 mg/kg) exerted positive inotropic, chronotropic, and dromotropic effects together with hypotension and reduced left ventricular end-diastolic pressure. An intravenous dose of 0.01 to 5 mg/kg results in a range of concentrations that are known to significantly inhibit rho-kinase (0.1 to 10 μM).[56]

Interestingly, these inhibitors appear to reduce BP more in diseased arteries rather than those with normal pressure. This may be because rho-kinase is upregulated in hypertension in spastic parts of endothelium such as occurs in vasospastic angina and during conditions of adverse cardiovascular remodeling such as post-myocardial infarction (MI).[56] In addition, growth factors such as transforming growth factor-β and macrophage inhibitory factor are upregulated post-MI and downregulated with a rho-kinase inhibitor.

Both fasudil and Y27632 impair thrombin-induced downregulation of eNOS expression[59,60]. However, in contrast to Y27632, fasudil increases basal eNOS expression without affecting basal rho-kinase activity, thus suggesting that fasudil has additional rho-kinase-independent effects on eNOS expression.

Pharmacokinetics of rho-kinase inhibitors

Y-27632 has successfully been given via inhalation (1 mM, 2 min), orally (humans and in drinking water for rats), intracavernosally, and intravenously. However, pharmacokinetics measures have not commonly been reported. However, peak plasma concentrations of Y-27632 of 10 to 20 ng/mL (0.03 to 0.06 μM) and 100 to 200 ng/mL (0.3 to 0.6 μM) have been reported in animal models after the intravenous administration of 0.01 and 0.1 mg/kg of Y-27632, respectively. There has been a noticeably greater reduction in BP with intravenous as compared to oral and inhalational therapy, suggesting that the hydrophilicity of Y27632 results in low oral availability.[56,61]

INDICATIONS

Hypertension

As rho-kinase is upregulated in hypertensive subjects but not in control normotensive subjects, rho-kinase inhibitors have predictably had more of a vasodilatory effect in hypertensive subjects.[62] These drugs are known to have a dose-dependent vasodilatory effect, but with their effects on vascular remodeling they also play a role in the pathogenesis of increased systemic vascular resistance long term.

In addition, fasudil increases upregulation of NO synthase and endothelial NO synthase-derived NO (which reduces the pathologic LV remodeling after MI in mice[63] and ameliorates endothelial dysfunction). Y27632 and hydroxyfasudil additionally upregulate NO synthetase, suggesting that it is a class effect.

Ventricular remodeling

Rho-kinase activation is involved in the pathogenesis of LV remodeling. Thus, rho-kinase inhibition would be expected to have a favorable effect on remodeling. In fact, after MI in an animal model of myocardial infarction fasudil suppressed the increases in LV end-diastolic pressure, the ratio of RV weight to body weight, and the ratio of lung weight to body weight. Fasudil is known to suppress the increased expression of several profibrotic cytokines (such as macrophage inhibitory factor, TGF-beta, IFN-gamma, monocyte chemoattractant protein-1, and angiotensin II) that occurs post-MI, reducing pathologic cardiac remodeling.[64]

Adverse effects

Potentially, rho-kinase inhibitors could cause symptomatic hypotension, especially if given intravenously. Phase I and II studies using both oral and intravenous doses with measurements of effect (as well as basic pharmacokinetic parameters such as plasma concentration, time to steady state, and area under the curve) will be required in order to decrease the likelihood of this problem. In fact, HA-1077 at a supratherapeutic dose has caused systemic hypotension in dehydrated animals (although no serious adverse side effects were reported).

In addition, it is known that protein kinases play a crucial role in the transduction of signals in cellular systems. Thus, although it is known that rho-kinase inhibitors do have some effect on other protein kinases (albeit with higher dissociation constants and lower potency) whether these effects translates into beneficial or detrimental effects on cell growth and proliferation long term is as yet unknown.

SUMMARY

Preclinical and early clinical studies of the rho-kinase inhibitors have shown that these agents have beneficial vasodilator and vascular remodeling effects in hypertension, coronary artery spasm, angina, hypercholesterolemia, and other noncardiovascular conditions such as erectile dysfunction, pulmonary hypertension, cerebral vasospasm, arteriosclerosis, bronchial asthma, glaucoma, and cancer. Further work is necessary regarding elucidation of the relationship between dose and effect and dose and plasma concentrations, as well as surveillance of long-term effects of these agents—especially with respect to their effects on growth and downstream markers of activation of other protein kinases.

REFERENCES

1. Nguyen G, Delarue F, Burckle C, Bouzhir L, Giller T, Sraer JD. Pivotal role of the renin/prorenin receptor in angiotensin II production and cellular responses to renin. *J Clin Invest* 2002;109:1417–27.

2. Fisher ND, Hollenberg NK. Is there a future for renin inhibitors? *Expert Opin Investig Drugs* 2001;10:417–26.

3. Hoover DJ, Lefker BA, Rosati RL, Wester RT, Kleinman EF, Bindra JS, et al. Discovery of inhibitors of human renin with high oral bioavailability. *Adv Exp Med Biol* 1995;362:167–80.

4. Fisher ND, Hollenberg NK. Renin inhibition: what are the therapeutic opportunities? *J Am Soc Nephrol* 2005;16:592–99.

5. Wood JM, Maibaum J, Rahuel J, Grutter MG, Cohen NC, Rasetti V, et al. Structure-based design of aliskiren, a novel orally effective renin inhibitor. *Biochem Biophys Res Commun* 2003;308:698–705.

6. Nussberger J, Wuerzner G, Jensen C, Brunner HR. Angiotensin II suppression in humans by the orally active renin inhibitor Aliskiren (SPP100): Comparison with enalapril. *Hypertension* 2002;39:E1–8.

7. Stanton A, Jensen C, Nussberger J, O'Brien E. Blood pressure lowering in essential hypertension with an oral renin inhibitor, aliskiren. *Hypertension* 2003;42:1137–43.

8. Gradman AH, Schmieder RE, Lins RL, Nussberger J, Chiang Y, Bedigian MP. Aliskiren, a novel orally effective renin inhibitor, provides dose-dependent antihypertensive efficacy and placebo-like tolerability in hypertensive patients. *Circulation* 2005;111:1012–18.

9. Simpson SA, Tait JF, Wettsein A, et al. Konstitution des aldosterons, des neuen mineralocorticoids. *Experientia* 1954;10:132–33.

10. Rocha R, Williams GH. Rationale for the use of aldosterone antagonists in congestive heart failure. *Drugs* 2002;62:723–31.

11. Liew D, Krum H. The role of aldosterone receptor blockade in the management of cardiovascular disease. *Current Opinion in Investigational Drugs* 2002;3:1468–73.

12. Brilla CG, Rupp H, Funck R, et al. The renin-angiotensin-aldosterone system and myocardial collagen matrix remodelling in congestive heart failure. *Eur Heart J* 1995;16(Suppl O):107–09.

13. Takeda Y, Miyamori I, Inaba S, et al. Vascular aldosterone in genetically hypertensive rats. *Hypertension* 1997;29:45–8.

14. Pitt B, Zannad F, Remme WJ, et al. The effect of spironolactone on morbidity and mortality in patients with severe heart failure. Randomized Aldactone Evaluation Study Investigators. *N Engl J Med* 1999;341:709–17.

15. Delyani JA. Mineralocorticoid receptor antagonists: the evolution of utility and pharmacology. *Kidney Int* 2000;57:1408–11.

16. Weinberger MH, Roniker B, Krause SL, et al. Eplerenone, a selective aldosterone blocker, in mild-to-moderate hypertension. *Am J Hypertens* 2002;15:709–16.

17. Pitt B, Reichek N, Willenbrock R, Zannad F, Phillips RA, Roniker B, et al. Effects of eplerenone, enalapril, and hypertrophy: The 4E-left ventricular hypertrophy study. *Circulation* 2003;108:1831–38.

18. Weinberger M, MacDonald T, Conlin PR, et al., on behalf of the Eplerenone 019 Investigators. Comparison of Eplerenone and Losartan in Patients with Low-Renin Hypertension. (Abstract). American Society of Hypertension 17th Annual Scientific Meeting, 2002 May 14–18; New York City, USA.

19. Flack JM, Oparil S, Pratt JH, et al. Efficacy and tolerability of eplerenone and losartan in hypertensive black and white patients. *J Am Coll Cardiol* 2003;41:1148–55.

20. Krum H, Nolly H, Workman D, et al. Efficacy of eplerenone added to renin-angiotensin blockade in hypertensive patients. *Hypertension* 2002;40:117–23.

21. Prisant LM, Krum H, Roniker B, Krause SL, Fakouhi K, He W. Can renin status predict the antihypertensive efficacy of eplerenone add-on therapy? *J Clin Pharmacol.* 2003;43:1203–10.

22. Pitt B, Remme W, Zannad F, et al. Eplerenone, a selective aldosterone blocker, in patients with left ventricular dysfunction after myocardial infarction. *N Engl J Med* 2003;348:1309–21.

23. Hartmann RW, Muller U, Ehmer PB. Discovery of selective CYP11B2 (aldosterone synthase) inhibitors for the therapy of congestive heart failure and myocardial fibrosis. *Eur J Med Chem* 2003;38:363–66.

24. Levin ER. Endothelins. *New Engl J Med* 1995;333:356–63.

25. Rubanyi GM, Polokoff MA. Endothelins: Molecular biology, biochemistry, pharmacology, physiology, and pathophysiology. *Pharmacol Rev* 1994;46:325–415.

26. Miyauchi T, Masaki T. Pathophysiology of endothelin in the cardiovascular system. *Annu Rev Physiol* 1999;61:391–415.

27. Simonson MS, Dunn MJ. Cellular signalling by peptides of the endothelin gene family. *FASEB J* 1990;4:2989–3000.

28. De Nucci G, Thomas R, D'Orleans-Juste P, Antunes E, Walder C, Warner TD, et al. Pressor effects of circulating endothelin are limited by its removal in the pulmonary circulation and by the release of prostacyclin and endothelium-derived relaxing factor. *Proc Natl Acad Sci USA* 1988;85:9797–9800.

29. Dupuis J, Stewart DJ, Cernacek P, Gosselin G. Human pulmonary circulation is an important site for both clearance and production of endothelin-1. *Circulation* 1996;94:1578–84.

30. Krum H, Viskoper RJ, Lacourciere Y, Budde M, Charlon V. The effect of an endothelin-receptor antagonist, bosentan, on blood pressure in patients with essential hypertension. Bosentan Hypertension Investigators. *New Engl J Med* 1998;338:784–90.

31. Nakov R, Pfarr E, Eberle S. HEAT Investigators. Darusentan: An effective endothelin A receptor antagonist for treatment of hypertension. *Am J Hypertens* 2002;15(7 Pt 1):583–89.

32. Wada A, Tsutamoto T, Ohnishi M, Sawaki M, Fukai D, Maeda Y, et al. Effects of a specific endothelin-converting enzyme inhibitor on cardiac, renal, and neurohumoral functions in congestive heart failure: Comparison of effects with those of endothelin A receptor antagonism. *Circulation* 1999;99:570–77.

33. Tabrizchi R. SLV-306. Solvay. *Curr Opin Investig Drugs* 2003;4(3):329–32.

34. Packer M, McMurray J, Massie BM, Caspi A, Charlon V, Cohen-Solal A, et al. Clinical effects of endothelin receptor antagonism with bosentan in patients with severe chronic heart failure: Results of a pilot study. *J Card Fail* 2005;11(1):12–20.

35. Teerlink JR. Recent heart failure trials of neurohormonal modulation (OVERTURE and ENABLE): Approaching the asymptote of efficacy? *J Card Fail* 2002;8(3):124–27.

36. Ravalli S, Szabolcs M, Albala A, Michler RE, Cannon PJ. Endothelin-1 peptide expression in transplant coronary artery disease. *Transplant Proc* 1997;29:2577–78.

37. Bartholomeusz B, Hardy KJ, Nelson AS, Phillips PA. Bosentan ameliorates cyclosporine A-induced hypertension in rats and primates. *Hypertension* 1996;27:1341–45.

38. Ergul S, Parish DC, Puett D, Ergul A. Racial differences in plasma endothelin-1 concentrations in individuals with essential hypertension. *Hypertension* 1996;28:652–55 (published erratum appears in *Hypertension* 1997;29:912).

39. Burnett JC Jr. Vasopeptidase inhibition: A new concept in blood pressure management. *J Hypertens Suppl* 1999;17:S37–43.

40. Gilbert RE, Kelly DJ, Atkins RC. Novel approaches to the treatment of progressive renal disease. *Curr Opin Pharmacol* 2001;1:183–89.

41. Campese VM, Lasseter KC, Ferrario CM, Smith WB, Ruddy MC, Grim CE, et al. Omapatrilat versus lisinopril: Efficacy and neurohormonal profile in salt-sensitive hypertensive patients. *Hypertension* 2001;38:1342–48.

42. Eisenstein EL, Nelson CL, Simon TA, Smitten AL, Lapuerta P, Mark DB. Vasopeptidase inhibitor reduces inhospital costs for patients with congestive heart failure: Results from the IMPRESS trial. Inhibition of Metallo Protease by BMS-186716 in a Randomized Exercise and Symptoms Study in Subjects With Heart Failure. *Am Heart J* 2002;143:1112–17.

43. Ferdinand K, Saini R, Lewin A, Yellen L, Barbosa JA, Kushnir E. Efficacy and safety of omapatrilat with hydrochlorothiazide for the treatment of hypertension in subjects nonresponsive to hydrochlorothiazide alone. *Am J Hypertens* 2001;14:788–93.

44. Kostis JB, Packer M, Black HR, Schmieder R, Henry D, Levy E. Omapatrilat and enalapril in patients with hypertension: The Omapatrilat Cardiovascular Treatment vs. Enalapril (OCTAVE) trial. *Am J Hypertens* 2004;17:103–11.

45. Messerli FH, Nussberger J. Vasopeptidase inhibition and angio-oedema. *Lancet* 2000;356:608–09.

46. Packer M, Califf RM, Konstam MA, Krum H, McMurray JJ, Rouleau JL, et al. Comparison of omapatrilat and enalapril in patients with chronic heart failure: The Omapatrilat Versus Enalapril Randomized Trial of Utility in Reducing Events (OVERTURE). *Circulation* 2002;106:920–26.

47. Cirillo I, Martin NE, Brennan B, Barrett JS. The effect of food on the pharmacokinetics of a dual angiotensin-converting enzyme/neutral endopeptidase inhibitor, M100240. *J Clin Pharmacol* 2004;44:1379–84.

48. Mukai Y, Shimokawa H, Matoba T, et al. Involvement of Rho-kinase in hypertensive vascular disease: A novel therapeutic target in hypertension. *FASEB J* 2001;15:1062–64.

49. Masumoto A, Mohri M, Shimokawa H, et al. Suppression of coronary artery spasm by the rho-kinase inhibitor fasudil in patients with vasospastic angina. *Circulation* 2002;105:1545–47.

50. Hirata K, Kikuchi A, Sasaki T, et al. Involvement of rho p21 in the GTP-enhanced calcium ion sensitivity of smooth muscle contraction. *J Biol Chem* 1992;267:8719–22.

51. Hattori T, Shimokawa H, Higashi M, et al. Inhibition of rho-kinase suppresses left ventricular remodelling after myocardial infarction in mice. *Circulation* 2004;109:2234–39.

52. Shimokawa H. Rho-kinase as a novel therapeutic target in treatment of cardiovascular diseases. *J Cardiovasc Pharmacol* 2002;39:319–27.

53. Higashi M, Shimokawa H, Hattori T, et al. Long-term inhibition of rho-kinase suppresses angiotensin II-induced cardiovascular hypertrophy in rats in vivo: Effect on endothelial NAD(P)H oxidase system. *Circ Res* 2003;93:767–75.

54. Shimokawa H, Seto M, Katsumata N, et al. Rho-kinase-mediated pathway induces enhanced myosin light chain phosphorylations in a swine model of coronary artery spasm. *Cardiovasc Res* 1999;43:1029–39.

55. Uehata M, Ishizaki T, Satoh H, et al. Calcium sensitization of smooth muscle mediated by a rho-associated protein kinase in hypertension. *Nature* 1997;389:990–94.

56. Davies S, Reddy H, Caivano M, et al. Specificity and mechanism of action of some commonly used protein kinase inhibitors. *Biochem J* 2000;351:95–105.

57. Kandabashi T, Shimokawa H, Miyata K, et al. Inhibition of myosin phosphatase by upregulated rho-kinase plays a key role for coronary artery spasm in a porcine model with interleukin-1b. *Circulation* 2000;101:1319–23.

58. Sugiyama A, Hashimoto K. Effects of gastrointestinal prokinetic agents, TKS159 and cisapride, on the in situ canine heart assessed by cardiohemodynamic and electrophysiological monitoring. *Toxicol Appl Pharmacol* 1998;152:261–69.

59. Takemoto M, Sun J, Horoki J. Rho-kinase mediates hypoxia-induced down-regulation of endothelial nitric oxide synthase. *Circulation* 2002;106:57–62.

60. Eto M, Barandier C, Rathgeb L, et al. Thrombin suppresses endothelial nitric oxide synthase and upregulates endothelin-converting enzyme-1 expression by distinct pathways: Role of rho/ROCK and mitogen-activated protein kinase. *Circ Res* 2001;89:583–90.

61. Iizuka K, Shimizu Y, Tsukagoshi H, et al. Evaluation of Y-27632, a rho-kinase inhibitor, as a bronchodilator in guinea pigs. *European Journal of Pharmacology* 2000;406:273–79.

62. Masumoto A, Hirooka Y, Shimokawa H, et al. Possible involvement of rho-kinase in the pathogenesis of hypertension in humans. *Hypertension* 2001;38:1307–10.

63. Scherrer-Crosbie M, Ullrich R, Bloch K, et al. Endothelial nitric oxide synthase limits left ventricular remodelling after myocardial infarction in mice. *Circulation* 2001;1286–91.

64. Matsumoto Y, Uwatoku T, Oi K, et al. Long-term inhibition of Rhokinase suppresses neointimal formation after stent implantation in porcine coronary arteries: Involvement of multiple mechanisms. *Arterioscler Thromb Vasc Biol* 2004;24:181–86.

Chapter

86

Fixed Low-Dose Antihypertensive Therapy

Ryan M. Woodham and Suzanne Oparil

Key Findings

- Prevalence of hypertension in the U.S. population is increasing.

- Monotherapy is inadequate in ≈70% of patients.

- Fixed low-dose combination therapy (defined as a combination in a single tablet of low doses of antihypertensive agents whose mechanisms of action are complementary) is an effective, safe, and cost-effective method of decreasing blood pressure (BP) in most patients with essential hypertension.

- Many neurohormonal and cellular mechanisms cause hypertension, making defining a specific etiology and creating a cause-specific treatment plan difficult.

- Many antihypertensives work by affecting fluid and sodium balance, blocking the renin-angiotensin-aldosterone system or sympathetic nervous system, and decreasing systemic vascular resistance by blocking L-type calcium channels.

- Combinations of angiotensin-converting enzyme (ACE) inhibitors, angiotensin receptor blockers (ARB) diuretics, and calcium channel blockers (CCB) have additive effects in controlling BP and minimizing adverse effects of individual components.

- The "polypill" concept promises to increase compliance, decrease multiple CV risk factors, and decrease morbidity and mortality with cardiac disease.

Hypertension is a major clinical problem, with an increasing prevalence.[1] Increased BP is an important modifiable risk factor for cardiovascular disease (CVD), the most common cause for death and disability in developed and developing countries. Its control significantly reduces these risks.[2]

Observational studies have shown that mortality and morbidity from ischemic heart disease and stroke in persons 40 to 89 years of age increases in log linear fashion with increases in both SBP and DBP.[3] For each increase in SBP of 20 mmHg or in DBP of 10 mmHg over the entire range from 115/75 mmHg to 185/115 mmHg, there is a twofold increase in mortality related to coronary disease and stroke. SBP and, accordingly, the prevalence of hypertension increase with age throughout life, whereas DBP decreases after age 60.[4,5]

A cohort study using data collected from the Framingham Heart Study from 1990 to 1999 revealed that the rate of BP control, defined as a SBP <140 mmHg and a DBP <90 mmHg, was only 32.4% of the cohort as a whole.[4] Control rates decreased with age and were lowest (23%)

in women >80 years of age. Poor BP control in the elderly is a particularly serious problem because hypertension is most prevalent in this age group. In the Framingham cohort, 74% of those >80 years old were hypertensive, compared to 63% of those aged 60 to 79 years and 27% of those <60 years old. Importantly, only 38% of patients in the oldest age group were receiving more than one antihypertensive medication. Previous studies (Figure 86–1) have demonstrated that between 2 to 4 agents on average are required to meet the current JNC 7 goal of SBP <140 mmHg and/or DBP <90 mmHg.

Clinical trial data indicate that lowering BP with antihypertensive drugs effectively reduces risk of a variety of CVD outcomes, including cardiovascular death and total mortality[2,6–10] (Figure 86–2). Meta-analyses of data from randomized controlled trials have not shown significant differences in total major CVD outcomes between regimens based on ACE inhibitors, CCBs, or diuretics or BBs, although there were some differences in cause-specific outcomes.[2,9,10] For outcomes other than heart failure, differences in achieved SBP lowering were related to the extent of risk reduction.[2] Thus, for the universe of hypertensive patients BP reduction appears to be more important than choice of antihypertensive drug(s) for reducing CVD risk.

For persons with BP >20/10 mmHg above goal (stage 2 hypertension), initial treatment with 2 drugs, usually including a thiazide-type diuretic, is recommended by the seventh report of the Joint National Committee on Prevention, Detection, Evaluation and Treatment of High Blood Pressure (JNC 7) because of the high risk of this patient group (Figure 86–3).[11,12] Randomized controlled trials have shown that single drug treatment usually is not adequate to achieve goal BPs in most hypertensive patients, particularly those with systolic hypertension (Figure 86–1). For example, in the very large Antihypertensive and Lipid Lowering Treatment to Prevent Heart Attack (ALLHAT) trial (n=42,418) less than 30% of participants achieved goal BP (<140/90 mmHg) on monotherapy.[13]

Fixed-dose combination drugs have been available for the treatment of hypertension for over 40 years. Agents marketed in the 1960s included reserpine/dihydralazine/hydrochlorothiazide (Unipres) and methyldopa/hydrochlorothiazide (Aldoril).[14] Importantly, the very earliest outcome trial of antihypertensive therapy in the United States, the Veteran's Administration Cooperative Study on Antihypertensive Agents, demonstrated dramatic reduc-

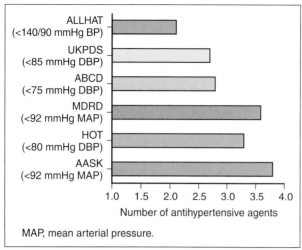

MAP, mean arterial pressure.

Figure 86–1. Average number of antihypertensive agents needed to achieve the current JNC 7 BP goals. MAP, mean arterial pressure. (Data from Bakris GL, Williams M, Dworkin L, et al. Preserving renal function in adults with hypertension and diabetes: A consensus approach. National Kidney Foundation Hypertension and Diabetes Executive Committees Working Group. *Am J Kidney Dis* 2000;36:646–61 and Cushman WC, Ford CE, Cutler JA, et al. Success and predictors of blood pressure control in diverse North American settings: The Antihypertensive and Lipid-Lowering treatment to prevent Heart Attack Trial (ALLHAT). *J Clin Hypertens* 2002;4:393–404.)

Box 86–1

Advantages of Fixed-dose Combination Therapy

- Increased compliance, simplified titration, and convenience of use
- Potentiation of antihypertensive effects of a single compound
- Additive or synergistic effect
- Enhancing effect in specific populations
- Diuretic with an ACE inhibitor, ARB, or beta blocker
- Attenuation in adverse events
- Decrease in diuretic-induced metabolic changes with ACE inhibitors or ARBs
- Decrease in calcium channel antagonist-related peripheral edema with ACE inhibitors
- Improved overall results, greater BP response, and lower cost when co-payments and pharmacy filling fees are considered

---

tions in CVD outcomes with a combination of hydrochlorothiazide, reserpine, and hydralazine compared to placebo.[15] Fixed-dose combination antihypertensive drugs later fell out of fashion because of a perception of increased toxicity compared to monotherapy. However, a large variety of fixed-dose combination agents have been developed in recent years, in part in response to the realization that older higher-risk hypertensive patients require multiple antihypertensive agents for BP control. A list of currently available fixed low-dose combination therapies can be found in Table 86–1.

FIXED LOW-DOSE COMBINATION THERAPY: ADVANTAGES AND DISADVANTAGES

Advantages

Fixed low-dose combination therapy (defined as a combination in a single tablet of low doses of antihypertensive agents whose mechanisms of action are complementary) is an efficacious, safe, and cost-effective method of decreasing BP in most patients with essential hypertension.[14] Initiating therapy with more than one agent offers the potential advantages of achieving BP control more rapidly and avoiding dose-related adverse effects of individual drugs by producing greater BP reductions at lower doses of the component agents. Fixed-dose combinations have several advantages that do not currently reside in any single molecule (Box 86–1). Fixed low-dose combination therapies enjoy these desirable characteristics, in part because combining agents with different but additive mechanisms of action helps to maximize antihypertensive potency while minimizing dose-related adverse effects.

The greater efficacy of combination agents with different (and complementary) mechanisms of action relates to their ability to antagonize more than one of the many mechanisms of the pathogenesis of hypertension, as well as the ability of one component to block counterregulatory responses to the other. For example, diuretics activate the renin-angiotensin-aldosterone system (RAAS), reduce volume, and make BP more angiotensin dependent. Concomitant administration of an ACE inhibitor or an ARB blocks angiotensin II generation or action, minimizing the compensatory pressor effect of diuretic-induced RAAS activation and producing an additive BP-lowering effect.

Fixed-dose combinations offer convenience for the patient because they can usually be administered once daily. It has been shown that multiple daily doses of medications are associated with decreased adherence.[16] Further, elderly patients usually suffer from a variety of medical conditions for which they require multiple medicines. In particular, elderly hypertensive patients frequently have target organ damage/concomitant CVD conditions that require treatment. Fixed-dose combination antihypertensive drugs are often useful in treating more than one such condition (e.g., ACE-inhibitor/diuretic or ARB/diuretic combinations for both heart failure and hypertension, and ACE-inhibitor/CCB combinations for both angina and hypertension). Thus, fixed-dose combinations can enhance patient adherence by simplifying medical regimens. An additional aid to medication adherence for most patients is low cost. Fixed-dose combinations have cost benefits that relate to the requirement for only a single co-payment and dispensing fee, as well as more competitive pricing in comparison to the individual components when purchased separately on most insurance plans.[17]

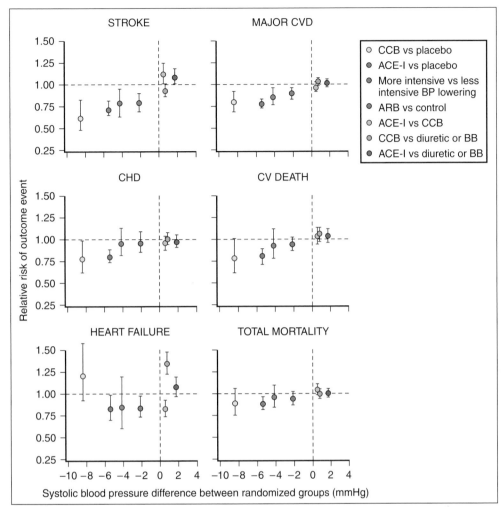

Figure 86–2. Associations of BP differences between groups with risks of major vascular outcomes and death. The circles are plotted at the point estimate of effect for the relative risk for every event type and the mean follow-up BP in the first listed group compared to the second listed group. Vertical lines are 95% CIs. CHD, coronary heart disease. CVD, cardiovascular disease. (Redrawn from Turnbull F, Neal B, Algert C, et al. Effects of different blood-pressure-lowering regimens on major cardiovascular events: Results of prospectively-designed overviews of randomized trials. Blood Pressure Lowering Treatment Trialists Collaboration. *Lancet* 2003;362:1527–35 with permission from Elsevier.)

Studies comparing low-dose combination therapy to monotherapy generally show a decreased incidence of dose-related adverse events with combination therapy.[14] This is due in part to packaging of the components in doses lower than are usually seen in monotherapy. In addition, in many of the combinations one agent compensates for the adverse effects caused by the another (e.g., ACE inhibitors decrease the incidence of peripheral edema associated with dihydropyridine CCBs and the hypokalemia associated with diuretics).

Disadvantages

Fixed-dose combinations may not be well tolerated in patients at risk for orthostatic hypotension. Some older persons, diabetic patients, and persons with autonomic dysfunction may experience profound hypotension (particularly orthostatic hypotension) when therapy is initiated

with more than one agent.[6,12,13] On the other hand, some fixed-dose combinations do not contain sufficient doses of the constituent drugs to provide BP control or to manage illnesses that commonly coexist with hypertension.[14] For instance, the doses of BBs found in combination antihypertensive therapy may not be large enough to treat concomitant angina and coronary artery disease adequately. Similarly, the doses of ACE inhibitors and ARBs in combination therapy may be too low to manage heart failure effectively.

Fixed-dose combination therapy has been faulted for a lack of flexibility in titrating doses of individual components. This problem may be more theoretical than real, however, in that it is uncommon for physicians to use the full dose range of individual antihypertensive drugs.[14] Most commonly, physicians begin treatment with the usual starting dose of an antihypertensive drug and rarely up-titrate.

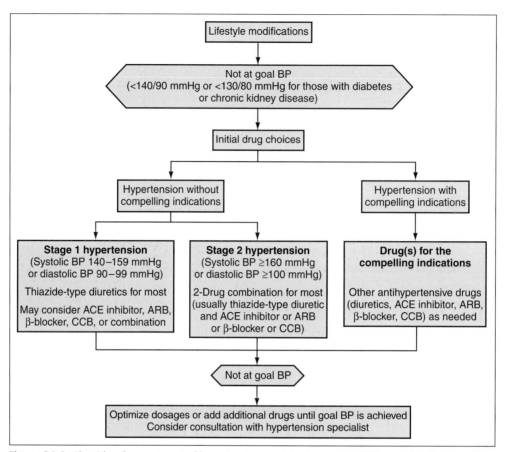

Figure 86–3. Algorithm for treatment of hypertension. BP, blood pressure; ACE, angiotensin-converting enzyme; ARB, angiotensin-receptor blocker; and CCB, calcium channel blocker. (Modified from Chobanian AV, Bakris GL, Black HR, et al. Seventh Report of the Joint National Committee on Prevention, Detection, Evaluation and Treatment of High Blood Pressure. *JAMA* 2003;289:2560–72 and Chobanian AV, Bakris GL, Black HR, et al. Seventh Report of the Joint National Committee on Prevention, Detection, Evaluation, and Treatment of High Blood Pressure. *Hypertension* 2003;42:1206–52.)

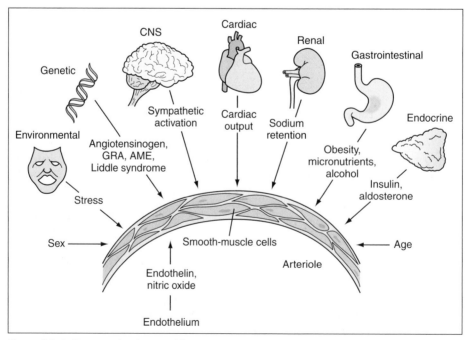

Figure 86–4. Hypertension is caused by a number of different mechanisms. Renal mechanisms are likely the primary cause of hypertension, but other mechanisms likely moderate this response.

CURRENTLY AVAILABLE COMBINATION ANTIHYPERTENSIVES			
Class	**Combination**	**Trade Name**	**Approval Date**
ACE inhibitors and diuretics	Benazepril 5-20 mg/HCTZ 6.25-25 mg	Lotensin HCT	Feb-92
	Captopril 25-50 mg/HCTZ 15-25 mg	Capozide	Oct-84
	Enalapril 5-10 mg/HCTZ 12.5-25 mg	Vaseretic	Oct-86
	Lisinopril 10-20 mg/HCTZ 12.5-25 mg	Zestoretic; Prinzide	Jul-1989; Feb-1989
	Fosinopril 10-20 mg/HCTZ 12.5 mg	Monopril HCT	Nov-04
	Quinapril 10-20 mg/HCTZ 12.5-25 mg	Accuretic	Dec-1999
	Moexipril 7.5-15 mg/HCTZ 12.5 mg-25 mg	Uniretic	Jun-97
ARBs and diuretics	Losartan 50 mg/HCTZ 12.5-25 mg	Hyzaar	Apr-95
	Valsartan 80-160 mg/HCTZ 12.5-25 mg	Diovan HCT	Mar-98
	Irbesartan 150-300 mg/HCTZ 12.5 mg	Avalide HCT	Sep-97
	Telmisartan 40-80 mg/HCTZ 12.5-25 mg	Micardis HCT	Nov-00
	Olmesartan 20-40 mg/HCTZ 12.5-25 mg	Benicar HCT	Jun-03
	Candesartan 16-32 mg/HCTZ 12.5 mg	Atacand HCT	Sep-00
	Eprosartan 600 mg/HCTZ 12.5-25 mg	Teveten HCT	Nov-01
Potassium sparing diuretics and HCTZ	Amiloride 5 mg/HCTZ 50 mg	Moduretic 5-50	Oct-81
	Spironolactone 25-50 mg/HCTZ 25-50 mg	Aldactazide	Jan-78
	Triamterene 37.5-75 mg/HCTZ 25-50 mg	Dyazide; Maxzide	Dec-1965; Oct-1984
Calcium channel blockers and ACE inhibitors	Amlodipine 2.5-10 mg/Benazepril 10-20 mg	Lotrel	Mar-95
	Felodipine 2.5-5 mg/Enalapril 5 mg	Lexxel	Dec-96
	Verapamil 180-240 mg/Trandolapril 1-4 mg	Tarka	Oct-96
Beta blockers and diuretics	Atenolol 50-100 mg/Chlorthalidone 25 mg	Tenoretic	Jun-84
	Bisoprolol 2.5-10 mg/HCTZ 6.25 mg	Ziac	Mar-93
	Nadolol 40-80 mg/Bendroflumethiazide 5 mg	Corzide	May-83
	Propranolol 40-80 mg/HCTZ 25 mg	Inderide	Oct-86

Table 86–1. Currently Available Combination Antihypertensives

MECHANISMS OF ACTION AND THE RELATIONSHIPS TO COMBINATION ANTIHYPERTENSIVE THERAPY

Antihypertensive drugs work by antagonizing neurohormonal and cellular mechanisms that promote BP elevation.[18] The complex pathophysiology of hypertension makes it difficult to define a specific etiology, and therefore to construct a cause-specific treatment plan in any individual patient. The use of combination therapies allows modulation of different pathways involved in the pathogenesis of hypertension and its complications.

There are multiple mechanisms of BP elevation that are interrelated. These include a genetic predisposition, increased renal sodium (Na$^+$) retention, sympathetic nervous system (SNS) activation, endothelial dysfunction, and activation of the RAAS (Figure 86–4).[19–21] It is also likely that abnormal renal sodium handling plays a primary role in hypertension, whereas other mechanisms (e.g., SNS activation, vascular remodeling, and endothelial dysfunction) may amplify or sustain the renal pressor effect.[19–21]

The RAAS is the best studied mechanism of BP and volume regulation, and development of pharmacologic antagonists to its various components has proved useful in the treatment of hypertension and related target organ damage (Figure 86–5).[21] Importantly, the primary mechanism by which the RAAS contributes to acute changes in BP and volume homeostasis is by regulating renin release into the circulation.[22] Circulating renin levels, as indexed by plasma renin activity (PRA), have been found to be an independent risk factor for myocardial infarction in hypertensive patients.[23,24]

As renal mechanisms play a primary role in the pathogenesis of hypertension,[19] and because of their extensive track record in preventing CVD outcomes in randomized controlled trials of antihypertensive treatment, thiazide diuretics are often recommended as first-line therapy for essential hypertension.[11,12] Thiazide diuretics work by inhibiting NaCl reabsorption by the Na/Cl transporter in the distal convoluted tubule and thus block 5 to 7% of the reabsorption of the glomerular filtrate.[25] This leads to a reduction in water and salt reabsorption and there-

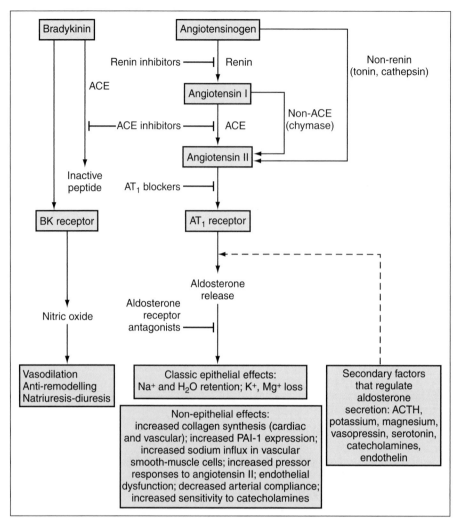

Fig. 86–5. The renin-angiotensin-aldosterone system. Multiple steps in the RAAS have been targeted to lower BP effectively. (Redrawn from Zaman MA, Oparil S, Calhoun DA. Drugs targeting the renin-angiotensin-aldosterone system. *Nat Rev Drug Discov* 2002; 1:621–36.)

fore a decrease in plasma and extracellular volume (Figure 86–6). Thiazide diuretics have flat dose-response curves, and exceeding the maximum dose recommended for any given agent increases adverse effects with little further reduction in BP.[14] It is likely that the impaired glucose tolerance seen with the thiazides is in part related to the reduction in serum potassium levels caused by this drug class and may be prevented or reversed by better potassium management.[26,27] Hypokalemia can be prevented by either supplementing potassium or combining thiazide diuretics with potassium-sparing agents.

The RAAS is an important mediator of hypertension and related target organ damage. This important physiologic/ pathophysiologic cascade can be inhibited pharmacologically at 5 distinct steps in the pathway: renin release, renin-angiotensinogen interaction, ACE action, the AT1 receptor, and the aldosterone (mineralocorticoid) receptor (Figure 86–5). As will be discussed later, BBs lower BP (at least in part) by inhibiting renin release from the juxtaglomerular apparatus.[28] Direct renin inhibitors, currently under development for clinical use, compete with angio-

tensinogen for the catalytic site of the renin molecule and thereby inhibit generation of Ang I.[29] ACE inhibitors inhibit the conversion of Ang I to Ang II and decrease the degradation of bradykinin, resulting in increased levels of bradykinin that in turn lead to NO and prostacyclin release.[30] Decreased Ang II production reduces stimulation of the AT1 receptor, resulting in arterial and venodilation and lowered systemic vascular resistance.

Blocking the RAAS may also prevent endothelial dysfunction and atherosclerosis by increasing levels of NO— a potent vasodilator, inhibitor of platelet aggregation, and suppressor of vascular smooth muscle cell migration[18,31] In hypertensive patients, NO production and/or action may be diminished. In this situation, blocking Ang II generation halts activation of NAD(P)H oxidase, causing a decrease in superoxide anion generation and leading to increased NO bioavailability and thus improvement in endothelial function.[32] The Study to Evaluate Carotid Ultrasound Changes in Patients Treated with Ramipril and Vitamin E (SECURE), a pilot study for the Heart Outcomes Prevention Evaluation (HOPE) trial, measured

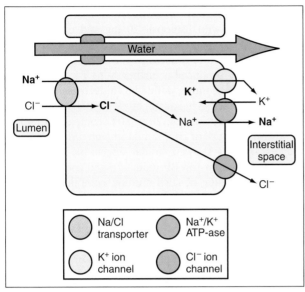

Figure 86–6. Thiazide diuretics work by blocking the Na/Cl transporter and decreasing Na ion transport in the distal convoluted tubule. This in turn leads to decreased water absorption. Note: Bolded ions refer to higher concentrations.

the effectiveness of ramipril compared to a placebo in reducing the mean maximum intimal-medial thickness of the study patients' carotid arteries over a 5-year period.[33] SECURE demonstrated a statistically significant 37% reduction in progression of atherosclerosis with high-dose ramipril treatment compared to placebo. The mechanism responsible may be related to Ang II inhibition and increased bradykinin stimulation with concomitant NO release. Most importantly, the HOPE trial showed that the ramipril regimen reduced CVD outcomes, including myocardial infarction, stroke, heart failure, and cardiovascular death—confirming the clinical significance of ACE-inhibitor-induced vasoprotection.[34]

As discussed previously, ACE inhibitors have fairly flat dose-response curves, and administration of higher-than-recommended doses does not result in improved BP control. However, because the duration of ACE inhibition with a given ACE inhibitor is dose dependent over a wide dose range, higher doses can prolong the duration of the BP response and thus offer clinically meaningful advantages.[35] The most common adverse effect of ACE inhibitors is cough, which is thought to be secondary to inhibition of bradykinin degradation.[30] ACE-inhibitor-induced cough is characteristically dry and nonproductive, but may be disturbing to the patient and usually requires discontinuation of the drug. It is not dose related and can occur in up to 35% of patients.[36] Angioedema is a less frequent but more serious and even deadly adverse effect particularly common in blacks.[30,37,38] Acute renal failure secondary to decreased glomerular filtration rate can also occur with ACE inhibitors, particularly in the patient who is overdiuresed or has renal artery stenosis or decompensated heart failure.[39–41] Hyperkalemia is a common dose-dependent adverse effect of ACE inhibitors, particularly when administrated to patients with diabetes and/or chronic kidney disease.

ARBs lower BP by blocking the action of Ang II at the AT1 receptor. The effects of ARBs on the circulation appear to be similar to those of the ACE inhibitors. However, some evidence has suggested that ARBs may be less effective in reversing endothelial dysfunction and in preventing coronary events.[42] These issues are currently being debated, and definitive evidence supporting an advantage for either drug class is lacking.[43] The Ongoing Telmisartan Alone and in Combination with Ramipril Global Endpoint Trial (ON TARGET) will provide the first head-to-head comparison of ACE inhibitor versus ACE-inhibitor/ARB combination treatment in high-risk patients with underlying CVD.[44] Pending the results of ON TARGET, compelling indications for the use of ACE inhibitors or ARBs in hypertensive patients are largely overlapping.[11,12] The major advantage of the ARB class is that its side effect profile resembles that of placebo. Acute renal failure, hyperkalemia, and angioedema are rare with the ARBs.[45,46]

Aldosterone is a product of the RAAS that increases BP mainly by causing renal sodium retention and stimulating sympathetic outflow from the central nervous system.[47] It also has pro-inflammatory and pro-fibrotic effects on the heart and vasculature that cause adverse structural remodeling, in part independently of BP. The mineralocorticoid receptor antagonists spironolactone and eplerenone lower BP and reverse the previously cited structural changes. Despite pharmacologic blockade of ACE and the AT1 receptor, levels of aldosterone will return to pretreatment levels over time—a phenomenon known as aldosterone rebound.[48] When upstream components of the RAAS are blocked, other mechanisms (such as elevated potassium levels and increased sympathetic nervous system activity) stimulate aldosterone secretion. The major dose-dependent adverse effect of mineralocorticoid receptor antagonists, particularly when combined with ACE inhibitors or ARBs, is hyperkalemia. The side effects of spironolactone (a nonselective mineralocorticoid receptor antagonist)—including decreased libido, impotence, and gynecomastia—are secondary to blockade of androgen receptors. Eplerenone is more selective for mineralocorticoid receptors and lacks these adverse effects.

CCBs block the voltage-dependent L-type calcium channel and thus block the influx of calcium into cardiac myocytes and smooth muscle cells, preventing actin-myosin interactions and leading to vasodilation and negative inotropic effects.[49] The CCBs are divided into two major classes: the dihydropyridines (which have mainly vascular effects) and the nondihydropyridines (which have mainly myocardial effects). Nondihydropyridines can further be subdivided into phenylalkylamine (verapamil)-like and benzothiazepine (diltiazem)-like drugs. The major dose-dependant adverse effect of the dihydropyridines is peripheral edema related to the mismatch between arteriolar and venular dilation, leading to fluid extravasation into tissues of the lower extremity. Other common adverse events include gingival hyperplasia and headache. Adverse events of nondihydropyridines (including bradycardia, A-V conduction abnormalities, constipation, and lethargy) are all dose related.

BBs lower BP by complex mechanisms that are not fully understood. In part, these relate to blockade of the sympathetic nervous system contribution to hypertension.[50] BBs reduce cardiac output and plasma volume, inhibit the RAAS and norepinephrine release, reset baroreceptor levels, and attenuate the pressor response of catecholamines to exercise and stress. Various BBs differ in their pharmacokinetics as well as their selectivity for beta receptor subtypes. Common adverse events noted with this class include bronchospasm, increased insulin resistance, bradycardia, and decreases in HDL cholesterol. A growing body of evidence has shown that BB monotherapy lacks efficacy in both reducing BP and preventing hypertension-related target organ damage and CVD morbidity and mortality.[51,52] Thus, BBs should no longer be considered first-line therapies for most hypertensive patients but may still be used in fixed-dose combinations with diuretics (as indicated in material following).

CURRENTLY AVAILABLE FIXED-DOSE ANTIHYPERTENSIVE COMBINATIONS

ACE inhibitor- or ARB-diuretic combinations

ACE inhibitor- or ARB-diuretic combinations are the most commonly used fixed-dose combination antihypertensive agents because of an additive effect on BP reduction related to complementary mechanisms of action of the components and the favorable metabolic/cardio-, vaso-, and renoprotective effects of the ACE inhibitors and ARBs.[11,12,53,54] The natriuretic/diuretic action of the thiazides reduces extracellular fluid volume, cardiac output, and BP—activating the RAAS and enhancing the Ang II dependence of BP, thus potentiating the antihypertensive efficacy of the ACE inhibitors or ARBs.[55,56] Importantly, combination with a thiazide greatly enhances the antihypertensive efficacy of ACE inhibitors and ARBs in patient groups weakly responsive to ACE/ARB monotherapy (e.g., African Americans and the elderly, particularly elderly women[11,12,57]). The proven benefits of RAAS blockers in patients with concomitant CVD [including heart failure, post myocardial infarction, established atherosclerotic vascular disease (including stroke), diabetes, and renal disease] are so great that first-line use of these agents is recommended by JNC 7 for hypertensive patients with these "compelling conditions" (Figure 86–3).[11,12] The increasing prevalence of these concomitant conditions and the emergence of treatment-resistant hypertension in the aging population, with its multiple medication requirements, have played a major role in increasing the use of ACE inhibitor- and ARB-diuretic combinations in clinical practice.

Randomized controlled clinical trials that compared the combination versus monotherapy with either ACE inhibitor or HCTZ have generally demonstrated greater BP-lowering efficacy with low-dose combinations over higher-dose monotherapy with either single agent.[58] In a representative trial, following a 4-week placebo washout period patients were randomized to 8 weeks of placebo,

lisinopril 10 mg, HCTZ 12.5 mg, HCTZ 25 mg, or combination therapy with lisinopril 10 mg and either HCTZ 12.5 mg or 25 mg.[59] Monotherapy with either agent lowered DBP by 6 to 8 mmHg over placebo, and combination therapy produced a further 6- to 7-mmHg reduction in DBP. BP control, defined as a decrease in DBP of >10 mmHg or achieving a goal of <90 mmHg, was highest with combination therapy: 70 to 80% compared to 40 to 50% with lisinopril or HCTZ monotherapy. Most similarly designed studies showed similar effects of combination versus monotherapy on BP reduction and control rates.[58]

Similarly, studies of ARB-diuretic combinations have demonstrated significantly greater reductions in SBP and DBP with combination compared to monotherapy with either individual agent.[58] A representative factorial study evaluated the efficacy of regimens that included either olmesartan 10 to 40 mg a day, HCTZ 12.5 or 25 mg a day, placebo, or the combinations of olmesartan and HCTZ.[60] At the end of this 8-week trial the greatest effect on BP was noted in the arm receiving 40 mg of olmesartan and 25 mg of HCTZ, in which SBP decreased by 10.8 mmHg and DBP by 7.3 mmHg more than with olmesartan 40 mg monotherapy (Figure 86–7). Control (SBP <140 mmHg and DBP <90 mmHg) rates were greater in patients taking the highest dose of the combined agents than in those taking the highest doses of monotherapies.

Use of ACE inhibitor- or ARB-diuretic combinations decreases the incidence of metabolic side effects of the individual components.[58] Thiazides waste potassium, whereas ACE inhibitors and ARBs tend to conserve potassium and thus may cause hyperkalemia. By combining these agents, the incidence of both hyper- and hypokolemia can be decreased. This concept was well demonstrated in a study that used a factorial design to evaluate the effects of various doses of quinapril and HCTZ on serum potassium levels.[61] In this study, patients were randomized to HCTZ 6.25 to 25 mg or quinapril 2.5 to 40 mg as either monotherapy or combination therapy. Serum potassium was measured at baseline and at the final visit, with a significant change in serum potassium defined as a decrease of ≥0.5 mmol/L. Thirty percent of patients receiving 25 mg HCTZ developed a significant fall in potassium, whereas combining 10 mg of quinapril with 25 mg HCTZ reduced this figure to 15%.

Thiazides dose dependently increase serum glucose, insulin resistance, and new-onset diabetes.[26] Although this problem is not as great as in earlier years (when thiazides were administered in doses higher than are commonly used today), it remains an important issue for clinicians. Reports differ as to whether diuretic-induced impaired glucose tolerance/diabetes has the same adverse effect on CVD outcomes as naturally occurring disorders of glucose metabolism.[27,62,63] Randomized controlled trials such as ALLHAT have failed to demonstrate an increase in CVD events with diuretic treatment within the trial period despite substantial increases in new-onset diabetes.[64] This suggests that the importance of better BP control may outweigh the added risk that would be expected to accompany the adverse metabolic effects of these agents, at least over a relatively brief 5-year follow-up period.

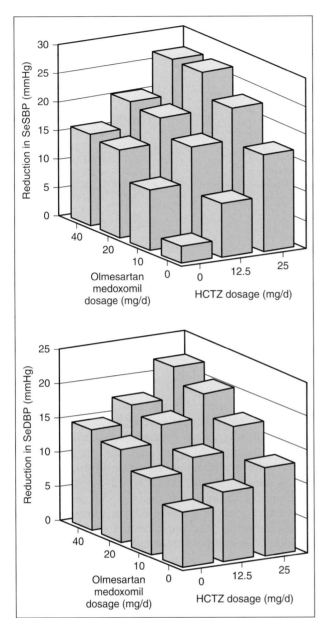

Figure 86–7. Reduction (model fitted) in seated systolic blood pressure (seSBP) (Top) and seated diastolic blood pressure (seDBP) for 12 groups in the factorial design by olmesartan medoximil and hychlorothiazide (HCTZ) dosage. (Redrawn from Chrysant SG, Weber MA, Wang AC, Hinman DJ. Evaluation of antihypertensive therapy with combination of olmesartan medoxomil and hydrochlorothiazide. *Am J Hypertens* 2004;17:252–9 with permission from *The American Journal of Hypertension Ltd.*)

In contrast to the adverse metabolic effects of diuretics, agents that antagonize the RAAS (such as ACE inhibitors and ARBs) have been shown in randomized controlled trials to uniformly increase insulin sensitivity and prevent new-onset diabetes.[65,66] Reductions of 20 to 30% in new-onset diabetes have been reported with ACE inhibitor or ARB-based therapy compared to placebo or therapy based on diuretics, BBs, or CCBs (Figure 86–8). This difference is preserved even when a diuretic is added to an ACE inhibitor or ARB to facilitate BP control. These findings provide a strong conceptual basis for use of fixed-dose ACE inhibitor- or ARB-diuretic combinations in antihypertensive treatment.

Potassium-sparing diuretic-thiazide combinations

Fixed-dose combination products containing a moderately high dose of a thiazide (e.g., 25 or 50 mg of HCTZ) and a potassium-sparing agent have been available since the 1980s.[14] The advantage of these is the ability to deliver a major BP-lowering dose of thiazide without the penalty of potassium and magnesium loss. Hypokalemia or hypomagnesemia induced by a diuretic may increase the frequency of cardiac arrhythmias and resultant mortality in patients with CVD.[67–69] This point was demonstrated by a controlled study in which lethal consequences (primary cardiac arrest) of antihypertensive treatment were seen with unopposed moderate- to high-dose thiazide diuretic use but not with combinations that included a potassium-sparing diuretic.[67]

ACE inhibitor- or ARB-CCB combinations

ACE inhibitor- or ARB-CCB combinations have additive antihypertensive effects and in some cases offer the added advantage of minimizing adverse effects of individual components (e.g., edema with dihydropyridine CCBs).[14] When used as monotherapy, CCBs lower BP and thus activate the RAAS—making BP more dependent on Ang II. Adding an ACE inhibitor or ARB blocks this compensatory mechanism, leading to improved BP reductions. Many CCBs that are used in combined preparations have more favorable pharmacokinetic/pharmacodynamic profiles than their RAAS blocking partners, extending the duration of antihypertensive action of the combinations.

The Anglo-Scandinavian Cardiac Outcomes Trial-Blood Pressure Lowering Arm (ASCOT-BPLA) presented evidence that a CCB-ACE inhibitor combination is more effective in lowering BP and reducing risk of mortality and major CVD events than traditional therapy with a BB-thiazide diuretic combination.[70,71] This large trial involved 19,257 patients randomly assigned to either amlodipine-based treatment (with the option of adding perindopril, followed by agents from other drug classes as needed for BP control) or to atenolol-based treatment (with the option of adding bendroflumethiazide and then agents from other classes if the BP was not controlled). Control was defined as BP <140/90 mmHg in patients without diabetes and BP <130/80 mmHg in diabetics. The CCB-ACE inhibitor combination lowered BP by an average of 2.7/1.9 mmHg more than the BB-diuretic combination throughout the 5.5-year median follow-up period. The trial was stopped early because of excess mortality and morbidity in the atenolol-based arm. Significant reductions in a number of outcomes (includ-ing all-cause mortality, fatal and nonfatal stroke, CVD mortality, nonfatal myocardial infarction, and new-onset diabetes) were noted with CCB +/– ACE inhibitor compared to BB +/– diuretic treatment. Overall, throughout the trial 50% of participants were taking amlodipine plus perindopril and 55% were taking atenolol plus bendroflumethiazide as assigned. Importantly, by the end of the trial only 15 and 9% of participants

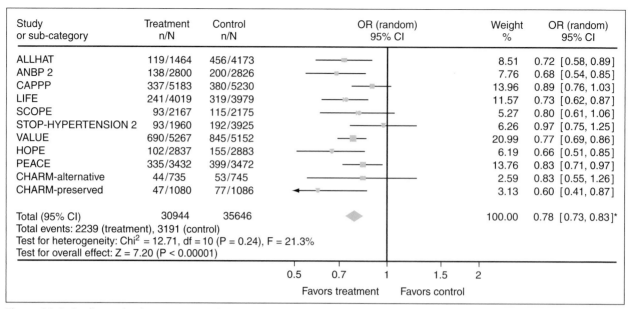

Figure 86–8. Studies evaluating new onset of type II diabetes mellitus. Absolute risk reduction = 1.7 (5% CI 1.3 to 2.1). (Redrawn from Gillespie EL, White CM, Kardas M, et al. The impact of ACE inhibitors or angiotensin II type 1 receptor blockers on development of new-onset type 2 diabetes. Copyright 2005 American Diabetes Association. From *Diabetes Care*:28:2261–66. Reprinted with permission from The American Diabetes Association.)

were taking amlodipine or atenolol monotherapy, respectively—providing additional evidence for the inadequacy of monotherapy for BP control in older higher-risk hypertensive patients.

The most bothersome adverse effect of dihydropyridine CCBs and the most common reason for discontinuation of therapy is peripheral edema.[72] This dose-related adverse effect is due to arteriolar dilation without complementary venodilation. The incidence of peripheral edema is decreased by 50 to 90%, depending on the study and the definition of edema, when ACE inhibitors/ARBs are combined with dihydropyridine CCBs.[73–75] The mechanism of this protective effect is thought to be complementary venodilation due to inhibition of the RAAS. A study of 1500 patients in a community practice setting who had peripheral edema while taking dihydropyridine CCB monotherapy demonstrated improvement of edema in 85% of subjects and complete resolution in 42% when placed on combination therapy that included an ACE inhibitor.[73] The particular drug combination tested in this study, amlodipine plus benazepril, has become the most commonly used CCB-ACE inhibitor combination in clinical practice because of its proven efficacy and tolerability.

BETA-BLOCKER/DIURETIC COMBINATIONS

BBs can be combined with diuretics to produce an additive effect on BP.[14,76] For example, the 12-week VA Cooperative Study demonstrated decreases in SBP of 10.5 mmHg with nadolol monotherapy, 17.4 mmHg with bendroflumethiazide monotherapy, and 25.3 mmHg with the combination—supporting the concept that the BB-diuretic combination has additive effects on BP reduction.[76] BBs in this combination blunt the activation of the RAAS and sympathetic nervous system that is seen with

unopposed diuretic treatment, whereas diuretics attenuate BB-induced sodium retention.[58] Studies have demonstrated a 50% reduction in plasma renin activity during BB monotherapy, and it is likely that this mechanism accounts for a substantial proportion of the antihypertensive effects of the BB class.[28]

Although combining low doses of BBs and diuretics may reduce some of the dose-related adverse effects of the monotherapies, the long-term usefulness of this combination is limited by adverse metabolic effects (hyperglycemia, insulin resistance, dyslipidemia, hyperuricemia) and sexual dysfunction.[58] For example, combining BB and thiazide treatment in the VA Cooperative Trial was associated with greater increases in serum glucose than either monotherapy.[76] Similarly, the ALLHAT study (which used the BB atenolol as a second-step antihypertensive agent) showed an increase in new-onset diabetes mellitus of 11.6% in the group randomized to a thiazide-like diuretic compared to 9.8% in the amlodipine arm and 8.1% in the lisinopril arm.[64] Further, ASCOT showed a 30% increase in new-onset diabetes in the BB/thiazide arm compared to the CCB/ACE inhibitor arm.[70] Major outcome trials have shown that BB-diuretic combinations are less effective than a variety of comparators (ARB-diuretic, ACE inhibitor-CCB) in preventing fatal and nonfatal CVD events.[70,77] This, in addition to their unfavorable adverse effect profile, has dampened enthusiasm for use of BB-diuretic combination in antihypertensive therapy.

"POLYPILL"

Control of multiple risk factors, including elevated BP and elevated LDL cholesterol, significantly decreases global CVD risk.[78] A review of published randomized controlled trials demonstrates that by treating hypertension, decreas-

EFFECTS OF THE "POLYPILL" ON THE RISK FOR CHD AND STROKE AFTER 2 YEARS OF TREATMENT IN PATIENTS AGES 55 TO 64					
Risk Factors	Agent	Reduction in Risk Factor	% Reduction in Risk (95% CI)		
			CHD Event	Stroke	Source
LDL cholesterol	Statin	70 mg/dL	61 (51–71)	17 (9–25)	Law et al.[79]
Blood pressure	Three antihypertensive agents	11 mmHg diastolic BP	46 (39–53)	63 (55–70)	Law et al.[79]
Serum homocysteine	Folic acid (0.8 mg/day)	3 µmol/L	16 (11–20)	24 (15–33)	Wald et al.[78]
Platelet function	Aspirin (75 mg/day)	Not quantified	32 (23–40)	16 (7–25)	
Combined effect	All		88 (84–91)	80 (71–87)	

Table 86–2. Effects of the "Polypill" on the Risk for CHD and Stroke After 2 Years of Treatment in Patients Ages 55 to 64

ing LDL cholesterol, decreasing homocystine, and inhibiting platelet dysfunction with aspirin it is possible to reduce CVD risk by 80% (Table 86–2). The "polypill" concept involves combining low doses of compounds that treat these risk factors in a single pill that can be taken by everyone at increased risk for CVD or stroke. In theory, this method could potentially decrease ischemic heart disease (IHD) by 88% and stroke by 80% and increase life span by approximately 12 years (with few adverse effects).[78] This strategy could be employed in large numbers of persons at risk for CVD, possibly even all persons >55 years of age.

The estimates of benefit of polypill therapy for hypertension on global CVD risk are based on a meta-analysis of 354 trials designed to determine the average reduction in BP, prevalence of adverse effects, and reduction in risk of stroke and CVD events produced by the five main categories of BP-lowering agents (CCBs, BBs, ACE inhibitors, ARBs, and diuretics) according to dose—singly and in combination.[79] It was shown that all five categories of antihypertensive agents produced similar reductions in BP. None of the studies used more than 2 drugs in combination, but the authors of the meta-analysis assumed that combining 3 agents would have an additive effect. They calculated that reducing SBP by 20 mmHg and DBP by 11 mmHg would result in a 46% reduction in CVD risk and a 63% reduction in risk of stroke. The proposed "polypill" includes a combination of 3 BP medications from the five major categories of antihypertensive agents at half standard dose to achieve better BP control without increasing dose-related adverse effects.

The Amlodipine/Atorvostatin Gemini study tested the efficacy of single-pill therapy with this CCB-statin combination in the treatment of concomitant hypertension and dyslipidemia in a total of 1220 patients with uncontrolled hypertension at baseline.[80] After 14 weeks of treatment, both BP and LDL cholesterol goals were achieved in almost 58% of participants. Only 5% discontinued therapy due to adverse events. The Gemini study is the first large-scale trial to examine the clinical-practice utility of single-pill therapy for the simultaneous treatment of more than one CVD risk factor. Its favorable outcome enhances the probability that this approach will be taken with additional drug combinations in the near future.

CONCLUSIONS

Fixed-dose combination antihypertensive drugs have been available for over 40 years but for a time lost favor due to the perception that they resulted in increased toxicity. More recently, it has become apparent that few hypertensive patients (particularly those who are older and at high cardiovascular risk) can be controlled with monotherapy. Therefore, combination therapy has been recommended by treatment guidelines and has become widely accepted by health care providers as either initial or maintenance therapy of hypertension. Low-dose fixed-dose combination agents, because of convenience and favorable side effect profiles, have become widely used in recent years. Most of the newer combination agents include ACE inhibitors, ARBs, or BBs in combination with diuretics. Less commonly, ACE inhibitors or ARBs are combined with CCBs.

To be approved for clinical use, a combination agent must be shown to have a greater antihypertensive effect than either of its components. This is accomplished by combining agents with complementary mechanisms of action. Further, in many cases the effects of one of the components may attenuate the adverse effects of the other (e.g., ACE inhibitors and ARBs tend to prevent hypokalemia and new-onset diabetes induced by diuretics). Fixed low-dose combination antihypertensives may also be more cost effective because they require only one co-pay and the component agents are usually marketed at a lower price when combined in a single pill. Combination medications are easier to take than monotherapies, as they can be taken as a single tablet once a day (thus increasing compliance).

The polypill concept embraces administration of multiple medications in a single pill to treat multiple CV risk factors. The first available agent (Caduet) has shown promise in reducing CV risk by producing significant improvements in both BP and LDL cholesterol levels. It has been suggested that a pill containing low doses of a statin, aspirin, folic acid, and multiple antihypertensive agents with complementary mechanisms of action could be used safely, effectively, and at relatively low cost to reduce CVD risk in entire at-risk populations (e.g., all persons over age 55 years and those with established CVD). Use of the polypill would exploit all of the advantages of low-dose fixed-dose combination therapy discussed in this chapter and would obviate the need for complicated dosing regimens and for multiple costly pharmaceutical agents prescribed individually.

REFERENCES

1. Fields LE., Burt VL, Cutler JA, et al. The burden of adult hypertension in the United States 1999 to 2000: A rising tide. *Hypertension* 2004;44: 398–404.
2. Turnbull F, Neal B, Algert C, et al. Effects of different blood-pressure-lowering regimens on major cardiovascular events: Results of prospectively-designed overviews of randomized trials: Blood Pressure Lowering Treatment Trialists Collaboration. *Lancet* 2003;362: 1527–35.
3. Lewington S, Clarke R, Qizilbash N, et al. Age-specific relevance of usual blood pressure to vascular mortality: A meta-analysis of individual data for one million adults in 61 prospective studies. Prospective Studies Collaboration. *Lancet* 2002;360:1903–13.
4. Lloyd-Jones DM, Evans JC, Levy D. Hypertension in adults across the age spectrum: Current outcomes and control in the community. *JAMA* 2005; 294:466–72.
5. Franklin SS, Gustin W, Wong ND, et al. Hemodynamic patterns of age-related changes in blood pressure: The Framingham heart study. *Circulation* 1997;96:308–15.
6. Franco V, Oparil S, Carretero OA. Hypertensive therapy: Part II. *Circulation* 2004;109:3081–88.
7. Collins R, Peto R, MacMahon S, et al. Blood pressure, stroke, and coronary heart disease. Part 2, short-term reductions in blood pressure: Overview of randomized drug trials in their epidemiological context. *Lancet* 1990; 335:827–39.
8. Neal B, MacMahon S, Chapman N, et al. Effects of ACE inhibitors, calcium antagonists, and other blood-pressure-lowering drugs: results of prospectively designed overviews of randomized trials. Blood Pressures Lowering Treatment Trialists' Collaboration. *Lancet* 2000;356:1955–64.
9. Staessen JA, Wang JG, Thijs L. Cardiovascular protection and blood pressure reduction: A meta-analysis. *Lancet* 2001;358:1305–15.
10. Staessen JA, Li Y, Thijs L, Wang JG. Blood pressure reduction and cardiovascular prevention: an update including the 2003-2004 secondary prevention trials. *Hypertens Res* 2005; 28:385–407.
11. Chobanian AV, Bakris GL, Black HR, et al. Seventh Report of the Joint National Committee on Prevention, Detection, Evaluation and Treatment of High Blood Pressure. *JAMA* 2003; 289:2560–72.
12. Chobanian AV, Bakris GL, Black HR, et al. Seventh Report of the Joint National Committee on Prevention, Detection, Evaluation, and Treatment of High Blood Pressure. *Hypertension* 2003;42:1206–52.

13. Cushman WC, Ford CE, Cutler JA, et al. Success and predictors of blood pressure control in diverse North American settings: The Antihypertensive and Lipid-Lowering treatment to prevent Heart Attack Trial (ALLHAT). *J Clin Hypertens* 2002;4:393–404.
14. Sica DA. Rationale for fixed-dose combination in the treatment of hypertension: The cycle repeats. *Drugs* 2002;62:443–62.
15. Veterans Administration Cooperative Study on Anti-hypertensive Agents: Effects of treatment on morbidity in hypertension. Results in patients with diastolic blood pressures averaging 115 through 129 mmHg. *JAMA* 1967;202: 1028–34.
16. Osterberg L, Rudd P. Medication adherence for antihypertensive therapy. In: *Hypertension: A Companion to Brenner and Rector's the Kidney, Second Edition.* Oparil S, Weber MA (eds.), Philadelphia, PA: Elsevier Saunders 2005:430–46.
17. Neutel JM, Smith DH, Weber MA. Low-dose combination therapy: An important first-line treatment in the management of hypertension. *Am J Hypertens* 2001;14:286–92.
18. Oparil S, Zaman MA, Calhoun DA. Pathogenesis of hypertension. *Ann Intern Med* 2003;139:761–76.
19. Guyton AC. Blood pressure control-special role of the kidneys and body fluids. *Science* 1991;252:1813–16.
20. Brook RD, Julius S. Autonomic imbalance, hypertension, and cardiovascular risk. *Am J Hypertens* 2000;13:112S–122S.
21. Zaman MA, Oparil S, Calhoun DA. Drugs targeting the renin-angiotensin-aldosterone system. *Nat Rev Drug Discov* 2002;1:621–36.
22. Oparil S, Haber E. The renin-angiotensin system. *N Engl J Med* 1974;291: 389–401,446–57.
23. Brunner HR, Laragh JH, Baer L, et al. Essential hypertension: renin and aldosterone, heart attack and stroke. *N Engl J Med* 1972;286:441–49.
24. Alderman MH, Madhavan S, Ooi WL, et al. Association of the renin-sodium profile with the risk of myocardial infarction in patients with hypertension. *N Engl J Med* 1991;324:1098–1104.
25. Knepper MA, Kleyman T, Gamba G. Diuretics: Mechanisms of action. In: *Hypertension: A Companion to Brenner and Rector's the Kidney, Second Edition.* Oparil S, Weber MA (eds.), Philadelphia, PA: Elsevier Saunders 2005:638–52.
26. Wilcox CS. Metabolic and adverse effects of diuretics. *Semin Nephrol* 1999;19:557–68.
27. Ramsay LE, Yeo WW, Jackson PR. Diabetes, impaired glucose tolerance and insulin resistance with diuretics. *Euro Heart J* 1992;13(Suppl G):68–71.
28. Saunders E, Weir MR, Kong BW, et al. A comparison of the efficacy and safety of a beta blocker, a calcium channel

blocker, and a converting enzyme inhibitor in hypertensive blacks. *Arch Intern Med* 1990;150:1707–13.
29. Gradman AH, Schmieder RE, Lins RL, et al. Aliskiren: A novel orally effective renin inhibitor, provides dose-dependant antihypertensive efficacy and placebo-like tolerability in hypertensive patients. *Circulation* 2005;111:1012–18.
30. Brown NJ, Vaughan DE. Angiotensin-converting enzyme inhibitors. *Circulation* 1998;97:1411–20.
31. Tiefenbacher CP, Friedrich S, Bleeke T, et al. ACE inhibitors and statins acutely improve endothelial dysfunction of human coronary arterioles. *Am J Physiol Heart Circ Physiol* 2004;286:1425–32.
32. Carey RM, Siragy HM. Newly recognized components of the renin-angiotensin system: Potential roles in cardiovascular and renal regulation. *Endocr Rev* 2003; 24:261–71.
33. Lonn EM, Yusuf S, Dzavik V, et al. Effects of ramipril and vitamin E on atherosclerosis: The Study to Evaluate Carotid Ultrasound changes in patients treated with Ramipril and vitamin E (SECURE). *Circulation* 2001;103: 919–25.
34. Yusuf S, Sleight P, Pogue J, et al. Effects of an angiotensin converting-enzyme inhibitor, ramipril, on cardiovascular events in high risk patients: The Heart Outcomes Prevention Evaluation (HOPE) study investigators. *N Engl J Med* 2000;342:145–53.
35. Elung-Jensen T, Heisterberg J, Kamper AL, et al. Blood pressure response to conventional and low-dose enalapril in chronic renal failure. *Br J Clin Pharmacol* 2003;55:139–46.
36. Israili ZH, Hall WD. Cough and angioneurotic edema associated with angiotensin-converting enzyme inhibitor therapy: A review of the literature and pathophysiology. *Ann Intern Med* 1992;117:234–42.
37. Brown NJ, Ray WA, Snowden M, Griffin MR. Black Americans have increased rate of angiotensin converting enzyme inhibitor-associated angioedema. *Clin Pharmacol Ther* 1996;60:8–13.
38. Kostis JB, Packer M, Black HR, et al. Omapatrilat and enalapril in patients with hypertension: the Omapatrilat Cardiovascular Treatment Vs. Enalapril (OCTAVE) trial. *Am J Hypertens* 2004; 17:103–11.
39. Hricik DE, Browning PJ, Kopelman R, et al. Captopril-induced functional renal insufficiency in patients with bilateral renal-artery stenosis or renal artery stenosis in a solitary kidney. *N Engl J Med* 1983;308:373–76.
40. Dzau VJ. Renal effects of angiotensin-converting enzyme inhibitor in cardiac failure. *Am J Kidney Dis* 1987;10(Suppl 1):74–80.
41. Murphy BF, Whitworth JA, Kincaid-Smith P. Renal insufficiency with combination of angiotensin converting

enzyme inhibitors and diuretics. *Br Med J (Clin Res Ed)* 1984;288:844–45.

42. McDonald MA, Simpson SH, Ezekowitz JA, et al. Angiotensin receptor blockers and risk of myocardial infarction: systematic review. *BMJ* 2005;331:873–77.

43. Blood Pressure Lowering Treatment Trialists' Collaboration. The comparative effects of angiotensin converting enzyme inhibitors and angiotensin receptor blockers on stroke, myocardial infarction and heart failure; (in press).

44. Teo K, Yusuf S, Sleight P, et al. Rationale, design and baseline characteristics of 2 large, simple, randomized trials evaluating telmisartan, ramipril, and the combination in high-risk patients: The Ongoing Telmisartan Alone and in Combination with Ramipril Global Endpoint Trial/Telmisartan Randomized Assessment Study in ACE Intolerant Subjects with Cardiovascular Disease (ONTARGET/TRANSCEND) trial. *Am Heart J* 2004;148:52–61.

45. Abdi R, Dong VM, Lee CJ, Ntoso KA. Angiotensin II receptor blocker-associated angioedema: on the heels of ACE inhibitor angioedema. *Pharmacotherapy* 2002;22:1173–75.

46. Burnier M. Angiotensin II type 1 receptor blockers. *Circulation* 2001;103:904–12.

47. McMahon EG. Eplerenone, a new selective aldosterone blocker. *Curr Pharm Des* 2003;9:1065–75.

48. Mckelvie RS, Yusuf S, Pericak D, et al. Comparison of candesartan, enalapril and their combination in congestive heart failure: Randomized Evaluation of Strategies for Left Ventricular Dysfunction (RESOLVD) pilot study. The RESOLVD pilot study investigators. *Circulation* 1999;100:1056–64.

49. Abernethy DR, Schwartz JB. Calcium-antagonist drugs. *N Engl J Med* 199; 341:1447–57.

50. Frishman WH. Beta adrenergic blockers. In: *Hypertension: A Companion to Brenner and Rector's the Kidney, Second Edition*, Oparil S, Weber MA (eds.), Philadelphia, PA: Elsevier Saunders 2005:653–59.

51. Carlberg B, Samuelesson O, Lindholm LH. Atenolol in hypertension: Is it a wise choice? *Lancet* 2004;364: 1684–49.

52. Lindholm LH, Carlberg B, Samuelsson O. Should beta blockers remain first choice in the treatment of primary hypertension? A meta-analysis. *Lancet* 2005;366:1545–53.

53. Weir MR, Dzau VJ. The renin-angiotensin-aldosterone system: A specific target for hypertension management. *Am J Hypertens* 2001; 12(Suppl 1):177S–181S.

54. Lewis EJ, Hunsicker LG, Bain RP, Rohde RD. For the collaborative study group: The effect of angiotensin-converting-enzyme inhibitor on diabetic nephropathy. *N Engl J Med* 1993;329: 1456–62.

55. Singer DR, Markandu ND, Sugden AL, et al. Sodium restriction in hypertensive patients treated with a converting

enzyme inhibitor and a thiazide. *Hypertension* 1991;17:798–803.

56. Welsh L, Ferro A. Drug treatment of essential hypertension: The case for initial combination therapy. *Int J Clinic Pract* 2004;58:956–63.

57. Veterans Administration Co-operative Study Group on Antihypertensive Agents: Racial differences in response to low dose captopril are abolished by addition of hydrochlorothiazide. *Br J Clin Pharmacol* 1982;14(Suppl 2):97S–101S.

58. Sica DA, Ripley E. Low-dose fixed-combination antihypertensive therapy. In: *Hypertension: A Companion to Brenner and Rector's the Kidney, Second Edition*. Oparil S, Weber MA (eds.), Philadelphia, PA: W.B. Saunders 2000:497–504.

59. Chrysant SG. Antihypertensive effectiveness of low-dose lisinopril-hydrochlorothiazide combination. *Arch Intern Med* 1994;154:737–43.

60. Chrysant SG, Weber MA, Wang AC, Hinman DJ. Evaluation of antihypertensive therapy with combination of olmesartan medoxomil and hydrochlorothiazide. *Am J Hypertens* 2004;17:252–59.

61. Canter D, Frank GJ, Knapp LE, et al. Quinapril and hydrochlorothiazide combination for control of hypertension: assessment by factorial design. *J Hum Hypertens* 1994;8:155–162.

62. Verdecchia P, Reboldi G, Angeli F, et al. Adverse prognostic significance of new diabetes in treated hypertensive subjects. *Hypertension* 2004;43:963–69.

63. Kostis JB, Wilson AC, Freudenberger RS, et al. Long-term effect of diuretic based therapy on fatal outcomes in subjects with isolated systolic hypertension with and without diabetes. *Am J Cardiol* 2005;95:29–35.

64. The ALLHAT Officers and Coordinators for the ALLHAT Collaborative Research Group. Major Outcomes in high-risk hypertensive patients randomized to angiotensin-converting enzyme inhibitor or calcium channel blocker vs. diuretic: The Antihypertensive and Lipid-Lowering Treatment to Prevent Heart Attack Trial (ALLHAT). *JAMA* 2002;288:2981–97.

65. Abuissa H, Jones PG, Marso SP, O'Keefe JH. Angiotensin-converting enzyme inhibitors or angiotensin receptor blockers for prevention of type 2 diabetes: A meta analysis of randomized clinical trials. *J Am Coll Cardiol* 2005;46:821–26.

66. Gillespie EL, White CM, Kardas M, et al. The impact of ACE inhibitors or angiotensin II type 1 receptor blockers on development of new-onset type 2 diabetes. *Diabetes Care* 2005;28: 2261–66.

67. Siscovick DS, Raghunathan TE, Psaty BM, et al. Diuretic therapy for hypertension and the risk of primary cardiac arrest. *N Engl J Med* 1994;330:1852–57.

68. Davidov ME, Becker FE, Hollifield JW. Serum magnesium and potassium levels in hypertensive patients after a therapeutic switch from

hydrochlorothiazide plus a potassium supplement to maxzide. *Am J Med* 1987;82(Suppl 3A):48–51.

69. Dyckner T, Wester PO. Potassium/magnesium depletion in patients with cardiovascular disease. *Am J Med* 1987;82(Suppl 3A):11–17.

70. Dahlof B, Sever PS, Poulter NR, et al. Prevention of cardiovascular events with antihypertensive regimen of amlodipine adding perindopril as required versus atenolol adding bendroflumethiazide as required, in the Anglo-Scandinavian Cardiac Outcomes Trial-Blood Pressure Lowering Arm (ASCOT-BPLA): A multicenter randomized controlled trial. *Lancet* 2005;366:895–906.

71. Poulter NR, Wedel H, Daholf B, et al. Role of blood pressure and other variables in the differential cardiovascular events rates noted in the Anglo-Scandinavian Cardiac Outcomes Trial-Blood Pressure Lowering Arm (ASCOT-BPLA). *Lancet* 2005;366:907–13.

72. Pedrinelli R, Dell'Omo G, Melillo E, Mariani M. Amlodipine, enalapril, and dependent leg edema in essential hypertension. *Hypertension* 2000;35: 621–25.

73. Messerli FH, Weir MR, Neutel JM. Combination therapy of amlodipine/benazepril versus monotherapy of amlodipine in a practice-based setting. *Am J Hypertens* 2002;15:550–56.

74. Jamerson KA, Nwose O, Jean-Louis L, et al. Initial angiotensin-converting enzyme inhibitor/ calcium channel blocker combination therapy achieves superior blood pressure control compared with calcium channel blocker monotherapy in patients with stage 2 hypertension. *Am J Hypertens* 2004;17: 495–501.

75. Gradman AH, Cutler NR, Davis PJ, et al. Combined enalapril and felodipine extended release for systemic hypertension. *Am J Cardiol* 1997;79:431–35.

76. Veterans Administration Cooperative Study Group on Hypertensive Agents. Efficacy of nadolol alone and combined with bendroflumethiazide and hydralazine for systemic hypertension. *Am J Cardiol* 1983;52:1230–37.

77. Dahlof B, Devereux RB, Kjeldsen SE, et al. Cardiovascular morbidity and mortality in the Losartan Intervention For Endpoint reduction in hypertension study (LIFE): A randomized trial against atenolol. *Lancet* 2002;359:995–1003.

78. Wald NJ, Law MR. A strategy to reduce cardiovascular disease by more than 80%. *BMJ* 2003;326:1419–22.

79. Law MR, Wald NJ, Morris JK, Jordan RE. Value of low dose combination treatment with blood pressure lowering drugs: Analysis of 354 randomised trials. *BMJ* 2003;326:1427–35.

80. Blank R, LaSalle J, Reeves R, et al. Single-pill therapy in the treatment of concomitant hypertension and dyslipidemia (the amlodipine/atorvastatin gemini study). *J Clin Hypertens (Greenwich)* 2005;7:264–73.

Chapter

87

Interactions Between Antihypertensive Drugs and Other Medications

Nigel J. Langford and Anthony Cox

Key Findings

- Drug interactions are a significant cause of morbidity and mortality.
- Polypharmacy, common in hypertensive treatment and in an aging population, increases the potential for drug interactions.
- Many drug interactions, including those leading to adverse events, are avoidable.
- Interactions between hypertension agents and other drugs can be pharmacokinetic or pharmacodynamic in nature.
- As herbal treatments and health foods become increasingly popular, the clinician should be aware of the potential for significant interactions with prescribed drugs.
- Non-cardiac drugs such as NSAIDs, including those bought over the counter, should also be considered a source of potential interactions.
- Although antihypertensive agents are often prescribed in combination, there exists the potential for deleterious drug interactions—in particular from arrhythmias and electrolyte disorders.
- Although electronic decision support tools can create awareness of potential drug interactions, they can make it difficult to differentiate between clinically significant and non-significant interactions.

An interaction is said to occur when effects of one drug are changed by the presence of another substance.[1] The outcome may be harmful, beneficial, or insignificant. In those patients receiving treatment for hypertension, it is estimated that only 50% of patients will achieve target blood pressures on monotherapy.[2] Consequently, in the management of hypertension we commonly use a combination of drugs to obtain a target blood pressure. With the increasing prevalence of hypertension associated with increasing age, there is an increase in co-morbidities. Consequently, the practice of prescribing multiple medications for all these individual problems is common. Such a practice is referred to as "polypharmacy."

Polypharmacy may be deleterious not only because of the increased potential for side effects and drug interactions but because taking unnecessary or borderline therapies reduces patient compliance and concordance with effective drugs. There is also an increased risk of drug interactions. The number of potential interactions occurring can be calculated as the binomial coefficient of the number of drugs prescribed. For example, with a patient taking six drugs there are $5 + 4 + 3 + 2 + 1 = 15$ possible combinations of individual drugs that have to be examined for drug interactions.[3] Such interactions may be further complicated by regional, ethnic, and pharmacogenetic differences in response to antihypertensive agents.

Such concerns are not just theoretical. In one English study it was estimated that 15 to 19% of hospital admissions owing to adverse events were secondary to interacting drugs,[4] whereas other studies estimated the rate to be between 20 and 25% of adverse drug reactions.[5]

Harmful interactions are obviously to be avoided. Prescribers need a holistic approach to the prescribing of medication, taking account of co-morbidities, previously and currently prescribed medications, and the patient's lifestyle (including potential illicit agents). This chapter looks at harmful interactions that may result when using medications and antihypertensive therapy. Those combinations of antihypertensive agents used synergistically to achieve a beneficial effect are considered elsewhere.

DRUG INTERACTIONS

Conventionally, drug interactions may be split between pharmacokinetic interactions and pharmacodynamic interactions. Those interactions that affect the processes of absorption, distribution, metabolism, and excretion are known as pharmacokinetic interactions. Those interactions where the effect of one drug is changed by the presence of another drug at its site of action are known as pharmacodynamic. In addition, there are pharmaceutical interactions that require consideration.

Pharmaceutical considerations

Within most developed countries drug regulatory authorities and manufacturers have strict quality control checks in place to ensure purity and consistency of product. In less well developed countries such checks may be less vigorous. Alternatively, when these checkpoints fail there can be discrepancies between alleged product and actual product, leading to problems of overdose or to problems of underdosing and treatment failure.

Inappropriate storage of product prior to dispensing or administration can lead to degradation of product. This can result in reduction of the actual active ingredient or of the compounds' excipients, leading to failure of drug release or absorption.

Pharmacokinetic interactions

These interactions can occur at any time during the passage of the drug through the body, starting with ingestion and absorption. Some drugs mimic naturally occurring dietary agents and are actively absorbed into the body. Others rely on passive absorption across the mucosal membrane, mainly in the jejunum and ileum. Lipid-soluble drugs are more readily absorbed. Those drugs that ionize are less well absorbed. Drug interactions can interfere significantly with drug absorption. Examples include alterations in gastric pH, affecting release of sustained release preparations; the formation of chelates, the proposed mechanism of interaction between ferrous compounds and methyldopa; and alterations in gastric motility. Slowing gastric motility (although potentially increasing the amount of a drug absorbed) may increase the amount of drug that can be broken down in the stomach or metabolized by the intestinal wall, as with levodopa.

The presence of food in the gastrointestinal tract may unpredictably alter absorption. With some drugs, the presence of food may enhance absorption (as with hydrochlorthiazide). Food can also reduce the amount of first-pass metabolism, increasing the bioavailability of drugs such as propranolol and metoprolol. Consequently, it is not always easy to predict the result of such an interaction.

Once absorbed through the intestinal wall, the drug enters the portal circulation and is transported via the liver to the systemic circulation. The drug may be subject to metabolism anywhere along this route. The initial metabolism, also known as phase I reactions, refers to a set of reactions that result in relatively small chemical changes that make compounds more hydrophilic. The principal reactions are hydrolysis, hydroxylation, oxidation, dealkylation, or deamination—leading to the formation of more polar compounds. Following phase I metabolism, phase II modification may occur as a large polar group is added to the compound by transferase enzymes. In most cases, phase II metabolism follows phase I metabolism because the functional group generated in phase I is needed for attachment of the polar group. However, in some cases in which the parent drug has an appropriate site phase II metabolism can occur first.

Most important phase I reactions are catalyzed by the cytochrome P450 microsomal enzymes, a set of hem-containing proteins localized primarily in the heptocytes and intestine. There are six main groups of isoenzymes important in drug metabolism. These groups are CYP1A2, CYP2C9, CYP2C19, CYP2D6, CYP2E1, and CYP3A4. Individuals have different amounts of these isoenzymes. Therefore, an interaction that occurs in one individual may vary significantly from another depending on the relative proportions of the enzyme available. Any agents that interfere with the CYP450 system have the potential to alter drug metabolism and hence drug action.[6] Drug action is altered via enzyme inhibition (reducing the rate of drug metabolism and increasing the amount of the parent drug in circulation) or via enzyme induction. Enzyme induction usually accelerates rates of metabolism, thereby reducing the amounts of parent compound in circulation. The chemical components are then distributed throughout the body before being excreted. The degree and extent this occurs depends on regional blood flow and the ability of the drug, or its metabolites, to diffuse across the cell membrane. The changes in regional blood flow are highly variable, depending on disease state as well as age and other drugs administered. Renal failure can lead to prolonged duration of action of certain agents, requiring dose alteration.

Within the circulation, many drugs bind loosely with plasma proteins. However, for a chemical agent to exert a pharmacologic effect it must be in its free form to either cross a membrane or bind with its receptor. The extent to which a drug is protein bound varies, depending on circumstances. In hypoalbuminemic states, acidic drugs are less well bound. Alternatively, basic drugs undergo increased binding with increased inflammatory responses. Often the changes in available drug are transient. However, if highly protein-bound drugs are given in reduced albumin states the effects the drug exerts can be significantly more pronounced.

Compounds may be passively or actively removed from the plasma by the kidney as they are excreted in the urine or in the bile. Interference of normal excretory pathways by drugs in the renal tubule can cause alterations in rates of drug excretion.

Pharmacodynamic interactions

Pharmacodynamic interactions are where the actions of one drug are changed in the presence of another. There are four main groups of pharmacodynamic interactions, all of which are important with antihypertensive medications.[1] The variability of such interactions may be further complicated owing to significant genetic differences between individuals. The first main group of pharmacodynamic interactions is of *synergistic interactions*. The action of an index drug is enhanced by another, such as the hypotensive action of one antihypertensive agent being enhanced when a second antihypertensive agent is given concurrently. The second group of interactions are labeled *antagonistic*, when the main action of an index drug is opposed by another, such as between beta-adrenoreceptor antagonists and beta agonists. The third group of pharmacodynamic interactions are *interactions secondary to changes in drug transport mechanisms*, such as occur at adrenergic nerve terminals when the actions of adrenergic neurone-blocking drugs such as guanethidine may be blocked by phenothiazine-type drugs or other indirectly acting sympathomimetic amines and tricyclic antidepressants (thereby negating their antihypertensive actions). The final group of pharmacodynamic interactions are *interactions due to disturbances in fluid and electrolyte balance*. Significant interactions with antihypertensive agents involve the thiazide diuretics and lithium. Thiazide diuretics block the secretion and excretion of lithium into the renal tubules, leading to increased lithium concentrations and subsequent toxicity.

Incidence of interactions

Adverse drug interactions occur commonly. Pirmohamed and colleagues found in their study of Liverpool hospitals that adverse drug-related events accounted for 6.5% of admissions. Drug interactions accounted for 16.6% of these admissions and were responsible for 50% of deaths recorded.[4] An American study looking at hypertensive patients and their medication estimated that between 23 and 48% of their patients had a potential drug interaction of a high significance.[7] However, it is estimated that between 50 and 84% of adverse drug events are avoidable.

Interacting agents
Food products

Food intake can have a significant impact in hypertensive patients, altering the efficacy of their prescribed antihypertensive medication. Dietary foods can have pharmacokinetic and pharmacodynamic interactions. Grapefruit juice, and to a lesser extent Seville orange juice, may interact significantly with certain calcium channel antagonists such as felodipine and nifedipine (as well as with other medications metabolized via the CYP3A4 pathway and P-glycoprotein pathway).[8] Orange juice has also been linked to reduction in the bioavailability of celiprolol.[9] Reduction in alcohol consumption can be beneficial in hypertensive patients. More recently, with concerns over salt consumption and links with hypertension alternative salt substitution preparations have become available—often containing significant concentrations of potassium chloride. Ray et al. advise close questioning of patients with unexplained hyperkalemia to avoid the inappropriate cessation of treatments such as ACE inhibitors due to patients taking potassium containing salt substitutes.[10]

Herbal and nonprescription products

Nonprescription products are commonly used in patients with cardiovascular problems. The most commonly used groups of agents are vitamins and mineral supplements, analgesics, and herbal remedies.[11] Commonly interacting herbal remedies include Saint-John's-wort and ephedrine containing compounds such as Ma Huang. Saint-John's-wort is well known to affect CYP3A4 and to interfere with the P-glycoprotein pathway. Consequently, the impact on other drugs is often difficult to predict (in particular because the impact of the Saint-John's-wort shows significant intra- and interindividual variability). It should also be noted that considerable variation occurs between differing manufacturers of herbal preparations, as well as variation due to the parts of the plant used and the weather conditions during the growing season.

The use of licorice has been linked to hypokalemia. The major component of licorice, glycyrrhizin, induces the retention of sodium and water, increases potassium excretion, and increases blood pressure. Doses of licorice between 150 and 250 mg daily for several weeks are enough to cause hypokalemia, even if ingested in the form of sweets.[12] Overconsumption should be avoided in those taking potassium-depleting diuretics.

Beta-adrenoreceptor antagonists

Epinephrine and norepinephrine are endogenous catecholamines involved in the regulation of virtually every organ system. They act via adrenergic receptors and can have a profound influence on morbidity and mortality. More specifically, the pharmacodynamic effects of beta-adrenoreceptor antagonists can be attributed to the high affinity for the beta-adrenoceptors in various organs—where a receptor-antagonist complex is formed that fails to activate the receptor. All beta-adrenoreceptor antagonists in present use are competitive antagonists.

Pharmacokinetic interactions involving beta-adrenoreceptor antagonists vary according to physicochemical properties. For example, lipid-soluble beta-adrenoreceptor antagonists such as metoprolol, bisoprolol, and carvedilol commonly involve the CYP2D6 enzyme in their metabolism. Those individuals who have reduced concentration of this enzyme are at increased risk of both adverse reactions and drug interactions. However, these individuals will be unaffected if prescribed water-soluble beta-adrenoceptor antagonists such as atenolol, nadolol, or sotalol because these drugs undergo less or no metabolism within the liver and are excreted primarily by the kidney. The liver can also give rise to further interactions via alterations in hepatic blood flow. Beta-adrenoceptor antagonists commonly reduce hepatic blood flow. This may lead to a decline in the rates of metabolism and clearance of other hepatically metabolized drugs, increasing their potential toxicity. Metoprolol and propranolol have been found to reduce lidocaine clearance by such a mechanism.[3]

In the Vaughan-Williams classification of antiarrhythmic agents, beta-adrenoceptor antagonists are class II agents. However, their actions also impinge on classes I and III. This gives a potential for interactions with antiarrhythmic agents from these classes leading to arrhythmias. Despite these theoretical concerns, the number of case reports involving beta-adrenoreceptor antagonists and other class I antiarrhythmic agents are surprisingly few. The reactions are usually pharmacokinetic in nature. For example, both concurrent propafenone and quinidine administration with a beta-adrenoceptor antagonist result in an increase in the beta-adrenoceptor concentration. A far more sinister interaction may occur between beta-adrenoceptor antagonists (such as sotalol) and concurrent drugs that cause lengthening of the QTc interval. Despite this, beta-adrenoceptor antagonists can be used beneficially with some class III agents such as amiodarone. Patients should be warned of the potential for hypotension, bradycardia, ventricular fibrillation, and asystole.

Macrolides, particularly erythromycin and clarithromycin (and the newer fluoroquinolones—moxifloxacin, sparfloxacin and grepafloxacin), potentially prolong the QTc interval. Concurrent administration of beta-adrenoceptor antagonists with similar properties has the potential to cause torsade de pointes. Although the risk is low,[13] the two groups of drugs should be rarely prescribed and only if there is no feasible alternative.[14] QTc prolongation is also seen with antimalarial therapy. Halofantrine, quinine, and quinidine all have the ability to prolong QTc intervals at therapeutic doses.[15] Mefloquine and artemether are less likely to alter ventricular repolarization, although a single case report exists of an interaction between propranolol and mefloquine resulting in cardiac arrest (the causality remains unproven).

Newer non-sedating antihistamines such as terfenadine and mizolastine also have the potential to prolong the QTc interval. Consequently, concurrent use with beta-adrenoceptor antagonists with similar properties can lead to significant arrhythmias.[16]

Beta-adrenoreceptor antagonists and antipsychotic or antidepressant medication have the potential to interact. For example, propranolol and chlorpromazine can both cause hypotension. This effect appears to be potentiated with concurrent administration. The probable mechanism of action appears to be mutual inhibition of metabolism of each other, thereby increasing each other's plasma concentration. A similar interaction may occur between propranolol and thioridazine, with resultant hypotension. Other lipid-soluble beta-adrenoceptor antagonists may be affected.

Amisulpride, the phenothiazine group of drugs, pimozide, sertindole, and the tricyclic antidepressants all have the potential to prolong the QTc interval. Consequently, concurrent administration with beta-adrenoceptor antagonists with similar properties may predispose to torsade. These combinations should be avoided unless no alternative agents are available.

Concurrent use of beta-receptor antagonists and calcium-channel-blocking agents are common. Beta-adrenoreceptor antagonists interact significantly with all groups of calcium-channel-blocking agents. They are used synergistically with group II calcium-channel-blocking agents the dihydropyridines. With class I antagonists, such as verapamil, they can induce heart block. Although studies have shown that diltiazem can be used safely with beta-adrenoreceptor antagonists, case reports of life-threatening bradycardia have been published.[17] The mechanism of action varies between beta-adrenoreceptor antagonists. For example, with metoprolol the proposed pharmacokinetic mechanism of action is that metoprolol reduces the systemic clearance of verapamil (whereas verapamil increases metoprolol bioavailability, necessitating a lower dose of metoprolol).[18]

A single case report exists of a renal transplant patient stabilized on atenolol and ciclosporin, whose beta-adrenoreceptor antagonist was changed to carvedilol. After 3 months of treatment, his ciclosporin dose was reduced by 20%.[19] Other beta-adrenoreceptor antagonists have not been recorded to produce such an effect. However, the observation that ciclosporin has the potential to worsen hypertensive disease is not uncommon. The exact mode of action is uncertain.

The combination of beta-adrenoreceptor antagonists and clonidine has been used therapeutically to treat hypertension. Sudden withdrawal of clonidine can lead to severe rebound hypertension and hypertensive crisis. The mechanism of action is believed to be secondary to unopposed alpha-adrenoceptor activity. Consequently, it is recommended that beta-adrenoreceptor antagonist withdrawal should occur slowly prior to clonidine withdrawal.

When used with beta-adrenoreceptor antagonists, diuretics often produce an enhanced hypotensive effect. A potential concern with their use is hypokalemia. Arrhythmias are more likely to result if used concurrently with beta-adrenoceptor agents with class III activity.

Moxisylyte is an alpha-1 and alpha-2 antagonist used in the treatment of erectile dysfunction. Although administered via an intra-cavernosal route it can produce systemic effects, resulting in significant orthostatic hypotension.

Non-steroidal anti-inflammatory drugs are well known to exacerbate hypertensive disease. However, some agents interact specifically with beta-adrenoceptor antagonists. Indometacin has been shown to interact with propranolol, oxprenolol, atenolol, and labetalol—causing an increase in mean blood pressure. The effect may be even more marked in the treatment of pre-eclampsia. The exact mechanism by which this increase in blood pressure occurs is uncertain, although it has been postulated that it occurs via prostaglandin (PGA and PGE) inhibition. Piroxicam also appears to increase blood pressure, albeit to a lesser extent. The other NSAID agents (such as diclofenac, ibuprofen, sulindac, and tenoxicam) do not interact significantly.

Predictably, beta-adrenoceptor antagonists will have a pharmacodynamic interaction with beta-adrenoceptor agonists. Patients taking nonselective beta-adrenoreceptor antagonists have experienced severe hypertension following administration of epinephrine, norepinephrine, or phenylephrine. These results have not been seen consistently and appear to occur most commonly in those patients taking nonselective beta-adrenoreceptor antagonists compared with cardioselective agents.[20-22] It is proposed that this occurs via unopposed alpha activity that leads to vasoconstriction and hypertension (which may be followed by a marked bradycardia). Interaction between beta-2 agonists and beta-adrenoceptor antagonists is well documented. Severe adverse effects may result, and deaths have occurred following the concurrent administration of propranolol and salbutamol. Similarly, topical nonselective beta-adrenoreceptor antagonists can also have severe adverse effects in asthmatics by blocking the normal action of beta-2 agonists. Uses of cardioselective beta-adrenoceptor antagonists are less likely to have such severe adverse effects, but even these agents have the potential to cause such effects because their beta-blockade is less selective at high doses.

Vasodilators

Vasodilators are potent antihypertensive agents that can cause a significant reduction in blood pressure in their own right. Specific drug interactions are limited. However, caution is advised with concurrent use of other agents that lower systemic blood pressure. They are often used in combination with beta-adrenoceptor antagonists and a thiazide diuretic.

Diazoxide and hydralazine, both vasodilator agents, interact significantly—resulting in severe hypotension. In a number of cases this has led to fatalities despite the use of pressor agents.

A single report exists of hydralazine interacting with iopamidol in a 60-year-old woman following urography, causing a cutaneous vasculitis. The mechanism of such an interaction is postulated to occur owing to hydralazine's ability to induce LE-like syndromes.[23] Certain studies have indicated that the normal antihypertensive action of hydralazine may be opposed with concurrent use of either indometacin or diclofenac.

Hydralazine appears to increase the bioavailability of those beta-adrenoreceptor antagonists that undergo extensive first-pass metabolism.[24] The water-soluble beta-adrenoreceptor antagonists appear to be largely unaffected. Despite significant increases in bioavailability, the clinical effects appear to be largely unchanged.

Minoxidil has been used in the treatment of hypertension in patients who have received organ transplantation and are concurrently receiving ciclosporin. Using this combination of drugs in certain patients has resulted in hypertrichosis, which has resolved following minoxidil withdrawal. The mechanism of action is unknown.

Centrally acting antihypertensive drugs

In common with all antihypertensive agents, these drugs may be antagonized or potentiated by drugs that affect blood pressure. The mechanisms of those reported with clonidine and methyldopa follow no pattern. Methyldopa acts centrally, probably via a number of different mechanisms, to reduce blood pressure.

Early reports suggested that the combination of haloperidol and methyldopa could result in dementia. Such reports were reinforced, in that symptoms resolved following haloperidol withdrawal. However, the combination has since been used without problems.

The antihypertensive effects of methyldopa may be significantly decreased following coadministration of iron-containing compounds.[25,26] The amount absorbed is significantly reduced, probably owing to the formation of iron-methyldopa chelates.[26] However, with other elements (such as lithium) the reverse can occur. Raised lithium concentrations leading to intoxication have been reported to occur with concurrent administration.[27,28] The exact mechanism of action is uncertain.

Methyldopa is widely used in the treatment of hypertension in pregnancy. Salbutamol is occasionally used as a tocolytic. Case reports have suggested that concurrent use can cause severe adverse events, possibly as a result of increased fluid retention.[29]

Clonidine acts primarily as a presynaptic CNS alpha-2 agonist, stimulating receptors in the nucleus *tractus solitarii* of the *medulla oblongata*. This inhibits sympathetic outflow, which results primarily in a reduction of sympathetically mediated vasoconstriction, cardiac inotropy, and chronotropy. It also has peripheral alpha1-agonist activity.

A significant fall in blood pressure was recorded in a patient receiving clonidine who also received intramuscular haloperidol. However, other reports of patients receiving clonidine and antipsychotic medication have failed to detect such effects. Consequently, caution is recommended in this group of patients. The normal antihypertensive action of clonidine may also be reduced, or completely abolished, following concomitant use with the tricyclic antidepressants.[30] Indeed, in some reports the blood pressure actually increased. Control of blood pressure with clonidine may be unaffected by the tetracyclic antidepressants such as mianserin.

Clonidine and beta-adrenoreceptor antagonists have been previously discussed. However, in addition there are reports of paradoxical increases in blood pressure in patients receiving combinations of clonidine and sotalol, and clonidine and propranolol.[31] Exactly why such a reaction should occur is uncertain. Few interactions occur with calcium-channel-blocking agents, but care should be taken with verapamil in light of two isolated case reports of complete heart block.

Mirtazapine is a newer tetracyclic antidepressant whose action occurs secondarily to stimulation of the noradrenergic system through antagonism at central alpha-2-inhibitory receptors. Concomitant use of mirtazapine and clonidine in a patient resulted in a significant alteration of blood pressure control. The reaction is postulated to occur following central alpha-adrenoreceptor competition between the two agents.[32]

Like other centrally active antihypertensive medications, moxonidine and beta-adrenoreceptor antagonist combination may lead to rebound hypertension upon drug withdrawal. Therefore, manufacturers advise that patients taking the combination should withdraw the beta-adrenoreceptor antagonist first to try to limit rebound hypertension. Owing to its centrally acting mode of action, moxonidine has the potential to interact with other sedatives and hypnotics and potentiate their actions. Such effects can be seen with the benzodiazepine group of drugs that lead to mild cognitive impairment and sedation. In addition, with benzodiazepines the hypotensive effects of moxonidine may be enhanced.

Adrenergic neurone-blocking drugs

Guanethidine and the related drugs debrisoquine and betanidine act by preventing the release of noradrenaline from post-ganglionic adrenergic neurones. Although not widely used in the United Kingdom, interactions[33] causing enhanced drops in blood pressure have been recorded with ethanol, general anesthetics, benzodiazepines, other muscle relaxants (such as baclofen and tizanidine), and other centrally acting and vasodilating antihypertensive agents. Its antihypertensive effects may also be antagonized by antipsychotic agents such as haloperidol and chlorpromazine, as well as by other directly and indirectly acting sympathomimetic agents such as norepinephrine, phenylephrine, oxymetazoline, phenylpropranoline, pseudoephedrine, and xylometazoline.

Alpha-adrenoreceptor antagonists

Alpha-adrenoceptor antagonists with selectivity for the post-synaptic alpha-1 adrenoceptor are a group of antihypertensive agents having high specificity in blocking sympathetic impulses to resistance and capacitance vessels. They cause lowering of blood pressure by reducing tone in arteriolar resistance vessels and by dilating venous capacitance vessels. Consequently, they have the potential to interact with other vasodilating agents such as ethanol potentiating their antihypertensive effects. Indeed, with most other groups of antihypertensive agents there may be an increased incidence of first-dose hypotension. This effect may be less with doxazosin and tamsulosin.

Phosphodiesterase type-5 inhibitors have a relaxing effect on vascular smooth muscle. These agents have been shown to cause an overall reduction in both systolic and diastolic blood pressure. Consequently, when these drugs are used concurrently hypotension may result. Presently, the manufacturers of sildenafil recommend caution with concurrent administration of alpha-adrenoreceptor antagonists. Tadalafil is contraindicated with alpha-adrenoreceptor antagonists except for 0.4 mg tamsulosin, and vardenafil is contraindicated with all alpha-adrenoreceptor antagonists.

Diuretics

Diuretics (in particular, thiazides) are widely used in hypertension, and as such their potential for drug interactions with other medications is of particular importance (especially given the likelihood of other cardiac co-morbidities, and associated treatments, in the hypertensive population). The majority of significant interactions associated with diuretic use are related to their effects on plasma electrolytes. Interference with potassium, sodium, and calcium concentrations can lead to adverse effects, but the most troublesome effects are related to changes in potassium concentrations.

The risk of diuretic-induced hypokalemia can be worsened by the prescribing of other drugs associated with potassium loss, leading to the deleterious effects of hypokalemia (such as muscle weakness and cardiac arrhythmias). Drugs that can decrease potassium levels include acetazolamide, amphotericin, beta-2 agonists, corticosteroids, itraconazole, and theophylline.

Alternatively, the arrhythmogenic potential of other drugs (cardiac and non-cardiac) can be aggravated by the presence of diuretic-induced hypokalemia. Cardiac drugs whose arrhythmogenicity can be increased by diuretics include the antiarrhythmics quinidine, sotalol, and flecainide.

Diuretic-induced potassium loss, exacerbating potassium loss from myocardial cells, increases the sensitivity of the myocardium to digoxin. Although there has been debate about the importance of this interaction, it is currently believed that the use of furosemide and bumetanide in combination should be carefully monitored. However, non-cardiac drugs with arrhythmogenic potential (such as tricyclic antidepressants, erythromycin, and terfenadine) are also potentially dangerous in the presence of diuretic-induced hypokalemia.

Hyperkalemia

Potassium-sparing diuretics such as spironolactone, amiloride, and triamterene all have the potential to cause hyperkalemia. This risk is increased when used in association with potassium supplements and salt substitutes, as previously noted. The risk of hyperkalemia with spironolactone increases threefold if used with potassium supplements. The use of concurrent loop diuretics does not guarantee that hyperkalemia will not occur. Potassium supplements should be avoided, except under very close supervision, in those taking

potassium-sparing diuretics. The use of the immunosuppressants ciclosporin and tacrolimus with potassium-sparing diuretics or aldosterone antagonists also increases the risk of hyperkalemia.

Pharmacokinetic absorption

Furosemide's absorption can be markedly reduced by the coadministration of the anionic exchange resins colestyramine and colestipol. This can have a significant effect on the diuretic effect of furosemide, and it is advised that doses should be given 2 to 3 hours before using these agents. Similar effects are seen when combining thiazides with exchange resins, and it is recommended that doses be separated by 4 hours (although this is not likely to prevent the effect completely).

Furosemide's diuretic effect can be reduced by as much as 50% if phenytoin is used concurrently. This is demonstrated regardless of the route of administration (both intravenous and oral doses of furosemide are affected). Increased doses of furosemide may be required.

NSAIDs versus diuretics

The concurrent use of NSAIDs with loop diuretics can lead to a reduction in the hypertensive and diuretic effects of the loop diuretic. Although evidence for some NSAIDs is stronger (indometacin, diclofenac, piroxicam, and naproxen), all NSAIDs carry some risk. It is thought that NSAIDs interfere with the production of renal prostaglandins, leading to reduced renal blood flow and sodium and water retention. The combination does not necessarily need to be avoided, but should be monitored. Those at greatest risk include the elderly and those with renal problems, cardiac failure, or renal insufficiency. Although most evidence is with furosemide, similar problems can present with bumetanide. High-dose aspirin has been shown to have some effect on bumetanide,[34] but low-dose aspirin is unlikely to have a significant clinical effect.

A well-established interaction exists between thiazides and indometacin or naproxen. Ibuprofen may also interact similarly, but evidence for other NSAIDs is limited. Again, interference with renal prostaglandins is the proposed mechanism.

Glycosides and diuretics

Both loop diuretics and aminoglycosides exhibit ototoxicity at high doses. The British National Formulary advises that an increased risk of ototoxicity can occur with the coadministration of loop diuretics and aminoglycosides (such as gentamicin, kanamycin, and tobramycin). Concerns also exist that such combinations may lead to nephrotoxicity. Nonetheless, three randomized controlled trials have failed to find an increased risk of ototoxicity.[35] In addition, furosemide has the potential to increase aminoglycoside concentrations by inhibiting renal excretion. Aminoglycosides are thought to increase the permeability of cell membranes in the inner ear, which may allow loop diuretics to obtain access at lower doses. Several case reports have been reported, one of which involved the use of once-daily gentamicin with a single dose of furosemide

20 mg IV after the second day's dose.[36] This led to profound bilateral hearing loss.

Toxicity is more common in those with severely reduced renal function who receive high doses of loop diuretics at rates faster than 4 mg per minute. By monitoring aminoglycoside levels and renal function, and by being alert for symptoms of ototoxicity, normal use should not pose a great risk.

Spironolactone can significantly impair digoxin clearance,[37] although the extent of this interaction is variable. However, coupled with the interference of spironolactone with digoxin assays[38] monitoring of combined use is prudent to avoid digoxin intoxication.

Other interactions with diuretics

Both loop diuretics and thiazides can cause a compensatory increase in proximal tubular reabsorption, leading to an increase in serum lithium concentrations. Toxic lithium concentrations may occur within 3 to 5 days following commencement of a diuretic. Some advocate a 25- to 50% reduction in the lithium dose if diuretics are started in a patient stabilized on lithium.[39]

A population-based study has shown that those who take lithium and are commenced on loop diuretics are six times more likely to be hospitalized with lithium toxicity. Although the study did not show that thiazides increased risk independently, care should be taken.[40] The reduced urinary excretion of calcium caused by thiazide diuretics can cause hypercalcemia and metabolic alkalosis when given in combination with high doses of vitamin D. This interaction is important both in those using vitamin D for osteoporosis and those being treated for hypothyroidism. The ingestion of high doses of calcium carbonate alone, present in some over-the-counter remedies for indigestion, in the presence of thiazides may also precipitate significant changes in serum calcium. Although this is not an absolute contraindication, calcium levels should be monitored to avoid excessive calcium levels.

ACE inhibitors

Commonly prescribed, ACE inhibitors have a number of interactions with other drugs, many of which are related to their effects on electrolytes or their effect on the renal system. NSAIDs, including aspirin, have been reported to attenuate the hypotensive action of ACE inhibitors due to their sodium- and water-retaining properties. At high doses, aspirin has been shown to reduce the blood-pressure-lowering effects of ACE inhibitors. At lower doses (75 mg) evidence is less clear, but there have been suggestions that outcome was poorer in post-infarction patients who received aspirin combined with ACE inhibition. Although studies have given conflicting information about the significance of this interaction, the well-established benefits of both ACE inhibitors and aspirin (particularly in patients with heart failure associated with ischemic heart disease) has led to recommendations that combined treatment not be withheld.[41] A systematic review gave a similar conclusion.[42]

More recently, an epidemiologic study in 24,012 patients showed that aspirin was associated in a reduction in risk of death, regardless of the co-prescription of ACE inhibitors.[43]

NSAIDs and ACE inhibitors can interact variably within the kidney. Patients with underperfused kidneys may see further deterioration. Other patients with adequately perfused kidneys may benefit from combining an NSAID with an ACE inhibitor. Rarely, NSAIDs and ACE inhibitors may cause hyperkalemia when used in combination.

Concern has been raised about hypotension caused by the use of anesthetic agents in patients taking ACE inhibitors. Although care should be taken, there is debate about whether ACE inhibitors should be discontinued prior to surgery. Some evidence suggests that these risks are outweighed by the problems of controlling postoperative hypertension—at least following a coronary artery bypass graft.[44]

ACE and lithium toxicity

Lithium toxicity has been reported in a number of patients co-prescribed ACE inhibitors. Lithium concentrations can be raised by 35% and clearance of lithium reduced by 26%. One in five patients can develop signs and symptoms suggestive of lithium toxicity. Case reports have included captopril, enalapril, and lisinopril, but it is likely to be a class effect. The mechanism is suspected to be related to fluid depletion and ACE inhibition of the constriction of efferent renal arterioles. This prevents a compensatory increase in the glomerular filtration rate and hence reduced lithium concentrations. Although not of clinical importance in all individuals, at-risk groups such as the elderly and those with heart failure, renal problems, or volume depletion should generally avoid this combination. A population study of 10,615 elderly patients in Canada, of whom 413 were hospitalized with lithium toxicity, found that the use of ACE inhibitors in the month prior to hospitalization was associated with a significantly increased risk of hospitalization with lithium toxicity.[45]

ACE inhibitors and blood dyscrasias

The use of ACE inhibitors and azathioprine has been associated with blood dyscrasias. Anemia has been reported in kidney transplant patients taking enalapril or captopril when switched from ciclosporin to azathioprine. The interaction is not pharmacokinetic in nature. The anemia appears to be due to the erythropoietin-lowering effect of ACE inhibitors, which increases the risk of anemia.[46]

A small number of case reports of leukopenia associated with the combination of captopril and azathioprine has been reported. Despite this limited evidence, manufacturers of captopril suggest that concomitant administration of ACE inhibitors with immunosuppressants may lead to an increased risk for leukopenia—particulary with higher doses.

Captopril has also been reported to increase the risk of neutropenia when used in combination with procainamide, with reported cases of neutropenia and serious infection. There is no evidence of a pharmacokinetic interaction. It is recommended that this combination be used with caution—especially in those with impaired renal function. Again, the manufacturers of other ACE inhibitors warn of the possible risk. Serious infections and neutropenia have also been reported using captopril with allopurinol.

Captopril has been associated with neutropenia in association with allopurinol. Although rare, it would seem that patients should be carefully monitored for signs of neutropenia on this combination. A number of manufacturers of other ACE inhibitors also warn of an increased risk of leukopenia when ACE inhibitors and allopurinol are used in combination.

ACE inhibitors and hypersensitivity

Hypersensitivity reactions to combined therapy with allopurinol and ACE inhibitors have also been reported. This has ranged from fatal Stevens-Johnson syndrome to fever, myalgia, and renal failure. No pharmacokinetic reaction has been shown in healthy volunteer studies. There has been one case of myocardial infarction related to severe coronary spasm induced by acute anaphylaxis with combined use of enalapril and allopurinol. Symptoms started within 20 minutes of allopurinol being given.[47] It should be noted that both drugs are able to cause hypersensitivity reactions alone, and in the case of allopurinol impaired renal function is an important risk factor. Although the validity of these reactions is unclear, vigilance of hypersensitivity reactions is advisable.

ACE inhibitors and clozapine

The atypical antipsychotic clozapine has been reported to interact with ACE inhibitors. Cases of syncope have been reported, with symptoms being seen within 5 hours of taking a dose. A patient on clozapine started on lisinopril had marked increases in clozapine levels. Behavioral changes were exhibited, including increasing disorganization, angry outbursts, and irritability. Sleep disturbances (frequent waking and nightmares) occurred, and the patient developed sialorrhea. Raised levels of the metabolite of clozapine (norclozapine) indicate possible impairment of renal excretion. After switching from lisinopril to diltiazem, clozapine concentrations decreased, as did sleep disturbances and irritability.[48]

ACE inhibitors and antacids

Antacids are suggested to reduce the absorption of ACE inhibitors, and captopril, enalapril, and fosinopril are named in the British National Formulary. Although pharmacokinetic studies do show reduced bioavailability of both captopril and fosinopril in the presence of aluminium- and magnesium-based antacids, there is no evidence that the blood pressure effect of these agents was impaired, and it seems likely that any interaction is clinically unimportant.

Ace inhibitors and loop diuretics

The administration of an ACE inhibitor to patients prescribed loop diuretics is widely known to increase the risk of profound hypotension after the first dose. This effect is exacerbated by patient factors such as heart failure, renovascular hypertension, dialysis, and diarrhea and vomiting. Doses of 80 mg of furosemide (or higher) are a particular risk. Temporary withdrawal or reduction in the dose of diuretic will also reduce the potential for this interaction. If this regimen is not possible, doses of ACE should be given under close supervision. The hypotension is thought to occur because of diuretic-induced hypovolemia, exaggerating the hypotensive effect of the ACE inhibitor.

ACE inhibitor renal impairment can be potentiated by loop diuretics,[49] and in 10 cases of renal deterioration linked to enalapril use 9 were linked to concurrent loop- or thiazides- use.[50] This underlines the importance of monitoring renal function in patients taking these drugs together.

ACE inhibitors and potassium-sparing diuretics

Due to the potassium-sparing nature of ACE inhibitors, clinicians have generally avoided prescribing these agents with potassium-sparing agents. Serious hyperkalemia is common, particularly in older people. Patients can exhibit severe symptoms of hyperkalemia, including heart block and ventricular fibrillation (and deaths have been reported). Cases have been reported with both spironolactone and other potassium-sparing drugs, such as amiloride. The increasing use of the aldosterone antagonist spironolactone in heart failure means that this combination is increasingly prevalent. Although the low-dose (25 mg) spironolactone prescribed in heart failure did not show significant increases in the incidence of hyperkalemia in the initial clinical trial,[51] evidence has been accumulating that the real-world use of low-dose spironolactone carries a significant risk of hyperkalemia.[52,53] The risk of hyperkalemia is also seen with eplerenone, which had a statistically significant increase in cases of hyperkalemia compared to placebo when used in heart failure,[54] and which has been advocated for use in low-renin hypertension.[55] Doses of spironolactone used to treat Conn's syndrome (between 100 and 400 mg) should not be used with ACE inhibitors.

Another area of controversy is whether ACE inhibitors can interfere with hypoglycemic agents such as the sulfonylureas and insulin. The evidence consists of varied case reports of hypoglycemia, some of which are significant. However, an interaction is not firmly established. Given the potential benefits of ACE inhibition, withholding ACE inhibitors is not necessary. Patients should be warned that such interactions are rare but should be watched for. Patients affected may be managed by reducing the dose of the hypoglycemic agents.

Angiotensin II receptor antagonists

Angiotensin II receptor antagonists share some common attributes with ACE inhibitors. Although their adverse effects are considered negligible by some commentators, they do share the potential for some similar interactions seen with ACE inhibitors. As would be expected, enhanced hypotensive effects will be seen when these are used in combination with other antihypertensive agents.

There have been case reports of lithium intoxication occurring in patients following the addition of candesartan,[56] losartan,[57] or valsartan[58] to their therapy. The mechanism may be similar to that for ACE inhibitors.

The potassium-retaining properties of angiotensin II receptor antagonists also mean that there is a potential for hyperkalemia with other potassium-retaining drugs. As with ACE inhibitors, concomitant ciclosporin use may increase the risk of hyperkalemia. Care should also be taken when ciclosporin is used with diuretics to avoid hypotensive episodes.

An area of concern has been over the use of angiotensin II receptor antagonists with beta-adrenoreceptor antagonists and ACE inhibition. In the ValHeFT study, valsartan was added to standard therapy and reduced the combined end-point of death or hospitalization for heart failure.[59] Patients taking valsartan with both an ACE inhibitor and a beta-adrenoreceptor antagonist appeared to have a reduced survival, although some caution is advocated with such subgroup analyses. The CHARM-Added trial used candesartan with ACE inhibition and showed a reduction in cardiovascular events[60] even in those taking beta adrenoreceptor antagonists.

Losartan may interact with ritonavir and nelfinavir, which may inhibit CYP2C9 metabolism and lead to increased plasma concentrations of losartan. Rifampicin's induction of the P450 isoenzymes CYP2C9 and CYP 3A4 is thought to be behind reduced losartan concentrations and an attenuation of the antihypertensive effect of losartan.

Indometacin use has been shown to attenuate the anti-hypertensive effect of losartan, candesartan, and valsartan. However, no evidence exists that aspirin has this effect. As with ACE inhibitors, an increased risk of renal effects is possible when angiotensin II receptor antagonists are given with NSAIDs and aspirin in doses above 300 mg.

Calcium-channel-blocking agents

This structurally varied group of drugs primarily acts on L-type Ca^{2+} channels in the tissues. Although the calcium-channel-blocking agents have common effects, they bind to distinct yet allosterically interacting receptors in the L-type Ca^{2+} channel—leading to differences in pharmacologic activity. This variation in activity is due to differences in specific tissues' reliance on exogenous Ca^{2+}, varied affinities of L-type Ca^{2+} channels to particular calcium-channel-blocking agents, and the varied distribution of those channels in body tissues. This is of importance when considering possible interactions.

The calcium-channel-blocking agents significantly vary in their cardio-depressant effects. The phenylalkylamine verapamil, and the benzothiazepine diltiazem to a lesser extent, have significant cardio-depressant effects—making them more likely to be involved in pharmacodynamic interactions with other hypertensive agents. This effect is largely absent in the dihydropyridine calcium antagonists such as nifedipine, which have no significant effects on the atrio-ventricular node.

The dangers of combining beta-adrenergic receptor agents and calcium-channel-blocking agents have been covered already in this chapter, but interactions can occur with other cardiovascular agents. The combination of verapamil or diltiazem with amiodarone is advised against on a theoretical basis because of the additive effects of the drugs on myocardial contractility and on the atrioventricular node, although one case of sinus arrest and hypotension with combined amiodarone and diltiazem has been reported.[61] Dihydropyridine calcium channel antagonists such as nifedipine and amlodipine should pose little risk.

A combined effect of digoxin and calcium-channel-blocking agents on the atrio-ventricular node is possible, although usually concern is focused on the effect of calcium-channel-blocking agents on digoxin serum levels. Verapamil is a particular concern and has been the cause of a number of deaths. The addition of verapamil to a patient previously stable on digoxin can cause severe (40 to 80% depending on the dose of verapamil) increases in serum digoxin concentrations over short periods (within 2 to 7 days), with patients exhibiting marked digoxin toxicity. Pre-emptive digoxin dose reduction by up to 50% is advocated by some. The proposed mechanism is reduced renal and biliary clearance of digoxin. Diltiazem can cause similar rises, although changes are more inconsistent. Care should be taken in patients with pre-existing renal conditions or serum digoxin concentrations at the higher end. Felodipine, nisoldipine, lacidipine, and nicardipine may produce clinically unimportant increases. Amlodipine and nimodipine do not interact.

As well as interactions involving the cardio-depressant activity of calcium-channel-blocking agents, interactions can also occur because calcium-channel-blocking agents are hepatically metabolized by the P450 cytochrome isoenzyme system. Their clinical effect can be reduced or increased by inhibitors and inducers, depending on the interacting drug present.

Ankle swelling is a well-known adverse effect of the dihydropyridine calcium channel blockers and may be aggravated by azole antifungals such as fluconazole and itraconazole. Case reports have been seen with felodipine, nifedipine, and isradipine. The mechanism is thought to be inhibition of the P450 CYP3A isoenzymes in the gut wall, which are involved in the metabolism of calcium-channel-blocking agents. Dosage reductions may be necessary.

P450 CYP3A isoenzymes are also thought to be involved in an interaction between felodipine and erythromycin. A treatment dose of erythromycin given to healthy volunteers taking felodipine showed significantly increased concentrations of felodipine. There is no evidence of a similar reaction with other calcium-channel-blocking agents.

Verapamil, diltiazem, and most dihydropyridine-type calcium-channel-blocking agents are CYP3A4 substrates that can lead to reductions in plasma concentrations of calcium-channel-blocking agents or an increase in plasma concentrate of competing substrate. Amlodipine may be an exception, with no clinical relevant interactions related to CYP3A4.

Grapefruit juice is a CYP3A4 inhibitor that can have major effects on the bioavailabilities of felodipine, nicardipine, nifedipine, nimodipine, nisoldipine, nitrendipine, and also amlodipine to a lesser extent. There is no evidence that diltiazem is affected. Management can involve either a down-titration of the dose of the calcium antagonist or the cessation of grapefruit juice drinking. Patients who complain of adverse drug reactions linked to raised doses of calcium channel blockers should be asked questions about their diet. Felodipine may interact,[62] but amlodipine appears to have no significant reaction.[63]

Diltiazem and nifedipine serum concentrations are increased when given with cimetidine. Recommended dosage reductions are 30 to 35% with diltiazem and 40% with nifedipine. The mechanism is inhibition of oxidative metabolism in the liver. Although other calcium channel blockers may interact, the interaction is thought to be clinically insignificant.

Calcium channel blockers have been reported to interact with statins. Both diltiazem and verapamil have been implicated as increasing the risk of muscle breakdown with both atorvastatin and simvastatin.[64] There is also an increased risk of myopathy with simvastatin if given with verapamil. Diltiazem, isradipine, and verapamil inhibit cytochrome P450 isoenzyme CYP 3A4, which is involved in the metabolism of atorvastatin, sinvastatin, and lovastatin. Fluvastatin and pravastatin are not significantly metabolized by this isoenzyme.

The calcium-channel-blocking agents have significant interactions with ciclosporin. Verapamil, diltiazem, and nicardipine all increase ciclosporin concentrations. At the same time, they are thought to have a renoprotective effect and contribute to immunosuppression. Dose reductions of between 30 and 60% may be required with diltiazem, and both verapamil and nicardipine have both doubled or tripled serum ciclosporin concentrations in transplant patients. Although careful monitoring should be undertaken, this interaction has also been exploited in order to reduce the costs of ciclosporin therapy.[65]

Nifedipine, amlodipine, and felodipine are less likely to interact. Isradipine, lacidipine, and nitrendipine appear not to.

The plasma concentration of tacrolimus is possibly increased by felodipine, and is increased by diltiazem and nifedipine. The mechanism is thought to be inhibition of P450 isoenzyme CYP3A4 and glycoprotein. Knowledge about other calcium channel blockers is limited, but tacrolimus levels should be monitored closely and dosages adjusted if necessary.

Anticonvulsants are a particular problem with calcium-channel-blocking agents, which can undermine epilepsy treatment and in turn have their own effects attenuated by anticonvulsants. Carbamazepine concentrations can be significantly increased, causing toxicity (by diltiazem use)—although nifedipine and amlodipine appear to be safe alternatives. Alternatively, the dose of carbamazepine may be halved. Verapamil has a similar effect on carbamazepine. Elevated phenytoin levels have been reported with diltiazem, and in one case with nifedipine. Retrospective studies appear to suggest that nifedipine's interaction with phenytoin may be rare.

The anticonvulsants carbamazepine, phenobarbital, and phenytoin can all reduce felodipine and nimodipine levels. Phenobarbital and phenytoin can also reduce verapamil levels. Increased doses of calcium-channel-blocking agents may be required in epileptic patients.

Rifampicin increases the metabolism of some calcium-channel-blocking agents in the gut wall. These agents can become therapeutically ineffective unless dosages are increased. The main drugs of concern are nifedipine, verapamil, and to a lesser extent diltiazem. Evidence for other calcium-channel-blocking agents is more limited.

Coadministration of ritonavir and indinavir with either amlodipine or diltiazem can cause sharp increases in the plasma concentrations of the calcium-channel-blocking agents. If co-prescribed, lower initiation doses should be used.

SUMMARY

As prescribing increasingly becomes electronic, so decision support networks alert the prescriber to the possibility of an interaction occurring. All too often interactions are noted that have no practical significance.[67]

Drug interactions are common. Although the easiest way to avoid such interactions would be use of monotherapy, as target blood pressures continue to drop so the need for multiple antihypertensive agents is increased. Unfortunately, with an aging population there is also an increased risk of co-morbidities also requiring treatment. As more medications become available and more conditions are deemed preventable or treatable, so the patient's prescription list continues to lengthen. Drug interactions are of increasing importance, and their adverse effects are a significant cause for hospitalization. Increasing awareness of drug interactions will obviously help to prevent such problems.

REFERENCES

1. Stockley I. *Stockley's Drug Interaction. Sixth Edition.* London: Pharmaceutical Press, 2002.
2. Materson B, Reda D, Cushman W, Massie B, Fries E, Mahendr S, et al. Single-drug therapy for hypertension in men-a comparison of six antihypertensive agents with placebo. *New England Journal of Medicine* 1993;328:914–921
3. Maas R, Böger R. Antihypertensive therapy: Special focus on drug interactions. *Expert Opin Drug Saf* 2003;2(6):549–79.
4. Pirmohamed M, James S, Meakin S, Green C, Scott A, Walley T, et al. Adverse drug reactions as cause of admission to hospital: Prospective analysis of 18820 patients. *Br Med J* 2004;329:15–19.
5. Levy M, Kewitz H, Altwein W, Hillebrand J, Eliakim M. Hospital admissions due to adverse drug reactions in hospitalised patients: A meta-analysis of prospective studies. *Eur.J Clin Pharmacol* 1980;17(1):25–31.
6. Flockhart DA, Tanus-Santos JE. Implications of cytochrome P450 interactions when prescribing medication for hypertension. *Arch Intern Med* 2002;162(4):405–12.
7. Carter BL, Lund BC, Hayase N, Chrischilles E, Carter BL, Lund BC, et al. A longitudinal analysis of antihypertensive drug interactions in a Medicaid population. *Am J Hypertens* 2004; 17(5 Pt 1):421–27.
8. Malhotra S, Bailey DG, Paine MF, Watkins PB. Seville orange juice-felodipine interaction: Comparison with dilute grapefruit juice and involvement of furocoumarins. *Clin Pharmacol Ther* 2001;69(1):14–23.
9. Lilja JJ, Juntti-Patinen L, Neuvonen PJ. Orange juice substantially reduces the bioavailability of the beta-adrenergic-blocking agent celiprolol. *Clin Pharmacol Ther* 2004;75(3):184–90.
10. Ray K, Dorman S, Watson R. Severe hyperkalaemia due to the concomitant use of salt substitutes and ACE inhibitors in hypertension: A potentially life threatening interaction. *J Hum Hypertens* 1999;13(10):717–20.
11. Ackman ML, Campbell JB, Buzak KA, Tsuyuki RT, Montague TJ, Teo KK. Use of nonprescription medications by patients with congestive heart

failure. *Ann Pharmacother* 1999; 33(6):674–79.

12. Hussain RM. The sweet cake that reaches parts other cakes can't! *Postgrad Med J* 2003;79:115–16.

13. Culley C, Lacy M, Edwards B. Moxifloxacin:Clinical efficacy and safety. *Am J Health-Syst Pharm* 2001;58:379–88.

14. Liu B, Juurlink D. Drugs and the QT interval-Caveat Doctor. *N Engl J Med* 2004;351(11):1053–56.

15. Touze JE, Heno P, Fourcade L, et al. The effects of antimalarial drugs on ventricular repolarisation. *Am J Trop Med Hyg* 2002;67(1):54–60.

16. Feroze H, Suri R, Silverman DI. Torsades de pointes from terfenadine and sotalol given in combination. *Pacing Clin Electrophysiol* 1996;19(10):1519–21.

17. Yust I, Hoffman M, Aronson RJ. Life-threatening bradycardic reactions due to beta blocker-diltiazem interactions. *Israel Journal of Medical Sciences* 1992;28:292–94.

18. Bauer L, Horn J, Maxon M, Easterling T, Shen D, Strandness DJ. Effect of metprolol and verapamil administered separately and concurrently after single doses on liver blod flow and drug disposition. *J Clin Pharmacol* 2000; 40:533–43.

19. Kaijser M, Johnsson C, Zezina L, Backman U, Dimeny E, Fellstrom B. Elevation of cyclosporin A blood levels during carvedilol treatment in renal transplant patients. *Clin Transplant* 1997;11(6):577–81.

20. Myers MG. Beta adrenoceptor antagonism and pressor response to phenylephrine. *Clin Pharmacol Ther* 1984;36(1):57–63.

21. Reeves RA, Boer WH, DeLeve L, Leenen FH. Nonselective beta-blockade enhances pressor responsiveness to epinephrine, norepinephrine, and angiotensin II in normal man. *Clin Pharmacol Ther* 1984;35(4):461–66.

22. Foster CA, Aston SJ. Propranolol-epinephrine interaction: A potential disaster. *Plast Reconstr Surg* 1983;72(1):74–8.

23. Reynolds NJ, Wallington TB, Burton JL. Hydralazine predisposes to acute cutaneous vasculitis following urography with iopamidol. *Br J Dermatol* 1993;129(1):82–5.

24. McLean AJ, Skews H, Bobik A, Dudley FJ. Interaction between oral propranolol and hydralazine. *Clin Pharmacol Ther* 1980;27(6):726–32.

25. Campbell NR, Hasinoff BB. Iron supplements: A common cause of drug interactions. *Br J Clin Pharmacol* 1991;31(3):251–55.

26. Greene RJ, Hall AD, Hider RC, Greene RJ, Hall AD, Hider RC. The interaction of orally administered iron with levodopa and methyldopa therapy. *J Pharm Pharmacol* 1990;42(7):502–04.

27. Byrd GJ, Byrd GJ. Lithium carbonate and methyldopa: Apparent interaction in man. *Clin Toxicol* 1977;11(1):1–4.

28. Yassa R, Yassa R. Lithium-methyldopa interaction. *CMAJ* 1986;134(2): 141–42.

29. Whitehead MI, Mander AM, Hertogs K, Williams RM, Pettingale KW. Acute congestive cardiac failure in a hypertensive woman receiving salbutamol for premature labour. *Br Med J* 1980; 280(6225):1221–22.

30. Briant RH, Reid JL, Dollery CT, Briant RH, Reid JL, Dollery CT. Interaction between clonidine and desipramine in man. *Br Med J* 1973;1(5852):522–23.

31. Warren SE, Ebert E, Swerdlin AH, Steinberg SM, Stone R, Warren SE, et al. Clonidine and propranolol paradoxical hypertension. *Arch Intern Med* 1979;139(2):253.

32. bo-Zena RA, Bobek MB, Dweik RA. Hypertensive urgency induced by an interaction of mirtazapine and clonidine. *Pharmacotherapy* 2000;20(4):476–78.

33. Ober KF, Wang RI, Ober KF, Wang RI. Drug interactions with guanethidine. *Clin Pharmacol Ther* 1973;14(2): 190–95.

34. Kaufman J, Hamburger R, Matheson J, Flamenbaum W. Bumetanide-induced diuresis and natriuresis: Effect of prostaglandin synthetase inhibition. *J Clin Pharmacol* 1981;21:663–67.

35. Smith CR, Lietman PS. Effect of furosemide on aminoglycoside-induced nephrotoxicity and auditory toxicity in humans. *Antimicorb Agents Chemother* 1983;23:133–37.

36. Bates DE, Beaumont SJ, Bayliss BW. Ototoxicity induced by gentamicin and furosemide. *Ann Pharmacother* 2002;36(3):446–51.

37. Waldorff S, Waldorff S, Andersen JD, Heeboll-Nielsen N, Nielsen OG, Moltke E, et al. Spironolactone-induced changes in digoxin kinetics. *Clin Pharmacol Ther* 1978;24(2):162–67.

38. Steiner w, Muller C, Eber B. Digoxin assays: frequent, substantial and potentially dangerous interference by spirolactone, canrenone, and other steroids. *Clin Chem* 2002;48(3):2405–06.

39. Beeley L. Drug interactions with lithium. *Prescribers' J* 1986;26:160–63.

40. Juurlink DN, Mamdani MM, Kopp A, Rochon PA, Shulman KI, et al. Drug-induced lithium toxicity of in the elderly: A population based study. 2004. *Journal of the American Geriatrics Society* 2004;52:794–98.

41. National Prescribing Centre. Aspirin and ACE inhibitor combination in patients with heart failure and CHD: Is there a problem? *Merec Extra* 2002;4:1.

42. Teo KK, et al. Effects of long-term treatment with angiotensin-converting-enzyme inhibitors in the presence or absence of aspirin: A systematic review. *Lancet* 2002;360:1037–43.

43. Masoudi FA, Wolfe P, Havranek EP, Rathore SS, Foody JM, Krumholz HM. Aspirin use in older patients with heart failure and coronary artery disease. *Journal of the American College of Cardiology* 2005;46(6):955–62.

44. Pigott DW, Nagle C, Allman K, Westaby S, Evans RD. Effect of omitting regular ACE inhibition before cardiac surgery on haemodynamic variable and vasoactive drug requirements. *Br J Anaesth* 1999;83(5):715–20.

45. Juurlink DN, Mamdani MM, Kopp A, Rochon PA, Shulman KI, et al. Drug-induced lithium toxicity of in the elderly: A population based study. 2004. *Journal of the American Geriatrics Society* 2004;52:794–98.

46. Gossman J, Thurmann P, Bachmann T, Weller S, Kachel, Schoeppe W, et al. Mechanism of angiotensin converting enzyme inhibitor-related anaemia in renal transplant recipients. *Kidney Int* 1996;50(3):973–78.

47. Ahmad S. Allopurinol and enalapril: Drug induced anaphylactic coronary spam and acute myocardial infarction. *Chest* 1995;108:586.

48. Abraham G, Grunberg B, Gratz S. Possible interaction of clozapine and lisinopril. *American Journal of Psychiatry* 2001;158:969.

49. Mandel AK, Market RJ, Saklayen MG, Manjus RA, Yokokawa K. Diuretics potentiate angiotensin converting enzyme inhibitor-induced acute renal failure. *Clin Nephrol* 1994;42:170–74.

50. Speirs CJ, Dollery CT, Inman WHW, Rawson NSB, Wilton LV. Postmarketing surveillance of enalapril II: Investigation of the potential role of enalapril in deaths with renal failure. *BMJ* 1988; 297:830–32.

51. Pitt B, Zannad F, Remme WJ, et al. The effect of spironolactone on morbidity and mortality in patients with severe heart failure. *N Engl J Med* 199; 341:709–17.

52. Anton C, Cox AR, Watson RDS, Ferner RE. The safety of spironolactone treatment in patients with hearty failure. *Journal of Clinical Pharmacy and Therapeutics* 2003;28:285–87.

53. Juurlink DN, Mamdani MM, Lee DS, Kopp A, Austin PC Laupacis A, Redelmeier DA. Rates of Hyperkalemia after Publication of the Randomized Aldactone Evaluation Study. *N Engl Med* 2004;351:543–51.

54. Pitt B, Remme W. Zannad F, et al. Eplerenone, a selective aldosterone blocker, in patients with left ventricular dysfunction after myocardial infarction. *N Engl J Med* 2003;348:1308–21.

55. Weinberger MH, White WB, Ruilope LM, et al. Effects of eplerenone versus losartan in patients with low-renin hypertension. *Am Heart J* 2005;150(3):426–33.

56. Zwanzger P, et al. Lithium intoxication after administration of AT1 blockers. *J Clin Psychiatry* 2001;62:208–09.

57. Blanche P, et al. Lithium intoxication in an elderly patient after combined treatment with losartan. *Eur J Clin Pharmacol* 1997;52:501.

58. Leung M, Remick RA. Potential drug interaction between lithium and valsartan. *J Clin Psychopharmacol* 2000; 20:392–93.

59. Cohn JN, Tognoni G. A randomized trial of the angiotensin-receptor blocker valsartan in chronic heart failure. *N Engl J Med* 2001;345:1667–75.

60. McMurray JJV, et al. Effects of candesartan in patients with chronic heart failure and reduced left-ventricular systolic function taking angiotensin-converting-enzyme inhibitors: The CHARM-Added trial. *Lancet* 2003;362:767–71.

61. Lee TH, Friedman PL, Goldman L, Stone PH, Antman EM. Sinus arrest and hypotension with combined amiodarone-diltiazem therapy. *Am Heart J* 1985; 109(1):163–64.

62. Bailey DG, Malcolm J, Arnold O, Spence JD. Grapefruit juice-drug interactions. *Br J Clin Pharmacol* 1998;46:101–10.

63. Josefsson M, Zackrisson AL, Ahlner J. Effect of grapefruit juice on the pharmacokinetics of amlodipine in healthy volunteers. *Eur J Clin Pharmacol* 1996;51:189–93.

64. ADRAC Reaction. *http://www.csmwm.org/reaction/29.pdf.*

65. Kumana CR, Tong MKL, Li C-S, Lauder IJ, Lee JSK, Kou M, et al. Diltiazem co-treatment in renal transplant patients receiving microemulsion cyclosporin. *British Journal of Clinical Pharmacology* 2003;56(6):670–78.

66. Glesby MJ, Aberg JA, Kendall MA, Fichtenbaum CJ, Hafner R, Hall S, et al. Adult AIDS Clinical Trials Group A5159 Protocol Team. Pharmacokinetic interactions between indinavir plus ritonavir and calcium channel blockers. *Clin Pharmacol Ther* 2005;78(2):143–53.

67. Li Wan Po A. Drug-drug interactions and adverse drug reactions:the bollards and flashing lights syndrome. *J Clin Pharm Ther* 2005;30:97–9.

Chapter

88 Lipid-Lowering Therapy

Ian S. Young and Brona V. Loughrey

Key Findings

- Hyperlipidemia is a key risk factor for atherosclerosis, and elevated lipids should be treated in all patients at high risk of cardiovascular disease.

- The primary target in lipid management is low-density lipoprotein (LDL) cholesterol. Important secondary targets include high-density lipoprotein (HDL) cholesterol, non-HDL cholesterol, and triglycerides.

- A statin is the first-choice lipid-lowering agent for the overwhelming majority of patients.

- Combinations of lipid-lowering drugs may be required to achieve lipid targets in high-risk patients.

INTRODUCTION

The key pathophysiologic features of atherosclerosis are lipid deposition and inflammation within the arterial wall.[1] The majority of important cardiovascular risk factors operate by increasing one or both of these processes. Oxidation of lipids deposited within the arterial intima represents an important inflammatory stimulus, and thus prevention of lipid deposition provides a mechanism of inhibiting both of these pathways. Arterial wall lipids mainly derive from lipid circulating in serum, and it is not surprising that there is overwhelming evidence that serum lipids are strong independent risk factors for the development of cardiovascular disease.

LIPIDS AND VASCULAR RISK

An enormous body of clinical and experimental research unequivocally identifies elevated plasma cholesterol as a causative factor in the progression of atherosclerosis.[2] Many prospective epidemiologic studies have identified a strong correlation between total cholesterol and increased incidence of cardiovascular disease (CVD). In general, the greater the level of total cholesterol the greater the risk of CVD, with no clear lower limit for cholesterol below which CVD risk no longer falls. The risk of CVD begins to increase more steeply above a total cholesterol level of approximately 5.0 mmol/L (200 mg/dL).

Some epidemiologic studies have suggested that very low levels of cholesterol may be associated with an increase in total mortality, attributable to a greater risk of death from cancer and other noncardiovascular causes. However, it is now generally felt that low cholesterol is a

consequence of the biochemical acute phase response present in any severely ill patient rather than a cause of increased risk. Since about 80% of total cholesterol in serum is contained in the LDL fraction, it is not surprising that LDL cholesterol has a similar relationship with CVD risk as total cholesterol. In the case of LDL cholesterol, risk increases more steeply above a level of approximately 3.0 mmol/L (120 mg/dL), but again there is no clear lower limit for LDL cholesterol below which risk no longer decreases.

In contrast to total cholesterol, LDL cholesterol, and triglycerides, HDL cholesterol concentration has an inverse association with CVD. The anti-atherogenic properties of HDL have been accounted for by the involvement of HDL in reverse cholesterol transport. However, HDL has numerous functions independent from lipid metabolism, which are protective against atherogenesis (including anti-inflammatory properties and an ability to protect LDL against oxidation[3]).

Serum triglycerides have a much weaker relationship with CVD risk than total or LDL cholesterol. Indeed, epidemiologic studies have often failed to identify an association between elevated total plasma triglyceride concentrations with greater cardiovascular risk. In part, the difficulties encountered identifying a strong correlation between triglycerides and CVD are due to the wide fluctuations in triglyceride concentrations throughout the day, the heterogeneity of triglyceride-rich lipoproteins, and the inseparable correlations between triglycerides and other CVD risk factors. However, meta-analyses of population-based prospective studies carried out by Austin et al.[4] conclusively identified raised triglyceride concentrations as a strong independent risk factor for CVD, estimating that raised triglyceride levels were associated with a 13% increase in CVD risk in men and a 37% increase in women following adjustment for confounding factors.

Triglycerides were found to have a strong inverse correlation with HDL-C, although the association between triglycerides and CVD was independent of this relationship. A more sophisticated approach to examining the physiologic impact of triglycerides is to analyze the individual triglyceride-rich lipoproteins (TRLs), which include a heterogeneous population of particles with wide-ranging atherogenic potential. Accumulating evidence suggests that elevated plasma triglycerides, in the form of TRL, are independent cardiovascular risk factors (with an atherogenic potential comparable to raised LDL[5]). TRL is a broad term encompassing chylomicrons, very low-density lipoproteins (VLDL), and their partially metabolized remnant lipoproteins. In view of the strong relationships between lipids and cardiovascular risk outlined previously, it is not surprising that abnormal lipids are a major cause of vascular disease (with, for instance, more than 30% of myocardial infarctions in hypertensive patients being explained by total cholesterol above 200 mg/dL).

CAUSES OF DYSLIPIDEMIA

Elevated lipid levels are mainly due to a combination of lifestyle and genetic factors. More than 50% of adults in most Western societies have a total cholesterol level above 200 mg/dL, reflecting a lifetime of a relatively high-fat diet along with a high prevalence of overweight and obesity and too little exercise. The genetic contribution to dyslipidemia most commonly takes a polygenic form, but there are several well-defined dyslipidemic conditions with a much stronger genetic contribution. The most important of these is familial hypercholesterolemia, a condition with an autosomal dominant pattern of inheritance due to a defect in the LDL receptor or apoB genes.

Familial hypercholesterolemia affects approximately one in five hundred individuals in most Western countries and if untreated is associated with a high incidence of premature cardiovascular disease. It should be suspected in families with a strong history of coronary heart disease affecting individuals aged less than 60 years.[6] Testing is most easily done by measuring total and LDL cholesterol in family members, but increasingly genetic testing is also available. Type III hyperlipidemia should be suspected in individuals with markedly elevated cholesterol and triglycerides. It is associated with the apoE phenotype E2/2. Other inherited diseases of lipid metabolism are less common.

Dyslipidemia is also a secondary feature of other medical conditions and it is important to consider testing for these in hyperlipidemic individuals. Undiagnosed hypothyroidism is a particular pitfall, and is associated with increased total cholesterol. Any decision about treating the cholesterol level should be deferred until normal thyroid function is restored. Fasting glucose should always be measured in individuals with high triglycerides, as the incidence of undiagnosed diabetes in this population is relatively high. Other conditions that may be associated with dyslipidemia include obesity, alcohol abuse, renal disease (particularly nephrotic syndrome), liver disease (especially cholestatic liver disease), and the use of certain drugs.

MECHANISMS OF ACTION

To understand the mechanisms of action by which pharmacologic agents reduce cholesterol it is first necessary to understand the main pathways of lipid metabolism.[7] The main lipids present in serum are cholesterol and triglycerides, with smaller amounts of phospholipids and free fatty acids. Cholesterol is in the form of free cholesterol or cholesterol esterified to fatty acids. The vast majority of serum lipids are present in particles known as lipoproteins, which also include proteins known as apolipoproteins. The arrangement of lipids in lipoproteins follows a common pattern, with particles containing more hydrophobic lipids such as triglycerides and cholesterol esters in their core, with more hydrophilic lipids (free cholesterol and phospholipids) on the outside.

The amount of lipid differs significantly between different particles, with the largest particles (chylomicrons) containing most lipid and the smallest particles (high-density lipoproteins) containing the least (Table 88–1). In contrast, apolipoproteins differ between lipoprotein classes and determine the metabolic fate of lipoprotein particles by acting as receptor ligands or by activating or inhibiting enzymes involved in lipid metabolism. The key properties and features of different lipoproteins are summarized in Table 88–2. Lipid metabolism can be considered according to three main mechanisms:[7] the exogenous pathway, the endogenous pathway, and reverse cholesterol transport.

CLASSIFICATION OF LIPOPROTEINS[a]			
Lipoprotein	Density (g/mL)	Mean Particle Diameter (nm)	Electrophoretic Mobility
Chylomicrons	<0.95	500	Origin
Very-low-density lipoproteins (VLDLs)	0.95–1.006	43	Pre-beta
Intermediate-density lipoproteins (IDLs)	1.006–1.019	27	Beta-1
Low-density lipoproteins (LDLs)	1.019–1.063	22	Beta
High-density lipoproteins (HDLs)	1.063–1.21	8	Alpha

a. Particle density increases and particle size decreases from chylomicrons to HDL. Agarose electrophoresis separates lipoproteins according to their characteristic electrophoretic mobility and is determined by particle charge and size.

Table 88–1. Classification of Lipoproteins[a]

APOLIPOPROTEIN FUNCTIONS AND ASSOCIATED LIPOPROTEINS[a]		
Apolipoprotein	**Main Functions**	**Associated Lipoprotein**
Apo AI	Ligand for HDL, cofactor for lecithin cholesterol acyl transferase	Chylomicrons, HDL
Apo AII	Ligand for HDL, cofactor for lecithin:cholesterol acyltransferase	Chylomicrons, HDL
Apo AIV	Ligand for HDL, activates lecithin cholesterol acyl transferase	Chylomicrons, HDL
Apo (a)	Provides structural integrity for Lp(a)	Lp(a)
Apo B_{48}	Provides structural integrity for chylomicrons	Chylomicrons
Apo B_{100}	Provides structural integrity for VLDL, IDL, and LDL; ligand for LDL receptor	VLDL, IDL, LDL
Apo CI	Activates lecithin cholesterol acyl transferase, activates lipoprotein lipase	Chylomicrons, VLDL, IDL, HDL
Apo CII	Activates lecithin cholesterol acyl transferase, activates lipoprotein lipase, inhibits lipoprotein lipase	Chylomicrons, VLDL, IDL, HDL
Apo CIII	Inhibits hepatic lipase, modulates uptake by lipoprotein related receptor (via binding to proteoglycans)	Chylomicrons, VLDL, IDL, HDL
Apo D	Unknown	HDL
Apo E	Ligand for Apo B/E receptor, Apo E2 receptor, and lipoprotein-related receptor	Chylomicrons, VLDL, IDL, LDL
Apo J	Implicated in cell membrane protection	HDL

a. Apolipoprotein composition is important for the characterization of plasma lipoproteins. In addition to providing structural integrity, these apolipoproteins are implicated in lipoprotein transport and enzyme activity.

Table 88–2. Apolipoprotein Functions and Associated Lipoproteins[a]

Exogenous lipid metabolism

Dietary lipids are absorbed by the mucosal cells of the intestine, which re-esterify cholesterol and free fatty acids to produce triglycerides and cholesterol esters. These lipids, along with phospholipids and unesterified cholesterol, are packaged together with apo B_{48} to form the largest triglyceride-rich lipoproteins (nascent chylomicrons). Chylomicrons are characterized by the presence of apo B_{48}, which is a low-molecular-weight form of apo B_{100}. This apoprotein is specifically produced by the intestine[8] and only contains residues 1 through 2152 (48%) of apo B_{100}, thus preventing chylomicrons from interacting with the LDL receptor.

Nascent chylomicrons are rapidly metabolized following their secretion into the general circulation. An exchange of apoproteins occurs between chylomicrons and HDL, and the chylomicrons acquire apo C and E apoproteins in exchange for apo A proteins. Chylomicron remnants become relatively deplete in triglycerides due to the hydrolysis of the particles' triglyceride core by lipoprotein lipase, an enzyme anchored to the endothelium. In addition, cholesterol ester is transferred from mature HDL to the chylomicrons in exchange for triglyceride by cholesteryl ester transfer protein (CETP)[9].

Chylomicron remnants are rapidly cleared from the circulation by hepatic receptors specific for apo E. The exogenous pathway efficiently delivers triglyceride to skeletal muscle and adipose tissue and deposits cholesterol for processing in the liver. Chylomicrons are normally undetectable following a 12-hour fast.[10]

Endogenous lipid metabolism

Fatty acids surplus to oxidative requirements are utilized by the liver for the synthesis of triglyceride and phospholipid. Cholesterol can also be produced endogenously by a pathway that includes the rate-limiting enzyme β-hydroxy-β-methylglutaryl-coenzyme. A reductase (HMG CoA reductase), subject to positive inhibition by the end product (cholesterol). Although the liver has the capacity to synthesize cholesterol and triglyceride, it is more efficient to utilize preformed lipids derived from the diet or excess stores in adipose tissue.

In the fasting (postabsorptive) state, VLDL replaces chylomicrons as the most abundant triglyceride-rich lipoprotein and the metabolism of VLDL is similar to that of chylomicrons. The liver packages triglyceride, cholesterol, cholesterol ester, and phospholipid together with C apoproteins, apo B_{100}, and apo E to form nascent VLDL (which is secreted into the bloodstream). Similarly to chylomicrons, nascent VLDL becomes relatively deplete in triglycerides following its interaction with lipoprotein lipase and cholesterol ester transfer protein. The particle also sheds apo C and E proteins to produce a "VLDL remnant" known as intermediate-density lipoprotein (IDL). Unlike chylomicron remnants, IDL can be taken up by the liver or may undergo further delipidation and loss of apoproteins to yield LDL.

The VLDL class encompasses an extremely heterogeneous population of lipoprotein particles that differ in size (80 to 1200 nm), composition, and metabolic fate. Large buoyant VLDL tends to be metabolized to IDL, which is subsequently cleared via apo B/E receptor-mediated uptake in the liver.[11] Conversely, smaller VLDL particles complete the metabolic cascade by producing IDL which ultimately yields LDL. LDL is removed by apo B_{100} receptor-mediated uptake in the liver, although LDL can also be utilized by extrahepatic tissue to provide cholesterol for normal cellular functions.

Reverse cholesterol transport

Reverse cholesterol transport incorporates HDL metabolism and involves the movement of cholesterol from extrahepatic tissue, including the vessel wall, to the liver for excretion.[12] The HDL lipoproteins are the smallest and most dense lipid particles. This heterogeneous population can be divided into two subclasses by ultracentrifugation: HDL_2 (1.063 to 1.125 g/mL) and HDL_3 (1.125 to 1.21 g/mL). Plasma concentrations of the HDL_3 subclass are more abundant than HDL_2 (3:1). The major apoprotein constituents of HDL are the A apoproteins (AI, AII, AIV), which are responsible for modulating HDL metabolism. The A apoproteins function as acceptors of cellular cholesterol (LCAT), serve as cofactors for lecithin cholesterol acyl transferase, and act as ligands for HDL receptors.

The liver and intestine synthesize and secrete nascent discoid HDL, which consists mainly of apo E, apo Cs, phospholipids, and free cholesterol. The particle acquires apo A proteins, which provides the lipoprotein with the capacity to utilize LCAT and adenosine triphosphate-binding cassette protein A1 (ABCA-1). This transporter protein regulates the concentration of plasma HDL and the levels of intracellular cholesterol. The ABCA-1 transporter protein facilitates the efflux of intracellular cholesterol through an interaction with apo AI on lipid-deplete HDL. Following this, LCAT catalyzes the esterification of HDL cholesterol (and the hydrophobicity of the sterol-ester results in its relocation from the surface of the lipoprotein to the hydrophobic core of the particle). The surface of HDL is available to accept more free cholesterol, forming mature spherical HDL particles.

In addition, HDL functions as a chaperone for the transfer of cholesterol ester to the liver. The scavenger receptor class B1 (SR-B1) modulates the selective uptake of HDL cholesterol ester by hepatocytes. HDL complexes with SR-B1 and is endocytosed. Cholesterol ester is hydrolyzed by cholesterol ester esterase and secreted as biliary cholesterol or utilized to produce steroid hormones. The SR-B1 receptor is distributed predominately on hepatocytes, but SR-B1 is also expressed on macrophages (where it may influence cholesterol efflux). Alternatively, CETP promotes the transfer of cholesterol ester from HDL to the apo-B-containing lipoproteins in exchange for triglyceride, yielding a small and more dense HDL particle.

MECHANISMS OF ACTION AND PHARMACOKINETICS OF INDIVIDUAL DRUG CLASSES

Statins

The first drug of this class, lovastatin, went on the United States market in 1987 and since then statins have come to dominate the field of lipid-lowering therapy. Statins are competitive inhibitors of the enzyme hydroxymethylglutaryl coenzyme A (HMG CoA) reductase, which catalyzes the formation of mevalonate from HMG CoA[13] (Figure 88–1). This is the rate-limiting step on the biosynthetic pathway of cholesterol in the liver. The affinity of statins for this enzyme is several thousand times that of its physiologic substrate, although this inhibition is partly offset by increased expression of HMG CoA reductase. Reduction of endogenous cholesterol synthesis leads to upregulation of the LDL receptor. Consequently, there is increased hepatic uptake of apoB-containing lipoproteins (especially LDL) and a reduction in the corresponding circulating cholesterol fractions. Triglycerides are reduced to a lesser extent. There is also a modest increase in HDL by a mechanism that is not well understood at present.

There are now several of this class of drug available, all given by mouth once daily (although the recommended dosages vary;[14] Table 88–3). Cholesterol-lowering potency has increased as newer agents have been developed. Lovastatin and simvastatin are pro-drugs, whereas pravastatin, fluvastatin, atorvastatin, and rosuvastatin are active in themselves. All undergo hepatic first-pass metabolism, as is appropriate for drugs whose main

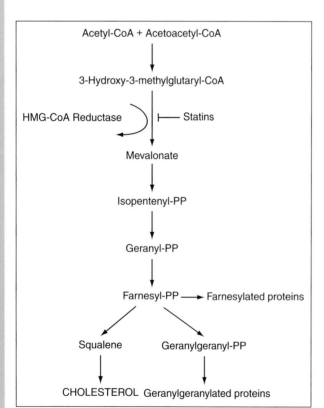

Figure 88–1. Cholesterol synthesis pathway showing point of action of statins. The synthesis of all intermediates distal to this point in the pathway is reduced.

TABLE 88-3

Drug	Reduction in TC (%)	Reduction in LDL-C (%)	Increase in HDL-C (%)	Reduction in TG (%)	Dosage Form Tablets (mg)	Metabolism	Protein Binding, (%)	T 1/2, h	Hydrophilic
Atorvastatin	25–45	26–60	5–13	17–53	10, 20, 40, 80	CYP3A4	98	13–30	No
Fluvastatin	16–27	22–36	3–11	12–25	20, 40, 80	CYP2C9	98	0.5–3.0	No
Lovastatin	16–34	21–42	2–10	6–27	10, 20, 40	CYP3A4	>95	2–4	No
Pravastatin	16–25	22–34	2–12	15–24	10, 20, 40, 80	Sulfation	43–67	2–3	Yes
Rosuvastatin	33–46	45–63	8–14	10–35	5, 10, 20, 40	CYP2C9	88	19	Yes
Simvastatin	19–36	26–47	8–16	12–34	5, 10, 20, 40, 80	CYP3A4	95–98	1–3	No

Abbreviations: TC (total cholesterol), TG (triglycerides), and T1/2 (half-life).

Table 88-3.

site of action is the liver in order to limit systemic side effects. Simvastatin and atorvastatin are substrates of the cytochrome P450 isoenzyme CYP3A4, which gives rise to the possibility of interaction with other drugs metabolized by this pathway (such as cyclosporin and macrolide antibiotics). The newest agent, rosuvastatin, is partly metabolized by CYP2C9 (and there are reports that it can increase the anticoagulant activity of warfarin).

Fibrates

The fibrates have been in use as lipid-lowering agents for many years. Whereas the main target of statins is LDL, fibrates have more broadly beneficial effects on triglycerides and HDLc as well as modest LDLc-lowering effects. Clofibrate was the original member of this class, which now includes ciprofibrate, bezafibrate, fenofibrate, and gemfibrozil[15] (Table 88–4).

Administration of fibrates results in a decrease in circulating VLDL and LDL and an increase in HDL. The exact mechanisms underlying these effects are complex and still not well understood. What is known is that the fibrates are ligands for the peroxisomal-proliferator-activated receptor α (PPARα).[16] This is one of a family of nuclear thyroid or steroid hormone receptors that when activated act as transcription factors by binding to response elements on certain target genes. The many proteins whose expression is altered by PPARα agonists include apolipoproteins, lipoprotein lipase, and other enzymes involved in fatty acid uptake and metabolism.

In general, the fibrates are well absorbed orally and may be given once daily or in divided doses. Some modified-release formulations are available. They are extensively protein bound in plasma and undergo metabolism by the cytochrome P450 system before being excreted by the kidneys. There are a number of significant interactions. They enhance the effects of anticoagulants and hypoglycemic drugs, and fenofibrate should not be given along with ciclosporin because of the risk of renal impairment.

Nicotinic acid (niacin)

As with the fibrates, the vitamin nicotinic acid has been available for many years. However, there is renewed interest in it recently with the increasing recognition of the importance of HDL in cardiovascular risk. It is currently the single best available agent for raising HDL, and it has beneficial effects on LDL and triglycerides.[17] These do not become apparent until a dose at least 50 times the recommended daily intake of the vitamin is given. It undergoes extensive first-pass metabolism, but this is saturable such that there is greater systemic bioavailability with higher doses. There is now a modified-release preparation available to avoid the previous need for divided doses. Again, the mechanisms of action are not straightforward, but at least two are known: inhibition of lipolysis in adipose tissue and reduction of hepatic uptake of HDL.

Ezetimibe

Ezetimibe, given in a dose of 10 mg once daily, selectively inhibits intestinal cholesterol absorption. The main effect is a fall in circulating LDL, although there is also a small reduction in triglyceride levels. The exact mechanism of action is as yet unknown, although it appears that ezetimibe acts via the Niemann-Pick C1-Like 1 (NPC1L1) protein.[18] It has few side effects or contraindications, and has no known significant interactions, although at present coadministration with fibrates is not recommended due to a theoretical increased risk of hepatobiliary disease.[19] It is best used as an adjunct to statin therapy if targets are not achieved with monotherapy. A combined preparation of ezetimibe and simvastatin is now available.

Omega-3 fatty acids

A diet rich in oily fish is associated with a low incidence of cardiovascular disease even though the fat content is relatively high. Fish oil contains high levels of ω-3 fatty acids such as docosahexaenoic acid (DHA) and eicosapentaenoic acid (EHA), which when administered to humans lead to reduction in circulating triglycerides.[20] The exact mechanism behind this is not yet known, but it may be that they inhibit esterification and incorporation into VLDL of other fatty acids. They also appear to exert an antiarrhythmic effect on the myocardium. The maximal effect of fish oil is at a dose far beyond that which can be incorporated into even the most health-conscious Western diet, and there are supplements now available by prescription. The biggest problem with prescribing these is patient compliance, as the capsules are large and need to be taken several times daily for the treatment of hypertriglyceridemia.

PHARMACOKINETIC PROPERTIES OF FIBRATES					
Drug	Bezafibrate	Ciprofibrate	Clofibrate	Fenofibrate	Gemfibrozil
Oral bioavailability (%)	100	75	100	60	100
Volume of distribution (L)	17	[????]	14.5	0.89 L/kg	[????]
t ½ in healthy volunteers (h)	1.5-3.0	81	15	19-27	1.3
t ½ in patients with renal failure (h)	9.2	172	30-110	143	[????]
Protein binding (%)	95	99	96	>99	98
Route of elimination	Renal (unchanged)	Renal	Renal (metabolites)	Renal (glucuronide)	Renal (glucuronide)
Abbreviation: t½ = half-life.					

Table 88–4. Pharmacokinetic Properties of Fibrates

Plant stanols and sterol esters

Stanols are hydrogenated derivatives of plant sterols, which are components of plant cell membranes. These resemble cholesterol in structure and competitively inhibit intestinal absorption of cholesterol.[21] Margarines and other preparations containing plant stanols are available in supermarkets as an aid to cholesterol reduction.

Resins

Colestyramine and colestipol were among the first available lipid-lowering agents. These are orally active anion-exchange resins that bind and prevent the reabsorption of bile salts in the gut.[22] This impairs fat absorption and leads to increased uptake of circulating cholesterol by the liver for the synthesis of more bile acids. There is also, however, a compensatory increase in endogenous cholesterol synthesis by the liver such that the net fall in serum cholesterol is not as great as with other hypolipidemic drugs. Some patients also show increased hepatic triglyceride output. Poor palatability, frequent gastrointestinal side effects, and limited efficacy mean that the resins are no longer widely used.

INDICATIONS/CONTRAINDICATIONS AND OBJECTIVES

The main indication for the use of lipid-lowering therapy is to reduce risk of cardiovascular disease. Therapy is therefore indicated for any individual at significant risk of cardiovascular disease whose serum lipids are above target levels. The primary targets for lipid-lowering therapy are total and LDL cholesterol, but treatment goals for HDL cholesterol, triglycerides, and non-HDL cholesterol may also be considered. In practice, CVD prevention should focus on people with any form of established atherosclerotic CVD, people with diabetes mellitus, or people without established CVD but who have a combination of risk factors that puts them at high total risk of developing CVD for the first time.

In addition, certain individuals with particularly elevated single risk factors also require CVD prevention. This is likely to include individuals with elevated blood pressure >160 mmHg systolic or >100 mmHg diastolic, or lesser degrees of blood pressure elevation with target organ damage. Individuals with an elevated total: HDL cholesterol ratio of >6.0 or with an inherited dyslipidaemia will also generally require lipid-lowering treatment.[23] Individuals at high risk of CVD require a multifactorial approach to risk factor management, of which treatment for serum lipids will constitute only one part. Risk factor management will include both lifestyle change and pharmacologic management.

ESTIMATION OF TOTAL CARDIOVASCULAR RISK

The concept of using total cardiovascular risk to determine the need for lipid-lowering therapy in the asymptomatic population is widely accepted in Europe, the United States, and internationally. A variety of risk prediction engines are used, most frequently based on the Framingham study. The level of total CVD risk at which lipid-lowering treatment is considered justified varies from country to country. The main risk factors taken into account include age, sex, smoking status, total to HDL cholesterol ratio, and blood pressure.

The advantages of this approach are that the total effect of risk factors acting on an individual can be taken into account when making treatment decisions, and that unnecessary treatment of single risk factors in individuals at overall low risk can be avoided. In the UK, risk tables are used, which are color coded to represent total CVD risk as low, medium, or high. In the United States, a scoring system based on the Framingham offspring study is used in conjunction with the National Cholesterol Education Program (NCEP) ATP III recommendations.[24]

This predicts only risk of fatal and nonfatal myocardial infarction, the rationale being that this is closer to the endpoint used in the majority of large statin trials. The Joint European Societies' guidelines on CVD prevention use the Heartscore system, which has the advantage of being based on European prospective epidemiologic data.[25] Heartscore predicts fatal CVD risk rather than total CVD risk, and the risk threshold for treatment is therefore defined as >5% 10-year risk, rather than the 20% 10-year risk threshold used in the UK guidelines that employ total CVD risk.

TARGETS FOR TREATMENT

The primary targets for lipid-lowering therapy are total and LDL cholesterol. Relevant targets are defined in appropriate national and international guidelines, and are derived from intervention trials that have been predominantly carried out using statins. Older studies (4S,[26] WOSCOPS,[27] CARE[28]) clearly demonstrated the value of reducing total and LDL cholesterol with statins. More recent studies have tended to focus on reducing total and LDL cholesterol to progressively lower levels. For instance, in the lipid-lowering arm of the ASCOT study (in which 10,305 subjects participated) a decrease in LDL cholesterol from 130 to 90 mg/dL reduced the primary endpoint of nonfatal myocardial infarction and fatal CHD by 36%.[29] In the CARDS trial, performed in subjects with diabetes and no previous history of cardiovascular disease, reduction in LDL cholesterol from 116 to 81 mg/dL produced a 37% reduction in major cardiovascular events.[30]

Recent studies (including PROVE-IT[31], IDEAL,[32] and TNT[33]) have also focused on comparing different statin regimes. For instance, in the PROVE-IT study pravastatin 40 mg per day was compared to atorvastatin 80 mg per day. Pravastatin 40 mg resulted in an LDL cholesterol level of 97 mg/dL compared with an LDL cholesterol level of 62 mg/dL in the atorvastatin 80-mg group. Reduction in LDL cholesterol to the lower level was associated with an additional 16% reduction in major CVD events.

Meta-analysis of the major statin trials demonstrates an essentially linear relationship between the degree of total or LDL cholesterol reduction and reduction in CVD events.[34] The reduction in CVD events is largely independent of the starting cholesterol level, so that a reduction in LDL cholesterol of 40 mg/dL produces a reduction in CVD events of approximately 23%. Furthermore, there is no clear evidence for a lower level of total or LDL cholesterol below which CVD risk does not fall.

The selection of appropriate targets for total and LDL cholesterol therefore depends on a synthesis of the available evidence. Current European guidelines recommend a target of less than 174 mg/dL (4.5 mmol/L) for total cholesterol and less than 97 mg/dL for LDL cholesterol.[25] UK guidelines recommend that total cholesterol should be reduced to less than 155 mg/dL or by 25% (whichever is greater) and that LDL cholesterol should be reduced to less than 78 mg/dL or by 30%, whichever is greater.[23] The NCEP ATP III guideline (revised in 2004) recommends that LDL cholesterol should be less than 70 mg/dL in high-risk individuals.[24]

Although the main target for lipid-lowering treatment should clearly be total and LDL cholesterol, it is also worth considering other lipid targets. These include targets for HDL cholesterol, triglycerides, and non-HDL cholesterol. Measures to achieve such targets should be taken once targets for total and LDL cholesterol have been achieved. As discussed previously, epidemiologic evidence suggests that CVD risk is particularly elevated in men with HDL cholesterol less than 40 mg/dL and women with HDL cholesterol less than 50 mg/dL. In addition, triglycerides above 65 mg/dL appear to be associated with increased CVD risk. Elevated triglycerides and low HDL cholesterol tend to go together, and are particularly common in patients with the metabolic syndrome or type 2 diabetes. Such individuals also have a preponderance of small dense LDL particles of increased atherogenicity.[35]

In general, most guidelines do not recommend specific targets for HDL cholesterol or triglycerides. This is because there is a lack of studies with clinical endpoints that have specifically altered HDL cholesterol or triglycerides independently of other lipids. Fibrates and nicotinic acid are the drugs most commonly used to lower triglycerides and increase HDL cholesterol. Studies using fibrates (e.g., VA-HIT,[36] FIELD[37]) and nicotinic acid (e.g., Coronary Drug Project[38]) have demonstrated a reduction in coronary heart disease events. However, LDL and total cholesterol were also lowered in these trials and it is difficult to attribute the reduction in events unequivocally to changes in particular lipids.

On balance, it seems reasonable to consider measures to increase HDL cholesterol or reduced triglycerides in individuals in whom levels remain undesirable after total and LDL cholesterol targets are achieved. This may be particularly appropriate in younger individuals at very high risk. It is likely that future trials will attempt to specifically address the value of raising HDL cholesterol using new pharmacologic agents.

Non-HDL cholesterol (total cholesterol minus HDL cholesterol) includes all cholesterol contained in apolipoprotein particles (LDL particles and triglyceride-rich lipoproteins). Non-HDL cholesterol therefore contains all of the pro-atherogenic lipoproteins and has the advantage that it can be measured in nonfasting samples. An appropriate target for non-HDL cholesterol is less than 130 mg/dL.

LIPID-LOWERING INTERVENTIONS

Lifestyle and diet

Having identified individuals at high CVD risk using appropriate national or international guidelines, initial lifestyle interventions to improve the CVD risk profile are recommended. These should include interventions to promote smoking cessation, optimal control of hypertension, and treatment of diabetes. Such advice should be given to all individuals at high CVD risk. This will include measures to promote weight loss where appropriate. In reference to dyslipidemia, specific advice should also be given to reduce total dietary fat to less than 30% of energy intake and to reduce the dietary cholesterol intake to less than 300 mg per day.[24]

In addition, saturated fats should account for less than 10% of energy intake, and in order to achieve this saturated fats should be replaced by monounsaturated fats in the diet. At least five portions per day of fruit and vegetables should be recommended, along with regular intake of oily fish and other sources of omega-3 fatty acids (equivalent to at least two portions of oily fish per week).[39] Dietary advice should be accompanied by advice to carry out 30 minutes of aerobic exercise on most days of the week.

Lifestyle intervention of this type has the potential to reduce total and LDL cholesterol by approximately 10%, and to produce moderate increases in HDL cholesterol. There is significant variation in individual response to dietary intervention, and occasional individuals will achieve significantly greater cholesterol reduction. However, overall response to dietary intervention in terms of cholesterol reduction is usually insufficient to achieve targets and most individuals are likely to require pharmacologic treatment in addition to lifestyle intervention.

Incorporation into the diet of specific foodstuffs with lipid-lowering properties can produce greater effects. These include plant stanol and sterol esters, soluble fiber, and soy protein. A portfolio diet including a mixture of such active ingredients can produce an LDL cholesterol reduction of approximately 30%, equivalent to the starting dose of most statins.[40] However, long-term compliance with a diet of this type is likely to be acceptable to only a small minority of individuals.

Specific lipid-lowering agents
Statins

A statin is the first-choice lipid-lowering agent in the overwhelming majority of patients. As discussed previously, statins have consistently demonstrated across a wide variety of placebo-controlled clinical trials their ability to reduce total and LDL cholesterol and to prevent total and fatal cardiovascular disease events. Specifically, pravastatin, lovastatin, simvastatin, and atorvastatin have been used in clinical endpoint trials. Fluvastatin and rosuvastatin also reduce total and LDL cholesterol, and it is likely that the reduction in LDL cholesterol is predictive of their clinical efficacy. Among other differences, the available statins differ in how effectively they reduce total and LDL cholesterol.

In practice, the choice of statin in individual patients is unlikely to matter significantly so long as appropriate reductions in total and LDL cholesterol are achieved. Any of the available statins will achieve a total and LDL cholesterol reduction of approximately 25%. In individuals in whom a larger reduction in total or LDL cholesterol is required to achieve target, one of the more effective statins (atorvastatin or rosuvastatin) is likely to be required. In any case, it is important to use an adequate dose of the chosen statin. If necessary, a low dose can be initiated and titrated up to achieve appropriate total and LDL cholesterol values. Using the highest doses of atorvastatin (80 mg) or rosuvastatin (40 mg), reductions in total and LDL cholesterol of more than 50% can be achieved.

In general, statins produce a similar degree of reduction in non-HDL cholesterol as in total and LDL cholesterol. Moderate reductions in triglycerides are also produced (10 to 30%), along with minimal increases in HDL cholesterol (0 to 10%). In patients who are unable to tolerate a statin as a result of side effects (see material following), it is usually necessary to use a combination of other lipid-lowering drugs. This would often include ezetimibe along with a fibrate or nicotinic acid in the first instance.

Fibrates

Fibrates may be used to lower triglycerides and to increase HDL cholesterol. They can also be used in combination with statins or other agents to provide additional reduction in LDL cholesterol. In most individuals with fasting triglycerides greater than 450 mg/dL, elevated total cholesterol is mainly due to cholesterol in the VLDL fraction. A fibrate is a suitable first-line lipid-lowering agent in this setting, and will typically achieve a triglyceride reduction of 30 to 50%. This will be associated with a decrease in total cholesterol (20 to 40%) and an increase in HDL cholesterol (5 to 15%). There is also likely to be a modest decrease in LDL cholesterol.

In patients who have already been treated with a statin, addition of a fibrate will further lower triglycerides and increase HDL cholesterol, and will provide a small additional decrease in LDL cholesterol. Fenofibrate has less potential than other fibrates to interact with statins, and is therefore the best fibrate to use in statin-fibrate combination therapy.

Nicotinic acid

In the pre-statin era, nicotinic acid was used as a total and LDL cholesterol-reducing agent. However, it is also the most effective drug currently available for increasing HDL cholesterol, and in addition lowers triglycerides significantly. Prolonged release forms of nicotinic acid are associated with reduced side effects (see material following), and are therefore preferred. Typical reductions in total cholesterol range from 5 to 15%, and LDL cholesterol from 5 to 20%.

Triglycerides are reduced from 10 to 40%, and HDL cholesterol increased from 15 to 30% (see Table 88–3). It is important to titrate the dose of prolonged-release nicotinic acid slowly upward in order to minimize the side effects, and a typical maintenance dose is 1000 to 2000 mg per day. Nicotinic acid is predominantly used in combination with a statin to provide additional LDL cholesterol reduction or to increase HDL cholesterol and reduced triglycerides once total and LDL cholesterol targets have been achieved.

Ezetimibe

Ezetimibe has become the lipid-lowering drug of choice to use in combination with a statin in patients who do not achieve total and LDL cholesterol targets on the maximum tolerated dose of the most effective statin. When added to a statin, ezetimibe produces an additional 15 to 25% reduction in total cholesterol and a 20 to 25% reduction in LDL cholesterol. There is a modest decrease in triglyceride of the order of 10%, and little change in HDL cholesterol. A single tablet combination of ezetimibe and simvastatin is available.

Omega-3 fatty acids

Omega-3 fatty acids are used predominantly to lower triglycerides in patients with severe hypertriglyceridemia. A dose of 2 g twice per day is normally required to produce significant triglyceride reduction. This is often used in addition to a statin fibrate combination in patients with severe hypertriglyceridemia. Triglyceride reductions of 10 to 20% usually result, and this may be associated with a small increase in LDL cholesterol.

Resins

Resins are most often used in patients unable to tolerate other lipid-lowering drugs. They provide effective reduction of total and LDL cholesterol, but their use may be associated with a small increase in triglycerides. Up to six sachets per day of cholestyramine or colestid are required for maximal effect.

Plant stanol and sterol esters

Stanol and sterol esters from plant sources can be incorporated into spreads or other food sources, and if 2 to 3 g per day are ingested a reduction in total and LDL cholesterol of about 10% can be achieved. This effect seems to be additional to the effect of most other lipid-lowering drugs, with the exception of ezetimibe.

COMPLICATIONS

In general, lipid-lowering treatment is safe and well tolerated. Some early studies suggested that very low levels of cholesterol were associated with an increased risk of cancer or death from accident/suicide as a result of altered neurologic function. However, subsequent large studies have not supported these suggestions.[41] Epidemiologic studies consistently show that very low levels of cholesterol are associated with increased mortality from a variety of causes, but because cholesterol is a negative acute phase reactant this is likely to be a consequence of underlying illness rather than implying any causative role for low cholesterol.

Statins

Overall, statins are safe and well-tolerated drugs. In placebo-controlled trials, withdrawal rates due to adverse events are typically between 2 and 5%. The most important statin-related side effects are disturbances of liver function tests and effects on skeletal muscle.[42] Skeletal-muscle-related side effects of statins can be divided into two groups: myalgia (muscle aches or weakness without creatine kinase (CK) elevation) and myositis (muscle aches or weakness with a CK elevation).

Various lines of evidence confirm that the incidence of such side effects is very low. For instance, in the Heart Protection Study CK concentrations rose to between 4 and 10 times the upper limit of normal in 0.2% of the simvastatin 40-mg group compared with 0.13% of the placebo group. CK concentrations greater than 10 times the upper limit of normal occurred in 0.11% of simvastatin recipients versus 0.06% of placebo recipients.[43] Similar findings have been reported for most other statins. The most common statin-related muscular side effect is myalgia. Pooled data from 44 clinical trials in patients treated with various doses of atorvastatin reported an incidence of treatment-associated myalgia of 1.9% compared with 0.8% with placebo.[44] Again, similar figures have been reported for other statins.

The most serious presentation of statin-related myopathy is rhabdomyolysis, which involves severe skeletal muscle injury and cell death and is associated with dramatic elevations of CK, myoglobinuria, and renal insufficiency. The incidence of statin-associated rhabdomyolysis is probably about 1 per 100,000 prescriptions for all statins, with cases of fatal rhabdomyolysis having an incidence of less than one death per million prescriptions.

Myositis and rhabdomyolysis occur most frequently at higher statin doses for all statins. Other factors associated with an increased risk of statin-associated myopathy include age greater than 70, female sex, low body mass, multisystem disease (e.g., chronic renal insufficiency, heart failure), the perioperative period, and interactions with specific concomitant medications. The most important of these are listed in Box 88–1. In general, therefore, factors associated with increased circulating statin concentrations lead to an increased risk of muscle-related side effects. The risk of these can be minimized by using lower statin doses in these settings.

Opinion is divided as to whether it is advisable to monitor CK concentrations routinely in patients receiving statin treatment. There is not a good evidence base to guide this. Many clinicians will choose to measure CK at baseline before commencing treatment, and only to measure CK subsequently if the patient complains of relevant symptoms.

Adverse statin effects on the liver predominately relate to the elevation of aspartate transaminase (AST) and alanine transaminase (ALT). There are isolated case reports of acute liver failure associated with statin treatment, but

---

Box 88–1

Important Statin Interactions

- Fibrates (especially gemfibrozil)
- Nicotinic acid
- Warfarin
- Ciclosporin
- Tacrolimus
- Protease inhibitors
- Grapefruit juice

---

the major statin trials have not reported any cases of cholestasis or severe hepatitis, suggesting that these must be extremely rare. Clinically significant elevations of AST or ALT (greater than three times the upper limit of the reference range) have typically been reported in about 1% or less of patients receiving statin treatment. The incidence is likely to be somewhat greater (up to 3%) in patients on high doses of the most effective statins. Minor elevations of transaminases are very common in the general population, most often due to nonalcoholic fatty liver disease, but there is no evidence that patients with minor disturbances of transaminases are any more likely to develop significant liver dysfunction after starting on statin treatment.

It is generally recommended that AST and ALT should be measured at baseline before starting statin treatment, and subsequently at about six weeks to three months after commencing treatment or after dose titration. Provided AST and ALT remain less than three times above the upper limit of the reference interval, treatment can be continued. However, statin treatment should be stopped if the transaminases exceed these limits.

Fibrates

Like statins, fibrates are generally well tolerated, with few significant side effects. The most common reasons for discontinuation of treatment are minor gastrointestinal side effects. Occasionally, muscle-related side effects or abnormal liver function tests are observed, but these are less common than with statins. Fibrates increase biliary cholesterol concentrations, and are contraindicated in patients with gallstones.

Fibrates increase serum creatinine concentrations by 10 to 15%. This is not associated with any decline in renal function and the change is reversible when the fibrate is discontinued. The likely mechanism is an effect on renal tubular creatinine transport.[45] Fibrate treatment also produces a significant increase in plasma homocysteine concentration. It is currently unclear whether this has any clinical significance.

Statin fibrate combination therapy is widely used in specialist lipid clinics. It has been suggested that such treatment may be associated with an increased risk of muscle-related side effects.[46] This is likely to be less of a problem when fenofibrate is used. It seems reasonable to warn any patient on combination statin fibrate treatment that they should discontinue the treatment if they experience unusual muscular aches and pains or weakness.

Nicotinic acid

The most common significant side effect of nicotinic acid is flushing. This occurs in approximately 75% of patients, even with prolonged-release forms of nicotinic acid. Mainly as a result of flushing, tolerability of nicotinic acid is relatively poor compared with other lipid-lowering agents. If patients can be encouraged to persist with nicotinic acid, flushing will decrease with time. To minimize the risk of significant flushing, prolonged-release forms of nicotinic acid should be used. Intact tablets can be taken before bedtime with a light snack. Excessive consumption of alcohol or spicy foods should be avoided, and aspirin taken shortly before the nicotinic acid tablet is also helpful.

Use of nicotinic acid is associated with minor deterioration of metabolic control in diabetes. This is generally not sufficiently severe to be a clinical problem,[47] but may be more marked in occasional patients. Higher doses of nicotinic acid can be associated with the development of hyperuricemia and gout. Minor gastrointestinal side effects are also relatively common.

Ezetimibe

Ezetimibe is generally well tolerated and is associated with few side effects. Minor gastrointestinal side effects occur rarely, and there have been occasional reports of disturbed liver function tests (predominately a cholestatic pattern) and muscle-related side effects.

Omega-3 fatty acids

Omega-3 fatty acids are generally well tolerated, apart from minor gastrointestinal side effects such as nausea and dyspepsia.

Resins

The most common side effects associated with resins are related to the gastrointestinal system, and constipation in particular may occur. Because resins may interfere with the absorption of fat-soluble vitamins, the diet may require supplementation with vitamins A, D, and K during high-dose treatment. Hypercholoremic acidosis has been reported very rarely after prolonged use of resins.[48]

SUMMARY

Hyperlipidemia is an important risk factor for atherosclerotic cardiovascular disease, and it is important that serum lipids should be treated in high-risk patients. This includes patients with established cardiovascular disease or with diabetes mellitus or healthy patients at high risk of cardiovascular disease as a result of risk factors. The primary target for treatment is total and LDL cholesterol. Secondary targets include non-HDL cholesterol, HDL cholesterol, and triglycerides. The main aim of treating hyperlipidemia is reduction of cardiovascular risk. Treatment of hyperlipidemia should therefore occur in the context of addressing all cardiovascular risk factors.

Lifestyle and dietary advice should be given to all patients for whom reduction of serum lipids is considered necessary. However, this will rarely be sufficient to achieve lipid target levels. A statin is the first-line drug of choice to reduce total and LDL cholesterol in the vast majority of patients for whom lipid-lowering therapy is considered necessary. Other lipid-lowering drugs can be used in combination with a statin or alone to achieve targets if necessary (Box 88–2). In general, lipid-lowering treatment is well tolerated and is associated with few side effects. Future developments are likely to focus on the development of new agents with greater potential to increase HDL cholesterol, such as cholesterol ester transfer protein inhibitors,[49] and studies assessing the value of therapies to increase HDL cholesterol may lead to the establishment of firm HDL cholesterol targets in addition to current LDL cholesterol targets.

Box 88–2

Use of Pharmaceutical Agents to Manage Dyslipidemia

Primary Target
- LDL cholesterol
  - Statin
  - Ezetimibe
  - Nicotinic acid/fibrate/resin

Secondary Targets
- HDL cholesterol
  - Nicotinic acid/fibrate
- Triglycerides
  - Fibrate
  - Statin
  - Nicotinic acid/omega-3 fatty acids

REFERENCES

1. Kromhout D. Epidemiology of cardiovascular diseases in Europe. *Public Health Nutr* 2001;4(2B):441–57.

2. Goldberg RJ, Burchfiel CM, Benfante R, et al. Lifestyle and biologic factors associated with atherosclerotic disease in middle-aged men: 20-year findings from the Honolulu Heart Program. *Arch Intern Med* 1995;155:686–94.

3. Ansell BJ, Navab M, Watson KE, et al. Anti-inflammatory properties of HDL. *Rev Endocr Metab Disord* 2004; 5:351–58.

4. Austin MA, Hokanson JE, Edwards KL. Hypertriglyceridemia as a cardiovascular risk factor. *Am J Cardiol* 1998;81:7B-12B.

5. Hamsten A, Silveira A, Boquist S, et al. The apolipoprotein CI content of triglyceride-rich lipoproteins independently predicts early atherosclerosis in healthy middle-aged men. *J Am Coll Cardiol* 2005;45:1013–17.

6. Jansen AC, van Aalst-Cohen ES, Tanck MW, et al. Genetic determinants of cardiovascular disease risk in familial hypercholesterolemia. *Arterioscler Thromb Vasc Biol* 2005;25:1475–81.

7. Kwiterovich PO Jr. The metabolic pathways of high-density lipoprotein, low-density lipoprotein, and triglycerides: A current review. *Am J Cardiol* 2000; 86:5L-10L.

8. Guo Q, Avramoglu R, Adeli K. Intestinal assembly and secretion of highly dense/lipid-poor apolipoprotein B48-containing lipoprotein particles in the fasting state: Evidence for induction by insulin resistance and exogenous fatty acids. *Metabolism* 2005; 54:689–97.

9. de Grooth GJ, Klerkx AH, Stroes ES, et al. A review of CETP and its relation to atherosclerosis. *J Lipid Res* 2004; 45:1967–74.

10. Julius U. Influence of plasma free fatty acids on lipoprotein synthesis and diabetic dyslipidemia. *Exp Clin Endocrinol Diabetes* 2003;111:246–50.

11. Packard CJ, Demant T, Stewart JP, et al. Apolipoprotein B metabolism and the distribution of VLDL and LDL subfractions. *J Lipid Res* 2000;41:305–18.

12. von Eckardstein A, Hersberger M, Rohrer L. Current understanding of the metabolism and biological actions of HDL. *Curr Opin Clin Nutr Metab Care* 2005;8:147–52.

13. Stroes E. Statins and LDL-cholesterol lowering: An overview. *Curr Med Res Opin* 2005;21:S9–16.

14. Vaughan CJ, Gotto AM Jr. Update on statins: 2003. *Circulation* 2004;110: 886–92.

15. Despres JP, Lemieux I, Robins SJ. Role of fibric acid derivatives in the management of risk factors for coronary heart disease. *Drugs* 2004;64:2177–98.

16. van Raalte DH, Li M, Pritchard PH, Wasan KM. Peroxisome proliferator-activated receptor (PPAR)-alpha: A pharmacological target with a promising future. *Pharm Res* 2004; 21:1531–38.

17. McCormack PL, Keating GM. Prolonged-release nicotinic acid: a review of its use in the treatment of dyslipidaemia. *Drugs* 2005;65:2719–40.

18. Garcia-Calvo M, Lisnock J, et al. The target of ezetimibe is Niemann-Pick C1-Like 1 (NPC1L1). *Proc Natl Acad Sci USA* 2005;102:8132–37.

19. Kosoglou T, Statkevich P, Johnson-Levonas AO, et al. Ezetimibe: A review of its metabolism, pharmacokinetics and drug interactions. *Clin Pharmacokinet* 2005;44:467–94.

20. Bhatnagar D, Durrington PN. Omega-3 fatty acids: Their role in the prevention and treatment of atherosclerosis related risk factors and complications. *Int J Clin Pract* 2003;57:305–14.

21. Plat J, Mensink RP. Plant stanol and sterol esters in the control of blood cholesterol levels: Mechanism and safety aspects. *Am J Cardiol* 2005; 96:15D-22D.

22. Ast M, Frishman WH. Bile acid sequestrants. *J Clin Pharmacol* 1990; 30:99–106.

23. British Cardiac Society; British Hypertension Society; Diabetes UK; HEART UK; Primary Care Cardiovascular Society; Stroke Association. JBS 2: Joint British Societies' guidelines on prevention of cardiovascular disease in clinical practice. *Heart* 2005;91(5):v1–52.

24. Expert Panel on Detection, Evaluation, and Treatment of High Blood Cholesterol in Adults. Executive Summary of the Third Report of the National Cholesterol Education Program (NCEP) Expert Panel on Detection, Evaluation, and Treatment of High Blood Cholesterol in Adults (Adult Treatment Panel III). *JAMA* 2001; 285:2486–97.

25. De Backer G, Ambrosioni E, Borch-Johnsen K, et al. European guidelines on cardiovascular disease prevention in clinical practice. Third Joint Task Force of European and other societies on cardiovascular disease prevention in clinical practice (constituted by representatives of eight societies and by invited experts). *Arch Mal Coeur Vaiss* 2004;97:1019–30.

26. Randomised trial of cholesterol lowering in 4444 patients with coronary heart disease: The Scandinavian Simvastatin Survival Study (4S). *Lancet* 1994; 344:1383–89.

27. Shepherd J, Cobbe SM, Ford I, et al. Prevention of coronary heart disease with pravastatin in men with hypercholesterolemia: West of Scotland Coronary Prevention Study Group. *N Engl J Med* 1995;333:1301–7.

28. Pfeffer MA, Sacks FM, Moye LA, et al. Cholesterol and Recurrent Events: A secondary prevention trial for normolipidemic patients. *Am J Cardiol* 1995;76:98C-106C.

29. Sever PS, Dahlof B, Poulter NR, et al. Prevention of coronary and stroke events with atorvastatin in hypertensive patients who have average or lower-than-average cholesterol concentrations, in the Anglo-Scandinavian Cardiac Outcomes Trial, Lipid Lowering Arm (ASCOT-LLA): A multicentre randomised controlled trial. *Lancet* 2003;361: 1149–58.

30. Colhoun HM, Betteridge DJ, Durrington PN, et al. Primary prevention of cardiovascular disease with atorvastatin in type 2 diabetes in the Collaborative Atorvastatin Diabetes Study (CARDS): Multicentre randomised placebo-controlled trial. *Lancet* 2004;364: 685–96.

31. Cannon CP, Braunwald E, McCabe CH, et al. Pravastatin or Atorvastatin Evaluation and Infection Therapy-Thrombolysis in Myocardial Infarction 22 Investigators: Intensive versus moderate lipid lowering with statins after acute coronary syndromes. *N Engl J Med* 2004;350:1495–504.

32. Pedersen TR, Faergeman O, Kastelein JJ, et al. Incremental Decrease in End Points Through Aggressive Lipid Lowering (IDEAL) Study Group: High-dose atorvastatin vs usual-dose simvastatin for secondary prevention after myocardial infarction. The IDEAL study: A randomized controlled trial. *JAMA* 2005;294:2437–45. Erratum in *JAMA* 2005;294:3092.

33. LaRosa JC, Grundy SM, Waters DD, et al. Treating to New Targets (TNT) Investigators: Intensive lipid lowering with atorvastatin in patients with stable coronary disease. *N Engl J Med* 2005; 352:1425–35.

34. Baigent C, Keech A, Kearney PM, et al. Efficacy and safety of cholesterol-lowering treatment: Prospective meta-analysis of data from 90,056 participants in 14 randomised trials of statins. *Lancet* 2005;366:1267–78. Erratum in *Lancet* 2005;366:1358.

35. Nesto RW. Beyond low-density lipoprotein: Addressing the atherogenic lipid triad in type 2 diabetes mellitus and the metabolic syndrome. *Am J Cardiovasc Drugs* 2005;5:379–87.

36. Robins SJ, Collins D, Wittes JT, et al. Veterans Affairs High-Density Lipoprotein Intervention Trial: Relation of gemfibrozil treatment and lipid levels with major coronary events. VA-HIT: A randomized controlled trial. *JAMA* 2001;285:1585–91.

37. Keech A, Simes RJ, Barter P, et al. Effects of long-term fenofibrate therapy on cardiovascular events in 9795 people with type 2 diabetes mellitus (the FIELD study): Randomised controlled trial. *Lancet* 2005;366:1849–61.

38. Canner PL, Berge KG, Wenger NK, et al. Fifteen year mortality in Coronary Drug Project patients: Long-term benefit with niacin. *J Am Coll Cardiol* 1986;8: 1245–55.

39. Kris-Etherton PM, Harris WS, Appel LJ; AHA Nutrition Committee. Omega-3 fatty acids and cardiovascular disease: New recommendations from the American Heart Association. *Arterioscler Thromb Vasc Biol* 2003;23:151–52.

40. Jenkins DJ, Kendall CW, Marchie A, et al. Direct comparison of a dietary portfolio of cholesterol-lowering foods with a statin in hypercholesterolemic participants. *Am J Clin Nutr* 2005; 81:380–87.

41. Law MR, Thompson SG, Wald NJ. Assessing possible hazards of reducing serum cholesterol. *BMJ* 1994;308: 373–79.

42. Vasudevan AR, Hamirani YS, Jones PH. Safety of statins: Effects on muscle and

the liver. *Cleve Clin J Med* 2005;72: 990–93,996–1001.

43. Heart Protection Study Collaborative Group. MRC/BHF Heart Protection Study of cholesterol lowering with simvastatin in 20,536 high-risk individuals: A randomised placebo-controlled trial. *Lancet* 2002;360:7–22.

44. Newman CB, Palmer G, Silbershatz H, Szarek M. Safety of atorvastatin derived from analysis of 44 completed trials in 9,416 patients. *Am J Cardiol* 2003; 92:670–76.

45. Elisaf M. Effects of fibrates on serum metabolic parameters. *Curr Med Res Opin* 2002;18:269–76.

46. Jacobson TA, Zimmerman FH. Fibrates in combination with statins in the management of dyslipidemia. *J Clin Hypertens* (Greenwich) 2006;8:35–41.

47. Shepherd J, Betteridge J, Van Gaal L; European Consensus Panel. Nicotinic acid in the management of dyslipidaemia associated with diabetes and metabolic syndrome: A position paper developed by a European

Consensus Panel. *Curr Med Res Opin* 2005;21:665–82.

48. Scheel PJ Jr., Whelton A, Rossiter K, Watson A. Cholestyramine-induced hyperchloremic metabolic acidosis. *J Clin Pharmacol* 1992;32:536–38.

49. Forrester JS, Makkar R, Shah PK. Increasing high-density lipoprotein cholesterol in dyslipidemia by cholesteryl ester transfer protein inhibition: An update for clinicians. *Circulation* 2005;111:1847–54.

Chapter

89

Antithrombotic Therapy in Hypertension

Gregory Y. H. Lip

Key Findings

- Current guidelines suggest that antiplatelet therapy (in particular, low-dose aspirin) is recommended for secondary prevention in patients with previous cardiovascular events to reduce the risk of stroke and myocardial infarction, provided the patients are not at excessive risk of bleeding.

- In hypertensive patients, low-dose aspirin is beneficial as primary prevention in patients older than 50 years of age with moderate increase in serum creatinine or a 10-year total cardiovascular risk of greater than 20%.

- In all hypertensives, low-dose aspirin should be preceded by well-controlled blood pressure.

Hypertension is clearly associated with increased risk for stroke. In the Framingham study, the presence of hypertension as a risk factor increased the risk of stroke 3.4-fold. In comparison, the presence of atrial fibrillation (AF) increased the risk of stroke 4.8-fold.[1]

Although systemic (arterial) hypertension results in high intravascular pressure, the main complications of hypertension [coronary heart disease (CHD), ischemic strokes, and peripheral vascular disease (PVD)] are related to thrombosis rather than to hemorrhage. The association between hypertension and risk for stroke and CHD almost appears to have a dose-response relationship, with increasing risk for higher blood pressures.[2–4] In middle and old age, there is a direct relationship between blood pressure and the risk of cardiovascular death without any evidence of a threshold down to a blood pressure of at least 115/75 mmHg.[5] Correspondingly, blood pressure reduction trials have shown a reduction in CHD by 16% and stroke by 38%. It should not be forgotten that hypertension is a risk factor for both hemorrhagic and ischemic strokes.

Some of the complications related to hypertension, such as heart failure and AF, are themselves associated with stroke and thromboembolism.[6] Increasing evidence also points toward a prothrombotic or hypercoagulable state conferred by the presence of hypertension, as evidenced by abnormalities of coagulation, platelets, and endothelial function in such patients.[7] There is also the recognition that hypertension is associated with abnormalities of inflammation, which can "drive" the prothrombotic state and contribute to endothelial abnormalities in this condition.[8–9]

It therefore seems plausible that use of antithrombotic therapy may help to prevent thrombosis-related complications of hypertension.[6] The antiplatelet agent aspirin has been recommended but frequently underutilized in the treatment and secondary prevention of many of the complications of hypertension.[10] Until recently, limited information has been available on its role in the management of the asymptomatic hypertensive individual. Warfarin has also been found to be useful as thromboprophylaxis in hypertensive patients with AF.[11] However, if blood pressures remain uncontrolled such therapy carries significant risks, especially from intracranial hemorrhage.[11]

WHAT DO THE GUIDELINES TELL US?

The 2003 joint European Society of Hypertension and European Society of Cardiology Guidelines[12] for the management of arterial hypertension recommended antiplatelet therapy (in particular, low-dose aspirin) for patients with previous cardiovascular events to reduce the risk of stroke and myocardial infarction, provided the patients are not at excessive risk of bleeding. In hypertensive patients, low-dose aspirin was particularly beneficial in patients older than 50 years of age with moderate increase in serum creatinine or a 10-year total cardiovascular risk of greater than 20%. In all hypertensive patients, low-dose aspirin should be preceded by good blood pressure control.

Broadly similar recommendations are provided by the North American JNC-7[13] and the British Hypertension Society guidelines.[14] The latter recommends that "unless contraindicated, low-dose aspirin (75 mg/day) is (used) for all people needing secondary prevention of ischaemic cardiovascular disease (CVD), and primary prevention in people with hypertension over the age of 50 years who have a 10-year CVD risk ≥20% and in whom BP is controlled."

WHAT DO THE TRIALS TELL US?

In terms of secondary prevention, the Antithrombotic Trialists' Collaboration clearly shows the efficacy of antiplatelet therapy and vascular events in various high-risk groups, reducing stroke and vascular events by 22%.[15] In an earlier analysis from the Antiplatelet Trialists' Collaboration,[16] data in relation to diastolic blood pressure were provided and suggested that in patients with diastolic blood pressure >90-mmHg antiplatelet therapy reduced events from 20.2 to 18.1%, translating to a benefit of 41 per 1000 patients (Table 89–1). However, the benefits of aspirin as a secondary prevention post myocardial infarction may only be most apparent in the first 35 days, as subsequent death rate ratios beyond day 35 showed no significant difference between aspirin and placebo use and the survival curves beyond day 35 were essentially parallel.[17]

In the Primary Prevention Project,[18] open-label aspirin 100 mg a day was given to participants, 69% of whom where hypertensive. This trial showed a reduction of total cardiovascular events (relative risk 0.77), cardiovascular deaths (relative risk 0.56), myocardial infarction (relative risk 0.69), and stroke (relative risk 0.67).

The only randomized placebo-controlled trial designed to investigate the effects of antithrombotic therapy (aspirin) on cardiovascular events and hemorrhagic complication in treated hypertensive patients was the large Hypertension Optimal Treatment (HOT) study.[19] This trial was a primary prevention trial in patients with elevated blood pressure (DBP between 100 and 115 mmHg). The aspirin component of this trial was a double-blind placebo controlled design, aspirin 75 mg, or identical placebo tablets once daily. Major cardiovascular events were defined as fatal and nonfatal myocardial infarction, fatal and nonfatal stroke, and other cardiovascular deaths. Silent myocardial infarction was defined as new Q or QS waves without clinical signs of myocardial infarction.

In the HOT study,[19] aspirin 75 mg resulted in a 36% reduction in myocardial infarction ($p=0.02$), with 45 fewer myocardial infarction events in the aspirin group compared to placebo. Interestingly, there were no significant differences in stroke events, but as cerebral scans were not routinely reported the possibility remains that some strokes were hemorrhagic. In HOT, there were 52 more gastrointestinal bleeds in patients given aspirin ($n=107$) compared to placebo ($n=55$), with no significant difference between aspirin and placebo for major bleeds. In a subsequent analysis[20] of aspirin on major cardiovascular events, a favorable balance between benefit and harm of aspirin was found in patients with a higher global baseline

cardiovascular risk and baseline systolic blood pressure >180 mmHg or diastolic blood pressure >107 mmHg. Furthermore, patients with serum creatinine >1.3 mg/dL has significantly greater reduction in cardiovascular events and myocardial infarction.[20] Importantly, uncontrolled blood pressures did significantly increase the risk of bleeding. The "numbers needed to treat" (NNT) for cardiovascular events in the overall HOT study was 176, versus "numbers needed to harm" (NNH) for bleeding of 188, which are quite close to each other. In contrast, among "high-risk" patients the NNT was 86, compared to an NNH of 205.

The Thrombosis Prevention Trial[21,22] was a primary prevention trial in patients with high risk of ischemic heart disease. Data for subgroup analysis of patients treated with antihypertensive medication at entry or during trial was reported in a subsequent publication. In this trial,[22] the relative risk of major cardiovascular events (coronary heart disease and stroke) by systolic blood pressure analyzed according to treatment suggests that aspirin gives a relative risk of 0.59 with systolic blood pressures <130 mmHg, a relative risk of 0.68 for systolic blood pressures of 130 to 145 mmHg, and a relative risk of 1.08 in the strata of systolic blood pressure >145 mmHg. In this trial, 5 to 10 episodes of cerebral hemorrhage occurred in men with blood pressures >145 mmHg in the combined warfarin plus aspirin treatment group (reflecting in a relative risk of 1.74).

Stroke is a devastating manifestation of hypertensive target organ damage. In an analysis of acute stroke trials,[23] aspirin use in this setting can be detrimental because it results in a 22% increase in the risk of hemorrhagic transformation. However, aspirin reduced the risk of recurrent ischemic stroke by 23%. In the MATCH trial[24] of clopidogrel with or without aspirin in TIA or stroke survivors, the addition of clopidogrel to aspirin resulted in no significant effects on vascular events, heart attacks, or strokes—even among the hypertensive subgroup ($n=5945$), which showed no difference in vascular events. However, there was a substantial increase in bleeding events by the addition of clopidogrel to aspirin.

TABLE 89–1. ASPIRIN VERSUS CONTROL IN HYPERTENSION: SUBGROUP ANALYSIS IN ANTITHROMBOTIC TRIALISTS' COLLABORATION META-ANALYSIS 1994				
DBP (mmHg)	<90		90+	
	Aspirin	Control	Aspirin	Control
Vascular events	1168	1451	2700	1073
No. patients	8330	8421	21,136	5308
[%]	14.0	17.2	12.8	20.2
p	<0.0001		<0.0001	
DBP = diastolic blood pressure. (Adapted from Antithrombotic Trialists' Collaboration 1994.)				

Table 89–1. Aspirin Versus Control in Hypertension: Subgroup Analysis in Antithrombotic Trialists' Collaboration Meta-analysis 1994

WHAT DOES THE COCHRANE REVIEW TELL US?

A Cochrane systematic review on antithrombotic therapy use in hypertension[24] concluded that for primary prevention in patients with hypertension antiplatelet therapy with aspirin could not be recommended because the magnitude of benefit (a reduction in myocardial infarction) was negated by a harm of similar magnitude, with an increase in major hemorrhage. For secondary prevention in patient with hypertension, antiplatelet therapy was recommended because the magnitude of the benefit over risk was many times greater. The analysis from the Cochrane review[24] is summarized in the following section.

Aspirin versus placebo

All-cause mortality was reported in one trial (HOT[19]), where mortality was 3.0% in the aspirin-treated patients compared to 3.2% in the placebo control group and was not significantly different ($p=0.36$). The cardiovascular and non-cardiovascular mortality were also not significantly different.

Cardiovascular events were evaluated in two studies.[19,22] In the HOT trial, aspirin reduced myocardial infarction (ARR = 0.5%, NNT = 200) and major cardiovascular events (ARR = 0.57%, NNT = 176) compared to placebo. However, when all cardiovascular events (including silent MI) were considered the reduction failed to reach statistical significance. In the Thrombosis Prevention Trial, no significant difference was observed in the cardiovascular events in the hypertensive subgroup between the aspirin (8.5%) and placebo (7.5%). When the results of both studies were pooled for all cardiovascular events, there was no significant difference with aspirin compared to placebo (OR 0.93; 95% CI: 0.82 to 1.06). In the pooled results of two trials (HOT, Thrombosis Prevention Trial), there was no significant difference between the aspirin and the control group for ischemic strokes (OR 0.94, 95% CI: 0.76 to 1.17).

Hemorrhage

The hemorrhagic effects of aspirin alone when compared to placebo were evaluated in the HOT study.[19] There was a significant increase in major bleeds (ARI = 0.65%, NNH = 154) and minor bleeds (ARI = 0.73%, NNH = 137) with aspirin compared to placebo. The differences in these events were mainly gastrointestinal (72 versus 34 for major bleeds and 30 versus 18 for minor bleeds) and nasal bleeds (22 versus 12 for major bleeds and 66 versus 24 for minor bleeds) in the aspirin group. There were no significant differences in fatal hemorrhagic events (7 in aspirin group versus 8 in placebo group).

Aspirin versus clopidogrel

The composite endpoint of stroke, myocardial infarction or vascular death, has been evaluated in one study in hypertensive patients and was not different in patients taking aspirin, 12.1%, as compared to clopidogrel, 11.0%[26]. Data on all-cause mortality, cardiovascular mortality, all cardiovascular events, stroke, myocardial infarction, or haemorrhagic events were not reported.

IMPLICATIONS FOR ANTIHYPERTENSIVE DRUG TREATMENT

Antiplatelet therapy use may have implications for the drug management of hypertension. There has long been some concern that aspirin may reduce the efficacy of ACE inhibitors, especially in heart failure patients.[27] Aspirin also influenced the mortality benefits of ACE inhibitors in the SOLVD studies, as well as the effect of ramipril in cardiovascular risk prevention in the HOPE study.[28] For example, subjects who are not taking aspirin had a 40% reduction in endpoints in the HOPE study compared to a 15% reduction among aspirin users.[26]

Although low-dose aspirin does not significantly interfere with the blood-pressure-lowering effects of antihypertensive therapy,[29] aspirin use did influence major cardiovascular event rates. Patients never treated with an ACE inhibitor had a 21% reduction in major cardiovascular events, whereas patients treated with an ACE inhibitor at least during some part of the follow-up had a 13% reduction in major cardiovascular events.

ASSOCIATED CONDITIONS

Hypertension is clearly associated with conditions that may merit anticoagulation therapy. For example, AF is the most common cardiac arrhythmia, and hypertension is the most important medical condition associated with AF.[30] Hypertension features in major risk stratification criteria for thromboprophylaxis in AF, and the presence of hypertension is accumulated to other risk factors such as congestive heart failure, diabetes, or previous stroke in AF.[11] Heart failure is another condition associated with hypertension that has an excess risk of thromboembolism.[31] In the two studies,[32] the use of aspirin resulted in more hospitalizations (27%) compared to warfarin-treated patients, which was not seen in patients taking clopidogrel.

CONCLUSIONS

Stroke and cardiovascular disease are often thrombosis-related complications closely related to hypertension. Antiplatelet therapy plays some role in treating hypertension, at least in some cases. In essential hypertension, antiplatelet therapy should only be used for primary prevention if the patients are at high risk and blood pressure control is excellent. Current guidelines also recommend antiplatelet therapy as secondary prevention against further vascular events. Limited data exists for warfarin as primary or secondary prevention in patients with essential hypertension, who are in sinus rhythm.[24]

However, certain hypertensive patient subgroups merit greater consideration of antithrombotic therapy use. In AF, for example, antiplatelet therapy is useful in low-risk patients. However, warfarin is needed for high-risk subjects. In heart failure, aspirin may cause more hospitalizations due to an interaction with ACE inhibitors, but further data from other trials are required.

REFERENCES

1. Wolf PA, Abbott RD, Kannel WB. Atrial fibrillation as an independent risk factor for stroke: The Framingham Study. *Stroke* 1991;22(8):983–88.
2. Collins R, MacMahon S. Blood pressure, antihypertensive drug treatment and the risks of stroke and of coronary heart disease. *Br Med Bull* 1994;50(2):272–98.
3. Collins R, Peto R, MacMahon S, Hebert P, Fiebach NH, Eberlein KA, et al. Blood pressure, stroke, and coronary heart disease. Part 2, Short-term reductions in blood pressure: Overview of randomised drug trials in their epidemiological context. *Lancet* 1990;335(8693):827–38.
4. Collins R, Peto R, MacMahon S, Hebert P, Fiebach NH, Eberlein KA, et al. Blood pressure, stroke, and coronary heart disease. Part 1, Prolonged differences in blood pressure: Prospective observational studies corrected for the regression dilution bias. *Lancet* 1990;335(8692):765–74.
5. Prospective Studies Collaboration. Age-specific relevance of usual blood pressure to vascular mortality: A meta-analysis of individual data for one million adults in 61 prospective studies. *Lancet* 2002;360:1903–13.
6. Lip GYH, Edmunds E, Beevers DG. Should patients with hypertension receive antithrombotic therapy? *Journal of Internal Medicine* 2001;249:205–14.
7. Nadar S, Lip GY. The prothrombotic state in hypertension and the effects of antihypertensive treatment. *Curr Pharm Des* 2003;9(21):1715–32.
8. Bautista LE. Inflammation, endothelial dysfunction, and the risk of high blood pressure: Epidemiologic and biological evidence. *J Hum Hypertens* 2003;17:223–30.
9. Boos CJ, Lip GY. Elevated high-sensitive C-reactive protein, large arterial stiffness and atherosclerosis: A relationship between inflammation and hypertension? *J Hum Hypertens* 2005;19(7):511–13.
10. Stafford RS, Monti V, Ma J. Underutilization of aspirin persists in U.S. ambulatory care for the secondary and primary prevention of cardiovascular disease. *PLoS Med* 2005;2(12):e353.
11. Lip GY, Boos C. Antithrombotic therapy for atrial fibrillation. *Heart* 2005;Sept. 13 [E-pub ahead of print].
12. European Society of Hypertension-European Society of Cardiology Guidelines Committee. 2003 European Society of Hypertension-European Society of Cardiology guidelines for the management of arterial hypertension. *J Hypertens* 2003;21(6):1011–53.
13. Chobanian AV, Bakris GL, Black HR, Cushman WC, Green LA, Izzo JL Jr., et al. National Heart, Lung, and Blood Institute Joint National Committee on Prevention, Detection, Evaluation, and Treatment of High Blood Pressure; National High Blood Pressure Education Program Coordinating Committee. The Seventh Report of the Joint National Committee on Prevention, Detection, Evaluation, and Treatment of High Blood Pressure: The JNC 7 report. *Hypertension* 2003;42:1206–52.
14. Williams B, Poulter NR, Brown MJ, Davis M, McInnes GT, Potter JF, et al. British Hypertension Society. Guidelines for management of hypertension: Report of the fourth working party of the British Hypertension Society, 2004-BHS IV. *J Hum Hypertens* 2004;18(3):139–85.
15. Antithrombotic Trialists' Collaboration. Collaborative meta–analysis of randomised trials of antiplatelet therapy for prevention of death, myocardial infarction, and stroke in high risk patients. *BMJ* 2002;324:71–86.
16. Antiplatelet Trialists' Collaboration. Collaborative overview of randomised trials of antiplatelet therapy. I: Prevention of death, myocardial infarction, and stroke by prolonged antiplatelet therapy in various categories of patients. *BMJ* 1994;308(6921):81–106.
17. Baigent C, Collins R, Appleby P, Parish S, Sleight P, Peto R. ISIS-2: 10 year survival among patients with suspected acute myocardial infarction in randomised comparison of intravenous streptokinase, oral aspirin, both, or neither. The ISIS-2 (Second International Study of Infarct Survival) Collaborative Group. *BMJ* 1998;316(7141):1337–43.
18. de Gaetano G. Low-dose aspirin and vitamin E in people at cardiovascular risk: A randomised trial in general practice. Collaborative Group of the Primary Prevention Project. *Lancet* 2001;357(9250):89–95. Erratum in: *Lancet* 2001;357(9262):1134.
19. Hansson L, Zanchetti A, Carruthers SG, Dahlof B, Elmfeldt D, Julius S, et al. for the HOT Study Group. Effects of intensive blood-pressure lowering and low-dose aspirin in patients with hypertension: Principle results of the Hypertension Optimal Treatment randomised trial. *Lancet* 1998;351:1755–62.
20. Zanchetti A, Hansson L, Dahlof B, Julius S, Menard J, Warnold I, et al. for the HOT Study Group. Benefit and harm of low-dose aspirin in well-treated hypertensives at different baseline cardiovascular risk. *J Hypertens* 2002;20(11):2301–07.
21. The Medical Research Council's General Practice Research Framework. Thrombosis prevention trial: Randomised trial of low-intensity oral anticoagulation with warfarin and low-dose aspirin in the primary prevention of ischaemic heart disease in men at increased risk. *Lancet* 1998;351(9098):233–41.
22. Meade TW, Brennan PJ. Determination of who may derive most benefit from aspirin in primary prevention: Subgroup results from a randomised controlled trial. *BMJ* 2000;321:13–17.
23. CAST (Chinese Acute Stroke Trial) Collaborative Group. CAST: Randomised placebo-controlled trial of early aspirin use in 20,000 patients with acute ischaemic stroke. *Lancet* 1997;349(9066):1641–49.
24. Felmeden DC, Lip GY. Antithrombotic therapy in hypertension: A Cochrane systematic review. *J Hum Hypertens* 2005;19(3):185–96.
25. Diener HC, Bogousslavsky J, Brass LM, Cimminiello C, Csiba L, Kaste M, et al. for the MATCH investigators. Aspirin and clopidogrel compared with clopidogrel alone after recent ischaemic stroke or transient ischaemic attack in high-risk patients (MATCH): Randomised, double-blind, placebo-controlled trial. *Lancet* 2004;364(9431):331–37.
26. CAPRIE Steering Committee. A randomised, blinded, trial of clopidogrel versus aspirin in patients at risk of ischaemic events (CAPRIE). *Lancet* 1996;348(9038):1329–39.
27. Harjai KJ, Nunez E, Turgut T, Newman J. Effect of combined aspirin and angiotensin-converting enzyme inhibitor therapy versus angiotensin-converting enzyme inhibitor therapy alone on readmission rates in heart failure. *Am J Cardiol* 2001;87(4):483–87.
28. Cleland JG. Is aspirin "the weakest link" in cardiovascular prophylaxis? The surprising lack of evidence supporting the use of aspirin for cardiovascular disease. *Prog Cardiovasc Dis* 2002;44(4):275–92.
29. Zanchetti A, Hansson L, Leonetti G, Rahn KH, Ruilope L, Warnold I, et al. Low-dose aspirin does not interfere with the blood pressure-lowering effects of antihypertensive therapy. *J Hypertens* 2002;20(5):1015–22.
30. Boos CJ, Lip GY. Targeting the renin-angiotensin-aldosterone system in atrial fibrillation: From pathophysiology to clinical trials. *J Hum Hypertens* 2005;19(11):855–59.
31. Lip GYH, Gibbs CR. Antiplatelet agents versus control or anticoagulation for heart failure in sinus rhythm (Cochrane Review). In: *The Cochrane Library, Volume 4*. Chichester, UK: John Wiley & Sons, 2001:CD003333.
32. Cleland JG, Ghosh J, Freemantle N, Kaye GC, Nasir M, Clark AL, et al. Clinical trials update and cumulative meta-analyses from the American College of Cardiology: WATCH, SCD-HeFT, DINAMIT, CASINO, INSPIRE, STRATUS-US, RIO-Lipids and cardiac resynchronisation therapy in heart failure. *Eur J Heart Fail* 2004;6(4):501–08.

Chapter

90

Control of Blood Glucose and Insulin Resistance

Kathleen Wyne and George L. Bakris

Key Findings

- People with diabetes have an increased risk of high blood pressure and cardiovascular disease.

- Insulin resistance and hyperglycemia independently contribute to the development of cardiovascular disease.

- Reducing insulin resistance reduces cardiovascular disease risk if the treatment is begun early enough in the disease process.

- Inhibition of the renin-angiotensin system improves glucose utilization and reduces insulin resistance.

- Aggressive identification of diabetes in people with hypertension is needed to decrease the morbidity and mortality seen in this population.

Hypertension is estimated to be present in at least 73% of the people in the United States who have diabetes, but less than 40% are at goal.[1] Many of these people are diagnosed with hypertension prior to having been diagnosed with diabetes. As noted in both the ADA and JNC 7 guidelines, one should screen for diabetes at the time of diagnosis of hypertension and repeat screening on an annual basis.

The rationale for aggressive diagnosis and treatment of diabetes in people with hypertension is that the combination is associated with an increased risk of cardiovascular events. In the first few years of the U.K. Prospective Diabetes Study Group (UKPDS), the morbidity and mortality was much higher in the 40% of the cohort who had been diagnosed with hypertension prior to the diagnosis of diabetes. This prompted the addition of the blood pressure control substudy, which showed that blood pressure control had a significant impact on decreasing both microvascular and macrovascular disease.[2–4]

Although blood pressure control is clearly important, it does not prevent all complications related to hyperglycemia. The long-term evaluation of the Diabetes Control and Complications Trial (DCCT) cohort has shown that intensive glucose control has delayed benefits in preventing macrovascular disease in patients with type 1 diabetes.[5] Thus, treatment must address the underlying disease and prevent any elevation in glucose.

The studies designed to investigate prevention of the complications of diabetes have focused on studying people who already have diabetes and then improving glucose control to prevent development of additional complications. These short-term studies have shown that improving hyperglycemia prevents microvascular events but not macrovascular events.[6,7] One exception has been the overweight subgroup in the UKPDS study, in which treatment with metformin was associated with a statistically significant decrease in myocardial infarctions (the significance of which is unknown).[8] In a recent clinical study, treatment of diabetes with agents that improve insulin resistance in patients with established diabetes and vascular disease did not result in a decrease of composite vascular endpoints, but did decrease some secondary macrovascular endpoints.[9]

Given the length of time required to see this benefit in people with type 1 diabetes, it is possible that the window of opportunity has already been lost when type 2 diabetes is diagnosed (as most of these people have had a prolonged period of hyperglycemia prior to their diagnosis). Studies are now ongoing to understand the disease process (i.e., the insulin resistance and the changes in the vasculature) to allow development of therapies that will be effective once the hyperglycemia is diagnosed. Simultaneously, strategies are being developed to diagnose type 2 diabetes earlier to prevent the morbidity and mortality associated with the disease.

The metabolic changes that are associated with insulin resistance, abnormal glucose regulation, and ultimately the hyperglycemia used to identify type 2 diabetes begin long before the sugar is elevated. This is likely why the studies designed to prevent the complications associated with diabetes have not been very successful. Animal studies have shown that there are abnormalities in fat metabolism that begin long before the sugar rises, which leads to an elevation of circulating free fatty acids (FFAs). These lead to the production of inflammatory cytokines.

These cytokines are initially involved in local changes in the vasculature in the adipose tissue that alter insulin and angiotensin II signaling. Over time, the excess FFAs are deposited (termed ectopic fat deposition) in nonadipose tissues, which leads to lipotoxicity.[10,11] This ectopic fat deposition can lead to abnormal cell function and potentially to cell death, but can also result in further inappropriate production of inflammatory cytokines and thus exacerbate the miscommunication between the vasculature and the adipose tissue.

LIPOTOXICITY

The metabolic abnormalities that occur in the adipose tissue are a combination of environmental (i.e., excess delivery of nutrients for storage) and genetic factors (i.e., an inability to store or metabolize the excess of nutrients). Although healthy lifestyle is one proven method of preventing this process, people appear to have different levels of sensitivity for developing the early stages of lipotoxicity. As the adipocyte enlarges, while trying to store the excess nutrients it also tries to metabolize them to minimize the mechanical stress on the cell. These changes, in addition to the intracellular energy fluxes, disrupt cellular homeostasis and lead to intracellular stress responses. One of these has been termed the endoplasmic reticulum (ER) stress response, which occurs when the intracellular stress alters the homeostasis in the endoplasmic reticulum, leading to activation of a signal transduction system linking the ER lumen with the cytoplasm and nucleus.

Intracellular signaling pathways are then activated or deactivated to preserve the cell's basic metabolic functions. These pathways lead to alterations in the activity of enzymes such as AMP-kinase and the c-Jun N-terminal kinase (JNK), which then affects the phosphorylation status of the insulin receptor and IRS-1 and in turn facilitates insulin resistance in the cell.[12] Insulin is then not able to activate its receptor to prevent lipolysis, and the unregulated release of FFAs results in an alteration of the circulating levels of the adipose-derived cytokines (which are also called adipocytokines).

These include adiponectin, leptin, TNF-alpha, Interleukin-6 (IL-6), and resistin. The enlarged adipocytes then secrete less adiponectin and more leptin and TNF-α as a form of communication to the nonadipose tissues to stimulate fatty acid oxidation with a goal of depleting the whole-body load of fatty acids. Teleologically, this would appear to be an appropriate response. However, if the nonadipose tissues are not able to respond appropriately to these adipocytokines and store the fatty acids instead of metabolizing them insulin resistance may also develop in other tissues throughout the body.

These adipocytokines also have other functions involved in responding to inflammation to provide adequate nutrition in the presence of stress (i.e., viral or bacterial infection). For example, TNF-alpha also stimulates preadipocytes to produce monocyte chemoattractant protein-1 (MCP-1). The local endothelial cells respond by also secreting MCP-1. This is compounded by the fact that the increased secretion of leptin by the adipocytes stimulates transport of macrophages to adipose tissue. The decreased production of adiponectin by adipocytes may also contribute to adhesion of macrophages to the endothelial cells.

Once these cells are activated, they contribute to perpetuating a cycle of macrophage recruitment, production of inflammatory cytokines, and impairment of adipocyte function (which results in alterations in insulin action).[13,14] Consequently, the altered pattern of adipocytokines

(which were probably originally generated as a protective mechanism to initiate an inflammatory process) impacts the endothelium throughout the body and the nonadipose tissues. The activation of the macrophages and endothelial cells is associated with an increase in production of ROS and oxidative stress, which then leads to the vascular abnormalities associated with cardiovascular disease. These are compounded by the direct toxicity of glucose in the form of the advanced glycation end products (AGEs).

GLUCOSE TOXICITY: AGES AND RAGE

In the presence of any amount of hyperglycemia, nonenzymatic glycoxidation of proteins and lipids leads to the formation of a series of products (AGEs). The AGEs are the result of a nonenzymatic reaction of reducing sugars with primary amino groups of proteins called the Maillard reaction. AGEs have been shown to act directly to induce protein cross links, which are protease resistant and cause irreversible damage to cells and tissues.

Through cell surface receptors, such as the receptors for AGEs (RAGE), AGEs also induce the release of cytokines that lead to activation of cells such as monocytes/macrophages, vascular smooth muscles cells, and endothelial cells (resulting in the production of reactive oxygen species, ROSs, which induce the oxidation of DNA and peroxidation of membrane lipids). Inhibition of RAGE is associated with an attenuation of diabetes associated atherosclerosis in animal models. An endogenous soluble truncated form of RAGE (esRAGE) has been found, which apparently functions to bind circulating AGEs and neutralize them.[15]

The inability of the body to clear the AGEs contributes to both the direct toxicity to the vessel wall and the indirect toxicity through their ability to increase inflammatory cytokines. The direct effect is one of pure mechanical dysfunction caused by AGE cross-bridges established between macromolecules. This prevents the structural proteins from moving properly during vascular contraction and dilation, thus transforming vessel walls into stiff inelastic tubes and disturbing basement membrane adhesion properties. This may result in high blood pressure, leaky vessels, and in the case of the heart stiffness in the form of diastolic dysfunction. AGE accumulation may also damage the blood vessels by trapping proteins (i.e., immunoglobulins and lipoproteins) and cells in the vessel wall, thus stimulating the immune and inflammatory response that has been described in atherosclerosis.[16]

The pathways that may be affected by the binding of the AGEs to the cell surface RAGEs include the generation of inflammatory cytokines and growth factors, leading to intimal proliferation and an overproduction of extracellular matrix (which may also contribute to the stiffness of the vessel). This process could possibly then be exacerbated by the events occurring in the adipose tissue, the presence of oxidized lipoproteins, and perhaps infectious events (either viral or bacterial). The constitutive presence of AGE receptors on resting T lymphocytes (CD4, CD8) has led to the hypothesis that their activation in the vessel wall may trigger a low-grade sustained inflammatory state that could be accelerated by any elevation in glucose. Studies are ongoing to develop therapeutic agents to neutralize the toxic effect of AGEs. At this time, the only available therapeutic strategy to prevent the glucose toxicity is to prevent any elevation in plasma glucose (thus minimizing the production of AGEs).

MANAGEMENT OF HYPERGLYCEMIA AND INSULIN RESISTANCE

The inflammatory state initiated by the hyperglycemia and the insulin resistance must be treated by addressing each component of the disease process. Treatment now involves the combined use of agents with complimentary pharmacologic mechanisms (Table 90–1). Some agents treat only one aspect, whereas others impact multiple components of the aforementioned processes. Thus, the combined use of agents that maximally decrease sugar, insulin resistance, and inflammation should theoretically have the lowest incidence of CV events. Although data from observational studies support this contention, ongoing trials will help to definitively determine whether this assertion is valid.

GLUCOSE LOWERING

Treatment of type 2 diabetes

The currently available classes of antidiabetic agents reduce plasma glucose levels by targeting four processes: (1) replacing the relative insufficiency of the pancreatic beta cells by either stimulating it to produce more insulin (sulfonylureas, non-sulfonylurea secretagogues, incretin mimetics) or replacing it with exogenous insulin and/or replacing amylin deficiency, (2) stimulation of glucose uptake by muscle and adipose tissues (thiazolidinediones), (3) reduction of glucose output by the liver (biguanides, thiazolidinediones), and (4) reduction of glucose absorption by the gut (alpha-glucosidase inhibitors). As seen in Figure 90–1, these agents target the various pathophysiologic mechanisms of type 2 diabetes.[17,18]

It should be noted, however, that diet and exercise remain the cornerstone for management of type 2 diabetes. As was noted in the DPP study, weight loss related to exercise yielded a much lower incidence of new-onset diabetes than metformin. Thus, caloric restriction, weight loss, and exercise can enhance insulin sensitivity and glycemic control. Early in the course of type 2 diabetes, anything that can enhance insulin sensitivity will result in prolonged time for the need of exogenous insulin. This results from exercise-associated enhanced insulin sensitivity and more efficient insulin utilization by the body. In spite of these lifestyle measures, everyone at sometime in the course of their diabetes will need medication to control their glucose level. The following section provides a brief overview of the available classes of the glucose-lowering agents.

GLUCOSE-LOWERING AGENTS	
Class	Trade Name
Alpha-glucosidase inhibitors: acarbose and miglitol	Precose Ultraset
Biguanides: metformin Incretin mimetics	Glucophage, generic
Exenatide	Byetta
Insulin	Humulin, Novolin, Lantus Humalog, Novolog
Insulin secretagogues: sulfonylureas	Diabeta, Glucotrol, Amaryl, generic
glyburide, glipizide nonsulfonylurea repaglinide, nateglinide	Prandin, Starlix
Pramlintide	Symlin
Thiazolidinediones: rosiglitazone	Avandia
pioglitazone	Actos
Fixed-dose Combinations Metformin/Secretagogue glyburide/metformin	Glucovance, generic
glipizide/metformin	Metaglip
Metformin/Thiazolidinedione rosiglitazone/metformin	Avandamet
pioglitazone/metformin	ACTOplus met

Table 90–1. Glucose-lowering Agents

Secretagogues

Glucose lowering can be achieved by increasing insulin secretion using secretagogues or augmenting glucose-stimulated insulin secretion using incretin mimetics. The secretagogues can be separated into two groups: sulfonylureas and non-sulfonylurea secretagogues. A number of sulfonylureas are available, in that this is one of the oldest classes of antidiabetic agents.[19] The two adverse events most commonly associated with sulfonylureas are hypoglycemia and weight gain. The newer (second-generation) sulfonylureas (i.e., glyburide, glipizide, glymepiride) are more effective and are associated with lower incidences of adverse events than the older agents.

The non-sulfonylurea secretagogues are a newer class and include two currently available products: nateglinide (a phenylalanine derivative) and repaglinide, a benzoic acid derivative. They have shorter half-lives than sulfonylureas and a reduced risk of hypoglycemia. Because of their brief half-lives, resulting in shorter duration action, the non-sulfonylurea secretagogues are administered at meals to improve postprandial glycemic control. The short half-life and short duration of action may be particularly useful in patients who do not eat three meals daily or eat at irregular times (including geriatric patients, those with renal disease, and high school or college students). Their function is to lower glucose but they do not impact insulin resistance or inflammation.

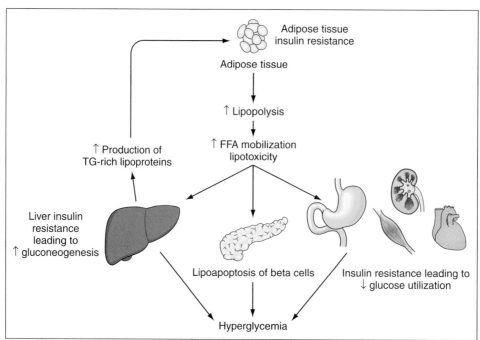

Figure 90–1. The pathophysiology of type 2 diabetes mellitus. (Adapted from DeFronzo R, Bonadonna R, Ferrannini E. Pathogenesis of NIDDM: A balanced overview. Copyright 1992 American Diabetes Association. From *Diabetes Care*:15(3):318–368. Reprinted with permission from The American Diabetes Association.

Incretin mimetics

The insulin secretory capacity of the pancreatic beta cell can also be augmented by the incretin mimetics. The enhanced insulin response to oral over intravenous glucose is known as the incretin effect. This physiologic observation led to the discovery of compounds now called incretins, such as glucagon-like peptide-1 (GLP-1), produced by the gastrointestinal (GI) tract in response to glucose. GLP-1 and other incretins enhance glucose-dependent insulin secretion and exhibit other anti-hyperglycemic actions following their release into the circulation from the gut.[18] Synthetic compounds have been developed that have some of the activities of the naturally occurring incretins, and have been named incretin mimetics.

The prototype of this class is exenatide, which has been shown to bind and activate the human GLP-1 receptor *in vitro*. Exenatide mimics certain antihyperglycemic actions of GLP-1, including promoting insulin release from beta cells in the presence of elevated blood glucose concentrations.[20] Exenatide has been approved for use in combination with sulphonylureas and/or metformin. Use with other agents (including non-sulfonylurea secretagogues, thiazolidinediones, or insulin) will require studies to optimize such regimens.

Nausea is a common side effect (~30%) at initiation of exenatide. This is decreased by starting at a low dose and waiting at least a month before increasing the dose and resolves over time. However, one study of dialysis patients given a single low dose found that they did not tolerate the nausea, suggesting that exenatide will require extensive studies to determine how (if it all) it should be dosed

in such a population. Exenatide should not be used in stage 4 or 5 CKD, as the renal clearance is reduced at least tenfold at this stage and studies have not been done to determine dosing in this population.

Amylinomimetics

Another addition to the armamentarium of glucose management is the injectable agent pramlintide. Pramlintide is a synthetic analog of human amylin, a naturally occurring neuroendocrine hormone synthesized by pancreatic beta cells that contributes to glucose control during the postprandial period. Pramlintide complements the effects of insulin in postprandial glucose regulation by decreasing glucagon secretion. Pramlintide exhibits linear pharmacokinetics, and peak serum levels are reached within 30 minutes of administration. The drug is predominantly eliminated by the kidneys, with a mean elimination half-life of 30 to 50 minutes. Clinical trials have shown that pramlintide suppresses post-meal glucagon secretion, slows gastric emptying, reduces postprandial glucose levels, and improves glycemic control while managing weight loss.[21,22]

Pramlinitide is approved for mealtime dosing as an adjunct to insulin in patients with type 1 diabetes mellitus who have not achieved control and in patients with type 2 diabetes mellitus who use mealtime insulin, with or without concurrent sulfonylurea and/or metformin, who have not achieved desired control. In patients with diabetes mellitus who are using pramlintide in addition to their insulin, the dose does not need to be modified in stage 3 or 4 CKD but it is not recommended for use in stage 5 CKD and it has not yet been studied in dialysis patients. Pramlintide has been associated with an increased risk of insulin-induced severe hypoglycemia. Other adverse events include nausea, anorexia, fatigue, and vomiting. Pramlintide is not a substitute for insulin and should only be used in combination with insulin.

Thiazolidinediones

Rosiglitazone and pioglitazone are the only two currently available thiazolidinediones in the United States. Therapeutic benefits of using thiazolidinediones early in the treatment of type 2 diabetes include the preservation of beta-cell function, augmentation of insulin sensitivity, and minimization of hypoglycemic adverse events.[19] Studies suggest that the thiazolidinediones increase the responsiveness of beta cells by reducing external factors (i.e., glucose and free fatty acids) that impair insulin secretion. Studies have also shown that treatment with thiazolidinediones significantly reduces proinsulin-to-insulin levels, indicating improved beta-cell function.

Preservation of beta-cell function and improvement of insulin sensitivity are the major efficacy rationales for the use of thiazolidinediones as first-line therapy, especially because current evidence suggests that deterioration of beta-cell function and resistance to insulin begin long before the diagnosis of diabetes. These data suggest that because thiazolidinediones preserve beta-cell function and improve insulin sensitivity, their use from the time of diagnosis of diabetes (or even before diagnosis) may improve glycemic control and prevent diabetic complications.

Rosiglitazone and pioglitazone have been proven safe and effective for long-term therapy in a number of clinical trials. The thiazolidinediones are rarely associated with hypoglycemia, and severe hypoglycemia (as can occur with sulfonylureas or insulin) is no longer a barrier to achieving glycemic targets. Using an agent that would minimize the occurrence of this adverse event is a good way to ensure compliance from the initiation of therapy, particularly in patients who have experienced hypoglycemic events on other therapies. Thiazolidinediones may cause weight gain and edema when initiated at high doses.

The thiazolidinediones have been associated with fluid retention and dilutional anemia, which is due to an increase in plasma volume, and are not recommended for use in patients with New York Heart Association class 3 or 4 cardiac status. Combination use with insulin may increase the incidence of cardiac failure.[23] Troglitazone, an older thiazolidinedione, was removed from the market because of hepatotoxicity. Studies show that hepatic failure is not a class effect with these agents. Rosiglitazone and pioglitazone have a more favorable hepatic safety profile than troglitazone or placebo. Scheduled monitoring of liver function tests is no longer required by the United States Food and Drug Administration (FDA).

Biguanides

The primary action of biguanides is to reduce the production of glucose by the liver. Metformin is the only biguanide available in the United States. Because the mode of action does not increase pancreatic insulin secretion, hypoglycemia is generally not associated with biguanides. However, lactic acidosis (a serious metabolic complication) has very rarely been reported with the use of metformin, particularly in individuals with renal dysfunction or advancing age. There may be some vitamin B12 and folate malabsorption with metformin use, and thus it may be prudent to measure a hemoglobin, hematocrit with red blood cell indices, and vitamin B12 and folate levels at initiation and at least annually.

Certain drugs such as cimetidine and ranitidine may increase metformin blood levels by competing for common renal tubular transport systems. Metformin is excreted unchanged in the urine (primarily through tubular secretion) and does not undergo hepatic metabolism. In patients with decreased renal function (i.e., <50 to 70 mL/min, based on measured creatinine clearance), the plasma and blood half-life of metformin is prolonged and the risk for lactic acidosis (which is fatal in 50% of cases) increases significantly. For this reason, the precautions recommended by the FDA should be carefully followed in all patients. Importantly, serum creatinine should be monitored routinely in all patients receiving a biguanide.

The FDA recommends that a creatinine clearance be measured prior to initiating therapy in patients 80 years of age or older.[24] A more conservative approach would be to measure the creatinine clearance in any patient who is 70 years of age or older at the time of initiating therapy. The most common adverse events include abdominal pain, nausea, and diarrhea, which can be minimized by dosing after meals and by initiating therapy at low doses and increasing slowly.

Alpha-glucosidase inhibitors

Acarbose and miglitol are alpha-glucosidase inhibitors that act by delaying carbohydrate absorption in the small intestine. These agents are taken by patients at the beginning of each main meal. The main advantage of the alpha-glucosidase inhibitors is that they are only minimally absorbed and are rarely associated with hypoglycemia and weight gain. However, they frequently cause loose stools and flatulence when used at the recommended doses (i.e., 100 mg acarbose three times daily). When used in low doses (i.e., 12.5 to 25 mg acarbose once or twice daily), the side effect of loose stools may be useful in a patient preoccupied with constipation.

Post hoc analysis of the STOP-NIDDM trial database suggests that treatment of patients who have IGT with acarbose is associated with a reduction in the risk of cardiovascular disease and hypertension.[25] These data will need to be confirmed in a prospective, randomized, controlled clinical trial. Because of their mechanism of action, these drugs are contraindicated in patients with diseases of the gastrointestinal tract (e.g., inflammatory bowel disease). These agents are poorly absorbed, with less than 2% of an oral dose recovered in the urine as active (i.e., parent compound and active metabolite) drug.

Pharmacokinetic studies showed that patients with renal impairment (creatinine clearance <25 mL/min/1.73m^2) attained about 5 times higher peak plasma concentrations of acarbose than volunteers with normal renal function. Consequently, alpha-glucosidase inhibitors are not recommended for use in patients with severe renal impairment (serum creatinine >2 mg/dL) because this population has not yet been studied. The concern is that the risk of drug accumulation in renal impairment through the increased plasma levels may have the potential for hepatotoxicity. However, when used in very low doses (i.e., 12.5 to 25 mg acarbose once or twice daily) it is possible this will be less or a risk but studies are needed in the population with stage 4 or 5 chronic kidney disease. These agents do lower glucose, but it is not yet clear whether they have any beneficial impact on the underlying disease process.

Fixed-dose combinations

Fixed-dose combination pills for the management of type 2 diabetes have recently been introduced in the United States. The advantages include better efficacy with lower doses of each component, improved compliance, increased adherence, fewer complications (i.e., less hypoglycemia) due to lower dosing, and the financial advantage of the tablets usually priced at the same cost as the more expensive component alone. The currently available combinations include metformin/glyburide, metformin/glipizide, metformin/rosiglitazone, and metformin/pioglitazone.

There is also a rosiglitazone/glymepiride combination pill undergoing regulatory evaluation by the FDA. One strategy for utilizing these fixed-dose combination pills is to combine the different combination pills such that the patient receives a low dose of a secretagogue, a low dose of a thiazolidinedione, and the highest tolerable dose of metformin. This can be done by giving one combination tablet in the morning and a different one at night.

Insulin use in type 2 diabetes

Optimizing or initiating insulin requires careful attention to detail by both the patient and the diabetes educator. Initiation of insulin can be done very slowly (i.e., insulin glargine 10 units at bedtime or premixed insulin, 70/30 or 75/25, 5 units twice daily before meals). The patient can then adjust the insulin regimen using a simple algorithm once or twice a week, as shown in Table 90–2. The typical insulin dose per day, in the absence of kidney disease, is 0.4 to 1.0 units/kg in type 1 diabetes and 1 to 2 units/kg in type 2 diabetes. For example, a 70-kg person with type 2 diabetes would typically require at least 70 to 140 units

INSULIN TITRATION ALGORITHMS		
Fasting Glucose or Pre-dinner Glucose (mg/dL)	Pre-mix Insulin Dose Adjustment	Glargine Insulin Dose Adjustment
<80	−2 units	−2 units
80–100	No change	No change
101–140	+2 units	+2–4 units
141–180	+4 units	+4–6 units
>180	+6 units	+6–8 units

Table 90–2. Insulin Titration Algorithms

insulin/day. Using patient-managed algorithms allows the patient to slowly increase the dose and to have control over their insulin.[26]

Does insulin have any benefits beyond glucose lowering?

Although insulin has been assumed for many years to have a detrimental effect on the vasculature by virtue of its growth factor-like effect, recent data have shown that insulin exerts desirable actions on the vasculature. It does so primarily by amplifying endothelium-dependent vasodilation, increasing endothelial constitutive nitric oxide synthase (eNOS) gene expression and activity (and therefore NO bioavailability), which in turn exerts a wide array of antiatherogenic actions.[14] Endothelial dysfunction is characterized by impaired endothelium-dependent vasodilation, which is caused by a reduction of the bioavailability of vasodilators (in particular, NO). The inappropriate elevation of plasma FFAs seen in insulin resistance is associated with a decrease in circulating levels of most amino acids, including l-arginine, which may reduce the substrate for NO formation.

Direct inhibition of NO synthesis by FFA has also been reported. The cellular changes that occur due to excess accumulation of FFAs are associated with overproduction of reactive oxygen species, resulting in increased oxidative stress. By reacting with NO, reactive oxygen species may reduce vascular NO bioavailability and promote cellular damage. Hence, increased oxidative stress is considered a major mechanism involved in the pathogenesis of endothelial dysfunction and may serve as a common pathogenic mechanism of the effect of risk factors on the endothelium.

Given the relationship between endothelial dysfunction and atherosclerosis, it is likely that the status of endothelial function may reflect the propensity of an individual to develop atherosclerotic disease. Consequently, the beneficial effect of insulin on decreasing endothelial activation (thereby improving endothelial dysfunction) raises the possibility that insulin therapy should be initiated much earlier in the disease process than it has been under traditional diabetes management.

Does treating the insulin resistance impact hypertension?

Studies of patients who are insulin resistant but do not have DM provide the opportunity to assess whether altering the dysregulation of FFA metabolism will impact individual CV risk factors such as hypertension. The thiazolidinediones have been shown to produce small but usually statistically significant reductions in blood pressure in diabetic patients and nondiabetic insulin-resistant.

One study has shown that treatment of insulin resistance in nondiabetic hypertensive patients was associated with restoration of the normal circadian pattern of blood pressure on continuous ambulatory blood pressure monitoring.[27] Although the mechanism of the reduction in blood pressure with improving insulin resistance is not known, it is likely related to improving the lipotoxicity in the kidney and improvements in endothelial function.

Does treating insulin resistance in people with hypertension prevent diabetes?

There are now a number of analyses from trials that utilized traditional therapies for lowering blood pressure or lipids, which found in post hoc analysis that active treatment with an angiotensin-converting enzyme (ACE) inhibitor, an angiotensin II receptor blocker (ARB), a peroxisome proliferator-activated receptor (PPAR) ligand, or some but not all statin agents was associated with a decreased likelihood of being diagnosed with diabetes while participating in the respective trial (Table 90–3).[28–30]

The decrease in being diagnosed with diabetes in the Antihypertensive and Lipid-Lowering Treatment to Prevent Heart Attack Trial (ALLHAT) is likely due to the benefit from the ACE inhibitor therapy and is probably an underestimate, as some were offset by the increased likelihood of diabetes in the presence of thiazide therapy. The incidence of newly diagnosed diabetes was a pre-specified endpoint in the HPS and the VALUE trials. The effect of simvastatin on newly diagnosed DM was not statistically significant in the HPS, which is consistent with the lack of basic science data to support a mechanism for such an effect of the statins.

Treatment with valsartan was associated with a significant decrease in the likelihood of being diagnosed with diabetes, as compared to amlodipine therapy, in the VALUE trial. This finding is not unexpected due to the data showing that angiotensin II signaling can interfere with insulin receptor signaling in the endothelial cell. In addition, the ARB telmisartan has been shown to improve the profile of adipocytokines released from adipose tissue in rodents.[31] Last, it should be noted that although blockers of the renin angiotensin system can clearly reduce the incidence of insulin resistance outcome

trials with thiazide diuretics extending over a duration of five years demonstrate a mortality benefit in spite of not reducing the incidence of new-onset diabetes. Thus, lowering blood pressure to targets (and other risk factors) still confers benefit.

Whether these observations are of clinical utility is now being tested in two large international trials: DREAM (Diabetes Reduction Assessment with Ramipril and Rosiglitazone Medication) and NAVIGATOR (Nateglinide and Valsartan in Impaired Glucose Tolerance Outcomes Research).[32,33] These trials will test whether inhibition of the renin angiotensin system by either an ACE inhibitor (DREAM) or an ARB (NAVIGATOR) will impact the progression from IGT to type 2 diabetes. Their comparators treat either the insulin resistance or the beta-cell defect, respectively.

SUMMARY

The combination of hypertension and diabetes is associated with significant morbidity and mortality. Treatment of hypertension in people at risk for diabetes should include agents that modify the renin-angiotensin system, as this may help slow the progressive insulin resistance and loss of beta-cell function. Preventing hyperglycemia is also important to prevent the glucose toxicity to the vasculature. Treating insulin resistance directly can also decrease endothelial activation and attenuate ongoing inflammation. Insulin therapy directly improves endothelial function and should be considered in all people with diabetes whose HbA1c is not at guideline goal using oral agents. Aggressive combination therapy is now warranted in the person with hypertension and diabetes to prevent complications.

ANALYSIS OF THE LIKELIHOOD OF BEING DIAGNOSED WITH DIABETES DURING HYPERTENSION OR LIPID THERAPY TRIALS				
Study (yrs.)	Follow-up	Incidence of New T2DM in Treated (%)	Incidence of New T2DM in Controls (%)	P Value Decrease	% Likelihood
ALLHAT	4.9	2.0	3.1	<0.001	35
ALPINE	1.0	0.5	4.1	0.03	88
CAPP	6.1	6.5	7.3	0.03	11
CHARM	3.1	6.0	7.4	NS	—
HOPE	4.5	3.6	5.4	<0.0001	33
LIFE	4.8	6.0	8.0	<0.0001	25
SCOPE	3.7	4.3	5.3	0.09	19
SOLVD	2.9	5.9	22.4	<0.0001	74
STOP-2	6.0	4.7	4.9	NS	—
WOSCOPS	4.9	1.9	2.7	0.042	30%
HPS	5.0	4.6	4.0	0.10	—
BIP	6.2	42.3	54.4	0.04	22
HPS	5.0	4.6	4.0	0.10	—
VALUE	4.2	13.1	16.4[a]	<0.0001	23

a. Control group received amlodipine-based therapy.
Abbreviations: T2DM = type 2 diabetes mellitus; NS = not significant.

Table 90–3. Analysis of the Likelihood of Being Diagnosed with Diabetes During Hypertension or Lipid Therapy Trials

REFERENCES

1. Saydah SH, Fradkin J, Cowie CC. Poor control of risk factors for vascular disease among adults with previously diagnosed diabetes. *JAMA* 2004; 291(3):335–342.

2. UK Prospective Diabetes Study Group. Cost effectiveness analysis of improved blood pressure control in hypertensive patients with type 2 diabetes: UKPDS 40. *BMJ* 1998;317(7160):720–726.

3. UK Prospective Diabetes Study Group. Efficacy of atenolol and captopril in reducing risk of macrovascular and microvascular complications in type 2 diabetes: UKPDS 39. *BMJ* 1998; 317(7160):713–720.

4. UK Prospective Diabetes Study Group. Tight blood pressure control and risk of macrovascular and microvascular complications in type 2 diabetes: UKPDS 38. *BMJ* 1998;317(7160): 703–713.

5. The Diabetes Control and Complications Trial/Epidemiology of Diabetes Interventions and Complications Research Group. Intensive diabetes therapy and carotid intima-media thickness in type 1 diabetes mellitus. *N Engl J Med* 2003;348(23):2294–2303.

6. The Diabetes Control and Complications Trial Research Group. The effect of intensive treatment of diabetes on the development and progression of long-term complications in insulin-dependent diabetes mellitus. *N Engl J Med* 1993; 329(14):977–986.

7. UK Prospective Diabetes Study Group. Intensive blood-glucose control with sulphonylureas or insulin compared with conventional treatment and risk of complications in patients with type 2 diabetes (UKPDS 33). *The Lancet* 1998; 352(9131):837–853.

8. UK Prospective Diabetes Study Group. Effect of intensive blood-glucose control with metformin on complications in overweight patients with type 2 diabetes (UKPDS 34). *The Lancet* 1998; 352(9131):854–865.

9. Dormandy JA, Charbonnel B, Eckland DJ, et al. Secondary prevention of macrovascular events in patients with type 2 diabetes in the PROactive Study (PROspective pioglitAzone Clinical Trial in Macrovascular Events): A randomised controlled trial. *The Lancet* 2005; 366(9493):1279–1289.

10. Tomas E, Kelly M, Xiang X, et al. Metabolic and hormonal interactions between muscle and adipose tissue. *Proc Nutr Soc* 2004;63(2):381–385.

11. Unger RH. Lipid overload and overflow: Metabolic trauma and the metabolic syndrome. *Trends Endocrinol Metab* 2003;14(9):398–403.

12. Hotamisligil GS. Role of endoplasmic reticulum stress and c-Jun NH2-terminal kinase pathways in inflammation and origin of obesity and diabetes. *Diabetes* 2005;54(2):S73–S78.

13. Wellen KE, Hotamisligil GS. Obesity-induced inflammatory changes in adipose tissue. *J Clin Invest* 2003; 112(12):1785–1788.

14. Hotamisligil GS. Inflammatory pathways and insulin action. *Int J Obes Relat Metab Disord* 2003;27(3):S53–S55.

15. Yonekura H, Yamamoto Y, Sakurai S, Watanabe T. Roles of the receptor for advanced glycation endproducts in diabetes-induced vascular injury. *J Pharmacol Sci* 2005(97):305–311.

16. Koyama H, Shoji T, Yokoyama H, et al. Plasma level of endogenous secretory RAGE is associated with components of the metabolic syndrome and atherosclerosis. *Arterioscler Thromb Vasc Biol* 2005;25(12):2587–2593.

17. DeFronzo R, Bonadonna R, Ferrannini E. Pathogenesis of NIDDM: A balanced overview. *Diabetes Care* 1992;15(3): 318–368.

18. D'Alessio DA, Vahl TP. Glucagon-like peptide 1: Evolution of an incretin into a treatment for diabetes. *Am J Physiol Endocrinol Metab* 2004;286(6): E882–E890.

19. Inzucchi SE. Oral antihyperglycemic therapy for type 2 diabetes: Scientific review. *JAMA* 2002;287(3):360–372.

20. Kolterman OG, Kim DD, Shen L, et al. Pharmacokinetics, pharmacodynamics, and safety of exenatide in patients with type 2 diabetes mellitus. *Am J Health Syst Pharm* 2005;62(2):173–181.

21. Chapman I, Parker B, Doran S, et al. Effect of pramlintide on satiety and food intake in obese subjects and subjects with type 2 diabetes. *Diabetologia* 2005;48(5):838–848.

22. Ceriello A, Piconi L, Quagliaro L, et al. Effects of pramlintide on postprandial glucose excursions and measures of oxidative stress in patients with type 1 diabetes. *Diabetes Care* 2005;28(3): 632–637.

23. Nesto RW, Bell D, Bonow RO, et al. Thiazolidinedione use, fluid retention, and congestive heart failure: A consensus statement from the American Heart Association and American Diabetes Association. *Diabetes Care* 2004;27(1): 256–263.

24. Bristol-Myers Squibb Company. Glucophage/Glucophage XR prescribing information. Princeton, NJ: Bristol-Myers Squibb Company, 2004.

25. Chiasson J-L, Josse RG, Gomis R, Hanefeld M, Karasik A, Laakso M. Acarbose treatment and the risk of cardiovascular disease and hypertension in patients with impaired glucose tolerance: The STOP-NIDDM trial. *JAMA* 2003;290(4):486–494.

26. Raskin P, Allen E, Hollander P, et al. Initiating insulin therapy in type 2 diabetes: A comparison of biphasic and basal insulin analogs. *Diabetes Care* 2005;28(2):260–265.

27. Raji A, Seely EW, Bekins SA, Williams GH, Simonson DC. Rosiglitazone improves insulin sensitivity and lowers blood pressure in hypertensive patients. *Diabetes Care* 2003;26(1):172–178.

28. Scheen AJ. Prevention of type 2 diabetes by inhibition of the renin-angiotensin system: Meta-analysis of randomized clinical trials. *Diabetes* 2004;53(2):363–PD.

29. MRC/BHF Heart Protection Study of cholesterol-lowering with simvastatin in 5963 people with diabetes: A randomised placebo-controlled trial. *The Lancet* 2003;361(9374): 2005–2016.

30. Julius PS, Kjeldsen PSE, Weber PM, et al. Outcomes in hypertensive patients at high cardiovascular risk treated with regimens based on valsartan or amlodipine: The VALUE randomised trial. *The Lancet* 2004; 363(9426):2022–2031.

31. Clasen R, Schupp M, Foryst-Ludwig A, et al. PPARγ-activating angiotensin type-1 receptor blockers induce adiponectin. *Hypertension* 2005;46(1):137–143.

32. Gerstein HC, Yusuf S, Holman RR, Bosch J, et al. Design and baseline characteristics of the DREAM (Diabetes Reduction Assessment with Ramipril and Rosiglitazone Medication) trial. *Diabetes* 2004;53(2):2022–PO.

33. Simpson RW, Shaw JE. The prevention of type 2 diabetes: Lifestyle change or pharmacotherapy? A challenge for the 21st century. *Diabetes Res Clin Pract* 2003;59(3):165–180.

Chapter

91

Target Blood Pressure in Hypertension Treatment: The J-shaped Curve Controversy

N. C. Shah and Chim C. Lang

Key Findings

- The target blood pressure is obviously the one associated with the greatest impact on cardiovascular and renal morbidity and mortality.

- Whereas the goal of 140/90 mmHg seems appropriate for relatively low-risk hypertensive patients, more intensive therapy to reach a goal below 130/80 mmHg is indicated for those with high-risk hypertension (including those with diabetes or renal insufficiency).

- There is no definite evidence of an increase in risk of aggressive treatment (a J-curve) unless diastolic blood pressure is lowered to less than 65 mmHg in elderly patients with isolated systolic hypertension.

It is well established that controlling blood pressure (BP) through the use of antihypertensive drugs reduces morbidity and mortality. It has been further demonstrated that lowering systolic BP (SBP) as well as diastolic BP (DBP) confers benefit. Recent evidence has emphasized the importance of optimal BP control, particularly in patients with high cardiovascular (CV) risk, such as those with diabetes mellitus and renal disease.[1-3] In patients with diabetes mellitus, the available data suggest that a BP below 130/85 mmHg reduces the incidence of CV events. In patients with slowly progressive chronic renal failure excreting more than 1 to 2 g of protein per day, reducing the BP to 130/80 or even to 125/75 mmHg might slow the rate of loss of renal function.[1-3]

Epidemiologic studies have shown that after adjustment for other risk factors, treated hypertensive patients with "normal" BP are still at higher risk for CVD than normotensive persons.[4] Moreover, in clinical trials the observed risk reduction for coronary events has been smaller than would be expected from the log-linear relationship between BP and risk according to epidemiologic data.[5] Clinical trials have reported a 5- to 6-mmHg difference between DBP of treatment and control groups. The risk reduction of 14% for coronary events contrasts with the 20 to 25% reduction noted in epidemiologic reports. It has been argued that these discrepancies may be related to the existence of a J-shaped relationship between BP and risk in which treated patients with low BP are at increased risk for events. This chapter discusses the optimal target BP and reviews the controversy relating to the J-shaped relationship between BP and mortality in treating hypertensive patients.

THE OPTIMAL TARGET BP IN GUIDELINES

Elevations in SBP and DBP are established CVD determinants that have been designated major components of CVD risk estimation algorithms.[6-8] These guidelines have noted the incomplete evidence on optimal targets for BP lowering, with better evidence for DBP targets than SBP targets—although for patients above the age of 50 years it is recognized that SBP is a more important prognostic determinant of adverse CVD outcome.[9] The goal of 140/90 mmHg has been set for relatively low-risk hypertensive patients. More intensive therapy is aimed at reaching a goal below 130/80 mmHg for those with high-risk hypertension, including those with diabetes or renal insufficiency. Indeed, the British Hypertension Society guidelines state that "the overwhelming evidence for an optimal BP supports a 'lower the better policy' without any convincing evidence of a J-curve relationship."[7] Although these recommendations are accepted by many, there are some who may not agree because of disputed allegations suggesting that low DBP may be associated with an excess of cardiac events (i.e., the existence of a J- or U-curve relation between DBP and death).

THE J-SHAPED CURVE: DOES IT EXIST?

Whether such a J-curve exists has long been a debated topic. A plethora of reports has described the shape of the relationship between BP and risk, some concluding that there is a J-curve relation to one or another clinical outcome. Others have reported a linear relation. Population-based longitudinal studies of hypertension have usually shown a continuous and positive relationship between BP and mortality. In a recent meta-analysis by the Prospective Studies Collaboration[10] involving more than 1 million individuals, it was reported that death from both ischemic heart disease and stroke increases progressively and linearly from BP levels as low as 115 mmHg systolic and 75 mmHg diastolic upward (Figure 91–1). Below these levels, there is little evidence of further benefit. It should be noted that the relation of BP to CVD and mortality is subject to considerable random fluctuation, especially in the "normotensive" BP range (where CVD incidence is low). Indeed, with correction for "regression dilution" the meta-analysis by the Prospective Studies Collaboration did reveal a statistically significant modest increase in CVD mortality for DBP <80 mmHg.

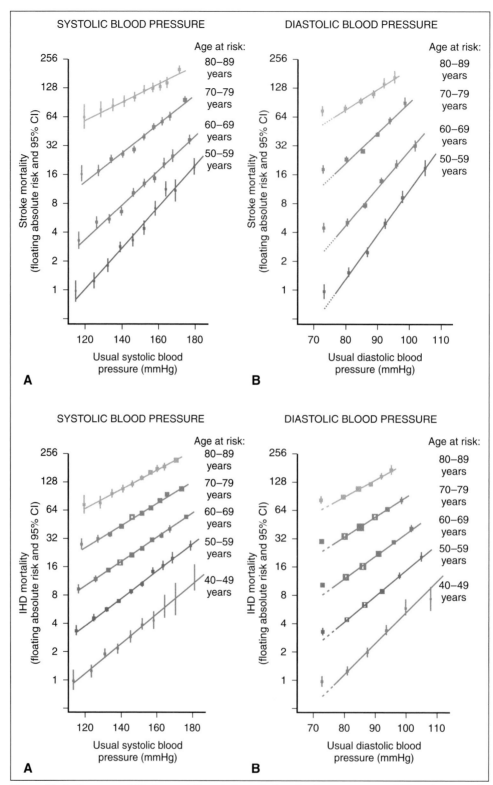

Figure 91–1. *Upper panel:* Stroke mortality rate in each decade of age versus usual BP at the start of that decade. *Lower panel:* Ischemic heart disease mortality rate in each decade of age versus usual BP at the start of that decade. (Reproduced from Lewington S, Clarke R, Qizilbash N, et al. Age-specific relevance of usual blood pressure to vascular mortality: A meta-analysis of individual data for one million adults in 61 prospective studies. *Lancet* 2002;360:1903–13, with permission from Elsevier.)

Early reports of the J-curve

It should be noted that reports of a J-shaped relationship had been reported previously. The reports of a J-shaped relationship have come from longitudinal cohort studies of treated patients.[11–15] There is also evidence from clinical trial data on antihypertensive treatment groups, and in some trials from control groups.[16–18]

Interpretation of the J-curve

Interpretation of these results has varied (Box 91–1). Several mechanisms have been suggested. It is possible that patients with occult coronary disease do worse at these lower BP levels because most coronary filling occurs during diastole. Similarly, underlying left ventricular hypertrophy can impair coronary reserve by diminishing the ability of the vessels to dilate as the coronary perfusion pressure is reduced.[19,20] In one study,[20] for example, progressively lowering the systemic BP with nitroprusside led to decreased coronary flow in hypertensive patients with left ventricular hypertrophy but not in normotensive individuals or hypertensive patients without left ventricular hypertrophy. Observations from the Framingham Study[21] are compatible with the potential importance of underlying coronary disease. A J-shaped curve for coronary deaths was noted for patients who experienced a myocardial infarction but not for those who had not. However, two additional findings are important. First, the increase in risk was noted only at relatively low DBPs (<75 mmHg). Second, the J-curve was independent of the use of antihypertensive drug therapy, suggesting that it was the combination of coronary disease and a low DBP that was important.

It should be emphasized that several authors have criticized the conclusions drawn from the results of the previously cited studies, arguing that the methods used were nonrandomized and the studies were uncontrolled, open, and retrospective.[22,23] Arguments against a J-curve that have been put forward include uncontrolled confounding factors related to poor health (such as heart failure and malignancy).[24,25] With aging, atheromatous arteries are associated with a wide pulse pressure and low DBP. Thus, a low DBP is a reflection of, rather than a cause of, increased risk.[26] With respect to pulse pressure, Kannel et al.[27] recently examined this in an analysis of the combined original and offspring Framingham cohorts and found an increasing tendency for a J-curve relation of CVD incidence to DBP with successive increments in accompanying SBP. In both males and females, a statistically significant excess of CVD events was observed at a DBP <80 mmHg only when accompanied by an SBP >140 mmHg that persisted after adjustment for age and associated risk factors. Thus, it appears at least from this analysis that the excess CVD risk at low DBP is largely confined to patients who also have an elevated SBP, implying that it is elevated pulse pressure (or isolated systolic hypertension) that is responsible for the excess risk observed at low BP.

A similar relation of pulse pressure with primary outcome was recently reported in the INVEST trial, a 22,000-patient trial in which all patients had hypertension and CAD.[28] In INVEST, low DBP was distinctly associated with increased risk of MI but not stroke. It should also be noted that following the early reports of the J-curve several reports appeared indicating that hypertensive or normotensive patients who were elderly or who had CAD failed to demonstrate such a J-shaped curve with treatment even if diastolic pressure was <90 mmHg.[29–31] Furthermore, there is little evidence from any of the previously mentioned studies suggesting a J-curve for the systolic BP. The risk of cardiovascular disease generally declines continuously at least to an SBP of 130 to 145 mmHg.[12] In a prospective evaluation[32] of more than 6000 patients for 9 years, a J-curve appeared only in patients with mild to moderate hypertension whose DBP was lowered more than 25 mmHg from the baseline value. Optimal results were seen at an SBP below 134 mmHg in men and approximately 140 mmHg in women.

The benefit of lower BPs might also apply to patients who already have end-organ damage. One study monitored 5362 patients with a history of a myocardial infarction.[33] During the first 2 years of follow-up, there was no detectable association between SBP and the coronary mortality rate. During the ensuing 14 years, however, linear associations were noted between the risk of coronary death and both SBPs and DBPs. Patients with lower BPs were at lower risk. In addition, analysis of over 300,000 MRFIT screenees showed a continuous linear relationship between DBP and relative risk of CAD.[34] Thus, it appeared that the J-curve controversy had resolved at the end of the 1990s.

REAPPEARANCE OF THE J-CURVE

It should be noted that the J-curve reappeared in the late 1990s. Two studies suggested a J-curve for stroke when already low normal diastolic levels are inadvertently lowered further by antihypertensive drug therapy of isolated systolic hypertension. During average follow-up of 4.7 years of 2351 hypertensive patients older than 55 years (average

---

Box 91–1

Arguments for and Against the J-Shaped Relationship Between BP and Mortality in Hypertensive Patients

Arguments for (and proposed mechanisms):
- Diastolic hypotension reduces coronary filling pressure.
- Underlying left ventricular hypertrophy can impair coronary reserve as the coronary perfusion pressure is reduced in diastolic hypotension.

Arguments against:
- Studies reporting J-shaped curve were open, retrospective, and nonrandomized. Inadequate statistical methods with large losses to follow-up.
- Other analyses have not found a J-shaped relationship.
- Lower DBP attributed to uncontrolled confounding factors related to deteriorating health (heart failure or malignancy).
- The low DBP is a marker for widened pulse pressure.

age 71.5 years), those who received antihypertensive drug therapy experienced a progressive decrease in the incidence of stroke as their DBPs were lowered to between 65 and 74 mmHg but a significant increase in stroke when DBPs were lowered to less than 65 mmHg.[35] Reanalysis of the data from the Systolic Hypertension in the Elderly Program[36] involving 4736 patients with initial average BPs of 177/77 mmHg found a 14% increase in the risk of stroke in patients whose DBPs were inadvertently reduced by 5 mmHg with active drug therapy.

Patients being treated who did not have a cardiovascular event had an average DBP of 68 mmHg. Those who had an event had an average DBP of 65 mmHg. The risks were still less in patients whose DBPs were lowered than in those receiving placebo, whose systolic levels remained elevated. However, there are some concerns regarding both studies. In the study by Voko et al.,[35] we do not know

whether the low pressures were actually induced by antihypertensive treatment. The authors did not exclude the possibility of selection bias or low pressures resulting from interim occult cardiovascular damage, which could have predisposed those patients to stroke.

In a reanalysis of the SHEP trial,[36] the numbers of patients who achieved DBP <55 mmHg were small and a careful reading of this study suggests that levels of 45 mmHg were not deleterious. These phenomena were noted in the treatment arm but not in the placebo arm. It is not clear whether the increased event rate associated with low DBP in the treatment arm was a direct result of diastolic hypotension or the result of some subclinical disease that was unmasked by antihypertensive therapy. Importantly, the event rate in those patients in the active treatment arm with diastolic hypotension was still lower than the event rate of patients in the placebo arm. The authors had concluded that

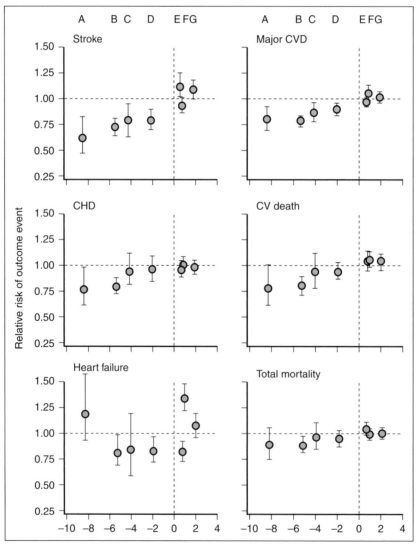

Figure 91–2. Associations of BP differences between groups with risks of major vascular outcomes and death. (Reproduced from the Blood Pressure Lowering Trialists' Collaboration. Effects of different blood-pressure lowering regimens on major cardiovascular events: Results of prospectively-designed overviews of randomised trials. *Lancet* 2003;362:1527–35, with permission from Elsevier.)

patients who achieve DBP levels of about 55 to 60 mmHg deserve more careful monitoring and more aggressive treatment of other CV risk factors.

TARGET BP AND J-CURVE: ANSWERS FROM PROSPECTIVE INTERVENTION TRIALS

It is clear that the only way to resolve the issue is to have specially designed prospective randomized studies of the potential benefits or drawbacks of intensive antihypertensive treatment that will help define the maximum benefit from antihypertensive therapy. There have been two studies of this nature. The BBB study[37] was conducted in hypertensive patients with no signs of IHD and showed no increase in cardiovascular events at DBP <80 mmHg. However, the power of the study was not sufficient to express a difference in the parameter.

The more important study was the Hypertension Optimal Treatment trial,[38] which was initially designed to settle the controversy over whether the J-curve exists in patients with combined systolic and diastolic hypertension by comparing outcomes in 19,000 patients (average pretreatment BP of 170/105 mmHg) randomized to three different DBP goal groups: less than or equal to 90, less than or equal to 85, or less than or equal to 80 mmHg. Treatment was begun with the long-acting dihydropyridine calcium channel blocker felodipine, 5 mg once a day. Either an angiotensin-converting enzyme inhibitor or a beta blocker was added if the target BP was not obtained with initial therapy. Further therapeutic options included increasing the doses of these agents or adding a diuretic.

After average follow-up of approximately 4 years, 78, 41, 28, and 22% of patients were taking felodipine, an angiotensin-converting enzyme inhibitor, a beta-blocker, and a diuretic, respectively. A significant problem emerged that reduced the power of this study: less separation in the DBP was achieved in the three target groups than had been planned. Mean DBPs attained for the less-than-or-equal-to 90, less-than-or-equal-to 85, and less-than-or-equal-to 80 mmHg groups were 85.2, 83.2, and 81.1 mmHg, respectively. This close degree of BP reduction in the three groups did not provide the power to detect any difference in protection with varying degrees of BP lowering. The data therefore did not disprove the existence of a J-curve. Analysis of the correlation between adverse cardiovascular events and BPs achieved with antihypertensive drug therapy revealed that the fewest major events and the lowest cardiovascular mortality rate were noted at average BPs of 138/83 and 139/86 mmHg, respectively.

Interestingly, a recent subgroup analysis of the HOT study[39] suggests that a J-shaped curve may exist for current smokers only. Once smokers were excluded, the reduction of DBP to an average of 82 mmHg rather than 85 mmHg significantly reduced the major cardiovascular events not only in diabetics but in patients at high and very high risk, as well as in patients older than 65 years.

The last round of analyses by the Blood Pressure Lowering Treatment Trialists' Collaboration[40] had examined the effects of strategies targeting different BP goals (i.e., examining "more intensive versus less intensive regimens." It should be noted that the trials included in the analysis were the HOT study[38] (DBP≤80 versus ≤85 or ≤90 mmHg), AASK study[41] (MAP≤92 versus 102 to 107 mmHg), ABCD (H)[42] (DBP≤75 versus ≤90 mmHg), ABCD (N)[43] (DBP 10 below baseline versus 80 to 89 mmHg), and UKPDS-HDS[1] (DBP <85 versus <105 mmHg). The data showed that for every outcome other than heart failure larger reductions in BP produce larger reductions in risk (Figure 91–2). It was argued that the finding with heart failure may be due to the divergent effects of calcium-antagonist-based regimens on this outcome—an effect that seemed to be determined mainly by factors other than reduction in BP. The same observation was made with regard to doxazosin on the risk of heart failure in the ALLHAT study.[44] Nonetheless, it should also be noted that collected data on heart failure in clinical trials is problematic because of problems related to case definition and validity of diagnosis.[45]

CONCLUSIONS

The optimal goal of antihypertensive drug therapy in most patients who are not at high risk with combined SBP and DBP is, as recommended by the guidelines,[6–8] a BP of less than 140/90 mmHg. In elderly patients with isolated systolic hypertension, it is fair to say that caution is advised if DBPs inadvertently fall below 65 mmHg. Based on the available evidence, more aggressive therapy to attain a DBP of 80 mmHg or even lower might be desirable in some patients, notably (1) in patients with diabetes mellitus and (2) in patients with slowly progressive chronic renal failure excreting more than 1 to 2 g of protein per day.

REFERENCES

1. UK Prospective Diabetes Study Group. Tight blood pressure control and risk of macrovascular and microvascular complications in type 2 diabetes: UKPDS 38. *BMJ* 1998;317:703–13.

2. Peterson JC, Adler S, Buckart JM, et al. Blood pressure control, proteinuria, and the progression of renal disease. The Modification of Diet in Renal Disease Study. *Ann Intern Med* 1995;123:754–62.

3. Lazarus JM, Bourgoignie JJ, Bukalew VM, et al. for the Modification of Diet in Renal Disease Study Group. Achievement and safety of a low blood pressure goal in chronic renal disease. *Hypertension* 1997;29:641–50.

4. Isles CG, et al. Mortality in patients of the Glasgow Blood Pressure Clinic. *J Hypertens* 1986;4:141–56.

5. Collins R, Peto R, MacMahon S, et al. Blood pressure, stroke, and coronary heart disease. Part 2, Short-term reductions in blood pressure: Overview of randomised drug trials in their epidemiological context. *Lancet* 1990;335:827–38.

6. Chobanian AV, Bakris GL, Black HR, et al. The Seventh Report of the Joint National Committee on Prevention, Detection, Evaluation, and Treatment of High Blood Pressure: The JNC 7 report. *Hypertension* 2003;42:1206–52.

7. Williams, B., Poulter NR, Brown MJ, et al. British Hypertension Society guidelines for hypertension management 2004 (BHS-IV): Summary. *BMJ* 2004;328:634–40.

8. 2003 European Society of Hypertension-European Society of Cardiology guidelines for the management of arterial hypertension. *J Hypertens* 2003;21:1011–53.

9. Kannel WB. Elevated systolic blood pressure as a cardiovascular risk factor. *Am J Cardiol* 2000;85:251–55.

10. Lewington S, Clarke R, Qizilbash N, et al. Age-specific relevance of usual blood pressure to vascular mortality: A meta-analysis of individual data for one million adults in 61 prospective studies. *Lancet* 2002;360:1903–13.

11. Stewart, IM. Relation of reduction in pressure to first myocardial infarction in patients receiving treatment for severe hypertension. *Lancet* 1979;1(8121):861–65.

12. Cruickshank JM, Thorp JM, Zacharias FJ. Benefits and potential harm of lowering high blood pressure. *Lancet* 1987;1:581–84.

13. Alderman MH, Ooi WL, Madhavan S, et al. Treatment induced blood pressure reduction and the risk of myocardial infarction. *JAMA* 1989;262:920–24.

14. Fletcher, AE, Beevers DG, Bulpitt CJ, et al. The relationship between a low treated blood pressure and IHD mortality: A report from the DHSS Hypertension Care Computing Project (DHCCP). *J Hum Hypertens* 1988;2(1):11–15.

15. Samuelsson OG, Wilhelmesen LW, Pennert KM, et al. The J-shaped relation between coronary heart disease and achieved blood pressure level in treated hypertension. *J Hypertens* 1990;8:547–55.

16. Cooper SP, Hardy RJ, Labarthe DR, et al. The relation between degree of blood pressure reduction and mortality among hypertensives in the Hypertension Detection and Follow-Up Program. *Am J Epidemiol* 1988;127:387–403.

17. Staessen J, Bulpitt C, Clement D, et al. Relation between mortality and treated blood pressure in elderly patients with hypertension: Report of the European Working Party on High Blood Pressure in the Elderly. *BMJ* 1989;298:1552–56.

18. Coope J, Wareender TS. Randomised trial of treatment of hypertension in elderly patients in primary care. *Br Med J (Clin Res Ed)* 1986;293:1145–51.

19. Cruickshank JM. Coronary flow reserve and the J curve relation between diastolic blood pressure and myocardial infarction. *BMJ* 1988;297:1227–30.

20. Polese A, DeCesare N, Montorsi P, et al. Upward shift of the lower range of coronary flow autoregulation in hypertensive patients with hypertrophy of the left ventricle. *Circulation* 1991;83:845–53.

21. D'Agostino RB, Belanger AJ, Kannel WB, et al. Relation of low diastolic blood pressure to coronary heart disease death in the presence of myocardial infarction: The Framingham Study. *BMJ* 1991;303:385–89.

22. McInnes GT. The J-curve: A sceptic's viewpoint. *Dialogues Cardiol* 1989;1:1–8.

23. Hansson L. How far should blood pressure be lowered? What is the role of the J-curve? *Am J Hypertension* 1990;3:248–54.

24. Glynn RJ, Field TS, Rosner B, et al. Evidence for a positive linear relation between blood pressure and mortality in elderly people. *Lancet* 1995;345:825–29.

25. Fletcher AE, Bulpitt CJ. How far should blood pressure be lowered? *N Engl J Med* 1992;326:251–54.

26. Bots ML, Witteman JC, Hofman A, et al. Low diastolic blood pressure and atherosclerosis in elderly subjects. The Rotterdam study. *Arch Intern Med* 1996;156:843–48.

27. Kannel WB, Wilson PW, Nam BH, et al. A likely explanation for the J-curve of blood pressure cardiovascular risk. *Am J Cardiol* 2004;94:380–84.

28. Messerli FH, Kupfer S, Pepine CJ. J curve in hypertension and coronary artery disease. *Am J Cardiol* 2005;95:160.

29. SHEP Cooperative Research Group. Prevention of stroke by antihypertensive drug treatment in older persons with isolated systolic hypertension: Final results of the Systolic Hypertension in the Elderly Program. *JAMA* 1991;265:3255–64.

30. Pfeffer MA, Braunwald E, Moye LA, et al. Effect of captopril on mortality and morbidity in patients with left ventricular dysfunction after myocardial infarction: Results of the survival and ventricular enlargement trial. *N Engl J Med* 1992;327:669–77.

31. SOLVD Trial Investigators. Effects of enalapril on survival in patients with reduced left ventricular ejection fraction and CHF. *N Engl J Med* 1991;325:293–302.

32. Bulpitt CJ, Palmer AJ, Fletcher AE, et al. Optimal blood pressure control in treated hypertensive patients: Report from the Department of Health Hypertension Care Computing Project (DHCCP). *Circulation* 1994;90:225–33.

33. Flack JM, Neaton J, Grimm R, et al. for the Multiple Risk Factor Intervention Trial Study Group. Blood pressure and mortality among men with prior myocardial infarction. *Circulation* 1995;92:2437–45.

34. McMahon S, Peto R, Cutler J, et al. Blood pressure, stroke and coronary heart disease. Part 1. Prolonged differences in blood pressure: Prospective observational studies corrected for the regression dilution bias. *Lancet* 1990;335:765–74.

35. Vokó Z, Bots ML, Hofman A, Koudstaal PJ, Witteman JC, Breteler MM. J-shaped relation between blood pressure and stroke in treated hypertensives. *Hypertension* 1999;34:1181–85.

36. Somes GW, Pahor M, Shorr RI, et al. The role of diastolic blood pressure when treating isolated systolic hypertension. *Arch Intern Med* 1999;159:2004–09.

37. Hannson L for the BBB Study Group. The BBB Study: The effect of intensified antihypertensive treatment on the level of blood pressure, side-effects, morbidity and mortality in "well-treated" hypertensive patients. Behandla Blodtryck Battre. *Blood Press* 1994;3:248–54.

38. Hansson L, Zanchetti A, Carruthers SG, et al. Effects of intensive blood-pressure lowering and low-dose asprin in patients with hypertension: Principal results of the Hypertension Optimal Treatment (HOT) randomised trial. *Lancet* 1998;351:1755–62.

39. Zanchetti, A, Hansson L, Clement D, et al. Benefits and risks of more intensive blood pressure lowering in hypertensive patients of the HOT study with different risk profiles: Does a J-shaped curve exist in smokers? *J Hypertens* 2003;21(4):797–804.

40. Blood Pressure Lowering Trialists' Collaboration. Effects of different blood-pressure lowering regimens on major cardiovascular events: Results of prospectively-designed overviews of randomised trials. *Lancet* 2003;362:1527–35.

41. Wright J, Bakris G, Green T, et al. Effect of blood pressure lowering and antihypertensive drug class on progression of hypertensive kidney disease: Results from the AASK Trial. *JAMA* 2002;288:2421–31.

42. Estacio R, Jeffers B, Hiatt W, et al. The effect of nisoldipine as compared with enalapril on cardiovascular outcomes in patients with non-insulin dependent diabetes and hypertension. *N Engl J Med* 1998;338:645–52.

43. Schrier R, Estacio R, Esler A, et al. Effects of aggressive blood pressure control in normotensive type 2 diabetic patients on albuminuria, retinopthay and strokes. *Kidney Int* 2002;61:1086–97.

44. ALLHAT Officres and Coordinators for the ALLHAT Collaborative Research Group. Major cardiovascular events in hypertensive patients randomized to doxazosin vs chlorthalidone: The Antihypertensive and Lipid-Lowering Treatment to Prevent Heart Attack Trial (ALLHAT). *JAMA* 2000;283:1967–75.

45. Remes J, Miettinen H, Reunanen A, et al. Validity of clinical diagnosis of heart failure in primary health care. *Eur Heart J* 1991;12:315–21.

PHARMACOLOGIC AND NONPHARMACOLOGIC INTERVENTIONS:
PHARMACOLOGIC TREATMENT

Chapter

92

Adherence, Quality of Life, Cost Effectiveness, and the Role of the Pharmacist

Barry L. Carter

Key Findings

- Hypertension control is poor in many populations due to physician inertia, inadequate systems of care, poor patient adherence, and other factors.
- Quality of life is generally better in patients with well-controlled blood pressure (BP) regardless of medication.
- In contrast to common beliefs, quality of life is frequently better with diuretics than with other agents or even placebo.
- Adherence to medications often requires multiple strategies. Pharmacists can assist physicians with monitoring for adverse reactions or poor adherence and recommend strategies to modify therapy to improve BP control.

Several chapters in this book and national organizations describe the problem of poor BP control in the United States.[1] Clinical trials, however, have shown that BP control rates of 70 to 80% can be achieved by forced medication titration and close monitoring.[2-5] There are many reasons for poor BP control, but one common problem is clinical inertia or lack of aggressive treatment by physicians.[6-8] One study found that "resistant hypertension" was due to poor patient adherence in 13% of cases and due to suboptimal treatment regimens in 61% of cases.[9] However, adherence and quality of life can impact BP control. This chapter examines patient adherence, quality of life, and the cost of medications. Strategies for improving BP control, including the role of the pharmacist in assisting the physician, are also explored.

ADHERENCE

Various studies have found discrepancies regarding long-term persistence with antihypertensive medications, which may relate to the patient population being studied. Patients with long-established treated hypertension tend to have medication persistence rates as high as 97% and 82% after 1 and 4.5 years of observation, respectively.[10] However, persistence may be as low as 45% for newly diagnosed patients.[10-12] It is clear, however, that some patients fail to adhere to lifestyle modifications, omit medication doses, forget to take medications, or discontinue therapy.

These behaviors contribute to poor BP control and may lead to increased complications, hospitalizations, and cost.[13] Importantly, when patients adhere to lifestyle modifications they are much more likely to have an antihypertensive withdrawn.[14]

Evaluating medication adherence

The assessment of adherence by clinicians is frequently superficial and inadequate. Often, the patient is only asked: "What medications are you taking?," "How are you taking your medications?" or "Are you taking your medications?" These questions do not adequately assess adherence.

There are strategies that can be used to improve the information, but no method of assessing adherence is ideal.[15] Several adherence assessments used in research studies such as pharmacy databases are not practical for assessing an individual patient. All methods of assessing adherence can be time consuming or expensive.

A self-reported questionnaire has been validated in patients with hypertension, and the questions are shown in Box 92–1.[16] This questionnaire had a strong predictive validity for BP control when evaluated in 290 patients. Although this questionnaire has been validated, these are all closed-ended questions. This author prefers to change the wording of the first question to an open-ended question such as "How many times in the last week have you missed {medication name}?" This question is then repeated for each medication and explored further when the patient admits to missing any doses.

Box 92–1

Self-reported Adherence Questionnaire

1. Do you ever forget to take your medicine?
2. Are you careless at times about taking your medicine?
3. When you feel better do you sometimes stop taking your medicine?
4. Sometimes if you feel worse when you take the medicine do you stop taking it?

From Morisky DE, Green LW, Levine DM. Concurrent and predictive validity of a self-reported measure of medication adherence. *Med Care* 1986;24(1):67–74.

There are several other questionnaires that have been used to evaluate adherence or ability to take antihypertensive medications, including the Brief Medication Questionnaire,[17] the Medication Adherence Self-Efficacy Scale,[18] and the Hill-Bone Compliance to High Blood Pressure Therapy Scale.[19] All of these tools have been good predictors of BP control. Self-report, however, tends to overestimate adherence. However, it is the most convenient approach for the clinical setting.[15,20]

Once in awhile a patient will firmly and repeatedly deny that they miss doses but the clinician may be suspicious based on BP trends. In these cases, pharmacy refill records may be revealing and explain poor BP control.[15,21,22] These refill records can usually be obtained by contacting the patient's pharmacist. As with all methods for assessing adherence, refill records have limitations. Refill records may overestimate adherence if patients fill their medications but do not take them (stockpiling). Alternatively, refill records may underestimate adherence if the physician tells the patient to lower a dose or cut pills in half or if the patient is given samples that are not documented in the medical record.

Other strategies used in clinical trials include performing pill counts or using automated devices with electronic caps.[15,23,24] Pill counts are not practical in most clinical situations because they require a precise knowledge of fill dates, dosage, and directions that may not be consistent. Electronic caps are required for each bottle, and are generally too costly to use when treating patients. For most clinical trials, it is suggested that two methods be used to assess adherence, which will provide a better overall picture of adherence than using just one method.[15]

Barriers to adherence

Several barriers to good patient adherence have been identified and are outlined in Box 92–2.[13,18,25–27] Most studies have found that older individuals adhere better to medication regimens than younger patients, but these findings have not been consistent.[10,12,21,28] There are also conflicting data about adherence in men and women, but most studies have found women tend to adhere better than men.[10,13]

Some patients have negative beliefs about treating their hypertension, inaccurate perceptions about medications, or lack knowledge about the BP goal. Thus, their adherence is lower than other patients.[18,27] Some patients have a vague but real fear that medications may cause adverse reactions in the future or that they should not take too much medication. These beliefs can interfere with adherence. Patients living in large urban centers, those with low socioeconomic status, or those with depression and substance abuse are much more likely to have poor medication adherence.[28,29]

Patients who take complex medication regimens and multiple daily doses may have major barriers to adherence.[18,26,27,30] Generally, complex regimens should be avoided. Although it may be counterintuitive, some studies have found that patients taking greater numbers of medications or those with multiple chronic conditions adhere better than patients with less complex conditions.[10,21,31] This finding is likely explained by the Health Belief Model, which suggests that patients who believe they are sicker may tend to adhere better to their treatment.[21]

Strategies for facilitating adherence

One Cochrane review of the literature and an expert panel on compliance from the American Heart Association provided recommendations based on scientific evidence to support strategies to improve adherence.[32,33] It is important to recognize that patient education alone is not sufficient to improve adherence. There are several facilitators to good patient adherence, some of which can be modified. Facilitators to adherence are displayed in Box 92–3.[13,18,26,27]

Box 92–2

Patient Barriers to Adherence

- Insufficient knowledge
- Negative beliefs about hypertension or its treatment
- Poor self-efficacy or lack of control
- Younger age, male gender, minority race
- Cognitive impairment
- Active depression
- Alcohol or substance abuse
- Smokers
- Large-city dwellers
- Low socioeconomic status
- Lack of single medical provider
- Complicated or costly medication regimens
- Adverse drug reactions
- Rapid lowering of BP or excessive initial medication dose

Box 92–3

Adherence Facilitators

- Female gender
- Higher education and/or higher socioeconomic status
- Married
- Multiple chronic conditions, especially a prior cardiovascular event
- Higher levels of BP
- Strong patient-provider relationship
- Patients who are involved with their treatment decisions
- Patient knows BP goal
- Self-monitoring of BP
- Monotherapy or combination therapy
- Clinic and refill reminders, pill boxes, adherence aids

Some patients intentionally decide not to adhere to their medications based on the risks and benefits as they perceive them.[34] Additional education or adherence aids may not benefit these patients, and the clinician may have success by evaluating the patient's culture or health beliefs. It may be possible to improve adherence by including the patient in treatment decisions or in performing self-monitoring. Patients should be taught to accurately measure their BP and keep a log of BP values.

Patients who have stronger social and family support systems have better adherence. Behavioral strategies that empower patients to improve their ability to take medications (self-efficacy) and include family or other individuals (social support) may improve adherence.[18]

When designing an antihypertensive regimen, lower starting doses and slower dosage increases may cause fewer side effects and may improve adherence.[1,35,36] However, it is important to achieve goal BP within the first 6 months of therapy and thus dosage should be titrated frequently.

Many patients can effectively adhere to twice-daily regimens, but once-daily therapy is generally preferred.[5,37,38] Regimens that include three or four doses per day, including medications for other indications, should be avoided because most patients have great difficulty adhering to such a regimen. If regimens become too complex, it may be possible to switch some of the medications to combination pills.[1,32] When patients have problems remembering to take their medications, pill boxes, unit-of-use packaging, administration routines (e.g., taking medication with breakfast or brushing teeth), and refill reminders are important strategies.[18,32,39]

QUALITY OF LIFE IN HYPERTENSION

There has been a great deal of discussion about adverse reactions or quality of life when patients take various classes of antihypertensive medications. Quality of life is much more comprehensive than just adverse reactions, as discussed in the following sections.

Adverse effects with antihypertensives

It is frequently assumed that diuretics and beta blockers are poorly tolerated, whereas newer medications [such as angiotensin-converting enzyme inhibitors (ACEIs), calcium channel blockers (CCBs), or angiotensin receptor blockers (ARBs)] have far fewer side effects. Complicating these impressions is the commonly held belief that hypertension is asymptomatic. A further problem is that patients with hypertension have a higher prevalence of confounding conditions such as depression or impotence attributable to medications.[29,40] Patients receiving treatment for hypertension have lower quality of life scores than non-hypertensive controls.[41] Interestingly, quality of life scores were higher in hypertensive patients with controlled BP than in those with uncontrolled BP. Treated patients with a BP of >140/90 mmHg had more symptoms and lower quality of life than treated patients whose BP was controlled. This and other studies suggest that hypertension is not an asymptomatic condition and that quality of life

improves in large populations when BP is controlled.[42]

Studies that examine persistence with antihypertensives by class of agent have had conflicting results, with some finding no difference in persistence and other studies suggesting that some drug classes are better tolerated.[11,12,22,43,44] These studies usually suffer from potential selection bias. A meta-analysis of 190 studies and 28,922 patients found the highest rate of discontinuation due to adverse events occurred with CCBs (dihydropyridine 6.9% and non-dihydropyridine 5.7%) and alpha-adrenergic blockers (6.0%), ACEI (4.7%), beta blocker (4.5%), and placebo (4.3%).[45] The lowest rates of discontinuation for adverse events were seen with diuretics (3.1%) and angiotensin receptor blockers (3.1%). This study found that adverse reactions and adherence following treatment with beta blockers was similar to placebo, whereas these rates were better with diuretics and angiotensin receptor blockers. Only CCBs and alpha-adrenergic blockers were worse than placebo or the other drugs.

One well-controlled study found that a diuretic (1.1%), beta blocker (2.2%), or ACEI (4.8%) was associated with lower adverse reactions than placebo (6.5%), a CCB (6.5%), clonidine (10.1%), or prazosin (13.8%).[46] Hydrochlorothiazide treatment was associated with the lowest rate of adverse reactions and had the fewest rates of discontinuation due to adverse events, including fewer than those receiving placebo. This study demonstrates the importance of placebo-controlled trials when evaluating adverse reactions.

The Treatment of Mild Hypertension Study (TOMHS) treated patients with placebo (n=234), chlorthalidone (n=136), acebutolol (n=132), doxazosin (n=134), amlodipine (n=131), or enalapril (n=135).[42] Patients whose BP was not controlled had another antihypertensive added (chlorthalidone; except in the chlorthalidone group, who received enalapril), and in fact 33% of those on placebo received chlorthalidone. Chlorthalidone and acebutolol both had significant improvements in quality of life scores compared to placebo. The other drug groups tended to have improvements over placebo that were not statistically significant. Again, this study demonstrates the importance of evaluating placebo-controlled trials when considering adverse reactions or quality of life changes over time.

Of course, patients and physicians frequently attribute symptoms to an antihypertensive drug. It often does not matter if this assessment is accurate because the patient may refuse to continue the medication either way. If the patient believes the medication is causing a side effect, the clinician will need to address the matter and this frequently requires changing doses or agents. Frequent follow-up is important, especially early in therapy or with patients newly diagnosed with hypertension because these patients are at high risk of discontinuing therapy or dropping out of the health care system. If patients are going to discontinue their medication, this is most likely to occur early in therapy.[10]

Quality of life assessments

The foregoing observations make an assumption that there is a relationship among adverse reactions, quality of life, and medication adherence (which is not necessarily true). Validated quality of life instruments typically measure physical health, bodily pain, vitality, social functioning, role limitations, mental health, and general health. Thus, adverse reactions to medications do not necessarily correlate well with quality of life measures. What about the relationship between quality of life and adherence? Intuitively, one would assume there should be a relationship but the data are not compelling. One study evaluated this relationship in 100 patients with hypertension, 199 patients at high risk for medication problems, and 365 elderly patients.[47] They studied six different quality of life instruments. Correlations between quality of life and adherence were very weak, and the weakest correlations occurred in the patients with hypertension. Although very weak, there was a negative correlation between physical and mental domains on quality of life instruments and adherence to antihypertensive medications, which the authors speculated may be related to adverse drug reactions.

In summary, quality of life scores appear to improve when BP is controlled—suggesting that hypertension may not be asymptomatic after all. Quality of life does not correlate well with adverse reactions or adherence. This is likely due to the fact that quality of life questionnaires are much more comprehensive than simply measuring adverse reactions. Quality of life may not correlate well to adherence for several reasons. Research has demonstrated that patients who perceive themselves as very sick may adhere better to their therapy (Health Belief Model). In this case, their scores for perception of their health, role limitations, or bodily pain may be low. However, because of these symptoms they may adhere to their medications.

COST EFFECTIVENESS OF ANTIHYPERTENSIVE TREATMENT

Whenever possible, inexpensive regimens should be designed. This can be accomplished using evidence-based treatment strategies. The cost of medications, including co-payments, is a significant predictor of adherence.[1,18,48,49] An interesting study evaluated nonadherence to medications as a function of drug affordability between 1997 and 2002.[48] The authors found that self-reported nonadherence to medications due to cost increased from 4.7% in 1997 to 5.9% in 2002. Blacks (8.4%) and Hispanics (6.7%) reported more nonadherence due to cost than did whites (5.5%) ($p<0.001$). As expected, health insurance coverage was strongly associated with medication nonadherence due to cost. Those with private insurance reported much lower rates of nonadherence than those without insurance (3% versus 18%, $p<0.001$). Interestingly, patients who were dually eligible for both Medicare and Medicaid were more likely to be nonadherent due to cost (11.4%) than overall Medicare beneficiaries (7.0%). These authors estimated that 16.6 million Americans were unable to purchase a prescribed medication in 2002. Obviously, cost-effective strategies should be employed to improve patient adherence and BP control.

In many areas of medicine there is often a trade-off between cost and efficacy. However, this is not true in hypertension—where the least costly medications (thiazide diuretics) are at least as effective in overall cardiovascular outcomes, and superior for select outcomes, when compared to more expensive medications.[50] An economic analysis found that 40% of 2.05 million prescriptions for antihypertensive drugs could have been for less costly agents based on scientific evidence.[50] Even when the potential need for laboratory monitoring was included in the analysis, these changes would have saved $11.6 million (or about one-fourth of the overall costs). If Medicaid pricing were used, the savings could have been $20.5 million. Replacing thiazides for CCBs resulted in the largest reduction in cost. The authors estimated that $1.2 billion could be saved nationally if prescribing patterns followed national guidelines and scientific evidence.

Many patients require two or more medications to manage hypertension, and some require alternative agents to manage coexisting conditions. The most versatile and cost-effective regimen is a thiazide-like diuretic (hydrochlorothiazide or chlorthalidone) and a generic ACEI such as lisinopril.[50,51] Many patients can have their BP and/or proteinuria effectively managed with this regimen, and as noted previously it is very well tolerated. For patients who require additional agents or who do not tolerate this regimen, there are many other options available that include low-cost medications. Any regimen that includes a CCB or angiotensin receptor blocker will be much more costly and should only be considered for specific indications in select patients.

ROLE OF THE PHARMACIST

Pharmacists in a wide variety of settings can be a valuable resource for physicians in assisting with patient management and improving BP control. Pharmacists have performed a wide variety of functions, including screening and referral, monitoring for adverse reactions and nonadherence, making recommendations to the physician for alterations in therapy, and disease-state management. Pharmacists can assist the physician with several items (listed in Box 92–3), including: (1) reinforcing the physician's BP goal with the patient, (2) teaching the patient to use BP monitoring devices sold in the pharmacy, (3) recommending regimen redesign to reduce complexity, adverse reactions, or cost, and (4) providing refill reminders, pill boxes, adherence aids, or other strategies for improving adherence.

In addition to community pharmacies, clinical pharmacists are frequently located in academic clinics, VA medical center clinics, and even private physician offices. In some of these settings, pharmacists assist physicians with managing hypertension or provide pharmacist-managed hypertension services.[52] Approximately 40 states have enacted legislation or rules that allow physicians and pharmacists to establish collaborative relationships, and the pharmacist can manage certain chronic conditions via protocol.[53] Although most of these collaborations occur in structured settings such as academic clinics, some include community pharmacies. The following sections discuss these areas as a function of the type of setting in which the pharmacist practices.

Community pharmacies

Although most community pharmacies continue to provide traditional services (medication dispensing and counseling), it is increasingly common to find pharmacies that provide more advanced services. Many patients visit their community pharmacy nearly once a month. If the physician and pharmacist have a good working relationship, the pharmacist can assist with screening and referral of patients with elevated BP, monitoring for adverse reactions and poor adherence, and making recommendations to the physician for overcoming these problems. The pharmacist can also assist the physician by providing patient education and counseling about the medications and strategies to improve BP control in an effort to reinforce the physician's treatment plan.

Several studies have been conducted in community pharmacies in which pharmacists measured BP and made recommendations to the physician to modify therapy.[54–56] McKenney conducted an intervention in which the community pharmacist collaborated with two physicians in an urban health center.[56] The pharmacist met with the physicians in their office and reviewed study patients' medical records. The pharmacist assessed patients monthly and made recommendations to the physicians. The control group had a deterioration in physician-measured BP (163/93 to 166/101 mmHg), whereas the BP in the intervention group improved (157/99 to 146/90 mmHg) and the difference between groups was significant ($p<0.001$). The intervention group, but not the control group, experienced significant improvements in medication adherence and knowledge of hypertension. One of the fascinating features of this study was that BP control and adherence deteriorated once the service was discontinued.

Carter performed an evaluation of a similar intervention except that the community pharmacy was a clinic pharmacy within the building of a private rural clinic.[54] Because of the close proximity of the pharmacists and physicians, the pharmacists reviewed medical records and made face-to-face recommendations to the physicians. Following monthly evaluations with the pharmacist, BP measured in the physician's office was significantly reduced at 6 months in the intervention group (146/83 versus 135/75 mmHg, $p<0.001$) but not the control group (147/82 versus 142/82 mmHg). In this study, several measures of quality of life improved in the intervention group but not the control group. In addition, a blinded peer review panel evaluated the quality of prescribing. There was no change in the quality of prescribing in the control group but the appropriateness of the BP regimen ($p<0.01$), potential benefit of the regimen ($p<0.05$), and assessment of the patient for adverse reactions ($p<0.001$) were all improved in the intervention group.

Even though the above were small studies, they all demonstrated improved BP control and medication adherence when community pharmacists provided these services. Although these collaborative programs are uncommon in community pharmacies, they are increasing nationwide.

Primary care clinics

Most examples of advanced services provided by pharmacists are found in academic family medicine clinics, internal medicine clinics, or in Veterans Affairs medical centers.[52] One study was conducted in a managed care setting and evaluated physician/pharmacist co-management of hypertension.[57] Patients were randomized to either usual care ($n=99$) or the co-managed group ($n=98$). BP was reduced more in the co-managed group than in the usual care group at 6, 9, and 12 months (22 versus 9, 25 versus 10, and 22 versus 11 mmHg, respectively; $p<0.001$).

Several other studies have found similar results.[58–64] In another study, a pharmacist worked with physicians in a medical residency training program.[58] The pharmacist role was to assist physicians with improving BP control. Patients ($n=95$) were randomized to a control or intervention group. Systolic BP declined 11 mmHg in the control group and 23 mmHg in the intervention group ($p<0.001$). Physicians accepted 93% of the 162 recommendations made by the pharmacist. Medication charges *increased* by $6.50 in the control group but *decreased* by $6.80 in the intervention group.

One study in a VA found that not only was BP significantly reduced when management was assisted by a clinical pharmacist but BP control was sustained for 4 years following management by the pharmacist or a nurse.[59,60] In larger group practices and academic centers, there are typically nurses or nurse practitioners and perhaps physician assistants in addition to clinical pharmacists. Each setting must determine how to efficiently utilize the practitioners in the office. In this case, clinical pharmacists would be best suited to assist with patients who have BP that has been difficult to control; who have complex regimens, adverse reactions, or problems with adherence; or who need assistance with reducing medication costs.

In many primary care settings that employ clinical pharmacists, the pharmacist assists with programs for designing cost-effective medication regimens. Some patients do require more expensive therapies, and these pharmacists (or in some cases pharmacy technicians) assist with indigent programs offered by the pharmaceutical industry. One study found significant improvements in disease outcome with such a program.[65]

Kaiser Permanente of Colorado is one of the best-performing managed care organizations in the United States.[66] In this organization, hypertension management is an integrated program among physicians, nurse practitioners, clinical pharmacy specialists, and others. Although different clinics within the region have different structures, they all achieve high BP control rates. In one model, patients with regular hypertension visit a registered nurse, who sees the patient, gathers a history, and measures vital signs. When BP is above goal, the nurse consults with the clinical pharmacy specialist to determine if changes in medication therapy are needed. If so, the clinical pharmacy specialist develops a therapeutic plan based on national guidelines. This interdisciplinary approach has resulted in innovative practice models that are likely the reason this Kaiser region has the highest BP control rates of any Kaiser region and most other managed care organizations. Figure 92–1 displays a potential model for interdisciplinary management of hypertension.

Pharmacist-managed hypertension clinics

Pharmacist-managed hypertension clinics are not common and have primarily been developed in VA medical centers. One survey found that one-third of hypertension clinics in VA medical centers were managed by pharmacists.[67] These clinics still have a physician medical director and policies and procedures to ensure a structured evidence-based approach to treatment. One study used blinded judges to evaluate the medication regimens and found that pharmacists scored better than physicians when selecting appropriate antihypertensive drugs ($p<0.01$); selecting the proper quantity, dose, and directions ($p<0.05$); and avoiding drug interactions ($p<0.05$).[62] The studies by Monson and Bond, in which most of the management of hypertension was performed by clinical pharmacists, was conducted within renal or arthritis clinics in the Madison VA.[59,60]

Finally, a study was conducted in San Antonio in a largely indigent Hispanic population.[63] BP control was similar in the pharmacist or physician-managed groups but BP was controlled in 97% in the pharmacist group compared to 78% in the physician group ($p<0.05$).

The previously cited studies strongly suggest that BP and medication regimens can be improved and adverse reactions avoided when pharmacists assist physicians with managing hypertension. Pharmacists in any setting can assist with developing cost-effective treatment strategies, track prescription refill history, educate patients on the use of pill boxes or other devices, and help the physician by reinforcing treatment goals.

SUMMARY

Hypertension control is poor in many populations due to physician inertia, inadequate systems of care, poor patient adherence, and other factors. There are many provider and organizational quality improvement strategies that should be used to improve BP control in individual patients and within a panel of patients in a clinic. Table 92–1 displays these strategies. Quality of life is generally better in patients with controlled BP regardless of medication. In contrast to common beliefs, quality of life is frequently better with diuretics than with other more expensive agents or even placebo. Adherence to medications is challenging for some patients, and multiple strategies need to be used to support patients in their effort to correctly take their medications. Pharmacists can assist physicians with monitoring for adverse reactions or poor adherence and recommend strategies to modify therapy to improve BP control. In some settings, pharmacists may collaborate with physicians and nurses to optimize BP control.

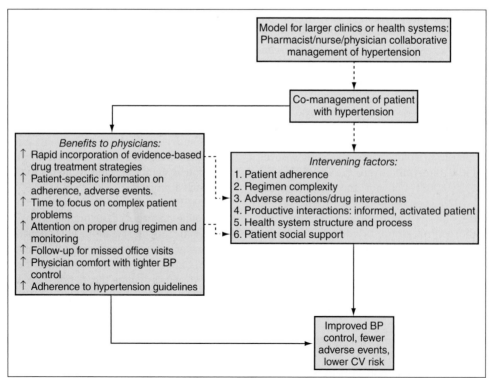

Figure 92–1. A potential model for interdisciplinary management of hypertension.

STRATEGIES FOR IMPROVING BP CONTROL	
Actions by Providers	**Strategies**
Foster effective communication with patients	
■ Provide clear, direct messages about importance of lifestyle modification or therapy ■ Include patients in decisions about prevention and treatment goals for BP ■ Incorporate behavioral strategies into counseling	■ Provide verbal and written instruction and rationale for treatments ■ Develop counseling skills ■ Use contracting strategies ■ Establish BP goals and a plan ■ Anticipate barriers or occasional low adherence and discuss solutions
Document BP goals and respond to patient's progress toward goals	
■ Create an evidence-based practice ■ Assess patient's adherence at each visit ■ Assess the patient's progress toward goal BP at each visit ■ Develop reminder systems to ensure identification and follow-up of patient status	■ Document the goal BP in the medical record ■ Determine methods of evaluating hypertension outcomes ■ Use self-report on adherence, pill counts, or electronic data ■ Contact pharmacist to obtain refill history ■ Use telephone follow-up
Actions by the Clinic or Office	**Specific Strategies**
Organization of the office or clinic must:	
■ Develop an environment that supports hypertension prevention and treatment interventions ■ Ensure continuity with one provider ■ Provide tracking and reporting systems ■ Benchmark BP control rates by provider or by clinic ■ Provide education and training of providers ■ Provide adequate reimbursement for allocation of time for all health care professionals ■ Rapidly and efficiently incorporate innovations into medical practice	■ Develop training in behavioral science and office set-up for all personnel ■ Use pre-appointment and refill reminders ■ Use telephone follow-up ■ Schedule evening/weekend office hours ■ Provide group counseling for patients and families ■ Develop computer-based systems such as electronic medical records ■ Require continuing education courses in communication, behavioral counseling ■ Hire behavioral counselors to provide adherence counseling ■ Develop incentives tied to desired patient and provider outcomes ■ Incorporate nurse and/or pharmacist case management of hypertension ■ Effectively store and document BP data obtained from patient self-monitoring ■ Provide continuous quality improvement training
Adapted from [33, 37, 68].	

Table 92–1. Strategies for Improving BP Control

REFERENCES

1. Chobanian AV, Bakris GL, Black HR, et al. The Seventh Report of the Joint National Committee on Prevention, Detection, Evaluation, and Treatment of High Blood Pressure. *Hypertension* 2003;42(6):1206–52.
2. Grimm RH Jr., Margolis KL, Papademetriou VV, et al. Baseline Characteristics of Participants in the Antihypertensive and Lipid Lowering Treatment to Prevent Heart Attack Trial (ALLHAT). *Hypertension* 2001;37(1):19–27.
3. Hansson L, Zanchetti A, Carruthers SG, et al. Effects of intensive blood-pressure lowering and low-dose aspirin in patients with hypertension: Principal results of the Hypertension Optimal Treatment (HOT) randomised trial. HOT Study Group. *Lancet* 1998;351(9118):1755–62.
4. Black HR, Elliott WJ, Neaton JD, et al. Baseline Characteristics and Early Blood Pressure Control in the CONVINCE Trial. *Hypertension* 2001;37(1):12–18.
5. Carter BL, Frohlich ED, Elliott WJ, et al. Selected factors that influence responses to antihypertensives: Choosing therapy for the uncomplicated patient. *Arch Fam Med* 1994;3(6):528–36.
6. Hyman DJ, Pavlik VN. Characteristics of patients with uncontrolled hypertension in the United States. *N Engl J Med* 2001;345(7):479–86.
7. Berlowitz DR, Ash AS, Hickey EC, et al. Inadequate management of blood pressure in a hypertensive population. *N Engl J Med* 1998;339(27):1957–63.
8. Oliveria SA, Lapuerta P, McCarthy BD, et al. Physician-related barriers to the effective management of uncontrolled hypertension. *Arch Intern Med* 2002;162(4):413–20.
9. Garg JP, Elliott WJ, Folker AC, et al. Resistant hypertension revisited. *Am J Hypertens* 2005;18:619–26.
10. Caro JJ, Salas M, Speckman JL, et al. Persistence with treatment for hypertension in actual practice. *CMAJ* 1999;160(1):31–7.

11. Degli Esposti E, Sturani A, Di Martino M, et al. Long-term persistence with antihypertensive drugs in new patients. *J Hum Hypertens* 2002;16(6):439–44.

12. Degli Esposti L, Degli Esposti E, Valpiani G, et al. A retrospective, population-based analysis of persistence with antihypertensive drug therapy in primary care practice in Italy. *Clin Ther* 2002;24(8):1347–1357; discussion 1346.

13. Flack JM, Novikov SV, Ferrario CM. Benefits of adherence to anti-hypertensive drug therapy. *Eur Heart J* 1996;17(Suppl A):16–20.

14. Espeland MA, Whelton PK, Kostis JB, et al. Predictors and mediators of successful long-term withdrawal from antihypertensive medications. TONE Cooperative Research Group. Trial of Nonpharmacologic Interventions in the Elderly. *Arch Fam Med* 1999;8(3):228–36.

15. Grymonpre RE, Didur CD, Montgomery PR, Sitar DS. Pill count, self-report, and pharmacy claims data to measure medication adherence in the elderly. *Ann Pharmacother* 1998;32(7/8):749–54.

16. Morisky DE, Green LW, Levine DM. Concurrent and predictive validity of a self-reported measure of medication adherence. *Med Care* 1986;24(1):67–74.

17. Svarstad BL, Chewning BA, Sleath BL, Claesson C. The Brief Medication Questionnaire: A tool for screening patient adherence and barriers to adherence. *Patient Educ Couns* 1999;37(2):113–24.

18. Ogedegbe G, Mancuso CA, Allegrante JP, Charlson ME. Development and evaluation of a medication adherence self-efficacy scale in hypertensive African-American patients. *J Clin Epidemiol* 2003;56(6):520–29.

19. Kim MT, Hill MN, Bone LR, Levine DM. Development and testing of the Hill-Bone Compliance to High Blood Pressure Therapy Scale. *Prog Cardiovasc Nurs* 2000;15(3):90–6.

20. Dunbar-Jacob J DK, Dunning J. Compliance with antihypertensive regimen: A review of the research in the 1980s. *Ann Behav Med* 1991;13:31–9.

21. Billups SJ, Malone DC, Carter BL. The relationship between drug therapy noncompliance and patient characteristics, health-related quality of life, and health care costs. *Pharmacotherapy* 2000;20(8):941–49.

22. Monane M, Bohn RL, Gurwitz JH, et al. The effects of initial drug choice and comorbidity on antihypertensive therapy compliance: Results from a population-based study in the elderly. *Am J Hypertens* 1997;10(7 Pt 1):697–704.

23. Choo PW, Rand CS, Inui TS, et al. Validation of patient reports, automated pharmacy records, and pill counts with electronic monitoring of adherence to antihypertensive therapy. *Med Care* 1999;37(9):846–57.

24. Lee JY, Kusek JW, Greene PG, et al. Assessing medication adherence by pill count and electronic monitoring in the African American Study of Kidney Disease and Hypertension (AASK) Pilot Study. *Am J Hypertens* 1996;9(8):719–25.

25. Ockene IS, Ockene JK. Barriers to lifestyle change, and the need to develop an integrated approach to prevention. *Cardiol Clin* 1996;14(1):159–69.

26. Ogedegbe G, Harrison M, Robbins L, et al. Reasons patients do or do not take their blood pressure medications. *Ethn Dis* 2004;14(1):158.

27. Ogedegbe G, Harrison M, Robbins L, et al. Barriers and facilitators of medication adherence in hypertensive African Americans: A qualitative study. *Ethn Dis* 2004;14(1):3–12.

28. Vaur L, Vaisse B, Genes N, et al. Use of electronic pill boxes to assess risk of poor treatment compliance: results of a large-scale trial. *Am J Hypertens* 1999;12(4 Pt 1):374–80.

29. Kim MT, Han HR, Hill MN, et al. Depression, substance use, adherence behaviors, and blood pressure in urban hypertensive black men. *Ann Behav Med* 2003;26(1):24–31.

30. Nuesch R, Schroeder K, Dieterle T, et al. Relation between insufficient response to antihypertensive treatment and poor compliance with treatment: A prospective case-control study. *BMJ* 2001;323(7305):142–46.

31. Knight EL, Bohn RL, Wang PS, et al. Predictors of uncontrolled hypertension in ambulatory patients. *Hypertension* 2001;38(4):809–14.

32. Schroeder K, Fahey T, Ebrahim S. How can we improve adherence to blood pressure-lowering medication in ambulatory care? Systematic review of randomized controlled trials. *Arch Intern Med* 2004;164(7):722–32.

33. Miller NH, Hill M, Kottke T, Ockene IS. The multilevel compliance challenge: Recommendations for a call to action. A statement for healthcare professionals. *Circulation* 1997;95(4):1085–90.

34. Bernardini J. Ethical issues of compliance/adherence in the treatment of hypertension. *Adv Chronic Kidney Dis* 2004;11(2):222–27.

35. Flack JM, Yunis C, Preisser J, et al. The rapidity of drug dose escalation influences blood pressure response and adverse effects burden in patients with hypertension: The Quinapril Titration Interval Management Evaluation (ATIME) Study. ATIME Research Group. *Arch Intern Med* 2000;160(12):1842–47.

36. Cohen JS. Adverse drug effects, compliance, and initial doses of antihypertensive drugs recommended by the Joint National Committee vs the Physicians' Desk Reference. *Arch Intern Med* 2001;161(6):880–85.

37. Carter BL, Zillich A.J. Management of essential hypertension . In: Schumock GT, Brundage DM, Chessman KH, et al. (eds.), *The Pharmacotherapy Self-Assessment Program, Fifth Edition.* Kansas City: The American College of Clinical Pharmacy; 2004:129–63.

38. Eisen SA, Miller DK, Woodward RS, et al. The effect of prescribed daily dose frequency on patient medication compliance. *Arch Intern Med* 1990;150(9):1881–84.

39. Murray MD, Birt JA, Manatunga AK, Darnell JC. Medication compliance in elderly outpatients using twice-daily dosing and unit-of-use packaging. *Ann Pharmacother* 1993;27(5):616–21.

40. Wang PS, Bohn RL, Knight E, et al. Noncompliance with antihypertensive medications: The impact of depressive symptoms and psychosocial factors. *J Gen Intern Med* 2002;17(7):504–11.

41. Erickson SR, Williams BC, Gruppen LD. Perceived symptoms and health-related quality of life reported by uncomplicated hypertensive patients compared to normal controls. *J Hum Hypertens* 2001;15(8):539–48.

42. Neaton JD, Grimm RH Jr., Prineas RJ, et al. Treatment of Mild Hypertension Study: Final results. Treatment of Mild Hypertension Study Research Group. *JAMA* 1993;270(6):713–24.

43. Alderman MH, Madhavan S, Cohen H. Antihypertensive Drug Therapy: The effect of JNC criteria on prescribing patterns and patient status through the first year. *Am J Hypertens* 1996;9(5):413–18.

44. Benson S, Vance-Bryan K, Raddatz J. Time to patient discontinuation of antihypertensive drugs in different classes. *Am J Health Syst Pharm* 2000;57(1):51–4.

45. Ross SD, Akhras KS, Zhang S, et al. Discontinuation of antihypertensive drugs due to adverse events: A systematic review and meta-analysis. *Pharmacotherapy* 2001;21(8):940–53.

46. Materson BJ, Reda DJ, Cushman WC, et al. Single-drug therapy for hypertension in men: A comparison of six antihypertensive agents with placebo. The Department of Veterans Affairs Cooperative Study Group on Antihypertensive Agents. *N Engl J Med* 1993;328(13):914–21.

47. Cote I, Farris K, Feeny D. Is adherence to drug treatment correlated with health-related quality of life? *Qual Life Res* 2003;12(6):621–33.

48. Kennedy J, Coyne J, Sclar D. Drug affordability and prescription noncompliance in the United States: 1997–2002. *Clin Ther* 2004;26(4):607–14.

49. Raji MA, Kuo YF, Salazar JA, et al. Ethnic differences in antihypertensive medication use in the elderly. *Ann Pharmacother* 2004;38(2):209–14.

50. Fischer MA, Avorn J. Economic implications of evidence-based prescribing for hypertension: Can better care cost less? *JAMA* 2004;291(15):1850–56.

51. Carter BL, Ernst ME, Cohen JD. Hydrochlorothiazide versus chlorthalidone: Evidence supporting their interchangeability. *Hypertension* 2004;43(1):4–9.

52. Carter BL, Zillich AJ, Elliott WJ. How pharmacists can assist physicians with controlling blood pressure. *J Clin Hypertens* 2003;5(1):31–7.

53. Hammond RW, Schwartz AH, Campbell MJ, et al. Collaborative drug therapy management by pharmacists 2003. *Pharmacotherapy* 2003;23(9):1210–25.

54. Carter BL, Barnette DJ, Chrischilles E, et al. Evaluation of hypertensive patients after care provided by community pharmacists in a rural setting. *Pharmacotherapy* 1997;17(6):1274–85.

55. Park JJ, Kelly P, Carter BL, Burgess PP. Comprehensive pharmaceutical care in the chain setting. *J Am Pharm Assoc (Wash)* 1996;NS36(7):443–51.

56. McKenney JM, Slining JM, Henderson HR, et al. The effect of clinical pharmacy services on patients with essential

hypertension. *Circulation* 1973;48(5):
1104–11.

57. Borenstein JE, Graber G, Saltiel E, et al.
Physician-pharmacist comanagement
of hypertension: A randomized,
comparative trial. *Pharmacotherapy*
2003;23(2):209–16.

58. Bogden PE, Abbott RD, Williamson P,
et al. Comparing standard care with a
physician and pharmacist team approach
for uncontrolled hypertension. *J Gen
Intern Med* 1998;13(11):740–45.

59. Monson R, Bond CA, Schuna A. Role of
the clinical pharmacist in improving
drug therapy: Clinical pharmacists in
outpatient therapy. *Arch Intern Med*
1981;141(11):1441–44.

60. Bond CA, Monson R. Sustained
improvement in drug documentation,
compliance, and disease control:
A four-year analysis of an ambulatory
care model. *Arch Intern Med* 1984;
144(6):1159–62.

61. Erickson SR, Slaughter R, Halapy H.
Pharmacists' ability to influence
outcomes of hypertension therapy.
Pharmacotherapy 1997;17(1):140–47.

62. McGhan WF, Stimmel GL, Hall TG,
Gilman TM. A comparison of
pharmacists and physicians on the
quality of prescribing for ambulatory
hypertensive patients. *Med Care* 1983;
21(4):435–44.

63. Hawkins DW, Fiedler FP, Douglas HL,
Eschbach RC. Evaluation of a clinical
pharmacist in caring for hypertensive
and diabetic patients. *Am J Hosp Pharm*
1979;36(10):1321–25.

64. Mehos BM, Saseen JJ, MacLaughlin EJ.
Effect of pharmacist intervention and
initiation of home blood pressure
monitoring in patients with uncontrolled
hypertension. *Pharmacotherapy* 2000;
20(11):1384–89.

65. Schoen MD, DiDomenico RJ, Connor SE,
et al. Impact of the cost of prescription

drugs on clinical outcomes in
indigent patients with heart disease.
Pharmacotherapy 2001;21(12):1455–63.

66. Anon. The State of Health Care Quality
2004. The National Committee for
Quality Assurance, Washington, D.C.
http://www.ncqa.org. Accessed
November 12, 2004.

67. Alsuwaidan S, Malone DC, Billups SJ,
Carter BL. Characteristics of ambulatory
care clinics and pharmacists in Veterans
Affairs medical centers. IMPROVE
investigators. Impact of Managed
Pharmaceutical Care on Resource
Utilization and Outcomes in Veterans
Affairs Medical Centers. *Am J Health Syst
Pharm* 1998;55(1):68–72.

68. Carter BL. Management of essential
hypertension. In: Bertch K, Dunsworth T,
Fagan S, et al. (eds.), *The Pharmacotherapy
Self-Assessment Program, Fourth Edition.*
Kansas City: The American College of
Clinical Pharmacy, 2001:1–39.

Chapter

93

Nonpharmacologic Management of Hypertension

Saverio Stranges and Francesco P. Cappuccio

Key Findings

- Nonpharmacologic interventions represent an essential approach to the primary prevention of high blood pressure and an important component of the treatment of hypertension.

- Current lifestyle modifications that effectively lower blood pressure include weight reduction; reduction of dietary sodium intake; increased potassium intake; moderation of alcohol consumption; adoption of a diet rich in fruit, vegetables, and low-fat dairy products with a reduced content of saturated and total fat; and regular aerobic exercise.

- Obesity is an important determinant of cardiovascular disease, and the relationship between obesity and hypertension is well documented.

- Weight gain, even of a modest magnitude, is itself an important risk factor for the development of hypertension in adulthood. In contrast, average reductions of 4.4/3.6 mmHg for systolic and diastolic blood pressure, respectively, are reported for a 5-kg weight loss.

- The amount of dietary sodium is an important determinant of blood pressure levels and of hypertension risk both in individuals and populations, and conversely, the reduction of dietary sodium intake reduces blood pressure and helps control hypertension.

- Several antihypertensive drugs blocking the renin-angiotensin system (e.g., angiotensin-converting enzyme inhibitors, beta-blockers, and angiotensin II receptors antagonists) have an additive effect on blood pressure reduction in those patients already on a reduced salt diet.

- The risk of hypertension is 30-50% higher in individuals who are physically inactive, and aerobic exercise is associated with a significant reduction in systolic and diastolic blood pressure of 3.8/2.6 mmHg, respectively.

Cardiovascular diseases (CVDs) are the leading cause of mortality, morbidity, and disability worldwide.[1] Although CVDs are proportionally more relevant in developed countries, currently 70% of the total number of cardiovascular deaths occur in developing countries. In fact, in the past several decades, the process of changes in patterns of diseases and their interaction with the socio-economic transformation, known as "epidemiologic transition,"[2] has caused an increasing burden of CVD in many developing countries. Thus, preventing CVD represents a formidable public health challenge not only in developed but also in developing countries.

The strategy for the primary prevention of CVD resides in the detection and management of major risk factors. Seventy-five percent of the global burden of CVD results from smoking, high blood cholesterol, and high blood pressure or a combination of these factors. Globally, excess blood cholesterol causes more than 4 million premature deaths a year, tobacco causes almost 5 million, and high blood pressure causes 7 million.[1] In particular, hypertension affects approximately 1 billion individuals worldwide, thus representing the most common cardiovascular condition in both developed and developing countries as well as the number one attributable risk for death throughout the world.[3] Indeed, according to a recent World Health Organization report, about 62% of cerebrovascular disease and 49% of ischemic heart disease are attributable to suboptimal blood pressure levels (systolic blood pressure >115 mmHg) with little variation by gender.[1]

The burden of hypertension-related diseases is likely to increase as the population ages, as suggested by recent data from the Framingham Heart Study, whereby normotensive individuals at 55 years of age have a 90% lifetime risk to develop hypertension.[4] Accordingly, prevention and treatment of hypertension are increasingly regarded as a public health priority in both developed and developing countries. In developed countries, because of the magnitude of the incidence of CVDs and the potential benefits of hypertension prevention; in developing countries, because of the rising magnitude of CVD incidence given the size of the populations, limited resources available, increase in hypertension prevalence, and marked trend to urbanization with the subsequent epidemiologic transition.[5]

Nonpharmacologic interventions, also termed "lifestyle modifications," represent an essential approach to the primary prevention of high blood pressure and an important component of the treatment of hypertension. They represent as well cost-effective measures in the context of a multifaceted public health strategy to reducing blood pressure at a population level. The current lifestyle modifications that effectively lower blood pressure include weight reduction if overweight or obese; reduction of dietary sodium intake; increased potassium intake; moderation of alcohol consumption; adoption of a dietary plan based on the DASH (Dietary Approaches to Stop Hypertension) diet, that is, a diet rich in fruit, vegetables, and low-fat dairy products with a reduced content of saturated and total fat; and regular aerobic exercise.[6] These lifestyle modifications are effective in reducing blood pressure, increasing the efficacy of pharmacologic therapies, and reducing the global risk of CVD.

In this chapter, we will review the available literature and discuss the importance of these nonpharmacologic measures, for which the current evidence consistently demonstrates their efficacy in lowering blood pressure. In addition, we will evaluate the appropriateness of recommendations at a population level regarding some of these measures (i.e., reduction of dietary sodium intake) and the different approaches to intervention needed to implement a successful strategy to prevent hypertension in developing and developed countries.

WEIGHT REDUCTION

Obesity is a worldwide public health priority.[7] In the United States, the prevalence of obesity, defined as body mass index (BMI) of 30 kg/m^2 or more, as well as of overweight (BMI ≥ 25 kg/m^2) has steadily increased since the second half of the last century as the population has aged. Data from the U.S. National Health and Nutrition Examination Survey (NHANES), obtained in 2003–2004, indicate that 32.2% of American adults (20 years or older) are obese whereas only one-third (33.7%) are in the range of normal weight (BMI < 25 kg/m^2).[8] The obesity trends in the United Kingdom have been similar; recent prevalence data indicate that over half of women and about two-thirds of men are either overweight or obese.[9] Obesity and overweight are becoming increasing public health issues in many developing regions as well (e.g., Latin America, Middle East) and represent major contributors to the global burden of disease.[10]

Obesity is an important determinant of CVD, and is strongly associated with several cardiovascular risk factors such as diabetes, high cholesterol, and high blood pressure. In fact, obesity is an independent risk factor for coronary heart disease, stroke, and total cardiovascular morbidity and mortality.[11]

The relationship between obesity and hypertension is very well documented. Blood pressure is strongly correlated with BMI. In the INTERSALT study, the relationship between BMI and blood pressure was examined in over 10,000 men and women, from 20 to 59 years of age, sampled from 52 centers around the world.[12] BMI was linearly associated with systolic and diastolic blood pressure, independent of age, alcohol intake, smoking habits, and sodium and potassium excretion. The prevalence of obesity-related hypertension varies with age, ethnicity, and gender of the population studied.[13] Approximately one-third of cases of hypertension are attributable to obesity, although in young adults (under 45 years of age) the figures may be substantially higher. For example, in the sample of young adults of the Framingham Offspring Study, 78% of cases of hypertension in men and 64% in women were attributable to obesity.[14] Additionally, variations have been observed by ethnic group. For example, results from the Atherosclerosis Risk in Communities Study suggest the association to be stronger in whites than in African Americans.[15]

Not only is obesity associated with high blood pressure, but weight gain, even of a modest magnitude, is itself an important risk factor for the development of hypertension in adulthood. This effect seems to be independent of baseline BMI and baseline blood pressure, present in both genders, stronger in young adults, and weaker in people of black African ancestry; conversely, weight loss reduces the risk of hypertension.[16–18]

While many of the earlier studies examined the association between obesity and blood pressure relying on BMI as an indicator of relative weight, more recent investigations have emphasized the importance of body fat distribution in this association. Specifically, abdominal adiposity has been reported as a stronger determinant of hypertension risk than relative weight.[15,19–21] In epidemiologic studies, several anthropometric measures have been used as proxy measures for body fat distribution, such as waist-to-hip circumference ratio, waist circumference, and abdominal sagittal diameter. Current clinical guidelines propose waist circumference as a reference measure of central adiposity in adults because its measurement is the least affected by observer bias.[22]

Given the overwhelming evidence on the relationship between body weight and blood pressure, weight reduction has been proposed as a measure to reduce blood pressure in both individual patients and the community at large. Over the past three decades, several randomized controlled clinical trials have reported on the beneficial effects of weight loss interventions on the prevention and treatment of hypertension. For example, the results of the multicenter randomized clinical Trials of Hypertension Prevention (TOHP), Phases I and II, indicate that both short- and long-term weight loss is successful in reducing blood pressure. In TOHP I, an 18-month intervention was significantly associated with 77% reduction in the incidence of hypertension after a 7-year follow-up.[23] Likewise, in TOHP II, a longer-term intervention of 36 months resulted in significant reductions in systolic and diastolic blood pressures and in a lower incidence of hypertension even in presence of modest weight loss.[24]

In the latest published meta-analysis of 25 randomized controlled trials, which included only trials based on weight reduction through energy restriction, increased physical activity, or both, average reductions of 4.4/3.6 mmHg for systolic and diastolic blood pressure, respectively, were reported for a 5-kg weight loss[25] (Figure 93–1). A dose–response relationship was observed, that is, the greater the weight loss, the greater the blood pressure reduction. Furthermore, the lowering effect of weight reduction on blood pressure was independent of age, gender, and initial BMI, although the effect appeared greater in patients on antihypertensive medication. This meta-analysis also highlights the problem of lack of compliance during long-term interventions because the maximal effect was reached before the end of the trials. Additionally, the long-term effects of weight reduction on blood pressure are not fully understood; however, they seem to be in magnitude less than those reported in short-term trials. In fact, a recent systematic review, based on studies with follow-up of 2 or more years, demonstrated decreases of 6.0/4.6 mmHg

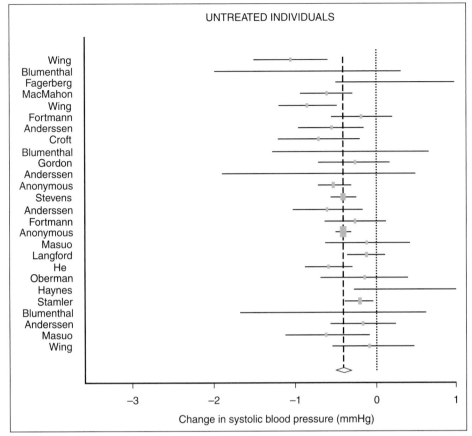

A

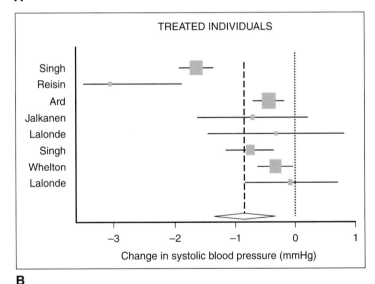

B

Figure 93–1. Short-term effect of weight reduction on systolic in untreated (**A**) and treated (**B**) individuals. (Data from Neter JE, Stam BE, Kok FJ, Grobbee DE, Geleijnse JM. *Hypertension* 2003;42:878–84.)

for systolic and diastolic and blood pressure, respectively, for 10-kg weight loss, about half of that predicted from the short-term trials.[26] Several factors such as initial blood pressure, length of follow-up, medication changes, and physiologic restrictions may contribute to this reduced effect in the long-term studies. Nevertheless, weight loss programs represent an essential component of a multi-

faceted nonpharmacologic intervention to manage hypertension; in addition, they are adjuvant measures to pharmacologic therapies, as they decrease the dosage of antihypertensive medication needed to reach blood pressure control.[27] Indeed, clinical trials have reported on the efficacy of combined lifestyle interventions including weight loss, hypo-caloric/low-salt diet, and regular exercise in reducing blood pressure levels to an extent comparable to that achieved with antihypertensive medication.[28,29]

Several biological mechanisms may explain the link among obesity, weight change, and blood pressure. In particular, an overactivity of the renin-angiotensin-aldosterone system has been regarded as a possible key mechanism of the hypertensive response in obese individuals, whose circulating levels of renin activity and aldosterone are higher than in nonobese subjects. Recent data support this mechanism suggesting that the overactivity of this system in obese individuals can be lowered by a reduction in body weight.[30] Further mechanisms may reside in inhibition of the natriuretic peptides system, which is critical to prevent excess salt and water retention, promote vascular relaxation, and inhibit sympathetic outflow; increased activity of the sympathetic nervous system; reduced insulin sensitivity; and hyperinsulinemia.[31]

Overall, the current evidence from clinical trials and observational studies strongly supports the notion that prevention of weight gain in normal-weight individuals and weight loss in overweight and obese individuals, in combination with other lifestyle modifications (e.g., hypocaloric diet, salt reduction, moderation in alcohol consumption and increased physical activity), are highly effective strategies for the prevention and management of hypertension both in individuals and population at large.[6]

DIETARY SODIUM REDUCTION

Epidemiologic evidence

Numerous animal studies, ecologic analyses, observational epidemiologic investigations, and clinical trials have supported a relationship between salt (sodium chloride) intake and blood pressure. The amount of dietary sodium is an important determinant of blood pressure levels and of hypertension risk both in individuals and populations. This relationship is direct and progressive without an apparent threshold. Thus, the reduction of dietary sodium intake is one of the most important and effective lifestyle modifications to reduce blood pressure and control hypertension.[6,32]

That habitual sodium intake could be associated with blood pressure levels was suggested several millennia ago, in the history of human mankind, after the transition from food gathering to food producing with the addition of salt to preserve food and the consequent shift to a high-salt diet.[33] Above and beyond earlier anecdotal observations, the relationship between dietary sodium and blood pressure has become the focus of intensive scientific scrutiny over the past decades. One of the earlier epidemiologic studies to address this question was also the INTER-SALT study.[34] This study tested both the within- and cross-population association between 24-hour urinary sodium excretion, reflecting the amount of sodium intake, and blood pressure levels. The within-center results showed a significant, positive, independent and linear association between 24-hour urinary sodium excretion and blood pressure levels. Specifically, a 100-mmol per day higher sodium intake (about 2.3 g/day) would predict a 3- to 6-mmHg higher systolic and up to 3 mmHg higher diastolic blood pressure. Similar results were obtained in different subgroup analyses: men, women, young, elderly, and for participants without hypertension. In the cross-population analysis, significant, independent relations were found between 24-hour urinary sodium excretion and median systolic and diastolic blood pressure, prevalence rate of hypertension, and rise of systolic and diastolic blood pressure with age. These results were further supported by findings from the Multiple Risk Factor Intervention Trial. In this cohort of more than 11,000 participants followed up for 6 years, sodium intake, as assessed by questionnaire, was significantly, directly, and independently related to systolic and diastolic blood pressure in both individuals receiving and not receiving antihypertensive medication.[35]

In addition to these observational investigations, over 50 randomized clinical trials have supported more persuasively a role of salt intake reduction in the prevention and management of high blood pressure. In the largest of

these trials, DASH, 412 participants were randomly allocated to two dietary regimens: one following a control diet, which was representative of the average diet in the United States; and one following the DASH diet, rich in fruit and vegetables, low-fat or fat-free diary products, and reduced in saturated and total fat content. Inside each arm of the trial, participants were randomly assigned to three groups with increasing amounts of sodium intake. As estimated from 24-hour urinary collections, the three sodium levels (lower, intermediate, and higher) provided 65, 107, and 142 mmol per day, respectively, which correspond approximately to intakes of 1.5, 2.5, and 3.3 g of sodium per day, respectively.[36] In this trial, a sodium reduction alone from a high to a low level was associated with a blood pressure reduction of 8.3/4.4 mmHg among hypertensive individuals and 5.6/2.8 mmHg among normotensive individuals. Moreover, the combination of this amount of sodium reduction and the DASH diet further reduced blood pressure by 11.5/5.7 mmHg and 7.1/3.7 mmHg, respectively, among those with and without hypertension. In subgroup analyses, significant effects of sodium reductions on blood pressure levels were present in both genders, and all racial and age groups, although they were more marked among African Americans, women (for systolic blood pressure), and persons aged more than 45 years.[37]

Pooled estimates from meta-analyses of clinical trials on the effects of salt reduction on blood pressure levels indicate a fall in systolic and diastolic blood pressure of 7.1/3.9 mmHg, respectively, in hypertensive individuals and 3.6/1.7 mmHg in normotensive individuals per 100 mmol reduction of 24-hour urinary sodium excretion (about 6 g salt/day). For example, He et al.[38] estimated blood pressure reductions of 5.0/2.7 mmHg in hypertensives and 2.0/1.0 in normotensives for a median reduction in urinary sodium of 78 mmol per day (Figure 93–2). In the latest published meta-analysis of 40 randomized trials, an average reduction in urinary sodium excretion of 77 mmol per day was associated with a reduction in blood pressure levels of 2.5/2.0 mmHg.[39] Blood pressure response was significantly larger in hypertensive than normotensive individuals (systolic: –5.2 vs. –1.3 mmHg; diastolic: –3.7 vs. –1.1 mmHg).

Accordingly, findings from randomized clinical trials have supported a role for reduction in dietary sodium in the primary prevention and management of hypertension. For example, in the Trials of Hypertension Prevention, phase II, a sodium reduction of 100 mmol per day, alone or combined with weight loss, prevented hypertension by 20% throughout 48 months of intervention in overweight adults.[40] Likewise, in the Trial of Nonpharmacologic Interventions in the Elderly (TONE), a sodium reduction of ~40 mmol per day was associated with a 30% decrease in the need for antihypertensive medication after 3 months of intervention in hypertensive individuals aged 60 to 80 years.[28]

The response of blood pressure to dietary changes in sodium intake, as to other environmental stimuli, may vary among individuals. This phenomenon has been called "salt sensitivity,"[41] and it is likely to be due to the

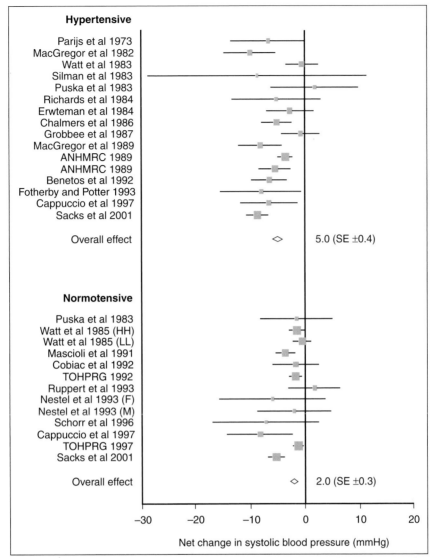

Figure 93–2. Effect of reduced sodium intake on systolic pressure in hypertensive and normotensive individuals. SE, standard error. (Reprinted by permission from Macmillan Publishers Ltd: He FJ, MacGregor GA. *J Hum Hypertens* 2002;16:761–70.)

degree of response of the renin-angiotensin system.[42,43] The weaker the response of this system to a change in sodium intake, the larger the response of the blood pressure will be. This phenomenon explains why the blood pressure–lowering effect of sodium reduction is larger in hypertensive individuals, elderly, and "low-renin" black populations. These groups are all characterized by weaker responses of the renin-angiotensin system to changes in the amount of sodium ingested, showing a greater blood pressure fall as a result of a reduction of dietary sodium. Indeed, although a significant reduction of blood pressure induced by reduced sodium intake has been observed in children and adolescents as well,[44] this response increases with age and is largest in the elderly. For example, in a double-blind randomized trial, a modest reduction in sodium intake in people over age 60 induced a significant reduction in blood pressure without untoward effect, irrespective of the initial blood pressure.[45] Further-more, the blood pressure fall observed in the elderly as a

result of a dietary sodium reduction may reduce the need for antihypertensive medication.[31] These observations are relevant to the prevention of hypertension-related diseases in developed countries, where the majority of strokes occur in the elderly and individuals with blood pressure levels below the treatment threshold for hypertension.[46] Nevertheless, several antihypertensive drugs blocking the renin-angiotensin system (e.g., angiotensin-converting enzyme inhibitors, beta-blockers, and angiotensin II–receptor antagonists) have an additive effect on blood pressure reduction in those patients already on a reduced salt diet.[47]

Furthermore, people of black African origin often show a greater blood pressure response when dietary salt is reduced.[36,43,48] For example, the efficacy of a moderate reduction in salt intake has recently been tested in two short-term trials in both urban and rural areas of West Africa, namely Nigeria and Ghana, where the prevalence of hypertension is increasing.[49,50] In both studies a moderate reduction in salt intake was associated with a significant reduction in blood pressure comparable to that seen in white populations. In areas such as sub-Saharan Africa, the prevalence of hypertension is increasing and health care resources are scarce, and thus the identification of people with hypertension is still haphazard. The effectiveness of a reduction in salt intake at a population level might prove extremely important for policymakers.

Finally, there is growing evidence on the genetic determinants of blood pressure sensitivity to sodium as well as its ethnic variations. Recently, genes involved in the regulation of the renin-angiotensin system, in transmembrane ion exchange, and in the modulation of sympathetic activity have been the focus of intense research. For example, in a study on a large population sample of white middle-aged men, an association between the Gly40Ser mutation of the glucagon receptor gene and an increased sodium reabsorption at the proximal tubule was observed,[51] which suggested a possible genetic contributor to the blood pressure sensitivity to salt. However, this genetic variant is almost absent in other ethnic groups, particularly in those of black African origin who are known to be most "salt sensitive."[52] Conversely, the C(–344)T polymorphic variant of the aldosterone synthase gene (CYP11B2) has been shown to modulate the relationship of blood pressure and plasma aldosterone levels with age.[53] Overall, the associations among functional mutations related to altered renal sodium handling and changes in sodium intake have not been clearly explained yet. A reasonable hypothesis seems to be that each functional mutation has an influence in the individual response of blood pressure to sodium intake.

Given the overwhelming evidence of the efficacy of dietary sodium reduction in the prevention and management of hypertension, the debate is currently based on issues regarding the long-term outcome benefits, and thereafter the appropriateness of a population-wide strategy to reduce dietary salt intake. The major benefit of sodium reduction is the lowering of blood pressure. It has been argued that the blood pressure reduction realistically achievable at a population level (i.e., 1 to 3 mmHg in systolic blood pressure) is small, not clinically significant, and with long-term benefits remaining unclear.[54] However, in a recent meta-analysis of 61 prospective studies, it has been estimated that even a reduction of 2 mmHg in systolic blood pressure would determine a 10% reduction in stroke mortality and a 7% reduction in mortality from coronary heart disease or other cardiovascular causes, meaning a large number of premature deaths and disabilities avoided.[55] Other results corroborate these estimates, and suggest that the benefits of such a small reduction in blood pressure, induced by salt reduction, in the population would be almost immediate.[38] Moreover, although the principal benefit of salt reduction is the blood pressure reduction, it is not the only one. There is a large body of evidence that supports other benefits: regression of left ventricular hypertrophy, reduction in proteinuria and glomerular hyperfiltration, reduction in bone mineral loss with age and osteoporosis, protection against stomach cancer and stroke, and protection against asthma attacks and possibly against cataracts.[56] Conversely, some potentially harmful effects have been reported following severe short-term sodium reductions, such as increased levels of renin, aldosterone, catecholamines, serum cholesterol and triglycerides.[57] However, these effects are likely caused by an acute volume concentration and are not detected after a moderate long-term sodium reduction.

In light of the present evidence, reduction of dietary salt intake appears to be a plausible population-wide recommendation for the prevention and treatment of hypertension.[6,32] A decrease of dietary sodium to no more than 100 mmol per day (2.3 g sodium or 5.8 g sodium chloride) represents a reasonable goal at a population level given the current dietary patterns of high levels of salt intake worldwide. However, this reduction will be only feasible in Western societies if efforts are made by the food industry, manufacturers, and restaurants to decrease the amount of salt added to processed food. In fact, in these societies, a large proportion of sodium intake (75% to 80%) comes from processed food and bread.[58] On the contrary, in developing countries where the prevalence of hypertension continues to increase, more traditional health promotion strategies would be applicable and nutritional education might have an important effect in these settings.[46,50,59]

Public health strategies to reduce salt intake in developed countries

In developed countries, the estimated prevalence of hypertension is, on average, 28% in North America (Canada and United States) and 44% in Western Europe.[60] The elevated prevalence of hypertension is a major public health concern in these countries as it accounts for 72% of cerebrovascular diseases and more than 50% of coronary heart diseases.[1] Community-based intervention trials to reduce blood pressure by means of salt reduction are scanty. For example, a community-based intervention trial in Portugal over 2 years involved a whole town to receive a health education program to reduce salt intake while another town was not given any advice and used as a control.[61] In the two towns, initial salt intake was high and 30% of persons were hypertensive. In the intervention community, a reduction of the population average blood pressure was achieved with a reduction in salt intake. Specifically, average blood pressure fell by 3.6/5.0 mmHg at 1 year and 5.0/5.1 mmHg at 2 years, due to a general distribution shift. By contrast, in the control community systolic/diastolic blood pressures either increased or remained stable, respectively. The difference in trends between the two communities was highly significant. However, in developed countries a sustained and long-term reduction in salt intake based on educational and behavioral interventions only is likely to be unsuccessful in reducing blood pressure at a population level, because the majority of an individual's salt intake is not added by the person but is already present in foods. Indeed, given that 75% to 80% of salt intake comes from salt added to bread and processed foods,[58] a population-wide strategy involving the food industry would be more effective in the long term. The North Karelia Project is a meaningful example to support this concept. This program was launched in 1972 in Finland to prevent noncommunicable diseases and, primarily, to reduce mortality and morbidity from CVDs.[62] The interventions implemented during this trial were extensive: collaborations with the community, the health services, and the food industry were added to a mass media campaign. The results have been outstanding. Over 25 years, the age-adjusted mortality rate from CVD among men aged 25 to 64 years fell by 73%.

These results clearly show that a comprehensive and collaborative program involving the food industry and health and community services is essential to successfully implement strategies of primary prevention of CVDs in developed countries. Moreover, the cost-effectiveness analysis of the North Karelia Hypertension Program, which was part of the overall project, showed that hypertension treatment represents a cost-effective treatment.[63] However, it would be even more cost-effective if hypertension could be treated as effectively without medications. This analysis showed that a comprehensive intervention is likely to improve the population's health and save money. The program included information campaigns, development of new industry food products with less salt, welfare losses from taxes/subsidies on food production with little salt, and, assuming a 2-mmHg reduction of systolic blood pressure, the cost of avoided treatment for myocardial infarction and stroke, cost of avoided antihypertensive treatment, hospital costs in additional life-years and productivity gains from reduced morbidity and mortality.

A recent global and regional analysis of population interventions including government cooperation with the food industry and change of legislation on salt content of processed food consistently showed cost-effectiveness in limiting CVDs.[64] This strategy has been adopted recently by the UK Department of Health, the Food Standard Agency, and the food industry showing a simple way of implementing a nonpharmacologic measure to limit the burden of CVDs in developed countries.

A complementary approach to lower salt intake, in developed countries, may reside in the use of salt substitutes. The American Heart Association recommends the use of non-chloride salts of sodium as they do not increase blood pressure.[65] This recommendation has been supported by results of clinical trials. For example, in a double-blind randomized placebo controlled trial including 100 men and women aged 55 to 75 years with untreated mild-to-moderate hypertension, a significant decrease in blood pressure of 7.6/3.3 mmHg was observed in individuals using a mineral salt substitute (sodium:potassium:magnesium, 8:6:1). The effect was sustained as long as the patients used the salt substitute.[66]

In conclusion, in developed countries comprehensive population strategies to reduce average levels of salt intake are required. Indeed, the expected benefits of a modest reduction in blood pressure across the whole population would be significant, especially on stroke, coronary heart disease, and all other cardiovascular conditions for which high blood pressure is a causative risk factor. The benefits would be greater in the elderly,

because they have a much higher stroke incidence (greater absolute risk); additionally, in this age group, the majority of strokes occur at levels of blood pressure not always requiring drug therapy (more stroke events attributable to the effect of blood pressure).

Public health strategies to reduce salt intake in developing countries

In developing countries, noncommunicable diseases are increasingly becoming an important threat to the health of populations.[1] Worldwide, stroke is second only to ischemic heart disease as a cause of death, and most of these deaths occur in developing countries.[10] For example, data from Tanzania suggest a high burden of stroke, comparable to that observed in developed countries.[67] Likewise, in areas like sub-Saharan Africa the prevalence of hypertension is elevated and comparable to figures from developed regions.[3,59] Thus, preventing the impending epidemic of CVD in these countries is critical as they are facing a dramatic demographic change and already experiencing a "double" burden of disease, that is, communicable and noncommunicable. In fact, in the 30-year period from 2000 to 2030, the population of elderly persons is projected to double in many sub-Saharan African countries. The repercussion of these changes will be substantial on the prevalence of CVDs given that age is an independent predictor of cardiovascular mortality and morbidity. Moreover, the burden of diseases attributable to hypertension (e.g., stroke, heart and renal failure) is much greater in sub-Saharan Africa than in the Western societies since competing risk factors like tobacco smoking and high serum cholesterol are not highly prevalent yet.[10] Likewise, many developing countries in Asia are facing the emergence of a CVD epidemic; the prevalence of hypertension varies among countries and between rural and urban settings from 5% to 35%.[3] Furthermore, in other developing areas, like the former socialist countries of Eastern Europe, a CVD epidemic is already in place.

Salt consumption in developing countries is becoming more common as urbanization increases. However, interventions to reduce salt intake at a population level have not been extensively studied in these countries. The population approach to reduce salt consumption is particularly relevant in developing countries due to the cost-effectiveness of these measures.[68] Furthermore, in countries of sub-Saharan Africa where effective health-care provision for chronic diseases is haphazard, a population strategy to limit salt consumption might prove extremely effective. It can be predicted that the same reduction in salt intake obtained with a behavioral intervention will be more effective in black African–origin populations than in Caucasian populations due to the higher salt sensitivity of black African–origin populations and because most of the salt ingested is added to food by the consumer, whereas processed food is used relatively scarcely compared to developed countries.[46] Two short-term trials in sub-Saharan Africa have confirmed that simple, cost-effective, and culturally adapted behavioral and educational interventions to reduce blood pressure can be successfully implemented[49,50] (Figure 93–3). Concerns

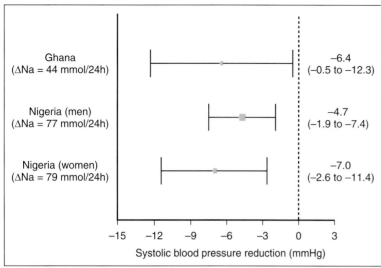

Figure 93–3. Trials on sodium reduction and systolic blood pressure in Africa. (Data from Adeyemo AA, Prewitt TE, Luke A, et al. *Ethn Dis* 2002;12:207–12; and Cappuccio FP, Kerry SM, Micah FB, Plange-Rhule J, Eastwood JB. *BMC Public Health* 2006;6:13.)

about population-wide strategies to limit salt consumption in developing countries pertain to the perceived risk of counteracting worldwide policies directed to the prevention of iodine-deficiency disorders through universal salt iodization. There is an urgent need to consider alternative vehicles for the deliveries of iodine to populations. In the meantime, an increase in the proportion of iodine fixed to salt could be considered.

The proportion of a disease that can be attributed to a specific risk factor in a population (i.e., population attributable risk) is a function of the incidence of the disease and the strength of the association between disease and a specific risk factor. Thus, when we consider the prevalence and relative risks of traditional risk factors for stroke such as modifiable risk factors (i.e., hypertension and smoking), atrial fibrillation, and other risk factors (i.e., diabetes, coronary heart disease or obesity) contributing to the overall incidence of stroke, the proportion of disease in populations that can be attributed to these risk factors varies from developed to developing regions.

To illustrate this concept we chose to compare aggregated data from developed countries and data available from sub-Saharan Africa.[69] A reduction in salt intake that prevented 10% of hypertension would have a greater impact in a sub-Saharan population than in a Western population. In fact, in sub-Saharan Africa 11 times more strokes are estimated to be prevented in people under age 65 when compared with developed countries. The benefit of a public health intervention aiming at reducing salt intake, thereby reducing the prevalence of hypertension, would be substantial in developing countries (almost a 20% reduction in the incidence of stroke in people under age 65). Given the size of the populations in sub-Saharan Africa, and considering that the incidence of stroke in people under 65 is estimated to be approximately seven times greater in this region compared with developed countries, one might expect the benefits of such an inter-

vention to be significantly greater in this region than in developed countries.

In conclusion, in developing countries, which are experiencing an increasing burden of CVD, multiple risk factor interventions and community-based programs of primary prevention should be encouraged. In particular, public health measures to promote dietary changes such a reduction in salt intake should be strongly recommended given that the prevalence of hypertension is likely to increase in these countries.

DIETARY POTASSIUM INCREASE

There is an established inverse association between dietary potassium intake and blood pressure levels. The evidence is supported by findings of animal studies, observational epidemiologic investigations, and clinical trials. In addition, meta-analyses of randomized controlled trials on the efficacy of potassium supplementation (Table 93–1) in reducing blood pressure levels in both normotensive and hypertensive individuals consistently demonstrate this inverse relationship.

Specifically, in an early meta-analysis including 19 clinical trials with both normotensive and hypertensive individuals, an overall effect of potassium supplementation of –5.9 mmHg (95% confidence interval [CI], –6.6 to –5.2) and –3.4 mmHg (95% CI, –4.0 to –2.8) was reported for systolic and diastolic blood pressure, respectively. The magnitude of the blood-pressure lowering effect of potassium supplementation was greater in individuals with high blood pressure (–8.2 mmHg, 95% CI, –9.1 to –7.3, for systolic, and –4.5 mmHg, 95% CI, –5.2 to –3.8, for diastolic blood pressure) and appeared to be more pronounced the longer the duration of the supplementation.[70] Likewise, in a later meta-analysis including 33 randomized controlled trials, potassium supplementation was associated with a significant reduction in mean systolic and diastolic blood pressure of –3.1 mmHg (95% CI, –1.9 to –4.3) and –2.0 mmHg (95% CI, –0.5 to –3.4), respectively.[71] The average effect size was larger in trials conducted in hypertensive individuals (–4.4 and –2.5 mmHg for systolic and diastolic blood pressure, respectively). Furthermore, in this meta-analysis, the blood pressure–lowering effect of potassium supplementation was greater in studies in which participants were simultaneously exposed to a high intake of sodium. Finally, a recent meta-analysis by Geleijnse et al.[39] including 27 potassium trials showed a significant, inverse association between increased potassium intake (median 44 mmol/24 h) and blood pressure levels, although the effect size reported was slightly smaller than that previously published, that is a decrease in systolic and diastolic blood pressure of –2.4 mmHg (95% CI, –1.1 to –3.7) and –1.6 mmHg (95% CI, –0.5 to –2.6), respectively. Consistent with the two previously published meta-analyses, blood pressure response was larger in hyper-

META-ANALYSES OF POTASSIUM SUPPLEMENTATION				
All Trials	**Systolic Blood Pressure**		**Diastolic Blood Pressure**	
	Net Change[a]	95% CI	Net Change	95% CI
Cappuccio et al. (1991)[70]	–5.9	–5.2 to –6.6	–3.4	–2.8 to –4.0
Whelton et al. (1997)[71]	–3.1	–1.9 to –4.3	–2.0	–0.5 to –3.4
Geleijnse et al. (2003)[39]	–2.4	–1.1 to –3.7	–1.6	–0.5 to –2.6

[a]Mean net systolic/diastolic blood pressure changes.
CI, confidence interval.

Table 93–1. Meta-Analyses of Potassium Supplementation

tensive than normotensive individuals (systolic –3.5 vs. –1.0 mmHg, $p=0.089$; diastolic: –2.5 vs. –0.3 mmHg, $p=0.074$) (Table 93–1).

The hypothesis of an inverse association between dietary potassium intake and blood pressure levels originated from findings of population studies showing that the prevalence of hypertension may be low in populations consuming high potassium diets. The INTERSALT cooperative study was one of the earlier epidemiologic investigations to estimate the effect of potassium intake on blood pressure levels. This study tested both the within- and cross-population association between 24-hour urinary sodium, potassium, and sodium/potassium ratio, reflecting the amount of dietary intake of these micronutrients, and blood pressure levels. In these centers, a reduction in systolic and diastolic blood pressure of 3.4/1.9 mmHg was related to a higher potassium intake of 50 mmol per day. Furthermore, the sodium/potassium ratio was positively and significantly related to the blood pressure levels of individuals in both men and women. These relationships were more marked with increasing age.[34] Moreover, two large prospective studies on American cohorts of health professionals examined the association between dietary potassium intake and prevalence of hypertension. Specifically, Ascherio et al.[72] analyzed a cohort of 30,681 U.S. male professionals, aged 40 to 75 years, without diagnosed hypertension for a follow-up period of 4 years. A significant, inverse association was found between potassium intake and risk of hypertension after adjustment for energy intake, age, relative weight, and alcohol consumption. When adjusted additionally for dietary fiber and magnesium intake, the association was no longer significant. The same result was observed before in a large cohort of women, the Nurses' Health Study cohort.[73] These results are not surprising given the high correlation between potassium and other micronutrients (e.g., calcium and magnesium), because they are present simultaneously in foods such as fruit, nuts, vegetables, cereals, and dairy products. Indeed, these results underscore the difficulty in differentiating the importance of the potassium effect when adjusted for other micronutrients in epidemiologic studies, and the need for randomized trials to determine whether there is a protective role of a specific dietary micronutrient in the regulation of blood pressure.[74]

Numerous clinical trials have reported on the effect of potassium supplementation on blood pressure levels in both normotensive and hypertensive individuals. Although results have not been always consistent, pooled estimates from meta-analyses consistently support a significant inverse association between potassium intake and blood pressure levels[39,70,71] in both normotensive and hypertensive individuals, as previously mentioned (Table 93–1). The lowering effect of potassium supplementation on blood pressure levels seems to be independent of the baseline potassium status, since it has been shown in individuals with low dietary potassium intake[75] and in individuals consuming normal/high potassium diets.[76] Moreover, this effect appears similar in women and men, whereas it is stronger among hypertensive individuals and individuals of black African origin, as also confirmed by pooled estimates of a published meta-analysis.[71] For example, findings from two intervention trials in participants of black African origin show, on average, a larger reduction in blood pressure levels after potassium supplementations than that reported in other ethnic groups.[75,77] Furthermore, the lowering effect of potassium supplementation on blood pressure is dependent on the concurrent intake of dietary sodium and vice versa. This means that the effect is larger in individuals on a high-sodium diet and smaller in individuals on a low-sodium diet; conversely, the lowering effect of a reduction in dietary sodium intake on blood pressure is larger in individuals on a low-potassium diet and smaller in individuals on a high-potassium diet.[32] Accordingly, the ratio of urinary sodium–potassium excretion is more closely related to changes in blood pressure levels than either urinary sodium or potassium excretion individually.[34,71] For example, in a study examining racial differences in the role of salt sensitivity in the development of high blood pressure, a high-potassium supplementation attenuated the rise in blood pressure levels following an increased dietary sodium intake in 24 normotensive black men and less markedly in 14 normotensive white men.[78] Moreover, in a 2×2 factorial trial examining the individual and simultaneous effects of reduced dietary sodium intake and increased potassium intake on blood pressure in 212 hypertensive individuals, the lowering effects on blood pressure levels were similar for either a reduced sodium intake or an increased potassium intake, individually.

However, when both interventions were implemented together, there was no further lowering effect on blood pressure levels.[79] Thus, these data suggest sub-additive effects of reduced salt intake and increased potassium intake on blood pressure.

Fruit, vegetables, and nuts are the main sources of dietary potassium in the form of inorganic or organic salts. These foods, especially fruit and vegetables, are rich in potassium as well as in other essential micronutrients; therefore, diet is a suitable strategy to increase the levels of potassium intake and prevents the need for supplements. Several randomized controlled trials have reported on the lowering effects on blood pressure of dietary interventions providing large intakes of potassium. For example, in the Dietary Approaches to Stop Hypertension (DASH) trial, the two groups that increased fruit and vegetable consumption, with larger amounts of potassium as a result, experienced significant reductions in blood pressure levels.[36] Likewise, in another trial examining the effects of fruit and vegetable consumption on plasma antioxidant concentrations and blood pressure, a significant reduction in blood pressure levels was detected.[80] Furthermore, the results of a recent randomized controlled trial conducted in 59 volunteers suggest that a substantial reduction in mean arterial blood pressure levels (i.e., 7.0 mmHg) may occur even at low-dose potassium supplementations (24 mmol of slow-release KCl per day) equivalent to the content of five portions of fresh fruit and vegetables per day.[76] Not only does the increase in dietary potassium help to reduce blood pressure, but it is a feasible and effective measure to reduce the need for antihypertensive medication. In 1991, Siani et al.[81] found that after dietary advice, which specifically aimed at increasing potassium intake, the intervention group increased potassium intake compared to the control group. More importantly, as a result of the dietary intervention, blood pressure could be controlled using less than 50% of the initial pharmacologic therapy in 81% of the patients in the intervention group compared with 29% of the patients in the control group. Thus, an increase in potassium intake from natural dietary sources may be a feasible and effective measure to reduce antihypertensive medication.

The mechanisms responsible for the lowering effect of increased potassium intake on blood pressure are not fully understood. Several hypotheses have been put forward.[82] High-potassium intake might exert a vascular protective effect and reduce the development of atherosclerosis. It may also reduce arteriolar thickening in the kidney. Moreover, potassium infusion increases acetylcholine-induced vasodilatation, and this effect is inhibited by the consequent infusion of the nitric oxide synthase inhibitor L-NMMA (L-nitromonomethylarginine). This suggests that potassium could lower blood pressure by a nitric oxide–dependent vasodilatation. Conversely, potassium depletion in humans is accompanied by sodium retention and calcium depletion, and also by an altered response to vasoactive hormones. These metabolic effects together with the direct vasoconstrictive effects of hypokalemia might be the cause of the

augmentation in blood pressure during a decrease of potassium intake.

Given the existing evidence, the adoption of a high-potassium diet is a reasonable, effective nonpharmacologic measure to improve blood pressure control in hypertensive individuals and to reduce the risk of hypertension in the general population. The level of intake that should be recommended is still a controversial issue depending on the levels of potassium status in a specific population, and the presence of conditions or drug therapies that can impair potassium excretion. However, a recent statement from the American Heart Association sets the recommended level of potassium intake, among healthy individuals, as 4.7 g/day (120 mmol/day).[32] This level of intake has been based primarily on findings from clinical trials,[71] and the potassium content of the DASH diet.[36] Indeed, in Western populations current levels of potassium intake are generally much lower than this recommended level. Moreover, in individuals affected by disease conditions impairing potassium excretion (e.g., diabetes, chronic renal insufficiency, end-stage renal disease, severe heart failure, and adrenal insufficiency) or on drug therapies that may interfere with potassium excretion (e.g., ACE inhibitors, angiotensin-receptor blockers, non-steroidal anti-inflammatory agents, and potassium-sparing diuretics), a lower level of intake (i.e., <4.7 g/day [120 mmol/d]) is recommended to prevent the risk of hyperkalemia.[83] In conclusion, an increase in potassium intake from natural dietary sources is a feasible and effective measure of preventing and treating hypertension.

MODERATION OF ALCOHOL CONSUMPTION

Extensive epidemiologic evidence suggests that heavy alcohol consumption is associated with elevated blood pressure and increased risk of hypertension, independent of age, gender, ethnic group, and other potential confounders.[84-86] For example, findings from the multinational INTERSALT study showed that heavier drinkers of both sexes had higher mean systolic and diastolic blood pressures than nondrinkers.[85] The increased risk of hypertension occurs at levels of consumption above two drinks per day in men and above one drink per day in women and lighter-weight individuals.[6,32] The observational data have been corroborated by findings of randomized controlled trials showing a blood pressure–raising effect of alcohol, which is reversible in both normotensive and hypertensive individuals.[87,88] In a recent meta-analysis of 15 randomized controlled trials, the authors estimated a reduction in systolic and diastolic blood pressure of 3.3/2.0 mmHg, respectively, for a median 76% reduction in alcohol consumption from a baseline of three to six drinks per day[89] (Figure 93–4). Blood pressure reductions were similar in hypertensive and normotensive individuals. Importantly, the relationship between reduction in mean percentage of alcohol and decline in blood pressure was dose dependent. Findings from this meta-analysis also suggest that the reduction in blood pressure following a reduction in alcohol intake can be sustained

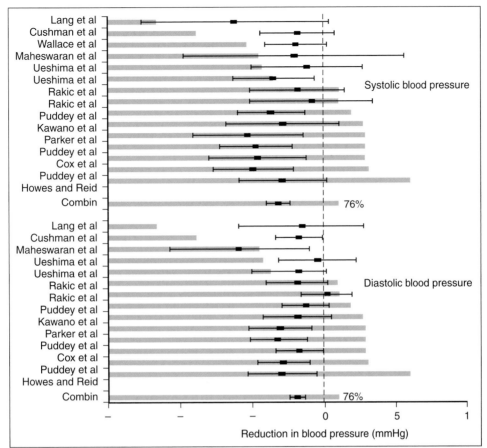

Figure 93–4. Effect of alcohol reduction on systolic and diastolic blood pressure. (Data from Xin X, He J, Frontini MG, Ogden LG, Motsamai OI, Whelton PK. *Hypertension* 2001;38:1112–17.)

over time. Therefore, altogether these results reinforce recommendations for moderation of alcohol consumption to prevent and treat hypertension.

There are still open questions, however, about this relationship. For example, it remains unclear whether, in the range of low-to-moderate alcohol consumption, the association is linear, or J-shaped, or whether there is a threshold effect. In the Kaiser-Permanente Study,[84] there was no difference in hypertension-related hospitalization between nondrinkers and light drinkers (i.e., less than two drinks per day), which suggests a threshold effect. Conversely, findings from the INTERSALT study suggest a continuous relationship between alcohol consumption and blood pressure in men and, if anything, a weaker relation at levels below 300 mL per week.[85] However, recent findings from the Nurses' Health Study II showed a J-shaped association between alcohol consumption and risk of developing hypertension, with light drinkers demonstrating a modest decrease in risk and more regular heavy drinkers demonstrating an increase in risk.[86] Other open questions concern the possible effect of different patterns of alcohol consumption on blood pressure elevation. Indeed, increasing, although not conclusive, evidence suggests that the association between alcohol consumption and blood pressure levels is a function not only of the average quantity consumed but also of the pattern in which alcohol is consumed. These patterns

include beverage preference, frequency and intensity of consumption, and drinking in relation to food consumption. For beverage preference, findings from observational studies are inconsistent[86,90]; moreover, a recent randomized controlled trial did not detect a beverage-specific effect on the association between alcohol consumption and blood pressure.[91] For frequency and intensity of consumption, some studies suggest that episodic heavy drinking may be associated with elevated blood pressure levels compared to regular drinking.[85,92,93] For example, in a crossover study of hospitalized hypertensive patients, heavy alcohol intake (4 pints of beer per day) significantly raised blood pressure, whereas alcohol withdrawal was associated with a significant fall in blood pressure.[92] More recently, findings from a study on the health consequences of binge drinking in 1154 men and women aged 18 to 54 years, showed that consumption of eight or more drinks on one occasion was associated with a significant increased risk of coronary heart disease and hypertension compared to a regular pattern of drinking.[93] However, no effect on the risk of other CVD was observed. Episodic drinking produces greater differences in blood pressure compared to regular drinking. This result is corroborated by the conclusions of the INTERSALT study.[85] Additionally, the effects on blood pressure of daily heavy drinking are more prominent than those of weekend heavy drinking.[94] However, other studies have reported inconsistent findings.[86,95] Furthermore, two population-based cross-sectional studies have examined the association between drinking pattern in relation to food consumption and hypertension risk.[90,96] Trevisan et al.,[96] in a large sample of adult men and women from the Italian Nine Communities Study, found that drinkers of wine with and without meals experienced significantly higher systolic blood pressure levels and a higher prevalence of hypertension than wine drinkers mostly with food, even after adjustment for differences in volume of alcohol consumption among the various drinking pattern categories. This association was similar in the two sexes. These findings were recently replicated in an analysis of 2609 white male and female healthy individuals from the Western New York Health Study.[90] Specifically, individuals reporting drinking mostly without food exhibited a significantly higher risk of hypertension than those drinking mostly with food, after adjustment for several confounders including total volume of alcohol consumed in the past 30 days. More interestingly, in this study drinking without food was associated with a significantly 45% increased risk of hypertension even in individuals with light to moderate alcohol intake (i.e., less than 2 drinks per day). This finding suggests that drinking without food may counteract the benefits associated with moderate alcohol use on the cardiovascular system. However, longitudinal studies are needed to support these findings and clarify the role of drinking pattern in the relationship between alcohol consumption and blood pressure.

In conclusion, moderation of alcohol consumption is a well-documented and effective recommendation to lower blood pressure among habitual drinkers. Currently, the recommended threshold is two or fewer alcoholic drinks per day in men and one or less per day in women and lighter-weight persons (one unit is equivalent to half a pint of beer, one glass of wine, or one measure of spirits).[6,32] Extended recommendations should pertain to the way in which alcohol is consumed among habitual drinkers. Specifically, a regular consumption versus a heavy episodic drinking pattern, preferably in relation to mealtimes, appears a reasonable, additional lifestyle behavior that should be adopted by habitual drinkers.

IMPORTANCE OF DIETARY PATTERNS

Diet plays a major role in the regulation of blood pressure and is one of the most important determinants of blood pressure levels in both individuals and populations. There are large variations in dietary patterns across populations that are likely to account for a considerable part of the observed differences in mean blood pressure levels, with populations consuming mostly plant-based diets having lower blood pressure than populations in industrialized countries. Additionally, even within industrialized countries, individuals consuming diets with increased intakes of fruit and vegetables and decreased intake of saturated fats tend to have, on average, lower blood pressure than individuals following more typical Western diets.[97] Differences from cross-cultural analyses have been corroborated by findings of numerous observational epidemiologic

investigations and randomized controlled trials, which have reported on the important role of dietary patterns in the development of hypertension. In this section, we will focus on two dietary patterns, for which the current evidence is consistent with regard to their efficacy in lowering blood pressure: the vegetarian diet and the DASH diet.

Vegetarian diet

Observational data clearly support the benefits on blood pressure levels derived from the adherence to a vegetarian dietary regimen with no or very small quantities animal-based products.[97] Many epidemiologic investigations have been conducted in selective population subgroups, in which a vegetarian diet is part of a multifaceted lifestyle including proscription of alcohol, tobacco use, and other "unhealthy" behaviors. The Seventh-Day Adventists represent one of the most studied population subgroups. Their members are expected, by religious belief, to abstain from alcohol and tobacco, and to follow a vegetarian diet supplemented with eggs and milk. Overall, they tend to have lower mortality from cancer, heart disease, and diabetes than non-Adventists living in the same communities. However, within this group, dietary patterns are not completely homogeneous and may resemble more typical Western habits. For example, in a cross-sectional analysis of a large cohort of 34,192 California Seventh-Day Adventists, the prevalence of hypertension was nearly double among Adventists who followed a diet similar to a typical American diet than in vegetarian Adventists.[98] These findings emphasize the independent role of dietary patterns in the risk of hypertension within this group of individuals characterized otherwise by common lifestyle behaviors. Furthermore, the age-dependent rise in blood pressure levels typically experienced by individuals living in industrialized countries, may be largely attenuated by long-term adherence to a vegetarian dietary regimen.[99] Overall, available data from observational studies indicate that vegetarians have lower systolic (3 to 14 mmHg) and diastolic (5 to 6 mmHg) blood pressure, and lower prevalence of hypertension than nonvegetarians (2% to 40% vs. 8% to 60%, respectively).[97]

Additionally, randomized controlled trials have reported on the blood pressure–lowering effects of vegetarian diets in both normotensive and hypertensive individuals, independently of common nondietary and dietary determinants of blood pressure. Indeed, a recent meta-analysis of 24 randomized placebo-controlled trials to estimate the effect of fiber supplementation on blood pressure overall and in population subgroups showed a moderate but significant reduction in blood pressure levels.[100] Specifically, fiber supplementation (average dose, 11.5 g/day) changed systolic blood pressure by –1.1 mmHg (95% CI, –2.5 to 0.2) and diastolic blood pressure by –1.3 mmHg (95% CI, –2.0 to –0.5), with larger reductions in older individuals (>40 years) and in hypertensive subgroups. The main characteristics of a vegetarian diet include a higher intake of fiber, potassium, and polyunsaturated and monounsaturated fatty acids, and a lower intake of alcohol, animal proteins, and saturated fats, which are all plausible contributors to the lower mean blood pressure levels in vegetarians, as compared to the general population. However, the lowering effects on blood pressure derived from a vegetarian diet are likely due as well to other nondietary factors (e.g., increased physical activity) that tend to cluster with dietary components as part of a comprehensive "vegetarian" lifestyle.

Dietary approaches to stop hypertension Diet

The Seventh Report of the Joint National Committee on Prevention, Detection, Evaluation, and Treatment of High Blood Pressure[6] and a recent "scientific statement" from the American Heart Association[32] emphasize the importance of adopting a dietary regimen resembling the so-called DASH diet as one major lifestyle modification to prevent and treat hypertension. The DASH dietary plan provides large intakes of fruit, vegetables, and low-fat dairy products; includes whole grains, poultry, fish, and nuts; and has limited amounts of red meat, sweets, and sugar-containing beverages. Thus, in comparison with habitual diets of Western societies, the DASH dietary pattern provides higher intakes in potassium, magnesium, calcium, fiber, and proteins, and lower intakes in total fat, saturated fat, and cholesterol.[101]

The blood pressure–lowering effect of this diet is the result of the combined effects of these nutrients when consumed together in food, rather than of the specific effect of a single nutrient. Indeed, the DASH trial was designed to test the effects on blood pressure of a change in dietary patterns, rather than the effects of a change in a single nutrient, as generally tested in previous trials.[102] This trial was an 11-week feeding program including 459 adults with ($n=133$) and without hypertension ($n=326$). For 3 weeks, participants followed a control diet that was low in fruit, vegetable, and dairy products. The fat content was representative of average consumption in the United States. Then, for the next 8 weeks, participants were randomly allocated in three groups and each group was fed three different diets. One group was fed the same control diet; the second group a diet richer in fruit and vegetables but similar to the control diet for other nutrients; and the third group was fed the DASH diet, that is, a diet rich in fruit and vegetables, low-fat or fat-free dairy products and reduced saturated and total fat content (in other words, a diet high in potassium, magnesium, calcium, fiber, and protein). The sodium intake was held constant in the three groups. Alcohol intake and body weight did not change during the trial or among the groups. Overall, findings indicated a gradient in the reduction in blood pressure among the diets. The DASH diet significantly reduced systolic and diastolic blood pressure by 5.5/3.0 mmHg, respectively, compared to the control diet, whereas the "fruit and vegetables" diet significantly reduced systolic and diastolic blood pressure by 2.8/1.1 mmHg, respectively, compared to the control diet. Among subjects with hypertension, the blood pressure reductions in the DASH group were more marked, that is 11.4/5.5 mmHg for systolic and diastolic blood pressure,

respectively, compared to the control diet. Interestingly, the blood pressure–lowering effects of the DASH diet occurred within the first 2 weeks of the trial. Further subgroup analyses showed significant effects of the DASH diet in all major subgroups (e.g., gender, race, age, body mass index, etc.), although the effects were more marked among African Americans (6.9 and 3.7 mmHg) than in whites (3.3/2.4 mmHg).[103]

In 2001, findings from a further trial on the same population testing the effects of the DASH trial in combination with a reduction in sodium intake were published.[36] A total of 412 participants were randomly allocated to two dietary regimens, one following a control diet representative of the average diet in the United States and one following the DASH diet. Within these two dietary regimens, participants were randomly assigned to three decreasing levels of salt consumption, defined as high (150 mmol/day, 3.5 g of sodium/day, reflecting typical consumption in the United States), intermediate (100 mmol/day, 2.3 g of sodium/day, reflecting the upper limit of the current recommendations), and low (50 mmol/day, 1.6 g of sodium/day). Each feeding period lasted 30 consecutive days.

Overall, findings indicate that (1) the DASH diet may lower blood pressure independent from the level of sodium intake, (2) the blood pressure–lowering effect of a reduction in sodium intake may occur by reducing the sodium intake even to levels below the currently recommended limit (i.e., 100 mmol/day); (3) the effects of sodium reductions are observed in all major subgroups; and (4) greater lowering effects on blood pressure may derive from the combination of the two interventions than from adopting either the DASH diet or low-sodium diet individually. In fact, the difference in systolic blood pressure between the DASH low-sodium group and the control high-sodium group was a substantial reduction of 7.1 mmHg in participants without hypertension and 11.5 mmHg in participants with hypertension. The last finding resembles the effect of a single-drug therapy in hypertensive individuals. Thus, the combination of the DASH diet and reduced sodium intake represents an alternative to drug therapy for individuals with mild hypertension and willing to comply with long-term dietary changes.

More recently, findings from the Optimal Macronutrient Intake Trial to Prevent Heart Disease (OmniHeart) have extended the observations derived from the DASH trials.[104] In fact, OmniHeart investigators examined the effects of three dietary patterns with documented lowering effects on blood pressure and serum lipids, among 164 adults with pre-hypertension or stage-1 hypertension. One diet, resembling the DASH diet, was rich in carbohydrates (58% of total calories); the other two dietary regimens partially replaced carbohydrates with either a higher content of proteins (about half from plant sources) or a higher content of unsaturated fats (predominantly monounsaturated fats). The feeding periods lasted 6 weeks and body weight was held constant. Systolic blood pressures were lowered in each of the three intervention groups compared with baselines. However, blood pressures were further lowered in the two dietary regimens providing a partial substitution of carbohydrates (10% of total kilocalories) with either proteins or unsaturated fats (1.4 and 1.3 mmHg, respectively). Thus, these findings indicate that, along with known determinants of blood pressure (i.e., micronutrients [sodium and potassium], body weight, alcohol consumption, and the DASH diet), macronutrients and the qualitative composition of diet are also important factors to consider for the prevention and management of hypertension. Finally, the role of dietary macronutrients on blood pressure was investigated in the International Study on Macronutrients and Blood Pressure (INTERMAP) study. This was a large cross-sectional epidemiologic study of 4680 persons, aged 40 to 59 years, from four countries.[105,106] The study found that vegetable protein intake was inversely related to blood pressure, consistent with recommendations that a diet high in vegetable products be part of a healthy lifestyle for prevention of high blood pressure and related diseases. The effect on blood pressure with a higher vegetable protein intake of 2.8% kilocalories was –2.14 mmHg systolic and –1.35 mmHg diastolic ($p<0.001$ for both); after further adjustment for height and weight, these differences were –1.11 mmHg systolic ($p<0.01$) and –0.71 mmHg diastolic ($p<0.05$).

REGULAR AEROBIC EXERCISE

Engaging in regular aerobic exercise represents an essential component of lifestyle modification to reduce cardiovascular risk, and is an important part of current recommendations for the prevention and treatment of high blood pressure.[6] It has been estimated that the risk of hypertension is 30% to 50% higher in individuals who are physically inactive.[107] At least 30 minutes per day of aerobic activity of moderate intensity (e.g., quick walking) on five or more occasions per week is the recommended level set by current guidelines for the prevention and management of high blood pressure.[6] Aerobic exercise comprises activities like walking, running, cycling, or swimming. Although all forms of dynamic exercise seem to be effective in reducing blood pressure, adherence to the intervention program is crucial to be successful in achieving and maintaining the benefit. In a recent meta-analysis of 54 randomized controlled trials including 2419 participants, aerobic exercise was associated with a significant reduction in systolic and diastolic blood pressure of 3.8/2.6 mmHg, respectively[107] (Figure 93–5). Blood pressure reductions induced by aerobic exercise were observed in both normotensive and hypertensive individuals and in normal-weight and overweight subgroups. Although the blood pressure–lowering effect of aerobic exercise can be considered clinically moderate, it constitutes, however, a valuable public health strategy for the prevention and treatment of high blood pressure. In fact, a modest reduction in the population's blood pressure levels would translate into a significant decrease in the incidence of hypertension-related diseases.

Conversely, resistance training, also know as isometric or static exercise (e.g., weight training or body building),

is not included in current recommendations for the prevention and management of high blood pressure because of the lack of conclusive evidence on its effectiveness in lowering blood pressure and the potential for long-term hypertensive effects. However, two recent meta-analyses of randomized controlled trials indicate that resistance training is not associated with chronic elevations of blood pressure and, instead, may induce a moderate reduction of blood pressure levels in healthy adults, whereas its efficacy in lowering blood pressure in hypertensive individuals and the elderly is still a controversial issue.[108,109] Currently, the evidence suggests that moderate-intensity resistance training could be performed in combination with aerobic exercise in the context of a comprehensive exercise program to prevent CVD in healthy adults.[110]

Furthermore, a few trials have examined the efficacy of the simultaneous implementation of current lifestyle recommendations, including regular exercise, to prevent and treat high blood pressure. For example, in the Diet, Exercise, and Weight Loss-Intervention Trial (DEW-IT), 44 hypertensive overweight adults on monotherapy for hypertension were randomly allocated to either a control group or comprehensive lifestyle intervention group.[29] The intervention comprised a low-sodium and hypocaloric version of the DASH diet, for 9 weeks, along with a supervised moderate-intensity exercise program three times per week. The control group received no intervention. At the end of the trial, in the intervention group the average total weight loss was 4.9 kg, and the differences in 24-hour ambulatory systolic and diastolic blood pressures were 9.5/5.3 mmHg, respectively, whereas the differences in daytime blood pressures were 12.1/6.6 mmHg, respectively. Thus, this trial clearly emphasized the efficacy of comprehensive lifestyle modifications as adjuvant therapy in hypertensive adults who are already on drug therapy; moreover, blood pressure reductions of the magnitude observed in this study resemble blood pressure reductions obtainable by means of pharmacologic therapy. These findings were extended by recent results of the PREMIER clinical trial, which examined the combined effects of the DASH diet with "established" recommendations, comprising weight loss, exercise, and restriction of sodium and alcohol.[111] Participants were 810 adults with above-optimal blood pressure, including stage-1 hypertension (120 to 159 mmHg systolic and 80 to 95 mmHg diastolic), and who were not on antihypertensive medications. They were randomly allocated to one of three intervention groups: (1) "established," a behavioral intervention that implemented established recommendations; (2) "established plus DASH," which also implemented the DASH diet; and (3) an "advice-only" control group. At the end of the trial (after 6 months) in the group assigned to lifestyle modification only, the mean net reduction in blood pressure was 3.7/1.7 mmHg, compared to the control group, whereas for the group that followed the established recommendations together with the DASH diet, the mean net reduction in blood pressure was 4.3/2.6 mmHg, compared to the control group. Thus, these findings indicate the feasibility of comprehensive lifestyle modifications

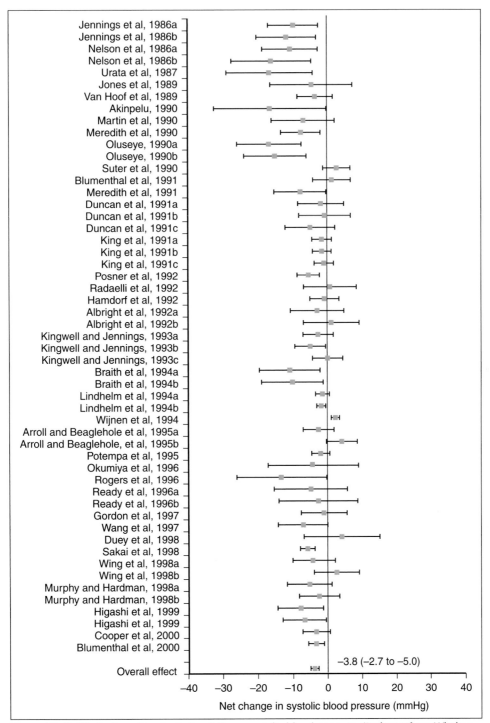

Figure 93–5. Effect of aerobic physical activity on systolic blood pressure. (Redrawn from Whelton SP, Chin A, Xin X, He J. Effect of aerobic exercise on blood pressure: a meta-analysis of randomized, controlled trials. *Ann Intern Med* 2002;136:493–503.)

and their beneficial effects on blood pressure for both nonhypertensive individuals with above-optimal blood pressure and hypertensive individuals who are not receiving medication therapy.

Several mechanisms are likely responsible for the blood pressure–lowering effects induced by regular exercise.[112] For example, a "hemodynamic" mechanism would involve the reduction of both resting cardiac output and peripheral vascular resistance. Furthermore, a "humoral" mechanism would determine the reduction of the activity of the renin-angiotensin-aldosterone system and of the sympathetic nervous system activity and an increase in prostaglandins with vasodilator effect. Finally, recent findings suggest that an enhancement in insulin sensitivity may represent a further mechanism for the beneficial effects of physical activity on blood pressure and hypertension risk.[113]

CONCLUSIONS

Extensive and consistent evidence provides the scientific basis for clinical and public health strategies directed to long-term lifestyle modifications to prevent and reduce the burden of disease related to high blood pressure in both individuals and populations. The current lifestyle modifications that effectively lower blood pressure include weight reduction if overweight or obese, reduction of dietary sodium intake, increased potassium intake, moderation of alcohol consumption among regular drinkers, adoption of a dietary plan based on the DASH (Dietary Approaches to Stop Hypertension) diet, and regular aerobic exercise.

In the clinical setting, a comprehensive lifestyle intervention represents a cost-effective therapeutic option among nonhypertensive individuals with above-optimal blood pressure levels, as well as among hypertensive individuals who are not receiving medication therapy and are compliant with sustained lifestyle changes. In addition, comprehensive lifestyle modifications represent an essential adjuvant therapy in hypertensive individuals who are already on drug treatment.

In the public health arena, there is an urgent need to develop and implement population-wide strategies aimed at substantial "societal" changes to tackle the current epidemic of hypertension in both developed and developing countries. However, these changes will be realistic only if collaborative initiatives are implemented at multiple levels: governments, manufacturers, health-care providers, researchers, and the general public. In particular, the increasing burden of hypertension is a serious public health challenge in developing countries due to the lack of resources. Nevertheless, community-based strategies of health promotion (e.g., salt reduction) are warranted in these settings.

REFERENCES

1. World Health Organization. *The World Health Report 2002—Reducing Risks, Promoting Healthy Life*. Geneva: World Health Organization, 2002–2.
2. Omran AR. The epidemiologic transition: a theory of the epidemiology of population change. *Milbank Mem Fund Q* 1971;49:509–38.
3. Kearney PM, Whelton M, Reynolds K, Muntner P, Whelton PK, He J. Global burden of hypertension: analysis of worldwide data. *Lancet* 2005; 365:217–23.
4. Vasan RS, Beiser A, Seshadri S, Larson MG, Kannel WB, D'Agostino RB, et al. Residual lifetime risk for developing hypertension in middle-aged women and men: the Framingham Heart Study. *JAMA* 2002; 287:1003–10.
5. Cappuccio FP. Commentary: epidemiological transition, migration, and cardiovascular disease. *Int J Epidemiol* 2004;33:387–88.
6. Chobanian AV, Bakris GL, Black HR, Cushman WC, Green LA, Izzo JL Jr, et al. The Seventh Report of the Joint National Committee on Prevention, Detection, Evaluation, and Treatment of High Blood Pressure: the JNC 7 report. *Hypertension* 2003;42:1206–52.
7. World Health Organization. *Obesity: Preventing and Managing the Global Epidemic*. WHO Technical Report Series no. 894. Geneva. World Health Organization, 2000
8. Ogden CL, Carroll MD, Curtin LR, McDowell MA, Tabak CJ, Flegal KM. Prevalence of overweight and obesity in the United States, 1999–2004. *JAMA* 2006;295:1549–55.
9. National Audit Office. *Tackling Obesity in England*. London: Stationery Office, 2001.
10. Lopez, Mathers CD, Ezzati M, Jamison DT, Murray CJL. Global and regional burden of disease and risk factors, 2001: systematic analysis of population health data. *Lancet* 2006;367:1747–57.

11. Mokdad AH, Ford ES, Bowman BA, Dietz WH, Vinicor F, Bales VS, et al. Prevalence of obesity, diabetes, and obesity-related health risk factors, 2001. *JAMA* 2003;289:76–79.
12. Dyer AR, Elliott P, Shipley M. Body mass index versus height and weight in relation to blood pressure. Finding for the 10,079 persons in the INTERSALT Study. *Am J Epidemiol* 1990;131: 589–96.
13. MacMahon S, Cutler J, Brittain E, Higgins M. Obesity and hypertension: epidemiological and clinical issues. *Eur Heart J* 1987;8:57–70.
14. Garrison RJ, Kannel WB, Stokes J, Castelli WP. Incidence and precursors of hypertension in young adults: the Framingham Offspring Study. *Prev Med* 1987;16:235–51.
15. Harris MM, Stevens J, Thomas N, Schreiner P, Folsom AR. Associations of fat distribution and obesity with hypertension in a bi-ethnic population. The ARIC study: Atherosclerosis Risk in Communities Study. *Obes Res* 2000; 8:516–24.
16. Huang Z, Willett WC, Manson JE, Rossner B, Stamper MJ, Speizer FE, et al. Body weight, weight change, and risk for hypertension in women. *Ann Intern Med* 1998;128:81–88.
17. Bakx JC, van den Hoogen HJ, van den Bosch WJ, van Schayck CP, van Ree JW, Thien T, et al. Development of blood pressure and the incidence of hypertension in men and women over an 18-year period: results of the Nijmegen Cohort Study. *J Clin Epidemiol* 1999;52:531–38.
18. Wilsgaard T, Schirmer H, Arnesen E. Impact of body weight on blood pressure with a focus on sex differences: the Tromso Study, 1986–1995. *Arch Intern Med.* 2000; 160:2847–53.
19. Siani A, Cappuccio FP, Barba G, et al. The relationship of waist circumference to blood pressure: the Olivetti Heart Study. *Am J Hypertens* 2002;15:780–86.

20. Canoy D, Luben R, Welch A, Bingham S, Wareham N, Day N, et al. Fat distribution, body mass index and blood pressure in 22,090 men and women in the Norfolk cohort of the European Prospective Investigation into Cancer and Nutrition (EPIC-Norfolk) study. *J Hypertens* 2004; 22:2067–74.
21. Stranges S, Trevisan M, Dorn JM, Dmochowski J, Donahue RP. Body fat distribution, liver enzymes, and risk of hypertension: evidence from the Western New York Study. *Hypertension* 2005;46:1186–93.
22. National Institutes of Health. Clinical Guidelines on the Identification, Evaluation, and Treatment of Overweight and Obesity in Adults—The Evidence Report. *Obes Res* 1998; 6:51S–209S.
23. He J, Whelton PK, Appel LJ, Charleston J, Klag MJ. Long-term effects of weight loss and dietary sodium reduction on incidence of hypertension. *Hypertension* 2000;35:544–49.
24. Stevens VJ, Obarzanek E, Cook NR, Lee IM, Appel LJ, Smith West D, et al. Long-term weight loss and changes in blood pressure: results of the Trials of Hypertension Prevention, Phase II. *Ann Intern Med* 2001;134:1–11.
25. Neter JE, Stam BE, Kok FJ, Grobbee DE, Geleijnse JM. Influence of weight reduction on blood pressure: a meta-analysis of randomized controlled trials. *Hypertension* 2003;42:878–84.
26. Aucott L, Poobalan A, Smith WC, Avenell A, Jung R, Broom J. Effects of weight loss in overweight/obese individuals and long-term hypertension outcomes: a systematic review. *Hypertension* 2005;45:1035–41.
27. Mulrow CD, Chiquette E, Angel L, Cornell J, Summerbell C, Anagnostelis B, et al. Dieting to reduce body weight for controlling hypertension in adults. *Cochrane Database Syst Rev* 2000; CD000484.

28. Whelton PK, Appel LJ, Espeland MA, Applegate WB, Ettinger WH Jr, Kostis JB, et al. Sodium reduction and weight loss in the treatment of hypertension in older persons: a randomized controlled trial of nonpharmacologic interventions in the elderly (TONE). TONE Collaborative Research Group. *JAMA* 1998;279:839–46.

29. Miller ER III, Erlinger TP, Young DR, Jehn M, Charleston J, Rhodes D, et al. Results of the Diet, Exercise, and Weight Loss Intervention Trial (DEW-IT). *Hypertension* 2002;40:612–18.

30. Engeli S, Böhnke J, Gorzelniak K, Janke J, Schling P, Bader M et al. Weight loss and the renin-angiotensin-aldosterone system. *Hypertension* 2005;45:356–62.

31. Wofford MR, Hall JE. Pathophysiology and treatment of obesity hypertension. *Curr Pharm Des* 2004;10:3621–37.

32. Appel LJ, Brands MW, Daniels SR, Karanja N, Elmer PJ, Sacks FM, et al. Dietary approaches to prevent and treat hypertension: a scientific statement from the American Heart Association. *Hypertension* 2006; 47:296–308.

33. Ruskin A. *Classics in Arterial Hypertension.* Springfield, IL: Charles C. Thomas, 1956.

34. Elliott P, Dyer A, Stamler R. The INTERSALT study: results for 24-hour sodium and potassium, by age and sex. INTERSALT Co-operative Research Group. *J Hum Hypertens* 1989;3:323–30.

35. Stamler J, Caggiula AW, Grandits GA. Relation of body mass and alcohol, nutrient, fiber, and caffeine intakes to blood pressure in the special intervention and usual care groups in the Multiple Risk Factor Intervention Trial. *Am J Clin Nutr* 1997;65:338S–65S.

36. Sacks FM, Svetkey LP, Vollmer WM, et al. Effects on blood pressure of reduced dietary sodium and the Dietary Approaches to Stop Hypertension (DASH) diet. DASH-Sodium Collaborative Research Group. *N Engl J Med* 2001;344:3–10.

37. Vollmer WM, Sacks FM, Ard J, et al. Effects of diet and sodium intake on blood pressure: subgroup analysis of the DASH-sodium trial. *Ann Intern Med* 2001;135:1019–28.

38. He FJ, MacGregor GA. Effect of modest salt reduction on blood pressure: a meta-analysis of randomized trials: implications for public health. *J Hum Hypertens* 2002;16:761–70.

39. Geleijnse JM, Kok FJ, Grobbee DE. Blood pressure response to changes in sodium and potassium intake: a meta-regression analysis of randomised trials. *J Hum Hypertens* 2003;17:471–80.

40. Effects of weight loss and sodium reduction intervention on blood pressure and hypertension incidence in overweight people with high-normal blood pressure: the Trials of Hypertension Prevention. Phase II: the Trials of Hypertension Prevention Collaborative Research Group. *Arch Intern Med* 1997;157:657–67.

41. Weinberger MH, Miller JZ, Luft FC, Grim CE, Fineberg NS. Definitions and characteristics of sodium sensitivity and blood pressure resistance. *Hypertension* 1986;8(part 2):II–127–II–134.

42. Cappuccio FP, Markandu ND, Sagnella GA, MacGregor GA. Sodium restriction lowers high blood pressure through a decreased response of the renin system—direct evidence using saralasin. *J Hypertens* 1985;3:243–47.

43. He FJ, Markandu ND, Sagnella GA, MacGregor GA. Importance of the renin system in determining blood pressure fall with salt restriction in black and white hypertensives. *Hypertension* 1998;32:820–24.

44. Simons-Morton DG, Obarzanek E. Diet and blood pressure in children and adolescents. *Pediatr Nephrol* 1997;11:244–49.

45. Cappuccio FP, Markandu ND, Carney C, Sagnella GA, MacGregor GA. Double-blind randomised trial of modest salt restriction in older people. *Lancet* 1997;350:850–54.

46. Cappuccio FP. Salt and blood pressure. Issues for population-based prevention and public health strategies. *Public Health Med* 2000;2:57–61.

47. Cappuccio FP, Siani A. Nonpharmacologic treatment of hypertension. In: Crawford MH, DiMarco JP, Paulus WJ, eds. *Cardiology.* Mosby, 2004:523–32.

48. Poulter N, Cappuccio FP, Chaturvedi N, Cruickshank K. *High Blood Pressure and the African-Caribbean Community in the UK.* Birmingham: MediNews Limited, 1997.

49. Adeyemo AA, Prewitt TE, Luke A, et al. The feasibility of implementing a dietary sodium reduction intervention among free-living normotensive individuals in south west Nigeria. *Ethn Dis* 2002;12:207–12.

50. Cappuccio FP, Kerry SM, Micah FB, Plange-Rhule J, Eastwood JB. A community programme to reduce salt intake and blood pressure in Ghana (ISRCTN 88789643). *BMC Public Health* 2006;6:13.

51. Strazzullo P, Iacone R, Siani A, et al. Altered renal sodium handling and hypertension in men carrying the glucagon receptor gene (Gly40Ser) variant. *J Mol Med* 2001;79:574–80.

52. Barbato A, Russo P, Venezia A, Strazzullo V, Siani A, Cappuccio FP. Analysis of Gly40Ser polymorphism of the glucagon receptor (GCGR) gene in different ethnic groups. *J Hum Hypertens* 2004;17:577–79.

53. Russo P, Siani A, Venezia A, et al. Interaction between the C(−344)T polymorphism of CYP11B2 and age in the regulation of blood pressure and plasma aldosterone levels: cross-sectional and longitudinal findings of the Olivetti Prospective Heart Study. *J Hypertens* 2002;20:1785–92.

54. Hooper L, Bartlett C, Davey SG, Ebrahim S. Systematic review of long term effects of advice to reduce dietary salt in adults. *BMJ* 2002;325:628.

55. Prospective Studies Collaboration. Age-specific relevance of usual blood pressure to vascular mortality: a meta-analysis of individual data for one million adults in 61 prospective studies. *Lancet* 2002;360:1903–13.

56. Cappuccio FP, MacGregor GA. Dietary salt restriction: benefits for cardiovascular disease and beyond. *Curr Opin Nephrol Hypertens* 1997; 6:477–82.

57. Graudal NA, Galloe AM, Garred P. Effects of sodium restriction on blood pressure, renin, aldosterone, catecholamines, cholesterols, and triglyceride: a meta-analysis. *JAMA* 1998;279:1383–91.

58. Mattes RD, Donnelly D. Relative contributions of dietary sodium sources. *J Am Coll Nutr* 1991; 10:383–93.

59. Cappuccio FP, Micah FB, Emmett L, et al. Prevalence, detection, management and control of hypertension in Ashanti, West Africa. *Hypertension* 2004;43:1017–22.

60. Wolf-Maier K, Cooper RS, Banegas JR, et al. Hypertension prevalence and blood pressure levels in 6 European countries, Canada, and the United States. *JAMA* 2003;289:2363–69.

61. Forte JG, Miguel JM, Miguel MJ, de Padua F, Rose G. Salt and blood pressure: a community trial. *J Hum Hypertens* 1989;3:179–84.

62. Pekka P, Pirjo P, Ulla U. Influencing public nutrition for non-communicable disease prevention: from community intervention to national programme—experiences from Finland. *Public Health Nutr* 2002;5:245–51.

63. Nissinen A, Tuomilehto J, Kottke TE, Puska P. Cost-effectiveness of the North Karelia Hypertension Program, 1972–1977. *Med Care* 1986;24:767–80.

64. Murray CJ, Lauer JA, Hutubessy RC, et al. Effectiveness and costs of interventions to lower systolic blood pressure and cholesterol: a global and regional analysis on reduction of cardiovascular-disease risk. *Lancet* 2003;361:717–25.

65. Kotchen TA, McCarron DA. Dietary electrolytes and blood pressure: a statement for healthcare professionals from the American Heart Association Nutrition Committee. *Circulation* 1998;98:613–17.

66. Geleijnse JM, Witteman JC, Bak AA, den Breeijen JH, Grobbee DE. Reduction in blood pressure with a low sodium, high potassium, high magnesium salt in older subjects with mild to moderate hypertension. *BMJ* 1994;309:436–40.

67. Walker RW, McLarty DG, Kitange HM, Whiting D, Masuki G, Mtasiwa DM, et al. Stroke mortality in urban and rural Tanzania. *Lancet* 2000;355: 1684–87.

68. Murray CJ, Lauer JA, Hutubessy RC, Niessen L, Tomijima N, Rodgers A, et al. Effectiveness and costs of interventions to lower systolic blood pressure and cholesterol: a global and regional analysis on reduction of cardiovascular-disease risk. *Lancet* 2003;361:717–25.

69. Gomez GB, Cappuccio FP. Dietary salt and disease prevention: a global perspective. *Curr Med Chem* 2005; 5:13–20.

70. Cappuccio FP, MacGregor GA. Does potassium supplementation lower blood pressure? A meta-analysis of published trials. *J Hypertens* 1991; 9:465–73.

71. Whelton PK, He J, Cutler JA, et al. Effects of oral potassium on blood pressure. Meta-analysis of randomized controlled clinical trials. *JAMA* 1997; 277:1624–32.

72. Ascherio A, Rimm EB, Giovannucci EL, et al. A prospective study of nutritional factors and hypertension among US men. *Circulation* 1992;86:1475–84.

73. Witteman JC, Willett WC, Stampfer MJ, et al. A prospective study of nutritional factors and hypertension among US women. *Circulation* 1989;80:1320–27.

74. Cappuccio FP. The epidemiology of diet and blood pressure. *Circulation* 1992;86:1651–53.

75. Brancati FL, Appel LJ, Seidler AJ, Whelton PK. Effect of potassium supplementation on blood pressure in African Americans on a low-potassium diet: a randomized, double-blind, placebo-controlled trial. *Arch Intern Med* 1996;156:61–67.

76. Naismith DJ, Braschi A. The effect of low-dose potassium supplementation on blood pressure in apparently healthy volunteers. *Br J Nutr* 2003;90:53–60.

77. Matlou SM, Isles CG, Higgs A, et al. Potassium supplementation in blacks with mild to moderate essential hypertension. *J Hypertens* 1986;4:61–64.

78. Morris RC Jr, Sebastian A, Forman A, Tanaka M, Schmidlin O. Normotensive salt sensitivity: effects of race and dietary potassium. *Hypertension* 1999;33:18–23.

79. Chalmers J, Morgan T, Doyle A, Dickson B, Hopper J, Mathews J, et al. Australian National Health and Medical Research Council dietary salt study in mild hypertension. *J Hypertens Suppl* 1986;4:S629–37.

80. John JH, Ziebland S, Yudkin P, Roe LS, Neil HA, for the Oxford Fruit and Vegetable Study Group. Effects of fruit and vegetable consumption on plasma antioxidant concentrations and blood pressure: a randomised controlled trial. *Lancet* 2002;359:1969–74.

81. Siani A, Strazzullo P, Giacco A, Pacioni D, Celentano E, Mancini M. Increasing the dietary potassium intake reduces the need for antihypertensive medication. *Ann Intern Med* 1991;115:753–59.

82. Krishna GG. Role of potassium in the pathogenesis of hypertension. *Am J Med Sci* 1994;307(Suppl 1):S21–25.

83. Saggar-Malik AK, Cappuccio FP. Potassium supplements and potassium-sparing diuretics. A review and guide to appropriate use. *Drugs* 1993;46:986–1008.

84. Klatsky AL, Friedman GD, Siegelaub AB, Gerard MJ. Alcohol consumption and blood pressure: Kaiser-Permanente Multiphasic Health Examination data. *N Engl J Med* 1977;296:1194–2000.

85. Marmot MG, Elliott P, Shipley MJ, Dyer AR, Ueshima H, Beevers DG, et al. Alcohol and blood pressure: the INTERSALT study. *BMJ* 1994;308:1263–67.

86. Thadhani R, Camargo CA Jr, Stampfer MJ, Curhan GC, Willett WC, Rimm EB. Prospective study of moderate alcohol consumption and risk of hypertension in young women. *Arch Intern Med* 2002;162:569–74.

87. Puddey IB, Beilin LJ, Vandongen R, Rouse IL, Rogers P. Evidence for a direct effect of alcohol consumption on blood pressure in normotensive men. A randomized controlled trial. *Hypertension* 1985;7:707–13.

88. Puddey IB, Beilin LJ, Vandongen R. Regular alcohol use raises blood pressure in treated hypertensive subjects. A randomised controlled trial. *Lancet* 1987;1:647–51.

89. Xin X, He J, Frontini MG, Ogden LG, Motsamai OI, Whelton PK. Effects of alcohol reduction on blood pressure: a meta-analysis of randomized controlled trials. *Hypertension* 2001;38:1112–17.

90. Stranges S, Wu T, Dorn JM, Freudenheim JL, Muti P, Farinaro E, et al. Relationship of alcohol drinking pattern to the risk of hypertension: a population-based study. *Hypertension* 2004;44:813–19.

91. Zilkens RR, Burke V, Hodgson JM, Barden A, Beilin LJ, Puddey IB. Red wine and beer elevate blood pressure in normotensive men. *Hypertension* 2005;45:874–79.

92. Potter JF, Beevers DG. Pressor effect of alcohol in hypertension. *Lancet* 1984;1:119–22.

93. Murray RP, Connett JE, Tyas SL, et al. Alcohol volume, drinking pattern, and cardiovascular disease morbidity and mortality: is there a U-shaped function? *Am J Epidemiol* 2002;155:242–48.

94. Seppa K, Laippala P, Sillanaukee P. Drinking pattern and blood pressure. *Am J Hypertens* 1994;7:249–54.

95. Rakic V, Puddey IB, Burke V, Dimmitt SB, Beilin LJ. Influence of pattern of alcohol intake on blood pressure in regular drinkers—a controlled trial. *J Hypertension* 1998;16:165–74.

96. Trevisan M, Krogh V, Farinaro E, Panico S, Mancini M. Alcohol consumption, drinking pattern and blood pressure: analysis of data from the Italian National Research Council Study. *Int J Epidemiol* 1987;16:520–27.

97. Berkow SE, Barnard ND. Blood pressure regulation and vegetarian diets. *Nutr Rev* 2005;63:1–8.

98. Fraser GE. Associations between diet and cancer, ischemic heart disease, and all-cause mortality in non-Hispanic white California Seventh-day Adventists. *Am J Clin Nutr* 1999;70:532s–38s.

99. Melby CL, Goldflies DG, Toohey ML. Blood pressure differences in older black and white long-term vegetarians and nonvegetarians. *J Am Coll Nutr* 1993;12:262–69.

100. Streppel MT, Arends LR, van't Veer P, Grobbee DE, Geleijnse JM. Dietary fiber and blood pressure. *Arch Intern Med* 2005;165:150–56.

101. Karanja NM, Obarzanek E, Lin PH, McCullough ML, Phillips KM, Swain JF, et al. Descriptive characteristics of the dietary patterns used in the Dietary Approaches to Stop Hypertension Trial: DASH Collaborative Research Group. *J Am Diet Assoc* 1999;99:S19–27.

102. Appel LJ, Moore TJ, Obarzanek E, Vollmer WM, Svetkey LP, Sacks FM, et al. A clinical trial of the effects of dietary patterns on blood pressure: DASH Collaborative Research Group. *N Engl J Med* 1997;336:1117–24.

103. Svetkey LP, Simons-Morton D, Vollmer WM, Appel LJ, Conlin PR, Ryan DH, et al. Effects of dietary patterns on blood pressure: subgroup analysis of the Dietary Approaches to Stop Hypertension (DASH) randomized clinical trial. *Arch Intern Med* 1999;159:285–93.

104. Appel LJ, Sacks FM, Carey VJ, Obarzanek E, Swain JF, Miller ER 3rd, et al. Effects of protein, monounsaturated fat, and carbohydrate intake on blood pressure and serum lipids: results of the OmniHeart randomized trial. *JAMA* 2005;294:2455–64.

105. Elliott P, Stamler J, Dyer AR, Appel L, Dennis B, Kesteloot H, et al. Association between protein intake and blood pressure: the INTERMAP Study. *Arch Intern Med* 2006;166:79–87.

106. Stamler J, Elliott P, Dennis B, Dyer AR, Kesteloot H, Liu K, et al. INTERMAP: background, aims, design, methods, and descriptive statistics (nondietary). *J Hum Hypertens* 2003;17:591–608.

107. Whelton SP, Chin A, Xin X, He J. Effect of aerobic exercise on blood pressure: a meta-analysis of randomized, controlled trials. *Ann Intern Med* 2002;136:493–503.

108. Kelley GA, Kelley KS. Progressive resistance exercise and resting blood pressure: a meta-analysis of randomized controlled trials. *Hypertension* 2000;35:838–43.

109. Cornelissen VA, Fagard RH. Effect of resistance training on resting blood pressure: a meta-analysis of randomized controlled trials. *J Hypertens* 2005;23:251–59.

110. Braith RW, Stewart KJ. Resistance exercise training: its role in the prevention of cardiovascular disease. *Circulation* 2006;113:2642–50.

111. Writing Group of the PREMIER Collaborative Research Group. Effects of comprehensive lifestyle modification on blood pressure control: main results of the PREMIER clinical trial. *JAMA* 2003;289:2083–93.

112. Pescatello LS, Franklin BA, Fagard R, Farquhar WB, Kelley GA, Ray CA. American College of Sports Medicine, position stand: exercise and hypertension. *Med Sci Sports Exerc* 2004;36:533–53.

113. Foy CG, Foley KL, D'Agostino RB Jr, Goff DC Jr, Mayer-Davis E, Wagenknecht LE. Physical activity, insulin sensitivity, and hypertension among US adults: findings from the Insulin Resistance Atherosclerosis Study. *Am J Epidemiol* 2006;163:921–28.

Chapter

94

Multidisciplinary Management of Hypertension and the Role of the Nurse

Cheryl R. Dennison and Martha N. Hill

Description

- Multidisciplinary teams, including nurses, physicians, and other health care providers, achieve effective control of hypertension in many practice settings.

Key Features

- The skills and clinical judgment of multidisciplinary team members contribute to a more comprehensive approach with increased individualization of hypertension care.

- Improving the processes and outcomes of hypertension care requires that the multidisciplinary team demonstrate the following five core competencies: (1) patient-centered care, (2) partnering, (3) quality improvement, (4) information and communication technology, and (5) public health perspective.

Clinical Implications

- The benefits of multidisciplinary teams, including nurses who participate in or lead hypertension care, have been demonstrated in a wide variety of studies from uncontrolled community- and clinic-based surveys to randomized multisite clinical trials, and in developing as well as developed countries.

- The roles of the nurse and NP in multidisciplinary hypertension management involve all aspects of hypertension management, including detection, referral, and follow-up; medication management; patient education, counseling, and skill building; coordination of care; and managing the clinic or office.

The management of hypertension requires long-term, effective collaboration among health care professionals, patients, and communities. A multidisciplinary team approach has consistently produced effective control of hypertension in clinical trials and many practice settings.[1-6] Since the late 1960s, when the detection, evaluation, and treatment of hypertension became a public health mandate, nurses have contributed to improved care and outcomes for patients with hypertension. The benefits of nurses participating in or leading hypertension care has been demonstrated in a wide variety of studies from uncontrolled community- and clinic-based surveys to randomized multisite clinical trials, and in developing as well as developed countries.[1,7-20] The proactive involvement of nurses, and other providers such as pharmacists, nutritionists, social workers, and community health workers, allows flexibility in matching patient needs with the competencies of providers and staff members who have different yet complementary skills and interests.

Nurses are the largest health profession; they practice in all settings where patients are seen including specialty clinics, private practice offices, worksite settings, primary care clinics, hospitals, and community centers. Patients with hypertension are identified, evaluated, and treated in all of these settings as well as hypertension specialty clinics. As the health care environment is challenged across the world by increasing rates of chronic illness, aging populations, and concerns about escalating health care costs, awareness is increasing that a team approach to chronic illness, such as hypertension management, is needed. Physicians working in collaboration with other health care professionals and communities can help patients develop the knowledge and skills required to control their hypertension and to optimize their health. In this chapter, we describe the multidisciplinary team approach and the specific roles of the nurse and nurse practitioner in hypertension management in outpatient or ambulatory settings and provide examples of their effectiveness.

DESCRIPTION OF TECHNIQUE

Multidisciplinary team management of hypertension

Multidisciplinary team management of hypertension can be conceptualized in steps as delineated in Table 94–1. The first step involves screening for detection of hypertension and referral for hypertension management. Step 2 involves patient education, counseling, and skill building, as well as coordination of care across the care continuum. Step 3 involves diagnostic testing and medication management. Steps 2 and 3 are iterative and often are addressed concurrently. Various members of the multidisciplinary hypertension care team are best prepared, in terms of skills, education, and licensure, to implement each of the steps.

The number of patients with chronic conditions, such as hypertension, is rapidly increasing. To engage patients as active participants, rather than passive recipients, and to provide effective care, the hypertension management team must demonstrate the following five core competencies:

MULTIDISCIPLINARY TEAM MANAGEMENT OF HYPERTENSION	
Steps in Management of Hypertension	**Multidisciplinary Team Interventionists**
Step 1 Screening, detection, and referral	Nurse, community health worker, community resource (e.g., drug store BP check), other health care professionals
Step 2 Patient education, counseling, and skill building and coordination of care	Nurse/nurse practitioner, health educator, nutritionist, physician, pharmacist, social worker, community health worker, other health care professionals
Step 3 Diagnostics and medication management	Physician, nurse practitioner

Table 94–1. Multidisciplinary Team Management of Hypertension

(1) patient-centered care, (2) partnering, (3) quality improvement, (4) information and communication technology, and (5) public health perspective[21] (Box 94–1). First, the multidisciplinary hypertension team needs to organize care around the patient or, in other words, adopt a patient-centered approach. This requires interviewing and communicating effectively, assisting changes in health-related behaviors, supporting patient self-management, and using a proactive approach. Second, providers need communication skills that enable them to collaborate with patients, work closely with other providers, and to join with communities to improve outcomes for patients with hypertension. Third, they need skills to ensure that the safety and quality of patient care are continuously improved. Fourth, competencies in information and communication technology that can assist them in monitoring patients across time, and in using and sharing information, are needed. Finally, the team must adopt a public health perspective in their daily work, including a systems view across the continuum of care. Education and skill building within the team may be necessary.

To achieve effective management of hypertension, in addition to engaging the patient as an active partner in care, it is essential that all team members understand the value of their own contribution, and the roles and skills of other professionals, as well as the importance of multidisciplinary collaboration. When pharmacists, nutritionists, social workers, community health workers, and others join nurses and physicians, the expertise of each discipline supplements and complements that of the others. In addition, involving family, friends, community resources, and other health professionals can assist patients in modifying lifestyle behaviors and maintaining these changes over time.

Case conferences, chart review sessions, and journal clubs are effective strategies to assemble the hypertension management team and to improve the quality of hypertension care. Team case conferences are an ideal forum for discussion of guidelines and the extent to which they need to be modified, if at all, for implementation at the individual patient level. Selecting a case with particularly complex and challenging issues for the conference can be an effective method to gain input from the multidisciplinary team in revising the plan of care to assist the patient in achieving blood pressure control. Sample questions to guide a multidisciplinary hypertension management team case conference[22] are provided in Box 94–2. Journal clubs can provide a forum to increase team awareness of new or revised treatment guidelines as well as newly published research findings that may lead to changes in practice patterns and improved patient outcomes.

Classic hypertension care and control clinical trials, such as HDFP,[9] MRFIT,[12] SHEP,[23] and TOMHS,[24] demonstrated that extensive and continuous interventions provided by multidisciplinary teams improved adherence and outcomes. These and other studies of multidisciplinary

---

Box 94–1

Core Competencies of Multidisciplinary Hypertension Management Team

1. Patient-centered care
   Interviewing and communicating effectively
   Assisting changes in health-related behaviors
   Supporting self-management
   Using a proactive approach
2. Partnering
   Partnering with patients
   Partnering with other health care providers
   Partnering with communities
3. Quality improvement
   Measuring care delivery and outcomes
   Learning and adapting to change
   Translating evidence into practice
4. Information and communication technology
   Designing and using patient registries
   Using computer technologies
   Communicating with partners
5. Public health perspective
   Providing population-based care
   Systems thinking
   Working across the care continuum
   Working in primary health care–led systems

From World Health Organization. *Preparing a Health Care Workforce for the 21st Century: The Challenge of Chronic Conditions.* Geneva: World Health Organization, 2005 (publication 11500621).

<table>
<tr><td>

Box 94–2

Questions for Management Case Conference of Multidisciplinary Hypertension Team

- Have blood pressure goals been set, clearly communicated to the patient and all members of the care team, and achieved?
- What type(s) of care does the patient require (e.g., aggressive titration of medications, behavior modification counseling)?
- What team members are skilled and licensed to provide the various elements of care?
- What team members provide the various elements of care in the most effective and efficient manner?
- Does this patient need to be referred to specialty medical care, social work, nutritionist, or others?
- What are the barriers to hypertension control? What is the plan for overcoming barriers to blood pressure control?
- Does the patient have family or others who offer social support and assist the patient with blood pressure control behaviors? How can this support be engaged?
- Does the patient have the resources to pay for the needed care, including prescription medications? If not, what is the plan to activate the necessary resources?

</td></tr>
</table>

team interventions designed to meet patient, provider, and organizational needs, and minimize barriers to blood pressure control have been effective in a variety of clinical and community settings.[1,5,6,19] In addition, the clinical effectiveness as well as cost effectiveness of a multidisciplinary team approach to care compared to physician care alone for chronic illness, including hypertension, have been demonstrated.[5]

One innovative program in which a nurse practitioner–led, multidisciplinary team addressed patient's beliefs and concerns in a multifaceted manner, providing outreach, follow-up, feedback, and free medication, if needed, has been highly successful.[1] In this randomized clinical trial with 309 hypertensive urban black men aged 21 to 54 years, Hill and colleagues[1] evaluated the effectiveness of a more-intensive (MI) comprehensive educational-behavioral-pharmacologic intervention by a nurse practitioner-community health worker-physician (NP/CWH/MD) team and a less-intensive (LI) education and referral intervention in controlling blood pressure (BP) and minimizing progression of left ventricular hypertrophy (LVH) and renal insufficiency.[1] At 36 months, the mean systolic BP (SBP)/ diastolic BP (DBP) change from baseline was −7.5/−10.1 mmHg for the MI group and +3.4/−3.7 mmHg for the LI group ($p=0.001$ and 0.005 for between-group differences in SBP and DBP, respectively). The proportion of men with controlled BP (<140/90 mmHg) was 44% in the MI group and 31% in the LI group ($p=0.045$). Left ventricular mass was significantly lower in the MI group than in the LI

group (274 g, MI; 311 g, LI; $p=0.004$). There was a trend towards slowing of the progression of renal insufficiency (incidence of 50% increase in serum creatinine) in the MI group compared to the LI group (5.2%, MI; 8.0%, LI; $p=0.08$).

The role of the nurse

Nurses have demonstrated the necessary critical clinical judgment to provide high-quality hypertension management. The roles of nurses include all aspects of hypertension management (Box 94–3), although the role of any individual nurse may vary by education, staffing needs of the practice site, and needs of the patients. For example, in a physician private practice office, the nurse's involvement may be limited to measurement of vital signs before the patient is seen by the physician. Alternatively, in another setting the nurse may not only measure blood pressure when assessing vital signs, but also assess adherence with the prescribed treatment regimen and barriers to optimal adherence, provide counseling regarding risk factor modification, such as smoking cessation or dietary sodium reduction, and as the patient visit concludes, the nurse may assess the need for prescription renewals and finally reinforce the recommended treatment plan. Nurse involvement in hypertension management provides an ideal example of nurse specialty practice with a variety of potential roles.

In managing a cohort of patients in a hypertension clinic, the nurse may be responsible for taking a thorough medical history and for ordering appropriate diagnostic tests. This allows physicians to devote their efforts during a subsequent visit to performing the physical examination and formulating an appropriate treatment plan based on extensive information and diagnostic data provided by the nurse. In settings in which the nurses do not have advanced practice credentials, physicians are responsible for making the diagnosis of hypertension and for determining secondary causes, which may influence decisions about appropriate treatment. Physicians help to formulate a treatment plan and provide consultation to nurses in managing complex cases.

The role of the nurse practitioner/ Advanced practice nurse

Nurse practitioners (NPs) are registered nurses who have acquired the expert knowledge base, complex decision-

<table>
<tr><td>

Box 94–3

Roles of Nurses and Nurse Practitioners in Hypertension Management

- Detection, referral, and follow-up
- Diagnostics and medication management
- Patient education, counseling, and skill building
- Coordination of care
- Management of clinic/office

</td></tr>
</table>

making skills, and clinical competencies for expanded practice.[25] In addition to advanced education and clinical training, the role function that distinguishes an NP from other nurses is the legal authority to write prescriptions. The legal aspects of practice, including required continuing education, credentialing, and scope of practice, including prescribing medication, are regulated by government and depend on local custom and requirements.

With the increasing emphasis on health promotion and disease prevention, and recognition of the benefits of a multidisciplinary approach to care, NPs are part of the solution to care. It has been established in developed countries that 60% to 80% of primary and preventive services traditionally performed by physicians can be provided by nurses with similar or better clinical outcomes, high levels of patient and provider satisfaction, and at lower cost.[26,27] This cost effectiveness is explained by a variety of factors relating to lower salary, cost of liability insurance, and cost of education of NPs compared to physicians.[26] Furthermore, in a randomized trial comparing physician primary care (*n*=510) to NP primary care (*n*=806), Mundinger and colleagues[28] found that at 6 months there were no differences in patients' health status, health care utilization, or satisfaction, and for patients with hypertension, diastolic blood pressure was significantly lower for NP patients (82 vs. 85 mmHg, *p*=0.04).

Depending on local practice regulations, NPs caring for patients with hypertension can practice independently, using protocols developed jointly with the collaborating physician. NPs follow the same hypertension treatment guidelines as do physicians. The effective implementation of guidelines requires not only dissemination and awareness but a commitment by all providers and staff to set expectations for the new standards, encourage implementation, create and explain incentives for adoption, build skills, and provide resources (i.e., tools). Nurses and NPs play an important role in enforcing the use of hypertension treatment guidelines.

INDICATIONS/CONTRAINDICATIONS AND OBJECTIVES

Specific roles

The roles of the nurse and NP in hypertension management involve all aspects of hypertension management,[29–31] including detection, referral, and follow-up; diagnostics and medication management; patient education, counseling, and skill building; coordination of care; and managing the clinic or office.

Detection, referral, and follow-up

Nurses routinely measure blood pressure in most health care settings as part of initial and ongoing assessments of each patient. In addition, nurses lead blood pressure screening and verification initiatives in community, worksite, church, school, and other settings. Once blood pressure is measured and recorded, the nurse analyzes the data to determine if the readings are in the normal, prehyper-

tensive, or hypertensive range per site protocol. A system to flag charts can help ensure that uncontrolled hypertension is recognized and treated. In addition, the nurse assesses the patient's level of cardiovascular risk. There are a number of tools, such as the interactive tool found on the National Heart, Lung, and Blood Institute website, that are helpful in guiding healthcare providers as they assess cardiovascular risk; these tools also can be used in patient education efforts.[32] It may be necessary to refer the patient for specialist evaluation for persistent uncontrolled blood pressure despite intervention or for abnormal renal or vascular findings. The nurse plays an important role in implementing referrals and educating patients regarding the purpose and importance of referral.

Follow-up between visits via telephone and/or mail can be effective to reinforce goals and enhance provider–patient relationship. Moreover, it is essential to follow up on missed appointments to maintain contact with the patient and to reinforce the importance of achieving blood pressure goals. Nurses often are the first health professionals to detect hypertension, and therefore have a key role in communicating with patients and other health professionals to enforce treatment guidelines through development and appropriate revision of the patient's treatment plan.

Diagnostics and medication management

Nurses or NPs may also be responsible for the diagnostic and pharmacologic aspects of hypertension management. Using well-defined protocols based on national treatment guidelines such as the seventh report of the Joint National Committee on Prevention, Detection, Evaluation, and Treatment of High Blood Pressure (JNC VII), NPs can prescribe and titrate medications to achieve blood pressure control.[33] Nurse management of antihypertensive medication has been demonstrated to result in greater rates of blood pressure control than those achieved with standard care.[1,2,8,28,34] These improved outcomes have resulted from nurses placing a greater number of patients on medications, altering drug regimens more frequently in response to inadequate blood pressure control, and placing a higher proportion of patients on multiple drug regimens in order to achieve greater control.[1,2,8,28,34] Greater use of antihypertensive medications may produce higher costs initially, as noted in a study conducted by Logan and colleagues.[35] However, if the goals of a clinic are to keep patients in treatment and achieve greater adherence and blood pressure control rates, then prescribing the most effective regimen is paramount.[36] In addition to management of hypertension, nurses have been shown to effectively manage other cardiovascular risk factors, such as diabetes[18–20] and dyslipidemia.[37]

Patient education, counseling, and skill building

In the majority of hypertension clinics as well as in other settings, nurses provide the education, counseling, and skill building necessary to ensure that patients are undertaking lifestyle changes that may favorably influence blood pressure. A combination of strategies is required to maximize long-term adherence and blood pressure control by actively engaging patients in care and preventing, recognizing, and responding to adherence problems. Effective, evidence-based strategies to promote blood pressure control are identified in Box 94-4, and are clustered under the following general approaches: (1) identify knowledge, attitudes, beliefs, and experiences, (2) educate about conditions and treatment, (3) individualize the regimen, (4) provide reinforcement, (5) promote social support, and (6) collaborate with other professionals.[22,34,38] It is important to consider that patient education is a means to an end. That is, knowledge is necessary but insufficient to bring about desired behaviors without development of skills and multiple other reinforcing factors. The ultimate goal is for the patient to have the necessary skills and resources, including knowledge,

to follow treatment recommendations and achieve and sustain blood pressure control.

Box 94-4

Strategies to Promote Blood Pressure Control

Identify Knowledge, Attitudes, Beliefs, and Experience
- Assess patient's understanding and acceptance of the diagnosis and expectations of being in care.
- Discuss patient's concerns and clarify misunderstandings.

Educate about Conditions and Treatment
- Inform patient of blood pressure level.
- Agree with patients on a goal blood pressure.
- Inform patient about recommended treatment, providing specific oral and written information.
- Elicit concerns and questions and provide opportunities for patient to state specific behaviors to carry out treatment recommendations.
- Emphasize need to continue treatment, that patient cannot tell if blood pressure is elevated, and that control does not mean cure.
- Teach self-monitoring skills.

Individualize the Regimen
- Include patient in decision making.
- Simplify the regimen.
- Incorporate treatment into patient's daily lifestyle.
- Set, with the patient, realistic short-term objectives for specific components of the treatment plan.
- Encourage discussion of side effects and concerns.
- Encourage self-monitoring of blood pressure.
- Prioritize critical aspects of the regimen.
- Implement treatment plan in steps.
- Modify dosages or change medications to reduce side effects.
- Minimize cost of therapy.
- Indicate that you will ask about adherence at next visit.
- When weight loss is established as a treatment goal, discourage quick weight-loss regimens, fasting, or unscientific methods, since these are associated with weight cycling that may increase cardiovascular morbidity and mortality.

Box 94-4—cont'd

Provide Reinforcement
- Provide feedback regarding blood pressure level.
- Ask about behaviors to achieve blood pressure control.
- Give positive feedback for behavioral and blood pressure improvement.
- Hold exit interviews to clarify regimen.
- Make appointment for next visit before patient leaves the office.
- Use appointment reminders and contact patients to confirm appointments.
- Schedule more frequent visits to counsel nonadherent patients.
- Contact and follow-up patients who missed appointments.
- Consider clinician–patient contracts.
- Consider home visits.

Promote Social Support
- Educate family members to be part of the blood pressure control process and provide daily reinforcement.
- Suggest small-group activities to enhance mutual support and motivation.

Collaborate with Other Professionals
- Draw on complementary skills and knowledge of nurses, pharmacists, dietitians, optometrists, dentists, and physician assistants.
- Recognize shared practice goals.
- Refer patients for more intensive counseling.

From Dennison CR, Hill MN. In: Battegay EJ, Lip GYH, Bakris GL, eds., *Hypertension: Principles and Practice.* Boca Raton, FL: Taylor & Francis Group, 2005.

Identify knowledge, attitudes, beliefs, and experience

A classic framework is useful in guiding nurses and other professionals to provide patient education, counseling, and skill building, and to facilitate patients' attainment of the following four critical behaviors that are necessary to achieve and sustain long-term blood pressure control: (1) make the decision to control blood pressure, (2) take medication as prescribed, (3) monitor progress toward the goal, and (4) resolve barriers that prevent reaching the goal.[39] The premise of this evidence-based framework is that the patient is an active participant, decision maker, and problem solver, with the nurse or other health professional functioning as advisor and guide favors successful management of hypertension. The patient's understanding and acceptance of the diagnosis and expectations of being in care are assessed, patient concerns addressed, and misunderstandings clarified.

Educate about conditions and treatment

Adequate knowledge of hypertension, consequences of uncontrolled hypertension, and treatment regimen is essential to achieve blood pressure control. It has been shown that patients who receive education and counseling on hypertension management exhibit increased adherence.[40] The nurse practices patient-centered care, engaging the patient in shared decision making and establishing mutually agreed upon blood pressure goals. The patient must always be informed of blood pressure and related diagnostic testing values. This provides an ideal opportunity to assess patient knowledge, educate, establish clear goals, and discuss progress toward goals with the patient. The nurse emphasizes the need to continue treatment even when blood pressure control has been achieved, that is, control does not mean cure. The nurse also plays a key role in educating patients regarding the necessary self-monitoring skills (e.g., home blood pressure monitoring). Patient knowledge is necessary but insufficient if appropriate action does not follow. In addition to patient education and skill building, effective communication, and a trustful relationship between the patient and nurse are of paramount importance to achieve sustained blood pressure control.

Individualize the regimen

Successful education and counseling to promote adherence to treatment regimen and blood pressure control require that nurses and other health professionals individualize care to maximize the patient's motivation to control their hypertension by remaining in care, maintaining a healthy lifestyle, taking prescribed medication, and monitoring progress toward goals. Nurse efforts to individualize the regimen should focus on patient response to the treatment regimen as well as self-care behaviors and skills necessary to hypertension control. The nurse can assist the patient to incorporate the treatment regimen into the patient's daily lifestyle that is required for long-term sustainability. The nurse works with the patient to mutually develop realistic outcomes-oriented goals and strategies for attaining the goals. Equally important, the nurse follows up with the patient frequently to assess progress toward goals and if necessary to revise strategies for attaining goals.

Nurses are trained to provide counseling regarding lifestyle modification, which is recommended for all hypertensive patients with lifestyle risk factors, such as obesity, excessive alcohol consumption, and high-sodium diet.[33] Weight loss, which may be the most successful nonpharmacologic technique for lowering blood pressure, requires behavior change in both diet and physical activity patterns.[33] Such nonpharmacologic approaches include helping patients to initiate or maintain an aerobic exercise program and to limit sodium intake and alcohol consumption to one to two drinks per day.[33] In addition, many hypertensive patients present with multiple risk factors for cardiovascular disease. The nurse also can provide education and counseling for smoking cessation and lipid reduction to help patients further lower their risk of cardiovascular disease. Modifying lifestyle behaviors requires many clinical interventions: assessment of an individual's baseline behaviors, education about how to make the appropriate changes, counseling to develop strategies such as setting short-term goals and self-monitoring that will ensure the achievement and maintenance of the changes, constant follow-up with the patient to determine whether adherence is a problem, working with patients to identify and resolve barriers to blood pressure control, and reinforcement of progress toward the goal of change in behavior.[41]

The extent to which patients are able to adhere to treatment recommendations is a major issue in blood pressure control and depends on many factors. Review of adherence in randomized controlled trials on cardiovascular disease prevention strategies identified the following successful approaches: signed agreements, behavioral skill training, self-monitoring, telephone/mail contact, spouse support, self-efficacy enhancement, contingency contracting, exercise prescriptions, external cognitive aids, persuasive communication, nurse-managed clinics, and work- or school-based programs.[42] Improving adherence to evidence-based guidelines is a multilevel challenge, and multiple strategies are required beginning with patient education, counseling, and skill building.[4]

Another important aspect of individualizing the regimen to promote blood pressure control involves assessing potential barriers to blood pressure control. Nurses are motivated and trained to assess common barriers to blood pressure control. Barriers may include: knowledge deficits, lack of health care or pharmacy insurance, inadequate communication with clinicians, cost of medication, complexity of the regimen, adverse effects of medication, transportation to and from the visit, work schedule, inconvenient clinic/office location or difficulty scheduling appointments, child or elder care, or other competing life demands.[43,44] Following identification of barriers, the nurse works with the patient and collaborating health professionals to minimize or eliminate the barriers, thereby promoting blood pressure control.

Provide reinforcement

It is important to work with individual patients to ensure that they understand what is necessary to achieve treatment goals and that they participate in treatment decisions. Nurse responsiveness to patient concerns with joint problem solving to prevent or minimize barriers to care and treatment as well as reinforcement and support are crucial. Provision of reminders, outreach, and follow-up services are beneficial. Follow-up between visits via telephone and/or mail can be an effective method to reinforce goals and enhance the provider–patient relationship. It is essential to follow up on all missed appointments to maintain contact with the patient and to reinforce the importance of achieving blood pressure goals. Success in implementing the treatment regimen to achieve blood pressure control requires frequent monitoring of blood pressure, modification of the treatment regimen, and interaction with the patient. These roles require training and dedicated time to provide the education and counseling necessary to build skills for and reinforce successful behavior change.

Promote social support

Nurses can also be effective in educating family members and/or friends to participate in the blood pressure control process. Family members can play a fundamental role by providing daily reinforcement of the patient's efforts to achieve blood pressure control. If the patient desires greater family participation, the nurse should encourage the patient to invite family members to attend and participate in clinic visits. In addition, some patients may benefit from small group activities, such as clinic support groups or group visits, to enhance social support and motivation.

Collaborate with other professionals

In planning care, the nurse works in conjunction with the patient, physician, and other members of the multidisciplinary hypertension management team. Nurse-supervised community health workers, nurse case managers, and nurse practitioners, in collaboration with physicians and other health professionals, in a variety of settings have effectively improved the outcomes of patients with hypertension.[1-6,19] Involving family, friends, community resources, and other health professionals can help patients to achieve and sustain blood pressure control.

Achieving and sustaining goal blood pressure levels over time requires continuous educational and behavioral strategies, an individualized regimen, and reinforcement so that patients have the knowledge, skills, motivation and resources to carry out treatment recommendations. Successful blood pressure control requires that patients know what steps to take and develop skills in problem identification and problem solving to address barriers. Strategies to help patients develop these skills need to be adapted so that they are culturally salient and feasible for staff to implement.

Coordination of care

Long-term maintenance of hypertension control requires regular monitoring of blood pressure, refilling of prescriptions, providing counseling and reinforcement of behavior change efforts, and titrating therapy as indicated. Each patient's management must be individualized with costs minimized. Patients often see different providers at several settings for various health problems, fill prescriptions in more than one pharmacy, receive inconsistent messages, and experience interruption of therapy and inadequate communication among providers. Nurses are skilled at building and maintaining both informal and formal collaborative linkages among providers, resources, and services within and external to their practice setting. Nurses can assist patients in understanding complex treatment regimen and navigating through the complex, challenging, and commonly confusing health care structure.[45]

Manage the clinic/office

A nurse may be in the position of managing or planning for the initiation of a hypertension clinic. Nurses frequently direct and/or coordinate the efforts of other team members who are working within the clinic or providing direct consultation. To enhance consistency and quality of care and to facilitate adherence to treatment guidelines, decision support systems (electronic and paper), such as flow sheets and feedback reminders, may be developed. In addition, it may be the responsibility of the nurse to hire, supervise, and train the community health workers, to deliver appropriate intervention strategies, and other staff, such as office assistants and receptionists, to take blood pressures, schedule appointments, make reminder telephone calls, obtain laboratory results, and enter data to support evaluation of clinical outcomes.[36] Nurses influence utilization of resources including appropriate length of visit and caseload size as well as optimizing reimbursement for services in the hypertension clinic setting.

It is imperative that all health professionals who measure blood pressure use correct measurement technique.[46,47] In addition to ensuring proper blood pressure measurement technique among staff, nurses often are responsible for ensuring that blood pressure measurement equipment is properly calibrated and functioning.[46]

Documentation of clinical outcomes is becoming increasingly important and necessary. Often it is the nurse in the hypertension care setting who has responsibility for tracking process and outcome measures for quality improvement efforts. Integrated systems with continuous quality improvement approaches enhance provider's delivery of care and patient outcomes. Tracking blood pressure, frequency of visits, medications, patient adherence, hospitalizations, and emergency room visits, using informatics technologies enables timely evaluation of clinical outcomes and the costs incurred in providing antihypertensive treatment.

COMPLICATIONS

The advantages of multidisciplinary management of hypertension, involving nurses, are numerous. Nurses provide effective hypertension care by adhering to treatment guidelines and protocols resulting in improved outcomes, including patient satisfaction and retention in care, and physician satisfaction.

The barriers to optimal implementation of multidisciplinary team management of hypertension include inadequate awareness of the role of nonphysician health care professionals in hypertension care, lack of time and resources, and lack of incentives and reimbursement. Inadequate financial reimbursement for patient education and counseling is a critical barrier that must be addressed at the policy level. In some settings, the barriers also include lack of practical implementation tools, such as decision support systems, and local social norms and ethics that preclude nurses from assuming greater responsibility for patient care and outcomes. A major barrier to nurse practitioners' practice in some provinces or states involves practice regulations or reimbursement plans.

SUMMARY

The prevalence and asymptomatic nature of hypertension and the need for lifelong treatment to prevent complications pose challenges that require professional expertise beyond that of physicians. Nurses and other health care professionals are critical to optimal hypertension management. A multidisciplinary team approach with collaborative partnerships, based on recognition of the roles of nurses and other health professionals and a supportive environment, are essential to successful multidisciplinary management of hypertension. Improving the processes and outcomes of hypertension care requires that the

multidisciplinary team demonstrate the following five core competencies: (1) patient-centered care, (2) partnering, (3) quality improvement, (4) information and communication technology, and (5) public health perspective. The meaningful implementation of multidisciplinary team management of hypertension involves bringing nurses, physicians, and other health professionals together to improve patient care, investing in team development, and influencing health policy.

REFERENCES

1. Hill MN, Han HR, Dennison CR, Kim MT, Roary MC, Blumenthal RS, et al. Hypertension care and control in underserved urban African American men: behavioral and physiologic outcomes at 36 months. *Am J Hypertens* 2003;16(11):906–13.
2. Reichgott MJ, Pearson S, Hill MN. The nurse practitioner's role in complex patient management: hypertension. *J Natl Med Assoc* 1983;75(12):1197–204.
3. Ginsberg GM, Viskoper JR, Fuchs Z, Drexler I, Lubin F, Berlin S, et al. Partial cost-benefit analysis of two different modes of nonpharmacological control of hypertension in the community. *J Hum Hypertens* 1993;7:593–7.
4. Miller NM, Hill MN, Kottke T, Ockene IS. The multilevel compliance challenge: Recommendations for a call to action: a statement for health care professionals. *Circulation* 1997; 95:1085–90.
5. Litaker D, Mion L, Planavsky L, Kippes C, Mehta N, Frolkis J. Physician-nurse practitioner teams in chronic disease management: the impact on costs, clinical effectiveness, and patients' perception of care. *J Interprof Care* 2003;17(3):223–37.
6. Norby SM, Stroebel RJ, Canzanello VJ. Physician–nurse team approaches to improve blood pressure control. *J Clin Hypertens* 2003;5:386–92.
7. Alderman MH, Schoenbaum EE. Detection and treatment of hypertension at the work site. *N Engl J Med* 1975; 293:65–8.
8. Logan AG, Milne BJ, Achber C, Campbell WP, Haynes RB. Work-site treatment of hypertension by specially trained nurses. *Lancet* 1979;1175–8.
9. Hypertension Detection and Follow-up Program Cooperative Group. Five-year findings of the Hypertension Detection and Follow-up program. I. Reduction in mortality of persons with hypertension, including mild hypertension. *JAMA* 1979;242:2562–71.
10. Viskoper RJ, Silverberg DS. Community control in Israel: cardiovascular risk factor control. In: Bulpitt CJ, ed. *Handbook of Hypertension*. Vol. 6: Epidemiology of Hypertension. Amsterdam: Elsevier Science Publishers, 1985.
11. Curzio JL, Rubin PC, Kennedy SS, Reid JL. A comparison of the management of hypertensive patients by nurse practitioners compared with conventional hospital care. *J Hum Hypertens* 1990;4:665–70.

12. SHEP Co-operative Research Group. Prevention of stroke by antihypertensive drug treatment in older persons with isolated systolic hypertension. *JAMA* 1991;265:3255–64.
13. Medical Research Council Working Party. Medical Research Council trial of treatment of hypertension in older adults: principal results. *BMJ* 1992; 304:405–12.
14. Becker DM, Yook RM, Moy TF, Blumenthal RS, Becker LC. Markedly high prevalence of coronary risk factors in apparently healthy African-American and white siblings of persons with premature coronary heart disease. *Am J Cardiol* 1998;82(9):1045–51.
15. Montgomery A, Fahey T, Peters T, MacIntosh C, Sharp D. Evaluation of computer based clinical decision support system and risk chart for management of hypertension in primary care: randomized controlled trial. *BMJ* 2000;320:686–90.
16. Rice VH, Stead LF. *Nursing Interventions for Smoking Cessation* (Cochrane Review). Oxford: Cochrane Library, 2002.
17. McPherson CP, Swenson KK, Pine DA, Leimer L. A nurse-based pilot program to reduce cardiovascular risk factors in a primary care setting. *Am J Manag Care* 2002;8(6):543–55.
18. Denver EA, Barnard M, Woolfson RG, Earle KA. Management of uncontrolled hypertension in a nurse-led clinic compared with conventional care for patients with type 2 diabetes. *Diabetes Care* 2003;26:2256–60.
19. Gary TL, Bone LR, Hill MN, Levine DM, McGuire M, Saudek C, et al. Randomized controlled trial of the effects of nurse case manager and community health worker interventions on risk factors for diabetes-related complications in urban African-Americans. *Prev Med* 2003;37:23–32.
20. New JP, Mason JM, Freemantle N, Teasdale S, Wong LM, Bruce NJ, et al. Specialist nurse-led intervention to treat and control hypertension and hyperlipidemia in diabetes (SPLINT). A randomized controlled trial. *Diabetes Care* 2003;26:2250–5.
21. World Health Organization. *Preparing a Health Care Workforce for the 21st Century: The Challenge of Chronic Conditions*. Geneva: World Health Organization, 2005.
22. Dennison CR, Hill MN. The role of nurses and nurse practitioners in hypertension management. In: Battegay EJ, Lip GYH,

Bakris GL, eds. *Hypertension: Principles and Practice*. Boca Raton, FL: Taylor & Francis Group, 2005.
23. Grimm RH, Cohen JD, Smith WM, Falvo-Gerard L, Neaton JD. Hypertension management in the Multiple Risk Factor Intervention Trial (MRFIT). Six-year intervention results for men in special intervention and usual care groups. *Arch Intern Med* 1985;145(7):1191–9.
24. Treatment of Mild Hypertension Study Research Group. Treatment of mild hypertension study: final results. *JAMA* 1993;270:713–24.
25. International Council of Nurses. *Nurse Practitioner/Advanced Practice Network: Definition and Characteristics of the Role*. http://icn–apnetwork.org. Accessed December 1, 2006.
26. American Nurses Assocation. *Advanced Practice Nursing: A New Age in Health Care*. Washington, DC: American Nurses Association, 1993.
27. Horrocks S, Anderson E, Salisbury C. Systematic review of whether nurse practitioners working in primary care can provide equivalent care to doctors. *BMJ* 2002;324:819–23.
28. Mundinger MO, Kane RL, Lenz ER, Totten AM, Tsai W, Cleary PD, et al. Primary care outcomes in patients treated by nurse practitioners or physicians. A randomized trial. *JAMA* 2000;283:59–68.
29. Curzio JL, Beevers M. The role of nurses in hypertension care and research. *J Hum Hypertens* 1997;11:541–50.
30. Bengtson A, Drevenhorn E. The nurse's role and skills in hypertension care. *Clin Nurse Specialist* 2003;17:260–8.
31. Oakeshott P, Kerry S, Austin A, Cappuccio F. Is there a role for nurse-led blood pressure management in primary care? *Fam Pract* 2003;20: 469–73.
32. National Cholesterol Education Program. Third Report of the Expert Panel on Detection, Evaluation, and Treatment of High Blood Cholesterol in Adults (Adult Treatment Panel III). Risk assessment tool for estimating 10-year risk of developing hard CHD (myocardial infarction and coronary death). Available at: *http://hin.nhlbi.nih.gov/atpiii/calculator. asp?usertype=prof*. Accessed October 14, 2005.
33. National Institutes of Health. *The Seventh Report of the Joint National Committee on Prevention, Detection, Evaluation, and Treatment of High Blood Pressure*

(JNC VII). National High Blood Pressure Education Program. Bethesda, MD: National Institutes of Health, National Heart, Lung and Blood Institute, 2003.

34. Runyan KW Jr. The Memphis Chronic Disease Program. Comparisons in outcome and the nurse's extended role. *JAMA* 1975;231:264–7.

35. Logan AC, Milne BJ, Flanagan PT, Haynes RB. Clinical effectiveness and cost-effectiveness of monitoring blood pressure of hypertensive employees at work. *Hypertension* 1983;5:828–36.

36. Miller NM, Hill MN. Nursing clinics in the management of hypertension. In: S. Oparil, M. Weber, eds. *Hypertension*, 2nd ed. Philadelphia: WB Saunders, 2004.

37. Debusk RF, Miller NH, Superko HR, Dennis CA, Thomas RJ, Lew HT, et al. A case-management system for coronary risk factor modification after acute myocardial infarction. *Ann Intern Med* 1994;120:721–9.

38. National Institutes of Health. The Fifth Report of the Joint National Committee

on Prevention, Detection, Evaluation, and Treatment of High Blood Pressure (JNC V). National High Blood Pressure Education Program. Bethesda, MD: National Institutes of Health, National Heart, Lung and Blood Institute, 1993.

39. Working Group to Define Critical Patient Behaviors in High Blood Pressure Control. Patient behavior for blood pressure control. Guidelines for professionals. *JAMA* 1979;241:2534–7.

40. Levine DM, Green LW, Deeds SG, Chwalow J, Russell RP, Finlay J. Health education for hypertensive patients. *JAMA* 1979;241:1700–3.

41. Miller NH, Taylor CB. *Lifestyle Management for Patients with Coronary Heart Disease. Current Issues in Cardiac Rehabilitation*. Monograph 2. Champaign, IL: Human Kinetics, 1995.

42. Haynes RB. Improving patient adherence: state of the art, with a special focus on medication taking for cardiovascular disorders. In: Burke LE, Ockene IS, eds.

Compliance in Healthcare and Research. Armonk, NY: Futura Publishing Company, 2001:3–21.

43. Eaton LE, Buck EA, Catanzaro JE. The nurse's role in facilitating compliance in clients with hypertension. *Med Surg Nurs* 1996;5:339–64.

44. Hill MN, Bone LR, Kim MT, Miller DJ, Dennison CR, Levine DM. Barriers to hypertension care and control in young urban black men. *Am J Hypertens* 1999; 12:951–8.

45. Aminoff UB, Kjellgren KI. The nurse—a resource in hypertension care. *J Adv Nurs* 2001;35:582–9.

46. Beevers G, Lip GY, O'Brien E. ABC of hypertension. Blood pressure measurement. Part I—sphygmomanometry: factors common to all techniques. *BMJ* 2001;322(7292): 981–5.

47. World Hypertension League. Measuring your blood pressure. Available at: *http:www.mco.edu/org/whl/bloodpre.html*. Accessed October 14, 2005.

Chapter

95

World Health Organization/ International Society of Hypertension (WHO/ISH): Hypertension Guidelines and Statements

Judith A. Whitworth

Hypertension is a major contributor to global mortality and disease burden. The *World Health Report 2002: Reducing Risks, Promoting Healthy Life* quantified the disease burden consequent on elevated blood pressure at 4.5%.[1] To quote Derek Yach who was executive director, Noncommunicable Disease and Mental Health, World Health Organization [WHO], the 2002 report "focuses on cardiovascular and other risks to global health and quantifies the substantial public health gains for populations and individuals as a result of a reduction in cardiovascular and other health risks. The report also highlights the fact that a large segment of the world population is at high cardiovascular risk due to one or more cardiovascular risk factors, including hypertension. As such, and to improve the health outcomes of populations at risk in a cost-effective and equitable manner, countries should, in the future, implement population and individual-based strategies in a complementary manner. The corporate view of WHO is that there is a need to establish comprehensive guidelines for the management of cardiovascular risk which will inform policy-makers, public health experts and clinicians ... to bring about a much needed paradigm shift from treating cardiovascular risk factors in isolation to a more holistic multiple risk factor approach and also facilitate key policy decisions that are integral to implementation of population-based strategies for reduction of cardiovascular risk."

The *World Health Report* showed that above a theoretical minimum of 115 mmHg, the association of systolic blood pressure with cerebrovascular disease (CVD), risk for stroke, ischemic heart disease, hypertensive disease, and other cardiac disease was continuous. Approximately 62% of CVD and 49% of ischemic heart disease globally was attributable to suboptimal blood pressure (systolic blood pressure >115 mmHg). Importantly, blood pressure ranks third as a risk for global burden of disease, after underweight and unsafe sex, and before tobacco, alcohol, unsafe water, cholesterol, and overweight. The report estimated that hypertension causes over 7 million premature deaths, 4.5% of the global disease burden, and 64 million disability-adjusted life years lost.[1]

WHO and the International Society of Hypertension (ISH) have collaborated over decades to produce several guidelines and statements on management of hypertension. The WHO/ISH Guidelines on hypertension were published in 1983,[2,3] 1986,[4,5] 1989,[6–8] 1993,[9] and 1999.[10–12] The collaboration has also given rise to statements, most notably the 2003 Statement on hypertension,[13] but also to statements on prevention of hypertension[14] and on the risk profile of calcium antagonists.[15]

The WHO/ISH Guidelines are intended to have wide publication and distribution and are not subject to copyright. Accordingly, this chapter contains extensive quotes from the 1999 Guidelines. The 2003 Statement is appended in full (see Appendix).

1999 WHO/ISH GUIDELINES

The 1999 WHO/ISH Guidelines were extensive and comprehensive and written for specialists in clinical practice; a shorter version was also prepared for family practitioners.

The 1999 Guidelines were very close to the 1993 Guidelines in the key areas of goals of therapy and antihypertensive choice. These 1999 Guidelines were reinforced by subsequent meta-analyses indicating that blood pressure lowering (as opposed to specific drug class)[16] is fundamental in reducing cardiovascular mortality and morbidity and a large body of evidence suggesting blood pressure goals should be modified downward.[17–22]

Key points from 1999 WHO/ISH Guidelines

Key points from the 1999 guidelines are summarized in Boxes 95–1 through 95–12, and Table 95–1.

WHO/ISH Statement 2003

In 2000, WHO decided to formalize methodology for clinical management guidelines using standardized methods for grading evidence. In 2001, a working group was set up under the auspices of the WHO/ISH Guidelines and Liaison Committees to update the 1999 Guidelines in three areas:

1. The ascertainment of overall cardiovascular risk to establish both the thresholds for initiation of

Box 95–1

The 1999 WHO/ISH Guidelines

- These Guidelines provide recommendations that are based on the collective expert interpretation by the WHO-ISH Guidelines Subcommittee of the available evidence from epidemiologic studies and clinical trials.
- The primary aim is to offer balanced information to guide clinicians, rather than rigid rules that would constrain their judgment about the management of individual patients, who will differ in their personal, medical, social, ethnic, and cultural characteristics.
- The WHO-ISH Guidelines are written for a global audience from communities that vary widely in the nature of their health system and availability of resources.
- It is hoped that national and regional experts will use them as a basis for drawing up recommendations that are specifically designed for management of patients in their own region.

Box 95–2

Hypertension versus Normotension (WHO/ISH 1999)

- Blood pressure levels are continuously related to the risks of cardiovascular disease and the definition of hypertension (or raised blood pressure) is, therefore, arbitrary.
- Much blood pressure–related disease occurs among individuals who would normally be considered normotensive.
- Most of the evidence about the benefits and risks of lowering blood pressure comes from studies in patients selected on the basis of high blood pressure.
- It is not clear whether estimates of treatment effect obtained from trials in hypertensives can be extrapolated to individuals with lower blood pressure levels.
- There is a strong rationale for expecting high-risk patients without hypertension to benefit from blood-pressure lowering and trials are required to investigate this possibility.

Box 95–3

Contribution of Blood Pressure and Other Factors to Cardiovascular Disease Risk (WHO/ISH 1999)

- Among patients with mild hypertension, differences in the risks of cardiovascular disease are determined not only by the level of blood pressure, but also by the presence or levels of other risk factors.
- For example, a man aged 65 years with diabetes, a history of transient ischemic attacks, and a systolic/diastolic blood pressure of 145/90 mmHg will have an annual risk of a major cardiovascular event that is more than *20 times greater* than that in a man aged 40 years with the same blood pressure but without either diabetes or a history of cardiovascular disease.
- In contrast, a man aged 40 years with a systolic/diastolic blood pressure of 170/105 mmHg will have a risk of a major cardiovascular event that is about two or three times greater than that of a man of the same age with a systolic diastolic blood pressure of 145/90 mmHg and similar other risk factor levels.
- Thus differences in the absolute level of cardiovascular risk between patients with hypertension will often be determined to a greater extent by other risk factors than by the level of blood pressure.

Box 95–4

Underestimation of Effects of Blood Pressure–Lowering Treatment in Randomized Controlled Trials (WHO/ISH 1999)

- Estimates of treatment effects in the trials of blood pressure lowering regimens generally provide conservative estimates of the full potential effects of treatment.
- In the trials, there was considerable crossover between treatment groups:
  Proportion of patients assigned to active therapy groups stopped treatment
  Proportion of those assigned to control groups began active treatment
- Such crossover is likely to have reduced the average difference in diastolic blood pressure between groups by 1 to 2 mmHg, in which case, the full relative effects of treatment on stroke and coronary heart disease would be somewhat greater than the effects observed.
- The average duration of treatment in the trials was only about 5 years, and it is possible that longer-term treatment over many years, as is usual for hypertensive patients, might have led to larger relative risk reductions.
- Low-risk patients were recruited to many trials, and the absolute effects of treatment among higher-risk patients seen in broader clinical practice are, therefore, likely to be greater than those typically observed (see Box 95–5).

treatment and the goals for treatment of people with hypertension in general and for various subgroups

2. The appropriate treatment strategies for both nondrug and drug therapies
3. The cost effectiveness of drug treatment

In other areas the 1999 Guidelines would remain current. Subsequently the work done by the guidelines group was incorporated into a WHO/ISH statement.[13] The 2003 statement superseded the 1999 Guidelines in the three

Box 95–5

Relative and Absolute Effects of Treatment (WHO/ISH 1999)

- The relative effect of treatment reflects the proportional difference between treatment groups in the incidence of disease events:

  In the Systolic Hypertension in the Elderly (SHEP) trial,[22] the incidence of major coronary heart disease (CHD) events over 4.5 years in patients assigned active treatment was 4.4% while in those assigned the placebo it was 5.9%. This represents a relative risk of 0.73 or a relative risk reduction of 27%.

- The absolute effect of treatment is generally of greatest interest to doctors and patients:

  In the SHEP trial, the absolute reduction in CHD risk over 4.5 years was 1.4%. This indicates that 14 events were prevented among every 1000 patients assigned active treatment, and that one major CHD event was avoided among every 71 patients assigned active treatment.

- Estimates of *relative* treatment effects from randomized trials provide a guide to the likely relative effects of treatment in other nonstudy patient populations. However, estimates of *absolute* treatment effects from trials of blood pressure lowering are of limited generalizability because of complex inclusion and exclusion criteria frequently resulted in the recruitment of patients at lower average risk than those seen in broader clinical practice.

- The best predictor of absolute treatment effects for any individual patient will be provided by application of the estimate of the relative risk reduction from trials to an estimate of the absolute disease risk for the individual in question.

- A simple table for estimating the absolute cardiovascular disease risk of individual hypertensive patients is provided for use with these guidelines.

Box 95–6

Situations in Which Ambulatory Blood Pressure Monitoring Should Be Considered (WHO/ISH 1999)

- Unusual variability of blood pressure over the same or different visits.
- Office hypertension in subjects with low cardiovascular risk.
- Symptoms suggesting hypotensive episodes.
- Hypertension resistant to drug treatment.

Box 95–7

Isolated Office ("White-Coat") Hypertension (WHO-ISH 1999)

- In some patients, office blood pressure is persistently elevated whereas daytime blood pressure outside the clinic environment is not.
- This condition is widely known as "white-coat" hypertension, although the term "isolated office" hypertension is preferable because the office-daytime blood pressure difference presumably depends on multiple factors, and does not correlate with the pressor response to blood pressure measurements by the doctor, the so-called "white-coat" effect.
- It is likely that only a small fraction of the hypertensive population exhibits isolated office hypertension, if the diagnosis is restricted to subjects whose ambulatory systolic/diastolic blood pressure measurements are truly normal (below 125/80 mmHg).
- Furthermore, there is continuing debate as to whether isolated office hypertension is an innocent phenomenon or whether it carries an increased burden of cardiovascular risk.
- Physicians should aim at its identification (by use of home or ambulatory blood pressure measurements) whenever clinical suspicion is raised.
- The decision to treat or not should be based on the overall risk profile and the presence or absence of target-organ damage. Close follow-up is essential for subjects with isolated office hypertension whom the physician chooses not to treat.

Box 95–8

Lifestyle and Blood Pressure (WHO-ISH 1999)

- It is important that lifestyle measures be instituted within the framework of a structured plan that includes the use of counseling and monitoring by appropriate health professionals such as nurses, dieticians, clinical psychologists, and other therapists, as well as the responsible physician.
- Recommendations should be tailored for each individual and greater use should be made of modern and well-validated counseling techniques.
- Lifestyle measures that are widely agreed to lower the blood pressure and that should be considered in all patients in whom they may apply are weight reduction, reduction of excessive alcohol consumption, reduction of high salt intake, and increase in physical activity.
- Particular emphasis should be placed on cessation of smoking and on healthy eating patterns that contribute to the treatment of associated risk factors and cardiovascular diseases.

Box 95–9

Benefits of Drug Treatment (WHO-ISH 1999)

- All classes of antihypertensive drugs have specific advantages and disadvantages for particular patient groups.
- There is as yet no evidence that the main benefits of treating hypertension are due to any particular drug property rather than to lowering of blood pressure *per se*.
- The randomized trials conducted to date have not provided any clear evidence of differential effects on outcome of different agents producing the same blood pressure reduction.
- However, most individual studies have been too small to detect plausibly modest differences in important outcomes such as stroke or myocardial infarction.

Box 95–10

Absolute Effects of Treatment on Cardiovascular Risk (WHO-ISH 1999)

- From the results of randomized controlled trials, it appears that each reduction of 10–14 mmHg in systolic blood pressure and 5–6 mmHg in diastolic blood pressure confers about two-fifths less stroke, one-sixth less coronary heart disease and, in Western populations, one-third less major cardiovascular events overall.
- In patients with grade 1 hypertension, monotherapy with most agents will produce reductions in systolic/diastolic blood pressure of about 10/5 mmHg. In patients with higher grades of hypertension, it is possible to achieve sustained blood pressure reductions of 20/10 mmHg or more, particularly if combination drug therapy is used.
- The estimated absolute effects of such blood pressure reductions on cardiovascular disease (CVD) risks (fatal plus nonfatal stroke or myocardial infarction) are as follows:

Patient group	Absolute risk (CVD) events over 10 years	Absolute treatment effects (CVD) events over 10 years prevented 10/5 mmHg	20/10 mmHg
Low-risk patients	<15%	<5	<9
Medium-risk patients	15–20%	5–7	8–11
High-risk patients	20–30%	7–10	11–17
Very-high-risk patients	>30%	>10	>17

- Between these strata, the estimated absolute treatment benefits will range from less than five events prevented per 1000 patient years of treatment (low risk) to more than 17 events prevented per 1000 patient years of treatment (very high risk).
- The absolute benefits for stroke and coronary heart disease will be augmented by smaller absolute benefits for congestive heart failure and renal disease.
- These estimates of benefit are based on relative risk reductions observed in trials of about 5 years' duration. Longer-term treatment over decades could produce larger risk reductions (see Box 95–4).

areas it considered. The full statement follows this chapter (see Appendix).

The WHO/ISH guidelines and statement differ from other major guidelines, particularly the European[23] and U.S. guidelines,[24] in their purpose and in their target audience. Global capacity to assess and manage hypertension is very different from that in Europe and the United States. A WHO global capacity assessment of 167 countries found that 61% had no national hypertension guidelines, 45% did not have health professionals appropriately trained to manage hypertension, in 25% antihypertensives were unaffordable, in 12% basic drugs were unavailable, and in 8% basic equipment for managing hypertension was unavailable.[25]

The classification of hypertension used in all guidelines is arbitrary, and reflects a simplified dichotomous approach of normotension versus hypertension when the reality is that blood pressure–related risk is continuous. It is now recognized that CVD prevention should be comprehensive rather than focused on single risk factors, and that comprehensive risk management should focus on lowering blood pressure rather than the old notion of simply treating hypertension. Accordingly the WHO/ISH statement emphasizes risk stratification. It should be noted that, as emphasized in the European guidelines, risk in this context means *added* risk, that is, low risk means low added risk. There is general agreement in contemporary documents on thresholds for treatment and targets for blood pressure lowering. Thresholds given are 140/90 mmHg systolic in low- to medium-risk and less than 130/80 mmHg in high-risk patients.

All guidelines recommend lifestyle measures for prevention and management of hypertension. These include weight loss in the overweight, increased physical activity, moderation of alcohol intake, healthy diet (fruit, vegeta-

bles, and low saturated fat), reduction of dietary sodium, and increased dietary potassium intake.

There is a very large literature on choice of initial therapy in hypertension management. To a significant degree, however, this emphasis is outdated. An equally large body of data suggests most patients will not be controlled on monotherapy. The WHO/ISH statement emphasizes that

Box 95–11

Monotherapy versus Combination Therapy (WHO-ISH 1999)

Drug Monotherapy

When drugs from the main classes available are used as monotherapy at the recommended doses, they produce very similar blood pressure reductions. In general, the sizes of the blood pressure reductions increase with the initial level of blood pressure, but typically the placebo-adjusted reductions average about 4% to 8% for both systolic and diastolic blood pressure. Thus for patients with blood pressures of about 160/95 mmHg, the usual reduction produced by monotherapy would be about 7 to 13 mmHg systolic and 4 to 8 mmHg diastolic. Clearly, for many patients with hypertension, such reductions in blood pressure would not restore optimal or even nonhypertensive blood pressure levels.

Drug Combination Therapy

Combination therapy of several of the available drug classes has been shown to produce blood pressure reductions that are greater than those produced by any group of individual agents used alone. The Hypertension Optimal Treatment (HOT) study in which blood pressure was lowered to below 90 mmHg in over 90% of patients, demonstrated that combination therapy was necessary in 70% of participants. Combinations with fully additive hypotensive effects will deliver blood pressure reductions that are around twice as great as those obtained with a single drug, of the order of 8% to 15%, or 12 to 22 mmHg systolic and 7 to 14 mmHg diastolic for patients with blood pressure of 160/95 mmHg.

Effective Drug Combinations

Diuretic and β-blocker
Diuretic and angiotensin-converting enzyme (ACE) inhibitor (or angiotensin II antagonists)
Calcium antagonist (dihydropyridine) and β-blocker
Calcium antagonist and ACE inhibitor
α-blocker and β-blocker
Effective drug combinations use drugs from various classes in order to obtain the additive hypotensive effect that comes from combining drugs with different primary actions, while minimizing the compensations that limit the fall in blood pressure. Combinations of limited value generally result from combining drugs that work through similar mechanisms so that their hypotensive actions may be less than additive, or drugs that have similar side effects so that the risk of adverse effects is increased.

Box 95–12

Causes of Refractory Hypertension (WHO-ISH 1999)

- Unsuspected secondary cause (e.g., renal and endocrine)
- Poor adherence to therapeutic plan
- Continued intake of drugs that raise blood pressure (e.g., nonsteroidal anti-inflammatory drugs)
- Failure to modify lifestyle including:
  Weight gain
  Heavy alcohol intake (e.g., binge drinking)
- Volume overload due to:
  Inadequate diuretic therapy
  Progressive renal insufficiency
  High sodium intake

Causes of Spurious Refractory Hypertension

- Isolated office (white-coat) hypertension
- Failure to use large cuff on large arm

benefits of hypertension treatment largely derive from blood pressure reduction, but also recognizes the strong evidence that specific agents benefit patients with compelling indications. For patients without such compelling indications, on the basis of comparative trial data, availability, and cost, the WHO/ISH statement recommends that (low-dose) diuretics be considered for first-line therapy.

The WHO/ISH statement places significant emphasis on feasibility and cost effectiveness, which are of great impor-tance globally in the context of limited health budgets. Cost effectiveness encompasses benefits for expenditure and differs from affordability, which relates to prevalence and cost of treatment in a particular country setting. It follows that where resources are limited, cost-effective treatment may not be affordable, and priority for drug therapy should be given to those at higher risk. The State-ment noted that in many (but not all) settings, thiazide diuretics are the cheapest available drugs and most cost effective. However, where compelling indications are present, drug classes providing additional benefits, even if more expensive, may be more cost effective. Where added risk is low, whether treatment is cost effective will depend on drug cost, but in high-risk patients with large benefits from treatment, more expensive drugs may be more cost effective.

The WHO/ISH 2003 Statement joins the 2002 *World Health Report* and the WHO/ISH 2000 Statement on preven-tion[14] in stressing that population strategies to reduce blood pressure are very cost effective worldwide. The WHO/ISH statement indicates that both population-based and high-risk group strategies are needed for prevention of CVD, with comprehensive targeting of unhealthy lifestyle (diet, tobacco, inactivity), hypertension, glucose intolerance, hyperlipidemia; and CVD management.

Prevention and control of the global epidemic of cardio-vascular disease requires a comprehensive program directed toward both populations and high-risk individuals, and focused on comprehensive risk factor reduction.

ACKNOWLEDGMENT

Amanda Jacobsen provided expert secretarial assistance.

STRATIFICATION OF RISK TO QUANTIFY PROGNOSIS (WHO-ISH 1999)			
	Blood Pressure (mmHg)		
Other Risk Factors and Disease History	Grade 1 (mild hypertension) SBP 140–159 or DBP 90–99	Grade 2 (moderate hypertension) SBP 160–179 or DBP 100–109	Grade 3 (severe hypertension) SBP ≥180 or DBP ≥110
I: no other risk factors	Low risk	Medium risk	High risk
II: 1–2 risk factors	Medium risk	Medium risk	Very high risk
III: 3 or more risk factor or target-organ damage or diabetes	High risk	High risk	Very high risk
IV: Associated clinical conditions	Very high risk	Very high risk	Very high risk
DBP, diastolic blood pressure; SBP, systolic blood pressure.			

Table 95–1. Stratification of Risk to Quantify Prognosis (WHO-ISH 1999)

REFERENCES

1. World Health Organization. *World Health Report 2002: Reducing Risks, Promoting Healthy Life.* Geneva: World Health Organization, 2002.
2. Guidelines for the treatment of mild hypertension. Memorandum from a WHO/ISH meeting. *Hypertension* 1983;3:394–7.
3. Guidelines for the treatment of mild hypertension. Memorandum from a WHO/ISH meeting. *Bull World Health Organ* 1983;1:53–6.
4. 1986 Guidelines for the treatment of mild hypertension: memorandum from a WHO/ISH meeting. *J Hypertens* 1986;3:383–4.
5. 1986 Guidelines for the treatment of mild hypertension: memorandum from a WHO/ISH meeting. *Bull World Health Organ* 1986;1:31–5.
6. 1989 Guidelines for the management of mild hypertension: memorandum from a WHO/ISH meeting. *J Hypertens* 1989;8:689–93.
7. 1989 Guidelines for the management of mild hypertension: memorandum from a WHO/ISH meeting. *Bull World Health Organ* 1989;5:493–8.
8. 1989 Guidelines for the management of mild hypertension: memorandum from a WHO/ISH meeting. *Clin Exp Hypertens* A 1989;11:1203–16.
9. 1993 Guidelines for the management of mild hypertension. Memorandum from a World Health Organization/International Society of Hypertension meeting. Guidelines Subcommittee of the WHO/ISH Mild Hypertension Liaison Committee. *Hypertension* 1993;22:392–403.
10. Guidelines Subcommittee 1999 World Health Organization-International Society of Hypertension Guidelines for the Management of Hypertension. *J Hypertens* 1999;17:151–83.
11. Guidelines Subcommittee 1999 World Health Organization-International Society of Hypertension Guidelines for the Management of Hypertension. *Blood Press* 1999;8(Suppl 1):9–43.
12. Guidelines Subcommittee 1999 World Health Organization-International Society of Hypertension Guidelines for the Management of Hypertension. *Clin Exp Hypertens* 1999;21:1009–60.
13. World Health Organisation-International Society of Hypertension Writing Group. 2003 World Health Organisation (WHO)/International Society of Hypertension (ISH) statement on management of hypertension. *J Hypertens* 2003;21:1983–92.
14. Chockalingam A, Chalmers J, Lisheng L, Labarthe D, MacMahon S, Martin I, et al. Prevention of cardiovascular diseases in developing countries: agenda for action (statement from a WHO-ISH Meeting in Beijing, October 1999). *J Hypertens* 2000;18:1705–8.
15. Alderman M, Arakawa K, Beilin K, Chalmers J, Cohn J, Collins R, et al. Effects of calcium antagonists on the risks of coronary heart disease, cancer and bleeding. *J Hypertens* 1997;15:105–15.
16. Blood Pressure Lowering Treatment Trialists' Collaboration. Effects of ACE inhibitors, calcium antagonists, and other blood-pressure–lowering drugs. *Lancet* 2000;356:1955–64.
17. Van den Hoogen PCW, Feskens EJM, Nagelkerke NJD, Menotti A, Nissinen A, Kromhout D, for the Seven Countries Study Research Group. The relation between blood pressure and mortality due to coronary heart disease among men in different parts of the world. *New Engl J Med* 2000;342:1–8.
18. Vasan RS, Larson MG, Keip JC, O'Donnell CJ, Kannel WB, Levy D. Impact of high-normal pressure on the risk of cardiovascular disease. *New Engl J Med* 2001;345:1291–7.
19. The Heart Outcomes Prevention Evaluation Study Investigators. Effects of an angiotensin-converting-enzyme inhibitor, ramipril, on cardiovascular events in high-risk patients. *N Engl J Med* 2000;324:145–153.
20. Progress Collaborative Group. Randomized trial of a perindopril based blood pressure lowering regimen among 6105 individuals with previous stroke or transient ischaemic attack. *Lancet* 2001;358:1033–41.
21. PATS Collaborating Group. Post-stroke antihypertensive treatment study. A preliminary result. *Chin Med J* 1995;108:710–7.
22. SHEP Co-operative Research Group. Prevention of stroke by antihypertensive drug treatment in older persons with isolated systolic hypertension: final results of the Systolic Hypertension in the Elderly Program (SHEP) *JAMA* 1991;265:3255–64.
23. ESH/ESC Hypertension Guidelines Committee. 2003. Practice guidelines for primary care physicians: 2003 ESH/ESC hypertension guidelines. *J Hypertens* 21:1779–86.
24. The Seventh Report of the Joint National Committee on Prevention, Detection, Evaluation and Treatment of High Blood Pressure: JNC 7 report. *Hypertension* 2003;42:1206–52.
25. Alwan A, Maclean D, Mandil A. *Assessment of National Capacity for Non-communicable Disease Prevention and Control.* The report of a global survey 2001. WHO/MNC/.01.2. Geneva: World Health Organization, 2001.

APPENDIX: 2003 WORLD HEALTH ORGANIZATION (WHO)/INTERNATIONAL SOCIETY OF HYPERTENSION (ISH) STATEMENT ON MANAGEMENT OF HYPERTENSION

World Health Organization/International Society of Hypertension Writing Group

ABSTRACT

Objective

Hypertension is estimated to cause 4.5% of current global disease burden and is as prevalent in many developing countries as in the developed world. Blood pressure–induced cardiovascular risk rises continuously across the whole blood pressure range. Countries vary widely in capacity for management of hypertension, but worldwide the majority of diagnosed hypertensives are inadequately controlled. This statement addresses the ascertainment of overall cardiovascular risk to establish thresholds for initiation and goals of treatment, appropriate treatment strategies for nondrug and drug therapies, and cost effectiveness of treatment.

Conclusions

Since publication of the WHO/ISH Guidelines for the Management of Hypertension in 1999, more evidence has become available to support a systolic blood pressure threshold of 140 mmHg for even "low-risk" patients. In high-risk patients there is evidence for lower thresholds. Lifestyle modification is recommended for all individuals. There is evidence that specific agents have benefits for patients with particular compelling indications, and that monotherapy is inadequate for the majority of patients. For patients without a compelling indication for a particular drug class, on the basis of comparative trial data, availability, and cost, a low dose of a diuretic should be considered for initiation of therapy. In most places, a thiazide diuretic is the least costly option and thus most cost effective, but for compelling indications where other classes provide additional benefits, even if more expensive, they may be more cost effective. In high-risk patients who attain large benefits from treatment, expensive drugs may be cost effective, but in low-risk patients treatment may not be cost effective unless the drugs are inexpensive.

Keywords: blood pressure lowering, hypertension, prevention, treatment, International Society of Hypertension, World Health Organization

INTRODUCTION

Cardiovascular disease (CVD) is responsible for one-third of global deaths and is a leading and increasing contributor to the global disease burden.[1] Importantly, CVD is eminently preventable. In order to achieve significant reductions in the avoidable CVD burden, a combination of population-based and high-risk strategies is necessary. These strategies should target lifestyle-related risk factors such as unhealthy diet, physical inactivity, and tobacco use, as well as the inter-mediate manifestations of these lifestyles, including hypertension, glucose intolerance, and hyperlipidemia. In addition, strategies aimed at improving management of those already affected by CVD should be an integral component of a comprehensive approach for the prevention and control of CVD.

Hypertension is already a highly prevalent risk factor for CVD throughout the industrialized world. It is becoming an increasingly common health problem worldwide because of increasing longevity and prevalence of contributing factors such as obesity, physical inactivity, and an unhealthy diet.[2,3] The current prevalence in many developing countries, particularly in urban societies, is already as high as those seen in developed countries.[4,5] Worldwide hypertension is estimated to cause 7.1 million premature deaths and 4.5% of the disease burden (64 million disability-adjusted life years). The proportion of global disease burden attributable to hypertension is substantial[1] (Figure 95A–1).

Hypertension plays a major etiologic role in the development of cerebrovascular disease, ischemic heart disease, and cardiac and renal failure. Treating hypertension has been associated with about a 40% reduction in the risk of stroke and about a 15% reduction in the risk of myocardial infarction.[6] Although the treatment of hypertension has been shown to prevent CVD and to extend and enhance life, hypertension remains inadequately managed everywhere.[7–13] In addition, hypertension often coexists with other cardiovascular risk factors such as tobacco use, diabetes, hyperlipidemia, and obesity, which compound the cardiovascular risk attributable to hypertension. Worldwide, these coexistent risk factors are inadequately addressed in patients with hypertension resulting in high morbidity and mortality.[7–9]

It has become increasingly evident that risks of stroke, ischemic heart disease, and renal failure are not confined to a subset of the population with particularly high levels of blood pressure but rather that risk occurs in a con-

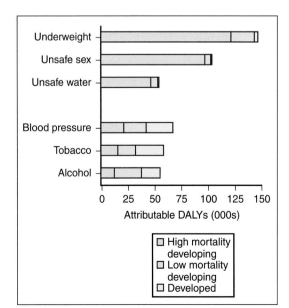

Figure 95A–1. Global distribution of disease burden attributable to six major risk factors.

tinuum, affecting even those with below average levels of blood pressure.[14] Globally, data indicate that about 62% of cerebrovascular disease and 49% of ischemic heart disease are attributable to suboptimal blood pressure (systolic blood pressure >115 mmHg).[1]

A global capacity assessment survey conducted by WHO shows that there is wide variation in the capacity for management of hypertension in various countries.[15] Of the 167 countries surveyed, national hypertension guidelines were not available in 61%, health professionals were not trained to manage hypertension in 45%, antihypertensives were not affordable in 25%, and basic equipment and drugs for the management of hypertension were not available in primary health care in 8% and 12% of countries, respectively.

This statement addresses the following issues: (1) the ascertainment of overall cardiovascular risk to establish both the thresholds for initiation of treatment and the goals of treatment for people with hypertension in general and for various subgroups, (2) the appropriate treatment strategies for both nondrug and drug therapies, and (3) the cost effectiveness of drug treatment.

ASSESSMENT OF RISK

Decisions about the management of hypertensive patients should not only take blood pressure levels into account, but also the presence of other cardiovascular risk factors, target-organ damage, and associated clinical conditions (Table 95A–1). The risk stratification table from the 1999 WHO/ISH Guidelines[16] has been minimally amended to indicate three major risk categories with progressively increasing absolute likelihood of developing a major cardiovascular event (fatal and nonfatal stroke and myocardial infarction) within the next 10 years: (1) low risk—less than 15%, (2) medium risk—15% to 20%, and (3) high risk—greater than 20% (Table 95A–2). The simplicity of the

method enables a rapid preliminary assessment of cardiovascular risk and provides a flexible risk stratification system that can be customized to a range of practice settings with varying levels of resources. However, the categorical method used is less accurate than those using continuous variables, and this is a limitation of this risk stratification chart. Other techniques to assess individual patients' risk status have been published[17–21] and may provide more accurate estimates. These risk charts use risk prediction equations derived from the Framingham heart study.[19] It should be noted that while the Framingham equations provide an acceptable prediction of risk in northern European populations, their predictive validity in other ethnic groups is less clear.

The risk charts and tables differ in the age categories used, duration of risk assessment and risk factor profiles used. The current New Zealand and Joint British charts[20,21] are similar in concept. While the former assess 5-year risk of all cardiovascular disease in eight discrete categories, the latter assess 10-year risk of coronary heart disease in three risk categories. Several recent studies have formally evaluated these charts for their comparative accuracy and patient preference.[22]

Threshold for blood pressure lowering in hypertensive patients at low and medium risk

Before 1999 when the WHO/ISH Guidelines on Management of Hypertension were published,[16] evidence of the benefits of initiating drug therapy to lower blood pressure at thresholds less than 160 mmHg systolic pressure was limited to observational data. While some evidence from early randomized controlled trials (RCTs) did support an intervention threshold of 90 mmHg diastolic blood pressure, almost all trials confirmed the benefits of treatment at levels of 160 mmHg systolic and 100 mmHg diastolic and above.[6,23] Both new clinical trial evidence and obser-

FACTORS INFLUENCING PROGNOSIS		
Risk Factors for Cardiovascular Disease	**Target-Organ Damage**	**Associated Clinical Conditions**
Levels of systolic and diastolic blood pressure (grades 1–3)	Left ventricular hypertrophy (electrocardiogram or echocardiogram)	Diabetes
Males >55 years	Microalbuminuria (20–300 mg/day)	Cerebrovascular disease
Females >65 years	Radiologic or ultrasound evidence of extensive	Ischemic stroke
Smoking	atherosclerotic plaque (aorta, carotid,	Cerebral hemorrhage
Total cholesterol >6.1 mmol/L	coronary, iliac and femoral arteries)	Transient ischemic attack
(240 mg/dL) or LDL cholesterol	Hypertensive retinopathy grade III or IV	Heart disease
>4.0 mmol/L (160 mg/dL)[a]		Myocardial infarction
HDL cholesterol M <1.0, F <1.2 mmol/L		Angina
(<40, <45 mg/dL)		Coronary revascularization
History of cardiovascular disease in		Congestive heart failure
first-degree relatives before age 50		Renal disease
Obesity, physical inactivity		Plasma creatinine concentration:
		females >1.4, males >1.5 mg/dL (120,
		133 μmol/L) Albuminuria >300 mg/day
		Peripheral vascular disease

[a]Lower levels of total and LDL cholesterol are known to delineate increased risk but they were not used in the stratification table.

Table 95–A1. Factors Influencing Prognosis

STRATIFICATION OF RISK TO QUANTIFY PROGNOSIS			
Other Risk Factors and Disease History	Blood Pressure (mmHg)		
	Grade 1 SBP 140–159 or DBP 90–99	Grade 2 SBP 160–179 or DBP 100–109	Grade 3 SBP ≥180 or DBP ≥110
I: No other risk factors	Low risk	Medium risk	High risk
II: 1–2 risk factors	Medium risk	Medium risk	High risk
III: 3 or more risk factors, or target-organ damage, or associated clinical conditions	High risk	High risk	High risk
DBP, diastolic blood pressure; SBP, systolic blood pressure.			

Table 95–A2. Stratification of Risk to Quantify Prognosis

vational data published since 1999 support the lowering of the systolic blood pressure threshold.[24–28] While there has been no new clinical trial evidence to support lowering thresholds to below 160 mmHg systolic and 90 mmHg diastolic in hypertensive patients at low risk, observational data published since 1999 do support the lowering of the systolic threshold.[24,25] These observational data suggest that even low-risk patients with blood pressure ≤140 mmHg systolic and/or ≤90 mmHg diastolic are likely to benefit from lower pressures. Although women are at lower absolute risk of cardiovascular disease for a given level of blood pressure and RCT evidence includes a greater proportion of men than women, the treatment threshold should be the same in both men and women.

Absolute risk of cardiovascular disease for any given level of blood pressure rises with age, but only limited RCT evidence is currently available about the benefits of treating those aged over 80 years. For now, the treatment threshold should be unaffected by age at least up to 80 years. Thereafter, judgment should be made on an individual basis and therapy should not be withdrawn from patients over 80 years of age. This is suggested by a meta-analysis of data from patients above 80 years of age in which the group on antihypertensive treatment showed a significant reduction in stroke incidence compared to the control group.[29]

Thresholds for blood pressure lowering in hypertensive patients at high risk

Since 1999, several new trials in high-risk patients[26–28] have demonstrated morbidity and mortality benefits of lowering blood pressures from thresholds significantly below 160 mmHg systolic and/or 90 mmHg diastolic. These trials[26–28] support the hypothesis that additional blood pressure lowering in high-risk complicated patients, irrespective of initial blood pressure results in a reduction in the number of cardiovascular events. Similarly, other smaller trials that evaluated the effect of angiotensin II receptor blockers (ARBs) on the progression of nephropathy also suggest that treatment for such patients should begin at lower thresholds.[30–32] As with the uncomplicated patients, this seems likely to be the case for older or female hypertensive patients.

Targets for blood pressure lowering in hypertensives at low and medium risk

No new trial evidence about blood pressure targets in medium-risk hypertensive patients is available beyond that known in 1999 from the Hypertension Optimal Treatment (HOT) trial, which found optimal reduction of major cardiovascular events at about 139/83 mmHg.[33] However, HOT trial data suggested that most of the benefit was achieved by lowering the systolic blood pressure to about 150 mmHg and the diastolic blood pressure to about 90 mmHg in nondiabetic patients.

However, clinic- and population-based survey data continue to suggest that the lower the blood pressure levels achieved, the lower the cardiovascular event rate.[34,35] In those over age 55, the systolic level assumes greater importance,[36] so the primary goal of therapy is to lower systolic blood pressure and the pragmatic target of below 140 mmHg is reaffirmed. This also has strategic value because aiming at below 140 mmHg as a systolic blood pressure target makes it more likely that more patients will reach values at or slightly above 140 mmHg. There is no apparent reason to modify this target for women or older patients with uncomplicated hypertension.

Targets for blood pressure lowering in hypertensive patients at high risk

Effective blood pressure control has considerable and immediate benefits in patients with established cardiovascular disease (CVD), diabetes, and renal insufficiency.[36–28,30–32] While several new trials[26–28] have shown clear cardiovascular benefits associated with lowering blood pressure significantly below 160/90 mmHg, none of these trials has attempted to identify the optimal blood pressure target for such patients. However, several trials have shown that in patients with diabetes reduction of diastolic blood pressure to about 80 mmHg and of systolic blood pressure to about 130 mmHg was accompanied by a further reduction in cardiovascular events or diabetes-related microvascular complications, as compared to patients with less stringent blood pressure control.[37,38] Based on clinical trial evidence, and also on extrapolation from epidemiologic studies, a target of <130/<80 mmHg seems appropriate. There is no evidence of a need to modify these target blood pressures for female or older patients with hypertension.

Feasibility and resource implications

The blood pressure thresholds for treatment discussed above will result in as many as 25% of all adults—and more than 50% of those over the age of 65—in some populations requiring antihypertensive therapy. Further, less than half of all hypertensive patients will attain the blood pressure targets recommended above with monotherapy.[33,39,40] Most will need at least two antihypertensive drugs, and as many as 30% of patients will need three or more drugs in combination to attain target blood pressure levels. Even in healthcare systems with generous resources, control of blood pressure is often unsatisfactory. One-half of all patients may drop out of care entirely within 1 year of diagnosis.[40] Of those who continue under medical supervision, only about half tend to adhere to their prescribed medication[41] and adherence is significantly influenced by drug choice, comorbidity, and health services' utilization.[41]

Further, numerous surveys have shown that about three-quarters of all patients with hypertension do not have optimal blood pressure control.[10–12] The reasons for this are complex, but include failure to detect hypertension, failure of patients or doctors to initiate and/or continue with treatment, incomplete adherence to treatment by patients and to guidelines by doctors, and lack of adequate therapy to control blood pressure.[10–12,40,41]

The high prevalence of hypertension and the difficulties in attaining and maintaining blood pressure targets outlined above pose particular problems for healthcare systems that have very limited resources. The cost of drug therapy can be kept low by using the least expensive drugs and generic formulations. Priority for drug therapy where resources are limited should be given to all hypertensive patients with high and then medium cardiovascular risk (Table 95A–2). In those with low cardiovascular risk (Table 95A–2), the decision to treat or monitor without treatment should be based on estimated cardiovascular risk and patients' choice. Although some patients in the blood pressure range of 140 to 159/90 to 99 mmHg have a 10-year cardiovascular risk higher than 20% (Table 95A–2), and should be treated, many patients are at low cardiovascular risk, albeit substantially higher than those with optimal BP. Low-risk patients have a correspondingly lower chance of gaining benefits from treatment (Table 95A–3). These patients should be given lower priority for treatment when resources are limited.

Regarding blood pressure targets where resources are limited, it should be remembered that recommendations are not based on robust clinical trial data. Furthermore, although based on a *post-hoc* analysis, the data from the HOT trial[33] suggest little disadvantage associated with a systolic blood pressure target of less than 150 mmHg. This is therefore a reasonable "fallback" target when resources are limited or adequate treatment fails to attain target values. It is also important to remember that even partial control of blood pressure provides substantial protection against cardiovascular complications.

It must be noted that in all parts of the world, population strategies to reduce blood pressure are very cost effective.[1] Legislative action and voluntary agreements with industry to ensure reduction of salt in processed food can lead to substantial reductions in salt intake resulting in significant shift of population blood pressure levels to a more optimal distribution (Figure 95A–2). Therefore high-risk approaches to management of hypertension should always be complemented with population-wide approaches.

TREATMENT STRATEGIES

Value of lifestyle modifications

A variety of lifestyle modifications have been shown in clinical trials to lower BP[42] and to reduce the incidence of hypertension.[43] These include weight loss in the overweight,[44] physical activity,[45] moderation of alcohol intake,[46] a diet with increased fresh fruit and vegetables and reduced saturated fat content,[47] reduction of dietary sodium intake,[47–49] and increased dietary potassium intake.[50]

Other lifestyle changes have not been found in multiple clinical trials to have a significant or lasting antihypertensive effect. These include calcium[51] and magnesium supplements,[52] reduction in caffeine intake,[53] and a variety of techniques designed to reduce stress.[54]

The overall antihypertensive effect of effective lifestyle interventions varies with the patient's adherence to therapy.

CHANCE OF PREVENTING CARDIOVASCULAR EVENT DURING 5-YEAR ANTIHYPERTENSIVE TREATMENT	
10-Year Cardiovascular Risk (%)	5-Year Number Needed to Treat (Assuming BP Reduction of 10/5 mmHg and Relative Risk Reduction by Treatment of 25%)
30	27
20	40
15	53
10	80
5	160
2	400

Table 95–A3. Chance of Preventing Cardiovascular Event during 5-Year Antihypertensive Treatment

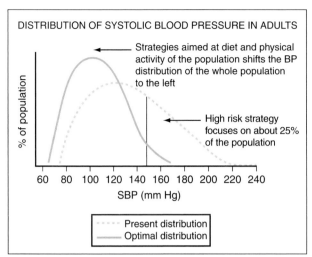

Figure 95A–2. Present and optimal systolic blood pressure distribution of the population. These smoothed curves portray the present distribution (interrupted lines) and the optimal distribution (continuous line) of systolic blood pressure in adults. A combination of population and high-risk strategies of blood pressure control is necessary to achieve the optimal blood pressure distribution.

When adherence is optimal, systolic blood pressure has been reduced by more than 10 mmHg,[47] but in less controlled clinical practice more modest effects have been seen.[42] Trials to evaluate the effects of lifestyle interventions on levels of blood pressure have not been designed or powered to evaluate reductions in overall or cardiovascular mortality or morbidity. Nonetheless, these lifestyle modifications are recommended for all patients with hypertension since even small reductions in blood pressure are associated in long-term, large-scale population studies with a reduced risk of cardiovascular diseases.[55]

In addition to their possible influence on blood pressure, observational studies have found that other lifestyle modifications, in particular cessation of smoking, have been found to reduce cardiovascular disease (CVD) mortality.[56] Moreover, weight reduction, dietary manipulation, and physical activity reduce the incidence of type 2 diabetes[57,58] and a low saturated-fat diet improves dyslipidemia.[59]

Therefore, regardless of the level of blood pressure, all individuals should adopt appropriate lifestyle modifications. The protective effects of modifying lifestyle include a reduction in the incidence of hypertension, diabetes, and dyslipidemia, a reduction in mortality by cessation of smoking, and a lowering of blood pressure that, in itself, is likely to reduce cardiovascular morbidity and mortality. Furthermore, unlike drug therapy, which may cause adverse effects and reduce the quality of life in some patients, nonpharmacologic therapy has no known harmful effects, improves the sense of well-being of the patient, and is often less expensive.

Choice of initial drug therapy

Data from more than 20 RCTs have been published since 1967 comparing diuretics, β-blockers, and calcium channel blockers (CCBs) against a placebo in hypertensive patients.[6,23,60] The data conclusively demonstrate reductions in both mortality and morbidity with these three drug classes. A meta-analysis of data from RCTs comparing two newer classes, that is, angiotensin-converting enzyme inhibitors (ACEIs) and CCBs, against older classes, that is, diuretics and β-blockers, in almost 75,000 hypertensive patients was published in 2000.[23] For the endpoints of total cardiovascular mortality, the meta-analysis shows no significant convincing differences between drug classes or between groups of old and new drugs. However, the available data do not exclude small to modest differences between different classes or drugs on specific fatal or nonfatal outcomes. For instance, in these comparative trials, ACEIs were associated with a lower incidence of coronary heart disease than CCBs, whereas CCBs were associated with a lower incidence of stroke than diuretic ± β-blockers.[23]

Two other large trials have been published since the meta-analysis in 2000, the Antihypertensive and Lipid-Lowering Treatment to Prevent Heart Attack Trial (ALLHAT)[61] and the Second Australian National Blood Pressure Study (ANBP2).[62] In ALLHAT, over 42,000 hypertensives with an initial mean blood pressure of 146/84 (90% already receiving antihypertensive therapy) were randomly assigned to a diuretic (chlorthalidone), an α-blocker (doxazosin), an ACEI (lisinopril), or a CCB (amlodipine). The α-blocker limb was prematurely stopped because of increased risk of the secondary endpoint of combined cardiovascular disease (CVD) (to which heart failure was a major contributor), although there was no difference in coronary events or mortality.[63]

The effects of the other two choices in ALLHAT compared to diuretic on the primary endpoint of fatal and nonfatal coronary disease were identical. Some differences were seen in protection against various secondary endpoints, in particular a higher risk of stroke with the ACEI in the Afro-American enrollees and a higher risk of heart failure with both ACEI and CCB. The lesser protection with the ACEI may be attributed in large part to the 3-mmHg lesser fall in systolic blood pressure provided by that agent compared to diuretic.

In the ANBP2 trial,[62] a diuretic was compared to an ACEI in 6083 patients who were generally older but with fewer cardiovascular risk factors than the ALLHAT participants. Those assigned to an ACEI had fewer cardiovascular events, particularly the men, and despite equal reductions of blood pressure, differences were of borderline statistical significance only when events subsequent to the first event were included.

In the LIFE trial,[64] among patients with ECG-determined left ventricular hypertrophy, therapy based on an angiotensin II receptor blocker (ARB) was more protective against a composite cardiovascular endpoint than therapy based on a β-blocker despite very similar blood pressure reductions. In fact the benefits were largely attributable to a protection against stroke and were particularly striking in the diabetic subgroup.[65]

With the exception of ALLHAT, these trials typically included Caucasian patients in North America, Europe, and Australasia, and in recent trials most participants had multiple cardiovascular risk factors. It is likely, however, that these relative risk reductions would apply to all patients with hypertension. In no trial were all enrollees maintained on the initial one drug to which they were assigned and in most trials the majority received two or more drugs to achieve the predetermined goal of therapy. Despite these potential limitations, the available data conclusively document the value of antihypertensive therapy and suggest that the benefits are largely derived from their reduction in blood pressure.

For the majority of patients without a compelling indication for another class of drug, a low dose of a diuretic should be considered as the first choice of therapy on the basis of comparative trial data, availability, and cost.

As previously noted, some patients need to have their blood pressure reduced to lower levels than previously recognized and will often require more than one drug.[26,27,33,38,64] However, pending results of trials such as the Anglo-Scandinavian Cardiac Outcomes Trial (ASCOT),[66] there are no comparative RCT data on mortality or morbidity to guide selection of optimal combinations. In the absence of such data, and since a diuretic should enhance the efficacy of all classes, a diuretic most often will be a component of combination therapy. A diuretic is often available in single tablets combined with other classes of drugs. Where they are no more expensive, such combined formulations may be preferable, since they have advantages in terms of compliance and blood pressure–lowering efficacy. Other combinations of drugs with complementary actions may be appropriate for patients' needs.

Choice of drugs in different populations

Most drugs used to treat hypertension have also been evaluated for a number of specific indications. These include ACEIs, ARBs, β-blockers, CCBs, and diuretics in patients with concomitant diabetes, nephropathy, coronary and cerebrovascular disease, heart failure, and left ventricular hypertrophy. When studies have shown greater reduction in various fatal and nonfatal major-disease endpoints with one or another type of drug class, that class is considered to have a compelling indication for its use. Table 95A–4 indicates the clear and compelling indications for which certain drugs are preferred, based on greater reductions in either mortality or morbidity in large, long-term randomized trials.

In addition, comparisons have been made between the ability of different classes of drugs to regress left ventricular hypertrophy (LVH) and to slow the progression of nephropathies. For regression of LVH, CCBs, ACEIs, and ARBs have been found to be more effective than β-blockers and diuretics.[64,67,68] In two comparative studies, a greater reduction in proteinuria has been found with initial therapy with ACEIs or ARBs than with other classes, in particular CCBs.[31,69] Multiple placebo-controlled trials have shown significant reductions in proteinuria and a slowing of progression of renal damage in both nondiabetic and type 1 diabetic nephropathies with ACEIs[70] and in type 2 diabetic nephropathy with ARBs.[30-32] Whether ACE inhibitors and ARBs have similar benefits on the progression of renal damage as each other in type 1 and type 2 diabetic nephropathy remains untested, and whether they are superior to agents

COMPELLING INDICATIONS FOR SPECIFIC ANTIHYPERTENSIVE DRUGS			
Compelling Indications	Preferred Drug	Reference for Evidence	Primary Endpoint
Elderly with isolated systolic hypertension	Diuretic	71	Stroke
	DHPCCB	72	Stroke
Renal Disease			
Diabetic nephropathy (type 1)	ACEI	73	Progression of renal failure
Diabetic nephropathy (type 2)	ARB	30–32	Progression of renal failure
Nondiabetic	ACEI	70	Progression of renal failure
Cardiac Disease			
Post-myocardial infarction	ACEI	26,74	Mortality
Left ventricular dysfunction	β-blocker	75	Mortality
	ACEI	76	Heart failure
CHF (diuretics almost always included)	ACEI	76,77	Heart failure
	β-blocker	78	Mortality
Left ventricular hypertrophy	Spironolactone	79	Mortality
	ARB	64,65	Mortality
Cerebrovascular Disease			
	ACEI + diuretic	27	Recurrent stroke
	Diuretic	28	Recurrent stroke
ACEI, angiotensin-converting enzyme inhibitor; ARB, angiotensin receptor blocker; CHF, congestive heart failure; DHPCCB, dihydropyridine calcium-channel blocker.			

Table 95–A4. Compelling Indications for Specific Antihypertensive Drugs

CONTRAINDICATIONS AND CAUTIONS FOR SPECIFIC ANTIHYPERTENSIVE DRUGS			
Drug	**Contraindications**	**Drug**	**Cautions**
ACEIs, ARBs	Pregnancy	α-blockers	CHF
	Bilateral renal artery stenosis		
	Hyperkalemia	Clonidine	Withdrawal syndrome
β-blockers	High degree of heart block	Methyldopa	Hepatotoxicity
	Severe bradycardia <50/min		
	Obstructive airways disease	Reserpine	Depression
	Raynaud's syndrome		Active peptic ulcer
		CCBs	CHF
Diuretics	Gout		
ACEI, angiotensin-converting enzyme inhibitor; ARB, angiotensin receptor blocker; CCB, calcium channel blocker; CHF, congestive heart failure.			

Table 95–A5. Contraindications and Cautions for Specific Antihypertensive Drugs

other than β-blockers[64] in terms of preventing major cardiovascular events in this situation is not as yet clear.

In addition to these compelling indications, certain drugs may logically be chosen for other reasons. Thus, when used as monotherapy, a diuretic or CCB may lower blood pressure more in Afro-Americans and older patients than an ACEI or a β-blocker[80,81] and an α-blocker will relieve symptoms of prostatism.[82] Central α-agonists (e.g., clonidine), or peripheral adrenergic blockers (e.g., reserpine), may be used as inexpensive therapies in certain settings despite the absence of outcome data.

Specific drugs are either contraindicated or should be used with caution in certain conditions (Table 95A–5). A few of the contraindications such as use of ACEIs and ARBs in pregnancy are absolute, but most indicate that specific drugs could aggravate various conditions. The cautions indicate the greater propensity of certain drugs to induce side effects, but do not preclude their use if patients have strong indications for those drugs and if the patients are carefully monitored.

Cost effectiveness

Cost effectiveness is determined by the relationship between the benefits obtained for the expenditure. The prevalence of a condition and the total cost of treating it in a specific setting, on the other hand, determine affordability. Because of limited resources, cost-effective treatment may not be affordable. The two main determinants of cost effectiveness are the cost of drug therapy and the initial cardiovascular risk of the patient.

An overview of the totality of trial evidence suggests that the major classes of antihypertensive drugs are largely equivalent in efficacy and safety. In most places, a diuretic is the cheapest option and is, therefore, most cost effective. However, for certain compelling indications (Table 95A–4), other classes will provide additional benefits; even if they are more expensive, they may be more cost effective. For equivalent blood pressure lowering within each class, the least expensive is the most cost-effective drug.

It should be noted that in very high-risk patients who attain large benefits from treatment, treatment with multiple drugs, even those drugs that are expensive might be cost effective. Conversely, the treatment of patients with low risk may not be cost effective unless the antihypertensive drugs used are inexpensive.[83]

ACKNOWLEDGMENT

Contributors to this statement are listed below. Contributors were recommended by WHO and by the WHO/International Society of Hypertension Liaison Committee. The deliberations were chaired by S. Mendis and J.A. Whitworth who appointed two additional members, N.M. Kaplan and N. Poulter, to the writing committee. The Writing Group was comprised of Norman Kaplan, Shanthi Mendis, Neil Poulter, and Judith Whitworth.

Contributors: *Imran Afridi, Karachi; Judy Canny, World Health Organization, Geneva; Yao Chonghua, Beijing Municipal Office of CVD Control, Beijing; Bo Christensen, Department of General Practice, University of Aarhus; Richard S. Cooper, Loyola Medical School, Maywood; Solomon Kadiri, University College Hospital, Ibadan; Suzanne Hill, University of Newcastle, Australia; Norman Kaplan, University of Texas Southwestern Medical Centre; Emilio Kuschnir, Universidad Nacional de Cordoba; Joel Lexchin, University of Toronto; Giuseppe Mancia, Universita Degli Studi, Monza; Shanthi Mendis, World Health Organization, Geneva; Neil Poulter, Imperial College of Science, Technology and Medicine, London; Bruce M. Psaty, University of Washington, Seattle; Karl-Heinz Rahn, University of Munster; Sheldon G. Sheps, Mayo Clinic, Rochester; Judith Whitworth, Australian National University, Canberra; Derek Yach, World Health Organization, Geneva; Rafael Bengoa, World Health Organization, Geneva; Larry Ramsay, Sheffield.*

REFERENCES

1. World Health Organization. *World Health Report 2002: Reducing Risks, Promoting Healthy Life*. Geneva: World Health Organization, 2002.

2. Singh RB, Suh IL, Singh VP, Chaithiraphan S, Laothavorn P, Sy RG, et al. Hypertension and stroke in Asia: prevalence, control and strategies in developing countries for prevention. *Hum Hypertens* 2000;14:749–63.

3. Yusuf S, Reddy S, Ounpuu S, Anand S. Global burden of cardiovascular diseases. Part I: General considerations, the epidemiologic transition, risk factors, and impact of urbanization. *Circulation* 2001;104:2746–53.

4. Khor GL. Cardiovascular epidemiology in the Asia-Pacific region. *Asia Pac J Clin Nutr* 2001;10:76–80.

5. Vorster HH. The emergence of cardiovascular disease during urbanisation of Africans. *Public Health Nutr* 2002;5:239–43.

6. Collins R, Peto R, MacMahon S, Hebert P, Fiebach NH, Eberlein KA. Blood pressure, stroke, and coronary heart disease. Part 2: Short-term reductions in blood pressure: overview of randomized drug trials in their epidemiological context. *Lancet* 1990;335:827–38.

7. Godley P, Pham H, Rohack J, Woodward B, Yokoyama K, Maue SK. Opportunities for improving the quality of hypertension care in a managed care setting. *Am J Health Syst Pharm* 2001; 58:1728–33.

8. Klungel OH, de Boer A, Paes AH, Seidell JC, Nagelkerke NJ, Bakker A. Under treatment of hypertension in a population-based study in the Netherlands. *J Hypertens* 1998;16:1371–8.

9. Trilling JS, Froom J. The urgent need to improve hypertension care. *Arch Fam Med* 2000;9:794–801.

10. Psaty BM, Manolio TA, Smith NL, Heckbert SR, Gotdiener JS, Burke GL, et al. Time trends in high blood pressure control and the use of antihypertensive medications in older adults. The Cardiovascular Health Study. *Arch Intern Med* 2002;162:2325–32.

11. Marques-Vidal P, Tuomilehto J. Hypertension awareness, treatment and control in the community. Is the "rule of halves" still valid? *J Hum Hypertens* 1997;11:213–20.

12. Primatesta P, Brookes M, Poulter NR. Improved hypertension management and control. Results from the Health Survey for England 1998. *Hypertension* 2001;38:827–32.

13. Mancia G, Bombelli M, Lanzarotti A, Grassi G, Cesana G, Zanchetti A, et al. Systolic vs diastolic blood pressure control in the hypertensive patients of the PAMELA population. *Arch Intern Med* 2002;162:582–6.

14. MacMahon S, Peto R, Cutler J, Collins R, Sorlie P, Neaton J, et al. Blood pressure, stroke and coronary disease. Part 1. Prolonged differences in blood pressure: prospective observational studies corrected for the regression dilution bias. *Lancet* 1990;335:765–74.

15. Alwan A, Maclean D, Mandil A. *Assessment of National Capacity for Noncommunicable Disease Prevention and Control*. The report of a global survey 2001. Geneva: World Health Organization, 2001.

16. 1999 World Health Organization/ International Society of Hypertension Guidelines for the management of hypertension. *J Hypertens* 1999; 17:151–83.

17. Wood D, Durrington P, Poulter N, McInnes G, Rees A, Wray R, for the British Cardiac Society, British Hyperlipidaemia Association, British Hypertension Society, and British Diabetic Association. Joint British recommendations on prevention of coronary heart disease in clinical practice. *Heart* 1998;80(Suppl 2):S1–29.

18. Expert Panel on Detection, Evaluation, and Treatment of High Blood Cholesterol in Adults. Executive summary of the third report of the National Cholesterol Education Program (NCEP) expert panel on detection, evaluation, and treatment of high blood cholesterol in adults (Adult Treatment Panel III). *JAMA,* 2001;285:2486–97.

19. D'Agostino RB, Russell MW, Huse DM, Ellison RC, Silbershatz H, Wilson PW, Hartz SC. Primary and subsequent coronary risk appraisal. New results from Framingham Study. *Am Heart J* 2000;139:272–81.

20. Jackson R. Updated New Zealand cardiovascular disease risk-benefit prediction guide. *BMJ* 2000;320:709–10.

21. Assmann G, Culler P, Schulte H. The Munster heart study (PROCAM). Results of follow-up at 8 years. *Eur Heart J* 1998;19:A2–11.

22. Jones AF, Walker J, Jewkes C, Game FL, Bartlett WA, Marshall T, et al. Comparative accuracy of cardiovascular risk prediction methods in primary care patients. *Heart* 2001;85:37–43.

23. Blood Pressure Lowering Treatment Trialists' Collaboration. Effects of ACE inhibitors, calcium antagonists, and other blood-pressure-lowering drugs. *Lancet* 2000;356:1955–64.

24. Van den Hoogen PCW, Feskens EJM, Nagelkerke NJD, Menotti A, Nissinen A, Kromhout D, for the Seven Countries Study Research Group. The relation between blood pressure and mortality due to coronary heart disease among men in different parts of the world. *N Engl J Med* 2000;342:1–8.

25. Vasan RS, Larson MG, Leip EP, Evans JC, O'Donnell CJ, Kannel WB, et al. Impact of high-normal pressure on the risk of cardiovascular disease. *N Engl J Med* 2001;345:1291–7.

26. The Heart Outcomes Prevention Evaluation Study Investigators. Effects of an angiotensin-converting-enzyme inhibitor, ramipril, on cardiovascular events in high-risk patients. *N Engl J Med* 2000;342:145–53.

27. Progress Collaborative Group. Randomized trial of a perindopril based regimen on blood pressure lowering among 6105 individuals with previous stroke or transient ischaemic attack. *Lancet* 2001;358:1033–41.

28. PATS Collaborating Group. Post-stroke antihypertensive treatment study. A preliminary result. *Chin Med J* 1995;108:710–7.

29. Gueyffier F, Boutitie F, Boissel JP, Pocock S, Coope J, Cutler J, et al. The effect of antihypertensive drug treatment on cardiovascular outcomes in women and men. Results from a meta-analysis of individual patient data in randomised controlled trials. *Ann Intern Med* 1997;126:761–7.

30. Parving HH, Lenhert H, Brochner-Mortensen J, Gomis R, Andersen S, Arner P. Irbesartan in Patients with Type 2 Diabetes and Microalbuminuria Study Group. The effect of Irbesartan on the development of diabetic nephropathy in patients with types 2 diabetes. *N Engl J Med* 2001;870:78.

31. Brenner BM, Cooper ME, de Zeeuw D, Keane WF, Mitch WE, Parving HH, et al., for the RENAAL Study Investigators. Effects of Losartan on renal and cardiovascular outcome in-patients with type 2 diabetes and nephropathy. *N Engl J Med* 2001;345:861–9.

32. Lewis EJ, Hunsicker LG, Clarke WR, Berl T, Pohl MA, Lewis JB, et al. Renoprotective effect of the angiotensin-receptor antagonist Irbesartan in patients with nephropathy due to type 2 diabetes. *N Engl J Med* 2001;345:851–60.

33. Hansson L, Zanchetti A, Carruthers SG, Dahlöf B, Elmfeldt D, Julius S, et al. Effects of intensive blood-pressure lowering and low-dose aspirin in patients with hypertension. Principal results of the Hypertension Optimal Treatment (HOT) randomized trial. *Lancet* 1998;351:1755–62.

34. Andersson OK, Almgren T, Persson B, Samuelsson O, Hedner T, Wilhelmsen L. Survival in treated hypertension: Follow-up to study after two decades. *BMJ* 1998;317:167–71.

35. Gamble G, MacMahon S, Culpan A, Ciobo C, Whalley G, Sharpe N. Atherosclerosis and left ventricular hypertrophy: persisting problems in treated hypertensive patients. *J Hypertens* 1998;16:1389–95.

36. Kannel WB. Elevated systolic blood pressure as a cardiovascular risk factor. *Am J Cardiol* 2000;85:251–5.

37. Zanchetti A, Ruilope LM. Antihypertensive treatment in patients with type 2 diabetes mellitus: what guidance from recent randomized controlled trials? *J Hypertens* 2002;20:2099–110.

38. UKPDS Prospective Diabetes Study Group. Tight blood pressure control and risk of macrovascular and microvascular complications in type 2 diabetes: UKPDS 38. *BMJ* 1998;317:703–13.

39. Boner G, Cao Z, Cooper ME. Combination antihypertensive therapy in the treatment of diabetic nephropathy. *Diabetes Technol Ther* 2002;4:313–21.

40. Okano GJ, Rascati KL, Wilson JP, Remund DD, Grabenstein JB, Brixner DI. Patterns of antihypertensive use among patients in the US Department of Defense database initially prescribed an angiotensin converting enzyme inhibitor or calcium channel blocker. *Clin Ther* 1997;19:1433–5.

41. Monane M, Bohn RL, Gurwitz JH, Glynn RJ, Levin R, Avorn J. The effects of initial drug choice and comorbidity on antihypertensive therapy compliance:

results from a population-based study in the elderly. *Am J Hypertens* 1997;10:697–704.

42. Ebrahim S, Smith GD. Lowering blood pressure: a systematic review of sustained effects of non-pharmacological interventions. *J Public Health Med* 1998;20:4441–8.

43. Stevens VJ, Obarzanek E, Cook NR, Lee IM, Appel LJ, Smith West D, et al. Long-term weight loss and changes in results of the Trials of Hypertension Prevention, Phase II. *Ann Intern Me* 2001;134:1–11.

44. Leiter LA, Abbott D, Campbell NRC, Mendelson R, Ogilvie RI, Chockalingam. A recommendation on obesity and weight loss. *CMAJ* 1999;160(Suppl 9):S7–11.

45. Hagberg JM, Park JJ, Brown MD. The role of exercise training in the treatment of hypertension: an update. *Sports Med* 2000;30:193–206.

46. Xin X, He J, Frontini MG, Ogden LG, Motsamai OI, Whelton PK. Effects of alcohol reduction on blood pressure: a meta-analysis of randomized controlled trials. *Hypertension* 2001;38:1112–7.

47. Sacks FM, Svetkey LP, Vollmer WM, Appel LJ, Bray GA, Harsha D, et al. Effects on blood pressure of reduced dietary sodium and the Dietary Approaches to Stop Hypertension (DASH) diet. DASH Sodium Collaborative Research Group. *N Engl J Med* 2001;344:3–10.

48. Cutler JA, Follmann D, Allender PS. Randomized trials of sodium reduction: an overview. *Am J Clin Nutr* 1997;65(Suppl):643S–51S.

49. Whelton PK, Appel LJ, Espeland MA, Applegate WB, Ettinger WH Jr, Kostis JB, et al. Sodium reduction and weight loss in the treatment of hypertension in older persons: a randomized controlled trial of non-pharmacological interventions in the elderly (TONE). *JAMA* 1998; 279:839–46.

50. He J, Whelton PK. What is the role of dietary sodium and potassium in hypertension and target organ injury. *Am J Med Sci* 1999;317:152–9.

51. Griffith LE, Guyatt GH, Cook RJ, Bucher HC, Cook DJ. The influence of dietary and non-dietary calcium supplementation on blood pressure. An updated meta-analysis of randomized controlled trials. *Am J Hypertens* 1999;12:84–92.

52. Kawano Y, Matsuoka H, Takishita S, Omae T. Effects of magnesium supplementation in hypertensive patients. Assessment by office, home, and ambulatory blood pressures. *Hypertension* 1998;32:260–5.

53. Jee SH, He J, Whelton PK, Suh I, Klag MJ. The effect of chronic coffee drinking on blood pressure. A meta-analysis of controlled clinical trials. *Hypertension* 1999;33:647–52.

54. Spence JD, Barnett PA, Linden W, Ramsden V, Taenzer P. Lifestyle modifications to prevent and control hypertension. Recommendations on stress management. *CMAJ* 1999;160(Suppl 9):S46–50.

55. Cook NR, Cohen J, Hebert PR, Taylor JO, Hennekens CH. Implications of small reductions in diastolic blood pressure for primary prevention. *Arch Intern Med* 1995;155:701–9.

56. Kawachi I, Colditz GA, Stampfer MJ, Willett WC, Manson JE, Rosner B, et al.

Smoking cessation and time course of decreased risks of coronary heart disease in middle-aged women. *Arch Intern Med* 1994;154:169–75.

57. Tuomilehto J, Lindström J, Eriksson JG, Valle TT, Hamalainen H, Ilanne-Parikka P, et al. Prevention of type 2 diabetes mellitus by changes in lifestyle among subjects with impaired glucose tolerance. *N Engl J Med* 2001;344:1343–50.

58. Knowler WC, Barrett-Connor E, Fowler SE, Hamman RF, Lachin JM, Walker EA, et al. Reduction in the incidence of type 2 diabetes with lifestyle intervention or metformin. *N Engl J Med* 2002;346:393–403.

59. Stefanick ML, Mackey S, Sheehan M, Ellsworth N, Haskall WL, Wood PD. Effects of diet and exercise in men and postmenopausal women with low levels of HDL cholesterol and high levels of LDL cholesterol. *N Engl J Med* 1998;339:12–20.

60. Psaty BM, Smith NL, Siscovick DS, Koepsell TD, Weiss NS, Heckbert SR, et al. Health outcomes associated with antihypertensive therapies used as first-line agents. A systematic review and meta-analysis. *JAMA* 1997;277:739–45.

61. ALLHAT Collaborative Research Group. Major outcomes in high-risk hypertensive patients randomized to angiotensin-converting enzyme inhibitor or calcium channel blocker vs diuretic: the Antihypertensive and Lipid-Lowering Treatment to Prevent Heart Attack Trial (ALLHAT). *JAMA* 2002;288:2981–97.

62. Wing LM, Reid CM, Ryan P, Beilin LJ, Brown MA, Jennings GL, et al. A comparison of outcomes with angiotensin-converting-enzyme inhibitors and diuretics for hypertension in the elderly. *N Engl J Med* 2003;348:583–92.

63. ALLHAT Collaborative Research Group. Major cardiovascular events in hypertensive patients randomized to doxazosin versus chlorthalidone. The antihypertensive and lipid-lowering treatment to prevent heart attack trial (ALLHAT). *JAMA* 2000;283:1967–75.

64. Dahlöf B, Devereux RB, Kjeldsen SE, Julius S, Beevers G, Faire U, et al. Cardiovascular morbidity and mortality in the Losartan Intervention for endpoint reduction in hypertension study (LIFE). A randomized trial against Atenolol. *Lancet* 2002;359:995–1003.

65. Lindholm LH, Ibsen H, Dahlöf B, Devereux RB, Beevers G, de Feure U, et al. Cardiovascular morbidity and mortality in patients with diabetes in the Losartan Intervention for endpoint reduction in hypertension study (LIFE). A randomized trial against Atenolol. *Lancet* 2002;359:1004–10.

66. Sever PS, Dahlöf B, Poulter NR, Wedel H, Beevers G, Caulfield M, et al. Rationale, design, methods and baseline demography of participants of the Anglo Scandinavian Cardiac Outcomes Trial. *J Hypertension* 2001;19:1139–47.

67. Schmieder RE, Schlaich MF, Klingbeil AU, Martus P. Update on reversal of left ventricular hypertrophy in essential hypertension (a meta-analysis of all randomized double-blind studies until December 1998). *Nephrol Dial Transplant* 1998;13:564–9.

68. Devereux RB, Palmieri V, Sharpe N, De Quattro V, Bella JN, de Simone G, et al. Effects of once-daily angiotensin-converting enzyme inhibition and

calcium channel blockade-based antihypertensive treatment regimens on left ventricular hypertrophy and diastolic filling in hypertension. The prospective randomized enalapril study evaluating regression of ventricular enlargement (preserve) trial. *Circulation* 2001;104:1248–54.

69. Agodoa LY, Appel L, Bakris GL, Beck G, Bourgoignie J, Briggs JP, et al. Effect of ramipril versus amlodipine on renal outcomes in hypertensive nephrosclerosis. A randomized controlled trial. *JAMA* 2001;285:2719–27.

70. Jafar TH, Schmid CH, Landa M, Giatras I, Toto R, Remuzzi G, et al. Angiotensin-converting enzyme inhibitors and progression of nondiabetic renal disease. A meta-analysis of patient-level data. *Ann Intern Med* 2001;135:138–9.

71. SHEP Cooperative Research Group. Prevention of stroke by antihypertensive drug treatment in older persons with isolated systolic hypertension. Final results of the Systolic Hypertension in the Elderly Program (SHEP). *JAMA* 1991;265:3255–64.

72. Staessen JA, Fagard R, Thijs L, Celis H, Arabidze GG, Birkenhager WH, et al. Randomised double-blind comparison of placebo and active treatment for older patients with isolated systolic hypertension. The Systolic Hypertension in Europe (Syst-Eur) Trial Investigators. *Lancet* 1997;350:757–64.

73. Lewis EJ, Hunsicker LG, Bain RP, Rohde RD. The effect of angiotensin-converting enzyme inhibition on diabetic nephropathy. The Collaborative Study Group. *N Engl J Med* 1993;329:1456–62.

74. Domanski MJ, Exner DV, Borkowf CB, Geller NL, Rosenberg Y, Pfeffer MA. Effect of angiotensin converting enzyme inhibition on sudden cardiac death in patients following acute myocardial infarction. A meta-analysis of randomized clinical trials. *J Am Coll Cardiol* 1999;33:598–604.

75. Freemantle N, Cleland J, Young P, Mason J, Harrison J. β blockades after myocardial infarction. Systematic review and regression analysis. *BMJ* 1999;318:1730–7.

76. The SOLVD Investigators. Effect of enalapril on survival in-patients with reduced left ventricular ejection fractions and congestive heart failure. *N Engl J Med* 1991;325:293–302.

77. Flather MD, Yusuf S, Kober L, Pfeffer M, Hall A, Murray G, et al. Long-term ACE-inhibitor therapy in patients with heart failure or left-ventricular dysfunction. A systematic overview of data from individual patients. ACE-Inhibitor Myocardial Infarction Collaborative Group. *Lancet* 2000;355:1575–81.

78. Metra M, Nodari S, D'Aloia AD, Bontempi L, Boldi E, Cas LD. A rationale for the use of β-blockers as standard treatment for heart failure. *Am Heart J* 2000;139:511–21.

79. Pitt B, Zannad F, Remme WJ, Cody R, Castaigne A, Perez A, et al. The effect of spironolactone on morbidity and mortality in patients with severe heart failure. Randomized Aldactone Evaluation Study Investigators. *N Engl J Med* 1999;341:709–17.

80. Cushman WC, Reda DJ, Perry HM, Williams D, Abdellatif M, Materson BJ.

Regional and racial differences in response to antihypertensive medication use in a randomized controlled trial of men with hypertension in the United States. Department of Veterans Affairs Cooperative Study Group on Antihypertensive Agents. *Arch Intern Med* 2000;160:825–31.

81. Radevski IV, Valtchanova ZP, Candy GP, Hlatswayo MN, Sareli P. Antihypertensive effect of low-dose hydrochlorothiazide alone or in combination with quinapril in black patients with mild to moderate hypertension. *J Clin Pharmacol* 2000;40:713–21.

82. Oesterling JE. Benign prostatic hyperplasia. Medical and minimally invasive treatment options. *N Engl J Med* 1995;99:109.

83. Lindholm L, Hallgren CG, Boman K, Markgren K, Weinehall L, Ogren JE. Cost-effectiveness analysis with defined budget. How to distribute resources for the prevention of cardiovascular disease? *Health Policy* 1999;48:155–70.

Chapter

96

Treatment Guidelines: The United States JNC7

Daniel W. Jones

The seventh report of the Joint National Committee on Prevention, Detection, Evaluation and Treatment of High Blood Pressure was published in 2003, first in an express version[1] and then in a comprehensive version.[2] The express version was published to facilitate application by busy clinicians. The comprehensive version was intended to provide more detail and careful documentation necessary for researchers and professionals focusing more deeply on hypertension. This 2003 report (JNC7) was a revision of the sixth report published in 1997 (JNC6).[3]

These reports have been prepared for more than three decades by the National Heart, Lung, and Blood Institute through the National High Blood Pressure Education Program, a coalition of 39 major professional, public, and voluntary organizations, and seven federal agencies. The work of the Joint National Committee was led by a 10-member executive committee appointed from the National High Blood Pressure Education Program Coordinating Committee membership. The report is an evidence-based report except where evidence does not exist to provide guidance. In those instances the report was consensus based.

CLASSIFICATION OF BLOOD PRESSURE

The JNC7 report departed from historical approaches and from other guidelines in its approach to classification of blood pressure. The classification added a new term, "prehypertension," for those at risk for developing hypertension. Table 96–1 shows the classification of blood pressure for adults as detailed in the JNC7 report. There is also a departure from the JNC6 report in that the classification which is used to make decisions regarding initial drug therapy does not take into consideration other risk factors but only measured blood pressure as a determination for treatment decisions.

BLOOD PRESSURE MEASUREMENT

The JNC7 and previous reports outlined the need for careful measurement of blood pressure. Recommendations for the use of a properly calibrated and validated instrument are noted. Recommendations from the most recent American Heart Association guidelines for the measurement of blood pressure again were used as the basis for recommendations.[4]

The JNC7 guidelines offered information on ambulatory blood pressure monitoring and self measurement of blood pressure as well. The report suggests that ambulatory blood pressure monitoring is warranted for evaluation of "white-coat" hypertension in the absence of target-organ injury; to assess patients with apparent drug-resistant hypotensive symptoms with antihypertensive medications; episodic hypertension; and autonomic dysfunction. The report notes that self-measurement of blood pressure might be beneficial in evaluating response to antihypertensive medication, improving patient adherence with therapy, and for evaluating possible "white-coat" hypertension.

PATIENT EVALUATION

Few changes were made in the recommendations for patient evaluation from previous reports. Routine laboratory and diagnostic tests recommended before initiating therapy in the report include an electrocardiogram, urinalysis, blood glucose, hematocrit, serum potassium, creatinine (or the corresponding estimated glomerular filtration rate), calcium, lipid profile after a 9- to 12-hour fast that includes a high-density lipoprotein cholesterol and low-density lipoprotein cholesterol and triglycerides. Optional tests for the clinician to consider include measurement of urinary albumin excretion for the albumin/creatinine ratio.

TREATMENT

The goal of therapy for most patients with hypertension is to reduce systolic blood pressure to below 140 mmHg and diastolic blood pressure to less than 90 mmHg. In patients with hypertension and diabetes or renal disease, the blood pressure goal is <130/80 mmHg.

Lifestyle therapy recommended in the report includes "weight reduction in those individuals who are overweight or obese, adoption to the Dietary Approaches to Stop Hypertension (DASH) eating plan, dietary sodium reduction, physical activity and moderation of alcohol consumption." Table 96–2 shows the recommended lifestyle

BLOOD PRESSURE CLASSIFICATION			
BP Classification	SBP (mmHg)		DBP (mmHg)
Normal	<120	and	<80
Prehypertension	120–139	or	80–89
Stage 1 hypertension	140–159	or	90–99
Stage 2 hypertension	≥160	or	≥100
BP, blood pressure; DBP, diastolic blood pressure; SBP, systolic blood pressure.			

Table 96–1. Blood Pressure Classification

LIFESTYLE MODIFICATIONS	
Modification	**Approximate SBP Reduction (Range)**
Weight reduction	5–10 mmHg/10 kg
Adopt DASH eating plan	8–14 mmHg
Dietary sodium reduction	2–8 mmHg
Physical activity	4–9 mmHg
Moderation of alcohol consumption	2–4 mmHg

DASH, Dietary Approaches to Stop Hypertension; SBP, systolic blood pressure.

Table 96–2. Lifestyle Modifications

modifications with expected reductions in systolic blood pressure.

Pharmacologic therapy is perhaps the most controversial part of the JNC7 report. There are some subtle differences here with other guidelines including the European guidelines.[5] The JNC7 guidelines note that five classes of drugs have evidence of reducing complications of hypertension, including angiotensin-converting enzyme (ACE) inhibitors, angiotensin receptor blockers, beta blockers, calcium channel blockers, and thiazide diuretics. The report also suggests that "thiazide type diuretics should be used as initial therapy for most patients with hypertension either alone

or in combination with one of the other classes demonstrated to be beneficial in randomized controlled outcome trials.... If a drug is not tolerated or is contraindicated then one of the other classes proven to reduce cardiovascular event should be used instead." An algorithm summarizing the recommendations is shown in Figure 96–1. Of note, the European guidelines do not give any priority to thiazide diuretics but simply recommend that clinicians choose among the five classes known to reduce mortality.[5]

Evidence supports "compelling indications" that require certain antihypertensive drug classes for high-risk conditions. Table 96–3 shows the classes recommended for several compelling indications.

COMPARISON OF JNC7 GUIDELINES TO EUROPEAN GUIDELINES

When the JNC reports were initially released, some of the differences vis-à-vis European guidelines generated considerable debate. In reality there are many more similarities than differences. In general, the U.S. and European guidelines are similar where the evidence is strong and different where the evidence is weaker. The guidelines certainly agree on lifestyle therapy for all and that lowering blood pressure to goal is the most important part of treatment. Both guidelines recommend selecting among classes with certain mortality benefit including thiazide diuretics, ACE inhibitors, angiotensin receptor blockers, beta blockers, and

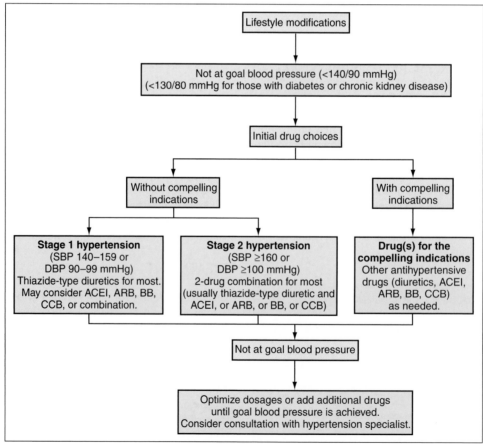

Figure 96–1. Algorithm for treatment of hypertension.

calcium channel blockers. Both guidelines suggest beginning with a combination in some patients, particularly those with higher levels of hypertension. Both guidelines call for specific classes in some circumstances, and both guidelines call for a goal blood pressure of 140/90 mmHg in most and 130/80 mmHg or lower in some patients.

There are differences in the guidelines in classification. The JNC7 guidelines use a new classification with a simplified approach to staging hypertension and the addition of "pre-hypertension." The guidelines also include some subtle differences regarding blood pressure level at which to initiate lifestyle therapy. The JNC7 guidelines call for initiation of lifestyle therapy at a blood pressure of 120/80 mmHg and the European guideline at 130/80 mmHg. The JNC7 report calls for initiation of drug therapy based on the level of blood pressure alone and for all at 140/90 mmHg and above.

The European guidelines call for initiation of drug therapy based on total cardiovascular risk and level of blood pressure, and consider antihypertensive therapy optional for "low-risk" individuals at 140 to 159/90 to 99 mmHg. As noted earlier, the U.S. guidelines suggest "thiazide type diuretics for most." The European guideline suggests that clinicians choose among the five classes of antihypertensive agents.

SUMMARY

The JNC7 guidelines are based on the best available evidence and provide guidance to clinicians for management of patients with hypertension. A stronger adherence to guidelines would lead to better treatment and control rates and lower cardiovascular disease rates in the future.

COMPELLING INDICATIONS FOR INDIVIDUAL DRUG CLASSES		
Compelling Indication	**Initial Therapy Options**	**Clinical Trial Basis**
Heart failure	THIAZ, BB, ACEI, ARB, ALDO ANT	ACC/AHA Heart Failure Guideline, MERIT-HF, COPERNICUS, CIBIS, SOLVD, AIRE, TRACE, ValHEFT, RALES
Post–myocardial infarction	BB, ACEI, ALDO ANT	ACC/AHA Post-MI Guideline, BHAT, SAVE, Capricorn, EPHESUS
High CAD risk	THIAZ, BB, ACE, CCB	ALLHAT, HOPE, ANBP2, LIFE, CONVINCE
Diabetes	THIAZ, BB, ACE, ARB, CCB	NKF-ADA Guideline, UKPDS, ALLHAT
Chronic kidney disease	ACEI, ARB	NKF Guideline, Captopril Trial, RENAAL, IDNT, REIN, AASK
Recurrent stroke prevention	THIAZ, ACEI	PROGRESS
CAD, coronary artery disease.		

Table 96–3. Compelling Indications for Individual Drug Classes

REFERENCES

1. Chobanian AV, Bakris GL, Black HR, et al. The seventh report of the Joint National Committee on Prevention, Detection, Evaluation, and Treatment of High Blood Pressure: the JNC7 Report. *JAMA* 2003;289:2560–72.
2. Chobanian AV, Bakris GL, Black HR, et al. Seventh report of the Joint National Committee on Prevention, Detection,

Evaluation, and Treatment of High Blood Pressure. *Hypertension* 2003;42:1206–52.
3. National High Blood Pressure Education Program. The sixth report of the Joint National Committee on Prevention, Detection, Evaluation, and Treatment of High Blood Pressure. *Arch Intern Med* 1997;157:2413–46.

4. Perloff D, Grim C, Flack J, et al. Human blood pressure determination by sphygmomanometry. *Circulation* 1993;88:2460–70.
5. 2003 European Society of Hypertension—European Society of Cardiology guidelines for the management of arterial hypertension. *J Hypertens* 2003;21:1011–53.

Chapter

97

The 2003 Guidelines for the Management of Hypertension of the European Society of Hypertension and European Society of Cardiology

Alberto Zanchetti

Key Findings

- The 2003 guidelines are the first specifically prepared in the area of hypertension management by European scientific organizations. They have an informative and educational purpose rather than a prescriptive one.

- Hypertension is defined in the context of a stratification of total cardiovascular risk that takes into account not only the levels of systolic and diastolic blood pressures, but also the presence or absence of other risk factors, target-organ damage, diabetes, and cardiovascular or renal disease.

- Because of the importance of subclinical damage in determining total cardiovascular risk, noninvasive procedures (such as ultrasound cardiac and vascular assessment, and search for microalbuminuria) are encouraged whenever these procedures may help in profiling the cardiovascular risk of the individual patient.

- Initiation of antihypertensive therapy is decided on the basis of total cardiovascular risk. Accordingly, grade 1 hypertension (systolic blood pressure [SBP] 140–159 or diastolic blood pressure [DBP] 90–99 mmHg) without any additional risk or disease may be managed by lifestyle changes only for several months before recurring to drug therapy, while high normal blood pressure (SBP 130–139 or DBP 85–89 mmHg) accompanying diabetes or clinical disease usually benefits from antihypertensive agents.

- The main benefits of antihypertensive therapy are due to lowering blood pressure *per se*. Therefore, all major classes of antihypertensive agents are considered suitable for initiation and maintenance of antihypertensive therapy. However, specific drug classes differ in some effect or in special groups of patients. Drugs also differ in terms of adverse disturbances, with important reflections on patients' compliance to treatment.

- To reach target blood pressure (at least below 140/90 mmHg in all hypertensive patients, and below 130/80 in diabetics and renal patients), a large proportion of subjects will require combination therapy with more than one agent. Combination therapy with two agents at low doses can also be used to initiate therapy in some patients.

- In patients at high risk, antihypertensive therapy may be beneficially associated with lipid lowering and antiplatelet therapies.

FIRST EUROPEAN GUIDELINES

The 2003 guidelines are the first ones prepared in the area of hypertension management by European scientific organizations.[1] Until that time, the European Society of Hypertension did not draw up specific guidelines on hypertension but chose to endorse guidelines previously prepared by the World Health Organization (WHO) and the International Society of Hypertension (ISH), and to incorporate them, with some adaptation, into joint recommendations of various European scientific societies for the prevention of coronary heart disease. However, in 2003 it was considered that the WHO/ISH guidelines are obviously written for a global audience from countries that vary widely in the extent of healthcare provision and the availability of resources. On the other hand, Europe was a much more homogeneous community, with populations with greater longevity but a higher incidence of chronic cardiovascular disease despite a high proportion of resources being devoted to disease prevention. The Councils of both the European Society of Hypertension and the European Society of Cardiology thought that preparation of European guidelines was a rational response to the suggestion of the WHO/ISH guidelines that national experts draw up recommendations specifically directed to patients in their own region. Giuseppe Mancia was asked to convene a representative group of European experts (28-member Guidelines Committee), and I chaired the Writing Committee consisting of R. Cifkova, R. Fagard, S. Kjeldsen, G. Mancia, N. Poulter, K.H. Rahn, J.L. Rodicio, L.M. Ruilope, J. Staessen, P. Van Zwieten, B. Waeber, and B. Williams.

PURPOSE OF GUIDELINES

The European guidelines are introduced by a statement that, in the Committee's opinion, guidelines should have an informative and educational purpose rather than a prescriptive one (Box 97–1). In the frame of this view, an extensive document with critical discussion of all relevant evidence available was first prepared,[1] which was later complemented by a brief set of practice recommenda-

Box 97–1

Purpose of European Guidelines

- ESH and ESC feel that guidelines, to be effective, should have an educational purpose rather than a prescriptive one.
- Therefore, the two societies have first prepared a detailed document discussing all evidence available, and then have prepared succinct recommendations for the practicing physician.
- The ESH/ESC guidelines intend to leave a reasonable margin of choice to the individual doctor treating individual patients.

ESH, European Society of Hypertension; ESC, European Society of Cardiology.

Box 97–2

Values and Limitations of Event-Based Randomized Trials

Values

- Randomization is the safest procedure to avoid bias.
- Large number of patients guarantee power to detect differences in primary endpoints.
- Endpoints are well-defined events of clinical relevance.

Limitation

- Selection of patients (most often patients at elevated cardiovascular risk) makes extrapolation to patients at a different risk level doubtful.
- Most trials are not powered for secondary endpoints.
- Therapeutic programs in trials often diverge from those followed in clinical practice.
- Compliance of patients is much higher than in clinical practice.
- Controlled randomized trials last for 4 to 5 years, whereas life expectancy in middle-aged hypertensives is of 20 to 30 years.

tions[2] directed to those practitioners wishing to receive concise advice. This marks, perhaps, the most important difference from other guidelines, as the European document intends to provide information on all the complexities of hypertension management, and although providing some simple, but not oversimplified, paradigm of decision, leaves a reasonable margin of choice to the individual doctor treating individual patients. In accordance with this view, the European Guidelines Committee considered that, although large randomized controlled trials and meta-analyses provide the strongest evidence about several aspects of therapy, scientific evidence is drawn from many sources, and where necessary all sources of evidence and information were used, without rigid classification of recommendations according to strength of available evidence (Box 97–2).

DEFINITION AND CLASSIFICATION OF HYPERTENSION

The European guidelines consider that the continuous relationship between the level of blood pressure (both systolic and diastolic values) and cardiovascular morbidity and mortality makes any numerical definition and classification of hypertension arbitrary, and to quote a 30-year-old definition by Geoffrey Rose,[3] "Hypertension should be defined in terms of a blood pressure level above which investigation and treatment do more good than harm," in order to indicate that any numerical definition must be a flexible one resulting from evidence of risk and availability of effective and well-tolerated drugs.

For practical reasons, however, a numerical classification is useful, and is indeed used by all available guidelines. The 2003 European guidelines have retained, with few modifications, the classification of the 1999 WHO/ISH guidelines. This classification is reproduced in Table 97–1. There are two differences between this classification and that provided by the Joint National Committee Report 7 (JNC 7) for the United States.[4] A likely minor one concerns the subdivision of hypertension into three grades, whereas JNC 7 lumps grades 2 and 3 into a single

group (stage 2), although it is felt that the division in three grades may be useful in order to better convey the concept of a continuous increase in risk with an increase in blood pressure. The other difference is more substantial: the European guidelines have not followed JNC 7 in classifying the very large number of subjects with blood pressures of 120 to 139/80 to 89 mmHg as prehypertensives, and have preferred to keep them split into two groups—normal blood pressure (120–129/80–84 mmHg) and high-normal blood pressure (130–139/85–89 mmHg). This avoids medicalization of millions of people, while preserving the concept that subjects with "high-normal

DEFINITIONS AND CLASSIFICATION OF BLOOD PRESSURE LEVELS (mmHG)		
Category	**Systolic**	**Diastolic**
Optimal	<120	<80
Normal	120–129	80–84
High normal	130–139	85–89
Grade 1 hypertension (mild)	140–159	90–99
Grade 2 hypertension (moderate)	160–179	100–109
Grade 3 hypertension (severe)	≥180	≥110
Isolated systolic hypertension	≥140	<90

Notes: When a patient's systolic and diastolic blood pressures fall into different categories, the higher category should apply. Isolated systolic hypertension can also be graded (grades 1, 2, 3) according to systolic blood pressure values in the ranges indicated, provided that diastolic values are <90.

Table 97–1. Definitions and Classification of Blood Pressure Levels (mmHg)

blood pressure" have a greater likelihood to develop hypertension in the subsequent 10 years than those with "normal blood pressure," as shown by the Framingham study.[5]

Apart from the merits of the different terms given to the numerical classification and subdivision of hypertension, an important feature of the European guidelines is that decisions about the management of patients with hypertension should rarely be made on blood pressure alone, but also on the presence or absence of other risk factors, target-organ damage, diabetes, and cardiovascular or renal disease, as well as on other aspects of the patient's personal, medical, and social situation. An algorithm for stratification of total cardiovascular risk is illustrated in Table 97-2. The terms low, moderate, high, and very high added risk are calibrated to indicate an approximate absolute 10-year risk of cardiovascular disease of less than 15%, 15% to 20%, 20% to 30% and more than 30%, respectively, according to Framingham criteria,[6] or an approximate absolute risk of fatal cardiovascular disease of less than 4%, 4% to 5%, 5% to 8%, and more than 8% according to the SCORE chart.[7] These categories can also be used as indicators of relative risk, leaving the doctors free to use one or the other approach without the constraint of arbitrary absolute thresholds of risk that are more friendly to health providers than to patients. Indeed, the guidelines call attention to the danger that intervention thresholds based on rather short-term absolute risk may lead to concentrating most resources on the oldest subjects, easily classified at high absolute risk, while young subjects at high relative risk may remain untreated, even though their treatment may exert benefits through a much longer potential life span. Accordingly, European guidelines suggest basing decisions on relative risk for subjects younger than 60 and on absolute risk levels for older patients.

Finally, as seen in Table 97-2, European guidelines give particular importance to target-organ damage, diabetes mellitus, and associated clinical conditions (such as a previous myocardial infarction or stroke). Presence of these most often implies a high or very high added risk even in subjects with "normal" or "high-normal" blood pressure, thus substantiating the concept that the definition of hypertension (i.e., the blood pressure level deserving to be actively lowered) is a variable, flexible one, depending on the individual's total cardiovascular risk.

DIAGNOSTIC EVALUATION

As in all guidelines, the European guidelines diagnostic procedures comprise repeated blood pressure measurement, medical history, physical examination, and laboratory and instrumental investigations. The value of various methodologies for measuring blood pressure is summarized in Box 97-3. As to laboratory and instrumental investigations, it is apparent from Box 97-4 that European guidelines have taken a rather liberal attitude in recommending, if expertise and resources are available (as

---

Box 97-3

Methods for Blood Pressure Measurements

- Blood pressure values measured in the doctor's office should commonly be used as references.
- Twenty-four–hour ambulatory blood pressure monitoring may be considered when:
  Office blood pressure values are considerably variable.
  Blood pressure is high in the office in subjects at low total cardiovascular risk.
  There is large discrepancy between office and home blood pressure.
  Resistance to drug therapy is suspected.
- Self-measurement of blood pressure at home should be encouraged in order to:
  Provide more information for the doctor's decision.
  Improve patient's compliance.
- Normal values are different for office (<140/90 mmHg), 24-hour ambulatory (<125/80 mmHg) and home (<135/85 mmHg) blood pressure.

STRATIFICATION OF RISK TO QUANTIFY PROGNOSIS					
			Blood Pressure (mmHg)		
Other Risk Factors and Disease History	**Normal** SBP 120–129 or DBP 80–84	**High Normal** SBP 130–139 or DBP 85–89	**Grade 1** SBP 140–159 or DBP 90–99	**Grade 2** SBP 160–179 or DBP 100–109	**Grade 3** SBP ≥ 180 or DBP ≥ 110
No other risk factors	Average risk	Average risk	Low added risk	Moderate added risk	High added risk
1–2 risk factors	Low added risk	Low added risk	Moderate added risk	Moderate added risk	Very high added risk
≥3 risk factors, target-organ damage, or diabetes	Moderate added risk	High added risk	High added risk	High added risk	Very high added risk
Associated clinical conditions	High added risk	Very high added risk	Very high added risk	Very high added risk	Very high added risk
DBP, diastolic blood pressure; SBP, systolic blood pressure.					

Table 97-2. Stratification of Risk to Quantify Prognosis

Box 97–4

Diagnostic Evaluation: Laboratory Investigations

Routine Tests

- Plasma glucose (preferably fasting)
- Serum total and HDL cholesterol; fasting serum triglycerides
- Serum creatinine
- Serum uric acid
- Serum potassium
- Hemoglobin and hematocrit
- Urinalysis (dipstick test and urinary sediment)
- Electrocardiogram

Recommended Tests

- Echocardiogram
- Carotid ultrasound
- Postprandial plasma glucose (when fasting value ≥6.1 mmol/L)
- Microalbuminuria
- Quantitative proteinuria (if dipstick test positive)
- Funduscopy (in severe hypertension)

they commonly are in Europe), a series of investigations in addition to the strictly necessary (or routine) ones. Echocardiography is recognized as much more sensitive than electrocardiography in diagnosing left ventricular

hypertrophy and predicting cardiovascular risk. The availability of echocardiography has increased in Europe, and when treatment decisions are uncertain, an echocardiographic examination may help in more precisely classifying the overall risk of the hypertensive patients and in directing therapy. The same is recognized to be the case for ultrasound examination of the carotid arteries with measurement of the intima-media thickness and detection of plaques, and for microalbuminuria (obligatory investigation in all diabetic patients, but also recommended in nondiabetic hypertensives).

THERAPEUTIC APPROACH

When to initiate antihypertensive treatment

Decisions on initiation of antihypertensive treatment are based not only on the blood pressure values repeatedly measured on several occasions but on stratification of total cardiovascular risk. Accordingly, Table 97–3 has been drawn on the same pattern as Table 97–2. When blood pressure is in the normal or high-normal range and no other risk factor is present (average risk), no intervention is recommended, but if one or two additional risk factors are associated, lifestyle changes are recommended. In the presence of target organ damage, diabetes, or clinical conditions, antihypertensive drugs should be prescribed even when blood pressure is lower than 140/90 mmHg, particularly if it is in the high-normal range. This recommendation is based on evidence from the PROGRESS (Perindopril Protection Against Recurrent Stroke Study),[8]

	INITIATION OF ANTIHYPERTENSIVE TREATMENT				
			Blood Pressure (mmHg)		
Other Risk Factors and Disease History	**Normal** SBP 120–129 or DBP 80–84	**High Normal** SBP 130–139 or DBP 85–89	**Grade 1** SBP 140–159 or DBP 90–99	**Grade 2** SBP 160–179 or DBP 100–109	**Grade 3** SBP ≥ 180 or DBP ≥ 110
No other risk factors	No intervention	No intervention	Lifestyle changes for several months, then drug treatment if preferred by the patient and resources available	Lifestyle changes for several months, then drug treatment	Immediate drug treatment and lifestyle changes
1–2 risk factors	Lifestyle changes	Lifestyle changes	Lifestyle changes for several months, then drug treatment	Lifestyle changes for several months, then drug treatment	Immediate drug treatment and lifestyle changes
≥3 risk factors, target-organ damage, or diabetes	Lifestyle changes	Drug treatment and lifestyle changes	Drug treatment and lifestyle changes	Drug treatment and lifestyle changes	Immediate drug treatment and lifestyle changes
Associated clinical conditions	Drug treatment and lifestyle changes	Immediate drug treatment and lifestyle changes	Immediate drug treatment and lifestyle changes	Immediate drug treatment and lifestyle changes	Immediate drug treatment and lifestyle changes

DBP, diastolic blood pressure; SBP, systolic blood pressure.

Table 97–3. Initiation of Antihypertensive Treatment

HOPE (Heart Outcomes Prevention Evaluation),[9] and ABCD (Antihypertensive Therapy in Type 2 Diabetes: Implications of the Appropriate Blood Pressure Control in Diabetes) trials.[10,11] Within the traditional hypertensive range, and particularly for patients with grade 1 hypertension, if the added total cardiovascular risk is low or moderate, treatment should be started with lifestyle changes and drugs added after several weeks or a few months if blood pressure does not reach the goal. When total risk is higher, drug treatment should be immediate but always accompanied by lifestyle recommendations. Lifestyle changes are an important component of antihypertensive treatment, but in many patients they are only effective when implemented with a structured behavioral program. Therefore, lifestyle changes cannot be considered as an easy and cheap approach to management of hypertension.[12]

Goal of treatment

According to the concept that what really matters is to achieve reduction in the total risk of cardiovascular morbidity and mortality, guidelines recommend treatment of all reversible risk factors and not only lowering of the raised blood pressure (Box 97–5). As to target blood pressure, it is recommended that both systolic and diastolic blood pressures be intensively lowered, at least below 140/90 mmHg and to lower values if tolerated, in all hypertensive patients, and below 130/80 mmHg in diabetics. However, guidelines acknowledge that these values may be difficult to achieve, particularly in the elderly, and that strong evidence in favor of reducing blood pressure below 140/90 is available only for diabetics and patients with a previous cardiovascular event, and that in diabetics only one study, ABCD-NT,[11] has shown significant benefit (stroke reduction) by achieving systolic blood pressures slightly below 130 mmHg.

Lifestyle measures

Lifestyle measures play an important role in the treatment of hypertension as well as in the correction of associated risk factors or disease; detailed recommendations are given in the European guidelines, as summarized in Box 97–6. It is pointed out, however, that lifestyle measures have not yet been shown to prevent cardiovascular complications in hypertensive patients, and should never delay unnecessarily the initiation of drug treatment, especially in patients at higher levels of risk, nor should such measures detract from compliance with drug treatment.

Pharmacologic treatment

The European guidelines have chosen to have recommendations about pharmacological therapy preceded by analysis of the available evidence of the benefits obtained by antihypertensive therapy and of the comparative benefits obtained by the various classes of agents. It is obviously acknowledged that the strongest type of evidence is that provided by large randomized trials based on fatal and nonfatal events. It is, however, recognized that even event-based trials have some limitations (Box 97–2), and randomized studies using intermediate endpoints (i.e., subclinical organ damage changes) have also been evaluated. Admittedly, evidence that regression or retardation of subclinical organ damage is associated with reduction of cardiovascular events is indirect, but it is also known that at least some of these alterations have predictive value of subsequent fatal and nonfatal events. Treatment-induced alterations of metabolic parameters, or induction or worsening of the metabolic syndrome or diabetes have also been considered as they may have an impact during the course of the patient's life and are taken into account when assessing total cardiovascular risk.

Regarding the choice of antihypertensive drugs, the European guidelines conclude that a very large number of randomized trials, both those comparing active treatment with placebo (Figure 97–1) and those comparing active treatment regimens based on different compounds, clearly show that the main benefits of antihypertensive therapy are due to lowering of blood pressure *per se*. However, there is evidence, often from studies of intermediate outcomes, that specific drug classes may differ in some effect or in special groups of patients, and this may help determine the choice in particular situations. Drugs also differ in terms of adverse disturbances, particularly in individual patients, with important reflections on patients' compliance

---

Box 97–5

Goal of Treatment

- Treatment should be directed to all reversible risk factors identified, including smoking, dyslipidemia, or diabetes, and the appropriate management of associated clinical conditions, as well as treatment of the raised blood pressure.
- It can be recommended that systolic and diastolic blood pressure be intensively lowered, at least below 140/90 mmHg and to definitely lower values if tolerated in all hypertensive patients, and below 130/80 mmHg in diabetics and renal patients.
- However, systolic blood pressure below 140 mmHg may be difficult to achieve, particularly in the elderly.

Box 97–6

Lifestyle Changes

- Lifestyle measures should be instituted whenever appropriate in all patients, including subjects with high normal blood pressure and patients who require drug treatment.
- The lifestyle measures to be considered include:
  Smoking cessation
  Weight reduction
  Reduction of excessive alcohol intake
  Physical exercise
  Reduction of salt intake

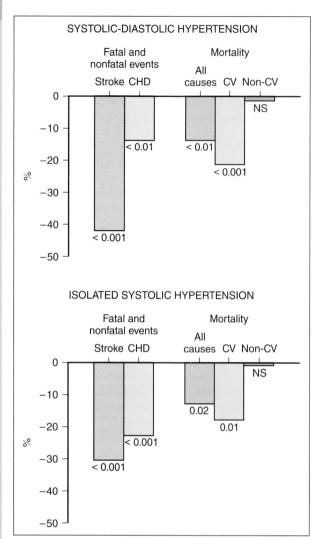

Figure 97–1. Risk reduction of fatal and combined fatal and nonfatal event in patients with active antihypertensive treatment versus placebo. CHD, coronary heart disease; CV, cardiovascular.

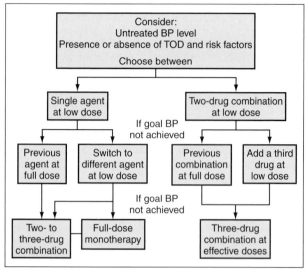

Figure 97–2. Choice between monotherapy and combination therapy. BP, blood pressure; TOD, target-organ damage.

tensive patients, especially in the elderly, but whenever important damage or clinical disease is present, treatment should be prompt and target pressure achieved in a few weeks, rather than months. The two-drug combinations found to be effective and well tolerated are indicated in Figure 97–3.

Therapeutic approaches in special conditions

European guidelines separately discuss therapeutic approaches in the elderly; diabetic patients; patients with renal disease, concomitant cerebrovascular or coronary disease or congestive heart failure; and pregnancy hypertension. For the elderly, it is pointed out that specific trials have clearly shown that reduced mortality and morbidity

to treatment. In principle, all major classes of antihypertensive agents—diuretics, β-blockers, calcium antagonists, angiotensin-converting enzyme (ACE) inhibitors and angiotensin receptor antagonists—are considered suitable for the initiation and maintenance of antihypertensive therapy. These conclusions are also illustrated in Box 97–7.

Table 97–4 summarizes indications and contraindications for the major classes of antihypertensive agents. Guidelines also recognize that, to reach target blood pressure, a large proportion of patients will require combination therapy with more than one agent. While the traditional approach to antihypertensive therapy has been that of starting with monotherapy and then resorting to combination therapy only when monotherapy fails, European guidelines suggest that when physicians think combination therapy is likely to become necessary (high initial blood pressure values, target-organ damage present), they can start therapy with a two-drug combination preferably at low doses (Figure 97–2). In general, antihypertensive therapy should be started gradually in most hyper-

---

Box 97–7

Choice of Antihypertensive Drugs

- The choice of drugs will be influenced by many factors including:
  Previous experience of the patient
  Cost of drugs (not to predominate over efficacy and tolerability)
  Risk profile, organ damage, clinical cardiovascular or renal disease or diabetes
  Renal disease or diabetes
  Patient's preference
- The physician should tailor the choice of drugs to the individual patient, after taking all these factors, together with the patient's preference, into account.
- Particular attention should be given to adverse events, even to subjective disturbances, as these may be an important cause of noncompliance.
- Patients should always be asked about adverse events, and drugs or dose changed accordingly.

INDICATIONS AND CONTRAINDICATIONS FOR MAJOR CLASSES OF ANTIHYPERTENSIVE DRUGS

Class	Conditions Favoring Use	Contraindications Compelling	Possible
Diuretics (thiazides)	Congestive heart failure Elderly hypertensives Isolated systolic hypertension	Gout	Pregnancy
Diuretics (loop)	Renal insufficiency Congestive heart failure		
Diuretics (antialdosterone)	Congestive heart failure Postmyocardial infarction	Renal failure Hyperkalemia	
β-Blockers	Angina pectoris Postmyocardial infarction Congestive heart failure (up-titration) Pregnancy Tachyarrhythmias	Asthma Chronic obstructive pulmonary disease A-V block (grade 2 or 3)	Peripheral vascular disease Glucose intolerance Athletes and physically active patients
Calcium antagonists (dihydropyridines)	Elderly patients Isolated systolic hypertension Angina pectoris Peripheral vascular disease Carotid atherosclerosis Pregnancy		Tachyarrhythmias Congestive heart failure
Calcium antagonists (verapamil, diltiazem)	Angina pectoris Carotid atherosclerosis Supraventricular tachycardia	A-V block (grade 2 or 3) Congestive heart failure	
ACE inhibitors	Congestive heart failure Left ventricular dysfunction Postmyocardial infarction Nondiabetic nephropathy Type 1 diabetic nephropathy Proteinuria	Pregnancy Hyperkalemia Bilateral renal artery stenosis	
Angiotensin II–receptor antagonists (AT1-blockers)	Diabetic nephropathy Diabetic microalbuminuria Proteinuria Left ventricular hypertrophy ACE-inhibitor cough	Pregnancy Hyperkalemia Bilateral renal artery stenosis	
α-Blockers	Prostatic hyperplasia (BPH) Hyperlipidemia	Orthostatic hypotension	Congestive heart failure

ACE, angiotensin-converting enzyme.

Table 97–4. Indications and Contraindications for Major Classes of Antihypertensive Drugs

are achieved by blood-pressure lowering. For patients with diabetes or with nondiabetic renal disease, intensive lowering of blood pressure is necessary and this will require combination therapy, regularly including an agent blocking the renin-angiotensin system, especially when proteinuria is present. The finding of microalbuminuria in diabetics is an indication for antihypertensive therapy, irrespective of blood-pressure values. Previous cerebrovascular and coronary heart diseases also require intensive blood-pressure lowering.

In prevention of congestive heart failure, calcium antagonists appear to be less effective than thiazide diuretics and ACE inhibitors. In pregnancy, the goal of treating hypertension is to reduce maternal risk, but the agents selected must be safe for the fetus. Methyldopa, labetalol, calcium antagonists, and β-blockers are the drugs of choice, although the β-blockers appear to be less effective than calcium antagonists. ACE inhibitors and

angiotensin-II antagonists should not be used in pregnancy, and diuretics are inappropriate in pre-eclampsia, which is generally associated with reduced plasma volume.

Treatment of associated risk factors or disease

The emphasis given in the European guidelines to assessment of total cardiovascular risk is paralleled by intervention recommendations. Box 97–5 indicates that the goal of treatment is to achieve reduction in total risk of cardiovascular morbidity and mortality. Therefore, guidelines recommend lipid-lowering (statins)[13] and antiplatelet (low-dose aspirin)[14] therapies in hypertensive patients, even in the absence of overt cardiovascular disease, if estimated 10-year cardiovascular risk is greater than 20% (high risk in the stratification algorithm of Table 97–2). However, low-dose aspirin administration should be preceded by good blood pressure control.[14] In diabetic

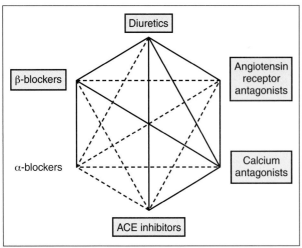

Figure 97–3. Possible combinations of different classes of antihypertensive agents. The most rational combinations are represented as thick lines. The frames indicate classes of antihypertensive agents proven to be beneficial in controlled interventional trials. ACE, angiotensin-converting enzyme.

patients, achieving satisfactory control of glycemia is also important: treatment goals are set to ≤6.0 mmol/L (110 mg/dL) for plasma preprandial glucose concentration and to less than 6.5% for HbA_{1c}.

IMPLEMENTATION OF GUIDELINES

Guidelines acknowledge that despite major efforts to diagnose and treat hypertension, this condition remains a leading cause of cardiovascular morbidity and mortality worldwide, and goal blood pressure levels are seldom achieved. This unsatisfactory delivery of care should be improved. The availability of guidelines should not only help clinicians to make decisions in everyday practice, but also make the health authorities in all countries aware of the critical points to consider in order to improve hypertension management. A powerful instrument for implementation is acceptance of guidelines by national hypertension societies and their dissemination in national languages. It is also acknowledged, however, that in order to be accepted by practicing physicians, guidelines should avoid being excessively prescriptive: European guidelines humbly recognize that guidelines provide information and advice concerning a disease or medical condition in general, whereas individual physicians are dealing with individual patients differing in their personal, medical, and cultural characteristics.

REFERENCES

1. Guidelines Committee. 2003 European Society of Hypertension–European Society of Cardiology guidelines for the management of arterial hypertension. *J Hypertens* 2003;21:1011–53.
2. Practice Guidelines Writing Committee. Practice guidelines for primary care physicians. 2003 ESH/ESC hypertension guidelines. *J Hypertens* 2003;21:1779–86.
3. Evans JG, Rose G. Hypertension. *Br Med Bull* 1971;27:37–42.
4. JNC 7 Express. The seventh report of the Joint National Committee on Prevention, Detection, Evaluation and Treatment of High Blood Pressure. *JAMA* 2003;289:2560–71.
5. Vasan RS, Larson MG, Laip EP, et al. Assessment of frequency of progression to hypertension in non hypertensive participants in the Framingham Heart Study: a cohort study. *Lancet* 2001; 358:1682–6.
6. Anderson KM, Wilson PW, Odell PM, Kannel WB. An update coronary risk profile. A statement for health professionals. *Circulation* 1991; 83:356–62.
7. Conroy RM, Pyörälä K, Fitzgerald AP, et al. Prediction of ten-year risk of fatal cardiovascular disease in Europe: the SCORE project. *Eur Heart J* 2003; 24:2070–1.
8. PROGRESS Collaborative Study Group. Randomised trial of perindopril based blood pressure-lowering regimen among 6105 individuals with previous stroke or transient ischaemic attack. *Lancet* 2001;358:1033–41.
9. Heart Outcomes Prevention Evaluation Study Investigators. Effects of an angiotensin-converting-enzyme inhibitor, ramipril on cardiovascular events in high-risk patients. *N Engl J Med* 2000;342:145–53.
10. Estacio RO, Jeffers BW, Hiatt WR, et al. The effect of nisoldipine as compared with enalapril on cardiovascular outcomes in patients with non-insulin dependent diabetes and hypertension. *N Engl J Med* 1998;338:645–52.
11. Schrier RW, Estacio RO, Esler A, Mehler P. Effects of aggressive blood pressure control in normotensive type 2 diabetic patients on albuminuria, retinopathy and strokes. *Kidney Int* 2002;61:1086–97.
12. Zanchetti A. Costs of implementing recommendations on hypertension management given in recent guidelines. *J Hypertens* 2003;21:2207–9.
13. Sever PS, Dahlöf B, Poulter NR, et al. for the ASCOT investigators. The prevention of coronary events and stroke by atorvastatin in hypertensive subjects with or below average cholesterol levels. The Anglo-Scandinavian Cardiac Outcomes Trial: Lipid-Lowering Arm (ASCOT:LLA). *Lancet* 2003;361:1149–58.
14. Hansson L, Zanchetti A, Carruthers SG, et al. Effects of intensive blood-pressure lowering and low-dose aspirin in patients with hypertension: principal results of the Hypertension Optimal Treatment (HDT) randomised trial. *Lancet* 1998;351:1755–62.

Chapter

98 Treatment Guidelines: The Developing World

Kolli Srinath Reddy, Nitish Naik, and Dorairaj Prabhakaran

Key Findings

- Hypertension is one of the leading causes of death and disability both in the Third World and developed countries.

- The same protection is afforded from blood pressure control as in developed countries.

- There is a wide heterogeneity in the burden of hypertension in the Third World countries.

- While it would be difficult to make hypertension management guidelines for each country, it would be pragmatic to use an approach similar to the World Health Organization Risk Factor Surveillance (STEPS) surveillance program.

- The guiding principles that should be considered in developing guidelines for therapy should include (1) knowledge of available strategies for the prevention and management of hypertension, (2) capacity to detect and manage hypertension, (3) barriers to prevention and management of hypertension at an individual level, (4) best available evidence for the various drug classes, (5) optimal first line of therapy, and (6) ethnic variability in response to drugs.

- In many low-income countries, at their current level of health expenditure, risk assessment may need to be entirely clinical, based on patients' blood pressure level, age, gender, smoking status, body mass index, and previous history of cardiovascular illness.

Hypertension is one of the leading causes of death and disability both in the Third World and developed countries. It plays a major etiologic role in the occurrence of cerebrovascular diseases, coronary heart disease (CHD), and cardiac and renal failure.[1] Worldwide, hypertension contributes to 49% of the population attributable fraction of ischemic heart disease.[2] In a large majority of Third World countries, similar to developed countries, hypertension is emerging as a major contributor to mortality and morbidity. Further, the contribution of hypertension to CHD risk appears to be similar across all ethnicities.[3] Given higher population growth in developing countries, it is expected that by 2020 these nations will account for 84% of the world's population. Therefore, not only is the burden of hypertension high among these nations, with increasing population, economic progress, and the epidemiologic transition underway, developing countries are likely to witness a manifold increase in the burden of hypertension by 2020.

Although this high burden is alarming, there are immense opportunities for prevention and appropriate management of hypertension. Several clinical trials involving drugs and lifestyle therapy have demonstrated the feasibility and success in the management of hypertension. Control of hypertension results in approximately 40% reduction in the risk of stroke and a smaller but meaningful (approximately 15%) reduction in CHD.[4] However, most of these have been based on data gathered from developed countries. The same protection is likely, afforded from blood pressure control in developing countries, but resource constraints in Third World or developing countries merit consideration, especially when new, expensive drug classes are promoted.

Awareness and optimal management of hypertension are inadequate worldwide.[5] Therefore, several attributes of hypertension should be considered while formulating guidelines. These include the burden of hypertension in a given country, its co-occurrence with other cardiovascular disease (CVD) risk factors such as diabetes and obesity, the available capacity to detect and manage hypertension, and the resource constraints of the country being studied. In this chapter we address these issues and discuss the need and basis for specific guidelines among developing countries.

DISEASE BURDEN

In 2000 there were approximately 972 million patients with hypertension worldwide[6]; 639 million of them resided in Third World countries. Modeled projections indicate an increase to 1.15 billion hypertensive patients by 2025 in Third World nations, which is an increase of 80% compared to 2000.[6] In India, the absolute number of people with hypertension is expected to rise from the current estimated figure of approximately 118 million to over 200 million by 2025. Similar trends are expected in China.[7]

There is a great heterogeneity in the burden of hypertension in the Third World countries. Although systematic national data on prevalence are not available from most of the Third World, the highest prevalence rates of hypertension have been reported from the Latin American countries such as Mexico, Paraguay, and Venezuela, where prevalence rates vary from 32% to 36.9%.[6] Lower rates of hypertension have been reported in some parts of sub-Saharan Africa with an estimated prevalence of 14%.[6] Countries such as China and India have intermediate prevalence in urban areas (approximately 20% to 30%).[6] Even within a given region, wide variations have been reported. Recent studies in urban India report a prevalence of 30% to 40% in adults, while the prevalence of hypertension in rural regions is about 12% to 17%.[8] Local practices have also been shown to influence the prevalence of hypertension. For example, in the predominantly rural setting of Assam, India, providing salt to tea garden workers has resulted in high rates of hypertension compared with other CVD risk factors.[9]

Time series trends also suggest a rising prevalence of hypertension. In China, the third national hypertension survey reported an increase in the overall prevalence of hypertension from 7.8% in 1979–1980 to 11.4% in 1991. The last survey in 2000–2001 (conducted by the International Collaborative Study of Cardiovascular Disease in ASIA [InterASIA]) reported a further increase to 27.2%.[10] Similar trends in hypertension prevalence have been reported in India. Rising population-based, mean blood pressure parallels the increase in prevalence of hypertension. For example, the World Health Organization's *Atlas of Heart Disease and Stroke* profiled a sustained increase in the mean systolic blood pressure level in India, from a low of 120 mmHg in 1942 to 130 mmHg in 1997.[11] Compounding this high burden is lack of awareness and insufficient and ineffective treatment. In urban Chennai, in India, the prevalence of hypertension was 22.8% and 19.7% in men and women, respectively. However, only 37.3% of hypertensives were aware of their hypertension status, and only half of these were on any kind of drug therapy. Only 40% of those who were treated had adequate blood pressure control.[12] Even where educational levels are high, as in worksite settings, awareness and treatment status are suboptimal. Prabhakaran et al.[13] reported awareness of hypertension in only one-third of survey participants, and in this group blood pressure was adequately controlled in only 38%, although more than two-thirds (66.4%) of those surveyed had graduate (university or college) or higher level education. Similarly, in a large community survey in China, only 42.6% were aware of their hypertension, and 6.6% of hypertensives had adequate control of blood pressure.[7] In this study, rates of awareness, treatment, and control were higher in women than in men, and higher in urban than in rural areas.

The awareness, treatment, and control status of hypertension in Africa is similarly unsatisfactory. Two recent surveys in Tanzania indicate that less than 20% of hypertensives were aware of their diagnosis, and approximately 10% of these reported receiving treatment and less than 1% were adequately controlled.[14] In South Africa awareness among women was higher than among men (47% vs. 20%), and treatment and control status among women was marginally better. Thus, given the resource constraints of these countries it is important to identify high-risk populations for hypertension and to target treatment programs on these groups.

ETHNIC VARIATIONS

Although disease patterns in the developing world are likely to mirror and follow the same patterns seen in developed nations, variations in disease manifestation, severity, and response to treatment are expected due to variations in both genetic and environmental influences.[15]

It has been demonstrated that the prevalence of hypertension is higher in African Americans as well as people of Afro-Caribbean descent than in white Americans.[16] This condition also occurs at an earlier age, is more severe, and is more often associated with target organ damage than among white Americans. Similar variations have been described among ethnic minorities settled in developed nations.[17] Variations in therapeutic response to antihypertensive drugs have also highlighted ethnic diversity. The response of African Americans to angiotensin receptor blockers (ARBs) has been suggested to be far less than that in whites; however, the differences are not as substantial upon accounting for sodium intake. Of note, the largest source of variation in blood pressure response, for example, to ACE inhibitors, is within racial/ethnic groups and not between them, as discussed in Chapter 57. Similarly, beta-blockers may be less effective in African Americans. Conversely, African Americans often respond better to diuretics than whites. These variations in therapeutic response have relevance when planning treatment guidelines as they affect patient safety, therapeutic response, and quality of life.

These racial/ethnic influences on blood pressure are established early on in life, with blood pressure following a higher and an earlier trajectory. In one such study conducted in California, a higher prevalence of blood pressure was noted in Asian girls, suggesting increased predisposition for earlier hypertension.[18] Recent data from a national survey performed on 5641 children aged 5 to 14 years in Pakistan reported overall prevalence of high blood pressure at 12.2% (95% CI 11.3% to 13.1%).[19] This is considerably higher than the 5% prevalence of hypertension reported in the U.S. Third National Health and Nutrition Examination Survey (NHANES III), conducted in 1988 to 1994. Results in the previous survey were even more significant upon consideration that the Pakistani children had significantly lower body mass index values than their Western counterparts.

Studies of ethnic minority children in the United Kingdom have also shown higher levels of blood pressure among children of South Asian descent compared to the white population. Indian, Pakistani, and Bangladeshi boys had higher systolic blood pressure than their white counterparts in the Health Survey for England 1999.[20] After controlling for age and height, Pakistani boys had a higher mean systolic blood pressure than a comparable general population. Indian, Pakistani, and Bangladeshi girls had higher diastolic pressure than girls in the general population. These results suggest the need for targeting children and teenagers to develop primordial prevention strategies in these populations.

NEED FOR TREATMENT GUIDELINES IN THE DEVELOPING WORLD

Guidelines are based on research evidence or consensus among experts, and are intended to help healthcare providers in choosing appropriate therapy and to create awareness among the general public for self-referral and screening. The need for guidelines in increasing awareness cannot be overemphasized, considering the success of the U.S. National High Blood Pressure Education Program (NHBPEP), which has been in place for 34 years. The program has been one of the most successful endeavors in public health. It has significantly increased awareness in the general population as well as medical and paramedical professionals about the importance of documenting blood pressure and the need for appropriate therapy. According to the NHANES, 73% of U.S. adults were aware of hypertension in 1988–1991, compared to 53% in 1960–1962.[21] In addition, better control of hypertension has been partly responsible for improved survival in the U.S. population, with reductions in age-related mortality for coronary artery disease and stroke. Hypertension prevalence also declined in the community due to adoption of healthier lifestyles. The success of this program spurred the development of public education programs for coronary artery disease, diabetes, and cholesterol, among others. Many nations have adopted similar programs to enhance physician and public awareness about the need to recognize and treat hypertension. Such programs need to be developed and integrated with other health programs in developing countries.

Therapy guidelines developed in the West are very strong on evidence but are not necessarily context-specific and resource sensitive. Detection, diagnosis, and evaluation guidelines are based on resource-intensive settings, some of which may not be relevant to developing country settings. Therefore, such guidelines are not widely used by physicians in developing countries. A global assessment survey conducted by the World Health Organization (WHO) shows that there is wide variation in the capacity for management of hypertension.[22] Of the 167 countries surveyed, there were no national guidelines in 102 countries. Further, in 45% of the countries surveyed, health professionals were not adequately trained to manage hypertension, and antihypertensive drugs were not affordable in 25% of the countries. A consensus statement from the South Asian Association for Regional Cooperation suggests that patients are unlikely to comply with prescribed therapy if the cost of drugs is more than 5% of their disposable income.[23] Therefore, optimal implementation of therapy guidelines requires high resource sensitivity. While it would be difficult to make guidelines for each country, it would be pragmatic to use an approach similar to WHO's surveillance program.[24]

The WHO STEP wise approach to Risk Factor Surveillance (STEPS) is a simple, standardized method for collecting, analyzing, and disseminating data for NCD risk factors in a strategic, coordinated, cost-effective, and sustainable manner.[24] STEPS is a sequential process, starting with data collection on key risk factors via questionnaires (Step 1), followed by measurement of simple physical measurements (Step 2) and collection of blood samples for biochemical assessment (Step 3). STEPS provide collection of standardized data and sufficient flexibility for use in various country situations and settings; thus, it provides opportunities for making inter-country comparisons.

Similar to the STEPs program, treatments and investigations identified as essential can be implemented at all levels. Those classified as expanded or ideal could be used in secondary or tertiary care settings where such resources

may be available. To identify therapies that could be added to the STEPS approach (core, expanded, and ideal therapies), we reviewed recommendations by the Joint National Committee on Prevention, Detection, Evaluation, and Treatment of High Blood Pressure (JNC 7), American College of Cardiology/American Heart Association, European Society of cardiology, and British Heart Foundation for management of hypertension. Using these recommendations as a framework and based on costing and feasibility of administration, we suggest a simple classification as illustrated in Table 98–1. Thus, for example, advice on reduced salt intake could be provided by a nonphysician health care provider, and the resource-intensive investigations and multiple drug therapies could be restricted to individuals with severe hypertension (e.g., >160/110 mmHg) and provided by physicians or cardiologists from secondary or tertiary care centers.

Principles in establishing guidelines for developing countries

Guiding principles in developing guidelines for therapy should include (1) available strategies for the prevention and management of hypertension, (2) capacity to detect and manage hypertension, (3) barriers to prevention and management of hypertension at an individual level, (4) best available evidence for the various drug classes, (5) the optimal first line of therapy, and (6) ethnic variability in response to drugs.

WHY TARGET HYPERTENSION?

As mentioned previously, high blood pressure is believed to contribute to nearly 2 million deaths annually in high-mortality developing countries. Worldwide, hypertension accounts for nearly 13% of all deaths. At least 21 million years of productive life will be jeopardized due to cardiovascular diseases in countries such as Brazil, China, India, Mexico, and South Africa. Despite these disturbing figures, noncommunicable diseases have not yet emerged as a disease priority for launching preventive public health programs in many developing countries. This is invariably the consequence of inadequate resources due to intensive budgeting of scarce fiscal resources for public health programs focused on communicable diseases. However, it must be realized that hypertension management represents the ideal "entry program" for cardiovascular disease control due to the following factors:

1. It is widely perceived by the general public as well as health care professionals as providing a recognized "clinical" demand, thereby eliciting stronger motivation.
2. Clinicians from a wide range of specialties (such as internists, cardiologists, nephrologists, endocrinologists, neurologists, obstetricians, ophthalmologists, etc.) deal with hypertension in their practice and can therefore recognize and address hypertension.
3. It is unlikely to face resistance from powerful lobbies as, for example, a tobacco control program would.
4. The program can serve as a platform for comprehensive cardiovascular disease reduction from which ancillary programs such as diabetes control, obesity control, and tobacco control, among others, can be initiated.

MANAGEMENT OF HYPERTENSION AND FEASIBILITY: VARIOUS MODALITIES AT DIFFERENT LEVELS OF CARE				
	Drug/Investigations	Recommending Guidelines	Feasibility in Different Settings		
			Primary	Secondary	Tertiary
Drugs					
Core	Dietary advice and other lifestyle changes	WHO/ISH, JNC VIII	Yes	Yes	Yes
Core	Diuretics	WHO/ISH, BHS, JNC VII	Yes	Yes	Yes
Core	Angiotensin-converting enzyme inhibitors	WHO/ISH, BHS, JNC VII	Yes	Yes	Yes
Core	Calcium channel blocker	WHO/ISH, BHS, JNC VII	Yes	Yes	Yes
Core	Beta-blockers	WHO/ISH, BHS, JNC VII	Yes	Yes	Yes
Expanded	Angiotensin receptor blockers	WHO/ISI, BHS, JNC VII	—	Yes	Yes
Ideal	Consult for difficult cases		—	Yes	Yes
	Detailed investigations		—	Yes	Yes
	Prescription of multiple drugs			Yes	Yes
	Risk stratification	WHO/ISI, BHS	Yes	Yes	Yes
Investigations					
Core	Sphygmomanometer		Yes	Yes	Yes
Expanded	Ultrasound		—	Yes	Yes
Ideal	Advanced investigations (microalbuminuria, echocardiography, radionuclide studies, renal angiography, etc.)		—	—	Yes
Who Should Be Providing Diagnosis/Care					
Core	Diagnosis by nonphysician health care provider		Yes	Yes	Yes
Core	Physician evaluation			Yes	Yes
Core	Lifestyle management advice (by non-physician health care providers)		Yes	Yes	Yes
Core	Initiation of therapy by physician		Yes if available	Yes	Yes

BHS, British Heart Society; JNC VII, Joint National Committee on Prevention, Detection, Evaluation, and Treatment of High Blood Pressure, 7th report; WHO/ISH, World Health Organization/International Society of Hypertension.

Table 98–1. Management of Hypertension and Feasibility: Various Modalities at Different Levels of Care

Potential strategies for intervention in developing countries

Hypertension control requires both a community-based approach as well as personal interventions to appropriately target hypertension. A community-based approach attempts to address hypertension through general measures by adopting healthy lifestyles such as restricting excessive salt consumption, preventing obesity, smoking cessation, increased physical activity, and so on. Even small reductions in blood pressure achieved through such interventions have large effects on hypertension-related morbidity and mortality. It has been projected that even a 5-mmHg reduction in systolic blood pressure in the community can reduce stroke mortality by 14%, mortality due to coronary artery disease by 9%, and all-cause mortality by 7%.[25]

Evidence for community-based interventions

Community-based interventions do not attempt to treat hypertension in isolation; instead, they are packaged to affect all major conventional CHD risk factors including diabetes and lipid abnormalities. The effectiveness of community-based programs for cardiovascular disease prevention has largely been based on the experience of

the North Karelia Project in Finland,[26] the first public health cardiovascular disease prevention program. In the 1970s, the Finnish population ranked very high globally in rates of cardiovascular mortality. The program targeted blood pressure as well as other cardiovascular risk factors including smoking and elevated cholesterol. Outcomes included a 28% decrease in smoking in the intervention group along with a 3% decrease in blood cholesterol and blood pressure as compared to the control group. These changes in risk factors had a tremendous impact on cardiovascular events—there was a 22% reduction in age-adjusted cardiovascular disease–related mortality in the intervention group. In addition, coronary artery disease–related mortality rates across Finland fell by 11%. Although the results were encouraging, in view of the simultaneous decline in CHD mortality rates in other parts of Finland, the utility of community-based programs has been questioned. A pooled analysis by Ebrahim et al.[27] suggested that community-based programs have limited utility in reducing the CHD burden. However, it is likely that community-based programs may perform differently in developing countries due to the rapidly increasing burden of hypertension and other CHD risk factors and the low level of awareness of these risk factors.

Several community-based intervention programs have been attempted in developing nations to control risk factors. These have been modeled on similar programs in the developed world. The Tianjin Project in China, launched in 1984, was a major noncommunicable disease prevention project.[28] This intervention program focused on reducing salt intake, decreasing smoking, and controlling hypertension among nearly 9 million urban residents. This public health program resulted in significant reductions in salt intake with reductions in prevalence of hypertension and smoking. The Mirame Project in Chile was initiated in the metropolitan region of Chile when surveys demonstrated high-risk behavior in children, even among those in lower socioeconomic groups.[29] Prevalence of smoking was estimated to be 84%, 30% were physically inactive, 15% were obese, and 8% had elevated blood pressure. Three years of intervention significantly lowered risk factor prevalence in these school children and their families. In Mauritius, a switch in the use of cooking medium from palm oil to soybean oil resulted in dramatic reductions in serum cholesterol due to lowered intake of saturated fats.[30] This low-cost public health policy measure, introduced by government-initiated legislation, has had significant long-term effects on overall cardiovascular mortality and morbidity in Mauritius.

Thus, integrated community-based strategies that target lifestyle-related risk factors could be effective tools if strategies are meticulously planned and the target population appropriately defined. These require participation from international bodies such as the World Health Organization, national and local government bodies, health ministries, food and allied industries, nongovernmental organizations, and various other sectors, and may also need enabling legislation where appropriate. While some of these programs in their entirety can be initiated by at least the low middle-income developing countries, it may still be out of reach currently for low-income developing countries at their current level of health care infrastructure and organization. In the latter countries, along with policy level initiatives to promote healthy lifestyle (enhanced tobacco taxation, promotion of consumption of locally available fruits and vegetables by influencing marketing policies and managing potassium additives to salt) thoughtfully designed multiple risk-factor intervention programs that target specific populations such as employees at worksites and school children may be useful.

Issues in management of hypertension at individual level

Pharmacologic intervention to control hypertension requires awareness about the disease as well as the patient's motivation to continue therapy. Physicians are responsible for counseling patients about the need to adopt lifestyle measures, as well as tailoring therapy to individual patients' needs, achieving target goals, and stratify patients based on risk factor profile. As care of hypertension is delivered across a wide spectrum of medical specialties ranging from doctors armed with only bachelor degrees in medicine to specialists in medicine and cardiologists, treatment algorithms that are simple and offer rational choice of antihypertensive therapy are also key inputs for the success of

national programs in low-income developing countries. Even low-cost, off-patent antihypertensive drugs will be prohibitively expensive for some countries in this category even though in countries that have a well-organized pharmaceutical industry, such as India, the cost of antihypertensive drugs is a fraction of the cost in the West. Due to lower input costs, these countries are better positioned to afford a variety of drug classes. However, even in these countries, national programs will only be able to maintain the most basic drug formulary. Thus, physician education through national treatment guidelines will help curb indiscriminate drug prescription patterns. The feasibility of such a program in a low-resource setting has been demonstrated in Cuba where hypertension awareness and control improved significantly due to concerted efforts at the primary health care level.[31]

Cost effectiveness of treatment guidelines is also affected by two other important factors. While the Western world has lowered the threshold for drug and lifestyle intervention in hypertension, such an approach will not be cost effective for much of the developing world. While hypertension represents a continuum of risk with no absolute "normal" and "abnormal" levels, absolute risk of a cardiovascular event due to high blood pressure is governed by blood pressure level, as well as but also the presence or absence of other cardiovascular risk markers. Thus, while the JNC VII guidelines have adopted a strategy of a blood pressure cut-off to initiate therapy, the treatment guidelines advocated by New Zealand Heart Foundation and the British Hypertension Society place emphasis on assessing absolute CDV risk before initiating drug therapy. Based on this approach, it was estimated that blood pressure treatment should be restricted to those with absolute levels of 170/100 mmHg or higher, and those with blood pressure levels between 150/90 to 169/99 mmHg and a predicted 5-year CVD risk of 15%. Such an approach would be cost neutral, and could prevent up to one-third additional adverse events than the approach of treating all those with BP > 140/90 mms of mercury without accounting for other risk factors.[32]

The cost effectiveness of guidelines aimed at evaluating absolute CVD was recently evaluated by Gaziano et al.[33] They assessed the cost effectiveness of current South African guidelines for hypertension in the setting of a developing country. The authors evaluated the cost of therapy and its effectiveness by using two levels of blood pressure (160/95 mmHg and 140/90 mmHg) and four levels of absolute CDV risk (>40%, 30%, 20%, and 15% 10-year probability) to initiate pharmacotherapy. Using this model, the incremental cost effectiveness of treating hypertension in those with a 10-year CVD risk of more than 40% was $700 versus $11,000 for those with an absolute risk of 15%. Thus, for national treatment guidelines to be more cost-effective in low-income developing countries, both absolute blood pressure level as well as absolute CVD risk should be determined. The recent revision of the South African guidelines according to a model based on absolute risk is a step in this direction. This form of risk assessment would help identify and treat high-risk individuals who would otherwise be inadequately treated and at the same time prevent scarce funds being diverted for pharmacotherapy of patients at low risk, with little absolute benefit in terms of lower CVD events in the population. However, for such a strategy to be successful, low-cost algorithms that are resource sensitive and incorporate clinical data and relevant point-of-care investigations need to be developed and validated in these countries.

In many low-income countries, given the prevailing level of health expenditure, risk assessment may need to be entirely clinical, based on the patient's blood pressure level, age, gender, smoking status, body mass index, and previous history of CVD. Intervention may be initiated with aspirin, beta-blocker, diuretic, and a generic low-dose statin, even in a polypill form, to improve compliance. Legislators and government officials must be persuaded to increase public sector expenditure on noncommunicable diseases in these countries if the United Nations' millennium development goals are to be realized.

Issues in health care delivery

Stumbling blocks in hypertension control in developing nations are summarized in Box 98–1. These include the absence of nationwide programs and low levels of robust primary health care services, physician knowledge about the choices and goals of therapy, lack of continuing medical education programs, knowledge of risk stratification, motivation to impart patient education, and government participation in noncommunicable disease prevention, and absence of national programs. All these issues have to be addressed using novel and innovative approaches. For example, strategies such as using nonphysician health care providers in detecting hypertension, providing lifestyle advice, and follow-up of those on monotherapy, where adequate numbers of physicians are not available, is likely to be acceptable, especially in cases where physicians are reluctant to relocate to remote areas. Further development of simple training modules to target multiple risk factors and estimating the absolute risk for an individual patient would be very useful to physicians overloaded with clinical and administrative

care. A simple example is the development of risk assessment charts similar to the one created by the New Zealand Heart Foundation.[34] If sufficient data for development of such charts are not available, adopting an existing tool used in a country that is similar in demography or race/ethnicity.

DRUG CLASSES: EVIDENCE

Most national and international guidelines advocate thiazide diuretics as the first-line therapy in mild hypertension cases as stand-alone therapy or in combination with beta-blockers, calcium channel blockers, angiotensin-converting enzyme (ACE) inhibitors, or ARBs. These guidelines continue to be promoted despite concerns about the development of diabetes in patients on these classes of drugs (as in the ALLHAT study).[35] However, their extremely low cost compared to all other therapies, as well as efficacy, makes them attractive initial options for the Third World. Although beta-blockers have been first-line treatment for decades, the utility of these drugs has recently been questioned, especially after the Anglo-Scandinavian Cardiac Outcomes Trial (ASCOT).[36] In this trial, despite equivalent reductions in blood pressure, patients in the amlodipine-perindopril arm had a mortality advantage over the atenolol-thiazide arm, which led to premature termination of the trial. In a meta-analysis, Carlberg et al.[37] questioned the effectiveness of atenolol in reducing strokes, where it was shown to be only marginally superior to placebo. This and other concerns regarding the development of diabetes and adverse effects on libido and lipid profile challenge the long-accepted practice of prescribing beta-blockers as first-line therapy in hypertension. However, their cost advantage makes them a better choice than other classes of drugs for use as antihypertensive drugs in the developing world, especially in patients with overt CVD. The newer long-acting calcium channel blockers have rapidly gained favor for hypertension management. They are effective in blacks, elderly patients, and patients with isolated systolic hypertension, and are also marginally better than other drugs in preventing stroke. ACE inhibitors and ARBs have been shown to be effective in patients with hypertension and heart failure, prevent renal damage in patients with diabetes mellitus, and in prevention of stroke (ACE inhibitors with diuretics). In most low-income developing countries, their use will be restricted due to high cost.

First-line therapies in developing nations

Recent evidence suggests that beta-blockers are harmful as compared to ACE inhibitors and calcium channel blockers, and diuretics should not be the first-line therapy in individuals prone to diabetes. Since beta-blockers are cheap options in many developing countries, and should be considered if there are no contraindications and if other drugs are prohibitively expensive. Where generic versions of several classes of drugs are cheap and easily available, physicians could adhere to the most contemporary evidence-based recommendations. In people with high risk for diabetes and metabolic syndrome, such as South Asians, it would be prudent to avoid beta-blockers as the first-line therapy. Similarly, extrapolating from the evidence con-

---

Box 98–1

Stumbling Blocks for Hypertension Control in Developing Nations

- Lack of robust primary health care services
- Lack of physician knowledge about goals of therapy and choice of therapy
- Lack of motivation to impart patient education
- Aberrant physician practices resulting from influence of medical representatives
- Lack of knowledge of risk stratification
- Lack of continuing medical education programs
- Lack of government participation in non-communicable diseases
- Lack of national programs

cerning African Americans in the United States, black people living in sub-Saharan Africa and South Africa are less likely to benefit from beta-blocker or ACE inhibitor monotherapy, and diuretics and calcium channel blockers should be considered as first-line therapy. Where necessary, there should be no hesitation in using multiple drug therapies.

CONCLUSIONS

Hypertension is a major cardiovascular risk factor in both the developing and the developed world. Lack of adequate public and physician awareness of the significance of hypertension attest to the increasing relevance of formulating nation-wide programs for hypertension education and control in the developing world. National programs along with clinical guidelines can provide a framework to prescribe, monitor, and implement necessary educational and clinical activities to promote control of hypertension, and this can favorably influence clinical practice and reduce costs of hypertension control. Emphasis should also be laid on promoting societal changes to reduce mean blood pressure at a population level. It has been estimated that a population-level reduction of blood pressure by 2% can reduce the incidence of stroke and ischemic heart disease by 10% in Asia alone.[38] A concerted effort by health care practitioners, professional organizations, education and vocational institutions, print and electronic media, nongovernmental organizations, and governments may be needed to increase awareness of lifestyle modifications in preventing hypertension.

REFERENCES

1. Chobanian AV, Bakris GL, Black HR, et al. The Seventh Report of the Joint National Committee on Prevention, Detection, Evaluation, and Treatment of High Blood Pressure: the JNC 7 Report. *Hypertension* 2003;42:1206–52.
2. Ezzati M, Hoorn SV, Rodgers A, Lopez AD, Mathers CD, Murray CJ. Comparative Risk Assessment Collaborating Group. Estimates of global and regional potential health gains from reducing multiple major risk factors. *Lancet* 2003;362:271–80.
3. Yusuf S, Hawken S, Ounpuu S, et al. Effect of potentially modifiable risk factors associated with myocardial infarction in 52 countries (the INTERHEART study): case–control study. *Lancet* 2004;364:937–52.
4. Collins R, Peto R, MacMahon S, Hebert P, et al. Blood pressure, stroke, and coronary heart disease. Part 2, Short-term reductions in blood pressure: overview of randomized drug trials in their epidemiological context. *Lancet* 1990;335:827–38.
5. Marques-Vidal P, Tuomilehto J. Hypertension awareness, treatment and control in the community: is the "rule of halves" still valid? *J Hum Hypertens* 1997;11:213–20.
6. Kearney PM, Whelton M, Reynolds K, et al. Global burden of hypertension: analysis of worldwide data. *Lancet* 2005;365:217–23.
7. Wang Z, Wu Y, Zhao L, et al. Trends in prevalence, awareness, treatment and control of hypertension in the middle-aged population of China, 1992–1998. *Hypertens Res* 2004;27:703–709.
8. Gupta R. Trends in hypertension epidemiology in India. *J Hum Hypertens* 2004;18:73–78.
9. Reddy KS, Prabhakaran D, Chaturvedi V, et al. Methods for establishing a surveillance system for cardiovascular diseases in Indian industrial populations. *Bull World Health Organ* 2006;84:461–69.
10. Kearney PM, Whelton M, Reynolds K, Whelton PK, He J. Worldwide prevalence of hypertension: a systematic review. *J Hypertens* 2004;22:11–19.

11. Mackay J, Mensah GA. *The Atlas of Heart Disease and Stroke*. Geneva: World Health Organization, 2004.
12. Deepa R, Shanthirani CS, Pradeepa R, Mohan V. Is the rule of halves in hypertension still valid? Evidence from the Chennai Urban Population Study. *J Assoc Physicians India* 2003;51:153–57.
13. Prabhakaran D, Shah P, Chaturvedi V, et al. Cardiovascular risk factor prevalence among men in a large industry of northern India. *Natl Med J India* 2005;18:59–65.
14. Edwards R, Unwin N, Mugusi F, et al. Hypertension prevalence and care in an urban and rural area of Tanzania. *J Hypertens* 2000;18:145–52.
15. Brown MJ. Hypertension and ethnic group. *BMJ* 2006;332:833–36.
16. Cooper R, Rotimi C. Hypertension in blacks. *Am J Hypertens* 1997;10:804–12.
17. Primatesta P, Bost L, Poulter NR. Blood pressure levels and hypertension status among ethnic groups in England. *J Hum Hypertens* 2000;14:143–48.
18. Hohn AR, Dwyer KM, Dwyer JH. Blood pressure in youth from four ethnic groups: the Pasadena Prevention Project. *J Pediatr* 1994;125:368–73.
19. Jafar TH, Islam M, Poulter N, et al. Children in South-Asia have higher body-mass adjusted blood pressure levels than white children in the United States. *Circulation* 2005;111:1291–97.
20. Agyemang C, Bhopal R, Bruijnzeels M. Do variations in blood pressures of South Asian, African and Chinese descent children reflect those of the adult population in the UK? A review of the cross-sectional data. *J Hum Hypertens* 2004;18:229–37.
21. Burt VL, Cutler JA, Higgins M, et al. Trends in the prevalence, awareness, treatment, and control of hypertension in the adult US population. Data from the health examination surveys, 1960 to 1991. *Hypertension* 1995;26:60–69.
22. Alwan A, Mclean D, Mondel A. Assessment of National Capacity for Non-Communicable Disease Prevention and Control. The Report of a Global Survey 2001. Geneva: World Health Organization, 2001.

23. Nishtar S. Preventing Coronary Disease in South Asia. Islamabad, Pakistan, 2005. Available at: heartfile.org/append.htm.
24. World Health Organization. STEPwise Approach to Surveillance (STEPS). Home page, 2006. Available at: www.who.int/chp/steps/en/.
25. Whelton PK, He J, Appel LJ, et al. Primary prevention of hypertension: clinical and public health advisory from the National High Blood Pressure Education Program. *JAMA* 2002;288;1882–88.
26. Puska P, Tuomilheto J, Nissinen A, Salonen J. Ten years of the North Karelia project. *Acta Med Scand Suppl* 1985;701:66–71.
27. Ebrahim S, Davey Smith G. Multiple risk factor interventions for primary prevention of coronary heart disease. *Cochrane Database Syst Rev* 2000;2CD001561.
28. Schooler C, Farquhar JW, Fortman P, Flora JA. Synthesis of findings and issues from community prevention trials. *Ann Epidemiol* 1997;7(Suppl):S54–68.
29. Nissinen A, Berrios X, Puska P. Community-based noncommunicable disease interventions: lessons from the developed countries to the developing ones. *Bull World Health Organ* 2001;79:963–70.
30. Uusitalo U, Feskens EJ, Tuomilheto G, et al. Fall in total cholesterol concentration over five years in association with changes in fatty acid composition of cooking oil in Mauritius: cross-sectional survey. *BMJ* 1996;313:1044–46.
31. Ordunez-Garcia P, Munoz JL, Pdraza D, et al. Success in control of hypertension in a low-resource setting: the Cuban experience. *J Hypertens* 2006;24:845–49.
32. Baker S, Priest P, Jackson R. Using thresholds based on risk of cardiovascular disease to target treatment of hypertension: modeling events averted and number treated. *BMJ* 2000;320:680–85.
33. Gaziano TA, Steyn K, Cohen DJ, Weinstein MC, Opie LH. Cost-effectiveness analysis of hypertension guidelines in South Africa. Absolute risk versus blood pressure level. *Circulation* 2005;112:3569–76.

34. Core Services Committee. *Guidelines for the Management of Raised Blood Pressure in New Zealand*. Wellington: Ministry of Health, 1995.

35. ALLHAT Collaborative Research Group. Major outcomes in high-risk hypertensive patients randomized to angiotensin-converting enzyme inhibitor or calcium channel blocker vs diuretic. The Antihypertensive and Lipid Lowering Treatment to Prevent Heart Attack Trial (ALLHAT). *JAMA* 2002;288:2981–97.

36. Dahlof B, Sever PS, Poulter NR, et al. Prevention of cardiovascular events with an antihypertensive regimen of amlodepine adding perindopril as required versus atenolol adding bendroflumethiazide as required, in the Anglo-Scandinavian Cardiac Outcomes Trial—Blood Pressure Lowering Arm (ASCOT—BPLA): a multicentre randomized controlled trial. *Lancet* 2005;366:895–906.

37. Carlberg B, Samuelsson O, Lindholm LH. Atenolol in hypertension: is it a wise choice? *Lancet* 2004;364:1684–89.

38. Rodgers A, Lawes C, MacMahon S. Reducing the global burden of blood pressure-related cardiovascular disease. *J Hypertension* 2000;18(Suppl):S3–6.

Page numbers followed by *f* indicate figure(s); *t*, table(s); *b*, box(es).